PRIMARY CARE FOR PHYSICIAN ASSISTANTS

CLINICAL PRACTICE GUIDELINES

SECOND EDITION

PRIMARY CARE FOR PHYSICIAN ASSISTANTS

CLINICAL PRACTICE GUIDELINES

SECOND EDITION

Editor

Rodney L. Moser, PA-C, PhD

Physician Assistant
Sutter Pediatric Medical Group, Roseville, CA
Course Coordinator/Family Medicine
Arizona School of Health Sciences, Phoenix, AZ

Assistant Editor

Anne Heinly, PA-C, MMS, MPS

Physician Assistant
Major, USAF, BSC, Chief of Emergency Services
Offutt AFB, Nebraska

McGraw-Hill
MEDICAL PUBLISHING DIVISION

New York Chicago San Francisco Lisbon London Madrid Mexico City
Milan New Delhi San Juan Seoul Singapore Sydney Toronto

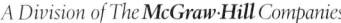

McGraw-Hill

*A Division of The **McGraw·Hill** Companies*

PRIMARY CARE FOR PHYSICIAN ASSISTANTS: CLINICAL PRACTICE GUIDELINES
Second Edition

Copyright © 2001, 1998 by *The McGraw-Hill Companies,* Inc. All rights reserved. Printed in the United States of America. Except as permitted under the United States Copyright Act of 1976, no part of this publication may be reproduced or distributed in any form or by any means, or stored in a data base or retrieval system, without prior written permission of the publisher.

1234567890   KGP KGP   09876543210

ISBN 0-07-137014-5

This book was set in Times New Roman by TechBooks.
The editors were Sally Barhydt, Katherine P. McCullough, and Scott Kurtz.
The production supervisor was Richard Ruzycka.
The cover designer was Eve Siegel Design.
The index was prepared by Steve Scheiner.

Quebecor World/Kingsport was printer and binder.

This book is printed on acid-free paper.

Library of Congress Cataloging in Publication Data

Primary care for physician assistants/Rodney L. Moser.—2nd ed.
    p. cm.
  Includes bibliographical references and index.
  ISBN 0-07-137014-5
    1. Physicians' assistants—Training of.   2. Physicians' assistants—Examinations, questions, etc.   3. Primary care (Medicine)—Examinations, questions, etc.   4. Medical personnel—In-service training.   I. Moser, Rod.
R847.P75 2001
616—dc21

                                                                 00-049622

*Dedicated to the thousands of medical professionals
who proudly have "PA" written after their names,
and to the growing number of enthusiastic students
longing to add these distinguished letters.*

CONTENTS

Section 3 EAR, NOSE, AND THROAT 113

Section 4 EMERGENCY MEDICINE 145

Section 5 ENDOCRINOLOGY 175

Section 6   GASTROENTEROLOGY   197

Section 7   GENETICS   271

Section 8   HEMATOLOGY   279

Section 9 INFECTIOUS DISEASES 295

Section 10 MUSCULOSKELETAL 361

Section 11   NEUROLOGY   431

Section 12   OBSTETRICS/GYNECOLOGY   465

Section 13   ONCOLOGY   505

Section 14   OPHTHALMOLOGY   533

Section 15   PEDIATRICS   553

Section 16   PSYCHIATRY   599

Section 17   RESPIRATORY   665

Section 18   UROLOGY   707

Color plates fall between pages 122 and 123.

CONTRIBUTORS

KATHERINE ADAMSON, PA-C, MMS
Clinical Coordinator/Instructor
Interservice Physician Assistant Program
Fort Sam Houston, Texas
(Chapters 1-5, 1-12, 9-5)

GAIL ALLISON, CNM, MSN, MPH
Certified Nurse Midwife
Adjunct Instructor
Samuel Merritt College
School of Nursing
Oakland, California
(Chapter 12-1)

DAVID P. ASPREY, PhD, PA-C
Associate Professor/Program Director
University of Iowa Physician Assistant Program
Staff Physician Assistant
Division of Pediatric Cardiology
University of Iowa Hospitals and Clinics
Iowa City, Iowa
(Chapters 1-2, 15-3, 15-8, 15-9)

CLAIRE BABCOCK O'CONNELL, MPH, PA-C
Associate Professor/Clinical Coordinator
Physician Assistant Program
Rutgers University
Piscataway, New Jersey
(Chapters 4-1, 4-2, 4-3, 9-1, 9-2, 9-8, 9-9, 17-6)

GARY J. BOUCHARD, EdM, PA-C
Senior Preclinical Coordinator
Physician Assistant Program
Weill Medical College of Cornell University
New York, New York
(Chapters 9-28, 9-29, 11-11, 11-12)

STEPHANIE D. BOWLIN, PA-C, EdD
Director
Physician Assistant Program
Western University School of Health Sciences
Pomona, California
(Chapters 3-15, 18-7)

KIMBERLY BROWN, MS, RD, PA-C
Brunswick Community Hospital
Department of Emergency Medicine
Wilmington, North Carolina
(Chapters 5-12, 11-7, 15-1)

MICHAEL BURNEY, MS, PA-C
Chair, Health Professions Education Program
Assistant Professor of PA Education
Western University School of Health Sciences
Pomona, California
(Chapter 10-21)

ROSSLYN S. BYOUS, DPA, PA-C
Assistant Professor
Physician Assistant Program
Western University School of Health Sciences
Pomona, California
(Chapter 9-20)

JAMES CANNON, DrPH, PA-C
Director
Native American Physician Assistant Program
Arizona School of Health Sciences
Phoenix, Arizona
(Chapter 4-10)

LAURA CAPOZZI, PhD, PA-C
Physician Assistant
LMC Inc.
Midland, Michigan
(Chapter 11-9)

BARRY CASSIDY, PhD, PA-C
Associate Dean, Professor
Director of Physician Assistant Program
College of Health Sciences
Arizona Midwestern University
Glendale, Arizona
(Chapters 17-5, 17-8)

R. SCOTT CHAVEZ, PhD (CANDIDATE), MPA, PA-C
Vice President
National Commission on Correctional Health Care
Bolingbrook, Illinois
(Chapters 9-31, 11-8)

SARAH CLARKE, PA
Physician Assistant
University of Iowa Hospitals and Clinics
Iowa City, Iowa
(Chapter 16-3)

STEPHEN M. COHEN, MS, MPAS, PA-C
Assistant Dean
College of Allied Health
Physician Assistant Program
Nova Southeastern University
Fort Lauderdale, Florida
(Chapters 10-12, 10-17)

GLEN E. COMBS, PA-C, MA
President
American Academy of Physician Assistants
Associate Professor, Program Director
Physician Assistant Program
Wake Forest University School of Medicine
Winston-Salem, North Carolina
(Chapters 9-6, 9-13, 12-15, 12-16)

CECILY COSBY, FNP, PA-C, PhD
Assistant Professor
Director, Family Nurse Practitioner Program
Samuel Merritt College
Oakland, California
(Chapters 1-3, 9-14, 9-22, 9-27)

JEANE MARIE COVINO, PA-C, MPA
Professor
Physician Assistant Program
Rutgers University
Holmdel, New Jersey
(Chapters 9-24, 10-9, 12-8, 12-10)

RANDY DANIELSON, MPAS, PA-C
Associate Professor/Chair
Physician Assistant Program
Arizona School of Health Sciences
Phoenix, Arizona
(Chapter 15-7)

RICHARD DAVIS, JR., PA-C
Senior Physician Assistant
Division of Gastroenterlogy, Hepatology,
   and Nutrition
University of Florida
Gainesville, Florida
(Chapter 9-30)

MEREDITH DAVISON, PhD
Professor and Director
Physician Assistant Program
Midwestern University
Downer's Grove, Illinois
(Chapters 11-10, 16-1)

JO ANN DEASY, PA-C, MPH
Faculty
Physician Assistant Program
Pace University Lenox Hill Hospital
New York, New York
(Chapters 6-14, 8-1, 8-7, 8-10, 9-4, 9-11,
   9-12, 9-15, 17-7)

RICHARD DEHN, MPA, PA-C
Clinical Professor, Assistant Director
Physician Assistant Program
University of Iowa
Iowa City, Iowa
(Chapters 3-4, 9-10, 9-16 through 9-18, 9-21, 9-23, 10-5,
   15-2, 15-5, 18-3)

MORTON A. DIAMOND, MD, FACP, FACC, FAHA
Professor and Medical Director
Physician Assistant Program
Professor of Public Health
Adjunct Professor of Law
Nova Southeastern University
Fort Lauderdale, Florida
(Chapters 1-1, 1-7, 1-8, 1-11)

MICHELLE O. DiBaise, MPAS, PA-C
Physician Assistant, Clinical Research Coordinator
Division of Dermatology
University of Nebraska Medical Center
Omaha, Nebraska
(Chapters 2-5, 2-18, 2-19, 2-23)

KATHLEEN J. DOBBS, PA-C
Faculty Development Specialist
College of Osteopathic Medicine
Michigan State University
Farmington, Michigan
(Chapters 3-13, 13-3)

SUSAN S. ENG-MA, MPH, RPA-C
Assistant Professor
Philadelphia University Physician
   Assistant Program
Point Pleasant, New Jersey
(Chapters 15-13, 17-12)

TIMOTHY C. EVANS, MD, PhD
Assistant Professor of Medicine
Medical Director of Medex NW
MEDEX Physician Assistant Program
University of Washington
Seattle, Washington
(Chapters 5-2 through 5-6, 5-9 through 5-11)

WILLIAM H. FENN, PhD, PA-C
Professor
Physician Assistant Program
Western Michigan University
Kalamazoo, Michigan
(Chapters 2-16, 2-17, 2-29, 9-26)

KATHRYN FRAKE, MPAS, PA-C
Physician Assistant/Assistant Professor
Physician Assistant Program
Central Michigan University
Mount Pleasant, Michigan
(Chapter 9-32)

DANA M. GALLAGHER, PA-C, MPH
Medical Writer/Physician Assistant
Carmel, California
(Chapters 3-11, 9-25, 12-4, 12-7, 12-9, 12-19, 12-22)

NOEL J. GENOVA, PA-C
Physician Assistant
Portland, Maine
(Chapter 12-12)

ANITA D. GLICKEN, MSW
Associate Professor of Pediatrics
Child Health Associate/Physician
   Assistant Program
University of Colorado
Denver, Colorado
(Chapter 16-4)

ROY GUIZADO, MS, PA-C
Program Director
Assistant Professor of Physician Assistant Education
Western University School of Health Sciences
Pomona, California
(Chapter 15-14)

VIRGINIA McCOY HASS, FNP-C, PA-C, MSN
Faculty
Physician Assistant/Nurse Practitioner Program
University of California at Davis
Sacramento, California
(Chapter 16-11)

ANNE P. HEINLY, PA-C, MMS, MPS
Major, US Air Force
BSC/Flight CC, Chief of Emergency Services
Offutt Air Force Base
Nebraska
Assistant Editor, *Primary Care for Physician Assistants*
(Chapters 6-1, 6-2, 6-4, 6-6, 6-7, 6-8, 6-10, 6-11, 6-12, 6-15
    through 6-21, 9-3, 13-1)

JANICE HERBERT-CARTER, MD, MGA, FACP
Associate Professor
Department of Medical Education
Morehouse School of Medicine
Atlanta, Georgia
(Chapters 5-1, 5-7, 5-8)

LAURA HESS, MSN, ANP
Adult Nurse Practitioner
Sutter Health Medical Group
Orangevale, California
(Chapter 12-17)

CATHERINE J. HEYMANN, PA-C, RD, CDE
Physician Assistant
Burlingame, California
(Chapters 1-4, 1-6, 17-3)

KATHERINE D. HOCUM, BS, PA-C
Physician Assistant
Community Manager, MayoClinic.com
Rochester, Minnesota
(Chapters 3-5, 3-7)

THERESA HORVATH, PA-C, MPH
Program Director/Assistant Professor
Graduate Program in Physician Assistant Studies
Mercy College
Dobbs Ferry, New York
(Chapters 10-20, 15-15)

PAT C. H. JAN, MS, PA-C
Adjunct Faculty
Internal Medicine Physician Assistant
China Square Clinic
Chicago, Illinois
(Chapters 6-3, 6-13, 6-22, 6-25, 6-26)

PATRICIA KELLY, MHS, PA-C, EdD
Assistant Professor/Director
Physician Assistant Program
Central Michigan University
Mount Pleasant, Michigan
(Chapters 13-4 through 13-6, 13-8
    through 13-13)

LANCE A. KIRBY, MS, PA-C
Staff Physician Assistant
Ingalls Memorial Hospital
Harvey, Illinois
(Chapter 12-6)

RICKY KORTYNA, MMS, PA-C
Instructor
Physician Assistant Program
Chatham College
Allegheny General Hospital
Department of Neurosurgery
Pittsburgh, Pennsylvania
(Chapters 10-6, 15-12)

DEBORAH KORTYNA, MMS, PA-C
Academic Coordinator
Chatham College
Physician Assistant Program
Pittsburgh, Pennsylvania
(Chapter 10-6)

NADINE KROENKE, PA-C
Staff Physician Assistant
Emergency Medicine Specialists
St. Michael Hospital
Milwaukee, Wisconsin
(Chapters 3-8, 3-9, 4-5)

DAVID A. LUCE, EdM, PA-C
Faculty
Physician Assistant Program
Midwestern University
Downer's Grove, Illinois
(Chapter 17-1)

SANDRA J. MARTIN, DPM, PA
Assistant Clinical Professor
Department of Orthopaedics
Medical Center
University of California at Davis
Sacramento, California
(Chapters 2-10, 10-18)

MARQUITA S. MAYFIELD, MEd, PA-C
Assistant Professor
Physician Assistant Program
School of Medicine
Emory University
Atlanta, Georgia
(Chapters 1-9, 6-5, 6-23)

MATTHEW McQUILLAN, MS, PA-C
Assistant Professor
Physician Assistant Program
Rutgers University
Piscataway, New Jersey
(Chapter 6-27)

CARMEN MERIDITH, MMS, PA-C
Associate Professor, Associate Director
Arizona School of Health Sciences
Phoenix, Arizona
(Chapter 18-5)

GREG J. METE, SR., PA-C, MPAS
Physician Assistant
Kodiak Island Medical Associates
Kodiak, Alaska
(Chapter 17-4)

JOE R. MONROE, PA-C, MPAS
Physician Assistant
Springer Clinic
Founder
Society of Dermatological Physician Assistants
Tulsa, Oklahoma
(Chapters 2-2 through 2-4, 2-6, 2-8, 2-9, 2-12, 2-13, 2-14, 2-20, 2-24 through 2-26)

LINDSEY MOSER, PA-C
Physician Assistant
Sutter Health Medical Group
Orangevale, CA
(Chapter 12-14)

RODNEY L. MOSER, PA-C, PhD
Editor, *Primary Care for Physician Assistants*
Physician Assistant
Sutter Medical Group/Roseville Pediatrics
Roseville, California
Course Coordinator/Family Practice
Arizona School of Health Sciences
Phoenix, Arizona
(Chapters 2-30 through 2-32, 3-2, 3-10, 3-14, 18-6)

WILLIAM A. MOSIER, MPAS, EdD, PA-C
Major, USAFR
Associate Director of Academic Curriculum
Physician Assistant Program
Assistant Professor of Health Care Sciences
School of Medicine and Health Sciences
George Washington University
Washington, DC
(Chapters 7-1, 10-10, 11-1, 11-2, 12-5, 13-2, 15-11, 16-2, 16-8, 18-2)

PAMELA MOYERS-SCOTT, MPAS, PA-C
Physician Assistant
Brierwood Medical Center
Lewisburg, West Virginia
(Chapters 3-12, 10-3, 10-4, 10-8, 10-19, 17-10)

NINA MULTAK, PA-C, MPAS
Clinical Assistant Professor
Physician Assistant Program
University of Florida
Gainesville, Florida
(Chapter 12-20, 12-21)

AMELIA NACCARTO-COLEMAN, MAS, PA-C
Assistant Professor
Western University Physician Assistant Program
Irvine, California
(Chapters 12-13, 13-7)

KAREN A. NEWELL, PA-C
Academic Coordinator
Physician Assistant Program
Emory University
Atlanta, Georgia
(Chapters 4-8, 4-9, 6-24, 10-2)

MAUREEN MacLEOD O'HARA, PA-C
Physician Assistant
Los Angeles, California
(Chapters 17-2, 17-11)

WESLEY T. OTA, OD, FAAO
Staff Optometrist
Sacramento VA Medical Center
Sacramento, California
Assistant Clinical Professor
School of Optometry
University of California Berkeley
Berkeley, California
Clinical Instructor
School of Medicine
(Chapters 14-1 through 14-14, 14-16)

PATTI PAGELS, MPAS, PA-C
Assistant Professor
Physician Assistant Program
University of North Texas
Colleyville, Texas
(Chapter 10-15)

LORI PARLIN PALFREYMAN, MS, PA-C
Assistant Professor
Physician Assistant
New York Hospital Medical Center of Queens
Department of OB/GYN
Queens, New York
University of Medicine and Dentistry of New Jersey and Rutgers University
Piscataway, New Jersey
(Chapter 12-18)

ALLAN PLATT, PA-C
Program Coordinator
Georgia Comprehensive Sickle Cell Center
Atlanta, Georgia
(Chapter 8-3)

TIMOTHY F. QUIGLEY, MPH, PA-C
Assistant Professor
Physician Assistant Program
Wichita, Kanasa
(Chapters 17-13, 18-8)

DANIEL P. RADAWSKI, MD, PHD
Medical Director
Physician Assistant Program
Central Michigan University
Mount Pleasant, Michigan
(Chapter 10-16)

JILL REICHMAN, MPH, PA-C
Co-Director/Associate Professor
Physician Assistant Program
Rutgers University
Robert Wood Johnson Medical School
Piscataway, New Jersey
(Chapter 15-6)

RALPH RICE, MPAS, PA-C
Faculty/Academic Coordinator
Physician Assistant Program
Southwest Missouri State University
Springfield, Missouri
(Chapters 4-4, 9-19)

ALLAN R. RIGGS, MS, PA-C
Faculty/Assistant Professor
Physician Assistant Program
Physician Assistant, Student Health Services
Central Michigan University
Mount Pleasant, Michigan
(Chapter 18-4)

DON ST. JOHN, MA, PA
Physician Assistant
University of Iowa Behavioral Health
Iowa City, Iowa
(Chapters 16-3, 16-5 through 16-7, 16-9)

BARBARA L. SAULS EdD, PA-C
Clinical Director
Physician Assistant Program
King's College
Wilkes-Barre, PA
(Chapters 2-1, 2-7, 2-15, 2-21, 2-22, 2-27, 2-28)

VIRGINIA FALLOW SCHNEIDER, PA-C
Director
Physician Assistant Program
Baylor College of Medicine
Houston, Texas
(Chapters 7-2, 15-10)

THOMAS SCHYMANSKI, PA-C
Physician Assistant
Lorton, Virginia
(Chapter 15-4)

DONALD J. SEFCIK, DO, RPH
Faculty/Medical Director
Physician Assistant Program
Midwestern University
Downer's Grove, Illinois
(Chapters 4-7, 18-1)

FREDDI SEGAL-GIDAN, PA, PhD
Director, Stroke Rehabilitation
Los Amigos National Rehabilitation Center
Downey, California
(Chapters 2-11, 6-9, 11-4, 11-5)

HOWELL J. SMITH III, PA-C, MMS
Staff Physician Assistant
Department of Surgery
Orthopaedic Service
James A. Haley Veterans Hospital
Tampa, Florida
(Chapters 10-7, 10-14)

JEFFREY R. SMITH, PA-C, MMS
Physician Assistant
Rockwood Clinic PS
Spokane, Washington
(Chapters 1-10, 4-6)

FRANCIS S. SOUSA, MD
Department of Ophthalmology
University of California Davis Medical Center
Sacramento, California
(Chapters 14-1 through 14-14, 14-16)

CHRISTOPHER STEPHANOFF, MA, PA-C
Academic Coordinator
Medical University of South Carolina
North Charleston, South Carolina
(Chapter 11-6)

GLORIA STEWART, EdD, PA-C, ATC
Program Director
Physician Assistant Studies Program
School of Medicine
University of South Dakota
Vermillion, South Dakota
(Chapter 10-1)

RANDY TRUDEAU, PA-C
Physician Assistant/Family Medicine
St. Luke's Hospital
Mission Valley Health Center
St. Ignatius, Montana
(Chapter 17-9)

DONNA TULLY, PA-C, MSW
Assistant Professor/Academic Coordinator
Physician Assistant Program
Samuel Merritt College
Oakland, California
(Chapter 16-10)

PEGGY VALENTINE, EdD, PA-C
Program Director/Associate Professor
Physician Assistant Program
Howard University
Washington, DC
(Chapters 12-2, 12-3, 12-11)

SUZANNE WARNIMONT, PA-C, MPH
Program Director
Physician Assistant Program
University of Detroit Mercy
Detroit, Michigan
(Chapters 3-3, 3-6, 14-15)

ANDREA G. WEISS, PA-C
Physician Assistant/Emergency Medicine
Richmond, California
(Chapter 11-3)

KAREN A. WRIGHT, MSA, PA-C
Academic Coordinator
Physician Assistant Program
College of Pharmacy, Nursing, and Allied Health Sciences
Howard University
Washington, DC
(Chapter 3-1)

DIANE S. WRIGLEY, BS, PA-C
Physician Assistant/Emergency Department
Blue Hill Memorial Hospital
Blue Hill Maine
(Chapters 8-2, 8-4 through 8-6, 8-8, 8-9, 8-11, 9-7)

DAVID ZINSMEISTER, PA-C
Physician Assistant
Universal City, Texas
(Chapters 10-11, 10-13, 10-14)

PREFACE

This second edition of *Primary Care for Physician Assistants* is designed for the practicing physician assistant and physician assistant student. Other primary care clinicians, such as nurse practitioners, medical students, and other allied health providers, will also surely benefit from this thorough, reader-friendly text.

The book is divided into 18 sections covering major primary care systems. Within each section are carefully selected topics that one may encounter in a primary care clinical setting. The consistent chapter structure, index, and cross-references allow easy access to its content. Although quite comprehensive, this book is not intended to replace the encyclopedic works of medicine. Rather, the focus is to offer the clinician or student a concise, relevant, and current overview of a broad spectrum of medical topics, either as a rapid clinical reference or as a study guide.

Primary Care for Physician Assistants has an excellent companion question/answer book called *Primary Care for Physician Assistants: Self-Assessment and Review.* The purpose of the review book is to prepare students for the Physician Assistant National Certification Examination (PANCE), to prepare practicing clinicians for the Physician Assistant National Recertification Examination (PANRE), and to help all practicing clinicians assess their primary care competency. This expanded second edition contains over 1000 **new** referenced questions and detailed explanations, covering 282 clinical topics that appear in this book. The majority of the questions have been written *by the authors* of the corresponding chapter in the text and referenced accordingly. They have been carefully edited and selected for their clinical relevancy.

ACKNOWLEDGEMENTS

The book has changed (not just the cover). One might think that the countless hours sitting at a computer assembling and editing the first edition of *Primary Care for Physician Assistants* would have solidified the statement, "Well, I'll never do *that* again!" One also might assume that a "second edition" would be easier and less stressful, since topics only need to be updated. WRONG again. The first edition had 249 chapters; the second edition has 33 more, making a total of 282 chapters. The first edition had 70 contributors; the second edition has 90 carefully selected (and arm-twisted) contributors. As editor of the second edition, I guess I have not learned my lesson. This book has changed. It is bigger *and* better.

Medicine (and everything else) has changed. Like PAs in the job market, medicine is ever-changing. In order for the printed word to be absolutely current, the ink must still be wet. Every contributor in this book has carefully researched their topics right up until the presses were rolling, making last-minute changes. Many of our contributors have changed jobs (myself included), changed careers, changed last names, and changed lives. Many of our first-edition contributors are still with us and many others have joined our diverse team. When I started the first edition, I was working clinically for an HMO in Sacramento, CA. When the HMO went bankrupt, I packed up my computer and moved to Michigan to be the clinical coordinator for the Central Michigan University Physician Assistant Program. Two years and two snow shovels later, we

returned to our old Sacramento home again, where I commuted 200 miles a day to the new Samuel Merritt College Physician Assistant Program in Oakland. Two years and two cars later, I am back working clinically in pediatric clinical practice a few miles from my home, working in the *same* building that housed the defunct and bankrupt HMO. And they say you can't come home again. I hope to stay put for a while.

Contributors and editors are changing. Each time that I have the opportunity of reading and editing these topics, I am truly humbled by the talent in our midst. There are some incredible clinicians among you. Be proud. There are also some very talented editors and authors. Major Anne Heinly is one of the most prolific writers that I know. I was pleased that she agreed to become my Assistant Editor for the second edition, even *after* being moved by the Air Force to a base in Korea and then back to Nebraska again. I am grateful for her countless hours of dedicated editing and writing. I could not have done the second edition without her help. Claire Babcock O'Connell constructively commented (complained) about the test questions in the first edition of the review book. Her skill as a test writer was promptly put to work as an Assistant Editor for the second edition. Numerous people can write chapters, but it takes a real talent to write "good questions." I am truly blessed to have her talent, skills, and guidance for this second round.

How do you adequately thank 90 contributors? Certainly not with a meager honorarium that mimics my dollar-an-hour rate. You thank them by telling them that you have read their chapter in this book and telling them how wonderful it is. It is this peer recognition that is priceless. I just edit their work. The contributors are the stars and deserve the collaborative credit for this fine work. It should be noted that most of the contributors donated their honoraria to the *Physician Assistant Foundation.*

Families are changing. I would like to thank my PA wife, Lindsey, for putting up with another edition and not divorcing me. Our five kids are mostly out of the house now, but two grandchildren now share our home. I would like to thank Shelby (age 7) for all of the times I missed playing with her, and Dylan (age 3) for not destroying my computer. The oldest child, Joshua, has returned to Sacramento from Dallas; Benjamin is finishing law school and joined the Navy. Alexander is an engineer, Ryan is in nursing school, and the photogenic Kristin lives in DC and has appeared on the cover (and centerfold) of *Tattoo Review* #82. Our dog had five puppies in our bedroom, and our formerly male parrot started laying eggs.

PAs are changing (and getting older). It has been 28 years now since I graduated from Alderson-Broaddus and moved to sunny California. The only time that I don't feel old anymore is when I see Bill Stanhope, the founding President of the American Academy of Physician Assistants walk by. He was one of *my* instructors and he is still going strong in a neurosurgical practice in San Francisco. Classmate (and chapter contributor) Glen Combs decided to do another term as President of the AAPA. I guess I am not the only one who goes for a second "edition." This year (2001) will be the twenty-fifth anniversary of the California Academy of Physician Assistants. As the founding president of this fine organization, I hope to share some words of wisdom with a growing rank of PAs and students who were yet to be born when I put on my first pair of sterile gloves. Old PAs never die . . . they just stay home and write books.

Students are changing. Students are smarter and more talented than we ever were. As one of the original "dinosaur PAs," I am truly pleased how PA programs have evolved. The future of our profession is indeed in the healing hands of our students and new graduates. Today's PA students are absolutely awesome, and I will proudly take off my stethoscope someday and allow them to care for me: Graduate PAs are students as well, migrating to masters and doctoral programs across the country. I have masters' students on the Internet, through the Arizona School of Health Sciences distance-learning program, that I have never personally met, yet I feel that I am having an intimate role in their graduate education. As PAs, we will *always* be students.

Patients are changing. Today's patients are more informed. Nearly ALL of my patients have computers and use them on a regular basis. When I am not editing these books, I am running the Ear Disorders board for WebMD, answering hundreds of poignant inquiries every year. Patients demand that their providers remain current in all aspects of treatment. We hope this book helps address this ongoing need for up-to-date medical information.

On behalf of our 90 contributors, my assistant editors, and the incredible editorial and support staff at McGraw-Hill, I humbly present this second edition of *Primary Care for Physician Assistants* to my beloved profession, and ultimately, to the patients we serve.

Rodney L. Moser

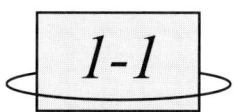

CONGESTIVE HEART FAILURE

Morton A. Diamond

DISCUSSION

Heart failure is the only cardiovascular disorder that has increased in frequency in the last decade. Approximately 2 million Americans have this disorder, and it develops in another 400,000 each year. Congestive heart failure (CHF) is best defined in terms of its clinical presentation. The cardinal features include dyspnea, edema, and fatigue. *Congestive heart failure* is a poor diagnostic term; it does not refer to patients with significant ventricular dysfunction who have no cardiac symptoms, yet those patients can benefit from therapy.

Pathophysiology

CHF patients, regardless of the underlying etiology, can be divided into those with *systolic* failure and those with *diastolic* failure. This classification enables a physician assistant to make an increased correlation between the pathology and the clinical presentation.

Systolic failure is a contractile impairment, a defect in the ability of fibrils to shorten against the load of arterial pressure. An example of pure systolic failure is a patient with CHF secondary to viral myocarditis. Other examples include patients with reduced viable myocardium after infarction and patients with aortic or mitral regurgitation. Patients with systolic failure have a low cardiac output that is manifested as fatigue, weakness, and mental obtundation with the signs of cool skin and reduced blood pressure ("forward failure").

Diastolic heart failure represents an inability of the ventricle to dilate normally during the relaxation phase. The ventricle is abnormally stiff. The problem, therefore, lies in ventricular filling, not in ventricular ejection. The stiff left ventricle leads to elevated atrial and pulmonary venous pressures without a loss of contractile function. The patient is dyspneic but does not have the symptoms of low cardiac output. Hypertrophy causes a permanent increase in stiffness. In contrast, myocardial ischemia produces a transient increase in stiffness. Examples of pure diastolic failure include hypertrophic cardiomyopathy and infiltrative myocardial diseases such as amyloidosis. It must be recognized that individual patients may manifest concomitant systolic and diastolic impairment.

In CHF, neurohumoral changes occur as a result of the hemodynamic abnormalities in heart failure: increased atrial pressure and reduced cardiac output. These neurohumoral changes relate primarily to the sympathetic nervous system and the renin-angiotensin-aldosterone system. Initially, these compensatory mechanisms are beneficial, since they work to sustain a satisfactory blood pressure and cardiac output. However, the same mechanisms ultimately are destructive and hasten cardiac death.

Risk Factors

Determinants that favor the development of heart failure include increasing age, hypertension, coronary artery disease, diabetes mellitus, obesity, cigarette smoking, and left ventricular hypertrophy of any cause. Both systolic and diastolic forms of hypertension are associated with an increased risk of heart failure. It is noteworthy that these factors have additive risk.

Etiology of Heart Failure

CHF may be caused by coronary artery disease, hypertension, congenital heart disease, cardiomyopathy, rheumatic heart disease, cor pulmonale, and high-cardiac-output states. Regardless of the cause of heart failure, the same underlying pathophysiologic mechanisms—systolic and diastolic dysfunction—are evident.

Precipitating Factors

Many factors may be responsible for the onset of CHF. The primary question a physician assistant must also address when caring for a heart failure patient is whether the cardiac disorder is due to myocardial ischemia. If ischemia is the provocation, therapy must increase myocardial perfusion and effect hemodynamic improvement.

A very common precipitating factor is the reduction or cessation of medication intake by a cardiac patient. The medication withdrawal may be due to a sense of well-being or to economic distress. Increased sodium intake, often in the form of snack foods, places an increased burden on the heart and frequently precipitates heart failure. Similarly, medications that increase salt and water retention, for example, nonsteroidal anti-inflammatory drugs, estrogens, and corticosteroids, may initiate clinical heart failure.

Acute hypertension in a previously normotensive patient or a sudden increase in blood pressure in a previously stable hypertensive patient is often responsible for the onset of heart failure.

In caring for a heart failure patient, a physician assistant must also consider anemia, infection, and pulmonary embolism as precipitating factors.

Exposure to an uncomfortably high temperature or acute emotional distress in a patient may be responsible for cardiac failure.

Finally, myocardial contractile impairment resulting from acidosis or medications such as beta blockers and doxorubicin may be responsible. Consideration of the precipitating event in heart failure is a primary factor in patient management.

SYMPTOMS AND SIGNS OF LEFT VENTRICULAR FAILURE

The reduced cardiac output in systolic heart failure causes the patient to experience undue fatigue and weakness. As left atrial pressure rises, the patient will note dyspnea and often a nonproductive cough. The breathlessness may initially be present only after effort. As the atrial pressure continues to increase, the patient will note orthopnea, later paroxysmal nocturnal dyspnea, and finally life-threatening pulmonary edema. A pulmonary edema patient coughs up copious quantities of white frothy sputum that may be tinged with blood.

Physical findings in heart failure patients correlate with the degree of hemodynamic compromise. There is generally evidence of increased adrenergic activity manifested as tachycardia, cool skin, and sweating. With mild failure, the patient may be pink and comfortable. With severe failure, the patient is in severe distress and is pale and cyanotic. The blood pressure in a heart failure patient is very variable and is dependent on prior blood pressure, cardiac output, and adrenergic tone. Central venous pressure is normal. Moist pulmonary rales are heard at the lung bases in patients with mild failure. More severe pulmonary congestion causes diffuse rales and pleural effusion. Palpation of the precordium will reflect anatomic and physiologic abnormalities. An apex displaced to the left and downward indicates left ventricular dilation, while a ventricular lift or heave signifies ventricular hypertrophy. A palpable presystolic (S_4) or protodiastolic (S_3) gallop may be noted. Cardiac auscultation may reveal an S_4 gallop when the atrium contracts more vigorously to fill the stiff left ventricle. A protodiastolic (S_3) gallop and a mitral regurgitant murmur may be heard in a patient with significant ventricular dilation. Peripheral edema reflects the increased sodium and water retention related to increased aldosterone secretion in heart failure patients. In high-cardiac-output failure, the patient is warm and flushed; this is indicative of peripheral vasodilatation. The pulse pressure is widened, pulses are bounding, and the precordium is active.

SYMPTOMS AND SIGNS OF RIGHT-SIDED HEART FAILURE

Right-sided heart failure most commonly is due to coexistent left-sided CHF. Other important causes include cor pulmonale, pulmonary hypertension caused by congenital disease or another disease, pulmonary valve stenosis, and right ventricular infarction.

Symptoms include weakness and peripheral edema and the symptoms related to hepatic congestion: nausea, anorexia, abdominal discomfort, and increased abdominal girth resulting from ascites. Physical examination reveals increased central venous pressure, hepatomegaly caused by congestion, hepatojugular reflux, signs of ascites, and peripheral edema. Precordial palpation may reveal the left parasternal lift of right ventricular hypertrophy and the gallop rhythm indicative of systolic or diastolic dysfunction.

HIGH-OUTPUT CARDIAC FAILURE

Cardiac pump function may be supranormal yet inadequate when metabolic demands or requirements for blood flow are excessive. Causes include anemia, arteriovenous fistula (from trauma or arteriovenous shunts), hyperthyroidism, Paget's disease of bone, and beriberi heart disease. The physiologic response of the heart is increased left ventricular volume. Stroke volume is increased, but the ejection fraction may be reduced. Symptoms include breathlessness and peripheral edema. Sinus tachycardia, widened pulse pressure, active precordial movements, and gallop rhythm are common physical signs.

FUNCTIONAL CLASSIFICATION OF FAILURE

The New York Heart Association (NYHA) has defined four categories that assist physician assistants in patient management and clarify the conclusions reached in clinical heart failure studies:

Class I: no cardiac symptoms with ordinary activity
Class II: cardiac symptoms with marked activity but asymptomatic at rest
Class III: cardiac symptoms with mild activity but asymptomatic at rest
Class IV: cardiac symptoms at rest

LABORATORY TESTS

A complete blood count may reveal anemia that may be causing high-output failure or exacerbating underlying cardiac dysfunction. Determination of blood urea nitrogen (BUN) and serum creatinine may demonstrate prerenal azotemia or chronic renal insufficiency causing hypertensive heart disease. Studies of thyroid and liver function and, if recent infarction is suspected, cardiac enzymes should be obtained.

Cardiac biopsy and other tests must be considered when an unusual form of cardiomyopathy is suspected.

An electrocardiogram (ECG) demonstrates arrhythmia, signs of ischemia or infarction, and intraventricular conduction abnormalities.

RADIOLOGIC AND IMAGING STUDIES

A chest x-ray will define the size and shape of the heart, giving information on any underlying heart problem. Examination of the lung fields may demonstrate equalization of blood vessel size at apexes and bases, a sign of early failure, or interstitial (Kerley B lines) or intra-alveolar edema. Bilateral or unilateral right effusion is often present. Echocardiography reveals the cardiac chamber size, wall thickness, systolic function (ejection fraction), diastolic (filling) properties of the heart, valvular disease, and pericardial effusion.

TREATMENT

Proper therapy for the patient includes the removal of precipitating factors, education related to diet and activity, medication, and possibly surgery. The severity of the patient's clinical condition will determine whether hospitalization is indicated. Hospitalization generally is recommended for the patient's initial episode of heart failure, for failure related to ischemia or arrhythmia, for those whose symptoms are rapidly accelerating, and for patients who require parenteral therapy.

The patient should be instructed to follow a low-sodium diet, usually 1.5 to 2.0 g daily, engage in moderate activity, and avoid extremes in temperature and humidity. Daily weight measurement can be invaluable in assessing the response to therapy and in early detection of recurrent water retention. Patients with moderate heart failure should receive oxygen and be placed on restricted activity.

Pharmacologic Management

The use of multiple medications, "polypharmacy," is now the accepted principle of treatment for CHF. The standard triple therapy for systolic CHF includes diuretics, the inotropic agent digoxin, and afterload reducing agents such as angiotensin converting enzyme (ACE) inhibitors. After 200 years of argument, it is now generally accepted that digoxin is valuable in therapy for systolic but not diastolic CHF. The usual dosage is 0.125 to 0.25 mg per day, with adjustment based on concurrent medication, renal function, weight, and any underlying ECG conduction abnormality. Side effects include nausea, vomiting, weakness, and arrhythmias.

Diuretics relieve the breathlessness and edema commonly associated with heart failure. While symptomatic improvement is important, it is noteworthy that these agents do not affect survival favorably. Diuretics lower the cardiac output. Therefore, a heart failure patient taking a diuretic will note lessened dyspnea but increased fatigue. In combination with other agents, diuretics are most efficacious in patients with NYHA class III or class IV failure. Depending on the agent, diuretics have multiple adverse reactions, including hyperglycemia, hyperuricemia, hypercholesterolemia, and hypokalemia. Furosemide and bumetanide produce fewer undesirable metabolic effects. Patients with severe volume overload or significant renal insufficiency should be treated with a loop diuretic.

ACE inhibitors reduce symptoms and lower morbidity and mortality rates in CHF patients. Further, recent studies of patients after a myocardial infarction who had a left ventricular ejection fraction under 40 percent and in whom an ACE inhibitor was started 3 to 16 days after the ischemic event demonstrated a reduction in both recurrent heart failure and mortality rate. All patients receiving diuretics for systolic heart failure should receive an ACE inhibitor. Renal function studies and electrolytes should be checked before the initiation of ACE inhibitor therapy and rechecked at appropriate intervals, since this class

TABLE 1-1-1. Medications Used in the Treatment of Heart Failure

DRUG	INITIAL DOSE mg	RECOMMENDED MAXIMUM DOSE, mg
Thiazide diuretics		
Hydrochlorothiazide	25 qd	50 qd
Chlorthalidone	25 qd	50 qd
Loop diuretics		
Furosemide	10–40 qd	240 bid
Bumetanide	0.5–1.0 qd	10 qd
Ethacrynic acid	50 qd	200 bid
Thiazide-related diuretic		
Metolazone	2.5*	10 qd
Potassium-sparing diuretics		
Spironolactone	25 qd	100 bid
Triamterene	50 qd	100 bid
Amiloride	5 qd	40 qd
ACE inhibitors		
Enalapril	2.5 bid	20 bid
Captopril	6.25–12.5 tid	100 tid
Lisinopril	5 qd	40 qd
Quinapril	5 bid	20 bid
Digoxin	0.125 qd	As needed
Hydralazine	10–25 tid	100 tid
Isosorbide dinitrate	10 tid	80 tid

*Given as a single test dose initially.
ACE = angiotensin converting enzyme; bid = twice a day; qd = once a day; tid = three times a day.
SOURCE: MA Konstam et al (eds): Heart failure: Evaluation and care of patients with left ventricular systolic dysfunction. Clinical Practice Guidelines No. 11. Rockville, MD, Department of Health and Human Services Public Health Service, Agency for Health Care Policy and Research, 1994. AHCPR Publication no. 94-0613.

of medication may adversely affect BUN, creatinine, and serum potassium. In certain patients, stable elevations in BUN and creatinine are acceptable for their symptomatic and clinical benefit. Potassium supplements should not be ingested, and potassium-sparing diuretics must be used with caution. Other side effects include cough, which may occur in approximately one-third of these patients. The medication should be discontinued only after other causes of cough have been excluded and the patient finds the cough intolerable. Other potential side effects include rash, hypotension, and the rare but serious angioneurotic edema. The initial doses of these agents should be low, with incremental increases considered at several-day intervals.

Oral vasodilator therapy in the form of hydralazine or nitrates may be used in addition to or in place of ACE inhibitors. The vasodilator agents are particularly recommended for heart failure patients who are unable to tolerate the ACE inhibitors. The initial doses should be low and should be increased on the basis of the patient's hemodynamic and symptomatic response.

In chronic CHF, other medications appear to be of clinical value. The β-adrenergic blocker, metoprolol, when taken with a diuretic and an ACE inhibitor, has been reported to reduce rates of sudden cardiac death and death from progressive heart failure. The initial dose of the slow-release metoprolol is 12.5 mg per day, with titration up to 200 mg per day. Carvedilol, a nonselective beta blocker with α-adrenergic blocking properties and antioxidant effects, has also been found to be a beneficial adjunctive therapy in severe chronic systolic heart failure. The dosage of carvedilol is initially 3.125 mg bid, with titration up to 25 mg bid as tolerated.

When added to standard triple therapy, the potassium-sparing diuretic spironolactone, in a dosage range of 25 to 50 mg per day, has been noted to reduce mortality in chronic heart failure.

Angiotensin II receptor antagonists are now being actively studied as therapy in systolic failure. Losartan, with a titrated dose up to 50 mg once daily, seems to be equivalent in effect to captopril in elderly patients with chronic failure and is better tolerated. Other angiotensin II receptor antagonists under investigation include telmisartan, candesartan, irbesartan, and valsartan. ACE inhibitors should be the initial therapy in CHF, but angiotensin II receptor antagonists should be given to patients who are unable to tolerate ACE inhibitor–induced side effects, particularly cough.

Other agents now being tested include antagonists to endothelin and tumor necrosis factor.

A patient with acute pulmonary edema should be treated with oxygen and, if necessary, intubation and assisted ventilation. Intravenous medication generally includes morphine, diuretics, and nitroprusside or nitroglycerine when blood pressure is preserved. For a patient in pulmonary edema associated with hypotension, the intravenous inotropic agents dopamine and dobutamine should be infused.

Table 1-1-1 summarizes the medications commonly used to treat heart failure. Heart transplantation should be considered in patients with intractable failure.

OTHER TREATMENT CONSIDERATIONS

Verapamil, nifedipine, and diltiazem should not be used to treat systolic heart failure. However, in pure diastolic failure these medications are of value, for they reduce ventricular stiffness. A diastolic heart failure patient may also receive an ACE inhibitor to reverse hypertrophy and a beta blocker to slow the heart rate.

Anticoagulation is indicated in an atrial fibrillation patient who is in CHF.

BIBLIOGRAPHY

Committee on Evaluation and Management of Heart Failure: Report to the American College of Cardiology/American Heart Association Task Force on Practice Guidelines: Guidelines for the evaluation and management of heart failure. *J Am Coll Cardiol* 26: 1376–1398, 1995.
Mair FS: Management of heart failure. *Am Fam Physician* 54:245–254, 1996.
Parmley WW: Surviving heart failure: Robert L. Frye lecture. *Mayo Clin Proc* 75(1):111–118, 2000.

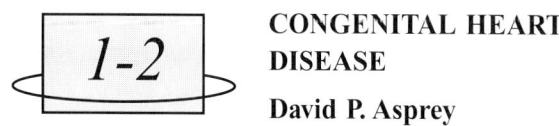

CONGENITAL HEART DISEASE
1-2
David P. Asprey

DISCUSSION

The incidence of congenital heart disease in the general public is approximately 1 percent (estimates vary from 6 to 12 per 1000 liveborn infants). Consequently, most clinicians will be responsible for providing care to several patients with congenital heart disease during their careers. Most children with significant congenital heart disease are diagnosed during the first 6 months of life. However, mild forms of congenital heart disease and occasionally some significant forms may not be detected until after 1 year of age.

When a child is diagnosed with congenital heart disease, subsequent siblings have a threefold increase in the likelihood of being affected. Studies have indicated that the probability of recurrence is substantially higher when the mother is the affected parent.

There are more than 30 different specific forms of congenital heart defects. This chapter addresses only the most common noncyanotic defects that are likely to be encountered by primary care clinicians. Specifically, it addresses ventricular septal defects (VSDs), which account for approximately 25 percent of all congenital heart defects. Patent ductus arteriosus (PDA) accounts for approximately 10 percent of all congenital heart defects, pulmonary stenosis (PS) accounts for 8 percent, atrial septal defects (ASDs) and coarctation of the aorta (COA) account for 8 percent each, and aortic stenosis (AS) accounts for 5 percent.

Among the most common cyanotic congenital heart lesions are tetralogy of Fallot (8 percent) and transposition of the great arteries (5 percent). While the cyanotic forms of congenital heart defects are not included in this chapter, this should not be misinterpreted as meaning that these lesions are unimportant. Rather, these important forms of congenital heart disease require considerable more attention than can be afforded in this chapter. Individuals with these defects require frequent evaluation by a pediatric cardiology clinician.

While many environmental and genetic factors are known to contribute to congenital heart disease, the specific etiology is unknown in approximately 90 percent of cases. Consequently, prevention of congenital heart disease is extremely difficult.

VENTRICULAR SEPTAL DEFECT

Pathology

VSDs are the single most common congenital heart defect, accounting for approximately 25 percent, of all these defects. VSD refers to the presence of a communication between the left ventricle and the right ventricle. This defect occurs as a result of incomplete partitioning of the ventricles during cardiac development. VSDs can occur in numerous places within the ventricular septum. The most common location is the perimembranous region (near the tricuspid valve), followed by the muscular or trabecular region of the ventricular septum.

The size of the defect can vary dramatically from a relatively large defect that presents with symptoms of congestive heart failure and pulmonary hypertension to a very small defect that is hemodynamically insignificant and presents with a murmur but no other signs or symptoms. In all patients with VSDs, pulmonary blood flow is increased above normal. If the amount of increased pulmonary blood flow is significant, it may result in increased pulmonary vascular resistance within the pulmonary arteries, leading to pulmonary hypertension. When the volume of pulmonary blood flow is twice as great as the systemic blood flow or more, the patient is at risk of developing pulmonary hypertension. Pulmonary hypertension develops secondary to the excessive pulmonary blood flow and may become irreversible if it is not corrected by 2 years of age. This pulmonary hypertension can become progressive and ultimately develop into Eisenmenger syndrome, which occurs when the right heart pressures exceed the left heart pressures and the blood begins to shunt from right to left, resulting in systemic cyanosis.

Signs and Symptoms

Often the diagnosis of a VSD is not made during the newborn period but several weeks after birth. This delayed diagnosis occurs in newborns because pulmonary vascular resistance remains high as a result of increased smooth muscle mass in the pulmonary arterioles, atelectasis, and alveolar hypoxia until a few weeks after birth. Clinical symptoms are dependent on the degree of shunting, which is determined by the pulmonary vascular resistance and/or the size of the defect. If the VSD is large and the pulmonary vascular resistance is low, the ratio of pulmonary blood flow to systemic blood flow will be high (greater than 2:1). This results in congestive heart failure that in children is manifested as tachypnea, tachycardia, poor feeding, poor weight gain and growth, diaphoresis with feedings, dependent edema, and decreased exercise tolerance.

Objective Findings

The most characteristic objective finding associated with VSDs is the grade 1 to 5/6 holosystolic murmur that is heard maximally at the middle to lower left sternal border. Often the VSD is small and restrictive (this means that the defect is small enough that it maintains a significant pressure difference between the right and left ventricles during systole), and the characteristic holosystolic murmur is accompanied by a palpable thrill. If the degree of left-to-right shunting is large (the pulmonary blood flow is twice the systemic flow or more), a diastolic flow rumble typically will be present at the lower left sternal border. When the pulmonary artery pressure is significantly elevated, the pulmonary component of S_2 will become increased in intensity.

Diagnostic Considerations

Often a skilled clinician can make the diagnosis of a VSD on the basis of the history and physical examination data alone. While in many instances this diagnosis can be made with a high degree of certainty by the history and physical examination alone, it is prudent to confirm the diagnosis by echocardiography if it persists beyond 2 years of age.

Laboratory Studies

Electrocardiographic (ECG) findings are useful in grossly quantifying the degree of left-to-right shunting. If the degree of shunting is small, the ECG will be normal. If there is moderate shunting, it may reveal a mild degree of left ventricular hypertrophy (LVH). If the degree of shunting is large, the ECG may demonstrate combined ventricular hypertrophy. In addition, if pulmonary hypertension develops, right ventricular hypertrophy (RVH) will be present.

Radiologic Studies

The chest x-ray findings may vary from normal heart size to cardiomegaly and from normal to increased pulmonary vascular markings based on the degree of increase in pulmonary blood flow. The echocardiogram is useful in establishing the diagnosis of VSD. In addition, it is instrumental in documenting the location of the VSD and estimating right ventricular (RV) pressures and the ratio of pulmonary to systemic blood flow.

Other Diagnostic Studies

In very large VSDs or in children with a VSD in combination with other types of congenital heart defects, cardiac catheterization may be indicated to further delineate the cardiac anatomy and hemodynamics.

Treatment

In the majority of cases, no specific interventions, either medical or surgical, are necessary. However, all individuals who have a confirmed VSD should observe subacute bacterial endocarditis (SBE) prophylaxis.

MEDICAL   In addition to SBE prophylaxis, patients with signs and symptoms of congestive heart failure should be treated with digitalis and/or diuretics.

SURGICAL   In patients with a ratio of pulmonary flow to systemic flow greater than 2:1 or pulmonary hypertension, surgical closure of the defect is indicated before 2 years of age. In addition, patients who have congestive heart failure and delayed growth rates are candidates for an elective surgical closure.

Patient Education

Patients with a VSD need to be advised to observe SBE prophylaxis. The parents of newborn infants diagnosed with VSD should be advised of the signs and symptoms that indicate congestive heart failure and should be advised to have their children evaluated by a clinician if those symptoms occur.

Disposition

Approximately one-half of all VSDs undergo spontaneous closure by 2 years of age. Forty percent remain patent but do not require surgical intervention, and the remaining 10 percent require surgical closure.

Complications and Red Flags

Infants who develop congestive heart failure, growth delay, or pulmonary hypertension that is resistant to medical management should be referred for surgical closure of the defect.

Pearls

When a murmur is absent in a newborn and then is detected for the first time at 6 to 8 weeks of life or later, a VSD should be considered.

ATRIAL SEPTAL DEFECT

Pathology

An ASD is any communication or defect in the atrial septum that normally separates the right atrium and left atrium. This communication can occur in one of three different regions of the atrial septum. The most common region for an ASD is the secundum or middle portion of the septum (accounting for approximately 65 percent of all ASDs). This type of defect occurs in the same anatomic location as the foramen ovale, which is the structure that allows the majority of the pulmonary circulation to bypass the lungs in the fetal circulation. In conjunction with the changes that occur in the circulation after birth, the foramen ovale closes and prevents any further right-to-left shunting of the pulmonary blood flow.

The second most common type is the primum ASD, which accounts for approximately 30 percent of all ASDs. This defect occurs in the lower portion of the atrial septum and results in a coinciding defect (cleft) in the mitral valve. The primum ASD is typically part of a defect known as an endocardial cushion defect, also referred to as atrioventricular canal defect. The endocardial cushion defect can be either partial (primum ASD with cleft mitral valve) or complete (primum ASD, cleft mitral valve, and VSD).

Finally, the ASD can occur at the upper region of the atrial septum near the entrance of the superior vena cava. This defect is known as a sinus venosus ASD and accounts for approximately 5 percent of all ASDs. This particular type of ASD often is associated with a defect known as partial anomalous pulmonary venous return.[1]

In all types of ASDs, left-to-right shunting of blood occurs through the defect. This shunting results in excess blood flow through the right atrium, right ventricle, and pulmonary arteries. The degree of shunting can vary dramatically and is dependent on the size and the pressure difference between the right atrium and left atrium. If the degree of excess pulmonary blood flow is significant (ratio of pulmonary blood flow to systemic blood flow greater than 2:1), pulmonary hypertension may develop later in adult life, eventually resulting in Eisenmenger syndrome.

Signs and Symptoms

In the vast majority of cases, the patient will be asymptomatic. Occasionally patients report that they fatigue more easily than do their peers when the degree of left-to-right shunt is significant.

Objective Findings

In patients with a significant left-to-right shunt, cardiomegaly will result. This may be evident on physical examination by the presence of a slight prominence of the left hemithorax. This finding is most noticeable by examining the contour of the patient's right and left chest in the supine position, with the examiner standing at the foot of the examining table. Typically, the second heart sound will be widely split and fixed (without variation throughout the respiratory cycle). A systolic ejection murmur, typically grade 2 or 3/6, will be present at the upper left sternal border. If the degree of left-to-right shunt is significant, a diastolic flow rumble will be audible at the lower left sternal border.

Diagnostic Considerations

Patients with an ASD are often asymptomatic, and their physical examination findings are rather subtle; thus, the diagnosis of small ASDs can be very difficult to make. Consequently, it is important that the clinician maintain a high index of suspicion when examining a patient with a systolic ejection murmur in the pulmonary area and/or a fixed, split second heart sound. When these findings are present, an ASD must be ruled out.

Laboratory Studies

The ECG findings may include right axis deviation, right bundle branch block, right ventricular hypertrophy, or an rSr′ pattern in V_1. This pattern in V_1 is indicative of volume overload of the right ventricle.

Radiologic Studies

The chest x-ray findings may include cardiomegaly, prominence of the main pulmonary artery segment, and increased pulmonary vascular markings that are dependent on the degree of left-to-right shunting. The echocardiogram will reveal the presence of the ASD and its specific location. The right atrium, right ventricle, and pulmonary artery may be enlarged.

Other Diagnostic Studies

If the defect is difficult to visualize by echocardiography or if other associated defects are suspected, a cardiac catheterization may be required to further assess the cardiac anatomy and hemodynamics.

Treatment

MEDICAL Patients with an ASD do not require SBE prophylaxis unless they have other associated abnormalities, such as mitral insufficiency (with primum ASDs) or valvular pulmonary stenosis. Studies are being conducted utilizing nonsurgical closure of ASDs, with devices placed into the ASD through a cardiac catheter. When properly placed, these devices can effectively prevent left-to-right shunting across the ASD, thus eliminating the need for surgical repair.

SURGICAL Once the presence of an ASD has been confirmed beyond the newborn period, surgical closure is indicated. When small, the defect may be closed directly with sutures; a larger defect may necessitate closure with a patch sewn in place over the defect. Typically, this repair is recommended before the patient enters school (4 to 5 years of age).

Patient Education

It is important to help the patient and the patient's parents understand that the primary reason for recommending closure of the ASD is preventive. Typically, the child is completely asymptomatic, and it is difficult for the parents to understand the need for surgery. However, uncorrected ASDs may result in pulmonary hypertension, which will not be detected until well into adulthood. Surgical closure is recommended before school age because the patient is of adequate size to make the procedure safe and it will not interfere with school.

Pearls

Patients with a systolic ejection murmur in the pulmonary region and a fixed, split second heart sound should be considered as having an ASD until proved otherwise.

PATENT DUCTUS ARTERIOSUS

Pathology

The ductus arteriosus is an important vascular structure in the fetal circulation that serves to connect the right and left sides of the circulation by allowing a communication between the main pulmonary artery and the descending aorta. In a fetus, this structure allows blood flow to bypass the nonfunctioning lungs. Normally, the ductus arteriosus undergoes closure shortly after birth, thus separating the right and left circulations of the heart. PDA is more common in infants who are born prematurely.

The amount of left-to-right shunting is dependent on the size of the PDA and the degree of pressure difference between the aorta and the pulmonary artery. In patients with significant left-to-right shunting, pulmonary vascular resistance can become elevated, resulting in the development of pulmonary hypertension.

Signs and Symptoms

The presence or absence of symptoms is dependent on the size of the PDA. If the PDA is small and the amount of left-to-right shunting is insignificant, there will be no symptoms. Conversely, if the PDA is large and the resulting degree of shunting is significant, signs of congestive heart failure may result.

Objective Findings

Typically there is a grade 1 to 3/6 continuous "to-and-fro" murmur at the upper left sternal border. A diastolic rumble may be present at the left lower border in patients who have a moderate to large left-to-right shunt. Accentuated (bounding) peripheral pulses may be noted on examination.

Diagnostic Considerations

PDA typically can be diagnosed by physical examination along with laboratory data. Echocardiography utilizing color flow Doppler is very sensitive in detecting the presence of a PDA.

Laboratory Studies

ECG findings may vary from normal in a small PDA to LVH or even combined ventricular hypertrophy in a large PDA.

Radiologic Studies

The chest x-ray also varies, depending on the size of the PDA and its subsequent shunting. In a PDA with a small degree of shunting, the chest x-ray may be normal. In a large PDA, there may be cardiomegaly and increased pulmonary vascular markings. The echocardiogram is very sensitive and can detect PDAs that are not evident by physical examination alone.

Other Diagnostic Studies

Typically, there is no need to perform a cardiac catheterization when surgical closure is the chosen treatment. However, some centers are now treating PDAs by closure with a spring or coil device that is placed in the PDA through the catheter. When this treatment is considered, a catheterization also serves as a diagnostic tool to establish the size of the PDA and select the correct size of the closure device.

Treatment

MEDICAL   Patients with a PDA require SBE prophylaxis at times when they are at risk. In children who develop congestive heart failure, digitalis and diuretics may be indicated.

Studies are being conducted utilizing nonsurgical closure of PDAs with devices placed into the PDA through a cardiac catheter. When properly placed, these devices can effectively prevent left-to-right shunting across a PDA.

SURGICAL   Once the presence of a PDA has been confirmed after the newborn period, surgical ligation and division are indicated. Typically, this repair is recommended after 1 year of age and before the patient enters school (4 to 5 years of age) or at the time of diagnosis in older children.

Patient Education

It is important to help the patient and the patient's parents understand that the primary reason for recommending closure of a PDA is preventive. Closure of a PDA will eliminate the need to observe SBE prophylaxis and reduce the risk of developing SBE. Also, uncorrected PDAs may result in pulmonary hypertension later in life.

Disposition

Once the patient has the PDA closed and has recovered from the surgical procedure, he or she is effectively cured. SBE prophylaxis can be discontinued 6 months after the repair.

Pearls

The continuous murmur that is characteristic of a PDA can be mimicked by a venous hum (a type of innocent murmur). Be certain you have distinguished between the two murmurs during the physical examination.

AORTIC STENOSIS

Pathology

AS results when there is an area of obstruction to the blood flow out of the left side of the heart through the aorta. This obstruction most often occurs at the level of the aortic valve but also may occur above (supravalvular) or below the valve (subvalvular). When this obstruction is present, it results in increased left ventricular pressure. This elevated pressure is necessary to create adequate blood flow through the aorta to ensure perfusion of the brain and body. The increased left ventricular pressure results in the development of increased left ventricular muscle mass or left ventricular hypertrophy.

Valvular aortic stenosis is the most common form of AS and occurs when the valve is thick and stiffened or when the valve is defective, such as a bicuspid aortic valve, which is the most common form of valvular AS. Subvalvular AS can occur as a discrete membrane or as a result of more generalized excessive muscle mass, which is the case in idiopathic hypertrophic subaortic stenosis. Supravalvular AS results when the portion of the aorta immediately above the valve has a discrete narrowing.

Signs and Symptoms

At the time of presentation, most patients with mild to moderate AS are asymptomatic. Infants with severe AS may present with the signs and symptoms of congestive heart failure. Children with moderate to severe AS may report decreased exercise tolerance, chest pain, or even syncope.

Objective Findings

Infants with severe AS will have findings consistent with congestive heart failure. Children with AS will have a systolic ejection murmur that is heard maximally at the upper right sternal border. This murmur may be accompanied by a thrill either in the suprasternal notch or over the aortic region of the precordium. In addition, if the stenosis is valvular, there typically will be a systolic ejection click present that is heard best at the apex. The presence of a high-pitched diastolic murmur is indicative of the aortic insufficiency that may accompany this defect.

Laboratory Studies

ECG findings vary from normal in children with mild AS to LVH in patients with moderate to severe AS.

Radiologic Studies

The chest x-ray findings typically are normal in patients with mild AS. In moderate to severe cases of AS, the ascending aorta may appear enlarged as a result of the poststenotic dilatation that results from the turbulent blood flow created by the stenosis. The pulmonary vascular markings will be normal. If cardiomegaly is present, one should consider aortic insufficiency. The echocardiogram is very useful in establishing the diagnosis along with the location of obstruction. An estimation of the degree of stenosis can be made by utilizing Doppler measurements of the velocity of the blood flow through the aorta. This test is also useful in screening for the presence of associated aortic insufficiency and for measuring the left ventricle's dimensions.

Other Diagnostic Studies

In infants and children with moderate to severe AS, a cardiac catheterization may be indicated to directly measure the degree of obstruction and quantify the degree of associated aortic insufficiency.

Treatment

MEDICAL Patients with AS should be advised to observe SBE prophylaxis during times of risk. Patients with moderate to severe AS should be advised to avoid strenuous physical exertion. Some centers are attempting to treat valvular AS with balloon dilatation valvuloplasty during the cardiac catheterization, with varying degrees of success.

SURGICAL In infants and children with severe AS, surgical treatment may be necessary. There are multiple surgical options available, varying from an aortic valve commissurotomy, to replacing the aortic valve with the patient's pulmonary valve and then placing the aortic valve or a pulmonary homograft in the position of the pulmonary valve (Ross procedure), to artificial valve placement.

Patient Education

AS is a significant and typically progressive form of congenital heart disease. Once a patient has been diagnosed with AS, he or she should be counseled to consider selecting sporting activities and careers that will not require him or her to perform isometric exercise or to be placed in a situation where he or she might continue to exercise or work despite experiencing chest pain or discomfort. It is essential that children with AS practice good oral hygiene and observe SBE prophylaxis when indicated.

Disposition

Patients with AS should be monitored frequently during periods of rapid growth. Patients who have significant aortic insufficiency in addition to AS require careful monitoring.

Pearls

AS affects males approximately four times as often as females. In infants and children with confirmed supravalvular AS, consider the diagnosis of William syndrome.

PULMONARY STENOSIS

Pathology

PS results when there is an area of obstruction to the blood flow out of the right side of the heart through the pulmonary artery. This obstruction most often occurs at the level of the pulmonary valve but also may occur above the valve (supravalvular) or below the valve (subvalvular). When the valve is affected, it may be thickened and stiff or dysplastic. When this obstruction is present, it results in increased right ventricular pressure. This elevated pressure is necessary to create adequate blood flow through the narrowed pulmonary artery. The increased right ventricular pressure results in increased right ventricular muscle mass development or RVH. In addition, the turbulent high-velocity jet of blood that results when the blood is forced through the narrowing causes poststenotic dilatation of the pulmonary artery distal to the area of stenosis.

Signs and Symptoms

At the time of presentation, most patients with mild to moderate PS are asymptomatic. Infants with severe PS may present with cyanosis, tachycardia, and tachypnea. Children with moderate to severe PS may report decreased exercise tolerance and dyspnea on exertion.

Objective Findings

A systolic ejection murmur is typically present and is heard maximally at the upper left sternal border. If the stenosis is moderate or severe, the murmur may be accompanied by a thrill that is palpable at the upper left sternal border. The murmur often will radiate to the lung fields. When the stenosis is valvular, a systolic ejection click will be present at the upper left sternal border. The presence of a high-pitched diastolic murmur suggests pulmonary insufficiency.

Laboratory Studies

ECG findings vary from normal in mild forms of PS to the presence of RVH in moderate PS and right atrial enlargement and RVH in more severe PS.

Radiologic Studies

Chest x-ray findings are normal in mild PS. The main pulmonary artery segment typically will be dilated in patients with moderate to severe PS as a result of poststenotic dilatation. The pulmonary vascular markings are normal; however, in infants who have severe PS, the pulmonary vascular markings may appear diminished. The echocardiogram can be utilized to confirm the specific site of stenosis, assess the pulmonary valve anatomy, and estimate the degree of stenosis through the use of Doppler.

Other Diagnostic Studies

Rarely, a cardiac catheterization is necessary to further define the cardiac anatomy and hemodynamics.

Treatment

MEDICAL Infants and children with PS should observe SBE prophylaxis. Balloon dilatation valvuloplasty is a very effective treatment for severe PS. If this treatment is performed at the time of catheterization, it can achieve a significant reduction in the pressure gradient across the pulmonary artery.

SURGICAL In infants and children who do not respond to balloon dilatation valvuloplasty, consideration should be given to surgical treatment. This treatment may consist of pulmonary valvulotomy or the placement of a patch across the right ventricular outflow tract to widen it and thus relieve the obstruction.

Patient Education

It is important for patients with valvular PS to observe SBE prophylaxis. Children with mild PS typically do not progress to severe forms of PS.

Disposition

Children with PS that is not severe should be allowed to participate in all forms of physical activity to their own comfort level.

Pearls

Children with PS and a murmur that is grade 3/6 or less typically have a mild degree of stenosis (less than a 30 mmHg gradient across the pulmonary valve).

COARCTATION OF THE AORTA

Pathology

COA refers to a narrowing in the descending aorta that occurs during development. When the narrowing is significant, it results in obstruction of blood flow from the heart to the lower half of the body. The degree of narrowing can vary dramatically from trivial to critical in cases where there is a nearly complete interruption of the descending aorta. The body attempts to compensate for the low blood pressure distal to the coarctation (as detected by the renal system) by increasing the systemic blood pressure. This results in systemic hypertension when the blood pressure is measured proximal to the site of the coarctation (i.e., the right arm). It is this elevated blood pressure that often results in the detection of COA.

COA affects approximately twice as many males as females. Infants born with severe COA present with the signs and symptoms of congestive heart failure and require immediate medical and surgical management. The discussion in this chapter is limited to children who present with few or no symptoms.

Signs and Symptoms

Most children who do not have critical COA report few or no symptoms. Occasionally these children report a feeling of weakness, fatigue, or even leg pain with vigorous exercise.

Objective Findings

The most consistent finding in children with COA is a differential in the blood pressures obtained between the upper and lower extremities. In association with this finding the majority of children with COA have a right arm blood pressure that exceeds the ninety-fifth percentile for age. The lower extremity pulses will vary depending on the severity of the coarctation and the degree of collateral formation. Collateral arterial blood vessels will enlarge and provide a mechanism for blood to bypass the site of the coarctation. If the coarctation is severe and the collaterals are poorly developed, the lower extremity pulses may be absent. If the coarctation is mild to moderate or the collateral formation is extensive, the lower extremity pulses will be decreased but palpable. In addition, when the pulses are palpable, there will be a delay in the femoral pulse when it is compared in timing to the radial pulse; this finding is known as femoral lag.

A grade 1 to 3/6 systolic murmur typically is audible at the middle left sternal border and in the infrascapular region of the back. Because of the high association of aortic valve disease with this condition, AS or a bicuspid aortic valve also may be present.

Diagnostic Considerations

The findings of the physical examination in patients with a mild COA are often subtle, and therefore a high index of suspicion must be maintained. Patients with mild hypertension or unequal upper and lower extremity pulses must be evaluated carefully for the presence of COA.

Laboratory Studies

The ECG may range from normal to findings of LVH if the degree of obstruction is severe.

Radiologic Studies

The chest x-ray findings are often subtle but may include mild cardiomegaly. Rib notching may be detectable if a child is of school age or older. The rib notching occurs as the collateral arteries enlarge to accommodate the additional blood flow bypassing the coarctation site. Echocardiography is useful in assessing the coarctation site and estimating the degree of narrowing.

Other Diagnostic Studies

Occasionally the coarctation site will be very difficult to visualize by echocardiography, and a magnetic resonance imaging (MRI) study may be useful to identify the anatomy of the aortic arch. In other instances, an aortogram may be required to define the arch anatomy clearly.

Treatment

MEDICAL Children with confirmed systemic hypertension should undergo pharmacologic treatment until the defect is repaired and the blood pressure returns to normal. Some institutions are attempting to treat discrete sites of coarctation with balloon dilatation angioplasty, with modest long-term success. SBE prophylaxis should be observed.

SURGICAL Asymptomatic patients with confirmed COA and a mild to moderate degree of obstruction can be treated electively at a convenient time. Children with profound hypertension should be considered for repair as soon as possible on a nonemergency basis.

Options for surgical treatment are end-to-end anastomosis and patch repair. The end-to-end anastomosis consists of completely dividing the aorta at the site of the coarctation, resectioning the defect, and then resuturing the aorta together. The patch repair consists of making a longitudinal slit across the site of the defect and placing a patch in the area of the defect to widen the lumen of the aorta. This patch can be made of a surgical material such as Teflon or from a portion of the left subclavian artery.

Patient Education

Patients with COA should be advised to monitor their blood pressure closely and be given guidelines on the indications for notifying the clinician. Postoperatively, patients may require pharmacologic treatment to control their systemic hypertension.

Disposition

Postoperative patients need routine follow-up for assessment of blood pressure. In addition, if patients are treated surgically before the completion of their growth, they should have their upper and lower extremity blood pressures checked periodically to assess the possibility of a pressure gradient recurring. The recurrence of a gradient suggests that the coarctation is recurring.

Pearls

Most children diagnosed with coarctation of the aorta also have abnormalities of the aortic valve and/or mitral valve. Estimates suggest that as many as 85 percent of patients with coarctation have an associated abnormality of the aortic valve.

REFERENCE

1. Park MK: *The Pediatric Cardiology Handbook,* 2d ed. St. Louis, Mosby, 1997.

BIBLIOGRAPHY

Adams FH, Emmanouilildes GC, Reimenschneider TA (eds): *Moss' Heart Disease in Infants, Children and Adolescents,* 4th ed. Baltimore, Williams & Wilkins, 1989.

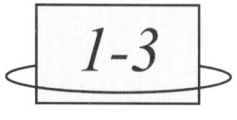

CEREBROVASCULAR ACCIDENT AND TRANSIENT ISCHEMIC ATTACK

Cecily Cosby

DISCUSSION

Cerebrovascular accident (CVA), or "stroke," is the third leading cause of death in industrialized countries after heart disease and cancer and is the leading cause of serious, long-term disability in the United States.[1] More than 500,000 new cases occur each year in the United States, resulting in 150,000 deaths.[1] The most devastating aspect of this disease is the physical and emotional impact on survivors and their families, along with the economic impact on the health care system and the nation in general. The annual cost of stroke in the United States is $30 billion. Roughly 60% of this figure involves direct medical costs, while the remainder is due to lost wages and productivity.

Medical and surgical treatments have little or no effect on a completed stroke. These interventions are intended only to limit the damage, restore as much function as possible, and reduce the risk of recurrence. Therefore, the focus in altering this disease process is twofold. The first focus is prevention, both primary and secondary. With many recognized modifiable risk factors and predisposing

conditions for stroke, it is estimated that 70 percent of all CVAs can be prevented.[1] Second, early recognition of the signs and symptoms of stroke will avoid needless delays and allow timely access to potentially outcome-enhancing care.[2] Public education is an essential part of this strategy.

A stroke is defined as a neurologic deficit that lasts more than 24 h and is due to infarction of brain tissue. Focal deficits that clear completely within 24 h are called transient ischemic attacks (TIAs); however, they usually last only minutes to a few hours. Events of intermediate duration (24 h to 1 week) may be called reversible ischemic neurologic deficits (RINDs). This term is seldom used, since a deficit lasting that long almost certainly is due to infarction, and such a fine distinction in regard to duration does not change the approach to the patient. These definitions are by convention only, helping to classify a particular event, and not all patients fit precisely into one group. What may be a TIA by the strict definition may actually be a small infarction that is well compensated. Surrounding brain tissues may resume the functions of the infarcted area, resulting in a rapid resolution of symptoms.

About 10 percent of all strokes are preceded by TIAs, while TIAs precede 50 to 75 percent of strokes caused by carotid artery thrombosis. Among those who have had one or more TIAs, about 36 percent will later have a stroke. Approximately one-third of patients who experience a TIA will experience a cerebral infarction within 5 years. A person who has had one or more TIAs is 9.5 times more likely to have a stroke than is someone of the same age and sex who has not.[1] For these reasons, TIAs are extremely important warning signs. Patients should be counseled to seek immediate medical attention after any suggestive signs or symptoms.

It is important for a physician assistant in the primary care setting to identify patients at risk for stroke and be well versed in modifiable risk reduction strategies. Understanding the initial presentation and management of stroke and appreciating the complications and long-term-care requirements of patients who have suffered a stroke are also important.

A basic knowledge of cerebrovascular anatomy and physiology is crucial in understanding the various mechanisms of stroke. The cerebral blood flow is abundant, receiving 750 mL/min at rest, supplied by four principal vessels: the paired vertebral and carotid arteries. The carotid arteries supply the anterior cerebral circulation, while the vertebrals supply the posterior circulation (see Fig. 1-3-1)

Aortic Arch

Three main arteries stem from the aortic arch: the so-called great vessels:

1. The innominate artery (or brachiocephalic trunk) divides to become the right subclavian artery and the right common carotid artery (CCA).
2. The left common carotid artery.
3. The left subclavian artery.

There are well-known congenital anomalies of the great vessels, usually affecting their origins, but they only rarely play a role in stroke.

CAROTID ARTERIES Each CCA courses upward in the neck, where it branches at the level of the thyroid cartilage to become the external and internal carotid arteries. The external carotid artery (ECA) supplies the face and scalp but also serves as an important source of collateral blood flow around the eye in cases of severe narrowing or occlusion of the internal carotid artery (ICA). Blood flow is capable of reversing direction in the ophthalmic artery, providing an indirect (collateral) source of blood to the brain.

The ICA travels upward behind the angle of the jaw, passes into the base of the skull, and emerges from the temporal bone to take an

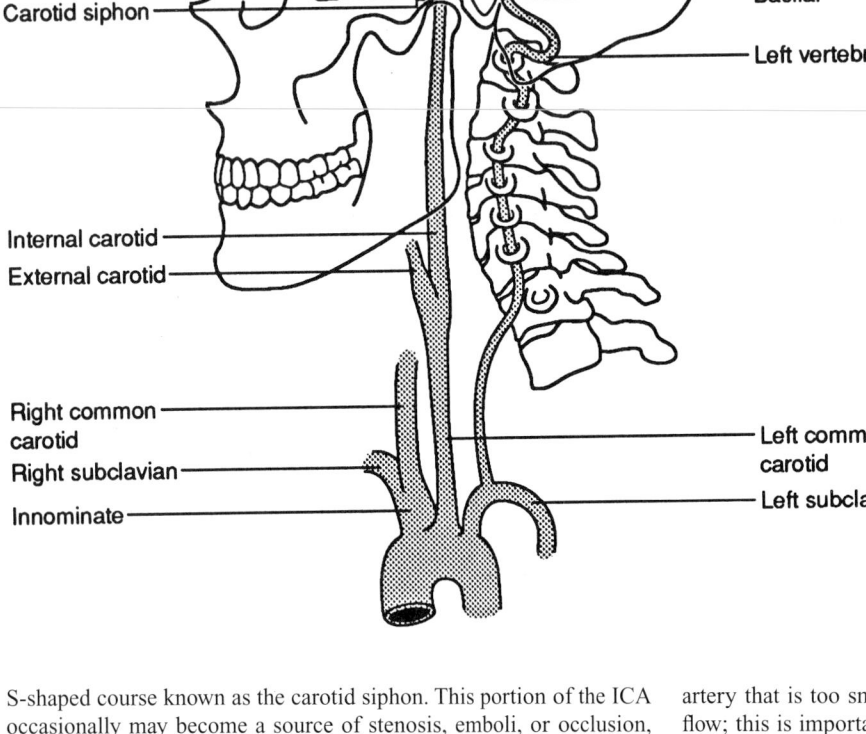

FIGURE 1-3-1. Cerebrovascular anatomy and aortic arch.

Anterior cerebral

Ophthalmic

Carotid siphon

Internal carotid

External carotid

Right common carotid

Right subclavian

Innominate

Middle cerebral

Posterior communicating

Posterior cerebral

Basilar

Left vertebral

Left common carotid

Left subclavian

S-shaped course known as the carotid siphon. This portion of the ICA occasionally may become a source of stenosis, emboli, or occlusion, resulting in cerebral ischemia. The ICA continues to the base of the cerebral hemispheres, where it joins the circle of Willis, but just before this structure it gives rise to the ophthalmic artery, which supplies the eye and the surrounding structures. Impaired flow in this vessel or the terminal branches of the retinal artery may result in the transient visual loss known as amaurosis fugax.

CIRCLE OF WILLIS   A unique vascular structure, the circle of Willis is the most important source of collateral blood flow to the brain when any of the principal feeding vessels become diseased. It lies at the base of the cerebral hemispheres, anterior to the brainstem and encircling the pituitary gland. A single anterior communicating artery (ACOM) and paired posterior communicating arteries (PCOMs) allow for "crossing over" of blood from one hemisphere to the other or from the anterior circulation to the posterior circulation if needed (see Fig. 1-3-2). Numerous anatomic variants exist in the circle of Willis, with only 20 percent of the population having the "classic" anatomy described above. Ten to 25 percent of the population has a small or functionally absent ACOM or PCOM, severely limiting potential pathways for collateral blood flow.

VERTEBROBASILAR SYSTEM   Each vertebral artery originates from its respective subclavian artery, traveling posteriorly and cephalad through the transverse processes of the cervical vertebrae before entering the foramen magnum at the base of the skull. The two arteries then course anterior to the brainstem before joining to become the single basilar artery, which ultimately becomes continuous with the circle of Willis. Ten percent of the population has at least one vertebral

artery that is too small to contribute significantly to brainstem blood flow; this is important if the other vertebral artery becomes diseased. Narrowing of the vertebral artery origins is common but rarely causes cerebral ischemia in and of itself.

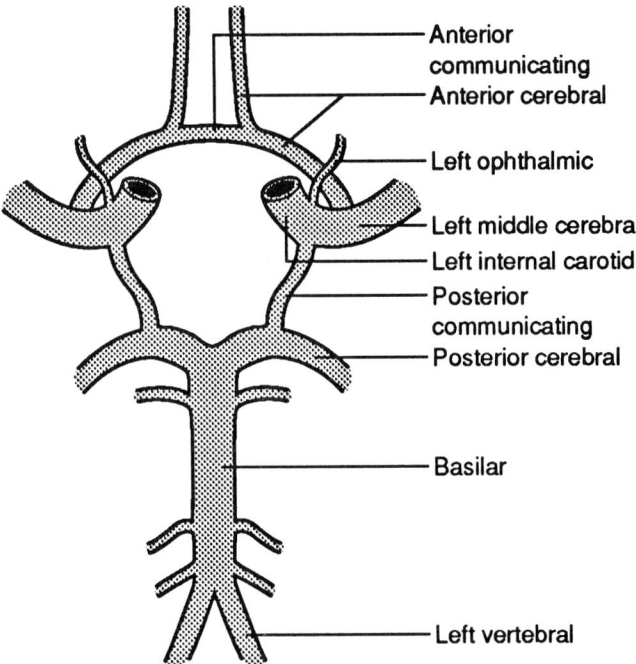

Anterior communicating

Anterior cerebral

Left ophthalmic

Left middle cerebral

Left internal carotid

Posterior communicating

Posterior cerebral

Basilar

Left vertebral

FIGURE 1-3-2. The circle of Willis as seen from below.

RISK FACTORS

The major risk factors for stroke are similar to those for heart disease, while others are unique to cerebrovascular disease (see Table 1-3-1). Most CVAs occur in the elderly (over 65 years old) as a result of the increased incidence of atherosclerosis in that group. In the young, the etiology is quite different, usually being due to congenital maladies such as aneurysms and arteriovenous malformations (AVMs), trauma, arterial dissection, or drugs such as cocaine and amphetamines. Stroke is slightly more prevalent in males than in females, and whites have more TIAs, with stroke rates 58 percent higher among blacks compared to whites.[3]

The most important modifiable risk factor is hypertension, which plays a crucial role in most causes of stroke and is the primary risk factor in certain types of CVA, such as lacunar infarcts and intra-cerebral hemorrhage. The important contribution of hypertension was shown in the SHEP study, where lowering the blood pressure of men and women age 60 and older with isolated systolic hypertension (<160 mmHg) resulted in a 36 percent reduction in stroke over 4 years.[4]

Heart disease is also important because it relates to cardiogenic emboli, which cause one-third of all strokes. Every form of cardiac disease carries an increased risk of stroke, but the single most important one is atrial fibrillation, which accounts for roughly 50 percent of all cardiogenic emboli. Recent myocardial infarctions (usually in the first few weeks) cause approximately 20 percent of these emboli as a result of local wall motion abnormalities, where an intramural thrombus may form and enter the arterial circulation. Cardiac valve abnormalities (from rheumatic disease) may result in the valvular vegetations that cause approximately 10 percent of all cardiogenic emboli. The remainder can be attributed to prosthetic cardiac valves and relatively rare causes of stroke such as endocarditis and septal defects.

A stroke risk is associated with female smokers who have a history of migraine headaches and also take oral contraceptive pills (OCPs). This presumably is due to cerebral vasospasm induced by migraines coupled with a hypercoagulable state brought on by OCPs and smoking. The degree of increased risk is not clear, but it is certainly quite small. One group of investigators estimated 19 strokes per 100,000 women with migraines.[5] From a primary care point of view, it is important to recognize that atherosclerosis is the underlying cause of most CVAs, and risk factor modification should be directed at preventing its occurrence.

TABLE 1-3-1. Risk Factors for Cerebrovascular Disease

Prior stroke or TIA
Hypertension
Diabetes
Smoking
Hyperlipidemia
Obesity
Hypercoagulable states
Alcohol
Drugs (amphetamines, cocaine)
Migraines
Family history
Gender
Ethnicity
Acquired immune deficiency syndrome (AIDS)
Cardiac disease
   Atrial fibrillation/flutter
   Recent myocardial infarction
   Valvular disease
   Endocarditis
   Ventricular aneurysm
   Septal defects
   Tumor (atrial myxoma)

PATHOPHYSIOLOGY

There are numerous etiologies for stroke, each with its own mechanism, treatment, and prognosis, but they generally may be classified as ischemic or hemorrhagic in nature (see Table 1-3-2). The brain maintains an appropriate cerebral blood flow at a given instant through autoregulation that it can sustain until the mean arterial pressure falls to near 60 mmHg, at which point cerebral perfusion depends on gravity. Isolated episodes of hypotension caused by syncope or orthostasis usually do not result in significant cerebral ischemia or infarction. However, the prolonged hypotension that occurs in cardiac arrest may result in infarction of poorly perfused "watershed" areas between major vascular territories.

Ischemic Stroke

Approximately 85 percent of all strokes are due to ischemia caused by arterial or cardiac pathology. The most common causes of ischemic stroke relate directly or indirectly to atherosclerosis. Atherosclerotic plaques have a predilection for arterial curves, branches, and origins. Severe stenoses may form in the extracranial or intracranial vessels, resulting in ischemia caused by low flow, thrombosis, or embolization. Plaques may rupture, causing embolization by showering debris downstream or by becoming a nidus for platelet and fibrin deposition, which also may embolize.

Atherosclerosis may lead to stroke indirectly through coronary artery disease, resulting in myocardial infarction, arrhythmias, and some forms of valvular disease.

The heart is the most common source of emboli to the brain, with ICA ("artery-to-artery") emboli being somewhat less common. Roughly 80 percent of cerebral emboli travel to the middle cerebral artery (MCA) distribution, 10 percent go to the posterior cerebral artery (PCA), and the remainder go to the vertebrobasilar system.

Lacunar infarctions cause 20 to 25 percent of all ischemic strokes. They are due to ischemia in small penetrating vessels of the deep white matter that arise from the vertebral and basilar arteries, the circle of Willis, and the MCA. Disease in these very small vessels usually is due to lipohyalinization caused by chronic hypertension. Lacunar infarcts also are found in patients with carotid disease and diabetes.

A TIA is an important clinical entity because it gives the clinician an opportunity to offer treatment before a more devastating CVA can occur. However, fewer than half of all patients with ischemic stroke have premonitory TIAs. Among patients with a TIA, 33 percent will suffer a stroke within 5 years, with no way to predict its severity. The risk of subsequent stroke is highest in the first month after an initial TIA and gradually tapers over the ensuing months. Amaurosis fugax is a monocular visual loss that results from ischemia within the retinal artery caused by low flow, occlusion, or emboli within the ipsilateral (occurring on the same side) ICA. The risk of subsequent CVA is slightly lower in amaurosis fugax than it is in hemispheric TIA, and permanent visual loss is rare. The mechanisms for TIA and CVA are the same.

TABLE 1-3-2. Stroke Classifications

Ischemic (85%)
   Embolic
      Cardiogenic
      Artery-to-artery
      Unknown source
   Thrombotic
Hemorrhagic (15%)
   Subarachnoid hemorrhage
      Saccular aneurysm
      Arteriovenous malformation
      Other
   Intracerebral hemorrhage

Hemorrhagic Stroke

Approximately 15 percent of all strokes are due to intracranial hemorrhage. Nontraumatic subarachnoid hemorrhage (SAH) most often is due to the rupture of an intracranial saccular or "berry" aneurysm, usually presenting between ages 30 and 65. The vast majority (85 percent) of these hemorrhages form in the anterior cerebral circulation, usually at the junction of the anterior cerebral artery and the ACOM. Bleeding into the subarachnoid space may cause vasospasm of nearby cerebral vessels, resulting in further ischemia. Saccular aneurysm rupture has a poor prognosis, with a 10 percent mortality rate in the first 24 h and 25 percent more over 3 months. Twenty percent rebleed within 2 weeks, and at least half the survivors will have severe neurologic deficits.

The majority of the remainder of SAHs are due to AVMs, which involve an abnormal tangle of vessels between the arteries and veins. They are more common in males, have a heritable component, and primarily affect the young. The highest risk of rupture is at ages 10 to 30, but AVMs occasionally may present as late as age 50 years. SAH caused by an AVM carries a slightly better prognosis than does a saccular aneurysm rupture, as the rate of rebleeding and vasospasm is lower.

An intracerebral hemorrhage (ICH) usually is due to large hypertensive hemorrhages that are not necessarily associated with exertion and most commonly occur during the daytime hours. Other causes of ICH include intracerebral AVMs and aneurysms, blood dyscrasias, trauma, neoplasms, and anticoagulation medications. They may result in mass effects and increased intracranial pressure, with a generally poor prognosis ranging from a 30 percent to an 80 percent mortality rate.

SIGNS AND SYMPTOMS

Perhaps the most common presentation is actually asymptomatic ischemia or infarction. Many so-called silent infarcts are found incidentally on computed tomography (CT) scans, and the patient has no recollection of these infarcts. Similarly, some people are found to have entirely occluded carotid arteries without neurologic sequelae. This is a testament to the rich collateral blood flow to the brain in most individuals. Cerebrovascular disease usually manifests as a focal neurologic deficit affecting motor, sensory, visual, or communication functions. The presenting signs and symptoms reveal which portion of the brain is affected and may suggest a mechanism for the injury. All strokes may vary in severity from nearly asymptomatic to fatal, depending on the location, the extent of injury, and collateral flow.

Hemispheric Stroke

Ischemia and infarction of the cerebral hemispheres constitute the most common presentation for stroke and depend on which cerebral vessel is affected and to what degree. The most common signs and symptoms are contralateral hemiparesis, hemiplegia and hemisensory loss of the face and limbs, homonymous hemianopia, conjugate eye deviations, and ipsilateral monocular visual loss. Aphasia may occur if the dominant hemisphere is affected (the left hemisphere in right-handed individuals and more than 75 percent of left-handed persons). Anosognosia, or hemineglect, is caused by ischemia of the nondominant hemisphere, while dysarthria may result from ischemia in either hemisphere (see Table 1-3-3). Strokes resulting from emboli usually have an abrupt onset of symptoms with a maximal deficit, whereas strokes with thrombotic or other causes may develop more gradually. Embolic strokes also have a tendency to show fluctuating symptoms as the embolus lyses, migrates, or partially occludes a vessel.

TIAs may present with the symptoms described above but with complete, rapid resolution of the deficit. Amaurosis fugax usually is described as a "shade" coming down or across the visual field or

TABLE 1-3-3. Common Terms and Definitions in Cerebrovascular Disease

TERM	DEFINITION
Hemiparesis	Muscular weakness on one side of the body
Hemiplegia	Paralysis on one side of the body
Ataxia	Lack of muscle coordination
Aphasia	Defect in the expression of language, including speech, reading, and writing, resulting from a central nervous system injury
Diplopia	Seeing two images instead of one; eyes may be unable to move to one side (ocular palsy) or may not move synchronously (dysconjugate gaze)
Dysarthria	Imperfect articulation of speech caused by loss of muscle control in the forming of words
Dysphagia	Difficulty swallowing
Homonymous hemianopia	Defective vision or blindness in half the visual field, occuring in the same location in each eye
Anosognosia	An inability to perceive a defect, especially hemiplegia, on one side of the body
Hemineglect	An impaired response to stimuli from one side of the body

occasionally as a loss of peripheral vision. Patients also may complain of facial or limb numbness (usually the arm).

Lacunar infarctions usually have a rapid onset but may present over hours to days. Recovery tends to occur quickly. There are many well-known lacunar syndromes, the most common of which are pure motor hemiparesis, pure sensory hemiparesis, dysarthria and hand weakness, and ataxia and leg weakness. Patients also may present with sensorimotor deficits that are more typical of hemispheric stroke.

Ischemia or infarction in the posterior cerebral (vertebrobasilar) circulation may affect the brainstem, cerebellum, temporal lobes, or occipital lobe. This manifests most commonly as dizziness, vertigo, diplopia, and ataxia (usually without weakness). It also may present with nystagmus, dysarthria, dysphagia, cranial nerve palsies, hemiplegia, eye movement paralysis, pupillary changes, hoarseness, various visual changes, and visual hallucinations. Hemiparesis is rare in patients with posterior infarcts. Since the cranial nerves originate in this region, these infarctions may present with cranial nerve signs contralateral to somatic signs, for instance, left facial numbness and right arm clumsiness.

Cerebellar and brainstem infarctions may rapidly result in respiratory arrest because of brainstem compression, since the posterior fossa of the skull does not allow for much swelling. Edema in this area may cause hydrocephalus, brainstem compression, coma, and death. Early signs and symptoms of this impending disaster may be subtle, consisting only of gait disturbances (inability to stand or walk) or changes in the level of consciousness.

Syncope is usually a manifestation of hypotension or cardiac disease (arrhythmias, aortic stenosis) and usually is not seen in someone presenting with an ischemic stroke or TIA. Similarly, vertigo or dizziness without any other brainstem, cerebellar, or occipital signs is not considered consistent with posterior ischemia. Instead, it usually is due to eighth cranial nerve or labyrinthine disease.

Severe narrowing or occlusion of the subclavian artery proximal to the origin of the vertebral artery causes subclavian steal syndrome. When the arm on the ipsilateral side is exercised, the patient may experience symptoms of vertebrobasilar insufficiency (dizziness, diplopia, gait disturbances). This occurs because the vertebral artery undergoes a reversal of flow, becoming a source of blood for the upper extremity, in effect "stealing" blood from the posterior cerebral circulation. Although this phenomenon may be demonstrated in many people by ultrasound examination, it rarely results in ischemia or infarction.

Stroke in evolution, also known as "stuttering stroke," represents a medical emergency in which a neurologic deficit is found to be progressing in a stepwise fashion over minutes or hours. It frequently is due to a severely stenotic or acutely occluded vessel, and a devastating stroke may be averted if rapid medical or surgical therapy is initiated.

Hemorrhagic Stroke

Hemorrhagic strokes from all causes commonly present with headache but also may show signs of increased intracranial pressure (ICP). Rupture of an intracranial saccular aneurysm usually presents as "the worst headache in my life" and frequently is accompanied by a sudden, temporary loss of consciousness. However, headache may be the only presenting complaint. Patients may have a prodromal phase of headache or cranial nerve signs as the enlarging aneurysm compresses nearby structures.

Intracranial hemorrhage also has a rapid onset and may be accompanied by headache and signs of elevated ICP, including nausea, vomiting, and changes in mental status. Focal neurologic deficits, if present, depend on the site of the bleeding as brain tissues are dissected by an expanding hematoma.

OBJECTIVE FINDINGS

A full history and a physical examination are essential in a patient who is undergoing a routine screening examination or one whose symptoms have been present for over 3 h.

A careful patient history may uncover past episodes of minor cerebral ischemia that may have been disregarded by the patient or the patient's family as unimportant or "just due to old age." Direct inquiries should be made about numbness, weakness, or clumsiness of facial and limb movements; changes in vision; "splotches" or "shades" in one eye; clumsiness in writing or handling objects; dizziness and vertigo; and slurring of speech.

Physical examination of the patient should rule out potential cardiac causes of stroke, such as atrial fibrillation and valvular disease. A thorough eye examination should be done, including pupillary responses to light, extraocular movements (to check for nystagmus and gaze paralysis or deviations), visual fields by confrontation (some patients may be unaware of a visual field cut because of hemineglect), and a funduscopic examination to look for small-vessel disease of hypertension and diabetes and rule out papilledema caused by increased ICP. A search for arterial bruits should be done. Supraclavicular and carotid bruits are the most frequently encountered, with a high-pitched systolic bruit fading into diastole arousing suspicion of a high-grade stenosis. However, not every bruit is caused by a significant narrowing, and the absence of one does not rule out significant stenosis. The lesion may be so severely stenotic or even occluded that no bruit is generated. A full neurologic exam should be performed to document any subtle deficits and serve as a baseline if the condition worsens. Elements of the neurologic examination should include mental status (assessment of language, memory, comprehension, etc.), cranial nerves, reflexes, and motor, sensory, and cerebellar functions such as gait and fine movements.

For a patient who presents with acute stroke signs or symptoms, initial triage is directed to assess ABCs (airway, breathing, circulation), determine the onset of symptoms, and arrange for a neurologic consultation with diagnostic studies, typically in the emergency department. Early recognition and treatment of stroke have been identified as essential factors in the stroke chain of survival and recovery.[6,7] Mild signs or symptoms may go unnoticed, and many stroke victims deny the presence of symptoms. This delay in care may limit the benefit from the newest therapies, such as thrombolytics, which must be instituted within 3 h of the onset of symptoms. The Prehospital Stroke Scale developed in Cincinnati[8] evaluates three major physical findings: facial droop,

TABLE 1-3-4. Differential Diagnosis for Stroke

Cardiac
  Arrhythmias
  Mural thrombus
  Septal defects
  Valvular disease
  Infectious

Vascular
  Atherosclerotic
  Dissection
  Compression
  Lipohyalinosis
  Inflammatory (granulomatous, arterities, etc.)
  Vasospasm (drugs, migraines, SAH)
  Aneurysm/AVM

Hematologic
  Hypercoagulable states (systemic lupus erythematosus, pregnancy, polycythemia, etc.)
  Blood dyscrasias, clotting abnormalities (warfarin therapy, etc.)

Other conditions causing focal neurologic changes
  Intracranial tumor
  Metabolic (hypoglycemia, hyperglycemia, drug overdose)
  Subdural hematoma
  Migraine headache
  Focal seizure
  Trauma
  Infectious (tuberculosis, fungal, HIV/AIDS)

motor arm weakness, and speech abnormalities. These findings can help identify a stroke patient who requires rapid transport to the hospital.

DIAGNOSTIC CONSIDERATIONS

The differential diagnosis for stroke is vast (see Table 1-3-4), but if the most common causes are excluded, most of the other etiologies will present in a way that suggests a diagnosis. For example, a patient with stroke symptoms, fever, bacteremia, and intracranial abscesses on CT will suggest septic emboli secondary to bacterial endocarditis.

LABORATORY TESTS

The basic laboratory tests required for the initial presentation of stroke include a complete blood count (hematocrit, hemoglobin, platelets, white and red cell indexes), electrolytes, blood urea nitrogen, creatinine, serum glucose, prothrombin and partial thromboplastin times, electrocardiography (ECG), and chest x-ray. Serum cholesterol should be checked for the purpose of general risk-factor modification. Other tests should be ordered as indicated by each situation, for instance, a toxicology screen if cocaine is suspected, special tests to differentiate hypercoagulable states, and the erythrocyte sedimentation rate (ESR) in patients with vasculitis and other inflammatory conditions. Serologic tests for syphilis, antiphospholipid antibodies, and blood cultures may be ordered for the evaluation of cerebral infarction.[9]

RADIOLOGIC STUDIES

In the acute CVA presentation, CT examination of the head should be performed to rule out structural problems (such as mass-occupying lesions, dural hematomas, old infarcts, and acute hemorrhages) or if one is considering anticoagulation. CT scans are a good first choice because of their relatively low cost and accessibility in most communities. To avoid confusing blood with contrast medium, the CT is performed without contrast enhancement. However, these studies have deficiencies in some instances. Detection of small hemorrhages (approximately 1 cm) is possible very early, but CT is much less sensitive in finding an early infarction. In acute stroke, CT scans detect infarcts only 5 percent of the time in the first 4 h, 50 percent in the first 24 h, and 95 percent by the eighth day. They also may miss cortical infarcts, lacunar infarcts, and small infarcts in the posterior fossa or brainstem as a result of bony interference.

Magnetic resonance imaging (MRI) is much more sensitive in detecting early infarctions as well as visualizing the entire brain, including the cortex, the lacunae of the deep white matter, and the posterior fossa. However, it is generally more expensive and less commonly found and has contraindications to its use, such as pacemakers, other implanted metal devices, and external equipment such as ventilators.

Angiography is considered the gold standard for evaluating the patency of the carotid and intracranial vessels. It is not an entirely benign procedure, carrying a 2 to 12 percent risk of bleeding, infection, catheter-related trauma, or stroke, and therefore is done only in special clinical situations at the direction of a surgeon, neurologist, or interventional radiologist.

OTHER DIAGNOSTICS

Duplex ultrasonography of the carotid, subclavian, and intracranial vessels is a valuable diagnostic tool. It provides not only physical information such as the locations and severity of stenoses but also physiologic information such as the direction of flow in a given vessel to indicate collateralization. It is also inexpensive and carries none of the risks of an invasive diagnostic procedure. Important potential deficiencies of ultrasound include stenoses in the mild to moderate range (near 60 percent) and very severely narrowed or preocclusive lesions of the carotid artery, which may be misinterpreted as total occlusions.

A lumbar puncture (LP) is recommended for patients with a high clinical suspicion of SAH and a negative CT scan, as it may reveal blood in the cerebrospinal fluid (CSF).[10] Approximately 5 percent of patients with subarachnoid hemorrhage have a normal CT.[11] Such patients usually have a small bleed and are alert without focal neurologic findings. If the patient has altered consciousness or focal findings, LP is deferred until CT evaluation. If CT demonstrates bleeding in a patient with SAH, an LP is contraindicated because it may precipitate a herniation syndrome in patients with a large hematoma. Performing a LP will also prohibit the later use of thrombolytic therapy.

Echocardiography (transthoracic or transesophageal) is performed commonly to evaluate possible cardiogenic causes of stroke. Valvular vegetations, mural thrombus, and wall motion abnormalities are easily detected by this study.

TREATMENT

Stroke Prevention

The focus of primary care should be on altering modifiable risk factors such as hypertension, diabetes, hyperlipidemia, atrial fibrillation, obesity, and smoking. Other treatments are tailored to specific causes of stroke, such as known carotid lesions and structural heart abnormalities.

Anticoagulants

Systemic heparinization is controversial in acute stroke because of the risk of hemorrhage into the infarct zone and probably should be used only under the direction of a neurologist. It is an extremely useful and potent medication for use in recurrent emboli, arterial dissection, and acutely thrombosed vessels and in preparation for surgery as well as for hypercoagulable states in which long-term warfarin (Coumadin) therapy is initiated.

Warfarin has been clearly shown to reduce the risk of stroke in patients with atrial fibrillation. An International Normalized Ratio (INR) of 2 to 3 is recommended for this indication. Warfarin also may be used in situations where antiplatelet agents have failed or are contraindicated (nonsteroidal anti-inflammatory drug sensitivities, gastric irritation, etc.) and in special circumstances such as complete carotid occlusion, in which the uppermost end of the occlusion may serve as

an embolic source to the cerebral circulation. Warfarin also may be used in symptomatic patients for whom surgery is contraindicated.

Antiplatelet Agents

Aspirin and ticlopidine (Ticlid) have been shown to decrease the risk of subsequent stroke in patients with a minor completed stroke. Aspirin is the primary antiplatelet agent used in stroke prevention since it is inexpensive and is well tolerated by most people. It is used primarily for asymptomatic carotid stenosis or for symptomatic stenosis in the mild to moderate range. The most effective dose is controversial, ranging from 80 to 325 mg daily. Ticlopidine is as effective as aspirin in stroke reduction but is considerably more expensive and is associated with side effects, including diarrhea and gastrointestinal upset, and is occasionally associated with neutropenia. Therefore, it requires monitoring of white blood cell counts every 2 weeks for the first 3 months of therapy. The usual dose is 250 mg twice daily. It generally is reserved for patients who have contraindications to aspirin.

Thrombolytics

The use of intraarterial and intravenous thrombolytic agents such as tissue plasminogen activator (TPA), streptokinase, and urokinase has been evaluated in stroke patients in clinical trials.[12,13] The U.S. Food and Drug Administration (FDA) has approved intravenous TPA for use in selected patients with ischemic stroke based on the positive results of an NINDS trial.[12] In the NINDS trial, patients treated with TPA within 3 h of the onset of symptoms were at least 30 percent more likely to have minimal or no disability at 3 months compared with those treated with placebo. Thrombolytic therapy is not recommended unless the diagnosis of acute ischemic stroke is established by a physician experienced in evaluating CT scans and diagnosing stroke.[11] It carries the real risk of major bleeding, and its use in children requires further study. See the American Heart Association guidelines recommendations and checklist for thrombolytic therapy.[14]

Carotid Endarterectomy

Three randomized studies have shown the superiority of carotid endarterectomy to aspirin alone in preventing subsequent stroke in symptomatic patients with greater than 70 percent carotid stenosis. In asymptomatic patients, the Asymptomatic Carotid Atherosclerosis Study (ACAS) has shown a slightly decreased risk of stroke over 5 years in patients with greater than 60 percent stenosis if the surgical risk is 3 percent or less.[15] The ACAS study determined the degree of stenosis by angiography, which means that the combined risk of angiography and surgery must not exceed 3 percent for a benefit to be seen. Severe asymptomatic stenoses (greater than 80 percent) may be at increased risk of embolization and therefore may benefit from surgery coupled with aggressive risk-factor modification if a patient is a good surgical risk and has a life expectancy that is thought to extend beyond 5 years.

ASYMPTOMATIC CAROTID BRUITS

Carotid bruits are commonly found in elderly patients and those with risk factors for atherosclerosis. The first step in their management is to determine the degree of narrowing by duplex ultrasonography. All patients with carotid plaques probably should be instructed to take at least 80 mg of aspirin daily for overall risk reduction. Severe stenoses should be referred to a vascular surgeon for evaluation. Otherwise, periodic examinations and follow-up ultrasound should be performed to determine whether the plaque is stable or progressing. Patients and their family members should be educated about stroke and TIA symptoms and instructed to notify the practitioner immediately if they occur.

MANAGEMENT OF ACUTE STROKE

Management of an acute CVA patient depends on the severity of the presentation. It is recommended that a neurologist be involved in all but the most minor CVAs for a thorough evaluation and documentation of the neurologic deficits and to maximize the treatment and rehabilitation potential of the patient. The intricacies of stroke treatment are beyond the scope of this chapter, but some fundamental knowledge is presented here. As always, the initial step is addressing the ABCs of airway, breathing, and circulation. Difficulty handling secretions is common in stroke patients because of dysphagia or an impaired gag reflex, and so airways should be protected to prevent aspiration. One should bear in mind that cardiac arrhythmias can be the cause of or can result from a CVA.

Hypertension is commonly seen in acute stroke, with diastolic pressure as high as 115 mmHg. Treatment for this is controversial, but in most cases the blood pressure should not be lowered. This is a protective mechanism induced by the brain to maintain blood flow to the poorly perfused infarct zone. Treatment of hypertension generally should be undertaken only if signs of end organ damage are present, such as angina, congestive heart failure, papilledema, hematuria, and retinal hemorrhages. In large intracranial hemorrhages caused by severe hypertension, the blood pressure may gingerly be lowered by about 25 percent over the first 24 h, but this must be done slowly, as the brain requires a high perfusion pressure. It is also important to control pyrexia, which occurs in one-third of stroke patients, with acetaminophen because of the increased metabolic demands this places on the brain. Hyperglycemia should be kept to 150 mg/dL or less because excess glucose is converted to lactic acid, which may exacerbate tissue damage.

Stroke in evolution is a medical emergency that should involve a neurologist immediately to determine its cause, which is frequently acute occlusion of an intracranial or extracranial vessel. Anticoagulation, surgery, and thrombolytic therapies are controversial in acute or evolving stroke patients but may avert a devastating or fatal stroke if applied early and appropriately. These patients should be kept flat in bed to maximize cerebral blood flow.

All subarachnoid hemorrhages require neurosurgical consultation to determine whether cerebral angiography or surgery is required. These patients should be kept in a dark, quiet room with adequate analgesia. These measures are intended to prevent rebleeding while a patient is awaiting neurosurgical evaluation.

Large intracranial hemorrhages resulting in increased ICP also may require neurosurgical consultation for decompression if they are anatomically accessible. Patients with infarcts in the posterior fossa can deteriorate rapidly because of brainstem compression. Neurosurgical consultation should be obtained early in these patients if signs of increased ICP are present. All patients with intracerebral hemorrhages should be kept with the head of the bed elevated 30 degrees to prevent cerebral edema.

Future Developments

When a thrombolytic drug is used to lyse a blood clot, blood flows into oxygen-deprived areas of brain tissue. Granulocytes are drawn into the injured tissue, where they adhere to the vessel walls and release protein-dissolving enzymes and free radicals. This can cause more extensive injury or reperfusion injury. Adhesion of granulocytes to the cell wall also brings about a partial reocclusion of the arteries. New drugs that block granulocyte binding or neutralize antibodies and free radicals are being developed. These neuroprotective agents may slow the tissue damage and extend the window of time for the successful treatment of ischemic stroke.[16]

REFERENCES

1. *1997 Heart and Stroke Statistical Update.* Dallas, American Heart Association; 1996.
2. Hazinski MF: Demystifying recognition and management of stroke. *Currents in Emergency Cardiac Care,* Winter, 6–7, 1996.
3. American Heart Association: *Stroke Statistics: Chronic Diseases and Their Risk Factors,* http://www.americanheart.org/HeartandStroke_A_ Z_Guide/asa.html.
4. SHEP Cooperative Research Group: Prevention of stroke by antihypertensive drug treatment in older persons with isolated systolic hypertension: Final results of the Systolic Hypertension in the Elderly Program (SHEP). *JAMA* 265:3255–3264, 1991.
5. Tzourio C, et al: Case-controlled study of migraine and risk of ischaemic stroke in young women. *BMJ* 310(6983):830–833, 1995.
6. Grotta JC. The importance of time, in *Proceedings of the National Symposium on Rapid Identification and Treatment of Acute Stroke.* National Institute of Neurological Disorders and Stroke, in press.
7. Pepe PE: The chain of recovery from brain attack: Access, prehospital care, and treatment, in *Proceedings of the National Symposium on Rapid Identification and Treatment of Acute Stroke.* National Institute of Neurological Disorders and Stroke, in press.
8. Kothari R, Hall K, Broderick J, Brott T: Early stroke recognition: Developing an out-of hospital stroke scale. *Acad Emerg Med* 1997.
9. Tierney L, McPhee SJ, Papadakis M (eds): *Current Medical Diagnosis and Treatment.* Stamford, CT, Appleton & Lange, 1999.
10. Mayberg MR, Batjer HH, Dacey R, et al: Guidelines for the management of aneurismal subarachnoid hemorrhage: A statement for healthcare professionals from a special writing group of the Stroke Council, American Heart Association. *Circulation* 90:2592–2605, 1994.
11. Adams HP, Brott TG, Furlan AJ, et al: Guidelines for thrombolytic therapy for acute stroke: A supplement to the guidelines for the management of patients with acute ischemic stroke. A statement for healthcare professionals from a special writing group of the Stroke Council, American Heart Association. *Circulation* 27:1711–1718, 1996.
12. The National Institute of Neurological Disorders and Stroke rt-PA Stroke Study Group: Tissue plasminogen activator for acute ischemic stroke. *N Engl J Med* 333:1581–1587, 1995.
13. Hacke W, Kaste M, Fieschi C, et al: Intravenous thrombolysis with recombinant tissue plasminogen activator for acute hemispheric stroke: The European Cooperative Acute Stroke Study (ECASS). *JAMA* 274:1017–1025, 1995.
14. American Heart Association: *Advanced Cardiac Life Support: Acute Stroke,* Dallas, TX 1997.
15. Executive Committee for the Asymptomatic Carotid Atherosclerotic Study: Endarterectomy for asymptomatic carotid artery stenosis. *JAMA* 273(18):1421–1459, 1995.
16. Barinaga M: Finding new drugs to treat stroke. *Science* 272:664–666, 1996.

ACKNOWLEDGMENTS

The editor wishes to acknowledge Dennis Loudenback, the author of this chapter in the first edition of *Primary Care for Physician Assistants,* whose work is included significantly in this update.

BIBLIOGRAPHY

Bronner LL, Kanter DS, Manson JE: Primary prevention of stroke. *N Engl J Med* 333:1392–1399, 1995.

Dobkin B: The economic impact of stroke. *Neurology* 45(Suppl 1):S6–S9, 1995.

Fauci AS, Braunwald E, Isselbacher KJ, et al (eds): *Harrison's Principles of Internal Medicine,* 14th ed. New York, McGraw-Hill, 1998, pp 2325–2348.

Gorelick P: Stroke prevention. *Arch Neurol* 2:347–355, 1995.

Pryse-Phillips W, Yegappan MC: Management of acute stroke: Ways to minimize damage and maximize recovery. *Postgrad Med* 96(5):75–85, 1994.

Roth GJ, Calverley DC: Aspirin, platelets, and thrombosis: Theory and practice. *Blood* 83(4):885–898, 1994.

Rowland LP (ed): *Merritt's Textbook of Neurology,* 9th ed. Media, PA, Williams & Wilkins, 1995, pp 227–285.

Rutherford RB (ed): *Vascular Surgery,* 4th ed. Philadelphia, Saunders, 1995, pp 1456–1660.

Schwartz GR, Cayten CG, Mangelsen MA, et al (eds): *Principles and Practice of Emergency Medicine,* 3d ed. Malvern, PA, Lea & Febiger, 1992, pp 1523–1533.

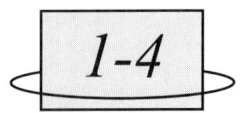

ATHEROSCLEROSIS

Catherine J. Heymann

DISCUSSION

Derived from the Greek *athero* ("porridge" or "gruel") and *sklerosis* ("hardening"), atherosclerosis is one of the leading causes of death in the United States. Atherosclerotic vascular disease (ASVD) affects the endothelial and intimal layers of the artery, resulting in plaque formation, narrowing of the lumen, decreased elasticity, alterations in contractility, and reduced blood flow.

A positive correlation between elevated serum lipid levels and atherosclerotic plaque formation is firmly established in the literature. Total cholesterol (TC) is divided into five general lipoprotein subclasses according to the density of each particle. Each lipoprotein subclass has a distinct chemical structure, specific role in lipid metabolism, and implications for ASVD (see Chap. 1-7). It is important to remember that atherosclerotic plaque formation may exist even if the TC is within "normal" ranges. This paradox has now focused attention on the role of low-density lipoprotein cholesterol (LDL-C) subclasses, intermediate lipoproteins, and remnant particles in plaque formation.

A strong correlation has also been established between several other risk factors and ASVD. If known risk factors are treated, the incidence of ASVD may be reduced and the progression slowed or regressed. Risk factors are classified as nonreversible or reversible (see Table 1-4-1). Fortunately, a "nonreversible" risk factor may be ameliorated by intensive management of treatable risk factors.

PATHOGENESIS

A three-layer permeable pipe, the artery is metabolically active. It maintains and repairs its structural components by secreting fatty acids, cholesterol, phospholipids, triglycerides, growth factors, and enzymes. A free exchange of fluids and solutes in blood takes place through the arterial membrane (see Table 1-4-2).

ASVD begins in early childhood and slowly progresses to symptomatic disease in the adult. Disease begins with the formation of a "fatty streak" within the arterial wall. Smooth muscle cells gradually surround the fatty streak, forming a fibrous cap. Through the years, the lesion fills with fibromuscular and/or fibrolipid material. As unhealthy lipid levels and risk factors persist, the lesion continues to grow in size and eventually encroaches into the arterial lumen. If the lesion ruptures and

TABLE 1-4-1. Risk Factors for Atherosclerotic Vascular Disease (ASVD)

NONREVERSIBLE	REVERSIBLE
Age	Cigarette smoking
Gender	Hypertension
Family history of premature CAD	Hyperlipidemia
Hyperinsulinemia (insulin resistance)	HDL-C <35 mg/dL
Genetic factors	Elevated lipoprotein(a) LDL-C >160 mg/dL Homocystinemia Diabetes mellitus Carbohydrate intolerance Abdominal obesity with a waist/hip ratio >0.8 in women and 1.0 in men Sedentary lifestyle

TABLE 1-4-2. Normal Artery Physiology

Intima

    Inner lining of artery
    Permeable and allows passive transport of LDL-C to subepithelial space
    Able to secrete several chemical factors needed for blood flow

Media

    Composed of smooth muscle cells bound by elastic and fibrous tissue
    Secondary site of atherosclerotic plaque formation as disease progresses

Adventitia

    Artery's outermost layer

forms a thrombosis, partial or complete occlusion of the artery will occur producing ischemia, infarction, or sudden death.

Plaque formation has overlapping yet distinct developmental phases—lipid deposition, cellular transport, and plaque thrombosis (see Figure 1-4-1).

Lipid Deposition

Atherosclerosis begins with the deposition of LDL-C in the subepithelial (intimal) space of the arterial wall. Once inside the subepithelial space, the oxidation of LDL-C produces *foam cells.* The foam cells eventually form a fatty streak in the vessel wall and are the earliest manifestation of the atherosclerotic process. A fatty streak has little clinical sequelae and does not encroach into the arterial lumen.

Cellular Transport

Smooth muscle cells migrate to and proliferate around the fatty streak, eventually forming a fibrous plaque. Ultimately, the lesion protrudes into the arterial lumen, causing stenosis. Vessels with up to a 90% occlusion may remain patent, be relatively asymptomatic, and provide an adequate blood supply to distal tissues.

Plaque Thrombosis

It is the soft, unstable lesion of 50 to 60 percent stenosis that is more likely to rupture and cause thrombus formation, occlusion, ischemia, and infarction of distal tissues. Calcified plaque is more stable, less likely to rupture or regress in size. Plaque progression may also result in an arterial wall weakness or aneurysm, especially in the abdominal aorta.

MICROBIOLOGY

No viral or bacterial pathogens have been identified in ASVD. One recent study found *Chlamydia pneumoniae* in up to 90% of arteries of patients with atherosclerotic plaque and in only about 4% of arteries of control subjects. Science is currently debating whether the bacteria causes the plaque formation or invades the plaque after its formation. The use of antibiotics to prevent plaque formation is now being evaluated. Numerous studies will be needed to define the organism's role, if any, in ASVD.

SIGNS AND SYMPTOMS

Sudden death may be the first and last symptom of ASVD. Atherosclerotic plaque produces few perceivable symptoms until the stenosis reaches critical levels or ruptures suddenly. Location of the occlusive lesion will usually determine any symptomatology. Patients may report a slow onset of angina, dyspnea, intermittent claudication, fatigue, cold extremities, arrhythmias, or transient ischemic attacks.

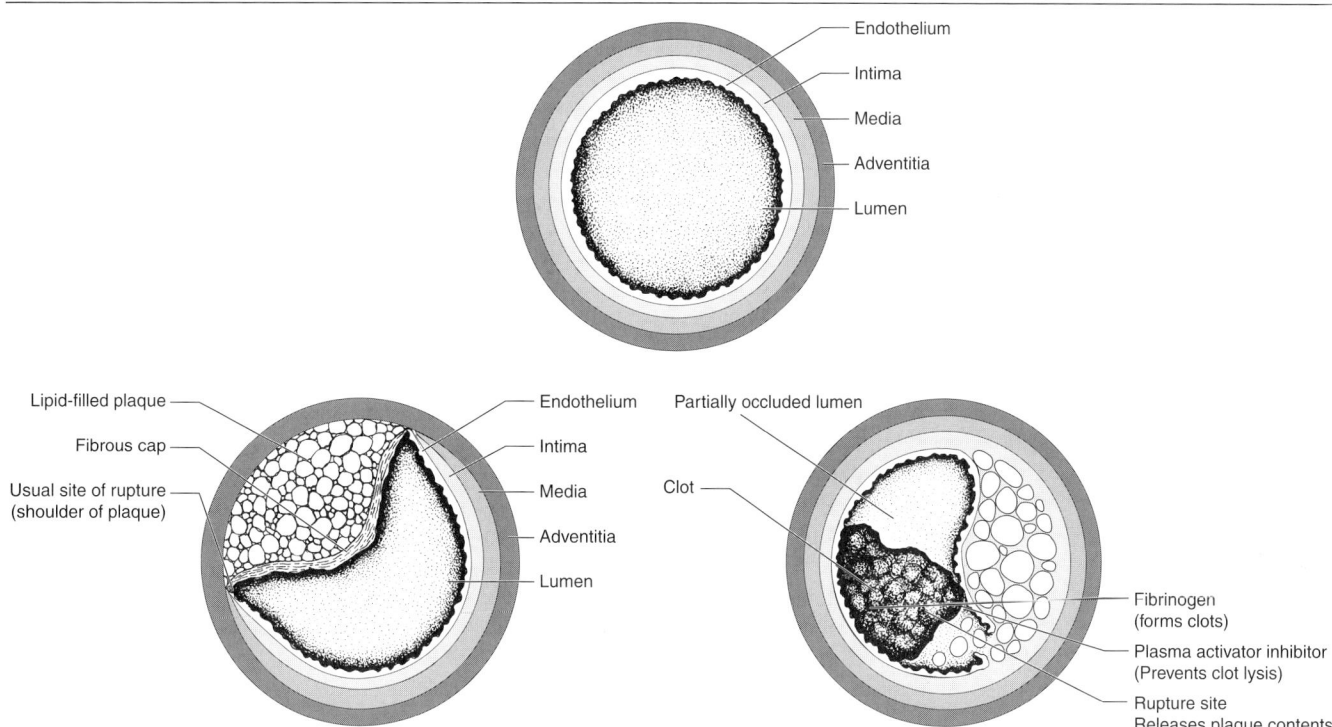

FIGURE 1-4-1. Stages of plaque formation.

OBJECTIVE FINDINGS

Subtle clues during history taking and physical examination may suggest the presence of ASVD, but a definitive diagnosis requires the use of angiography and/or various radiologic modalities. Disease may be surprisingly localized or widely diffuse. Each major organ system should be carefully evaluated for evidence of atherosclerosis (see Table 1-4-3). Laboratory data, chest radiography, electrocardiography, or exercise stress testing may provide additional evidence for ASVD. Referral to a cardiologist or vascular surgeon may be appropriate.

DIAGNOSTIC CONSIDERATIONS

Diagnosis of ASVD is often presumptive and based on the functional, physiologic, or metabolic effects of a narrowed arterial lumen. Differential diagnoses of common presenting symptoms—fatigue, dyspnea, chest pain, claudication, peripheral edema—should be considered (see Table 1-4-4).

Etiologies unrelated to atherogenesis may also result in a decreased arterial lumen diameter. Therefore, the course of disease and treatment modalities in such cases may be substantially different from those involving plaque formation, stenosis, and occlusion.

Mönckeberg's sclerosis consists of focal deposits of calcium in the smooth muscle cells of the medial layer of the artery causing rigid arteries that are easily visible on radiograph, readily palpable, and tortuous. The exact cause is not known, but long-term use of corticosteroids, smoking, or poorly controlled diabetes may be implicated. Arterial stenosis is seen only if ASVD coexists.

Arteriolosclerosis is a degeneration and hyalinization of the arteries/arterioles of major organs such as the spleen, pancreas, kidney, and adrenal glands. Hypertension is often present. Disease results in arteries that are hyperplastic, elastic, fibrous, or necrosed. Leriche's syndrome is a chronic obstruction of the aortic bifurcation from arteriosclerosis. Intermittent claudication in the buttocks, impotence, and absent femoral pulses are the usual symptoms.

A diffuse proliferation of smooth muscle cells and cholesterol esters in the medial layer of the artery cause age-related thickening of the arterial wall. The amount of cholesterol deposition is thought to be directly related to circulating plasma lipid levels. Resulting defects include rigidity; increased arterial wall width, dilation, and elongation; tortuous contour; and focal arterial wall weakness that may result in aneurysms. Atherosclerotic plaque formation is a separate process but often coexists. Small vessel disease secondary to diabetes, renal insufficiency, autoimmune disorders, hypersensitivity, or congenital structural defects may also result in dysfunctional vasculature.

SPECIAL CONSIDERATIONS

Diabetes mellitus (DM) is associated with an increased risk of atherogenesis and peripheral vascular disease in both insulin- and non-insulin-dependent states. The role of altered carbohydrate metabolism is unclear but thought to be multifactorial. The increase in circulating insulin due to insulin resistance often observed in DM type 2 may contribute to the increased incidence of atherosclerosis. Whatever the mechanism, there is no histologic difference in atherosclerotic lesions found in diabetic individuals and in persons with normal glucose tolerance. The Diabetes Control and Complications Trial has implied that blood glucose control resulting in a glycosylated hemoglobin within one percentage point of "normal" (<7%) may reduce the risk of ASVD (see Chap. 5-1).

Obesity alone has not proved to be an independent risk factor for atherosclerosis. However, abdominal adiposity with a waist/hip ratio greater than 0.8 in women and 1.0 in men is strongly correlated with the development of diabetes and/or cardiac disease. Gluteal and femoral obesity are not associated with increased risk. If carbohydrate intolerance, hypertension, hyperlipidemias, or insulin resistance syndrome accompany obesity, increased rates of ASVD are noted (see Chap. 5-12).

Hypertension is associated with many forms of cardiovascular disease including ASVD. Thiazides and beta blockers, often used in hypertensive therapy, may potentiate increases in plasma lipid or glucose levels, both ASVD risk factors. However, current information

TABLE 1-4-3. Clues to ASVD on Physical Exam

Funduscopic Exam

"Silver wire" veins
Altered artery/vein ratio
A-V "nicking"
Hollenhorst plaque

Cardiac

New onset murmurs
Arrhythmias
S_3 (atrial gallops) or S_4 (ventricular gallops)
Heart sounds
Cardiomegaly
Shift in cardiac axis
Electrocardiogram changes
Neck vein distention
Carotid bruits
Paradoxical pulse

Pulmonary Exam

Basilar rales
Wheezes

Abdominal Exam

Aortic, renal, or iliac bruits
Pulsating abdominal mass
Palpable aorta wider than 5 cm

Extremity Exam

Cyanosis or clubbing of nails
Cool feet or hands
Decreased or absent pulses
Poor capillary refill
Edema
Arterial insufficiency

Skin Exam

Cool, dusky, mottled, pale skin
Abnormally dry flaking or thickened skin
Plantar or malleolar ulcerations
Erythema or rubor of the skin
Shiny, hairless skin
Xanthomas of tendon sheaths
Xanthomas in skin creases of hands, eyelids, or elbows

TABLE 1-4-4. Differential Diagnosis

Edema

venous insufficiency or obstruction
lymphatic obstruction
tumor invasion or compression
surgical damage
physical trauma
lymphedema
cor pulmonale
malnutrition
liver or renal disease
myxedema
volume overload or alterations in vascular permeability
adverse reaction to drugs

Dyspnea

pneumothorax
pulmonary edema
pulmonary emboli
trauma
sepsis
pneumonia
tuberculosis
emphysema
asthma
lung cancer
interstitial lung disease
pulmonary hypertension
pleural effusions
gastric or foreign body aspiration
noxious gas inhalation
acute anemia
metabolic acidosis

Chest Pain

skin and subcutaneous lesions
breast lesions
bruised or fractured rib
mitral valve prolapse
periosteal hematoma
costochondritis
intercostal myositis
muscular strain
shoulder bursitis, strain, tendinitis
cervical disk herniation
osteoarthritis
thoracic outlet syndrome
neuralgias
pericardial diseases
mediastinal disorders
pulmonary disease
gastroesophageal reflux
gastritis
peptic ulcer disease
cholecystitis
pancreatitis
psychogenic sources

Arrhythmias

hyperthyroidism
anxiety
hyperventilation
anemia
fever
volume depletion
postural hypotension
hypoglycemia
adverse drug reaction
other cardiac disorder

is controversial concerning the duration of any metabolic change and the actual long-term risk-versus-benefit ratio of utilizing these medications (see Chap. 1-12).

Family history of early coronary artery disease (CAD) or death from myocardial infarction may indicate a genetic abnormality of lipid metabolism. Although the role of genetic mechanisms are not completely understood, early detection and management of treatable risk factors seems prudent. Even if lipids are within normal ranges, a strong family history of early cardiac disease warrants further investigation to diagnose and treat genetic dyslipidemias.

Chronic cigarette smoking or exposure to secondhand tobacco smoke is a well-established risk factor for ASVD. Increased risk for development or progression of ASVD appears to be reversible with smoking cessation.

LABORATORY TESTS

No blood test for atherosclerosis exists. Laboratory testing is directed toward discovery of accompanying metabolic disorders, evaluation of genetic susceptibility, and evaluation of efficacy of treatment. See Chap. 1-6 on hyperlipidemia for recommendations on laboratory testing.

RADIOLOGIC STUDIES

Radiologic visualization by angiography is the "gold standard" for diagnosis and evaluation of ASVD. Several other less invasive testing methods are available, including Doppler studies, ultrafast computed tomography scans (CINE-CT), magnetic resonance imaging (MRI), positron emission tomography (PET), radionuclide imaging, coronary angiography, intravascular ultrasound (IVUS), angioscopy, arterial scans, and echocardiograms. Each technique has its advantages, disadvantages, risk factors, costs, availability, and diagnostic value.

A chest radiograph may detect calcification of the aorta or arteries, congestive heart failure, cardiomegaly, aneurysm, or other abnormalities associated with ASVD. However, atherosclerotic plaque is not always calcified and the extent of calcification noted on x-ray will not always correlate with the severity of disease.

OTHER DIAGNOSTICS

An electrocardiogram (ECG) is inexpensive and the least invasive and readily available study for detection of myocardial ischemia. Nonspecific S-T changes, Q waves, arrhythmias, or left ventricular hypertrophy may indicate the need for further diagnostic testing. Young women may have a "false positive" ECG with nonspecific S-T wave changes that may not be indicative of cardiac disease. The decision for more intensive testing relies on apparent risk factors, family history, laboratory data, symptoms, and current medical status. Ambulatory electrocardiographic monitoring (Holter monitor) may demonstrate cardiac ischemic changes in the asymptomatic patient. Remember, a normal ECG *does not* exclude ASVD or cardiac disease.

TREATMENT

Therapy is directed to reducing lipids and managing the symptoms of vessel stenosis, including angina pectoris, hypertension, claudication, congestive heart failure, and arrhythmias. Additional therapy should focus on the reduction of treatable risk factors such as hyperglycemia, smoking, obesity, physical inactivity, and stress.

Pharmacologic Management

There is no direct pharmacologic treatment for atherosclerotic plaque although new modalities are under investigation. Partial regression of plaque size has been documented with tight lipid management by several studies. See Chap. 1-6 for discussion of pharmacologic management of hyperlipidemias.

Aspirin therapy (81 mg/d) has been shown to be an effective tool in lowering coronary artery and cerebrovascular events by reducing platelet aggregation. Enteric-coated aspirin may be used in individuals with a history of gastric irritation.

Therapy with statins may reduce endothelial inflammation and dysfunction as well as lipid levels, theoretically reducing the progression of plaque formation. Many patients will need combination therapy with statins, fibrates, niacin, etc.

Surgical Treatment

Numerous invasive procedures may be utilized to reduce or remove vessel stenosis. Percutaneous transluminal angioplasty (PCTA), atherectomy, endarterectomy, laser therapy, intravascular stents, coronary artery bypass surgery (CABS), and arterial graft surgeries are widely available. PCTA is indicated in patients with angina, ischemia, thrombosis, or acute myocardial infarction. Atherectomy removes, rather than stretches, the obstructing plaque. Current technology includes directional coronary atherectomy (DCA), rotational ablation, transluminal extraction (TEC), and lasers. Atherectomy is often utilized for difficult lesions or chronic restenosis. Stents are coiled or interwoven metal tubes that provide an internal supporting structure to hold a vessel open against its elastic recoil.

Revascularization may also be achieved through bypass or graft surgery. CABS is usually reserved for severe or multiple vessel disease. Grafting techniques may be utilized in the repair of aneurysms, major artery stenosis, and cerebral revascularization. Unfortunately, reocclusion is a frequent complication. Studies indicate revascularization procedures are required in approximately 50% of patients within 5 to 10 years. Grafted vessels are three to six times more likely to restenose. Fortunately, medication, diet, and lifestyle modifications have been shown to prolong the time to restenosis significantly.

Supportive Measures

The preferred treatment modality, prevention, is classified as either primary or secondary. In primary prevention, measures to avoid the development of ASVD are initiated. Secondary prevention focuses on arresting the progression of ASVD after clinical disease is evident. The treatment and prevention of ASVD involve the triad of medical therapy, pharmacologic management, and lifestyle modifications.

Life-style modifications include smoking cessation, dietary changes, increased physical activity, and stress reduction. Each component is essential in reducing the risk of or limiting the progression of ASVD. Smoking cessation and obesity have been discussed earlier in this text. Current recommendations for dietary modification of hyperlipidemias are reviewed in Chap. 1-6. Moderate use of red wine or alcohol may reduce the risk of ASVD. The exact mechanism is not clearly understood, but it may include increases in protective high-density lipoprotein cholesterol (HDL-C) or the antioxidant properties of the bioflavonoids (phenols) in grapes. Careful counseling on drug/alcohol interactions should be included in any recommendations for alcohol consumption.

Numerous studies have confirmed the benefits of physical activity in the treatment of obesity, stress, hypertension, diabetes, and cardiac disease. Exercise appears to have a favorable impact on serum cholesterol levels (HDL-C, TC), improves physical conditioning, and facilitates weight (fat) loss. Any aerobic activity enjoyed by the individual should be encouraged with the emphasis placed on frequency and duration rather than intensity. An exercise prescription should include a gradual conditioning process and should not be so intense as to discourage compliance. Ultimate goals include one-half hour of aerobic exercise three to five times per week within target heart rate (THR) ranges or target training zones on the Borg Scale of Perceived Exertion. Individuals at risk for ASVD should be carefully evaluated before beginning any exercise program.

$$THR = (220 - age) \times .60 \text{ to } .80.$$

Conditioning should begin at 60 percent of THR and advance to 80 percent.

The Borg Scale of Perceived Exertion is a scale of 0 to 20 upon which a patient bases his or her perceived level of exertion. Lower numbers correlate with a minimum exercise level and higher numbers with maximal exertion level.

The role of stress is not clearly understood, but stress may be capable of precipitating an acute cardiac episode in a susceptible individual. Knowledge of a patient's personality and lifestyle is helpful when referring to sources for counseling on stress modification.

PATIENT EDUCATION

Education should describe the disease process and treatment modalities while empowering the patient to make life-style modifications. Information is essential if an individual is to understand the expected benefit, methodology, or potential adverse effects and risks of a treatment modality. Compliance will usually increase in direct proportion to effective patient education. The local affiliate of the American Heart Association is one of many organizations that can provide educational materials to the practitioner and the patient. Regular follow-up to evaluate for complications, progression of disease, and reassessment of the treatment plan may improve the patient's compliance and quality of life. Referral to a cardiologist or vascular surgeon for evaluation and consultation may be appropriate. Education and medical nutrition therapy by a registered dietitian is important for successful dietary modification. Utilizing an exercise physiologist, physical therapist, or cardiac rehabilitation program may enhance exercise compliance.

COMPLICATIONS AND RED FLAGS

The medical practitioner must be alert to the signs and symptoms of disease progression or reocclusion. A patient who is noncompliant with necessary life-style changes or has suboptimal control of a comorbid disease should be monitored closely. Careful questioning and history taking will help elicit information on recurrent symptoms in a timely fashion.

NOTES AND PEARLS

Research on future treatment for atherosclerosis is concentrating on preventing as well as curing ASVD. Gene therapy, direct drug delivery systems, advanced pharmacologic agents, new laboratory testing procedures, and innovations in surgical technology are on the horizon. Innovative utilization of "old" drugs such as estrogen, nitrous oxide, folate, vitamin B$_6$, L-arginine, and vitamin E are promising.

Laboratory tests can now identify and quantitate specific lipoprotein subclasses thought to be atherogenic. A lipid panel alone may not be sufficient to diagnose a patient prone to ASVD. The Framingham Study showed that individuals with elevated cholesterol levels are at higher risk for heart disease; however, nearly 80 percent of those individuals developing heart disease maintained TC levels similar to those who did not. Possibly one of the most sensitive indicators for current or future development of atherosclerosis is an elevation in C-reactive protein (hs-CRP) coupled with dyslipidemia. Increased levels of hs-CRP may indicate endothelial inflammation or dysfunction, an early phase in atherosclerotic plaque formation. Elevated levels of plasminogen activator inhibitor-1 (PAI-1) and fibrinogen may also be markers of cardiovascular disease. Although numerous new modalities are on the horizon, individuals will still need to maintain a healthy lifestyle utilizing diet, exercise, stress reduction, and smoking cessation to reduce the development of cardiovascular disease.

BIBLIOGRAPHY

FORRESTER JS: Efficacy of risk factor management. *J Am Coll Cordiol* 27:964–1047, 1996.

HAFFNER S et al: Insulin sensitivity in subjects with type 2 diabetes. *Diabetes Care* 22(4): 562–568, 19xx.

ISSELBACHER KJ et al: *Harrison's Principles of Medicine*, 14th ed. New York, McGraw-Hill 1994.

MUHLESTEIN JB et al: Increased incidence of *Chlamydia* species within the coronary arteries of patients with symptomatic atherosclerotic versus other forms of cardiovascular disease. *J Am Coll Cardiol* 27:1555–61, 1996.

SKILLINGS J, HOWES DG: Recertification series hyperlipidemia and atherosclerosis, part I. *Physician Assistant* 7:32–68, 1996.

SKILLINGS J, HOWES DG: Recertification series hyperlipidemia and atherosclerosis, part II. *Physician Assistant* 8:32–62, 1996.

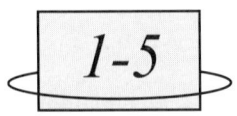

COR PULMONALE

Katherine Adamson

DESCRIPTION

The term *cor pulmonale* refers to enlargement or malfunction of the right ventricle secondary to pulmonary hypertension. The antecedent pulmonary hypertension may result from disease of the lung parenchyma or pulmonary vasculature or from diseases that affect the mechanics of respiration. Cor pulmonale may occur acutely secondary to massive pulmonary emboli. This chapter addresses the more common chronic process.

In the United States, chronic obstructive pulmonary disease (COPD) is by far the most common etiology of cor pulmonale. An estimated 47 million people in this country suffer from COPD; more than half of these individuals have evidence of cor pulmonale. In terms of prevalence, approximately 5 to 10 percent of adult heart disease can be attributed to cor pulmonale.

PATHOGENESIS

To understand the pathophysiology associated with cor pulmonale, it is vital that one appreciate the marked differences in pressure normally found in the pulmonary circulation compared with the systemic circulation. The pulmonary circulation is best thought of as a very compliant reservoir with vascular resistance approximately one-tenth that of the systemic circulation. This relatively easy compliance allows for minute-to-minute changes in flow volume with a minimal increase in pulmonary artery pressure. For pulmonary hypertension to result in cor pulmonale, a significant disturbance in the form of diffuse pulmonary vasoconstriction or occlusion of the pulmonary arterial system has to have occurred. As was stated above, COPD leads the list of the etiologies of cor pulmonale. Table 1-5-1 summarizes other common causes.

The pulmonary vessels course through pulmonary parenchymal tissue. With COPD, the alveoli enlarge and place direct pressure on the very thin peripheral vessels. These vessels respond to this external pressure with compression and eventual shunting of blood away from the periphery of the lung and toward the more central regions. Added to this abnormal situation is a relative degree of hypoxia-induced vasoconstriction. The result is an increase in pulmonary artery pressure. This increase in right ventricular afterload causes the right ventricle to compensate by increasing its muscle mass, leading to right ventricular hypertrophy (RVH).

SYMPTOMS

Chronic cor pulmonale does not exist by itself. These patients present with symptoms of the underlying process that resulted in RVH and eventual failure. The clinician should quantify the type and degree of pulmonary disease process and then be alert for the development of cor pulmonale. Typically, the patient complains of an increase in chronic respiratory distress in the form of progressive easy fatigability, an increase in dyspnea and sputum production, and the symptoms of right-sided heart failure, particularly peripheral edema.

OBJECTIVE FINDINGS

The examiner must be aware that the classic abnormal findings associated with right ventricular failure may be obscured by the physical alterations that are common in patients with COPD. For example, the left parasternal heave noted in RVH may not be palpable because

TABLE 1-5-1. Etiologies of Cor Pulmonale

Diseases of the lung parenchyma
  Emphysema
  Chronic bronchitis
  Absence of lung tissue secondary to trauma and/or surgical resection
  Cystic fibrosis

Diseases of pulmonary vasculature
  Primary pulmonary hypertension
  Acute massive pulmonary emboli causing acute cor pulmonale
  Recurrent small emboli resulting in chronic cor pulmonale

Infiltrative processes
  Connective tissue diseases such as sarcoidosis, rheumatoid arthritis, and systemic lupus erythematosus
  Malignant and/or metastatic disease

Processes that affect the mechanics of respiration
  Morbid obesity
  Thoracic malformations such as kyphoscoliosis
  Sleep apnea syndromes

of pulmonary hyperinflation and the development of a barrel-shaped thorax. With that caveat in mind, physical examination findings may include the following. The patient will be dyspneic and often will show signs of central cyanosis. Examination of the neck veins will demonstrate distention and prominence of the *a* and *v* waves. (Recall that the *a* wave corresponds to atrial contraction, while the *v* wave relates to atrial filling.) Inspection and palpation of the precordium may reveal a parasternal lift caused by the hypertrophied right ventricle. Upon auscultation, the examiner often notes a systolic murmur along the left lower sternal border that changes with respiration. This is the murmur of tricuspid regurgitation resulting from stretch on the valve annulus by the dilated and hypertrophied right ventricle. When the heart sounds are not too obscured by pulmonary disease, one may appreciate the accentuated closure of the pulmonic valve (loud P_2 or S_2), which is considered diagnostic of pulmonary hypertension. A right-sided S_3 gallop frequently is heard along the left sternal border or in the epigastrium. Abdominal examination may disclose ascites and tenderness in the right upper quadrant from an enlarged liver. Peripheral edema is sure to be found in the sacrum, the pretibial areas, or both.

DIAGNOSTIC CONSIDERATIONS

Chronic cor pulmonale results from any disease process that interferes with adequate ventilation and perfusion from the pulmonary valve to the entry of the pulmonary veins into the left atrium. This chapter has listed several etiologies for cor pulmonale. It is important that the clinician be aware of the relation between these various processes and the development of RVH and eventual ventricular dysfunction.

LABORATORY TESTS

Pulmonary function studies are markedly abnormal with marked airflow obstruction. Arterial blood gases reflect the hypoxia and hypercarbia of the underlying COPD.

RADIOLOGIC STUDIES

Interpretation of chest radiographs may present a challenge because of the hyperinflation that is invariably present. The chest x-ray often shows enlarged central pulmonary vessels and a marked decrease in or even absence of peripheral vessel markings that also is known as pruning.

OTHER DIAGNOSTICS

A standard 12-lead electrocardiogram may demonstrate right ventricular hypertrophy (right axis deviation and an unusual prominence of the R wave in leads V_1 and V_2 in the presence of a QRS of normal duration). Another typical electrocardiographic finding is a "P pulmonale," a prominent peaked P wave in leads II, III, and aVF. P pulmonale is indicative of right atrial enlargement, a frequent companion of RVH. It is not at all unusual for a patient with cor pulmonale to be in a supraventricular dysrhythmia such as atrial fibrillation.

Accurate interpretation of echocardiography in a patient with cor pulmonale often is confounded by the all too common presence of pulmonary hyperinflation. Doppler echocardiography may confirm the enlargement of the right ventricle and the presence of tricuspid valve regurgitation.

Magnetic resonance imaging (MRI) is now considered the preferred method for determining right ventricular dimensions. Many clinicians are now using serial MRIs to evaluate the effects of therapy. Economic considerations may limit the use of this diagnostic tool.

On occasion a patient with cor pulmonale may require cardiac catheterization. The right side of the heart is accessed through the venous system, with blood/oxygen samples and pressure readings taken at various points along the catheter route. This procedure is often technically difficult because of the pathology present. Since pulmonary artery wedge pressure is a reflection of left atrial pressure, it is usually normal.

TREATMENT

Pharmacologic Management

The treatment must focus on the underlying disease process. Since this most often involves chronic bronchitis and/or emphysema, the use of bronchodilators, antibiotics, and beta agonists is common. Every effort should be made to decrease the pulmonary arterial hypertension that is at the root of cor pulmonale. Hypoxia-induced vasoconstriction may be improved with chronic oxygen administration. For this reason, oxygen may be the most important medication in the clinician's arsenal against cor pulmonale. Caution must be exercised in the prescription of oxygen therapy, as a large number of patients with cor pulmonale are carbon dioxide retainers. Oxygen can depress the ventilatory drive in this subset of patients, worsening their hypercapnia.

There is much discussion in the literature regarding the use of vasodilators, specifically nifedipine (Procardia), in the treatment of cor pulmonale. The consensus seems to be that vasodilator therapy is a useful adjunct acutely but that the resultant decrease in pulmonary vascular resistance and the concomitant increase in right ventricular stroke volume are seen only briefly. Most authors recommend that vasodilators, including directly acting vasodilators such as hydralazine, as well as calcium channel blockers be reserved for patients who do not respond to more conventional COPD treatment. The hypotension that often accompanies vasodilation places further limitations on its routine use.

Diuretics may be useful in the treatment of cor pulmonale for the relief of systemic edema. The practitioner needs to be alert for resultant electrolyte disturbances, particularly if the patient is taking a cardiac glycoside such as digitalis. Digitalis may be employed in patients with cor pulmonale, especially if a patient presents in uncontrolled atrial fibrillation or concomitant left ventricular failure, but the routine use of digitalis-type medications is controversial at best. While digitalis may increase the force of right ventricular contraction, this drug also produces some degree of pulmonary vasoconstriction.

Long-term prostacyclin administration through a permanent intravenous infusion mechanism has been approved by the U.S. Food and Drug Administration for the treatment of patients with severe primary pulmonary hypertension. This potent pulmonary vasodilator and inhibitor of platelet aggregation has demonstrated significant benefit in this category of patients. Trials are under way to evaluate the utility of this treatment for patients with pulmonary hypertension of collagen vascular etiology. However, this treatment is complicated by severe side effects and may be encountered only in the subset of patients waiting for heart-lung or lung transplantation.

Another exciting therapeutic modality for critically ill patients with cor pulmonale is the inhaled administration of nitric oxide (NO). NO has long been identified as a potent pulmonary vasodilator. Therapeutic studies are in progress to assess the efficacy of chronic inhaled NO therapy.

Supportive Measures

Maintaining a clear airway is perhaps the most important supportive measure one can offer a patient with cor pulmonale. The patient and his or her caretakers need to be skilled in the various modalities of pulmonary toilet, including chest physical therapy, breathing exercises, and the employment of airway suction devices.

Patient Education

Prevention of cor pulmonale is centered on the prevention of COPD. Patients deserve access to effective smoking cessation programs. Asthma support groups can be helpful in encouraging patients to maintain a difficult but effective medication regimen. One should alert patients to the signs and symptoms of right-sided heart failure so that they can be dealt with on a timely basis. These patients often develop a reactive erythrocytosis, which, when combined with a sedentary lifestyle, may precipitate the development of deep venous thrombophlebitis

(DVT). Patients need to be alert for the telltale signs of DVT, such as lower extremity discomfort and/or unilateral lower extremity swelling.

Disposition

The prognosis in cor pulmonale associated with chronic lung disease is intimately related to the underlying disease process. Emphysema carries a poorer prognosis than does bronchitis. It is clear that the prognosis improves after the administration of long-term oxygen therapy.

COMPLICATIONS AND RED FLAGS

Patients with pulmonary hypertension and resultant RVH are prone to dysrhythmias. Aberrant rhythms often overtax an already compromised cardiovascular system, leading to dangerous decreases in cardiac output and aggravation of hypoxia. A careful history and physical that uncover the signs of dysrhythmia should be a part of every clinician-patient encounter. Remember to ask about palpitations, syncope and near syncope, and the telltale discomfort of cardiac ischemia.

NOTES AND PEARLS

Providers learn to focus on the underlying disease, but often at the risk of overlooking the primary problem's sequelae. Chronic cor pulmonale is best viewed as a result of long-standing pulmonary parenchymal or vessel insult. The usually low-pressure right heart cannot deal effectively with these increases in pressure. Long-term compensation in the form of right ventricular dilatation, hypertrophy, and eventual dysfunction will follow. Awareness of the pathophysiologic process will enable a clinician to anticipate and recognize the symptoms of cor pulmonale when they occur.

BIBLIOGRAPHY

Braunwald E: Cor pulmonale, in Fauci AS, et al (eds): *Harrison's Principles of Internal Medicine,* 14th ed. New York, McGraw Hill, 1998, pp 1324–1328.
Georgiou D, Brundage BH: Pulmonary hypertension, in Kloner RA (ed): *The Guide to Cardiology,* 3d ed. Greenwich, CT, Le Jacq, 1995, pp 607–625.
Gratz I: Pulmonary hypertension. *Anesthesiol Clin North Am* 17:693–707, 2000.
Palevsky HI: Therapeutic options for severe pulmonary hypertension. *Clin Chest Med* 18:595–609, 1997.
Wiedemann HP, Matthay RA: Cor pulmonale, in Braunwald E (ed): *Heart Disease: A Textbook of Cardiovascular Disease,* 5th ed. Philadelphia, Saunders, 1997, pp 1604–1625.

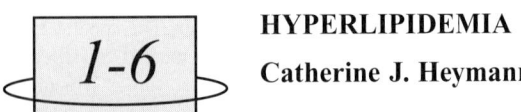

1-6 HYPERLIPIDEMIA
Catherine J. Heymann

DISCUSSION

Cholesterol, triglycerides, and phospholipids are the major lipids in the human body. Hyperlipidemias (or dyslipidemias) are the result of abnormal transport, accelerated synthesis, and/ or retarded degradation of lipid particles in the plasma, vascular endothelial cells, or liver. Lipid metabolism varies with gender, age, genetics, and environment. Chemically, cholesterol is not fat, but rather a molecule from the sterol family with a lipid-like structure. Cholesterol is an essential nutrient utilized in cell wall membranes, in the formation of steroid hormones, in the synthesis of vitamin D, as a component of bile acids, and throughout the nervous system. Triglycerides (TGs) are the body's long-term storage of excess energy in the form of adipose tissue. An integral part of cholesterol metabolism, TGs are composed of three free fatty acids (FFAs) held together by a glycerol molecule. Phospholipids resemble fat in appearance. They

are incorporated into the outer coating of a lipid molecule to assist with solubility.

In order to transport lipids (oil particles) in the bloodstream (aqueous solution), the body produces a single cell coating called an apoprotein to encompass the particle (see Fig. 1-6-1). The body produces many forms of apoproteins, each with a unique sequence. During lipid metabolism, apoproteins are readily altered or exchanged to facilitate metabolic, cell synthesis, or transportation requirements.

There are five general lipoprotein subclasses (see Table 1-6-1). The three most frequently assayed are high-density lipoprotein (HDL), low-density lipoprotein (LDL), and TGs. They are categorized by their lipid composition, weight, particle size, electric charge, and apoprotein coating. Abnormal lipid metabolism may result in an increased risk of atherosclerotic vascular disease (ASVD), coronary artery disease (CAD), pancreatitis, or stroke.

PATHOGENESIS

The two metabolic pathways for lipid synthesis are exogenous (dietary sources) and endogenous (within the body). Each pathway may cause dyslipidemias independently or in synergism with each other. Dyslipidemias are genetically predetermined abnormalities in lipid metabolism, which affect the amount, type, or metabolic pathway of cholesterol particles, cholesterol subtypes, lipid remnants, or TGs. While total cholesterol levels may not be elevated, the subclassifications of lipid molecules may have highly atherogenic properties.

SYMPTOMS

Mild hyperlipidemias do not produce symptoms until complications of ASVD become apparent. Angina, dyspnea, claudication, fatigue, transient ischemic attacks (TIAs), or cardiac arrhythmias may be the first indication of vascular damage caused by preexisting abnormal lipid metabolism (see Chap. 1-4).

Elevated TG levels are now considered an independent risk factor for cardiovascular disease. With significant TG elevations, patients may report recurrent abdominal pain, nausea, or vomiting related to pancreatitis. As the level of TGs increases, the blood becomes lipemic, thick, and sludgelike. The lipemic blood cannot flow easily through the fine capillaries of the pancreas, resulting in organ damage, inflammation, fibrosis, and pain.

Joint pain due to gouty arthritis may result from the high uric acid levels associated with elevated TGs. Although the first joint of the great toe is the classic site of gout, any joint may be affected. Migratory polyarthritis resulting from hyperlipidemias may produce warm, erythematous, or swollen joints. The onset is sudden, lasts a few days to weeks, and produces no articular damage.

OBJECTIVE FINDINGS

Extreme elevations of cholesterol or TGs may produce skin eruptions (xanthomas or xanthelasmas), lipemic (pale and creamy) blood samples, pale white retinal vessels (lipemia retinalis), hepatomegaly, splenomegaly, elevated uric acid levels, or foam cell infiltration of bone marrow. Table 1-6-2 summarizes some of the physical findings of hyperlipidemias.

Skin lesions called *xanthomas* may bring the patient to the practitioner for cosmetic reasons. Small yellow-white or yellow-orange papules with an erythematous "halo" may appear on pressure sensitive areas such as the buttocks, elbows, or knees. Larger tuber-like growths may appear on the Achilles, patellar, elbow, or digital extensor tendons. The lesions will usually disappear when the underlying lipid abnormality is corrected.

Yellow-orange discoloration in the creases around the eyelids is called *xanthelasmas.* Plane xanthomas present as flat yellow-orange patches on the palms of the hands, in palmar creases, on the face and upper trunk,

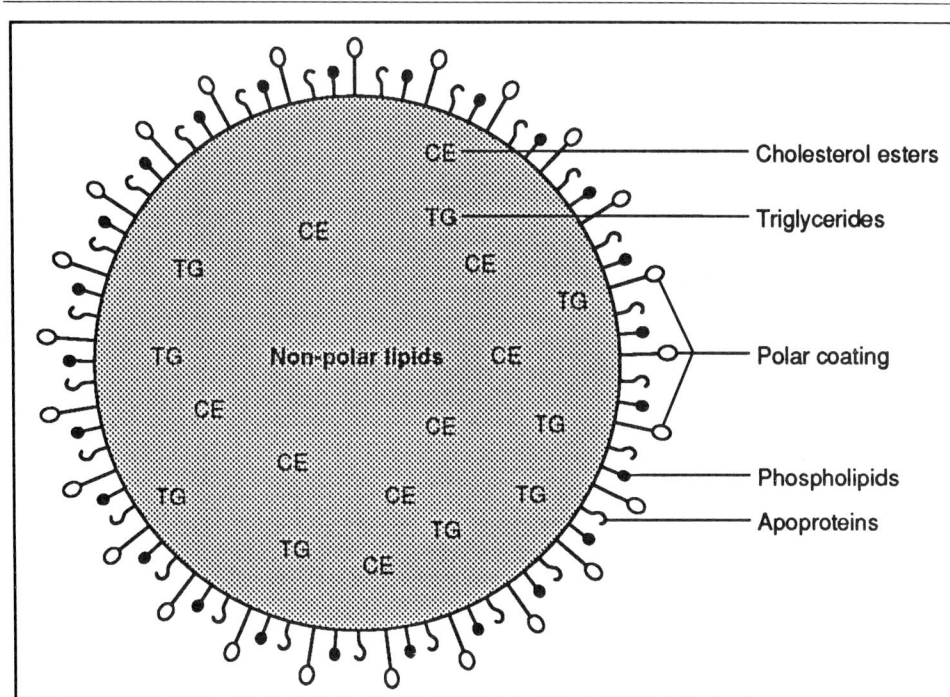

FIGURE 1-6-1. Lipoprotein molecule.

Cholesterol esters

Triglycerides

Polar coating

Phospholipids

Apoproteins

or in scar tissue. Subtler in presentation than large disfiguring tuber xan-thomas, they should alert the practitioner to a potentially lethal abnor-mality of lipid metabolism. Abdominal exam may reveal an enlarged liver or spleen from chronic inflammation due to congested lipemic blood flow observed in hypertriglyceridemia (TGs >1000 mg/dL).

DIAGNOSTIC CONSIDERATIONS

Abnormal lipid metabolism that is linked to a genetic anomaly is des-ignated as *primary. Secondary* hyperlipidemias may be associated with several metabolic abnormalities, pharmacologic agents, or ex-cessive alcohol consumption. Primary hyperlipidemias include sev-eral familial hyperlipoproteinemias. Single or multiple variant genes, each with a specific impact on lipids, are often present. Genetically linked abnormalities of lipid metabolism may be associated with in-appropriate apoprotein production, various lipid enzyme or receptor site deficiencies, abnormalities of fat metabolism (lipodystrophy), hy-popituitarism (dwarfism), and glycogen storage disease. Environ-mental factors such as obesity, diet, comorbid illnesses, smoking, and physical inactivity play a major role in the expression of a genetic disorder of lipid metabolism.

Numerous chronic illnesses that may induce secondary hyperlipid-emias include diabetes, insulin resistance syndrome (syndrome X or dysmetabolic syndrome), hypothyroidism, hepatic diseases, pancre-atitis, biliary obstruction, renal disease, nephrotic syndrome, preg-nancy, physical/emotional stress, anorexia nervosa, acromegaly, autoimmune disorders, porphyria, Cushing's syndrome, uremia, or obesity. The underlying disorder must be addressed before the hyper-lipidemias can effectively be treated (see Table 1-6-3).

Drug-induced hyperlipidemias may result from oral contraceptives, estrogens, androgens, glucocorticoids, thiazides, beta blockers, 13-*cis*-retinoic acid (isotretinoin, Accutane), or alcohol consumption (see Table 1-6-3).

LABORATORY TESTS

The National Cholesterol Education Program II recommends all adults (20 years or older) be routinely screened for hyperlipidemias by a total serum cholesterol level (see Table 1-6-4). Since cholesterol levels are not affected by the preceding meal, a random check may be obtained at a routine office visit. If results are <200 mg/dL, the test should be repeated every 5 years. If the total cholesterol (TC)

TABLE 1-6-1. Lipoprotein Subclasses

LIPOPROTEIN	ROLE IN METABOLISM	ROLE IN DISEASE
Chylomicrons	Transport dietary TGs (exogenous)	Precursor to TGs
Very-low-density lipoprotein (VLDL-C)	Transports endogenous TGs	Precursor to IDL-C and LDL-C
Intermediate-density lipoprotein (IDL-C)	Precursor to LDL-C	Intermediate step in lipid metabolism; the remnants produced in this step may be the most atherogenic component of lipid metabolism
Low-density lipoprotein (LDL-C) or β-lipoproteins	Transports cholesterol to cells	Highly atherogenic—may be either small and dense (pattern B, most atherogenic) or light and fluffy (pattern A). LDL-C oxidation is a key step in atherosclerotic plaque formation.
High-density lipoprotein (HDL-C)	Transports cholesterol from cells to liver	Protective—returns cholesterol to liver where it is degraded

ABBREVIATION: TGs, triglycerides.

TABLE 1-6-2. Physical Findings of Hyperlipidemias

PHYSICAL FINDING	HYPERCHOLESTEROLEMIA	HYPERTRIGLYCERIDEMIA
Abdominal pain (recurrent)		X (usually >1000 mg/dL)
Eruptive or plane xanthomas	X	X
Xanthelasma	X	X
Hepatosplenomegaly		X
Lipemia retinalis		X
Atherosclerosis	X	Unknown
Glucose intolerance (associated with certain familial hyperlipidemias)		X

is >200 mg/dL, a complete lipid assessment, including fasting TC, LDL-C, HDL-C, and TGs, should be obtained. Triglyceride and chylomicron levels are affected by the preceding meal; therefore, a fasting sample should be obtained. Further decisions on management and treatment may be based on several indices including LDL-C, TGs, current disease, comorbid disease, and genetic cardiac risk factors.

LDL-C (and possibly the intermediate products of LDL-C metabolism) may be the most predictive single laboratory test of future disease. Desirable levels for the general population is <160 mg/dL. If there are significant risk factors but no current evidence of cardiac or vascular disease, acceptable ranges are decreased to 100 to 130 mg/dL. A LDL-C level of <100 mg/dL has been recommended for all patients with CAD, ASVD, and/or diabetes.

HDL-C_2 is responsible for "reverse cholesterol transport" or removal of excess LDL-C from the blood. Acceptable ranges are >35 mg/dL for males and >50 mg/dL for females. A HDL-C_2 level above 70 mg/dL is considered cardioprotective.

Hypertriglyceridemia is now considered an independent risk factor for ASVD. Newer recommendations advise TG levels <150 mg/dL in all patients. Ratios of lipid subclasses are often utilized to evaluate a patient's risk of developing ASVD. The most frequently used cardiac risks ratios are TC:HDL-C (<4.5 indicates average risk) or LDL-C:HDL-C (<3.5 denotes average risk). The validity of risk ratios is questionable and best utilized if one lipid subclass is unusually high or low. For example, a patient with TC of 285 mg/dL may be

considered high risk; however, if the HDL-C is 95 mg/dL, then the TC:HDL-C ratio is 3:1 or low risk. The generous amount of HDL-C counterbalances the elevation in TC.

There are no "normal" ranges for serum lipids or lipid subclasses, only desirable levels *thought* to prevent or retard atherosclerotic disease (see Table 1-6-4). It is important to remember that a "desirable" range in the United States still produces one of the highest rates of CAD in the world. Epidemiological studies have documented an increase in ASVD as immigrants come to the United States and adopt our sedentary lifestyle and poor dietary habits.

Tests for additional markers of genetic disorders of lipid metabolism are now available and will soon be the gold standard. Currently utilized laboratory tests are inadequate to diagnose the majority of genetic abnormalities, which are responsible for approximately 80 percent of cardiac and vascular diseases. Risk or genetic predisposition to ASVD may be better evaluated with specific assessments of lipid subclasses, LDL particle size (A is large and B is small, dense), apoproteins, homocysteine metabolism, apo E isoforms, C-reactive proteins, plasma activating factor (PAI-1), fibrinogen, and/or enzyme deficiencies. Each of these tests denotes a genetic abnormality of lipid metabolism and is essential in selecting appropriate treatment options.

The laboratory testing described above is relatively new. The cost of such testing has declined in the last few years but is still expensive. Some medical plans are beginning to reimburse these assays with appropriate supporting data, but they are not yet appropriate screening tools for the general population. A family history (genetic map) should alert the practitioner to those patients who could benefit from specialized testing procedures. Any patient with CAD should undergo advanced testing methods for abnormal lipid metabolism to detect treatable genetic disorders and reduce further ASVD.

TABLE 1-6-3. Potential Causes of Abnormal Lipids

DISORDER OR SUBSTANCE	RESULTING LIPID ABNORMALITIES
Hypothyroidism	High TC, high LDL-C
Nephrotic syndrome	High TC, high LDL-C
Chronic renal failure	High TGs
Diabetes (uncontrolled)	High TGs
Insulin resistance (dyslipidemia or syndrome X)	High TGs, low HDL-C, high LDL-C
Systemic lupus erythematosus	High TGs
Porphyria	High LDL-C
Oral contraceptives	High TGs
Progesterones	Low HDL-C
Alcohol	High TGs
Beta blockers	High TGs, high LDL-C, low HDL-C
Tobacco smoke	Low HDL-C
Thiazides	High TGs, high TC, high LDL-C

ABBREVIATIONS: HDL, high-density lipoprotein; LDL, low-density lipoprotein; TC, total cholesterol; TGs, triglycerides.

RADIOLOGIC STUDIES

There are no radiologic studies to employ unless CAD, atherosclerosis, or peripheral vascular or cerebrovascular disease is suspected.

OTHER DIAGNOSTICS

Classically, the Fredrickenson and Levy phenotyping system has been used to classify specific abnormal patterns of lipid metabolism. Currently, additional genotypes have been identified through more sophisticated testing methods mentioned above, which may soon render this classification system obsolete. See Table 1-6-5 for a summary of hyperlipidemia phenotypes, expected lab values, and treatment modalities.

TREATMENT

Before initiating treatment, other medical conditions or pharmacologic agents that may cause or contribute to hyperlipidemias must be

TABLE 1-6-4.   Cholesterol, Triglyceride, and Lipid Subclass Levels

DESIRABLE RANGES		NO RISK FACTORS	TWO OR MORE RISK FACTORS FOR ASVD	ASVD PATIENT WITH DIABETES MELLITUS
	TC	<200 mg/dL	<200 mg/dL	<200 mg/dL
	HDL	>35 mg/dL (male) >50 mg/dL (female)	>35 mg/dL (male) >50 mg/dL (female)	>35 mg/dL (male) >50 mg/dL (female)
	LDL	<160 mg/dL	<130 mg/dL	<100 mg/dL
	TGs	<200 mg/dL	<150 mg/dL	<100 mg/dL

ABBREVIATIONS: ASVD, atherosclerotic vascular disease; HDL, high-density lipoprotein; LDL, low-density lipoprotein; TC, total cholesterol; TGs, triglycerides.

considered (see Table 1-6-3). Dietary management and life-style modifications should always be the first line of treatment for hyperlipidemias. If therapy fails after an appropriate trial, medications may be added. Currently, numerous governmental, private, and research organizations recommend a diet that meets the following criteria:

Maintain a reasonable body weight; 30 percent or fewer calories from fat; reduction of saturated fats to <10 percent of calories; cholesterol intake of <300 mg/day; plenty of fresh fruit and vegetables; and increased intake of whole grains, beans, and legumes.

The type of fat ingested may be just as important as the amount. Fats may be saturated, monounsaturated fatty acids (MUFAs), or polyunsaturated fatty acids (PUFAs). Each type of fat has a distinct impact on lipid metabolism. Saturated fats are implicated in accelerating the production of cholesterol in its most potentially lethal form, LDLs. Always solid at room temperature, saturated fats are found in animal fats, coconut oil, and palm kernel oil. MUFAs are thought to be effective in lowering LDL-C and increasing HDL-C. Always liquid at room temperature, sources are olive, canola, and many nut oils. PUFAs were once thought to be cardioprotective. Although they may reduce TC, PUFAs increase the amount of LDL-C and may produce a form more prone to oxidation. PUFAs also decrease cardioprotective HDL-C. They are always liquid at room temperature. Solid margarine is made by the partial saturation of hydrogenated liquid oils. Recent research has questioned whether the hydrogenation process may indeed produce a more atherogenic rather than a beneficial dietary fat source.

The impact of dietary cholesterol on the lipid profile is variable but usually minimal. A portion of chicken, pork, fish, or beef has essentially the same cholesterol content; however, they vary significantly in the saturated fat content. Complex interactions among saturated fats, endogenous/exogenous cholesterol metabolism, and genetics influence serum lipid levels. Cholesterol is found only in animal sources, primarily in the flesh of animals, fish, poultry, organ meats, dairy products, and eggs.

Dietary modifications are successfully implemented only with intensive education, counseling, family support, and realistic goal-setting. The American Dietetic Association has a consumer information hotline (800-366-1655) and referral service.

Pharmacologic Management

Medications for hyperlipidemias fall into four basic categories: bile acid–binding resins, 3-hydroxy-3-methylglutaryl coenzyme A (HMG-CoA) reductase inhibitors, fibric acid derivatives, and nicotinic acid (see Table 1-6-6). All have numerous adverse effects that may affect patient compliance. Effectiveness depends not only on patient compliance with the medication but also on adherence to a healthy diet, regular exercise, smoking cessation, and stress reduction.

TABLE 1-6-5.   Phenotypes of Hyperlipidemias (Frederickenson/Levy Classification System)

PHENOTYPE	LABORATORY DATA	PHYSICAL SYMPTOMS AND COMPLICATIONS	TREATMENT
Type I	Increased circulating chylomicrons	Pancreatitis	Dietary—low fat, low simple carbohydrate, no alcohol
Type IIa	Elevated TGs Elevated LDL-C	Accelerated atherosclerosis Xanthomas Early myocardial infarction	Niacin and/or statin
Type IIb	Lipids may be normal Elevated LDL-C	Atherosclerosis	Life-style changes Niacin plus a resin and/or statin
Type III	Increased intermediate lipoproteins	Obesity Hypothyroidism Xanthomas	Low-cholesterol diet Estrogen replacement therapy if post-menopausal Weight reduction Treatment of hypothyroidism Fibric acid derivatives
Type IV	Elevated cholesterol Elevated TGs	Obesity Caloric excess Poorly controlled diabetes Alcohol consumption	Dietary—low calorie, low simple carbohydrate, no alcohol If TGs >1000 mg/dL, use a fibric acid derivative or niacin
Type V	Elevated chylomicrons Elevated very-low-density lipoproteins	Abdominal pain Pancreatitis Glucose intolerance Hepatosplenomegaly Xanthomas	No alcohol Dietary—low calorie, low fat, low carbohydrates

TABLE 1-6-6. Pharmacologic Treatment of Hyperlipidemias

MEDICATION	EFFECTS ON LIPIDS	ADVERSE EFFECTS	POSSIBLE DRUG INTERACTIONS	CONTRAINDICATIONS
Bile acid–binding resins	Lowers LDL Lowers TC	GI intolerance Epigastric pain May raise TGs Headache	Digoxin Thyroxine Tetracycline Coumadin Thiazides Vitamins A, D, K Folic acid Glipizide Gemfibrozil Iopanoic acid Phosphates Piroxicam Propranolol	Peptic ulcers Diverticulitis Allergic reaction Pregnancy Lactation
Fibric acid derivatives	Lowers TGs Raises HDL Lowers VLDL Lowers TC	Flulike illness Sore muscles Cholelithiasis Abnormal liver enzymes GI distress	Coumadin Cyclosporine Statins Insulin Sulfonylureas	Liver disease Pregnancy Allergic reaction Gall bladder disease
HMG-CoA reductase inhibitors	Lowers LDL-C Raises HDL-C Lowers VLDL-C Lowers TGs Lowers TC	Sore muscles Abnormal liver enzymes Rash GI distress	Cyclosporine Fibric acid derivatives Erythromycin Warfarin Gemfibrozil Niacin	Pregnancy Allergic reaction Liver disease Lactation
Nicotinic acid (niacin)	Lowers LDL-C Lowers TGs Lowers VLDL-C Lowers TC Raises HDL-C	Rash Flushing Abnormal liver enzymes Gout (hyperuricemia) Skin discoloration Migraines Decreased vision Glucose intolerance GI intolerance Dyspepsia Peptic ulcers	Aluminum-containing medications	Liver disease Arrhythmias Peptic ulcers Irritable bowel syndrome Gout Tartrazines allergy

ABBREVIATIONS: GI, gastrointestinal; HDL, high-density lipoprotein; HMG-CoA, 3-hydroxy-3-methylglutaryl coenzyme A; LDL, low-density lipoprotein; TC, total cholesterol; TGs, triglycerides; VLDL, very-low-density lipoprotein.

Bile acid–binding resins reduce LDL-C by forming an insoluble compound with bile acids in the intestine, restricting their reabsorption and limiting cholesterol production. These drugs are often used in conjunction with HMG-CoA reductase inhibitors for a synergistic effect.

HMG-CoA reductase inhibitors competitively limit LDL-C formation early in cholesterol biosynthesis. The exact mechanism is still not completely understood, but a decrease in very-low-density lipoprotein (VLDL-C), LDL-C, and TGs and an increase in HDL-C are usually noted. The most effective time to administer the medication appears to be with dinner or at bedtime, as the majority of cholesterol synthesis takes place during the night. This class of drugs is nicknamed the *statins*—lovastatin, pravastatin, simvastatin, atorvastatin, etc.

Fibric acid derivatives reduce hepatic TG and VLDL-C production while increasing the synthesis of HDL-C. Clofibrate is infrequently used in the United States due to the increased incidence of intestinal tumors associated with its use.

Nicotinic acid (niacin) reduces TC, VLDL-C, LDL-C, and TGs and increases HDL-C. The effect appears to be dose dependent. Niacin is often combined with a bile acid sequestrant to further reduce LDL-C. An inexpensive medication, compliance is dependent on patient tolerance of unpleasant side effects. Slow titration or the addition of aspirin 30 minutes before the niacin is ingested may help reduce the annoying cutaneous flushing and itching. There are slow-release forms of niacin available now, which may help reduce the unpleasant symptoms. Doses of >1000 mg to 1500 mg per day may affect glucose tolerance or diabetic control.

Estrogen replacement therapy in postmenopausal women is believed to reduce the incidence of CAD, possibly by maintaining higher HDL-C levels. Progesterone therapy must also be utilized to reduce the risk of uterine cancer if the woman has a uterus.

Medications may be combined to increase the lipid-lowering effect. Most CAD patients have more than one genetic abnormality of lipid metabolism that may need separate treatment modalities.

Patient Education

Assessment, education, therapy, and monitoring of life-style modifications require a significant amount of the practitioner's time as well as unique skills. Use of ancillary professionals such as nurse practitioners, dietitians, social workers, psychologists, and physical therapists can facilitate the education and support process. Knowing what symptoms to expect, the risks and benefits of a medication, and coping mechanisms for any unpleasant side effects of therapy will help promote patient compliance. Before beginning an exercise program, patients should be evaluated for ischemic cardiac or atherosclerotic disease. The only effective exercise program is one the patient can comply with on a regular basis. Suggest nontraditional forms of exercise if needed rather than insisting on something the patient cannot or will not attempt.

COMPLICATIONS AND RED FLAGS

Pancreatitis, peripheral vascular disease, cardiac disease, cerebrovascular disease, major vessel disease, and disability or death are the most frequently seen complications of elevated lipids. A family history combined with appropriate laboratory assessment of serum lipids may alert the practitioner to patients at potential risk. Chapter 1-4 includes information on the detection and evaluation of atherosclerosis.

Dyslipidemia is now thought to be a genetic disorder. Although we have made significant strides in understanding the atherogenic potential of lipids, it would be premature to think we have all the answers. Certainly, ASVD involves more than hypercholesterolemia, and the solution involves considerably more than a diet. New laboratory tests, lipid management protocols, medications, surgical techniques, gene therapy, and vitamin/mineral supplementation are on the horizon. Numerous well-respected studies have shown that currently utilized therapies can reduce cardiac events up to 30 percent; inversely, up to 70 percent of coronary events are not prevented! Hopefully, future technology will reduce the incidence of ASVD—the leading cause of death and disability in the United States.

BIBLIOGRAPHY

Skillings J, Howes DG: Recertification series hyperlipidemia and atherosclerosis, part I. *Physician Assistant* 7:32–68, 1996.
————: Recertification series hyperlipidemia and atherosclerosis, part II. *Physician Assistant* 8:32–62, 1996.
Surperko HR: New aspects of risk factors for the development of atherosclerosis, including small low-density lipoprotein, homocysteine, and lipoprotein (a). *Curr Opin Cardiol* 10:347–354, 1995.

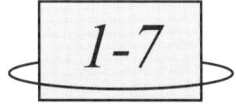

ISCHEMIC CORONARY ARTERY SYNDROMES

Morton A. Diamond

DISCUSSION

Coronary atherosclerosis is the most common cause of ischemic heart disease. Less frequently, myocardial ischemia may be a result of nonatheromatous coronary disease, such as Prinzmetal's variant angina and microvascular angina (syndrome X), or of myocardial hypertrophy, either idiopathic or secondary to aortic valvular disease. This chapter focuses on ischemic coronary syndromes caused by atherosclerosis (see Chap. 1-4).

The atheromatous plaque represents the cardinal substrate of coronary artery disease. The central features of atheroma formation are endothelial injury and low-density lipoprotein (LDL) excess. Increased endothelial permeability to LDL results in subintimal deposition. The LDL is oxidized, attracting macrophages. The macrophages engulf the LDL and become foam cells. In turn, the foam cells elaborate growth factors, free radicals, lipases, and proteinases. The growth factors cause smooth muscle cells to multiply and secrete collagen, with resultant atheroma formation. Inflammation appears to promote the development of atherosclerosis, and high levels of C-reactive protein and fibrinogen are associated with increased risk of acute coronary events. Chronic infection has been found to be significantly associated with the development of atheromata, with its attendant clinical manifestations, including angina pectoris, acute myocardial infarction, and stroke. However, no specific causal relationship has been established between an organism and atheroma formation. The infectious agents with the most evidence to suggest an association with atherosclerosis are *Chlamydia pneumoniae* and cytomegalovirus. Future studies will further define the relationship between chronic infection and this degenerative process.

TABLE 1-7-1. Factors Favoring the Development of Coronary Atherosclerosis

Increasing age
Sex (male< female)
Genetics: family history of coronary disease doubles risk
Smoking
Hypertension
Diabetes mellitus
Dyslipidemia
Emotional stress
Obesity
Sedentary life-style

Superimposed thrombosis is the primary cause of acute coronary syndromes: unstable angina, acute myocardial infarction, and sudden death. Thrombosis is precipitated by endothelial denudation or plaque rupture. Platelets then adhere to the injured endothelium, and this is followed by fibrin deposition, resulting in an occlusive or nonocclusive thrombus. The composition of the atheromatous plaque is the most important determinant of the development of thrombus-mediated unstable angina, myocardial infarction, and sudden death. Thrombosis does not occur until mature plaques are present. Myocardial infarction results from an acute total thrombotic occlusion, while unstable angina usually is due to mural (incomplete) thrombus development.

Since ischemic coronary artery syndromes represent a spectrum of the same pathophysiologic process, they will be considered together rather than as separate disease entities.

Risk Factors

The factors favoring the development of coronary atherosclerosis are listed in Table 1-7-1.

STABLE (CHRONIC) ANGINA PECTORIS

Chronic angina occurs when myocardial oxygen demand outstrips oxygen delivery by the coronary circulation. Angina typically occurs during physical exertion, emotional upset, fever, and tachyarrhythmias. The frequency of anginal discomfort does not accurately reflect the anatomic or functional severity of the atherosclerotic process. Angina is still a diagnosis made by history.

SIGNS AND SYMPTOMS

The discomfort typically is described as tightness or pressure and is most commonly felt in the chest or arms. Frequently, however, the discomfort may be noted in the neck, jaw, gums, upper back, and even the umbilical area. Sharp or jabbing pain is not suggestive of angina; discomfort affected by breathing, body position, or swallowing is similarly not characteristic of angina. Cardiac patients who describe only exertional dyspnea must have the etiology of the breathlessness clearly defined, for in some patients the dyspnea represents myocardial ischemia (anginal equivalent). An anginal patient may experience other cardiac symptoms related to cardiac function, such as peripheral edema, palpitations, and fatigue.

The physical examination in a stable anginal patient is variable. Cardiac examination in a resting asymptomatic patient may be normal or may demonstrate evidence of antecedent myocardial dysfunction. A patient examined during myocardial ischemia often manifests a presystolic (S_4) gallop and/or a transient mitral regurgitant murmur as a result of papillary muscle dysfunction.

Diagnostic Considerations

Esophageal, chest wall, and breast disorders as well as intraabdominal diseases must be considered in a patient who experiences chest discomfort. A careful history and physical examination, complemented by laboratory and imaging studies, will enable a physician assistant to define the correct diagnosis.

Laboratory and Radiologic Studies

There are no laboratory tests that specifically assist in the diagnosis of angina. However, clinical risk factors should be sought, for example, hyperglycemia, anemia, dyslipidemia, hyperthyroidism, and hypoxemia. A chest x-ray may provide information concerning heart size and left ventricular function.

Other Diagnostic Tests

A resting electrocardiogram (ECG) indicates rhythm, the presence of atrioventricular or intraventricular conduction defects, evidence of a previous infarction, and hypertrophy or ischemia. In the majority of stable anginal patients, the resting ECG is normal when the patient is asymptomatic.

Treatment

Treatment consists of the following:

- Modify risk factors: Patients require weight reduction, smoking cessation, dyslipidemia or diabetes treatment, and control of hypertension.
- Modify activity: Patients should avoid heavy lifting, sudden bursts of running, and extremes of temperature.
- Assess risk: Since the frequency of anginal attacks does not correlate with anatomic abnormality, patients should undergo exercise or pharmacologic stress testing to define the risk for a cardiac event, that is, an acute myocardial infarction or sudden death. A low-risk patient is treated medically; a high-risk patient is referred for coronary angiography and revascularization.

Pharmacologic Management

NITROGLYCERIN   Sublingual or inhaled nitroglycerin is used both in the treatment of an acute anginal attack and as a prophylactic to prevent episodes. For patients having more than four or five attacks per week, long-acting oral or transdermal agents should be added. An 8- to 10-h nitrate-free interval helps prevent nitrate tolerance. The dose of the nitrate is variable, depending on resting blood pressure and concomitant medication intake.

ASPIRIN   Aspirin, 160 mg/d or 325 mg every other day, should be prescribed unless a contraindication exists, since this agent reduces cardiac mortality rate.

BETA BLOCKERS AND CALCIUM CHANNEL BLOCKERS   The appropriate choice of a beta or calcium channel blocker depends on the presence of concomitant medical conditions. These disorders, which influence the choice of medication, include resting heart rate, atrioventricular conduction disturbances, arrhythmias, chronic lung disease, congestive heart failure, lipid abnormalities, valvular heart disease, hyper- or hypoglycemia, and peripheral arterial vascular disease. In general, beta blockers are preferred in an anginal patient with resting sinus tachycardia or a history of ventricular tachycardia. A selected calcium channel blocker is prescribed for patients with sinus bradycardia, hyper- or hypoglycemia, congestive heart failure, peripheral vascular disease, and hypercholesterolemia.

Important side effects of beta blockers include congestive heart failure, unrecognized hypoglycemia, atrioventricular block, and exacerbation of bronchospastic symptoms or peripheral claudication. Calcium channel blockers may precipitate congestive heart failure or orthostatic hypotension. The dose of each agent is variable. One should start low, increasing the medication dose as clinically appropriate.

Clinical Pearls

When talking to a patient with ischemic symptoms, one should use the term *discomfort*, not *pain.* A patient with angina will often respond negatively when asked whether he or she has chest pain but affirmatively when asked about discomfort. If a patient with a presumptive diagnosis of angina does not respond to nitroglycerin, one should reexamine the diagnosis. However, an anginal patient may not be receiving the proper dose of the medication.

A simple and effective clinical test is performed by serially measuring blood pressure for 3 min after sublingual nitroglycerin administration. A systolic blood pressure decrease of 10 mmHg is the desired hemodynamic effect. If the patient's systolic pressure does not demonstrate this hypotensive effect, one should increase the tablet dose. Nitroglycerin should be taken while the patient is sitting down. If the patient is unable to sit, leaning against a stationary object may lessen the risk of significant orthostatic hypotension.

Angina lasts continuously for at least 1 min and is experienced in an area at least the size of a silver dollar. One should emphasize to the patient that it is important to take nitroglycerin immediately upon the onset of angina.

Do not allow the patient to " see if I really need it." Further, the patient should be instructed to notify their medical provider if there is a change in the pattern of angina, specifically including the appearance of nocturnal angina, angina at rest, or angina with lessened exertion.

UNSTABLE ANGINA PECTORIS

Unstable angina is defined as symptomatic myocardial ischemia occurring at rest or abruptly increasing in frequency in a previously stable anginal patient or new-onset angina.

Signs and Symptoms

Dyspnea, palpitations, and fatigue are the commonly associated symptoms. Single-vessel coronary artery disease is found in 40 to 50% of these patients, and multivessel disease in 45 to 50%. An acute, nonocclusive thrombus is found in the majority of these patients. The angiogram is normal in the remaining patients.

Physical examination may be normal or may demonstrate transient presystolic (S_4) gallop or mitral regurgitant murmur.

Laboratory and Radiologic Tests

The chest x-ray will define heart size and, if present, evidence of congestive heart failure. An ECG is performed to look for evidence of ischemia, myocardial injury, or infarction. Serum creatine kinase (CPK) and its MB isoenzyme should be obtained serially over 24 h in order to determine whether myocardial necrosis has occurred. Troponin T and troponin I appear to be more specific and sensitive than creatine kinase and its MB isoenzyme, CK-MB. This greater sensitivity allows for diagnosis of lesser degrees of myocardial necrosis characteristic of acute ischemic coronary syndromes and can identify patients who are at high risk of cardiac death despite normal CK-MB levels and electrocardiographic findings.

Treatment

Patients experiencing rest angina or worsening angina associated with ECG changes should be urgently hospitalized, placed on bed rest with cardiac monitoring and control of precipitating factors [see "Stable

(Chronic) Angina Pectoris," above], and started on medication. Referral to a physician is indicated.

Pharmacologic Management

Treatment of unstable angina includes oral aspirin, intravenous unfractionated heparin (bolus followed by continuous infusion) to maintain the partial thromboplastin time (PTT) at 1.5 to 2.5 times control, intravenous nitroglycerin, and a beta blocker. Thrombolytic agents are not of clinical value in treating unstable angina. Low-molecular-weight heparins have advantages over unfractionated heparin in that they include better bioavailability, more predictable effect, twice-daily subcutaneous administration, and lack of need to monitor effect and adjust dose. At present, either unfractionated heparin or low-molecular-weight heparin may be used in therapy of unstable angina pectoris.

Glycoprotein IIb/IIIa receptor inhibitors act by competitive inhibition in the final common pathway of platelet aggregation. These agents are most effective in high-risk patients, e.g., those with elevated serum markers and those who are to undergo percutaneous coronary intervention. Glycoprotein IIa/IIIb inhibitors are indicated in those patients whose ischemic symptoms are resistant to therapy with heparin, aspirin, and beta blockers; patients with persistent ST- segment depression; and those with planned coronary invasive procedures. Currently available agents include abciximab, tirofiban, and eptifibatide. Direct comparisons of these agents are not extant. In these patients, careful control of heparin anticoagulation is essential in order to reduce bleeding complications. Contraindications include thrombocytopenia and history of bleeding diathesis. Rarely, these inhibitors may cause severe thrombocytopenia.

ACUTE MYOCARDIAL INFARCTION

Myocardial infarction is the most frequent cause of death in the United States. Approximately 1.5 million heart attacks occur annually. With modern therapy, hospital mortality rate is 15%. Half the deaths occur in the first hour as a result of ventricular fibrillation; the other deaths generally are due to cardiogenic shock or congestive heart failure and occur within 2 days of hospitalization. While atherosclerotic disease is the overwhelming cause of acute myocardial infarction (AMI), it is important to recognize that there are other, nonatherosclerotic etiologies of infarction. In a young adult, cocaine abuse may precipitate an acute, nonthrombotic AMI.

Signs and Symptoms

The patient usually has experienced continuous severe ischemic discomfort for at least 30 min. In some patients, the discomfort may wax and wane ("stutter"). In the elderly, AMI may not be associated with discomfort; instead, the patient will present with syncope or left ventricular congestive heart failure or weakness.

Physical examination often reveals an anguished expression on the patient's face. The skin may be moist and cool from adrenergic discharge associated with heart failure. Peripheral cyanosis is noted in AMI patients with cardiogenic shock. The blood pressure and pulse are variable, depending on sympathetic tone and left ventricular function. Precordial palpation may reveal a presystolic impulse correlating with an auscultatory S_4 gallop. Anterior or lateral infarction may be associated with a systolic impulse in the third, fourth, or fifth interspace along the left sternal border. A systolic murmur may be heard near the cardiac apex, indicating mitral regurgitation from papillary muscle dysfunction. A pericardial friction rub is heard in approximately 15% of AMI patients.

Diagnostic Considerations

The differential diagnosis includes pericardial and pleural pain, pulmonary embolism, aortic dissection, and intraabdominal diseases, including peptic ulcer disease, cholecystitis, and pancreatitis.

Laboratory and Radiologic Tests

Total creatine kinase (CK) is abnormal 4 to 8 h after the onset of symptoms and returns to normal in 2 to 3 days. The MB isoenzyme is not entirely specific for myocardium, but an increased MB fraction in the absence of trauma or surgery involving the intestine, uterus, or prostate is indicative of AMI. CK-MB isoforms are most efficient for early diagnosis of AMI, within the first 2 or 3 h of symptom onset. Troponin T and I may not be detectable in serum for up to 6 h after onset of chest symptoms. In the patient who has sustained an AMI, troponin T may be elevated for 10 to 14 days, and troponin I for up to 7 days, after the infarction. Therefore, measurement of troponins is preferable to measurement of lactate dehydrogenase and its isoenzymes in patients who seek medical attention more than 24 to 48 h after onset of symptoms.

Serial ECGs generally reveal abnormalities in an infarction. It is important, however, to realize that a normal ECG at the patient's initial presentation in the emergency department is not uncommon. Classic ECG changes include the development of Q waves with ST-segment elevation (Q-wave infarction). Frequently, ECGs demonstrate ST-segment depression and/or T-wave inversion (non-Q-wave infarction). In the non-Q-wave group, the diagnosis of AMI rests more on clinical findings and elevation of enzymes than on the ECG.

Treatment

The physician assistant in the emergency department must urgently evaluate patients who experience chest pain to identify those who require perfusion therapy. A history of ischemic discomfort and the standard ECG represent the primary data for patient management.

Patients should be promptly attached to a cardiac monitor, receive nasal oxygen, and have an intravenous 5% dextrose-in-water infusion started.

All patients with an acute coronary syndrome should chew an adult aspirin tablet, and thereafter oral aspirin should be continued indefinitely. Glycoprotein IIa/IIIb inhibitors have been found to be of greater benefit to those patients who have elevated cardiac-specific troponin levels, yet without ST-segment elevation, compared to those patients without elevated troponin levels. Intravenous glycoprotein inhibitors may be used in the acute phase of AMI without ST-segment elevation.

If the ECG shows 1 mm or more ST elevation in contiguous leads, intravenous thrombolytic therapy should be given quickly unless a contraindication is present. A patient whose ECG demonstrates ST depression and/or T-wave inversion should not be considered for thrombolytic therapy. Thrombolytic agents activate plasminogen, converting it to plasmin, which causes dissolution of a thrombus by digesting the supporting fibrin network. There has been considerable interest in the efficacy of the various thrombolytic agents. The agents most commonly administered are tissue plasminogen activator (tPA), anistreplase, streptokinase, and reteplase. The most important consideration in thrombolytic therapy appears to be early administration, rather than any specific advantage of a particular medication. Table 1-7-2 lists indications for and contraindications to thrombolytic therapy in AMI patients.

Anticoagulation with intravenous unfractionated heparin is continued for at least 24 h after tPA and reteplase, but is optional in patients receiving streptokinase.

Compared to unfractionated heparin, low-molecular-weight heparins have the advantage of high bioavailability and a predictable effect on coagulation. Enoxaparin has been demonstrated to be superior to unfractionated heparin in patients with unstable angina pectoris and non-Q-wave AMI. Clinical trials utilizing low-molecular-weight heparins in AMI are continuing.

Intracranial hemorrhage is the most serious complication of thrombolytic therapy. More common, though relatively minor, is bleeding at vascular puncture sites. Most patients exposed to streptokinase and APSAC will develop antibodies to these agents. Therefore, a patient with AMI should not be treated with streptokinase if he or she has received that agent within the last year.

TABLE 1-7-2. Patient Selection for Thrombolytic Therapy

Indications

    Ischemic chest pain for more than 30 min
    Electrocardiogram
        ST-segment elevation greater than 1 mm in two contiguous leads or new left bundle branch block
    Time window
        < 6 h: most beneficial
        6–12 h: less effective but still beneficial
        >12 h: high-risk, continued chest pain
    Special subsets (treat in absence of other contraindications)
        Remote (more than 6 months) history of nonhemorrhagic stroke
        Past history (more than 2 months) of gastrointestinal bleeding
        Hypotension or moderate hypertension
        Cardiopulmonary resuscitation

Contraindications

    Absolute

        Major surgery or trauma in last 2 weeks
        Active internal bleeding (excluding menses)
        Prior intracranial bleed or cerebral neoplasm
        Cerebrovascular events or head trauma (within last 6 months)
        Known allergy to a drug considered for use

    Relative

        Active peptic ulcer
        Pregnancy or within 1 month postpartum
        Severe, persistent hypertension (systolic/diastolic blood pressure greater than 200/110 mmHg)
        Current use of anticoagulants

Analgesia utilizing intravenous morphine or meperidine is effective. Morphine has vagomimetic effects, and meperidine has an atropine-like effect. Oral nitroglycerin should be given as long as the systolic blood pressure is greater than 90 mmHg and there is no evidence of inferior infarction with associated right ventricular infarction. (Right ventricular infarction should be considered when patients with inferior infarction exhibit signs of low cardiac output and elevated central venous pressure.) Intravenous nitroglycerin is most beneficial if the patient is in congestive heart failure or continues to have ischemic discomfort. Close monitoring of blood pressure is essential.

Patients seen within 4 h of the onset of symptoms as well as those with sinus tachycardia or hypertension should receive an intravenous beta blocker as long as no contraindication is present. Contraindications include congestive heart failure, bronchospasm, hypotension, sinus bradycardia, and heart block. At the time of discharge, oral beta blocker therapy should be continued if no contraindication exists. Angiotensin converting enzyme (ACE) inhibitors also play an important role in AMI therapy. Elderly patients, those with an anterior infarction or a previous infarction, and asymptomatic patients with an ejection fraction of 40% or less should receive lifelong ACE inhibitor therapy. The calcium channel blockers verapamil and diltiazem should not be routinely used.

Complications

Major complications of AMI may be arbitrarily divided into two categories: pump failure and electrical instability. Left ventricular dysfunction continues to be the single most important predictor of death after an AMI. Physiologically, the heart failure may be systolic with a resultant decrease in cardiac output. Alternatively, there may be coexistent systolic and diastolic failure with pulmonary venous congestion and dyspnea.

Heart failure is most effectively treated by a reduction in afterload through the administration of diuretics and nitrates. ACE inhibitors may be added. For severe heart failure not responsive to these agents, beta receptor agonists such as dopamine and dobutamine may be infused.

Digitalis is generally reserved for AMI patients with superimposed supraventricular arrhythmia and those whose heart failure is refractory to vasodilator medication, diuretics, and beta agonists.

The most severe manifestation of left ventricular heart failure is cardiogenic shock caused by extensive myocardial damage. These patients exhibit a clouded sensorium, cool skin, and peripheral cyanosis related to a severe reduction in cardiac output. Medical management includes beta agonists, intraaortic balloon counterpulsation, and in selected cases emergency coronary bypass surgery. Despite therapy, the mortality rate remains high at approximately 60 to 70%.

AMI is associated with frequent abnormalities in heart rhythm, both supraventricular and ventricular in origin. Sinus tachycardia, sinus bradycardia, atrial fibrillation and flutter, paroxysmal supraventricular tachycardia, ventricular premature beats, ventricular tachycardia, and ventricular fibrillation are common. The hemodynamic consequences of arrhythmia primarily relate to the fact that both tachycardia and bradycardia lower cardiac output. Loss of atrial contraction in atrial fibrillation further reduces cardiac output because of lessened ventricular filling. Transient atrioventricular block is common after AMI; the resultant bradycardia may require temporary cardiac pacing. It is more common after inferior than anterior AMI, since in 90% of individuals, a branch of the right coronary artery perfuses the AV node. First-degree, Mobitz I (Wenckebach), and complete heart block are common, but generally transient, in inferior AMI. A patient who has inferior wall infarction with first-degree block should preferably receive meperidine rather than morphine for analgesia since meperidine has an atropine-like effect while morphine has a vagal effect. If complete heart block is present, the underlying escape rhythm is usually stable. Temporary cardiac pacing is indicated for symptomatic bradycardia. Permanent cardiac pacing is rarely required in patients who have had inferior AMI. In contrast, patients who have anterior wall AMI complicated by complete heart block have an unstable, wide QRS escape rhythm. Cardiac pacing is indicated, but prognosis is poor because of the extensive myocardial necrosis in these patients. AMI patients whose course is complicated by arrhythmia require prompt physician consultation.

The treatment of arrhythmia requires careful evaluation of an AMI patient. Therapy may include not only antiarrhythmic drugs and electrical intervention (cardioversion, defibrillation, pacemaker insertion) but also correction of electrolyte and acid-base abnormalities, anemia, and hypoxemia.

Other Complications

Recurrent chest discomfort in a patient with a recent infarction may be due to ischemia (angina or infarct expansion) or nonischemic causes (pericarditis, pulmonary embolism). Careful physical examination, ECG comparison, and the response to nitroglycerin are early measures that may be supplemented with echocardiography or perfusion scans. Pericarditis occurs in transmural infarction, with pain present as early as the first or second day. The pain is typically longer in duration than is that caused by ischemia. The pericardial discomfort is increased during recumbency and deep inspiration and eased when the patient leans forward when sitting.

A transient pericardial friction rub is heard frequently. The echocardiographic presence of a pericardial effusion generally is considered an indication to discontinue anticoagulants. Aspirin in higher doses than are prescribed regularly after an infarction is usually effective and is preferable to corticosteroids and nonsteroidal anti-inflammatory agents. Mural left ventricular thrombi are common in AMI patients who are not anticoagulated. The incidence of mural thrombi has decreased dramatically in patients receiving thrombolytic agents with heparin or heparin therapy alone. Echocardiography is the most accurate method for diagnosing left ventricular mural thrombi. If they are present, anticoagulation with warfarin for 3 to 6 months generally is recommended.

Predischarge Considerations

A low-level exercise test (5 to 6 Mets) frequently is performed before hospital discharge to identify those at risk for another cardiac event. The provocative test is done to detect ventricular arrhythmia and myocardial ischemia. Those who have a normal hemodynamic and ECG response to low-level testing have a 1 to 2% annual mortality rate. In contrast, recurrent cardiac events are likely in patients who cannot perform the test or who demonstrate ischemic ST-segment depression or significant ventricular arrhythmia. Patients who demonstrate ischemia may be referred for coronary angiography. Electrophysiologic studies may be indicated for those who exhibit exercise-induced ventricular arrhythmia.

Assessment of left ventricular systolic function, frequently ejection fraction determination by echocardiography, has important therapeutic and prognostic significance. Those whose ejection fraction is 40% or less have a significantly higher cardiac mortality rate. However, recent clinical trials have demonstrated the therapeutic benefit of long-term ACE inhibitor therapy in these patients.

At the time of hospital discharge, preventive measures include instruction in diet, activity level, weight control, smoking cessation, treatment of dyslipidemia, and, if no contraindication is present, indefinite aspirin and beta blocker therapy.

CORONARY HEART DISEASE IN WOMEN

In the United States, 230,000 women die annually from AMI, and 87,000 die from an acute cerebrovascular accident. Coronary heart disease (CHD) is the leading cause of death in both sexes. It is the leading cause of death in men by age 45 years and in women by age 65 years. There are significant gender differences in the character of CHD.

The risk factors for development of CHD in women are the same as in men, namely, age, family history of premature heart disease, dyslipidemia, cigarette smoking, hypertension, diabetes mellitus, and obesity. Diabetes is a much more potent risk factor for the development of CHD in women than in men. Diabetes obviates the cardiovascular protective effects of estrogen. Further, diabetes removes the normal sex-related differences in the prevalence of CHD. In persons 50 to 59 years of age, diabetes is a greater risk factor for CHD in women than in men. The risk of coronary events, unstable angina pectoris, acute myocardial infarction, and sudden cardiac death is two times greater in diabetic women than in diabetic men. The risk of cardiovascular death in women with diabetes is 3 to 7 times greater than in nondiabetic women. Smoking confers a greater risk in diabetic women than in diabetic men.

Acute Myocardial Infarction in Women

While 1 in 3 women in the United States over age 65 years has CHD, the onset is delayed in nondiabetic women by an average of 10 years when compared to men. There is a less favorable outcome for women than men in AMI. The in-hospital mortality for young women with acute infarction is significantly higher than in men. Under age 50 years, mortality for women is two times greater than in men of the same age. Mortality at 6 weeks post-AMI is greater in women. Further, 44% of women die within 1 year following AMI, compared to a 27% mortality in men. The reasons for women faring worse in AMI include women being older at the time of infarction; having a higher incidence of co-existent diabetes mellitus and hypertension; being more likely to manifest pump failure, including cardiogenic shock; and responding less well to thrombolytic agents.

Efficacy of Medicines to Treat AMI in Women

Aspirin and beta-sympathetic blockers are of significant value in reducing mortality in AMI in both women and men. Thrombolytic agents are not as effective in women as in men. In the GUSTO I trial, overall mortality at 30 days in women was 11.3% and in men, 5.5%, despite patency rates of coronary arteries and ventricular function being equal in both sexes. While women in this clinical trial were older and more likely to have hypertension, diabetes, and dyslipidemia, nonetheless, gender was still an independent predictor of death.

Prevention of CHD in Women

Aspirin is of significant and equal value in women and men in the *secondary* prevention of CHD, resulting in a 25% reduction in overall cardiovascular mortality and nonfatal infarction. Presently, there are no data related to the efficacy of aspirin in the *primary* prevention of ischemic cardiac disease. Pravastatin, an HMG-coenzyme A reductase inhibitor agent ("statin"), has been demonstrated to be of significant value in women in the *secondary* prevention of CHD. Lovastatin significantly reduced acute coronary events in a *primary* prevention clinical trial.

The Heart and Estrogen/Progestin Replacement Study (HERS study) was the first large, randomized, placebo-controlled clinical trial of hormones and CHD in women. This secondary prevention study included 2763 postmenopausal women having an average age of 66.7 years. All had an intact uterus. The hormone-treated group received daily conjugated equine estrogen (CEE) and daily medroxyprogesterone acetate (MPA). The treated group had an 11% reduction in LDL-C and a 10% increase in HDL-C. Unexpectedly, the CEE/MPA group showed a 50% increased risk of coronary events during the first year of hormonal therapy. After 4.1 years, the CHD rates did not differ in women assigned to active versus placebo treatment. The frequency of revascularization procedures and of all causes of mortality was the same in both groups. There was an increased risk of venous thrombosis in the CEE/MPA cohort during each year of the study. In contrast to the statin agents, initiation of estrogen alone, or in combination with a progestin, is unjustified at this time in the prevention of ischemic coronary events in women with and without CHD.

The Women's Health Initiative, a primary prevention trial in postmenopausal women, is in progress. This placebo-controlled study has two study groups; women with an intact uterus will receive CEE/MPA versus placebo, and women without a uterus will receive CEE versus placebo.

SILENT ISCHEMIA

Silent ischemia is myocardial ischemia that occurs in the absence of symptoms. These patients are at increased risk for myocardial infarction and have an increased mortality rate. Silent ischemia is more common in diabetic patients.

The diagnosis is established by defining ischemic ST-segment changes during ambulatory electrocardiography or during treadmill testing in a patient who is not experiencing cardiac symptoms. Silent ischemia may occur in patients who have never had ischemic discomfort. Moreover, silent ischemic episodes are very common in patients who also have anginal discomfort. In fact, the majority of ischemic episodes in this group are asymptomatic.

The presence of ischemic ST-segment depression during an exercise test confers an increased risk of subsequent cardiac events regardless of whether anginal discomfort occurred during the test.

In considering the management of silent ischemia, it is significant that medications that prevent anginal discomfort also prevent silent ischemia. Therefore, aspirin, beta blockers, and nitrates may be prescribed.

SUDDEN CARDIAC DEATH

Sudden cardiac death (SCD) is arguably the primary problem in contemporary cardiology. Approximately 400,000 sudden deaths occur annually in the United States. In one-quarter the sudden death is the initial expression of heart disease. In the majority of cases SCD is due to ventricular fibrillation. Three subsets of patients are at highest risk of sudden cardiac death. The most common substrate of sudden death is myocardial ischemia. In only a small percentage of cases, however, is there associated myocardial infarction. Additionally, patients with left ventricular dysfunction of any etiology and patients with left ventricular hypertrophy are at increased risk. The last subset includes hypertrophic cardiomyopathy, a major cause of sudden death in young adults.

A bifold approach has been taken to this major public health problem. First is the identification of known heart disease patients at greatest risk of sudden death. These patients often demonstrate malignant ventricular arrhythmia. Some of these patients are survivors of sudden cardiac death ("cardiac arrest") who undergo implantation of an automatic defibrillator.

The second approach is the public health measure of placing external defibrillators in public places, e.g., sports arenas, with attendant training of nonmedical personnel to be used on those who suddenly collapse and are pulseless. Pilot programs are under way to determine the efficacy of such efforts.

BIBLIOGRAPHY

ACC/AHA Guidelines for the Management of Patients with Acute Myocardial Infarction. A Report of the American College of Cardiology/American Heart Association Task Force on Practice Guidelines (Committee on Management of Acute Myocardial Infarction). 1999. http://www.acc.org/clinical/guidelines/nov96/1999/

Falk E et al: Coronary plaque disruption. *Circulation* 92:657–671, 1995.

Hulley S, Grady D: Randomized trial of estrogen plus progestin for secondary prevention of coronary heart disease in postmenopausal women. *JAMA* 280(7):605–613, 1998.

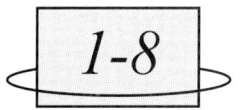

PERICARDIAL DISEASE
Morton A. Diamond

DISCUSSION

Pericardial disease is increasingly recognized because patients with cancer, renal disease, and connective tissue disease are living longer. Patients with disease of the pericardium may present with acute pericarditis, pericardial effusion, or constrictive pericarditis. When a physician assistant establishes a diagnosis of pericardial disease, the determination must be made whether a causative systemic illness is present. In the United States, cancer spreading to the pericardium is now the most common cause of disease of the pericardium.

ACUTE PERICARDITIS

Pathophysiology

Pericardial inflammation may be caused by a variety of infectious agents and other disorders (Table 1-8-1). The most common is idiopathic pericarditis that is thought to be due to viruses, usually coxsackievirus and echovirus. Purulent pericarditis is most often due to *Pneumococcus* and *Staphylococcus* from an adjacent intrathoracic infection. Gram-negative organisms and fungi also may produce purulent inflammation. Tuberculous pericarditis is increasing in frequency because of an increase in cases of drug-resistant disease. Tuberculous pericarditis usually occurs in the absence of demonstrable pulmonary disease. AIDS patients may develop acute pericarditis from a wide variety of opportunistic infectious agents. Vasculitis connective tissue

TABLE 1-8-1. Causes of Acute Pericarditis

Idiopathic
Viral
Purulent
Tuberculosis
Uremia
Myocardial infarction
Acute pericarditis
Post–myocardial infarction syndrome
Neoplastic disease
Radiation therapy
Vasculitis—connective tissue disorders
Invasive medical procedures
Medication
Sarcoid
Inflammatory bowel disease

diseases associated with acute pericarditis include systemic lupus erythematosus (SLE), scleroderma, and polyarteritis. SLE must be ruled out in any female patient presenting with acute pericarditis. Uremic pericarditis is common and is dramatic in onset. Its clinical manifestations are similar to those of idiopathic inflammation. Pericardial involvement from neoplasia most frequently is due to lymphoma or contiguous spread from breast or lung cancer. Invasive medical procedures, including heart surgery, pacemaker insertion, and cardiac catheterization, are increasingly common causes of acute pericarditis.

Medications that cause acute inflammation include isoniazid, hydralazine, penicillin, phenylbutazone, procainamide, diphenylhydantoin, and doxorubicin. Aortic root dissection into the pericardium is a rare cause but may quickly cause life-threatening cardiac tamponade.

Signs and Symptoms

The cardinal symptoms and signs of acute pericarditis include chest pain and friction rub. The pain may be precordial or retrosternal and commonly radiates to the neck. The discomfort may be sharp or dull and typically is aggravated by recumbency, inspiration, and body motion. Dyspnea may be noted since the patient is unable to take a full inspiration because of chest pain. The physician assistant must differentiate pericardial pain from that caused by myocardial ischemia. A pericardial friction rub establishes the diagnosis. However, the rub may be transitory, and therefore frequent auscultation is necessary.

Post–myocardial infarction syndrome (Dressler's syndrome), which is manifested by chest pain, malaise, fever, and both pleural and pericardial effusions, is thought to be an autoimmune disorder but is lessening in frequency. Though pericardial effusions may be large, tamponade is rare. Recurrences of Dressler's syndrome are common, but the prognosis of the initial infarction is not altered. Therapy includes nonsteroidal anti-inflammatory drugs (NSAIDs) and, if necessary, corticosteroids.

Laboratory and Radiologic Studies

In idiopathic pericarditis, mild leukocytosis and an elevation of the erythrocyte sedimentation rate are common. Pericarditis associated with SLE frequently reveals leukopenia and a positive antinuclear antibody response. Significant elevation of the white blood cell count, particularly when associated with a leftward shift, suggests bacterial infection. Renal function studies will confirm uremic pericarditis.

The chest x-ray is usually normal unless the pericarditis is associated with significant pericardial effusion or an intrathoracic neoplasm is present. In acute pericarditis, the echocardiogram commonly demonstrates increased pericardial fluid but may be normal.

Electrocardiogram

When not associated with myocardial infarction, the electrocardiogram (ECG) demonstrates ST-segment and T-wave changes without alteration of the QRS complex. The elevated ST segments have a concave upward character and are noted in all leads except V_1 and aV_R. There is no reciprocal ST-segment depression as is noted in myocardial injury or infarction. In pericarditis the T wave inverts after the ST segments have returned to baseline, while in myocardial infarction T-wave inversion occurs while ST segments are still elevated. The ECG changes of acute pericarditis also must be differentiated from those of early repolarization. In early repolarization, ST-segment elevation may be diffuse but serial changes are not noted.

PERICARDIAL EFFUSION

Pericardial effusion may be caused by many disorders, including infectious, neoplastic, metabolic, and autoimmune etiologies (Table 1-8-2). The rate of pericardial fluid accumulation determines the clinical state of the patient. Because the pericardium is compliant, a slowly enlarging effusion may contain 2000 mL of fluid without hemodynamic compromise. In contrast, a rapidly developing small effusion may cause life-threatening tamponade related to inadequate cardiac filling. Effusions may be associated with chest pain when they are related to an inflammatory process or may be painless, as may occur in neoplasia.

Clinical Features

Idiopathic pericarditis usually occurs in a young adult who has had an upper respiratory infection during the preceding weeks. The onset of chest pain is often dramatic. The diagnosis is made by friction rub, ECG changes, and echocardiographic demonstration of pericardial effusion. No underlying disease is found. NSAIDs commonly suppress the pain within 24 h. Corticosteroids may be given to a patient whose symptoms are resistant to the initial therapy. While effectively suppressing clinical manifestations, corticosteroids may promote exacerbations of inflammation. The illness usually lasts 1 to 3 weeks and is self-limited. In fewer than 5% of cases, a recurrence of acute pericarditis will occur. Rarely, tamponade may develop. Bacterial pericarditis should be suspected when a patient has high fever, chills, and night sweats. Suspicion of this disease requires diagnostic pericardiocentesis. If it is present, therapy includes antibiotics and surgical drainage. Mortality rates

TABLE 1-8-2 Causes of Pericardial Effusion

Neoplasia
Infection
Idiopathic
Myocardial infarction
Congestive heart failure
Trauma
Vasculitis—connective tissue disorders
Medication
Uremia
Nephrotic syndrome
Hypothyroidism

range from 55 to 75% and are particularly high when pericarditis is associated with gram-negative organisms. If pericarditis is mistaken for myocardial infarction, thrombolytic therapy can have life-threatening consequences. Pericarditis is a relative contraindication to both thrombolytic and anticoagulant agents. In transmural myocardial infarction, pericarditis is usually manifest on the second or third day. This pain must be clinically differentiated from myocardial ischemia and infarct extension. Therapy with NSAIDs is generally effective.

Pericardial involvement in AIDS, characterized by moderate or large effusion, occurs in approximately 15% of cases. Tamponade, however, is rare, occurring in only 2%. Echocardiography should be performed in the AIDS patient who has tuberculosis or other pulmonary infection, congestive heart failure, or Kaposi's sarcoma.

Signs and Symptoms

Symptoms and signs are primarily related to the underlying disorder unless tamponade is present. A small effusion may be present in an asymptomatic patient who has a normal cardiac examination. The effusion may be demonstrated only on echocardiographic study. Large effusions may cause cough and dyspnea as a result of compression of adjacent lung tissue and often are associated with muffled heart tones. Tamponade occurs when rapidly developing effusions reduce filling of the heart and subsequently cardiac output. The patient complains of dyspnea, cough, and weakness. Central venous pressure is universally elevated. Tachycardia, tachypnea, paradoxical pulse, and hypotension are very common. Paradoxical pulse—the exaggeration of the normal difference in systolic pressure between inspiration and expiration—can be defined only in a patient in sinus rhythm. The most common cause of a paradoxical pulse is obstructive lung disease.

Radiologic Studies

Radiographic signs in effusion are variable, depending on the size of the fluid accumulation and the presence of an intrathoracic neoplasm. Small effusions are associated with a normal cardiac appearance, while large effusions produce the "water bottle" enlarged cardiac silhouette. The echocardiogram is the best diagnostic tool for the diagnosis of effusion. Tamponade, which is characterized by increased intrapericardial pressure, is diagnosed by demonstration of diastolic collapse of the right atrium and right ventricle.

Management

Therapy is dependent on the presence or absence of hemodynamic compromise. Tamponade requires immediate pericardiocentesis, preferably with catheter drainage. Otherwise, effusion management is related to treatment of the underlying cause. Physician referral is indicated in all cases of pericarditis associated with systemic disease or effusions resulting in hemodynamic impairment.

CONSTRICTIVE PERICARDITIS

Constrictive pericarditis is a tightening vise around the heart. The three most common identifiable causes are cardiac surgery, pericarditis, and mediastinal irradiation, usually for Hodgkin's disease or breast carcinoma. Other causes include connective tissue disease, uremia, sarcoidosis, and neoplasia.

The pericardial constriction becomes evident an average of 13 years after radiotherapy, but may occur as early as 1 year or as long as 40 years posttherapy. When constriction is due to virulent pericardial infection or, uncommonly, to pericardial neoplasia, clinical presentation may occur over weeks.

Physiologically, constriction is associated with increased cardiac filling pressure and decreased cardiac output.

Signs and Symptoms

Typical symptoms include fatigue, dyspnea, nausea, chest discomfort, and weakness. Physical examination reveals distended neck veins from elevated central venous pressure, congestive hepatomegaly, ascites, peripheral edema, and often atrial arrhythmias. The lung fields are typically clear. Kussmaul's sign—loss of the inspiratory decrease in jugular venous pressure—is common, but paradoxical pulse is noted in a minority of patients. The physician assistant must differentiate this disorder from right ventricular heart failure and restrictive cardiomyopathy.

Radiologic Studies

The chest x-ray may show pericardial calcification. Echocardiography, as well as computed tomography and magnetic resonance imaging can demonstrate pericardial thickening and small heart chambers.

Electrocardiogram

The ECG generally reveals low-voltage and diffuse T-wave inversion. Atrial fibrillation and atrioventricular and intraventricular conduction defects are common.

Differential Diagnosis

The differentiation of constrictive pericarditis from restrictive cardiomyopathy is still a major diagnostic challenge. Sarcoidosis, hematochromatosis, and amyloid disease of the heart also reduce ventricular filling. Therefore, the clinical appearance of patients in both cardiac disorders is similar. Cardiac catheterization with endomyocardial biopsy is employed to help make the correct diagnosis. Thoracotomy may still be necessary to establish the diagnosis. If constriction is found, pericardiectomy is performed.

BIBLIOGRAPHY

Ling LH et al: Constrictive pericarditis in the modern era. *Circulation* 100: 1380–1386, 1999.

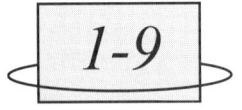

PERIPHERAL VASCULAR DISEASE

Marquitha S. Mayfield

DISCUSSION

Peripheral vascular disease (PVD) is a broad term encompassing a variety of disorders that affect the arteries, veins, and lymphatics. Specifically included in this category of diseases are vessels providing peripheral circulation to the extracranial cerebral vasculature (carotid and vertebrals), the extremities, and the organs of the thoracic and abdominal cavity. Diseases of the peripheral vasculature are common. Of the adult population, 20% suffer from varicose veins. Approximately 5% of patients over 70 years have symptomatic arterial disease. Each year approximately 2 million cases of venous thrombosis and 2000 cases of aortic aneurysms are diagnosed in the United States. PVD is a leading cause of death and limb loss in the country. Most patients are middle aged or elderly. Table 1-9-1 reviews the types of peripheral vascular disease.

As the patient population continues to age, the prevalence of disorders involving the peripheral vasculature will continue to increase. Many patients with mild to moderate symptoms of chronic vascular disease can be safely managed conservatively in the primary care setting. Others with severe or acute symptoms of vascular disease will require intensive diagnostic evaluation and management, often involving the expertise of subspecialty consultants. The primary care provider

TABLE 1-9-1. Types of Peripheral Vascular Disease

Arterial Disease
Arterial insufficiency
Atherosclerotic peripheral vascular disease
Acute arterial insufficiency
Nonatherosclerotic arterial occlusive disease
Aortic aneurysm and dissection
Venous Disease
Varicose veins
Chronic venous insufficiency
Venous stasis and venous ulcers
Venous thrombosis
Deep-venous thrombosis
Superficial thrombaphlebitis
Lymphatic Disease
Lymphedema
Lymphangitis

must be able to differentiate between these two patient population groups to render proper clinical management.

DEFINITIONS
Atherosclerosis

This is a progressive, systemic disease characterized by deposition of lipoprotein along the intimal layer of the arterial wall. These deposits become thrombotic, fibrotic, and calcified, forming an atheroma. Atheromatous plaques build up over time and progressively occlude the lumina of arteries. Atherosclerosis may also cause the medial layer of the vessel wall to degenerate, increasing the risk for developing aneurysms. Because atherosclerosis is a multisystemic disease, many patients also have coexisting coronary and/or cerebral vascular disease (see also Chap. 1-3).

Thrombosis

Thrombosis involves the formation of a clot that remains attached to the vessel wall. Clots usually form at sites of previous injury, vessel narrowing, or anastomosis. Clots can occlude the lumina of vessels, diminishing arterial blood supply or obstructing venous return. Distal tissues become ischemic from arterial occlusion or edematous from venous obstruction.

Thromboembolism

This is the detachment or fragmentation of a proximal thrombus (clot) into the bloodstream. This material travels to a distal site, producing vessel occlusion. Both arteries and veins may be affected by embolic phenomenon. An embolic event in the arterial tree can precipitate severe ischemia and tissue necrosis (gangrene) from acute arterial insufficiency. In the venous circulation, a pulmonary embolus can result, with catastrophic results.

Aneurysms and Varicosities

When arterial walls weaken and dilate, aneurysms form. These same changes in veins produce varicosities. Increased intravascular pressure can distend the vessel lumen, weakening vessel walls. Congenital defects can weaken vessel walls as well.

Vasculitis

Infection or inflammation of the vessel wall, vasculitis, can occur. Bacteria introduced into the circulation can seed previously damaged areas of blood vessels. Inflammatory disorders of arteries and veins increase the incidence of thrombosis and vascular obstruction.

Vascular Trauma

The placement of catheters into the lumina of arteries and veins for diagnostic and therapeutic purposes can injure the vessel wall, precipitate the formation of clots that obstruct flow, or cause severe vasospasm with vessel occlusion. Vessels may also be transected in a variety of injuries, both major and minor.

Vasospasm

Vasospasm may produce transient vascular occlusion, sometimes with marked distal tissue ischemia. Small arteries are usually affected. Vasospastic disorders may be primary in origin (Raynaud's disease) or iatrogenic (induced by arterial cannulation procedures).

Congenital Malformations

Congenital malformations include narrowing of the aorta (coarctation) and abnormal connections between arteries and veins (arteriovenous fistulas). These abnormalities produce turbulent flow through vessel lumina, increasing the incidence of thrombosis and embolism.

ARTERIAL DISEASE: ATHEROSCLEROTIC PERIPHERAL VASCULAR DISEASE

DISCUSSION

An occlusive process that reduces or completely obstructs blood flow to the distal tissues causes arterial insufficiency. The vascular occlusion may be acute or chronic in origin. Occlusion of 50% of the arterial lumen (75% of the vessel diameter) produces clinically significant reduction in blood flow, resulting in tissue hypoxia and ischemia. Severe ischemia can result in tissue necrosis with gangrenous changes and limb loss or distal organ failure. The most common cause for arterial occlusive disease is atherosclerosis. Atheromatous plaques often develop at points of vascular bifurcation (branching), abrupt curvature, or narrowing because of the shearing forces and turbulent blood flow associated with these areas. Lower extremities are affected more often than upper extremities because of the higher arterial pressures in the legs. Common sites for vessel occlusion include the aorta-iliac bifurcation, common and superficial bifurcation, femoral-popliteal transition, popliteal-tibial-peroneal trifurcation, and common carotid bifurcation.

Because atherosclerosis is a chronic, slow process, collateral circulation develops around areas of chronic occlusion. With adequate collateral flow, patients may be asymptomatic or have minimal symptoms. With time, however, these collateral vessels also become diseased and occluded. Risk factors for the development of arterial occlusive disease include smoking, hypercholesterolemia, diabetes mellitus, hypertension, family history, and male sex.

SIGNS AND SYMPTOMS

Pain is the principal symptom of arterial insufficiency. Intermittent claudication is a classic finding in chronic arterial insufficiency. Claudication may be described as a cramping discomfort, weakness, or tired sensation induced by lower extremity exertion (e.g., walking, biking) and relieved with minimal rest. The calves are most commonly affected, although symptoms of claudication can also occur in the thighs or buttocks. The area of vascular occlusion is proximal to the site of claudication (e.g., thigh claudication would correlate with iliac arterial disease). Claudication may become progressive over months or years, and decreasing levels of patient ambulation and activity can indicate increasing severity.

Rest pain is a more ominous sign of severe occlusive disease. Pain is continuous and severe from constant inadequate tissue perfusion

through a severely stenotic artery. It occurs in the foot and is classically described as a burning or aching discomfort in the forefoot that is most intense at night. Dangling the foot on the side of the bed may bring some relief because of enhanced tissue perfusion with gravity. The presence of rest pain is consistent with impending tissue necrosis and is a major indication for surgical intervention.

In males impotence can be a presenting symptom when aorta-iliac disease is present. Its presence suggests occlusion of the internal iliac artery or distal aorta, as seen in Leriche's syndrome. Thigh and/or buttock claudication may also occur.

Transient ischemic attacks (TIAs) may be manifestations of occlusive disease of the carotid arteries. Amaurosis fugax (transient monocular blindness often described as a "shade" or "curtain" descending over one eye) is a classic symptom of transient occlusion of the ophthalmic branch of the internal carotid artery. An atheromatous embole from a diseased carotid artery is commonly the cause. Other symptoms suggestive of TIAs are reviewed in Chap. 1-3.

OBJECTIVE FINDINGS

Patient examination should be tailored to look specifically for the following clinical features seen in chronic occlusive disease.

1. *Diminished or absent peripheral pulses.* Compare pulses in both extremities and look for asymmetry. Conduct this exam both before and after exercise since pulses distal to the occlusion may diminish after exercise.
2. *Bruits* heard over the carotid, aortic, renal, iliac, or femoral vasculature. When vessels are severely stenotic, bruits may be absent.
3. *Ischemic skin changes* such as pallor on leg elevation followed by erythema on dependency, poor capillary refill, or digital cyanosis.
4. *Trophic changes* such as loss of hair on the extremity (especially the feet and toes), shiny atrophic skin, and thickened toenails.
5. *Collapsed superficial veins* consistent with poor arterial inflow.
6. *Painful ischemic ulcers* that bleed minimally located on the distal aspect of digits or the heel of the foot. Gangrenous changes (wet or dry) of the distal extremity may also be noted.

DIFFERENTIAL DIAGNOSES

The differential diagnosis for *chronic* arterial insufficiency includes trauma, arterial embolism, arterial aneurysm or dissection, atherosclerotic vascular disease, and nonatherosclerotic disorders such as Berger's disease. A variety of disorders can mimic the pain of claudication, including:

• Degenerative disk disease and spinal stenosis
• Osteoarthritis of the hip or knee
• Diabetic neuropathy
• Nocturnal leg cramps

Additionally, neuropathic ulcers and venous ulcers may be confused with ischemic ulcers of arterial disease.

LABORATORY AND RADIOLOGIC TESTS

In the primary care setting, baseline lab studies to detect and evaluate pertinent risk factors (i.e., hypertension, diabetes, and hyperlipidemia) should be ordered.

OTHER DIAGNOSTICS

Handheld Doppler devices provide a quick, easy method for detecting nonpalpable pulses in the office. When combined with the use of a blood pressure cuff, an ankle/brachial ratio or index (ABI) can be measured to provide more information about the severity of vascular occlusion. ABIs >0.9 are considered normal. ABIs of 0.5 to 0.9 are consistent with arterial claudication. ABIs <0.4 are seen with rest pain and severe arterial stenosis. Measurements should be recorded before and after exercise (e.g., walking down the hall). Patients suspected of having significant arterial insufficiency should be referred to a vascular lab to have a complete segmental arterial Doppler flow study performed.

Diabetics and patients with renal failure frequently have falsely elevated ABIs due to calcified vessel walls as well as small vessel disease. Segmental plethysmography measures changes in pulse volume instead of pressures and provides a better evaluation in these patients. Obtaining digital (toe) pressures may also be useful.

Arterial duplex scanning combines Doppler with ultrasound imaging to visualize the vessel wall for defects and atheromas as well as to evaluate blood flow. It is extremely useful in evaluating the carotid artery and its branches for stenotic lesions.

Arteriography can be used to determine the precise location and extent of vascular occlusion. However, because of the attendant risk for contrast-induced renal failure, hematoma, or vascular dissection, it should be reserved for those patients in whom surgical intervention is anticipated.

TREATMENT

Medications

Pentoxifylline (Trental) or cilostazol (Pletal) may help some patients with intermittent claudication. Pentoxifylline alters the red blood cells, enhancing their flexibility and flow through stenotic vessels. Cilostazol enhances vasodilation and has antiplatelet effects. Gastrointestinal side effects are common with the use of pentoxifylline, and the medication is contraindicated in patients with recent cerebral or retinal hemorrhages. Headache is a common side effect of cilostazol, and it is contraindicated in patients with congestive heart failure. The dosage for pentoxifylline is 400 mg tid. Cilostazol is given 100 mg bid. Patients should be warned that it might take as long as 2 to 3 months to achieve significant results, and not all patients see a significant reduction in their claudication.

In patients with thrombotic/embolic events or carotid artery disease, treatment with buffered aspirin or clopidogrel (Plavix) may be beneficial. Both medications inhibit platelet aggregation and diminish clot formation. Aspirin is administered in small doses (80 to 325 mg/d). Clopidogrel is given 75 mg daily.

Pharmacologic measures to control hypertension, diabetes, and hyperlipidemia should be employed also. Anticoagulants (heparin, Coumadin, etc.) have no role in the management of chronic arterial occlusive disease.

Supportive Measures

Patients with a history of mild to moderate claudication, midrange ABIs, and no rest pain or ischemic changes may benefit from conservative management. A program of daily walking to the point of claudication followed by 2- to 30-min rest periods repeated throughout the day is the most effective way to enhance the development of collateral vessels and improve circulation. Patients on an exercise program can increase their walking distance by as much as 50% or more after 3 months of activity. The benefits of exercise as well as smoking cessation should be explained to the patient. Instructions on proper foot care should also be given. Patients placed on an exercise program should be instructed to try to "walk through" their period of claudication a little more each day. They should also be instructed to avoid medications that may constrict the arterial vasculature (e.g., ergotamine derivatives, alpha agonists).

Other Treatment Modalities

Vascular reconstruction or angioplasty may be indicated for patients with debilitating claudication, rest pain, or evidence of severe occlusion. The best candidates are those with proximal occlusive disease and patent distal vessels. Arterial grafts (prosthetic or saphenous vein) are usually employed to bypass the occluded vessel(s). Thromboendarterectomy is also useful in repairing diseased carotid, iliac, and femoral arteries. Transluminal angioplasty is often utilized in short segmental disease and is a cost-effective alternative to bypass surgery. Amputation of affected limbs may be warranted in patients with gangrenous changes or in patients who are nonambulatory with severe rest pain or are poor surgical candidates for vascular reconstruction.

Disposition

Follow-up visits for patients with uncomplicated stable disease may be conducted at 2–3-month and 6-month intervals. Consultative evaluation with a vascular surgeon should be obtained for any patient with progressive, refractory, or debilitating symptoms, or for patients whose quality of life has been significantly affected.

COMPLICATIONS AND RED FLAGS

Secondary infections of ischemic ulcers, cellulitis, and tissue necrosis with wet or dry gangrene are complications that may be prevented with appropriate assessment and management. Red flags include new-onset rest pain, ischemic ulceration, tissue necrosis, and any symptoms suggestive of acute occlusive disease.

OTHER NOTES AND PEARLS

Patients with diabetes mellitus develop atherosclerosis more frequently and earlier than nondiabetic persons do. Although large and small vessels may be involved, occlusion of smaller vessels (especially tibial arteries) is more common, making surgical management more difficult. Ischemic ulcers, when present, are more likely to be painless due to neuropathy secondarily infected with multiple organisms and are slow to heal. These patients require close supervision and consultative management.

ACUTE ARTERIAL INSUFFICIENCY

DISCUSSION

Arterial insufficiency may occur acutely as a result of thrombosis or embolization. The most common cause for acute arterial insufficiency is an embolus from the heart. Abnormalities affecting the left side of the heart, such as atrial fibrillation or flutter, mitral stenosis, and transmural infarction, can produce clots that embolize. Other causes include trauma, aneurysmal embolization or thrombosis, hypercoagulable states, and arterial cannulation procedures. Embolic obstruction of vascular flow is 10 times more likely in the lower extremities than upper. The superficial femoral artery is the most common site. When vessel occlusion occurs acutely, severe ischemia develops rapidly because collateral blood vessels have not had time to develop. Acute arterial occlusion represents a vascular emergency. Final outcome for limb salvage is dependent on the duration of tissue ischemia. There is a 4- to 6-h "golden window" in which limb loss can be minimized by prompt restoration of blood flow.

SIGNS AND SYMPTOMS

Patients often present with an acute onset of severe pain, loss of pulses, and ischemic changes in the extremity (cool limbs, +/− cyanosis). Symptoms are usually unilateral and may affect only the digits initially. In some patients the first manifestation may be that of a stroke, ischemic colitis, or organ failure (e.g., renal insufficiency).

TABLE 1-9-2. The "Five Ps" of Acute Arterial Insufficiency

Pain—constant and aggravated by any movement

Pallor—occurs initially and is followed by cyanosis

Pulselessness—often associated with a cold limb

Paresthesias—caused by anoxia to peripheral nerves

Paralysis—caused by necrosis of muscular tissue and motor nerves

In gathering the patient history, look for the following:

- Time of onset of the initial symptoms
- Previous history of cardiac disease (cardiac arrhythmias, valvular heart disease, or myocardial infarction)
- Previous history of atherosclerotic PVD
- Recent episode of hypotension

OBJECTIVE FINDINGS

Table 1-9-2 lists the "five Ps" of acute arterial insufficiency—the most common objective findings. These findings are distal to the site of vascular occlusion. Both paresthesias and paralysis are relatively late and grave signs seen with tissue necrosis and impending limb loss.

DIFFERENTIAL DIAGNOSES

The most important consideration for the differential diagnosis is whether the acute loss of blood flow is embolic or thrombotic in origin since the treatment modality is different for each.

Additional diagnostic considerations include:

- Arterial transection due to trauma or vascular procedure
- Aortic dissection with occlusion of peripheral vessels
- Severe arteriospasm
- Acute deep-venous thrombosis with massive swelling that obstructs arterial flow
- Severe hypotension

LABORATORY AND RADIOLOGIC TESTS

A standard workup should include the following:

- Chest x-ray to check for evidence of cardiac disease or thoracic aortic aneurysm
- Echocardiogram to rule out mural thrombus, myxoma, or valvular vegetation that can serve as sources of emboli
- Electrocardiogram to rule out arrhythmias
- Arteriogram if a noncardiac etiology is suspected and surgical intervention is anticipated
- Serum creatine kinase and urine myoglobin tests to check for evidence of muscle necrosis
- Prothrombin time (PT) and partial thromboplastin time (PTT) for baseline monitoring of anticoagulant therapy
- Abdominal and popliteal ultrasound to rule out aneurysmal disease.

TREATMENT

Time is a critical factor in patient management. Unless contraindicated, immediate anticoagulation with heparin should be started to prevent further propagation of the clot. Heparin is given intravenously first as a bolus (5000 to 10,000 U), followed by 1000 U/h to 1500 U/h, titrated to maintain a PTT at 1.5 to 2 times the normal range. The patient remains heparinized until the etiology is clearly established. A surgical consult is indicated for further patient management. If cardiac emboli are the source, often long-term management with oral anticoagulants (warfarin) is needed.

Noncardiac thrombi may also be treated with intraluminal clot lysis using tissue plasminogen activator to restore blood flow or with an emergent embolectomy/thrombectomy, depending on the duration of tissue ischemia. Low-molecular-weight heparin (Lovenox, Fragmin) in the management of acute arterial insufficiency is not efficacious.

Supportive Measures

One should provide appropriate postoperative care for vascular surgical patients. Patients on anticoagulants should be closely monitored for symptoms and signs suggestive of bleeding diathesis (e.g., hematuria, rectal bleeding, easy bruising, epistaxis). Patients with a history of hypertension, diabetes, or hyperlipidemia should be encouraged to follow treatment recommendations for control of their disease. Smokers should be encouraged to quit and provided with needed support. Patients placed on long-term anticoagulation thereby should be instructed to report any symptoms of easy bruising or bleeding. Aspirin, nonsteroidal agents, and alcohol should be avoided.

COMPLICATIONS

Limb loss, organ failure, compartment syndrome, and reperfusion syndrome are major complications that increase in incidence the longer the affected tissues remain ischemic. Vessels may also reocclude, or attempts to remove the offending clot may fail. Overall prognosis for patients with acute occlusive disease is poor. Many patients also have significant cardiac disease. The average survival despite treatment is 3.1 years.

NONATHEROSCLEROTIC ARTERIAL INSUFFICIENCY

DISCUSSION

Although less common, nonatherosclerotic causes for arterial insufficiency may occur. Patients tend to be much younger at the time of onset (twenties to forties). Most patients have symptoms and signs suggestive of chronic arterial occlusive disease; however, acute presentations do occur. The upper extremities are often involved. The most common disorders in this category are described below.

SIGNS AND SYMPTOMS

Cystic Medial Necrosis

This disease affects primarily young men. Degenerative changes occur in the medial layer of the vessel wall, resulting in aneurysmal formation or aortic dissection. Except for the symptoms associated with arterial aneurysm or aortic dissection, patients are typically asymptomatic. Physical exam findings are the same as found in aneurysmal disease or aortic dissection.

Buerger's Disease (Thromboangiitis Obliterans)

In this chronic, occlusive disease, inflammation of the medium and small arteries and veins is followed by healing and thrombosis, resulting in vascular obstruction. Ischemic ulcerations that lead to gangrene may occur. The hands and feet are commonly affected. Smoking is directly related to these changes. Migratory thrombophlebitis is also common. Pain and tenderness of the affected part constitute the chief complaint. On physical exam one may see rubor or cyanosis. The skin may be thin and shiny and nails thick and dystrophic. Peripheral pulses are usually palpable and symmetrical. In advanced disease, gangrenous changes of the digits may be noted.

Raynaud's Disease and Phenomenon

Raynaud's disease is an arteriospastic disorder that produces occlusion of small subcutaneous and cutaneous arteries and arterioles, usually of the hands and feet. The disease is characterized by a triphasic color change of the digits (white turns to blue and then red) as well as paresthesias. In Raynaud's disease, arteriospasm may be precipitated by exposure to cold, smoking, or emotional upset. Arteriospasm is paroxysmal and transient, rarely resulting in significant tissue ischemia. Fingertips and fingers are usually affected bilaterally, with the thumb spared. Rarely are the toes affected. The disease occurs almost exclusively in women between the ages of 15 and 45 years. The cause is idiopathic.

In Raynaud's phenomenon, an underlying vasculitis produces arteriospasm. Digital cyanosis is prolonged and gangrenous ulcers are more common. Raynaud's phenomenon is often associated with a connective tissue disorder such as systemic sclerosis, lupus, or rheumatoid arthritis. Males are more commonly affected than females.

Patients complain of trasient numbness, tingling of digits associated with a classic description of the triphasic color change. Physical exam may be completely normal during symptom free periods. Peripheral pulses are intact.

In both Raynaud's disease and Buerger's disease, patients may present with clinical manifestations of single or multiple digital involvement.

Disposition

Patients with non-atherosclerotic arterial insufficiency should be managed in consultation with a vascular surgeon. A rheumatology consult may also be warranted in patients with Raynaud's phenomenon.

DIFFERENTIAL DIAGNOSIS

The differential diagnosis includes arterial thrombosis, acute arterial insufficiency, thoracic outlet syndrome, and vascular trauma.

LABORATORY AND RADIOLOGIC TESTS

Arterial dopplers to obtain digital pressures and evaluate digital blood flow should be ordered. Arterial dopplers may be used occasionally in patients with transient ischemic events, and vasospasm may have to be induced in the lab by exposing the digits to precipitating factors (i.e., cold) to confirm the diagnosis. Digital plethysmography may be helpful in differentiating Raynaud's disease from Raynaud's phenomenon. Occasionally, an arteriogram is performed if the above studies are positive.

TREATMENT

The most important part of treatment for Buerger's disease is cessation of cigarette smoking. Patients with Raynaud's should be advised to avoid exposing their digits to extreme cold. Gloves may present ischemic alters. For both Buerger's disease and Raynaud's disease and phenomenon, vasodilators (e.g., calcium channel blockers, beta blockers) may be given to relieve vasospasm. In refractory vasospasm, a sympathectomy may be warranted.

AORTIC ANEURYSMS AND DISSECTIONS

DISCUSSION

Degeneration of the medial layer of the arterial wall results in the formation of aneurysms. Any artery can be affected, most commonly the aortic (abdominal and thoracic), popliteal, and femoral arteries (in order of decreasing frequency). Aneurysms may be fusiform or saccular in shape. Over 95 percent of aortic aneurysms are caused by atherosclerosis. Hypertension is a major risk factor, and men are more frequently affected than women are.

Although aneurysm formation can affect any part of the aorta, most are abdominal, with 90 percent originating below the level of the renal arteries. The aorta below the renal arteries averages 2 cm in diameter. An aneurysm is said to be present when the diameter equals or exceeds 4 cm. Other aneurysms in the peripheral arteries often coexist, with the popliteal artery most frequently involved. Aneurysms may also affect any portion of the thoracic aorta from the aortic valve to the descending segment, with the descending aorta most frequently affected. In addition to atherosclerosis, deceleration trauma and cystic medial necrosis are other common causes for thoracic aneurysms.

Aneurysms, have a natural history for expanding in size and rupturing. The larger the aneurysm, the greater the risk for spontaneous rupture. At 6 cm in diameter the rate of rupture rapidly increases, with 43% of aneurysms this size rupturing within 1 to 2 years. The mortality rate for aortic rupture is extremely high, approaching 90% in some populations. Most patients die before they reach the operating room.

Although the term *dissecting aortic aneurysm* is often used, an aortic dissection is not technically an aneurysm. Both may have the same etiology, however. Aortic dissection is caused by extravasation of blood into and along the layers of the arterial wall through an intimal tear that produces a false lumen. The dissection does not extend around the circumference of the vessel but rather along the length of the vessel. This extension can partially or completely occlude any branch vessel in its path, producing loss of peripheral pulses and multiple organ ischemia and failure. Dissection may affect any part of the aorta, but the thoracic aorta is most frequent: 60% of intimal tears occur in the proximal ascending aorta, 20% in the descending aorta, 10% in the aortic arch, and the rest in the abdominal aorta. In addition to anatomic location, aortic dissections may be classified according to extension of the dissection. Type I dissections originate in the ascending aorta and extend distally to the abdominal aorta. Type II dissections are confined to the ascending aorta. Type III dissections begin in the descending aorta and may extend distally to the level of the iliac arteries. The most common cause for proximal aortic dissections is cystic medial necrosis. Atherosclerosis is the most common cause for distal aortic dissections. Deceleration trauma, as with high-speed motor vehicle accidents, has been implicated in the etiology of some cases of aortic dissection.

SYMPTOMS

Most aneurysms are asymptomatic and are detected as incidental findings on a routine physical exam or chest x-ray. The appearance of symptoms is usually an ominous sign indicating acute aneurysmal expansion that will likely lead to intrathoracic or retroperitoneal bleeding or impending rupture. Occasionally, clots formed along the wall of the aneurysm may embolize, producing symptoms of acute arterial insufficiency. When patients are symptomatic the most common complaint is abdominal or back pain for abdominal aneurysms and substernal, back, or neck pain in thoracic aneurysms. Pain intensity may vary from mild to severe and may be constant or intermittent.

In addition to pain, thoracic aortic aneurysms may produce other compressive symptoms such as dysphagia, hoarseness, cough, stridor, or dyspnea.

Unlike aneurysms that may be silent, the clinical manifestations for aortic dissection tend to be sudden and intense. Patients classically present with sudden onset of severe, tearing pain that is well localized initially but radiates as the dissection extends. Pain beginning in the chest and then radiating to the abdomen or back is frequently described. Partial or complete occlusion of the branch arteries arising from the aorta may lead to symptoms of syncope, renal failure, bowel obstruction or infarction, hemiplegia, or paralysis of the lower extremities.

OBJECTIVE FINDINGS

A pulsatile midabdominal mass in the umbilical region is the most common finding in abdominal aneurysms. A bruit may also be present. With thoracic aneurysm, distended neck veins and edema in the neck and arms may be seen if the superior vena cava is obstructed. A murmur of aortic regurgitation may also occur with involvement of the aortic valve. Peripheral pulses may be normal, diminished, or absent. Signs of acute arterial insufficiency may be present if a mural thrombus along the aneurysm wall has embolized.

An aortic dissection rarely presents as a pulsatile mass. Instead, classic findings on physical exam include clinical signs of shock in the face of frank hypertension, signs of heart failure, a diastolic murmur with retrograde involvement of the aortic valve, and ischemic changes in the lower extremities due to occlusion of the iliac artery by extension of the dissection.

DIFFERENTIAL DIAGNOSES

The differential diagnosis includes aortic compression caused by an intrathoracic or abdominal tumor and aortic trauma with partial or complete transection. Occasionally, complete disruption of the arterial wall with extravascular accumulation of clotted blood forming a "false aneurysm" may occur. These "pseudoaneurysms" are commonly a consequence of vascular trauma due to angiograms, intraarterial thrombolytic therapy, arteriovenous fistulas, infection of vascular grafts, or bleeding at the site of surgical vascular anastomosis. Treatment is primarily surgical.

LABORATORY AND RADIOLOGIC TESTS

Computed tomography (CT) scan using contrast media is the gold standard for diagnosing both abdominal and thoracic aortic aneurysms. It is highly sensitive and specific, providing information on the size and exact location of the aneurysm. An abdominal ultrasound is a good noninvasive test for screening and monitoring abdominal aneurysms. Plain-film radiography often demonstrates calcifications in the wall of the aneurysm that appear as an "eggshell" pattern. Chest films may show a thoracic aneurysm as a widened mediastinum. A transesophageal echocardiogram (TEE) is also a good tool for diagnosing thoracic aneurysms. Aortograms often fail to detect an aneurysm when an intraluminal clot exists, thrombosing the false lumen but preserving the true lumen. They should be reserved for preoperative evaluation. Patients with an aneurysm of the ascending aorta should have studies of their aortic valve and coronary arteries completed since these structures may also require surgical repair.

In aortic dissection, laboratory studies may provide evidence of end organ failure (abnormal liver function tests) and renal insufficiency. Chest x-rays may show a widened superior mediastinum. An echocardiogram will reveal a dilated aortic root, pericardial effusion, or fluctuating intimal flap. Although CT scans with contrast media and magnetic resonance imaging are sensitive tests, spiral CT scans are rapid, widely available, and often the test of choice. A TEE is useful in hemodynamically unstable persons. An aortogram is indicated preoperatively to determine the precise location and extent of dissection.

TREATMENT

Asymptomatic aortic aneurysms, >4 cm in diameter if abdominal and >6 cm in diameter if thoracic, may be electively repaired. Control of hypertension may slow the progression of some aneurysms. Symptomatic patients should have surgical repair regardless of aneurysm size. A ruptured aneurysm is a surgical emergency. Management of aortic dissection is primarily surgical with preoperative control of blood pressure, pain, and hemodynamic monitoring. The mortality rate is highest for acute dissections (<2 weeks in duration), with aortic rupture as the most frequent cause of death.

Disposition

Patients with small (diameter <4 cm) and asymptomatic aortic aneurysms are often followed with abdominal ultrasound every 6 to 12 months to monitor the aneurysm for expansion. All patients with a documented aortic aneurysm or dissection should be managed in collateral with a thoracic or vascular surgeon and cardiologist if the thoracic aorta is involved.

COMPLICATIONS

The vast majority of aneurysms will continue to expand until they rupture. Digital or leg ischemia secondary to microemboli from an aneurysmal clot is another common complication. Other complications include renal insufficiency from renal artery ischemia or occlusion, ischemic colitis from inferior mesenteric artery occlusion or poor collateral flow paraplegia caused by spinal ischemia, and chylous ascites or chylothorax when the lymphatic vessels leak postoperatively.

VENOUS DISEASE

Venous circulation has three subsystems in the lower extremities:

1. *The superficial venous subsystem* includes superficial veins that drain blood from the skin, subcutaneous tissue, and feet. Two primary veins and their tributaries comprise this venous network: the greater saphenous vein (GSV) that drains the medial aspect of the thigh and lower leg and the lesser saphenous vein (LSV) that drains the posterolateral aspect of the calf.
2. *The deep-venous subsystem* drains most of the venous blood from the legs. Located within intramuscular tissue, these deep veins run parallel with arteries and are named accordingly (e.g., femoral vein, popliteal vein, etc.).
3. *The communicating (perforating) subsystem* is a network of vascular channels and smaller veins that connect the deep and superficial systems.

Venous blood normally flows in one direction, from the superficial to the deep system via the perforators and then toward the inferior vena cava. Veins from the superficial venous subsystem also connect directly to the deep-venous subsystem at the sapheno-femoral and sapheno-popliteal junction. Venous valves are present in all three subsystems to prevent retrograde flow of blood from one system to the next and within the same system. Veins have thinner and structurally different walls than arteries and are not directly affected by some disorders that damage arteries, such as atherosclerosis and vasospasm.

Pathophysiologic changes affecting the venous vasculature commonly involve the development of thrombosis that can obstruct venous return; destruction or incompetence of the venous valves, allowing reflux of blood; or dilatation of the venous lumen due to persistent elevation of intraluminal venous pressures. Venous disorders commonly treated by primary care providers include varicose veins, chronic venous insufficiency (with or without venous stasis ulcers), and thromboembolic disease.

VARICOSE VEINS

DISCUSSION

Varicose veins are caused by incompetence of the saphenous veins, their tributaries, or the connecting perforators. Increased intravascular pressure or defective valves cause the GSVs and LSVs to stretch, elongate, and become tortuous. The vessel walls also weaken and thin out. Varicosities occur principally in the superficial veins of the medial and anterior thigh, calf, and occasionally ankle. Contributing factors include heredity, prolonged standing, pregnancy, and previous thrombophlebitis. Varicose veins are very common, affecting 10 to 20% of the adult population. Varicosities are more common in females, often due to pregnancy.

SIGNS AND SYMPTOMS

Aside from the unsightly appearance of varicosities, most patients with varicose veins are asymptomatic. Symptoms when present include a tiredness or heaviness of the legs, local aching or burning, itching ankle edema, or easy bruising from minor leg trauma. Standing or sitting for prolonged periods and obesity may aggravate these symptoms.

OBJECTIVE FINDINGS

Inspection for varicose veins in the legs is best performed from behind the patient, with the patient standing. Standing allows any varicosities to fill with blood and dilate. Look for tortuous vessels that are easily compressed. Mild ankle edema may occasionally be noted. Ulcers are rare and when present suggest problems of the deep-venous system.

DIFFERENTIAL DIAGNOSIS

The differential diagnosis includes thrombophlebitis, venous insufficiency, arterial insufficiency, peripheral neuritis, and arthritis.

LABORATORY AND RADIOLOGIC TESTS

The diagnosis of varicose veins can usually be made by history and physical exam. Noninvasive vascular testing is not routinely completed unless an associated venous insufficiency or obstruction or arterial occlusive disease is also suspected, or pre-op evaluation for vein ligation or stripping is needed.

OTHER DIAGNOSTICS

When varicose veins are present, a manual compression test and/or Trendelenburg's test may be useful in determining whether the valves in the saphenous system or communicating veins are competent. For the manual compression test, feel the dilated vein while the patient is standing. Using your fingertips, compress the vein at its proximal end with one hand and feel for an impulse transmitted to the fingers of your other hand at the distal end of the vessel. Incompetent valves in the saphenous system allow blood to backflow, creating a palpable thud at the distal end. In Trendelenburg's test, elevate the patient's leg to drain venous blood. Next, occlude the saphenous vein in the upper thigh manually or with a tourniquet, and then have the patient stand. Watch for the direction of venous filling with the vein occluded and with the tourniquet removed. Normally, the saphenous vein fills slowly from below. Rapid filling from below is seen with incompetent valves of the perforators. Rapid filling from above once the tourniquet is removed is seen with incompetence of the sapheno-femoral junction. These two exam modalities will help determine whether the patient may benefit from surgical therapy.

TREATMENT

Varicose veins may be managed conservatively with custom vascular support stockings. Support stockings sold in department stores do not give proper fit and give inadequate compression. Below-the-knee stockings are preferred. Patients should be instructed to replace their stockings within 6 months or whenever compression is lost. Tight garments that restrict venous return in the thigh should be avoided. Prolonged standing should be avoided, and legs should be elevated when sitting. An exercise routine that includes daily walking is encouraged. Obese patients should be given support to lose weight. Saphenous vein ligation and stripping is the mainstay of surgical therapy. It is warranted in patients with large varicosities. Sclerotherapy uses a sclerosing agent injected into a vessel to scar and shrink down varicosities. It is a useful alternative treatment plan for small varicosities.

COMPLICATIONS AND RED FLAGS

Long-term varicosities may precipitate valve incompetence secondary to chronic stretching in the vessel wall. This can result in chronic venous insufficiency. Superficial thrombophlebitis may also occur. Additionally, varicosities may enlarge to the point the overlying skin becomes thin and friable; they may spontaneously bleed and become thrombotic or secondarily infected.

CHRONIC VENOUS INSUFFICIENCY

DISCUSSION

Previous inflammation or thrombosis can destroy the valves of the deep veins, promoting bidirectional flow of blood and creating incompetent venous perforators. Incompetence of the perforating veins allows blood to backflow from the deep system to the superficial venous system. Chronic elevation of venous pressures develops over time and results in fluid transudation into the surrounding soft tissue. Chronic edema ensues, which promotes skin breakdown and the formation of *stasis ulcers.* Skin ulcers commonly develop along the medial aspect of the leg above the medial malleolus, due to the large number of venous perforators in this area. Hemosiderin from stagnant blood and tissue death turns the skin dark (*stasis dermatitis*). Postphlebitic syndrome is the most common cause for chronic venous insufficiency. In some patients congenital weakness of venous valves may be a precipitating factor.

SIGNS AND SYMPTOMS

The most common complaint seen in chronic venous insufficiency is edema. Leg edema usually advances above the ankles and may be bilateral. Both of the patient's legs should be measured at the ankle, midcalf, and above and below the knees and a comparison made of the results to document edema. Any edema present should also be examined for pitting and graded accordingly. The skin may have a "brawny" discoloration. Look for evidence of ulceration and any associated signs of cellulitis, both of which are often painless.

DIFFERENTIAL DIAGNOSES

For unilateral leg edema, the differential diagnosis includes deep-venous thrombosis, lymphatic obstruction, cellulitis, and trauma. For bilateral leg edema, it includes congestive heart failure, nephrotic syndrome, severe malnutrition, liver failure, and lymphedema (rare).

LABORATORY AND RADIOLOGIC TESTS

Venous ultrasound to rule out the presence of deep-venous thrombosis should be completed. In patients with bilateral leg edema, order a urinalysis and blood urea nitrogen and serum creatinine tests to rule out renal disease; liver function tests, serum albumin, and a coagulation profile to rule out liver disease; and a chest film for evidence of heart failure.

TREATMENT

Treatment of venous insufficiency is directed primarily at reducing and controlling leg edema and preventing the occurrence of leg ulcers. Bed rest with leg elevation is recommended in the acute presentation. The foot of the bed should be elevated or the leg propped on pillows. When upright, patients should recline rather than sit, with the leg(s) elevated higher than the hips. The addition of diuretics (hydrochlorothiazide 50 mg qid) may also help reduce recalcitrant edema.

Once the edema resolves, the mainstay of therapy is the use of custom-fitted vascular elastic support hose (e.g., Jobst or Juzo stockings) to maintain an appropriate venous pressure gradient. TED hose and stockings exert an inadequate amount of vascular compression (<20 mmHg) for reducing lower extremity edema and should be avoided. Vascular support stockings minimally should be knee high and should be worn at all times when the patient is erect. Dryness of the skin should be prevented to reduce ulcer formation. Moisturize the skin daily with lotions or other topical lubricants (e.g., Eucerin, Lubriderm, Vaseline).

Management of venous stasis ulcers includes leg elevation and compression dressings. Stasis ulcers that are secondarily infected require treatment with oral antibiotics to eradicate *Staphylococcus* and gram-negative rods. Moisturizing gels such as hydrogel dressings should be changed every other day. Occlusive wound care dressings (DuoDerm, Tegaderm, Epigard, etc.) in combination with Ace compression bandages are commonly applied. These dressings should be changed following manufacturers' guidelines (usually every 3 to 7 days) or as needed for draining ulcers. A medicated compression boot, the "Unna boot," or multilayered compression bandage boots (Profore) may also be applied to the lower leg. The boot keeps compression on the lower extremity so that edema does not occur. These boots are changed weekly or as needed for draining ulcers. Uncomplicated ulcers may take up to 3 to 4 weeks to heal. Deep or extensive ulcers may require local wound debridement with or without skin grafting.

Always perform a complete arterial assessment when evaluating venous disease. Venous ulcers will not heal without adequate arterial inflow and surgery may be indicated to improve blood supply.

Supportive Measures

Once the ulcer heals, edema of the leg must be controlled throughout life to prevent ulcers from forming in the future. The mainstay of preventive therapy is the use of custom-fitted vascular support hose. Patients wearing support hose should be instructed to wear them throughout the day, putting them on upon arising and removing them just before retiring at bedtime. Routine follow-up is required on a weekly or biweekly basis until uncomplicated edema resolves, then every 3 to 6 months thereafter. Patients with stasis ulcers should be seen every 3 to 7 days for dressing changes until the ulcer heals. Refractory edema or recurrent or nonhealing ulcers require consultation with a vascular surgeon. Saphenous vein stripping may be indicated in cases that do not respond adequately to conservative management.

COMPLICATIONS AND RED FLAGS

Venous stasis ulcers may become secondarily infected if not treated promptly. Cellulitis may also develop. Venous stasis ulcers in patients with an associated arterial insufficiency or diabetes may take a long time to heal. Any ulcer that fails to heal after 6 months to 1 year of therapy should be biopsied to rule out an underlying skin cancer.

VENOUS THROMBOSIS

DISCUSSION

Superficial thrombophlebitis is an inflammation of the superficial veins of the upper or lower extremities due to thrombus formation.

Superficial thrombophlebitis of the arms is a common inpatient problem caused by intravenous catheters. The most common cause for lower extremity involvement is varicose veins and trauma.

Deep-venous thrombosis (DVT) is thromboembolic disease of the veins of the deep-venous system. Conditions that produce venous stasis (surgery, postoperative immobilization, pregnancy), endothelial injury of the vessel wall (trauma, fractures, central intravenous infusions), and hypercoagulable states (cancer, estrogen use, nephrotic syndrome, thrombocytosis, and antithrombin III deficiency, protein C and S deficiency) precipitate the formation of clots in the venous vasculature. Within 7 to 10 days, clots formed adhere to the vessel wall. They are subsequently dissolved by the fibrinolytic system over the next 3 to 4 months. During the first 3 to 4 days, clots are more likely to embolize and the risk for pulmonary embolism is high. Most clots form in the small veins of the calf where they are unlikely to embolize. A small percentage, however, may propagate proximally to the deep veins of the knee and thigh where the risk for pulmonary embolization markedly increases. Patients with clots in the ileofemoral or pelvic veins are at greatest risk for a pulmonary embolus. DVT of the upper extremities rarely occurs unless a central venous catheter is present.

SIGNS AND SYMPTOMS

Patients with superficial thrombophlebitis usually complain of dull, aching, or burning pain in the area of the involved vein. Fever, chills, and malaise may occur if a secondary septic phlebitis is also present. Patients with DVT may be asymptomatic. Clinicians must have a high index of suspicion, as the first symptoms may be those associated with a pulmonary embolus (PE). The most reliable symptom if present is the acute onset of unilateral persistent swelling of the involved extremity. Additional symptoms include fever and calf or thigh pain.

OBJECTIVE FINDINGS

In superficial thrombophlebitis, look for tenderness, erythema, increased warmth, and slight swelling along the length of the vein on physical exam. Sometimes the vein is palpable as a subcutaneous venous cord. Patients with indwelling venous catheters are more likely to be febrile as well. Unless there is an associated DVT, edema of the extremity rarely occurs.

Physical exam findings in DVT include increased warmth and tenderness of the affected extremity. Homans' sign (calf pain on dorsiflexion of the foot) is an unreliable exam clue. The most reliable sign is unilateral edema that is distal to the site of the clot. Classically, a calf vein DVT produces edema of the ankle and foot, a femoral vein DVT results in edema extending up to the thigh, and a DVT in the iliac vein produces edema of the entire leg. The superficial veins may also be dilated due to collateral flow around the deep-venous obstruction. Fever is common. Peripheral pulses are usually palpable except for the rare case of edema massive enough to compromise arterial flow.

DIFFERENTIAL DIAGNOSES

The differential diagnosis for superficial thrombophlebitis includes cellulitis, erythema nodosum, sarcoidosis, and Kaposi's sarcoma. The differential diagnosis for DVT includes cellulitis, lymphedema, a ruptured Baker's cyst, arthritis, venous compression by tumor, and severe muscle strain or sprain.

LABORATORY TESTS

A white cell count can rule out leukocytosis and blood cultures in patients with suspected septic superficial thrombophlebitis. Cultures of IV fluids given may also be warranted. Order coagulation studies—prothrombin time (PT), partial thromboplastin time (PTT), antiplatelet factor levels, and anticoagulant factors (proteins C and S, antithrombin III)—in patients suspected of having an associated coagulopathy.

RADIOLOGIC TESTS

Color flow or duplex ultrasound with venous Doppler is a noninvasive, highly sensitive test for detecting obstruction of blood flow. It is much more sensitive in detecting DVT at or above the knee (popliteal and femoral) than below. A venogram is considered the gold standard (high specificity and sensitivity) for confirming the location and extent of venous thrombosis. An invasive test with associated risks, it should be reserved for an equivocal venous Doppler report. A ventilation/perfusion (V/Q) scan is warranted if a PE is suspected. Look for a V/Q mismatch that is "highly suspicious" for PE. The test is not always diagnostic, and a pulmonary arteriogram may be indicated to confirm the diagnosis in symptomatic patients with equivocal test results. Venous plethysmography measures changes in venous blood volume from the leg. It is as accurate as duplex ultrasound in detecting popliteal and femoral DVTs and is a widely available, less expensive alternative.

TREATMENT

The clinical course for superficial thrombophlebitis is usually benign and conservative therapy is recommended. Treatment includes elevation of the extremity, warm compresses, and ambulation to prevent the development of DVT and the use of support stockings once the initial inflammation resolves. Analgesics [acetaminophen or nonsteroidal anti-inflammatory drugs (NSAIDs)] may also be given for pain relief. The best treatment for DVT is prevention. Early ambulation in the postoperative period helps prevent venous stasis, a major contributing factor for thrombus formation. Low doses of aspirin (<325 mg qid) may also have some prophylactic value. Patients considered at high risk for DVT (those scheduled for orthopedic procedures, trauma surgery, or lengthy general surgical procedures) should be anticoagulated during the perioperative period. Low-molecular-weight heparin (LMWH; e.g., Enoxaparin/Lovenox, Dalteparin/Fragmin) has been shown in clinical trials to provide superior anticoagulation in the prevention of DVT in postoperative patients. LMWH is administered by subcutaneous injections using weight-adjusted dosing. LMWH is usually given within 2 h before surgery and continued for 5 to 10 days after surgery. Unfractionated heparin may also be given as a "minidose" (5000 U bid subcutaneously) 2 h preoperatively and continued during the immediate postoperative period.

Patients with DVTs distal to the popliteal vein can be treated conservatively on an outpatient basis. A 1- to 5-day course of bed rest with elevation of the edematous extremity should be started along with anticoagulants using LMWH or oral warfarin (Coumadin).

Patients with popliteal or ileofemoral DVTs should be hospitalized initially. Strict bed rest with elevation of the edematous extremity by raising the foot of the bed is implemented. Anticoagulant therapy is also begun immediately. Unfractionated heparin (5000 to 10,000 U) is given, initially as an intravenous bolus followed by 1000-U/h continuous intravenous infusion. Heparin is then titrated in dosages to maintain the PTT at 1.5 to 2 times normal. Within 1 to 3 days, patients are also started on warfarin (Coumadin), 5 to 10 mg qid for oral maintenance therapy. Heparin is discontinued once a therapeutic level of Coumadin is reached (usually INR 2.0 to 3.0). Recent studies suggest that LMWHs are an effective and safe alternative to heparin/Coumadin therapy for management of acute proximal venous thrombosis in patients who do not have clinically overt pulmonary embolism. Home treatment throughout the entire course of therapy or after a few days in the hospital is being utilized in many clinical settings. LMWHs are administered subcutaneously in weight-adjusted dosages one or twice daily, and although more expensive, they do not require monitoring of coagulation panels (PT, PTT, or INR).

Outpatient anticoagulant therapy should continue for 3 months or until follow-up vascular studies document resolution of the clot. Patients with massive edema obstructing arterial blood flow may require an emergent venous thrombectomy. Patients with a contraindication to anticoagulation [those with a history of gastrointestinal (GI) bleeding, bleeding coagulopathy, etc.] or a history of recurrent pulmonary emboli may require placement of a venous filter in the vena cava to "capture" emboli before they reach the lungs.

Complications relative to the use of anticoagulants (e.g., epistaxis, GI bleeding, hematuria) should also be observed, particularly in patients on Coumadin. There is a lower risk for bleeding with LMWH use. Coumadin is a known teratogen and is contraindicated in pregnancy. LMWH is contraindicated in patients with heparin or pork allergies.

PATIENT EDUCATION

All patients with extremity edema should be instructed to elevate the affected part. The upper extremity should be elevated above heart level using several pillows. The foot of the bed should be elevated for leg edema. Reclining instead of sitting upright is recommended, with the leg elevated higher than the hip. Prolonged sitting or standing is discouraged. Walking is encouraged unless an acute DVT is suspected. Vascular support hose should be worn throughout the day. Patients who have been placed on anticoagulants should be warned of the possible side effects and to avoid concurrent use of aspirin, NSAIDs, and alcohol. They should also be encouraged to return for regular monitoring of the coagulation panel.

COMPLICATIONS AND RED FLAGS

Complications for DVT include:

- *Pulmonary embolus* may occur as late as 1 week after a patient's surgery.
- *Phlegmasia cerulea dolens* is a painful, acute arterial insufficiency secondary to massive edema. Cyanosis, loss of distal pulses, and limb loss are of major concern.
- *Postphlebitic syndrome* and its the accompanying inflammation may destroy the venous valves with subsequent development of chronic venous insufficiency and secondary varicose veins.

Complications for superficial venous thrombosis are rare. When they do occur, the most common would be extension of the clot into the deep-venous system with the associated risk of pulmonary embolism.

LYMPHATIC DISEASE

DISCUSSION

The lymphatic system is a special vascular system of lymphatic vessels and lymph nodes that run adjacent to arteries and veins. These lymphatic vessels drain excess tissue fluid back to the venous circulation by way of two lymphatic ducts in the chest, the right lymphatic duct and the thoracic duct, that empty into the subclavian veins. Normally blood flows from the arterial to the venous circulation through the capillary bed. Plasma seeps from the capillary bed into the interstitial tissue where the exchange of cellular nutrients, wastes, and gases occurs. Most of this interstitial fluid (lymph) is reabsorbed into the bloodstream at the venous end. However, approximately 3 L of fluid each day lags behind in the interstitial tissue and must eventually be returned to the cardiovascular system to maintain adequate blood volume. Lymph contains water and plasma proteins needed to maintain both hydrostatic and oncotic pressures within the vascular tree. Any pathologic process that obliterates or obstructs the lymphatic vessels will prevent drainage of that extremity.

Lymphedema, an abnormal accumulation of excess water and protein in the skin and subcutaneous tissue, can be primary or secondary. Primary lymphedema is rare and is caused by developmental abnormalities of the lymphatic system (hypoplasia, aplasia, or varicose dilatation). This condition is more commonly seen in young patients (<35 years.). Most cases of lymphedema result from secondary causes such as surgical ligature of lymphatic vessels, radiation therapy for tumors, cancer, trauma, or recurrent infections, all of which obliterate lymphatic vessels or nodes. The most common cause for lymphedema of the lower extremities is pelvic tumors.

Lymphedema is a chronic, progressive condition that is frequently exacerbated by recurrent episodes of secondary infection. In some cases the extremity may become so edematous that clothing and shoes may be difficult to wear—so-called elephantiasis.

Lymphatic vessels may also become inflamed or secondarily infected producing acute lymphangitis. Extension of staphylococci or beta-hemolytic streptococci bacteria from a local infection is the most common cause. In 15–20% of cases of lymphedema, lymphangitis occurs secondarily.

SIGNS AND SYMPTOMS

Patients with lymphangitis present with pain, malaise, and lassitude of acute onset. Patients with lymphedema classically present with painless, unilateral edema that starts in the foot or hand and progresses proximally. Unlike edema from other causes, elevation of the extremity provides little relief. In some cases, both lower extremities may be involved.

OBJECTIVE FINDINGS

In lymphangitis, look for red streaks that follow the course of lymphatic collecting ducts. Multiple, fine erythematous lines are seen streaking up an extremity and may extend from a local wound or area of cellulitis. Regional lymph nodes are usually enlarged and tender. Skin overlying the area may be indurated and tender as well. The edema of lymphatic obstruction has a brawny discoloration and is firm, rubbery, and nonpitting. However, unlike the edema of venous insufficiency, ulceration and the hyperpigmentation of stasis dermatitis do not occur. The overlying skin in lymphedema is usually thickened and indurated and may have a *peau d'orange* appearance. Signs of lymphangitis may also be present.

DIFFERENTIAL DIAGNOSES

The differential diagnosis for lymphangitis includes cellulitis, superficial thrombophlebitis, and cat-scratch disease. The differential diagnosis for lymphedema includes chronic venous insufficiency, lipedema, DVT, and postphlebitic syndrome.

LABORATORY AND RADIOLOGIC TESTS

Cultures of any exudative wound should be obtained in cases of lymphangitis. If the patient appears acutely ill or is also febrile, blood cultures should also be obtained. Lymphoscintigraphy involves injection of a small amount of radioactive isotope into the lymphatic channels of the interdigital web spaces and imaging the extremity for delayed transport of lymph. The test has few adverse side effects, is simple to perform on an outpatient basis, and is the preferred test for diagnosing lymphedema. Lymphangiography is an alternative test that uses radiopaque contrast media to visualize the lymphatic circulation. The test is difficult to perform and complication rates are high. Nevertheless, it may be useful in differentiating primary from secondary causes of lymphedema. CT scan of the pelvis and abdomen are frequently ordered to rule out malignancy in newly diagnosed lymphedema.

TREATMENT

Antibiotic therapy with penicillin G, nafcillin, a cephalosporin, or erythromycin is used to treat lymphangitis. A 2-week course of oral antibiotics may be given unless there is an associated cellulitis. Parenteral antibiotics may be indicated in patients who are acutely ill. Some patients with seasonal exacerbation or acute lymphedema may benefit from the use of diuretics.

The main objective of treatment for lymphedema is to eliminate as much edema as possible. External compression using a sequential air compression device (lymphedema pump) is very effective in "milking" the edema fluid from the extremity. Lymphedema pumps may be used on an outpatient basis. Once maximal reduction of edema is achieved, custom-fitted vascular support those with maximal compression should be worn throughout the day. Any localized abscess associated with lymphangitis should be incised and drained unless there is also an associated cellulitis.

Supportive Measures

Heating pads or hot, moist compresses and elevation of the affected extremity may provide some symptomatic relief in lymphangitis. Oral analgesics may also help with any discomfort. Patients with lymphedema should be instructed in proper foot care to minimize trauma and/or acute infections. Dietary restriction of sodium should also be encouraged. Any signs of associated lymphangitis or cellulitis should be reported promptly so that proper antibiotic therapy may be initiated.

COMPLICATIONS AND RED FLAGS

The most important complication seen in lymphangitis is sepsis due to delayed or inadequate treatment. Recurrent cellulitis and lymphangitis are common complications in lymphedema. Lymphangiosarcoma, a rare lymphatic cancer, may occur, particularly in cases of upper extremity postmastectomy lymphedema. Any patient with violaceous, maculopapular skin lesions that coalesce or ulcerate should be referred for biopsy and further evaluation.

BIBLIOGRAPHY

Barker LR et al (eds): *Principles of Ambulatory Medicine,* 4th ed. Baltimore, Williams Wilkins, 1995, pp 1298–1320.
Bick RL: Prevention of deep venous thrombosis and pulmonary embolus in surgery and trauma. *Surgical Physician Assistant* 500:22–39, 1999.
Davies R, Coady M: Low molecular weight heparin: An evaluation of current and potential utility in surgery. *Int J Angiol* 8:203–215, 1999.
Goroll AH et al (eds): *Primary Care Medicine: Office Evaluation and Management of the Adult Patient,* 4th ed. Philadelphia, J B Lippincott, 2000, pp 125–132, 236–248.
Tierney L et al: *Current Medical Diagnosis and Treatment.* New York, Lange Medical/McGraw-Hill, 2000, pp 467–493, 679–680.

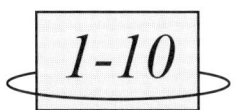

ACQUIRED VALVULAR HEART DISEASE

Jeffrey R. Smith

DISCUSSION

Valvular heart disease consists of two basic groups of disorders: *congenital* valvular anomalies and *acquired* valvular diseases. Acquired valvular diseases are further defined as *rheumatic* and *nonrheumatic* in origin. Valvular disease can further be classified as *regurgitant* (commonly referred to as "leaky" or "insufficient") and *stenotic* (commonly referred to as "narrowed"); components of both types may be present. Of the four cardiac valves (aortic, mitral, tricuspid, and pulmonic), attention is given in this chapter only to the mitral and aortic valves. The diseases of these two valves constitute the most common and significant disorders of acquired valvular disease.

RHEUMATIC VALVULAR HEART DISEASE

The frequency and intensity of rheumatic fever caused by group A β-hemolytic streptococcal bacterial infection has diminished, particularly in developed countries where antibiotics and treatment are readily available. Despite this fact, rheumatic fever continues to play an important role in the development of valvular disease. In fact, there was a resurgence of rheumatic fever in some areas of the United States in the 1980s.[1] If patients with acute rheumatic fever receive appropriate prophylactic antibiotic therapy, about 1% subsequently develop severe cardiac disease (class IV rheumatic heart disease) and 4% develop debilitating rheumatic heart disease.[2]

The pathogenesis of rheumatic valvular disease involves fibrotic scarring of the valve tissue, leading to thickening, retraction, and fusion of the valve leaflets after recovery from an episode of rheumatic fever. Actually, valvular stenosis of rheumatic origin progresses gradually throughout adult life, long after any evidence of rheumatic activity. It may take many years for the valvular disease to develop. The aortic and mitral valves are the most commonly affected.

NONRHEUMATIC VALVULAR HEART DISEASE

Aortic stenosis that occurs as an isolated lesion usually is a result of a congenital bicuspid valve or degenerative thickening and calcification of leaflets that were originally normal.

Pure nonrheumatic aortic regurgitation is usually a result of dilation of the aortic root. Myxomatous changes in the aortic leaflets that are similar to changes seen in the mitral valve are found in many cases as well. These changes may cause severe aortic regurgitation without dilation of the aortic root (floppy aortic valve syndrome).[3] Marfan's syndrome, bacterial endocarditis, and in some cases severe trauma are other potential causes of aortic regurgitation.

Mitral regurgitation generally is caused by one of two basic pathogenic sources. The first is coronary artery disease and is related to papillary muscle dysfunction resulting from ischemia or infarction. The second is a prolapsing mitral valve caused by an idiopathic pathologic process typically characterized by loss of fibrous tissue in the chordae tendineae.

Other nonrheumatic causes of valvular disease include damage to valves from radiation therapy.[4] Methysergide, which is used to treat migraine and cluster headaches, has been observed to affect cardiac valves.[5] Rheumatoid arthritis occasionally produces severe valve disease when large rheumatoid nodules involve the leaflets.[6]

SIGNS AND SYMPTOMS

Understanding the anatomy and physiology of stenosis and regurgitation is essential for recognizing the signs and symptoms of these disorders. Valvular stenosis obstructs blood flow through the heart. This generally results in elevated pressures in the chamber proximal to the stenosis (in aortic stenosis, left ventricular systolic pressure is elevated; in mitral stenosis, left atrial pressure is elevated above left ventricular diastolic pressure). In aortic stenosis, the increase in pressure load thickens the ventricular wall without affecting the size of the chamber and, combined with a fibrotic myocardium, causes a decrease in diastolic compliance. Over time, the left ventricular chamber dilates and contraction weakens. In mitral stenosis, the left atrium becomes hypertrophied because of pressure loads similar to those seen in aortic stenosis. This leads to atrial dilation, decreased atrial con-

traction, and elevated left atrial pressure. This elevated pressure eventually affects the pulmonary system.

In valvular regurgitation, an amount of blood flows back into the left atrium (mitral regurgitation) each time the ventricle contracts and back into the left ventricle (through an incompetent aortic valve) during diastole. Because the stroke volume of the affected ventricle is increased, systemic flow is kept at nearly normal rates. This produces overwork for the ventricle and eventually dilation of the ventricle (or the atrium in mitral disease) without an increase in wall thickness (differing from stenosis, where there is an increase in wall thickness). Ultimately, ventricular performance decreases, ejection fraction is reduced, and because of longstanding volume overwork the ventricle fails (or the atrium dilates). In combined cases of stenosis and regurgitation, there is an additive affect of strain from overwork and increased pressures.

Most patients with aortic stenosis characteristically present with dyspnea with exertion, angina pectoris, and syncope, any or all of which may be present. Patients with aortic regurgitation may present with symptoms very similar to those of aortic stenosis. Dyspnea, angina pectoris, and palpitations are the most common symptoms.

Angina is seen in both aortic stenosis and aortic regurgitation secondary to a decrease in diastolic perfusion combined with an increase in myocardial oxygen consumption.

In mitral stenosis, the most important symptom is dyspnea, which indicates left atrial pressures high enough to produce transudation of fluid into pulmonary capillaries. Because of this, hemoptysis is also commonly seen. Other signs and symptoms include cough, orthopnea, and paroxysmal nocturnal dyspnea.

Mitral regurgitation often is asymptomatic until the disease becomes very severe. Once that level of severity occurs, the most common presenting symptoms include fatigue, dyspnea with exertion, and palpitations.

OBJECTIVE FINDINGS

Auscultation of the heart is the cornerstone of the detection of valvular heart disease. Knowledge of the location and characteristics of the auscultated murmur is critical to an accurate diagnosis. Understanding how cardiac murmurs should be described is essential in properly communicating physical findings to colleagues.

Aortic stenosis is primarily distinguished from other valvular disorders by its characteristic loud, harsh systolic ejection murmur, heard best at the second intercostal space on the right sternal border and radiating into the carotid arteries. Other classic physical findings include narrow pulse pressure, sustained apical pulse, a paradoxically split S_2, a soft S_2, and a present S_4.

In aortic regurgitation, the classic murmur is known as a high-pitched, decrescendo diastolic murmur that begins immediately after the second heart sound and is best heard at the second intercostal space on the right sternal border. Physical findings that are commonly seen include visible bounding and forceful peripheral pulses (Corrigan's pulse), pulsations in the capillary beds of nails (Quincke's pulse), and a systolic ejection murmur resulting from increased flow across the valve area.

Patients with mitral stenosis have a typical murmur that can be recognized by the characteristic opening snap and diastolic rumbling murmur. Patients with longstanding and severe mitral stenosis are often quite thin and frail. Jugular venous distention is seen frequently. Auscultation of the lungs may reveal fine crackles in the bases.

A harsh holosystolic murmur heard best at the apex (left fifth intercostal space, midclavicular line) with radiation into the axilla is the hallmark murmur of mitral regurgitation. Other findings include a laterally displaced and diffuse apical pulse, a widely split S_2, and a present S_3.

DIFFERENTIAL DIAGNOSES

In acquired valvular heart disease, there is no differential diagnosis per se. The challenge during history taking and physical examination lies in differentiating between the different intracardiac possibilities. There may be concurrent processes occurring, such as myocardial infarction, chronic obstructive pulmonary disease, and/or congestive heart failure.

LABORATORY TESTS

No laboratory tests are helpful in securing an accurate diagnosis of valvular heart disease. A discussion of pertinent electrocardiogram (ECG) findings is in the next section.

RADIOLOGIC STUDIES

While the history and physical examination remain the cornerstones for the diagnosis of acquired valvular heart disease, radiographic studies such as echocardiography (using a transesophageal transducer or a standard precordial transducer) and color flow Doppler studies confirm the diagnosis and provide vital information in regard to the severity of disease. Most would agree that the transesophageal echocardiography approach provides more sophisticated images, but it is certainly a more invasive procedure.

In aortic stenosis, echocardiographic studies reveal thickened and calcific valve leaflets with reduced mobility. Pressure gradients and the aortic valve area are calculated by using Doppler studies. These values also can be obtained through invasive procedures such as heart catheterization. Hemodynamically significant stenosis is associated with gradients of about 50 mmHg. An aortic valve area less than 1.0 cm^3 is considered significant in most adults. Other studies include chest x-ray, which generally reveals some prominence of the ascending aorta but usually little enlargement of the heart unless significant congestive heart failure is present. Abnormal ECG findings include left ventricular strain patterns such as QRS and T-wave changes that reflect left ventricular hypertrophy.

Echocardiographic findings in aortic regurgitation reveal an incompetent valve during diastole and may include a characteristic flutter-like movement in the anterior mitral leaflet that occurs during diastole. Chest x-ray shows cardiac silhouette enlargement, with the apex being displaced to the left and downward. ECG findings may show signs of left ventricular strain and hypertrophy.

Echocardiographic findings in mitral stenosis generally reveal decreased movement of the mitral leaflets. As in aortic stenosis, the valve area and the diastolic pressure gradient are important in determining the severity of disease and can be calculated with heart catheterization and/or Doppler studies. Gradients of 10 mmHg or more generally suggest the presence of severe stenosis. Chest x-ray almost always reveals left atrial enlargement and also may show pulmonary congestion in the form of Kerley B lines (dilated pulmonary lymphatics that become visible as transverse lines in the lower lung fields). ECG findings consistent with left atrial enlargement as well as atrial fibrillation are often present.

Mitral regurgitation is best seen as a regurgitant jet in systole on echocardiography. Quantitative two-dimensional echocardiography can provide a more precise calculation of the severity of regurgitation. A new method—the proximal isovelocity surface area method—measures the size of the regurgitant orifice by quantitating the velocity of regurgitant blood. This technique provides an estimate of the severity of the valvular abnormality that does not depend on hemodynamic variables such as afterload and contractility.[7] Chest x-ray may reveal pulmonary congestion, but this is much less commonly seen than it is in mitral stenosis. Atrial fibrillation may also be seen on ECG.

TREATMENT

Treatment can be divided into nonsurgical and surgical components. General nonsurgical medical management includes treatment of atrial arrhythmias, warfarin therapy to decrease the risk of embolism from the left atrium, and the use of antibiotics to prevent infective endocarditis. Vasodilator therapy used to treat congestive heart failure also may prove valuable. It may be used in severe but asymptomatic aortic regurgitation with the goal of slowing the development of left ventricular dysfunction and delaying the need for valve replacement.[8]

General surgical treatment involves either repair or replacement. Nonreplacement (repair) procedures play a role in the treatment of valvular disorders, particularly operations such as mitral commissurotomy for the repair of noncalcific forms of aortic valve stenosis.[9] Surgical repair has become the procedure of choice for most patients with floppy valve syndrome and for many patients with other anatomic types of mitral regurgitation.[10] Valve replacement is the other surgical option, and there are over 30 different models of mechanical and tissue-type valves. The most frequently used prosthetic valves are the Starr-Edwards, CarboMedics, and St. Jude valves.[11,12] Homograft aortic valves and porcine aortic valves are the tissue-type valves used for replacement.

Deciding whether a patient is a candidate for surgical or nonsurgical treatment remains challenging and must include factors such as severity of disease, age, social and environmental concerns, patient compliance, and patient understanding of the disease process. A delay in surgical treatment may be risky in some patients because of the irreparable damage that may occur to the left ventricle.

DISPOSITION

Meticulous medical management in both nonsurgical and surgical (especially in the postoperative phase) treatment is absolutely crucial to achieving positive outcomes.

Patients who have their cardiac valves replaced are subject to a variety of long-term complications and potential medical problems. Prevention of arterial embolism and monitoring of anticoagulation are probably the most frustrating problems for both the patient and the medical team.

The outcome of valvular replacement surgery is favorable in patients with few comorbid factors and those who are motivated to participate in their own care.

PEARLS

Do not be fooled by the intensity of the murmur in aortic stenosis, either soft or loud. The duration of the murmur and a later peak of intensity suggest more severe aortic obstruction.

Typically, in mitral regurgitation, the murmur radiates into the axilla. An exception is the murmur produced by rupture of the chordae tendineae of the posterior papillary muscle. The murmur produced in this case radiates into the aortic area and neck and mimics the murmur of aortic stenosis.

The single most important predictor of outcome in a patient undergoing cardiac surgery is the ejection fraction.

REFERENCES

1. Bisno AL: Group A streptococcal infections and acute rheumatic fever. *N Engl J Med* 325:783, 1991.
2. Mlandenovic J (ed): *Primary Care Secrets.* St. Louis, Mosby, 1995, p 121.
3. Agozzino L et al: Non-inflammatory aortic root disease and floppy aortic valve as cause of isolated regurgitation: A clinico-morphologic study. *Int J Cardiol* 45:129, 1994.
4. Chenu PC et al: Bilateral coronary ostial stenosis and aortic valvular disease after radiotherapy. *Eur Heart J* 15:1150, 1994.
5. Austin SM et al: Mitral valve disease associated with long-term ergotamine use. *South Med J* 86:1179, 1993.
6. Mullins PA et al: Rheumatoid heart disease presenting as acute mitral regurgitation. *Am Heart J* 122:242, 1991.
7. Enriquez-Sarano M et al: Effective mitral regurgitant orifice area: Clinical use of the proximal isovelocity surface area method. *J Am Coll Cardiol* 125:703, 1995.

8. Scognamiglio R et al: Nifedipine in asymptomatic patients with severe aortic regurgitation and normal left ventricular function. *N Engl J Med* 331:689, 1994.

9. Shapira N et al: Aortic valve repair for aortic stenosis in adults. *Ann Thorac Surg* 50:110, 1990.

10. Cohn LH et al: Long term results of mitral valve reconstruction for regurgitation of the myxomatous mitral valve. *J Thorac Cardiovasc Surg* 107:143, 1994.

11. Copeland JG III et al: Four year experience with the CarboMedics valve: The North American experience. *Ann Thorac Surg* 58:630.

12. Ibrahim M et al: The St. Jude medical prosthesis: A thirteen year experience. *J Thorac Cardiovasc Surg* 108:221, 1994.

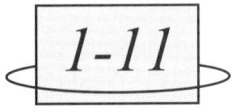

CARDIAC ARRHYTHMIAS
Morton A. Diamond

DISCUSSION

Arrhythmias are electrical disturbances in heart rhythm. They may be asymptomatic, or, when the patient is aware of heart action, palpitations may be noted. Palpitations are often described as pounding, thumping, fluttering, or pausing. Moreover, arrhythmias may cause secondary symptoms such as dyspnea, anginal discomfort, faintness, syncope, and congestive heart failure.

Cardiac rhythm disturbances may occur in the absence or presence of underlying structural heart disease. Their varied causes include ingestion of caffeine, alcohol, or over-the-counter medications; electrolyte imbalance; hypoxemia; acid–base disturbances; tobacco use; prescribed medications; and emotional stress as well as organic congenital and acquired heart disease. Finally, in some patients, the etiology of cardiac rhythm disturbance is not defined.

Both the prognosis and the treatment of a patient's arrhythmia depend on the clinical setting in which it occurs. Arrhythmias are more common in older patients and may have more significant hemodynamic effects because of underlying left ventricular dysfunction.

Cardiac rhythm disturbances are classified as supraventricular (SV) and ventricular. SV arrhythmias include sinus bradycardia, sinus tachycardia, atrial premature beats, paroxysmal supraventricular tachycardia, atrial fibrillation, and the Wolff–Parkinson–White syndrome (WPW). A patient with sick sinus syndrome usually manifests a supraventricular bradyarrhythmia intermingled with episodes of atrial flutter or atrial fibrillation. Ventricular rhythm abnormalities include ventricular premature beats, ventricular tachycardia, and ventricular fibrillation. In addition, arrhythmias may be due to atrioventricular conduction disturbances (AV block). First-, second-, or third-degree (complete) heart block may occur.

PHYSIOLOGIC BASIS OF ARRHYTHMIAS

The mechanisms underlying rhythm disturbances include disorders of automaticity, impulse conduction, reentry, and triggered activity. In brief, reentry is the mechanism for many premature beats as well as most paroxysmal tachycardias. Conduction abnormalities are due to prolongation of the refractory periods of cardiac tissue. Triggered activity may be the mechanism responsible for ventricular tachycardia in patients with congenital or acquired long QT intervals.

ARRHYTHMIA EVALUATION

A physician assistant must not only define the presence and character of a rhythm disorder but also establish a causal relationship between the arrhythmia and the patient's symptoms. Patients with life-threatening conditions—such as out-of-hospital sudden death, arrhythmia-induced seizures, and congestive heart failure—receive inpatient cardiac monitoring. Outpatients who have palpitations have an ECG taken as the initial diagnostic test. Outpatient 24-h ambulatory monitoring, often with an event recorder, is indicated in patients with palpitations or symptoms consistent with arrhythmia. In selected patients, provocative stress testing is indicated to determine the presence of ischemia-induced conduction disturbance or ectopy. Signal-averaged ECG and electrophysiologic testing may be indicated after referral to a cardiologist.

THERAPEUTIC PRINCIPLES

Therapeutic options in the treatment of cardiac rhythm disorders include medication, cardioversion, pacemakers, automatic implantable cardioverter defibrillators, and cardiac surgery. The physician assistant and the consulting cardiologist determine the appropriate treatment.

Antiarrhythmic medications have been arbitrarily classified into four classes. Class I agents are further subdivided into subsets Ia, Ib, and Ic. Class Ia agents include quinidine, procainamide, disopyramide, and moricizine. Class Ib medications include lidocaine, mexiletine, phenytoin, and tocainide. Class Ic includes flecainide and propafenone. Class II medications consist of the beta-sympathetic blockers acebutolol, esmolol, metoprolol, and propranolol. Class III includes amiodarone, sotalol, and bretylium.

The calcium channel blockers diltiazem and verapamil are class IV antiarrhythmic agents. A physician assistant must be aware that these agents must be used with caution. They may have side effects superimposed on limited efficacy. For example, flecainide, moricizine, and encainide demonstrated worsening ventricular arrhythmia in postmyocardial infarction patients with asymptomatic ventricular arrhythmia.

SUPRAVENTRICULAR ARRHYTHMIAS

Sinus Bradycardia

In sinus bradycardia, the heart rate is below 60 beats per minute. Each normal P wave is followed by a normal QRS complex unless there is a preexisting intraventricular conduction defect. Sinus bradycardia may be entirely normal in well-conditioned athletes, but may occur transiently during periods of increased vagal tone. Other common causes include medication (beta blockers, calcium channel blockers, parasympathomimetic medications, lithium), hypothyroidism, and sinus node disease. This rhythm disturbance should be treated only if it causes symptoms such as weakness and confusion. If necessary, cardiac pacing appears preferable to sympathomimetic agents and atropine-like medication.

Sinus Arrhythmia

A gradual increase in heart rate during inspiration and a gradual decrease during expiration are characteristic of sinus arrhythmia in young patients. In contrast, nonphasic sinus arrhythmia, in which the changing heart rate is not related to respiration, occurs in the elderly and in diabetic patients. Sinus arrhythmia does not require treatment.

Sinus Tachycardia

A heart rate greater than 100 beats per minute, in which a normal P wave is followed by a normal QRS complex, is characteristic of sinus tachycardia. This arrhythmia may be a normal response to emotional stress, fever, anemia, hypotension, congestive heart failure, hyperthyroidism, myocardial ischemia, cardiogenic or hemorrhagic shock, medication, or foods containing caffeine. Treatment depends on the underlying cause.

Atrial Premature Contractions

Atrial premature contractions (APCs) occur in patients with normal or diseased hearts. APCs commonly are noted in patients with infection, myocardial ischemia, and congestive heart failure (CHF). They may also be found in those who have ingested caffeine products or alcohol and those who smoke tobacco products. In a patient with a history of paroxysmal supraventricular tachycardia, APCs may be a harbinger of recurrent tachyarrhythmia. This patient should be treated with a beta blocker, digoxin, or a calcium antagonist. In a cardiac patient who has recently gained weight, APCs may be an important sign of incipient clinical CHF. These patients should receive more vigorous therapy depending on whether systolic or diastolic ventricular dysfunction is present.

Paroxysmal Supraventricular Tachycardia

Paroxysmal supraventricular tachycardia (PSVT) is the most common paroxysmal tachyarrhythmia. It occurs in both normal and diseased hearts. Attacks typically are of abrupt onset and termination. Heart rate is generally in the range of 160 to 220 beats per minute. In PSVT, the P wave may precede, be within, or follow the QRS complex. If the arrhythmia is due to digitalis intoxication, an AV block is also present. Treatment is directed toward termination of the acute episode and prevention of subsequent tachycardia. Carotid sinus massage may be effective in aborting the tachycardia. It should be applied on one carotid artery at a time and never in the presence of carotid bruits. A 6-mg bolus of intravenous adenosine, followed if necessary 1 to 2 min later by a bolus of 12 mg, is often successful in terminating the rhythm disturbance. Adenosine should not be used in asthmatic patients. Theophylline products inhibit the action of adenosine. In contrast, patients receiving dipyridamole are highly sensitive to adenosine. In these patients, one should start with a 1-mg intravenous bolus followed 2 min later, if necessary, by a 3-mg bolus. Intravenous verapamil in incremental doses up to a total of 20 mg in 15 min is also an excellent therapeutic option. Intravenous diltiazem and the short-acting beta blocker esmolol may be appropriate therapeutic options. Cardioversion may be urgently applied in cases of hemodynamic compromise. Further, it may be used if medicinal therapy proves ineffective.

A physician assistant has many therapeutic choices in the prevention of recurrent attacks. Oral digoxin (maintenance dose generally 0.125 to 0.5 mg daily) and oral verapamil (maintenance dose generally 120 to 360 mg daily), alone or in combination, are effective. Verapamil increases digoxin blood levels. Additionally, beta blockers are effective. Less frequently, class Ia, class Ic, and class III agents are prescribed. Radiofrequency catheter ablation therapy is considered the treatment of choice in PSVT patients in whom reentry is the underlying mechanism promoting recurrent tachycardia.

Atrial Flutter

In atrial flutter, the atrial rate is generally 250 to 350 beats per minute with an abnormal contour to the atrial wave (classically a "sawtooth" appearance). The ventricular rate in an untreated patient is generally in the range of 100 to 150 beats per minute. The QRS complex is normal unless there is a preexisting bundle branch block or the ventricular rate is so fast that aberrant intraventricular conduction is evident. Flutter is rarely found in a normal heart and is rarely chronic. This arrhythmia occurs in many congenital and acquired cardiac disorders as well as in constrictive pericarditis, chronic obstructive lung disease, and postoperative cardiac surgery patients. Because pharmacologic control of the ventricular response may be difficult, electrical cardioversion to normal sinus rhythm is usually advisable. The risk of thromboembolism is thought to be low. Nonetheless, anticoagulation is considered advisable in patients with mitral valve disease who are considered for elective cardioversion.

Atrial Fibrillation

Atrial fibrillation (AF) is the most commonly encountered arrhythmia in clinical practice. Its prevalence increases with age; approximately

10 percent of the population over age 80 years has this rhythm disorder. AF may be acute (paroxysmal) or chronic. It may occur in both normal and diseased hearts. AF is common in rheumatic heart disease, coronary atherosclerotic heart disease, pericarditis, hypertension, atrial septal defect, mitral valve prolapse, congestive and hypertrophic cardiomyopathy, and hyperthyroidism. AF is found in 20 percent of patients with acute myocardial infarction. Further, acute attacks may be precipitated by cardiac surgery, alcohol ingestion, and medications.

The most recognized hazard of AF is the increased risk of stroke. In patients aged 50 to 59 years, atrial fibrillation accounts for 0.5 percent of all strokes; in contrast, in octogenarians, AF is thought responsible for approximately 25 percent of acute cerebrovascular accidents. There is no difference in stroke risk when patients with paroxysmal AF are compared with those with chronic AF. The more serious sequela of AF is the increased mortality associated with this arrhythmia. Compared to age-matched controls without AF, follow-up of male and female patients with AF revealed a significantly higher mortality in the AF population.

Atrial activity is very fast, with 400 to 600 impulses per minute reaching the atrioventricular node (AVN). In an untreated patient, the ventricular response is approximately 80 to 180 beats per minute. Fast ventricular rates, especially in patients with underlying organic heart disease, may produce ischemic coronary syndromes, hypotension, or CHF.

The principal goals of therapy for AF are control of ventricular rate, restoration of sinus rhythm in patients with paroxysmal arrhythmia, prevention of recurrent episodes, and prevention of stroke and systemic embolism

Control of Ventricular Rate

Rate control signifies the attainment of ventricular rates that are physiologically appropriate to the patient's level of activity. The physician assistant must note the ventricular response not only at rest but also with activity. Cardiac exercise testing or ambulatory cardiac monitoring may be performed in the AF patient in order to evaluate ventricular response during activity.

In the absence of CHF or preexcitation syndrome, verapamil, diltiazem, and beta-sympathetic blockers are more effective than digoxin for long-term control. In a patient with an uncontrolled ventricular rate, verapamil may be given intravenously in a dose of 5 to 10 mg over 3 min and repeated in 30 min if necessary. When rate control has been achieved, oral verapamil may be given in a dose range of 40 to 120 mg tid. Intravenous diltiazem 20 mg or 0.25 mg/kg may be administered over 2 min. If necessary, 25 mg or 0.35 mg/kg may be given 15 min later. Oral diltiazem usually is prescribed in a dose of 60 to 120 mg PO tid. Calcium channel blockers are preferred in patients with bronchospasm, diabetes mellitus, and peripheral arterial vascular disease.

When digoxin is the therapeutic option, an intravenous dose of 1.0 to 1.5 mg is given over 24 h in incremental doses of 0.25 to 0.5 mg. The oral maintenance digoxin dose is 0.125 to 0.5 mg daily. One must remember that digoxin blood levels are of little value in assessing an adequate dose. Digoxin must be used cautiously in patients with renal disease. When it is used jointly with verapamil to control the ventricular rate, the verapamil raises serum digoxin levels. Intravenous propranolol is given of 1.0 mg every 2 min until the heart rate is controlled or until a total dose of 7 mg has been injected. The oral maintenance dose is in a wide range of 10 to 120 mg PO bid or tid. Propranolol in low doses may be added to digoxin therapy.

In selected patients who do not respond to medicinal therapy, radiofrequency catheter ablation of the atrioventricular node, coupled with rate-responsive pacemaker implantation, is indicated.

Restoration of Sinus Rhythm

The physician assistant and the consulting cardiologist must determine which patients will undergo efforts toward the restoration of normal rhythm. There are, however, patients in whom ventricular rate control and anticoagulation are clearly the preferred therapy.

In a patient with acute AF lasting less than 48 h, pharmacologic or electrical cardioversion may be attempted after control of the ventricular rate has been attained. Class Ia or class Ic agents may be used. However, close cardiac monitoring is essential. Electrical transthoracic cardioversion, using direct current, may be performed urgently in a patient in severe hemodynamic distress. For a patient who has been in atrial fibrillation less than 48 h, electrical cardioversion can be performed without anticoagulant therapy. If fibrillation has been present more than 48 h, the patient should receive, in addition to medication to control heart rate, warfarin therapy for 3 to 4 weeks before cardioversion. The dose of warfarin should maintain the International Normalized Ratio (INR) at 2.0 to 3.0. Those receiving digoxin should have this medication discontinued 24 h before cardioversion. After a successful return to sinus rhythm, warfarin therapy should be continued for a minimum of 4 to 6 weeks. Alternatively, transesophageal echocardiography may be performed to exclude atrial thrombi so that early cardioversion can be accomplished safely. A physician assistant should be cognizant that this clinical approach is not universally accepted. In selected cases, elective cardioversion is performed using an internal cardiac catheter.

The physician assistant may opt for pharmacologic cardioversion rather than electrical conversion of AF. Ibutilide, 2 mg over 30 minutes, or 10 mg/kg of intravenous procainamide is more effective for recent-onset AF than for more protracted episodes. These agents must be used with caution, for they may precipitate torsades de pointes. Magnesium sulfate, 1 to 2 g intravenously, may be used to treat drug-induced torsades.

Pharmacologic cardioversion can also be achieved in new-onset AF with a single oral 600-mg dose of propafenone or a single oral 300-mg dose of flecainide. These medications must be avoided in AF patients with ischemia or structural heart disease. Additionally, these agents should follow a medication that slows atrioventricular conduction, in order to prevent an abrupt increase in ventricular rate if AF converts to atrial flutter. When a decision is made to attempt pharmacologic cardioversion, the physician assistant and cardiologist must decide whether that procedure is to be attempted on an outpatient or inpatient basis. Procainamide, amiodarone, and disopyramide are not FDA approved for AF therapy.

Prevention of Recurrent Episodes

No available medication has been proved to be clearly superior in maintaining patients in sinus rhythm. All medications, however, have adverse side effects and potential toxicity. Therefore, the choice of chronic antiarrhythmic therapy for AF prevention is empiric. The goal is to reduce the frequency of AF recurrences and to abbreviate the duration of those episodes. Beta blockers, calcium channel blockers, and digoxin are frequently prescribed. Amiodarone, 100 to 200 mg daily after the loading dose, appears to be valuable in those patients who have failed class I drug therapy.

Nonpharmacologic Therapy in Atrial Fibrillation

In selected patients, AV node ablation, coupled with cardiac pacemaker implantation, is performed to affect heart rate control. Additionally, the maze procedure, in which incisional lines in the atria are produced by cryoablation or radiofrequency current, may be performed in selected patients who have problematic AF recurrences. This operation may be done alone or in conjunction with aortocoronary bypass or mitral valve operations. An implantable atrial defibrillator is presently undergoing clinical evaluation.

Prevention of Stroke and Systemic Embolism

Cerebral infarction in an AF patient is thought to result from embolization of intracardiac thrombi. Patients with both valvular and nonvalvular heart disease are at risk for this complication. Those with atrial fibrillation and valvular disease, including persons with prosthetic valves, should receive chronic warfarin therapy unless a contraindication exists.

Nonvalvular AF is thought to be the most common cardiac disorder causing cerebral embolism. Studies of patients with paroxysmal and chronic nonvalvular AF have demonstrated six independent predictors of risk for embolism. These high-risk categories include hypertension, diabetes mellitus, previous stroke or transient ischemic attack, history of CHF, left atrial dimension greater than 2.5 cm/m^2, and age above 65 years. In these patients, warfarin reduces ischemic stroke by 70 percent. These patients should receive warfarin to achieve an INR of 2.0 to 3.0. Warfarin should not be discontinued if the patient returns to normal sinus rhythm for a period of time. An adult-dose aspirin should be given daily to noncompliant patients and to those who have a contraindication to warfarin. Patients with lone atrial fibrillation—that is, those with atrial fibrillation without underlying structural heart disease or the risk factors listed above—have a very low incidence of stroke. Patients with lone atrial fibrillation under age 60 years do not require anticoagulation or antiplatelet therapy. Those between the ages of 60 and 75 years should take 325 mg aspirin daily. After age 75 years, lone atrial fibrillation patients preferably should receive warfarin therapy.

WOLFF–PARKINSON–WHITE SYNDROME

Wolff–Parkinson–White syndrome (WPW) represents the primary example of preexcitation syndrome, in which atrial impulses may reach the ventricles early via anatomic accessory AV conducting fibers. In preexcitation, the atrial impulse may not traverse the normal AV nodal conducting tissue. Therefore, the heart is prone to the development of AF with an extremely fast ventricular response. This may deteriorate into ventricular fibrillation, accounting for the sudden death observed in these patients. The typical ECG pattern in WPW includes a PR interval less than 120 ms, a QRS complex greater than 120 ms with slurred upstroke, and secondary ST-T wave changes. Anatomic variants of the preexcitation syndrome manifest different ECG patterns.

The most common tachycardia found in WPW patients is regular at a rate of 150 to 250 beats per minute with a normal QRS complex. More serious is AF with atrial impulses conducted to the ventricles without the normal rate-modulating effect of AV nodal conduction tissue. The ventricular rate in these patients may reach 300 beats per minute. Syncope may result from inadequate cerebral blood flow. Sudden death may occur if the rhythm deteriorates into ventricular fibrillation. The physician assistant and the consulting cardiologist must identify WPW patients who are at risk for AF.

TREATMENT

In an adult patient with the ECG abnormality of WPW but without a history of tachyarrhythmia, no investigation or therapy is necessary. For a patient with a history of tachyarrhythmia, electrophysiologic testing is indicated. Radiofrequency catheter ablation of an accessory pathway is now considered the treatment of choice in these patients.

For the termination of an acute episode of tachycardia that is regular and has a *normal QRS complex,* intravenous adenosine or the intravenous calcium channel blockers verapamil and diltiazem may be administered. An external defibrillator must be immediately available if necessary. For the termination of AF with a *wide QRS complex,* medications that slow conduction in both the accessory pathway and the AV nodal tissues are employed. Procainamide may be given intravenously. Class Ic and class III antiarrhythmic medications may be indicated, but the physician assistant is advised to seek cardiology consultation. For a patient exhibiting hemodynamic collapse, electrical cardioversion is the initial treatment.

SICK SINUS SYNDROME

Also known as the brady-tachy syndrome, sick sinus syndrome (SSS) is commonly found in elderly patients. It is characterized by intermittent bradycardia—for example, sinus bradycardia or sinus pauses—interspersed with AF, atrial flutter, or PSVT. The underlying cause is sinus node disease and cardiac conduction abnormalities. However, digoxin, beta blockers, calcium channel blockers, and other antiarrhythmic agents may cause transient SSS. Coronary artery disease is an uncommon cause of SSS. The syndrome's initial presentation may be light-headedness, syncope, angina pectoris, or CHF associated with bradycardia or symptoms related to tachycardia with uncontrolled ventricular rates.

Initial therapy consists of the removal of any offending medication. Further treatment includes the insertion of a permanent cardiac pacemaker to prevent bradycardia and an antiarrhythmic agent to prevent paroxysmal tachycardia.

VENTRICULAR ARRHYTHMIAS

Ventricular Premature Beats

Ventricular premature beats (VPBs) are characterized by an early QRS complex that is not preceded by a P wave. They are ubiquitous, found in both normal and diseased hearts. They may be symptomatic or asymptomatic. The importance and treatment of ventricular premature beats depend on the clinical setting in which they occur. In normal hearts, VPBs tend to disappear with exercise. A patient without heart disease who exhibits these premature beats should be treated with reassurance and withdrawal of any offending agents, such as caffeine-containing products. Only a symptomatic patient without heart disease should receive antiarrhythmic medication. Beta blockers are usually efficacious in this setting. VPBs resulting from sinus bradycardia should be treated with medications that increase heart rate, such as parasympatholytic or sympathomimetic agents, or even with cardiac pacing. A hypertensive patient with VPBs but without coexistent left ventricular dysfunction would generally benefit from beta blocker therapy. In the setting of acute myocardial infarction, patients who have VPBs that are close to the preceding T wave, occur more frequently than six times per minute, are of multiform contour, or occur in salvos of two or more should be treated with intravenous lidocaine (1 mg/kg bolus, followed by an infusion of 2 mg/min). If lidocaine is ineffective, intravenous procainamide, or beta blockers, may be given. Consideration must be given to the hemodynamic status of the patient.

Ventricular Tachycardia

Ventricular tachycardia (VT) is defined as three or more VPBs in a row. The VT rate may vary between 70/min (nonparoxysmal) and 250/min (paroxysmal). VT is rarely found in normal hearts. It occurs commonly in patients with ischemic heart disease, rheumatic heart disease, congestive cardiomyopathy, myocarditis, and digitalis toxicity. The physician assistant should seek provocative causes for tachycardia onset, such as hypoxemia, acute ischemia, and hypokalemia. It may be difficult even for an experienced electrocardiographer to differentiate between VT and SV tachycardia associated with aberrancy.

VT is classified as nonsustained if the arrhythmia lasts less than 30 s and is asymptomatic. VT is sustained when the tachycardia lasts more than 30 s (symptomatic or asymptomatic) or causes hemodynamic collapse within 30 s.

Nonsustained ventricular tachycardia associated with acute myocardial infarction is treated with intravenous lidocaine (1-mg/kg bolus followed by 2-mg/min infusion). In patients whose ventricular ectopy is refractory to the lidocaine, infusion rate may be increased to 4 mg/min. Side effects include tremor, twitching, anxiety, confusion, seizures, and respiratory depression. Intravenous procainamide, amiodarone, or bretylium may be administered in patients whose ectopy is persistent.

The treatment of chronic, recurrent, nonsustained VT is controversial because the efficacy of antiarrhythmic medication has not been established. It is known that patients with nonsustained VT who have left ventricular dysfunction are at increased risk of sudden death. Electrophysiologic studies of left ventricular dysfunction patients may demonstrate those with inducible VT. This subset of patients should be treated. Class Ia, class II, and class III (sotalol and amiodarone) agents have been prescribed for these patients. Recent studies suggest that in patients with atherosclerotic heart disease who have reduced ejection fractions and asymptomatic nonsustained VT, implantable cardioverter defibrillators are superior to pharmacologic therapy in reducing the risk of sudden cardiac death.

Sustained VT occurs most frequently in patients with an acute or old myocardial infarction. Sustained VT in an acutely infarcted patient is treated with intravenous lidocaine, intravenous procainamide, or, if necessary for a patient in hemodynamic collapse, DC cardioversion. Because of the high risk of sudden death in these patients, electrophysiologic (EPS) studies are frequently performed. The purpose of an EPS study is to determine whether any antiarrhythmic agent can prevent inducible VT in the laboratory. A medication found to be effective on EPS appears to have clinical efficacy. However, implantable cardioverter defibrillators appear to be superior to medication in prevention of sudden cardiac death in these high-risk patients.

Patients with symptomatic or asymptomatic sustained VT who do not respond to pharmacologic agents should receive an implantable cardioverter defibrillator. The device is constructed so that many VT episodes can be terminated via overdrive pacing without need for a cardiac shock. If overdrive pacing is unsuccessful, or the patient goes into ventricular fibrillation, the implanted device delivers a shock to the heart. In selected patients with recurrent sustained VT, catheter ablation or surgical aneurysmectomy procedures are performed.

Ventricular Fibrillation

In acute myocardial infarction, ventricular fibrillation (VF) occurs in two clinical settings. Primary VF occurs very early in the illness and typically is not associated with severe left ventricular dysfunction. If it is treated quickly, the patient does not have a negative long-term prognosis. Secondary VF typically occurs on the second or third day and is associated with severe left ventricular mechanical dysfunction. The prognosis is poor in these patients. This arrhythmia is further addressed in the section on sudden death in Chap. 1-7.

Torsade de Pointes

Torsade de pointes is a polymorphic VT in which the QRS complexes change in amplitude around the isoelectric axis. It is typically associated with a long QT interval on ECG. Torsade may be associated with a congenitally long QT interval in which the child frequently collapses during physical exertion. Therapy in the congenital group includes beta blockers, a left stellate ganglion block, or a cervical/high-thoracic ganglionectomy. An acquired long QT interval usually is due to class Ia antiarrhythmic agents, but some class Ic and antidepressant agents also may be precipitants. With class Ia medicines, the QT prolongation most frequently occurs within 96 h of the initiation of therapy. It is widely accepted that patients started on class Ia medicines should be under hospital cardiac monitoring during this time period. Torsade occurring at a later time in patients taking these medications frequently is due to complicating hypokalemia or hypomagnesemia. Treatment includes withdrawal of the offending medication and, if necessary, electrolyte replacement, infusion of magnesium sulfate (1 to 2 g intravenously), or temporary cardiac pacing.

ATRIOVENTRICULAR BLOCK (HEART BLOCK)

Heart block is classified as first-degree, second-degree, or third-degree. In first-degree block, every atrial impulse is conducted to the ventricles with a PR interval greater than 0.20 s. In second-degree block, some atrial impulses are not conducted to the ventricles when the block is not due to physiologic interference. Second-degree AV block is further subdivided into Mobitz type I (Wenckebach) and Mobitz type II. Type I is characterized by progressive PR prolongation culminating in a nonconducted P wave. Type I block typically occurs at the level of the AV node so that the QRS complex is narrow. In Mobitz II block, the PR interval is constant before the blocked P wave. The conduction disorder often is in the His-Purkinje system, with a resultant bundle-branch QRS complex. Third-degree heart block (complete heart block) may be due to a conduction abnormality at the AV node or in the His-Purkinje system.

First-degree and Mobitz I blocks may occur transiently in normal persons who experience heightened vagal tone. Other possible causes include digitalis toxicity, myocardial ischemia, inferior myocardial infarction, acute rheumatic fever, myocarditis, conducting tissue calcification, and degenerative conduction disease. Medications including digoxin, calcium channel blockers, and beta blockers may cause these rhythm disturbances. Treatment of first-degree block generally consists of discontinuation of the offending medication. Mobitz I conduction delay is treated by medication withdrawal and, if the ventricular rate is slow enough to cause symptoms, the insertion of a temporary pacemaker.

Mobitz II AV block is not caused by digitalis toxicity. It most commonly is due to acute myocardial infarction, degenerative conduction system disease, or myocarditis. Mobitz II is an unpredictable rhythm, and urgent pacing is required because of its propensity to advance to complete heart block or sudden death. In complete heart block, the ventricular rate is usually 30 to 40 beats per minute. Important causes include digitalis or potassium toxicity, acute infarction, chronic ischemic heart disease, and infiltrative cardiac disease. Complete heart block associated with inferior infarction is associated with a stable junctional (AV nodal) rhythm at a rate of 30 to 60 beats per minute. This conduction defect is typically of short duration (e.g., hours to days), and temporary pacing suffices. In anterior infarction, Mobitz II or complete heart block may occur. Escape rhythm is usually idioventricular and unstable in character. Temporary cardiac pacing is indicated, but the mortality rate remains at approximately 80 percent because of the associated severe myocardial damage. Chronic complete heart block caused by structural disease is treated with permanent cardiac pacing.

BIBLIOGRAPHY

Buxton AE, Duc J, et al. Ventricular arrhythmias. Nonsustained ventricular tachycardia. *Cardiol Clin* 18:327–336, 2000.

Miller JM, Coppess MA, et al. Ventricular arrhythmias. Management of postinfarct ventricular tachycardia. *Cardiol Clin* 18:293–308, 2000.

Reiffel JA. Selecting an antiarrhythmic agent for atrial fibrillation should be a patient-specific, data-driven decision. *Am J Cardiol* 82:72N–81N, 1998.

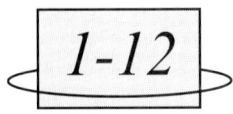

HYPERTENSION
Katherine Adamson

DISCUSSION

Systemic hypertension is one of the most common health problems in this country, affecting as many as 50 million Americans.[1] It is a chronic condition that afflicts more blacks than whites and is found in greater numbers among those in the lower socioeconomic strata. Hypertension results in more office visits to primary care providers than does any other chronic illness, with only one in four hypertensive Americans

controlling their hypertension to below 140/90 mmHg.[2] Hypertension is a well-established major risk factor for the development of coronary artery disease and is the most important risk factor for cerebrovascular disease. The Sixth Joint National Committee on Detection, Evaluation and Treatment of High Blood Pressure (JNC-VI)[1] published guidelines in 1997 that differed from their predecessors in that JNC-VI relied on evidence-based medicine as well as expert consensus to formulate recommendations. JNC-VI emphasizes absolute risk and benefit and adds risk stratification as a treatment strategy. Once again, beta blockers and diuretics are recommended as an initial choice when medication for hypertension becomes a necessity. This report recognizes the appropriateness of choosing other classes of medications for the initial treatment of essential hypertension as patients' circumstances dictate.

For years clinicians have been taught that control of the diastolic blood pressure is paramount, but it has been confirmed that systolic elevations in blood pressure carry as much significance, if not more, than do diastolic elevations. This awareness prompted JNC-V to formulate new parameters for the classification of blood pressure in the adult population. JNC-VI modified those parameters only slightly, combining stage 3 with the relatively infrequently found stage 4 (see Table 1-12-1).

Those who have practiced medicine for a while note that the tolerance level for elevations of blood pressure is changing. It is now recognized that the vast majority of individuals with hypertension fall into the "mild," or stage 1, category. One must not be misled by the assumption that a mild label equals a minimal outcome. Patients with stage 1 hypertension constitute the majority of all hypertensives, and all stages of elevated blood pressure are associated with an increased risk of both fatal and nonfatal cardiovascular events.

It is also important to view hypertension from an etiologic perspective. Over 90 percent of all patients with hypertension seen in the United States fall into the category of primary hypertension. Primary hypertension may be referred to as "essential" or even "idiopathic." This nomenclature underscores the fact that we have not identified the cause of the vast majority of cases of hypertension. The exact causality in essential hypertension may be elusive, but factors involved in the development of essential primary hypertension have been well established: advancing age, ethnicity, gender, family history, sodium intake, excessive alcohol ingestion, socioeconomic status, tobacco abuse, and the presence of high levels of emotional stress.

The term *secondary hypertension* implies that the patient has a clearly identifiable and often treatable cause for the elevation in blood pressure. Secondary hypertension, while rare, usually results from problems in the endocrine system or renal system. Approximately 4 percent of cases of hypertension in the general population

TABLE 1-12-1. Classification of Blood Pressure for Adults Age 18 and Older Not Taking Antihypertensive Drugs and Not Acutely Ill

CATEGORY	SYSTOLIC, mmHg		DIASTOLIC, mmHg
Optimal	<120	and	<80
Normal	<130	and	<85
High normal	130–139	or	85–89
Hypertension			
Stage 1	140–159		90–99
Stage 2	160–179		100–109
Stage 3	≥180	or	≥110

SOURCE: Adapted from *Sixth Report of the Joint National Committee on Detection, Evaluation and Treatment of High Blood Pressure*, National Institutes of Health Publication No. 98-4080.[1]

can be related to disease of the kidney and/or renal vasculature, with another 2 percent related to an endocrine pathway, such as primary aldosteronism, Cushing's syndrome, pheochromocytoma, hyperthyroidism, hyperparathyroidism, acromegaly, and oral contraceptives.[3] One goal of the clinical evaluation of hypertensive patients is to identify the few individuals who need further investigation to determine the existence of an underlying treatable etiology for hypertension.

Malignant hypertension implies an extreme elevation in blood pressure that is associated with acute end organ damage or failure. This clinical emergency can occur in primary or secondary hypertensive patients.[4]

PATHOGENESIS

Sustained elevated levels of blood pressure result in an acceleration of atherosclerosis. This manifests as coronary artery disease, aortic dissection, peripheral vascular disease, cerebral infarction or hemorrhage, retinopathy, and renal failure. In addition, the heart compensates for the increased workload caused by hypertension by increasing left ventricular wall thickness. If the hypertension is not treated, the hypertrophied heart eventually will cease to compensate and congestive heart failure will ensue. These pathologic presentations are loosely referred to as end organ or target organ manifestations.

There is a direct relation between the level of blood pressure and the incidence of fatal and nonfatal cardiovascular events and renal disease. As the pressure increases, so does the incidence of end organ damage. From a physiologic point of view, the major factors involved in the maintenance of blood pressure are systemic vascular resistance and cardiac output. These two functions are controlled by a variety of neurohumoral mechanisms (sympathetic outflow) and the kidney (renin-angiotensin-aldosterone cascade).

CLINICAL EVALUATION

All health care professionals should measure the blood pressure of every patient at each visit. A diagnosis of hypertension should be made only if the blood pressure readings fall within the parameters shown in Table 1-12-1 for a minimum of three office visits over a 1-week to several-week period. If a patient's readings fall in the very severe category on a single occasion with no apparent causative event (e.g., acute cocaine intoxication), it is reasonable to make the diagnosis of hypertension on the basis of this single presentation.

The goals of clinical evaluation are to evaluate the extent of end organ manifestations and identify patients who require in-depth evaluation or referral for suspected secondary hypertension. All the cardiovascular risk factors should be searched for and properly addressed. This includes evidence of glucose intolerance or diabetes, hyperlipidemia, and life-style considerations.

SIGNS AND SYMPTOMS

Primary hypertension has long been referred to as a silent killer. Symptoms relating to elevated pressure alone are uncommon. Most symptomatology can be tied to long-standing pressure elevations and consequent target organ damage. A minority of patients may be diagnosed with hypertension when they present with occipital headache, dizziness, or epistaxis. In everyday practice, hypertension is uncovered when a patient's pressure is checked routinely as part of a physical examination or health maintenance screening program.

Primary hypertension often is first seen in middle-aged individuals with a strong family history of hypertension, whereas secondary hypertension often presents in relatively young patients (<35 years of age).[4] Since hypertension is a major cardiovascular and cerebrovascular risk factor, it is imperative that a thorough cardiac and neurologic review of systems be conducted. It is useful to direct both history and physical examination with the target organ system in mind.

All patients should be historically screened for secondary hypertension by determining the presence of episodic palpitations, headache, and diaphoresis (pheochromocytoma); polyuria, polydipsia, and muscle weakness (from the hypokalemia associated with primary aldosteronism); and mood swings and weight gain (Cushing's syndrome).[4]

PHYSICAL EXAMINATION

A thorough physical examination is mandatory in the evaluation of hypertension. The clinician needs to check the blood pressure readings personally, both supine and upright. The pressures in both upper extremities and one lower extremity pressure are necessary to rule out coarctation of the aorta. While performing a general inspection, one should look for the moon face associated with Cushing's syndrome. A careful funduscopic examination frequently will uncover the earliest physical evidence of uncontrolled hypertension. The Keith-Wagener-Baker classification of retinopathy is a useful reference for grading funduscopic changes.[4] Palpation and auscultation of the pulses are of paramount importance. The presence of a bruit will alert the examiner not only to a careful evaluation for accelerated atherosclerosis but also to a consideration of renovascular stenosis as a possible etiology for the hypertension. Examination of the neck must include inspection for venous distention and palpation of the thyroid. A palpable radial femoral pulse delay provides further evidence of aortic coarctation. The suspicion of left ventricular hypertrophy (LVH) on physical examination is significant. Left ventricular hypertrophy is an independent risk factor for cardiovascular disease, and when it is found, aggressive antihypertensive therapy is indicated.[4] One should look for and document the point of maximal impulse (PMI), especially if it is deviated laterally and inferiorly. The presence of an S_4 sound is not uncommon; however, an S_3, particularly in the setting of pulmonary rales, indicates ventricular dysfunction. Careful auscultation for the presence of cardiac murmurs and extra heart sounds in addition to the rate and rhythm cannot be overemphasized. Auscultation of the abdomen may rarely uncover the bruit of renal artery stenosis. Abdominal palpation should be directed at the discovery of organomegaly or masses, with particular attention paid to the kidneys. Palpation of the abdomen would be incomplete without a gross measurement of the aorta and an assessment of aortic pulsation. The neurologic examination should be thorough and should include a screen for focal deficits in addition to noting the patient's gait and balance.

LABORATORY STUDIES

All hypertensive patients should have the following laboratory diagnostics: complete blood count, urinalysis, serum glucose, potassium, calcium, creatinine, uric acid, lipid profile, and 12-lead electrocardiogram (ECG).[1,4] This relatively inexpensive battery of tests will assist in the evaluation of target organ status and cardiovascular risk factor analysis and the identification of individuals with secondary hypertension. If ventricular hypertrophy is suspected from the physical examination and/or ECG findings, it is prudent to obtain an echocardiogram. Evidence of heart failure should be further investigated with a chest x-ray. Additional diagnostic studies may be ordered as the situation mandates (see Table 1-12-2).

TREATMENT

The goal of treatment of hypertension is to reduce target organ damage while preserving the quality of life. Ideally, the blood pressure should be controlled with life-style modifications and, when necessary, medication. JNC-VI has reaffirmed the definition of hypertension as a blood pressure equal to or greater than 140/90. Therefore, a reasonable goal for blood pressure control is below this level.

TABLE 1-12-2. Considerations in the Evaluation of Secondary Causes of Hypertension

DIAGNOSIS	HISTORY	PHYSICAL EXAMINATION	DIAGNOSTIC TESTS
Aortic coarctation	Generally young at presentation with long history of hypertension	Diminished or absent lower extremity pulses; decreased lower extremity blood pressure; systolic murmur over precordium	Chest x-ray with rib notching and "3" sign of aortic compression with pre- and poststenotic dilatation; ECG with LVH; aortography is definitive test
Parenchymal renal disease	Frequent urinary tract infections		Elevation of blood urea nitrogen and creatinine
Renovascular disease	Young women have fibromuscular dysplasia variety; majority of cases found in older smokers	Abdominal bruits; hypertension refractory to treatment	Captopril-enhanced radionuclide renal scan, duplex Doppler flow studies are noninvasive; definitive diagnosis requires renal angiography
Polycystic kidneys	Often with family history; flank pain and hematuria may be present	Abdominal or flank masses	Elevated blood urea nitrogen and creatinine; urinalysis with proteinuria and hematuria, cysts identified on renal ultrasound
Hyperthyroidism	Nervousness, tremor, weight loss, heat intolerance, mood swings	Tachycardia and/or atrial fibrillation common, tremor, thyroid enlargement, exophthalmos	Thyroid function studies
Hyperaldosteronism	Weakness, polyuria, polydipsia	Nothing specific	Low serum potassium levels, often less than 3.5
Cushing's syndrome	Sexual dysfunction, depression, weight gain	Truncal obesity, hirsutism, striae, ecchymosis	Dexamethasone suppression test
Pheochromocytoma	Episodic headache, tremor, tachycardia, diaphoresis		24-h urine collection for metanephrines and catecholamines; computed tomography or magnetic resonance imaging required to localize tumor preoperatively

Life-Style Modifications

All patients diagnosed with hypertension must be counseled regarding a healthy life-style and strongly encouraged to adopt lifelong healthy habits. Life-style modifications should be viewed as adjunctive therapy for most patients and definitive therapy for some. These modifications are cost-effective and present little or no risk to the patient. Hypertension must be viewed as an independent cardiovascular risk factor, and many life-style modifications are aimed at improvement in cardiac risk factor status as well as direct reduction of blood pressure. One should encourage patients to attain and maintain ideal body weight, since there is a close correlation between obesity and hypertension. A weight loss program is enhanced by regular aerobic exercise, which of course improves cardiac fitness. The ideal diet is lean in fat and low in sodium while being rich in calcium, magnesium, and potassium. It goes without saying that tobacco must be eliminated from the patient's life. These patients should be instructed to keep alcohol consumption at moderate levels, generally defined as not exceeding 1 oz of ethanol daily (8 oz of wine, 24 oz of beer, or 2 oz of 100-proof whiskey).[3] The role of stress management strategies has not been defined clearly. Nonetheless, it is reasonable to counsel patients about the deleterious effects of sustained high levels of emotional stress.

Risk Stratification

An individual's risk for the development of cardiovascular disease is dependent on a number of risk factors in addition to hypertension. The clinician must determine the presence or absence of the well-known cardiovascular risk factors (smoking, hyperlipidemia, diabetes) and use this information to guide the therapeutic intervention. JNC-VI presented a risk stratification scheme that is very beneficial in guiding therapy (see Table 1-12-3).

Pharmacologic Management

Currently, more than 70 different pharmaceutical products are available for the treatment of hypertension, with many more agents on the horizon. With the exception of patients with severe hypertension, a prudent clinician will avoid prescribing medication without allowing a reasonable period of time for life-style modification to have an impact. Generally speaking, if life-style modifications alone are to be effective, this will occur within the first 3 to 6 months. Once it has been determined that medications are necessary, a prudent clinician will use as low a dose as possible to attain control. JNC-VI reaffirmed the recommendation from JNC-V stating, "When the decision has been made to begin antihypertensive therapy and if there are no indications for another type of drug, a diuretic or beta blocker should be chosen because numerous RCTs (randomized controlled trials) have shown a reduction in morbidity and mortality with these agents."[1] This recommendation continues to create significant controversy.[2,5] It may be reasonable to follow the treatment algorithm provided in Fig. 1-12-1, which includes the initial medication choice adjusted to a specific patient situation. The choice of initial therapy needs to be tailored to the patient, with recognition of the increased cost to the patient with the use of many of the newer agents. These cost considerations must be balanced against total cost; that is, it may be less cost-effective to prescribe a cheaper agent that will require more frequent laboratory follow-up, as may be the case with diuretic therapy and the need for frequent electrolyte measurement.

Because black Americans tend to have low renin levels, this subset of the population is more responsive to diuretics and calcium channel blockers than it is to angiotensin converting enzyme (ACE) inhibitors or beta blockers.[1] ACE inhibitors are known to delay the progression of diabetic nephropathy.[2] This property makes ACE inhibitors ideal agents for the treatment of diabetic hypertensives. There

TABLE 1-12-3.   Risk Stratification and Treatment

BLOOD PRESSURE STAGES, mmHg	RISK GROUP A (NO RISK FACTORS, NO TOD/CCD*)	RISK GROUP B (AT LEAST 1 RISK FACTOR, NOT INCLUDING DIABETES; NO TOD/CCD)	RISK GROUP C (TOD/CCD AND/OR DIABETES WITH OR WITHOUT OTHER RISK FACTORS)†
High normal (130–139/85–89)	Life-style modification	Life-style modification	Drug therapy‡
Stage 1 (140–159/90–99)	Life-style modification (up to 12 months)	Life-style modification (up to 6 months)	Drug therapy
Stages 2 and 3 (≥160/≥100)	Drug therapy	Drug therapy	Drug therapy

For example, a patient with diabetes and a blood pressure of 142/94 mmHg plus left ventricular hypertrophy should be classified as having stage 1 hypertension with target organ disease (LVH) and with another major risk factor (diabetes). This patient would be categorized as "stage 1, risk group C" and recommended for immediate initiation of pharmacologic treatment. Life-style modification should be adjunctive therapy for all patients recommended for pharmacologic therapy.

*Target organ disease/clinical cardiovascular disease.

†For patients with multiple risk factors, clinicians should consider drugs as initial therapy plus life-style modifications.

‡For those with heart failure, renal insufficiency, or diabetes.

SOURCE: Adapted from the *Sixth Report of the Joint National Committee on Detection, Evaluation and Treatment of High Blood Pressure,* National Institutes of Health Publication No. 98-4080.[1]

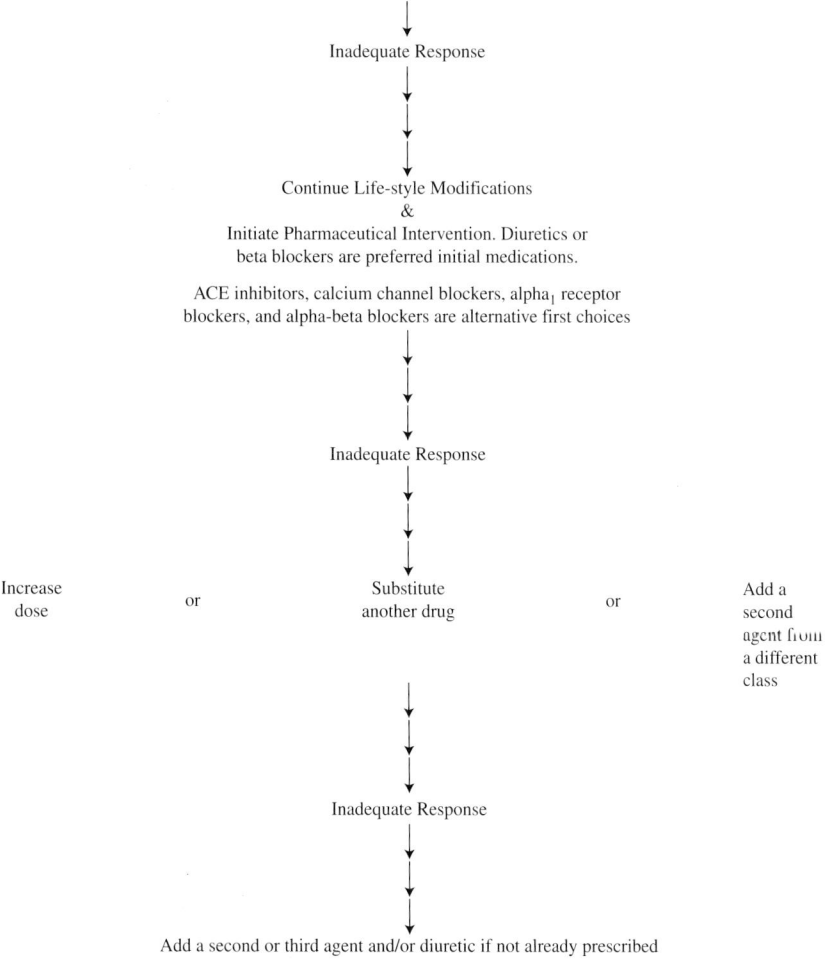

FIGURE 1-12-1. Treatment algorithm for hypertension. (Adapted from the *Sixth Report of the Joint National Committee on Detection, Evaluation, and Treatment of High Blood Pressure.* National Institutes of Health Publication No. 98-408-0.[1])

is substantial evidence that ACE inhibitors are effective in preventing congestive heart failure[2] and play a significant role in ameliorating postinfarction ventricular remodeling in patients with evidence of poor ventricular function.[6] In the author's experience, alpha[1] blockers have a higher incidence of untoward side effects than do the other suggested antihypertensives. However, the beneficial effect alpha[1] blockers have on benign prostatic hypertrophy (BPH) makes them ideal for an older male hypertensive with a history of BPH. Experienced clinicians are aware of the synergistic effect of low-dose thiazide diuretics combined with one of several other classes of antihypertensives. The untoward effects of thiazides on glucose, uric acid, and lipids appear to be both dose-related and time-limited.[2,5] Recognition of these metabolic effects leads one away from choosing diuretics as the initial therapy in a hypertensive patient with concomitant gout or glucose intolerance. A pharmaceutical approach that takes the whole patient into account is best. Many of these medications have impotence as a side effect. It is often necessary to question the patient directly about these personal issues so that adjustments in the medication regimen can be made to ensure higher rates of compliance.

COMPLICATIONS AND RED FLAGS

Hypertensive emergencies are situations in which acute organ damage takes place secondary to extreme elevations in blood pressure. Patients in this situation often present with encephalopathy, acute pulmonary edema, dissecting aortic aneurysm, unstable angina, or acute myocardial infarction. Obviously, these patients are cared for in intensive or coronary care units with parenteral medications.

Hypertensive urgency is defined as a diastolic blood pressure in excess of 120 mmHg with no evidence of acute end organ damage. These patients are often asymptomatic but require blood pressure reduction within 24 h. They can be handled in an outpatient setting by using oral medications (see Table 1-12-4).

NOTES AND PEARLS

A common practice in emergency rooms and outpatient settings throughout the country is to treat hypertensive urgencies with sublingual nifedipine. This is a practice that should be not only discouraged but abandoned. The sublingual route for nifedipine has never been approved by the U.S. Food and Drug Administration (FDA). This route is fraught with problems because absorption is unpredictable. There have been numerous reports of significant negative sequelae to this treatment approach.[7] Serious hypotensive episodes can result, with the induction of ischemia in the central nervous system or the heart. While ACE inhibitors are generally effective and well tolerated, a few caveats need to be remembered. ACE inhibitors carry a boxed warning from the FDA regarding teratogenicity. It is best to avoid this class of drugs in the treatment of hypertension in women of childbearing age. Also, ACE inhibitors in combination with low-dose thiazide diuretics are extremely effective, but one must prescribe the addition of diuretics to ACE inhibitor therapy in the correct sequence. The addition of ACE therapy for

TABLE 1-12-4. Management of Hypertensive Urgency: Outpatient Management with Close Follow-Up

Therapeutic goal is to lower blood pressure (BP) by 20% or to a diastolic BP < 120
Clonidine 0.1–0.2 mg PO, then 0.05 to 0.1 mg q 1 h up to 0.6 mg
Captopril 6.25–25 mg PO, repeat every 30 min as required
Labetalol 200–400mg PO, repeat every 2–3 h as needed
Observe at least 6 h before discharge
Discharge patient on same medication used for initial BP reduction

a patient on diuretics can result in extreme and dangerous episodes of hypotension. The reverse is not true, and so one must remember that it is acceptable to add a diuretic to an ACE but not to do the reverse.

The ACE-diuretic combination is attractive because of the potassium-sparing nature of ACE inhibitors. One must be aware of this effect and avoid using potassium-sparing diuretics in conjunction with ACE inhibitors.

Calcium channel blockers are also very effective antihypertensives. However, owing to an unresolved controversy regarding the possibility of increased cardiac mortality with the shorter-acting agents, those agents should be used with caution or not at all in the long-term treatment of hypertension.[5]

Hypertension is the most common chronic illness encountered in the primary care provider's office. We now have far more effective and better-tolerated forms of therapy, yet only one in four patients is controlled at goal blood pressure levels. These patients may be partially accountable in that noncompliance often is a problem. Ultimately, caregivers need to do a better job in educating patients and being sensitive to the social and economic cost of the therapy prescribed.

REFERENCES

1. *The Sixth Report of the Joint National Committee on Prevention, Detection, Evaluation, and Treatment of High Blood Pressure.* Bethesda, MD, National Institutes of Health; National Heart, Lung, and Blood Institute; National High Blood Pressure Education Program. NIH Publication 98-4080. November 1997.
2. Moser M: Management of hypertension, part I. *Am Family Phys* 53(57): 2295–2302, 1996.
3. Williams G: Hypertensive vascular disease, in Fauci AS, et al (eds): *Harrison's Principles of Internal Medicine,* 14th ed. New York, McGraw Hill, 1998, pp 1380–1394.
4. Griffith C: Hypertension evaluation and management. *Physician Assist* 19(9):25–42, 1995.
5. Moser M: Management of hypertension, part II. *Am Family Phys* 53(8):2553–2559, 1996.
6. Hagar J, Olson H, Kloner R: Acute myocardial infarction, in Kloner RA (ed): *The Guide to Cardiology,* 3d ed. Greenwich, CT, Le Jacq, 1995, pp 299–300.
7. Grossman E et al: Should a moratorium be placed on sublingual nifedipine capsules given for hypertensive emergencies and pseudoemergencies? *JAMA* 276(16):1328–1330, 1996.

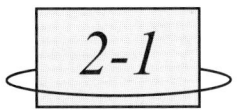

CONTACT DERMATITIS
Barbara L. Sauls

DESCRIPTION

Contact dermatitis is an inflammatory skin reaction of the dermis and epidermis to an external agent or toxin. When the agent directly damages the skin, it is called *irritant contact dermatitis*. If the reaction is immunologic in nature, it is called *allergic contact dermatitis*. Common offending agents are plants, cleaning chemicals, and metals (especially nickel and chromium) in jewelry or clothing. Reactions may range in severity from subacute to acute and chronic and can occur anywhere on the body, possibly even in the nose and mouth. The reaction may occur with the first exposure or may be delayed until the patient has been exposed several times.

The patient's history plays an important role in the diagnosis of contact dermatitis, with occupation, hobbies, changes in household products, and environmental exposures leading the list. Typical jobs that create risk for this disease are cleaning personnel, beauticians, chemists, painters, and workers in manufacturing plants that use chemicals. Hobbies at risk are model building, arts and crafts (from glue and paints), and gardening. Environmental risks are seen in hikers, mountain bikers, campers, and other outdoor enthusiasts. Persons with black skin seem to be less susceptible to contact dermatitis. Changes in soaps and detergents and the use of ointments and creams frequently are implicated in contact dermatitis. Even the long-established use of a certain product is not exempt, since manufacturers often change the chemical composition of their products without changing the brand names. Labels such as "new and improved" and "fresher smell" indicate that a chemical change probably has taken place.

Contact dermatitis (see Fig. 2-1-1) is not contagious to other individuals, a common point of contention between the practitioner and the patient. There is seasonal proclivity only for plant contact dermatitis such as poison ivy, poison oak, and poison sumac during the spring, summer, and fall, when these plants are growing. Collectively, these conditions are known as *Rhus dermatitis*. The offending allergen of the *Rhus* species is the urushiol contained in the oleoresin spots on the undersides of the leaves of these plants. The oleoresin is an extremely stable, oily agent and may be carried on inanimate objects such as unwashed clothing or shoes, firewood, and gardening tools and later cause a reaction when a person touches them even *years* later. Smoke from the burning of *Rhus* is highly allergenic from both contact and inhalation, commonly causing reactions in firefighters and onlookers.

SIGNS AND SYMPTOMS

Patients complain of burning and itching of the exposed skin areas. The skin may turn red, become edematous, and form weeping (serous fluid) areas. Patients commonly believe that this serous drainage is "the poison" that is contagious to others.

OBJECTIVE FINDINGS

Physical examination of the subacute reaction reveals areas of mild erythema and fine scales or papules. There may be mild desquamation of the skin. Acute reactions cause areas of erythema that are poorly demarcated and edematous, with vesicular lesions that may have progressed to crusting and drying. These areas of reaction are often linear when caused by direct plant exposure. A random pattern may occur from airborne contact such as the burning of plants. Airborne contact may cause a reaction to occur in the mucous membranes of the respiratory tract. The vesicles may ooze serous fluid. With chronic contact, dermatitis patients develop patches of dry, thickened, mildly red skin. Lichenification often is noted, which includes hyperkeratosis and deepening of skin lines. The pattern of chronic exposure is often in a specific pattern such as a ring or watchband or a sandal strap. See Fig. 2-1-2 (Plate 1) and Table 2-1-1.

DIAGNOSTIC CONSIDERATIONS

When a patient can relate a history of specific exposure followed by a reaction, it is almost impossible to miss the diagnosis, but identifying the actual offending agent can be an unrewarding, time-consuming task. Patch testing may be required to make a specific determination but is not necessary in most cases.

LABORATORY TESTS

It is not necessary to order laboratory tests to make the diagnosis of contact dermatitis. However, if a biopsy of the affected area was ordered, histiocyte and monocyte infiltration of the skin would indicate an allergic origin, whereas vesicles that contain polymorphonuclear leukocytes lead to a diagnosis of primary irritant dermatitis.

TREATMENT

The most important treatment is the recognition and removal of the offending agent. Occupational exposures may be limited by the use of proper protective gear. Hobby enthusiasts should protect their skin as well. Reactions to clothing, shoes, and jewelry are treated the same way. Patients may be able to get jewelry coated to avoid contact with a nickel-based metal or purchase nickel-free jewelry. Shoes may be replaced, or a reaction may be prevented through the use of socks. Hikers and campers should be shown photos of *Rhus* species plants so that they can try to avoid exposure, or at least they should cover their arms and legs while in the woods.

Topical steroids are used to treat contact dermatitis. Low-potency agents are appropriate for facial and intertriginous areas, middle-potency agents are good for nonfacial and nonintertriginous areas, and high-potency agents are useful on the soles and palms, where the skin is thick. Oral steroids in tapering doses may be needed for a generalized reaction or severe reactions on the face or other areas prone to atrophy from topical steroid use (axillae, groin). The use of steroids in the eyes may precipitate a preexisting fungal or herpetic infection, and so extreme care must be taken.

Table 2-1-2, although not meant to be complete, lists some commonly used topical steroids for steroid-sensitive dermatoses.

SUPPORTIVE MEASURES

Cool compresses or tepid baths with Aveeno oatmeal bath or baking soda or starch shakes often help relieve the symptoms, albeit temporarily.

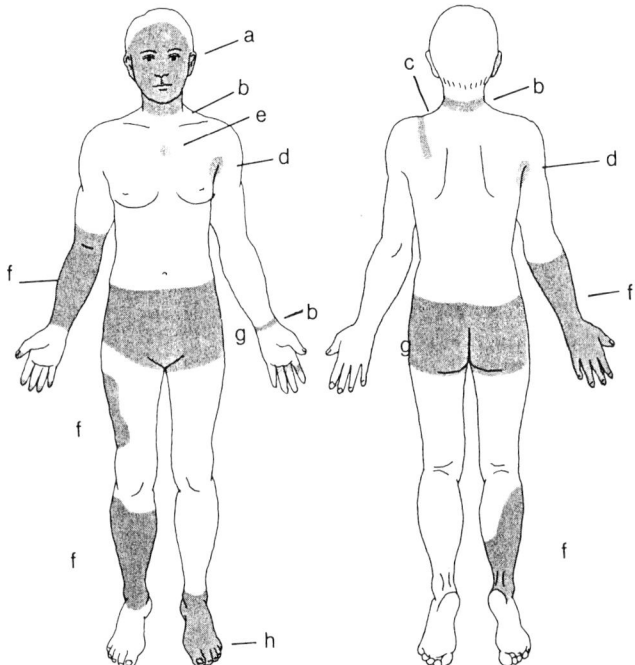

FIGURE 2-1-1. Eczematous dermatitis (contact). *a,* Airborne allergens, plants, pollens, sprays; *b,* jewelry, clothing, furs; *c,* clothing straps; *d,* deodorant, antiperspirant; *e,* metal tags; *f,* plants; *g,* trunks and panties; *h,* shoes or hose. *(From Fitzpatrick TB, et al: Color Atlas and Synopsis of Clinical Dermatology: Common and Serious Diseases, 2d ed. New York, McGraw-Hill, 1992, p 18. Used with permission.)*

Calamine lotion is sometimes helpful. Preparations containing topical diphenhydramine (Caladryl) may cause a sensitivity reaction and can worsen the skin reaction in some cases. Oral diphenhydramine hydrochloride (Benadryl) or other oral antipruritics may be used if the pruritus is severe, but they are not without well-known side effects, especially sedation. It is important to keep the patient's hands away from the affected area to limit secondary infections. There are no restrictions of activity, since this illness is not contagious and rest does not affect disease regression. Since these children often are excluded from school or day care, a note regarding their noncontagiousness may be required.

PATIENT EDUCATION

Patients must be educated about the avoidance of items that cause contact dermatitis reactions. Gloves and long pants and sleeves should be

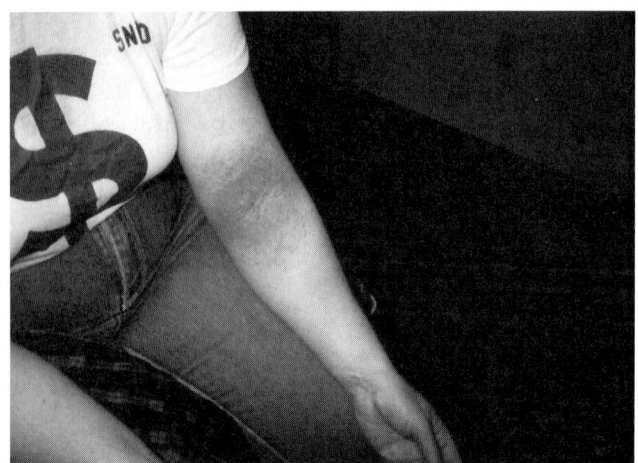

FIGURE 2-1-2 (PLATE 1). Acute contact dermatitis of the antecubital area. (*Courtesy of Harold Milstein, MD, The Dermatology Center, Hazleton, PA.*)

TABLE 2-1-1. Various Forms of Contact Dermatitis and Their Manifestations

	SUBACUTE	ACUTE	CHRONIC
Color	Mild redness	Erythema	Dark red
Scaling	Yes, small	No	No
Desquamation	Superficial	No	Excoriations
Edema	No	Yes	No
Vesicles	No	Yes	No
Pattern	Exposed area	Linear, random, or specific to exposed area	Shaped like item exposed to
Distribution	Often localized and isolated	Random, isolated, localized, or generalized	Usually localized

worn to limit contact with *Rhus* plants. *Rhus* dermatitis victims often claim that each subsequent reaction seems worse than the previous one. This may be due to an increasing intolerance to the oleoresin with repeated exposure. Those who burn brush should be instructed that the *Rhus* species' oleoresin becomes airborne and remains active. Anyone may be affected by downwind smoke exposure. It is possible to have severe *Rhus* dermatitis in the eyes as well as the entire respiratory tract.

Any inanimate items (boots, garden tools, etc.) that have come in contact with *Rhus* oleoresin as well as any exposed skin should be washed with an effective detergent soap (Fels Naphtha) that deactivates the oleoresin. Carefully wiping the skin, avoiding the face and mucous membranes, with isopropyl (rubbing) alcohol in a well-ventilated area will deactivate oleoresin if immediate soap and water washing is not possible. Immediate skin decontamination often prevents any reaction from occurring in a sensitized individual.

Bentoquatam 5% (Ivy Block) is a topical over-the-counter preparation that is available to protect individuals from *Rhus* dermatitis. It is applied 15 minutes before exposure and provides a protective barrier that eliminates or reduces the contact dermatitis reaction to *Rhus* species plants. It must be reapplied every 4 h.

DISPOSITION

Severe reactions, especially of the face, should be followed at least weekly, or sooner if the reaction worsens. Practitioners must monitor for secondary bacterial infections that may develop in areas the patient has excoriated. Patients initially treated with topical steroids may need a change to oral steroids if the reaction is not clearing. Full resolution may take up to 3 weeks.

COMPLICATIONS AND RED FLAGS

Severe *Rhus* dermatitis in the eyes typically affects the conjunctiva but may develop on the corneas, although this is a rare occurrence. This condition warrants a referral to an ophthalmologist to monitor for future scarring and vision loss.

Patients who develop respiratory tract lesions from the inhalation of a toxin or allergen should be considered for hospital admission. A hand-held nebulizer with a steroid preparation as well as oral or intravenous (IV) steroids may be needed.

In some individuals, future exposures to the same agent may cause more severe reactions with each subsequent contact. This does not occur in every patient.

Chronic contact dermatitis should lessen in severity once the offending agent is removed. Depending on the length of time the

TABLE 2-1-2. Topical Steroid Preparations*

POTENCY LEVEL	GENERIC	BRAND	DOSE	FREQUENCY	CAUTIONS
Superhigh	Halobetasol propionate	Ultravate	0.05% cream, ointment	Once or bid	Do not use more than 2 consecutive weeks Not for use in groin, axilla, or on face No occlusive dressings
	Betamethasone dipropionate	Diprolene	0.05% ointment	Once or bid	As above
High	Clobetasol propionate	Temovate	0.05% cream, ointment	Bid	As above
	Diflorasone diacetate	Psorcon	0.05% cream, ointment	Once to tid	As above
Medium	Amcinonide	Cyclocort	0.1% cream, ointment, lotion	Bid to tid	
	Mometasone furoate	Elocon	0.1% cream, ointment, lotion	Once daily	
	Diflorasone diacetate	Florone	0.05% ointment	Once to qid	
	Halcinonide	Halog	0.1% cream, ointment, lotion	Bid to tid	
	Fluocinonide	Lidex	0.05% cream, ointment, gel, solution	Bid to qid	
	Desoximetasone	Topicort	0.25% cream, ointment; 0.05% gel	Bid	
	Triamcinolone acetonide	Aristocort A	0.1% ointment	Tid to qid	
	Fluticasone propionate	Cutivate	0.005% ointment	Bid	
	Fluocinolone acetonide	Synalar	0.025% cream, ointment 0.01% cream, solution	Bid to qid	
	Hydrocortisone valerate	Westcort	0.2% cream, ointment	Bid to tid	
Low	Hydrocortisone	Hytone	1% cream, ointment, lotion 2.5% cream, ointment, lotion	Bid to qid	

*Although this list of topical steroids is not complete, the level of potency, brand and generic names, dosing, preparation type, frequency, and significant cautions are provided as a starting reference for treatment.

reaction has been present, the skin may never completely return to normal. These areas often remain slightly darker and with thickened skin. This does not cause complications but may be cosmetically disfiguring.

PEARLS

One of the old-time treatments for *Rhus* dermatitis was to take baths with bleach water or to put bleach directly on the affected areas. Some patients may still do this. One of the major problems with this treatment is the development of an alkali burn that results in a second problem. There is some basis to this treatment, since it has been observed that children with *Rhus* who swim in chlorinated pools seem to heal faster. Tell patients that it is all right to go swimming and that it may even help. The children will love it.

BIBLIOGRAPHY

General

Fauci AS, Braunwald E, Isselbacher KJ, et al (eds): *Harrison's Principles of Internal Medicine,* 14th ed. New York, McGraw-Hill, 1998.
Fitzpatrick TB, Johnson RA, Wolff K, et al: *Color Atlas and Synopsis of Clinical Dermatology: Common and Serious Diseases,* 3d ed. New York, McGraw-Hill, 1997.

Recommended Dermatology Texts

Arndt KA, Robinson JK, LeBoit PE, et al: *Cutaneous Medicine and Surgery.* Philadelphia, Saunders, 1996.
DuVivier A: *Dermatology in Practice.* Philadelphia, Lippincott, 1990.
Goldstein BG, Goldstein AO: *Practical Dermatology,* Primary Care Series. St. Louis, Mosby Year Book, 1992.

Weinberg S, Prose NS, Kristal L: *Color Atlas of Pediatric Dermatology,* 3d ed. New York, McGraw-Hill, 1998.

Advanced Reading

Shelley WB, Shelley ED: *Advanced Dermatology Diagnosis.* Philadelphia, Saunders, 1992.

Other Suggestions for Dermatology Education

INTERNET For those with Internet access, there are numerous dermatology-related sites that have dermatology information, educational courses, dermatologic drug research, and patient information. These sites often have hundreds of excellent photos. A high-resolution computer monitor will show even minute details.

To obtain an updated list of recommended dermatologic sites and dermatologic magazines, contact the Society of Dermatology Physician Assistants (SDPA): http://www.pacifier.com/~jomonroe Address: 6218 E 78 Place, Tulsa, OK 74136 Phone: 918-523-1992 FAX: 918-523-1920.

CD-ROMS

McLean D, Sober AJ: *Illustrated Dermatology: Synopsis of Diagnosis and Treatment.* 1-800-346-0085, ext 477, or fax 218-723-9433.
Reeves JRT: *Clinical Dermatology Illustrated: A Regional Approach.* Continuing Medical Education Associates, 4015 Hancock St., Suite 120, San Diego, CA 92110.

Research and Patient Support Groups

For a list of addresses or contacts for approximately a dozen skin disease patient support groups organized under the Coalition of Patient Advocates for Skin Disease Research (CPA-SDR), write to CPA-SDR at 710 C St, #11, San Rafael, CA 94901, 415-456-4644, fax 415-456-4274.

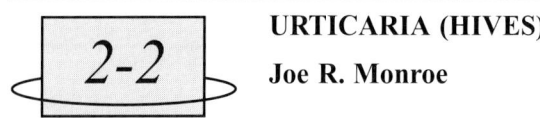

URTICARIA (HIVES)
Joe R. Monroe

DISCUSSION

Urticaria is a transient, blanchable, wheal-like erythematous dermal swelling of acute onset that is usually highly symptomatic (sting and/or itch). Urticaria is quite common, affecting 20 to 25 percent of all individuals during their lifetimes. The lesions appear suddenly as pale to red well-defined areas of focal, shallow dermal edema that vary from pinpoint to palm size. The individual round lesions frequently coalesce into annular or serpiginous plaques surrounded by an erythematous (or pallored) rim.

The fact that individual urticarial lesions seldom last more than 24 h is extremely useful in differentiating this condition from other hive-like conditions. Digital pressure on urticarial lesions produces a brief whitening effect, a phenomenon called blanching, which helps differentiate urticaria from vasculitis, a much more serious condition.

Acute urticaria, traditionally defined as being of less than 6 weeks' duration, is probably more common in children and young adults, whereas recurrent hives, predominately affecting adults, last longer and are termed *chronic.*

On a cellular level, urticaria is caused by the sudden release of histamine from affected mast cells, which leads to increased vascular permeability and subsequent leakage of serum into the tissues. At least 40 percent of cases are idiopathic, but known causes include food, drink, and medicines (e.g., peanuts, shellfish, wheat and eggs, penicillin, and sulfa drugs) and are more common in atopic (allergy-prone) individuals.

Among the non-allergy-related causes of urticaria are the so-called physical urticarias. These include urticarias caused by firm stroking of the skin (dermatographism) and exposure to cold, heat, water, sun, exercise, and vibration.

Urticarial lesions also can accompany diseases such as hepatitis A and B and infectious mononucleosis.

Angioedema is urticaria affecting deeper tissues, presenting with acute focal painless swelling of areas such as the lips, nose, eyelids, hands, feet, and genitals. Like urticaria, angioedema may be acute or chronic and may be seen in conjunction with urticaria or by itself.

Hereditary angioedema (HAE) is a potentially life-threatening form of urticaria that is transmitted in an autosomal dominant manner. Death from laryngeal edema can occur in up to 26 percent of cases of undiagnosed or untreated HAE, and so careful history taking is needed to identify a suggestive family history such as sudden unexplained deaths of apparent respiratory origin. Eighty-five percent of HAE patients have a deficiency of C_1 esterase, a substance whose level can be measured in most laboratories.

DIFFERENTIAL DIAGNOSIS

Fortunately, the evanescent nature of urticaria is extraordinarily helpful in its diagnosis. No other hive-like lesion goes away as abruptly. This distinguishes it from other hive-like conditions, such as urticarial vasculitis and erythema multiforme. Urticarial lesions can be seen in conjunction with other illnesses, such as rheumatoid arthritis, lupus erythematosus, viral hepatitis, and infectious mononucleosis, and so the clinical context in which the lesions appear needs to be taken into account.

LABORATORY

A diagnosis of urticaria usually requires no laboratory work, but a biopsy may be required to rule out systemic diseases presenting with urticaria, such as the vasculitides. Likewise, blood work may be called for, such as sedimentation rate, antinuclear antibodies (ANA), rheumatoid agglutinin (RA), liver function tests, mononucleosis test, and C_1 esterase levels, as the clinical context dictates.

TREATMENT

Treatment of urticaria involves the following steps:

- Identify and eliminate the cause, if possible.
- *Antihistamines.* First-generation H_1 blockers such as diphenhydramine hydrochloride (Benadryl and others) and hydroxyzine (Atarax and others), used at bedtime because of their sedative effects, adding second-generation H_1 blockers such as cetirizine (Zyrtec) for daytime use to avoid problems with sedation. H_2 blockers such as ranitidine can be added and may be helpful in some cases, though only in conjunction with the other agents.
- *Topicals.* Other than cool baths or compresses, topical agents are of little use in the treatment of urticaria.
- If these steps fail, the next step should be referral to a dermatologist not only for confirmation of the diagnosis and possible identification of the trigger but because that physician will have expertise with a variety of agents that have proved useful in treating urticaria, including calcium channel blockers and systemic corticosteroids, among many others.

PATIENT EDUCATION

Patient education should include the following points:

- When investigating chronic urticaria, teach patients about the need to keep an accurate record of food, drink, and medicine ingested.
- Educate patients about the early symptoms of anaphylaxis and the need to seek prompt medical attention.
- Instruct angioedema patients to quiz family members about a possible family history of sudden, unexplained death involving respiratory distress.
- Educate patients about the need to take prescribed antihistamines around the clock, not just "as needed."

PEARLS

Knowledge of the following points can contribute to a satisfactory patient outcome:

- A truly evanescent lesion, that is, one that leaves rapidly, is probably urticaria.
- Viral hepatitis and mononucleosis can present with urticaria.
- Over-the-counter medications, especially nonsteroidal anti-inflammatory drugs, can cause urticaria and frequently are overlooked by patients and providers, as are food additives such as dyes and preservatives.
- If the lesions will not blanch (turn white) with pressure, a biopsy probably is indicated to rule out entities such as vasculitis.

PROGNOSIS

Within a year 50 percent of these patients are disease-free, but 20 percent will have the condition for 10 years or more. HAE is fatal in up to 26 percent of cases if undetected. The combination of angioedema and urticaria lasts up to 5 years in 50 to 75 percent of cases.

BIBLIOGRAPHY

Arndt KA, Robinson JK, LeBoit PE, et al: *Cutaneous Medicine and Surgery.* Philadelphia, Saunders, 1996.

DuVivier A: *Dermatology in Practice.* Philadelphia, Lippincott, Gower, 1990.

Fitzpatrick TB, Johnson RA, Polano MK, et al: *Color Atlas and Synopsis of Clinical Dermatology: Common and Serious Diseases,* 3d ed. McGraw-Hill, New York, 1997.

Goldstein BG, Goldstein AO: *Practical Dermatology,* Primary Care Series. St. Louis, Mosby Year Book, 1992.

Shelley WB, Shelley ED: *Advanced Dermatologic Diagnosis.* Philadelphia, Saunders, 1992.

Weinberg S, Prose NS, Kristal L: *Color Atlas of Pediatric Dermatology,* 3d ed. New York, McGraw-Hill, 1998.

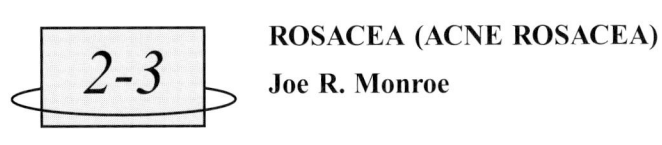

ROSACEA (ACNE ROSACEA)
Joe R. Monroe

DISCUSSION

Rosacea is a chronic inflammatory acneiform disorder that typically affects middle-aged or older adults, and is characterized by intermittent flushing erythema and the recurrent appearance of papules, pustules, and tiny permanent blood vessels called telangiectases that are seen primarily on the central cheeks, nose, brow, and chin. Symptoms of burning and itching are common, and there is a tendency toward progression unless they are treated.

Although the true cause of rosacea is unknown, clearly it is not a type of acne, since there is almost a complete absence of comedones (blackheads and whiteheads), a key diagnostic point. Perhaps the most persistent theory of etiology holds that rosacea is due to the inflammatory response generated by leakage of fluid through dilated vessel walls in certain individuals with vasomotor instability. After years of vasodilatation, the superficial blood vessels in the affected areas "lock in the open position," giving rise to multiple telangiectases, permanent redness, and eventually the formation of papules, pustules, and, on occasion, granulomatous nodules.

Twenty percent of skin biopsies will demonstrate the presence of *Demodex,* a genus of ectoparasitic mites found on all human faces, in the follicles. In rosacea, up to 200 of these organisms are seen in each follicle, compared with only 3 to 5 in unaffected individuals. However, treatment for *Demodex* with crotamiton or other pharmaceuticals does not appear to be very effective in most cases of rosacea, and so researchers are still searching for the true cause of rosacea.

Although the sexes are equally affected by this malady, more women than men request treatment for this condition, which typically begins between ages 30 and 50.

It can be complicated by eye involvement (blepharitis, episcleritis, and conjunctival hyperemia) and can progress to rhinophymatous changes, a bulbous appearance of the nose caused by sebaceous hyperplasia, especially in men.

DIFFERENTIAL DIAGNOSIS

Diseases such as acne vulgaris, seborrhea, pityriasis rubra pilaris, lupus erythematosus, syphilis, cutaneous tuberculosis, carcinoid, and sarcoid can all appear like rosacea. Other telangiectatic processes (e.g., scleroderma) may superficially simulate rosacea but usually can be readily distinguished on clinical and/or histopathologic grounds.

LABORATORY

Although generally not necessary, biopsy can be helpful, with a histopathologic picture that varies according to the type and stage of the disease process, typically showing a nonspecific lymphohistiocytic perivascular infiltrate and telangiectases. As with all biopsies, it is important to let the pathologist know the differential being considered.

TREATMENT
Oral

Tetracycline 250 mg, one or two capsules bid, for at least 2 months tapering over a 1- to 2-month period is remarkably effective, but recurrences are common. Side effects include the following: (1) potentially diminished effectiveness of birth control pills (must use a backup such as foam, condom, or sponge), (2) potential discoloration to a mottled brown of the permanent teeth of any fetus present during therapy, (3) possible neutralization of the effects of tetracycline by calcium-rich foods such as milk products and calcium-containing antacids (requires avoidance of these foods for 1 h before or after dose), since there is a marked affinity of tetracycline for calcium, (4) potential photosensitivity (sunburn-like rash) in a small but significant number of patients. Other oral antibiotics, such as erythromycin, amoxicillin, and even trimethoprim-sulfamethoxazole (Septra), have been used but are much less effective.

Topical

Metronidazole (MetroGel) used twice a day has been reported to be effective, but in this author's experience, it has been a very poor alternative to oral antibiotics and at best takes 6 to 8 weeks to begin working. A less drying cream form of topical metronidazole is now available.

Anything that is known to exacerbate facial flushing or blushing (e.g., hot foods, alcohol, stress) needs to be eliminated or reduced.

PATIENT EDUCATION

Patients need to know that ocular symptoms of grittiness or irritation may be secondary to the effects of rosacea and may require evaluation by an ophthalmologist. Stress the chronic nature of rosacea and the necessity of staying on medication for extended periods.

PEARLS

Knowledge of the following points can contribute to a positive patient outcome:

- "Acne" primarily affecting the nose is probably rosacea.
- Self-prescribed topical steroids are frequently used by these patients and are decidedly counterproductive in treating rosacea because of a rebound effect when they are stopped.
- The "typical" patient is perimenopausal with a history of being a blusher.
- Marked sparing of the periorbital area is common in rosacea.

PROGNOSIS

An excellent response to treatment is the rule, but maintenance therapy with as few as two to three capsules of 250-mg tetracycline a week is often necessary to prevent recurrences. Severe or unresponsive cases require referral to a dermatologist.

BIBLIOGRAPHY

Arndt KA, Robinson JK, LeBoit PE, et al: *Cutaneous Medicine and Surgery.* Philadelphia, Saunders, 1996.

DuVivier A: *Dermatology in Practice.* Philadelphia, Lippincott, Gower, 1990.

Fitzpatrick TB, Johnson RA, Polano MK, et al: *Color Atlas and Synopsis of Clinical Dermatology: Common and Serious Diseases,* 3d ed. New York, McGraw-Hill, 1997.

Goldstein BG, Goldstein AO: *Practical Dermatology,* Primary Care Series. St. Louis, Mosby Year Book, 1992

Shelley WB, Shelley ED: *Advanced Dermatologic Diagnosis.* Philadelphia, Saunders, 1992.

Weinberg S, Prose NS, Kristal L: *Color Atlas of Pediatric Dermatology,* 3d ed. New York, McGraw-Hill, 1998.

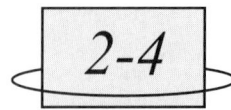

ALOPECIA AREATA
Joe R. Monroe

DISCUSSION

Alopecia areata (AA) is a localized, sharply defined loss of hair in round or oval areas without visible inflammation or significant skin symptoms. Thought to be an autoimmune disease, this condition may occur on any hair-bearing surface of the body and may progress to total scalp and brow hair loss (alopecia totalis) or even total loss of body hair (alopecia universalis).

Typically affecting younger adults and children, AA is not a sign of multisystem disease but may be associated with other autoimmune diseases, such as vitiligo and Hashimoto's thyroiditis, and can be brought on by emotional stress.

DIFFERENTIAL DIAGNOSIS

The differential diagnosis includes tinea capitis (which probably will demonstrate scaling and inflammation, may be potassium hydroxide (KOH)-positive, and may fluoresce) and secondary syphilis [appearance of moth-eaten patches in scalp or beard, with positive VDRL (Venereal Disease Research Laboratories test)]. The lack of scaling, redness, and sharply demarcated loss of hair usually make AA easy to distinguish from these other conditions.

LABORATORY

Punch biopsy shows infiltrates of mononuclear cells around hair bulbs, a fact that often is useful in establishing the correct diagnosis. Other laboratory tests can be obtained to rule out coexistent autoimmune diseases such as Hashimoto's thyroiditis (thyroid function tests), lupus erythematosus [antinuclear antibodies (ANA)], pernicious anemia [complete blood count (CBC), iron studies], and syphilis (VDRL).

TREATMENT

Treatment for AA is unsatisfactory. For small, solitary spots, intralesional triamcinolone acetonide 5 to 10 mg/cm^3 is temporarily very effective. No treatment has been shown to alter the ultimate course of this disease. Avoid systemic corticosteroids since any benefit inevitably will be lost upon discontinuing the drug.

PATIENT EDUCATION

Reassure the patient about the usually self-limiting nature of the disease. In severe disease, patients may require counseling to share their feelings about having permanent hair loss.

PEARLS

Knowledge of the following points can contribute to a positive patient outcome:

- Sharply demarcated total hair loss in a round configuration without epidermal skin changes (redness, scaling, etc.) is probably alopecia areata.
- There is no good evidence that treatment induces remission or affects the permanent course of the disease.
- Among all the indicators for a poor prognosis, onset at an early age is the most reliable, with involvement of occipital scalp being the next most reliable.

PROGNOSIS

The majority of AA patients recover without any treatment within 9 months. Predictors of a poor or guarded prognosis are onset at an early age, multiple patches, occipital hair loss, loss of eyebrow and eyelash hair, a history of previous attacks, associated atopic disease, and alopecia totalis/universalis.

BIBLIOGRAPHY

Arndt KA, Robinson JK, LeBoit PE, et al: *Cutaneous Medicine and Surgery.* Philadelphia, Saunders, 1996.

DuVivier A: *Dermatology in Practice.* Philadelphia, Lippincott, 1990.

Fitzpatrick TB, Johnson RA, Polano MK, et al: *Color Atlas and Synopsis of Clinical Dermatology: Common and Serious Diseases,* 3d ed. New York, McGraw-Hill, 1997.

Goldstein GB, Goldstein AO: *Practical Dermatology,* Primary Care Series. St Louis, Mosby Year Book, 1992.

Shelly WB, Shelly ED: *Advanced Dermatologic Diagnosis.* Philadelphia, Saunders, 1992.

Weinberg S, Prose NS, Kristal L: *Color Atlas of Pediatric Dermatology,* 3d ed. New York, McGraw-Hill, 1998.

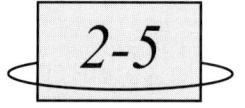

ARTHROPOD INFESTATIONS
Michelle DiBaise

DISCUSSION

Pediculosis Capitis (*Pediculus humanus* var. *capitis*): Head Lice

The head louse infests the scalp and neck of humans, most commonly at the occiput and postauricular areas but rarely in the beard or other hairy sites.[1-4] The louse deposits eggs, or "nits," on the emerging hair shaft. Head lice can occur in any age group but most commonly occur in school-age children. This condition is more common in whites and females than it is in others.[1-4] Head lice are not confined to any socioeconomic group and are not related to a patient's hygiene. The head louse can be transmitted via shared brushes, combs, hats, or bedding in addition to head-to-head contact.

Pediculosis Corporis (*Pediculus humanus* var. *corporis*): Body Lice

The body louse infests the hair-bearing surfaces of the body but lives and lays nits predominantly in the seams of clothing. It is relatively uncommon among affluent populations and is related to poor patient hygiene.[2-4] Unlike other lice, pediculosis corporis is a vector of diseases such as trench fever (*Rickettsia quintana*), typhus (*R. prowazekii*), and relapsing fever (*Borrelia recurrentis*).[2-4]

Pediculosis Pubis (*Phthirus pubis*): Pubic Lice, or Crabs

The pubic louse is the smallest of the lice species. It is found only on the human host and most commonly infests the hair-bearing areas of the pubic region but may infest the hair of the chest, axillae, eyebrows, and eyelashes.[1-4] Pubic lice occur in all age groups but are most common in young adults, being more commonly found in males.[1-4] This condition is spread by close contact, including sexual intercourse, sleeping in the same bed, and possibly sharing articles of clothing. Pubic lice are one of the most contagious sexually transmitted diseases.[2-4]

Scabies (*Sarcoptes scabiei*): Scabies

Sarcoptes scabiei is a mite that infests the skin. The female mite burrows into the stratum corneum about 2 to 3 mm over a 24-h period, usually at night, and lays eggs during the day.[1,3,4] She deposits fecal pellets, or scybala, in the burrow behind her. Scabies occurs in all age groups but is more common in children under 5 years, the institutionalized, and young adults, who often acquire the mites through sexual contact.[1,3,4] Scabies is transmitted by skin-to-skin contact but also by contact with infested bedding or clothing, since the mite can remain alive for more than 2 days after leaving the human host.

SIGNS AND SYMPTOMS

Pediculosis Capitis, Pediculosis Corporis, Pediculosis Pubis

The presenting complaint of the patient is pruritus of the infested area of the body. However, a patient with pubic lice may be asymptomatic. There also may be a complaint of nodularity of the pubic hairs.

Scabies

The first infestation of the scabies mite requires an incubation of 1 month before the onset of pruritus. This is due to the development of a hypersensitivity reaction to the mite. With recurrent infestations, pruritus will begin within 24 h. The pruritus is often described as generalized, intense, and intractable and may be disproportionate to the number of lesions. It often wakes the patient at night and generally spares the head and neck in adults. Frequently, other family members and close contacts complain of pruritus.

OBJECTIVE FINDINGS

Pediculosis Capitis

PRIMARY INFESTATION   In a majority of patients, there are only about 10 lice present, and they are rarely seen.[1,4] The nits are oval grayish-white capsules approximately 1 mm in length and are firmly cemented to the hairs (see Fig. 2-5-1 and Plate 2). New viable nits have a creamy yellow color, whereas empty nits are white.[1–4]

SECONDARY LESIONS   Excoriations, crusts, and impetiginized lesions commonly result from scratching and can potentially mask the presence of lice and nits. Secondary lesions may extend onto the neck, forehead, face, and ears. In severe cases, the hair can become matted with lice, nits, crusts, and purulent discharge. With secondary infection, there also may be associated occipital and/or cervical lymphadenopathy.

Pediculosis Corporis

PRIMARY INFESTATION   The host almost always has poor hygiene. Body lice visit the host only to feed; therefore, nits and lice are observed in the seams of clothing (see Fig. 2-5-2 and Plate 3). Sites of feeding may present as red macules or papules.

SECONDARY LESIONS   Primary lesions are commonly excoriated. In atopic individuals, an eczematous dermatitis can develop. These secondary lesions are commonly impetiginized. There also may be associated regional adenopathy present.

Pediculosis Pubis

PRIMARY INFESTATION   Pubic lice appear as 1- to 2-mm brownish gray specks in the involved hairy areas.[1–4] They are usually few in number. The nits appear as tiny white-gray specks. They can be few to numerous and appear initially at the hair-skin junction, predominantly in the pubic area and axillae but may be present on the perineum, thighs, lower legs, trunk, and periumbilical area. In hairy males, they may be found in the nipple areas and upper arms and rarely the wrists, beard, and mustache area. In children they can appear on the eyelashes and eyebrows and may not have pubic involvement (see Fig. 2-5-3 and Plate 4).[1–4] Eyelash infestation may be a sign of childhood sexual abuse.

SECONDARY LESIONS   Red macules or papules may be seen at sites of feeding, especially the periumbilical region. Rarely, the feeding sites become bullous. With scratching, secondary changes of lichenification and excoriations are common. These lesions can become impetiginized and lead to inguinal lymphadenopathy.

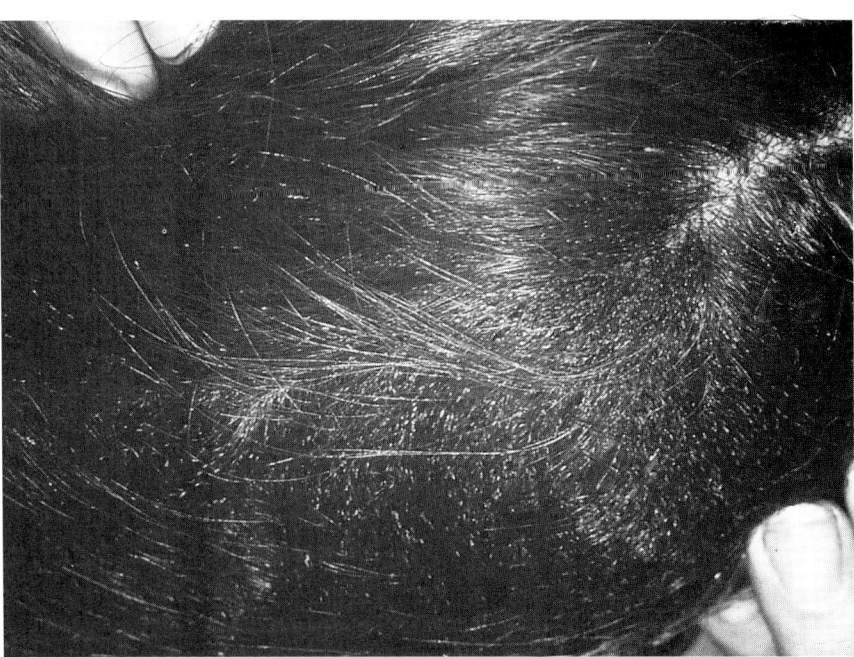

FIGURE 2-5-1 (PLATE 2). Nits. (*From Fitzpatrick, Johnson, Wolff, et al.*[1])

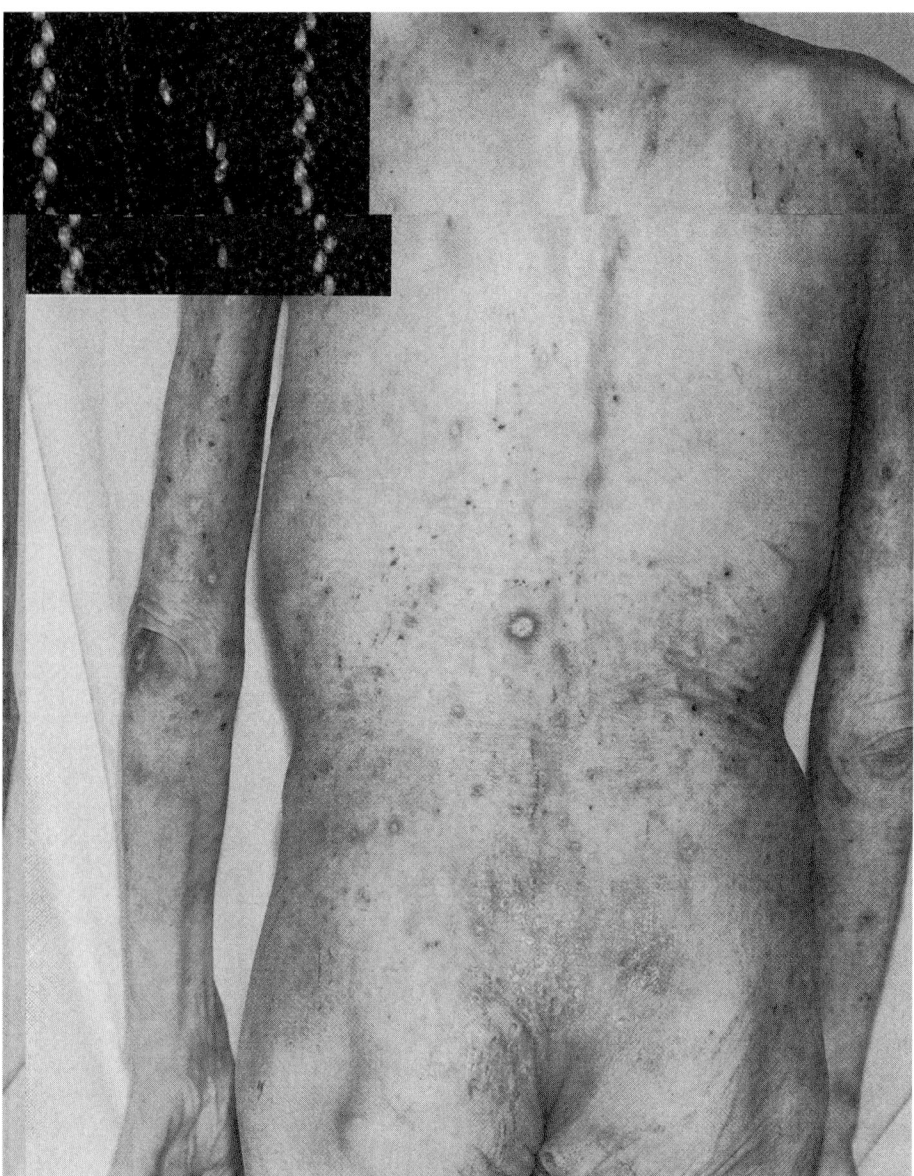

FIGURE 2-5-2 (PLATE 3). Pediculosis corporis. (*From Fitzpatrick, Johnson, Wolff, et al.*[1])

Scabies

PRIMARY INFESTATION   Burrows are in areas with few or no hair follicles where the stratum corneum is thin, such as the interdigital web spaces, wrists, elbows, buttocks, and axillae. In men, the penis and scrotum are usually involved, and in women, the breast, especially the areola and nipple, may be infested (see Fig. 2-5-4).

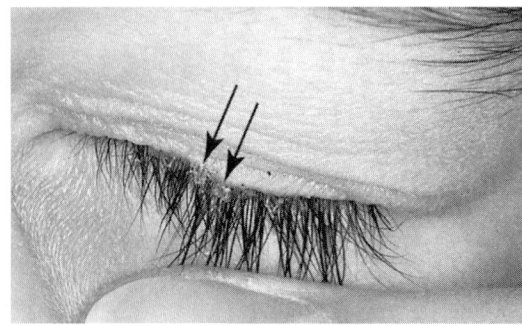

FIGURE 2-5-3 (PLATE 4). Pediculosis palpebrum. (*From Fitzpatrick, Robinson, Wolff, et al.*[1])

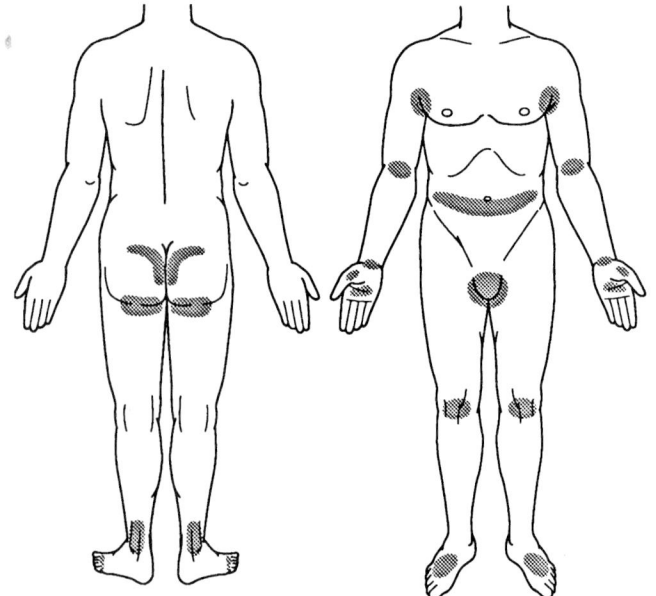

FIGURE 2-5-4. Distribution of scabies. (*Courtesy of Michelle DiBaise.*)

FIGURE 2-5-5 (PLATE 5). Nodular scabies. (*From Fitzpatrick, Johnson, Wolff, et al.*[1])

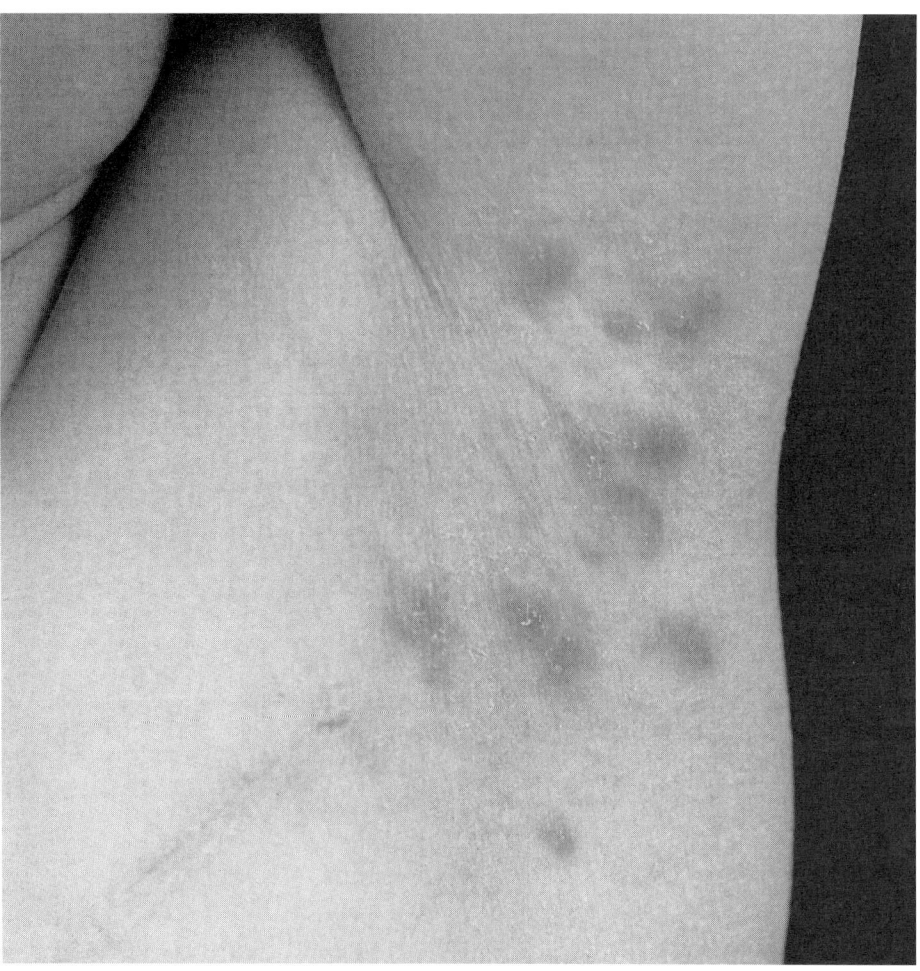

The burrow appears as gray or skin-colored ridges 0.2 to 10 cm in length, linear, curved, or S-shaped with a pinpoint vesicle, papule, and/or halo of erythema at the end of the burrow.[1–4] The mite may appear as a black speck at the end of the burrow.

The patient can develop signs of a hypersensitivity reaction, including pruritus and generalized small urticarial papules predominantly on the anterior trunk, thighs, buttocks, and forearms. In atopic individuals, an eczematous dermatitis can develop at the sites of infestation. With chronic scratching, multiple excoriations are commonly seen. In severe hypersensitivity reactions, the patient can become erythrodermic. Signs of secondary infection include impetiginization, ecthyma, folliculitis, abscess formation, lymphadenitis, and cellulitis

Nodular scabies is a variant that has been noted to develop in 7 to 10 percent of patients with scabies.[1–4] The nodules range from 5 to 20 mm in diameter and are pink, red, tan, or brown in color.[1–4] An early nodule may have a burrow noted on the surface (see Fig. 2-5-5 and Plate 5).

Norwegian, or crusted, scabies is another variant seen in immunocompromised persons or individuals with neurologic or mental disorders. Crusted scabies appears as well-demarcated markedly hyperkeratotic and/or crusted plaques. Itching may be absent or severe. It can begin as ordinary scabies or present initially with asymptomatic crusting. The distribution can be generalized, even involving the head and neck in adults, or it can be localized (see Fig. 2-5-6 and Plate 6).

Scabies in infants often is misdiagnosed because it can differ from adult infestations. In infants, there is often head and neck involvement. Infants may have multiple vesicles or pustules on the palms and soles. Nodules are seen in the axillae, the diaper area, and the lateral edge of the foot. Secondary eczematization and impetiginization are common and obscure the primary lesions (see Fig. 2-5-7 and Plate 7).

SECONDARY LESIONS Secondary lesions are common and result from scratching. Secondary lesions include pinpoint erosions, excoriations, eczematous dermatitis, and lichen simplex chronicus. With secondary infection, pustules may be seen as well as impetiginization. There also may be associated regional lymphadenopathy.

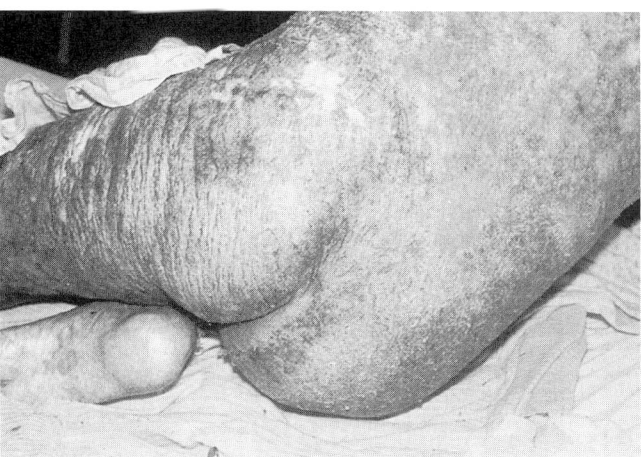

FIGURE 2-5-6 (PLATE 6). Crusted scabies. (*From Fitzpatrick, Johnson, Wolff, et al.*[1])

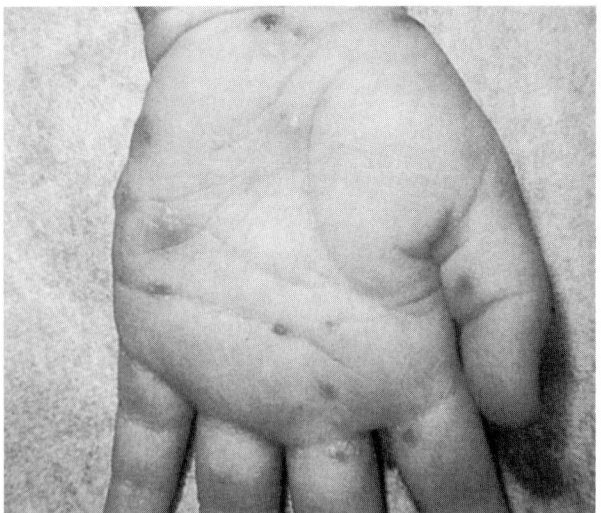

FIGURE 2-5-7 (PLATE 7). Scabies in infants. (*Courtesy of Ramon Fusaro.*)

DIAGNOSTIC CONSIDERATIONS

Pediculosis Capitis

The differential diagnosis of head lice includes the use of hair sprays and gels as well as seborrheic dermatitis (dandruff). These, however, are easily removed, whereas nits are firmly cemented and are difficult to remove.

Pediculosis Corporis

The differential diagnosis of body lice includes eczema, folliculitis, and lichen simplex chronicus.

Pediculosis Pubis

The differential diagnosis of pubic lice includes eczema, seborrheic dermatitis, tinea cruris, folliculitis, and molluscum contagiosum.

Scabies

The differential diagnosis of pruritus in scabies includes a cutaneous drug reaction, eczema, contact dermatitis, urticaria, pediculosis corporis or pubis, lichen planus, delusions of parasitosis, and metabolic pruritus. The differential diagnosis for nodular scabies includes urticaria pigmentosa (in young children), papular urticaria, Darier's disease, prurigo nodularis, and secondary syphilis. The differential diagnosis for crusted scabies includes psoriasis, eczematous dermatitis, and seborrheic dermatitis.

LABORATORY TESTS

Pediculosis Capitis and Pediculosis Corporis

On microscopy, the nits are oval, whitish eggs. A Wood's lamp examination will fluoresce live nits a pearly color but will not fluoresce dead nits. The louse is a wingless insect with six legs 1 to 4 mm in length and a translucent grayish-white body.[1-4] The louse becomes red or rust-colored when it is engorged with blood (see Fig. 2-5-8).

Pediculosis Pubis

On microscopy, the pubic louse has a short oval body and prominent claws resembling those of sea crabs (see Fig. 2-5-9).[1-4] Bacterial cultures should be considered if lesions appear secondarily infected. Patients should be questioned about risk factors for other sexually transmitted diseases.

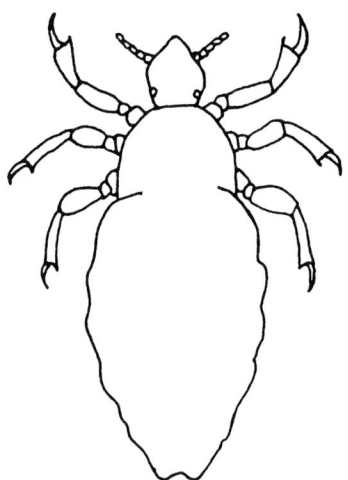

FIGURE 2-5-8. Body louse. (*Courtesy of Wendy Brunsman.*)

Scabies

A healthy adult has 6 to 10 mites infesting the body.[1-4] Therefore, it may be difficult to find a mite on skin scraping. The best yield is from a burrow on the finger web spaces, the volar aspect of the wrists, or the penis. To identify a burrow, place a drop of blue or black ink on the skin. The burrow will absorb the ink and be highlighted as a dark line. The surface ink is removed with an alcohol pad. A drop of mineral oil is placed over a burrow, and the burrow is scraped with a no. 15 blade. The scraping is placed on a microscope slide with a drop of mineral oil on it. It is diagnostic if the mite, eggs, or fecal pellets (scybala) are seen. The female mite is 0.3 mm long with a flattened oval body and eight legs, and the eggs are ovoid brown capsules (see Fig. 2-5-10).[1-4] Scybala are dark masses and are smaller than the eggs (see Fig. 2-5-11 and Plate 8).

TREATMENT

A hot, soapy bath is contraindicated before the application of any of these agents, since moisture increases the permeability of the epidermis and increases the chance for systemic absorption.[1-4] Sex partners and close personal or household contacts within the last month should be treated even if they are asymptomatic.

Pediculosis Capitis, Pediculosis Corporis, and Pediculosis Pubis

Permethrin 1% cream rinse (Nix) is applied to the affected areas and washed off after 10 min. It has less potential for toxicity in the event of inappropriate use. Pyrethrins with piperonyl butoxide are not completely ovicidal. Pyrethrins (RID, A-200, R&C) are applied to the affected areas and washed off after 10 min.

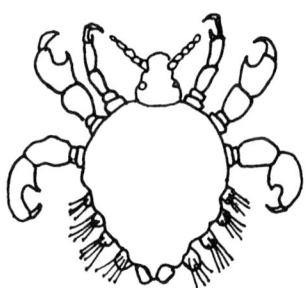

FIGURE 2-5-9. Pubic louse. (*Courtesy of Wendy Brunsman.*)

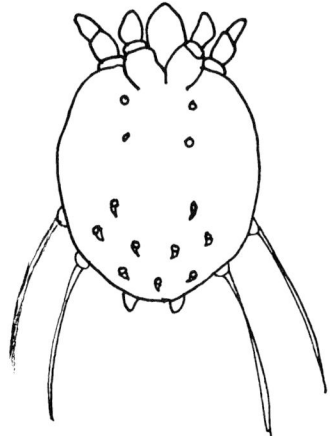

FIGURE 2-5-10. Scabies mite. (*Courtesy of Wendy Brunsman.*)

Lindane 1% shampoo, lotion, or cream (Kwell) is applied to the affected area and then thoroughly washed off after 4 min. Seizures and neurotoxicity in infants have occurred with the improper use of lindane.[1–4] Aplastic anemia also has been reported.[1–4] Lindane therefore is not recommended for pregnant or lactating women, children under 2 years of age, and individuals with extensive dermatitis. Lindane is the least expensive therapy.

Malathion 0.5% lotion (Ovide) is used for head lice. It is applied to the scalp for 8 to 12 h and then thoroughly washed off, after which the nits are removed with a comb. The treatment can be repeated in 7 to 9 days. It is not recommended for infants and neonates. Malathion was on the market in the past but was removed as a result of market failure, most likely because of the odor, flammability, and length of application time. It is an irreversible cholinesterase inhibitor but has no reported systemic adverse effects.[5] Because of its flammability, avoid its use near heat sources such as hair dryers and open flames. It

is rapidly ovicidal and pediculicidal in vitro, killing 100 percent of lice within 5 min and 95 percent of eggs within 10 min.[6] The application of petrolatum or another occlusive ophthalmic ointment to the eyelashes bid for 8 to 10 days or tid for 5 days should treat pediculosis palpebra. Alternatives include physostigmine ophthalmic preparations applied bid for 1 or 2 days, baby shampoo applied with a cotton swab tid for 5 days, and fluorescein drops.

Once treatment is complete, the nits must be removed with a tweezers or a fine-toothed nit comb. White vinegar on the hair for 15 min may loosen the nits and facilitate removal.

Because the incubation period of louse eggs is 6 to 10 days, the agents should be reapplied in 7 to 14 days.[1–4] Secondary bacterial infections generally are caused by *Staphylococcus aureus* or group A beta-hemolytic *Streptococcus* and should be treated with appropriate doses of erythromycin, dicloxacillin, topical mupirocin, or another effective antibiotic.

Scabies

For all agents, infants and young children should be treated on all body areas, including the head and neck, and patients with a relapse also should be treated from head to toe. Reapply any agent to the hands if the hands are washed. The nails should be cut short, and medication should be applied under them vigorously with a toothbrush.

Permethrin cream 5% (Elimite) has low toxicity. It is applied to all areas of the body from the chin down and is washed off after 8 to 14 h.

Lindane 1% lotion, cream, or shampoo is applied thinly to all areas of the body from the chin down and is washed off thoroughly, adults after 12 h and infants after 8 h. Resistance to this agent has been reported.[1–4,7,8] Infants should have lindane applied during the day and be fully clothed and observed to prevent licking of treated sites. If licking cannot be prevented, sulfur or permethrin should be used. With lindane, a repeated dose should be applied 1 week after the first treatment.

FIGURE 2-5-11 (PLATE 8). Burrow with scabies mite, eggs, and scybala (feces). (*From Fitzpatrick, Johnson. Wolff. et al.*[1])

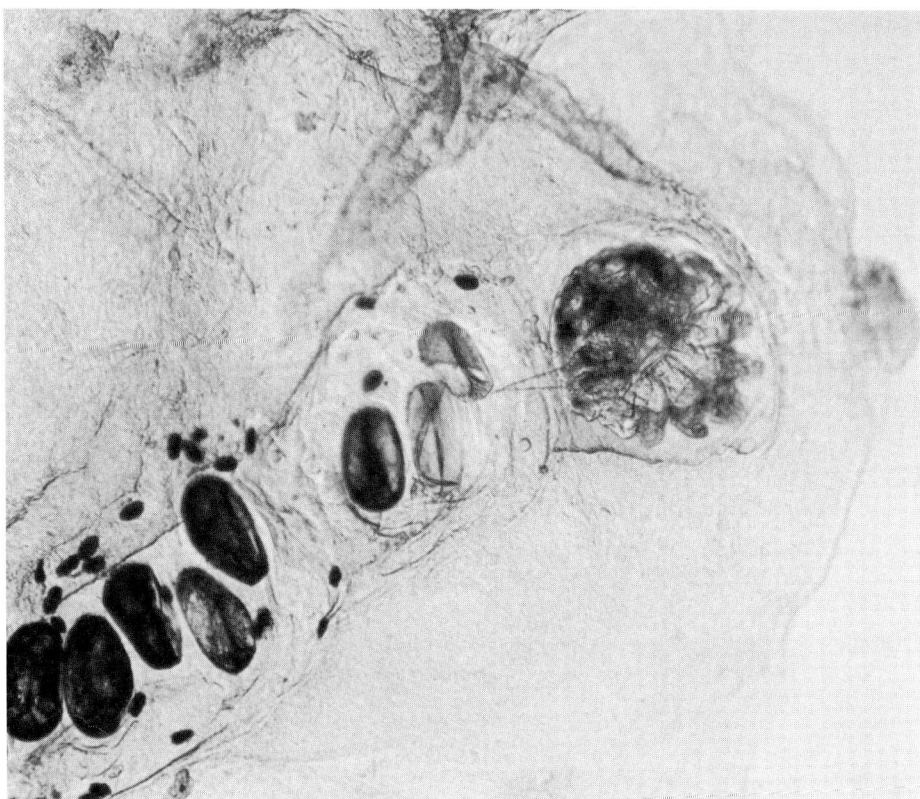

Crotamiton cream 10% (Eurax lotion) is applied thinly to the entire body from the chin down nightly for two consecutive nights and is washed off 24 h after the second application. The toxicity of crotamiton is unknown.

Sulfur ointment 6 to 10% in petrolatum or cold cream is applied to the entire body from the chin down for 2 to 3 days. The patient bathes 24 h after each application. These preparations are messy, have an unpleasant odor, stain, and cause dryness. The safety of topical sulfur has never been tested.

The pruritus often persists up to several weeks after successful eradication of mite infestation because it is a hypersensitivity reaction to the mite antigens. The pruritus can be treated with antihistamines such as hydroxyzine (Atarax) and diphenhydramine (Benadryl), topical corticosteroid ointments, and in severe cases a tapered course of prednisone for 1 to 2 weeks.

Scabetic nodules may persist for up to a year. Intralesional triamcinolone 5 to 10 mg/mL into each lesion is effective. In crusted scabies, a single application of a scabicide kills 90 to 95 percent of mites.[1,2,4] Multiple applications may be required, and in an HIV-infected individual eradication may be impossible. Ivermectin in a 200-μg/kg PO one-time dose is reported to be effective for crusted scabies in immunocompromised hosts.[1,2,4,9] The associated pruritus is rapidly controlled. Patients with thick, crusted lesions do better with a combination of ivermectin and a topical treatment such as permethrin cream.[9]

Secondary infections should be treated with mupirocin ointment or appropriate systemic antimicrobial agents that cover *Staphylococcus* and group A *Streptococcus*.

PATIENT EDUCATION

Patients should avoid contact with possibly contaminated items such as hats, headsets, clothing, towels, combs, hairbrushes, bedding, and upholstery. Bedding, linen, clothing, and headgear should be washed and dried on the hot cycle or removed from body contact for 72 h. Combs and brushes should be soaked in rubbing alcohol or Lysol 2% solution for 1 h. The environment should be vacuumed. Otherwise, coats, furniture, rugs, floors, and walls do not need to be cleaned in any special manner.

FOLLOW-UP

Patients should be evaluated after 1 week if symptoms persist. Subsequent treatments may be necessary if lice or nits are observed at the hair-skin junction or if mites and eggs are observed on repeat skin scraping. Patients who do not respond to one regimen should be re-treated with an alternative.

COMPLICATIONS AND RED FLAGS

Acute streptococcal glomerulonephritis has been reported to follow group A beta-hemolytic *Streptococcus* secondary infections of the skin.[1-4] Bacteremia and death have been reported after secondary *S. aureus* infection of crusted scabies in an HIV-infected individual.[1,4] Therefore, symptoms consistent with glomerulonephritis or bacteremia should be treated aggressively, especially in the presence of immunodeficiency.

REFERENCES

1. Fitzpatrick TB, Johnson RA, Wolff K, et al: *Color Atlas and Synopsis of Clinical Dermatology: Common and Serious Diseases.* New York, McGraw-Hill, 1997, pp 836–849.
2. Habif TP: *Clinical Dermatology: A Color Guide to Diagnosis and Treatment,* 3d ed. St. Louis, Mosby Yearbook, 1996, pp 445–456.
3. Arnold HL, Odom RB, James WD: *Andrews' Diseases of the Skin: Clinical Dermatology,* 8th ed. Philadelphia, Saunders, 1990, pp 512–515, 523–527.
4. Orkin M, Maibach HI: Scabies and pediculosis, in Fitzpatrick TB, Freedberg IM, Eisen AZ, et al (eds): *Dermatology in General Medicine,* 5th ed. New York, McGraw-Hill, 1993, pp 2677–2684.
5. *The Medical Letter on Drugs and Therapeutics,* vol. 41, issue 1059, The Medical Letter, Inc, August 1999.
6. Meinking TL, Taplin D, Kalter DC, et al: Comparative efficacy of treatmets for pediculosis capitis infestations. *Arch Dermatol* 122(3):267–271, 1986.
7. Purvis RS, Tyring SK: An outbreak of lindane-resistant scabies treated successfully with permethrin 5% cream. *J Am Acad Dermatol* 25:1015–1016, 1991.
8. Judd LE: Gamma benzene hexachloride resistant scabies. *N Z Med J* 106:61–63, 1993.
9. Meinking TL: The treatment of scabies with ivermectin. *N Engl J Med.* 333:26–30, 1995.

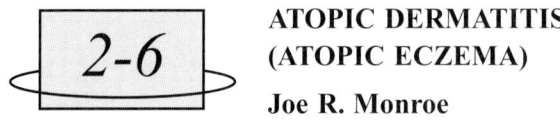

2-6 ATOPIC DERMATITIS (ATOPIC ECZEMA)
Joe R. Monroe

DEFINITION

Atopic dermatitis is a pruritic inflammation of the dermis and epidermis that frequently is associated with a personal or family history of hay fever, asthma, allergic rhinitis, or atopic dermatitis.

CLINICAL DISCUSSION

Atopic dermatitis (AD) is an IgE-mediated papulosquamous process with typical onset in the first 2 months of life, or by the end of the first year in 60 percent of patients, with a highly variable course after that time. It sometimes persists into adulthood and occasionally (fewer than 10 percent of patients) begins in adulthood; the sine qua non is pruritus, fueling an itch-scratch-itch cycle and manifesting as a symmetric papulosquamous patchy rash in flexural locations in adults (antecubital, popliteal, and neck, among others). In contrast, infantile AD tends to be more papulovesicular and affects facial and extensor skin as well as the locations involved in adult AD. Itching in AD is triggered by contact with wool, detergents, soaps, sweating, and stress but primarily by the act of scratching itself.

Associated clinical findings include xerosis, ichthyosis vulgaris, pigmentary changes (hypo- and/or hyperpigmentation), eye changes (cataracts, keratoconus), periorbital skin changes (scaling of lid skin, allergic shiners), and hand and foot dermatitis. Complications include increased colonization of affected skin with *Staphylococcus aureus,* which can trigger attacks; increased susceptibility to viral infections of the skin such as warts, molluscum, and herpes; increased susceptibility to fungal infections, especially in the hands and feet; generalized exfoliative erythroderma; mental or emotional dysfunction; and growth retardation.

Among the complications of AD, the most feared is the development of disseminated herpes (or, rarely, vaccinia) infection of AD-involved skin, called eczema herpeticum or Kaposi's varicelliform eruption, which can occur even in patients in AD remission. The virus colonizes eczematous and noneczematous skin, leading to a widespread eruption of discrete, tense vesicles surrounded by erythema. The patient may therefore be extremely ill and probably will require parenteral acyclovir. Atopic patients therefore should be advised to avoid individuals with an active herpes simplex infection.

DIFFERENTIAL DIAGNOSIS

In infants, seborrheic dermatitis (SD) can resemble AD but differs significantly in the following ways:

- AD itches, whereas SD is nonpruritic.
- AD is chronic, whereas SD lasts approximately 6 weeks.

- With AD there is usually a definite family history of atopy, whereas with SD there is none.
- SD involves the axillae and diaper area, areas seldom involved in AD.

Other common conditions mimicking AD include contact dermatitis and scabies. Certain rare metabolic disorders also can mimic AD and should be considered. These include gluten enteropathy, acrodermatitis enteropathica, glucagonoma syndrome, and phenylketonuria.

LABORATORY

Biopsy can be helpful in ruling out other conditions but is not pathognomonic for AD. Serum levels of IgE are often elevated, but not consistently enough to be helpful. Culture for herpes simplex virus (HSV) where indicated.

TREATMENT

The goals of treatment of AD are to (1) hydrate the skin, (2) identify and eliminate triggers, (3) decrease pruritus and inflammation, and (4) educate patients and their families about the nature of AD.

For children especially, worsening of AD can be related to stress, and so education of parents and patients is crucial. For example, they must understand that no treatment course, however carefully devised, can be effective if the problems of xerosis (dry skin) and scratching are not addressed.

To that end, hydration of the skin is a key element, especially after bathing, while the skin is still moist, using white petrolatum or products such as Eucerin cream and 12% ammonium lactate lotion (Lac Hydrin) but avoiding common hand lotions, especially those with artificial scent or color. The use of alkaline soaps in bathing should be kept to a minimum because of their drying effects.

AD patients are susceptible to all skin infections but especially to *S. aureus,* which can colonize or even mildly infect involved skin, producing minimal indications of overt infection but providing a powerful pruritic trigger. In fact, often the only sign is either a flare of AD or unresponsiveness to the usual AD treatments. A short course of oral antibiotics (erythromycin, dicloxacillin, or cephalosporin) and/or topical application of antibacterial ointment (mupirocin, bacitracin, or Polysporin) can make a dramatic difference.

Other triggers for AD flares include exposure to irritants such as sweat; environmental irritants, especially on the job (solvents, cleansers, etc.); or true allergens (airborne or food). Even though AD is not caused by a specific allergen, ongoing exposure to dust mites or seasonal allergens, for example, can be a key factor and needs to be identified and eliminated if possible.

Topical steroid use has revolutionized AD treatment, but there are potential problems with these drugs. Dermal atrophy and striae formation are caused by prolonged application and/or failure to match the concentration of the steroid preparation to the area being treated. The latter is particularly true of thin-skinned areas such as the face (especially the lids) and genitals but also applies to intertriginous skin, that is, skin that is rubbed or covered by adjacent skin, as in the axillae, groin, and intergluteal area. Systemic steroids seldom are indicated in AD patients because (1) they can be used for only brief periods (1 to 3 weeks), (2) potential side effects, especially in children, are numerous and potentially severe, and (3) withdrawal of the patient from oral corticosteroids can result in a dramatic rebound of AD. If the disease is unresponsive to routine therapy, referral to a dermatologist should be seriously considered.

Tar preparations were the mainstay of treatment for AD before the introduction of topical steroids in 1952, and even though tar's mode of action is not known, it is a potent anti-inflammatory, steroid-sparing topical agent. Commercial preparations such as Estar Gel and PsoriGel are available by prescription, or a pharmacist can compound a wide variety of tar-plus-ointment combinations.

The dermatologist to whom a physician assistant may refer more difficult patients has a wide variety of treatment modalities to choose from, including phototherapy, interferon gamma, cyclosporine, and thymopentin, among others, but referral has other values: (1) Seeing a dermatologist can be very reassuring to patients and their families. (2) As the primary care provider, a physician assistant can learn more about the management of AD from the dermatologist after following up on the referral. (3) The correct diagnosis can be confirmed or other diagnoses in the differential can be considered, since the diagnosis of AD is not always straightforward, sometimes requiring extraordinary expertise.

PATIENT EDUCATION

The following items can contribute to a positive patient outcome:

1. Encourage the parents and siblings to discuss any anxiety or feelings of aggression about having a child with AD.
2. Educate parents about increased anxiety in an affected child and how it can manifest through increased scratching that will worsen the disease.
3. Tell parents and siblings that frequent affectionate touching of atopic infants and young children not only will not hurt the child but will help alleviate anxiety for both the parents and the child.
4. Teach the parents that AD is a chronic, recurring condition that requires daily attention with lubricating lotions; avoidance of wool products, lanolin-containing creams, and other triggers; and adherence to treatment schedules with steroids, tar preparations, and others, with instructions given in writing.
5. Educate parents about the necessity for antibiotic therapy with flares or failure to respond to the usual treatments.
6. Explain how and why AD patients should not be exposed to the herpes simplex virus because of the risk of eczema herpeticum.

PROGNOSIS

Spontaneous resolution of AD frequently occurs during childhood but with occasional, more severe recurrences during adolescence. In most patients, the disease lasts 15 to 20 years.

BIBLIOGRAPHY

Arndt KA, Robinson JK, LeBoit PE, et al: *Cutaneous Medicine and Surgery.* Philadelphia, Saunders, 1996.
DuVivier A: *Dermatology in Practice.* Philadelphia, Lippincott, 1990.
Fitzpatrick TB, Johnson RA, Polano MK, et al: *Color Atlas and Synopsis of Clinical Dermatology: Common and Serious Diseases,* 3d ed. New York, McGraw-Hill, 1997.
Goldstein BG, Goldstein AO: *Practical Dermatology,* Primary Care Series. St Louis, Mosby Year Book, 1992.
Shelley WB, Shelley ED: *Advanced Dermatologic Diagnosis.* Philadelphia, Saunders, 1992.
Weinberg S, Prose NS, Kristal L: *Color Atlas of Pediatric Dermatology,* 3d ed. New York, McGraw-Hill, 1998.

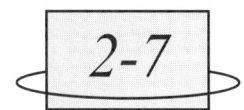

BASAL CELL CARCINOMA
Barbara L. Sauls

DESCRIPTION

Basal cell carcinoma (BCC) is the most common type of skin cancer and arises from the epidermal basal cells. These lesions are slow-growing, rarely metastasize, and are relatively easy to treat. The incidence of this cancer has risen over the years, particularly in the increasing aged population. Men have a higher incidence of basal cell carcinoma than

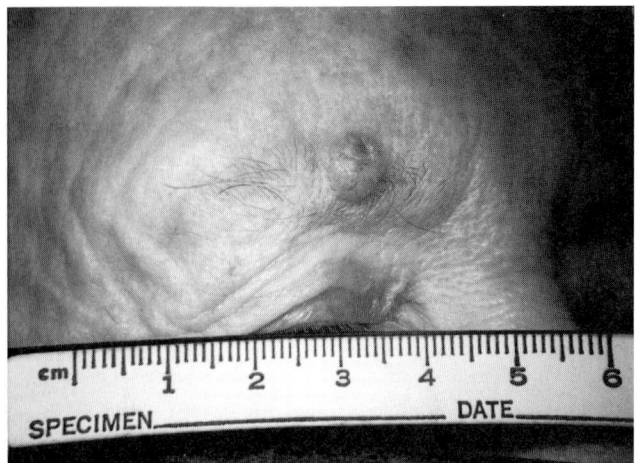

FIGURE 2-7-1 (PLATE 9). Classic presentation of nodular basal cell carcinoma. Note the small area of ulceration in the upper part of the lesion. (*Courtesy of Harold Milstein, MD, The Dermatology Center, Hazleton, PA.*)

do women, though the difference is decreasing. Risk factors include light-skinned persons, people with poor tanning capacity, previous x-ray therapy (such as for acne or cancer), occupations that require extensive exposure to the sun such as road workers and farmers, and increasing age. The most frequently affected skin areas are those exposed to the sun. Brown or black skin is protective.

SIGNS AND SYMPTOMS

The classic presentation of basal cell carcinoma is as a *nonhealing papule, asymptomatic nodule,* or *ulcer.* BCCs present less often in other forms, such as a scarlike lesion or flat scaly patches that often are misdiagnosed as a fungal infection and even as a deeply pigmented brown-to-black papule (see Fig. 2-7-1 and Plate 9).

OBJECTIVE FINDINGS

Physical examination reveals an isolated, elevated, firm papular or nodular area that often has a central depression. Lesions are round or oval with borders that are described as rolled in appearance. The lesion often looks "pearly" and may be black, red, or pink. Ulcerated lesions may develop that often have a crusting over them and also have

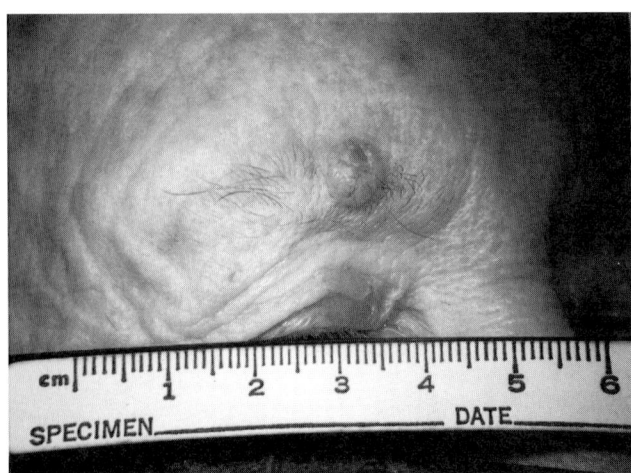

FIGURE 2-7-2 (PLATE 10). Small telangiectasias on left side of basal cell carcinoma. (*Courtesy of Harold Milstein, MD, The Dermatology Center, Hazleton, PA.*)

an elevated border; they are referred to as *rodent ulcers.* Close inspection may reveal telangiectasias over the surface of the BCC, which is often a useful diagnostic feature (see Fig. 2-7-2 and Plate 10).

DIAGNOSTIC CONSIDERATIONS

Nonulcerated nodular lesions look like dermal nevi or cysts but feel firmer.

LABORATORY TESTS

The diagnosis of BCC is made by means of shave or punch biopsy or excision.

TREATMENT

Eradication of BCC is best produced by surgical excision. Alternative therapies include cryotherapy, laser therapy, radiation therapy, and electrodesiccation. Topical chemotherapy may be used as well as intralesional interferon. The cure rate is high unless the lesions have been neglected and have deeply eroded. Excision in this case often produces a poor cosmetic result.

PATIENT EDUCATION

Patients must be counseled on the use of sunscreens and wide-brimmed hats, covering the arms and legs when outside, avoidance of the sun from 10 A.M. until 2 P.M., and avoidance of tanning salons.

DISPOSITION

Routine skin examination by a medical practitioner should be done on a regular basis, paying special attention to the face, ears, and neck. This examination should be performed every 6 months to 1 year for 5 years after a diagnosis of BCC. Patients should be instructed to report any nonhealing or new lesions. These lesions should be examined and possibly biopsied as soon as they are noted.

CONSIDERATIONS

Dermatologists best manage skin cancers. The initial biopsy may be done in the family practice office, but it is also appropriate to send the patient to the dermatologist for this initial biopsy. An excisional biopsy can be performed at this initial visit.

BIBLIOGRAPHY

Fauci AS, Braunwald E, Isselbacher KJ, et al (eds): *Harrison's Principles of Internal Medicine,* 14th ed. New York, McGraw-Hill, 1998.
Fitzpatrick TB, Johnson RA, Wolff K, et al: *Color Atlas and Synopsis of Clinical Dermatology: Common and Serious Diseases,* 3d ed. New York, McGraw-Hill, 1997.

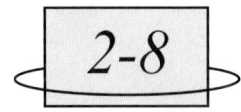

2-8 BULLOUS BLISTERING DISEASES
Joe R. Monroe

DEFINITION

Bullae are blisters (vesicles) larger than 0.5 cm, most often resulting from benign processes such as thermal burns, insect bites, contact dermatitis, and impetigo or as part of more serious diseases such as lupus erythematosus and dermatitis herpetiformis. Unfortunately, they can also be one of the first signs of a rather serious group of blistering diseases, including some that are potentially fatal, such as pemphigus vulgaris, and bullous pemphigoid.

CLINICAL DISCUSSION

The appearance of bullae is cause for real concern and should prompt an adequate and timely assessment. Unless the cause is obvious, one key element of such an assessment should be a punch biopsy preserved in special fixative (consult the pathology department) for immunofluorescent (IF) studies. Key clinical features of individual diseases are discussed below.

DIFFERENTIAL DIAGNOSES

See the discussion of the miscellaneous conditions presenting with bullae below.

LABORATORY

IF studies elucidate the precise histologic level at which abnormal antibodies are deposited, separation takes place, and blister formation occurs and are definitive for each disease entity. They greatly complement the history and physical examination, with the latter including Nikolsky's sign, which is said to be positive when the blister margin can be extended by digital pressure. A positive Nikolsky's sign indicates a shallow level of separation, suggesting a variant of pemphigus characterized clinically by flaccid, thin-walled bullae, whereas a negative test is consistent with bullous pemphigoid, a less serious disease marked by thick-walled, tense bullae, the roofs of which are composed of the entire epidermis.

TREATMENT

Treatment consists of systemic steroids, often with the addition of azathioprine, usually on long tapering doses (3 months or more) for pemphigus and bullous pemphigoid.

KEY CLINICAL FEATURES OF SELECTED BULLOUS DISEASES

Pemphigus vulgaris has the following features:

- It begins during the fourth or fifth decade.
- Flaccid, easily broken bullae often present with painful erosions.
- Initial areas of involvement often include mucous membranes in the mouth and genitals and then the face, trunk, and flexures.
- A positive Nikolsky's sign is exhibited.
- It may present as hoarseness.

Bullous pemphigoid has the following features:

- Involvement of elderly patients
- Usually very itchy
- Tense blisters with surrounding erythema
- Symmetric involvement of limbs and trunk
- A negative Nikolsky's sign

Dermatitis herpetiformis has the following features:

- Symmetric, grouped, excoriated papulovesicular rash
- Involves knees, elbows, buttocks
- Often associated with gluten enteropathy
- Alleviated by gluten-free diet and/or dapsone

Epidermolysis bullosa has the following features:

- 27 different types
- All genodermatoses

- Most common type EB simplex, also known as Weber-Cockayne syndrome, characterized by early onset, no extracutaneous involvement, blistering and hyperhidrosis of palms and soles, and autosomal dominant transmission

Features of erythema multiforme are listed in Chap. 2-12.
Toxic epidermal necrolysis (TEN, Lyell's syndrome) has the following features:

- Cutaneous and mucosal exfoliation, beginning with blisters
- Usually in response to drugs (penicillin, sulfa, etc.), also to infectious agents, but possibly idiopathic
- Potentially life-threatening
- Treated like a burn

Staphylococcal scalded-skin syndrome has the following features:

- Toxin-mediated epidermolytic disease
- Occurs mainly in newborns and infants
- Spectrum of disease ranges from localized bullous impetigo to generalized epidermal sloughing
- Caused by *Staphylococcus aureus* phage group II, type 71
- Treated like a burn

Porphyria cutanea tarda has the following features:

- Adults (age 30 to 50) present with complaint of "fragile skin" (bullae), especially on the dorsa of hands.
- Major triggers are ethanol and sun.
- Periorbital hypertrichosis.
- Orange-red fluorescence of urine (plus uroporphyrin).

Pediatric diseases that can present with bullae include varicella, urticaria pigmentosa, and chronic bullous disease of childhood (rare).

Miscellaneous conditions that can present with bullae include burns (thermal or chemical), contact dermatitis, drug reactions (fixed drug eruptions and others), insect bites (fleas, mosquitoes), lichen planus, lupus erythematosus, and pityriasis rosea.

PEARLS

Knowledge of the following points can contribute to a positive patient outcome:

- The appearance of bullous disease, especially in the very old or very young, should suggest possible referral to a dermatologist.
- Punch biopsies submitted in special fixative (*not* the usual formalin) can be crucial in the workup of bullous disease.
- Pemphigus can present with hoarseness (eroded laryngeal bullae) as the sole symptom.
- The symmetric distribution of a pruritic papulovesicular/bullous rash on the elbows, knees, and buttocks should suggest dermatitis herpetiformis.
- Porphyria cutanea tarda often is induced by alcohol.
- Many common, relatively benign dermatoses (e.g., lichen planus, erythema multiforme, pityriasis rosea) have bullous variants.

PROGNOSIS

Both pemphigus and bullous pemphigoid were quite lethal before the advent of steroids in 1952, with death rates of almost 75 percent. The clinical course was inexorably downward, with complications similar to those in burn patients, with fluid loss, overwhelming sepsis, and renal failure ultimately leading to death. Since 1952, the death rate has fallen to about 10 percent, but these disorders are still considered quite serious.

BIBLIOGRAPHY

Arndt KA, Robinson JK, LeBoit PE, et al: *Cutaneous Medicine and Surgery.* Philadelphia, Saunders, 1996.

DuVivier A: *Dermatology in Practice.* Philadelphia, Lippincott, 1990.
Fitzpatrick TB, Johnson RA, Wolff K, et al: *Color Atlas and Synopsis of Clinical Dermatology: Common and Serious Diseases,* 3d ed. New York, McGraw-Hill, 1997.
Goldstein BG, Goldstein AO: *Practical Dermatology,* Primary Care Series. St Louis, Mosby Year Book, 1992.
Shelley WB, Shelley ED: *Advanced Dermatologic Diagnosis.* Philadelphia, Saunders, 1992.
Weinberg S, Prose NS, Kristal L: *Color Atlas of Pediatric Dermatology,* 3d ed. New York, McGraw-Hill, 1998.

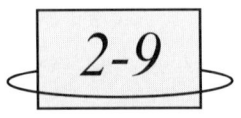

CELLULITIS (INCLUDING ERYSIPELAS)
Joe R. Monroe

DISCUSSION

Cellulitis is an acute infection of the skin and subcutaneous tissue, not involving muscle, that most often is caused by group A beta-hemolytic streptococci or *Staphylococcus aureus.* True erysipelas denotes cellulitis involving only the face and involves more superficial levels of the skin than does cellulitis.

Cellulitis can involve any area of skin, especially areas that have been traumatized or are lymphedematous, particularly the legs. A classic presentation of cellulitis is that of the dorsal forefoot starting from a tiny interdigital fissure, itself resulting from tinea pedis. Other risk factors include hematologic malignancies, intravenous (IV) drug use, diabetes mellitus, and immunocompromise. Cellulitis can rapidly produce significant symptomatology with localized tenderness and erythema as well as fever, chills, and malaise. Recurrences are common in areas of chronic lymphedema such as postmastectomy surgical sites.

Cellulitis is characterized by sharply demarcated, slightly elevated plaques with a fiery red to bluish-purple coloration. Lymphangitic streaking is fairly common, as is tender regional adenopathy.

Other organisms can cause variants of cellulitis. *Haemophilus influenzae* is one of the more common ones seen on the faces of children, as in periorbital cellulitis. Many other examples are seen in severely immunocompromised patients, such as cellulitis of cryptococcal origin.

Fortunately, most cases of cellulitis lend themselves well to clinical diagnosis. Exceptions to this include immunocompromised patients; so-called erysipeloid cellulitis of the hand or fingers, an indolent process typically seen as an occupational condition in those who handle fish, poultry, or meat; and necrotizing fasciitis, a rapidly evolving aggressive, centrally necrotic cellulitic process involving superficial fascia and subcutaneous tissue caused by a rather wide variety of potential pathogens.

DIFFERENTIAL DIAGNOSIS

Contact dermatitis, herpes zoster, stasis dermatitis, deep vein thrombophlebitis, gout, and other diseases can mimic cellulitis.

LABORATORY

Culture (needle aspirate, blister, blood) is only occasionally helpful. The peripheral white count and sedimentation rate may be elevated. Biopsy is only rarely indicated.

TREATMENT

If the organism is not known, treatment should cover both *Streptococcus* and *Staphylococcus,* for example, dicloxacillin 0.5 to 1.0 g q 6 h PO or erythromycin 500 mg q 6 h PO. Predisposing conditions such as lymphedema and tinea pedis need to be addressed.

PATIENT EDUCATION

Educate patients about the need to follow directions for antibiotics and other treatments.

PEARLS

Knowledge of the following points can contribute to a positive patient outcome:

- On feet, think of tinea pedis as a factor predisposing to cellulitis.
- Clearly demarcated, fiery red edematous plaques of skin are clearly suspicious for cellulitis.
- The sequelae of undiagnosed or mistreated cellulitis include hematogenous dissemination of infection, especially to abnormal heart valves.
- Cellulitis can present with a sudden onset of fever, chills, vomiting, and confusion, symptoms far worse than the skin findings would suggest.

PROGNOSIS

A dramatic response to antibiotics is typical with staphylococcal and streptococcal infections. When attacks are recurrent (e.g., postmastectomy sites), the patient may have to be placed on prophylactic antibiotics. A lack of response to common antibiotics should prompt a more thorough history (immunocompromised? occupational?) and possible punch or incisional biopsy sent for hematoxylin and eosin (H & E) as well as bacterial, fungal, and acid-fast cultures.

BIBLIOGRAPHY

Arndt KA, Robinson JK, LeBoit PE, et al: *Cutaneous Medicine and Surgery.* Philadelphia, Saunders, 1996.
DuVivier A: *Dermatology in Practice.* Philadelphia, Lippincott, 1990.
Fitzpatrick TB, Johnson RA, Wolff K, et al: *Color Atlas and Synopsis of Clinical Dermatology: Common and Serious Diseases,* 3d ed. New York, McGraw-Hill, 1997.
Goldstein BG, Goldstein AO: *Practical Dermatology,* Primary Care Series. St Louis, Mosby Year Book, 1992.
Shelley WB, Shelley ED: *Advanced Dermatologic Diagnosis.* Philadelphia, Saunders, 1992.
Weinberg S, Prose NS, Kristol L: *The Color Atlas of Pediatric Dermatology,* 3d ed. New York, McGraw-Hill, 1998.

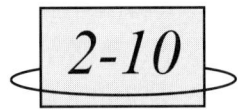

COMMON DERMATOLOGIC DISORDERS OF THE FEET
Sandra J. Martin

HYPERKERATOSES

DISCUSSION

Hyperkeratoses are areas of thickened epidermis that occur as a protective mechanism or reaction of the skin to repeated mechanical and shearing stress. The etiology can be friction from the ground when walking, which creates calluses on the bottom or side of the foot, or from shoes or adjacent toes as the skin is trapped over or between bony prominences. Long-term, chronic hyperkeratoses can cause permanent changes in skin architecture.

The most common plantar hyperkeratoses are caused by friction during weight bearing. They may be diffuse or more concentrated beneath specific pressure points such as metatarsal heads. They become symptomatic when they either become thick enough to cause symptoms or become fissured down to deeper, more sensitive epidermis closer to the dermis.

Diffuse hyperkeratoses on the plantar surface commonly are located beneath the metatarsal heads and around the heel. The calluses around the heel and on the plantar-medial aspect of the first metatarsal head frequently become so thick that they fissure and can bleed. They usually are seen in patients who wear open sandals or go barefoot.

TREATMENT

Common plantar hyperkeratoses may be debrided by the clinician, or patients may be taught self-care. Patients can use an emery board or sandpaper to debride a dry, hard callus or use a pumice type of stone to debride softened calluses. They should initially debride a little each day until the area has been adequately thinned. Then they should maintain the area by debriding once or twice a week as needed.

Dry or mildly hyperkeratotic, cracking plantar skin can be softened by placing petrolatum on the area, covering it with plastic wrap and a sock, and leaving this on all night. During the day, emollient creams may be used to maintain hydration of the skin. Lotions and creams containing a large amount of alcohol dehydrate the skin and should be avoided.

NUCLEATED HYPERKERATOSES

Some hyperkeratoses are nucleated and appear to have firm, hard, tender centers. These conditions may present a diagnostic challenge. In considering the differential diagnosis, it is necessary to consider the location of the lesion, the appearance of the lesion, and the movements that create pain.

Callus with discrete nucleated areas exhibits the following characteristics:

• Usually located in weight-bearing surfaces
• Skin lines through the lesion
• Tenderness with direct pressure
• No pinpoint bleeding with debridement

Plantar verruca (wart) has the following characteristics:

• May be in weight-bearing or non-weight-bearing areas
• Skin lines around the lesion
• Tender to lateral compression
• Pinpoint bleeding at the base with debridement

A foreign body may exhibit the following characteristics:

• Any location on plantar surface
• Skin lines through the lesion
• Frequently a single small puncture
• Tender with direct pressure more than lateral compression

TREATMENT

Nucleated hyperkeratotic lesions may be sharply debrided with a no. 15 blade. Debridement should be gradual, keeping the blade almost parallel to the surface of the skin. Avoid digging out the center, since this can result in cutting the patient. As the lesion is gently debrided parallel to the surface, the central area also becomes thinner. Appropriate padding with an aperture around the area can significantly retard recurrence of the lesion. Any insole can be used. The area directly under the lesion should be cut out. Padding directly beneath the lesion will cause it to become more painful. The foot can be marked with lipstick or any marking device that will transfer to the insole with pressure. Then the patient should put the marked foot in a shoe in which the insole has been placed. This delineates where the pressure points hit the insole so that area can be cut out (see Fig. 2-10-1).

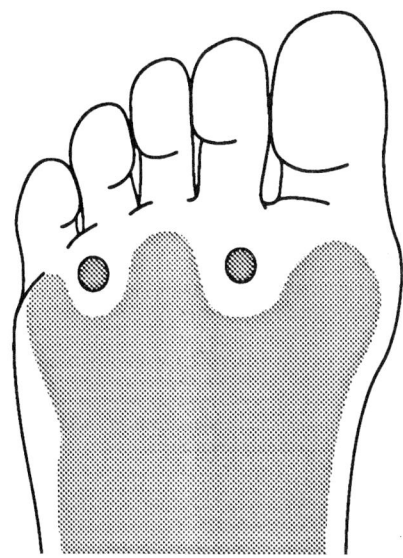

FIGURE 2-10-1. Padding around calluses or tender metatarsal heads.

PLANTAR WARTS

DISCUSSION

Similar to other warts, warts on the foot are caused by a virus that invades the skin. The most common is the human papillomavirus, which often is found on the plantar aspect of the foot. *Verrucae plantaris* are plantar warts, and they are often covered with hyperkeratotic tissue, raising them above the surrounding surface. They invade only the epidermis, which is very thick on the plantar aspect of the foot and makes the warts difficult to treat. Warts may present clinically as either singular lesions or multiple (mosaic) verrucae that coalesce with satellite lesions at the periphery. In debriding the hyperkeratotic covering of a plantar verruca, pinpoint bleeding that represents disruption of the small capillaries within the papilla is seen frequently.

TREATMENT

Plantar verrucae are difficult to treat because of the involved thicker epidermis. The lesions do not breach the dermis. Topical keratolytic acids may be used most successfully on solitary lesions, and care should be taken to protect the surrounding healthy tissue from the acid. Debride the hyperkeratotic tissue and then cautiously apply the acid to the lesion. It should be placed under occlusion with adhesive tape for 24 h. Caution patients that they may feel a burning sensation. Debridement and retreatment every few weeks should be continued until the lesion has resolved.

Avoid the use of liquid nitrogen on the plantar aspect of the foot because it does not penetrate to the deeper level of the epidermis and creates a painful blister that will make walking difficult.

Surgical excision of a verruca that is well demarcated and resistant to topical acids affords the best chance for resolution of the lesion. This involves incision and curettement of the lesion as follows:

1. Use a local anesthetic block with local infiltration or a regional block usually with 1% lidocaine plain and then infiltrate immediately beneath the lesion with a small amount of 1% lidocaine with epinephrine for hemostasis.
2. Using a no. 15 blade, incise the circumference of the lesion 1 to 2 mm beyond the visual border of the wart and skive it so that the wound is wider at the surface. The incision should be down to only the level of the dermal-epidermal junction.
3. Curette the lesion off the dermis. The lesion will shell out, leaving a glistening white dermis intact.

4. Cauterize the base of the lesion with 89% phenol, other chemocautery, or fulguration.

5. A dressing with antibiotic cream such as silver sulfadiazine should be applied. Be aware that this area may bleed liberally when the foot is put in a dependent position.

6. Have the patient remove the dressing in 12 to 24 h and soak in plain warm water for 30 min twice a day. The area should heal without scarring if the dermis has not been violated. The healing time depends on the size and location of the lesion.

PLANTAR FOREIGN BODIES

Foreign bodies of all different materials may be found embedded in the plantar aspect of the foot. If they go beneath the epidermis, they can be very painful and become infected. They frequently present with no known history of the patient stepping on something. Diagnosis of a foreign body may be difficult because conventional film x-ray will show only radiopaque objects. Foreign bodies may present like a hyperkeratotic lesion at the site of entry. The area will be tender to direct pressure. Other signs are variable.

Practitioners should not get caught up in a "search and destroy" mission for something they are unsure is present. If gentle debridement of the overlying hyperkeratosis does not yield a foreign body, it is best to refer the patient for further evaluation and treatment.

CORNS

Corns are of two general types: *soft* corns (heloma molle) and *hard* corns (heloma durum). Soft corns are present between the toes at the base of the digits in an area that is usually moist, thereby creating a macerated hyperkeratotic lesion. They occur from pressure on the skin by adjacent underlying bones. The most common sites for heloma molle are between the fourth and fifth toes or the third and fourth toes when hammertoes are present in a way that creates underlapping toes.

The best treatment is to separate the toes with some type of interdigital pad, especially when shoes are worn, and use antifungal powder sparingly before stockings are put on. This combination removes the pressure and allows the area to dry out. Acid pads should be avoided because they can create further irritation and encourage infection.

Heloma dura are found on the tops, ends, or sides of the toes and are hard because of the lack of moisture such as that seen in the interdigital spaces (see Fig. 2-10-2). They form over pressure points of bony prominences that are present because of an altered position of the toes (hammertoe, mallet toe, claw toe) or hypertrophy of the bone. Conservative treatment consists of debridement of the hyperkeratosis and appropriate padding or a change in shoe gear to alleviate pressure on the area. If this fails to relieve the symptoms, the patient may require referral for surgical intervention.

INGROWN TOENAILS (ONYCHOCRYPTOSIS)

DISCUSSION

Toenails become ingrown most frequently at the distal, lateral, or medial edges. Onychocryptosis on the distal edge of a toenail is usually the result of a nail that has previously been removed or lost regrowing into the distal soft tissue. Without the pressure on the nail bed, the distal nail bed becomes bulbous and the new nail must gradually press it down and flatten it out so that the nail can grow over it. Frequently the nail becomes embedded in the distal, bulbous soft tissue. This requires frequent debriding of the nail and pushing the soft tissue down so that the nail can grow over it.

Treatment in the office consists of using a very small tissue nipper to debride the distal edge of the nail. Then the patient should be encouraged to use a cuticle stick to push the skin away from the distal nail edge daily after bathing until the nail makes it over the top of the nail bed.

When the medial or lateral edges of a toenail become ingrown, the cause is usually improper trimming of the nail or pressure on the border from a tight shoe or the adjacent toe. Sometimes there is excessive (hypertrophic) soft tissue in the nail groove secondary to repeated irritation of the area by an ingrown or vertically growing nail border. A less common cause of an incurvated nail is a subungual exostosis that grows up from the distal tuft of the distal phalanx. Therefore, a nail can be simply ingrown, have a hypertrophic ungualabia, or be incurvated. The nail may be ingrown and asymptomatic, ingrown and tender, or ingrown and infected (paronychia).

The simple tender ingrown border that is secondary to improper cutting leaves a small spicule at the edge that will grow distally into the soft tissue and become symptomatic. Figure 2-10-3 illustrates this condition. The spicule acts like a foreign body, causing local inflammation, infection, and granuloma.

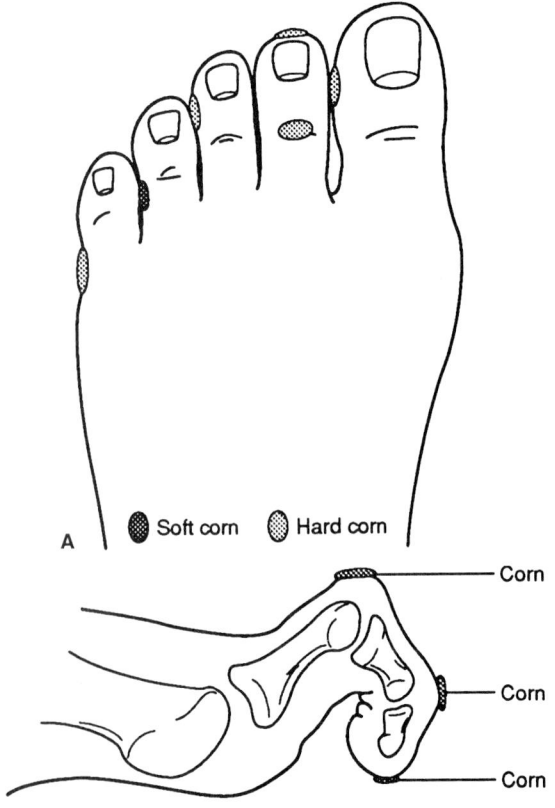

FIGURE 2-10-2. A. Soft and hard corns. **B.** Corns over bony prominences on a mallet toe.

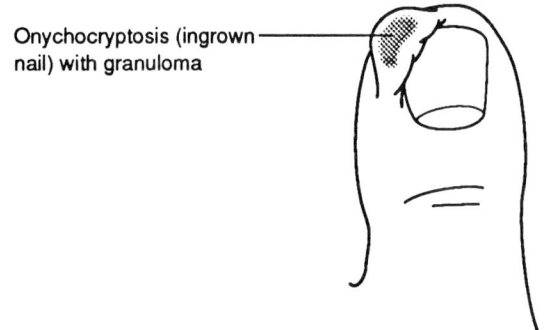

FIGURE 2-10-3. Onychocryptosis with granuloma.

The initial treatment of an ingrown nail border, infected or not, is to trim the nail border, thereby removing the offending foreign body. This should be trimmed to avoid leaving a new spicule proximally. It is not necessary to remove more than the distal offending edge as the initial conservative treatment. The patient should be encouraged to soak in warm water a few times a day until the symptoms have resolved.

If the symptoms do not resolve or if they return, permanent removal of the offending border is recommended. There is controversy regarding the appropriateness of doing a permanent procedure when a paronychia exists. There is always the chance of causing proximal extension of a localized infection when a matrixectomy is performed. It is this author's choice to resolve any gross infection before performing a chemical matrixectomy. Simply trimming the offending border and placing the patient on soaks twice a day frequently will resolve most of the localized infection. Oral antibiotics may also be used, depending on the severity of the infection and the general medical condition of the patient.

Some things to be aware of before performing a permanent removal of a nail border include the following:

1. Chronic paronychia may extend into an osteomyelitis in an immunocompromised patient such as a diabetic. In these patients, it is prudent to take x-rays of the toe to rule out possible bony involvement.
2. Check the vascular status of the patient before performing any minor surgical procedure. Patients who have peripheral vascular disease will experience slow healing and may even progress to more serious ischemic consequences.
3. Patient compliance in the postoperative period is essential to an uneventful postoperative course and a good result. Discuss this with the patient before performing any procedure.

The literature describes many different procedures with different approaches and techniques to treat paronychia. One that is technically simple, requires only a few special instruments, and has a favorable success rate is described here. There are many variations of the following procedure. Care should be taken not to remove so much nail that the patient is left with only a small central spicule, to remove as much of the matrix as possible, to avoid burning surrounding tissues with the phenol, and to provide a mechanism by which the area can drain (see Fig. 2-10-4).

TREATMENT

Phenol and alcohol partial matrixectomy has become the most widely used procedure to permanently remove all or part of a toenail. The procedure is simple, provides a good cosmetic result, has less postoperative

discomfort than other procedures, and has a relatively low recurrence rate. The phenol provides antisepsis, and many clinicians perform this procedure when infection is present. If there is a hypertrophied ungualabia, the excessive tissue can be removed with a tissue nipper and cauterized with the phenol during the procedure.

The following instruments are used:

• 1 Penrose drain, 1/4 in
• 2 straight hemostats
• 1 English anvil nail splitter
• 1 no. 61 miniblade and minihandle
• 1 curette, 2.0 mm
• 1 periosteal elevator or spatula/packer
• 1 tissue nipper

The following supplies are needed:

• Gauze: 2 × 2 and 4 × 4
• Phenol, 89% liquefied
• Cotton-tipped applicators with half the cotton removed or toothpicks with a small amount of cotton on the end
• Nu Gauze 1/4-in plain packing strips
• Silver sulfadiazine or another antibiotic cream (avoid ointments)
• Coban, 3 in

The procedure includes the following steps:

1. Use a local anesthetic block at base of the toe with approximately 3 mL (cc) 1% lidocaine plain (do not use epinephrine).
2. Apply a Penrose drain around the base of the toe to obtain hemostasis. Secure it with a hemostat and use a 2 × 2 between the drain and the skin to protect the skin. Make sure the patient does not have a medical condition that contraindicates the tourniquet.
3. Using the English anvil nail splitter, split the nail (Fig. 2-10-5) longitudinally just where it begins to become incurvated. Split the nail back to the cuticle.
4. Using the no. 61 miniblade, continue the longitudinal split in the nail beneath the cuticle until the tissue is felt to give, which should signify the proximal edge of the nail and matrix.
5. Undermine the portion of the nail to be removed with a packer or periosteal elevator.
6. Grasp the portion of the nail to be removed with a hemostat from distal to beneath the cuticle. Push proximally to loosen the nail border; then roll the hemostat with the border in it toward the center of the nail.
7. Use a curette and tissue nipper to remove any remaining nail matrix (pearly white tissue), granuloma, or fibrous tissue in the nail groove.
8. Apply the phenol. Using the cotton-tipped applicators or toothpicks, dip one in the phenol and then blot it to remove excess acid.

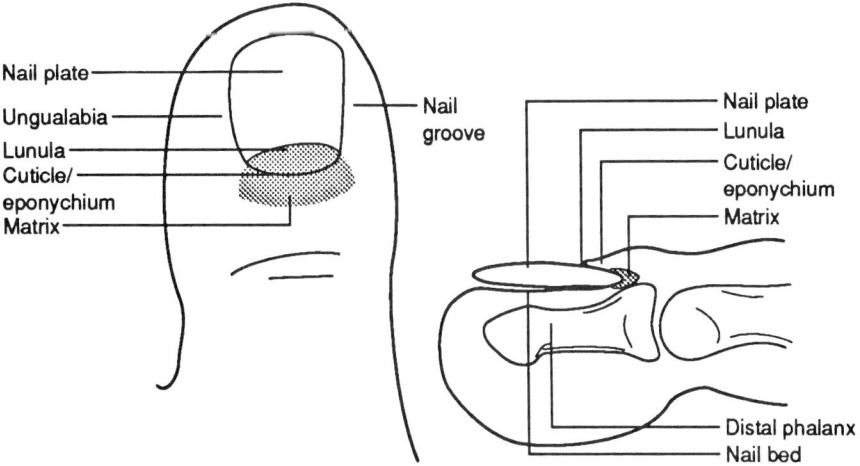

FIGURE 2-10-4. Nail anatomy.

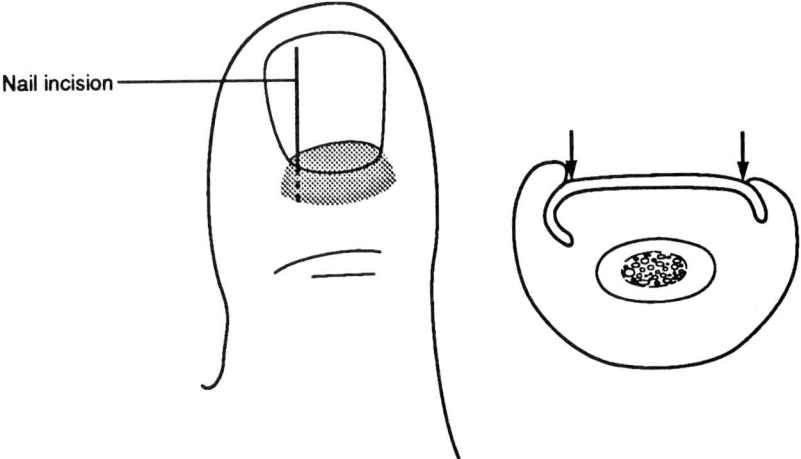

FIGURE 2-10-5. Area of nail to cut when performing a matrixectomy.

Apply to the matrix area beneath the cuticle and to the nail bed for 30 s. Repeat this for a total of three applications.

9. Flush the area with alcohol and remove the tourniquet. Place the silver sulfadiazine or antibiotic cream into the nail groove and loosely pack it with the 1/4-in packing so that the edge of the packing is free. Apply a dressing of 2 × 2 and Coban.

10. Prescribe an otic solution of neomycin, polymyxin B sulfates, and hydrocortisone or another antibiotic solution.

Postoperative instructions are as follows:

1. A clear, yellowish exudate will drain from the operative area for up to a few weeks. Explain this to the patient.

2. The patient should remove the dressing that evening and soak the toe in warm water for 30 min, leaving the packing in place. Pat the toe dry and apply a few drops of the Cortisporin otic solution to the area. Redress with a *loose* bandage. Letting air into the area is important to aid healing. Therefore, an occlusive dressing should be avoided.

3. Continue soaking and treating as in step 2, twice a day. The packing may be removed after 24 h. After the packing is removed, the patient should begin to debride the area gently with a soft toothbrush or a cotton-tipped applicator to tolerance. It is important to keep the nail groove clear of crusted exudate.

4. Soaking, debridement, and medication should continue until there is no more drainage.

The clinician should follow the patient a few days after the procedure and then every few weeks until the area is completely healed. When the nail groove is full of necrotic tissue or crusted exudate, gently debride the area with a curette.

The phenol and alcohol procedure described above also can be used for a total matrixectomy. Keep in mind that more phenol should be used and that it may take up to 6 weeks to achieve complete healing.

SUBUNGUAL HEMATOMA

Trauma to a nail can cause bleeding of the nail bed beneath the nail. The accumulation of blood in a closed area creates pressure and considerable pain. If the injury is recent and the blood beneath the nail is still liquid, placing a few holes in the nail will release the fluid and alleviate most of the discomfort. If the nail has been broken, it should be removed totally to allow the nail bed to heal. Simple soaks in warm water will provide comfort to the patient and aid healing of the nail bed.

If the trauma has been severe, an x-ray of the toe should be obtained to rule out a fracture. If the nail bed is lacerated, depending on the extent of the laceration, it can be sutured or steri-stripped. Counsel the patient that the new nail may have some deformity, depending on the damage to the nail bed and matrix.

ONYCHOMYCOSIS

DISCUSSION

Onychomycosis is an infection of the nail bed and nail by mycotic (fungal) organisms and may affect more than 20 percent of the adult population. Yeast and bacterial infections can mimic mycotic infections. The pathophysiology is more complicated than is commonly thought and usually begins with some type of trauma or disease process that affects the nail bed. This results in compromise of the area's resistance to colonization by microorganisms. A fungal infection of the nail frequently begins as a simple distal subungual onychomycosis in the nail grooves or beneath the nail's distal edge. The infection can then spread proximally, involving more and more of the nail bed and, subsequently, the nail. The result may be as severe as complete involvement of the nail plate with discoloration, crumbling, lifting of the nail plate, and the accumulation of a lot of malodorous subungual debris.

TREATMENT

Treatment has been a controversial subject for many years. This author believes that minimal nail involvement in an immunocompetent patient should be treated either with cosmetic methods or with topical treatments. Cosmetically, the nail can be improved greatly by filing with an emery type of file to both thin and shorten the nail plate. Even the most severely involved mycotic nail can be managed by filing it to keep it under control.

However, some patients dislike the appearance of a mycotic nail so much that they insist on treatment. They are willing to take systemic medications or even have the nail permanently removed. However, they may not like the cosmetic result of permanent nail removal, and it is quite tedious to permanently remove multiple mycotic nails.

If only a small distal portion or a portion of one of the sides is involved, some topical medications may control the infection, although a cure should not be anticipated. Liquid antifungals designed specifically for nails, such as Mycocide NS and Fungoid Tincture, used as directed, may accomplish significant clearing of the nail plate. However, fungal infections of the nails are usually resistant to topical treatment, and when the medication is discontinued, the onychomycosis usually will recur.

The most effective treatment for onychomycosis with the best possible chance for cure and a resultant normal nail is one of the newer oral antifungal agents: itraconazole (Sporanox) and terbinafine (Lamisil). Both have shown significant cure rates for onychomycosis. Fluconazole (Diflucan) also is used for the treatment of onychomycosis. These new oral antifungals have different side-effect profiles, drug interactions, and dosing schedules. Pretreatment liver function studies should be considered before these medications are used. Pulse dosing has been used effectively with all these medications, and patient compliance has been excellent during clinical trials. The effectiveness of treatment usually is first seen in clearing of the new, proximal nail. It may take a few months after the medication has been finished for complete clearing.

These oral antifungals are indicated for the treatment of onychomycosis of the toenail or fingernail resulting from dermatophytes. A positive culture of the nail should be obtained before initiating treatment with these medications. Proper culture technique is important and should be performed by taking the specimen proximal to the distal edge of the infected nail. It is essential that the nail clippings not come from the distal edge but instead be taken from a portion of nail on top of the nail bed and, if possible, some of the subungual debris for submission to the laboratory. Obtaining nail clippings of at least 3 mm will increase the chance for a positive culture. Do not submit specimens if the patient is currently undergoing antifungal therapy because this will often result in a negative culture. If the first culture is negative, a repeat culture is recommended, based on clinical impression.

BIBLIOGRAPHY

Odom RB: New therapies for onychomycosis. *J Am Acad Dermatol* 35:S26–S30, 1996.

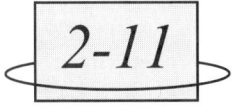

DECUBITUS ULCERS
Freddi Segal-Gidan

DISCUSSION

Decubitus ulcers (pressure sores) are caused by prolonged pressure on an area of skin that results in underlying tissue damage and loss of skin integrity. They usually occur over bony prominences, most commonly the hip, sacrum, lateral malleolus, and heel. With proper patient education, pressure sores usually, but not always, can be prevented. The elderly, paralyzed persons, and those with diabetes, peripheral vascular disease, or peripheral sensory neuropathy are the most likely to develop pressure sores.

PATHOGENESIS

Pressure, shear, and friction are the three primary underlying forces that influence the formation of pressure ulcers.[1] The presence of moisture increases the deleterious effects of these forces. When external pressure exceeds that of the venous system, total tissue pressure increases. This then causes increased capillary pressure, which results in transudation of fluid from the capillaries, producing tissue edema and autolysis of cells. Pressure also occludes lymphatic drainage, allowing toxic by-products of anaerobic metabolism to accumulate. The duration of pressure is a critical factor; the higher the pressure is, the less time is required to cause tissue damage.

Shearing forces result from sliding of adjacent surfaces. Such forces are created between body surfaces and that of a bed or chair. They produce stretching and angulation of blood vessels in the subcutaneous tissues, thus causing thrombosis and undermining of the dermis.

Frictional force is the primary factor leading to superficial skin breakdown. Moisture increases the friction between surfaces, thus exacerbating skin breakdown.

TABLE 2-11-1. Predisposing Conditions for Pressure Ulcer Development

Paraplegia
Quadriplegia
Diabetes mellitus
Peripheral vascular disease
Peripheral neuropathy (sensory)
Immobility

SYMPTOMS

Presentation is most typically with a painless open sore over an area of bony prominence or pressure. Detection requires a high index of suspicion for occurrence and frequent, regular complete skin examinations. Those predisposed to pressure sore development must be taught preventive techniques before skin breakdown ever occurs (see Table 2-11-1). Prevention of pressure ulcers requires assessment of the individual's overall physical health, medication use, nutritional status, functional problems, psychosocial factors, and pain. Medical conditions that affect peripheral circulation (diabetes, peripheral vascular disease), impair mobility (hip or other lower-extremity fracture, hemiplegia, paraplegia, or quadriplegia), or affect perception (dementia, neuralgia) increase the probability of developing pressure ulcers. Poor nutrition, especially low protein and serum albumin, predisposes to ulcer development and impairs healing. Medications that affect cognition and voluntary movements (sedatives) or pain perception (narcotics) may contribute to pressure sores, whereas other medications (steroids) impair healing. Knowledge about a patient's level of independent function and concomitant need for assistance may point to the need to incorporate others into any prevention or treatment program. Pressure ulcer formation and healing also are influenced by mental status; substance abuse; individual goals, values, and life-style; and available resources, such as caregivers, money, and equipment.

OBJECTIVE FINDINGS

A complete skin examination, with particular attention to areas prone to skin breakdown, should be performed routinely on all those prone to pressure sore development. This requires the routine removal of socks and shoes and, for wheelchair-bound individuals, visual inspection of the sacrum and buttocks. Bed-bound patients in a hospital or nursing home should have skin checks daily.

When a pressure sore is present, note its location and size, including the length, width, and depth. The National Pressure Ulcer Advisory Panel[2] has developed criteria to assess ulcers that are based on the level of tissue damage (see Table 2-11-2). Note the presence of any exudate or necrotic tissue. Examine the surrounding skin for erythema, maceration, and induration. Look for the presence of granulation and epithelization. The ulcer should be palpated gently, and the edges

TABLE 2-11-2. Clinical Staging of Pressure Ulcers

STAGE	DESCRIPTION
I	Nonblanchable erythema of intact skin
II	Partial-thickness skin loss involving epidermis and dermis. Presents as abrasion, blister, or shallow ulceration
III	Full-thickness skin loss. Damage or necrosis of subcutaneous tissue. May extend down, but not through, fascia
IV	Full-thickness skin loss with extensive destruction. Damage through fascia, often involving muscle and/or bone. Undermining and sinus tracts common

probed for undermining and/or sinus tract formation. Check the peripheral circulation, noting the presence or absence of pulses and capillary refill, since these factors will have an impact on healing.

DIAGNOSTIC CONSIDERATIONS

The differential diagnosis of skin ulcers lies primarily in determining the underlying etiology or predisposing factors.

SPECIAL CONSIDERATIONS

Pressure ulcer formation is much more common in the elderly and among residents of acute-care and long-term-care settings. Skin changes that accompany aging account for the susceptibility of the elderly to the development of pressure ulcers. Nearly two-thirds of all pressure ulcers occur in individuals over age 70, and most occur within a few weeks after an acute illness.

LABORATORY TESTS

Laboratory testing is essential for identifying etiologic conditions as well as factors that influence wound healing. Routine blood work, including complete blood cell count (CBC) with differential, erythrocyte sedimentation rate (ESR), serum electrolytes, creatinine, glucose, calcium, protein, and albumin, should be performed. Serum glucose is essential for the identification of undiagnosed diabetes. In diabetic patients, a serum hemoglobin A_{1c} provides indirect information about glucose control during the past 3 months. Serum protein and albumin levels are key indicators of current nutritional status.

Blood cultures are important to ascertain for the presence of sepsis. Tissue biopsy or needle aspiration should be performed when an infected ulcer is suspected. Surface swab cultures are inaccurate, may not reveal the true pathogens, and do not differentiate between infecting organisms and commensals.

RADIOLOGIC STUDIES

Routine radiographs are not warranted. If bone is exposed or the pressure ulcer is present for more than a month, one should suspect underlying osteomyelitis. A radiographic study of the underlying bony skeleton is warranted; it may show lytic lesions, reactive bone formation, and periosteal elevation associated with osteomyelitis.[3] Radionuclide scanning is sensitive, particularly in new lesion development, but has limited usefulness in following the clinical response to the therapy over time. Computed tomography (CT) scanning is useful for documenting the extent of underlying soft tissue injury.

TREATMENT

Optimal management of pressure ulcers involves prevention, early recognition, and aggressive treatment.[4]

Wound Care

Early pressure ulcer development, stage I or II, is best treated with local measures and pain relief (see below) to avoid further ulcer progression.

Debridement of necrotic tissue is essential for ulcer healing (see Table 2-11-3). It may be done mechanically or by instrumentation. Wet-to-dry dressings are the most common form of mechanical debridement. Wound irrigation and hydrotherapy are also forms of mechanical debridement. Sharp debridement involves the use of a scalpel, a scissors, or another sharp instrument. This is the most rapid form of debridement and is required when there are signs of advancing cellulitis or sepsis. Extensive ulcers require surgical debridement, which may be done at the bedside but more often requires an operating room because of the need for better management of the associated pain and bleeding.

TABLE 2-11-3. Debridement of Pressure Ulcers

TYPE	TECHNIQUE
Sharp	Use of scalpel, scissors, or another sharp instrument Often requires operating room and surgeon
Mechanical	Wet-to-dry dressings Wound irrigation Dextranomers
Enzymatic	Collagenase Santyl ointment
Autolytic	Wound Dress DuoDerm

Enzymatic debridement uses a topical agent to dissolve necrotic tissue. Agents must be applied according to the manufacturer's instructions. The process may be used alone to break down eschar, after sharp debridement, or in association with mechanical debridement. This is most appropriate when the patient is not a candidate for surgical debridement, such as a long-term-care resident or a homebound patient.

Synthetic dressings allow for autolytic debridement. The wound is covered, and devitalized tissues self-digest from enzymes normally present in the wound fluid. This is a slow and lengthy process that is most appropriate for individuals who cannot tolerate other debridement methods. Autolytic debridement is contraindicated when pressure ulcers are infected.

Optimal healing requires that all necrotic tissue, exudate, and waste be removed from the ulcer. Once the ulcer has been debrided, routine cleansing after each dressing change is necessary to decrease the risk of infection. As with all wounds, pressure ulcers should be cleansed gently and thoroughly. Normal saline is the preferred cleansing agent for most ulcers. Skin cleansers or antiseptics such as peroxide and povidone iodine should never be used since they are toxic to healing tissues. The ulcer should be irrigated with enough pressure to be effective (about 4 to 15 lb/in^2) without causing tissue trauma. The use of a large-capacity syringe (>25 mL) with a 17- to 19-gauge angiocatheter is very effective for wound irrigation. Whirlpool cleansings should be considered for pressure ulcers that contain thick exudate, slough, or necrotic tissue and should be discontinued when the ulcer is considered clean.

Dressings are used to keep the ulcer tissue moist to promote healing and keep the surrounding skin intact and dry. Dressings do not have to be sterile but must be clean.

Moist saline or occlusive dressings are optimal for stage I to III ulcers. In stage III or IV ulcers with cavity formation, the cavity needs to be gently filled with moist packing to wick away drainage. Avoid overpacking, which may cause additional damage from pressure on the wound surface.

Dressings should be monitored regularly and changed at least daily or more frequently, if necessary, because of drainage or soiling. Those near the anus are especially difficult to keep intact and clean. "Picture framing" the edges of a dressing may help secure it.

Electrical stimulation is the only currently recommended adjunctive therapy. It involves the application of surface electrodes to the wound site. It may be employed for stage III and IV pressure ulcers that have been unresponsive to conventional therapy and recalcitrant stage II pressure ulcers.

Other adjunctive therapies that have been tried but lack sufficient evidence to recommend include hyperbaric oxygen; infrared, ultraviolet, and low-energy laser irradiation; and ultrasound.

Surgical Treatment

Surgical intervention is often required for stage III and IV pressure sores to remove necrotic tissue and scar tissue that may delay healing. Resection of bony prominences that may contribute to recurrent ulceration also may be required. In the operating room, surgical closure of the ulcer through a myocutaneous flap or skin homograph may be accomplished. Limb amputation may be required when the ulcer is too large to cover with rotational flats or in the presence of extensive osteomyelitis or severe joint contractures.

Pharmacologic Management

Medication in the treatment of pressure ulcers should be aimed at pain control and any underlying conditions. Nonsedating analgesics used on a regular rather than an as-needed basis should be used if pain is an ongoing factor. Chronic pain that is unresponsive to analgesics often responds to an antidepressant such as nortriptyline. Proper treatment of diabetes with either oral hypoglycemic agents or insulin is essential to aid healing. Peripheral circulation may improve with the use of pentoxifylline (Trental). Systemic antimicrobial therapy is required if complications of sepsis or osteomyelitis are suspected.

Supportive Measures

Positioning is the key to preventing pressure ulcer formation. First, avoid pressure on any existing ulcer; second, reduce pressure on other bony prominences or other areas at risk for the development of pressure ulcers. Bed-bound and immobile individuals must be turned often, every 2 h, to avoid continuous pressure on any one area. The head of the bed should always be at the lowest elevation consistent with other medical conditions. Avoid positioning immobile individuals on their trochanters and use devices to relieve pressure on the heels. Foam pads or wedges and pillows should be used to prevent direct contact between an ulcer and the support surface and between areas at risk for breakdown, particularly bony prominences, and the support surface. Never use rigid doughnut-type ring cushions because they may cause pressure ulcers, not prevent them. When a pressure ulcer is on a sitting surface, avoid the sitting position; place patients on their side or prone.

Proper support surfaces are also essential in preventing pressure ulcer formation and promoting the healing of already formed ulcers. Selection should be based primarily on the therapeutic benefit of the product, but the clinical condition of the individual, characteristics of the care setting, and cost also must be considered. The goal is to provide a support surface that provides airflow to dry the skin. Simple mattress overlays include simple foam overlays and water flotation mattresses. These devices must be monitored for bottoming out. If less than 1 in of support material remains under the affected ulcer or other bony prominence, the overlay should be replaced. More complex bed support surfaces include an alternating-air mattress, a low-air-loss bed, and an air-fluidized bed. These surfaces are indicated primarily for large stage III and IV pressure ulcers on multiple sites.

Surface support also is required for sitting, especially in nonambulatory patients. Wheelchair cushions should be properly fitted to the chair and person. Again, doughnuts should never be used.

Paraplegics and other wheelchair-bound individuals should be taught pressure-relief maneuvers that they can perform regularly to prevent continued pressure on any one surface. Individuals who cannot perform their own pressure-relief maneuvers need to have their caregivers properly instructed in these techniques so that they are done without producing harm to the patient or caregiver.

PATIENT EDUCATION

Prevention is the key to pressure sore management. Patients, their families, and their caregivers must be engaged both to prevent their development and to promote proper healing. Individuals at risk for pressure sore development should be identified and given ongoing education about proper skin care, positioning, and overall health. The role of proper nutrition and hygiene to maintain circulatory and skin integrity should be emphasized and assessed routinely by the practitioner. If an ulcer develops, individuals should be instructed to contact their provider immediately. Individuals who are able should be instructed in the techniques for proper wound care and be active participants in daily dressing changes. Usually, however, it is the family or caregivers who must be educated about signs of pressure ulcer development and wound care techniques for an active pressure sore.

COMPLICATIONS AND RED FLAGS

Pressure ulcers that increase in size or fail to heal in the presence of an active wound care program should be referred for surgical evaluation. Surgical debridement is often needlessly delayed and usually is required to treat stage III and IV ulcers and sepsis.

PEARLS

The time invested in the early identification of individuals at risk for pressure ulcer development and the education of those persons and their families is both good medicine and cost-effective. Nursing staff in the office or hospital can provide the actual education. Videotapes that a patient or family can view and then discuss with the provider or a knowledgeable staff member are a very effective way to teach both prevention (pressure-release maneuvers, transfer techniques, skin assessment) and wound care (irrigation, dressing changes).

REFERENCES

1. Kertesz D, Chow AW: Infected pressure and diabetic ulcers. *Clin Geriatr Med* 8(4):835–852, 1992.
2. National Pressure Ulcer Advisory Panel: Pressure ulcers prevalence, cost, risk assessment: Consensus development conference statement. *Decubitus* 2:24, 1989.
3. Thornhill-Joyness M, Gonzales G, Stewart CA, et al: Osteomyelitis associated with pressure ulcers. *Arch Phys Med Rehabil* 67:314, 1986.
4. U.S. Department of Health and Human Services, Agency for Health Care Policy and Research: Treatment of pressure ulcers. Clinical Practice Guidelines, no. 15, 1994.

BIBLIOGRAPHY

Linder RM, Morris D: The surgical management of pressure ulcers: A systemic approach based on staging. *Decubitus* 3:32–54, 1990.
Mackelbust A, Sieggreen *M: Pressure Ulcers: Guidelines for Prevention and Nursing Management.* West Dundee, IL, S-N Publications, 1991.
U.S. Department of Health and Human Services, Agency for Health Care Policy and Research: Pressure ulcers in adults: Prediction and prevention. Clinical Practice Guidelines no. 3, 1994.

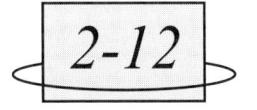

ERYTHEMA MULTIFORME
Joe R. Monroe

DEFINITION

Erythema multiforme (EM) is a relatively common self-limited inflammatory process of acute onset, often recurrent, that manifests initially as distinctive target-shaped papules with a characteristic histopathology.

CLINICAL DISCUSSION

Most commonly found on the extremities, especially the dorsa of the hands, palms, soles, knees, and dorsal feet, but also on the penis (50 percent) and vulva, EM lesions are frequently tender and can involve mucous membranes as well.

The morphology of EM lesions is somewhat variable, as the term *multiforme* suggests, but the typical picture is striking and thus readily identifiable. The sudden appearance of iris or target lesions is the hallmark; this is a round papule that displays concentric rings of different colors, with darker centers tending to vesiculate (blister), ranging from 1 to 3 cm in size, and distributed symmetrically in characteristic areas (see above).

Atypical lesions frequently resemble hives (urticaria) but, unlike hives, remain in one location for days.

EM is considered a hypersensitivity reaction pattern of an immune response to a variety of potential agents, the best documented of which are recurrent herpes simplex virus (HSV) infection, *Mycoplasma pneumoniae* infection, and drugs. Among drugs, the major offenders include the sulfonamides, anticonvulsant medications (phenytoin and barbiturates), penicillins, allopurinol, and nonsteroidal anti-inflammatory drugs (NSAIDs). Lesional HSV antigen frequently can be demonstrated by polymerase chain reaction, and intradermal injection of HSV antigen has reproduced the condition, facts that some take as proof that most EM, especially the recurrent form, is caused by hypersensitivity to HSV antigen. To the proponents of this concept, the other reported triggers for EM—sunlight, infection, foods, and progesterone—do so only because they are known to trigger overt or clinically inapparent HSV attacks.

EM traditionally is described in two forms that probably represent opposite extremes of a continuum. EM minor, which is characterized by a lack of bullae, mucosal lesions, or systemic symptoms, most often is caused by an outbreak of HSV. EM major, which usually is caused by drugs (see above), by definition involves mucous membranes and demonstrates extensive bullous formation, with fever and prostration. Many authors still use the term *Stevens-Johnson syndrome* as synonymous with EM major accompanied by erosion of less than 10 percent of the total epidermal surface, whereas the term *toxic epidermal necrolysis* (TEN) generally is reserved for a similar condition in which more than 10 percent of the epidermis is lost in sloughing of large sheets. Mortality rates from EM major and TEN are 20 to 30 percent, usually from sepsis.

Rare to begin with, EM major is rarely recurrent and also can be caused by *M. pneumoniae,* most often in children and young adults.

DIFFERENTIAL DIAGNOSIS

Fortunately, the diagnosis is usually easy with such distinctive lesions. However, EM can present with mucosal lesions as the only presenting sign; this should prompt the consideration of bullous disease or another disease affecting mucosal tissues, such as HSV. In the case of atypical dermal EM, the differential would include urticaria, insect bites, drug eruption, and viral exanthems, among others.

LABORATORY

Punch biopsy for routine hematoxylin and eosin (H & E) pathology can be very helpful, particularly for the bullous form.

TREATMENT

Treatment is largely symptomatic with EM minor. Topical steroids are of no use in the treatment of EM, since the problem is much too deep for them to reach. Suspected herpes triggers are treated with acyclovir. With EM major, the following steps are recommended: (1) Give priority to finding the trigger if possible and eliminating it, as in the case of drugs, or treating it, as with HSV. (2) Assess and treat potential complications (fluid loss, sepsis, ophthalmic pathology, nutritional deficits). Strong consideration should be given to hospitalization and, in severe cases, transfer to a burn unit.

PATIENT EDUCATION

Reassure the patient about the likely benign, self-limited nature of EM minor. Patients must be made aware of potential triggers in cases where the cause has not yet been found.

PEARLS

Consideration of the following points can contribute to a positive patient outcome:

- Target-like (iris) papules of acute onset are pathognomic for EM.
- HSV is the trigger for EM until proved otherwise, though 50 percent of cases are idiopathic.
- EM major is a potentially fatal condition that requires timely diagnosis and referral to a dermatologist experienced in treating it.
- Erythematous palmar or plantar lesions that are tender should suggest EM.

PROGNOSIS

The prognosis is self-limited, with EM minor lasting up to 4 weeks, whereas EM major can last 6 weeks, with new lesions, especially oral, appearing for weeks after that. The mortality rates from EM major and TEN are 10 to 20 percent, usually from sepsis.

BIBLIOGRAPHY

Arndt KA, Robinson JK, LeBoit PE, et al: *Cutaneous Medicine and Surgery.* Philadelphia, Saunders, 1996.

DuVivier A: *Dermatology in Practice.* Philadelphia, Lippincott, 1990.

Fitzpatrick TB, Johnson RA, Wolff K, et al: *Color Atlas and Synopsis of Clinical Dermatology: Common and Serious Diseases,* 3d ed. New York, McGraw-Hill, 1997.

Goldstein BG, Goldstein AO: *Practical Dermatology,* Primary Care Series. St Louis, Mosby Year Book, 1992.

Shelley WB, Shelley ED: *Advanced Dermatologic Diagnosis.* Philadelphia, Saunders, 1992.

Weinberg S, Prose NS, Kristal L: *Color Atlas of Pediatric Dermatology,* 3d ed. New York, McGraw-Hill, 1998.

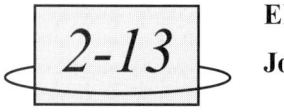

ERYTHEMA NODOSUM
Joe R. Monroe

DEFINITION

Erythema nodosum (EN) is an inflammatory reaction pattern in response to certain drugs, infections, or other disease states that is characterized by the bilateral appearance of subcutaneous tender erythematous nodules on extensor surfaces that represent an underlying process of septal panniculitis (acute inflammation of fat).

CLINICAL DISCUSSION

EN is the most common of the panniculitides and, except for certain well-defined causes, is idiopathic (cause unknown) in approximately 40 percent of cases. It presents as an acute process and spontaneously regresses, leaving no surface changes (scarring, ulceration, or atrophy) behind. Most commonly affecting lower extremities, EN also can appear on arms and the neck, and the lesions are quite tender. The lesions themselves are poorly defined, being bright red initially and tending toward more violaceous hues as they mature, sometimes becoming frankly ecchymotic before disappearing after 2 to 6 weeks. They often appear in crops and range in size from 2 to 20 cm. Before puberty, the incidence is the same in both sexes, but after that, the ratio of females to males rises to 3:1. Although 40 percent of cases are idiopathic, the rest have discernible causes, the most common of which are streptococcal infections, birth control pills, and sarcoidosis. Less common causes include primary tuberculosis (especially in children), sulfa drugs, coccidioidomycosis, ulcerative colitis, leprosy, and Behçet's syndrome. Most EN patients also complain initially of fever, malaise, and arthralgia but may have symptoms related to the causative disease, such as cough, sore throat, or gastrointestinal symptoms.

DIFFERENTIAL DIAGNOSES

The diagnosis is usually straightforward with such a striking presentation. Unfortunately, the trigger is often unclear. The most common misdiagnosis is cellulitis or another infectious process, but the latter is not likely to present with multiple subcutaneous lesions showing no break in the skin surface. This lack of epidermal skin change in EN is quite helpful in ruling out a number of other disease processes that might otherwise be considered, such as insect bites and folliculitis.

LABORATORY

For EN itself, a deep skin biopsy (well into the fat) is necessary to demonstrate the characteristic septal panniculitis. For the workup of possible triggering diseases, a basic battery of tests should include complete blood cell count (CBC), erythrocyte sedimentation rate (ESR), chemistry screen, chest films, antistreptolysin O (ASO) titer, purified protein derivative (PPD), and serum angiotensin converting enzyme (ACE) level.

TREATMENT

Find and treat the trigger if possible. Nonsteroidal anti-inflammatory drugs (NSAIDs), elevation of the affected limbs, and compression with elastic bandages all provide supportive relief while this self-limited disease slowly clears. Unresponsive cases often are treated with potassium iodide 300 to 600 mg tid PO for up to 4 weeks. Recurrent cases are not unusual and should be referred to a dermatologist.

PATIENT EDUCATION

Repeated reassurances are often necessary, since the initial presentation of this condition can be fairly impressive and therefore frightening in terms of both appearance and symptomatology.

PROGNOSIS

This disease is usually self-limited, lasting 3 to 6 weeks. The underlying trigger may not be benign; thus, a careful search for it is indicated.

PEARLS

Knowledge of the following points can contribute to a positive patient outcome:

- EN and bilateral hilar adenopathy may be the presenting signs of sarcoidosis, but this typically short-lived radiologic finding may be associated with EN in the absence of sarcoidosis.
- When biopsy is needed, a 6-mm punch or deep incisional biopsy that gets a specimen well into the fat is necessary to diagnose EN, since the actual disease process involves only the fibrotic septa of the subcutaneous adipose (fat) tissue, not the overlying skin.
- Given a choice, never biopsy thin anterior tibial skin, since healing is often a problem there.
- The three most common causes of EN in this country are streptococcal infections (especially in children), birth control pills, and sarcoidosis, but the list of reported triggers is enormous.
- The acute appearance of painful, subcutaneous erythematous nodules on the legs of young women represents EN until proved otherwise.
- As EN nodules resolve, they often go through the same color changes as bruises (erythema contusiformis).

BIBLIOGRAPHY

Arndt KA, Robinson JK, LeBoit PE, et al: *Cutaneous Medicine and Surgery.* Philadelphia, Saunders, 1996.
DuVivier A: *Dermatology in Practice.* Philadelphia, Lippincott, 1990.
Fitzpatrick TB, Johnson RA, Wolff K, et al: *Color Atlas and Synopsis of Clinical Dermatology: Common and Serious Diseases,* 3d ed. New York, McGraw-Hill, 1997.
Goldstein BG, Goldstein AO: *Practical Dermatology,* Primary Care Series. St Louis, Mosby Year Book, 1992.
Shelley WB, Shelley ED: *Advanced Dermatology Diagnosis.* Philadelphia, Saunders, 1992.
Weinberg S, Prose NS, Kristal L: *Color Atlas of Pediatric Dermatology,* 3d ed. New York, McGraw-Hill, 1998.

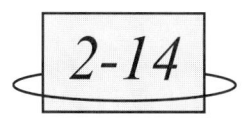

FOLLICULITIS

Joe R. Monroe

DISCUSSION

Folliculitis is inflammation of the hair follicle, usually by bacteria and sometimes by other organisms, resulting in the appearance of follicular pustules—that is, tiny pus-filled papules often pierced centrally by a hair. The term *folliculitis* traditionally is used to denote a relatively mild, superficial inflammatory process that heals without scarring. Occlusion of the skin by oils or by impervious dressings seems to be an etiologic factor, as does shaving. However, these discrete, superficial pustules also can evolve into furuncles, which involve deeper tissues and appear acutely as hot, red, tender nodules. Multiple furuncles can then coalesce into larger, even more tender fluctuant masses called carbuncles ("boils"), which are caused by *Staphylococcus.*

Apart from this classic presentation, folliculitis also can be caused by a large number of other agents in an equally wide variety of clinical contexts. A classic example is *Pseudomonas* folliculitis, also known as "hot tub folliculitis," a relatively common self-limited condition promoted by the superhydration inherent in using a hot tub (or sauna), making the follicle susceptible to infection by *Pseudomonas aeruginosa,* which is present in the tub in great numbers because of fecal contamination.

Candida albicans can cause a similar condition that is especially common in bed-fast, febrile patients. Folliculitis caused by dermatophytic fungal organisms is common, especially when tinea corporis, cruris, or pedis is mistreated with topical steroids, which in effect promote deeper and more vigorous fungal growth.

The follicular mite *Demodex* can cause folliculitis, usually on the face.

Pseudofolliculitis, a common condition often seen in black men, is caused by the sharp end of a shaved, curly hair that as it grows out, curls back in and actually reenters the follicle from which it came, provoking a chronic folliculitis.

Acne vulgaris (see Chap. 2-29) can evolve into a true folliculitis when it suddenly worsens because of superinfection with gram-negative organisms.

DIFFERENTIAL DIAGNOSIS

Folliculitis can be mistaken for acne, but multiple comedones (blackheads or whiteheads), which are missing in folliculitis, are seen in acne. Tiny flat warts, especially common on the face; tiny mollusca; and herpes simplex vesicles can all mimic folliculitis.

Inflamed inclusion cysts can do a good imitation of a carbuncle; they are relatively nontender and are characterized by modest erythema confined to the immediate perilesional skin, whereas a carbuncle is exquisitely tender ("sore as a boil") and hot to touch with a relatively large zone of erythematous blush around it.

LABORATORY

Gram stain of pustular material looking for clusters of gram-positive cocci and polymorphonuclear neutrophil leukocytes (PMNs), bacterial culture and sensitivity, potassium hydroxide (KOH) preparation for the pustule roof (the need for which should be suggested by the failure of antibacterial treatment), and punch biopsies can all be helpful but are seldom necessary in ordinary circumstances. In chronic furunculosis, consider checking the blood sugar for evidence of diabetes and doing a complete blood cell count (CBC) for neutropenia.

TREATMENT

For superficial mild folliculitis, use topical antibacterials such as mupirocin (Bactroban) plus warm soaks.

For acute furunculosis, hot packing and incision and drainage (I & D) usually suffice. The same is true for carbuncles if the incision and drainage are adequate. Systemic antibiotics are seldom necessary unless systemic symptoms (fever, chills, malaise) are present, suggesting the need for blood cultures before antibiotic treatment. Positive blood cultures suggest the need for intravenous (IV) antibiotic therapy.

For chronic furunculosis, long-term (2 to 3 months minimum) treatment with clindamycin 150 mg qid is often used, along with nightly swabbing of the nares with mupirocin and daily use of antibacterial bar soaps.

Pseudomonas folliculitis is usually self-limited and relatively asymptomatic; thus, no treatment is necessary unless pain, fever, or chills are present. Yeast or fungal folliculitis often requires treatment with oral antifungals (ketoconazole, fluconazole, itraconazole, or terbinafine), especially if inappropriate steroid treatment has encouraged infection deeper into the dermis.

Demodex folliculitis (diagnosed by KOH preparation) can be treated with crotamiton (Eurax) cream twice a day.

The best treatment for pseudofolliculitis barbae is to stop shaving. Gram-negative folliculitis, as a complication of acne, is commonly treated with long-term sulfa drugs. However, culture and sensitivity may be necessary to establish the best treatment as well as the diagnosis.

PATIENT EDUCATION

Stress the importance of home treatment measures such as hot packing and antibiotic ointment application. Educate diabetics and other immunocompromised patients about watching for the development of systemic symptoms. In hot tub folliculitis, after reassuring the patient about the usually benign course, refer the patient to the county health department for advice about how to prevent such problems in the future.

PEARLS

Knowledge of the following points can contribute to a positive patient outcome:

• Look for a pustule pierced by a hair when folliculitis is suspected.
• Suspect yeast or fungal folliculitis when antibacterial measures fail, topical steroid application makes things worse, or the patient is immunosuppressed.
• The morphologic appearance of *Pseudomonas* folliculitis lesions is distinctive:
  They are central tiny pustules surrounded by a 0.15- to 0.30-cm circle of bluish red, slightly edematous skin.
  They are more likely to be found on the skin under a bathing suit, are usually surprisingly asymptomatic, and do not always affect everyone who was in the hot tub.
• Suspect gram-negative folliculitis when acne formerly responsive to tetracycline suddenly gets out of control and starts to turn cystic.
• When boils begin with menarche and chronically recur in the axillae, groin, and intergluteal skin, it is probably hidradenitis suppurativa.

PROGNOSIS

The prognosis for folliculitis is self-limited in most cases, except as was noted above.

BIBLIOGRAPHY

Arndt KA, Robinson JK, LeBoit PE, et al: *Cutaneous Medicine and Surgery.* Philadelphia, Saunders, 1996.
DuVivier A: *Dermatology in Practice.* Philadelphia, Lippincott, 1990.
Fitzpatrick TB, Johnson JA, Wolff K, et al: *Color Atlas and Synopsis of Clinical Dermatology: Common and Serious Diseases,* 3d ed. New York, McGraw-Hill, 1997.
Goldstein BG, Goldstein AO: *Practical Dermatology,* Primary Care Series. St Louis, Mosby Year Book, 1992.
Shelly WB, Shelley ED: *Advanced Dermatologic Diagnosis.* Philadelphia, Saunders, 1992.
Weinberg S, Prose NS, Kristal L: *Color Atlas of Pediatric Dermatology,* 3d ed. New York, McGraw-Hill, 1998.

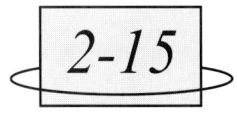

HAND-FOOT-AND-MOUTH DISEASE
Barbara L. Sauls

DISCUSSION

Hand-foot-and-mouth disease is a self-limiting viral infection that usually is caused by subtype A16 of the coxsackievirus family but also may result from another enteroviral infection. The most commonly affected individuals are children age 2 to 8 years. Infectiousness occurs in the manner of a typical virus with a tendency to pass to school or day care mates and siblings, though many contacts will be spared. This disease occurs most frequently in the spring months. A variant of this illness is herpangina (subtype A7), which has lesions limited to the pharynx.

SIGNS AND SYMPTOMS

The signs and symptoms of hand-foot-and-mouth disease are fairly classic. Children commonly develop a prodrome of anorexia, nausea, vomiting, and diarrhea with or without mild elevation of temperature. This is followed by the development of painful small oral vesicles that ulcerate, commonly found along the soft palate (see Fig. 2-15-1 and Plate 11). This results in a sore throat and dysphagia, with children

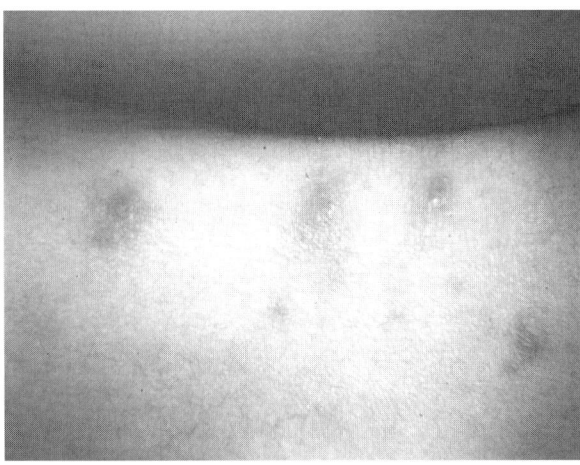

FIGURE 2-15-1 (PLATE 11). Typical lesions of hand-foot-and-mouth disease. Small vesicular papules or tiny ulcers with surrounding erythema. (*Photo courtesy of William H. Fenn. Used with permission.*)

often refusing everything by mouth for several days. A vesicular eruption also develops on the soles of the feet and the palms of the hands. These distal lesions usually do not ulcerate. The development of a rash on the soles and palms is unusual in other viral illnesses, since these areas are most often spared.

OBJECTIVE FINDINGS

Physical examination reveals a benign general picture except for the skin and pharynx. Temperature is often normal or is mildly elevated. Oral examination shows lesions in various stages beginning as small vesicles, whitish to gray in color, with a red halo; the lesions often are pinpoint in size. The oral lesions are seen along the soft palate, uvula, and tonsillar area but do not involve the buccal mucosa, lips, or tongue. These areas eventually ulcerate to form a shallow crater with a red base but do not progress further. Even though there is poor oral intake of fluids, there are usually no signs of dehydration unless the condition is accompanied by a more severe gastrointestinal (GI) illness. Infants and young children are more prone to dehydration.

The lesions on the soles and palms are often discrete. The vesicles are often very small and filled with a minimal amount of fluid. These lesions do not ulcerate and are not usually painful. The patient or parent often does not notice the lesions until the practitioner points them out. It is often difficult to distinguish these lesions clearly in very dark-skinned individuals.

DIAGNOSTIC CONSIDERATIONS

The differential diagnosis of the oral illness most commonly includes herpesvirus infection (see Chaps. 2-16 and 2-17), although these lesions commonly involve the lips, tongue, gingiva, and buccal mucosa, which are spared in coxsackievirus infection. A rash on the soles and palms may be seen in Rocky Mountain spotted fever, but this has a much more severe onset, is macular in appearance, and occurs on the trunk and extremities as well as the soles and palms. The lesions do not form vesicles in this disease.

LABORATORY TESTS

It is not usually necessary to order any laboratory tests for this illness, although it is possible to order serologic studies for coxsackievirus if the practitioner believes it is needed. Viral cultures are expensive and of limited value in the treatment of this disease.

TREATMENT

Treatment of hand-foot-and-mouth disease is supportive in nature; there is no specific cure for this illness. If the patient is able to swallow small amounts of fluid, it is usually possible to encourage small sips every half hour along with acetaminophen or ibuprofen for pain relief. Over-the-counter sore throat sprays (Chloraseptic) or gargles may offer some relief. Patients who are unable to swallow anything are given either viscous lidocaine to dab on specific areas with a cotton swab or lidocaine solution to swish, gargle, and spit. An alternative is "magic mouthwash," which is mixed by the pharmacist and is a combination of 2 oz Maalox, 1 oz viscous Xylocaine, and 15 mL liquid Benadryl. Some practitioners keep the ingredients on hand and mix it themselves for patients. Patients may swish, gargle, and spit several times daily. Swallowing the solution will not harm younger infants. The numbing effect allows patients to eat and drink adequate amounts. Counsel the parents to watch for signs of dehydration.

SUPPORTIVE MEASURES

Supportive measures include rest and increasing food intake as tolerated.

PATIENT EDUCATION

It is important to counsel patients that this illness may take up to 2 weeks to resolve fully. They should not expect the sore throat to go away overnight. Parents often call back in 2 days when their child is still not eating, but proper education helps them overcome their fears. Let them know that fluids are more important than solid food at this point.

DISPOSITION

Follow-up appointments are not necessary unless there is a need to monitor hydration status, as in the very young or in those with longer-lasting illness. Dehydration is an uncommon complication of this illness.

BIBLIOGRAPHY

Fitzpatrick TB, Johnson RA, Wolff K, et al: *Color Atlas and Synopsis of Clinical Dermatology: Common and Serious Diseases,* 3d ed. New York, McGraw-Hill, 1997.
Fauci AS, Braunwald E, Isselbacher KJ, Wilson JD, et al (eds): *Harrison's Principles of Internal Medicine,* 14th ed. New York, McGraw-Hill, 1998.

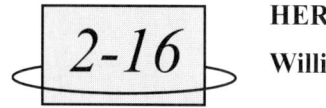

HERPES SIMPLEX
William H. Fenn

DISCUSSION

Herpes simplex viruses types 1 and 2 (HSV-1 and HSV-2) cause superficial mucocutaneous infections in humans. These vesicular eruptions range from the ubiquitous cold sore to the stigmatized genital herpes and together account for well over 100 million outbreaks yearly in the United States alone.

PATHOPHYSIOLOGY

Initial infection with either double-stranded DNA virus occurs after direct transmission from an infected person. Although standing water, such as on the side of a pool, has been shown to harbor the virus for short periods, the virus is incapable of infection via such a route. Inoculation requires direct contact from an infected person to mucous membranes or abraded skin. Most often this dispersion occurs from an active lesion; however, some asymptomatic persons actively shed the virus. As the virus penetrates epidermal cells, viral reproduction and host cell destruction occur with resulting intraepidermal vesicles. Symptoms occur after a 2- to 20-day incubation period, with 95 percent of patients developing symptoms within 2 weeks. After the initial acute episode, the virus migrates to the sensory or autonomic ganglia and becomes dormant, with reactivation possible after several reported factors, including stress, ultraviolet radiation, and certain foods.

Many conflicting reports attribute differing proportions of HSV-1 and HSV-2 to oropharyngeal versus genital sites. From a clinical point of view, there is no need to distinguish the two strains, since treatment is based on site and primary versus recurrent eruption. Therefore, it is not useful to get caught up in this issue. However, it is important to avoid drawing conclusions regarding the transmission source solely on the basis of viral subtype identification.

SIGNS AND SYMPTOMS

Patients complain of a painful eruption that sometimes is accompanied by fever, general malaise, and headaches. In some people, the

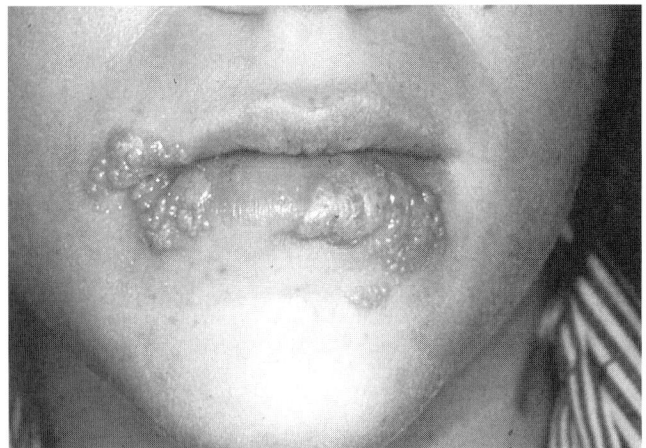

FIGURE 2-16-1 (PLATE 12). Herpes simplex lesions on the lips. Noted grouped vesicles on an erythematous base. (*Photo courtesy of William H. Fenn.*)

subjective symptoms precede the eruption, and for some individuals with recurrent disease, this prodrome is a reliable predictor of eruption. As a general rule, the discomfort of an initial eruption is more severe than that of subsequent recurrences, but this is far from universal.

OBJECTIVE FINDINGS

The classic eruption of herpes simplex is one of localized grouped vesicles on an erythematous base. However, these vesicles rapidly turn into pustules that rupture, resulting in a weeping erosive lesion that subsequently crusts. Recurrences may consist of a single small vesicle.

The most common location is at or near the vermilion border of the mouth, referred to as herpes labialis (see Fig. 2-16-1 and Plate 12). However, it is important to remember that HSV infection can occur anywhere on the skin. When it occurs on the trunk or extremities, it frequently takes on some characteristics of herpes zoster and is referred to as zosteriform herpes simplex. Herpes genitalis may occur anywhere on the genitals, but in females it is found most commonly on the labia. Low-grade fever is common, especially in primary infections. Regional lymphadenopathy is very common in primary and recurrent disease.

DIAGNOSTIC CONSIDERATIONS

As was noted above, truncal HSV may resemble zoster. Oral HSV may resemble aphthous stomatitis. Contact dermatitis is relatively less likely in the face of pain and systemic signs and symptoms. Impetigo may be ruled out by Gram stain. Genital lesions may suggest chancroid or lymphogranuloma venereum: A syphilitic chancre is relatively less likely in the face of pain.

SPECIAL CONSIDERATIONS

HSV in immunocompromised hosts has a much higher risk for complications, many severe, and therapy must be more aggressive. Although it is beyond the scope of this chapter, neonatal herpes is a dreaded condition. As there is a 50 percent rate of transmission if the virus is present at delivery and the results of infection are devastating, a cesarean delivery is indicated. Routine prenatal screening also is recommended owing to the high incidence of clinically inapparent infection. A more diffuse eruption, eczema herpeticum, may occur in patients with atopic dermatitis, especially children. Although the appearance is more dramatic and the course more prolonged, treatment is usually quite successful. Secondary bacterial infection is common.

LABORATORY TESTS

The definitive test remains the viral culture. Polymerase chain reaction (PCR) laboratory studies to identify HSV exist but are not widely available clinically. A number of antigen detection systems are available, with differing levels of sensitivity and specificity. Serologic testing is of limited value because of the retrospective nature of the result and the fact that more than 85 percent of adults have antibodies to HSV-1.

Gram stain will help distinguish a bacterial infection, and other serologic tests may be indicated if other disorders are under consideration.

Most protocols call for routine laboratory screening for other sexually transmitted diseases, including HIV testing with patient consent, any time a diagnosis of primary genital herpes is established.

RADIOLOGIC STUDIES

There are no appropriate radiologic studies for HSV.

OTHER DIAGNOSTIC CONSIDERATIONS

The Tzanck smear is a simple and useful office procedure. The lesion is unroofed (if needed), and the base is gently scraped with a blade. The material is placed on a slide and stained with Wright stain, Giemsa stain, or toluidine blue. A positive smear displays multinucleated giant cells (see Fig. 2-16-2 and Plate 13). The sensitivity of this test is variable, and so a negative test does not disprove the diagnosis. The test is specific only to herpes viruses in general and thus will not distinguish simplex from zoster.

TREATMENT

Medications

Therapy is aimed at controlling symptoms as well as reducing recurrences and sequelae. Although no treatment is available that eradicates infection, prompt institution of therapy has been shown to dramatically reduce the healing time and reduce viral shedding.

PRIMARY INFECTION   The treatment consists of acyclovir (Zovirax) 200 mg five times daily for 10 days or valacyclovir (Valtrex) 1 g bid for 10 days. Therapy should be instituted within 48 to 72 h of onset; after this time, treatment is of questionable benefit. Famciclovir (Famvir) has not been approved for initial infections but has been used. These agents are of approximately equal effectiveness; however, acyclovir is far less costly, while the others have increased compliance,

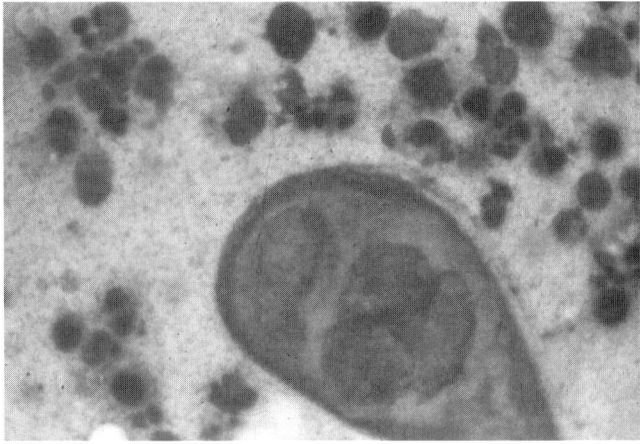

FIGURE 2-16-2 (PLATE 13). Positive Tzanck smear with arrow indicating giant multinucleated cell. (*Photo courtesy of William H. Fenn.*)

presumably because of simpler dosing schedules. Acyclovir ointment is much less effective and generally is not recommended.

RECURRENT INFECTION   Treatment consists of acyclovir 200 mg five times daily for 5 days, valacyclovir 500 mg twice daily for 5 days, or famciclovir 125 mg twice daily for 5 days.

Since prompt initiation of therapy is essential, patients should be given a single supply of medication to keep at home, with instructions to initiate a course of medication at the first sign of recurrent infection. Patients with predictable prodromal symptoms should begin the medication at the onset of the symptoms.

SUPPRESSION OF RECURRENCES   Current recommendations call for suppressive therapy in any patient who experiences six or more recurrent genital infections in a 12-month period. Acyclovir (400 mg twice daily), famciclovir (250 mg twice daily), or valacyclovir (500 mg to 1 g daily) administered for up to 1 year dramatically reduces the frequency and severity of infections but does not eliminate viral shedding.

SPECIAL CASES   Immunocompromised patients and other patients with acyclovir-resistant disease may require foscarnet or vidarabine.

Supportive Measures

Cool dressing or soaks may offer short-term relief from discomfort. Prescriptive analgesics may be warranted, depending on the site and extent of the eruption. A number of over-the-counter preparations for nongenital lesions are available. Although these preparations have not been subjected to objective clinical trials, sufficient anecdotal reports exist to suggest that they may be of symptomatic benefit.

Patient Education

Preventive measures must be discussed frankly. It is important to assist the patient in dealing with the stigma associated with this disease. Many areas have support groups, and the American Social Health Association maintains a herpes hotline. On-line support is available at www.herpes.net and www.herpes.org. The myths and realities of the sexual transmission of genital herpes must be explored, including the potential for transmission by asymptomatic patients. Many patients are not aware of this potential because their knowledge is based on information that is outdated. In the general population, the risk of contagion is reduced by condom use and increased by contact with multiple sexual partners.

COMPLICATIONS AND RED FLAGS

Autoinoculation to distant sites is possible. Herpetic keratitis, which is characterized by dendritic fluorescein staining, requires prompt ophthalmic evaluation. HSV-1 is a major etiologic agent for viral encephalitis. Uncommonly, HSV patients may develop erythema multiforme.

OTHER NOTES OR PEARLS

Several new antiviral medications for treating HSV infection are under development, with release imminent. Additionally, clinical trials of HSV-2 vaccines are under way. A successful vaccine program would change the approach to this infection dramatically.

BIBLIOGRAPHY

Fitzpatrick TB, Johnson RA, Wolff K, et al: *Color Atlas and Synopsis of Clinical Dermatology,* 3d ed. New York, McGraw-Hill, 1997, pp 792–809.
Goldstein BG, Goldstein AO: *Practical Dermatology,* 2d ed. St. Louis, Mosby, 1997, pp 237–240.

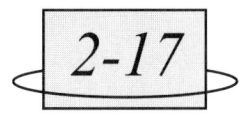

HERPES ZOSTER
William H. Fenn

DISCUSSION

Herpes zoster (shingles) is an acute painful vesicular eruption that occurs along the distribution of a dermatome in patients with a history of varicella. The incidence increases with age, with two-thirds of cases occurring after age 50 and fewer than 10 percent occurring before age 20. The lifetime risk is probably between 10 and 20 percent.

PATHOPHYSIOLOGY

Herpes zoster is the reactivation of latent varicella-zoster virus (VZV) from its latency in sensory ganglia. It occurs after primary VZV infection (varicella), usually many years later. The incidence increases with age, presumably as host immune response declines. Other causes of immune reduction, such as HIV infection, also increase the incidence. When reactivated, the virus migrates down the involved sensory nerve, causing prodromal symptoms of pain and pruritus to the skin, where the characteristic eruption ensues.

SIGNS AND SYMPTOMS

These patients complain of pain and altered sensation in the affected area, which may precede the eruption by 3 to 5 days. These symptoms may lessen somewhat with the onset of the eruption but generally persist throughout the course. A minority of patients may report associated headache, general malaise, and fever.

OBJECTIVE FINDINGS

The principal lesions are groups of vesicles and bullae on an erythematous base, but early presentation will show papules and late presentation will show only confluent crusting and weeping lesions (see Fig. 2-17-1 and Plate 14). The defining characteristic of the eruption is its distribution within a unilateral dermatome, although a few discrete lesions across the midline are not uncommon, presumably owing to small nerve fiber crossings. Occasionally infection occurs in adjacent dermatomes, and it occurs rarely in bilateral dermatomes. Occasionally zoster occurs without visible lesions. Regional lymphadenopathy is usual, and a low-grade fever may be present.

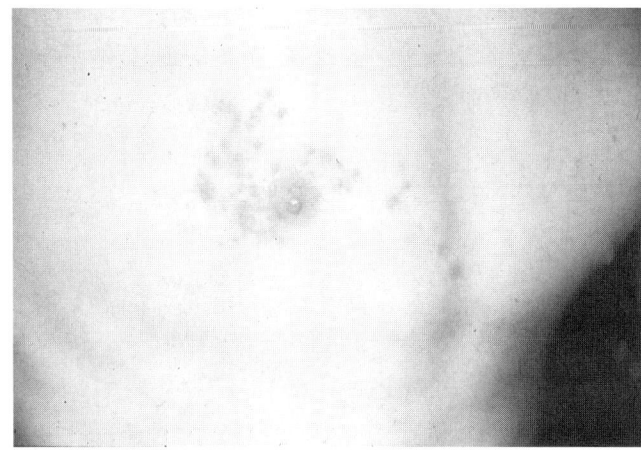

FIGURE 2-17-1 (PLATE 14). Herpes zoster (shingles) lesions on the chest. Note grouped vesiculations. (*Photo courtesy of William H. Fenn.*)

DIAGNOSTIC CONSIDERATIONS

Herpes simplex occasionally can appear in a dermatome pattern, and multiple recurrences suggest this diagnosis. The prodromal pain may suggest several different diagnoses, depending on the location. Involvement of cranial dermatomes may mimic migraine, thoracic dermatomes pleuritis, or myocardial infarction, and lumbar dermatome involvement may suggest a herniated nucleus pulposus. The onset of the eruption generally makes the diagnosis clear, but appropriate diagnostic measures to rule out underlying pathology should not be delayed pending the eruption.

SPECIAL CONSIDERATIONS

Involvement of the auditory or ophthalmic nerves warrants specialist evaluation. Vesicles on the tip of the nose indicate involvement of the nasociliary branch of the ophthalmic nerve.

Immunocompromised patients may develop disseminated zoster and visceral involvement.

LABORATORY TESTS

Generally testing is not necessary. Viral culture is definitive when needed. Direct immunofluorescence staining is also available. Tzanck smears are easily performed (see "Other Diagnostic Considerations" in Chap. 2-16) but do not distinguish between zoster and simplex eruptions.

RADIOLOGIC AND OTHER DIAGNOSTIC STUDIES

There are no appropriate radiologic or diagnostic studies for herpes zoster.

TREATMENT

Medications

Treatment consists of acyclovir (Zovirax) 800 mg five times daily for 7 to 10 days, valacyclovir (Valtrex) 1 g three times daily for 7 days, or famciclovir (Famvir) 500 mg every 8 h for 7 days.

Prompt institution of therapy reduces acute pain and healing time. Therapy does not appear to affect the incidence of postherpetic neuralgia (PHN), although famciclovir is reported to reduce its duration.

The use of potent analgesics is often warranted. Several recommendations have been made for the use of systemic steroids in older populations to reduce the risk of PHN; however, this benefit has not been confirmed, and such treatment is probably not worthwhile. Tricyclic antidepressant therapy, TENS, and topical capsaicin (Zostrix) may be useful in the management of PHN if it occurs.

Supportive Measures

The lesions should be kept clean to avoid secondary bacterial infection. Cool or astringent compresses may reduce weeping, but otherwise topical measures are generally ineffective.

Patient Education

Educate patients about the cause and course of the disease. Patients should be aware that in at least 30 percent of cases, they may transmit VZV to nonimmune persons, which will cause varicella, not zoster. This is particularly relevant in older patients who may be visiting grandchildren.

Patients should be aware that recurrence is possible, although the 5 percent recurrence rate is lower than most patients and health care personnel believe.

Disposition

Patients should be reexamined if the character of drainage changes or if symptoms are progressive. Persistence of pain after the lesions have resolved should prompt evaluation and discussion of PHN.

COMPLICATIONS AND RED FLAGS

PHN is the most likely complication. It is uncommon under age 40 but occurs in up to 65 percent of patients over age 60. The variation in incidence figures is due partly to the many definitions of PHN. Most commonly it is regarded as pain persisting longer than 1 month.

Treatment reduces symptoms in many patients, and 80 percent of patients with PHN are asymptomatic at 1 year. Radical therapies such as nerve destruction are, fortunately, seldom indicated.

OTHER NOTES OR PEARLS

The advent of vaccination to prevent varicella offers the possibility of a reduction in the incidence of herpes zoster. Proof of this, however, is lacking, and it will be some time before the effects of widespread immunization on zoster incidence are known. As the onset of zoster appears to be related to a reduction in immune status, it is also possible that a booster immunization of the varicella vaccine in aging patients with a history of varicella may reduce the incidence of zoster. The results of ongoing controlled studies are needed before such recommendations can be made.

BIBLIOGRAPHY

Fitzpatrick TB, Johnson RA, Wolff K, et al: *Color Atlas and Synopsis of Clinical Dermatology,* 3d ed. New York, McGraw-Hill, 1997, pp 810–825.

Goldstein BG, Goldstein AO: *Practical Dermatology,* 2d ed. St. Louis, Mosby, 1997, pp 240–243.

Levin MJ, Hayward AR: The varicella vaccine: Prevention of herpes zoster. *Infect Dis Clin North Am* 10(3):657–675, 1996.

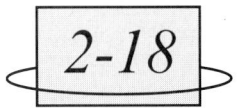

HUMAN PAPILLOMAVIRUS
Michelle DiBaise

DISCUSSION

The human papillomavirus (HPV) infects keratinized skin and is therefore limited to the epidermis. More than 60 HPV subtypes have been identified.[1–5] Some of those subtypes have been shown to play a role in skin and mucosal oncogenesis, predominantly squamous cell carcinoma. There is an increased incidence of all warts in immunocompromised individuals, as in the cases of HIV disease, organ transplantation, and the use of immunosuppressive agents. These warts tend to be larger, more numerous, and more difficult to eradicate.

Verruca Vulgaris

Known as the common wart, verruca vulgaris accounts for approximately 70 percent of all cutaneous warts.[1] As many as 5 to 20 percent of all school-age children will develop warts.[1,4,5] Verruca vulgaris is spread by skin-to-skin contact, especially through minor breaks in the skin from trauma or underlying dermatoses.

Verruca Plantaris

The plantar wart can occur on the palms as well as the soles. It accounts for approximately 30 percent of all warts and is most common in older children and young adults.[1] Like the common wart, it is spread by skin-to-skin contact. A phenomenon called "kissing warts" occurs in which two warts develop where skin surfaces touch.

Verruca Plana

The flat wart accounts for only about 4 percent of all cutaneous warts.[1] It is most common in children and adults. Like other warts, it is spread by skin-to-skin contact. More than other varieties of warts, it is commonly spread by shaving.

Condyloma Acuminata

The most common mucosal form of HPV is condyloma acuminata, or the genital wart.[1] It is the most prevalent sexually transmitted disease in all developed countries, including the United States.[1,3,6] It is estimated that 3 to 28 percent of women have condylomata.[1] Among females with condylomata, nearly 100 percent of their male sex partners are infected, and the majority of the lesions are subclinical.

Clinical warts are thought to be more infectious than the subclinical wart. Once infected, it may take weeks to months for an individual to develop lesions. The lesions of condylomata can last for months to years; however, there is some evidence that the infection may last throughout the individual's lifetime.

Condylomata in infants and children can imply sexual abuse. Studies show that up to 50 percent of genital HPV in infants and children actually is related to sexual abuse.[2,4] It may be difficult to prove abuse because there is a prolonged incubation period before the development of lesions. This hinders pinpointing the exact time of the infection. Also, HPV can be acquired from passage through the birth canal of an infected woman.[1,4,5] Common warts on the hands occasionally can be spread to the genitalia, mouth, or anal area from the child or a caretaker.[2,4,5]

SIGNS AND SYMPTOMS

Most warts are usually asymptomatic. They may cause cosmetic disfigurement and therefore affect the patient's self-esteem. They can be painful and interfere with normal daily activity. Plantar warts can be painful enough to interfere with walking. Recurrent trauma such as that which occurs with shaving or toileting can cause warts to bleed.

OBJECTIVE FINDINGS

Verruca Vulgaris

The common wart is a round, dome-shaped papule, firm to palpation, with thickening of the stratum corneum (hyperkeratosis) and measuring 1 to 10 mm in size.[1,5] The surface has vegetations and is clefted. It is generally flesh-colored and may have black dots that are actually thrombosed capillary loops within the wart. Lesions tend to be discrete but can at times coalesce into larger plaques (see Fig. 2-18-1 and Plate 15).

Previously treated warts can form around the area of the old wart in an annular or doughnut shape. The wart is commonly found in areas that are recurrently traumatized, such as the hands, fingers, and knees. When the wart involves the paronychia, it can extend underneath the nail plate. A variant of the common wart is the filiform wart, which generally occurs on the head and neck. It has a narrow base and fingerlike projections.

Verruca Plantaris

A plantar wart begins as a small, flesh-colored papule but eventually enlarges into hyperkeratotic plaques with multiple black dots. Warts on the palms and soles distort the normal skin lines of the finger or footprint and occur over weight-bearing areas such as the metatarsal heads and heel.

Verruca Plana

Flat warts are round or oval, flat, flesh-colored or light-brown papules measuring 1 to 5 mm in diameter and only 1 to 2 mm in thickness.[1–3,6] They are common on the face and dorsum of the hands [see Fig. 2-18-2 (Plate 16)]. In men, they frequently are spread in the beard area from shaving, and in women they spread on the legs. When they are spread through autoinoculation from shaving or scratching, they have a linear appearance.

Condyloma Acuminata

Condylomata begin as minute papules and may grow to soft, moist, large cauliflower- or grape-like lesions. If lesions are subclinical, they are best visualized by applying 5 to 7% acetic acid to the skin for 5 min (aceto-whitening), which turns the lesions white. Clinical

FIGURE 2-18-1 (PLATE 15). Verruca vulgaris. (*From Fitzpatrick, Johnson, Wolff, et al.*[1])

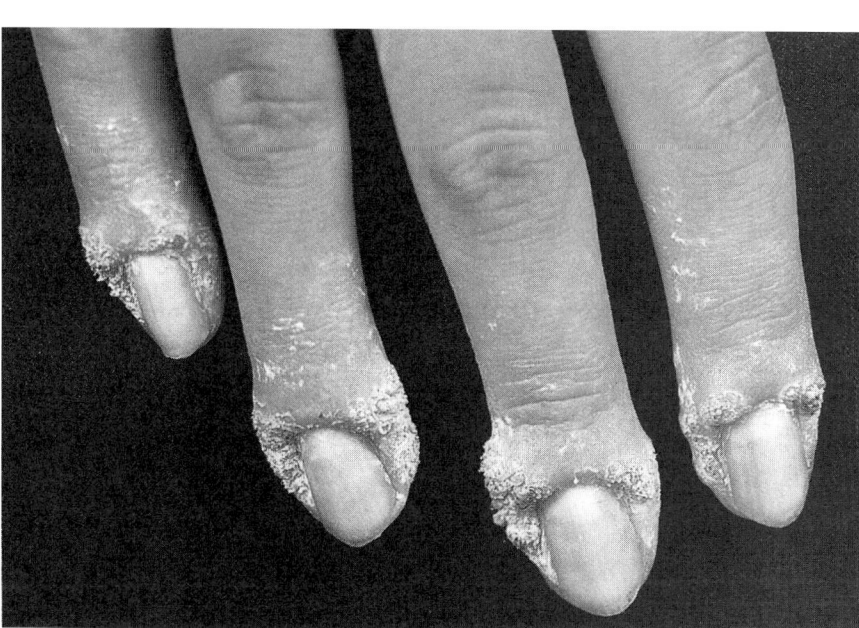

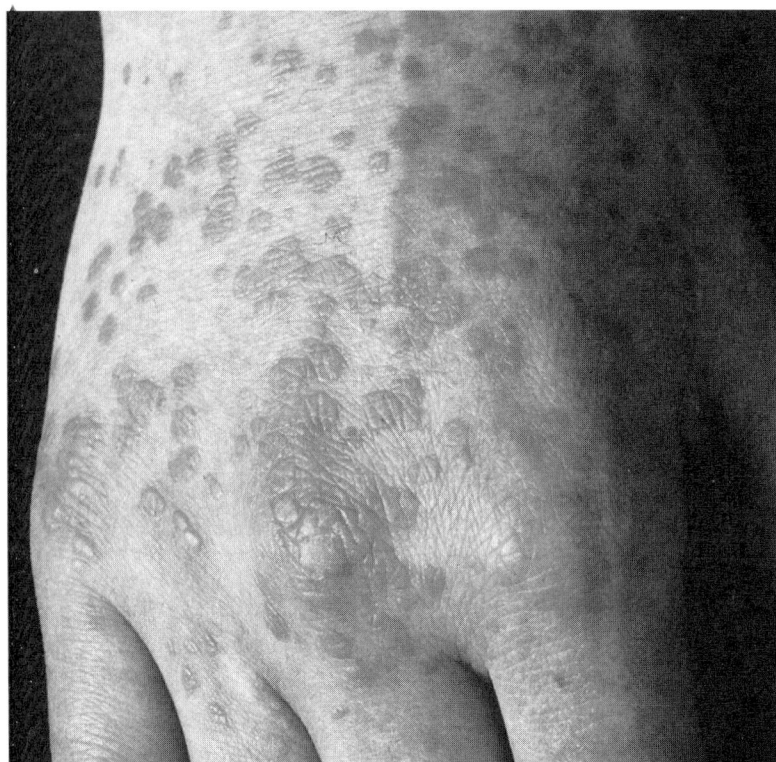

FIGURE 2-18-2 (PLATE 16). Verruca plana. (*From Fitzpatrick, Johnson, Wolff, et al.*[1])

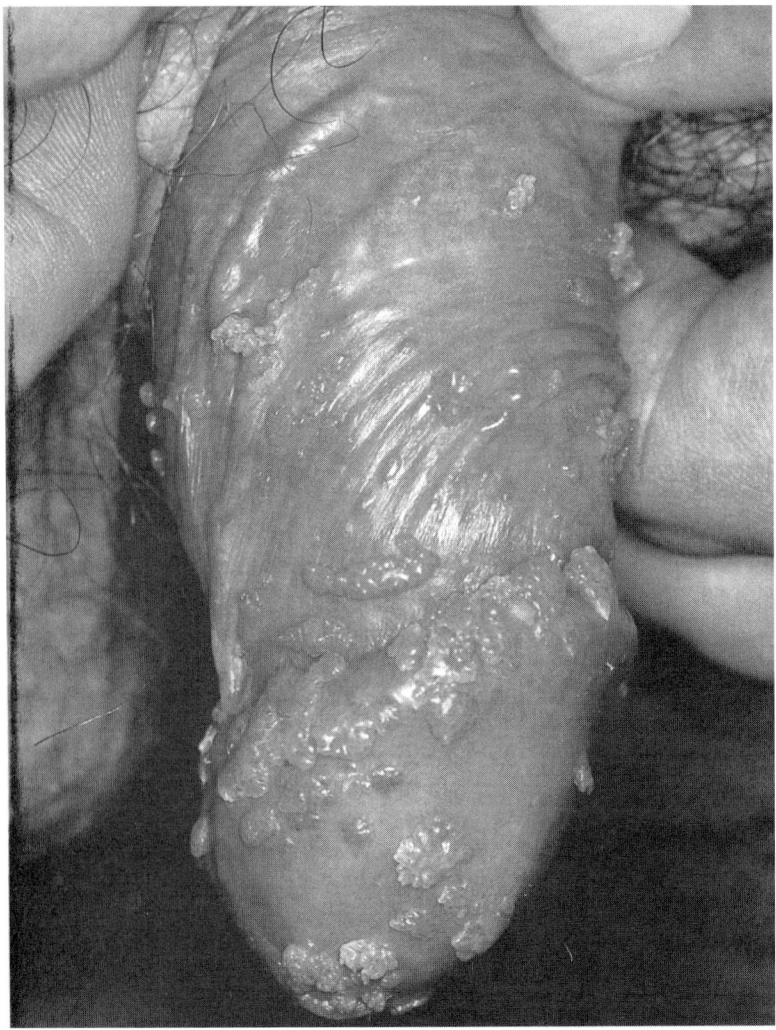

FIGURE 2-18-3 (PLATE 17). Condyloma acuminata. (*From Fitzpatrick, Johnson, Wolff, et al.*[1])

lesions are flesh-colored in general but can be pink or red. They usually occur in clusters and tend to occur on the penis and scrotum in men, the vagina and cervix in women, and the perineal area, perianal area, urethra, rectum, bladder, and oropharynx in both sexes [see Fig. 2-18-3 (Plate 17)].

DIAGNOSTIC CONSIDERATIONS

Verruca Vulgaris

The differential diagnosis of the common wart includes molluscum contagiosum, seborrheic keratoses, and callus. In a callus, the normal skin lines are maintained. In older individuals and immunosuppressed persons, the differential also includes basal cell carcinoma and squamous cell carcinoma.

Verruca Plantaris

The differential diagnosis for plantar warts includes callus, corns, and the shearing trauma that occurs in sports. Both a callus and a corn do not distort the normal skin lines or exhibit black dots.

Verruca Plana

The differential diagnosis for flat warts includes molluscum contagiosum, seborrheic keratoses, syringoma (when present on the face), closed comedones, and lichen planus.

Condyloma Acuminata

The differential diagnosis for condyloma acuminata includes condyloma lata (a manifestation of secondary syphilis), squamous cell carcinoma (invasive or in situ), molluscum contagiosum, bowenoid papulosis (see "Complications and Red Flags," below), lichen planus, seborrheic keratoses, skin tags, pearly penile papules (a benign variant seen on the corona of the penis and occasionally on the shaft), nevi, and sebaceous glands.

LABORATORY TESTS

Verruca Vulgaris and Verruca Plantaris

The diagnosis is almost always based on clinical findings. If there is doubt, a no. 15 blade can be used to gently pare the wart and confirm the presence of the black dots of the thrombosed capillaries.

Verruca Plana

The diagnosis usually is made by clinical examination. The linear distribution leads away from a diagnosis of seborrheic keratosis and toward that of flat warts.

Condyloma Acuminata

Clinical examination is usually sufficient to make the diagnosis. Subclinical lesions can best be discerned by aceto-whitening. Aceto-whitening is not specific for HPV. Other lesions that whiten with acetic acid include candidiasis, lichen planus, normal sebaceous glands, psoriasis, and areas of healing.[2] Because condylomata is a sexually transmitted disease (STD), the practitioner should consider testing for other STDs, such as syphilis and HIV. Women with condylomata and those whose partners have condylomata should have annual Pap smears because of the increased risk for cervical dysplasia and squamous cell carcinoma. Anoscopy or proctoscopy should be considered in the presence of perianal warts. The most common HPV types associated with malignant change include 6, 11, 16, 18, 31, and 33.[1–5] HPV subtyping can be performed in cases of sexual abuse.

TREATMENT

In an immunocompetent host, warts are self-limiting. Estimates are that between 35 and 65 percent of warts spontaneously resolve in 2 years.[3,5] They usually resolve with little or no intervention. It is best, therefore, to avoid overly aggressive treatments that risk scarring. Up to 20 percent of patients will have recalcitrant warts requiring more aggressive therapy.[2] An immunocompromised host will have warts that are very difficult to eradicate. These patients may require monthly visits in which the goal is controlling the bulk of the lesions, not eradication of the warts.

Verruca Vulgaris and Verruca Plantaris

Topical therapy includes over-the-counter medications that contain various strengths of salicylic acid 14 to 17% (Occlusol, DuoPlant, Compound W, and others). The medicine is painted on and allowed to dry every night. Resolution can be hastened by soaking the area for 10 to 15 min and gently paring the wart with an emery board. Care must be taken to use a new area of the emery board with each wart and dispose of the board when finished. The medicine is then applied to the pared wart. Cure rates have been reported at 70 percent for common warts and 84 percent for plantar warts.[6] The topical medications have a plaster variety with salicylic acid 40% (Mediplast, Duofilm, and others) that is applied directly to the wart and left in place for 24 to 48 h. The plaster is removed, the wart is pared down, and a new plaster is applied. This is repeated until the wart is gone. The plasters work best on larger warts because normal skin becomes macerated in the process.

Cryosurgery is an alternative for patients in whom topical medications used alone have failed. It can be used in conjunction with a topical medication as well. Liquid nitrogen is applied to the wart, using a cryospray or a cotton swab. The wart should be frozen until an ice ball forms on 1 to 2 mm of the surrounding normal skin. The area is allowed to thaw, and the procedure is repeated. The area may blister within 24 h. The patient is instructed not to rupture the blister. If the blister ruptures, it should be covered with antibiotic ointment and a dressing. The blister eventually will crust over in a few days. Once the crust falls off, if there is remaining wart, the topical medicine can be applied until the patient returns to the clinic. Repeat freezing usually occurs in 4-week cycles. Cryotherapy does not kill the virus but instead destroys the normal skin, sloughing the wart off in the process.

Electrocautery is an alternative to freezing. It is more effective than cryotherapy but has an increased incidence of scarring. The area can be anesthetized before the procedure by using EMLA (a topical anesthetic cream) or injecting lidocaine. HPV has been found in the plume of smoke from cautery and can cause infection of the airways.[1] Cure rates range from 60 to 80 percent.[6]

CO_2 laser surgery is also effective for recalcitrant warts. The area must be anesthetized. This treatment is expensive and potentially scarring. HPV has been found in the plume of smoke from laser procedures and can infect the airways.[1] Cure rates up to 90 percent have been reported.[6]

Surgical removal can be performed. The least scarring method is curettage. A shave procedure also may be performed. A surgical excision is not necessary, as the infection is limited to the epidermis.

Hyperthermia for plantar warts has been advocated.[1] It requires immersion in hot water for 30 to 45 min two to three times a week for up to 16 treatments.

Cimetidine (Tagamet) works as an immune modulator, most likely through the T-cell line, although the exact mechanism remains unclear. The dose necessary to show an effect is 400 mg tid in adults or an equivalent based on weight for children. Therapy must be continued for 3 months and be used in conjunction with a destructive method. The literature is mixed about whether the addition of cimetidine is effective compared to placebo.[4,7–12]

Interferon alpha (Intron-A, Alferon N) is reserved for warts that do not respond to conventional therapy and situations in which the disease process limits social and physical activity. The patient must be older than 18 years of age. It is given intralesionally three times a week, is extremely painful, and causes influenza-like symptoms. It is quite expensive. Regression has been reported in as many as 60 to 80 percent of lesions.[6]

Bleomycin sulfate is used intralesionally in cases of warts that have failed to respond to all forms of conventional therapy. It cannot be used in pregnant women. It has been shown to have a cure rate of 48 to 92 percent, depending on the location and size of the wart.[2,6] Side effects include pain, necrosis, and the development of Raynaud's phenomenon.

Contact immunotherapy uses agents such as dinitrochlorobenzene (DNCB), diphenylcyclopropenone, and squaric acid dibutylester. DNCB may be carcinogenic as well as mutagenic; therefore, its use should be avoided until further safety testing is available. Immunotherapy works by sensitizing the individual to the chemical in a remote site from the wart. The chemical agent is subsequently applied to the wart, causing immune destruction. Reported cure rates for DNCB were 80 percent in one study.[6]

Verruca Plana

Tretinoin (Retin A) has been shown to be effective for the treatment of flat warts. The doses available are 0.025, 0.05, and 0.1% cream and 0.01, 0.025, and 0.1% gel. Treatment may take several months and can produce irritation, excessive erythema, or scaling.

Light cryotherapy is an alternative but may require treatment over a large surface area.

Topical 5-fluorouracil (Efudex) is applied once or twice a day for approximately 1 month. It should be reserved for recalcitrant warts. It is irritating and may cause hyperpigmentation.

Condyloma Acuminata

Topical treatment can be performed either in the office or at home by the patient. In-office treatment is performed with podophyllin 10 to 25% in a tincture of benzoin compound. The solution is applied directly to the wart, avoiding normal skin. The amount applied can be no more than 0.5 mL or a surface area of 10 cm^2 per session. The solution is washed off completely within 1 to 4 h. The treatment can be repeated weekly. Systemic reactions have been noted, including renal effects, paresthesia, ileus, thrombocytopenia, leukopenia, polyneuritis, shock, and death.[2,3] If a biopsy is performed after therapy with podophyllin, the pathologist must be informed because the chemical changes may be mistaken for squamous cell carcinoma.[2] After six treatments, if warts persist, an alternative therapy should be considered.[1] Podophyllin cannot be used during pregnancy because of its effects on the fetus.[1,3]

The take-home treatment is podophyllin 0.5% (Podofilox, Condylox). The patient applies the solution to the warts twice a day for 3 days and then uses no treatment for the following 4 days. The cycle is repeated up to four times. The volume of solution should not be more than 0.5 mL per day or cover an area greater than 10 cm^2. Side effects include local pain, burning, inflammation, and erosion of the skin.[2] If the warts are still present after four cycles, an alternative form of therapy should be considered.[1] This treatment should not be used during pregnancy.

Trichloroacetic acid 25 to 90% can be used in the office. It is effective but potentially scarring with excessive application. The normal surrounding tissue is protected with petroleum jelly. The solution is applied directly to the wart, which reacts immediately by whitening. The excess acid is then neutralized with sodium bicarbonate. The warts can be treated weekly if necessary, but if they are present after six treatments, an alternative therapy should be considered.[1]

Cryotherapy is an inexpensive alternative performed in the office. The method is the same as that for common warts. It does not result in scarring; however, it is painful. Cryotherapy can be repeated monthly and also can be used in combination with topical at-home therapy.

Electrocautery is an effective method for the removal of warts. As in common warts, it requires anesthesia and is potentially scarring; HPV particles are potentially aerosolized in the smoke.

CO_2 laser is best reserved for extensive lesions and for those who have failed other treatment regimens. A "brush" technique has been developed that superficially coagulates normal-appearing skin in an attempt to eradicate subclinical lesions. This technique can be used on the mucosal surfaces.[2]

Interferon alpha (Intron-A, Alferon N), as in other varieties of warts, should be reserved for cases that have failed conventional therapy. However, it has been shown to clear approximately 36 to 54 percent of recalcitrant lesions.[2,4]

5% Imiquimod (Aldara) is reserved for recalcitrant warts mostly because of cost factors. Despite studies that show effectiveness of 5% imiquimod for various types of warts, the only U.S. Food and Drug Administration (FDA)-approved indication at this time is for condyloma acuminata. It is applied topically three times a week and induces the production of interferon alpha and other cytokines. Side effects include minor erythema and irritation but no evidence of scarring. In one large double-blind trial, 5% imiquimod was shown to provide complete clearing in 56 percent of tested patients, with a recurrence rate of 13 percent.[13]

Topical 5-fluorouracil (Efudex) also is reserved for recalcitrant warts. It is applied as a cream to external genital regions and in a suppository form for the vaginal area. The normal skin is protected by the use of petroleum jelly, zinc oxide paste, or hydrocortisone ointment.[2] It cannot be used on pregnant women since it may cause birth defects. Side effects include irritation, inflammation, and ulceration.

Phase I trials have been conducted on a *human papillomavirus vaccine* for use in the treatment of genital warts. The vaccines have been shown to be safe and to stimulate immune responses in test subjects.[14,15] It remains to be seen whether these vaccines will prove to be efficacious in eradicating HPV infection and protecting against dysplasia and carcinoma of the cervix.

FOLLOW-UP

In condyloma acuminata, women with HPV of the genitalia and those whose male sex partners are infected with HPV should have annual Pap smears. The patient should be encouraged to use condoms to prevent transmission of the virus to uninfected partners. Recurrence is more likely to be due to activation of subclinical infection in the individual than to reinfection from the patient's sex partner.[1,2]

COMPLICATIONS AND RED FLAGS

Verruca Plana

A rare hereditary disorder, epidermodysplasia verruciformis, mimics verruca plana. The lesions are numerous and large, and they coalesce into larger plaques. Between 30 and 80 percent of cases have been reported to become squamous cell carcinoma, both in situ and invasive, usually in sun-exposed areas.[4–6]

Condyloma Acuminata

Condylomata can undergo malignant change and become squamous cell carcinoma, both in situ and invasive. Any lesion that does not resolve with adequate therapy may warrant a biopsy. Squamous cell carcinoma can arise on any mucosal surface infected with HPV, including the oropharynx and the rectum. An uncommon variant is bowenoid papulosis or intraepithelial neoplasia and is caused by HPV subtype 16. It occurs in the genital area of sexually active adults. It is an erythematous or pigmented papule that resembles squamous cell carcinoma in situ. It may resolve spontaneously. Females with bowenoid papulosis and female partners of infected men should have annual Pap smears because of the risk of cervical dysplasia.

Laryngeal papillomatosis is a condition that occurs in infants and adults from the nasal passages to the lungs. It presents with stridor, hoarseness, and only rarely airway obstruction from HPV-associated papillomas.[4,5] It may be acquired in infants born to mothers with active HPV infection. It does not appear that passage through the birth canal is necessary to develop laryngeal papillomatosis, since there are reports of affected infants who were delivered by cesarian section.[2] Adult infection has occurred when HPV-infected smoke was inhaled during cautery or laser procedures.

REFERENCES

1. Fitzpatrick TB, Johnson RA, Wolff K, et al: *Color Atlas and Synopsis of Clinical Dermatology: Common and Serious Diseases,* 3d ed. New York, McGraw-Hill, 1997, pp 766–771, 899–909.
2. Habif TP: *Clinical Dermatology: A Color Guide to Diagnosis and Treatment,* 3d ed. St. Louis, Mosby Yearbook, 1996, pp 297–303, 325–334.
3. Lookingbill DP, Marks, Jr. JG: *Principles of Dermatology,* 2d ed. Philadelphia, Saunders, 1993, pp 66–72.
4. Seabury-Stone M, Lynch PJ: Viral warts, in Sams WM, Lynch PJ (eds): *Principles and Practice of Dermatology,* 2d ed. New York, Churchill-Livingstone, 1996, pp 127–133.
5. Lowry DR, Androphy EJ: Warts, in Fitzpatrick TB, Eisen AZ, Wolff K, et al (eds): *Dermatology in General Medicine,* 5th ed. New York, McGraw-Hill, 1999, pp 2484–2497.
6. Arnold HL, Odom RB, James WD: *Andrews' Diseases of the Skin: Clinical Dermatology,* 8th ed. Philadelphia, Saunders, 1990, pp 468–476.
7. Wargon O: Cimetidine for mucosal warts in an HIV positive adult. *Australas J Dermatol* 37(3):149–150, 1996.
8. Glass AT, Solomon BA: Cimetidine therapy for recalcitrant warts in adults. *Arch Dermatol* 132(6):680–682, 1996.
9. Yilmaz E, Alpsoy E, Basaran E: Cimetidine therapy for warts: A placebo controlled, double-blind study. *J Am Acad Dermatol* 34(6):1005–1007, 1996.
10. Ronna T, Lebwohl M: Cimetidine therapy for plantar warts. *J Am Podiatr Med Assoc* 85(11):717–718, 1995.
11. Choi YS, Hann SK, Park YK: The effect of cimetidine on verruca plana juvenilis: Clinical trials in six patients. *J Dermatol* 20(8):497–500, 1993.
12. Orlow SJ, Paller A: Cimetidine therapy for multiple viral warts in children. *J Am Acad Dermatol* 28(5):794–796, 1993.
13. Edwards L, Ferenczy A, Eron L, et al: Self-administered topical 5% imiquimod cream for external anogenital warts. *Arch Dermatol* 134(1):25–30, 1998.
14. Rowen D, Lacey C: Toward a human papillomavirus vaccine. *Dermatol Clin* 16(4):835–838, 1998.
15. Thompson HS, Davies ML, Holding FP, et al: Phase I safety and antigenicity of TA-GW: A recombinant HPV6 L2E7 vaccine for the treatment of genital warts. *Vaccine* 17(1):40–49, 1999.

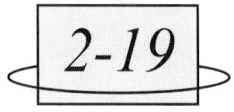

IMPETIGO AND ECTHYMA
Michelle DiBaise

DISCUSSION

Impetigo and ecthyma are common skin infections caused by *Staphylococcus aureus,* group A beta-hemolytic streptococci, or a combination of both. Impetigo occurs as superficial erosions, whereas ecthyma is a deeper infection. Both diseases can present as a primary or secondary infection.

Primary infection requires a minor trauma in which breaks in the skin allow bacteria to gain a portal of entry. In *S. aureus* infections, the patient may not remember a traumatic event. However, infection with group A beta-hemolytic streptococci requires more vigorous inoculation, usually from scratching.[1–3] Primary infections occur more often in children. Primary impetigo can be bullous or nonbullous. Bullous impetigo is due primarily to staphylococci that produce an exotoxin at the site of infection; the exotoxin produces cleavage within the epidermis. Bullous impetigo is seen more commonly in newborns and infants.[1–3]

Secondary infection occurs most commonly in inflammatory dermatoses (such as atopic dermatitis), bullous diseases, ulcers, burns, and trauma.[1–3] Lesions that are secondarily infected are said to be impetiginized. Secondary infections can occur at any age. Both primary and secondary lesions occur more commonly in warm temperatures, high humidity, overcrowded situations, individuals with poor hygiene, and persons with underlying dermatoses.[1–3]

With adequate treatment of impetigo, there is prompt resolution. Untreated lesions may last up to several weeks, but the majority resolve spontaneously. Some lesions, however, progress to areas of ecthyma, usually secondary to poor hygiene and neglect. Recurrence may occur because of failure to eradicate the organism or reinfection from a family member. Recurrent infection also may be an indication that the patient is a carrier of *S. aureus.* It is estimated that 20 to 40 percent of adult nasal passages are colonized with *S. aureus,* and approximately 20 percent of individuals are colonized on the perineum or axillae.[1,3] Among atopic individuals, 90 percent are colonized with *S. aureus* in areas of active lesions and 70 percent are colonized on apparently normal skin.[1,3]

SIGNS AND SYMPTOMS

Patients with impetigo may experience pruritus, especially in the presence of atopic dermatitis. They also may have mild discomfort in the area of the lesion. Individuals with ecthyma tend to experience more pain or tenderness. Systemic symptoms are not common, although the development of acute streptococcal glomerulonephritis has been reported.[1–4]

OBJECTIVE FINDINGS

Both bullous impetigo and nonbullous impetigo begin as vesicles with a very thin roof that is easily ruptured. Lesions can be found anywhere, but most often are located on the face. In bullous impetigo, the vesicles enlarge rapidly to form bullae. The bullous contents become cloudy. The center of the bulla umbilicates, whereas the periphery may retain fluid. A honey-colored crust appears in the center; if it is removed, an inflamed base is revealed that exudes serum. As the lesion enlarges, a scaling border replaces the bulla and eventually forms a crust. The lesions have minimal or no surrounding erythema. Individual lesions may increase in size to 2 to 8 cm [see Fig. 2-19-1 (Plate 18)].[2] In darker-skinned individuals, the lesions tend to heal with hyperpigmentation. Regional adenopathy is uncommon with staphylococcal impetigo.

In nonbullous impetigo, the small vesicle or pustule usually is not seen. The most commonly encountered finding is the honey-colored crust [see Fig. 2-19-2 (Plate 19)]. The lesions extend radially, and satellite lesions appear beyond the periphery. There is little surrounding erythema. The lesions average 1 to 3 cm in size.[1–3] The skin around the nose, the mouth, and the limbs are the sites most commonly affected.[1–4] The palms and soles are not affected. Regional adenopathy is more common with streptococcal impetigo and it is most common in children 5 to 7 years of age.[2,3]

Ecthyma is caused by group A beta-hemolytic streptococci. It is seen more commonly in excoriations, bites, and areas of trauma, especially in diabetic patients, the elderly, and alcoholic patients.[1–3] The presenting lesion is usually a crust, but the more important clinical feature is the depth of infection. In ecthyma, the infection is deep, and so when the crust is removed, an ulcer is noted. Because the ulcer of ecthyma

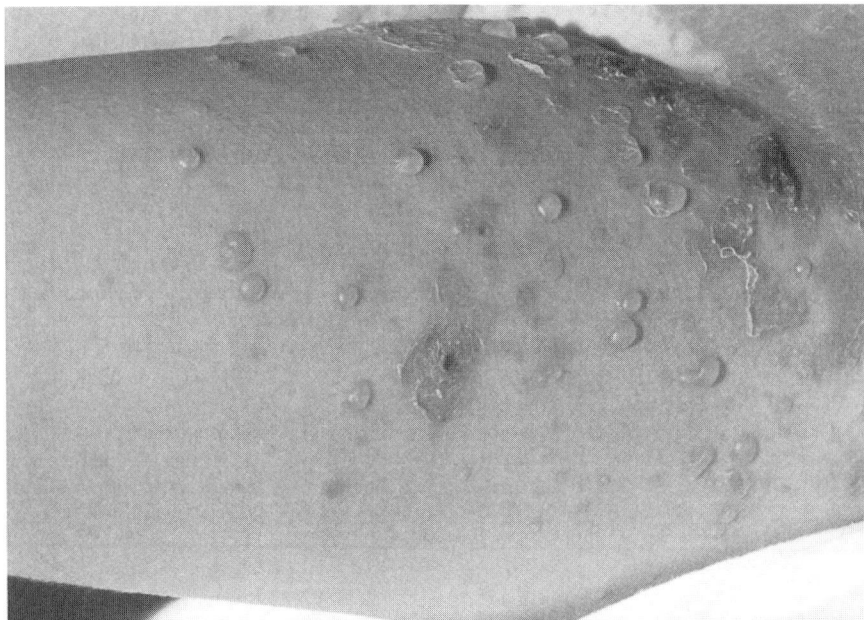

FIGURE 2-19-1 (PLATE 18). Bullous impetigo. (*From Fitzpatrick, Johnson, Wolff, et al.*[1])

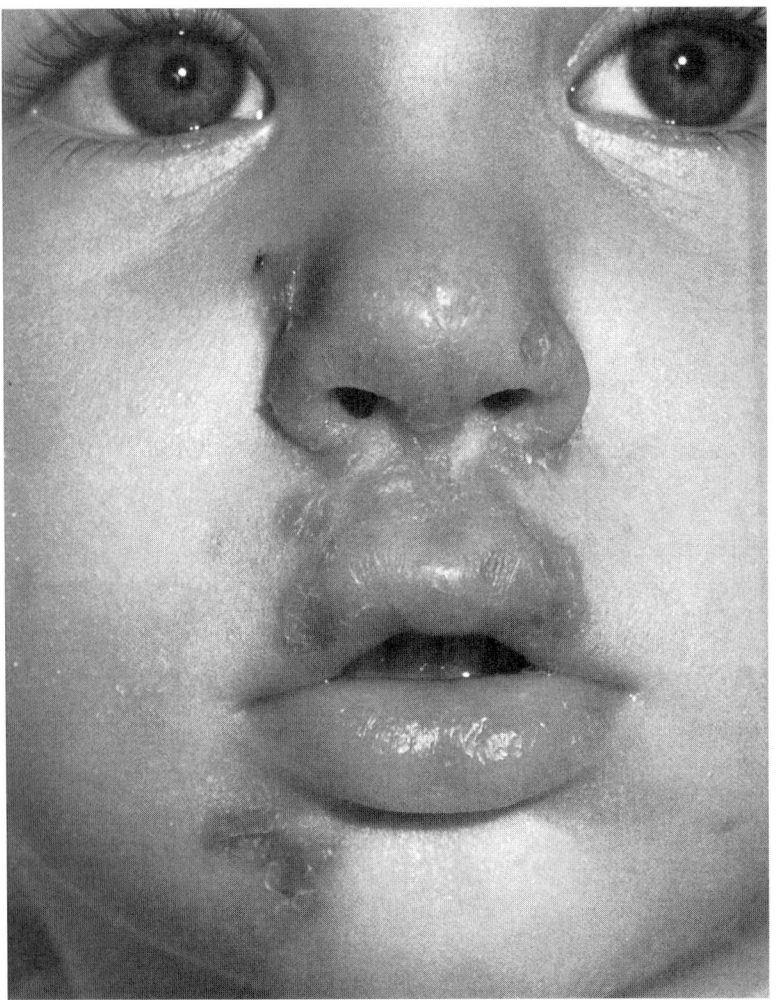

FIGURE 2-19-2 (PLATE 19). Non-bullous impetigo. (*From Fitzpatrick, Johnson, Wolff, et al.*[1])

extends into the dermis, it more often heals with scarring. The lesion of ecthyma may have a hemorrhagic crust and be indurated or tender. In streptococcal infection, the erythema surrounding the lesion may be moderate to severe. Ecthyma usually is found on the lower extremities [see Fig. 2-19-3 (Plate 20)]. There may be associated lymphadenopathy.

DIAGNOSTIC CONSIDERATIONS

The differential for nonbullous impetigo includes excoriation, perioral dermatitis, seborrheic dermatitis, allergic contact dermatitis, eczema, herpes simplex, arthropod infestations, and inflammatory fungal infections.

The differential for bullous impetigo includes allergic contact dermatitis such as to poison ivy, herpes simplex, herpes zoster, pemphigus vulgaris, burns, bullous pemphigoid, erythema multiforme, fixed drug eruptions, and dermatitis herpetiformis. When the patient presents with crusts, it may be difficult to differentiate impetigo from herpes simplex. A history of a prodrome that includes tingling, burning, or recurrence in the same areas and a history of clear vesicles on an erythematous base will favor a diagnosis of herpes. Potassium hydroxide (KOH) examination and fungal culture help differentiate fungal from bacterial infection.

The differential for ecthyma includes chronic herpetic ulcers, excoriated insect bites, neurotic excoriations, porphyria cutanea tarda if limited to the dorsa of the hands, and stasis ulcers if limited to the legs.

LABORATORY TESTS

A Gram stain will reveal gram-positive cocci in chains or clusters. Bacterial culture more commonly will grow *S. aureus* and less frequently group A beta-hemolytic streptococci. In obtaining material for Gram stain and culture, it is important to first remove the crust so that the specimen can be obtained from the base of the lesion.

Further testing in uncomplicated impetigo is costly and may not add information to the clinical picture. In suspected streptococcal impetigo or when symptoms of acute glomerulonephritis are present, serotyping may be necessary. The antistreptolysin O (ASO) titer does not rise to a significant level; however, anti-DNAse B rises to high levels and is a sensitive indicator of streptococcal impetigo.[2,4] Antihyaluronidase also increases significantly.[2,4] In acute glomerulonephritis, cultures of the pharynx and skin lesions should be performed and the serotype of the group A streptococci should be determined by typing with M-group and T-type antisera. The MT serotypes associated with acute glomerulonephritis are 2, 49, 55, 57, and 60.[2]

TREATMENT

Impetigo may resolve spontaneously, but it can become chronic and widespread. Studies show that 2% mupirocin ointment (Bactroban) is as effective as oral antibiotics and is associated with fewer side effects in the treatment of patients with nonbullous impetigo.[1–3] It is active against staphylococci, including methicillin-resistant strains, and group A beta-hemolytic streptococci. In superficial skin infections that are not widespread, mupirocin ointment is the treatment of choice. Mupirocin is applied three times a day until all lesions have cleared. The involved areas should be cleansed once or twice a day with an antibacterial soap. There is a debate about whether the crusts should be removed because they potentially block the penetration of antibacterial creams. It may be sufficient to soften the crusts by soaking

FIGURE 2-19-3 (PLATE 20). Ecthyma. (*From Fitzpatrick, Johnson, Wolff, et al.*[1])

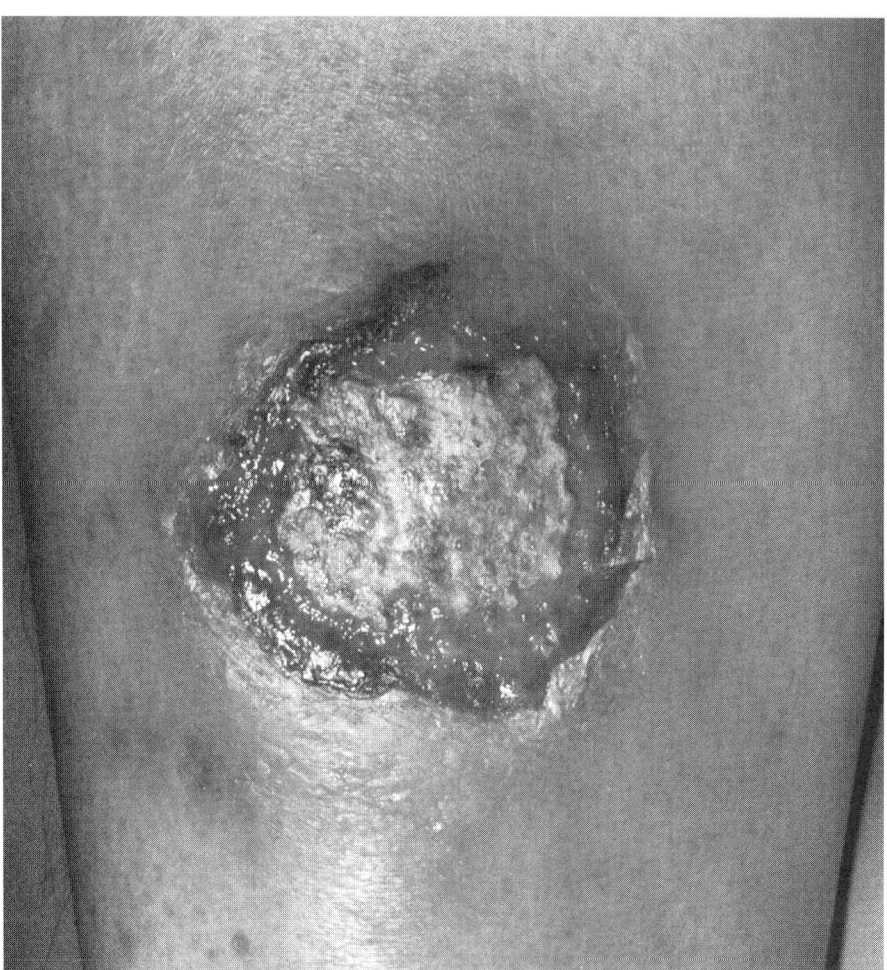

the area with a wet cloth compress. Local treatment does not affect evolving lesions in other areas. Infected children should be quarantined briefly until treatment is under way.

A 7- to 10-day course of an oral antibiotic such as cloxacillin, dicloxacillin, cephalexin (Keflex), or the newer macrolide antibiotics such as clarithromycin (Biaxin) and azithromycin (Zithromax) induces rapid healing.[1–3] Erythromycin may not be as effective because some strains of staphylococci are resistant.[2,3] Most *S. aureus* strains produce penicillinase, and so penicillin is also an inappropriate treatment.[2,5]

FOLLOW-UP

Patients with recurrent impetigo should be evaluated for carriage of *S. aureus.* The nares are the most common sites of carriage, but the perineum, axillae, and toe webs also may be colonized.[1–3] Mupirocin ointment (Bactroban) applied to the colonized area twice a day for 5 days reduces *S. aureus* carriage. Benzoyl peroxide wash also decreases colonization. Family members should be examined for signs of impetigo.

COMPLICATIONS AND RED FLAGS

Acute glomerulonephritis tends to occur when many individuals in a family have impetigo, mostly in the southern United States, with the highest incidence in children between 2 and 4 years of age.[2] Infants under 1 1/2 years of age rarely are affected by acute glomerulonephritis following impetigo. The overall incidence of acute glomerulonephritis with impetigo ranges from 2 to 5 percent, but when a nephritogenic strain is present, the rate ranges from 10 to 15 percent.[2] The period between the formation of the skin lesions and the onset of acute glomerulonephritis ranges from 1 week to 5 weeks, with an average of 10 days.[2]

The most common clinical features include hematuria with erythrocyte casts, proteinuria, and edema that varies with the amount of dietary sodium.[2] In the morning, there may be periorbital and lower extremity edema. Moderate hypertension is also common. Central nervous system (CNS) symptoms, congestive heart failure (CHF), and acute renal failure are less common.[2] There is usually marked improvement in most patients within 7 to 10 days.

Other complications of superficial skin infections with *S. aureus* and group A beta-hemolytic streptococci have been seen. Group A beta-hemolytic streptococcal impetigo may precipitate or flare an episode of guttate psoriasis. Primary or secondary impetiginous lesions can progress to cellulitis, erysipelas, or bacteremia. Osteomyelitis, septic arthritis, and pneumonia have been reported to occur in infants after episodes of impetigo.[6] Rheumatic fever has not been reported as a complication.[2]

REFERENCES

1. Fitzpatrick TB, Johnson RA, Wolff K, et al: *Color Atlas and Synopsis of Clinical Dermatology: Common and Serious Diseases,* 3d ed. New York, McGraw-Hill, 1997, pp 604–609.
2. Habif TP: *Clinical Dermatology: A Color Guide to Diagnosis and Treatment,* 3d ed. St. Louis, Mosby Yearbook, 1996, pp 236–242.
3. Lee PK, Weinberg AN, Swartz MN, et al: Pyoderma: *Staphylococcus aureus,* streptococcus and other gram-positive bacteria, in Fitzpatrick TB, Eisen AZ, Wolff K, et al (eds): *Dermatology in General Medicine,* 5th ed. New York, McGraw-Hill, 1999, pp 2182–2207.
4. Rajajee S: Post-streptococcal acute glomerulonephritis: A clinical, bacteriological and serological study. *Ind J Pediatr* 57:775–780, 1990.
5. Demidovich CW, Wittler RR, et al: Impetigo: Current etiology and comparison of penicillin, erythromycin and cephalexin therapies. *Am J Dis Child* 144:1313–1315, 1990.
6. Arnold HL, Odom RB, James WD: *Andrews' Diseases of the Skin: Clinical Dermatology,* 8th ed. Philadelphia, Saunders, 1990, pp 272–273.

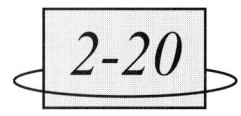

LICHEN PLANUS
Joe R. Monroe

DISCUSSION

Lichen planus (LP) is a relatively common inflammatory condition with a highly characteristic purple color, a distinctive papular morphology, and a characteristic histopathologic pattern. It is a curious disorder of unknown etiology that affects the skin, hair, scalp, mucous membranes, and nails. It affects slightly more women than men, especially those ages 30 to 60.

Attacks often begin suddenly with the appearance of 1- to 3-mm flat-topped (planar) discrete purplish papules, especially on the volar wrists, low back skin, legs, and genitals. More likely to itch than not, these papules sometimes coalesce into plaques up to 5 cm. Trauma, especially scratching, can cause arrangement of these papules along lines of trauma, an occurrence known as the Koebner phenomenon. The surfaces of the lesions also may exhibit fine parallel white striations called Wickham's striae, a useful fact for identifying LP lesions.

Dermatologic tradition holds that LP can be diagnosed easily in most cases by using the "Ps" of LP: papular, pruritic, planar (i.e., flat-topped), polygonal (i.e., multangular), plaque-like, penile, and puzzling.

Several variants of LP have been described, the most common of which is involvement of the buccal mucosa (40 to 60 percent of all LP patients), in which a white, lacy reticulated papular pattern is seen. This form of LP can become erosive and painful, affect the lips and tongue as well, and be very challenging to treat. LP also can affect scalp skin (atrophy and hair loss), and 10 percent of patients experience destruction of nails. Morphologic variants include bullous and annular forms, whereas on the legs, LP tends to present as hypertrophic, hyperpigmented plaques that can resemble psoriasis, especially in people with darker skin.

DIFFERENTIAL DIAGNOSIS

Contact dermatitis, drug eruptions, lupus erythematosus, and psoriasis are included in the differential diagnosis. In the mouth, the differential diagnosis includes thrush and oral hairy leukoplakia.

LABORATORY

A biopsy that shows a very characteristic histopathologic picture can be quite helpful, but the distinctive clinical presentation usually permits an easy diagnosis.

TREATMENT

Steroids (topical, intralesional, systemic) can be very effective in controlling pruritus. PUVA (psoralen), an oral drug, is used in combination with ultraviolet A (UVA) light exposure, especially for widespread eruptions. For oral LP, triamcinolone in Orabase and oral retinoids are used, but often require referral to a dermatologist is necessary.

PATIENT EDUCATION

Reassurance about the (usual) self-limited, benign nature of LP is helpful.

PEARLS

Knowledge of the following points can contribute to a positive patient outcome:

• Remember the "Ps," especially purple.
• The darker the skin, the darker the purple.

- Genital LP is surprisingly common.
- Pruritus is the rule with LP (80 percent).
- Add LP to the differential diagnosis for "fungal" fingernails.
- The quintessential LP presentation is highly pruritic purple papules on volar wrist skin.

PROGNOSIS

This disease is usually over in weeks but may persist for years, especially in the mouth and on the shins with the hypertrophic variety.

BIBLIOGRAPHY

Arndt KA, Robinson JK, LeBoit PE, et al: *Cutaneous Medicine and Surgery.* Philadelphia, Saunders, 1996.
DuVivier A: *Dermatology in Practice.* Philadelphia, Lippincott, 1990.
Fitzpatrick TB, Johnson RA, Wolff K, et al: *Color Atlas and Synopsis of Clinical Dermatology: Common and Serious Diseases,* 3d ed. New York, McGraw-Hill, 1997.
Goldstein BG, Goldstein AO: *Practical Dermatology,* Primary Care Series. St Louis, Mosby Year Book, 1992.
Shelley WB, Shelley ED: *Advanced Dermatologic Diagnosis.* Philadelphia, Saunders, 1992.
Weinberg S, Prose NS, Kristal L: *Color Atlas of Pediatric Dermatology,* 3d ed. New York, McGraw-Hill, 1998.

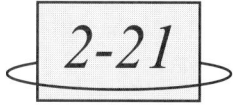

MALIGNANT MELANOMA
Barbara L. Sauls

DISCUSSION

Malignant melanoma is a primary cancer of melanocytes, the pigment-producing cells of the epidermis. Melanoma is a life-threatening condition because of the potential for rapid growth and metastases. Most lesions typically begin with a horizontal growth pattern, but all eventually have a vertical growth phase. One type of melanoma, the nodular form, does not have a horizontal growth phase, growing only vertically into a papule and into the skin. It is during the horizontal growth phase that lesions are detectable and more easily cured. Once deeper growth has occurred, the cure rate and longevity greatly decrease. Sun exposure, light skin, and poor tanning capability predispose an individual to melanoma. Individuals with red and blond hair are especially susceptible. Dark skin is protective. A history of previous, blistering sunburn, especially before age 5 years, has been statistically correlated with later development of melanoma, as has being immunocompromised. There seems to be a hereditary component, and the presence of a congenital melanocytic nevus or multiple melanocytic nevi is cause for concern. Metastases may occur in any tissue, with the brain and liver being favored sites; even the choroid of the eye has been affected.

Individuals of all ages are affected, but the average age of 40 is in marked contrast to other types of sun-caused cancer (basal cell carcinoma and squamous cell carcinoma), whose incidence increases with age. Women frequently develop melanoma on the back or lower legs, while the back is the most common site in men. Melanoma may develop on the palms, soles, and nail beds of those with dark skin, presumably owing to a lesser amount of pigment in that area. Three principal types of melanomas occur in persons with white skin: lentigo maligna melanoma, which is the least common; superficial spreading melanoma, which is the most common; and nodular melanoma. The nodular form has a propensity for rapid vertical growth. Acral lentiginous melanoma, which occurs on the soles, palms, and ungual areas, is found most frequently in those with dark skin, whereas whites typically have the superficial spreading form (see Figs. 2-21-1 to 2-21-3 and Plates 21 to 23).

SIGNS AND SYMPTOMS

Patients present with a lesion that has changed in color, has multiple colors, and exhibits irregular borders. Melanoma may develop in sites of a "mole," or nevus, that becomes larger and irregular and with colors ranging from black to blue, browns, reds, pink, and tan. There may be itching or bleeding associated with these lesions, but pain is not noted.

FIGURE 2-21-1 (PLATE 21). A C-shaped malignant melanoma of the abdomen. (*Courtesy of Harold Milstein, MD, The Dermatology Center, Hazleton, PA.*)

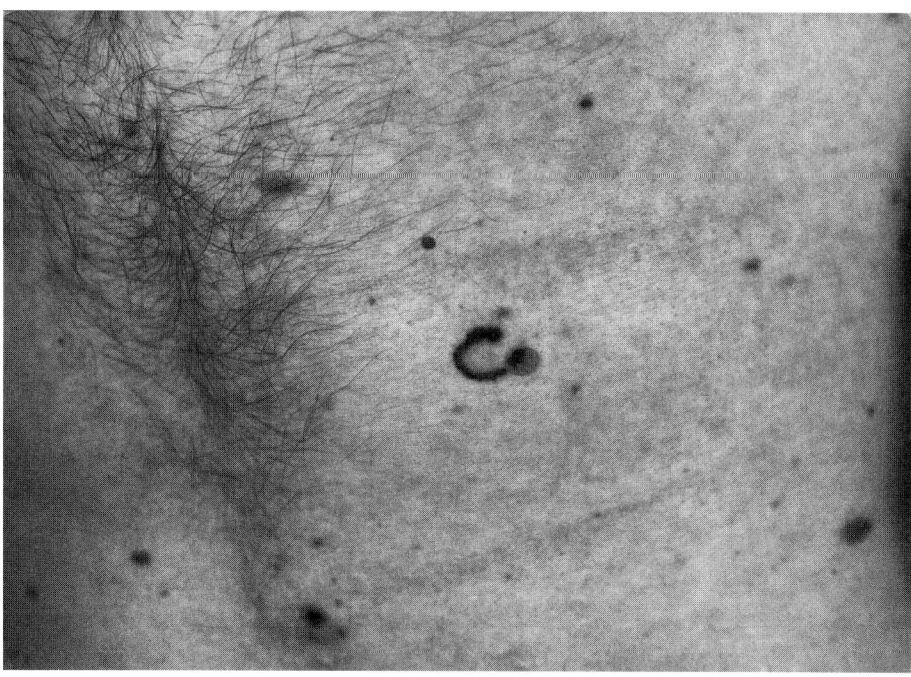

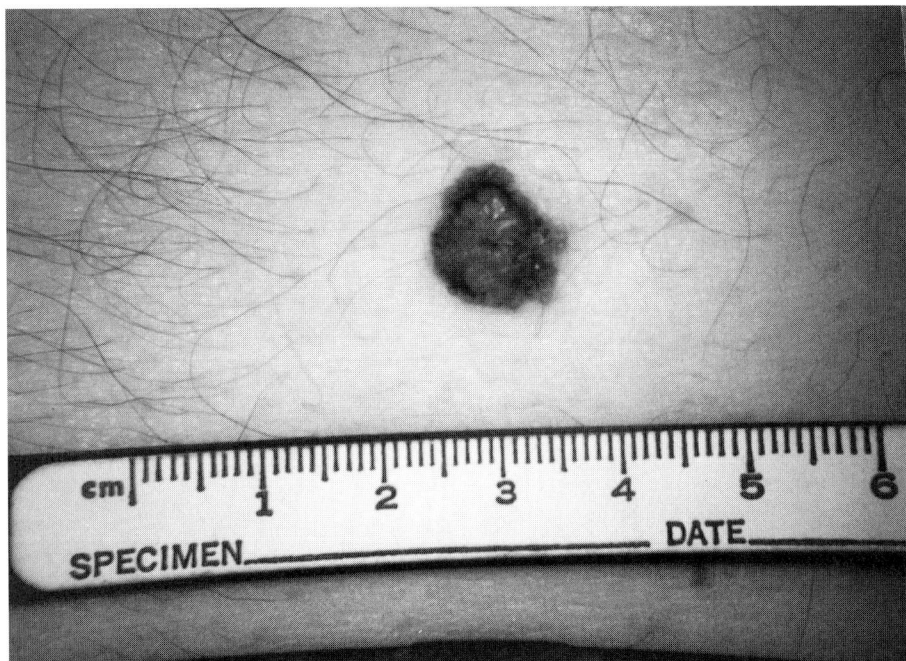

FIGURE 2-21-2 (PLATE 22). A nodular malignant melanoma of the abdomen. (*Courtesy of Harold Milstein, MD, The Dermatology Center, Hazleton, PA.*)

OBJECTIVE FINDINGS

Clinicians should be aware of the **ABCDEs** of malignant melanoma. Any or all of these conditions warrant further investigation.

A is for **asymmetry** of the lesion. The right side does not look like the left.

B is for **border** irregularity. This area can be deeply notched or scalloped or ill-defined in appearance.

C is for changing or multiple **colors,** or mottling.

D is for a **diameter** greater than 5 or 6 mm.

E is for **elevation,** which is almost always present. It is possible to note this with side lighting, but it may not be palpable. E may also be **enlarging.** Malignant melanomas have a propensity for fairly rapid growth.

S is for **shadowing,** the "bleeding" of the border of the lesions into the surrounding tissue. This appears lighter in color than the main lesion.

DIAGNOSTIC CONSIDERATIONS

The differential diagnosis of malignant melanoma includes various benign nevi, basal cell carcinoma, a tattoo from a lead (graphite) pencil, dye, another procedure or trauma, seborrheic keratosis, and other benign pigmented lesions. Most nevi are round or oval and have smooth borders, although this is not always the case. Seborrheic keratoses are dark, waxy, "stuck-on" lesions and are usually distinguishable on physical examination. However, if there is any question about the diagnosis, a biopsy is warranted. The patient may be able to remember a specific incident such as having a tattoo or getting a lead pencil stuck in the area.

SPECIAL CONSIDERATIONS

Immunocompromised individuals are at greater risk for the development of skin cancers of any type. Special care for prevention and periodic examination are essential.

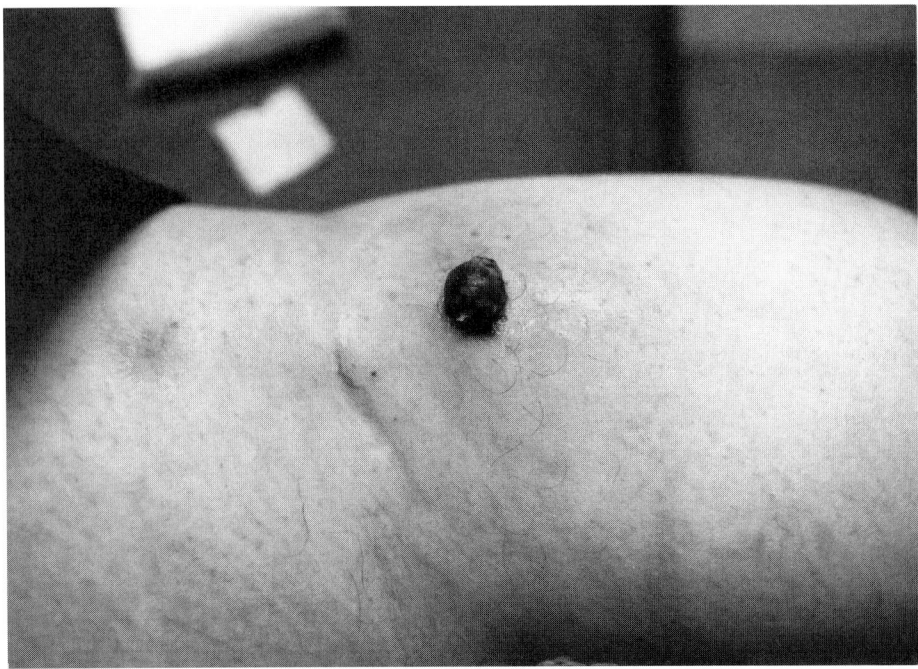

FIGURE 2-21-3 (PLATE 23). Malignant melanoma of the leg. (*Courtesy of Harold Milstein, MD, The Dermatology Center, Hazleton, PA.*)

Individuals born with a congenital nevomelanocytic or hairy nevus have a high incidence of melanoma in that area. The bigger, darker, and more irregularly shaped a lesion, the greater the risk of malignant transformation. It is recommended that all children be evaluated by a dermatologist and have lesions removed as soon as they are old enough to tolerate the procedure. Extensive lesions of this type often require skin grafting after removal.

LABORATORY TESTS

Prompt referral for excisional biopsy with thin margins is recommended to confirm the diagnosis. It is possible to perform a punch or incisional biopsy initially if an excisional biopsy cannot be performed, for example, if the lesion is quite large and would require extensive surgical removal. In this case, it is important to biopsy the darkest, most elevated portion of the lesion.

TREATMENT

Surgical excision is the treatment of choice. Because of the high rate of metastases of this cancer, all patients are staged depending on thickness, extension, node, and organ involvement. Some patients may be candidates for chemotherapy, interferon or other immunotherapy, or palliative radiation; however, metastatic disease generally is considered incurable, and so early detection and removal while the lesion is still thin are of the utmost importance.

PATIENT EDUCATION

As with all skin cancers, the avoidance of sun exposure is essential. Sunscreens, long-sleeved shirts and pants, and remaining in the shade from 10 A.M. to 2 P.M. daily are recommended. Patients should perform self-skin examination monthly and report any changing lesion immediately. Their partners should participate in this procedure, since it is difficult to examine all areas of the back and lower extremities completely.

DISPOSITION

After treatment, a fully unclothed skin examination by a medical provider should be performed every 3 months for 1 year, every 6 months for another year, and then yearly for the patient's lifetime.

COMPLICATIONS AND RED FLAGS

This condition is most appropriately referred to a dermatologist or plastic surgeon for initial evaluation, follow-up, and treatment. Plastic surgeons often perform excisional surgery for lesions on the face or if skin grafting may be required.

PEARLS

Always maintain an index of suspicion when examining lesions. Give patients the benefit of the doubt and biopsy any lesions that are not definitely and completely benign. In this case, a life may be saved. Be sure to keep the patient in mind during the examination; for instance, a redhead with heavily sun-damaged skin requires careful examination.

BIBLIOGRAPHY

Fauci AS, Braunwald E, Isselbacher KJ, et al (eds): *Harrison's Principles of Internal Medicine,* 14th ed. New York, McGraw-Hill, 1998.
Fitzpatrick TB, Johnson RA, Wolff K, et al: *Color Atlas and Synopsis of Clinical Dermatology: Common and Serious Diseases,* 3d ed. New York, McGraw-Hill, 1997.

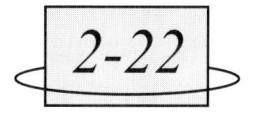

MOLLUSCUM CONTAGIOSUM

Barbara L. Sauls

DISCUSSION

Molluscum contagiosum, which is caused by a poxvirus, exhibits discrete, small papular lesions that are scattered and most commonly are found on the neck, trunk, and anogenital area. HIV infection may be associated with multiple (often hundreds) facial lesions that often become quite large. The lesions are seen more commonly in males but are found in both children and adults. Those seen in adults may have been sexually transmitted. Lesions commonly develop over a period of one to several months, and spontaneous resolution over months to years is not uncommon.

SIGNS AND SYMPTOMS

Other than the small, discrete papular lesions, there are no associated symptoms such as itching, pain, and burning. These lesions usually are pointed out during a routine visit. If they develop a secondary bacterial infection, they may become pruritic or tender. This may occur in sites of recurrent irritation such as collar areas and areas that are constantly rubbed from sitting or if they are picked at inadvertently by the patient.

OBJECTIVE FINDINGS

Physical examination shows one to many discrete round or oval papules that are pearly, flesh-colored, and umbilicated. They are usually 1 to 2 mm in diameter and are rarely larger. If seen in a patient with an HIV infection, they can be up to five times this size. These lesions are nontender to touch and are usually firm (see Fig. 2-22-1 and Plate 24).

DIAGNOSTIC CONSIDERATIONS

Differential diagnoses include basal cell carcinoma, which may present as a nodular area with central indentation, and keratoacanthoma, which is more like a crater with a central plug.

HIV infection should be suspected if an individual presents with a number of large lesions of this type. This may be their initial presentation.

Genital and perianal molluscum lesions in children are suspicious of sexual abuse and require further investigation.

LABORATORY TESTS

It is not necessary to biopsy these lesions, though a Giemsa stain of the core will reveal inclusion bodies called *molluscum bodies.* This sample may be obtained without local anesthesia, using the bevel of a needle or a pointed scalpel. With local anesthesia, a punch biopsy or curettage of the lesions may be done.

TREATMENT

Treatment is often unnecessary, since there is often spontaneous resolution of these lesions. If the lesions are in an area that is highly visible or frequently irritated, it is possible to lightly freeze or electrocauterize them with complete resolution. Curettage is also possible. It is unnecessary to treat the core completely; a light touch is all that is needed.

Destruction with a topical application of cantharone is used occasionally, particularly in children.

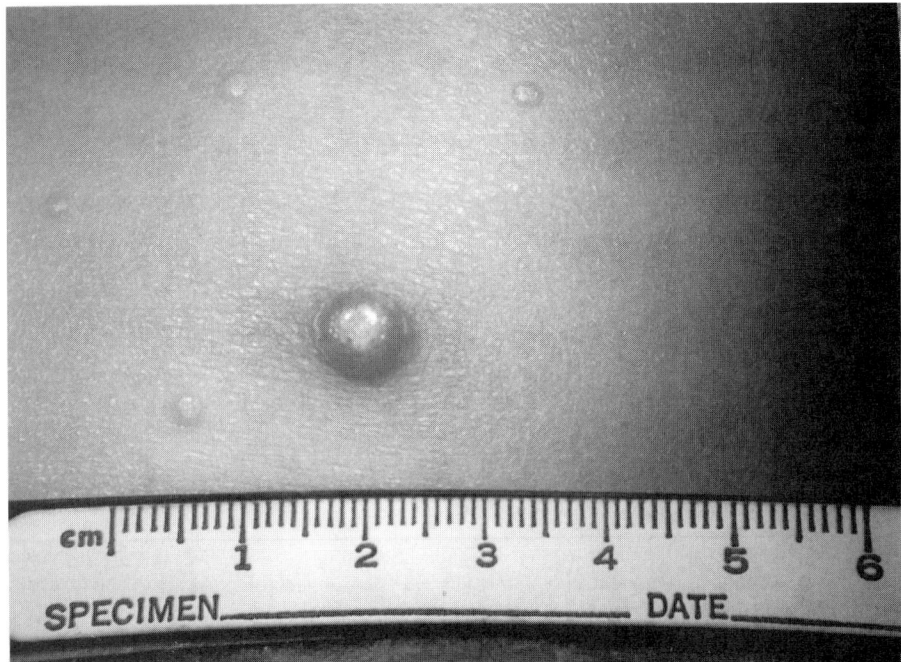

FIGURE 2-22-1 (PLATE 24). Several small molluscum lesions with one giant lesion on the chest. Note the central umbilication and the irritation associated with the larger lesion. In this case, it is appropriate to remove the lesions because of the irritation. (*Courtesy of Harold Milstein, MD, The Dermatology Center, Hazleton, PA.*)

PATIENT EDUCATION

Teach patients to leave the areas alone after treatment and to use a topical antibiotic ointment if they develop redness. Since this is a poxvirus infection, it is necessary to tell patients that this does not cure the viral infection and that lesions may develop in the future, though not necessarily in the same area. These lesions are not typically infectious but can be transmitted sexually.

Since children are seen routinely for health maintenance examinations, it is often possible to persuade parents to leave the lesions alone for the time being, with reassurance that future treatment will be available if they spread or do not resolve spontaneously. This prevents unnecessary stress to children, especially if they are young and uncooperative with the treatments.

BIBLIOGRAPHY

Fauci AS, Braunwald E, Isselbacher KJ, et al (eds): *Harrison's Principles of Internal Medicine,* 14th ed. New York, McGraw-Hill, 1998.

Fitzpatrick TB, Johnson RA, Wolff K, et al: *Color Atlas and Synopsis of Clinical Dermatology: Common and Serious Diseases,* 3d ed. New York, McGraw-Hill, 1997.

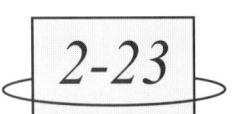

PITYRIASIS ROSEA
Michelle DiBaise

DISCUSSION

Pityriasis rosea is an acute papulosquamous dermatosis of unknown etiology. It is relatively common and is usually asymptomatic and self-limiting. Pityriasis rosea is characterized by the development of a single large lesion, the "herald patch," followed by a generalized eruption with a distinctive pattern, predominantly on the trunk. The majority of patients are between the ages of 10 and 35 years, but pityriasis rosea has been seen in all ages, from 4 months to 78 years.[1-4] There is evidence that pityriasis rosea is viral in origin. It demonstrates seasonal variation with a peak in the winter months. As many

as 20 percent of patients can relate a recent history of an infectious syndrome, including headache, fatigue, sore throat, lymphadenitis, and fever.[2,4] Small epidemics have been noted to occur on military bases and in fraternities.[2] However, despite these findings, pityriasis rosea is seen uncommonly among household contacts. Attempts to transmit the disease experimentally have been unsuccessful. A recent study found the presence of human herpes virus-7 (HHV-7) in the blood and skin tissue of individuals with acute pityriasis rosea compared to healthy controls.[5] Further testing is needed to prove whether HHV-7 is the causative agent of pityriasis rosea.

Pityriasis rosea appears to be more common among atopic individuals and slightly more common in women. The entire disease process resolves in approximately 6 to 8 weeks. About 2 percent of these patients have a recurrence.[1-4]

SIGNS AND SYMPTOMS

On presentation, the majority of patients are asymptomatic. The patient may relate a history of a recent viral syndrome followed by the development of a single lesion. Within a few days to weeks, the patient develops a generalized eruption. If the patient is symptomatic, the main complaint is pruritus. The pruritus of pityriasis rosea ranges from mild to moderate. Severe itching may accompany extensive eruptions.

OBJECTIVE FINDINGS

The herald patch usually can be identified by the patient as the first lesion to appear; however, it occurs only in about 80 percent of patients.[1-4] It is the largest of the lesions and ranges in size from 2 to 10 cm. It is an ovoid to round plaque with a fine scale at the periphery. The scale edge faces toward the center of the lesion and has been described as a trailing or inverse marginal collarette. The generalized eruption follows in a few days to weeks, with the average time ranging from 7 to 14 days.[1-4] The early lesions may be papular. In most cases, however, the lesions have the same appearance as the herald patch but are smaller in size at 1 to 2 cm. The lesions range in color from pink or salmon in those with light skin to hyperpigmented in those with darker skin. The multiple lesions are scattered and discrete, reach a peak in 1 to 2 weeks, and number from a few to hundreds. They appear mainly on the trunk and proximal extremities but can

FIGURE 2-23-1 (PLATE 25). Pityriasis rosea. (*From fitzpatrick, Johnson, Wolff, et al.*[1])

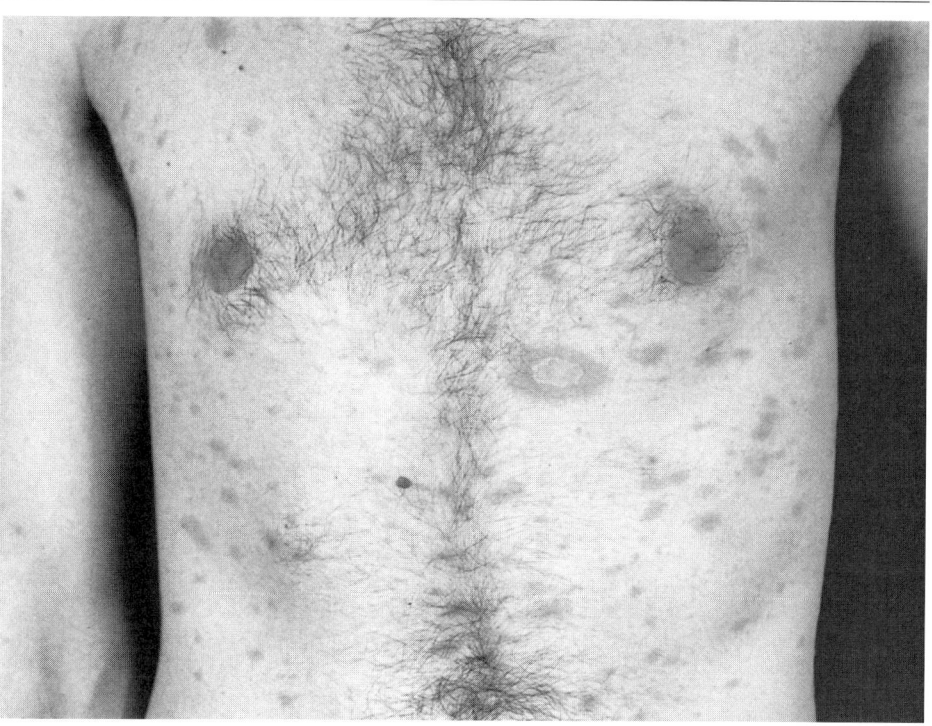

appear on the arms, legs, and face in severe cases [see Figs. 2-23-1 (Plate 25) and 2-23-2]. The long axis of the lesions follows the lines of cleavage of the skin in a pattern that has been called a Christmas tree. In children, pityriasis rosea can more commonly involve the face. A papular variant is seen more commonly in young children, pregnant women, and those with darker skin. Vesicles, purpura, pustules, and lesions that appear as erythema multiforme but occur in the typical distribution of pityriasis rosea are also seen and develop more commonly in infants and children. Oral lesions have been reported

and have a variety of appearances, including erythematous macules, hemorrhagic lesions, and small ulcerations.[1-4,6,7] The disease resolves spontaneously in 2 weeks to 2 months, with an average of 6 weeks.[1-4] Patients may have residual postinflammatory hyperpigmentation, especially those with darker skin. If pityriasis rosea has an atypical presentation, the practitioner should look for other causes of the eruption. Atypical manifestations include lesions on the face and neck only, the absence of a herald patch or a herald patch that is the only manifestation of the disease, lesions on the palms and soles, and a patient who

FIGURE 2-23-2. Distribution of pityriasis rosea.

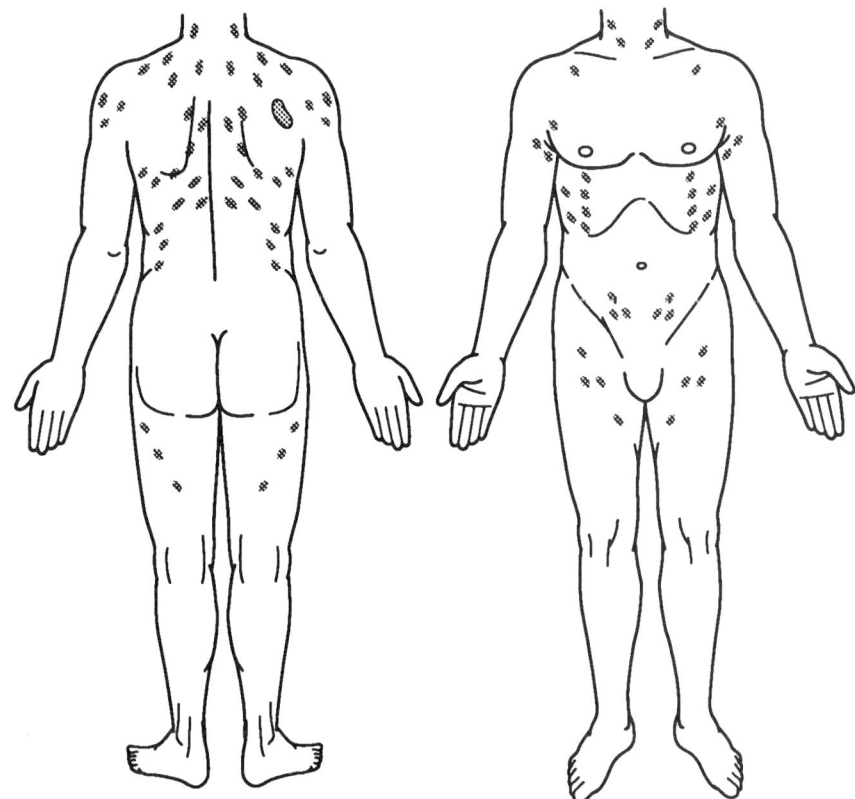

appears systemically ill. If the eruption persists for more than 6 to 8 weeks, a skin biopsy should be considered to rule out other disorders.

DIAGNOSTIC CONSIDERATIONS

The herald patch can be misdiagnosed as tinea corporis. A potassium hydroxide (KOH) preparation will not show the hyphae and spores consistent with a fungal infection.

Erythema chronica migrans is a solitary annular lesion associated with Lyme disease that extends from the periphery. It can be differentiated from a herald patch by the lack of scale. A central punctum where the tick bite occurred also may be noted.

Several disorders can mimic the generalized eruption of pityriasis rosea. Guttate psoriasis has a sudden onset with small, discrete lesions that have a distribution similar to that of pityriasis of rosea. The patient also may have a history of recent streptococcal pharyngitis. For the most part, the scale of psoriasis is thick and silvery and is distributed throughout the lesion. The course of guttate psoriasis is longer than that of pityriasis rosea.

Generalized lichen planus also can mimic pityriasis rosea in its distribution. The lesions of lichen planus are described as polygonal purple papules; this can help distinguish it from pityriasis rosea.

Pityriasis lichenoides chronica, also known as chronic or guttate parapsoriasis, is an uncommon disorder in which the lesions may be similar in appearance to those of pityriasis rosea, but this is a chronic rather than transient condition. Drug eruptions also should be considered in the differential diagnosis. Usually, a drug eruption is more confluent and erythematous, there is little or no scaling, and the eruption may be more symptomatic than that of pityriasis rosea. Nummular eczema may also mimic pityriasis rosea, but the onset tends to be more insidious and the course more prolonged.

In the presence of atypical pityriasis, the most important differential diagnosis to consider is secondary syphilis. A serologic test for syphilis should be ordered for all sexually active individuals.

AIDS-associated Kaposi's sarcoma demonstrates ovoid, purpuric lesions that follow the lines of cleavage of the skin (see Chap. 9-2). It should be considered in the differential of the purpuric variant of pityriasis rosea.

The differential diagnosis of the vesicular variant of pityriasis rosea should include other generalized bullous disorders, such as contact dermatitis to the toxicodendrons, generalized bullous impetigo, and, in older individuals, pemphigus vulgaris.

LABORATORY TESTS

The diagnosis is made predominantly by the clinical findings. A skin biopsy is nonspecific and rarely is indicated. If lesions persist longer than 6 to 8 weeks, a skin biopsy can help in diagnosing other conditions. A potassium hydroxide (KOH) test can be performed on the scale of the lesion to rule out tinea corporis. Serologic testing for syphilis should be considered for all sexually active individuals.

TREATMENT

This is a self-limited disease that usually does not require treatment. In instances where pruritus is present, antihistamines, topical corticosteroids, and emollients can help alleviate the symptoms. A group V topical steroid is usually sufficient to control symptoms. The rare severe case associated with intense pruritus can be treated with a 1- to 2-week course of prednisone. Ultraviolet B light (UVB) therapy has been shown to accelerate the resolution of pityriasis rosea. The treatment is most helpful when started within the first week of the eruption.[1–4]

COMPLICATIONS AND RED FLAGS

There are no complications with the exception of postinflammatory hypo- or hyperpigmentation, which resolves slowly over time, often

months. The residual skin changes are more common in darker-skinned individuals. In pregnant women, there is no documented risk to the fetus.[2]

REFERENCES

1. Fitzpatrick TB, Johnson RA, Wolff K, et al: *Color Atlas and Synopsis of Clinical Dermatology: Common and Serious Diseases.* New York, McGraw-Hill, 1997, pp 104–106.
2. Habif TP: *Clinical Dermatology: A Color Guide to Diagnosis and Treatment,* 3d ed. St. Louis, Mosby Yearbook, 1996, pp 218–220.
3. Arnold HL, Odom RB, James WD: *Andrews' Diseases of the Skin: Clinical Dermatology,* 8th ed. Philadelphia, Saunders, 1990, pp 231–232.
4. Bjornberg A, Tegner E: Pityriasis rosea, in Fitzpatrick TB, Eisen AZ, Wolff K, et al (eds): *Dermatology in General Medicine,* 5th ed. New York, McGraw-Hill, 1999, pp 541–546.
5. Drago F, Ranieri E, Malaguti F, et al: Human herpesvirus 7 in patients with pityriasis rosea: Electron microscopy investigations and polymerase chain reaction in mononuclear cells, plasma and skin. *Dermatology* 195(4): 374–378, 1997.
6. Vidimos AT, Camisa C: Tongue and cheek: Oral lesions in pityriasis rosea. *Cutis* 50:276–280, 1992.
7. Pierson JC, Dijkstra JW, et al: Purpuric pityriasis rosea. *J Am Acad Dermatol* 28:1021, 1993.

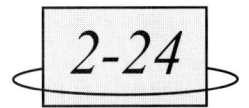

PSORIASIS
Joe R. Monroe

DISCUSSION

Psoriasis is the benign, focal acceleration of the normal production, upward migration, and shedding of epidermal skin. It is probably of genetic origin, and its course is influenced by a complex interaction of genetic and environmental factors. It is a common skin disease, affecting around 2 percent of the population of Western countries but a much lower percentage of the population elsewhere. Intensive ongoing research is starting to clarify its pathogenesis, but the exact cause remains elusive. It is fortunate for the patients whose lives are so deeply affected by this disease that treatment has improved tremendously over the last 30 years.

Men and women are affected equally by this disease, which occurs in all age groups. There is probably a multifactorial inheritance mode, the genetic component of which also is influenced by a variety of environmental factors. One-third of affected patients answer affirmatively when asked about a family history of psoriasis.

Exacerbations of psoriasis can be precipitated by drugs such as lithium, beta blockers, oral contraceptives, and nonsteroidal anti-inflammatory drugs (NSAIDs); pregnancy; alcohol; any type of skin trauma; stress; and streptococcal infections. Systemic corticosteroids also are considered an exacerbating factor because of a very marked and predictable tendency for psoriasis to rebound as these drugs are withdrawn.

Plaque-type psoriasis is morphologically characterized by the appearance of round to oval salmon-pink plaques covered by thick adherent silvery scales, tending toward symmetric involvement of the extensor surfaces and scalp. Other, lesser "stigmata" include umbilical and intergluteal involvement (so-called intergluteal pinking), pitting, and onycholysis of nails. The extent of involvement can vary a great deal and can favor one region (e.g., the scalp) over all others.

The fact that psoriasis also "koebnerizes," that is, forms along lines of trauma such as scratches, surgery, or even sunburns, can be diagnostically useful. However, many other dermatologic conditions koebnerize (warts, mollusca, lichen planus, and others).

CLINICAL PRESENTATION

The appearance of psoriasis can vary considerably, depending on the location and type, as follows:

- *Chronic plaque psoriasis (psoriasis vulgaris).* The most common morphologic type, described above.
- *Guttate psoriasis.* Characterized by the sudden appearance of multiple guttate, that is, drop-like, small psoriatic plaques over widespread areas of the body. Infection [streptococcal pharyngitis or viral upper respiratory infection (URI)] may precede it by 1 to 2 weeks and is suspected of being the trigger. An episode of guttate psoriasis, which is common in those under age 20, may be the first indication of the patient's propensity for the disease.
- *Generalized pustular psoriasis.* Also known as *Von Zumbusch psoriasis,* this type is characterized by a sudden appearance of widespread tiny pustules on a psoriatic base with progression toward coalescence. It is occasionally fatal, always difficult to treat, and, fortunately, unusual.
- *Psoriatic erythroderma.* With total involvement ("red man"), mostly in patients with previously diagnosed psoriasis, this form may come up with steroid withdrawal. Methotrexate often is needed in these cases.
- *Light-induced psoriasis.* This is exaggerated koebnerization to sun damage in a few unfortunate sun-sensitive individuals with preexisting psoriasis.
- *Scalp.* The scalp is a favored area for psoriasis. It can be mild or can present a particular treatment challenge. Often very disturbing to patients because of appearance and itching, it may spill over onto the forehead, ears, or neck. Psoriasis itself does not cause hair loss even with extensive scalp involvement, which may be the only manifestation of the disease. It often is mistaken for tinea capitis.
- *Psoriasis of palms and soles.* This may be part of generalized psoriasis but is often the only manifestation. It can look very eczema-like (brownish, maculopapular) or, more typically, psoriatic (whitish scales on a dusky red base). It is frequently mistaken for a fungal infection.
- *Pustular psoriasis of palms and soles.* Painful, tiny pustules accompanied by erythema and scaling distinguish this type.
- *Psoriasis of flexural folds.* Not uncommon, this is also known as inverse psoriasis. Shiny salmon-pink to dusky-red plaques in axillae, genitals, groin, and intergluteal and inframammary skin probably represent the process of koebnerization. Because of friction and moisture in these areas, scale is notably lacking, producing a confusing clinical picture.
- *Nail psoriasis.* This form includes tiny pits in the nail plate, color changes, onycholysis, subungual debris, and dystrophy. Similar changes can been seen in other diseases, such as eczema and lichen planus, but the finding of tiny "thimble" pits in nail plates can be very helpful in corroborating the diagnosis of psoriasis. This can be the patient's only manifestation of the disease and presents a particular treatment challenge. It is very commonly mistaken for fungal disease and affects fingernails more than toenails.
- *Psoriatic arthritis.* The incidence in the psoriatic population is 7 to 20 percent, with women slightly outnumbering men. The most common pattern is an asymmetric arthritis classically involving a single digit ("sausage finger"). Other types include a seronegative asymmetric polyarthritis resembling rheumatoid arthritis. The most severe form of psoriatic arthritis is called arthritis mutilans, involving osteolysis of the small bones of the hands and feet, leading to gross deformity and subluxation, similar to what is seen in rheumatoid arthritis. Psoriatic arthritis is common enough that routine history taking from psoriasis patients should always include questions about joint pain.

DIFFERENTIAL DIAGNOSIS

The differential diagnosis varies, depending on the location and type of disease, but includes seborrheic dermatitis, pityriasis rosea, dermatophyte infection, nummular eczema, secondary syphilis, monoarticular arthritis (seronegative), and skin cancers [mycosis fungoides (cutaneous T-cell lymphoma), squamous cell carcinoma, Paget's disease].

LABORATORY

Punch biopsy of skin lesions can be quite helpful in showing fusing and elongation of rete ridges, parakeratosis, lymphocytic perivascular infiltrate, or Munro's microabscesses. Biopsy of early psoriatic lesions is notoriously misleading since the changes listed above are incomplete. Moreover, so-called psoriasiform changes in biopsy reports can be quite nonspecific for psoriasis itself and are commonly found in many other diseases.

TREATMENT

Although no cure is currently available, a number of topical and systemic agents can be quite helpful. However, some attention must first be paid to eliminating possible exacerbating factors, such as medications (e.g., lithium, beta blockers), alcohol, stress, chronic infection, and scratching.

It is also advisable to determine the patient's expectations for treatment, since patients vary greatly in their tolerance for this disease. Some are very accepting of it and require little treatment, whereas others find it devastating and need ongoing expert treatment.

Other factors to consider before treating include the extent and visibility of affected areas, symptoms, type of psoriasis, function of the affected skin (e.g., hands and feet or genitals), the patient's age and health, and past treatment history, that is, what worked and what did not.

The primary care provider can safely attempt topical treatment but should have a very low threshold for referral to a dermatologist as the disease progresses. The dermatologist not only will have a better understanding of the disease and experience with difficult cases but also will have expertise with a wider variety of treatment modalities, particularly ultraviolet A and B (UVA and UVB) phototherapy, and powerful systemic medications. In short, there is no reason for a primary care provider to struggle with an unresponsive psoriasis patient.

Most topical treatments and some systemic medications are subject to the phenomenon called tachyphylaxis, in which continued use of the same agent, especially topical steroids, leads to progressive diminution of the therapeutic effect and is combatted by rotating treatment with different agents. It also should be noted that combinations of treatment agents and modalities often are used. For example, UVA and UVB plus tar and calcipotriene or methotrexate and psoralen plus UVA light treatment (PUVA) help avoid tachyphylaxis and reduce undesirable side effects such as skin cancer from UV modalities.

TREATMENT AGENTS

Emollients

Safe, effective, and inexpensive, these include petroleum jelly, Eucerin cream, mineral oil, and many other agents that can be very useful to hydrate, soften, and loosen scales.

TOPICAL CORTICOSTEROIDS

These are the mainstays of psoriasis treatment, especially plaque-type, because they have anti-inflammatory, antiproliferative, and antimitotic activity. They are much more effective when psoriatic scale has been removed with emollients or after the lesions have been soaked in warm water. They also work better under occlusion (with plastic wrap or hydrocolloid covering) because of enhanced hydration and decreased trauma.

The thicker the skin, the stronger the steroid preparation. For example, facial (especially eyelids), intertriginous, and genital skin is thinner than elbow, knee, and truncal skin. Thus, although the latter areas need strong preparations such as betamethasone valerate and clobetasol propionate ointments, the former require only 1 to 2.5% hydrocortisone because they could be adversely affected by the stronger preparations. Even on thicker skin, prolonged application (e.g., more than 2 weeks bid) of the stronger products can cause not only atrophy but also unsightly striae and telangiectases. The hands and palms, having the thickest skin on the body, can be treated longer and stronger than all other areas.

Tachyphylaxis is a problem, especially with the stronger steroid preparations, and if weekly use exceeds 50 g. Prolonged and widespread use of these agents can even cause adrenal suppression; therefore, steroid-sparing agents such as calcipotriene and anthralin are used instead for a time until they too become relatively ineffective.

Intralesional Steroids

For small but persistent psoriatic plaques (up to 3 cm), intralesional injection of triamcinolone acetonide (Kenalog and others) in an aqueous suspension of 5 mg/mL is quite effective. Possible side effects include local atrophy, systemic absorption, and adrenal suppression. *Note:* If the injection does not require a fair amount of force, the medicine probably is being placed too deeply in the tissue.

Other Topical Agents

These include anthralin (Lasan or Anthra-Derm, Drithocreme), calcipotriene ointment (Dovonex), and various tar-containing formulations used in combination with emollients, often under occlusion.

Systemic Corticosteroids

These are very rarely used except in the most extraordinary situations because of the previously mentioned tendency for psoriasis to rebound with a vengeance after the withdrawal of systemic corticosteroids. For this reason, the presence of psoriasis also constitutes a relative contraindication to the use of such agents for other disease states in a patient.

Other Systemic Agents

Methotrexate, cyclosporine, and sulfasalazine are powerful drugs that traditionally are reserved for use by dermatologists only in the most difficult cases. Some dermatologists believe that bacterial and/or fungal antigens drive psoriasis in certain difficult cases for which they give drugs such as Duricef and/or Diflucan on a long-term basis, but this is controversial.

Psoralen Plus UVA Light Treatment

The oral drug psoralen, a potent photosensitizer, is given, followed later by UVA light exposure on a regular basis as a very effective treatment for recalcitrant psoriasis. This mode requires special equipment and expertise and therefore is used only under the direction of a dermatologist, who will sometimes prescribe UVB treatment instead. For many patients, natural sunlight is quite beneficial.

TREATMENT OF SCALP PSORIASIS

Scalp psoriasis is particularly difficult to treat because of the hindrance that the hair presents both to local application of medications and in shielding the scalp from phototherapy. Scalp psoriasis quite frequently itches, leading to scratching, which produces even more scale, which must be removed or at least thinned before other medications (e.g., steroids) can reach the actual diseased skin. In that regard, the use of salicylic acid shampoos (T-Sal shampoo or 20% salicylic acid in mineral oil) is quite beneficial. Once the scale is removed, tar-based shampoos (Pentrax, T-gel) and topical steroid solutions (betamethasone valerate 0.1% or clobetasol propionate solution 0.05%) will reduce the itching, redness, and scale formation.

For long-term maintenance, patients must be convinced that they must shampoo daily with products such as Selsun, Head and Shoulders, and T-gel, rotating them to prevent tachyphylaxis. Patients must then be cautioned to refrain from scratching, since this will negate all treatment efforts.

TREATMENT OF NAIL PSORIASIS

Difficult at best, treatment of nail psoriasis should be left to dermatologists experienced in that area. Some dermatologist–nail specialists inject the matrices of involved fingers with triamcinolone. Other treatments used for nail psoriasis include topical agents such as 5-fluorouracil cream, urea paste, calcipotriene, and/or potent topical steroids.

TREATMENT OF OTHER FORMS OF PSORIASIS

Dermatologists have a number of effective agents available for the treatment of refractory plaque psoriasis, pustular psoriasis, and erythrodermic psoriasis. These include methotrexate (an anticancer drug), retinoids (vitamin A–derived, such as etretinate), hydroxyurea (an anticancer drug used in combination with UVA or UVB therapy), and cyclosporine (a powerful immunosuppressant), among others.

Phototherapy with various combinations of UVA and UVB lightwave exposure alone or in combination with tar, anthralin, and oral drugs such as psoralen is extremely useful in treating difficult cases of psoriasis.

PEARLS

Knowledge of the following points can contribute to a positive patient outcome:

- Thinking fungal? Think psoriasis first.
- Ask about a family history of psoriasis. Psoriasis patients often assume the practitioner knows about their disease. It's old hat to them.
- Acute exacerbation of psoriasis? Ask about (1) alcohol intake, (2) change in stress level, (3) change in medications, and (4) recent febrile illness.
- Is more than 10 percent of the body surface area affected? Strongly consider referral to a dermatologist.
- Psoriasiform changes in skin biopsy do not necessarily mean the patient has psoriasis. Expand the differential diagnoses.
- Intralesional steroid injections (triamcinolone acetonide 5 mg/cm^3) are especially useful for small plaques (smaller than 3 cm), especially in the scalp.
- Never use systemic corticosteroids for psoriasis and always ask about possible psoriasis before placing patients on it for other conditions.

PATIENT EDUCATION

Especially important for children and adolescents, it can include counseling, sick leave, and vacation (especially to sunny climates). There are special psoriasis camps for children.

Patients should be encouraged to join the National Psoriasis Foundation at 1-800-723-9166. Its Web site can be accessed at http://www.psoriasis.org.

Patients need to know exacerbating factors, and so the provider must spend the necessary time with them to make sure they understand their role in treating the disease.

PROGNOSIS

Psoriasis is a lifelong disease with genetic implications for offspring. Exacerbations and remissions characterize the clinical course, and even though treatment has vastly improved, practitioners are still unable to cure the disease.

BIBLIOGRAPHY

Arndt KA, Robinson JK, LeBoit PE, et al: *Cutaneous Medicine and Surgery.* Philadelphia, Saunders, 1996.
DuVivier A: *Dermatology in Practice.* Philadelphia, Lippincott, 1990.
Fitzpatrick TB, Johnson RA, Wolff K, et al: *Color Atlas and Synopsis of Clinical Dermatology: Common and Serious Diseases,* 3d ed. New York, McGraw-Hill, 1997.
Goldstein BG, Goldstein AO: *Practical Dermatology,* Primary Care Series. St Louis, Mosby Year Book, 1992.
Shelley WB, Shelley ED: *Advanced Dermatologic Diagnosis.* Philadelphia, Saunders, 1992.
Weinberg S, Prose NS, Kristal L: *Color Atlas of Pediatric Dermatology,* 3d ed. New York, McGraw-Hill, 1998.

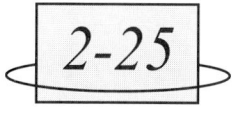

SEBORRHEIC DERMATITIS (SEBORRHEA)

Joe R. Monroe

DISCUSSION

Seborrheic dermatitis (SD) is found in 3 to 5 percent of adults and is a bit more common in men than in women. It is characterized by scaling and redness in areas of the face, scalp, skin folds, and presternal skin. The percentage of infants affected is unknown, but SD in babies is thought to be common. The cause is controversial.

Since it occurs mostly in areas of skin rich in oil glands also favored by the lipophilic commensal yeast *Pityrosporum ovale,* some practitioners point to that organism as the cause. As further proof, they correctly point out that SD worsens dramatically in patients with HIV disease. However, histologic sections through affected hair follicles show no more of these microorganisms than would be normally expected, and SD is often unresponsive to treatment with antifungal agents. Moreover, SD also occurs in oil-poor areas not favored at all by this organism.

Morphologically, SD in adults presents as scaly pinkish-orange patches in highly characteristic symmetric locations, especially alongside the nose, in the brows, behind the ears, and in the external auditory canal. Involvement of the scalp (dandruff) is almost universal in SD patients, with diffuse, fine scaling and faint erythema, if any. Patches often crop up in areas of the face covered by a mustache or beard.

As it moves off the face, SD tends to become more weepy and exudative, especially in the umbilicus. On occasion, it also can affect presternal, axillary, genital, upper intergluteal, and even interscapular skin. Seborrheic blepharoconjunctivitis and styes can accompany SD.

Adult SD often itches, very predictably in the scalp but variably elsewhere.

This is not the case with infants who have SD; they do not seem to be bothered at all by even moderately severe cases. Infant SD usually presents in the first 6 months of life and typically is gone by age 1 year, reappearing in late adolescence, if at all. Unlike adult SD, it favors the scalp, where thick, greasy scales develop (so-called cradle cap), but also is seen in the flexural creases and the diaper area. Its morphology is a little different from that of adult SD, being composed mostly of shiny, erythematous plaques with well-defined borders, often with florid intensity.

DIFFERENTIAL DIAGNOSIS

Face

Rosacea, unlike SD, is composed of papules, pustules, and telangiectases, and perioral dermatitis (affects mostly young women, appears acneiform, and frequently involves the inappropriate use of exacerbating topical steroids on the face) is part of the differential diagnosis.

Scalp

Psoriasis should be included in the differential diagnosis. SD is characterized by diffuse, fine scaling with minimal erythema, whereas psoriasis presents with focal heavy scaling on an erythematous base. Pediculosis should be included too; look for nits and for the telltale fine red rash on the nape of the neck seen with head lice.

Intertriginous

SD in these areas appears orange-pink and shiny, with little scaling, in contrast to SD imitators in these areas, such as fungal infection [potassium hydroxide (KOH)-positive], candidiasis (which will exhibit satellites, unlike adult SD), contact dermatitis, and psoriasis, which sometimes can be difficult to distinguish from SD.

LABORATORY

Biopsy is seldom necessary but occasionally can be helpful, showing spongiosis (intraepidermal edema), a nonspecific finding that is useful in distinguishing SD from psoriasis.

TREATMENT

Infants

Cradle cap responds well to a 2% salicylic acid in olive oil mixture, which breaks up the scale nicely.

Adults

The following steps are recommended:

1. Daily shampooing with an over-the-counter dandruff shampoo such as Head and Shoulders, Selsun, or T-gel, leaving it in place for 5 min before rinsing
2. Hydrocortisone 1% cream applied up to twice a day to the face as needed for itching and redness
3. T-sal (over-the-counter) shampoo to thin out heavy scale in the scalp (use carefully, according to directions)
4. For scalp itching, midstrength steroid solution, such as betamethasone valerate 0.1%, up to twice a day, for no more than 3 days in a row
5. For resistant cases, Nizoral (ketoconazole) shampoo for scalp and face or an oral antifungal such as fluconazole (Diflucan) 200 mg bid for a week (see package insert for drug interactions)

PATIENT EDUCATION

Teach patients about the following:

1. Daily shampooing is a necessity.
2. Limit hat wearing, which makes SD worse.
3. Make sure the patient understands that a cure is not possible and that control is the goal.
4. Educate patients about the noncontagious nature of SD.

PEARLS

Knowledge of the following points can contribute to a positive patient outcome:

- Pruritic patchy midsternal scaling and redness is probably SD, which responds well to antifungal creams in this area.
- Sudden appearance or exacerbation of SD suggests two possibilities: HIV disease or Parkinson's disease.
- SD in infants seems to be asymptomatic and thus does not require treatment except in the scalp.

PROGNOSIS

No permanent cure exists. SD tends to improve with age in adults. Infant SD associated with diarrhea and failure to thrive suggests an entity called Leiner's disease, which can be life-threatening. These children need prompt evaluation by a dermatologist or pediatrician.

BIBLIOGRAPHY

Arndt KA, Robinson JK, LeBoit PE, et al: *Cutaneous Medicine and Surgery.* Philadelphia, Saunders, 1996.
DuVivier A: *Dermatology in Practice.* Philadelphia, Lippincott, 1990.
Fitzpatrick TB, Johnson RA, Wolff K, et al: *Color Atlas and Synopsis of Clinical Dermatology: Common and Serious Diseases,* 3d ed. New York, McGraw-Hill, 1997.
Goldstein BG, Goldstein AO: *Practical Dermatology,* Primary Care Series. St Louis, Mosby Year Book, 1992.
Shelley WB, Shelley ED: *Advanced Dermatologic Diagnosis.* Philadelphia, Saunders, 1992.
Weinberg S, Prose NS, Kristal L: *Color Atlas of Pediatric Dermatology,* 3d ed. New York, McGraw-Hill, 1998.

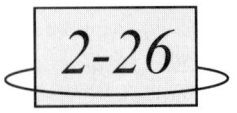

SEBORRHEIC KERATOSIS ("SENILE KERATOSIS")

Joe R. Monroe

DISCUSSION

Seborrheic keratosis is an extremely common, benign pigmented epidermal keratotic papular lesion that becomes more common with increasing age. It is not a disease at all but a name for the most common benign lesions found on human beings. Seborrheic keratoses are equally common between the sexes, and although their cause is unknown, a definite familial tendency exists. Although easily confused with precancerous actinic keratoses, they are not related to sun exposure.

These keratoses spare high-friction and moist areas such as palms, soles, and genitalia but can be found on any other area, predominating on the trunk and face.

The lesions, which usually appear in multiples, can vary quite a bit in color and configuration, with the "norm" being grayish brown, warty, and dry, with a "stuck-on" appearance. These lesions also can be yellowish and mostly flat or even jet black, greasy-looking, and impressively papular. The appearance of the lesions often typifies the patient's idea of how skin cancer ought to look.

In that regard, seborrheic keratoses are benign, with almost no potential for malignant degeneration. However, the sudden appearance of multiple lesions has been known to accompany the occult development of internal malignancy, especially of the gastrointestinal tract. This rare occurrence is called the Leser-Trélat sign.

On blacks, multiple tiny, soft dark brown to black papules develop with age on facial skin, especially around the eyes, and are termed papulosa nigra.

Seborrheic keratoses can be quite dry, tiny, and barely pigmented, especially on the legs and dorsal feet, where they are called stucco keratoses.

DIFFERENTIAL DIAGNOSES

Usually the epidermal (stuck-on) appearance makes the diagnosis clear, as does the multiplicity of lesions. Occasionally, though, punch or excisional biopsy is necessary to distinguish these from melanoma, warts, or pigmented basal cell carcinoma.

LABORATORY

No test is required except biopsy as described above.

TREATMENT

Liquid nitrogen or curettement is recommended, and excision is seldom indicated. Among those with darker skin, care needs to be exercised in treating facial seborrheic keratoses (e.g., papulosa nigra) because of a well-documented tendency for residual darkening in treatment locations that can take months to clear; this is called postinflammatory hyperpigmentation.

PATIENT EDUCATION

Reassure patients about the benign nature of these lesions and the almost total lack of malignant potential. For fair-skinned patients especially, use the opportunity to contrast these lesions to melanomas, which do not often come in multiples, are not epidermal in nature (i.e., tend to be more macular), and tend more toward black coloration.

PEARLS

Knowledge of the following points can contribute to a positive patient outcome:

- There is no law that says a melanoma cannot occur in the middle of several seborrheic keratoses.
- If it is warty, comes off in pieces, is one of several, and appears on a patient over age 35, it is probably a seborrheic keratosis.
- Liquid nitrogen treatment is often diagnostic as well as curative, since it highlights the pseudocysts (appearing as tiny pores) that pock the surfaces of the lesions.
- Seborrheic keratoses are exactly what patients imagine skin cancers look like.

PROGNOSIS

Treatment is very effective, but expect more lesions to appear.

BIBLIOGRAPHY

Arndt KA, Robinson JK, LeBoit PE, et al: *Cutaneous Medicine and Surgery.* Philadelphia, Saunders, 1996.
DuVivier A: *Dermatology in Practice.* Philadelphia, Lippincott, 1990.
Fitzpatrick TB, Johnson RA, Wolff K, et al: *Color Atlas and Synopsis of Clinical Dermatology: Common and Serious Diseases,* 3d ed. New York, McGraw-Hill, 1997.
Goldstein BG, Goldstein AO: *Practical Dermatology,* Primary Care Series. St Louis, Mosby Year Book, 1992.
Shelley WB, Shelley ED: *Advanced Dermatologic Diagnosis.* Philadelphia, Saunders, 1992.
Weinberg S, Prose NS, Kristal L: *Color Atlas of Pediatric Dermatology,* 3d ed. New York, McGraw-Hill, 1998.

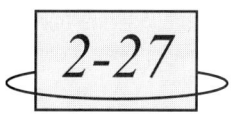

SQUAMOUS CELL CARCINOMA

Barbara L. Sauls

DISCUSSION

Squamous cell carcinoma is the second most common skin cancer after basal cell carcinoma. The lesions arise in the epithelial keratinized cells of the skin. This cancer is able to metastasize and grows rapidly, unlike basal cell carcinoma. The typical patient is older than 50 years and has light skin with a poor tanning capacity and a history of frequent sun exposure. Long-term smokers often develop lesions on the lower lip in the area where the cigarette, pipe, or cigar typically rests. These lip lesions have a high rate of metastasis. Exposure to arsenic and coal combustion by-products and chronic heat exposure also have been implicated in the development of squamous cell carcinoma. Dark-skinned individuals may get this disease from toxic agents rather than from sun exposure. Occupations at risk include individuals who work outdoors (e.g., farmers, construction workers, fishermen) and those with industrial exposure to chemical carcinogens. Individuals who travel to foreign countries on their own or with the military may have been exposed to arsenic in water sources.

Actinic keratosis, cheilitis, and leukoplakia are precursors of squamous cell carcinoma. Squamous cell carcinoma that arises in an actinic keratosis is believed to have a lesser potential for metastases. Bowen's disease is a form of squamous carcinoma that remains superficial, though this form occurs on sun-exposed and protected sites as well as internally. This lesion also is associated with arsenic exposure.

Patients with a previous diagnosis of certain subtypes of human papillomavirus (HPV) frequently develop squamous cell carcinoma of the anal area, penis, and cervix. Immunosuppression also promotes the development of both squamous and basal cell carcinomas.

SIGNS AND SYMPTOMS

Patients typically present with a slowly evolving, nonhealing, ulcerated or scaling lesion, though there is a wide variety of presentation. Presentation may simply be a scaly erythematous patch or a keratotic nodule.

OBJECTIVE FINDINGS

The most common presentation of squamous cell carcinoma is a nonhealing, elevated, ulcerated nodular lesion, but it also may present as a firm papule or plaque. Erosion may or may not be present. The lesion is usually reddish in color and isolated. Typical areas of occurrence are sun-exposed: tops of ears, nose, cheek, scalp in bald persons, tops of hands, and forearms. There also may be localized lymphadenopathy.

DIAGNOSTIC CONSIDERATIONS

The differential diagnoses of squamous cell carcinoma are few. Paget's disease, basal cell carcinoma, actinic keratoses, and eczematous lesions may resemble squamous carcinoma and need to be differentiated through biopsy. Bowen's disease may mimic psoriasis or nummular eczema.

SPECIAL CONSIDERATIONS

Smokers have a predisposition to lip and oropharyngeal lesions, often beginning as leukoplakia (see Fig. 2-27-1 and Plate 26). Squamous cell carcinoma of the lip is more aggressive and prone to spread than are other cutaneous squamous cell carcinomas. It is

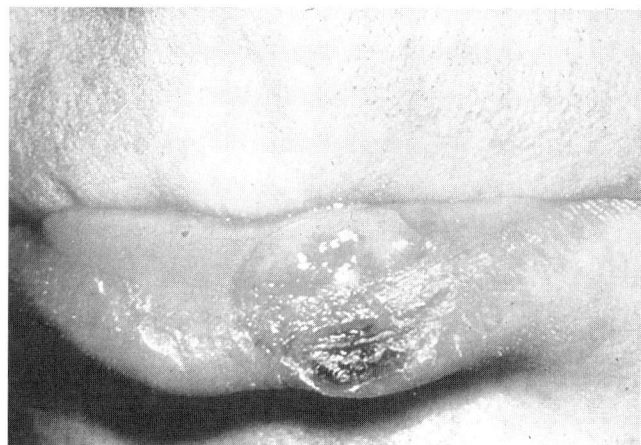

FIGURE 2-27-1 (PLATE 26). A classic squamous cell carcinoma of the lip found on a smoker. (*Photo courtesy of William H. Fenn. Used with permission.*)

common for smokers to develop leukoplakia on the buccal mucosa. Any leukoplakia should be biopsied when first observed and then monitored on a regular basis thereafter if the initial pathology report is benign.

LABORATORY TESTS

Biopsy is required for a definitive diagnosis of any suspicious skin lesions.

TREATMENT

Surgery and radiation are used for the treatment of squamous cell carcinoma. The choice depends on the location, size, and shape of the lesion as well as the age and overall condition of the patient.

Precancerous lesions such as actinic keratoses should be treated with topical chemotherapy such as 5-fluorouracil (5-FU) cream, cryotherapy, or surgical removal.

PATIENT EDUCATION

Since the majority of cases of squamous cell carcinoma are due to sun exposure, patients must be counseled to avoid the sun from 10 A.M. to 2 P.M. and to use a sunscreen, hat, long sleeves, and long pants when they are in the sun.

Routine skin examination is required, with close attention paid to developing lesions or areas of leukoplakia. Patients should be instructed to notify the practitioner of any new or changing lesions and not to wait until the next scheduled appointment to have those lesions evaluated.

COMPLICATIONS AND RED FLAGS

A dermatologist should treat these lesions. A prompt referral is needed after the initial diagnosis is made.

BIBLIOGRAPHY

Fauci AS, Braunwald E, Isselbacher KJ, et al (eds): *Harrison's Principles of Internal Medicine,* 14th ed. New York, McGraw-Hill, 1998.

Fitzpatrick TB, Johnson RA, Wolff K, et al: *Color Atlas and Synopsis of Clinical Dermatology: Common and Serious Diseases,* 3d ed. New York, McGraw-Hill, 1997.

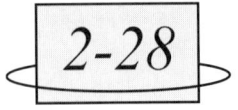

TINEA INFECTIONS OF THE SKIN (TINEA CORPORIS, TINEA CAPITIS, TINEA CRURIS, TINEA PEDIS, TINEA VERSICOLOR)

Barbara L. Sauls

DISCUSSION

Tinea is a term used to describe superficial dermatophyte infections of keratinized tissue such as the skin, nails, and hair. The most common causative organisms include *Trichophyton, Microsporum,* and *Epidermophyton* species. Tinea versicolor is an exception and is caused by the nondermatophyte fungus *Pityrosporum.* These infections are acquired from other individuals, from the skin of animals, and less commonly from the soil.

Tinea pedis occurs most commonly and often becomes a chronic condition. It is promoted by warm, wet environments and hot and humid weather. Individuals who bathe infrequently, sweat heavily, and do not dry themselves properly, especially between the toes, are at great risk for developing tinea infections of the feet and groin. Tinea capitis is most common in children. Tinea cruris usually is seen in adult male athletes and obese individuals in the warm, moist environment of body folds.

There is an increased incidence of tinea infections in the late spring and summer months, when the weather is more hot and humid. Adult blacks seem to have a lower incidence of fungal skin infections, whereas immunosuppressed persons have a higher incidence, and their infections are more difficult to treat.

SIGNS AND SYMPTOMS

Tinea Capitis

Patients most commonly report circular areas of alopecia with little or no pruritus.

Tinea Corporis

This also is referred to as *ringworm.* This infection presents as a reddish, raised pruritic lesion that grows into a circular (annular) shape. The center of the lesion often clears, and the border tends to be elevated and scaly. There may be more than one lesion present.

Tinea Pedis

This also is known as *athlete's foot.* Patients complain of burning, itching, and peeling of the skin of the feet. This most commonly occurs in the web spaces of the toes. Subacute or chronic conditions may have various stages from dry scaling to edema and maceration.

Tinea Cruris

This condition is also known as *jock itch* and presents as reddened, moist skin in the groin area with itching and burning, notably sparing the scrotum.

Tinea Versicolor

This condition also is known as pityriasis versicolor. Presentation in light-skinned individuals is usually as mildly scaling, well-demarcated, hyperpigmented areas. The lesions occasionally may be hypopigmented and confused with those of vitiligo. Persons with dark skin typically have hypopigmented lesions, though the lesions may barely be perceptible. No other skin symptoms are associated with this infection. Distribution over the shoulders, upper trunk, and arms is called "mantle" distribution and is a common characteristic.

OBJECTIVE FINDINGS

Tinea Capitis

Physical examination of the hair and scalp typically reveals hair shafts that are broken off close to the scalp (see Fig. 2-28-1 and Plate 27). This area feels fuzzy when it is rubbed, as opposed to alopecia, which does not. *Microsporum* infection usually causes broken hair shafts and is called *gray patch ringworm. Trichophyton* infection causes hair to break, appears as black dots, and is called *black dot ringworm.* Kerion has inflammatory pustular areas where hairs fall out when tugged. *Favus* is caused by a *Trichophyton* species. This type of fungal infection develops yellowish crusts and scales called scutula. It has areas of atrophy and scar formation that heal as scarring alopecia. There also may be a secondary bacterial infection of the scalp.

Tinea Corporis

Examination shows one or more lesions that began as red areas and expanded into raised, red borders with central clearing, giving justification to the name *ringworm* (see Fig. 2-28-2 and Plate 28). The border is often scaly. These lesions can become quite large and usually are well demarcated.

Tinea Pedis

Examination of the feet shows moist, macerated skin with whitish scales, erosions, vesicles, or bullae. The most common site of infection is the area between the third and fourth toes, which in untreated cases will often extend to the sole and other interdigital spaces. The sides and soles of the feet also may demonstrate a dry,

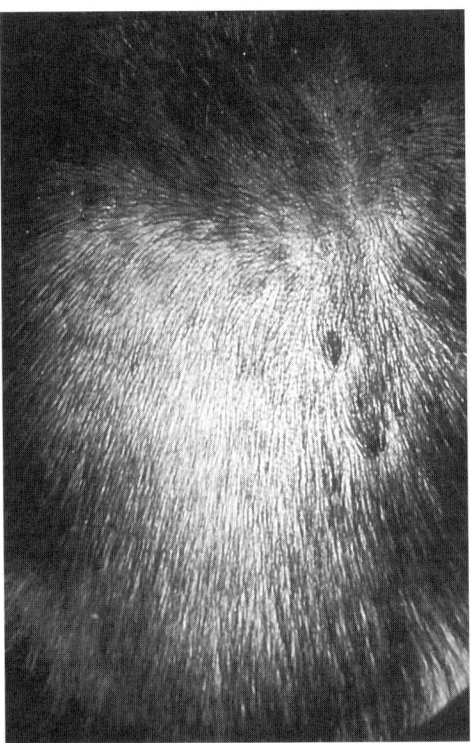

FIGURE 2-28-1 (PLATE 27). Typical area of alopecia from tinea capitis with kerion formation. Note broken hair shafts and pustules. (*Photo courtesy of William H. Fenn. Used with permission.*)

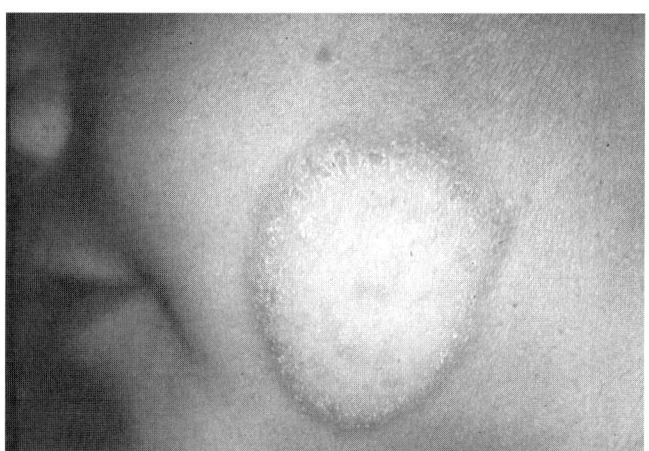

FIGURE 2-28-2 (PLATE 28). Typical circular, raised, well-demarcated red border of tinea corporis. Scaling is also present. Note central clearing. (*Photo courtesy of William H. Fenn. Used with permission.*)

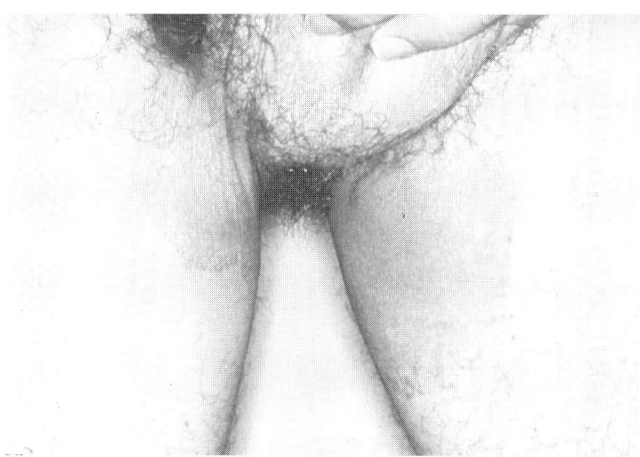

FIGURE 2-28-4 (PLATE 30). Typical tinea cruris with well-demarcated, moist red skin on the thighs. Note sparing of the scrotum. (*Photo courtesy of William H. Fenn. Used with permission.*)

scaly nonpruritic dermatitis. This is often seen in a "moccasin" pattern (see Fig. 2-28-3 and Plate 29).

Tinea Cruris

Physical examination often demonstrates a symmetric large red plaque with sharp margins that are slightly elevated with light scaling over the intertriginous area and inner thighs (see Fig. 2-28-4 and Plate 30). The scrotum usually is not affected by tinea infection, though this is not the case with a fungal infection of the groin caused by *Candida*. Satellite lesions are not seen. Pustules are seen occasionally.

Tinea Versicolor

Physical examination findings include sharply marginated macules that are scattered and discrete. Colors vary from normal skin and range from white to brown, with all shades in between. Caucasians usually have darker patches, whereas those with dark skin have lighter patches (see Fig. 2-28-5 and Plate 31). A fine scale may be present. The lesions

are most commonly found on the trunk, arms, abdomen, and thighs and rarely on the face.

DIAGNOSTIC CONSIDERATIONS

The following points should be considered in the diagnosis:

- *Tinea capitis.* Alopecia, trichotillomania (hair pulling), or bacterial folliculitis may resemble the various forms of tinea capitis.
- *Tinea corporis.* Psoriasis or cellulitis should be considered.
- *Tinea pedis.* In less severe cases, it is possible to confuse this infection with contact dermatitis.
- *Tinea cruris.* Cellulitis or candidiasis may resemble tinea cruris.
- *Tinea versicolor.* Hypopigmented lesions may be confused with vitiligo. The presence of scaling is more suggestive of tinea.

SPECIAL CONSIDERATIONS

Fungal infections are often the hallmark of an immunocompromised state such as diabetes or HIV and may require further investigation. Fungal infections are notoriously difficult to treat in immunocompromised patients. The course of treatment is often prolonged and complicated by other medications and therapies.

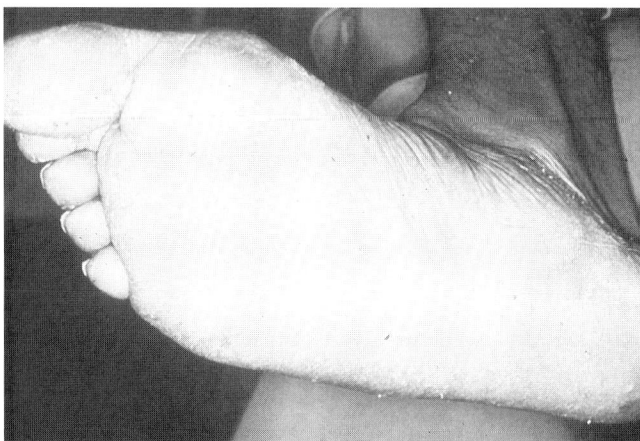

FIGURE 2-28-3 (PLATE 29). Moccasin pattern tinea pedis. The infection is present on the soles of the foot and along the sides and between the toes, where a moccasin-type shoe would touch the skin. The affected skin is dry and peeling, and these patients typically complain of burning and itching. (*Photo courtesy of William H. Fenn. Used with permission.*)

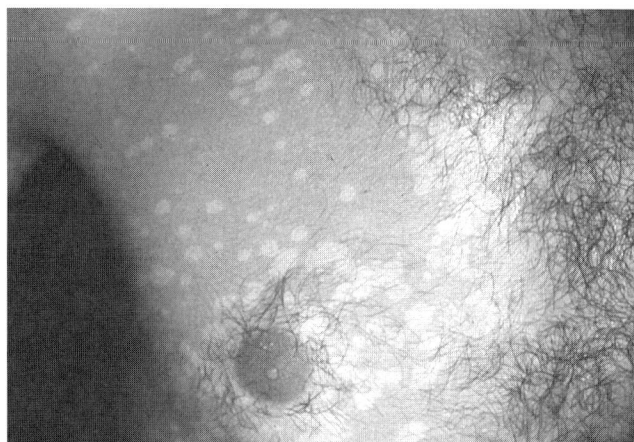

FIGURE 2-28-5 (PLATE 31). Tinea versicolor affecting the chest. Note areas of hypopigmentation. (*Photo courtesy of William H. Fenn. Used with permission.*)

Care should be taken when prescribing oral antifungal medications, since some are potentially hepatotoxic. Itraconazole (Sporanox) and terbinafine (Lamisil) have not been shown to be hepatotoxic.

LABORATORY TESTS

Many tinea skin infections can be diagnosed with a potassium hydroxide (KOH) preparation. This is performed by scraping a small amount of tissue from scales, hair shafts, or pustular areas with the edge of a scalpel onto a microscope slide. A drop or two of 10% KOH solution is placed on the scrapings to lyse the epithelial cells and make the hyphae and buds more easily visible. A glass cover slip is placed over the scrapings, and the slide is heated gently (not boiled). Examine under a microscope at low power. Look for the long filaments of *hyphae,* either straight or coiled together, and multiple *buds,* either alone or attached to the hyphae, like grapes.

A fungal culture will confirm these results and determine the exact organism causing the infection. Since cultures may take several weeks, treatment can be initiated pending the results.

A Wood's lamp is sometimes helpful in distinguishing tinea infections. Infections will fluoresce different colors, depending on the causative organism. Tinea capitis fluoresces bright or grayish green, tinea corporis will appear blue-green, and tinea versicolor tends to be yellow-green. Vitiligo will show reflected light and not fluoresce.

TREATMENT

The length of treatment varies for both topical and oral antifungal drugs (see Table 2-28-1). Package insert materials should be reviewed carefully.

Consider the following:

- *Tinea capitis.* Oral antifungal medications are required. Baseline liver function studies are suggested before oral therapy is initiated.
- *Tinea corporis.* Topical antifungals usually are all that is necessary. Persistent or widespread disease may require oral therapy.
- *Tinea pedis.* Topical antifungals plus hygiene: frequent washing with complete drying, the use of drying powders, and wearing only white cotton socks are beneficial. Resistant cases may require oral antifungal preparations.
- *Tinea cruris.* Topical antifungals are required, plus hygiene; bathe with complete drying and use drying powders. Encourage weight loss if obesity is a contributing factor. Resistant cases may require oral antifungal preparations.
- *Tinea versicolor.* Depending on the severity, oral or topical antifungal medication may be effective. Selenium sulfide applications also are used with varying success.

SUPPORTIVE MEASURES

Hygiene is a major factor in the management of tinea infections. Bathing followed by complete drying is essential. Reducing humidity is also beneficial but often difficult to accomplish. Powders with cornstarch may help control moisture. Absorbent cotton socks (white) are important for tinea pedis because the dyes in dark socks can promote fungal growth. Patients should alternate shoes or allow shoes to dry out between uses.

PATIENT EDUCATION

Fungal infections are contagious and can spread to close contacts. Other family members should be examined for similar infections,

TABLE 2-28-1. Summary of Tinea Infections and Effective Medications*

INFECTION	BRAND NAME	GENERIC	FREQUENCY	CAUTIONS
Tinea capitis	Grifulvin V, 250- or 500-mg tabs; 125 mg/5 mL susp.	Griseofulvin	500 mg daily in divided doses; children under 50 lb: 5 mg/lb daily	Use with care in liver disease; Oral antifungal may adversely react with other medications
	Fulvicin P/G 125-, 165-, 250-, and 330-mg tablets	Ultramicrosize Griseofulvin	375 to 750 mg daily in divided dose; children over 2 years: 3.3 mg/lb daily, divided	Above
	Nizoral, 200-mg tablets	Ketoconazole	One tab daily	Above
Tinea corporis	Lotrimin, 1% cream, lotion, solution	Clotrimazole	Twice daily	
	Nizoral, 2% cream	Ketoconazole	Once daily	
	Loprox, 1% cream and lotion	Ciclopirox olamine	Twice daily	
	Spectazole cream	Econazole	Once daily	
	Lamisil, 1% cream	Terbinafine hydrochloride	Once daily	
	Monistat Derm cream	Miconazole nitrate	Apply twice daily for 2 weeks	
Tinea pedis	See corporis		Treat for 1 month to 6 weeks	
	Lamisil, 1% cream	Terbinafine hydrochloride	bid	
Tinea cruris	See corporis			Above
Tinea unguium	See capitis		May require 6 to 12 months of treatment	Above
	Sporanox, 100-mg capsules	Itraconazole	Once daily for 3 months	
Tinea versicolor	Selenium sulfide, 2.5% lotion; use in conjunction with topical antifungals	Selsun	Apply once daily for 2 weeks; lather, leave on for 10 min, and rinse; repeat after 7 days to 2 weeks	

*Topical therapy that does not result in a complete response may require a change to oral therapy.

especially if a patient has recurrent infections. Pets such as dogs and cats suspected of having fungal infections should be examined by a veterinarian and treated appropriately. Most cases of tinea corporis in children are from animal vectors. Although this is obvious to medical practitioners, parents may need to be reminded that "ringworm" infections are not "worms."

DISPOSITION

Patient follow-up depends on the severity and type of infection and the choice of antifungal medications. Usually, patients on oral therapy should be monitored closely for adverse effects. Liver function studies are suggested every 2 months while patients are on oral antifungals. If enzyme levels rise, the medication should be discontinued. Liver enzymes usually return to normal after cessation of the medication.

COMPLICATIONS

Secondary bacterial infections are the most common complication of fungal infections and should be treated with an appropriate antibiotic.

PEARLS

Knowledge of the following points can contribute to a positive patient outcome:

- Skin scrapings are easy on a compliant patient, but children are often frightened. As an alternative to using a scalpel to scrape the skin, consider using a tongue depressor or the edge of a glass slide to obtain a specimen.
- If you put a drop of KOH on the slide immediately and use a cover slip, it is less likely that the scraping will be lost while being carried to the microscope.

BIBLIOGRAPHY

Fauci AS, Braunwald E, Isselbacher KJ, et al (eds): *Harrison's Principles of Internal Medicine,* 14th ed. New York, McGraw-Hill, 1998.

Fitzpatrick TB, Johnson RA, Wolff K, et al: *Color Atlas and Synopsis of Clinical Dermatology: Common and Serious Diseases,* 3d ed. New York, McGraw-Hill, 1997.

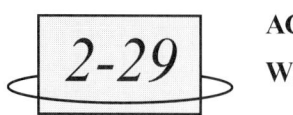

ACNE
William H. Fenn

DISCUSSION

Acne vulgaris is one of the most common skin disorders, affecting as much as 85 to 90 percent of the population at one time or another. Although peak incidence is during the adolescent years, some skin changes of acne are found as early as age 9 in many individuals, and lesions may persist or even initially appear between 20 and 40 years of age. So common is the disorder that almost all patients self-diagnose prior to presentation and many have attempted self-treatment.

PATHOPHYSIOLOGY

The lesions of acne are the result of a complex cascade of events. Stimulation of the pilosebaceous unit by androgens results in increased sebum production. It is assumed by many that the increased production of androgens with the onset of puberty accounts for this, but increased sensitivity of the sebaceous glands may be more important.

Obstruction of the follicular outlet by adherent keratinized cells, possibly also mediated by androgens, leads to plugging and a cyclical accumulation of keratinaceous debris. In this environment, anaerobic bacteria, especially *Propionibacterium acnes,* proliferate and contribute to the inflammatory process along with the release of free fatty acids. The exact mechanism of the bacterial contribution is controversial, with several competing theories being advanced. That *Propionibacterium acnes* plays a clinically significant role, however, is not in doubt. As observed in other skin disorders, significant stress (physical, emotional, or psychological) may exacerbate the eruption but is not a causative factor. It is also useful to note that, in general, diet and cleanliness do not play a significant role in the evolution or course of acne.

SIGNS AND SYMPTOMS

Patient complaints are principally related to the cosmetic aspect of the eruption. Some patients also note sensations of burning or pruritus, although these may also be related to attempts at self-therapy.

OBJECTIVE FINDINGS

The initial lesions of acne are the open and closed comedones, often referred to as blackheads and whiteheads, respectively. These may evolve into papules and pustules, and most patients will have all of these lesions simultaneously. In some patients, the disease course involves progression to multiple large scarring cysts and nodules that are often painful. The determinant of which patients suffer from nodular-cystic acne is most likely genetic. Lesions predominate on the face in most patients, with the upper back and trunk often involved.

DIAGNOSTIC CONSIDERATIONS

Diagnosis of acne is rarely in doubt. Steroid acne may result from high-strength topical preparations or systemic steroids. The eruption from systemic steroids tends to be more truncal, whereas that of topical steroids is limited to the area of application. Although history is generally revealing in the case of topical steroids and systemic steroids used for legitimate medical purposes, laboratory testing may be required if there is a high degree of suspicion of illicit steroid abuse.

Acne induced by halogenated occupational chemicals tends to have comedones as the predominant lesions. A sudden onset of adult acne may raise the consideration of dysfunction within the hypothalamic–pituitary–adrenal axis. In the older patient, rosacea is a consideration and may be excluded by the absence of telangiectasia.

SPECIAL CONSIDERATIONS

Neonatal acne is generally self-limited and does not require therapy. Comedones occurring in a geriatric population (sometimes referred to as senile acne) generally respond better to mechanical extraction than medication if treatment is desired.

LABORATORY TESTS

There are no relevant laboratory tests, unless secondary causes such as steroid abuse or hormonal disturbances are suggested by other findings.

TREATMENT
Medications

Multiple topical and systemic medications are available for the treatment of acne (see Table 2-29-1). A rational basis for selection focuses primarily on lesion type, along with patient compliance and risk

TABLE 2-29-1. Common Acne Medications

MEDICATION	DOSAGE REGIMEN	COMMENTS
Topical Agents		
Topical antibiotics (erythromycin, clindamycin, tetracycline)	Multiple preparations, generally applied twice daily	Little significant difference between medications. Topical tetracycline most efficacious in some studies, but availability limited, higher side-effect profile
Benzoyl peroxide preparations	2%, 5%, 10% strength lotions, creams, gels, washes	5% most useful strength. Washes of little or no use. Apply qd–bid. When used in combination with other topicals, apply alone qd. The only OTC medication of significant benefit
Azelaic acid (Azelex)	20% cream applied bid	May be used qd if skin irritation (common) occurs. Relatively new in U.S. but longer worldwide use. Mechanism uncertain, but may be antimicrobial against *P. acnes*
Topical retinoids, tretinoin (Retin-A, Renova), adapalene (Differin), tazarotene (Tazorac)	Multiple preparations of tretinoin. Most useful are 0.025% gel, Differin 0.1% gel. Daily application	Wash hands thoroughly after application. Increase in apparent acne prior to improvement. Adapalene more efficacious with fewer side effects
Oral Antibiotics		
Tetracycline	Initial: 500 mg bid, taper to lowest controlling dose (250–500 mg qd)	Need for empty stomach absorption limits adolescent compliance. Dental staining precludes use during pregnancy or prior to permanent teeth
Minocycline	Initial: 100 mg qd–bid, taper to 50 mg qd	If intolerant of or unresponsive to tetracycline
Erythromycin	Initial: 500 mg bid, taper to lowest controlling dose (250–500 mg qd)	If intolerant of or unresponsive to tetracycline. Newer macrolides have little advantage in acne, much higher cost
Oral Retinoids		
Isotretinoin (Accutane)	Multiple slightly differing dosing regimens	Drug of choice for nodulocystic acne. NOT indicated for mild-moderate acne vulgaris. High side-effect profile. Pregnancy category X. Use of this medicine by providers without extensive experience is discouraged. Refer likely candidates to qualified provider

factors. Severity, independent of lesion type, is not a useful basis for medication selection. Topical retinoids are the most effective agents for comedones, whereas topical or systemic antibiotics are more useful against inflammatory and pustular lesions. Providers and patients should expect some changes in medication(s) as the eruption changes. Although more than one preparation is usually beneficial, care should be exercised to ensure the simplest possible regimen.

Supportive Measures

Thoughtful selection of medications used for other reasons may benefit acne. The best example is the informed selection of an oral contraceptive agent in patients desiring such therapy. Rational selection among agents will also result in a reduction of acne lesions. Norgestimate/ethinyl estradiol (Tri-Cyclen) is the only oral contraceptive (OCP) specifically labeled for this situation, although other OCPs may also be useful. Although acne is not perceived as a serious disorder, it is important that the patient hear that the practitioner understands the psychosocial ramifications and takes those seriously. It may also be necessary to discuss this with the parents.

Patient Education

Patient education forms a critical portion of therapy for acne. Because the majority of patients are adolescents, it is very helpful to have both the patient and at least one parent present to boost compliance and avoid conflicting demands on the patient. Patients must be taught proper use of all therapeutic modalities prescribed, as well as proper use of cosmetics, cleansers, and other products. It is critical to tell patients that the medication(s) prescribed will control, not cure, the acne and that once the lesions have been eliminated, it is important to continue the medication(s) until they are told to discontinue them. Inevitably this leads to questions as to when the acne will go away permanently, and it is important to be honest and acknowledge that this cannot be predicted for each individual.

Teaching the patient how to read and interpret labels on cosmetics and skin and hair care products is not only good general education for patients, but beneficial for relief of the acne as well. Although avoidance of these products would be ideal from a clinical point of view, that is simply not a realistic goal in today's society. The use of any such product should be minimized while acne is present, and all cosmetics used should be labeled as noncomedogenic. Other terms, such as *dermatologist-tested* or *hypoallergenic,* are not appropriate guides for use.

Incorrect preexisting myths must be debunked; for example, patients must be taught that food products do not play a significant role in acne so long as a generally balanced diet is followed. Scrupulous avoidance of foods such as chocolate, nuts, or cheese will not improve acne. Some authors in the field acknowledge this, but believe that patient beliefs are so strong as to make it impractical to discuss. This author believes that it is important to dispense accurate information in a practical fashion and recognize that it is then up to the patient to use or not use the information. It is also important to note that "dirtiness" is not a factor in the development of acne, and basic good hygiene with twice-daily face washing with a mild soap will suffice. More frequent washing or the use of stronger cleansing preparations may actually aggravate acne. To assist patients (or parents) in understanding this, it may be helpful to remind them that acne is, at its root, a rash, and just as with other rashes, such as that of poison ivy, mechanical or chemical irritation is not beneficial.

Disposition

After starting initial therapy, reexamination at 8 to 10 weeks is useful to evaluate efficacy. Once efficacious control is obtained, follow-up every 6 months is reasonable, with instructions to return sooner should an extended period of exacerbation occur. Therapy for control may span many years, and it is necessary to periodically discontinue treatment to determine if remission has occurred. Although there is no right timing for this, a yearly trial off medications is probably warranted.

TABLE 2-29-2. Acne Chart with Sample Entries

	FACE	BACK
Comedones	1	0
Papules	2	2
Pustules	2	1
Cysts	0	0
Scars	0	1

Scale: 0 = None, 4 = extensive, to the point of confluence.

COMPLICATIONS AND RED FLAGS

With such a good prognosis, complications are limited. Although the cystic form of acne is inherently scarring, the more common form is not. The patient must understand that scars may nonetheless result from inappropriate picking, squeezing, or otherwise traumatizing acne lesions.

OTHER NOTES OR PEARLS

One difficulty often encountered is assessing the degree of improvement from visit to visit. Descriptors such as *mild, moderate,* and *severe* are not particularly evocative of the patient's appearance, and although the patient's input is helpful, it is highly subjective. The use of a photographic record is ideal, but is not practical for most general practices for a number of reasons, although progress in digital technology may soon change that. A better method is to record the findings in a manner such as that shown in Table 2-29-2, and purchasing a rubber stamp is helpful when treating significant numbers of acne patients. This type of charting allows for rapid recording of findings and a quick method of assessing interval change both in severity and lesion type, each of which may have a bearing on potential treatment changes.

BIBLIOGRAPHY

Cunliffe WJ, Caputo R, Dreno B, et al: Clinical efficacy and safety comparison of adapalene gel and tretinoin gel in the treatment of acne vulgaris: Europe and U.S. multicenter trials. *J Am Acad Dermatol* 36:S126–S134, 1997.

Fitzpatrick TB, Johnson RA, Wolff K, et al: *Color Atlas and Synopsis of Clinical Dermatology,* 3rd ed. New York, McGraw-Hill, 1997, pp. 2–7.

Goldstein BG, Goldstein AO: *Practical Dermatology,* 2nd ed. St. Louis, Mosby, 1997, pp. 46–51.

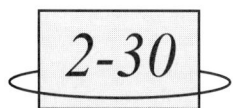

DIAPER DERMATITIS
Rodney L. Moser

DISCUSSION

Diaper dermatitis is one of the most common primary irritant contact dermatoses seen in pediatric practices. Prolonged contact to the sensitive skin by feces and/or urine contained in a diaper results in the breakdown of the natural protective barrier of the skin. The proteolytic enzymes in feces (especially diarrhea) appear to be a far greater primary irritant than urine, causing more erosive lesions.

Once the integrity of the skin has been breached, the warm, dark, moist, and contaminated environment of diapers leads to opportunistic, secondary infections by common bacterial skin pathogens and/or *Candida albicans.*

Chemical irritants, such as soaps, detergents, and fabric softeners, are often predisposing factors in cloth-diapered or training pants–wearing children. Frequency of diaper changes, neglect of hygiene, recent antibiotic use, and contact allergies are also primary factors to consider. Basically, some children tend to be more susceptible to diaper eruptions than others.

Diaper dermatitis is becoming less common since the advent of the new superabsorbent disposable diapers. Newer diapers contain highly absorbent polymer gels that can absorb up to 80 times their weight in water (or in this case, urine). Rash-preventing additives, like petrolatum, lessen friction with the wet surface and help protect the skin. Although disposable diapers pose some environmental concerns in landfills, these technological advances have drastically reduced the overall incidence of the common childhood malady. Cloth diapers are much less effective in preventing diaper-related dermatoses, and the energy and chemicals required to launder them poses equal, if not greater, environmental concerns. The bottom line is that the primary cause of diaper rash is simply diapers, since diapered adults in nursing homes exhibit similar cutaneous responses.

TYPES OF DIAPER DERMATITIS

Primary irritant dermatitis is the most common diaper dermatitis and is caused by repeated or prolonged contact of feces (usual cause) and urine in the diaper areas.

Allergic diaper dermatitis (caused by chemicals, soaps, topical medications, etc.) may mimic primary irritant dermatitis. Often a careful history may reveal a potential allergen. Since the chemical composition of many regular products used on children, such as diaper wipes, ointments, creams, and perfume-containing soaps, tends to change, it may be difficult to pinpoint a cause without systematic product elimination (and reintroduction). Words like "new and improved" or "even fresher smell" are clues of recent product modifications that may prompt allergic responses.

Candidal (monilial) diaper dermatitis is the most commonly seen fungal infection in children. Infants tend to harbor *C. albicans* in the lower intestine—feces is the primary source of this eruption. Recent antibiotic use and diarrhea (from any source) are other predisposing factors. This opportunistic fungus can appear 3 to 5 days after the onset of a primary irritant dermatitis. You must simultaneously treat candidiasis and contact irritation in order to control this condition.

SIGNS AND SYMPTOMS

The term "diaper rash" is not an isolated clinical entity but a dermatosis that can have a wide variety of clinical signs and symptoms, depending on the specific cause. Regardless of the cause, the act of defecating and urinating on raw, irritated skin can be exquisitely painful. Depending on the degree and duration of the irritant, the exposed skin will appear erythematous and macerated, and may even bleed. In more chronic cases, the skin may have a shiny, wrinkled, parchment-like appearance with areas of dry scaling.

In *primary irritant dermatitis,* the intertriginous folds may be spared, but exposed areas of the genital, perianal, and diaper borders will appear inflamed.

Allergic diaper dermatitis may mimic the appearance of primary irritant dermatitis. The skin may appear diffusely red or have papulovesicular responses with scaling.

Candidal (monilial) diaper dermatitis has a characteristic fiery-red (beefy) appearance with pinpoint pustulovesicular "satellite" lesions, mostly seen along the borders of the eruption and in the intertriginous areas. These satellite lesions are diagnostic of this most common primary and secondary invader. Confluent eruptions may have raised edges and sharp borders. Cutaneous candidiasis may also occur in association with oral thrush (see Chap. 3-13).

DIAGNOSTIC CONSIDERATIONS

Seborrheic dermatitis (see Chap 2-25) can occur in the diaper area, especially in infants who also have this common skin condition on the scalp, neck, and face. Like primary irritant dermatitis, this too can become superinfected with candidiasis or bacterial pathogens and must be treated accordingly.

Psoriasiform "napkin" dermatitis resembles psoriasis in appearance with sharply marginated, scaly plaques. It is often caused by a seborrheic/candidiasis superinfection and can lead to the development of true psoriasis in some cases (see Chap. 2-24). Because of the location, this can be very difficult to treat.

Atopic dermatitis (see Chap. 2-6) can occur in the diaper area. Because the diaper area is mostly covered, the appearance of the eruption lacks the usual excoriations caused by scratching.

Kawasaki disease (see Chap. 10-6), an acute multisystem inflammatory disease, can result in profound diaper reactions, especially with erythema and dryness at the diaper margins (tidewater dermatitis). A child with fever for more than 5 days, rash, swelling of hands or feet, conjunctivitis, lymphadenopathy, and mucosal changes should have laboratory testing for thrombocytosis, an elevated erythrocyte sedimentation rate, and an elevated C-reactive protein level.

Impetigo (see Chap. 2-19), *Staphylococcus* scalded skin syndrome, herpes simplex (see Chap. 2-16), and scabies (Chap. 2-5) should also be considered in the differential diagnoses for unusual or difficult-to-manage diaper eruptions.

LABORATORY STUDIES

Laboratory studies are indicated when the provider is uncertain of the diagnosis and in situations where other signs and symptoms warrant further investigation. Routine cultures for *C. albicans* are rarely done since the appearance is usually diagnostic. Direct microscopic examination (KOH and wet mount, Gram stains) may reveal large numbers of yeast, as budding hyphae or any stage of yeast growth. Bacterial cultures are rarely indicated in secondarily infected eruptions since skin pathogens are the most likely culprits and can be treated empirically.

TREATMENT

The ABCDEF acronym may be used to describe the therapeutic approach to generic diaper eruptions:

- **Air:** Attempts should be made to "air out" the diaper area periodically. Children can be undiapered during limited, monitored periods (such as nap time) to limit maceration caused by wetness. Direct sun exposure should be avoided since it may lead to sunburn in as little as 6 min.
- **Barrier:** There are many skin protectant products that can be safely used in the diaper area of children. The most widely used over-the-counter products contain petrolatum, zinc oxide, or both (A&D Ointment, Desitin), or add Burow's solution—aluminum acetate (Triple Paste by Summers Laboratory). These products are very safe and effective and will protect the affected skin. These products should be applied regularly and generously, especially after stooling.
- **Cleansing:** The diaper area should be carefully and thoroughly cleaned after defecation. Commercial diaper wipes are used most often by parents, although some products contain alcohol, which can sting irritated skin. A gentle bath with lukewarm water and mild soap (optional) may be needed if children are heavily soiled with adherent feces.
- **Diaper:** Superabsorbent disposable diapers are clearly superior to cloth diapers and should be used. Occasionally children are allergic to one or more of the diaper components. In this case, other brands should be tried. Diapers should be changed frequently.

- **Education:** Parents, especially new parents, should be educated about diaper dermatitis. Medical providers should furnish patients with easy-to-understand pamphlets on the prevention and home treatment of diaper dermatitis.
- **Fungus:** *C. albicans* is the most common fungal pathogen in the diaper area. It should be recognized early and treated appropriately with antifungal medications, some of which are now available over the counter: nystatin, miconazole (Micatin, Monistat), clotrimazole (Lotrimin), or econazole (Spectazole). Antifungal medications are typically used twice per day and may be used in combination with low-potency hydrocortisone and/or barrier products. Parents should use only small amounts worked into the affected skin (and a small amount beyond the rash area) before applying other topicals.

Disposition

Children with nonresolving or severe, recurrent dermatitis should be reexamined.

COMPLICATIONS AND RED FLAGS

Parents and child-care providers should be aware of potentially serious fecal contaminants in diaper-changing areas and appropriate disinfection procedures should be in place. Severe diaper dermatoses should alert the clinician to consider more serious causes, such as Kawasaki disease, impetigo, or cellulitis.

Although short-term use of the lowest-potency topical corticosteroids (hydrocortisone) are occasionally used alone or in combination with topical antifungal therapy, the use of potent topical corticosteroids is clearly contraindicated. Hydrocortisone cream (1%) may be safely applied several times per day for 5 to 7 days in moderate to severe diaper dermatitis. The use of potent steroids (like betamethasone) or combination topical steroid/antifungal preparations can be systemically absorbed, resulting in adrenal suppression (Cushing's syndrome) or cutaneous atrophy or striae.

PEARLS

Baby powders should be discouraged. Many commercially available baby powders contain perfumes that can cause allergic reactions. Aerosolized powders (talcum) and corn starch are well-known respiratory hazards that can cause severe pneumonitis from aspiration during careless use.

Not all home remedies and herbal preparations are safe. A barrier cream used for cow udders has been reported to cause precocious puberty when applied to the diaper area. Since the safety of topical herbal preparations in the diaper area has not been established, their use cannot be sanctioned.

Parents should be cautioned against using any nonprescribed steroid preparation in the diaper area.

Chronic, unresponsive diaper dermatitis is superinfected with either yeast or bacteria (or both) and should be carefully evaluated and appropriately treated. Topical antibacterial ointments (mupirocin/Bactroban) are useful when signs of bacterial infection are present. Systemic antistaphylococcal antibiotics may be necessary if pustules and bullae are present.

BIBLIOGRAPHY

Boiko S: Treatment of diaper rash. *Dermatol Clin* 17:235–240, 1999.
———: Making rash decisions in the diaper area. *Pediatr Ann* 29(1):50–56, 2000.
Hansen RC et al: Dealing with diaper dermatitis. *Contemporary Pediatrics* (special edition based on presentations at 7th annual Masters in Pediatrics meeting, Jan. 14–19, 1998, Key Biscayne, FL).
Mendenhall AK, Eichenfield LF: Back to the basics—caring for the newborn's skin. *Contemporary Pediatrics* 17(8):98–114, 2000.

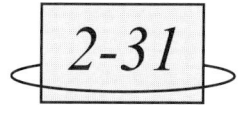

ERYTHEMA INFECTIOSUM (FIFTH DISEASE)

Rodney L. Moser

DISCUSSION

Erythema infectiosum (EI), also known as fifth disease, is caused by parvovirus B19 and is spread by respiratory and nasal droplets. EI has an incubation period of 4 to 18 days (average, 8 to 9 days) and a 25 to 50 percent "attack rate" in susceptible children. It usually occurs in children ages 5 to 11 during the 3- to 6-month period of late winter–early spring. It may occur in focal outbreaks or in communitywide epidemics, similar to rubella. Up to 35 percent of school-aged children will contact EI.

Children with EI are more contagious before the characteristic skin signs and are not considered particularly infectious when the rash is present, although the virus can be detected in the respiratory tract for up to 6 days after exposure.

SIGNS AND SYMPTOMS

Most children appear well but may have variable prodromal symptoms of headaches, chills, fever, sore throat, coryza, malaise, or myalgia during this viremic state (about 2 days). About 1 to 4 days later, children develop the classic bilateral, fiery-red "slapped cheek" facial eruption. There may be some circumoral pallor. The lesions are maculopapular and blanchable. The facial eruption is followed by another characteristic reticular (lace-like) erythema on the trunk and extremities. Red macules may be present on the buccal mucosa or palate. Pruritus also is reported.

Although the eruption lasts about a week, exposure to temperature change (hot baths, showers, traveling from the outside and/or inside, sunlight, etc.) as well as emotional upset may prompt a resurgence of the eruptions for several weeks or months after the acute state.

DIAGNOSTIC CONSIDERATIONS

EI often is misdiagnosed during the prerash, prodromal stage. It usually is recognized as a viral syndrome, but many children are unnecessarily treated with antibiotics, which complicates the clinical diagnosis by adding the possibility of a cutaneous drug eruption. Other childhood viral exanthems, such as rubella (see Chap. 9-21) and roseola (see Chap. 2-32), should be considered.

Erysipelas may present as a bright red facial eruption. Unlike well-appearing children with EI, children with erysipelas may be toxic-appearing and have a high fever. The lesions are also hot and tender, unlike EI (see Chap. 2-9). Other eruptions, such as scarlet fever, also should be entertained in an ill-appearing child.

LABORATORY TESTS

The diagnosis of EI is based primarily on clinical findings. IgM antibody assay is positive in 90 percent of cases by 3 to 4 days. IgG is present by a week and can last for years after the disease.

TREATMENT

The treatment of EI is symptomatic. Antipruritic medications (Atarax, Benadryl) or starch/colloidal oatmeal baths may be helpful.

Children with EI may attend school or day care during the often prolonged rash stage. They are not considered contagious at this point.

COMPLICATIONS AND RED FLAGS

Of particular risk during epidemics are first-trimester pregnant women who care for children (teachers, day care providers). Parvovirus B19 crosses the placenta and may cause intrauterine infection, hydrops fetalis, fetal death, and miscarriage. The pregnancies of EI-exposed women should be monitored carefully. A therapeutic abortion is not indicated for B19 infections. Since only 50 percent of women are seroprotected against B19, pregnant teachers and other child care workers should consider taking a leave of absence during epidemics.

Although rare in children and more common in adults, transient arthralgia or arthritis can occur, lasting only a few days.

High-risk groups for EI complications include patients with hemolytic anemias (sickle cell, etc.) and the immunocompromised (acute lymphocytic leukemia). An aplastic crisis could occur, requiring a transfusion.

BIBLIOGRAPHY

Fitzpatrick TB, Johnson RA, Wolff K, et al: *Color Atlas and Synopsis of Clinical Dermatology: Common and Serious Diseases,* 3d ed. New York, McGraw-Hill, 1997.

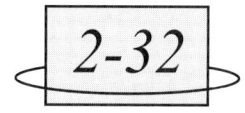

ROSEOLA INFANTUM (EXANTHEM SUBITUM)

Rodney L. Moser

DISCUSSION

Roseola, also known as exanthem subitum or sixth disease, is a viral exanthem caused by human herpes virus-6 (HHV-6) and possibly herpes virus-7 (HHV-7). It commonly occurs in children age 3 months to 3 to 4 years (peak incidence at 7 to 13 months); 90 percent of all cases occur by age 2. It is believed that roseola is transmitted by either respiratory secretions or the fecal-oral route. It has a highly variable incubation period from 5 to 15 days and can occur at any time of the year.

SIGNS AND SYMPTOMS

Roseola is characterized by an abrupt onset of high fever (often as high as 105°F) during the 3 to 5 days before the onset of the rash. The febrile stage can be alarming to parents, particularly new parents, and inexperienced pediatric providers. Unrecognized roseola often results in numerous laboratory studies and unnecessary treatments (usually antibiotics). Children's reaction to fever is quite variable; some will appear healthy and happy, while others will be irritable and appear sick. It is the later group that is more likely to get a diagnostic workup.

Defervescence is followed by a pale, discrete (or confluent), bright "rosy" macular eruption that lasts 1 or 2 days. The eruption initially occurs on the neck and trunk and then involves the arms, face, and legs and may be somewhat transient. At this point, the child is nonfebrile and appears quite well. Nonspecific lymphadenopathy, usually suboccipital, may be present.

The history is the key to the early diagnosis of roseola. Several days of high fever without a discernible cause followed by an erythematous, macular eruption at the cessation of the fever is usually diagnostic.

DIAGNOSTIC CONSIDERATIONS

Because fever (and viral skin eruptions) is so nonspecific in the roseola age bracket, the diagnostic considerations tend to be numerous. Other viral exanthems, such as rubella (see Chap. 9-21), measles (see Chap. 9-16), scarlet fever, and erythema infectiosum (see Chap. 2-31), should be considered. Kawasaki syndrome (see Chap. 10-6) tends to have a fever that is poorly responsive to antipyretics but should be included in the differential.

The rapid onset of fever characteristic of roseola can initiate a febrile seizure episode in some children, prompting further diagnostic consideration, such as meningitis (see Chap. 9-28) or encephalitis.

Children who are unnecessarily treated with antibiotics for "phantom" bacterial infections (otitis media, pharyngitis) during the febrile stage often are misdiagnosed as having a drug-related eruption when the rash develops. Since fever, especially the high fever associated with roseola, can cause the tympanic membranes to appear injected, it is easy to understand how these children may be treated as having an emerging otitis media. (see Chap. 3-2).

LABORATORY AND RADIOLOGIC STUDIES

A careful evaluation to rule out other treatable causes of fever is important. During the febrile stage of roseola, numerous laboratory (including a cerebrospinal fluid examination) and x-ray studies often are done. Although these tests are invariably normal, many may be warranted since the diagnosis is often unclear.

TREATMENT

None. Antipyretics may be helpful for patient comfort during the febrile stage.

DISPOSITION

Children may return to school or day care facilities when they are fever-free, even if the rash is still present.

COMPLICATIONS AND RED FLAGS

Because rapid hyperpyrexia can initiate a febrile seizure, these children may undergo a cerebrospinal fluid examination to rule out meningitis. There are no long-term neurologic sequelae to febrile seizure, but their presence prompts a higher degree of clinical uncertainty. About 5 to 10 percent of children will have a tonic-clonic seizure associated with fever.

PEARLS

In most cases, providers should avoid empirically treating normal, healthy children with undiagnosed febrile illnesses with antibiotics.

BIBLIOGRAPHY

Cherry JD: Roseola infantum (exanthem subitum), in Feigin RD, Cherry JD (eds): *Textbook of Pediatric Infectious Diseases,* 3d ed. Philadelphia, Saunders, 1997, vol. II, pp 1789–1791.

Fitzpatrick TB, Johnson RA, Wolff K, et al: *Color Atlas and Synopsis of Clinical Dermatology: Common and Serious Diseases,* 3d ed. New York, McGraw-Hill, 1997, pp 826–827.

Schwartz MW: *The 5 Minute Pediatric Consultant.* Baltimore. Williams & Wilkins, 1997, pp 674–675.

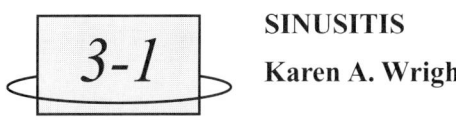

SINUSITIS

Karen A. Wright

DISCUSSION

Sinusitis is an infection or inflammation of one or more of the paranasal sinuses. It is encountered frequently in the health care industry and accounts for approximately 25 million office visits per year. More than $2 billion is spent annually for the medical management of this condition.[1] It affects both children and adults.

CLASSIFICATION

Sinusitis can be classified into four different groups, based on the duration of its symptoms:

1. *Acute sinusitis* has symptoms that last less than 4 weeks.
2. *Subacute sinusitis* involves symptoms lasting between 4 and 12 weeks.
3. *Recurrent sinusitis* is defined by four or more episodes of acute sinusitis per year with symptoms that last 7 to 10 days.
4. *Chronic sinusitis* involves persistence of symptoms for more than 12 weeks.

ANATOMY AND PHYSIOLOGY

The paranasal sinuses are four paired air-filled cavities (maxillary, ethmoid, sphenoid, and frontal) within the skull that surround the eye sockets. The sinuses are lined with respiratory mucosa and cilia that communicate with and drain into the nasal cavity. A mucous blanket coats each of the paranasal sinuses. The mucociliary clearance system keeps the cavities clean by propelling mucus toward the ostia (small sinus openings) to allow appropriate drainage. The direction of the mucous flow varies for each sinus. Under normal conditions, this clearance system allows the paranasal sinuses to remain sterile.

The maxillary and ethmoid sinuses are present at birth. The maxillary sinus is the largest paranasal sinus. The sphenoid sinuses develop during the first few years of life. The frontal sinuses, which are absent in approximately 10 percent of the population, develop during the first year of life. The anatomy of the paranasal sinuses varies from patient to patient because of anatomic variations and congenital abnormalities.

PATHOGENESIS

Mucosal swelling causes the ostia to narrow, leading to partial or complete obstruction. This in turn impedes drainage of the paranasal sinuses, resulting in an accumulation of mucus, and creates an environment conducive to bacterial overgrowth. Factors that lead to impaired or delayed mucociliary clearance or obstruction of the ostia can result in sinusitis. The most common site for ostial obstruction is the osteomeatal complex that drains the maxillary, frontal, and anterior ethmoid sinuses.

The most common cause of sinusitis is a viral upper respiratory infection. Other conditions that can predispose to sinusitis include

allergic and nonallergic rhinitis, anatomic anomalies (e.g., polyps and septal deviation), and immune deficiencies.

The maxillary sinuses have the greatest potential for infection and are the most common site of sinus infection. The ostia are in the upper portion of the sinus. Ciliary movements are against gravity and thus make it more difficult to propel the mucus for proper drainage.

MICROBIOLOGY

Pathogens isolated from the paranasal sinuses vary with the classification of the sinusitis and the age of the patient. Some of the pathogens that are responsible for acute otitis media play a role in sinusitis. *Streptococcus pneumoniae* and *Haemophilus influenzae* (nontypeable) account for approximately 75 percent of cases of acute community-acquired sinusitis in adults. There has been an increase in the prevalence of β-lactamase-producing *H. influenzae*. Other pathogens implicated in sinusitis include streptococci other than pneumococci, gram-negative bacteria, and anaerobes (usually associated with dental infections). *Staphylococcus aureus* is not a common cause of acute sinusitis in adults or children. *Streptococcus pneumoniae, Moraxella catarrhalis,* and *H. influenzae* are the most common causes of acute community-acquired sinusitis in children. Viral infection caused by rhinovirus, influenza, and parainfluenza also plays a role in community-acquired sinusitis. Viral sinusitis also may lead to secondary bacterial infection.

The bacteriology of chronic sinusitis in adults and children is not as clearly defined. *Staphylococcus aureus* and respiratory anaerobes are isolated more frequently in chronic sinusitis. Acute exacerbations with the classic pathogens of community-acquired sinusitis can occur.

Nosocomial sinusitis that most likely is due to nasotracheal intubation generally is caused by gram-negative enterics such as *Pseudomonas aeruginosa, Klebsiella pneumonia, Enterobacter* species, *Proteus mirabilis, Serratia marcescens,* and gram-positive cocci. Diabetic patients, cancer patients, patients receiving immunosuppressive therapy, and patients with immune deficiencies are prone to fungal sinusitis. *Aspergillus* is the most common cause of fungal sinusitis in immunosuppressed patients.[2]

SIGNS AND SYMPTOMS

Acute Sinusitis

Acute sinusitis usually follows an upper respiratory infection that has persisted for more than 7 days. Purulent nasal or postnasal drainage, headache, facial pain or pressure over the involved sinus (aggravated by lying down or bending over), nasal congestion, and cough are commonly present. Halitosis and low-grade fever also may be present.

Maxillary sinusitis may present with pain or pressure in the cheek or upper teeth (incisors, canines, or molars). It is important to elicit from the patient a recent history of dental extraction (usually upper molars), since the root is situated close to the floor of the maxillary sinus and may be a source of infection. The pain or pressure associated with ethmoid sinusitis usually is located between the eyes or retroorbitally, while that of frontal sinusitis usually is located above the eyebrows or in the region of the forehead. Sphenoid sinusitis pain, by contrast, may be felt retroorbitally or in the occipital area.

Chronic Sinusitis

Chronic sinusitis is caused by persistent inflammation or infection of one or more paranasal sinuses. The presentation of chronic sinusitis is not as obvious as that of acute sinusitis. Symptoms may be subtle, nonspecific, or attributed to another medical condition. It is important to determine whether the patient has underlying chronic diseases or immunosuppressive conditions that may predispose to sinusitis.

Purulent postnasal drainage, nasal congestion, headache, and sinus pressure may be present. Coughing, clearing of the throat (from postnasal drainage), sore throat, loss or decreased sense of smell, and malaise may be manifestations of chronic sinusitis as well. Fever is uncommon.

OBJECTIVE FINDINGS

The physical examination should include careful evaluation of the ear, nose, and throat (ENT); dentition (particularly the upper canines, incisors, and molars); lungs; and neurologic system. Examination of the anterior aspect of the nose with an otoscope is essential to observe for purulent drainage, nasal polyps, septal deviation, mucosal changes, and any other anomalies. The throat also should be inspected for evidence of purulent drainage. The ears should be examined for evidence of acute otitis media, especially in the pediatric population. Percussion over the frontal and maxillary sinuses may or may not elicit pain. Respiratory and neurologic examination should be performed to evaluate complaints of cough and headache. In patients with uncomplicated sinusitis, the respiratory and neurologic examinations should be unremarkable.

DIAGNOSTIC CONSIDERATIONS

Other conditions that may present with nasal congestion, facial pain, or headache and require consideration in the differential diagnosis include allergic and nonallergic rhinitis, otitis media, trigeminal neuralgia, optic neuritis, and dental disease.

It is important to keep in mind that several primary diseases or conditions may predispose the host to secondary sinus infection. Some of these conditions are allergic disease, cystic fibrosis, autoimmune deficiency syndrome, Wegener's granulomatosis, bronchiectasis, and changes in atmospheric pressure such as deep-sea diving and airplane travel.

SPECIAL CONSIDERATIONS

Immunocompromised patients are at increased risk for developing the complications of sinusitis. Management in a hospital setting usually is recommended.

Tobacco smokers, patients with chronic allergies, and asthmatic patients have an increased incidence of sinusitis. Cocaine abusers and chronic users of topical nasal medications also are predisposed to sinusitis.

LABORATORY STUDIES

Laboratory testing usually is not indicated in uncomplicated acute sinusitis. Cultures of nasal secretions should be obtained through puncture of the sinus to avoid contamination. This invasive procedure is indicated in recurrent and chronic sinusitis.

RADIOLOGIC STUDIES

In the majority of cases of acute uncomplicated sinusitis, a clinical diagnosis can be made from history and physical examination findings

alone. Sinus films may provide a definitive diagnosis. Standard sinus films include four views: Water's (maxillary), Caldwell (frontal), lateral (sphenoid), and submentovertical (ethmoid). Radiologic findings may include an air-fluid level, sinus opacification, and mucosal thickening. Sinus films may be normal despite clinical evidence of sinusitis. Abnormal sinus films may be seen in patients with transitory changes.

Computed tomography (CT) in the coronal plane is much more sensitive than plain sinus films and is similar in cost to a four-view sinus series. It provides an accurate view of the anatomy of the paranasal sinuses and the extent of disease involvement. Acute changes can be seen in asymptomatic patients as well as patients with the common cold. The use of CT scanning should be reserved for patients with recurrent sinusitis, complicated acute sinusitis, or chronic sinusitis and hospitalized patients. Full sinus scans are indicated for preoperative evaluation. Magnetic resonance imaging (MRI) is recommended for the evaluation of tumors and should be limited in use.

OTHER DIAGNOSTICS

Transillumination generally has not proved diagnostically helpful because of variations in soft tissue thickness and technique but is done occasionally during the office clinical assessment.

Sinus endoscopy performed by an ENT specialist allows for visualization of the nasopharynx and access for obtaining sinus secretions for nasal cultures.

TREATMENT

Pharmacologic Management

Management of sinusitis is directed at reducing mucosal edema, unblocking ostia to allow appropriate drainage of sinus secretions, and eliminating secondary bacterial infection. Several key factors must be considered before initiating treatment for sinusitis, including the following:

- Age of the patient
- Duration and frequency of infection
- Severity of the infection
- Underlying conditions that predispose to sinusitis
- History and response to previous treatments[3]

Table 3-1-1 describes recommended antibiotic treatment regimens for acute sinusitis. A 14-day course of antibiotic therapy is recommended. Longer treatment may be indicated. If there is no improvement in symptoms after 72 h of therapy, consider switching to another antibiotic. Anaerobic infections should be treated with clindamycin (500 mg PO tid) or a combination of amoxicillin or another antibiotic (guided by nasal cultures) and metronidazole. Fungal sinusitis usually requires surgical debridement and prolonged intravenous therapy with amphotericin B. Intravenous therapy also is recommended for nosocomial infections (initially with nafcillin and ceftriaxone) and in immunocompromised patients.

Chronic antibiotic therapy for sinusitis should be based on culture results and usually requires the use of broad-spectrum agents. Prolonged therapy for 3 to 6 weeks often is required. The majority of recurrent sinus infections respond to initial antibiotic therapy.

Adjunctive therapy for sinusitis includes oral or nasal decongestants, topical intranasal corticosteroids, and mucolytics (e.g., guaifenesin to thin secretions); this is helpful and improves the patency of the ostia. Systemic corticosteroids may be indicated in patients with allergies or chronic sinusitis. Antihistamines should be avoided because of their drying effects. One exception to this would be patients with allergies, and the use should be limited to the allergy season. Acetaminophen and ibuprofen are appropriate

TABLE 3-1-1. Antibiotics for Acute Sinusitis in Adults

ANTIBIOTIC	DOSAGE REGIMEN	COMMENTS
First-line choices:		
Amoxicillin (Amoxil)	250–500 mg PO tid	Drug of choice for initial therapy; low cost; well tolerated
Trimethoprim-sulfamethoxazole (Bactrim or Septra)	80–160 mg trimethoprim; 400–800 mg sulfamethoxazole, PO bid	Alternative initial therapy in penicillin-sensitive patients
Second-line choices:		
Amoxicillin-clavulanate (Augmentin)	250–500 mg PO tid	β-lactamase-inhibiting properties; good coverage for β-lactamase-producing *H. influenzae and M. catarrhalis*
Cefuroxime (Ceftin)	250–500 mg PO bid	High level of activity against intermediate-level resistant pneumococci; first-line choice among cephalosporins (alternative second- and third-generation cephalosporins can be used)
Clarithromycin (Biaxin)	250–500 mg PO bid	Alternative second-line therapy for penicillin-sensitive patients (alternative to azithromycin)
Levofloxacin	500 mg PO qd	Good broad-spectrum coverage; reserve for patients allergic or unresponsive to β-lactam agents (alternative fluoroquinolones can be used)

Note: All regimens should be continued for 14 days; longer treatment may be indicated.
SOURCE: Modified from Hansen M: Sinusitis, in Moser RL (ed): *Primary Care for Physician Assistants,* 1st ed. New York, McGraw-Hill, 1998, pp 111–112.

analgesics to manage the facial pain or headaches associated with sinusitis.

Supportive Measures

Nasal lavage with saline at least twice daily, steam inhalation, and drinking six to eight glasses of water daily help in clearing the secretions.

Surgical Management

Functional endoscopic sinus surgery (FESS) is performed to widen the occluded ostia and drain the sinus secretions and pus accumulation. Surgery is indicated in patients who have not responded to medical management for 4 to 6 months. Surgery may be indicated in cases of complicated or recurrent acute sinusitis, chronic sinusitis, for drainage of mucoceles (see "Complications and Red Flags," below), and for debridement in fungal sinusitis.

Patient Education

Environmental allergens should be avoided if possible. Tobacco smoke, whether direct or secondhand, should be avoided as well. The importance of medication compliance should be stressed, especially with the increased prevalence of antimicrobial resistance.

Disposition

Uncomplicated acute sinusitis can be managed on an outpatient basis. Follow-up should occur while the patient is still receiving antibiotic therapy to determine whether a longer course is required. Hospital admission is recommended for immunocompromised patients, patients with persistent symptoms despite prolonged medical therapy, those with sinus complications, and those with pansinusitis (involvement of multiple cavities).

COMPLICATIONS AND RED FLAGS

Improperly treated sinus infection has the potential to spread to neighboring structures. Appropriate antibiotic therapy and close follow-up are essential to reduce the risk of progression beyond the acute state. Osteomyelitis results from the spread of infection from the sinus (particularly the frontal sinus) to the surrounding bone or tissue. Treatment requires prolonged intravenous antibiotic therapy and excision of necrotic bone.

Intracranial complications of frontal or ethmoid sinusitis include brain abscess, subdural empyema, and meningitis. Neurologic damage or even death can result. The complications of ethmoid sinusitis also include periorbital cellulitis and orbital cellulitis.

Mucoceles, which result from prolonged obstruction, can become secondarily infected and require surgical removal. Another complication of sinusitis (sphenoid) is cavernous sinus thrombosis.

Frequent recurrences and persistent infection despite prolonged therapy are indications for referral to an otolaryngologist. Other indications include nosocomial infections, sinus complications, deterioration within 48 h, and immunocompromised patients.[1]

OTHER NOTES AND PEARLS

Pneumococcal vaccination should be considered in patients with recurrent and chronic sinusitis because of the high incidence of *S. pneumoniae*.

REFERENCES

1. Poole MD: A focus on acute sinusitis in adults: Changes in disease management. *Am J Med* 106(5A):38S–47S, 1999.
2. Wald ER: Microbiology of acute and chronic sinusitis in children and adults. *Am J Med Sci* 316(1):13–20, 1998.
3. Kaliner M: Medical management of sinusitis. *Am J Med Sci* 316(1):21–28, 1998.

ACKNOWLEDGMENT

The editor would like to acknowledge the significant contributions of Meredith Hansen, author of the "Sinusitis" chapter in the first edition of *Primary Care for Physician Assistants*.

BIBLIOGRAPHY

Durand M, Joseph M, Baker AS: Infections of the upper respiratory tract, in Fauci AS, Braunwald E, Isselbacher KJ, et al (eds): *Harrison's Principles of Internal Medicine,* 14th ed. New York, McGraw-Hill, 1998, pp 179–181.
Reinhardt S, Ransom J, Nogueira I, et al (eds): *Current Medical Diagnosis and Treatment,* 39th ed. New York, McGraw-Hill, 2000, pp 237–239.
Zinreich SJ: Functional anatomy and computed tomography imaging of the paranasal sinuses. *Am J Med Sci* 316(1):2–11, 1998.

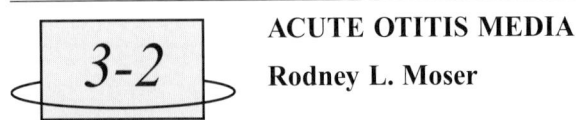

3-2

ACUTE OTITIS MEDIA
Rodney L. Moser

DISCUSSION

Middle-ear infections affect nearly 90 percent of all children before age 6 and result in frequent office visits and millions of prescriptions for antibiotics. The most common use of antibiotics in the United States is for the treatment of otitis media, resulting in an estimated 30 million office visits and $2 billion to $3 billion in health care–related costs. It is estimated that over 1 million tympanostomy tubes are inserted annually. Otitis media (OM) and otitis media with effusion (OME) are associated with conductive hearing loss, deficient verbal abilities, and cognitive learning problems.

Upper respiratory infection is the most common predisposing factor, followed closely by day care attendance. Children (especially very small children and infants) cared for in larger group settings are exposed to viral and bacterial pathogens at a higher rate than are children cared for at home. Although ear infections are not contagious, the predisposing upper respiratory infections are, and so children with high exposure are at a higher risk. Acute otitis media (AOM) peaks in the winter and spring: the traditional "cold and flu" season.

Anemic children appear to have a higher prevalence of AOM episodes, compared to nonanemic children. A recent study has shown a direct relationship between the degree of anemia and the number of AOM episodes.[1]

Bottle-fed babies lack the immunoprotective effects of human milk during the early months, and allergies associated with cow's milk may be more common than was previously recognized. Oligosaccharides in human milk may help fight OM. Feeding positions also have been implicated as predisposing factors, since breast-fed babies are fed at a more upright angle than are bottle-fed babies. Children given "crib bottles" and those who use pacifiers also tend to have higher rates of OM.

Allergic children, especially those with enlarged adenoids, are more prone to middle-ear effusions and infection. Children who are susceptible to OM are also prone to sinusitis. The pathogens responsible for most cases of AOM are virtually identical to those which cause acute sinusitis.

Parental behavior can increase the risk of otitis media in children. Maternal cigarette smoking and exposure to secondary smoke (including wood-burning stoves) are proven predisposing factors. Prenatal alcohol use can cause hearing loss and OME. The tendency to develop OM in childhood appears to have a familial link, with siblings having similar bouts. A low-income family is also a risk factor.

Boys and Native American children also have a higher incidence. The incidence of OM peaks between ages 6 months and 6 years. Children under age 2 have the highest incidence; OM occurs less often in later childhood and adulthood. Many adults who present with OM have a history of frequent childhood episodes.

Children with Down's syndrome, cleft palate, and immunocompromised disease (such as HIV) have a higher risk for developing OM.

PATHOGENESIS

Most cases of AOM occur when nasopharyngeal pathogens enter the warm, moist middle-ear space via the eustachian tube. Eustachian tubes in children under age 6 tend to be short, narrow, and more horizontal, resulting in poor middle-ear drainage and ventilation. The narrow lumens of the eustachian tubes are easily obstructed by enlarged adenoids, nasopharyngeal irritation and/or infection, and allergies. The presence of pathogens leads to mucosal swelling in the middle ear and inflammatory obstruction of the eustachian tube. The resultant purulence and pressure usually result in pain and fever. As children mature, the eustachian tube elongates and angles downward, improving drainage. This change, along with the strengthening of the pediatric immune system, accounts for the reduced incidence of AOM in later childhood.

OME is a painless (usually) middle-ear inflammation that can affect one or both ears, usually as a result of an abnormal or malfunctioning eustachian tube. The middle-ear effusion becomes viscous and sticky and often is referred to as "glue ear." This condition develops 3 to 16 weeks after an acute infection, can last several weeks or months, and is exacerbated by the same factors as AOM (secondhand smoke, viral infections, etc). Half of OME cases develop within the first year of life and remain a prime indication for myringotomy tubes.

MICROBIOLOGY

Middle-ear fluid in children, collected by tympanocentesis, often is polymicrobial, containing both bacterial and viral pathogens. Bacteria are detected in 70 percent or more of AOM cases and are a primary cause of infection. Among the main bacterial pathogens, *Streptococcus pneumoniae* causes about 40 percent of cases of AOM and is one of the most likely causes of persistent infections. Pneumococcal infections contribute to more morbidity and mortality than do other AOM pathogens and are the least likely to resolve spontaneously. *Haemophilus influenzae* causes about 25 percent of cases of AOM, followed by *Moraxella catarrhalis* (14 percent) (see Table 3-2-1).

Up to 25 percent of middle-ear cultures are reported as "sterile," but most are felt to be viral. Although the role of viruses in OM is unclear, respiratory syncytial virus (RSV) appears to be one of the more common viral pathogens in cases of OM.[1A] Although the presence of RSV in middle-ear fluid does not prove causation, some researchers feel that RSV may play a significant pathogenic role and may account for some antimicrobial failures. Influenza virus and rhinovirus also have been implicated as causative organisms.

Middle-ear pathogens may vary with the population and geographic location. There is strong empirical evidence that some middle-ear pathogens are becoming more drug-resistant. The emergence of drug-resistant strains of *S. pneumoniae* in the United States has not only complicated empiric treatment but led to increased numbers of treatment failures.[2] There has also been a steady increase in the incidence of β-lactamase-producing strains of *H. influenzae* and *M. (Branhamella) catarrhalis*. About 50 percent of *H. influenzae* produces β-lactamase, which inactivates ampicillin, amoxicillin, and first-generation cephalosporins. About 90 percent of *M. catarrhalis* strains produce β-lactamase (see Table 3-2-1).

SYMPTOMS

In a young child, nonspecific irritability, crying, malaise, fever, diminished appetite, and ear pulling may be observed. Upper respiratory infection (URI) and allergic symptoms (runny nose, congestion, conjunctival inflammation, etc.) are often present. Less commonly, associated symptoms may include purulent ear discharge (from a perforation) or systemic symptoms, such as diarrhea and/or vomiting. OM also may be relatively asymptomatic.

OM certainly has a variable, fluctuating effect on hearing. Mild to moderate temporary hearing loss is expected during bouts of AOM. A chronic OME-related hearing loss can retard language development and reading skills and has been associated with behavioral and social problems.

TABLE 3-2-1. Microbiologic Causes of Otitis Media

Streptococcus pneumoniae	35–40% (5% may be resistant strains)
Haemophilus influenzae	23–25% (up to 50% may be β-lactamase producers)
Moraxella (Branhamella) catarrhalis	14% (about 90 percent produce β-lactamase)
Beta-hemolytic *Streptococcus* group A	5–8% (most biologically common cause of spontaneous rupture of the tympanic membrane)
Viral (RSV and others)	25% or more

Previous experience with OM leads some parents to believe that virtually any mood change or incidence of ear pulling is OM until proved otherwise. In an older child or adult, well-localized otalgia is the most common symptom. Referred ear pain from dental infections, tonsillitis, or cervical lymphadenitis may mimic OM symptoms and should be ruled out by careful examination. Retropharyngeal carcinomas in adults (usually current or former smokers) may present with otalgia.

OBJECTIVE FINDINGS

On otoscopic examination, the tympanic membrane (TM) appears red, bulging, or opacified, with decreased motility and poorly visible landmarks. Strategic cerumen removal may be necessary for proper viewing. A pneumatic otoscopic test, using the proper soft pneumatic ear specula, should *always* be performed. Decreased motility of the TM appears to be more predictive than are color changes in diagnosing AOM. As OM develops, pain may precede eardrum redness. The TM may appear opaque or yellow in some cases of AOM. A scarred, thick, or opaque TM makes it difficult to distinguish between OM and OME.

The conductive hearing loss that occurs with middle-ear effusion can result in a 40-db hearing loss, roughly equivalent to the hearing loss that occurs when putting a finger in one's ear. This degree of hearing loss, if persistent, can lead to speech delays, learning disabilities, and behavior problems. An age-specific, objective assessment of hearing should be done as part of the routine OM examination and subsequent follow-up.

Because of increasing access to care, many children are examined before strong clinical signs are evident, and so OM often is diagnosed and treated simply on the basis of symptomatology, suspicion, and past medical history. This practice tends to result in an unnecessary overuse of antibiotics. Providers should avoid treating AOM in the presence of equivocal objective findings.

DIAGNOSTIC CONSIDERATIONS

Otalgia, or ear pain, may originate in the ear or from sources outside of the ear (referred pain).[3] In most cases of otalgia not associated with direct ear causes (otitis media, otitis externa, etc.), the source is identified in the pharynx (tonsillitis, pharyngitis). Any lesion or inflammation in the areas of the trigeminal, facial, glossopharyngeal, or vagus innervation can result in referred otalgia (see Table 3-2-2).

SPECIAL CONSIDERATIONS

As a result of infectious disease exposure, children in group care situations develop OM more often than do children cared for at home or

TABLE 3-2-2. Direct and Referred Sources of Otalgia

Otitis externa	Direct
Cerumen impaction/foreign body	Direct
Furunculosis/skin infections	Direct
Otitis media	Direct
Otitis media with effusion	Direct
Barotitis/pressure changes	Direct
Dental infections/molar impactions	Referred
Temporomandibular joint dysfunction	Referred
Trauma	Referred or direct
Sinusitis	Referred or direct
Cervical lymphadenitis	Referred
Tonsillitis/pharyngitis	Referred
Retropharyngeal tumors	Referred
Temporal arteritis	Referred
Trigeminal neuralgia (tic douloureux)	Referred

in smaller day care settings. Parents who smoke put their children at risk and should be encouraged to stop or never to smoke around children. Mothers should be encouraged to breast-feed or avoid propped bottles with the child in the supine position. Cleaning the ears with cotton-tipped applicators should be discouraged to avoid TM and ear canal trauma.

LABORATORY TESTS

Unless the child is toxic-appearing, no laboratory tests are needed in primary care settings. Tympanocentesis with culture may be done by an ear, nose, and throat (ENT) specialist in refractory cases. Concurrent pharyngitis can be screened for group A beta-hemolytic streptococci. Nasopharyngeal cultures may not correlate with middle-ear pathogens and are unnecessary in most cases. Allergy testing is indicated only in carefully selected allergic patients and never is done routinely. When milk allergy or other food allergies are considered, an elimination diet may be more cost-effective than allergy testing.

Children with frequent AOM should be evaluated for iron-deficiency anemia. If levels are lower than 10 g/dL iron supplementation should be started to achieve a level of at least 11 g/dL.[1]

RADIOLOGIC STUDIES

No routine radiologic or special imaging studies are necessary unless diagnostic considerations include mastoiditis, sinusitis, cholesteatomas, neoplastic disease, or other complications.

OTHER DIAGNOSTICS

A pneumatic otoscopic examination is quick, easy, and rarely uncomfortable for the patient and should be performed routinely as the standard of care. Tympanometry and acoustic reflex testing are important diagnostics that are underused in primary care settings. Gross hearing evaluation and whisper tests are commonly used screening tools in the clinical setting but should not replace audiometric studies if hearing loss is suspected. Video otoscopy with magnification may be available in some specialty practices. More specialized studies, such as computed tomography (CT) to show images of the middle ear and the surrounding bone structure and magnetic resonance imaging (MRI) to check for soft tissue problems, nerve damage, or tumors, are most often ordered by the ENT specialist.

TREATMENT

Pharmacologic Management

Primary antibiotic management is the standard, initial care in the United States, although there is growing evidence that early antibiotic intervention may be not always be necessary and actually may be counterproductive in many cases. Providers often feel pressured by patients and families into prescribing antibiotics whether they are needed or not. Since the vast majority of cases of uncomplicated AOM tend to resolve without the use of antibiotics, it may be prudent not to use antibiotics initially in mild or "evolving" infections. The emergence of certain antibiotic-resistant strains is related in part to the overuse of antibiotics for the treatment of OM.

Antibiotics are used less often in Europe for the management of AOM. In 1990, the Dutch College of General Practitioners adopted a guideline for the care of OM. For patients age 2 years and older, only symptomatic treatment (acetaminophen with or without decongestant nose drops) is given for the first 3 days.[4] If OM-related pain and fever continue after 3 days, reevaluation is required, and amoxicillin (unless contraindicated) is given for 7 days. As one might imagine, there are fewer drug-resistant strains in the European community because of the more conservative use of antimicrobials. This more conservative approach to AOM management has not been fully embraced by the American community, but the trend toward using fewer antibiotics appears to be growing.

Effectiveness, cost, safety, compliance, side effects, and knowledge of community strains are major considerations in choosing among the antibiotics used for treating OM (see Table 3-2-3). Practitioners often have their own individual preferences for selecting an antibiotic, usually based on prior experiences. Antibiotics with suitable pharmacokinetic and pharmacodynamic parameters should be chosen. Depending on the antibiotic selected, most practitioners use a 10-day course of therapy, although courses from 2 to 7 days have been cited as equally effective in select patients.[5] When clinically appropriate, a full 10-day course of therapy should be used in children under age 2 and in patients with minor complications such as a perforated tympanic membrane.

Amoxicillin tends to be the initial drug of choice in uncomplicated OM, depending on the prevalence of resistant strains in the community. Doubling the standard dose of amoxicillin from 40 mg/kg to 80 to 90 mg/kg has been proposed to improve the drug's efficacy, especially in areas where there is an increased risk of drug-resistant pneumococcal strains. Trimethoprim-sulfamethoxazole (Bactrim, Septra) is another effective first-line antibiotic choice. If OM fails to resolve with first-line antibiotics, a β-lactamase-producing organism often is involved either alone or in a polymicrobial mix that may involve viruses. Amoxicillin/clavulanate potassium (Augmentin) and a cephalosporin antibiotic are common next-line choices. The later generations of cephalosporins are highly effective in the management of OM, and some practitioners use cephalosporins as first-line drugs. Cephalosporins should be used with caution in penicillin-allergic individuals.

Most cases of otalgia usually resolve 8 to 24 h after the institution of an antibiotic. Patients should be essentially asymptomatic after 2 to 3 days, or an alternative medication may be considered. The practitioner should be wary of the common side effects (nausea, vomiting, diarrhea, rash, etc.) of the selected antibiotics and inform the patient or parent.

TABLE 3-2-3. Antibiotics for Otitis Media

ANTIBIOTIC	DOSE	COMMENTS
Amoxicillin (Amoxil)	20–40 mg/kg/d in divided doses tid × 7–10 days; doses as high as 80–90 mg/kg/d have been used in resistant cases	Most common, cost-effective first-line choice; well tolerated, available in suspension, chewable tablets, and capsules; few side effects; treatment failure could indicate resistant organism
Trimethoprim-sulfamethoxazole (Septra or Bactrim)	Based on 40 mg/kg/d divided bid × 10 days of sulfamethoxazole	Not for children under 2 months; twice-daily dosage convenient for day care; suspension does not require refrigeration; sulfa rash is common side effect
Trimethoprim (Primsol)	10 mg/kg daily in 2 divided doses every 12 h for 10 days	Not for children under 6 months; rash, GI upset, hematologic and renal effects; avoid large doses or prolonged use.
Erythromycin-sulfisoxazole (Pediazole)	50 mg/kg/d erythromycin and 150 mg/kg/d sulfisoxazole divided qid × 10 days	Not for children under 2 months; inconvenient qid dosage; gastrointestinal (GI) side effects common with erythromycin, and rash with sulfa
Amoxicillin-clavulanate (Augmentin)	40 mg/kg/d based on amoxicillin in divided doses tid × 10 days (twice-daily dosage form now available)	Available in tablets, chewables, and suspension; very effective but costly; diarrhea is common side effect that may be related to improper dosing
Cefaclor (Ceclor)	40 mg/kg/d in divided doses tid × 10 days; can be divided bid for convenience	Available in liquid suspension or tablets; costly; generally well tolerated and effective
Cefixime (Suprax)	8 mg/kg/d in single doses for 10 days	Available in suspension (100 mg per 5 mL) and 400-mg tablets; good once-a-day compliance; GI side effects most common
Cefprozil (Cefzil)	30 mg/kg/d in bid dosage	Well tolerated, with diarrhea and nausea the most common side effects; not used in children under 6 months
Cefuroxime (Ceftin)	30 mg/kg/d divided bid	Available in tablets and suspension; tablets taste terrible if chewed and must be swallowed whole; oral suspension more tolerable; diarrhea and/or vomiting most common side effects; used in children over 3 months
Loracarbef (Lorabid)	30 mg/kg/d divided bid	Best tasting of all oral suspensions for OM; side effects of diarrhea, vomiting, and nausea less than with other cephalosporins
Cefpodoxime (Vantin)	10 mg/kg/d	Convenient once-a-day dosage; side effects include diarrhea and diaper rash; not studied in infants under 5 months; bitter-tasting but works well
Ceftriaxone (Rocephin)	50 mg/kg in single IM injection	Efficacy, simplicity, and convenience of a single-dose therapy are desirable; cost, pain of injection, and lack of long-term studies are downside; IV for serious infections
Clarithromycin (Biaxin)	15 mg/kg/d divided bid for 10 days	Convenient dosage; GI side effects (diarrhea and vomiting) most common; tolerated well; reasonable price; suspension has objectionable taste to some children
Azithromycin (Zithromax)	10 mg/kg/d on first day, then 5 mg/kg/d on days 2–5	Once-per-day dosing for only 5 days; no refrigeration; only 1–2% GI side effects; reasonably priced
Ceftibuten (Cedax)	9 mg/kg/d for 10 days (1 tsp per 10 kg once per day)	Once-per-day dosing; GI side effects most common: 4% diarrhea and 2% vomiting
Cephalexin (Keflex)	75–100 mg/kg/d in 4 divided doses	Indicated for otitis media but not used very often in clinical practice in favor of other, more potent cephalosporins
Cephradine (Velosef)	75–100 mg/kg/d in 2–4 divided doses; max 4 g/d	For use in children over 9 months only
Cefdinir (Omnicef)	14 mg/kg every 24 h for 5–10 days	Pleasant-tasting with wide microbial coverage; not used in children under 6 months; possible GI side effects

Antibiotics with once- or twice-daily dosing are the preferred choices for children, especially those in school or day care. Some reconstituted oral antibiotics require refrigeration to maintain full potency. Medication noncompliance (missed or improperly measured doses, stopping prematurely, etc.) and improper storage are major factors in treatment failures, and so providers should try to strategically "match" the medication with the patient and the family situation.

Supportive Measures

Analgesia is very important in the overall management of OM and tends to be underused. Ibuprofen or acetaminophen will effectively control most OM-related pain in young children. Older children and adults may require codeine-containing analgesics. It is not necessary to treat simple fever, which is considered therapeutic.

Topical analgesics such as antipyrine and benzocaine (Auralgan) are also effective. One should fill the ear canal with body-temperature drops, insert a cotton plug, and repeat every 2 h if needed. One should not use Auralgan if the TM is perforated or myringotomy tubes are in place. Effectively controlling ear pain helps limit late-night calls and after-hours care and is very cost-effective in managed care settings. Since many OM cases resolve spontaneously, effective analgesia may postpone or eliminate the eventual need for antibiotics in some cases.

Oral decongestants or combination products have few or no benefits in the management of AOM. These products may be used safely if there is concurrent congestion, but many experts feel that they should *not* be used. A possible exception is the short-term use of decongestant nasal sprays to help prevent air travel–related barotitis in older children with OME. Decongestant nasal sprays are used more frequently in Europe for the initial treatment of AOM in lieu of primary antibiotic use. The overall value of decongestant sprays in the management of AOM is controversial.

Antihistamines are not recommended because of their drying effects and have limited value in allergy-complicated OM. Mucolytics may have some benefit in the management of AOE, but further studies are needed to confirm this.

The use of intranasal and/or systemic steroids in the management of AOM and OME remains controversial, although they may have some limited value in the management of allergic children over age 3 with concurrent eustachian tube dysfunction.

Patient Education

Patient education is vital in the comprehensive management of OM. Because parents expect and often demand antibiotics, this may be difficult for providers who elect to practice more conservative management. Intense educational efforts are necessary to curb antibiotic overuse. It is important to discuss risk factors and modify the ones that can be changed, particularly secondhand smoke exposure and day care. Suggesting a less populated day care setting (fewer than eight children) or smaller pods (such as home-based day care) will help limit pathogen exposures. Medication noncompliance can be limited by selecting antibiotics with fewer daily doses and fewer side effects. Proper measuring of doses is also important.

When properly instructed by the provider and encouraged, any parent can learn to use an inexpensive home otoscope.[6] Patient education and the use of a home otoscope may reduce unnecessary visits and allow the parent to participate more in the care of a child with OM. An educated parent may be less likely to solicit unnecessary antibiotics. Acoustic reflectometers are also available in the consumer market. There are many OM Internet sites available to parents (see "Patient Education and Internet Resources," below).

Prevention

Pregnant women should not smoke or use alcohol or expose their children to secondary smoke in any form. New mothers should be encouraged to breast-feed for at least 6 months. The use of pacifiers should be discouraged. Efforts to improve hygiene such as hand washing and routine surface disinfection may help prevent predisposing colds and influenza. Vaccination against pneumococcal or influenza strains should boost immune factors (see "Notes and Pearls," below).

Disposition

Patients on antibiotic therapy should be reexamined in 2 to 3 weeks or sooner if the patient is worse or is not responding to treatment. Earlier rechecks often reveal postinfection effusion that could be treated unnecessarily as a nonresolving infection. Some effusions can last 3 to 4 months and require careful monitoring. Children with AOM who are *not* initially treated with antibiotics should be monitored at closer intervals. A phone follow-up or a recheck appointment in 3 days may be prudent.

COMPLICATIONS AND RED FLAGS

Chronicity, recurrent infections, and temporary hearing loss are among the most common complications. If hearing loss is unilateral, it may go undetected for a long period. In preverbal children, middle-ear effusion (OME) can delay speech development. In older children, it can result in behavioral and learning difficulties and lead to a more permanent hearing loss. Hearing tests performed by an audiologist are recommended for patients with persistent OME and those with obvious hearing or language development problems.

Mastoiditis (see Chap. 3-12) is a relatively rare (in the United States) and potentially serious complication. Limiting the current overuse of antibiotics is unlikely to cause a resurgence of preantibiotic-era mastoiditis. Redness, tenderness, and swelling of the mastoid should be confirmed diagnostically by x-ray or CT. Treatment involves aggressive antibiotic therapy and occasionally surgical intervention. Meningitis (see Chap. 9-28), labyrinthitis (see Chap. 3-5), facial paralysis, and other intracranial complications can occur as a result of OM but are rare.

Chronic otitis media is a consequence of frequent bouts of AOM and can lead to conductive hearing loss, sclerosis, chronic TM perforations, and destruction of the ossicular chain. Continuous or intermittent purulent aural discharge is the most common symptom; otalgia is less common. Organisms such as *Pseudomonas aeruginosa, Proteus* species, and *Staphylococcus aureus* are common pathogens in chronic suppurative otitis media. Oral ciprofloxacin and/or topical fluoroquinolones are effective against *Pseudomonas* (see Chap. 3-14).

Prolonged eustachian tube dysfunction (with negative middle-ear pressure) and chronic otitis media can lead to cholesteatoma, a keratin-filled and chronically infected sac that appears as a retraction pocket. If untreated, cholesteatomas can erode the ossicular chain, eventually eroding the inner ear and facial nerve and leading to permanent hearing loss and/or dizziness. The treatment is surgical marsupialization of the sac or its complete removal.

Surgical Intervention and Tubes

A tympanocentesis is a diagnostic and a pain-relieving procedure that can be done if a patient is seriously ill or toxic-appearing. It is rarely necessary for effective treatment. A new office laser procedure provides an alternative to tubes. Laser-assisted myringotomy (LAM) uses a laser to create a small hole in the tympanic membrane that allows middle-ear ventilation for several weeks. This procedure is done without anesthesia and should help limit repeated antibiotic courses.

According to the 1994 U.S. Department of Health and Human Services Task Force on Otitis Media,[7] children age 1 to 3 with uncomplicated OME, especially those with hearing loss, should be evaluated for possible tympanostomy (myringotomy) tubes only after 4 to 6 months of watchful waiting. Tympanostomy tubes should be reserved for children who have failed on antibiotics and those with hearing loss and other complications. The tubes tend to last about a year, although they can extricate or obstruct at any time.

Complications of the procedure are very uncommon. Acute otorrhea through a tympanostomy tube (if not secondary to a cholesteatoma) usually is treated with ofloxacin or ciprofloxacin ear drops (see Chap. 3-14). Scarring and tympanic membrane perforation are other commonly reported problems. General anesthesia also poses calculated risks that should be considered.

Adenoidectomy is recommended for the surgical management of OME only when there is specific adenoidal pathology, such as obstruction or encroachment of the eustachian tubes, and in children over age 4. Tonsillectomy has no proven value in the management of OM.

Suppression Therapy for Chronic/Recurrent Otitis Media

When a child experiences three or more ear infections in a 6-month period or four or more within a year, chemoprophylaxis often is used. Antimicrobial chemoprophylaxis using daily doses of amoxicillin (20 mg/kg/d) or sulfisoxazole (50 mg/kg/d of Gantrisin) is most commonly used in primary care. Other prophylactic antibiotic regimens also have been used. Prescribing criteria range from daily doses for up to 6 months to 6-week bursts of therapy followed by an antibiotic-free "vacation." Suppression therapy often is timed to occur in the peak OM season. Many primary care providers feel that suppression therapy should be tried before myringotomy is considered, but others fear that subtherapeutic antimicrobial dosing promotes and encourages drug-resistant strains. Some studies favor myringotomy over suppression therapy. There appears to be a reduction in recurrent OM after the age of 16 months whether children are given preventive antibiotics or not.

NOTES AND PEARLS

Preliminary studies have shown a reduction in the incidence of OM after the administration of flu vaccine and/or pneumococcal vaccine, especially in children with asthma or other chronic respiratory problems.

A pneumococcal 7-valent conjugate vaccine (Prevnar) has been shown to be effective in preventing pneumococcal disease in infants and toddlers and in reducing the incidence of AOM. A study of 39,000 children in the Kaiser Permanente Vaccine Study Center found that the vaccine has a significant impact on OM. Children in the study were 7 percent less likely to have AOM, 20 percent less likely to need tubes, and 23 percent less likely to have recurrent AOM.[8] Since many of the invasive pneumococcal serotypes (4, 6B, 9V, 14, 18C, 19F, and 23F) also have been implicated in OM, Prevnar should be considered for all children, especially those in day care and those with recurrent or chronic OM.

Studies using a live, attenuated, trivalent intranasal influenza vaccine (Flu Mist) in children showed that the vaccine protected 93 percent against the flu and 98 percent against influenza-related OM.[9] Most important, there were 30 percent fewer episodes of febrile OM among the vaccinated children. The potential health and economic benefits of routinely administering influenza vaccine to all OM-prone children as part of a preventive program remain controversial.

The HIB vaccine appears to have little or no effect in preventing OM. Other bacterial or viral vaccines are being investigated, including new vaccines for RSV.

Children with frequent AOM should be evaluated for iron-deficiency anemia. Iron supplementations and dietary adjustments should be instituted to achieve a hemoglobin level of 11 g/dL or better.[1]

There are limited studies that show that children who chew gum or swallow syrup containing xylitol, a sugar alcohol, experience fewer ear infections. This may have limited value in children between 6 and 18 months, the primary age group for OM.

There is a growing trend to reduce the astronomic amounts of antibiotics used in the management of AOM. According to Culpepper and Fromm, in many routine cases, antimicrobial treatment may not be necessary.[10] The disturbing emergence of resistant strains of pneumococcal organisms in hospitals and day care centers is likely to continue. One can expect newer antibiotics and treatment modalities to combat these evolving microorganisms and a trend toward antimicrobial moderation in healthy children with uncomplicated OM.

REFERENCES

1. Goltz A, Netzer A, Goldenberg D, et al: Iron deficiency and recurrent AOM. Poster 6. Presented at the Annual Meeting of the American Academy of Otolaryngology, Sept 24–27, 2000, Washington, D.C.
1A. Heikkinen T, Thint M, Chonmaitree T: Prevalence of various respiratory viruses in the middle ear during acute otitis media. *N Eng J Med.* 340: 260–264, 1999.
2. Jacobs MR: Increasing importance of antibiotic-resistant *Streptococcus pneumoniae* in acute otitis media. *Pediatr Infect Dis J* 15:940–943, 1996.
3. Moser RL: Ear infections in children— controversies in care. *Physician Assist* 13:23–45, 1989.
4. Van Buchem FL, Peeters MF, Van'T Hof MA, et al: Acute otitis media— a new treatment strategy. *Br Med J* 290:1033–1037, 1985.
5. Paradise JL: Short-course antimicrobial treatment for otitis media. *JAMA* 278 (20):1640–1642, 1997.
6. Moser RL: *Ears: An Owner's Manual.* Ferndale, CA, Notoco, 1994 (www.earpain.com).
7. U.S. Department of Health and Human Services: *Otitis Media with Effusion in Young Children.* Washington, DC, AHCPR Publication No. 94-0622, 1994.
8. Black S, Shinefield H, Fireman B, et al: Efficacy, safety and immunogenicity of heptavalent pneumococcal conjugate vaccine in children: Northern California Kaiser Permanente Vaccine Study Center. *Pediatr Infect Dis J* 19(3):187–195, 2000.
9. Belshe R, Mendelman P, Treanor J, et al: The efficacy of live, attenuated, cold-adapted, trivalent, intranasal influenza virus vaccine in children. *N Engl J Med* 338(20):1405–1412, 1998.
10. Culpepper L, Fromm J: Routine antimicrobial treatment for otitis media: Is it necessary? *JAMA* 278(20):1644, 1997.

PATIENT EDUCATION INTERNET RESOURCES

Otitis Media Board: WebMD: www.webmd.com.
Home Otoscope and Consumer Otitis Media Information: Notoco, Ferndale, CA: www.earpain.com.

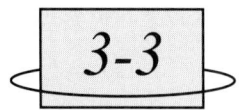

MONONUCLEOSIS
Suzanne Warnimont

DISCUSSION

Infectious mononucleosis (IM) is an acute illness that presents classically with sore throat, fever, and adenopathy. It usually is caused by the Epstein-Barr virus (EBV). IM affects people of all ages, particularly teenagers and young adults in the middle to upper socioeconomic classes. College students develop mononucleosis at an annual rate of 0.5 to 12 percent. EBV tends to infect children at an early age in lower socioeconomic groups, but symptomatic IM is uncommon in infants and young children.

Infectious mononucleosis is affectionately known as the "kissing disease," since the virus is transmitted by repeated intimate oral contact with an asymptomatic carrier who is shedding the virus through the saliva. EBV rarely is transmitted by transfusion of fresh blood or organ transplantation.

Infrequent (<10 percent) causes of mononucleosis include cytomegalovirus, human immunodeficiency virus (HIV), *Toxoplasma gondii,* and human herpes virus-6.

SIGNS AND SYMPTOMS

After an incubation period of 30 to 50 days (4 to 8 weeks), there is abrupt onset of fever, prominent malaise, and severe pharyngitis. IM also can present as fever and adenopathy *without* pharyngitis. The patient also may complain of chills, headache, photophobia, anorexia, dysphagia, myalgia, and distaste for cigarettes. The infection may be asymptomatic or may be manifested by a brief febrile illness in infants and young children. The acute phase of the illness lasts 1 to 3 weeks, with most patients experiencing recovery in 6 to 8 weeks.

OBJECTIVE FINDINGS

Physical findings include periorbital edema, enlarged tonsils with erythema and exudate, palatine petechiae, cervical adenopathy, and splenomegaly in the second week of illness. Less common findings include jaundice and hepatomegaly. A maculopapular rash develops in 5 percent of these patients, usually on the arms and trunk.

Ampicillin causes generalized macular rash in 90 percent of patients treated for acute infectious mononucleosis.

DIAGNOSTIC CONSIDERATIONS

Primary infection by HIV-1 causes a monolike illness that lasts 2 to 4 weeks. There is no exudative pharyngitis. In the overall management of IM, it is important to rule out the following diseases and conditions:

- *Bacterial disease:* streptococcal pharyngitis, mycoplasma, bacteremia
- *Viral disease:* cytomegalovirus, toxoplasmosis, respiratory viruses, viral hepatitis, rubella, mumps
- HIV, human herpes virus-6
- Drug reactions
- Hematologic malignancies: leukemia or lymphoma

LABORATORY TESTS

Specific laboratory abnormalities may not be present until the second or third week of clinical illness, as follows:

- Complete blood count (CBC): The white blood cell is elevated to 12 to 50,000/mm^3, with most of the increase in lymphocytes; 8 to 10 percent of the lymphocytes are atypical.
- Mild reduction of platelet count is seen in 50 percent of patients.
- Serum transaminases are elevated two to three times normal in more than 90 percent of patients.
- Serum heterophile antibodies (Monospot) are found in 75 percent of patients with EBV mononucleosis by the seventh day of illness and in 95 to 97 percent by the twenty-first day. The Monospot is usually positive for 3 to 6 months but can persist for 1 year.

RADIOLOGIC STUDIES

Routine radiologic studies are not indicated. A chest x-ray rarely shows infiltrates and possible elevated left hemidiaphragm in cases of mono-related splenic rupture.

TREATMENT

Uncomplicated mononucleosis requires only supportive therapy. Warm saline gargles and acetaminophen 650 to 1000 mg every 4 h for fever are used.

Antibiotic treatment is necessary for bacterial superinfection of the pharynx.

Pharmacologic Management

Corticosteroids (40 to 80 mg PO qd for 3 days and then tapered over 5 to 14 days) are useful in the management of airway obstruction, hemolytic anemia, and thrombocytopenia. Otherwise, steroids are not useful, since they have no effect on the clinical course.

Penicillin or erythromycin should be taken for 10 days to treat bacterial superinfection by group A beta-hemolytic streptococci (ampicillin and amoxicillin should be avoided, as they are likely to produce a rash).

Supportive Measures

The patient should avoid strenuous exercise and contact/collision sports to decrease the risk of splenic rupture. Patients should limit activity during acute illness and return to contact or collision sports only after complete recovery.

Patient Education

No contact sports for 4 to 8 weeks or as long as the spleen is palpable or is enlarged on x-ray (usually during the first month of illness). Intimate contact during acute illness is restricted to reduce transmission. Isolation is not necessary, as the virus in not likely to be transmitted by aerosols or fomites. Because viremia is present for several months after recovery, any blood donation should be postponed for at least 6 months.

Disposition

Symptoms resolve slowly, with 50 percent of patients symptom-free by 2 weeks, 80 percent symptom-free by 3 weeks, and 97 percent symptom-free by 4 weeks. Malaise and fever are the most persistent symptoms. Some patients remain so fatigued that they have difficulty returning to school or work for months after the infection.

COMPLICATIONS AND RED FLAGS

Complications are uncommon but include hemolytic anemia, immune thrombocytopenia, neutropenia, upper airway obstruction, pneumonia, myopericarditis, splenic rupture, severe hepatitis, bacterial superinfection, and central nervous system infections (encephalitis, aseptic meningitis, transverse myelitis, hearing loss, cranial nerve palsy, and peripheral neuropathy including Guillain-Barré syndrome). Rarely, symptoms of fever, malaise, pharyngitis, cervical adenopathy, or neuropsychiatric symptoms can recur months or years after acute EBV mononucleosis.

BIBLIOGRAPHY

Cohen JI: Epstein-Barr virus infections, including infectious mononucleosis, in Fauci A, Braunwald E, Isselbacher K, et al (eds): *Harrison's Principles of Internal Medicine,* 14th ed. New York, McGraw-Hill, 1998, pp 1089–1091.

Policar M: Mononucleosis clinical topics, in Ferri F (ed): *Clinical Advisor.* St Louis, Mosby Year Book, 1999, p 304.

Schooley RT: Epstein-Barr virus (infectious mononucleosis), in Mandell GL, Bennett JE, Dolin R (eds): *Principles and Practice of Infectious Diseases,* 4th ed. New York, Churchill Livingstone, 1995, pp 1364–1377.

Waterbury L, Zieve PD: Selected illnesses affecting lymphocytes, in Barker LR, Burton JR, Zieve PD (eds): *Principles of Ambulatory Medicine,* 4th ed. Baltimore, Williams & Wilkins, 1995, pp 624–626.

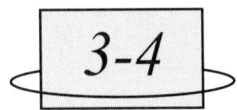

ALLERGIC RHINITIS
Richard Dehn

DISCUSSION

Allergic rhinitis is a disease that affects primarily the nasal mucous membranes. Allergic rhinitis is quite common, and it has been estimated that up to one-sixth of the U.S. population is affected. Symptoms usually begin by the fourth decade of life and tend to decrease with age. Most cases of allergic rhinitis are caused by airborne allergenic particles that initiate an IgE-mediated response in the nasal mucosa.

Patients presenting with allergic rhinitis usually can be classified into two subgroups depending on whether the symptoms are seasonal or perennial. The seasonal subgroup is the largest, and patients in this classification present with recurring symptoms that are limited to a certain time of the year every year. Spring and late summer are the most common times of presentation for seasonal allergic rhinitis, which is often called *hay fever.* Airborne plant pollens or mold spores usually trigger this type of allergic rhinitis; therefore, the symptoms follow the pollination season of the sensitizing plant or mold. Pollen cycles are often unique for each geographic area, and so symptoms present in a consistent annual pattern if the patient stays in the same environment. Allergenic plants often pollinate in the early-morning hours, and so symptoms can be worse in the morning. It is not uncommon for a patient to be allergic to more than one type of pollen. This complicates the identification of the allergen. The most common allergens are ragweed, grass, and tree pollens.

The perennial subgroup is sensitive to allergens that are present year-round. These allergenic agents are usually present in the home or work environment. The most common allergens are house dust, mites, animal dander, and mold spores. Occasionally chemical allergens from the home or work environment are the causative agent, with the most common being vapors released from construction materials or furniture. On very rare occasions, the allergen is contained in the patient's food.

PATHOGENESIS

Allergens in the environment enter the respiratory system through the nose, where they are trapped by the mucosal surfaces of the turbinates. The allergen elicits an IgE-mediated response that causes nearby mast cells to release histamine and other mediators. The effects of this release may occur within a few minutes or may take several hours to develop. Histamine release produces tissue edema and eosinophilic infiltration and indirectly stimulates sensory nerve receptors, resulting in a centrally mediated parasympathetic reflex that produces itching, sneezing, and increased nasal secretions. Histamine also increases mucosal cell permeability, which gives the allergen access to submucosal regions, where additional IgE-mediated responses are initiated.

SIGNS AND SYMPTOMS

The immune response resulting from the allergen's contact with the nasal mucosa produces the classic symptoms of allergic rhinitis. The most common of these symptoms are sneezing, increased nasal secretions, and nasal congestion. They often are accompanied by itching of the eyes, ears, nose, or throat. Severe cases may present with conjunctival inflammation with excessive tearing and mucoid discharge. Persistent postnasal drainage can result in sore throat and a productive cough. Recurrent or chronic allergic rhinitis also may present with fatigue, headache, irritability, ear pain, decreased hearing, and malaise.

The nasal mucosa appears edematous, boggy, and a pale or bluish color coated with clear secretions, though it is not uncommon for the mucosa to appear erythematous. Nasal polyps, which are hypertrophic areas of mucosa that appear as yellow masses, sometimes are seen on examination. Severe mucosal edema is often present and in severe cases can produce airway obstruction and compromise the visualization of the

nasal airway. Commonly the conjunctiva is somewhat injected, and a watery and clear discharge is present. In severe and chronic cases, periorbital edema may be present, with a pooling of venous blood around the eyes that produces a characteristic sign called *allergic shiners.* In response to chronic nasal itching, children often use the side of the hand to rub the nose in an upward motion known as the *allergic salute,* and this process over time can produce a horizontal mark across the bridge of the nose. The mucosa of the posterior pharynx can be inflamed in severe cases, and a postnasal drainage can be visualized. Irritation of the eustachian structures can lead to occlusion, which can produce a reduction of tympanic membrane mobility, serous otitis media, or acute otitis media.

SPECIAL CONSIDERATIONS

Allergic rhinitis often is found in individuals with a predisposition to chronic or recurrent sinusitis, atopic dermatologic conditions, otitis media, and asthma. Sometimes these conditions occur secondary to a flare-up of allergic rhinitis so that treatment of the allergic rhinitis will improve the secondary condition. In some cases, treatment that prevents the symptoms of allergic rhinitis reduces the number and frequency of occurrences of the secondary condition. Chronic allergic rhinitis can result in the development of nasal polyps, which can contribute to obstruction and the development of sinusitis.

DIAGNOSTIC CONSIDERATIONS

Allergic rhinitis must be distinguished from viral and bacterial infections of the nasal mucosa. This differentiation usually can be made by means of physical examination, since infections often present with erythematous mucosa. Additional information can be obtained by microscopically examining the nasal secretions, which will contain significant neutrophilia in an infectious process, in contrast to the eosinophilia seen with allergic rhinitis.

Allergic rhinitis also can be confused with vasomotor rhinitis, in which nasal secretions are due to functionally hyperactive mucosa. In vasomotor rhinitis, precipitating factors include sudden temperature change, strong odors, air-conditioning, alcoholic beverages, and even sexual activity. In patients with vasomotor rhinitis, itching and sneezing are usually absent, since the syndrome does not involve the release of histamine.

The chronic use of nasal decongestants (rhinitis medicamentosa) also can produce symptoms of allergic rhinitis. Rebound nasal congestion after overuse of these drugs can precipitate a purulent rhinitis in which the mucosa appears bright red. Obstructions also can contribute to the symptoms of allergic rhinitis. These symptoms can have many primary etiologies, such as septal deviation, tumors, foreign bodies, and adenoidal hypertrophy. Several endocrinologic states also can produce symptoms of allergic rhinitis, including hypothyroidism and pregnancy.

LABORATORY TESTING

Identification of significant eosinophilia from a swabbing of the nasal secretions is highly suggestive of allergic rhinitis. The presence of neutrophils in nasal secretions is more suggestive of sinusitis.

Radioallergosorbent testing (RAST) and skin testing are useful in identifying the specific allergens to which a patient is sensitive. A RAST test measures in vitro specific IgE present in the serum, while skin testing measures the skin's direct response to antigen exposure. Information from RAST or skin testing can be useful if the goal of therapy is allergen avoidance or immunotherapy.

TREATMENT

The treatment of allergic rhinitis involves allergen avoidance, pharmacologic therapy, and immunotherapy. Although allergen avoidance is the cheapest and least invasive form of therapy, pharmacologic therapy is the most commonly used first-line treatment since it does not require the identification of the offending allergen or allergens (see Table 3-4-1).

Color Plates*

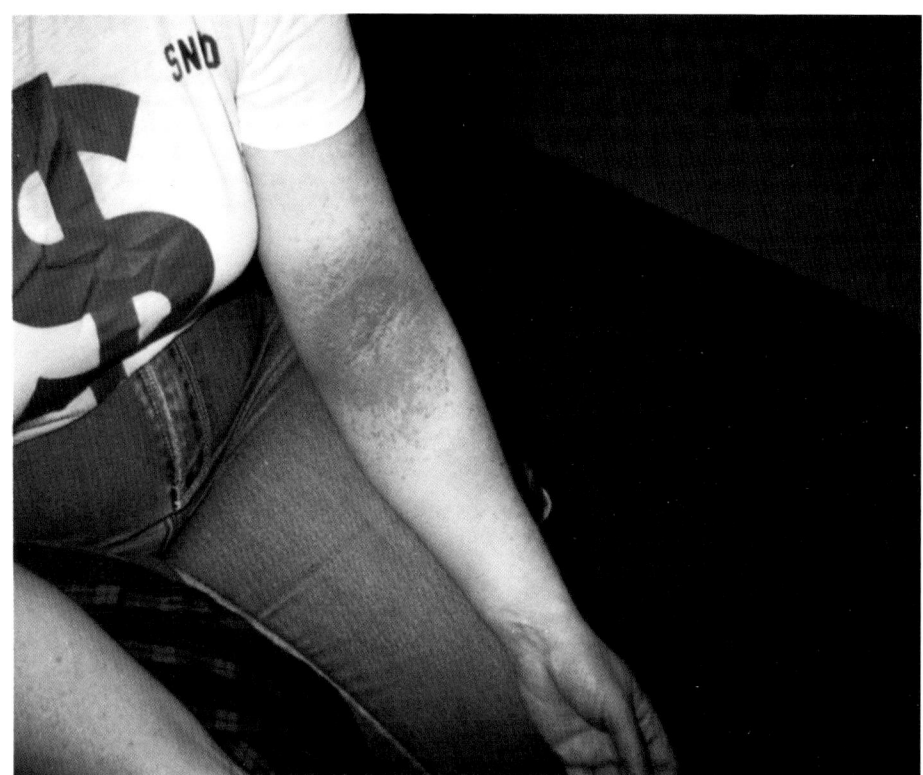

PLATE 1 (FIGURE 2-1-2). Acute contact dermatitis of the antecubital area. *(Courtesy of Harold Milstein, MD, The Dermatology Center, Hazleton, PA.)*

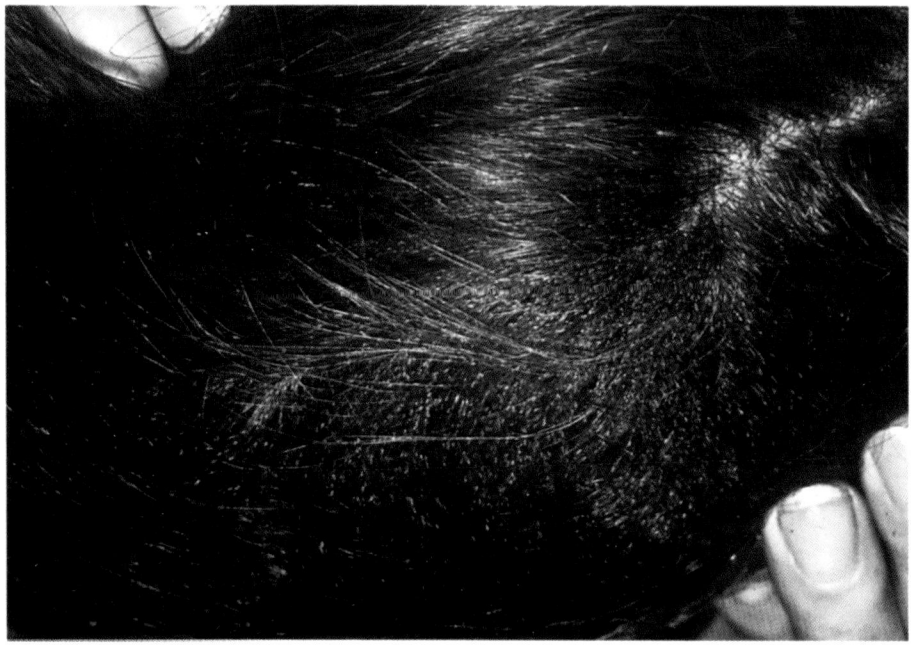

PLATE 2 (FIGURE 2-5-1). Nits. *(From Fitzpatrick, Johnson, Wolff, et al.[1])*

*The figures in parentheses following the Plate numbers have been double-numbered in order to indicate the chapter in which they are discussed and the order of their citation therein.

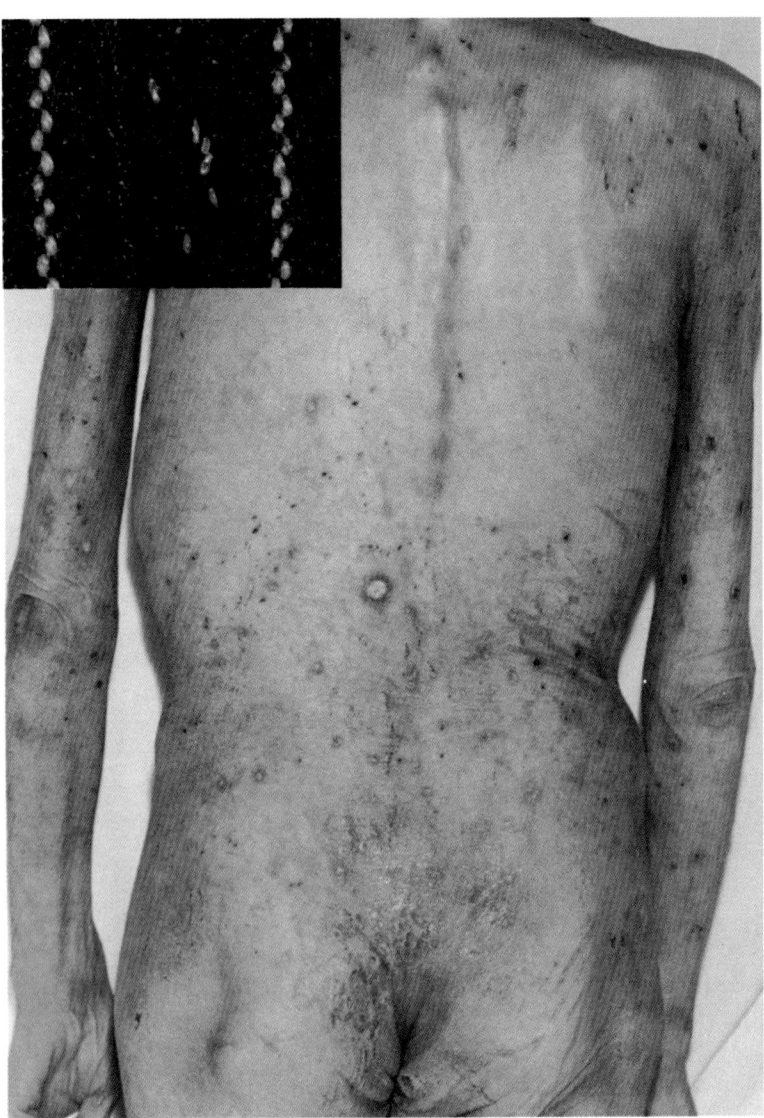

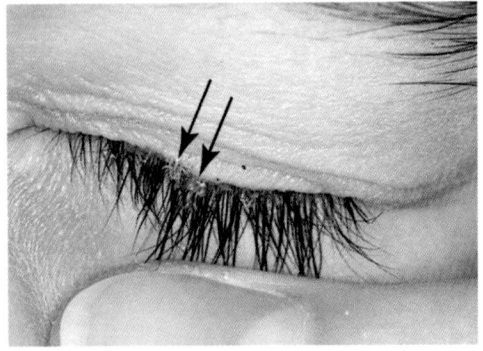

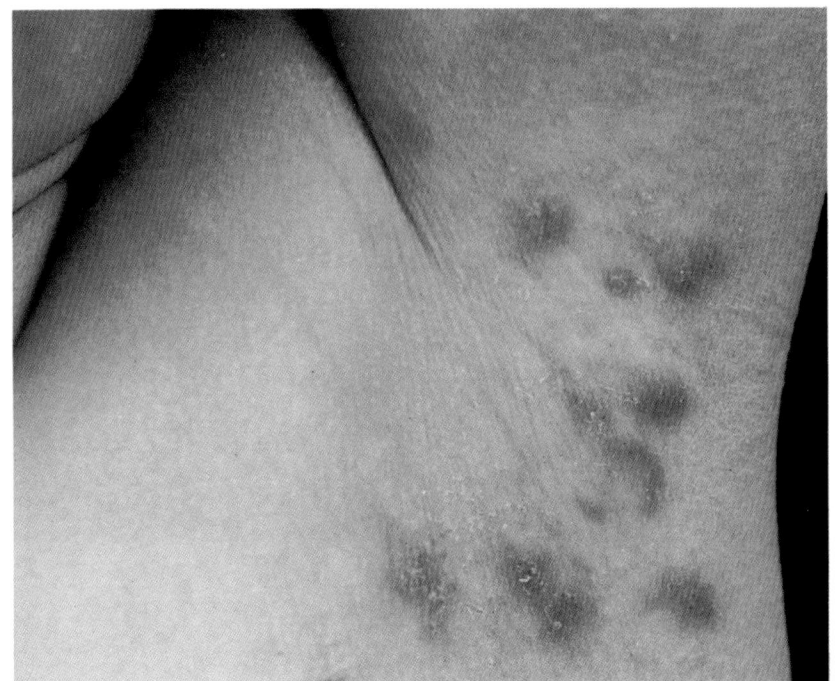

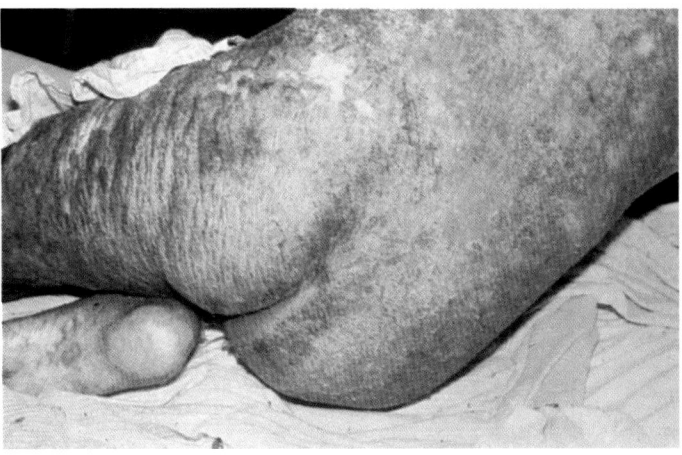

PLATE 6 (FIGURE 2-5-6). Crusted scabies. *(From Fitzpatrick, Johnson, Wolff, et al.[1])*

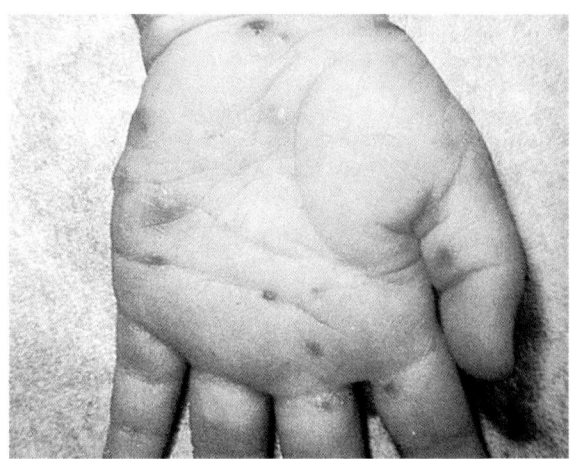

PLATE 7 (FIGURE 2-5-7). Scabies in infants. *(Courtesy of Ramon Fusaro.)*

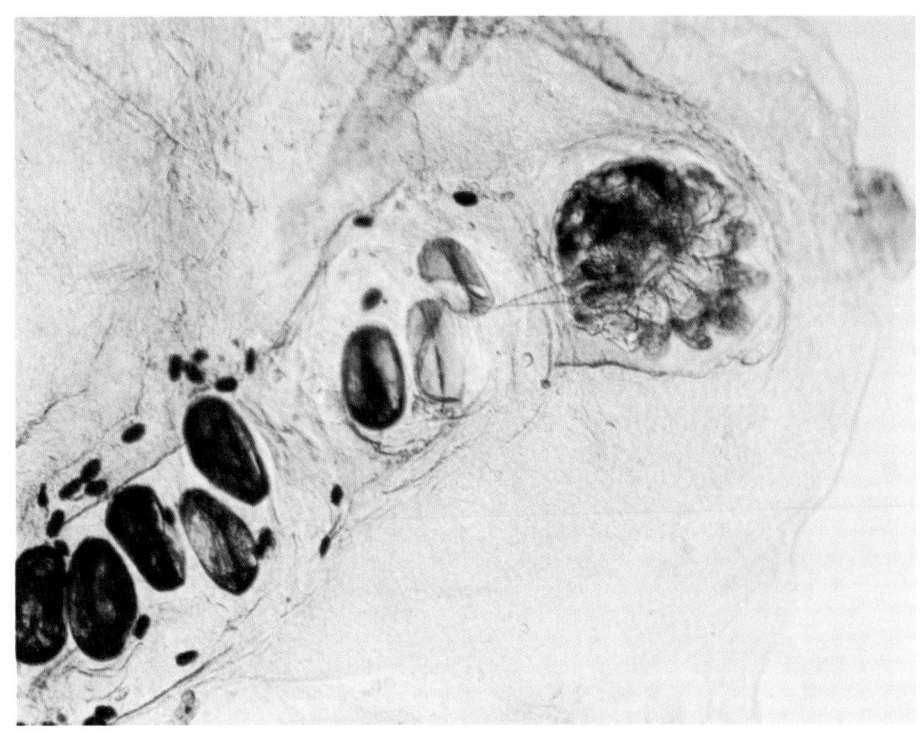

PLATE 8 (FIGURE 2-5-11). Burrow with scabies mite, eggs, and scybala (feces). *(From Fitzpatrick, Johnson, Wolff, et al.[1])*

PLATE 9 (FIGURE 2-7-1). Classic presentation of nodular basal cell carcinoma. Note the small area of ulceration in the upper part of the lesion. *(Courtesy of Harold Milstein, MD, The Dermatology Clinic, Hazleton, PA.)*

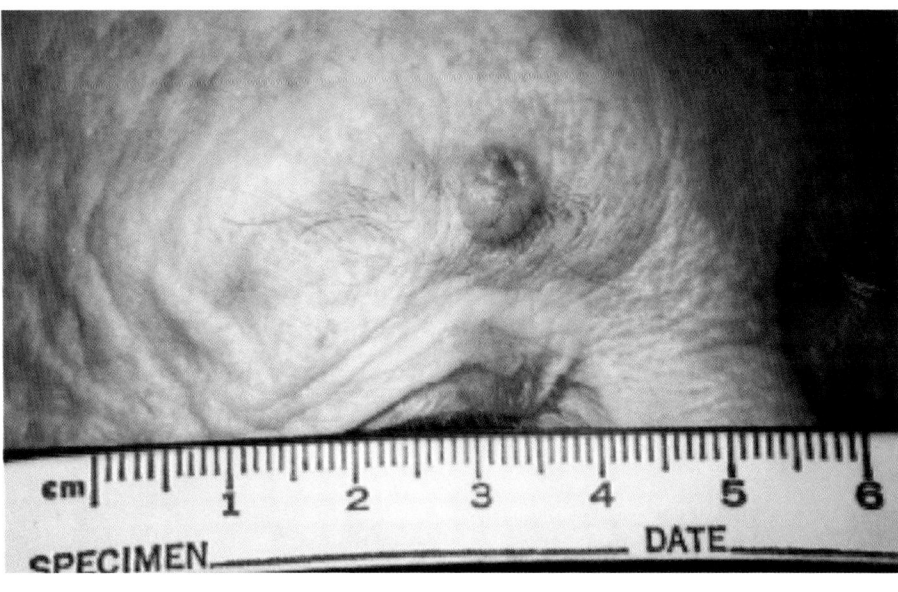

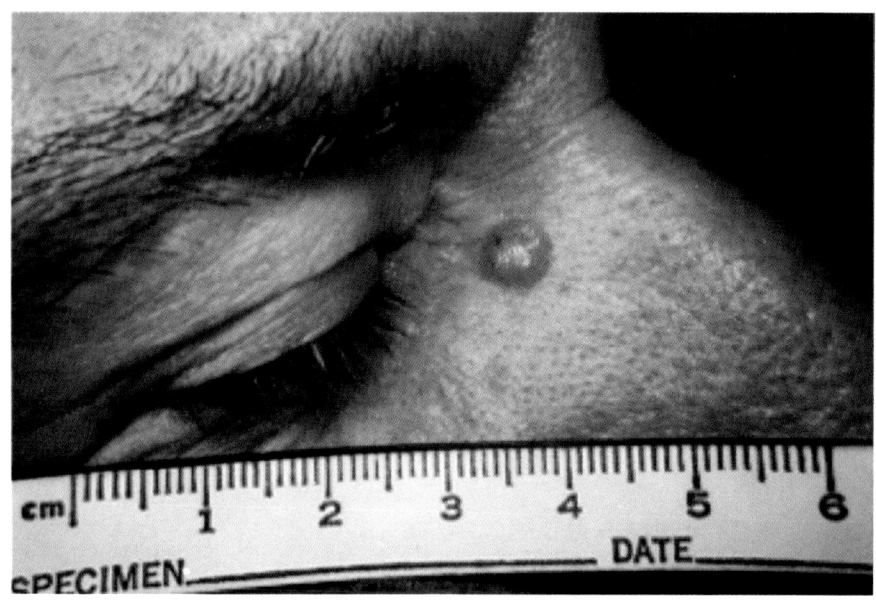

PLATE 10 (FIGURE 2-7-2). Small telang-iectasias on left side of basal cell carcinoma. *(Courtesy of Harold Milstein, MD, The Dermatology Clinic, Hazleton, PA.)*

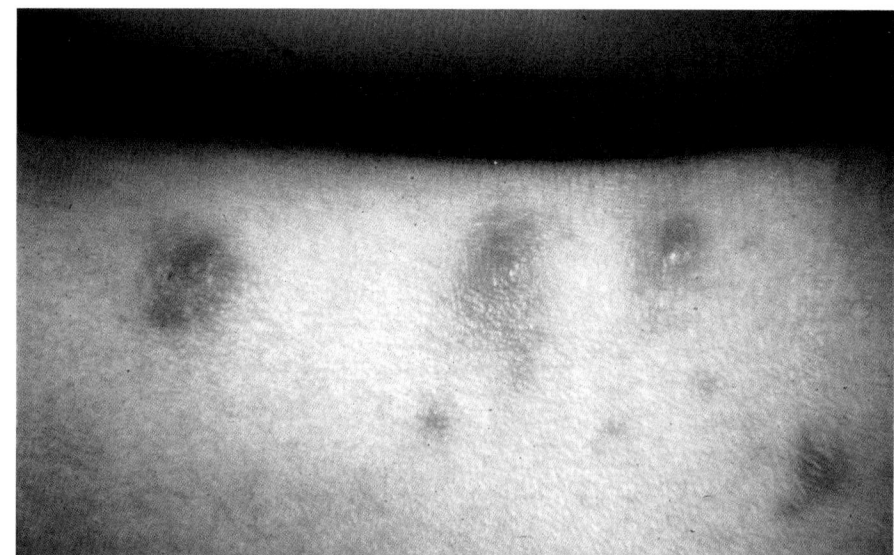

PLATE 11 (FIGURE 2-15-1). Typical lesions of hand-foot-and-mouth disease. Small vesicular papules or tiny ulcers with surrounding erythema. *(Photo courtesy of William H. Fenn. Used with permission.)*

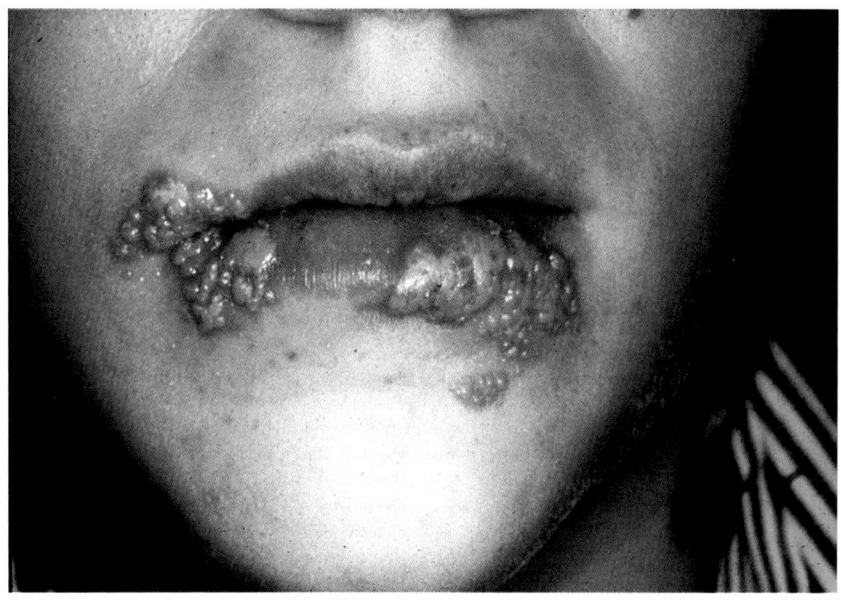

PLATE 12 (FIGURE 2-16-1). Herpes simplex lesions on the lips. Noted grouped vesicles on an erythematous base. *(Photo courtesy of William H. Fenn.)*

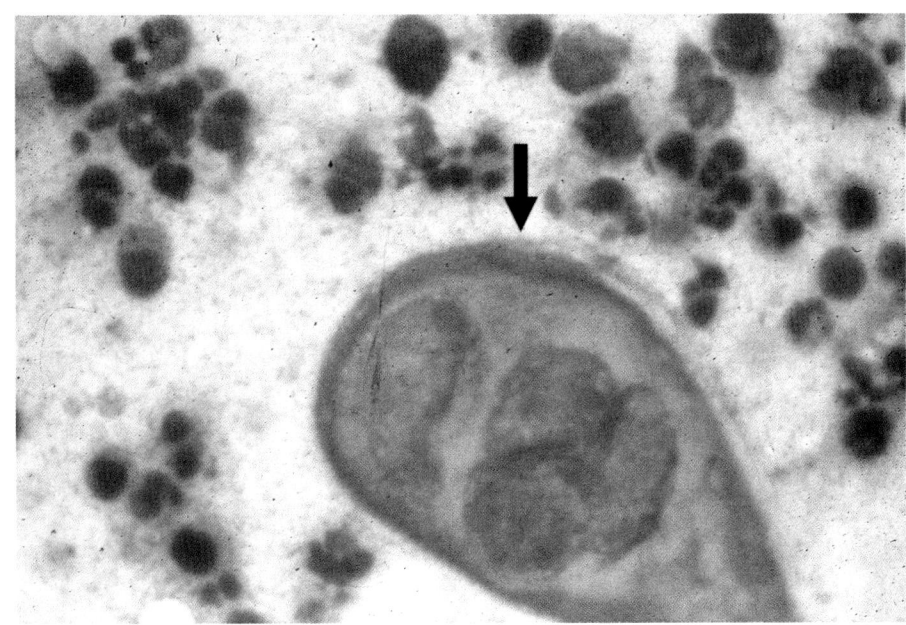

PLATE 13 (FIGURE 2-16-2). Positive Tzanck smear with arrow indicating giant multinucleated cell. *(Photo courtesy of William H. Fenn.)*

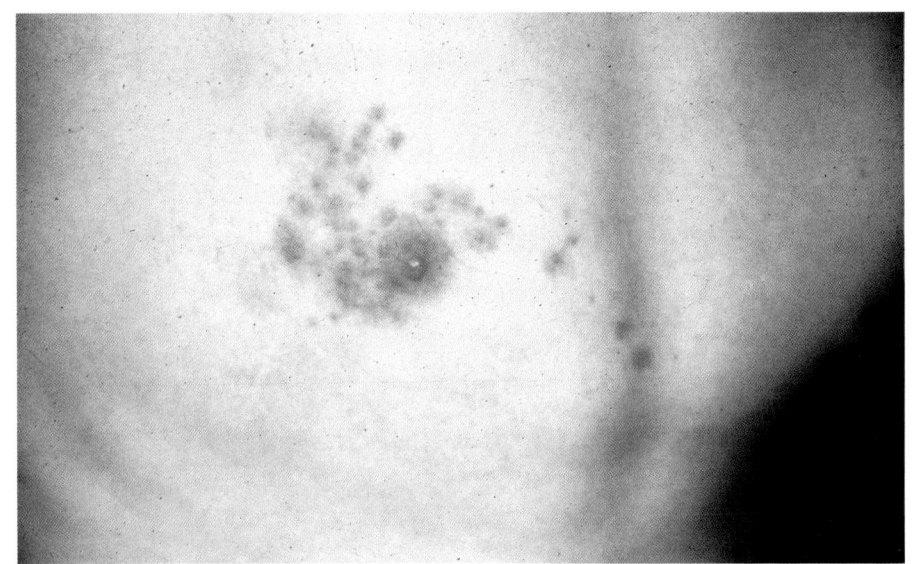

PLATE 14 (FIGURE 2-17-1). Herpes zoster sshingles) lesions on the chest. Note grouped vesiculations. *(Photo courtesy of William H. Fenn.)*

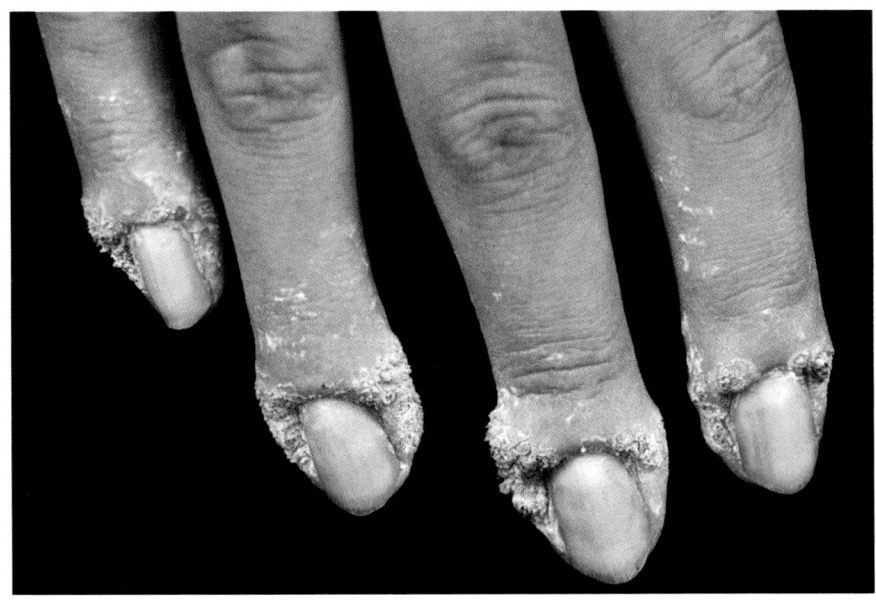

PLATE 15 (FIGURE 2-18-1). Verruca vulgaris. *(From Fitzpatrick, Johnson, Wolff, et al.[1])*

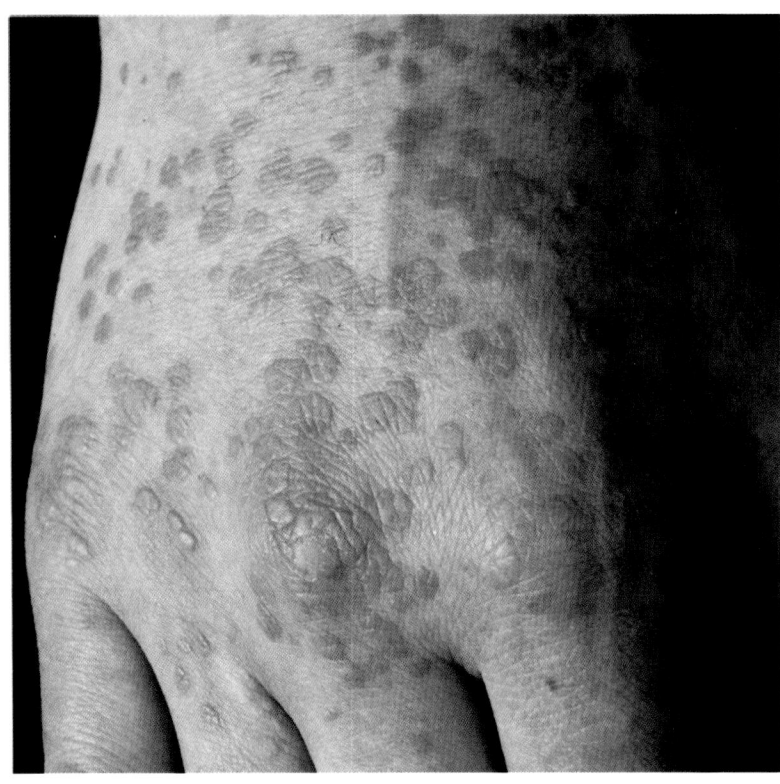

PLATE 16 (FIGURE 2-18-2). Verruca plana. *(From Fitzpatrick, Johnson, Wolff, et al.[1])*

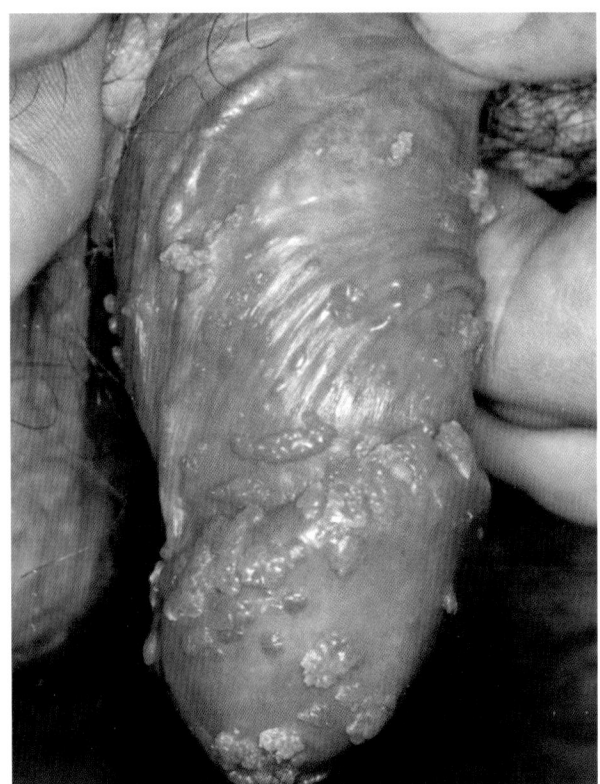

PLATE 17 (FIGURE 2-18-3). Condyloma acuminata. *(From Fitzpatrick, Johnson, Wolff, et al.[1])*

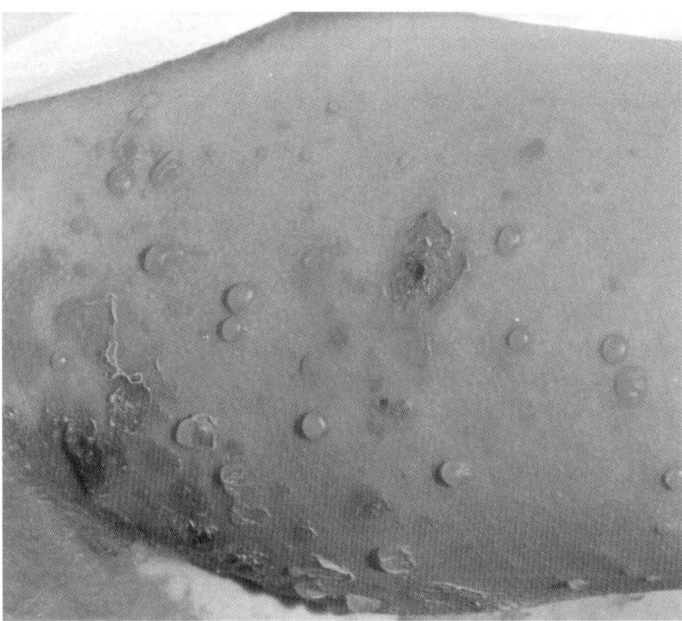

PLATE 18 (FIGURE 2-19-1). Bullous impetigo. *(From Fitzpatrick, Johnson, Wolff, et al.[1])*

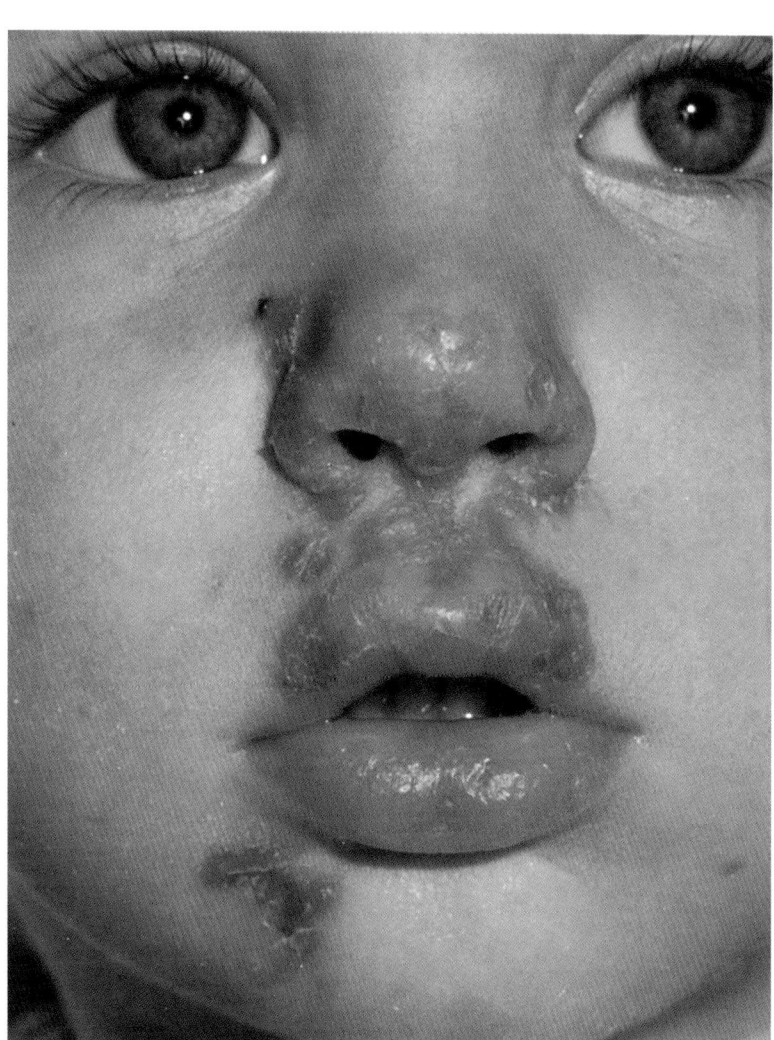

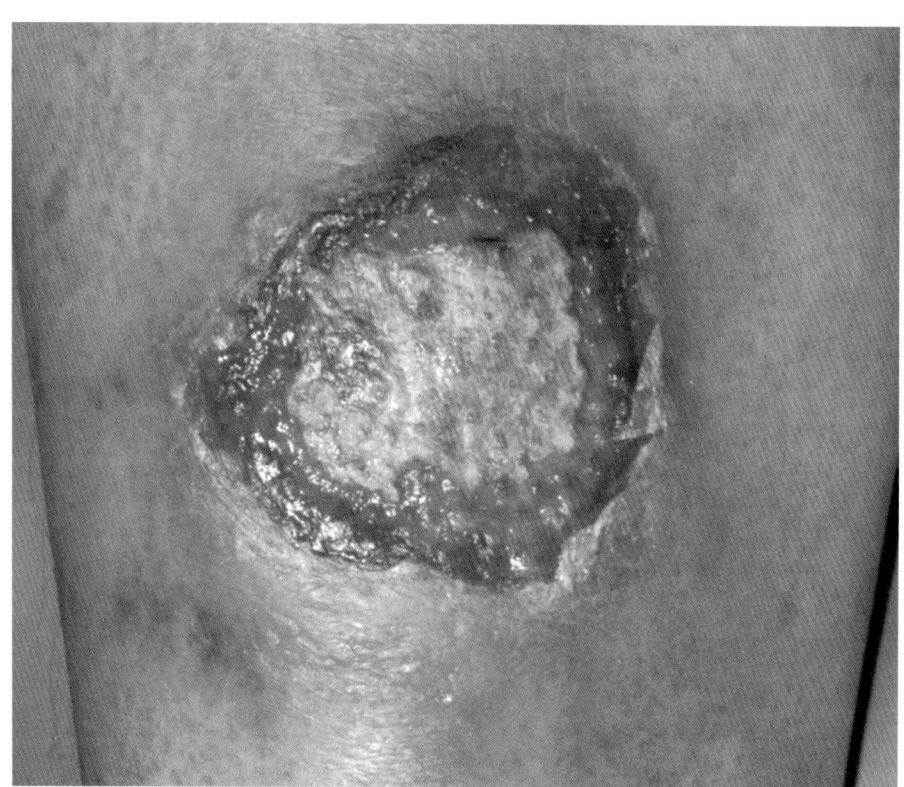

PLATE 19 (FIGURE 2-19-2). Nonbullous impetigo.
(From Fitzpatrick, Johnson, Wolff, et al.[1])

PLATE 20 (FIGURE 2-19-3). Ecthyma.
(From Fitzpatrick, Johnson, Wolff, et al.[1])

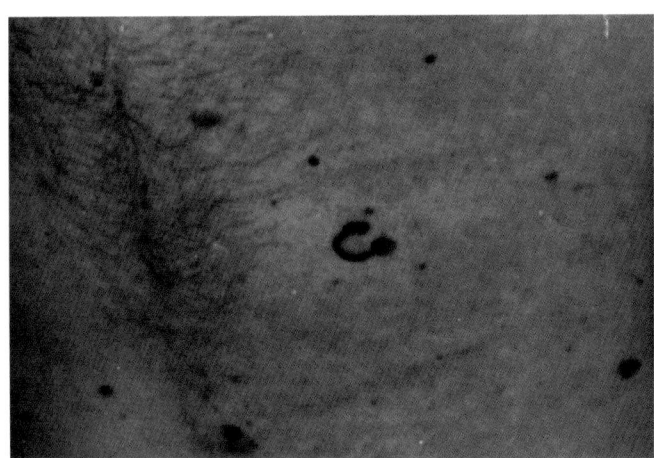

PLATE 21 (FIGURE 2-21-1). A C-shaped malignant melanoma of the abdomen. *(Courtesy of Harold Milstein, MD, The Dermatology Center, Hazleton, PA.)*

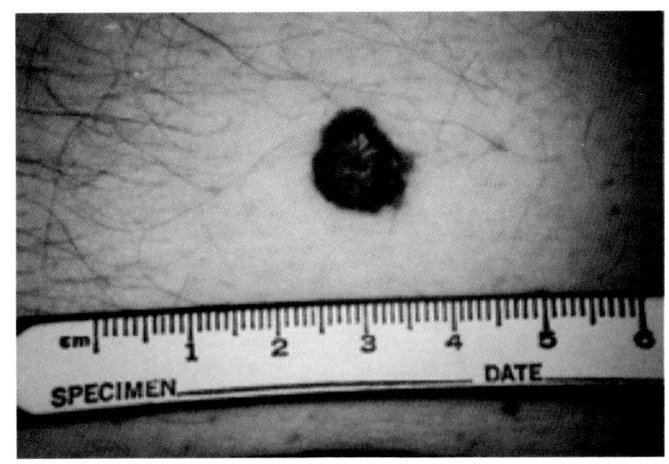

PLATE 22 (FIGURE 2-21-2). A nodular malignant melanoma of the abdomen. *(Courtesy of Harold Milstein, MD, The Dermatology Center, Hazleton, PA.)*

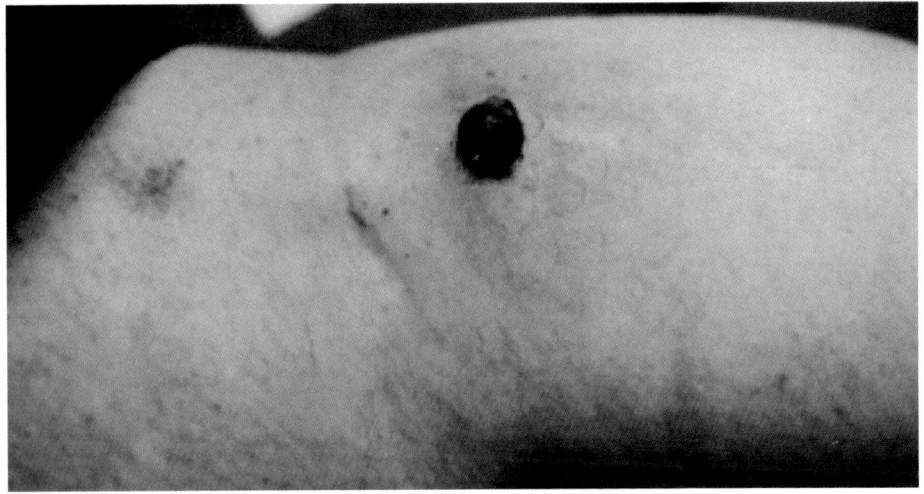

PLATE 23 (FIGURE 2-21-3). Malignant melanoma of the leg. *(Courtesy of Harold Milstein, MD, The Dermatology Center, Hazleton, PA.)*

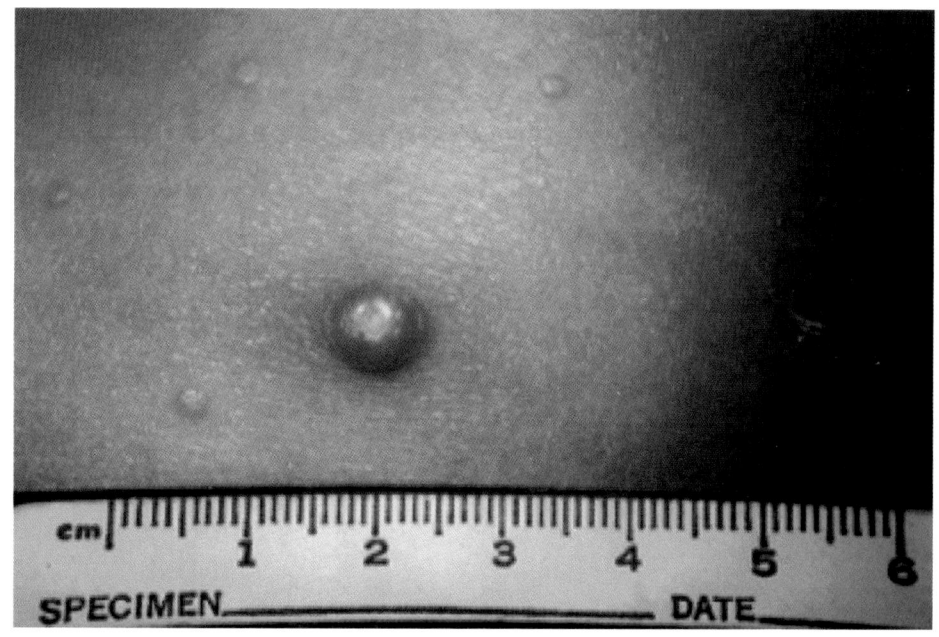

PLATE 24 (FIGURE 2-22-1). Several small molluscum lesions with one giant lesion on the chest. Note the central umbilication and the irritation associated with the larger lesion. In this case, it is appropriate to remove the lesions because of the irritation. *(Courtesy of Harold Milstein, MD, The Dermatology Center, Hazleton, PA.)*

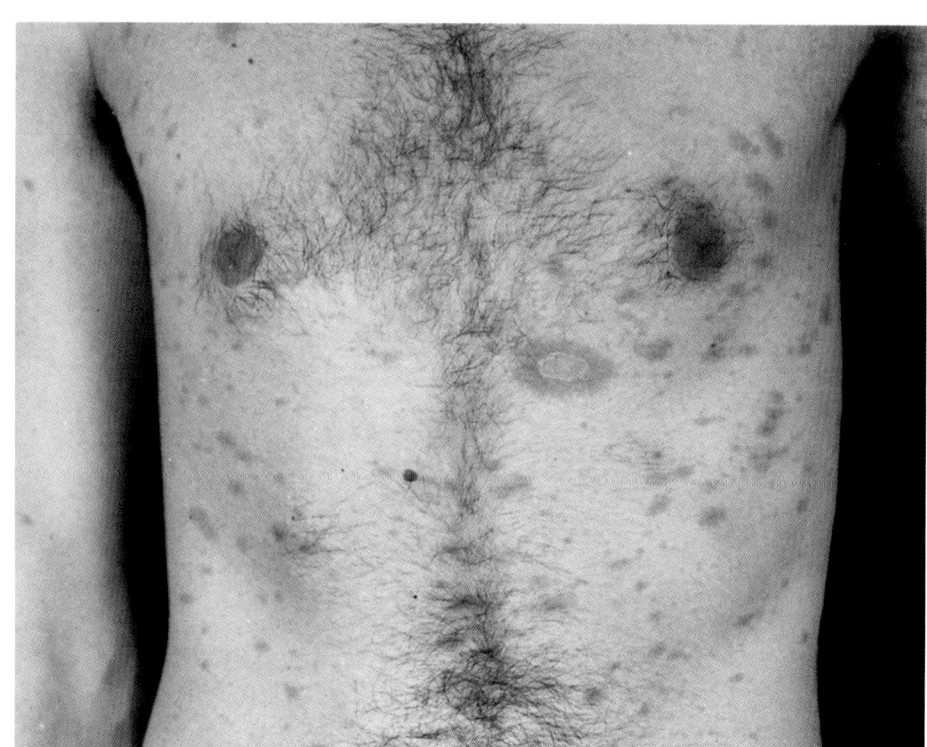

PLATE 25 (FIGURE 2-23-1). Pityriasis rosea. *(From Fitzpatrick, Johnson, Wolff, et al.[1])*

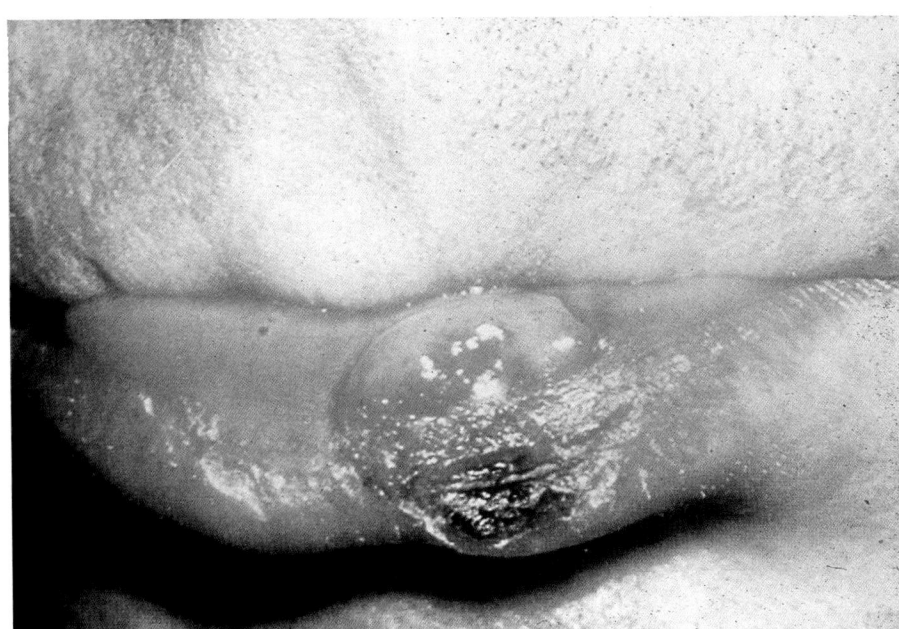

PLATE 26 (FIGURE 2-27-1). A classic squamous cell carcinoma of the lip found on a smoker. *(Photo courtesy of William H. Fenn. Used with permission.)*

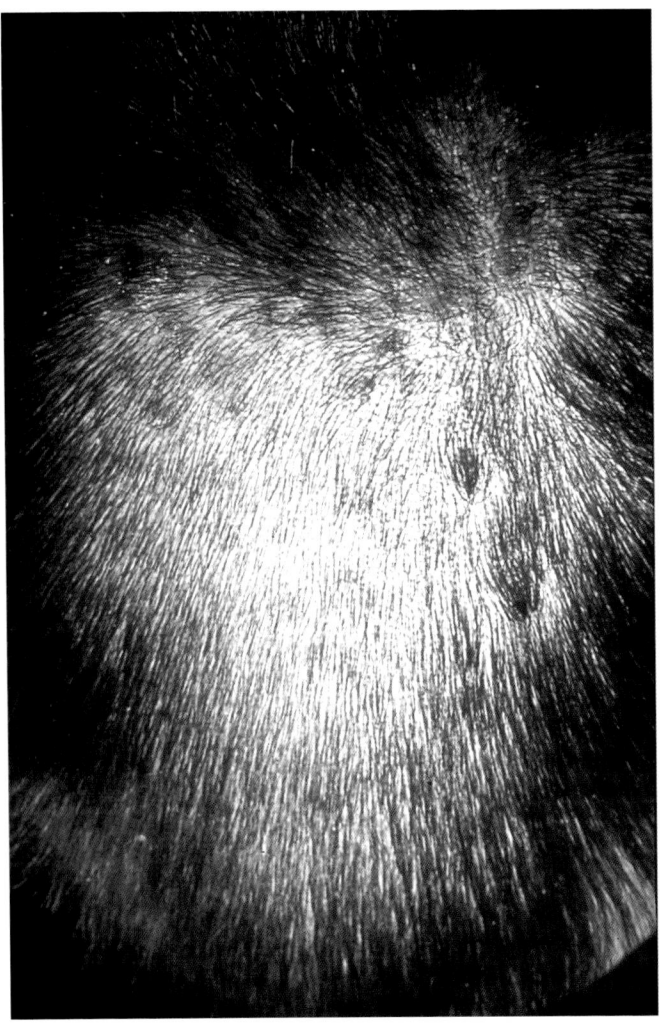

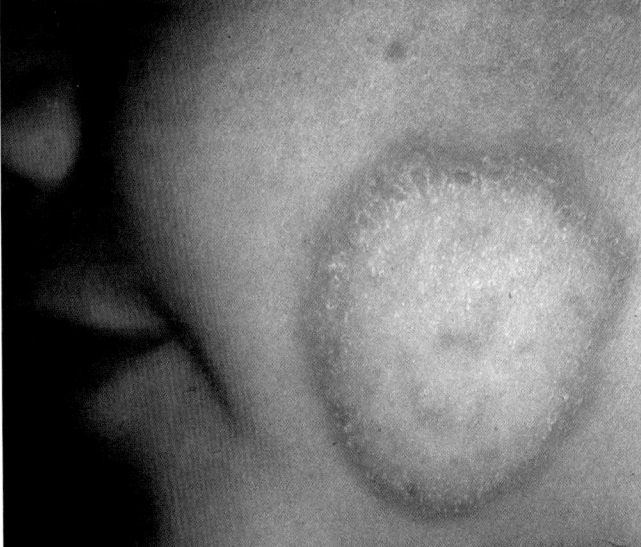

PLATE 28 (FIGURE 2-28-2). Typical circular, raised, well-demarcated red border of tinea corporis. Scaling is also present. Note central clearing. *(Photo courtesy of William H. Fenn. Used with permission.)*

PLATE 27 (FIGURE 2-28-1). Typical area of alopecia from tinea capitis with kerion formation. Note broken shafts and pustules. *(Photo courtesy of William H. Fenn. Used with permission.)*

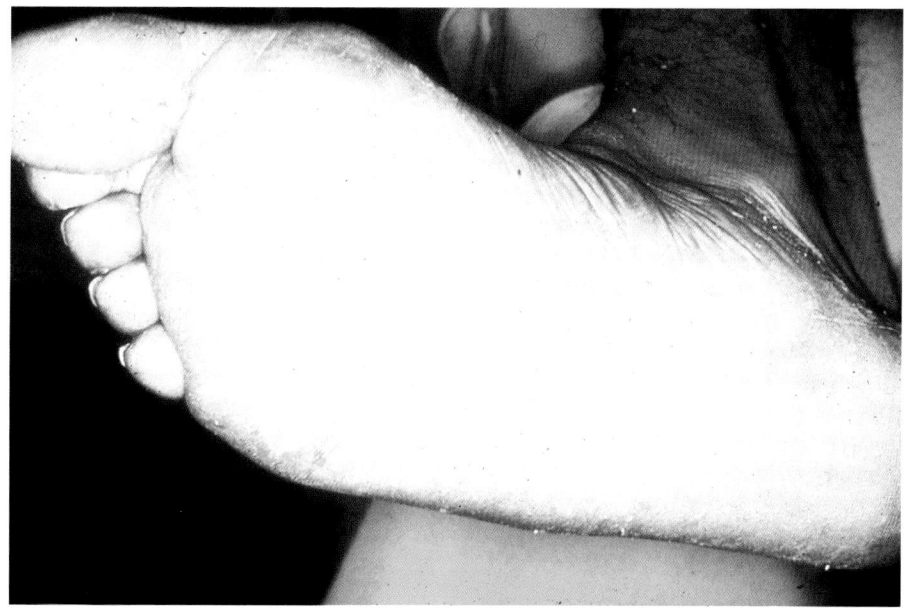

PLATE 29 (FIGURE 2-28-3). Moccasin pattern tinea pedis. The infection is present on the soles of the foot and along the sides and between the toes, where a moccasin-type shoe would touch the skin. *(Photo courtesy of William H. Fenn. Used with permission.)*

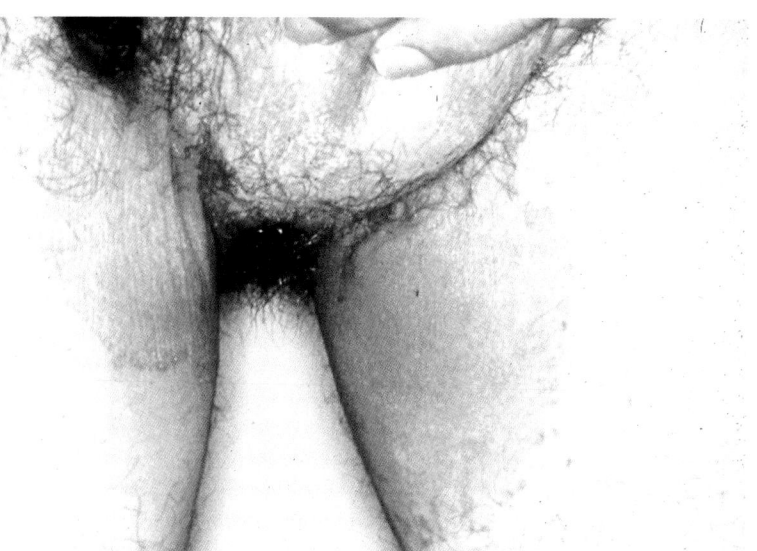

PLATE 30 (FIGURE 2-28-4). Typical tinea cruris with well-demarcated, moist red skin on the thighs. Note sparing of the scrotum. *(Photo courtesy of William H. Fenn. Used with permission.)*

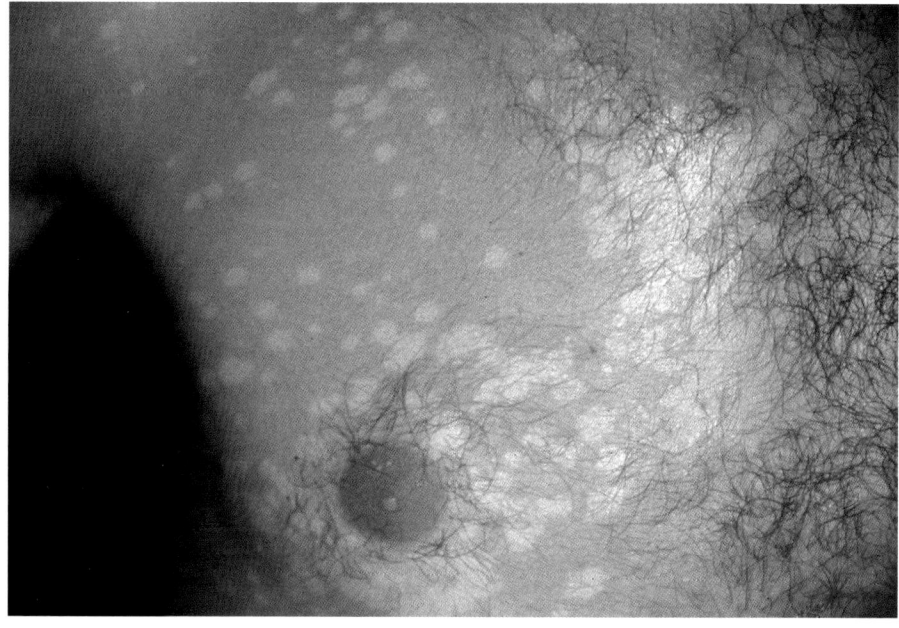

PLATE 31 (FIGURE 2-28-5). Tinea versicolor affecting the chest. Note areas of hypopigmentation. *(Photo courtesy of William H. Fenn. Used with permission.)*

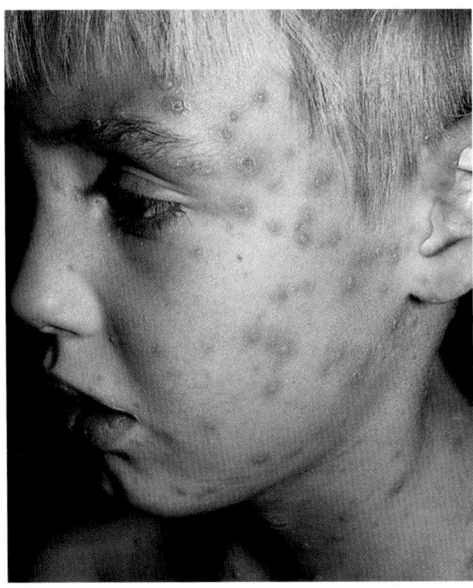

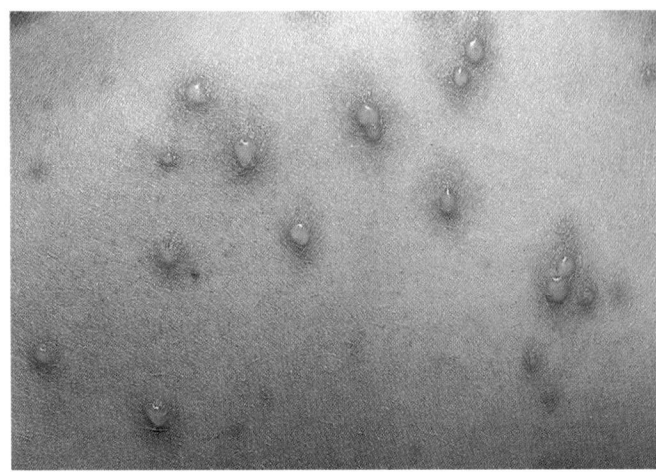

PLATE 33 (FIGURE 9-26-2). Close-up of varicella vesicles showing the characteristic "dewdrop on a rose petal" appearance. *(Photo courtesy of Rodney L. Moser. Used with permission.)*

PLATE 32 (FIGURE 9-26-1). Pediatric varicella with multiple vesicles and crusting. *(Photo courtesy of Rodney L. Moser. Used with permission.)*

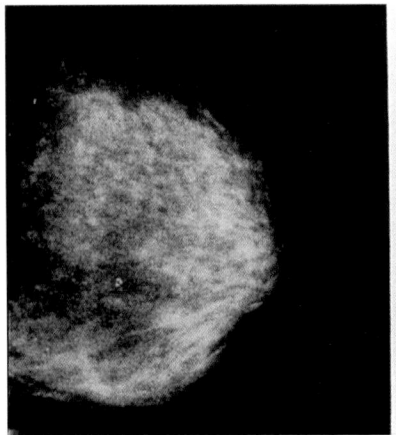
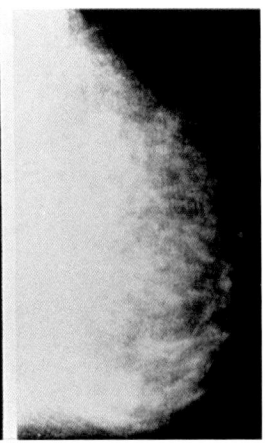

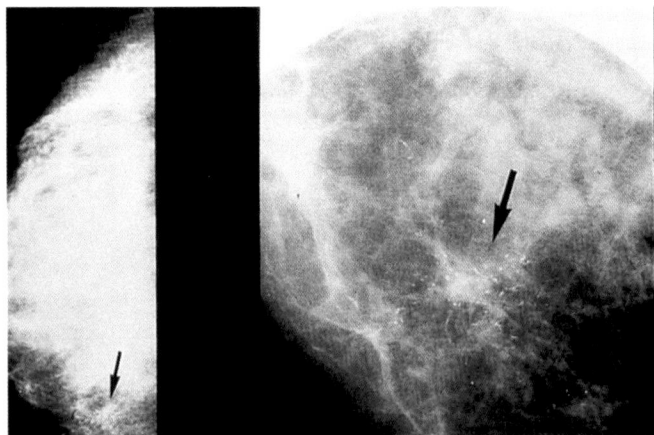

PLATE 34 (FIGURE 12-12-1). Quality assurance for mammography is critical. These images are of the same breast. The image on the left shows a breast that is not properly compressed. It could have mistakenly been read as a dense, glandular breast with no abnormality. The image on the right shows the same breast with proper compression. It is much easier to find a white density indicative of cancer on the right image than on the left image. *(From the American Medical Women's Association for the Breast and Cervical Cancer Education Project for Primary Care Providers, under a cooperative agreement with the Centers for Disease Control and Prevention.)*

PLATE 35 (FIGURE 12-12-2). The left side contains a density indicated by the black arrow. The cone compression view on the right reveals a finding even more ominous than the original film, illustrating how useful cone compression mammography can be. This finding represented carcinoma. *(From the American Medical Women's Association for the Breast and Cervical Cancer Education Project for Primary Care Providers, under a cooperative agreement with the Centers for Disease Control and Prevention.)*

PLATE 36 (FIGURE 12-12-3). On the left side, the radiologist has noted some white specks. These represent microcalcifications in the breast. Imaging them with a magnification view as shown on the right helps identify the sizes and shapes of the calcifications. These are highly suggestive of carcinoma because they are pleomorphic, that is, of different sizes and shapes. In general, cone compression mammography is used to evaluate densities further, and magnification views are done to identify and discern calcifications. *(From the American Medical Women's Association for the Breast and Cervical Cancer Education Project for Primary Care Providers, under a cooperative agreement with the Centers for Disease Control and Prevention.)*

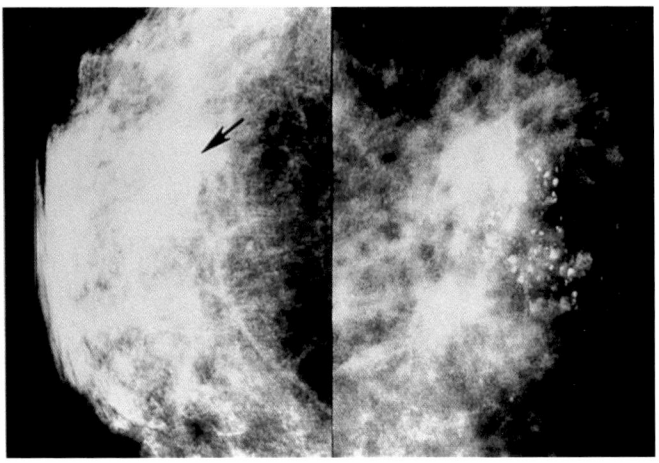

TABLE 3-4-1. Pharmacologic Treatment of Allergic Rhinitis

AGENT	DOSAGE (FOR ADULT UNLESS SPECIFIED)	COMMENTS
SEDATING ANTIHISTAMINES		
Chlorpheniramine (Chlor-Trimeton)	4 mg qd	Major side effects are sedation and anticholinergic effects Relatively inexpensive Available without a prescription
Brompheniramine (Dimetane)	4 mg qd	Same as for chlorpheniramine
Diphenhydramine (Benadryl)	25–50 mg qd	Same as for chlorpheniramine
NONSEDATING ANTIHISTAMINES		
Loratadine (Claritin)	10 mg qd	Low incidence of sedation and anticholinergic effects Expensive and available only by prescription
Astemizole, (Hismanal)	10 mg qd	Same as for loratadine Has produced QT-interval prolongation when taken with macrolide antibiotics, ketoconazole, or itraconazole and in patients with liver failure
Fexofenadine (Allegra)	60 mg bid	Same as for loratadine
Cetirizine (Zyrtec)	5–10 mg qd	Same as for loratadine
Azelastine (Astelin) topical nasal spray	2 sprays in each nostril bid	Same as for loratadine Topical administration avoids central effects Altered taste sensation after use
DECONGESTANTS		
Pseudoephedrine (Sudafed)	60 mg every 4 h	Can produce nervousness Sympathomimetic effects often raise blood pressure, increase heart rate, and cause coronary vasoconstriction Systemic side effects can be avoided by using topical preparations
Phenylpropanolamine	25 mg every 4 h	Same as for pseudoephedrine
Oxymetazoline (Afrin 12 Hour) topical nasal spray	2–3 sprays in each nostril every 12 h	Available without prescription Use should be limited to 5 days to avoid rhinitis medicamentosa
Phenylephrine (Neo-Synephrine) topical nasal spray	2–3 sprays in each nostril every 4 h	Available without prescription Use should be limited to 3 days to avoid rhinitis medicamentosa
ANTIHISTAMINE AND DECONGESTANT COMBINATIONS		
Wide variety of oral preparations available by prescription and over the counter	Specific for each combination	The side effects of these combination preparations are unpredictable from patient to patient, depending on how well drowsiness of antihistamine is balanced against nervousness of decongestant
CORTICOSTEROIDS		
Routes include topical nasal, oral, and intramuscular (IM)	Topical: many products available; dosing varies for each product Some improvement can be expected in 1 to 2 weeks; optimum effect apparent in 1 or 2 months Oral: prednisone 40–60 mg daily for 5–10 days before tapering off	Utilized when antihistamines and decongestants are not effective or are intolerable Topical preparations result in negligible systemic absorption Local side effects of stinging and epistaxis are not uncommon Work best if treated before mast cell degranulation Oral and IM routes reserved for difficult cases due to significant side effects
CROMOLYN		
Available over the counter as a 4% solution (Nasalcrom)	One spray in each nostril 3–4 times daily	Effective in inhibiting mast cell degranulation Most effective if treatment precedes mast cell contact with antigen Maximum effect noted after 4 to 6 weeks of regular use Not systemically absorbed but can cause local irritation and sneezing Not very effective when the nasal mucosa is thickened, and so efficacy can be increased by using a nasal decongestant before cromolyn application
ANTICHOLINERGIC PREPARATIONS		
Ipratropium bromide (Atrovent) 0.03%	Two sprays in each nostril bid or tid	Major side effects are nasal mucosal dryness, irritation, and bleeding
LEUKOTRIENE MODIFIERS		
Montelukast sodium (Singulair)	10 mg qd	Approved for use in asthma Reduces nasal congestion, rhinorrhea, and sneezing in allergic rhinitis Headache a frequent side effect Expensive
Zafirlukast (Accolate)	20 mg bid	Same as for montelukast sodium
Zileuton (Zyflo)	600 mg qd	Same as for montelukast sodium Recommended that hepatic transaminases be evaluated before and during therapy

Drug therapy is most appropriate for patients with seasonal or mild perennial allergic rhinitis. First-line drugs include antihistamines and decongestants. Antihistamines work by competitively blocking histamine at the H_1 receptor sites. The most commonly used sedating antihistamines are chlorpheniramine (Chlor-Trimeton), brompheniramine (Dimetane), and diphenhydramine (Benadryl). The major advantages of these antihistamines are low cost and nonprescription availability; however, there are major side effects of sedation and anticholinergic effects. Nonsedating antihistamines are available but cost significantly more and are available only by prescription. The most common nonsedating antihistamines are astemizole (Hismanal), loratadine (Claritin), fexofenadine (Allegra), and cetirizine (Zyrtec). The decision whether to use a sedating or a nonsedating medication is primarily a cost-benefit compromise, since the nonsedating drugs are expensive. Astemizole has been known to cause QT-interval prolongation when taken with macrolide antibiotics or the antifungal agents ketoconazole and itraconazole and in patients with liver failure.

Decongestants also are used as first-line therapy for allergic rhinitis. They work as sympathomimetics, producing vasoconstriction, and are available as both systemic and topical agents. The most common oral preparations are pseudoephedrine (Sudafed) and phenylpropanolamine. Systemic decongestants can produce nervousness as a side effect, limiting their use. Decongestants should be used carefully in patients with hypertension or cardiac disease, since the sympathomimetic effects often raise the blood pressure, increase the heart rate, and cause coronary vasoconstriction. Most of the systemic side effects can be avoided by using topical preparations, since a much smaller quantity of the drug is systemically absorbed. Commonly used topical decongestants include oxymetazoline (Afrin) and phenylephrine (Neo-Synephrine); however, the use of topical decongestants should be limited to 3 to 5 days to avoid rhinitis medicamentosa. Often oral over-the-counter and prescription preparations contain a formulation of both antihistamines and decongestants. The side effects of these combination preparations are unpredictable from patient to patient and depend on how well the drowsiness from the antihistamine is balanced against the nervousness from the decongestant.

Corticosteroid preparations are utilized when symptoms are more severe, are more chronic, or do not respond to antihistamines or decongestants and when the side effects of antihistamines or decongestants are intolerable. Corticosteroids work by reducing the release of histamine and other mediators from mast cells; this reduces eosinophilic migration and prevents the centrally mediated parasympathetic reflex. Corticosteroids work best if treatment begins before mast cell exposure to the allergen. Systemic oral or intermuscular corticosteroids are used occasionally; however, topical corticosteroid preparations are equally effective and do not have the side effects of systemic absorption. Several preparations of topical nasal corticosteroids are available. Treatment with topical nasal corticosteroids is primarily preventive; therefore, patients should not expect immediate improvement. A decrease in symptoms can be expected after 1 to 2 weeks of regular use, and the optimum effect can take 1 or 2 months. Severe cases may require increased dosing, though many patients are able to decrease to a small maintenance dose once the symptoms have been controlled. Since little systemic absorption occurs with the topical preparations, very few systemic side effects are reported; however, local side effects of stinging and epistaxis are not uncommon.

Cromolyn is effective in inhibiting mast cell degranulation. Intranasal cromolyn sodium is available over the counter as a 4% solution (Nasalcrom), and one spray should be used in each nostril three or four times daily. Similar to topical corticosteroids, cromolyn is most effective if treatment precedes mast cell contact with the antigen, and a maximum effect is noted after 4 to 6 weeks of regular use. Cromolyn is not systemically absorbed, but it can cause local irritation and sneezing. It is not very effective when the nasal mucosa is thickened, and so efficacy can be increased in those cases by using a nasal decongestant before the cromolyn application.

Anticholinergic preparations have been found to be effective in reducing the symptoms of allergic rhinitis. Ipratropium bromide (Atrovent) can be sprayed twice into each nostril bid or tid. The major side effect is nasal mucosal dryness.

Leukotriene modifiers work by decreasing leukotriene production; thus, they are used in asthma prevention. They are effective in decreasing nasal congestion, rhinorrhea, and sneezing in patients with allergic rhinitis. The major disadvantage of these medications is their high cost. Additionally, zileuton (Zyflo) requires the monitoring of liver function.

Allergen avoidance is important for the long-term management of allergic rhinitis in patients who are not responsive to or intolerant to medications. Occasionally a patient is able to identify the offending allergen; however, most of the time skin testing and/or RAST must be performed to identify the allergen or allergens responsible. Identification of the allergens will allow the patient to attempt to remove those substances from the environment. In the case of outdoor seasonal pollens, this may involve avoiding outdoor activity during the peak season or wearing a filtering mask while outside. Indoor allergens can be reduced substantially by cleaning of furniture and bedding frequently, placing mattresses and pillows in plastic cases, removing pets from the household, fixing areas where molds grow, and eliminating carpeting in favor of wood floors.

Patients with chronic and severe allergic rhinitis who are unable to avoid allergens are candidates for immunotherapy. With immunotherapy, or hyposensitization therapy, small quantities of allergen are regularly injected subcutaneously in increasing doses. Up to 80 percent of patients undergoing immunotherapy show improvement after 1 to 2 years of treatment. Successful immunotherapy requires careful identification of the allergen and a compliant patient, since treatment involves a significant investment of time and resources over a 4- or 5-year course. Practitioners capable of interpreting the reactions in order to adjust the doses appropriately should do the primary management of immunotherapy.

BIBLIOGRAPHY

Austen KF: Diseases of immediate type hypersensitivity, in Fauci AS, Braunwald E, Isselbacher KJ, et al (eds): *Harrison's Principles of Internal Medicine,* 14th ed. New York, McGraw-Hill, 1998, pp 1860–1869.

Baroody FM: Allergic rhinitis caused by inhalant factors, in Rakel RE (ed): *Conn's Current Therapy 2000.* Philadelphia, Saunders, 2000, pp 743–748.

DeShazo RD: Allergic rhinitis, in Goldman L, Bennett JC (eds): *Cecil Textbook of Medicine,* 21st ed. Philadelphia, Saunders, 2000, pp 1445–1450.

Dixon HS, Dixon BJ: *Common Problems of the Head and Neck Region.* American Academy of Otolaryngology, Head and Neck Surgery Foundation. Philadelphia, Saunders, 1992.

Jackler RK, Kaplan MJ: Ear, nose, and throat, in Tierney LM Jr, McPhee SJ, Papadakis MA (eds): *Current Medical Diagnosis and Treatment,* 39th rev. ed. New York, McGraw-Hill, 2000, pp 240–241.

Kishiyama JL, Adelman DC: Allergic and immunologic disorders, in Tierney LM Jr, McPhee SJ, Papadakis MA (eds): *Current Medical Diagnosis and Treatment,* 39th rev. ed. New York, McGraw-Hill, 2000, pp 784–788.

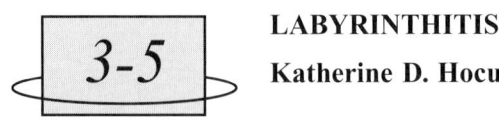

3-5

LABYRINTHITIS
Katherine D. Hocum

DISCUSSION

Acute labyrinthitis (vestibular neuronitis, inner-ear infection) is a benign condition that is more accurately described as a peripheral non-Ménière's vestibular disorder. While labyrinthitis may be caused by various bacteria (suppurative labyrinthitis), most often it is viral in origin and is more commonly known as vestibular neuronitis. Vestibular neuronitis (VN) is an acute unilateral infection or inflammation of the vestibular system. It is a common clinical condition that presents as severe vertigo, nystagmus, nausea, and vomiting. Symptoms such as tinnitus and hearing loss are most often absent. Patients often report a history of recent upper respiratory infection (URI). They also may have suffered recently from otitis media (OM) or sinusitis. Adolescents and young adults appear to be affected most often. A familial and/or seasonal component appears to be associated with this condition.

PATHOGENESIS

The pathophysiology of this syndrome appears to be secondary to a sudden unilateral disruption of the normal vestibular neural input to the brainstem and cerebral cortex. The brain erroneously interprets the altered neural input as violent head movement, and that misinterpretation is responsible for the vertigo. The vestibular symptoms are due in part to an isolated infection of the labyrinth or vestibular nerve by a virus after a recent URI. Paralysis of the vestibular nerve, as found in Bell's palsy, or inflammation of the nerve trunk has been suggested as a cause. After a viral URI, it appears that the virus may distribute itself into the ganglionic nuclei of the cranial nerves, where it remains latent for a short period. Upon replication, there is a sudden autoimmune reaction that causes inflammation and edema. Spontaneous reactivation of the virus is common after periods when inflammation is minimal. Inflammation and edema cause the vertigo.

SIGNS AND SYMPTOMS

The clinical features of vestibular neuronitis are severe rotational vertigo, nystagmus, nausea, and vomiting. There is an absence of tinnitus or hearing loss. Vertigo is persistent at first and then becomes paroxysmal. The patient also may present with ataxia. Nystagmus is horizontal-rotatory away from the affected ear. Central nervous system (CNS) deficits are not present. The condition lasts 7 to 10 days and is usually self-limiting. VN may occur as a single episode or, as in the majority of patients, paroxysmal episodes over 12 to 18 months. Generally, each subsequent attack is less severe and of shorter duration than the first.

OBJECTIVE FINDINGS

The evaluation of a patient presenting with a sudden onset of vertigo or dizziness poses a diagnostic challenge. Numerous disease states and conditions may cause vertigo, nystagmus, or ataxia. It is essential that the practitioner elicit an accurate and detailed history when evaluating a patient with dizziness. The diagnosis of VN is often a presumptive one that is based on the patient's history of sudden vertigo, nausea, and vomiting after a URI. While hearing loss and tinnitus usually are absent, disorders of the CNS or cardiovascular system and metabolic and psychiatric disorders should be considered (see Table 3-5-1).

The evaluation of any patient presenting with dizziness must include a complete physical examination of the head, eyes, ears, neck, nose, and throat. Hearing acuity and speech discrimination also should be tested. Examination of the tympanic membranes, unless the patient is suffering from OM, often is normal. Nystagmus is generally present and should be described accurately. Nystagmus should be horizontal-rotatory in nature and should move away from the affected side. A complete neurologic examination, including mental status, should be performed. Ataxia is not an uncommon finding in patients with VN. Evaluation of the endocrine, pulmonary, and cardiovascular systems should be included in any workup of a patient with dizziness.

DIAGNOSTIC CONSIDERATIONS

The initial step in the evaluation of the patient is to obtain an accurate description of the "dizziness." The vertigo associated with VN will

TABLE 3-5-1. Differential Diagnosis of Vestibular Neuronitis

Benign paroxysmal positional vertigo
Ménière's disease
Acoustic neuroma
Ototoxic medications
Vertebrobasilar insufficiency
Faintness and syncope
Vertiginous migraine
Hypo- and hypercapnia, hypoxia
Multiple sclerosis
Aortic stenosis
Anemia, hypovolemia
Depression, anxiety, another psychiatric illness
Epilepsy
Cervical spondylosis
Otosclerosis
Orthostatic blood pressure changes
Cerebellar disease
Space-occupying lesions
Trauma
Hyperventilation
Diabetes, hypoglycemia

remain present whether the patient opens or closes the eyes. Precipitating factors and the frequency or timing of vertigo should be elicited. Associated signs suggesting central vertigo (neurologic deficits) should be absent. There may be evidence of URI, OM, or sinusitis.

Benign paroxysmal positional vertigo (BPPV) and Ménière's disease are the diagnoses most likely to mimic VN. Ototoxicity and otosclerosis may present with similar symptoms. Acoustic neuroma should always be considered, although the lack of neurologic deficits should make this disorder unlikely. Metabolic disorders and psychiatric disorders also should be included in the differential diagnosis (Table 3-5-2).

SPECIAL CONSIDERATIONS

VN often follows a viral URI. Adolescents and young adults are the most frequently affected. There is often an occurrence of this disorder in members of the same family or during certain periods of the year. Patients with VN may have a past medical history of similar, more severe episodes.

TABLE 3-5-2. Differential Diagnosis of Dizziness

PERIPHERAL CAUSES	CENTRAL CAUSES	OTHER CAUSES
Benign paroxysmal positional vertigo	Vertebrobasilar insufficiency	Diabetes mellitus Anemia, hypovolemia
Labyrinthitis/vestibular neuronitis	Transient ischemic attack/ischemia	Psychiatric illness Orthostatic blood pressure changes
Trauma		
Ototoxic medications changes	Multiple sclerosis	
Otosclerosis	Tumors/neuroma	Medications
Neurosyphilis	Vestibular epilepsy	Aortic stenosis
Herpes zoster oticus	Cerebellar injury/disease	Migraine
	Cerebrovascular accident	

TABLE 3-5-3. Pharmacologic Management of Vestibular Neuronitis

AGENT	DOSE/ROUTE	COMMENTS
Diazepam (Valium)	5–10 mg IM or PO	Used most often for acute attacks
Trimethobenzamide hydrochloride (Tigan)	200 mg IM q12h	For severe nausea and vomiting
	250 mg PO q8h	For nausea and vomiting
Meclizine (Antivert)	25–50 mg PO q6h	Nausea and vomiting: 12.5 mg PO tid in elderly patients
Dimenhydrinate (Dramamine)	50 mg PO q6h	Do not operate machinery

LABORATORY TESTS

There is no laboratory test to confirm the diagnosis of VN.

DIAGNOSTICS

If the presence of neurologic signs associated with vertigo cannot be differentiated adequately, computed tomography (CT) and magnetic resonance imaging (MRI) are essential to rule out central lesions. Electronystagmography (ENG) also helps in the diagnosis of peripheral versus central vertigo.

TREATMENT

While VN is usually a self-limiting condition, the vertigo may be severe enough to require symptomatic treatment during the acute phase. Diazepam (Valium) 5 to 10 mg intramuscularly or orally may be helpful initially. Trimethobenzamide hydrochloride (Tigan) 200 mg intramuscularly every 12 h or 250-mg capsules orally every 8 h may relieve nausea and vomiting. Medications that sedate the vestibular system may be appropriate. Meclizine (Antivert) 25 to 50 mg orally every 6 h or dimenhydrinate (Dramamine) 50 mg orally every 6 h should relieve most patients. Patients who take vestibular sedatives should be advised about the drowsiness associated with these agents and should not operate machinery while under treatment. The use of steroids also has been successful in reducing inflammation of the vestibular nerve in some cases (see Table 3-5-3).

RED FLAGS

Isolated acute vertigo in an elderly patient may signify vascular disease (cerebral infarct, transient ischemic attack) in 25 percent of cases. Careful attention should be paid to the presence of neurologic signs and/or confusion. Diagnostic imaging studies (CT, MRI) are warranted in an elderly patient who presents with dizziness.

PEARLS

Most patients with VN require only reassurance and symptomatic treatment. Complications and sequelae are uncommon.

BIBLIOGRAPHY

Bates B, Bickley L, Hoekelman R (eds): *A Guide to Physical Examination and History Taking,* 6th ed. Philadelphia, Lippincott, 1995, pp 147–227.

Fauci AS, Braunwald E, Isselbacher KJ, et al (eds): *Harrison's Principles of Internal Medicine,* Harrison's on-line ed. New York, McGraw-Hill, 1999.

Gorroll AH, May L, Mulley A (eds): *Primary Care Medicine: Office Evaluation and Management of the Adult Patient.* Philadelphia, Lippincott, 1995, pp 985–1010.

Rakel RE: *Conn's Current Therapy.* Philadelphia, Saunders, 1999.

Shea JJ: Classification of Ménière's disease. *Am J Otolaryngol* 14(3):224–229, 1993.

Tran Ba Huy P: Physiopathology of peripheral non-Ménière's vestibular disorders. *Acta Otolaryngol* 513(Suppl):5–10, 1994.

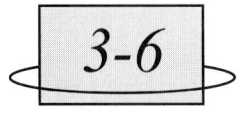

LARYNGITIS

Suzanne Warnimont

DISCUSSION

Laryngitis is an inflammation of the laryngeal mucous membranes. It is usually a viral disease that lasts a few days to a week. Adenoviruses and influenza are the most common causes of acute symptoms. Other causes include rhinovirus, coxsackievirus, and respiratory syncytial virus. Laryngitis often is associated with an upper respiratory infection (URI) and may persist even after other symptoms of the URI have resolved.

Bacterial causes include *Moraxella catarrhalis, Corynebacterium diphtheriae,* and *Haemophilus influenzae. Streptococcus pneumonia, Staphylococcus aureus,* and group A streptococci also may cause laryngitis associated with pharyngitis, sinusitis, or tonsillitis.

The history usually will determine the cause of laryngitis. It should include a history of vocal abuse, URI, trauma to the throat (including intubation), infectious or toxic exposure (including tobacco smoke, alcohol, fumes, smoke inhalation, and radiation), and gastrointestinal or pulmonary complaints.

SIGNS AND SYMPTOMS

Hoarseness and dysphonia (variation in vocal quality) are the most common symptoms. Occasionally, mild difficulty swallowing and/or an irritating cough are reported. Pain may be present, localized to the larynx or referred to the ear.

OBJECTIVE FINDINGS

Usually there are no objective findings. Fever with infectious causes may be present. There may be vesicles on the soft palate and lymphadenopathy. Indirect laryngoscopy reveals diffuse erythema, edema and vascular engorgement of the vocal folds, and perhaps mucosal ulcerations.

A thorough head and neck examination should be done. Indirect laryngoscopy should be done to look for inflammation, masses, vocal cord dysfunction, and structural abnormalities.

DIAGNOSTIC CONSIDERATIONS

Other causes of hoarseness should be ruled out. Persistent hoarseness that does not resolve after conservative treatment may be due to bronchogenic spread of tuberculosis, secondary or tertiary syphilis, rhinoscleroma, histoplasmosis, blastomycosis, coccidioidomycosis, candidiasis, aspergillosis, sporotrichosis, rhinosporidiosis, and parasitic infection.

It is important to rule out the following causes of persistent hoarseness:

- *Laryngeal polyps.* Caused by voice abuse or direct trauma (intubation). Appear as discrete polypoid growths on the true vocal cords.
- *Vocal nodules.* Also known as "singer's nodules" or "preacher's nodules." Caused by poor voice use or overuse. Seen as bilateral, discrete, pearly-white lesions at the junction of the anterior and middle third of the true vocal cords.

- *Laryngeal papillomatosis.* HPV types 6 and 11 can cause laryngeal and respiratory papillomatosis in young children and may be life-threatening. It usually is acquired from a maternal genital tract infection. In adults, it can be acquired by orogenital sexual contact and is usually mild. It is relatively uncommon in the United States but may be seen in immigrant populations.
- *Contact ulcers.* Caused by voice abuse. Occur as bilateral ulcerations at the tips of the vocal processes of the laryngeal cartilages, causing hoarseness and pain upon phonation. Biopsy is required to rule out carcinoma.
- *Hyperkeratosis* ("whiskey voice"). Associated with smoking and/or alcohol abuse. Vocal cords are thickened, rough, and covered with hyperkeratotic plaques, which often are premalignant. Refer for biopsy and follow-up.
- *Leukoplakia.* Related to voice and alcohol abuse and smoking. Appears as white, raised plaques at the anterior extremity of one vocal cord. It is premalignant, and biopsy with close follow-up is necessary.
- *Carcinoma.* The most serious cause of hoarseness. Any patient with a suspicious laryngeal lesion should be referred for direct laryngoscopy and biopsy.
- *Vocal cord paralysis.* Paralysis of one vocal cord can cause hoarseness. Patient should be referred for evaluation.

In young children, it is important to rule out epiglottitis, laryngotracheobronchitis, bacterial tracheitis, and foreign body aspiration (see Chaps. 17-4 and 4-5).

SPECIAL CONSIDERATIONS

Smoking and alcohol can aggravate simple laryngitis and are risk factors for more serious causes of persistent hoarseness.

LABORATORY TESTS

A white blood cell count with a differential should be done if infection is suspected. A culture from the throat or larynx is taken in certain cases.

RADIOLOGIC STUDIES

No radiologic studies are necessary unless there is evidence of airway compromise.

OTHER DIAGNOSTICS

Indirect or direct laryngoscopy is used to view the vocal cords. Biopsy may be necessary in selected cases.

TREATMENT

The underlying cause should be identified and treated. For most cases, voice rest, elimination of throat clearing, humidified air, and hydration will speed recovery. The condition is self-limiting.

Medications

Cough suppression may be necessary for irritative coughing. Relief of nasal congestion and humidified air may help. Other medications are given as indicated for bacterial infection or gastroesophageal reflux.

Patient Education

Patients should be instructed to use the voice as little as possible, since both shouting and whispering strain the vocal cords. If speaking is necessary, a normal tone of voice should be encouraged. Patients should avoid breathing extremely cold air. The use of tobacco and alcohol should be discouraged.

Disposition

Laryngitis is a self-limiting condition. Most patients recover their voices within 2 to 3 weeks or sooner. Chronic laryngitis or acute laryngitis that does not respond to treatment should be investigated further. Laryngeal polyps and vocal nodules require surgical removal. Patients with suspicious or premalignant lesions must be referred to an otolaryngologist for direct examination and biopsy.

COMPLICATIONS AND RED FLAGS

Voice abuse will cause repeated hoarseness. Speech therapy may be necessary to eliminate further abuse.

BIBLIOGRAPHY

Durand M, Joseph M, Baker AS: Infections of the upper respiratory tract, in Fauci A, Braunwald E, Isselbacher K, et al (eds): *Harrison's Principles of Internal Medicine,* 14th ed. New York, McGraw-Hill, 1998, pp 183, 1099.

Eason JV: Laryngitis clinical topics, in Ferri F (ed): *Clinical Advisor.* St. Louis, Mosby Year Book, 1999, pp 266.

Gwaltney JM: Acute laryngitis, in Mandell GL, Bennett JE, Dolin R (eds): *Principles and Practice of Infectious Diseases,* 4th ed, New York, Churchill Livingstone, 1995, pp 572–573.

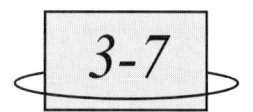

MÉNIÈRE'S DISEASE

Katherine D. Hocum

DISCUSSION

Ménière's disease (Ménière's syndrome, endolymphatic hydrops) is a pathologic condition of the inner ear that is characterized by episodic vertigo, tinnitus, and fluctuant sensorineural hearing loss. It is a poorly understood progressive disorder that affects over 2 million people in the United States. It is four times as prevalent as otosclerosis and more common than all carcinomas and tumors involving the larynx and salivary glands. It is seen most frequently in adults 20 to 60 years of age. The frequency with which Ménière's disease occurs in the right or left ear is equal. Similarly, there is no gender predilection; it occurs in males as often as it does in females. One in three patients may suffer from bilateral disease. While the triad of vertigo, tinnitus, and hearing loss dominates the clinical presentation, many patients may complain of a sensation of "fullness" in the affected ear. Vegetative symptoms such as nausea and vomiting are also reported commonly.

PATHOGENESIS

It is believed that the symptoms of Ménière's disease result from a malfunction of the endolymphatic sac in the inner ear. Although the etiology is often idiopathic, it has been postulated that the condition results from an imbalance between the amount of endolymph produced by the cochlea and the amount absorbed by the endolymphatic sac, leading to a consistent finding of endolymphatic hydrops. The increased hydrostatic pressure produced by the accumulation of endolymph subsequently causes dizziness and the sensation of aural fullness. As the hydrops becomes more extensive, hearing loss ensues. This chronic distention of the endolymphatic system results in a dysfunction of vestibular and cochlear hair cells that is presumed to cause the chronic disequilibrium and irreversible hearing loss reported by these patients. The etiologic basis of Ménière's disease appears to be multifactorial as well as inherited in many patients. Whites appear to be at increased risk, along with those with a history of allergy or excessive exposure to noise. While no single mechanism leading to endolymphatic hydrops can be identified, currently most clinical research and therapeutic measures focus on elimination of the hydrops and identification of viral, autoimmune, and metabolic factors (lipid disorders, allergy) that may lead to the formation of endolymphatic hydrops. Clearly, further research into the pathophysiology of Ménière's disease is necessary to develop stricter diagnostic criteria and suitable treatment modalities.

SIGNS AND SYMPTOMS

The clinical features of Ménière's disease have been described as a triad of symptoms: recurrent debilitating vertigo, progressive sensorineural hearing loss, and tinnitus. These patients also may complain of aural pressure or fullness in the affected ear as well as nausea and vomiting associated with vertiginous episodes. Usually these symptoms appear together, although it is not uncommon for tinnitus or diminution of hearing to precede the onset of vertigo. The onset of vertigo is usually sudden and often disabling. The vertigo may last minutes or hours but rarely lasts longer than 24 to 48 h. Persistent vertigo that lasts longer than this suggests a diagnosis other than Ménière's disease. Some patients may report loudness recruitment and diplacusis associated with this condition. Vestibular nystagmus may be present during attacks; however, neurologic signs such as loss of consciousness, aphasia, headache, aura, and paresthesias are clinically absent. Progressive loss of speech discrimination leads to an irreversible hearing loss that does not improve with the use of a hearing aid. Ménière's disease attacks, while unpredictable, are usually short-lived and self-limiting. Patients frequently are well between vertiginous episodes.

OBJECTIVE FINDINGS

A patient presenting with vertigo or dizziness can represent a diagnostic challenge. Numerous disease states and conditions may cause vertigo, deafness, tinnitus, disequilibrium, or a combination of these symptoms. It is essential that the practitioner elicit an accurate and detailed history when evaluating a dizzy patient. The diagnosis of Ménière's disease is often a presumptive one based on patient complaints of fluctuating sensorineural hearing loss, episodic vertigo, and tinnitus. It is also a diagnosis of exclusion, as conditions affecting the central nervous system and the cardiovascular system and metabolic or psychiatric disorders all may present with similar features and must be considered (see Table 3-7-1).

A complete physical examination of the head, eyes, ears, nose, neck, and throat is a must. Hearing acuity and speech discrimination should be tested. Examination often shows normal tympanic membranes (TMs), as no observable anatomic or morphologic changes are associated with the vertigo, hearing loss, tinnitus, and aural fullness of Ménière's disease. Nystagmus, if present, should be described accurately. A thorough neurologic examination, including reflexes, mental status, and gait, should be performed. Care should be taken to assess the cardiovascular, pulmonary, and endocrine systems adequately. Frequently, patients presenting with Ménière's disease have an unremarkable physical examination.

DIAGNOSTIC CONSIDERATIONS

The initial step in evaluating the patient is to obtain an accurate description of the "dizziness." True vertigo, as experienced in Ménière's disease, typically is described as a sensation of one's environment "spinning" or "everything moving." Precipitating factors, if any, and the frequency and timing of the vertigo should be elicited. The patient also should be encouraged to relate any other symptoms associated with the episodes. Vestibular vertigo may be central or peripheral in origin, and the practitioner should be aware of conditions that mimic Ménière's disease but arise from significantly different causes.

TABLE 3-7-1. Differential Diagnosis of Dizziness

Benign paroxysmal positional vertigo
Labyrinthitis or vestibular neuronitis
Ménière's disease
Acoustic neuroma
Ototoxic medications
Vertebrobasilar insufficiency
Faintness and syncope
Vertebrobasilar migraine
Hypo- and hypercapnia, hypoxia
Multiple sclerosis
Aortic stenosis
Anemia, hypovolemia
Depression, anxiety, other psychiatric illnesses
Epilepsy
Cervical spondylosis
Otosclerosis
Orthostatic blood pressure changes
Cerebellar disease
Space-occupying lesions
Temporal bone trauma, perilymphatic fistula
Hyperventilation
Diabetes, hypoglycemia

Typically, isolated vertigo with or without tinnitus and hearing loss arises from a peripheral lesion. In patients with central lesions, vertigo often is accompanied by neurologic deficits (see Table 3-7-2).

Benign paroxysmal positional vertigo (BPPV) is sudden isolated vertigo that is experienced when the head is moved into specific positions. The symptoms are self-limiting but may resume when the patient moves into a "trigger" position. BPPV may last up to 6 months, and recovery is often spontaneous and complete. Labyrinthitis, which sometimes is called vestibular neuronitis, develops in the inner ear after a viral upper respiratory infection (URI). Any vertigo, hearing loss, or tinnitus is temporary and usually resolves spontaneously within 3 to 6 weeks. Ototoxicity, otosclerosis, and herpes zoster oticus may have a similar presentation. Acoustic neuroma should always be considered, though the accompanying neurologic signs (decreased corneal reflex, ataxia) often make the diagnosis clear. Central causes of vertigo are often more worrisome. Multiple sclerosis (MS), vertebrobasilar insufficiency, and a decompensated cardiovascular system may present initially as vertigo. Often these conditions, like transient ischemic attacks (TIAs), are accompanied by other signs and symptoms, making the diagnosis of

TABLE 3-7-2. Central Versus Peripheral Vertigo

SIGNS OR SYMPTOMS	PERIPHERAL VERTIGO	CENTRAL VERTIGO
Severity of vertigo	Marked, spontaneous	Often mild, gradual
Tinnitus/hearing loss	Usually present	Usually absent
Vertical nystagmus	Never	Occasionally
Horizontal nystagmus	Uncommon	Common
Duration	Finite, intermittent	Variable, chronic
Central nervous system signs	None	Common

TABLE 3-7-3. Differential Diagnosis of Ménière's Disease

PERIPHERAL CAUSES	CENTRAL CAUSES	OTHER CAUSES
Benign paroxysmal positional vertigo	Vertebrobasilar insufficiency	Diabetes mellitus
Labyrinthitis/ vestibular neuronitis	Transient ischemic attack/ ischemia	Anemia, hypovolemia
Trauma	Multiple sclerosis	Psychiatric illness
Ototoxic medications	Tumors/neuroma	Orthostatic blood pressure changes
Otosclerosis	Vestibular epilepsy	Medications
Neurosyphilis	Cerebellar injury/ disease	Aortic stenosis
Herpes zoster oticus	Cerebrovascular accident	Migraine

Ménière's disease less likely. Psychiatric illness (depression, anxiety states) and metabolic disorders (hypoxia, drug overdose) also should be considered in evaluating a patient with dizziness (see Table 3-7-3).

SPECIAL CONSIDERATIONS

An elderly patient with vertigo is likely to be the most difficult to diagnose. Many geriatric patients complain of dizziness and suffer from one or more multisystem disorders (diabetes, TIA) that may make the diagnosis complicated.

LABORATORY TESTS

No single laboratory test or battery of tests can confirm the diagnosis of Ménière's disease. The diagnosis is often presumptive after a thorough history and physical examination.

RADIOLOGIC STUDIES

Computed tomography (CT) and magnetic resonance imaging (MRI) of the internal auditory canal and cerebellopontine angles should always be performed to rule out localized or space-occupying lesions.

OTHER DIAGNOSTICS

Electronystagmography (ENG) with warm and cold calorics differentiates between central and peripheral causes of vertigo. Audiologic testing to document hearing loss also is indicated. If neuroma of the eighth cranial nerve is suspected, brainstem auditory response testing should be performed. Electroencephalography (EEG) will aid in the diagnosis of epilepsy or migraine. Patients should not be medicated with vestibular sedatives during testing, as these agents may affect the response or invalidate the diagnostic study altogether.

TREATMENT

Treatment of Ménière's disease may be medical or surgical. While it is clear that there is no universally effective treatment for patients with this disease, most treatment modalities are aimed at reducing endolymphatic hydrops or symptomatically suppressing the vertigo. Until the definitive etiology of Ménière's disease is elucidated, treatment will remain only moderately effective in the majority of patients.

Pharmacologic Treatment

For an acutely disabled patient, diazepam (Valium) 5 mg intramuscularly or 10 mg orally may be helpful. Trimethobenzamide hydrochloride (Tigan) capsules 250 mg every 8 h (adults) or 100 mg every 8 h (children) may be administered to control nausea and vomiting. If the nausea and vomiting are severe, the intramuscular route, 200 mg every 12 h, should be considered. Medications that sedate

TABLE 3-7-4. Pharmacologic Management of Ménière's Disease

AGENT	DOSE/ROUTE	COMMENTS
Diazepam (Valium)	5–10 mg IM or PO	Used most often for acute attacks
Trimethobenzamide hydrochloride (Tigan)	200 mg IM q12h	For severe nausea and vomiting
Meclizine (Antivert)	25–50 mg PO q6h	For nausea and vomiting
Dimenhydrinate (Dramamine)	25–50 mg PO q6h	Nausea and vomiting: 12.5 mg PO tid in elderly patients
Hydrochlorothiazide (Hydro-Diuril)	50 mg PO tid	Do not operate machinery
Triamterene (Dyrenium)	25–50 mg PO / 50 mg PO	Check serum potassium / Check serum potassium

the vestibular system, such as meclizine (Antivert) and dimenhydrinate (Dramamine), are also effective. Antivert 25 to 50 mg orally every 6 h or Dramamine 50 mg orally every 6 h should relieve most patients. Both agents may cause considerable drowsiness. Patients should be warned against driving or operating machinery while medicated. Lower doses in elderly patients may be less sedating but equally effective. For a patient with an established diagnosis of Ménière's disease, treatment is aimed at preventing vertiginous episodes through diet modification and diuretics. Hydrochlorothiazide (Hydro-Diuril) 25 to 50 mg orally or triamterene (Dyrenium) 50 mg once a day is effective as a long-term treatment. Patients also are encouraged to maintain a low-salt diet (1 to 2 g sodium per day). Some clinicians believe that a vasodilating agent such as papaverine hydrochloride (Pavabid) 150 mg orally bid or cyclandelate (Cyclospasmol) 200 mg orally tid may aid endolymph resorption. The majority of patients with Ménière's disease, however, can be controlled adequately on diuretic therapy coupled with diet modification and vestibular sedatives as needed. Patients who are unresponsive to pharmacologic management may be candidates for surgical intervention (see Table 3-7-4).

Surgical Management

While medical therapies are the first-line treatment for patients with Ménière's disease, some patients do not respond to these conservative measures. Procedures designed to drain the endolymphatic system or ablate the eighth cranial nerve and/or labyrinth may be warranted in aggressive cases. Decompression of the endolymphatic sac and internal shunt placement may be achieved by means of sacculotomy or cochleosacculotomy. The results are highly variable with these procedures, and while they may reduce vertigo, they often precipitate sensorineural hearing loss. Labyrinthectomy is currently the gold standard in surgical treatment of Ménière's disease, relieving episodic vertigo in the majority of cases. Intratympanic instillation of ototoxic antibiotics such as gentamicin and streptomycin has been successful in relieving vertigo while preserving hearing in many patients. Surgical resection of the eighth nerve has had some success in controlling vertigo but is associated with postsurgical complications such as headache, hearing loss, and an incomplete vestibular response. Patients affected with bilateral disease make the choice of treatment a greater challenge, as preservation of hearing in at least one ear is desirable.

COMPLICATIONS AND RED FLAGS

Irreversible sensorineural hearing loss is the major complication of Ménière's disease. These patients are also at increased risk for falls and accidents secondary to vertigo, disequilibrium, and/or sedation associated with medical therapy. Patients on diuretic therapy should be encouraged to keep well hydrated, and practitioners may want to evaluate their serum potassium levels periodically.

OTHER NOTES AND PEARLS

Current management of Ménière's disease provides most patients with symptomatic relief only. Patients are advised to avoid caffeine, alcohol, and smoking. Stress reduction may help. Newer diagnostic tools such as electrocochleography (ECoG), inner-ear-specific immunoassays, and labyrinthine MRIs may be employed. Human genetic studies may one day allow gene manipulation therapy, making symptomatic treatment obsolete. Future diagnostic techniques and treatment modalities will require well-controlled, multicenter research studies.

BIBLIOGRAPHY

Bates B, Bickley L, Hoekelman R (eds): *A Guide to Physical Examination and History Taking,* 6th ed. Philadelphia, Lippincott, 1995, pp 147–227.

Fauci AS, Braunwald E, Isselbacher KJ, et al (eds): *Harrison's Principles of Internal Medicine,* Harrison's on-line ed. New York, McGraw-Hill, 1999.

Gorroll A, May L, Mulley A (eds): *Primary Care Medicine: Office Evaluation and Management of the Adult Patient.* Philadelphia, Lippincott, 1995, pp 985–1010.

Isenhower WD: The evaluation and diagnosis of the dizzy patient. *J S C Med Assoc* 90(10):517–522, 1994.

Merchant SN: Meniere's disease. *Eur Arch Otorhinolaryngol* 252:63–75, 1995.

Monsell EM: Therapeutic use of aminoglycosides in Ménière's disease. *Otolaryngol Clin North Am* 26(5):737–746, 1993.

Norrving B: Isolated vertigo in the elderly: Vestibular or vascular disease? *Acta Neurol Scand* 91:43–48, 1995.

Rakel RE: *Conn's Current Therapy 1999.* Philadelphia, Saunders, 1999, pp 858–878.

Rakel RE: *Textbook of Family Practice,* 5th ed. Philadelphia, Saunders, 1995, pp 441–480.

Shea JJ: Classification of Meniere's disease. *Am J Otolaryngol* 14(3):224–229, 1993.

Sullivan M: Psychiatric and otologic diagnoses in patients complaining of dizziness. *Arch Intern Med* 153(12):1479–1484, 1993.

Tran Ba Huy P: Physiopathology of peripheral non-Ménière's vestibular disorders. *Acta Otolaryngol* 513(Suppl):5–10, 1994.

Walker JS: Dizziness: The difficult diagnosis. *Emerg Med Clin North Am* 16(4):845–875, 1998.

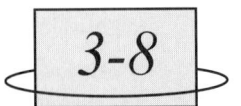

PERITONSILLAR ABSCESS
Nadine Kroenke

DISCUSSION

Peritonsillar abscess (PTA) is one of the most commonly seen abscesses of the head and neck area. PTA is a complication of tonsillitis, peritonsillar cellulitis (PTC), and mononucleosis. The abscess forms as a result of an infection extending from within the tonsil through its fibrous capsule into the peritonsillar space and then the peritonsillar fascial planes. The peritonsillar space is designated as the area of the neck between the capsule of the palatine tonsil medially and the fascia of the superior constrictor muscle laterally.

The classic onset of PTA symptoms usually begins only 3 to 5 days before patients seek treatment. Many patients are currently on appropriate antibiotics for a preceding tonsillitis.

PTC and abscess formation are fairly common occurrences in young adults, with the average patient's age being less than 30 years. It is relatively rare in young children and older adults. Occurrences in young children and older adults should alert the clinician to an underlying susceptibility to infection from immune deficiency, malnutrition, leukemia, or another systemic disease. There has been no agreement on sex distribution. PTA has the highest incidence in the winter months.

Peritonsillar abscess is most often polymicrobial, with anaerobic bacteria being recovered most often. The most common aerobic isolates are *Streptococcus pyogenes, S. milleri, Haemophilus influenzae,* and *S. viridans.* Generally, the abscess forms in the supratonsillar space of the soft palate immediately above the superior pole of the affected tonsil. The supratonsillar space initially becomes inflamed, and cellulitis begins. This results in pus formation in the supratonsillar space and the surrounding muscle, which produces trismus.

No reliable criteria exist for differentiating PTA from PTC on physical examination. A practitioner familiar with the procedure can differentiate the diagnosis of PTA and PTC by means of careful needle aspiration of the affected tissue. If aspiration in three loci yields negative findings, the patient is diagnosed as having PTC. Aspiration may be stopped after one positive aspirate. An otolaryngologist [ear, nose, and throat (ENT) specialist] may also make the diagnosis after the patient's clinical course has been followed.

SIGNS AND SYMPTOMS

The typical presentation of a patient with PTC or PTA occurs about 2 to 3 days after the onset of a sore throat. Many of these patients are on appropriate antibiotics for pharyngitis. Patients will describe the classic symptoms of pharyngitis, such as fever, sore throat, and odynophagia (pain on swallowing). They also may complain that the sore throat is much worse on the side of the abscess. Other symptoms include referred ear pain, headache, and malaise. Patients may complain of trouble handling secretions and may be actively drooling.

OBJECTIVE FINDINGS

Physical examination of a patient with PTA/PTC reveals a patient in mild to moderate distress secondary to pain. Low-grade fever and mild tachycardia is present. A distinctive "hot potato" voice is often noted during the history taking. Palpation of the neck reveals ipsilateral anterior chain lymph node enlargement. The patient may be drooling, spitting, or having trouble handling oral secretions. Trismus is noted in attempts to visualize the oral pharynx. Trismus is considered the leading clinical finding helpful in differentiating PTA/PTC from severe tonsillitis. Visualization of the oropharynx reveals a deviated uvula with unilateral peritonsillar swelling. The posterior pharynx will be diffusely erythematous. Exudate may or may not be present.

DIAGNOSTIC CONSIDERATIONS

Differential diagnosis for PTA includes pharyngitis, tonsillitis, PTC, and retropharyngeal abscess.

SPECIAL CONSIDERATIONS

All pediatric patients should be treated with a trial of intravenous hydration and antibiotics when no airway compromise is present and if no improvement is observed within 24 h. If symptoms worsen, surgery should be performed. It is not recommended to attempt a needle aspiration on a child without general anesthesia.

LABORATORY TESTS

Fluid aspirate culture from a PTA may be obtained, depending on the practitioner's preference. It is recommended in every immunosuppressed patient. Cultures often do not change patient management and outcome.

RADIOLOGIC STUDIES

Because the treatment of PTA and PTC are different and since needle aspiration is a painful invasive procedure, computed tomography scans of the neck and intraoral ultrasound are being used increasingly in some institutions to aid in the differential diagnosis.

TREATMENT

PTC can be treated with antibiotics alone, whereas a PTA should be drained. Treatment options when the abscess has already formed include incision and drainage, needle aspiration, and immediate tonsillectomy followed by intramuscular or intravenous penicillin. None of the surgical interventions has been identified as the optimal procedure for the drainage of a PTA. Tonsillectomy is considered the definitive treatment. There have been reports of recurrence with this method, however.

Pharmacological Management

Currently, penicillin is the recommended drug of choice: 1.2 million units of Bicillin LA administered intramuscularly. Other antibiotics, such as clindamycin, amoxicillin/clavulanic acid (Augmentin), and third-generation cephalosporins are appropriate. However, they should by administered only after consultation with an ENT specialist.

DISPOSITION

Primary outpatient management of PTA is recommended by present and prior studies. Patients appropriate for outpatient treatment are those who are nontoxic, compliant, without drooling or severe pain, and taking oral fluid well. Follow-up by an ENT specialist should be done within 24 h. The patient should be seen midway through the course of treatment and again 1 week after finishing antibiotics.

Patients should be admitted for incision and drainage under general anesthesia when they are dyspneic, in severe pain, have excessive trismus on physical exam, or are too young to undergo needle aspiration. Inpatient treatment is required in approximately 15% of cases, and an individual stay usually does not exceed an average of 2 days. Patients should be seen again promptly for any recurrence of symptoms.

COMPLICATIONS AND RED FLAGS

The most common complications are recurrent tonsillitis and recurrent PTA, which occur in about 10% of these patients. The factors related to the recurrence of PTA are unclear. The general time frame for recurrence is 3 months. An untreated PTA may rupture, leading to aspiration and pneumonia. Spreading infection of the parapharyngeal spaces can lead to mediastinitis and meningitis. Other complications of peritonsillar cellulitis and PTA are endocarditis, polyarthritis, cervical abscess, and sepsis. When the patient is treated early with appropriate incision and drainage and antibiotics, these complications can be avoided. Antibiotic treatment has led to rare complications and limited mortality.

BIBLIOGRAPHY

Ahmed K et al: Radiology in focus: The role of ultrasound in the management of peritonsillar abscess. *J Laryngol Otol* 108:610–612, 1994.
Blokmanis A: Ultrasound in the diagnosis and management of peritonsillar abscesses. *J Otolaryngol* 23:260–262, 1994.
Fauci AS et al (eds): *Harrison's Principles of Internal Medicine,* 14th ed. New York, McGraw-Hill, 1998, p 183.
Passy V: Pathogenesis of peritonsillar abscess. *Laryngoscope* 104:185–190, 1994.
Roberts J: Emergency department considerations in the diagnosis and treatment of peritonsillar abscess. *Emerg Med News* 2:4–7, 1996.
Sakaguchi M et al: Radiology in focus: Computed tomographic findings in peritonsillar abscess and cellulitis. *J Laryngol Otol* 109(5):449–451, 1995.
Strong E et al: Intraoral ultrasound evaluation of peritonsillar abscess. *Laryngoscope* 105:779–782, 1995.
Tintinalli J et al (eds): *Emergency Medicine: A Comprehensive Study Guide.* New York, McGraw-Hill, 1996, pp 1077–1078.

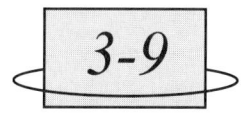

PHARYNGITIS/TONSILLITIS
Nadine Kroenke

DISCUSSION

Sore throat is one of the most frequently encountered outpatient complaints, accounting for over 40 million outpatient visits per year. Pharyngitis/tonsillitis is reported to be anywhere from the third to the seventh most common emergency department diagnosis. These statistics demand a well-structured treatment plan and follow-up.

The disease involves inflammation and infection of the oropharynx and the associated lymphoid tissue. Microbiology reveals that up to 80% of adult patients have pharyngitis/tonsillitis that is viral in etiology. Some of the more common viral agents are adenovirus and herpesvirus, which cause significant symptoms, and rhinovirus and coronavirus, which are more common and typically cause a milder course. Anywhere from 5 to 20% of bacterial infections are due to group-A β-hemolytic streptococci (GABHS) in adults. GABHS accounts for up to 50% of all cases of pediatric pharyngitis/tonsillitis, making this the most common bacterial pathogen in both the pediatric and the adult populations. GABHS has the most serious consequences to health; therefore, treatment is directed at GABHS. Other bacterial etiologic agents in adults are *Mycoplasma, Chlamydia,* and *Corynebacterium.*

Pharyngitis/tonsillitis is most commonly seen in children ages 5 to 15 years with no noted sex prevalence. This infection is most common in the winter and spring. Children are at increased risk because of exposure at school. The disease is spread through direct contact via droplet spread. The course of all types of pharyngitis/tonsillitis is about 1 week. Fever usually resolves in about 3 days, with improvement of the sore throat and other associated symptoms afterward. Lymph node enlargement and tonsillar hypertrophy may take several weeks to resolve.

SIGNS AND SYMPTOMS

The typical incubation period of streptococcal pharyngitis is 2 to 3 days. Classically, GABHS infection is described as the abrupt onset of sore throat and odynophagia (pain on swallowing). Other associated symptoms include headache, malaise, fever, anorexia, "sandpaper" rash, arthralgias, and myalgias. Nausea, vomiting, and abdominal pain are common complaints in children. It is important to remember that the sore throat complaint may be a minor component in the patient's presentation. Cough and rhinorrhea suggest a viral etiology. Viral pharyngitis has no distinguishing features to suggest a specific causative agent.

OBJECTIVE FINDINGS

Regardless of the specific etiology, the patient is likely to be moderately ill with tachycardia and fever, usually higher than 38.3°C (101°F). Examination of the throat reveals infection, erythema, and lymphoid hyperplasia of the posterior pharynx. The tonsils, if present, may be enlarged and erythematous, with or without exudate. Neck examination will reveal tender and enlarged anterior cervical chain lymph nodes. Patients who have had a tonsillectomy tend to experience a milder clinical course.

Fever is considered the most commonly occurring symptom in children with GABHS. The combination of fever, exudate, and tender, enlarged lymph nodes tends to be regarded as the most sensitive indicator of GABHS. Patients with these symptoms have positive throat cultures 30 to 45% of the time. Petechiae of the soft palate have a tendency to be found only in streptococcal infection. A scarlatiniform rash or "strawberry" tongue is also considered pathognomonic of streptococcal disease. Physical examination is considered unreliable in differentiating streptococcal infection from a viral or other bacterial infection. Even the best practitioners have been found to be correct on the basis of physical findings alone only about 50% of the time.

DIAGNOSTIC CONSIDERATIONS

While GABHS is the most common bacterial pathogen, other bacterial and viral causes should be considered in the differential diagnosis. *Chlamydia* occurs in adults predisposed by oro-genital sexual activity (see Chap. 9-6). *Mycoplasma* is associated with lower respiratory tract infections and headache. *Haemophilus influenzae,* which is more commonly found in pediatric patients, is usually found to cause pharyngitis, otitis media, laryngotracheitis, and epiglottitis. Diphtheria, which is rare in the current immunized population, is characterized by the presence of a gray exudative membrane that bleeds easily (see Chap. 9-10).

Mononucleosis should be considered in patients with exudative tonsillitis that is unresponsive to antibiotics, has a lingering course, and features posterior chain lymph node enlargement and abdominal pain (see Chap. 3-3). Noninfectious causes should be considered when the patient does not improve as expected; consider agranulocytosis, leukemia, and lymphoma (see Chaps. 8-2 and 13-11).

SPECIAL CONSIDERATIONS

Patients who are refractory to antibiotic therapy suggest a resistant bacteriologic or viral etiology. Therefore, other laboratory tests may be indicated at that time. In known streptococcal infections, the Infectious Diseases Society of America's guidelines recommend that treatment failure may be considered after no response at 3 to 5 days of therapy and alternative therapy, and diagnostics should be considered at that time. It is important to remember that lack of compliance accounts for a significant proportion of treatment failures—ascertain compliance before regarding a patient as a treatment failure.

LABORATORY TESTS

While 90% sensitive, the rapid strep latex agglutination test has a specificity of only about 80%. A negative strep screen does not indicate the absence of GABHS. Literature review recommends that all negative rapid strep screens be followed with routine culture. Obtaining this test depends on the individual clinical situation, compliance, and the availability of follow-up. Rapid strep screens are helpful when there are multiple children in the same family. The known presence or absence of GABHS can help determine the treatment of other family members if they become symptomatic. It is important to remember that a routine culture that is positive for GABHS may not always indicate the pathogen. Approximately 5 to 30% of all patients are considered chronic carriers of GABHS. Streptococcal carriers appear at no risk for rheumatic fever or suppurative complications or for transmission of infection to others.

A Monospot test may be obtained to rule out mononucleosis. This test is often negative in the early phase. In a complete blood count with differential, looking for reactive lymphocytes can by helpful. An anti-streptolysin O (ASO) titer may be obtained but is rarely useful in the acute setting.

RADIOLOGIC STUDIES

No radiology studies are indicated for routine pharyngitis/tonsillitis unless the diagnosis is unclear.

PHARMACOLOGIC MANAGEMENT

The treatment of pharyngitis is directed at preventing nonsuppurative complications of GABHS. Therapy may relieve signs and symptoms of infection and reduce the transmission risk. Penicillin remains the drug of choice (see Table 3-9-1). Steroids have recently become accepted adjuncts to the treatment of both bacterial and viral pharyngitis. Decadron, 10 mg intramuscularly, has been shown to provide quicker resolution of symptoms with no increased incidence of complications.

SUPPORTIVE MEASURES

Hydration, antipyretics, rest, and pain medications can provide supportive care. Aspirin should be avoided in children and teenagers because of the possibility of Reye's syndrome. Ibuprofen is an excellent choice for pain and inflammation in both adults and children.

PATIENT EDUCATION

Patients should be encouraged to complete the full course of antibiotics and maintain adequate hydration. A patient should be seen again if a rash or arthralgia develops or if symptoms are not progressively improving. Adults and children are no longer considered infectious after 24 h of continuous therapy and may return to work, day care, or school without restrictions while on medication. Virtually all these patients can be managed on an outpatient basis. Patients can return to their usual activities when they are improved.

COMPLICATIONS

Streptococcal pharyngitis is associated with two delayed nonsuppurative sequelae: acute rheumatic fever, which can be prevented by treatment up to 2 weeks after onset, and acute glomerulonephritis, which may occur regardless of treatment. Streptococcal infection of the pharynx may lead to acute otitis media and sinusitis. Other diseases that may develop secondarily to streptococcal infection include cervical lymphadenitis, retropharyngeal and parapharyngeal abscess, peritonsillar cellulitis and/or abscess, toxic shock syndrome, and scarlet fever.

TABLE 3-9-1. Treatment for Adults and Children

Adults

Bicillin LA, 1.2 million U intramuscularly
Penicillin VK, 250 mg or 500 mg qid for 10 days
Amoxicillin, 250 mg or 500 mg tid for 10 days
Erythromycin, 20–40 mg/kg per day divided bid or qid for 7–10 days (if the patient is allergic to penicillin)
Cephalexin (Keflex), 500 mg qid for 7–10 days
Cefadroxil (Duricef), 1–2 g divided qid or bid for 7–10 days
Cefaclor (Ceclor), 250 mg tid for 7–10 days
Cefuroxime (Ceftin), 250–500 mg bid for 7–10 days
Azithromycin (Zithromax), 500 mg daily for 5 days
Clarithromycin (Biaxin), 250–500 mg bid for 10 days
Cefixime (Suprax), 400 mg PO or 200 mg bid for 10 days
Ceftibuten (Cedax), 400 mg qd for 10 days

Children

Bicillin LA, 600,000 U intramuscularly for patients 27 kg or less
Penicillin VK suspension (or tablets), 125–250 mg qid for 10 days
Amoxicillin suspension, 40 mg/kg per day divided tid for 10 days
Erythromycin elixir, 30–50 mg/kg per day divided tid for 10 days
Pediazole suspension, 50 mg/kg per day divided qid for 10 days
Azithromycin (Zithromax) suspension, 12 mg/kg once daily for days 1 through 5
Ceftibuten (Cedax) suspension, 90 mg/day qid if 10 kg, 180 mg/day if 20 kg, 360 mg/day if 40 kg, 400 mg/day if 45 kg
Clarithromycin (Biaxin) suspension, 7.5 mg/kg bid for 10 days
Cefixime (Suprax) suspension, 8 mg/kg per day divided qid/bid

BIBLIOGRAPHY

Bisno, AL: Acute pharyngitis: Etiology and diagnosis. *Pediatrics* 97(supp l6): 949–954, 1996.

Bonilla J, Bluestone C: Pharyngitis: When is aggressive treatment warranted? *Postgrad Med* 97:61–69,1995.

Esposito S et al: Clinical comparison of cefaclor twice daily versus amoxicillin-clavulanate or erythromycin three times daily in the treatment of patients with streptococcal pharyngitis. *Clin Ther* 20(1):72–79, 1998.

Kaplan EL: Clinical guidelines for group A streptococcal throat infections. *Lancet* 350(9082):899–900, 1997.

Kearsely Nl et al: Comparison of clarithromycin suspension and amoxicillin syrup for the treatment of children with pharyngitis and/or tonsillitis. *Br J Clin Pract* 51(3):133–137, 1997.

Scaglione F et al: Optimum treatment of streptococcal pharyngitis. *Drugs* 53(1):86–97, 1997.

Tarlow MJ: Marcrolides in the management of streptococcal pharyngitis/tonsillitis. *Pediatr Infect Dis J* 16(4):444–448, 1997.

Thatai D, Turi ZG: Current guidelines for the treatment of patients with rheumatic fever. *Drugs* 57(4): 545–555, 1999.

Vukmir R: Adult and pediatric pharyngitis: A review. *Emerg Med Rev* 10: 607–616, 1992.

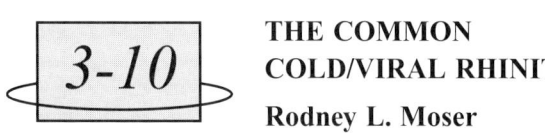

THE COMMON COLD/VIRAL RHINITIS

Rodney L. Moser

DISCUSSION

Viral upper respiratory illness (URI), or the common cold, is one of the most common community illnesses. In most cases, it is self-diagnosed and treated by the patient with a vast armada of over-the-counter medications designed for symptomatic relief. The economic impact of URI is staggering. Estimates of annual expenditures for medications used in therapy for the common cold exceed $2 billion annually.[1] Viral URIs are self-limiting—it is said that a cold lasts a week if it is treated, and 7 days if you leave it alone.

PATHOGENESIS

The common cold (URI) is caused by numerous serologic types of viruses. (see Table 3-10-1). The rhinoviruses account for 30 to 50 percent of the cases. Rhinoviruses have over 100 antigenically different, mutating types that easily find susceptible human hosts. Coronaviruses are the next most prevalent virus, accounting for 10 to 20 percent, followed by the adenoviruses (5 percent), parainfluenza viruses (5 percent), respiratory syncytial viruses (5 percent), influenza viruses (5 percent), and others.

Children from 6 months to 6 years of age average 6 to 10 "colds" per year, depending on their exposures. Children in day-care settings have a higher incidence of upper respiratory infections of all types. Adults tend to have 3 to 4 colds per year, mostly in fall and winter.

Influenza virus, parainfluenza virus, and adenovirus present with a more severe influenza-like syndrome often involving the lower respiratory tract, whereas rhinovirus and coronavirus present with the more common nasal mucosal irritation and scratchy, irritated sore throat. Seasonal peaks of URIs in the early fall and spring usually are caused by rhinovirus, while winter peaks are attributed to coronavirus.

It is difficult to distinguish between the various viruses from a clinical examination alone, and often the severity of the illness may be the only clue. Early fall peaks of the common cold are often attributed to the start of school and the spread of virus particles by schoolchildren. Contrary to popular belief, cold temperature (or temperature change) is not an important factor in the epidemiology of colds, although the crowding associated with colder weather does promote the spread of

TABLE 3-10-1. Etiologic Viruses in the Common Cold

VIRUS	FREQUENCY (%)	COMMENT
Rhinovirus	30–50	Most common cause—$\frac{1}{3}$ to $\frac{1}{2}$ of all colds; 100 serotypes; starts in Sept, peaks again in Feb/Mar; can occur all year
Coronavirus	10–20	Winter season; highest Dec/Jan; occurs often in older children
Parainfluenza	5	Fall/winter season; starts Oct/Nov
Influenza	5	Fall/winter; consider influenza vaccine
Respiratory syncytial	5	Fall/winter; major cause of croup in children
Adenovirus	5	All year; local epidemics occur; 45 serotypes; pharyngitis is most common adenovirus disease in children
Enterovirus	5–10	Causes "summer colds" in older children

viruses. Psychological stress has been shown to be a factor in the frequency of colds, probably through compromise of the immune system.

SYMPTOMS

Many of the symptoms of the common cold are the result of the body's defense mechanisms. URI symptoms vary from individual to individual, but usually include malaise, headache, nasal and sinus congestion, watery rhinorrhea, sneezing, and coughing. The nasal discharge is clear at first and may become purulent after a day or so. The presence of a purulent nasal discharge suggests secondary bacterial involvement and/or the simple stagnation of mucus. Pharyngitis is present in about two-thirds of cases. Adenoviruses cause most cases of pharyngitis in children. A primary differential diagnostic concern in a patient presenting with pharyngitis, especially exudative, is group A *Streptococcus*. Appropriate cultures should be obtained if indicated by the physical examination.

The most common predisposing factor to otitis media in children is a viral URI. Parents of otitis media–prone children often seek antibiotics early in the course of a common cold in an effort to prevent ear infections. Well-meaning clinicians often treat these children with antibiotics well before clinical signs or symptoms of otitis media appear. The overuse of antibiotics in the treatment of otitis media has been cited as a primary cause of resistant bacterial strains (see Chap. 3-2).

Cough can be prolonged in children and in patients who smoke, and may be dry or productive. Patients with comorbid conditions such as asthma, chronic lung disease, diabetes mellitus, or various immunocompromised diseases are susceptible to secondary infections in the paranasal sinuses, throat, and lungs. Bronchitis and pneumonia are often preceded by a viral URI.

Adenovirus presents with a more severe illness and is the etiologic agent in febrile pharyngoconjunctival illness. Respiratory syncytial virus (RSV) presents with a more severe illness and can be an important etiologic agent in day-care and nursery outbreaks (see Chap. 9-20).

OBJECTIVE FINDINGS

Objective findings may be few. Red irritated nasal mucosa, watery (or purulent-appearing) rhinorrhea, and a diffusely red pharynx are the most common physical signs. Mild respiratory wheezing can accompany some viral infections, especially in children, and can be precursors to exacerbations of asthma.

Sinus pain can be elicited in many patients with URIs. CT of sinuses during a recent study in patients with the common cold revealed that 60 percent had abnormalities of the ethmoid or maxillary sinuses and that 30 percent had abnormalities of the frontal sinuses.[2]

Cervical adenopathy and a low-grade fever may be present. Although fever is basically harmless and nonspecific in children, many will mount higher temperatures (102 to 104°F) with mild respiratory infections. Fever is therapeutic, but may be erroneously presumed to be harmful by some patients. Because of this, fevers are often aggressively self-treated with acetaminophen, ibuprofen, or both. Treating myalgia and headaches with these analgesic medications, however, is certainly appropriate.

DIAGNOSTIC CONSIDERATIONS

In patients with pharyngitis, the differential diagnosis should include beta-hemolytic *Streptococcus,* although the presence of coryza and cough is generally not consistent with streptococcal pharyngitis (see Chap. 3-9). Pharyngitis is the most common adenovirus disease in children.

Acute infections with mononucleosis (see Chap. 3-3) should be considered when the illness appears to be prolonged or unusually severe. Measles (Chap. 9-16), now rare in the United States, and chickenpox (Chap. 9-26) may present with the symptoms of the common cold in the early stages, resulting ultimately in the usual exanthems typical of the disease. This differential should be considered in unimmunized children if there is a concurrent community outbreak. Influenza (see Chap. 9-15) may present in the early stages with typical cold symptoms, but usually other constitutional symptoms (myalgia, severe malaise, high fevers), are present and the severity of the symptoms is greater.

Although one can have "back to back" viral upper respiratory infections (this is particularly true in day-care children), one should consider allergic rhinitis (see Chap. 3-4) among the differentials when the rhinitis, sneezing, and cough lasts longer than the expected number of days for a URI. Vasomotor rhinitis, commonly seen in pregnancy, can be mistaken for a viral URI.

SPECIAL CONSIDERATIONS

Complications of the common cold are relatively unusual if one considers the enormous number of infections. Complications tend to occur more often in patients who are prone to asthma. Viruses may be precursors to exacerbations of acute asthma attacks,[3] especially in children. Acute exacerbations may require corticosteroids to control bronchospasm. Newer therapies for the treatment or prevention of viral URIs could greatly reduce mortality and morbidity rates in this population (see Chap. 17-1).

Bacterial infections of the middle ear, and otitis media with effusion (see Chap. 3-2), are considerations, especially in children. Sinusitis (see Chap. 3-1) may appear at any time during the course of a URI and may require antibiotic therapy. There has been an increase in the frequency of pneumonia and bronchitis after URIs, especially in the debilitated and elderly populations.

LABORATORY TESTS

No specific laboratory tests are recommended for the common cold. Pharyngeal streptococcal screens may be appropriate for patients with severe pharyngitis and adenopathy. Viral cultures and immunoassays are generally unnecessary; however, in major outbreaks, such tests can indicate which virus is the prevailing type.

RADIOLOGIC STUDIES

There are no specific recommendations for radiologic studies. In patients with severe illness and wheezing, chest x-ray may be helpful in ruling out an underlying pneumonitis. In patients with sinus pressure or pain, an x-ray of the paranasal sinuses would be deemed appropriate.

TREATMENT

There is no specific treatment for a common cold, other than symptomatic measures. Sir William Osler was quoted as saying, "There is just one way to treat a cold . . . with contempt."

Most cases of the common cold are diagnosed and treated by the patient without medical intervention. Though billions of dollars are spent for over-the-counter preparations, many of these have shown to be ineffective and may actually prolong symptoms. Some clinicians feel that aspirin and acetaminophen may have a detrimental effect on URI therapy through neutralization of antibodies, which can result in an increase in nasal symptoms; however, naproxen has been shown to produce a significant reduction in the symptoms of the common cold without altering viral shedding[4] or prolonging the symptoms.

Antihistamines

Although they are frequently used for allergic rhinitis, antihistamines do not appear to be effective for viral URIs. Symptomatic relief by antihistamines such as diphenhydramine (Benadryl) or chlorpheniramine maleate (Chlor-Trimeton) may derive more from the sedative effect than from the actual local effect.[2] The mucosal drying effect of these medications may thicken secretions, making it more difficult to drain. Combinations of antihistamines and decongestants are the most common over-the-counter preparations. Some children taking antihistamines experience a paradoxical effect of stimulation and hyperactivity—certainly undesirable if given at bedtime.

The newer antihistamines, such as fexofenadine (Allegra), loratadine (Claritin), and cetirizine (Zyrtec) have less sedation and are primarily indicated for allergic and vasomotor rhinitis, and not for viral URIs.

Decongestants and Combination Drugs

The oral sympathomimetics (pseudoephedrine, phenylephrine) help reduce secretions from the nasal mucosa by neutralizing the effects of kinin production. Recently, nasal ipratropium was advocated as a local measure in colds to reduce nasal congestion and secretions. The mechanism of action is again a reduction in kinin production or neutralization.

Pseudoephedrine (Sudafed) is basically the only "pure" decongestant used in the management of nasal congestion. It is found in numerous cold products and is available in children's liquid preparations and adult tablets (in various strengths from 30 to 120 mg). Some of the major side effects of decongestants include palpitations, irritability, excitement, headaches, dizziness, and tachycardia. Providers should be wary of patients requesting unusual amounts of pseudoephedrine, because this product is used as a base for the home manufacture of methamphetamine.

The number of combination products for colds is staggering, with over 800 products on the market. Decongestants are more likely to be combined with antihistamines or other drugs to control the multi-symptomatology associated with colds. Medications such as expectorants (guaifenesin) and analgesics/antipyretics (acetaminophen, ibuprofen) are often found in combination products. Side-effect profiles of combination drugs include specific reactions to the individual components. Providers should become thoroughly familiar with a few favorites and use them exclusively.

Topical sympathomimetics (phenylephrine), such as Neo-Synephrine nasal sprays, should be used for very short periods. Because of the rebound effect and dependence resulting in chronic use, they should be used for only a few days.

The clinician should exercise extreme care when recommending combination cold medications to patients who have hypertension (especially those on beta blockers), diabetes mellitus, ischemic heart disease, hyperthyroidism, increased intraocular pressures, or prostatic hypertrophy, and to patients on MAOIs or tricyclic antidepressants. The elderly (over 60 years of age) are more likely to exhibit adverse reactions.

PPA (phenylpropanolamine)-containing products, such as Dimetapp, some Triaminic brands, and certain over-the-counter appetite suppressants, have been withdrawn from the market because of a higher incidence of stroke in some adult patients.

Saline Nasal Sprays

Saline nasal sprays and drops (Ocean Mist, Pediamist) are effective nasal moisturizers and help thin thick secretions. They may be used safely in patients of all ages, but are particularly helpful in infants and children or in patients where pharmacotherapeutics are contraindicated.

Cough Expectorants/Suppressants

Guaifenesin is one type of expectorant seen in cold and cough preparations. It increases the output of phlegm and bronchial secretions by reducing adhesiveness and surface tension. The increased flow of viscid secretions promotes the ciliary action and changes a dry, unproductive cough to one that is more productive and less frequent.

The use of cough suppressants in the management of URIs is controversial, because a functioning cough mechanism is essential to clear secretions from the bronchial tree and lungs. When the cough is persistent and interferes with daily activities or sleep, the limited use of these products will make the patient more comfortable during the duration of the cold. Many combination cough preparations contain expectorants, suppressants, and alcohol.

Codeine is an effective cough suppressant, and there are many codeine-containing cough products available. The duration of action is approximately 4 h, which may not be desirable for nighttime cough control. Codeine is a controlled medication and subject to abuse.

Pure dextromethorphan-containing cough suppressants (Delsym) can last 12 h, have less sedation and fewer gastrointestinal effects, and do not require a prescription. Many other products that have the abbreviation "DM", such as Robitussin DM, contain various amounts of dextromethorphan.

Antibiotics

Because more than 90 percent of all URIs are viral, antibiotics are not indicated. Patients often request antibiotics, and providers sometimes are pressured into prescribing these. As a result of the emergence of numerous strains of antibiotic-resistant bacteria, antibiotic use should be confined to cases of documented bacterial infection. The use of antibiotics to prevent "emerging" bacterial secondary infections is clearly controversial.

Humidity and Oral Hydration

Humidity and oral hydration is very helpful in the management of URIs. Humidity can be achieved with a cool mist humidifier or steam vaporizer. Cool mist humidifiers (especially the newer ultrasonic brands) are preferred and are safer with children. Steam vaporizers, once the mainstay of childhood, are also effective. Steam vaporizers carry a burn risk for children and the elderly, and the use of products containing menthol, camphor (Vicks), or eucalyptus oils is not recommended because prolonged use may cause nasal and respiratory irritation and worsen symptoms. Rubbing menthol and camphor-containing products on the chest or around the nasal orifices is another long-established home remedy with limited (albeit harmless) effects.

Patient should be encouraged to drink plenty of fluids. Water is the recommended choice, but fruit juices and various teas are used as well. Alcohol-containing beverages have no value in the overall management of colds, but patients often use "hot toddies" to relax and ease symptoms. Alcohol in moderation need not be discouraged if no harm is perceived.

Sleep and Rest

The value of sleep and rest during a severe cold cannot be overemphasized. Children who cannot adequately function in school or day-care due to the symptoms or side effects of medications should remain home. Most people with colds tend to carry on with their usual daily activities, however.

Natural Remedies

Home remedies for colds span the ages and all cultures. "Grandmother" remedies should be tactfully challenged by the provider to assure patient safety and should be permitted if there is no presumed harm. It is highly unlikely that one could know all of the vast array of herbal and natural pharmaceuticals that may be contained in ethnic concoctions, however. Keep in mind that these unknown products could contain potentially harmful chemicals.

The use of homeopathic, naturopathic, herbal, vitamins/minerals, and "natural" remedies is increasing. Many highly publicized claims are purely anecdotal and not based on scientific studies. The author does not intend to endorse or recommend any specific natural remedy.

The value of vitamin C (ascorbic acid) in large doses (1 to 6 g/day) has been used for over 20 years since the publication of Linus Pauling's *Vitamin C, the Common Cold and the Flu*. Although numerous medical studies have challenged faulty studies and dispute the value of vitamin C in the treatment of cold episodes, its use continues. Interestingly, some studies found that vitamin C reduced the duration of cold episodes by 1 day.

One of the more popular natural approaches to the common cold is the use of zinc and zinc lozenges. There is no scientific proof that supports this practice, but zinc is a critical micronutrient for immune system function. Further studies are needed to prove the benefits of zinc.

There are many herbs that claim to enhance the immune function. There have been hundred of studies (mostly European) that have investigated *Echinacea* sp. German physicians and pharmacist have prescribed millions of doses of *Echinacea* for the common cold and feel that infections are less severe and resolve more quickly. *Echinacea* is available in numerous herbal cold preparations.

Patient Education

To prevent antibiotic resistance, do not prescribe antibiotics indiscriminately, and educate patients about their appropriate use.[4] Patients should be instructed in good hand-washing techniques to prevent or reduce spread by surface contact or hand-to-hand contact. There is empirical evidence that increased surface disinfection (especially in day-care centers and schools) with an effective antiseptic product may reduce the incidence of viral spread. Children should be instructed not to touch the eyes and nose, important portals of entry for respiratory viruses.

Disposition

Patients should follow up if symptoms are prolonged—that is, if they last over 7 to 10 days. Fever appearing late in the illness may be a warning of a secondary bacterial infection such as sinusitis or pneumonia, particularly in a patient who is immunocompromised.

Viral upper respiratory infections routinely challenge our immune system, not unlike vaccinations. In most cases, the course of the illness cannot be modified. Patients often require ongoing reassurance that they will recover uneventfully and not develop more serious sequelae.

ACKNOWLEDGEMENT

The author and editor would like to acknowledge the contributions of John P. Donnelly, author of this chapter in the first edition of *Primary Care for Physician Assistants*.

REFERENCES

1. Spector SL: The common cold: Current therapy and natural history. *J Allergy Clin Immunol* 95:1133–1138, 1995.
2. Engel JP: Viral upper respiratory infections. *Semin Respir Infect* 10:3–13, 1995.
3. Abramson MJ, Marks GB, Pattermore PK: Are non-allergic environmental factors important in asthma? *Med J Aust* 163:542–545, 1995.
4. DeMasters, TA, Madara-Kelly K, Charan NB: An appeal to clinicians—don't prescribe antibiotics for acute URI. *JAAPA* 12:8; 37–45, 1999.

BIBLIOGRAPHY

Murray MT, Pizzorno J: *Encyclopedia of Natural Medicine,* 2nd ed. Rocklin, CA, Prima Publishing, 1998.
Pauling L: *Vitamin C, the Common Cold and the Flu.* San Francisco, Freeman, 1976.

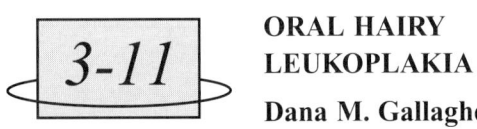

ORAL HAIRY LEUKOPLAKIA

Dana M. Gallagher

DISCUSSION

Oral hairy leukoplakia (OHL) is a white striated or corrugated mouth lesion that typically is found on the sides of the tongue, although it also may occur on the soft palate and the floor of the mouth. OHL may affect mere millimeters or cover the dorsum of the tongue entirely.

Although OHL was first observed in 1981 in homosexual males with HIV infection, it is not pathognomonic. Approximately 25 percent of people with HIV develop OHL[1]; it also has been found in people with iatrogenically induced immunosuppression (those with organ transplants or leukemia, asthmatics on steroids) and in three patients with no evidence of immunocompromise.[2] It is much less often seen in females with HIV than their male cohorts.[3] OHL occurs more frequently in smokers.

PATHOGENESIS

OHL is not a malignant or even a premalignant lesion. It is likely that cell turnover, as evidenced by the keratinization of the lesion, is actually reduced.[3] OHL is a signal of advancing HIV infection[4] and is not infectious.

Microbiology

OHL is caused by the Epstein-Barr virus (EBV)[1] and also has been associated with human papillomavirus (HPV) infection. The shedding of EBV from saliva to the mucosa maintains the leukoplakia. It has been noted that there are a variety of EBV types, strains, and variants. Coinfection and recombination of EBV are consistently found in those with OHL, regardless of their immune status.

SYMPTOMS

OHL is asymptomatic. Unlike another common HIV-related mouth condition, oral candidiasis (thrush), OHL does not cause pain, bad breath, unpleasant tongue sensations, or taste changes.

OBJECTIVE FINDINGS

A white corrugated lesion unilaterally or bilaterally on the tongue is visible on gross examination. In contrast to thrush, OHL cannot be scraped away with a tongue depressor or toothbrush.

DIAGNOSTIC CONSIDERATIONS

The diagnosis of OHL usually is made clinically and therefore is frequently treated presumptively. OHL often is seen in conjunction with oral candidiasis and can be confused with smoker's leukoplakia and oral cancers.

LABORATORY TESTS

Biopsy is the gold standard; however, in primary care settings, it usually is not performed until a treatment trial has failed. Unfortunately, viral cultures cannot be used to make the diagnosis.

RADIOLOGIC STUDIES

No radiologic studies are necessary.

TREATMENT

Pharmacologic Management

The following agents can be used.

1. Acyclovir, 800 mg orally five times a day, has been shown to be effective. Lesions probably will recur if the medication is stopped.
2. A one-time application of 25% topical podophyllin is efficacious[5,6] (this is not currently an FDA-approved use for podophyllin). Patients report minimal transient side effects, including a burning sensation, pain, and altered taste. Patient tolerance is high. Considerable short-term resolution of lesions can be expected.

Supportive Measures

Good mouth hygiene (tongue and mouth self-examinations, frequent brushing and flossing) is critical for all HIV-positive people.

Patient Education

Patients should be told the following facts:

- Kissing, sharing utensils, and drinking from the same cup cannot spread OHL. However, people with HIV should not share toothbrushes with others, since bleeding gums can theoretically spread the virus.
- Treating OHL is not mandatory (but often the patient will want to for cosmetic or psychological reasons). OHL can be treated but probably will recur when the treatment stops.
- If the patient is a smoker, a smoking cessation program should be recommended and instituted.

DISPOSITION

HIV-positive patients should have a mouth examination at every office visit. The finding of OHL on a routine examination should prompt testing in a patient whose HIV status is unknown.

NOTES AND PEARLS

Ganciclovir (DHPG), used in the treatment of cytomegalovirus infection, has simultaneously been used to treat OHL. The newer acyclovir-like drugs (famciclovir, valacyclovir) may prove useful in treatment.

REFERENCES

1. WALLING DM et al: Epstein-Barr virus co-infection and recombination in human immunodeficiency virus-associated oral hairy leukoplakia. *J Infect Dis* 171:1122, 1995.

2. ZAKRZEWSKA JM et al: Oral hairy leukoplakia in a HIV-negative asthmatic patient on systemic steroids. *J Oral Pathol Med* 24:282, 1995.
3. BARTON JC, BUCHNESS MR: Nongenital dermatologic disease in HIV-infected women. *J Am Acad Dermatol* 40(6 Pt 1):938–948, 1999.
4. GREENSPAN JS, GREENSPAN D: Oral complications of HIV infection, in MA Sande, PA Volberding (eds): *The Medical Management of AIDS,* 5th ed. Vienna, VA, W.B. Saunders, 1997, p 174.
5. SANFORD JP et al: *The Sanford Guide to HIV/AIDS Therapy.* Vienna, VA, Antimicrobial Therapy, 1996, p 33.
6. GOWDEY G et al: Treatment of HIV-related hairy leukoplakia with podophyllum resin 25% solution. *Oral Surg Oral Med Oral Pathol* 79:64–67, 1995.

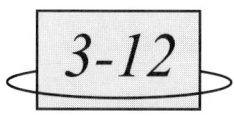

MASTOIDITIS

Pamela Moyers Scott

DISCUSSION

Mastoiditis is a bacterial infection that causes coalescence of the mastoid air cells by destroying the bony partitions between them. It is generally a complication of otitis media (see Chap. 3-2). The primary pathogens are *Streptococcus pneumoniae* (22 percent), *S. Pyogenes* (16 percent), *Staphylococcus* aureus (7 percent), *H. Influenzae* (4 percent), and *Pseudomonas Aeruginosa* (4 percent).[1]

In the preantibiotic era, acute mastoiditis complicated up to 20 percent of all cases of acute otitis media. With the advent of appropriate antibiotic therapies and early treatment of acute otitis media, the incidence of acute mastoiditis has declined to an estimated 0.2 to 2.0 percent.[2] A chronic subclinical mastoiditis is probably more prevalent than is acute mastoiditis in today's medical practice.

SIGNS AND SYMPTOMS

Acute mastoiditis is characterized by the return of otalgia, fever, and diminished hearing approximately 2 weeks after the initial onset of acute otitis media. Additionally, the patient generally complains of postauricular pain and swelling.

Chronic mastoiditis is asymptomatic, although the individual generally experiences frequent episodes of acute otitis media. Therefore, symptoms related only to the otitis media will be present.

OBJECTIVE FINDINGS

In acute mastoiditis, the tympanic membrane has the appearance of acute otitis media: erythematous, bulging, and with poorly distinguishable landmarks. If a perforation is present, a purulent creamy discharge usually is seen. Additionally, there are varying degrees of postauricular tenderness, erythema, and edema.

In chronic mastoiditis, there are no concomitant physical findings unless otitis media is also present.

DIAGNOSTIC CONSIDERATIONS

If there is marked postauricular edema, erythema, or tenderness, a careful examination is imperative to evaluate for the possibility of an associated fluctuant postauricular mass that indicates the presence of an abscess.

Chronic mastoiditis in adults frequently is associated with an underlying allergic condition.

LABORATORY TESTS

Unless a patient with acute mastoiditis appears toxic, no specific laboratory analysis is indicated.

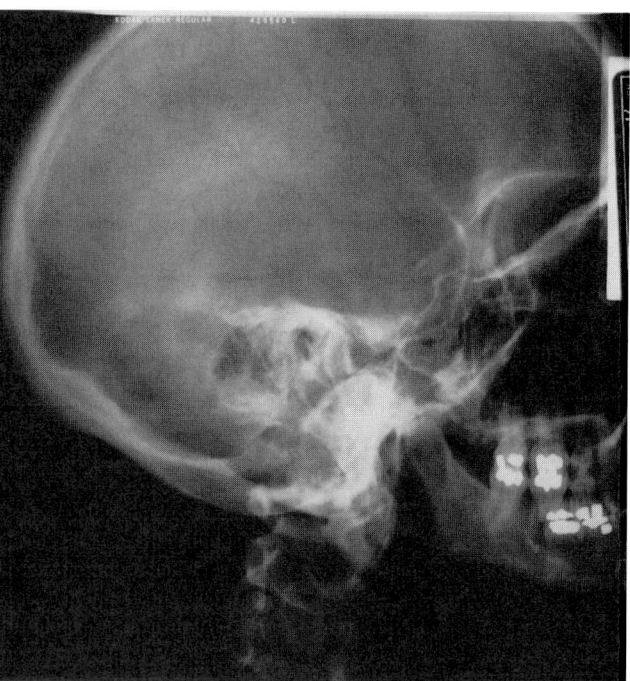

FIGURE 3-12-1. Cloudiness of the mastoid air cells and frank loss of the air cells as a result of destruction of the bony partitions between them are common radiographic findings in mastoiditis.

RADIOGRAPHIC STUDIES

Early in the course of acute mastoiditis, the mastoid x-ray can be normal or show minimal cloudiness of the mastoid air cells. As the disease progresses, the cloudiness increases. As mastoiditis becomes chronic, mastoid films reveal destruction of the bony partitions separating the mastoid air cells (see Fig. 3-12-1).

Computed tomography (CT) can reveal the cloudiness of the mastoid air cells and the destruction of the mastoid bony partitions that result in the coalescence of these air cells.

TREATMENT

Pharmacologic Management

If the patient is not toxic, does not have an abscess, and does not have a palsy of a cranial nerve, a trial of 24 to 48 h of oral antibiotics on an outpatient basis in a compliant patient is appropriate.

First-line therapy is generally the same as that for otitis media.[1] Appropriate antimicrobials to consider include the following:

- Amoxicillin (Amoxil) usual dose 250 to 500 mg q8h for adults or 40 to 45 mg/kg/day divided q8h or q12h for children
- Amoxicillin (Amoxil) high dose 500 mg q8h for adults or 80 to 90 mg/kg/day divided q8h or q12h for children
- Amoxicillin/clavulanate potassium (Augmentin) high dose 500 mg q8h or 875 mg q12h for adults or 80 to 90 mg/kg/day of amoxicillin component. (Must use plain amoxicillin along with the amoxicillin/clavulanate to keep clavulanate dose at approximately 10 mg/kg/day
- Cefuroxime axetil (Ceften) 500 mg q12h for adults or 30 mg/kg/ divided q12h for children.

However, in choosing an antibiotic for the treatment of acute mastoiditis, it is imperative to consider the frequency of methicillin-resistant *Staph. aureus* and β-lactamase-producing *H. influenzae* in your geographic region to make the empirical choice appropriate. All therapy should last for at least 14 days.

If the patient does not respond or worsens in the first 48 h, hospitalization with intravenous antibiotics and possibly surgery should be considered. Some providers feel that all patients with acute mastoiditis should be hospitalized initially.[2,3]

Surgical Interventions

If the patient does not respond to empirical antibiotic therapy and the tympanic membrane is intact, a tympanocentesis and myringotomy with or without tympanostomy tubes should be performed. This facilitates drainage of the middle ear and provides a specimen for culture and sensitivity testing. Again, some experts feel that this should be done immediately after the diagnosis.

If a patient with acute mastoiditis does not respond to treatment or has chronic mastoiditis, he or she needs some form of mastoidectomy, depending on the severity of the disease. The goals of a mastoidectomy include resolving the infection, preventing intracranial complications, improving hearing to preinfection levels, reventilating the middle ear, and allowing healing of the tympanic membrane if a perforation was present or myringotomy was performed.[4] The estimated success rate of a simple or modified radical mastoidectomy is approximately 80 percent.[5]

Supportive Measures

Pain relief is essential. Nonsteroidal anti-inflammatory drugs (NSAIDs) such as ibuprofen (Motrin) 800 mg tid to qid are generally effective. Occasionally, narcotic pain medications are required to alleviate the pain. Fever may be controlled with ibuprofen and/or acetaminophen.

Patient Education

If acute mastoiditis is treated on an outpatient basis, it is imperative that the patient understand the potential sequelae resulting from mastoiditis and the importance of frequent, regular follow-up visits as well as compliance with the antibiotic regime to minimize complications.

If a perforated tympanic membrane is present, the patient must be instructed in the proper use of earplugs, the importance of follow-up, and the potential need for surgical repair.

DISPOSITION

If outpatient therapy is chosen for a patient, that patient should be seen again in 24 to 48 h. Follow-up visit frequency depends on the response and whether perforation of the tympanic membrane is present.

COMPLICATIONS AND RED FLAGS

The complications of acute and chronic mastoiditis can be divided into intra- and extracranial conditions. Extracranial complications can consist of hearing loss, labyrinthitis, Bell's palsy, and Gradenigo's syndrome (characterized by otalgia, otorrhea, and paralysis of the ipsilateral sixth cranial nerve). A subperiosteal abscess and a deep neck abscess to the sternocleidomastoid muscle, secondary to the infection breaking the mastoid rim (Bezold's abscess), are possible if the infection tracks under the periosteum of the temporal bone.[6]

Intracranial complications from acute or chronic mastoiditis are the same as those from otitis media. They include meningitis, brain abscess, epidural abscess, lateral sinus thrombophlebitis, and otitic hydrocephalus.

The following situations require immediate referral to an otorhinolaryngologist for hospitalization:

• Presence of an abscess.
• Paralysis of the sixth or seventh cranial nerve.
• Failure to respond to antibiotic therapy in 24 to 48 h.

• Any patient who has incomplete resolution of all symptoms or develops chronic mastoiditis should be referred to an otorhinolaryngologist.

REFERENCES

1. Gilbert DN, Moellering RC Jr, Sande MA: *The Sanford Guide to Antimicrobial Therapy.* Hyde Park, VT, Antimicrobial Therapy, 13th ed., 2000, pp 7–8.
2. Giebink SG: Epidemiology and natural history of otitis media, in Lim D, Bluestone C, Klein J, Nelson J (eds): *Recent Advances in Otitis Media with Effusion.* Philadelphia, Decker, 1994, pp 5–9.
3. Bailey J, Struck C, Smith C: Otolaryngology, in Rakle R (ed): *Textbook of Family Practice,* 5th ed. Philadelphia, Saunders, 1995, pp 455–456.
4. Snow J: Surgical disorders of the ears, nose, paranasal sinuses, pharynx and larynx, in Sabinston D: *Textbook of Surgery,* 15th ed. Philadelphia, Saunders, 1997, pp 1275–1297.
5. Niparko J: Hearing loss and associated problems, in Barker LR, Burton J, Zieve P (eds): *Principles of Ambulatory Medicine,* 4th ed. Baltimore, Williams & Wilkins, 1995, pp 1410–1411.
6. Durand M, Joseph M, Baker AS: Infections of the upper respiratory tract, in Fauci AS, Braunwald E, Isselbacher KJ, et al (eds): *Harrison's Principles of Internal Medicine.* New York, McGraw-Hill, 1998, pp 179–184.

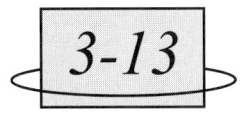

ORAL CANDIDIASIS
Kathleen J. Dobbs

DESCRIPTION

Oral candidiasis is the most common oral fungal infection, with prevalence in the general population of about 1%.[1] This number increases to 50% in HIV-positive individuals.[2] *Candida* is typically a harmless, dimorphic yeast that lives without producing disease in the oral cavities of up to 68% of normal individuals.[2–4] The opportunistic pathogen has also been cultured from other animals and birds. *C. albicans* is the most frequent cause of fungal disease in humans. *Candida* infections tend to affect the very young and the elderly. Anyone with candidal infection outside these age extremes requires detailed assessment to identify the underlying problem.

There are several types of *Candida* infections, which can be divided into acute, chronic, and mucocutaneous categories. This chapter will focus on acute and chronic pseudomembranous candidiasis or thrush in the newborn, infant, and adult; acute atrophic or erythematous candidiasis; angular cheilitis; chronic hypertrophic/hyperplastic candidiasis; and chronic mucocutaneous candidiasis.

PATHOGENESIS

Candida is an opportunistic pathogen and is considered normal flora of the oral and digestive tract. These organisms do not produce disease unless some change in the circumstances of the host lowers its natural defenses. It is possible that a change in phenotype may be required to produce disease. Usually the yeast must change to the pseudohyphal form for a clinical infection to occur, although hyphae can be found on tongue smears in a significant number of normal people.[5] Opportunistic fungal infections occur in individuals who are debilitated or immunosuppressed as a result of an underlying disease or treatment.

People colonized with *C. albicans* possess numerous complicated and often interdependent mechanisms to prevent the organism from establishing an infection. Efficient protection is believed to involve both humoral and cell-mediated immunologic mechanisms. Nonspecific mechanisms are also important, but it is well recognized that the contribution of particular elements to protection against mucosal, cutaneous, and deep-seated forms of candidiasis is different. Even trivial impairments of these mechanisms are often sufficient to allow *C. albicans,* the most pathogenic member of the genus, to establish a

TABLE 3-13-1. Predisposing Conditions for Oral Candidiasis

Medications

    Broad-spectrum antibiotics
    Multiple antibiotic regimes
    Corticosteroids, systemic or inhaled
    Cytotoxic agents
    Immunosuppressive agents
    Anticholinergics (xerostomia producing)

Endocrinopathies

    Diabetes mellitus
    Hypoadrenalism
    Hypoparathyroidism
    Hypothyroidism
    Polyendocrinopathy

Hematologic and Oncologic Disorders

    Aplastic anemia
    Agranulocytosis
    Lymphoma
    Leukemia
    Thymoma
    Advanced and widespread cancer

Nutritional Deficiencies

    Iron deficiency
    Folic acid deficiency
    Biotin deficiency
    Vitamin B deficiency
    Vitamin C deficiency
    Malnutrition
    Malabsorption

Immunodeficiency

    HIV disease
    Thymic alymphoplasia
    Thymic hypoplasia
    Severe combined immunodeficiency syndrome
    Hyperimmunoglobulinemia E syndrome
    Chronic mucocutaneous candidiasis

Leukocyte Disorders

    Myeloperoxidase deficiency
    Agranulocytosis
    Leukopenia
    Neutropenia

Other

    Radiation therapy
    Sjögren's syndrome
    Pregnancy
    Xerostomia
    Old age
    Infancy
    Denture use

SOURCE: From Muzyka and Glick.[11]

cutaneous or mucosal infection. More serious impairment of the host can lead to life-threatening deep-seated infection, often with less pathogenic *Candida* species.[6]

Numerous predisposing factors for oral candidiasis have been recognized, including metabolic, dietary, mechanical, and iatrogenic factors.[7] See Table 3-13-1.

CLINICAL EXAMINATION OF THE ORAL CAVITY

Candida infections may occur on any mucosal surface. Inspection of the mouth should include the lips, tongue, hard palate, soft palate, tonsils, vestibules, buccal mucosa, floor of the mouth, and teeth. Particular attention should be given to removal of dental prostheses, since *Candida* can be present under dental plates. Normal oral mucosa is

pink, ranging from whitish to reddish. A good light source and a tongue blade are essential.

Oral changes in aging are many: the mucosa thins and becomes drier; the epithelial turnover is slowed, leaving the mucosa more vulnerable to injury; the salivary glands become more fibrotic with fewer glandular elements; and over 50% of older adults have enlarged sublingual veins, also known as caviar tongue.[18] These changes may predispose the older adult to candidal infections.

SUBJECTIVE AND OBJECTIVE FINDINGS

Thrush or pseudomembranous candidiasis is the most common *C. albicans* infection. The soft, creamy white patches resembling milk curds are typically seen on the buccal mucosa, palate, and tongue. If the tongue is affected, the dorsum is depapillated, shiny, and smooth. Tongue movement is restricted and swelling results in trauma to the lateral borders if a natural dentition is present. The mouth is often so tender that the patient finds it difficult to tolerate solid food and hot or cold beverages.

The patches can be easily swabbed away leaving an erythematous base. If left untreated, the patches can form confluent plaques. The lesions are often painless, although mucosal erosion and ulceration may occur. The lesions may spread to involve the throat, leading to dysphagia.

It is important to distinguish this condition from chronic hyperplastic candidiasis (oral leukoplakia). The simplest test is to determine whether the white pseudomembrane can be dislodged. If it can, leaving an eroded, erythematous, bleeding surface, then this is diagnostic for acute pseudomembranous candidiasis.

Thrush is seen in healthy neonates, infants, and the elderly. It is unusual in healthy adults, and therefore the clinician should look for an underlying medical condition. Up to 80% of AIDS patients contract thrush (see Chap. 9-1).

Thrush is seen in 15% of newborns and is uncommon in babies delivered by cesarean section. Treating pregnant women before delivery dramatically decreases the risk of the infant contracting *Candida*. It is rare for any lesion to be visible in the first week. Typical sites of involvement include the tongue, soft palate, and buccal mucosa. In more severe cases, the posterior mouth may be involved, leading to apparent difficulties in feeding and swallowing and even breathing. Angular cheilitis often appears simultaneously because of drooling.

Thrush in both breast- and bottle-fed infants also occurs. The source is speculated to be the mother colonizing the infant by cleaning the bottle nipple or pacifier with her saliva. Clinical presentation and treatment is the same as for newborns.

Chronic oral candidiasis is synonymous with chronic pseudomembranous infection of the mouth. Angular cheilitis is often present. The major symptom is chronic pain and soreness of the mouth. Occasionally, patients develop esophagitis.

Acute atrophic candidiasis is the next most common type after thrush. Red atrophic patches, especially after antibiotic therapy, should suggest *Candida* as readily as a cheesy white patch does. In contrast to thrush, atrophic candidiasis is almost always painful. The tongue is most often involved and the treatment is identical to that for thrush.

Chronic atrophic candidiasis (erythematous or denture stomatitis) is the most common form of secondary oral candidiasis and is typically associated with oral prostheses, occurring in up to 60% of denture wearers. The condition is usually asymptomatic, but may present with an associated angular cheilitis. More often it is an incidental finding when the upper denture plate is removed for examination of the palate or a new prosthesis is needed. Lower dentures are seldom involved. The characteristic presenting signs are chronic erythema and edema of the portion of the palate that comes into contact with dentures. White patches are not seen. Look for this in diabetic patients.[8]

Angular cheilitis or perlèche often develops in association with other forms of oral candidiasis, in particular denture stomatitis, but it may occur without signs of other oral disease. The condition is common in patients with moist, deep folds at the corners of the mouth. These angular folds are often due to a decrease in facial height due to worn dentures. Angular cheilitis can occur in non–denture wearers, including AIDS patients. The characteristic presenting signs are soreness, erythema, and fissuring at the corners of the mouth.[6,9]

Chronic hyperplastic candidiasis or *Candida* leukoplakia is an important condition because the lesions can undergo malignant transformation. About 5% of all oral leukoplakias become malignant, but for *Candida* leukoplakia the figure is 15 to 20%. It remains unclear whether this condition is a hyperplastic lesion superinfected with *C. albicans* or the converse.

The most common site of chronic hyperplastic candidiasis is the inside surface of one or both cheeks or, less often, on the tongue. The lesion is usually asymptomatic and is often associated with smoking or local trauma due to dental neglect. Lesions range from small translucent white areas to large dense opaque plaques. Lesions that contain both red and white erythroplakia must be regarded with great suspicion, since malignant change is often present. In contrast to thrush, the lesions cannot be rubbed from the surface of the buccal mucosa. Biopsy is essential.

Chronic mucocutaneous candidiasis describes a group of uncommon conditions in which individuals with congenital immunologic or endocrinologic disorders develop persistent or recurrent mucosal, cutaneous, or nail infections with *C. albicans.* The disease often appears within the first 3 years of life. The mouth is the first site to be involved, but lesions then appear on the scalp, trunk, hands, and feet. The nails and sometimes the entire fingertip can be affected. Patients with chronic mucocutaneous candidiasis seldom develop deep-seated infection, despite their widespread or generalized cutaneous or mucosal lesions.[6]

DIAGNOSTIC CONSIDERATIONS

Key to the diagnosis of candidiasis is the clinical presentation. It is far more important than the microbiological studies. Differential diagnosis considerations include: lichen planus and some forms of leukoplakia, which can initially mimic thrush. The simple use of a tongue blade to remove the plaque should resolve this question. A white sponge nevus can also be mistaken for *Candida,* but the history clarifies the issue.[8]

It is best to provide the lab with scrapings of the lesion and tissue base; however, most clinicians tend to use swabs for various convenience factors. Swabs should be either moistened with sterile water or saline prior to taking the sample or sent to the lab in transport medium. Specimens must be processed as soon as possible after collection. Delay may result in the death of fastidious organisms, overgrowth of contaminants, and/or multiplication in the number of organisms present.[6]

Microscopic examination is the simplest and most helpful lab test. A culture may provide the definitive diagnosis, but it has limitations. There may be failure to recover the yeast, and it can take several weeks to get a definitive result. Serologic tests for the detection of fungal antibodies may be appropriate for deep-seated fungal infections but are not warranted for superficial oral infections.

Biopsy may be necessary if leukoplakia is suspected in cases that do not resolve after completing a course of therapy.

TREATMENT

Antifungal therapy has significantly improved in the past 10 years. Treatment should focus on two main areas: correction of the underlying condition and antifungal therapy.[10]

Antifungal therapeutics are used for all categories of candidiasis. Starting with the simplest treatment regimens and advancing as needed is prudent. The simplest treatments are topical: Nystatin pastilles (troches, lozenges) or suspension, amphotericin B lozenges (rarely used), or miconazole oral gel. It is important to keep the topical agents

in contact with the infected mucosa as long as possible. If a suspension is used in adults, proper swish, hold, and swallow maneuvers should be explained to the patient. In infants the suspension should be dropped into the mouth slowly to keep the medication in contact with the oral mucosa for as long as possible.

For more chronic forms of candidiasis or if there is accompanying esophagitis, it is necessary to use an orally absorbed drug such as ketoconazole 200 to 400 mg daily for 2 to 3 days in acute infections. Chronic infections may require the same dose for 3 to 5 weeks to achieve remission. Other choices include itraconazole 100 mg daily and fluconazole 50 mg daily.[11]

Prophylaxis is an evolving art with many regimens advocated, including alternate-day or weekly doses of oral imidazole or ketoconazole. Relapses occur when there are continuing immunologic defects, such as neutropenia, and it may not be possible to completely rid the mouth of organisms. In such patients treatment may be continuous or given in repeated courses. Resolution of the infection does not confer protection, and reinfection or reactivation may occur if host resistance is again lowered.[6]

REFERENCES

1. Root RK et al (eds.): *Clinical Infectious Diseases, a Practical Approach.* New York, Oxford University Press, 1999.
2. Hauman CHJ et al: Oral carriage of *Candida* in healthy and HIV-seropositive persons. *Oral Surgery* 76:570–572, 1993.
3. Soll DR et al: Developmental and molecular binding of switching in *Candida. Oral Surgery Oral Medicine Oral Pathology* 78:194–201, 1994.
4. Fetter A et al: Asymptomatic oral *Candida albicans* carriage in HIV-infections: Frequency and predisposing factors. *J Oral Pathol Med* 22: 57–59, 1993.
5. Wood NK, Goaz PW: *Differential Diagnosis of Oral Lesions,* St. Louis, MO, CV Mosby, 1997.
6. Richardson MD, Warnock DW: *Fungal Infection: Diagnosis and Management.* Oxford, Eng (UK), Oxford Blackwell Scientific, 1993.
7. Lynch DP: Oral candidiasis. History, classification, and clinical presentation. 78(2):189–193, 1994.
8. Bork K et al: *Diseases of the Oral Mucosa and Lips.* Philadelphia, Saunders, 1996.
9. Noble J (ed): *Textbook of Primary Care Medicine.* 2d ed. St. Louis, Mosby-Yearbook, 1996.
10. Jacobs PH, Nall L (eds): *Antifungal Drug Therapy: A Complete Guide for the Practitioner.* New York, Marcel Dekker, 1990.
11. Muzyka BC, Glick M: A review of oral fungal infections and appropriate therapy. *J Am Dent Assoc* 126:63–72, 1995.

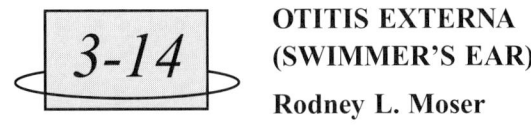

OTITIS EXTERNA (SWIMMER'S EAR)

Rodney L. Moser

DISCUSSION

Acute otitis externa (AOE), more commonly called "swimmer's ear," is a bacterial skin infection in the external auditory canal that occasionally involves the pinna and related structures. The skin in the bony portion of the canal lacks a subcutaneous layer and is attached directly to the periosteum, an important feature in the pathogenesis of invasive otitis externa.[1] The loss of the protective function of cerumen from swimming and/or the use of cotton-tipped applicators results in maceration of the skin from persistent moisture. Water exposure from showers or baths is implicated less frequently but does occur. This maceration predisposes the area to secondary bacterial infection. Other causes include trauma from self-instrumentation (paper clips, bobby pins, etc.), foreign bodies, contact dermatitis, eczema, and otorrhea through a chronic tympanic membrane perforation.

The most common pathogens found in AOE is *Pseudomonas aeruginosa* (about 95 percent of cases). *Staphylococcus aureus, Streptococcus* species, *Haemophilus influenzae, Moraxella catarrhalis, Proteus* species, and other skin organisms also are reported. In chronic cases, fungi also may be present, especially *Aspergillus niger, A. alba,* or *Candida albicans.*

SIGNS AND SYMPTOMS

Because of the rich innervation of the external auditory canal, AOE can be exquisitely painful and/or pruritic. Movement of the pinna or tragal pressure will cause increased pain and is one of the diagnostic hallmarks. The drainage and visible debris may be absent, minimal, or profuse, occasionally with dried, yellow crusts present at the os. Unless the occlusion is severe, hearing is usually affected minimally.

If the ear canal is grossly edematous and painful, the patient may resist an otoscopic inspection. In acute infections, it may be impossible to visualize deeper canal structures or the tympanic membrane.

More severe infections (cellulitis) may spread to the auricle, the periauricular area, and rarely to other parts of the body. Localized swelling and/or tenderness of the periauricular and cervical lymph nodes are common.

OBJECTIVE FINDINGS

Because of the stenosis caused by soft tissue swelling, it may be difficult or impossible to perform an otoscopic speculum examination. Since certain ototopical medications cannot be given safely in the presence of a nonintact tympanic membrane (TM), this unfortunate lack of visualization often drives antimicrobial selection toward antibiotics that are not known to be ototoxic (such as the fluoroquinolones). Pinna and/or tragal tenderness, visible swelling, and/or discharge are other supportive findings.

DIAGNOSTIC CONSIDERATIONS

Diagnostic considerations include acute otitis media (with otorrhea from a TM perforation), chronic otitis media (with long-standing perforation), cholesteatoma, eczema, contact dermatitis, seborrheic dermatitis, impetigo, herpes zoster, cellulitis, folliculitis, a retained foreign body, and trauma (from self-instrumentation during ear cleaning, a direct blow, or acoustic trauma). Although psoriasis may be present in and around the external auditory canal, this usually is not considered a cause of otitis externa. Clear, watery otorrhea after a severe head injury could indicate the presence of cerebrospinal fluid. Squamous and basal cell carcinomas can occur in the external auditory canal, and so atypical suspicious lesions should be biopsied.

SPECIAL CONSIDERATIONS

Immunocompromised and elderly patients are more prone to progressive infections and should be treated more aggressively in the early stages. Fungal pathogens should be investigated in refractory cases, and appropriate cultures should be taken. Neoplastic conditions are less common but also should be considered. Herpes zoster and simplex can occur in the external auditory canal, causing severe otalgia, often accompanied by ipsilateral facial paralysis (cranial nerve VII).

Invasive ("malignant") otitis externa is a potentially life-threatening infection, usually due to *P. aeruginosa,* that slowly invades from the external canal into adjacent soft tissues, mastoid, and temporal bone and spreads across the base of the skull. It occurs primarily in diabetic patients.[1]

LABORATORY TESTS

Routine cultures are rarely performed in uncomplicated cases, since otitis externa is highly responsive to antimicrobial therapy. Treatment failure and refractory cases should alert the provider to investigate other, less common pathogens, particularly fungi. In these cases, cultures should be taken before antimicrobial therapy begins.

RADIOLOGIC AND IMAGING STUDIES

None, unless there is acute head trauma or mastoid or neurologic involvement. Computed tomography (CT) and magnetic resonance imaging (MRI) studies are essential for defining the extent of bone and/or soft tissue involvement.

TREATMENT

Medications

Topical medications used for the treatment of AOE include ototopical antibiotics with or without topical steroids, topical ophthalmic antibiotics, and acidic preparations.

Cerumen helps maintain an acidic environment in the external auditory canal. When cerumen is absent or deficient, much of the protective effect is lost. Acidifying solutions (Otic Domeboro, VoSol, etc.) can be helpful in the management of mild otitis externa or for chronic preventive use. These acidic preparations are somewhat helpful in the long-term management or prevention of minor fungal infections.

Over-the-counter (OTC) preparations usually contain a combination of acetic acid and boric acid; some include alcohol as well. OTC preparations are more helpful for prevention than they are curative. Acceptable home remedies include a 50/50 solution of white vinegar and water and other alcohol and vinegar combinations.

Topical treatment has some distinct advantages over systemic therapy (see Table 3-14-1). Topical medication is delivered directly to the target area, bypassing the systemic circulation and safely reducing systemic antibiotic side effects. Short-term topical treatment has rarely been implicated in the creation of resistant organisms. A study done at the University of Pittsburgh[2] on 231 cases of AOE in which *P. aeruginosa* was isolated found that 99.6 percent showed sensitivity to polymyxin B, one of the antibiotics found in Cortisporin Otic. In spite of three decades of use of this medication, it remains quite effective. Systemic antibiotics often represent an "overkill."

The commonly used otic preparation Cortisporin Otic contains neomycin sulfate, polymyxin B (both of which are potentially ototoxic[3]), and hydrocortisone. This medication can be used safely when the TM is known to be intact. Aminoglycosides (gentamicin, tobramycin, streptomycin, etc.) also are known to be ototoxic, usually after high-dose parenteral administration. The potential for ototoxic complications from *topical* aminoglycosides is quite small. Only limited animal studies have shown ototoxic effects from topical aminoglycosides.[4]

Hypersensitization does not appear to be an important problem with topical antibiotics, although some sensitive patients (those with chronic dermatoses) may react to neomycin-containing products. These products should be discontinued if sensitivity is suspected.

If the status of the TM is unknown or if a perforation is present, nonototoxic antibiotics should be used first. Ciprofloxacin (Cipro) and ofloxacin (Floxin) are not known to be ototoxic and can be used by adults and children. The American Academy of Otolaryngology—Head and Neck Surgery (AAOHNS) recommends that these broad-spectrum fluoroquinolones be used first.[4] Cipro is nonsterile and is indicated for otitis externa only. Floxin is approved for use in the middle ear. Topical aminoglycosides can be used if the fluoroquinolones fail, which rarely occurs. Fluoroquinolone otic preparations have a very high cure rate.

Basically, topical antibiotics should be used alone. The use of systemic antibiotics in the management of AOE often depends on the immune status of the patient, the extent of the infection, the presence of cellulitis, and the propensity for further systemic involvement. Limiting the overuse of oral antibiotics may reduce the development of resistant bacterial strains.

TABLE 3-14-1. Otic Preparations Used to Treat Otitis Externa

MEDICATION	DOSE
Acetic preparations	
Otic Domeboro	*Acetic acid 2%:* instill 4–6 drops in affected ear every 2–3 h; contraindicated in TM perforations
Vosol	*Acetic acid 2%:* instill 5 drops in ear canal 3–4 times per day; indicated for bacterial and fungal infections; contraindicated in TM perforations
Vosol HC	*Acetic acid 2%* with hydrocortisone 1%: same dosage as Vosol; should not be used in presence of viral (herpetic) otic infections
Antibiotic/Steroid Combinations	
Cortisporin-TC Otic	*Colistin—neomycin—hydrocortisone:* instill 4 drops in ear canal 3–4 times per day, max. 10 days; contraindicated in presence of herpetic infection
Cortisporin Otic Suspension	*Polymyxin B—neomycin—hydrocortisone:* same dose and contraindications as Cortisporin-TC; *suspension* has a milky, aqueous/alcohol base and penetrates the canal easily; should be shaken well before each use
Cortisporin Otic Solution	Same as Cortisporin Otic Suspension; *solution* has a syrupy, glycerine base that may adhere better to the ear canal
Coly-Mycin S Otic	*Colistin—neomycin—hydrocortisone:* instill 5 drops in ear canal 3–4 times per day; contraindicated in presence of herpetic infection
Cipro HC	*Ciprofloxacin—hydrocortisone:* instill 3 drops bid for 7 days; not recommended for children under age 1; use of hydrocortisone is contraindicated in presence of herpetic infection
Floxin Otic	*Ofloxacin:* instill 5–10 drops in affected ear bid for 10 days; 14 days for chronic suppurative otitis media
Ophthalmic Steroid Preparations Used in the Ear	
Decadron Ophthalmic Solution	*Dexamethasone:* instill 3–4 drops 2–3 times per day for steroid-responsive inflammation; contraindicated in presence of herpetic, mycobacterial, or fungal infections

The use of corticosteroids in the management of uncomplicated otitis externa remains controversial, and so their use is an individual preference. In cases where there is a significant inflammatory response in the auditory canal, hydrocortisone-containing preparations are helpful. Stronger corticosteroids (i.e., dexamethasone) in an ophthalmic preparation have been used in the ear. Corticosteroids should not be used in the presence of herpetic infections such as herpes zoster, herpes simplex, or varicella. Prolonged use of corticosteroid preparations may result in overgrowth of fungi.

Management of fungal infections depends on the severity. Minor infections respond to the acidic preparations (i.e., VoSol); more extensive infections may require the use of antifungal dermatologic solutions. None of the topical antifungal agents have been well tested for otic use. Serious fungal infections, such as those in immunocompromised patients, may respond better to systemic antifungal agents. Persistent cases should be referred to a specialist.

Supportive Measures

Before topical therapy is instituted, an attempt should be made to remove excess cerumen and desquamated epithelium from the ear canal unless the canal is too edematous. This can be accomplished by using a gentle lavage with warm Burow's solution or normal saline or by mechanical suction with a device designed for this purpose.

A cellulose ear wick or laminaria can be used for the first few days to allow the ear drops to penetrate the swollen canal. The wick will facilitate the penetration of the medication deeper into the canal, allowing more contact with the infected skin surfaces. Most wicks are removed in 2 to 3 days, when clinical improvement is evident.

Otitis externa can be exquisitely painful, and so patients may be offered short-term oral analgesics such as codeine if OTC analgesics are not helpful. Topical analgesic preparations are not usually helpful for otitis externa.

Patient Education

All patients should be instructed in the proper use of topical otic preparations. After the proper dose has been instilled in the ear canal, the patient should remain in a reclining position for several minutes to allow adequate penetration of the drops.

Otic solutions should be brought up to "body temperature" before use. An acceptable temperature can be achieved by holding the room-temperature bottle in the hand for several minutes or placing the bottle in warm (approximately 100°F) water. Advise patients *not* to store drops in the refrigerator (a common error). The use of ice-cold otic preparations may precipitate a caloric response with dizziness, nausea, or vomiting.

Avoiding excessive water exposure from showers, baths, or swimming pools is important. During treatment and for prophylactic measures, patients should be advised to use occlusive earplugs.

Patients should understand the protective nature of cerumen and should be cautioned against the routine (often daily) use of cotton-tipped applicators. The use of self-instrumentation for cerumen removal (bobby pins, paper clips, etc.) should be highly discouraged.

Disposition

Although improvement usually is seen within 3 days, patients should be instructed to use the otic preparations for the full prescribed course (5 to 10 days or more), depending on the severity of infection, the individual response to therapy, and the type of medication prescribed. Patients should be advised to consult their provider if they do not respond to therapy within this period or experience the signs or symptoms of a progressive infection.

Patients should be cautioned against using left-over otic preparations chronically for prophylaxis, especially those which contain corticosteroids.

COMPLICATIONS AND RED FLAGS

Rare. The elderly, diabetic patients, and immunocompromised patients are more likely to exhibit signs and symptoms of malignant otitis externa. These patients tend to experience persistent fever and pain and have very friable granulomatous tissue in the external auditory canal. Atypical lesions in the auditory canal may be an indication of a squamous or basal cell carcinoma and should be biopsied. Osteomyelitis and mastoiditis are also rare complications.

OTHER NOTES AND PEARLS

Because the status of the TM cannot be observed easily, many providers use systemic antibiotics unnecessarily. Unless there are clinical indications of more extensive infection, the vast majority of cases can be exclusively treated with topical preparations.

REFERENCES

1. Durand M, Joseph M, Baker AS: Infections of the upper respiratory tract, in Fauci AS, Braunwald E, Isselbacher KJ, et al: *Harrison's Textbook of Medicine,* 14th ed. New York, McGraw-Hill, p 181.
2. Dohar JE, Kenna MA, Wadowsky RM: In vitro susceptibility of aural isolates of *P. aeruginosa* to commonly used ototopical antibiotics. *Am J Otolaryngol* 17:207–209, 1996.
3. Bluestone CD, Klein JO: *Otitis Media in Infants and Children.* Philadelphia, Saunders, p 155.
4. Bell EA: Topical antibiotics for treating ear infections, *Infect Dis Child* 13(6):59–61, 2000.

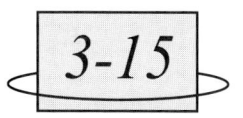

EPISTAXIS
Stephanie D. Bowlin

DISCUSSION

Epistaxis results from an interaction of factors, damaging the nasal epithelial lining and blood vessel walls. The most common cause of epistaxis is nose picking and accidental injury.[1,2] Other causes of epistaxis include environmental factors (humidity, temperature, and high altitude); local factors (trauma, foreign body, anatomic abnormalities, nasal or sinus infection, allergies); systemic factors (hypertension, platelet and coagulation abnormalities, renal failure, and alcohol abuse); and medications (prolonged use of nose drops, anticoagulants), nasally inhaled street drugs (methamphetamines, cocaine), and nonsteroidal anti-inflammatory drugs. Nasal septal deviation is common to the cause of epistaxis, but its role in epistaxis is unclear.[1,2]

Clot formation, which will occur due to an intact coagulation system, is required to stop the flow of blood from the nose.[1]

SIGNS AND SYMPTOMS

Patients presenting with epistaxis will have free-flowing blood originating from the nostrils. The frequency of nosebleeds may vary from once a month to several times per day.[2] If the blood is bright red, the bleeding site is usually close to the nasal opening. If the nosebleed is located deeper in the nasal cavity, the blood may appear dark red.

A brief history should be attained to determine the cause and duration of blood loss. The clinician should perform an inspection of entire oral cavity, nasopharynx, and face for the presence of deformities and ecchymosis. Palpation of the sinuses, orbits, and facial bones for tenderness or crepitus should also be performed. Examination of Kiesselbach's area may reveal a red and raw surface with fresh clots or old crust.[2,3] Orthostatic blood pressures should be taken if severe blood loss has occurred. Lightheadedness from blood loss, rapid heartbeat, black stool from swallowed blood, shortness of breath, and pallor occur only with a significant amount of blood loss.[1,4]

Table 3-15-1 shows the specific diseases and conditions that are associated with epistaxis.

LABORATORY TESTS

A baseline hematocrit should be performed. Complete lab work is only needed if the patient has a family history of a bleeding disorder, a past medical history of easy bleeding, a bleeding episode that lasts more than 30 min that will not clot with direct pressure, or if the patient is under 2 years of age. If a severe nosebleed has occurred, anemia may be present 6 to 12 h after the bleeding has ceased.

TABLE 3-15-1. Specific Diseases Associated with Epistaxis

Allergic rhinitis
Rheumatic fever
Scurvy
Scarlet fever
Hodgkin's disease
Atherosclerosis
Malaria
Typhoid fever
Hypertension
Bleeding disorders[a]

[a]Bleeding tendencies may also be associated with aplastic anemia, leukemia, hemophilia, thrombocytopenia, alcoholism, and liver disease.[1,4] These disease processes must be treated appropriately.

COMMON DIFFERENTIAL DIAGNOSIS

The most common differential diagnosis of epistaxis is allergic rhinitis (see Chap. 2-4). In allergic rhinitis the mucosa is inflamed and boggy. Epistaxis, in this condition, is a result of itching and rubbing the nose.[2]

COMPLICATIONS

Complications are rare in anterior bleeds, unless an underlying bleeding disorder exists. The only complication in routine epistaxis may be a mild anemia that responds to iron or nutritional therapy.

In severe, posterior bleeds, rare complications with posterior packs include respiratory failure, cardiac failure, and death.

TREATMENT

Epistaxis should be treated promptly. The patient should sit up and lean forward to prevent the swallowing of blood, which may cause dyspepsia and vomiting.

The treatment of epistaxis is directed at the bleeding site. If the bleeding site is anterior, the nose should be compressed over the area for a minimum of 5 to 10 min.[2,4] The patient should be instructed to breathe through the mouth. If bleeding does not subside during this time period, the pressure should be reapplied by adjusting the fingers on the compression site. If pressure treatment is unsuccessful, the clots should be removed by suction or blowing the nose. A good light source is needed to visualize the bleeding site. A compress that is moistened with 0.25% phenylephrine nose drops or 1% lidocaine with 1:1000 epinephrine should be inserted and placed near the identified bleeding site. Pressure is reapplied for another 10 min. These techniques are usually successful.[2]

Where available (usually in the emergency department), 1% cocaine may be used in the nose in place of the phenylephrine or lidocaine. This technique is very effective. Cocaine should be avoided in the elderly and in patients with a history of cardiovascular disease or of cocaine abuse. Patients should be informed that cocaine will be used in the event of a subsequent drug screen.

If bleeding is not controlled, the placement of an anterior pack such as the standard anterior nasal gauze pack is required and often performed by the otolaryngologist[4] or a provider trained in this procedure.

Posterior bleeds are more difficult to locate and treat. Posterior bleeds are often associated with hypertension and/or atherosclerosis in elderly patients who have decreased platelet and clotting functions. The treatment of a posterior bleed usually requires a posterior nasal pack, especially if the anterior pack did not stem the blood flow or if blood is actively flowing down the patient's throat. For the placement of posterior packs, hospitalization may be required.

In cases of severe epistaxis, otolaryngologists are effectively using a device called a *suction end*. The advantages of this device over other commonly used devices include its comfortable length for handling and the adequate diameter for effectively controlling severe hemorrhage. The device is also disposable, thereby reducing the risk of blood-borne transmission of disease.[3]

Electrocautery is sometimes used to treat severe cases of nosebleed; however, it is contraindicated in patients under 2 years of age.[2,4]

PREVENTIVE MEASURES

The use of a daily application of petroleum jelly or an antibiotic ointment, using a cotton-tipped applicator, for 5 days until no nosebleed has reoccurred, will keep the nasal cavity moist. If no nosebleed occurs in 5 days, the patient can then lubricate the nasal cavity weekly for 1 month. Humidification of the patient's room has proved helpful. The use of aspirin and hard blowing of the nose should be avoided.

Patients or parents (in the case of children) should be well educated on the causes of epistaxis and given first-aid instruction on routine management of future episodes.

REFERENCES

1. Tan L, Calhoun K: Epistaxis. *Med Clin North Am* 83:43–46, 1999.
2. Hay W, Groothuis J, Hayward A, Levin M, eds: *Current Pediatric Diagnosis and Treatment,* 12th ed. Norwalk, CT, Appleton & Lange, 1995, pp. 477–480.
3. Shehab Z, Pahor A: Short communications—A valuable device in the management of epistaxis. *J Laryngol Otol* 111:361,1997.
4. Health Library: Management of anterior and posterior epistaxis. *http://thriveonline.aol.com/assets/health.lookrule.gif.*

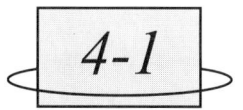

ACID-BASE DISORDERS
Claire Babcock O'Connell

DISCUSSION

Plasma pH constantly adjusts to changes in hydrogen ion content and the concentration of other substances, such as bicarbonate, carbon dioxide, and organic acids, that are inherently acidotic or alkalotic in nature. Through the adjustments made mainly by the lungs and the kidneys, extracellular pH is held relatively constant at 7.35 to 7.45. Intracellular pH is slightly lower because of cellular metabolism; for practical applications, the pH of the extracellular fluid is used for clinical assessment and evaluation.

Determination of pH is based on the Henderson-Hesselbach equation (see Fig. 4-1-1), which describes the relationship between bicarbonate and carbonic acid, which are the principal players in the acid-base balance of the extracellular fluid. Carbonic acid is very short-lived and readily converts to water and carbon dioxide (see Fig. 4-1-2). The overall pH is determined by the ratio of the concentrations of HCO_3^- to CO_2. The normal ratio is 20 HCO_3^- to 1 CO_2. When the ratio exceeds 22, the condition is alkalotic; a ratio below 18 is acidotic. The ratio changes with variations in the concentration of either substance. An increase in bicarbonate or a decrease in carbon dioxide will cause an increase in the ratio (alkalosis); a decrease in bicarbonate or an increase in carbon dioxide will cause a decrease in the ratio (acidosis). In general, the pH varies directly with changes in HCO_3^- and indirectly with changes in CO_2.

Regulation of pH balance is conducted by the lungs and kidneys, which continually respond to minute changes in ion concentration and bring the overall condition of the body back to equilibrium. The lungs affect pH by blowing off CO_2, a volatile gas that, through its release, decreases the concentration of hydrogen ion. Through changes in the rate and depth of respirations, the pH is finely adjusted. The blood-brain barrier is freely permeable to CO_2 and reacts rapidly to changes in the CO_2 content in the blood by stimulating or inhibiting respirations. High CO_2 (low pH) stimulates an increase in respiration; low CO_2 (high pH) inhibits respiration. This respiratory response to changes in pH is rapid but becomes blunted fairly quickly.

The kidneys are not as rapid as the lungs in their role in the maintenance of pH balance. The kidneys respond to changes in hydrogen ion concentration by adjusting their ability to retain HCO_3^- and excrete H^+. The kidneys are responsible for the more chronic adjustments through this alteration in renal function. High levels of HCO_3^- drive the bicarbonate–carbonic acid equation to the left, producing increased H^+. Acidosis (high H^+) stimulates hydrogen ion secretion and hence the production of ammonia. H^+ is then excreted as ammonium with new HCO_3^- produced and reabsorbed. Decreased CO_2 has the opposite effect. Alkalosis (low H^+) inhibits hydrogen secretion, reducing HCO_3^- generation. In alkalosis, there is already a high concentration of HCO_3^-, which results in increased HCO_3^- excretion.

LABORATORY

Acid-base status is clinically evaluated through the measurement of arterial blood gases. Pa_{O_2} (normally >80 mmHg), Pa_{CO_2} (normally 35 to 45 mmHg), and pH (7.35 to 7.45) are measured directly; HCO_3^- (normally 22 to 26 mmHg) is determined by using a nomogram. Proper technique is necessary to assure accurate blood-gas analysis. Specimens should be put on ice promptly; the CO_2 will rise over time, especially at room temperature, which will cause a fall in pH. Long delays in analyzing the specimen will cause lysis of cells, which will cause a false acidosis. Body temperature at either extreme will affect the gases: high fevers and hypothermia necessitate correction of the pH (increased in fever, decreased in hypothermia) and the Pa_{O_2} and Pa_{CO_2} (decreased in fever, increased in hypothermia). Large air bubbles caught in the specimen introduce additional O_2 into the specimen and therefore result in a relative reduction in Pa_{CO_2} and a falsely higher pH.

In general, metabolic disorders indicate a change in HCO_3^- and respiratory disorders indicate a change in CO_2. The clinical assessment of acid-base status for the most part can be done by using pH and Pa_{CO_2}. The suffix *emia* denotes the status of hydrogen ion in the blood; the suffix *osis* indicates the condition of the patient. Alkalemia occurs whenever there is a rise in HCO_3^- or a fall in CO_2; acidemia occurs whenever there is a rise in CO_2 or a fall in HCO_3^-. The pH rises in alkalemia and falls in acidemia. Compensation is carried out by the body in reaction to these changes in hydrogen ion concentration and pH. If the primary condition causing the imbalance is metabolic, the lungs will be the principal player in compensation; if the primary condition is respiratory in nature, the kidneys will attempt compensation.

EVALUATION

The first step in evaluating acid-base disorders in practice is the history and physical examination. Analysis of arterial blood bases confirms and quantitates the condition and helps direct and monitor treatment. However, the interpretation of the blood gases should not be complicated. Simply look at the pH first and determine whether it is normal, elevated, or low. Then look at the Pa_{CO_2}. If the pH is acidotic and Pa_{CO_2} is elevated, there is a *respiratory acidosis;* if the Pa_{CO_2} is low or normal, there is a *metabolic acidosis*. In this case, the HCO_3^- will be low; any decrease in Pa_{CO_2} represents respiratory compensation. Alternatively, if the pH is alkalotic and the Pa_{CO_2} is decreased, there is a respiratory alkalosis; if the Pa_{CO_2} is high or normal, there is a metabolic alkalosis. Here the HCO_3^- will be elevated, and an increase in Pa_{CO_2} represents respiratory compensation. Compensation may bring the pH back into the normal range (7.35 to 7.45) but will never move past the midline (7.4) and "overcompensate." Table 4-1-1 illustrates the major changes in acidosis/alkalosis.

METABOLIC ACIDOSIS

Bicarbonate loss or consumption underlies all metabolic acidosis. Bicarbonate is consumed whenever there is an increase in acid production (lactic acid, ketoacids, etc.) or a decrease in renal excretion of H^+. Bicarbonate loss results from renal dysfunction. Differentiation among the causes of metabolic acidosis is aided by the determination of the anion gap $[Na^+ - (Cl^- + HCO_3^-)]$. The major cation in plasma is sodium; the major "measured" anions are chloride and bicarbonate. The unmeasured anions (mainly albumin, phosphate, sulfate, lactate, and the salts of weaker acids) are collectively known as the anion gap. An increase in these unmeasured anions increases the anion gap.

$$pH = pk + \log \frac{(HCO_3^-)}{(H_2CO_3)}$$

$$pH = pk + \log \frac{(HCO_3^-)}{(H_2O + CO_2)}$$

FIGURE 4-1-1. The Henderson-Hesselbach equation.

Conditions of metabolic acidosis that are associated with an increased anion gap are known as high anion gap metabolic acidosis; those which do not are known as normal anion gap metabolic acidosis.

High anion gap metabolic acidosis is usually an acute process and is caused by increased production of nonvolatile acids [ketoacidosis (diabetes, starvation, alcohol), lactic acidosis (cardiopulmonary failure), and salicylate, methanol, or ethylene glycol poisoning] or by decreased acid excretion by the kidney (uremia, renal failure). Normal anion gap metabolic acidosis is more commonly a chronic process and is caused by renal tubular dysfunction or by the loss of bicarbonate (severe or prolonged diarrhea or malabsorption). The pH is low, and the HCO_3^- is low; respiratory compensation may be evident by a reduction in $Paco_2$.

Clinically, metabolic acidosis is manifested by dehydration, thirst, weakness, and restlessness. The patient may complain of fatigue, appear confused, and progress to stupor or coma. The respiratory rate commonly is increased in an effort to blow off CO_2 and raise the pH. Treatment should be directed at the underlying cause and is based on the patient's condition. Severe acidosis (generally below 7.10) should be treated with the administration of intravenous bicarbonate. The dose is based on body weight and base excess and is given in small increments as the pH is monitored. Indiscriminate use of bicarbonate may produce further lactate production and worsen the metabolic acidosis, and so bicarbonate should not be used unless the condition is severe. Overzealous administration of bicarbonate also may produce a rebound alkalosis, especially in chronic forms of metabolic acidosis such as renal tubular dysfunction.

METABOLIC ALKALOSIS

Metabolic alkalosis can be associated with volume depletion states (vomiting, gastric drainage, diuretics), hyperadrenocorticoid states that stimulate H^+ secretion (Cushing's syndrome, Bartter's syndrome, primary hyperaldosteronism), or abundance of alkali (iatrogenic overdose, milk-alkali syndrome, antacid abuse). The condition consists of increased pH and increased HCO_3^-. The bicarbonate level is elevated as a result of the gain of bicarbonate or the loss of hydrogen ion. Severe hypokalemia impairs renal tubular function by producing intracellular acidosis; this acidosis in turn stimulates bicarbonate retention and can lead to metabolic alkalosis. Vomiting causes a loss of H^+ and Cl^- as well as volume depletion; the kidneys respond by generating and retaining bicarbonate and excreting potassium.

Mineralocorticoids cause excess Na^+ retention with H^+ loss in exchange; mineralocorticoids also cause hypokalemia, further perpetuating the metabolic alkalosis.

Metabolic alkalosis does not produce many clinical signs. Apathy and confusion may occur. The diagnosis is based on history and laboratory values. A clue to the differential diagnosis of metabolic alkalosis is the measurement of urinary chloride. In volume-depletion causes of metabolic alkalosis, urinary chloride will be low; in hyperadrenocorticoid states or hypokalemia, urinary chloride will be high. Metabolic alkalosis rarely requires specific treatment. Volume-depleted states should respond to the administration of fluid and chloride salts.

$$H_2O + CO_2 \leftrightharpoons H_2CO_3 \leftrightharpoons H^+ + HCO_3^-$$

FIGURE 4-1-2. The bicarbonate–carbonic acid exchange system.

TABLE 4-1-1.   Common Acid-Base Disorders*

	ACIDOSIS (pH <7.35)	ALKALOSIS (pH >7.45)
Respiratory	⇑CO_2 [↑HCO_3^-]	⇓CO_2 [↓HCO_3^-]
Metabolic	⇓HCO_3^- [↓CO_2]	⇑HCO_3^- [↑CO_2]

*Bracketed ([ ]) values indicate compensation.

RESPIRATORY ACIDOSIS

Hypoventilation causes retention of CO_2, which drives the bicarbonate–carbonic acid equation to the right, increasing the concentration of H^+–respiratory acidosis. Acute respiratory acidosis can be caused by trauma, drugs, or cerebral dysfunction (i.e., cardiac arrest). The rapid rise in tissue acidosis is buffeted somewhat, but because the blood-brain barrier is easily permeated by carbonic acid, confusion, obtundation, asterixis, and papilledema indicating increased intracranial pressure rapidly develop. Chronic states of respiratory acidosis are seen most commonly in patients with chronic alveolar hypoventilation [chronic obstructive pulmonary disease (COPD), Pickwickian syndrome]. In chronic acidotic states, the kidneys increase the production of ammonia and enhance the excretion of ammonium; bicarbonate retention increases, and the urine becomes acidotic.

The diagnosis of respiratory acidosis depends on the history, evidence of hypoventilation, and increased $Paco_2$ with decreased pH. The bicarbonate level will be high in chronic states of respiratory acidosis as renal (metabolic) compensation becomes evident. It is necessary to correlate the changes in blood gases with the patient's history in order to direct treatment. In acute, severe respiratory acidosis, such as that which occurs in cardiac arrest, administration of bicarbonate with careful monitoring may be justified in addition to increasing ventilation. In cases of chronic hypoventilation and chronic respiratory acidosis, treatment of the underlying cause (i.e., increasing ventilation) is the sole means of treatment.

RESPIRATORY ALKALOSIS

Hyperventilation causes a reduction in $Paco_2$, which drives the bicarbonate–carbonic acid equation to produce alkalosis. Hyperventilation may be self-induced or occur in response to hypoxia. The decreased oxygen level in hypoxic states activates the respiratory centers in the brain to stimulate breathing. These centers also may be activated by anemia or severe hypotension in response to reduced oxygen delivery to the cells. Anxiety, sepsis, fever, pregnancy, and toxins also may excite the respiratory centers and lead to respiratory alkalosis.

Clinically, respiratory alkalosis is manifested by irritability, anxiety, vertigo, paresthesia, and numbness of the mouth, hands, and feet. In severe cases, confusion and loss of consciousness may occur. Tetany may develop with normal serum calcium because of the increased excitability of neuromuscular tissue. Electrocardiogram (ECG) recordings may show ST- or T- wave flattening. Arterial blood gases will reveal increased pH and decreased $Paco_2$; renal elimination of bicarbonate indicates compensation. The objective in the treatment of respiratory alkalosis is to remove the underlying cause. Assurance, sedation, and supplemental oxygen are usually sufficient to alleviate the symptoms. In the acute hyperventilation syndrome, rebreathing into a paper bag may help raise the $Paco_2$.

BIBLIOGRAPHY

Bongard FS, Sue DY (eds): *Current Critical Care Diagnosis and Treatment.* Norwalk, CT; Appleton-Lange, 1994.

Fluids and Electrolytes Made Incredibly Easy. Springhouse, PA, Springhouse Corporation, 1997.

Goldman L, Bennett JC (eds): *Cecil Textbook of Medicine,* 21st ed. Philadelphia; Saunders, 2000.

Hafstad L: Evaluation of acid-base disturbances. *Physician Assist* 16(3):17–45, 1992.

Williamson JC: Acid-base disorders: Classification and management strategies. *Am Family Physician* 52(2):584–590, 1995.

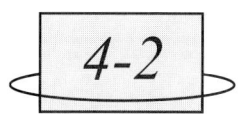

DISORDERS OF ELECTROLYTE BALANCE

Claire Babcock O'Connell

SODIUM

Sodium is the most abundant and important extracellular cation, accounting for 92 percent of the positive charge in the extracellular fluid (ECF). It is exchanged for potassium in cell depolarization and is returned to the extravascular space by active transport. The body content of sodium determines the ECF volume, including the plasma volume. Serum sodium and interstitial sodium are in equilibrium; therefore, the serum level represents ECF sodium. Normal serum sodium is 136 to 145 meq/L. This amount is kept relatively constant despite variations in intake.

The average American takes in about 3 to 6 g of sodium per day in the form of various sodium salts, mainly sodium chloride. The excess sodium is excreted in the urine. Sodium is filtered at the glomerulus; 70 percent is reabsorbed in the proximal tubule, and most of the remainder is reabsorbed in the distal tubule under the influence of aldosterone. Aldosterone accelerates the exchange of sodium and potassium in all cells and promotes the retention of sodium and the excretion of potassium in the kidney. Therefore, a deficiency in aldosterone results in excess loss of sodium and retention of potassium. Conversely, estrogen may cause a cyclic retention of sodium and loss of potassium, leading to menstrual bloating.

An increased concentration of sodium in the circulatory fluid stimulates the thirst mechanism and the release of antidiuretic hormone (ADH). Once osmolality decreases, ADH secretion is suppressed and sodium is excreted with water. If ADH is not suppressed, the body may retain excess water, increasing the ECF volume and leading to edema. The key to correcting the excess volume state is to treat the underlying cause [congestive heart failure (CHF), hepatic cirrhosis, nephrotic syndrome, etc.]. Sodium deficiency may prompt osmotic water excretion, leading to water depletion, decreased ECF, and clinical dehydration. Changes in the ECF volume (water) cause greater clinical effects than do changes in the absolute sodium content. Hyponatremia may exist with normal, high, or low absolute levels of sodium.

Hyponatremia

Hyponatremia exists whenever the ratio of solute to water is reduced (see Table 4-2-1). If water intake exceeds water loss or water loss is defective, a relative reduction in sodium to water content occurs. Total body water can be normal, reduced, or increased. Any condition that generates a reduction in effective circulatory volume will stimulate the release of ADH as a result of the diminished delivery to the diluting segments of renal tubules. ADH will prompt increased reabsorption of water beyond the amount of sodium reabsorbed, thereby producing hyponatremia. In chronic impaired water excretion states, the excess water is distributed between intracellular fluid (ICF) and ECF; no edema results. Generally, the clinical manifestations are more directly related to the volume state than to the sodium level.

Clinical manifestations of hyponatremia depend on the degree and rapidity of sodium loss. Acute rapid increases in body water relative to sodium concentration cause a rapid influx of water into cells. Swelling of cells in the central nervous system causes lethargy, confusion, stupor, or coma. A rapid reduction in sodium concentration causes hyperexcitability, which is evident by muscle twitching, irritability, and seizure activity. Chronic slower processes that lead to hyponatremia are handled better. The central nervous system is able to excrete inorganic ions (potassium and others) and produce idiogenic osmoles that assist in maintaining water balance within the central nervous system cells and preserving neurologic function. Moderate hyponatremia will cause increased salivation, lacrimation, and watery diarrhea in an attempt to rid the body of the excess water relative to sodium content.

Diagnosis is made through history, physical examination, and laboratory values. The history should concentrate on water intake and fluid losses. The physical examination will allow categorization into normal volume, excessive volume (fluid overload), and reduced volume (dehydration) states. The blood urea nitrogen (BUN) and creatinine levels are drawn to verify the suspected volume states: High values indicate dehydration or renal losses (or renal failure); normal or low values support fluid overload causes or normal volume states of hyponatremia.

Treatment of hyponatremia is targeted at the underlying cause. In most situations, the hyponatremia does not require specific treatment and can be corrected promptly by removal of the causative disorder. In the rare case of severe, acute hyponatremia, correction can be assisted by the infusion of hypertonic saline, with careful monitoring to avoid shrinkage of central nervous system cells in response to the osmotic gradient of the infused solution into the ECF.

Hypernatremia

In hypernatremia, the ratio of solute to water is increased. Excess sodium concentration can result from pure water losses, water and sodium loss (proportionally more water than sodium is lost), or states of excess sodium (see Table 4-2-2). Assessment of overall fluid status

TABLE 4-2-1. Common Causes of Hyponatremia

Volume depletion states (water and sodium depleted)
Diuretic abuse (loop diuretics, thiazides, other)
Proportionally greater loss of sodium than water (vomiting, diarrhea, burns, etc.)
Fluid overload states, edema
Congestive heart failure
Cirrhosis
Nephrotic syndrome
Normal volume states (or moderately increased volume states, no edema)
Syndrome of inappropriate ADH (SIADH)
Chronic renal failure
Endocrine disorders
Adrenal insufficiency
Hypothyroidism
Psychogenic polydipsia
Essential hyponatremia
Other
Oncotic losses (glucose, mannitol)
Artifactual (lab error, interference by proteins or lipids in sample)

TABLE 4-2-2. Common Causes of Hypernatremia

Pure water deficits
Extrarenal losses
Fever
Burns
Increased respiratory states
Renal losses
Diabetes insipidus
Hypothalamic disorders
Water and sodium loss (hypotonic loss)
Extrarenal loss
Sweating without adequate intake
Renal loss
Osmotic diuresis
DKA
Mannitol
Urea diuresis (high-protein diets)
Hyperosmolar nonketotic diabetic come (glucose diuresis)
Excess sodium states
Iatrogenic sodium overload
Adrenal hyperfunction (Cushing's syndrome)

is essential because treatment options will differ. Clinical manifestations resulting from the high concentration of sodium reflect the status of dehydration that often coexists with hypernatremia: decreased lacrimation, decreased salivation, dry mucous membranes, flushed skin, decreased skin turgor, restlessness, weakness, tachycardia, and hypotension. The high solute concentration causes an osmotic flow of water from the ICF into the ECF. The central nervous system is affected less inasmuch as it can counterbalance the osmotic loss with the production of idiogenic osmoles to help retain water in neurons. Changes in mental status, confusion, delirium, muscle twitching, seizures, obtundation, stupor, and coma may result as the sodium concentration rises above this ability to counter the increased osmotic pressure. Acute rapid increases in sodium concentration are more detrimental than are slower, more chronic increases because of the production of these idiogenic osmoles over 1 to 3 days.

Overall correction of hypernatremia relies on treatment of the underlying cause. In the acute setting, treatment decisions are based on whether the high sodium concentration is accompanied by volume loss, volume expansion, or normal volume states. Increased solute without expansion of volume necessitates solute diuresis with the accompanying replacement of obligate water losses. In states of diminished volume (loss of hypotonic fluid that results in overall hypertonic vascular fluid), both water and sodium must be replaced. Normal (isotonic) saline is hypotonic to the patient and usually is recommended as the first-line replacement fluid. After some expansion of ECF is evident, switch to half-normal saline or $D_5$1/2 NS to continue water replacement. Infusion of D_5W, which is solute-free, may correct the hypernatremic state too quickly; the osmotic forces may drive ECF into the ICF, causing swelling of the brain cells. Glucose carries the risk of hyperglycemia and therefore an osmotic diuresis, which would worsen the hypertonic state, and so it should be used with caution.

POTASSIUM

Potassium is the major cation of the ICF, accounting for 77 percent of all intracellular cations and providing the bulk of intracellular osmotic pressure. Of total body potassium, 98 percent is found within cells. The ratio of potassium to sodium is essential for cellular metabolism, proper membrane potential, and depolarization. Small changes in concentration can be detrimental to physiologic function. Serum potassium concentration is used as a rough indicator of overall potassium balance.

Obligate daily potassium losses are small. The kidneys excrete most of the dietary intake of potassium. Excretion of potassium is facilitated by high sodium levels and high intracellular concentrations of potassium; it is inhibited by low potassium filtration and low sodium loads in the distal nephron. The shift of potassium from the ECF to the ICF is enhanced by insulin, catecholamines, and metabolic alkalosis. Potassium is shifted out of the cells and into the ECF by metabolic acidosis, as in diabetic ketoacidosis (DKA). In DKA, the initial measurement of serum potassium may be increased but the actual body potassium may be normal or low.

Acid-base disorders upset potassium balance. Alkalosis causes hypokalemia by increasing renal secretion of potassium with the excess bicarbonate and also, to some extent, by trading extracellular potassium ions for intracellular hydrogen ions. Acidosis, as in DKA, causes a shift of potassium ions from the intracellular space to the extracellular space in exchange for hydrogen ion. The high potassium load presented to the kidney may cause excess potassium secretion, thereby producing true low total body potassium in the face of normal or high potassium levels. Correction of the acidotic state therefore may uncover hypokalemia.

Hypokalemia

True potassium deficits can occur through gastrointestinal (GI) losses or excessive renal excretion. A false potassium deficit may arise from any condition that causes a shift of potassium ions into cells without true overall body potassium depletion (see Table 4-2-3). Clinical

TABLE 4-2-3. Common Causes of Hypokalemia

GI losses
  Vomiting (metabolic alkalosis induces potassium wasting)
  Diarrhea (rarely severe enough to produce symptoms)
  Fistulas, laxative abuse, malabsorption

Renal losses
  Metabolic alkalosis
  Diuretics (thiazides, loop, carbonic anhydrase inhibitors)
  Osmotic diuresis (including DKA and hyperosmolar nonketotic
    diabetic coma)
  Excess mineralocorticoids
  Renal tubular diseases
  Magnesium depletion
  Post–renal transplant diuresis
  Nephritis

Hypokalemia without total body potassium depletion
  Insulin, hyperalimentation
  Alkalosis
  Catecholamines

Other
  Hyperaldosteronism
  Acute alcoholism
  Congestive heart failure
  Bartter's syndrome

manifestations of potassium depletion are influenced by the amount and rapidity of loss. Severe or abrupt potassium depletion can lead to neuromuscular losses, paralysis, rhabdomyolysis, myoglobinuria, diminished reflexes, and paralytic ileus. As the lack of potassium affects smooth muscles, anorexia, nausea, vomiting, decreased bowel sounds, and constipation occur. Impaired renal tubular function secondary to low potassium concentration in tubular fluid causes a decreased concentrating ability and may produce polyuria and polydipsia.

Cardiac manifestations of hypokalemia include a weak irregular pulse, flattening and inversion of T waves, prominence of U waves, and a sagging ST segment. Severe or rapid loss of potassium may precipitate cardiac arrest. Hypokalemia in the presence of digitalis can increase the likelihood of digitalis toxicity and produce arrhythmias.

Treatment of hypokalemia consists of potassium replacement. Oral potassium is preferred if it can be tolerated. Parenteral potassium is indicated in true potassium deficits if there is GI impairment or neuromuscular or cardiac manifestations that indicate a moderate to severe deficit. False hypokalemia does not necessitate potassium replacement. Treatment of the underlying cause of potassium shift should correct the hypokalemia. In instances where hypokalemia exists despite treatment of the underlying cause, potassium should be replaced.

Hyperkalemia

Excessive dietary intake of potassium should not cause hyperkalemia in persons with normal renal function. Renal excretion should be equal to dietary intake. However, the addition of excess potassium directly into the extravascular space by intravenous therapy or a reduced ability of the kidneys to excrete potassium loads may lead to hyperkalemia (see Table 4-2-4). Hyperkalemia is often asymptomatic until the potassium level has risen above 7.0 meq/L. Hyponatremia, hypocalcemia, and acidosis will potentiate the effects of increased potassium levels. Correction of these abnormalities will aid in the avoidance of hyperkalemic complications. The most common symptom of a rising potassium level is muscle weakness. Associated features of mild to moderate hyperkalemia include nausea, vomiting, diarrhea, and intestinal colic. As the weakness progresses, flaccid paralysis and respiratory disturbances may occur; cerebral function remains normal.

The most devastating effect of hyperkalemia is cardiac arrhythmia. Mild hyperkalemia (5.0 to 6.0 meq/L) produces peaked T waves. Potassium levels between 6.0 and 8.0 meq/L prolong the PR interval and

TABLE 4-2-4. Common Causes of Hyperkalemia

Inadequate potassium excretion
   Renal disorders
      Renal failure, acute or chronic (oliguria)
   Tubular disorders
      Systemic lupus erythematosus
      Amyloidosis
      Posttransplant rejection

Decreased effective circulatory volume (enhances reabsorption, inhibiting
   secretion)
   Hypoaldosteronism
      Adrenal disorders
      Hyporeninemia
   Potassium-sparing diuretics

Extracellular potassium addition
   Tissue damage (muscle crush, hemolysis, internal bleeding)
   Drugs that alter potassium uptake (succinylcholine, arginine, digitalis
      toxicity)
   Metabolic acidosis
   Hyperosmolality
   Insulin deficiency
   Hyperkalemia period paralysis

Excessive intake
   Iatrogenic overload

Pseudohyperkalemia
   Thrombocytosis
   Leukocytosis
   Hemolysis of sample in vitro
   Poor laboratory technique

produce heart block. Severe hyperkalemia (>8.0 meq/L) causes a loss of P waves, a widened QRS, ventricular fibrillation, and cardiac standstill. Patients suspected to be at risk for hyperkalemia should be followed with electrocardiography as well as laboratory measurements of potassium.

Correction of hyperkalemia hinges on the treatment of the underlying cause. Elimination of the cause of hyperkalemia will allow the body's metabolism to bring the potassium back to normal levels. In the acute setting, it is imperative to treat any concurrent volume deficit and acidosis and monitor the patient with serial electrocardiograms (ECGs) and plasma measurements. Calcium can be administered to directly counteract the effects of the potassium on cardiac tissue and prevent fatal arrhythmias. Specific measurements aimed at a rapid reduction in serum potassium include promoting potassium transfer from the ECF to the ICF (glucose with insulin, sodium bicarbonate, and beta agonists) and enhancing potassium elimination (non-potassium-sparing diuretics, dialysis, exchange resins).

CALCIUM

Much of the calcium in the human body is locked in bone. The ionized calcium in the ECF is important, though, for the proper functioning of muscles and neurons. Dietary calcium intake is important to maintain adequate body stores of calcium. Absorption of calcium in the GI tract is dependent on vitamin D. In a normal individual, about 30 percent of ingested calcium is absorbed. In times of deficient calcium status, absorption can rise to 90 percent. Children and pregnant women require higher daily intake of calcium to support skeletal growth. Prolonged immobilization precipitates bone loss and calcium efflux to the blood.

About half the nonbone calcium is bound to protein in the plasma; most of the remaining calcium is unbound, ionized calcium, and a small amount exists as calcium salts (citrates, phosphates). Laboratory analysis of total calcium levels must always be assessed in light of serum protein status. Hypoalbuminemia is associated with a measured hypocalcemia. Specimens for the measurement of the calcium level should be taken with the patient fasting and seated or recumbent to stabilize the

albumin. Alkalosis promotes calcium binding with protein, which results in a decrease in ionized calcium. Acidosis acts in the opposite direction.

Ionized calcium is filtered and reabsorbed in the kidney. Conditions that interfere with sodium and potassium reabsorption also affect the absorption of calcium and increase calcium excretion in the urine. Calcium balance is regulated by parathyroid hormone (PTH) and vitamin D [active metabolite 1,25-dehydroxycholecalciferol $(1,25\text{-}(OH)_2D_3)$]; increases in PTH cause the release of calcium from the bone, decreased calcium excretion from the kidney, and augmented reabsorption of calcium in the gut. PTH release is governed primarily by the serum calcium level. Calcitonin acts antagonistically to PTH; it promotes renal excretion of calcium and inhibits bone resorption and intestinal absorption.

Hypercalcemia

The vast majority of cases of hypercalcemia result from one of two causes: a defect in calcium regulation (hyperparathyroidism) or increased release of calcium from bone caused by endogenous parathyroid-like substances commonly produced in malignancy. High levels of calcium on routine blood screening and the manifestation of hypercalcemia (renal stones, bone pain) are often the earliest indicators of underlying disease (malignancy, hyperparathyroidism, Paget's disease, sarcoidosis, hyperthyroidism, adrenal insufficiency). Excessive vitamin D intake causes increased absorption of calcium and increased bone resorption, leading to hypercalcemia. Lithium therapy also is associated with hypercalcemia.

Hypercalcemia induces an osmotic diuresis and resultant polydipsia and polyuria. If the patient can maintain adequate fluid intake and functional kidneys, the high calcium levels may go undetected until other symptoms occur. If the high calcium levels and associated interference with ADH action continue for a prolonged period, permanent renal damage may occur, especially if there is a concomitant elevation in the phosphate level.

High levels of calcium affect the motility of GI tract, producing abdominal pain, nausea, vomiting, anorexia, decreased bowel sounds, and constipation. Acute pancreatitis is not uncommon in patients with hypercalcemia. Lethargy, fatigue, weakness, and hyporeflexia are encountered in hypercalcemia secondary to neuromuscular dysfunction. The QT interval may be shortened, and bradycardia may develop. Severe hypercalcemia (>15 mg/dL) is a medical emergency that can result in coma or cardiac arrest.

Diagnosis of the cause of hypercalcemia can for the most part be made through a medical history and PTH level. Asymptomatic individuals with a chronic increase in calcium most likely are exhibiting primary hyperparathyroidism. Decreased PTH with an acute presentation of hypercalcemia indicates malignancy. Low or normal levels of PTH with chronically elevated calcium warrant investigation for other causes, such as sarcoidosis, vitamin D excess, or conditions of high bone turnover.

Mild, asymptomatic hypercalcemia does not need to be treated. A search for and the treatment of the underlying cause of the hypercalcemia are warranted. Very high levels of serum calcium (>12 mg/dL) or hypercalcemia associated with symptoms should be treated while one is searching for the cause. Expansion of the extracellular volume with isotonic saline will result in a decreased reabsorption of sodium and calcium, thereby lowering the serum calcium level. The addition of furosemide will enhance this process. When hypercalcemia is due to pathologic losses from bone, pharmacologic therapy to enhance bone reuptake can be attempted (mithramycin, diphosphates). Calcitonin has short-lived effects but is used to promote renal excretion of calcium, inhibit bone breakdown, and slow GI absorption of calcium. Hemodialysis is effective for patients with inadequate renal function.

Hypocalcemia

Low levels of serum calcium must be assessed in view of the plasma proteins because the calcium that is measured in routine laboratory testing is protein-bound. If the serum albumin is low, the serum calcium level should be corrected by adding 0.75 mg/dL for every 1.0 g/dL below 3.5 g/dL of albumin. Hypocalcemia is a result of a lack of efficient PTH function. When the body detects deficient calcium levels, PTH secretion is increased within seconds; within days, there is evidence of increased biosynthesis of PTH, followed by parathyroid cell hyperplasia within weeks. This process is known as secondary hyperparathyroidism and causes an increase in renal secretion of 1,25(OH)$_2$D$_3$ and increased calcium flow into the blood from the intestinal lumen, bone, and renal tubules. Primary hypoparathyroidism (inherited or acquired) and hypomagnesia result in a severe depletion or absence of hormone. Whenever the responses to low calcium are weakened or blunted (either primarily or secondarily), hypocalcemia results. Additional, less common causes of hypocalcemia include inadequate dietary intake, malabsorption, pancreatic insufficiency, hypomagnesemia, alkalosis, and certain drugs, such as loop diuretics, phosphates, phenytoin, phenobarbital, and gentamicin.

Clinically, a low-calcium state is associated with increased neuromuscular excitability, which is first manifested as paresthesis in the fingers and toes and around the oral cavity. As the serum level drops lower, muscle cramping, carpopedal spasm, laryngeal stridor, and convulsions may occur. The appearance of symptoms is related to the degree and rate of calcium deficit. Latent tetany associated with calcium deficit may be demonstrated with Chvostek's sign (twitching of the upper lip after tapping on the facial nerve) and Trousseau's sign (carpal spasm after inflating a cuff above systole for 2 to 3 mins).

Low serum calcium also is associated with mental disturbances, including irritability, depression, and psychosis. Arrhythmias and ECG changes may occur. Papilledema may indicate increased intracerebral pressure. Cataracts may occur in long-standing calcium-poor states. Prolonged hypocalcemia also causes resorption of calcium from bone and other structures, which results in fractures, brittle nails, and dry skin and hair.

The diagnosis is based on the history and physical examination and confirmed by laboratory results. Hypocalcemia, hyperphosphatemia, and normal renal function support primary hypoparathyroidism; this is confirmed by low levels of PTH. Low calcium with normal or low phosphate indicates malabsorption of vitamin D; the PTH level will be elevated, and the patient's GI function should be evaluated.

Treatment of hypocalcemia is based on the underlying cause. In an acute situation, calcium can be administered intravenously. Replacement of magnesium may be necessary as well. Oral calcium supplementation is recommended for persons at risk of calcium loss or in need of excess calcium, including children, pregnant women, patients facing prolonged immobilization, and peri- and postmenopausal women.

PHOSPHORUS

Phosphorus is the major anion of the intracellular compartment. It is found in virtually all soft tissue, although the majority of it is in bone. Its functions include the building of cell membrane phospholipids, and it participates in various energy-producing reactions. It is absorbed in the gut under the influence of vitamin D and filtered and reabsorbed in the kidney. When phosphorus levels exceed a transport maximum (TmP), phosphorus will be excreted in the urine; an increase in PTH will inhibit renal phosphate reabsorption.

Hypophosphatemia

Low phosphate can result from either ion shift or depleted stores. Ingestion of a high carbohydrate load or alkalosis will cause a transient shift of phosphate into cells. More commonly, hypophosphatemia results from depleted stores. Poor intake and poor GI absorption (hyperalimentation, prolonged use of phosphate-binding antacids) account for some cases of depletion; more often hypophosphatemia is a result of inadequate renal reabsorption, which is seen in poorly controlled diabetes mellitus, in alcoholism, and in the recovery period after severe burns or starvation.

A sustained hypophosphatemia causes widespread cellular enzymatic dysfunction and a decline in phosphate-dependent energy sources. Phosphate deficiency causes changes in the cell membrane structure and function, depletes intracellular phosphorylated compounds such as adenosine triphosphate (ATP) and 2,3-diphosphoglycerate and increases the intracellular calcium levels. The effects are seen throughout several organ systems. There is weakness and possible paralysis, rhabdomyolysis, and cardiomyopathy; altered red blood cell (RBC) function including hemolytic anemia, impaired leukocyte function, and poor platelet aggregation; increased bone resorption, osteomalacia, and rickets; impaired hepatic and renal function; and metabolic encephalopathy and hypoglycemia.

Treatment is aimed at correcting the underlying disorder. In severe or symptomatic hypophosphatemia, the goal is to minimize urinary losses and enhance absorption from the gut. Supplemental phosphates given intravenously are associated with changes in other electrolytes, including calcium and magnesium, and therefore should be monitored closely. Oral phosphate supplements are associated with diarrhea, metabolic acidosis, hypertension, and loss of calcium from the gut.

Hyperphosphatemia

Increased renal reabsorption or reduced renal excretion of phosphate leads to hyperphosphatemia. With normally functioning kidneys, increased oral intake is only rarely associated with hyperphosphatemia; all excess phosphate will be excreted. Iatrogenic overload via intravenous phosphate can occur. A transient rise in phosphate levels will be seen in any state that causes rapid cell destruction.

High levels of phosphate will bind with calcium and deposit into soft tissue. This will cause a hypocalcemia and possibly tetany. Chronic hyperphosphatemia-hypocalcemia will cause a resultant secondary hyperparathyroidism. Phosphate also reduces the action of vitamin D and therefore reduces the amount of calcium absorption in the gut. Clinically, the signs and symptoms of hypocalcemia are more important than is the hyperphosphatemia. Correction of the underlying process will prompt a return to balance for both calcium and phosphate.

MAGNESIUM

Magnesium is the second most abundant intracellular cation after potassium. It is vital for proper enzymatic actions, including ATP, and, with calcium, proper neuromuscular functioning. One-quarter of serum magnesium is protein-bound. Hormones or acid-base status does not control magnesium distribution. Free magnesium is reabsorbed, and a steady state is readily established with a normal diet. Excess amounts of magnesium are not protein-bound and are excreted up to a limit imposed by the glomerular filtration rate.

Hypomagnesemia

Decreased intake and/or increased excretion account for the majority of cases of hypomagnesemia. Poor dietary intake is rarely a cause of low magnesium; conditions that affect GI absorption will cause hypomagnesemia. Severe diarrhea, steatorrhea, and familial malabsorption syndromes are associated with low body magnesium with low urinary magnesium. Renal magnesium loss is associated with normal to high urinary magnesium levels. Renal wasting can be divided into intrinsic renal disorders (familial or sporadic renal tubular disorders, Bartter's syndrome, nephrotoxic agents) and extrinsic renal disorders (volume expansion, hypercalcuria, diuretic abuse, diabetic ketoacidosis).

Other disorders associated with magnesium loss include thyrotoxicosis, pancreatitis, lactation, alcoholism, and severe burns. Acute myocardial infarction often is accompanied by hypomagnesemia, and treatment of this magnesium deficit will reduce the risk of ventricular arrhythmias greatly. Forty percent of patients found to be deficient in magnesium have a coexisting hypocalcemia and a refractory potassium depletion state. The addition of magnesium will rapidly assist in treatment.

Hypomagnesemia often is manifested clinically in association with hypokalemia and hypocalcemia. Weakness, anorexia, apathy, fasciculations, and tremors indicate neuromuscular dysfunction. Chvostek's and Trousseau's signs may progress to overt tetany. Ventricular arrhythmias occur, especially in the presence of digitalis toxicity. Rarely, patients may exhibit seizures resulting from low levels of magnesium.

Treatment of mild magnesium deficits that are asymptomatic consists of dietary recommendations. Symptomatic hypomagnesemia warrants replacement. It is important to note that only half the supplemental intravenous magnesium will remain in circulation; the remaining half will be excreted in the urine. Replacement of magnesium will greatly assist in alleviating the symptoms of hypocalcemia and hypokalemia. Ultimately, correction of the underlying cause of electrolyte deficiency is the best objective.

Hypermagnesemia

Increased dietary magnesium is virtually unknown to cause hypermagnesemia. Abuse of magnesium-containing laxatives and antacids and excess intravenous magnesium sulfate (as occurs in the treatment of preeclampsia-eclampsia) can cause magnesium overload. High loads of magnesium are presented to the renal tubules in an unbound form and will be excreted if there is ongoing sodium excretion. Only a set amount of magnesium is reabsorbed; any excess magnesium filtered will be excreted unless the glomerular filtration rate is impaired.

The symptoms and signs of hypermagnesemia are nonspecific: weakness, lethargy, nausea, and hyporeflexia. As the level of magnesium rises, the deep tendon reflexes are lost and the patient may exhibit flaccid quadriplegia. Acute, severe hypermagnesemia also may cause respiratory depression, hypotension, bradycardia, and, rarely, complete heart block and cardiac arrest.

Severe, symptomatic hypermagnesemia requires urgent treatment. Calcium is a direct antagonist of magnesium. Intravenous calcium gluconate or calcium chloride will block the effects of magnesium. Once the patient is stabilized, efforts to reduce the level of magnesium are needed. Any excess intake should be discontinued, and magnesium excretion should be maximized. With functional kidneys, furosemide with half-normal saline will increase the urine volume and maintain proper diuresis. In patients with impaired renal function or renal failure, hemodialysis is effective in removing excess magnesium.

BIBLIOGRAPHY

Bongard FS, Sue DY (eds.): *Current Critical Care Diagnosis and Treatment.* Norwalk, CT; Appleton-Lange, 1994.
Fluids and Electrolytes Made Incredibly Easy. Springhouse, PA, Springhouse Corporation, 1997.
Goldman L, Bennett JC (eds.): *Cecil Textbook of Medicine,* 21st ed. Philadelphia, Saunders, 2000.
Williamson JC: Acid-base disorders: Classification and management strategies. *Am Family Physician* 52(2):584–590, 1995.

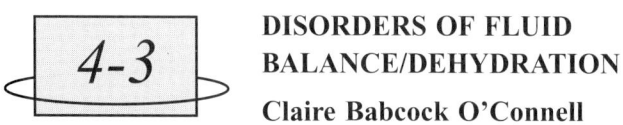

DISORDERS OF FLUID BALANCE/DEHYDRATION

Claire Babcock O'Connell

DISCUSSION

The human body is approximately 60 percent water, which is able to freely move among body compartments in response to solute concentration. In the average 70-kg person, there is approximately 40 L of water: two-thirds of this water is in the intracellular fluid (ICF) compartment (25 L), and one-third is in the extracellular fluid (ECF) compartment (15 L). Within the ECF two-thirds of the water is interstitial (10 L); one-third is in the plasma (5 L). The average hematocrit is 40 to 45 percent, therefore leaving about 2.5 L of fluid obtainable by venipuncture—most of which is water.

Daily water intake is about 2500 mL per day, mostly from food and fluid intake. Average daily water loss is about equal (2500 mL/day). Water is lost through skin (500 mL/day), expired air (350 mL/day), urine (1500 mL/day), and feces (150 mL/day). The balance of water intake and loss is maintained within close limits by sensitive thirst mechanisms and kidney regulation. Clinical manifestations occur as a result of problems affecting this balance: inability to swallow, vomiting, diarrhea, excessive urination or perspiration, starvation, fistulas, and so on.

Movement of water among compartments depends on the amount of solute in each compartment. Solute composition includes electrolytes, cells and cellular material, proteins, and organic acids. The ionic state of each compartment is kept in balance by the movement of ions; this requires energy (active transport). Water follows rapidly to balance each compartment, following osmotic gradients; no energy is required. The main determinant of ECF volume is sodium concentration. ICF volume is determined chiefly by potassium concentration. Large changes in cell volume can handicap or destroy cells. It is imperative to maintain optimum cell volume; active transport of ions against a concentration gradient and free osmotic movement of water in response to these changes ensure proper cell volume.

In the vascular space, hydrostatic pressure forces water out of the capillaries. The osmotic pressure of plasma proteins and solutes brings water back into the capillaries. Protection of the effective blood volume (ECF) is key to survival. Disturbances in osmolality cause a response via thirst mechanisms. High osmolality (low water/high solute) increases thirst and stimulates the release of antidiuretic hormone (ADH), which increases tubular water reabsorption, and therefore less water is excreted in the urine. Low osmolality (high water/low solute) inhibits thirst and ADH release, resulting in large volumes of dilute urine. Receptors in the kidney and elsewhere also respond to changes in effective blood volume. Low-volume states result in salt retention, thereby retaining water through the renin-angiotensin system. High-volume states stimulate the release of natriuretic hormones; water is pulled into the urine with the excess sodium through osmosis.

VOLUME EXCESS

Excess fluid volume is essentially excess water. Total body sodium is usually high as well. Volume excess is due to an intake of water and/or salt that exceeds the loss of water and/or salt. Common clinical causes of volume excess include congestive heart failure (CHF), the nephrotic syndrome, hepatic cirrhosis, mineralocorticoid or ADH overproduction, renal insufficiency, and iatrogenic fluid overload. The symptoms of volume excess are dyspnea, orthopnea, paroxysmal nocturnal dyspnea, and rapid weight gain caused by edema. Clinical signs reflect the fluid overload in the vascular space and include increased venous pressure, bibasilar rales, decreased breath sounds, an S_3 heart sound, dependent pitting edema, ascites, anasarca, hepatomegaly, and hepatojugular reflux. The main objective in the treatment of fluid overload states is to treat the underlying cause. Once the cause of the fluid overload is corrected, it is best to monitor the patient and provide supportive measures as needed. The body has a tremendous ability to return to hemostatic balance. Fluid and sodium restriction, diuretics, and digitalis are helpful during acute crises as the underlying cause is corrected.

VOLUME DEPLETION

Inadequate volume is a result of inadequate water or salt intake or excessive loss. As depicted in Table 4-3-1, there are three major causes of volume depletion: hormonal deficits, renal deficits, and extrarenal losses. Clinically, symptoms and signs of volume depletion depend on the magnitude, rate, and nature of the fluid loss coupled with the responsiveness of the vascular system. Water loss is equilibrated rapidly

TABLE 4-3-1. Common Causes of Volume Depletion

Hormonal deficits (loss of ADH or aldosterone)
   Pituitary diabetes insipidus
   Addison's disease
   Interstitial nephritis
   Hyporeninemic hypoaldosteronism

Renal deficits (impaired renal tubular sodium or water conservation)
   Renal tubular nephropathies
      Nephrogenic diabetes insipidus
   Diuretic abuse
   Osmotic diuresis
      Glucose (DKA, hyperglycemic hyperosmolar coma, hyperalimentation)
      Urea (burn patients)
      Mannitol, glycerol (iatrogenic)
   Chronic renal failure

Extrarenal losses
   Hemorrhage
   Cutaneous loss
   Gastrointestinal losses
      Fluid loss (vomiting, diarrhea, gastric drainage, GI fistulas)
      Sequestration (peritonitis, ascites)

through the ECF and ICF owing to osmosis. Vascular depletion results in circulatory collapse; intracellular loss leads to cellular damage and death, compromising physiologic functions.

It is important to assess the amount of fluid intake in any patient suspected to be volume-depleted. Fluid intake must be assessed in parallel to known fluid losses. On examination, general appearance and mental status are the keys to assessing volume status. Vital signs, the appearance of the skin and mucous membranes, and the ability to cry or sweat are good indicators of the approximate magnitude of loss. A quick patient assessment allows the examiner to decide whether the patient is mildly, moderately, or severely depleted. Table 4-3-2 outlines the general clinical guidelines for the assessment of dehydration.

Tears are lost at approximately 7 percent dehydration. Their presence or absence is the most reliable indicator of fluid status in children. Skin turgor is helpful in assessing children; it is not reliable in adults and the elderly. Pulse, blood pressure, capillary refill, and laboratory measurements are evaluated as a group; none of these measurements should be used alone in assessing fluid status. It is important to examine the complete picture in conjunction with the patient's history.

Severe volume depletion can result in end organ damage and death. Any comatose patient who is suspected of being volume-depleted should be challenged with 500 mL of normal saline over 1 to 3 h.

TABLE 4-3-2. General Guidelines for Dehydration Assessment

5% dehydration—mild dehydration
   Mild postural giddiness
   Postural mild tachycardia
   Weakness
   Thirst +/− dry mucous membranes
   Tears present
10% dehydration—moderate dehydration
   Decreased skin turgor
   Dry mucous membranes
   Tachycardia
   Orthostatic hypotension
   Decreased urine volume
   No tears produced
15% dehydration—severe dehydration
   Hypotension, shock
   Recumbent tachycardia
   Oliguria, anuria
   Coldness of extremities
   Mental status changes (lethargy, stupor, coma)

This fluid challenge both offers a clue to the underlying diagnosis and helps maintain effective circulating volume. Mild and moderate volume depletion can be remedied easily. The absolute treatment naturally is treatment of the underlying cause. While the definitive diagnosis and treatment protocol are being investigated, fluid should be restored to maintain effective circulatory volume and alleviate symptoms. Choice of fluid type, rate of infusion, and route of administration depend on the clinical scenario. Any patient who can be maintained on oral fluids should be. Patients who are more than mildly depleted, are suffering from protracted vomiting or diarrhea, or are candidates for surgical treatment may need intravenous replacement of fluids.

TREATMENT

Sodium-free solutions such as D_5W are equivalent to solute-free. The fluid will distribute uniformly in all body compartments. One liter of solute-free fluid will result in about 75 to 100 mL of fluid into the intravascular space, a 2 percent increase in intravascular volume. Sodium-containing solutions preferentially expand the ECF, although much of the water will flow into the interstitial space and into the ICF. One liter of normal saline will result in about 300 mL of fluid into the intravascular space, a 6 percent increase in intravascular volume.

Colloid-containing solutions (albumin, plasma) preferentially expand the ECF. The oncotic pressure provided by the colloid particles causes an osmotic flow of water from the ICF to the ECF. The large proteins cause a rapid expansion of intravascular volume. However, these solutions have relatively short half-lives and are expensive. They are used primarily in the treatment of burn patients and during acute circulatory collapse with severe fluid depletion.

Blood is the most potent expander of the intravascular space. One liter of packed red blood cells will remain entirely in the vascular space. This will cause an osmotic flow of water into the vessels and a rapid increase in the effective circulatory volume. In patients with acute hemorrhage or severe volume loss with changes in mental status, packed cells are administered along with normal saline or a colloid solution to enhance circulatory function.

The amount and rate of fluid replacement are guided by the patient's status and weight. Fluid orders must take into account maintenance fluid, any deficit, and any ongoing losses. Maintenance fluid is based entirely on body weight. A simple guide is to provide 100 mL of fluid per kilogram for the first 10 kg of body weight, 50 kg of fluid for the second 10 kg of body weight, and 20 kg of fluid for every remaining kilogram of body weight. Thus, for the average 70-kg person, 2500 kg of fluid is required per day for maintenance ($10 \times 100 = 1000$; $10 \times 50 = 500$; $50 \times 20 = 1000$; $1000 + 500 + 1000 = 2500$).

Deficits also are estimated on the basis of body weight. If a 70-kg person is assessed clinically as being 5 percent dehydrated, the deficit is estimated to be 3.5 L, or 3500 mL ($70 \times 0.05 = 3.5$). Total fluid requirements for this patient (if there are no ongoing losses) is 2500 mL + 3500 mL = 6000 mL. Because the patient is dehydrated, fluid replacement is necessary to improve the clinical status. Therefore, the objective is to get the fluid in as quickly as possible without overloading the system and risking complications. The general guideline is to infuse one-half of the total fluid needs in one-third of the time. In this case, the orders would be for 3000 mL of fluid in the first 8 h (375 mL/h) followed by 3000 mL of fluid in the following 16 h (188 mL/h). Throughout the replacement time, the patient should be monitored and the fluid rate should be adjusted according to the clinical status. If this patient is admitted without circulatory compromise, indicating that the deficit was throughout all body compartments, a dilute solute-containing solution such as half-normal saline will be appropriate. If the patient presents with signs of circulatory compromise, a crystalloid solution such as Ringer's lactate may be the appropriate starting fluid.

BIBLIOGRAPHY

Bongard FS, Sue DY (eds): *Current Critical Care Diagnosis and Treatment.* Norwalk, CT, Appleton-Lange, 1994.

Fluids and Electrolytes Made Incredibly Easy. Springhouse, PA, Springhouse Corporation, 1997.

Goldman L, Bennett JC (eds): *Cecil Textbook of Medicine,* 21st ed. Philadelphia; Saunders, 2000.

Williamson JC: Acid-base disorders: Classification and management strategies. *Am Fam Physician* 52(2):584–590, A 1995.

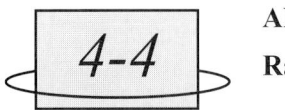

ANIMAL BITES

Ralph Rice

DISCUSSION

With more than 3 million occurrences every year, animal bites cause 1 percent of emergency room visits.[1] One in every two Americans will be bitten during his or her lifetime by an animal or another human being.[1,2] The annual health care cost for bite injuries is estimated to be in excess of $30 million.[1] Most animal bites come from dogs and cats. Other bites come from snakes, rodents, and other wild and exotic animals. Dog and cat bites are the primary focus of this chapter.

Dog bites account for 80 to 90 percent of all animal bites.[1] Among those bites, researchers estimate that between 2 and 20 percent become infected.[1,2] Dog bites occur most frequently in males and in persons between 2 and 19 years of age. The peak incidence of dog bites occurs during the warmer, summer months and between the hours of 4 and 6 P.M.[2,3] The most common site of injury is the hand and upper extremity.[4] However, children typically are bitten on the face. The victim in 70 to 90 percent of reported cases knows the dog. In the United States, domestic dogs kill 10 to 20 people per year.[5,6]

With an annual incidence of 400,000 bites per year, cats inflict 5 to 15 percent of all animal bites, the second most common source of bite injury in the United States.[1,2] In contrast to dog bites, cat bites occur most frequently in females. The upper extremity is the site most often bitten. The victim usually knows the cat. The infection rate of cat bites is more than double that of dog bites, with 30 to more than 50 percent becoming infected.

PATHOGENESIS

In general, animal bites may be classified as contaminated crush injuries or puncture wounds. A dog may generate as much as 450 lb/in^2 of pressure during the bite. As carnivores, they have teeth that have become adapted to tearing tissue. Their bites may result in devitalization, crushing, tearing, and avulsion of the tissue along with exposure of the victim to the oral flora of the dog.

Because cats' teeth are slender and extremely sharp, inoculation of potential pathogens deep into tissue may occur, along with easy penetration into the bone and joint space. As with any bite, this may result in osteomyelitis, sepsis, septic arthritis, or tenosynovitis.

Cellulitis, lymphangitis, and abscess formation may occur in any animal bite. Possibly the most feared potential consequence of any animal bite is rabies (see Chap. 9-19).

A thorough history is vital in assessing a person's risk of infection and determining optimal wound management. Time of injury is important because a treatment delay of more than 12 h increases the risk of infection. The circumstances surrounding the injury (was the attack provoked or unprovoked?) and the ownership, location, and immunization status of the animal, if known, are important items that should be asked about.

MICROBIOLOGY

Reflecting the oral cavity of the mouth, most dog and cat infections are polymicrobial. A median of five bacterial species per culture, including two anaerobic species, have been isolated from wound cultures.[6] Although the complete list of organisms recovered from infected dog and cat bites is extensive, the most commonly cultured organisms are noted in Table 4-4-1. In infected dog bites, *Pasteurella canis* is the most frequently cultured organism. In infected cat bites, *P. multocida* is the most commonly isolated organism.

Pasteurella multocida, along with *Bartonella henselae* and *Capnocytophaga,* deserves special attention. *Pasteurella multocida* is a gram-negative aerobic organism that is found in the majority of dog and cat mouths. More than 50 percent of cat bites and 30 percent of dog bites that become infected will have *P. multocida* recovered. *Pasteurella* infection causes an intense, rapid inflammatory reaction, normally occurring in less than 24 h, and may be associated with fever and/or a purulent discharge. In addition to osteomyelitis and septic arthritis, peritonitis, meningitis, and sepsis have occurred in *Pasteurella* infections.[5]

Cat-scratch disease (see Chap. 9-5) is caused by the gram-negative rod *B. henselae* and may be caused by a scratch or bite from either a cat or a dog. An erythematous papule forms at the primary site 3 to 10 days after the onset of injury, followed by the development of regional lymph node enlargement and fever. This disease is normally self-limiting.

Formally known by the Centers for Disease Control designation DF-2, *Capnocytophaga canimorsus* infection, which is thought to be rare, is associated with dog bites and has a 28 percent fatality rate.[5] Among victims who become seriously infected, 80 percent are immunocompromised or asplenic or have alcoholic liver disease. *Capnocytophaga* infection presents with signs of sepsis and is characterized by fever, leukocytosis, petechiae, disseminated intravascular coagulation, hypotension, and/or renal failure.

SYMPTOMS AND OBJECTIVE FINDINGS

In most cases, evidence of trauma presents as abrasions, punctures, and/or avulsions. A physical examination should include a description of the injury, including the type (avulsion, puncture, crush), location, and measurement. Diagrams can add clarity to a written description. Exploration of the wound to assess wound depth, exclude the presence of foreign bodies, and inspect for damage to underlying structures should be documented. Anesthetizing the area before exploration may be required, but this should be done only after the completion of a thorough neurovascular and musculoskeletal examination. If a joint space was penetrated or tendon damage was sustained, limited range of motion and/or decreased motor strength may be noted.

The initial symptoms of infection are inflammation, pain, and swelling in the localized area of the bite. Most infections are associated with a gray, malodorous serosanguineous discharge along with the cellulitis. Fever may be present in addition to regional lymphadenopathy.

SPECIAL CONSIDERATIONS

Variables that increase the risk of infection are listed in Table 4-4-2.

TABLE 4-4-1. Common Infecting Organisms in Bite Wounds

Streptococcus species
Staphylococcus species
Corynebacterium species
Pasteurella multocida
Pasteurella canis
Neisseria species
Moraxella species

TABLE 4-4-2. Risk Factors for Infection

A bite on hand or foot

Involvement of bone, joint, or tendon

Prosthetic heart valve

Wound in proximity of prosthetic joint

A bite on face or scalp of an infant

Patient age >50 years

Seeking treatment >12 h after injury

Immunosuppression: immune disorders, asplenism, corticosteroid use

Underlying medical disorders: diabetes, chronic alcohol abuse, vascular disease, malignancy

Cat bites

Puncture wounds

Severe crush injury and/or edema

LABORATORY TESTS

In general, laboratory tests are unnecessary for most bite injuries. However, if signs or symptoms of infection are present, several tests may be indicated. A complete blood count and sedimentation rate may be useful in a patient with suspected cellulitis. A Gram stain, though not useful or routine in clinically uninfected wounds, may be of value in infected wounds. Whether or not a Gram stain is done, all clinically infected wounds should have aerobic and anaerobic cultures collected. These cultures should be collected from deep in the wound. Because of the slow-growing nature of some pathogens, laboratory personnel should be instructed to hold the cultures for 7 to 10 days. In patients who present with sepsis, liver function and coagulation studies may be helpful in the management.

RADIOGRAPHIC STUDIES

If there is suspicion of a foreign body, most commonly part of a tooth, a radiograph of the area should be obtained. Some advocate routine radiographic studies of hand bites and any other bites potentially involving deep structures. When a bone or joint space may have been penetrated during the injury, a radiograph will provide a baseline reference for the evaluation of osteomyelitis. When an infection occurs in the proximity of a joint or bone, a radiograph should be obtained. If an infection is present, the presence of air in the tissue spaces should heighten suspicion for a necrotizing infection.

TREATMENT

The first step in proper treatment is cleaning the wound and the surrounding area. Adding 1% povidone iodine solution to the cleansing solution is acceptable, but because of its tissue toxicity, povidone iodine surgical scrub should be avoided. Irrigation of the wound with saline or Ringer's lactate should follow the wound cleansing. Wound cleansing using an 18- to 20-gauge angiocatheter and a 35-mL syringe will generate up to 10 lb/in² pressure and help remove foreign bodies from the wound. If there is devitalized, crushed tissue present, 1 to 2 mm of debridement of the wound margin should be undertaken. Particular care should be taken with debridement on the face. Debridement of puncture wounds, however, is not recommended.

Wound closure remains controversial. In general, all bite wounds without risk factors for infection should be sutured. Because of cosmetic considerations, all facial injuries should be closed by primary intention if they are less than 12 h old. Wounds that are closed should be loosely approximated to allow proper drainage to occur. For injuries not closed by primary intention, delayed primary closure may be considered in the absence of risk factors for infection. The wound should then be loosely bandaged and elevated.

Pharmacologic Treatment

Antibiotics should be used in the treatment of any infected wound and in cases in which risk factors for infection are present. Because of the high rates of infection from cat bites, antibiotic prophylaxis generally is recommended. Unless risk factors are present, most dog bites do not require antibiotic prophylaxis. If antibiotics are prescribed, the medication selected should be active against the normal oral flora of the animal, both aerobic and anaerobic; against normal skin flora; and against any possible environmental contaminants.

Because of its broad spectrum of activity, amoxicillin-clavulanate (Augmentin) is an acceptable first choice in the treatment of dog and cat bites.[7,8] The recommended dose for adults is 500 mg three times per day; in children, it is 40 mg/kg/day amoxicillin, divided into three equal doses and administered every 8 h. As an alternative, cefuroxime may be used, with an adult dose of 500 mg bid and a children's dose 30 mg/kg/day, divided equally and given bid.

Patients with an allergy to penicillin may require two or more antibiotics to have an effect against possible pathogens. This may include a combination of erythromycin and trimethoprim-sulfamethoxazole. In these cases, discussion with an appropriate consultant should help guide proper antibiotic selection.

Prophylactic antibiotics should be given for 3 to 5 days. If cellulitis is noted, antibiotics should be continued for 10 to 14 days. Patients with septic arthritis or osteomyelitis may require intravenous antibiotics and other treatment longer than 30 days. Hospitalization may be required in these cases.

Analgesics should be considered in the management plan. This is especially important for extensive injuries, injuries to the hands or feet, and injuries to children. Medications may range from over-the-counter anti-inflammatory medications to more potent agents such as codeine and oxycodone. The patient profile and the extent of the injuries should guide the caregiver in this selection.

Tetanus (see Chap. 9-23), though rarely acquired from animal bites, has been reported. If no booster injection has been given in the past 5 years, the standard of care should include the administration of tetanus toxoid.[9] Those who have never been fully immunized may require tetanus immunoglobulin in addition to the toxoid.

Since the 1940s and 1950s, when programs for the control of rabies in the United States intensified, the rate of human rabies has been reduced dramatically. Since 1980, a total of 36 cases of rabies have been reported to the Centers for Disease Control.[10] Local health departments should be contacted for information regarding rabies (see Chap. 9-19).

DISPOSITION

Most animal bite injuries can be treated on an outpatient basis. Clinical follow-up should be done 24 h after the initial evaluation. In some incidences, additional follow-up at 48 h may be appropriate. An intramuscular or intravenous dose of antibiotic may be instituted in select cases before outpatient management. All patients should be educated and advised to seek medical attention after the development of signs and symptoms of infection. Hospitalization should be considered in selected cases, using any of the criteria listed in Table 4-4-3.

TABLE 4-4-3. Hospitalization Criteria

Complicated wounds

Involvement of bone, joint, or tendon

Severe cellulitis

Rapidly advancing cellulitis

Cellulitis extending beyond one joint

Signs of systemic infection

Failure of outpatient management

PATIENT EDUCATION

Prevention of animal bites is the key to management. Animals should be avoided when they are eating. Strange animals and animals that exhibit erratic behavior also should be avoided. Nursing animals, even if they appear friendly or are pets, should be approached cautiously, if at all. As most bite injuries occur in children, parents should take an active role in educating their children not to tease animals and teaching them how to behave properly toward animals. Parents should not leave a child alone with any animal or pet. Simple measures such as these should reduce the incidence of animal bites.

REFERENCES

1. Griego RD, Rosen T, Orengo IF, Wolf JE: Dog, cat and human bites: A review. *J Am Acad Dermatol* 33(6):1019–1029, 1995.
2. Goldstein EJC: Bite wounds and infections. *Clin Infect Dis* 14:633–638, 1992.
3. Doan-Wiggins L: Animal bites and rabies, in Rosen P, Barkin RM, Braen GR, et al (eds): *Emergency Medicine: Concepts and Clinical Practice.* St. Louis, Mosby Year Book, 1992, pp 864–875.
4. Anderson CR: Animal bites: Guidelines to current management. *Postgrad Med* 92(1):134–147, 1992.
5. Lewis KT, Stiles M: Management of cat and dog bites. *Am Fam Physician* 52(2):479–485, 1995.
6. Talan DA, Citron DM, Abrahamian FM, et al: Bacteriologic analysis of infected dog and cat bites. *N Engl J Med* 340(2):85–92, 1999.
7. Sanford JP, Gilbert DN, Sande MA: Empirical antimicrobial therapy on clinical grounds, in Sanford JR (ed): *The Sanford Guide to Antimicrobial Therapy.* Dallas, TX, Antimicrobial Therapy, 1998, p 36.
8. Sanford JP, Gilbert DN, Sande MA: Recommended antimicrobial agents against selected organisms, in Sanford JR (ed): *The Sanford Guide to Antimicrobial Therapy.* Dallas, TX, Antimicrobial Therapy, 1998, pp 48–49.
9. Sanford JP, Gilbert DN, Sande MA: Anti-tetanus prophylaxis, wound classification, immunization, in Sanford JR (ed): *The Sanford Guide to Antimicrobial Therapy.* Dallas, TX, Antimicrobial Therapy, 1998, p 123.
10. Centers for Disease Control and Prevention: Human rabies: Prevention–United States 1999. *MMWR* 48(RR1):1–21, 1999.

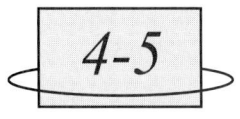

EPIGLOTTITIS: ACUTE SUPRAGLOTTIC LARYNGITIS

Nadine Kroenke

DISCUSSION

Epiglottitis is a true medical emergency. Although it is relatively rare, failure to diagnose and intervene accurately and quickly can lead to airway obstruction, respiratory arrest, and death.

Anatomically, this infection involves the epiglottis, the supraglottic structures, the lingular tonsillar area, the epiglottic folds, and the false vocal cords.

Until the late 1980s, epiglottitis was seen most commonly in the pediatric population, with a peak incidence in children 2 to 5 years old. Before 1990, *Haemophilus influenzae* type b was the most common organism, accounting for almost 80 to 90 percent of cases in both children and adults.

Since the introduction of the Hib-Imune vaccine in 1985, there has been a dramatic decline in the number of cases of epiglottitis. It is now most often seen in children with a median age of 7 years. The administration of the Hib-Imune vaccine has led to an ever-changing epidemiology, with other organisms, such as *Streptococcus pneumoniae, Staphylococcus aureus, Candida albicans,* and herpes simplex virus, increasingly being documented as the causative agents in adults. *Haemophilus influenzae* now accounts for only 25 percent of all cases.

Classically, epiglottitis is described in children with the acute onset over several hours of sore throat, fever, stridor, and drooling. Today epiglottitis is seen more frequently in adolescents and adults. The course is usually more indolent and progressive over 1 to 2 days. Presentation generally involves a complaint of a sore throat with pain out of proportion to the physical findings. Practitioners need to become more suspicious of this disease in older adults and those with less typical symptomatology.

Genetic predisposition leads to a predominance in white people and makes it relatively rare in Native American and Inuit populations. There is no agreed upon seasonal predisposition.

Various pathways are known for the approach and workup with a patient suspected of having epiglottitis. The method chosen depends on the clinical stability of the patient and the practitioner's airway expertise. Airway management is key. The diagnosis of epiglottitis remains primarily clinical and does not depend on direct visualization of a "cherry-red" epiglottis.

Epiglottitis protocols should be in place to quickly coordinate the appropriate staff to treat the patient. The primary care provider should recognize the disease and transfer the patient appropriately. The emergency physician provides initial care and closely observes the patient's airway, ready to provide an airway if needed while an otolaryngologist and anesthesiologist are notified. A patient with this diagnosis never should be left unobserved without appropriate airway management tools in close proximity.

SIGNS AND SYMPTOMS

The classic presentation of epiglottitis includes the abrupt onset of sore throat, drooling, stridor, anxiety, dysphagia, dysphonia, and high fever. Symptoms usually develop over several hours, and the patient usually appears toxic. Many of the objective findings may be absent in patients younger than 2 years old.

Adults, because of their larger airways, typically present with a complaint of sore throat, dysphagia, low-grade fever, and pain without significant physical findings.

OBJECTIVE FINDINGS

The textbook appearance of a patient with epiglottitis is an anxious, apprehensive, toxic older child or adult. Most patients will be febrile with readings of approximately 102.2°F (39°C), although up to 25 percent of patients have no documented fever. The absence of spontaneous cough is important to note. Tenderness of the pharynx sometimes is found in adults. Adults will have a preference for a sitting position since this is easier on the airway.

A child is typically found in the characteristic "sniffing" or "tripod" position, sitting up with the chin forward and the neck slightly extended. Children will resist lying prone and should not be laid down. Providers should attempt to reassure and calm the patient at all times. Children should be kept with a parent at all times and should not be agitated. Mouth examinations traditionally are avoided in children because of their potential to cause laryngospasm.

Later symptoms are noted by inspiratory stridor, active drooling, or trouble handling secretions by the patient.

DIAGNOSTIC CONSIDERATIONS

The following illnesses should be considered in the differential diagnosis:

- Pharyngitis/tonsillitis
- Peritonsillar abscess
- Retropharyngeal abscess
- Croup
- Foreign body obstruction
- Laryngeal tracheitis
- Bronchospasm

SPECIAL CONSIDERATIONS: AIRWAY MANAGEMENT AND INTUBATION

Airway management is the priority whether it is through continuous observation or immediate intervention with incubation. There is controversy among practitioners regarding the most appropriate management of these patients. If a child with symptoms highly suggestive of epiglottitis has a clinically unstable airway, it is necessary to intervene immediately with intubation. If the child has symptoms suggestive of the disease but has an airway that is patent and well maintained, the child should be transferred, if needed, and closely observed until operating room intervention is performed. Portable radiographs of the lateral neck soft tissues can be obtained, remembering that nothing should be done that could potentially irritate the child.

If airway compromise occurs before intervention, bag mask ventilation will maintain oxygenation. Mask ventilation is easily accomplished in most patients with epiglottitis since airway compromise usually is due to diaphragmatic fatigue, not complete airway obstruction from an enlarged edematous epiglottitis. Generally, unsuccessful mask ventilation indicates improper head positioning.

The role of intubation in the management of a stable adult with epiglottitis is unclear. Successful management is well documented with only observation, antibiotics, and supportive care. The decision to place an airway depends on the need for airway stabilization and the availability of personnel skilled in advanced airway management.

While adults can be managed with observation alone, all children with epiglottitis require intubation. The mortality rate is higher in children who are only monitored compared with children who are managed with intubation because of respiratory arrest.

LABORATORY TESTS

Laboratory tests should be delayed in children until after airway stabilization. Most practitioners agree that a complete blood count (CBC) with a differential and two blood cultures are recommended. A direct culture of the epiglottis may be obtained with intubation, and antigen testing also may be done.

A CBC with differential will show an increased white blood cell count with many polymorphonuclear leukocytes. Blood cultures will be positive 80 percent of the time in children and about 25 percent of the time in adults.

RADIOLOGIC STUDIES

Radiographs should not delay appropriate airway management or prevent adequate observations of the patient. Portable lateral soft tissue neck radiographs may be obtained in a stable patient. The best results are obtained when the film is taken during inspiration with the neck extended.

When one is viewing a soft tissue neck film, there are four things to consider and examine:

1. The epiglottis
2. The retropharyngeal or prevertebral space
3. The tracheal air column
4. The hypopharynx

In epiglottitis, soft tissue radiographs reveal an enlarged epiglottis and surrounding structures to form the "thumbprint" sign on the lateral view. In adults, accepted standards that are consistent with epiglottitis are epiglottic width greater than 8 mm, aryepiglottic folds larger than 7 mm, a decrease in the angle of the valleculae, and an increase in the ratio of the hypopharyngeal air column to the tracheal air column (see Fig. 4-5-1).

OTHER DIAGNOSTIC CONSIDERATIONS

It is important to look for concurrent infections such as pneumonia, otitis media, and upper respiratory tract infections. Approximately 25 percent of these children will have a secondary infection.

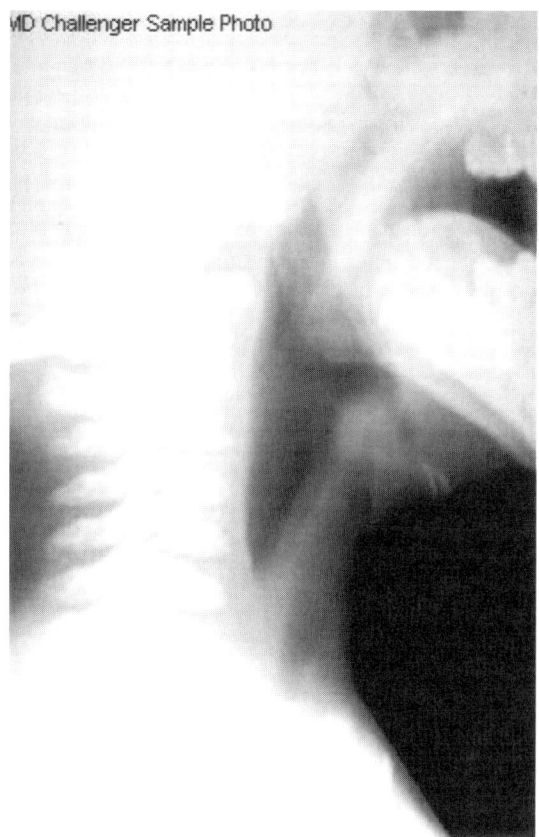

FIGURE 4-5-1. Lateral soft tissue neck with enlarged epiglottis, "thumbprint" sign, indicative of epiglottitis. *(Photo courtesy Challenger Corporation, Copyright. © 1997.)*

TREATMENT

Supportive Measures

The following should be included in supportive treatment:

• Humidified O_2 administered in accordance with pulse oximetry
• Intravenous (IV) hydration

Pharmacologic Management

Consideration of *H. influenzae* immunization status is important when planning antibiotic therapy, such as the following:

• Cefuroxime (Ceftin) 100 to 150 mg/kg/day divided in three doses.
• Chloramphenicol 100 mg/kg/day alternatively to cefuroxime if allergic.
• Cefotaxime (Clarforan) 50 to100 mg/kg/day every 6 to 8 h IV.
• Rocephin (ceftriaxone) 50 to 75 mg/kg/day every 12 h IV.
• Ampicillin-sullbactam (Unasyn) and trimethoprim-sulfamethoxazole (Bactrim/Septra) also are reasonable choices.
• In adults, cefazolin (Ancef) 1 g IV every 6 h often is added.

IV antibiotics are continued for 48 to 72 h, followed by a 10-day course of oral medication such as trimethoprim-sulfamethoxazole (Bactrim/Septra) or cefaclor (Ceclor).

Prophylactic antibiotics are recommended in the case of invasive *H. influenzae*. All nonpregnant household contacts over 4 years of age should receive a prophylactic daily dose of rifampin at 20 mg/kg for 4 days.

Racemic epinephrine is not beneficial in reducing stridor. Steroids remain controversial in regard to their role in reducing airway edema and are not currently recommended.

DISPOSITION

Patients with this diagnosis should be admitted to intensive care for observation, airway management and stabilization, and antibiotic therapy. An ear, nose, and throat (ENT) specialist and an anesthesiologist should be consulted for additional intervention and management. Resolution of symptoms generally takes place over 36 to 48 h.

COMPLICATIONS AND RED FLAGS

Complications involve those which result from airway obstruction secondary to swelling and edema of the epiglottis. If the airway is not managed, there is the potential for respiratory arrest, asphyxia, hypoxic brain damage, and death.

BIBLIOGRAPHY

Barkin R, Rosen P (eds): *Emergency Pediatrics: A Guide to Ambulatory Care.* St Louis, Mosby Year Book, 1994.

Rothrock S, Perkin R: Stridor: A review, update, and current management recommendations. *Pediatr Emerg Med Rep* 4:29–40, 1996.

Ryan M, Hunt M, Snowberger T: A changing pattern of epiglottitis. *Clin Pediatr,* September 1992, pp 532–535.

Saunders, C, Ho M (eds): *Current Emergency Diagnosis and Treatment.* Norwalk, CT, Appleton & Lange, 1992.

Schwartz G, Cayten C, Mangellsen M, Mayer T, Hanke B (eds). *Principles and Practice of Emergency Medicine.* New York, Lea & Febiger, 1992.

Tintinalli JE, Ruiz E, Krome RL (eds): *Emergency Medicine: A Comprehensive Study Guide.* New York, McGraw-Hill, 1996.

Wilson JD, Braunwald E, Isselbacher KJ (eds): *Harrison's Principles of Internal Medicine,* 14th ed. New York, McGraw-Hill, 1998.

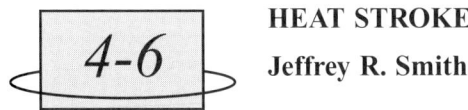

4-6 HEAT STROKE
Jeffrey R. Smith

DISCUSSION

High environmental heat and humidity contribute to a number of heat stress syndromes. It is important to recognize heat injury as a spectrum of disorders ranging from heat cramps to heat stroke, with heat stroke being the most serious and potentially lethal. Heat stroke occurs primarily when the ambient temperature is higher than 95°F for a day or two and the relative humidity is in the range of 50 to 75%.[1] High ambient temperature impairs heat loss via radiation, and the high ambient humidity limits heat dissipation by the evaporation of sweat.

The elderly tend to be most susceptible to sudden changes in heat, most likely due to thermoregulatory dysfunction, multiple medications (which may inhibit heat control), and socioeconomic factors. The urban poor are particularly susceptible to heat stroke, women are more affected than men, and infants also tend to be at risk. Other factors that may increase the risk of heat stroke include obesity, neurologic and cardiovascular disorders, diuretics, neuroleptic drugs, anticholinergic medications, and alcohol consumption.

A second form of heat stroke is caused by exercising in a hot and humid environment. The primary physiologic mechanism is heat production from exercising skeletal muscle. Affected by environmental factors and dehydration, the potential for heat stroke exists among football players, runners, cyclists, and triathletes. Those athletes who are less fit and/or do not replace fluids during training, races, or games are most likely to succumb to heat stroke. Although dehydration impairs thermoregulatory mechanisms during exercise, the intensity of exercise is a much more accurate predictor of exertional heat stroke.[2] Other factors include exposure to direct sunlight, lack of acclimatization to heat, and inappropriate heavy attire. In the United States, in addition to athletes, exertional heat stroke is seen in industrial workers and military recruits. In Saudi Arabia, both forms of heat stroke are particularly common during the annual pilgrimage to Mecca.[3]

Heat stroke is far from uncommon. Between 1979 and 1991, more than 5200 deaths in the United States were attributed to excess heat exposure.[4,5] In 1980 alone, a severe summer heat wave caused more than 1265 deaths in the United States.[6]

SIGNS AND SYMPTOMS

As with any patient, an accurate and thorough history proves invaluable. In the case of heat stroke, often a source of medical history from someone other than the patient, such as family or friends, is more valid. Past medical history, including current medications and doses, is important, as well as possible comorbid factors. Knowledge of duration and activity during heat exposure is valuable as well.

The major clinical signs and symptoms of both classic heat stroke and exertional heat stroke are similar despite differences in pathophysiology and epidemiology. An abrupt rise in body temperature is universal. In heat stroke, all of the mechanisms for body cooling have failed to the extent that core body temperature above 106°F (40 to 41°C) ensues.[1] Disordered mentation, ranging from lethargy to coma and seizures, soon follows. Irritability, aggressiveness, hysteria, and emotional lability often give way to apathy and a glassy stare. An unsteady gait or inability to ambulate also may occur. Anhidrosis, or failure of perspiration, is commonly seen, although sweating persists in up to 50% of exertional heat stroke cases. Pulmonary abnormalities such as pulmonary edema, adult respiratory distress syndrome, and aspiration pneumonia may be seen.

OBJECTIVE FINDINGS

The physical examination is initially focused around the core body temperature and evaluating the cardiovascular and neurologic status of the heat stroke patient. Once a core temperature above 105°F is determined, attention is given to the patient's cardiovascular status. Nearly all heat stroke victims have sinus tachycardia. Hemodynamic measurements generally reveal hypotension (from a low peripheral vascular resistance and probable low circulating volume) and a high cardiac output. ECG abnormalities include conduction disturbances and ST-segment changes.[7]

Impairment of the patient's neurologic status may range from lethargy to coma, seizures, and nuchal rigidity. It is critical (especially in the elderly patient) to know the patient's baseline mental status. The important objective finding of pupillary dilation does not always indicate brain death in cases of heat stroke.

Other body systems that give a wealth of information regarding the diagnosis are the hepatic and renal systems; serum glutamic-oxaloacetic transaminase (SGOT) and bilirubin levels are commonly elevated. It is generally considered a poor prognostic sign to have an SGOT level greater than 1000 IU. Coagulation abnormalities are more common in classic nonexertional heat stroke and are clinically evident by the presence of melena, hematuria, purpura, hemoptysis, and even disseminated intravascular coagulation (DIC).

Renal failure is seen in 25 to 30% of exertional heat stroke patients but only 5% of nonexertional heat stroke patients.[8] Turbid urine, myoglobulinuria, proteinuria, and casts are commonly seen along with oliguria.

DIFFERENTIAL DIAGNOSIS

A meticulous medical history is critically important in developing a complete differential. Since the diagnosis of heat stroke is to a certain extent a diagnosis of exclusion, ruling out other causes of high temperature and altered mental status is crucial. Encephalitis and meningitis can pass as heat stroke. A lumbar puncture can help differentiate between heat stroke and a central nervous system infection. If a patient has returned from travel to an area that is endemic for malaria, cerebral falciparum malaria should be considered. A thick and thin blood smear will help in the diagnosis.

Medication-induced heat illness should always be a consideration. Overdoses of such medications as anticholinergics, salicylates, and sympathomimetics like amphetamines and cocaine can all cause hyperpyretic syndromes. Haloperidol therapy is usually the causative agent in neuroleptic malignant syndrome, an uncommon disorder (occurring in fewer than 1% of patients receiving neuroleptic therapy) characterized by hyperthermia, severe dyskinesia, diaphoresis, and dyspnea. Phenothiazines, butyrophenones, and thioxanthenes, as well as withdrawal from amantadine, levodopa, and other dopaminergic medications, may also contribute to neuroleptic malignant syndrome.[9] Endocrine disorders like thyroid storm and pheochromocytoma may also present with symptoms that mimic heat stroke.

LABORATORY TESTS

Laboratory tests used for heat stroke are listed in Table 4-6-1.

TREATMENT

Rapid recognition of heat stroke followed by aggressive therapy can prevent permanent organ damage and death. Primary therapy consists of prompt lowering of the core body temperature. A rectal thermistor probe should be placed for monitoring of core temperature every 5 min. Methods used for lowering the core temperature are varied and somewhat controversial. Immersion in ice water remains the standard approach, although applying ice packs to the body may be just as effective and logistically an advantage. Both techniques produce cutaneous vasoconstriction, which potentially could impede the transfer of heat from the skin.

Despite this potential drawback, ice baths remain effective and relatively safe. In a study of 252 marine recruits whose therapy for exertional heat stroke included ice bath immersion, there were no fatalities.[10] Other cooling techniques used include ice water enemas and gastric lavage, and spraying the patient with a cool mist followed by cool air directed over the body from a large fan. Administration of room temperature intravenous fluids should be used as well. The high thermal conductivity of water usually allows reduction of the core temperature to 39°C within a period of 10 to 40 min. At this point cooling measures should be removed to prevent hypothermic overshoot.

TABLE 4-6-1. Laboratory Tests for Heat Stroke

TEST	COMMON FINDINGS
Complete blood count	Leukocytosis, hemoconcentration, thrombocytopenia
Electrolytes	Hypokalemia, hypocalcemia, hypophosphatemia
Liver panel	Elevated SGOT, hyperbilirubinemia
Renal panel	Elevated BUN and creatinine
Urinalysis	Proteinuria, hematuria, abundant granular casts
Coagulation studies	Prolonged bleeding time, elevated PT and PTT
Arterial blood gases	Respiratory alkalosis followed by metabolic acidosis
Drug screen	Sympathomimetics, anticholinergics, salicylates (important for differential)

ABBREVIATIONS: BUN, blood urea nitrogen; PT, prothrombin time; PTT, partial thromboplastin time; SGOT, serum glutamic-oxaloacetic transaminase.

Use of isopropyl alcohol sponge baths to facilitate cooling, especially in the young patient, should be avoided because of isopropanol poisoning reported in children. Fluid resuscitation is also a crucial element in treating the heat stroke patient. Oral rehydration is preferred, but in cases where that is not possible intravenous fluids with 5% dextrose 0.5% normal saline at 75 to 100 mL/h is sufficient.

In exertional heat stroke where patients participated in events lasting less than 4 h, the standard fluid replacement is 5% dextrose 0.5% normal saline; in events lasting longer than 4 h, the fluid of choice is D_5NS or lactated Ringer's solution. Administration of mannitol (12.5 g intravenously initially, followed by 12.5 g/L intravenous fluid) has been advocated to promote renal blood flow and prevent damage from myoglobinuria. It can also serve to treat cerebral edema. Urinary alkalinization with 2 ampules (100 meq) $NaHCO_3$ per liter of 5% dextrose in water, infused at a rate sufficient to maintain output of at least 50 mL/h, is indicated for myoglobinuria.[8] In comatose patients, endotracheal intubation for airway protection may be warranted. Benzodiazepines may be used to control seizures.

As with most medical conditions, prevention is the best treatment. Paying close attention to weather bulletins predicting heat waves, checking on elderly family members and friends regularly, staying cool with fans or air conditioners, maintaining proper hydration, and avoiding strenuous activity in direct heat are recommended. Acclimatization is an important concept in prevention of exertional heat stroke. Acclimatization is the body's compliance to heat stress over a period of time, and it involves modification in hormonal, neural, cardiovascular, and pulmonary physiology. Opinions as to the optimal amount of time needed for acclimatization varies. Most agree that at least 4 to 7 days with as little as 90 min of exposure to heat each day will allow the body to fully adapt to heat stress. Others claim that full acclimatization does not occur before 2 months of exposure. An informal interview with ultradistance triatheletes arriving in Kona, Hawaii, for a world championship race would probably reveal most athletes arriving for the race 7 to 10 days prior to competition. Appropriate fluid replacement during training and racing and during acclimatization is crucial. The American College of Sports Medicine currently recommends that runners drink 100 to 200 mL after every 2 to 3 km. This is a generality, however. At the extremes, it is interpreted that slow runners drink only 330 mL/h and faster runners should drink up to 2000 mL/h.[11]

DISPOSITION

Even with aggressive therapy, heat stroke has an appreciable mortality rate. However, most patients who do recover have a return to normal thermoregulatory mechanisms and heat tolerance.[12] Despite the dramatic central nervous system manifestation of extreme heat stroke, most patients who survive do not exhibit neurologic impairment.[13]

Patient education of causative factors remains the cornerstone of preventing further episodes of heat stroke.

PEARLS

Beware of athletes on nonsteroidal anti-inflammatory drugs (NSAIDs). If they exhibit signs and symptoms of heat stroke and yet do not have a core body temperature higher than 105°F, they still may be suffering from heat stroke but cannot register a high core temperature owing to the effects of the NSAID. Treat them as you would any other heat stroke victim, but be judicious in cooling techniques.

REFERENCES

1. American Academy of Orthopaedic Surgeons Editorial Board, Hunter-Griffen LY (chair): *Athletic Training and Sports Medicine,* 2d ed. Rosemont, IL, American Academy of Orthopaedic Surgeons, 1992, p 854.

2. Noakes TD et al: Metabolic rate, not percent dehydration, predicts rectal temperature in marathon runners. *Med Sci Sports Exerc* 23:443, 1991.

3. al-Harthi SS et al: Metabolite and hormonal profiles in heat stroke patients at Mecca pilgrimage. *J Intern Med* 228(4):343–346, 1990.

4. Heat-related deaths/United States. *MMWR* 42(28):558–560, 1993.

5. Heat-related deaths/Philadelphia and United States, 1993–1994. *MMWR* 43(25):453–455, 1994.

6. Heatstroke/United States, 1980. *MMWR* 30(23):277–279, 1981.

7. Akhtar MJ et al: Electrocardiographic abnormalities in patients with heat stroke. *Chest* 104:1498, 1993.

8. Yarbrough BE: Heat related disorders. *Hosp Med* 27(6):81–91, 1991.

9. Caroff SN, Mann SC: Neuroleptic syndrome. *Med Clin North Am* 77:185, 1993.

10. Costrini A: Emergency treatment of exertional heatstroke and comparison of whole body cooling techniques. *Med Sci Sports Exerc* 22:15, 1990.

11. Coyle EF, Montain SJ: Benefits of fluid replacement with carbohydrate during exercise. *Med Sci Sports Exerc* 24:325, 1992.

12. Armstrong LE et al: Time course of recovery and heat acclimation ability of prior exertional heat stroke patients. *Med Sci Sports Exerc* 22:36, 1990.

13. Sminia P et al: Effect of hyperthermia on the central nervous system: A review. *Int J Hyperthermia* 10:1, 1994.

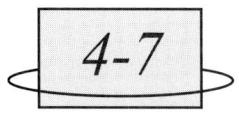

SHOCK
Donald J. Sefcik

DISCUSSION

Shock may be defined as inadequate cellular oxygenation secondary to insufficient tissue perfusion. The result is cellular dysfunction. The manifestations of shock range from subtle, nonspecific symptoms to the classic clinical presentation of altered mental status, cool extremities, tachycardia, tachypnea, and hypotension.

Although the etiologies of shock are numerous, they may be grouped into four major categories (see Table 4-7-1). Inadequate vascular volume, myocardial cellular dysfunction, obstruction of cardiac filling or emptying, and loss of vascular tone independently or in combination may cause the clinical syndrome of shock.

The body employs several compensatory mechanisms (e.g., cardiovascular, respiratory, metabolic) during shock. If they remain unrecognized or are treated suboptimally, irreversible cellular injury or death may occur.

PATHOGENESIS

To function normally, tissues require a mechanism to supply the necessary nutrients and oxygen. Organ perfusion is determined by two major factors: arterial blood pressure and tissue vascular resistance. If inadequate arterial pressure exists, the driving force behind tissue oxygenation is insufficient. When the vascular resistance is inappropriate (tone is reduced or distribution of blood flow is improper), the nutritional and oxygenation demands of tissues are not met. Subsequently, cellular metabolic dysfunction ensues, and the signs and symptoms of the shock syndrome begin.

Arterial blood pressure is the product of cardiac output (CO) and total peripheral resistance (TPR). Cardiac output is the product of stroke volume (SV) and heart rate (HR). Therefore, blood pressure is actually determined by three major variables: $BP = SV \times HR \times TPR$. A reduction in any of these variables may diminish systemic blood pressure and produce a relative or absolute state of hypoperfusion. Factors that may exert detrimental effects on systemic arterial pressure are multifactorial and include dysrhythmias, blood loss, myocardial cellular dysfunction, pericardial disorders, and mediators of vascular tone (see Table 4-7-2).

TABLE 4-7-1. Major Categories of the Shock Syndromes

Hypovolemic shock
  Hemorrhage
    Traumatic
    Nontraumatic
      Gastrointestinal hemorrhage
  Nonhemorrhagic
    Volume depletion
      Inadequate intake (e.g., anorexia)
      Excessive losses
        Gastrointestinal (vomiting, diarrhea)
        Urinary (polyuria)
    Extravascular ("third") spacing
      Peritoneal fluid
      Inadequate oncotic pressure

Cardiogenic shock
  Myocardial dysfunction
    Cellular ischemia or infarction
    Dysrhythmias
    Inflammatory disorders (myocarditis)
    Pharmacologic effects (negative inotropic or chronotropic agents)
  Valvular heart defects
    Significant stenotic lesions
    Significant insufficiency

Obstructive noncardiogenic shock
  Pericardial tamponade
  Tension pneumothorax
  Significant pulmonary embolism
  Left ventricular outflow obstruction

Distributive shock
  Septic shock
  Neurogenic shock
  Anaphylactic shock
  Drug-induced shock

The early stages of shock may be reversible. However, once cellular injury has occurred, the likelihood of irreversible shock increases, and even the most aggressive therapy may not save the patient.

SYMPTOMS

The classic clinical manifestations of shock—hypotension, tachycardia, a weak pulse, cool extremities, tachypnea, an altered mental status (confusion), and reduced urine output—are well known. The

TABLE 4-7-2. Causes of Hypotension

Reduced cardiac output
  Stroke volume
    Preload reduction
      Inadequate intravascular volume
      Inadequate atrial contractile state
    Myocardial cell dysfunction
      Cellular ischemia or infarction
      Dysrhythmias
      Altered heart rate or oxygen demand
      Pharmacologic agents
    Afterload abnormality
      Outflow tract disorder
  Heart rate
    Dysrhythmias
Total peripheral vascular resistance
  Reduction of arterial tone
    Pharmacologic sources (vasodilators)
    Metabolic products
    Exogenous products
      Endotoxins

more subtle presentations of shock, however, challenge the diagnostic acumen of even the most experienced clinician.

When one is presented with an altered mental status, a confusional state, a combative patient, or the comment from a family member that the patient is "just not himself," consideration must be given to a cerebral hypoperfusional state. Complaints of dizziness, especially when assuming an upright position, should be considered a sign of cerebral hypoperfusion and should be evaluated. Nonspecific complaints of weakness, fatigue, and generalized arthralgias or myalgias may represent a relative hypoperfusional state or the metabolic sequelae of inadequate tissue oxygenation.

Shortness of breath at rest, dyspnea on exertion, and palpitations may represent attempts at cardiovascular compensatory efforts. Complaints of reduced urine output and a concentrated-appearing or "strong" odor to the urine may be indications of attempted renal compensation secondary to hypoperfusion.

OBJECTIVE FINDINGS

A common feature in most shock syndromes is hypotension. Sustained systolic blood pressure values lower than 90 mmHg need to undergo diagnostic scrutiny. Keep in mind, however, that although a chronic hypertensive patient may present with what appears to be a normal blood pressure, a relative hypotensive state may in fact exist. Recent blood pressure values obtained from earlier charts may offer insight.

Tachycardia, especially in a resting state, must be evaluated. This usually represents an attempt by the body to compensate for a reduced cardiac output or a reduction in total peripheral resistance. Cool, sometimes cyanotic extremities are common features of a patient in shock and are manifestations of the body's increasing peripheral resistance through vasoconstriction. Catecholamine release is responsible for both the tachycardia and the cool extremities.

Reduced urine output often is noted, a result of nephron hypoperfusion. Renal attempts to elevate perfusion result in fluid reabsorption, which clinically manifests as oliguria. Tachypnea develops in an attempt to increase tissue oxygenation and compensate for the metabolic acidosis.

DIAGNOSTIC CONSIDERATIONS

Of paramount importance to the appropriate treatment of a patient in shock is discovering the etiology. Initial considerations should be directed toward establishing a general categorical diagnosis (see Table 4-7-1).

Hypovolemic causes of shock may be obvious (hemorrhage, trauma, etc.) or less obvious (third spacing of fluids, gastrointestinal losses, or diuresis). Generally, historical information and physical examination (dry membranes, altered skin turgor, reduction of urine output, etc.) will provide diagnostic insight.

Cardiogenic disorders may present more of a challenge. Acute myocardial cellular dysfunction (myocardial ischemia or infarct, valvular alteration, etc.) may be difficult to detect. Cardiac dysrhythmias may be easier to appreciate.

Although obstructive causes of shock may provide clues, astute diagnostic perception is required. Pericardial effusions may demonstrate muffled heart tones, jugular venous distention, and hypotension. However, failure to appreciate absent apical breath sounds (often a problem in a setting with significant background noise) may result in a missed diagnosis of tension pneumothorax. The diagnosis of a massive pulmonary embolism is at times elusive, but profound hypoxemia and a widened alveolar-arterial (Aa) gradient provide diagnostic clues.

Distributive forms of shock have many possible causes. After careful evaluation for the other types of shock, the etiologies of this group should be given consideration. The diversity of the causes of distributive shock challenges even the most experienced clinicians (see Table 4-7-1).

LABORATORY TESTING

Critical to the outcome of a patient in shock is hemodynamic monitoring (see "Treatment," below). Initial laboratory testing is directed toward those studies which are necessary for early intervention. The studies generally obtained include a complete blood cell count (CBC), serum chemistries [sodium, potassium, calcium, blood urea nitrogen (BUN), creatinine, and magnesium], and arterial blood gas (ABG). Additional testing should be directed toward the underlying process. Laboratory selection is guided by history, physical examination, and the patient's response to therapy. Additional tests to consider include cultures (blood, sputum, and urine), toxicology studies, liver enzymes, and cardiac enzymes. Other diagnostic information may be gained by reviewing chest x-rays, electrocardiograms (ECGs), echocardiograms, computed tomography (CT) scans, and nuclear radiologic studies.

Although each of these individual tests may prove useful, the benefit of obtaining serial laboratory studies to optimize patient therapy (assure the response to treatment and guide additional therapeutic interventions) cannot be overemphasized.

TREATMENT

As with any medical emergency, basic resuscitative measures are critical in the patient's treatment. These patients need to receive supplemental oxygen, have serial blood pressure measurements, receive intravenous fluids, be placed on cardiac monitors and pulse oximeters, and have a Foley catheter secured. Consideration must be given to an indwelling arterial catheter, both as a monitoring device and as a source for multiple arterial blood specimens, if necessary. A central venous catheter provides important hemodynamic information.

At least two intravenous catheters are placed, preferably large-bore (16 gauge or larger), since rapid fluid administration is a common requirement in the treatment of shock. Normal saline and lactated Ringer's solution are generally the crystalloid fluids of choice. Vasopressors (dopamine or norepinephrine) as well as volume expanders (albumin or dextran) may be required. Pneumatic antishock garments, also known as MAST (military antishock trousers), are useful in selected cases (especially hypovolemia).

Corticosteroids and opioid antagonists (naloxone) have been utilized in some shock situations (to reduce the effects of β-endorphins) but generally are not employed in most cases of shock. As a temporary measure for cardiogenic shock, an intraaortic balloon pump (IABP) is often useful.

COMPLICATIONS AND RED FLAGS

Major complications to anticipate in the course of treatment include the development of adult respiratory distress syndrome (ARDS), disseminated intravascular coagulation (DIC), and acute renal failure (ARF).

NOTES AND PEARLS

Be wary of a patient with hypotension and bradycardia. Suspect a primary myocardial disorder or an extracardiac etiology (i.e., pharmacologic agents) that is inhibiting the normally expected compensatory mechanism to hypotension. Also, be suspicious of a hypotensive patient with warm extremities. This may represent septic shock, also known as warm shock.

PROGNOSIS

If a patient in shock is identified early, the etiology of the problem is determined, and aggressive appropriate therapy is instituted, the prognosis is improved greatly. If, however, the early symptoms or signs go unnoticed, therapy is not directed at the underlying cause, or therapy is inadequate, the shock syndrome may reach a state of irreversibility and the outcome will be death.

BIBLIOGRAPHY

Ferguson DW: Shock, in *Cecil Textbook of Medicine,* 20th ed. Philadelphia, WB Saunders,1996, pp 477–496.

Parrillo JE: Shock, in Fauci AS, Braunwald E, Isselbacher KJ, et al (eds): *Harrison's Principles of Internal Medicine,* 14th ed. New York, McGraw-Hill, 1998, pp 214–222.

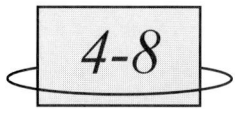

POISONING AND DRUG OVERDOSE
Karen A. Newell

EPIDEMIOLOGY

It is estimated that more than 4 million cases of poisoning or drug overdose occur each year in the United States. Most of these occur in children between the ages of 1 and 5 years and involve accidental ingestion. In adolescents and young adults, cases are secondary to drug experimentation and suicide attempts. The majority of the adult cases are intentional, with the remainder from occupational and household accidents.

INITIAL MANAGEMENT

As with any serious emergency, the clinician must address the ABCs of airway, breathing, and circulation. Specific airway considerations include determining the presence of oropharyngeal mucosal injury or edema and relieving obstruction (often from the tongue).

Next, any patient who presents unconscious or with signs of altered mental status should be given 50 mL of 50% dextrose, 0.8 to 2 mg of naloxone (1 to 2 mg repeated boluses to a total of 4 mg), and 100 mg of thiamine intravenously. In alcoholic patients, administration of glucose before thiamine can precipitate Wernicke-Korsakoff syndrome. Prior to arrival in the emergency department, the patient should be kept in the left lateral decubitus position to slow absorption in those with oral ingestions.

HISTORY AND PHYSICAL EXAMINATION

Attention to the identity and amount of the substance, when and why it was taken, association with other substances, and underlying medical conditions can be very helpful; however, this is often unreliable information. Monitor vital signs including temperature, blood pressure, respiratory pattern and rate, and pulse rate and rhythm. Check for odor on the breath and assess the skin for needle marks or tracks (linear scarring noted parallel to venous distribution, usually located on the forearms), diaphoresis, and skin color changes. Auscultate for pulmonary edema or cardiac dysrhythmia. Check for the presence or absence of bowel sounds, rigidity, distention, or organ enlargement. During the neurologic examination pay particular attention to mental status, pupillary size and reaction to light, presence of nystagmus, focal deficits, deep tendon reflexes, and presence or absence of gag reflex.

DIAGNOSTIC STUDIES

Complete blood cell count and serum toxicology are helpful for determining the presence of acetaminophen, salicylate, theophylline, lithium, lead, carbon monoxide, methemoglobinemia, alcohol, and digitalis. Perform an initial fingerstick glucose and tests for serum blood urea nitrogen (BUN), creatinine, serum glucose, and measured osmolality. Obtain urinalysis and urine toxicology, pulse oximetry, electrocardiogram (ECG), chest x-ray, and serum pregnancy test. Consideration is also given to arterial blood gases, abdominal x-ray, liver function studies, and gastric aspirate or emesis for toxicology.

TREATMENT
Skin Decontamination

Each of the following should be carried out when there has been cutaneous exposure; the examiner should observe universal precautions with gown and eye protection.

- Remove clothing and place in plastic bags.
- Brush off any powder or particulate matter prior to irrigation.
- Wash involved skin surfaces thoroughly with mild soap and water.

Gastrointestinal Decontamination

Unless contraindicated, the following three routes are used in gastrointestinal (GI) decontamination: gastric lavage, treatment with activated charcoal, and use of cathartics. In recent years, induced emesis has not been shown to improve the outcome of toxic patients and has been eliminated to avoid increased risk of adverse outcome.

GASTRIC LAVAGE   See Table 4-8-1 for the indications and procedure for gastric lavage.

Complications include pulmonary aspiration, gastric erosion or perforation, and esophageal tears.

ACTIVATED CHARCOAL   This is the gold standard for toxic ingestion. Activated charcoal will bind many toxic substances and is indicated after vomiting or lavage. It is not effective in those who have ingested ethanol, methanol, iron, lead, strong acids or bases, lithium, or cyanide. Contraindications include patients who should receive a specific oral antidote (activated charcoal may bind to the antidote and reduce its effectiveness) and patients who will require endoscopy (e.g., for caustic ingestion; activated charcoal will interfere with the visual inspection).

Procedure   Activated charcoal is diluted in four parts of water or sorbitol and given orally or by lavage. If this is vomited, it should be repeated. It

TABLE 4-8-1.   Indications and Procedure for Gastric Lavage

Indications

- Large ingestions of toxins that are known to be highly lethal
- Life-threatening ingestions without an antidote
- Life-threatening ingestions of a substance that is not bound by activated charcoal
- Ingested poisons in a patient who is unable to protect his or her airway (altered mental status, seizure activity)

Contraindication

- Patient has a history of ingesting strong acid or alkali

Procedure for tube placement

1. Select the proper size of nasogastric (NG) tube.
2. Use 28 to 40 Fr Ewald orogastric tube (16 to 26 Fr in children), since smaller-bore NG tubes are not effective for lavage. Typically, these patients are already intubated with either an endotracheal tube or nasotracheal tube.
3. Confirm tube placement by injecting 60 mL of air while listening over the gastric bubble or aspirate the gastric contents. If unclear, radiologic confirmation is absolutely necessary before lavage.

Take the following steps for gastric lavage:

1. Place the patient in the left lateral decubitus position.
2. Withdraw all stomach contents.
3. Place 200 to 300 mL of room-temperature tap water (50 to 100 mL in children) into the stomach through the tube.
4. Continue to inject and aspirate the fluid until clear; use 2 L in those who are initially clear.
5. Send the first 100 mL of aspirate for toxicology.
6. Massaging the left upper quadrant can help to dislodge any tablets or large particulate matter during aspiration.

is tasteless, but it is visually unpleasant and gritty. Select the proper dose: adults or children, 1 g/kg of body weight, minimum dose of 30 g.

Activated charcoal may be readministered every 4 to 6 h in those with ingestion of theophylline, phenobarbital, tricyclic antidepressants, phenothiazines, and digitalis to prevent later reabsorption.

CATHARTICS   The use of cathartics is controversial. Cathartics can be used to expedite the elimination of toxic substances through the bowel and may be indicated in those with life-threatening ingestions of sustained-release drugs, those who have ingested drug bags or packets, and those exposed to toxins not bound by activated charcoal. Contraindications include the following: infants, patients who received an oral antidote, adynamic ileus, severe diarrhea, intestinal obstruction, abdominal trauma, recent abdominal surgery. Sodium sulfate is contraindicated in patients with hypertension, severe left ventricular dysfunction, or congestive heart failure. Sodium phosphate (Fleet Phospho-Soda) is contraindicated in children and in ethylene glycol ingestion. Avoid magnesium-containing cathartics in patients with renal failure. Cathartic choices and dosages are found in Table 4-8-2. Avoid oil-based cathartics where there is a risk of pulmonary aspiration. Also, be aware that activated charcoal can bind to these agents and make them useless.

ENHANCED ELIMINATION   Enhanced elimination through diuresis may be useful in cases of isoniazid, bromide, or ethanol ingestion. It is contraindicated in patients with hypotension and pulmonary edema. The recommended medication is mannitol (20 to 100 g) and intermittent furosemide (20 mg). Monitor electrolytes to prevent hyponatremia and hypokalemia.

Alkaline diuresis of urine prevents reabsorption by the kidney and is useful in ingestion of phenobarbital, salicylates, lithium, or isoniazid. Use one or two ampules of intravenous sodium bicarbonate (slowly), then one or two ampules of sodium bicarbonate in 1 L of 0.25 to 0.45% normal saline constant intravenous infusion; maintain urine pH at 7.3 to 8.5. Furosemide is also helpful. Keep urine output at 5 to 7 mL/kg per hour. Complications include metabolic alkalosis, hypernatremia, hyperosmolality, and fluid retention. Make sure to adequately hydrate the patient prior to forcing alkaline diuresis, especially in salicylate ingestion.

Acid diuresis of urine prevents reabsorption by the kidney and, though controversial, is used after the ingestion of amphetamines, phencyclidine, quinidine or quinine, and fenfluramine. Use 500 mg to 1 g oral or intravenous ascorbic acid (initially), repeated every 6 h; ammonium chloride, 4 g every 2 h by nasogastric tube; or 1 to 2% solution per normal saline (NS) intravenously to maintain urine pH between 5.5 and 6.5. Furosemide and 0.45% normal saline given intravenously helps to keep urine output regulated at 5 to 7 mL/kg per hour. Patients with myoglobinuria (e.g., excessive seizure activity) should not undergo acid diuresis. Carefully monitor serum electrolytes.

DIALYSIS   Hemodialysis is the most effective procedure in severe poisonings, especially in nonorganic compounds not well bound by activated charcoal or peritoneal dialysis. Use after ingestion of ethylene glycol, methanol, or paraquat. Dialysis may be considered in severe ingestion of theophylline, lithium, salicylates, phenobarbital, bromide, and ethanol.

HEMOPERFUSION   During hemoperfusion the patient's blood is passed through a filter and replaced. It is used for severe toxicity from

TABLE 4-8-2.   Types of Cathartics Used

30 g magnesium sulfate (monitor carefully for fluid and electrolyte shifts)
30 g magnesium citrate (children, 4 mg/kg)
30 g sodium sulfate
100 to 150 mL of a 70% solution of sorbitol
15 to 30 mL sodium phosphate, diluted at 1:4 with water

substances including barbiturates, glutethimide, methaqualone, ethchlorvynol, meprobamate, and chloral hydrate. Complications include decreased platelets, plasma calcium, glucose, fibrinogen, or transient leukopenia.

RECOGNITION AND MANAGEMENT OF SPECIFIC DRUG POISONING

This is intended as a review of the more common clinical scenarios encountered and is not complete or exhaustive.

Narcotic Analgesics

These central nervous system (CNS) depressants and respiratory depressants are classified as follows:

- *Natural opiates:* opium, morphine, and codeine
- *Semisynthetics:* heroin, hydromorphone (Dilaudid), oxymorphone (Numorphan), hydrocodone (Vicodin), oxycodone (Percocet, Percodan, Tylox)
- *Synthetics:* meperidine (Demerol), methadone (Dolophine), butorphanol (Stadol), fentanyl, nalbuphine (Nubain), propoxyphene (Darvon), pentazocine (Talwin)

PRESENTATION   The patient may present with miotic pupils, bradycardia, decreased respirations, hypotension, hypothermia, decreased GI motility, and noncardiac pulmonary edema. Death from respiratory depression may occur.

TREATMENT   Use naloxone (Narcan) 0.8 to 2 mg intravenously every 5 min to a maximum of 10 mg (0.03 to 0.1 mg/kg for children); consider continuous infusion and/or oxygen.

HEROIN WITHDRAWAL   Symptoms occur at about 12 h after the last dose; patients may present with restlessness, lacrimation, rhinorrhea, piloerection, diaphoresis, mydriatic pupils, muscle cramps, nausea, vomiting, diarrhea, and/or hyperpyrexia. The condition resolves after 72 to 96 h. Treat with 10 mg oral or intramuscular methadone upon initial symptoms and every 8 to 12 h; taper dose by half every 2 days until resolution.

Barbiturates

These CNS depressants can be long acting (6 to 12 h), like phenobarbital or barbital; intermediate acting (3 to 6 h), like amobarbital; short acting (less than 3 h), like pentobarbital or secobarbital; or ultra short acting (20 min), like thiopental.

PRESENTATION   Early after ingestion there is drowsiness and dysarthria; later there is sedation, hypnosis, or coma. Patients have decreased respiration, hypothermia, decreased GI motility, and variation in pupillary responses (barbiturates are often coingested with ethanol, which potentiates sedation).

TREATMENT   Use oxygen, gastric lavage up to 8 h after ingestion, activated charcoal, alkaline diuresis, intravenous fluids, and supportive care; consider hemodialysis.

WITHDRAWAL   When seen it will occur 2 to 3 days after the last dose, the patient may present with restlessness, agitation, diaphoresis, delirium, auditory hallucinations, tremor, nausea, vomiting, hypotension, and seizure (resolves within 3 to 7 days). Treat initially with diazepam, then with tapered phenobarbital.

Amphetamines

Methamphetamine (speed) and MDMA (ecstasy) are examples of this class of drugs.

PRESENTATION   These CNS stimulants may cause agitation, confusion, tremor, diaphoresis, mydriatic pupils, tachypnea, tachycardia, cardiac arrhythmias, nausea, vomiting, hyperpyrexia, seizure, and coma.

TREATMENT   Use gastric lavage, acid diuresis (if not exhibiting seizures or hyperthermic activity), and supportive care; a benzodiazepine may be helpful. Consider hemodialysis or hemoperfusion in refractory cases.

Cocaine

This CNS stimulant may be taken intranasally, smoked as crack, or taken intravenously. Accidental ingestion by body "packers" and "stuffers" may also be seen.

PRESENTATION   The patient may present with agitation, tachycardia, cardiac arrhythmias, chest pain, hypertension, hyperthermia, seizures, nausea, or vomiting. Death may occur from respiratory failure or cardiac ischemia, infarction, and arrest.

TREATMENT   Give supportive care. Benzodiazepines may be helpful for agitation. Activated charcoal or whole-bowel irrigation may be helpful for body packers and stuffers. Avoid Class 1a antiarrhythmics (quinidine, procainamide, and disopyramide) and beta blockers as unopposed adrenergic activity may worsen hypertension or myocardial ischemia.

Hallucinogens

Hallucinogens like psilocybin, mescaline, 2,5-dimethoxy-4-methamphetamine (STP), and lysergic acid diethylamide (LSD) may be sniffed, ingested, or smoked. Onset of action is 20 to 30 min with duration from 1 to 6 h.

PRESENTATION   Acute presentation may include nausea, blurred vision, mydriatic pupils, tachycardia, hyperpyrexia, hyperreflexia, visual distortions, and hallucinations.

Chronic presentation may include flashbacks and intermittent psychosis.

TREATMENT   Give supportive care and "talk the patient down" with much reassurance; consider a benzodiazepine for severe agitation. Avoid phenothiazines because they can lessen the seizure threshold. GI decontamination procedures are unnecessary. Seizures can be treated with diazepam.

PCP   PCP is a frequently used adulterant in street drugs. PCP has a 2- to 3-min onset after smoking, with a presentation much more violent and bizarre (dissociative). Treatment of comatose patients may include GI decontamination, activated charcoal, and acid diuresis.

Benzodiazepines

These include anxiolytics, muscle relaxants, anticonvulsants, and drugs with hypnotic properties. Examples include diazepam (Valium), oxazepam (Serax), chlordiazepoxide (Librium), and lorazepam (Ativan).

PRESENTATION   The patient may present with drowsiness, ataxia, dysarthria, nystagmus, cardiac arrhythmias, and coma; death is possible but uncommon with oral ingestion unless coingested with other substances, such as ethanol.

TREATMENT   GI decontamination procedures including lavage and activated charcoal should be employed in those patients presenting with severe CNS depression. The antidote flumazenil should be given, 0.2 mg intravenously over 30 s; repeat if necessary with 0.3 mg, then increments of 0.5 mg every 60 s to a total dose of 3 mg. It is contraindicated in head injury, in children, and in those who have ingested other substances, since it can precipitate seizure activity. Remember to consider head trauma, stroke, hypoglycemia, metabolic abnormali-

ties, and carbon monoxide poisoning as potential etiologies in patients presenting with CNS depression. Withdrawal symptoms are similar to ethanol and barbiturates but less severe.

Ethanol

This sedative-hypnotic can cause the following blood alcohol levels:

- 25 mg/dL blood alcohol from an ounce of whiskey, one glass of wine, or one beer
- 100 mg/dL, which is associated with intoxication in nonchronic users
- >400 mg/dL, which is associated with lethality, although chronic users can survive with these levels and higher

The level naturally decreases about 20 to 30 mg/dL/h.

PRESENTATION   The patient may present with ataxia, dysarthria, visual impairment, lateral nystagmus, stupor, vomiting, hypotension, seizure, and/or coma.

TREATMENT   Give oxygen, thiamine, and supportive care. All intoxicated patients must be held in the emergency department until they are not a danger to themselves or others. This may require a physical or chemical restraint.

WITHDRAWAL   Withdrawal can bring on tremor. The patient may have visual or auditory hallucinations. Seizures can occur 12 to 48 h after the last ingestion. Delirium tremens occur 3 to 4 days after the last alcohol ingestion and is fatal in about 15% of cases. Treat with 10 mg diazepam intravenously followed by 5 mg diazepam every 5 min until sedated. Agitation can be treated with 2 to 5 mg haloperidol intramuscularly. Death can occur from respiratory depression.

Methanol

Also known as wood alcohol, methanol is found in paint thinner, antifreeze, and Sterno (fuel for cooking); it is very toxic. A lethal ingested dose can be as little as 15 to 30 mL in adults.

PRESENTATION   Presentation is similar to that with ethanol but with more drowsiness. Toxic metabolites (formaldehyde) can occur from 6 to 36 h after ingestion and can induce severe vomiting and upper abdominal pain, diarrhea, headache, dizziness, blurred vision, blindness, and seizures.

TREATMENT   Use gastric lavage and activated charcoal administration, with intravenous bicarbonate for acidosis. Maintain a continuous intravenous blood ethanol level (100 to 150 mg/dL) to compete with methanol and decrease amounts of metabolite. Folate 50 mg intravenously can also be given every 4 h to aid in detoxification. Consider hemodialysis in severe cases.

Ethylene Glycol

Colorless, odorless, and having a sweet taste, ethylene glycol is used as antifreeze. The lethal ingested dose is 1 to 1.5 mL/kg.

PRESENTATION   Between 30 min and 12 h after ingestion, the patient may present with ataxia, nystagmus, vomiting, hyporeflexia, severe acidosis, seizures, or coma. Between 12 and 14 h, tachypnea, tachycardia, cyanosis, and pulmonary edema may appear. From 24 to 72 h, flank pain and renal failure can occur secondary to acute tubular necrosis.

DIAGNOSTIC STUDIES   Check for severe acidosis, increased anion gap, hypocalcemia, calcium oxalate crystals in the urine (urine may fluoresce when placed under an ultraviolet light depending on brand, amount, and time from ingestion), and hematuria.

TREATMENT   Treatment is the same as for methanol intoxication. Consider fomepizole 15 mg/kg intravenous load, then 10 to 20 mg/kg every 12 h for 48 h in severe cases. Calcium gluconate may be given intravenously for hypocalcemia and seizures. Additionally, consider giving thiamine and pyridoxine 100 mg intravenously each day.

Isopropyl Alcohol

Alcoholic patients often use rubbing alcohol since it is less expensive and more readily available and it produces an intoxicated state more quickly and with less consumption than ethanol. The toxic dose of a 70% solution is roughly 1 mL/kg.

PRESENTATION   Presentation is similar to that with ethanol toxicity except with increased hemorrhagic gastritis. Diagnostic studies may demonstrate acetone in the urine, an elevated anion gap, and an elevated osmolar gap.

TREATMENT   Treatment includes supportive care, GI decontamination procedures, and bicarbonate to treat acidosis if noted; hemodialysis should be considered.

Cyanide

Cyanide can be found naturally in apple, apricot, peach, plum, cherry, and almond seeds. It is often used in industry.

PRESENTATION   Giddiness, ataxia, headache, dyspnea, nausea, vomiting, seizures, coma, and death can be signs of ingestion. Physical examination may reveal a bitter almond odor on the patient's breath.

TREATMENT   Initially crush an amyl nitrate pearl and have the patient inhale for 15 to 30 s. Next, give 10 mL of 3% sodium nitrate intravenously over 3 to 5 min (0.33 mL/kg for children, maximum of 10 mL) and 50 mL of 25% sodium thiosulfate intravenously over 10 mL (1.65 mL/kg for children, maximum of 50 mL). This may be repeated.

Carbon Monoxide

Carbon monoxide is a colorless, odorless gas; 5% of automobile exhaust is composed of carbon monoxide. It is also found in furnaces and charcoal fires.

PHYSICAL EXAMINATION   The clinician may detect a cherry red appearance of the skin, mucous membranes, and fingernails since carbon monoxide preferentially binds to hemoglobin molecules, limiting oxygen-carrying capacity.

DIAGNOSTIC STUDIES   A rapid initial test detects the presence of carboxyhemoglobin by diluting 1 mL of blood with 10 mL of water and adding 1 mL of 5% sodium hydroxide (a color change of straw or pink is considered positive, whereas brown is negative). The blood carboxyhemoglobin level can be assessed definitively.

TREATMENT   Less than 10% of patients are usually asymptomatic, requiring no treatment. Between 10 and 20% have mild headache and irritability; these patients can be treated with high-flow oxygen (100% nonrebreather mask) and observation. Between 20 and 40% have associated lightheadedness, confusion, dizziness, agitation, nausea, vomiting, and coordination difficulty; these patients require treatment with high-flow oxygen and hospital admission. Between 40 and 60% exhibit syncope, dyspnea, lethargy, coma, and respiratory or cardiac arrest. These patients require high-flow oxygen and hospital admission; hyperbaric oxygen may be helpful if available. Cerebral edema may be treated with dexamethasone, 4 to 6 mg intravenously every 6 h. Transfusion of erythrocytes remains controversial.

Selective Serotonin Reuptake Inhibitors (SSRIs)

Recent development and increase in the utilization of such agents as fluoxetine (Prozac), sertraline (Zoloft), paroxetine (Paxil), fluvoxamine (Luvox), and citalopram (Celexa) have contributed to a notable increase in serotonin syndrome usually related to multidrug interactions.

PRESENTATION   Cognitive-behavioral, autonomic nervous system, and neuromuscular changes may occur, including agitation, anxiety, sinus tachycardia, mild hypertension, hyperthermia, diaphoresis, diarrhea, and/or muscular rigidity. Diagnosis is based on clinical suspicion since no definitive confirmatory study currently exists.

TREATMENT   Overdose of SSRIs requires admission for supportive care. Most symptoms resolve spontaneously within 24 h. Give consideration to benzodiazepines for patient comfort. Cyproheptadine 4 to 8 mg orally may be helpful and may be repeated every 4 to 6 h (maximum of 0.5 mg/kg per day or 32 mg/d).

Tricyclic Antidepressants

Imipramine amitriptyline is one example of a tricyclic antidepressant. Tricyclic antidepressants are dangerous overdoses and the leading cause of death by intentional overdose by prescription medications (mortality rate is 2 to 5%).

PRESENTATION   CNS symptoms may include confusion, anxiety, delirium, hallucinations, hyperreflexia, seizures, and coma. Anticholinergic symptoms may include mydriatic pupils, hyperpyrexia, skin flushing, blurred vision, tachycardia, dehydration, urinary retention, decreased GI motility, and decreased secretions. Cardiac arrhythmia is characterized on ECG by increased intervals, abnormal QRS complexes, bigeminy, fibrillation, and cardiac arrest.

PEARL   "Hot as Hades, blind as a bat, dry as a bone, red as a beet, mad as a hatter" is indicative of anticholinergics.

DIAGNOSTIC STUDIES   The therapeutic dose of most tricyclic antidepressants is 2 to 4 mg/kg; more than 4 mg/kg is considered potentially toxic; more than 10 mg/kg is life-threatening.

TREATMENT   Aggressive treatment is necessary and includes gastric lavage, activated charcoal administration, consideration of cathartics, urinary alkalinization, and ACLS protocols (avoid class 1a antiarrhythmic agents, atropine, digoxin, and pressors other than norepinephrine as these may exacerbate the condition).

Lithium

Lithium is a common medication used in the treatment of manic-depressive disorders.

PRESENTATION   Sluggishness, drowsiness, tremor, muscle twitching, nausea, vomiting, diarrhea, polydipsia, and polyuria exhibit mild toxicity. Muscular rigidity, hyperreflexia, seizures, cardiac arrhythmia, hypotension, renal abnormalities, and coma exhibit serious toxicity.

DIAGNOSTIC STUDIES   The clinician may note hyponatremia and hypokalemia. The ECG may have ST-segment depression and T-wave inversion. There may be a prolonged QT interval if hypokalemic. Obtain serum lithium level where the therapeutic dose is 0.6 to 1.2 meq/L. Mild toxicity is 1.5 to 2.4 meq/L; serious toxicity is 2.5 to 3.5 meq/L; critical toxicity is over 3.5 meq/L.

TREATMENT   If the patient is hypotensive, give fluids and vasopressors; if the patient is normotensive, give 0.25 to 0.50% normal saline to prevent exacerbation of renal abnormalities and to correct fluids and electrolytes. Consider GI lavage if ingestion occurred within 4 h. Activated charcoal is helpful if there has been coingestion of other drugs, since it does not bind lithium. Avoid magnesium-based cathartics since they can exacerbate renal abnormalities. Alkaline diuresis is controversial. Consider hemodialysis in severe cases.

Neuroleptics

Phenothiazines, indoles, thioxanthenes, butyrophenones, and loxapine are classified as neuroleptics.

PRESENTATION   Anticholinergic symptoms include sedation, muscle rigidity, dystonia, seizures, hypotension, and cardiac abnormalities. Abdominal x-ray may be helpful since these drugs are radiopaque.

TREATMENT   Treatment is largely supportive. Use GI decontamination with activated charcoal, readministered every 4 to 6 h for up to 48 h. Diphenhydramine 0.5 to 1.0 mg/kg intramuscularly or intravenously for children (50 mg in adults) or benztropine mesylate (adults) 2 mg intravenously over 2 min or intramuscularly may help alleviate extrapyramidal effects. Class 1a antiarrhythmic agents are contraindicated.

Acetaminophen

Accidental ingestion is usually found in children. Adolescents and adults may take an intentional overdose. For adults with a single-dose ingestion, toxicity can occur at 7.5 g/24 h (23 regular or 15 extra-strength tablets).

PRESENTATION   Within 12 to 24 h, the patient may experience nausea, vomiting, and diaphoresis, then may appear to resolve. At 3 to 5 days, right upper quadrant pain, anorexia, nausea, vomiting, jaundice, encephalopathy, coagulopathy, metabolic acidosis, coma, and potential death can occur from hepatic or renal failure.

DIAGNOSTIC STUDIES   Liver function studies and acetaminophen blood level tests are recommended. Also helpful are electrolytes, arterial blood gases (ABGs), prothrombin time (PT), and bilirubin. Obtain acetaminophen blood level at 4 h after ingestion for use with nomograms.

TREATMENT   Use gastric lavage and activated charcoal administration if within 2 h of ingestion; in cases of potential toxicity use N-acetylcysteine (Mucomyst) 140 mg/kg orally, then 70 mg/kg every 4 h for 17 doses, from the Rumack-Matthews nomogram based on single-dose ingestion of regular-release acetaminophen. For improved taste, give 20% Mucomyst, which has 200 mg/mL of N-acetylcysteine, diluted 1:3 with fruit juice or soft drink. If vomited within the hour, repeat the dose or utilize a nasogastric tube for placement. This treatment is effective within the first 24 h and best within 8 to 16 h, but it can be given up to 24 h.

Salicylates (Aspirin)

PRESENTATION   CNS stimulation may present as confusion, anxiety, tinnitus, hyperpyrexia, tachypnea, tachycardia, nausea, vomiting, abdominal pain, dehydration, seizures, and coma. The toxic dose for adults is 150 mg/kg and the lethal dose is 480 mg/kg.

DIAGNOSTIC STUDIES   PT, partial thromboplastin time (PTT), and salicylate blood levels 6 h after ingestion and again at 8 to 10 h are recommended. Consider obtaining ABGs, glucose, electrolytes, calcium, complete blood count, liver function tests, and urine pH. One

quick test includes adding 10% ferric chloride to 1 mL of urine; a purple color change indicates as little as two aspirin ingested within the past several hours (however, this may be associated with false-positives from other medications).

TREATMENT   Treatment is based on 6-h salicylate levels. Those patients with less than 40 mg/dL can be discharged safely after gastric decontamination, those with 60 to 95 mg/dL should be admitted for observation and treatment, and those above 95 mg/dL require aggressive treatment. The Done nomogram may be helpful in acute adult ingestion if the time of ingestion is known. Use gastric decontamintion, activated charcoal administration, cathartics (avoid magnesium-containing cathartics, which can increase salicylate absorption), aggressive fluid correction with addition of glucose and potassium, intravenous bicarbonate for acidosis, oxygen, and alkalinization of urine once hypokalemia is corrected. Consider hemodialysis.

Digitalis (Digoxin, Digitoxin)

Digoxin and digitoxin are common medications used in the treatment of atrial fibrillation and heart failure.

PRESENTATION   The patient may present with mild confusion, visual disturbances (yellow halos), anorexia, nausea, vomiting, abdominal pain, diarrhea, bradycardia, hypotension, and variable ECG changes.

TREATMENT   Consider GI decontamination; correction of fluid and electrolytes, especially potassium; and correction of cardiac arrhythmias. Antidigoxin Fab fragments are useful in those with severe toxicity.

Beta-Adrenergic Antagonist (Beta Blocking) Agents

These class II antiarrhythmic drugs are used in the treatment of hypertension, cardiac dysrhythmias, and angina, and they include such drugs as propranolol, metoprolol, timolol, and pindolol.

PRESENTATION   In toxicity, patients may present with lethargy, delirium, hyperkalemia, hypoglycemia, bronchospasm, bradycardia, hypotension, pulmonary edema, AV block, and/or asystole. Symptoms may vary depending on the specific medication's cardioselectivity (e.g., β_1 antagonist leads to decreased sinus rate, contractility, conduction, and renin release; β_2 antagonist leads to increased smooth muscle contraction, altered insulin release, and triglyceride metabolism).

TREATMENT   Treatment consists of supportive and symptomatic care including gastric lavage and administration of activated charcoal. Non-magnesium-containing cathartics may be helpful. In those with symptomatic bradycardia or hypotension, glucagon may be helpful.

Calcium Channel Antagonist (Calcium Channel Blocking) Agents

These class IV antiarrhythmics are commonly used in the treatment of hypertension, dysrhythmia, angina, and migraine, and they include such drugs as verapamil, nifedipine, and diltiazem.

PRESENTATION   In toxicity, patients may present with nausea, vomiting, mild CNS symptoms, hyperglycemia, hypotension, and bradyarrhythmias.

TREATMENT   Gastric lavage and activated charcoal is the treatment of choice. Consider whole-bowel irrigation in those with sustained-release ingestions. Fluids should be given in those with hypotension. Symptomatic bradycardia can be treated with calcium (10 mL of 10%

calcium chloride or 30 mL of calcium gluconate, repeated every 15 to 20 min for up to 5 doses), atropine, glucagon (initially 5 to 10 mg in an intravenous bolus with continuous infusion at 5 mg/h), isoproterenol, epinephrine, and temporary pacing.

Theophylline

Theophylline is a mild stimulant used in the treatment of asthma.

PRESENTATION Agitation, tachycardia, cardiac dysrhythmias, and seizures are the most common symptoms.

DIAGNOSTIC STUDIES A single acute ingestion in which the serum levels range between 20 and 40 μg/mL suggests minimal toxic, 40 to 100 μg/mL suggests moderate toxicity, and greater than 100 μg/mL indicates severe cases.

TREATMENT Gastric decontamination procedures and elimination enhancement (charcoal hemoperfusion) if available are recommended.

RECOGNITION AND MANAGEMENT OF HEAVY METAL POISONING

Iron

Children frequently ingest iron because it is readily available.

PRESENTATION Phase 1 (1 to 6 h after ingestion) includes abdominal pain, vomiting, diarrhea, possible hematemesis (or bloody diarrhea), hypotension, lethargy, seizures, and coma. Phase 2 (12 to 24 h postingestion) includes apparent resolution of initial symptoms; some may skip this stage entirely. Phase 3 (12 to 40 h postingestion) includes severe metabolic acidosis and hepatic and/or renal failure. Phase 4 (2 to 8 weeks later) includes GI obstruction secondary to scarring.

DIAGNOSTIC STUDIES Draw blood 3 to 5 h after ingestion and test for serum iron and total iron binding capacity (TIBC). Abdominal x-ray may be helpful since iron is radiopaque.

TREATMENT Use GI decontamination procedures. Activated charcoal does not bind to iron but is helpful in cases of coingestion. Avoid magnesium-based cathartics because they can bind with iron to form GI concretions. Consider chelation therapy in severe cases with 40 to 90 mg/kg up to a total dose of 2 g per injection at 4- to 12-h intervals (up to 6 g per day) of deferoxamine mesylate administered intramuscularly.

Lead

Lead is ingested inorganically from painted metallic objects or inhaled organically from leaded gasoline.

PRESENTATION After inorganic ingestion, the patient may have nausea, vomiting, abdominal pain, convulsions, and coma. After organic inhalation, more CNS symptoms appear. The clinician may note lead lines on the gingiva or teeth in cases of chronic exposure. Neuropathy may be present.

DIAGNOSTIC STUDIES Check for anemia and red cell stippling on peripheral smear. Long bone and rib films may demonstrate densities at the ends. Radiopaque material may be seen within the gastrointestinal tract. Obtain blood lead levels and erythrocyte protoporphyrin level.

TREATMENT Use GI decontamination if there has been recent ingestion or the lead is radiologically evident. Give chelation therapy

consisting of dimercaprol [British antilewisite (BAL)], 3 to 5 mg/kg intramuscularly every 4 h, then *calcium disodium edetate* (EDTA) begun after the second dimercaprol dose, consisting of 250 mg intravenously every 6 h. Maintain urine output to prevent renal damage.

Mercury

Mercury used in industry and agriculture can be absorbed cutaneously or by inhalation or ingestion. (Thermometer mercury ingested requires no specific treatment because it is poorly absorbed.)

PRESENTATION The patient may report a metallic taste. If the mercury was inhaled, symptoms may include cough, dyspnea, chest discomfort, weakness, nausea, vomiting, and diarrhea. Ingestion of mercury causes tremor, nausea, vomiting, diarrhea, hematemesis, hematochezia, dehydration, altered mental status, seizure, and renal failure. Check blood and urine levels.

TREATMENT Use GI and skin decontamination procedures and activated charcoal administration. Avoid cathartics if diarrhea is present. Correct fluids and electrolytes. Perform chelation with dimercaprol, 3 to 5 mg/kg intramuscularly every 4 h for 7 to 10 days.

Arsenic

Inhalation or ingestion can absorb industrial or agricultural forms of arsenic.

PRESENTATION The patient may have garlic-like breath and may complain of a metallic taste. Nausea, vomiting, diarrhea, a burning sensation of the oropharynx, cardiac arrhythmias, hypotension, hepatic and/or renal failure, and coma may occur. Test the urinary arsenic level.

TREATMENT Use GI decontamination and avoid cathartics if there is severe diarrhea. One must correct fluid and electrolytes. Perform chelation with dimercaprol (BAL), 3 to 5 mg/kg intramuscularly, than 2.5 mg/kg every 8 h for three doses, then given every 12 to 24 h for 10 days.

RECOGNITION AND MANAGEMENT OF CORROSIVE HOUSEHOLD PRODUCT POISONING

Strong Acids

Strong acid examples include hydrochloric acid, sulfuric acid (battery acid), and nitric acid.

SKIN CONTACT When there has been skin contact, which can result in burns, irrigate copiously with water.

EYE CONTACT When there has been eye contact, flush copiously with water (pH testing before and after can guide irrigation) and use fluorescein stain for assessment of ocular damage.

INHALATION OF FUMES A patient who has inhaled fumes can present with a range of symptoms from mild respiratory irritation to complete laryngeal obstruction. Pulmonary edema can be delayed. Give supportive treatment (bronchodilators, oxygen, and possibly steroids).

INGESTION Presentation may include severe pain of oral, pharyngeal, and gastric mucosa; nausea; vomiting; and hematemesis. Avoid neutralization with water since this can cause an exothermic reaction. Some authors suggest nasogastric tube placement with aspiration followed by lavage with cold water; others do not wish to risk vomiting during placement of a nasogastric tube, which may expose tissue to further contact with substance.

Strong Alkali

A strong alkali is defined as a substance with a pH greater than 11.5. Included in this category are sodium and potassium hydroxide (detergents, lye, paint removers) and sodium hypochlorite (bleach).

SKIN OR EYE CONTACT   If there has been skin or eye contact, irrigate copiously and arrange for ophthalmology consultation.

INGESTION   After ingestion of a strong alkali, emesis, lavage, and activated charcoal are contraindicated. Most authors suggest dilution by oral ingestion of milk or water followed by consultation for endoscopy within 12 to 24 h. Chest and abdominal films are needed to assess for perforation.

Recognition and Management of Hydrocarbons, Petroleum Distillates, and Turpentine

Gasoline and kerosene fall into this category.

INGESTION   The patient may present with oral and pharyngeal burning, nausea, vomiting, and diarrhea. Aspiration can produce cough, dyspnea, bronchospasm, and hemoptysis; later, it can cause pulmonary pneumonitis.

INHALATION   The patient may present with euphoria, nausea, vomiting, ataxia, seizures, and coma. The patient may have the odor of the substance involved on his or her breath. Death can result from cardiac arrhythmia or respiratory depression.

TREATMENT   Intubation is recommended for serious respiratory compromise and terbutaline may be considered for bronchospasm. Gastric decontamination is controversial as it may increase the risk of aspiration.

Halogenated Hydrocarbons

Carbon tetrachloride and chloroform fall into this category.

PRESENTATION   The patient may present with headache, nausea, vomiting, hepatic and renal dysfunction, and coma.

TREATMENT   Use GI decontamination, oxygen, intravenous fluids, and vasopressors. Correct electrolytes.

Aromatic Hydrocarbons

Benzene, toluene, and xylene fall into this category.

ACUTE TOXICITY   Euphoria, dizziness, weakness, headache, blurred vision, tremor, ataxia, seizures, respiratory depression, and coma indicate acute toxicity.

CHRONIC TOXICITY   Bone marrow depression, leukemia, neoplasm, neuropathy, and renal damage indicate chronic toxicity (e.g., with benzene).

TREATMENT   Treatment is similar to that for halogenated hydrocarbons.

RECOGNITION AND MANAGEMENT OF INSECTICIDE POISONING

This category includes organophosphates (malathion), carbamates, organochlorines (DDT and lindane) and pyrethrins. Of all hospitalized cases for pesticide poisoning, 80% occur through exposure from the organophosphate group.

PRESENTATION   Early symptoms may include nausea, vomiting, diaphoresis, miotic pupils, blurred vision, abdominal cramping, dyspnea, bradycardia, salivation, lacrimation, urination, and diarrhea. Later the patient may develop mydriatic pupils, restlessness, anxiety, confusion, delirium, headache, ataxia, tremors, muscle fasciculation, weakness, paralysis, seizures, tachycardia, coma, or death.

DIAGNOSTIC STUDIES   Test for serum cholinesterase level.

TREATMENT   Conduct skin, ocular, and GI decontamination. Give atropine 2 to 4 mg intravenously, which may be repeated every 5 to 10 min depending on severity (0.015 to 0.05 mg/kg for children), and for organophosphate exposures, pralidoxime (2-PAM) 1 g in 100 mL of normal saline given intravenously at less than 500 mg/min (children, 25 to 30 mg/kg over 15 to 30 min). Dosage can be repeated every 20 min. Treat until symptoms are reversed (may take 12 to 24 h). Avoid atropine toxicity. Do not give morphine, aminophylline, phenothiazines, tetracycline, furosemide, or beta blockers to these patients as these may exacerbate the toxicity.

PEARL   The mnemonic for cholinergic is SLUDGE: salivation, lacrimation, urination, defecation, GI cramping, and emesis.

SUICIDAL ATTEMPTS AND GESTURES

Facts about suicide include the following: Of the general population, 2% have seriously considered suicide and 1% have attempted it. Suicide is the ninth leading cause of death in the United States. Suicide is the second leading cause of death in those younger than age 24 years. For every 1 successful suicide, there are 40 attempts. Males are two to three times more likely to complete suicide, but women are two to three times more likely to attempt suicide. Males (especially those over 45 years of age) often choose a more lethal method with less chance of rescue (see Chap. 16-7).

Treatment

The clinician should take every suicide attempt seriously. An attempted suicide necessitates psychiatric evaluation or hospital admission for observation. Remove all potentially lethal items from the patient's vicinity and have the patient supervised at all times. Any patient who wishes to leave the hospital against medical advice must be physically or chemically restrained. Characteristics of individuals at high risk for suicide are found in Table 4-8-3.

TABLE 4-8-3.   Risk Factors for Suicide

Individuals with a personal or familial history of previous suicide attempts
Persons with a psychiatric history (10% of all schizophrenic patients are eventually successful)
Excessive alcohol or drug users (alcoholics are at 50 times increased risk; 25% of all suicide cases are associated with alcohol)
Patients with little social support
Patients having conflict in personal relationships
Patients experiencing depression or serious medical problems
Homosexual youths without positive familial or social support
Patients who are unemployed
Patients of Caucasian or Native American descent

BIBLIOGRAPHY

Cline DM et al (eds): *Emergency Medicine: A Comprehensive Study Guide, Companion Handbook,* 5th ed. New York, McGraw-Hill, 2000, section 12, pp 511–597 and pp 941–942.

Jenkins JL, Braen GR: *Manual of Emergency Medicine,* 4th ed. Philadelphia, Lippincott Williams and Wilkins, 2000, section 65, pp 507–566 and pp 599–604.

Plantz SH, Adler JN: *NMS Emergency Medicine.* Baltimore, Williams & Wilkins, 1998, chap. 20, pp 605–637.

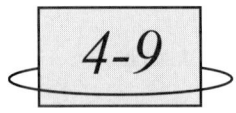

HYPOTHERMIA AND OTHER COLD INJURIES

Karen A. Newell

HYPOTHERMIA

DISCUSSION

Hypothermia can be defined as the condition at which human core temperature drops below 35°C, or 95°F. This temperature can be measured through tympanic methods, esophageal measurements using an endotracheal tube, or a rectal probe. It is important to recognize that the lowest temperature measured by some standard thermometers is 35°C (95°F), so specialized equipment may be required to accurately measure temperatures and monitor these individuals.

Two helpful equations used for converting Celsius and Fahrenheit are:

Celsius to Fahrenheit: $(°C \times 9/5) + 32 = °F$

Fahrenheit to Celsius: $(°F - 32) \times 5/9 = °C$

The following list categorizes the severity stages of hypothermia:

- *Mild:* Core temperature above 32°C (89.6°F) but below 35°C (95°F), associated with a 25% mortality rate
- *Moderate:* Core temperature between 26 and 32°C (78.8 and 89.6°F), associated with a 50% mortality rate
- *Severe:* Core temperature lower than 26°C (78.8°F), associated with a 60% mortality rate

Most cases reported in the United States occur in urban areas, especially during late summer and early fall nights. Mortality rates can be greater than 50% in those with serious underlying diseases. The susceptible populations are shown in Table 4-9-1. Hypothermia may occur in healthy populations as a result of exposure because of inadequate clothing in an unfavorable environment (e.g., skiers or hikers). These individuals may be inexperienced, exhausted, unprepared, or unknowledgeable with regard to wind chill and their own realistic limitations. Mortality rates in these individuals are significantly less, at about 5%.

These cases can often be best prevented through education and public awareness, including the following recommendations:

1. Encourage recreational activity with a buddy system.
2. Wear layered clothing consisting of natural wool or one of the many newer synthetic products (e.g., Gore-Tex); these materials tend to resist moisture more than down or cotton do.
3. Ensure adequate coverage of head, wrists, neck, hands, and feet. (An uncovered head can lose up to 70 to 80% of total body heat.)
4. Avoid cold water immersion (increases heat loss by 25 times) and wet clothing (increases heat loss by 5 times).
5. Consider using heat-insulating foils, which may be helpful.

TABLE 4-9-1.   Susceptible Populations for Hypothermia

Extremes of age (the very young have increased ratio of surface area to mass, and the elderly may not sense cold or may fail to take necessary adaptive action)

Individuals with mental or mobility impairment

Intoxicated persons (ethanol increases heat loss by peripheral vasodilation and interferes with heat production by inhibiting shivering; barbiturates are sometimes associated)

Individual taking certain medications (may interfere with thermoregulation by impairing centrally mediated vasoconstriction); examples: phenothiazines, benzodiazepines, tricyclic antidepressants

Persons with endocrine abnormalities (hypoglycemia, hypothyroidism, adrenal insufficiency, hypopituitarism)

Malnourished individuals

Persons with uremia or sepsis

Race (black-skinned people may be more susceptible to cold temperatures than lighter-skinned individuals)

SIGNS AND SYMPTOMS

Mild Hypothermia

A mildly hypothermic person may present with shivering, dysarthria, and ataxia; may exhibit difficulty with judgment; and may appear mildly confused. The shivering mechanism is maximized at 35°C (95°F) and can raise heat production 2 to 5 times. It can be effective for several hours until glycogen stores are depleted and fatigue appears. Shivering disappears at temperatures below 32°C (89.6°F).

Moderate Hypothermia

An individual presenting with moderate hypothermia may exhibit progressive mental status deterioration and may appear uncooperative or intoxicated. Many times hypothermia coexists with overdose and intoxication or may mimic other conditions such as cerebrovascular accident. In the elderly it may be confused with septicemia. Other signs may include atrial or ventricular arrhythmias, decreased pulse and respiratory rate, dilated and nonreactive pupils, loss of voluntary motor function, and loss of reflexes. In fact, the knee jerk, if present, may be the last to disappear and the first to reappear during rewarming.

Severe Hypothermia

The patient who presents in severe hypothermia may exhibit hypotension, ventricular fibrillation, or coma, or even appear deceased. At temperatures below 28°C (82.4°F), ventricular fibrillation occurs. At 19 to 26°C (66.2 to 78.8°F), the electroencephalogram (EEG) becomes flat line. At 15 to 18°C (59 to 64.4°F), asystole occurs. Because there are reported cases of individuals who were presumed dead who survived, *no one is considered dead until he or she is warm and dead.* Therefore, do not stop resuscitative efforts until the core temperature is greater than 35°C (95°F). Treatment is aimed at rewarming with attention to identification and treatment of underlying etiology.

Patients may appear cold and pale. They may have stiff to completely rigid or even decomposing extremities. They may appear to be in rigor mortis or opisthotonus (back arched from contraction of major muscle groups). Hands may be fixed in flexion at the interphalangeal joints and wrists with extension at the metacarpophalangeal joints. Mental status varies from mild confusion to coma. Neurologic assessment including the Glascow coma scale is unpredictable and unreliable for prognosis.

DIAGNOSTIC STUDIES

It is paramount to obtain continuous temperature measurements; most recommend a rectal thermistor probe placed between 5 and 15 cm with care taken not to place it into cold feces. In addition, take careful and frequent vital sign readings (counting pulse for at least 30 to 45 s). Also be aware that the respiratory rate may be asynchronous.

Exercise cervical spine precautions if the history is unknown or if the patient is unconscious until a full cervical spine series can be obtained. Avoid excessive movement of the patient so as to minimize cardiac arrhythmias due to increased cardiac irritability.

Blood work should include initial arterial blood gases (ABG), complete blood cell count (CBC), electrolytes [blood urea nitrogen (BUN), creatinine, glucose, calcium], toxicology screen, liver function studies, and amylase. Also consider obtaining serum cortisol, magnesium, lipase, prothrombin time (PT), partial thromboplastin time (PTT), fibrinogen, thyroid function studies (TFS), cardiac isoenzymes, and blood, urine, and cerebrospinal fluid (CSF) cultures. Realize that the initial unreliability of hematocrit, BUN, and creatinine is secondary to fluid shifts. Also note that most patients will have an elevated glucose (unless the hypothermia is due to hypoglycemia) because there is impairment of insulin secretion, cellular uptake, and effectiveness at low body temperatures. Do not attempt to rapidly correct pH or P_{co_2} based on initial blood gases as P_{o_2} and P_{co_2} may be falsely increased and pH may be falsely decreased secondary to the lowered temperature.

Some authors suggest that to correctly reflect true readings, 0.0147 should be added to the measured pH for each degree Celsius below 37°C. However, most current thought supports acid-base treatment without regard for temperature correction.

RADIOLOGIC AND OTHER DIAGNOSTIC STUDIES

Radiologic studies include plain films of the chest and abdomen. Continuous electrocardiogram (ECG) may demonstrate a variety of cardiac arrhythmias including the following:

- Tachycardia.
- Bradycardia, which may be effective in meeting oxygen demands; therefore be cautious since a rapid correction can precipitate ventricular fibrillation and asystole. Atropine is not effective in hypothermic patients. Cardiac pacing is controversial.
- Atrioventricular block.
- Atrial fibrillation, which is common at core temperatures below 32°C (89.6°F) and does not require treatment since it disappears with rewarming.
- Prolonged intervals (may affect all intervals).
- Osborn or J waves, which are sometimes noted at temperatures between 25 and 32°C (77 and 89.6°F). These appear as an extra upward deflection noted at the junction of the QRS and ST segments, especially in leads II and V_6 (see Fig. 4-9-1).

TREATMENT

Mild Cases

Because these patients are capable of endogenous thermogenesis, passive external rewarming (PER) techniques are employed:

1. Remove all clothing, cover the patient with warm blankets to prevent further heat loss, and place in a warm, dry environment.
2. Monitor core temperatures carefully; they should rise 0.5 to 2°C/h (0.9 to 3.6°F/h). If core temperatures do not rise, consider giving levothyroxine, 400 to 500 mg intravenously, and hydrocortisone, 100 mg intravenously.
3. Admission with cardiac observation for at least 24 h is suggested.

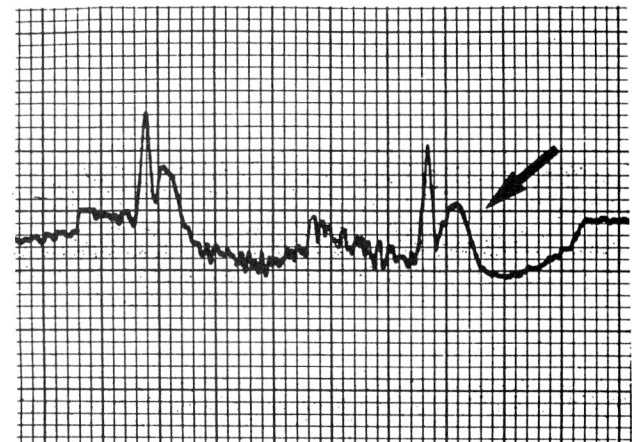

FIGURE 4-9-1. Rhythm strip from patient with temperature of 25°C (77°F), showing atrial fibrillation with a slow ventricular response, muscle tremor artifact, and Osborn (J) wave (arrow). (*From Tintinalli* et al., p 848. *Reprinted with permission from McGraw-Hill, Inc.*)

Moderate to Severe Cases

The following treatment is recommended:

1. Initially, as with all seriously ill patients, begin with the ABCs: airway, breathing, and circulation.
2. As with any unconscious patient, administer thiamine, 100 mg intravenously, and naloxone hydrochloride (Narcan), 2 mg intravenously.
3. Give 50 to 100 mL of 50% dextrose intravenously as well if the initial fingerstick glucose is low. The serum glucose level will serve as a guide when results of laboratory work become available.
4. An initial fluid challenge of 250 to 500 mL of heated (40 to 42°C or 104 to 107.6°F) normal saline with 5% dextrose may be helpful. This can easily be created with a 1-L bag of fluid placed in the microwave on high power for 2 min. Be sure to shake vigorously to redistribute any "hotspots," and avoid rapid central administration. Fluid warmers are also very helpful.
5. The remainder of fluid is given cautiously to avoid fluid overload. Lactated Ringer's solution should be avoided secondary to a potential increased lactate level.
6. Central venous pressure or Swan-Ganz monitoring may be necessary.
7. An indwelling urinary catheter may also be helpful for fluid monitoring and general assessment of renal function. However, it is not a reliable indicator of cardiovascular status secondary to "cold diuresis."
8. These patients may also require a nasogastric tube secondary to decreased gastric motility.

Although controversy exists, most authorities consider patients with core temperatures below 30°C (86°F) incapable of self-generating heat and requiring some type of active rewarming. Generally, there are two main types: active external rewarming (AER) and active core rewarming (ACR). AER consists of heated or electric blankets, heated water bottles, and warm water immersion. These methods are applied to the trunk first to prevent extremity vasodilatation and blood pooling which can further exacerbate shock since an already compromised cardiovascular system may not be able to handle the added load of total body rewarming. Similarly, if the entire body is rewarmed simultaneously, shunting cooler blood from the extremities to the trunk, a decrease in core temperature referred to as *afterdrop* can occur. A rapid washout of lactic acid from the periphery can also overload the patient, further complicating acidosis.

ACR may be indicated in those who are hemodynamically unstable and may consist of the following:

1. Inhaling heated (43°C or 109.4°F) humidified oxygen by mask or endotracheal tube
2. Infused heated (40 to 45°C or 104 to 113°F) crystalloid peritoneal lavage using an isotonic potassium-free dialysate with 1.5% dextrose at a rate of 6 L/h
3. Hemodialysis
4. Gastrointestinal tract lavage (gastric and colonic)
5. Bladder lavage
6. Extracorporeal blood rewarming (cardiopulmonary bypass techniques)
7. Mediastinal irrigation through chest tubes or open thoracotomy in extreme cases
8. Diathermy (ultrasonic and low-frequency microwave radiation in those without frostbite, burns, significant edema, metallic implants, or pacemakers)

Often endotracheal tube placement and ventilatory support may be necessary. However, the patient requires up to 50% less than what would normally be suggested. For every 10°C (18°F) decrease in temperature, oxygen consumption decreases two to three times, and similarly for every 8°C (14.4°F), CO_2 production decreases by about half. Attempt to maintain P_{CO_2} at 40 mmHg. Hyperventilation should be avoided to decrease the chance of serious cardiac arrhythmias.

Defibrillation is usually not effective at core temperatures less than 28 to 30°C (82.4 to 86°F). Cardiopulmonary resuscitation (CPR) rate is controversial. However, the American Heart Association suggests the same rate as for the normothermic patient. Most believe it should be administered if pulselessness is established, despite the possibility of inducing lethal cardiac arrhythmias in a patient with an undetected yet viable pulse rate.

Most of the cardiac drugs, including lidocaine, may not be effective at lower core temperatures and may even exacerbate cardiac irritability. Therefore, treatment in these situations is aimed at warming the patient first, then treating the specific conditions as they occur. Also be aware that markedly increased doses of medication may be necessary to obtain a response; however, during rewarming the patient may become toxic. Bretylium may be helpful in preventing ventricular fibrillation.

COMPLICATIONS AND RED FLAGS

Too rapid rewarming can precipitate disseminated intravascular coagulopathy, pulmonary edema, hemolysis, or acute tubular necrosis.

LOCAL COLD INJURIES

DISCUSSION

Local cold injury usually involves the extremities, particularly the hands and feet. At temperatures below 25°C (77°F), tissue metabolism is decreased, producing a cyanotic appearance. At 15°C (59°F), tissue metabolism is markedly decreased and skin may appear pink secondary to dissociation of oxyhemoglobin. It is at and below this temperature that actual tissue damage occurs.

Chilblain, or pernio, results from vasoconstriction which produces dermal edema and mild vasculitis, ultimately resulting in lesions. Anatomic locations commonly include the face and dorsal surface of the hands and feet. It presents more often in women and occurs especially in susceptible individuals (collagen vascular disorders, Raynaud's disease).

SIGNS AND SYMPTOMS

Despite no actual freezing of the tissue, signs and symptoms include erythema, edema, blistering, mild pain, and pruritus. Later, ulcerative lesions may appear and can persist for months. These lesions resolve with warmer weather changes but may recur seasonally.

TREATMENT

Treatment is symptomatic. Some studies suggest nifedipine (20 mg orally tid) and topical corticosteroids (0.025% fluocinolone cream) or short-course oral corticosteroids (prednisone) may be of benefit. Do not rub or massage the injured tissues and do not apply heat or ice since tissue destruction can be exacerbated. Protect the area from excessive pressure or trauma to prevent further injury (e.g., avoid tight footwear). Prevention obviously eliminates the need for treatment. Patient education and public awareness may decrease the incidence of this condition.

TRENCH FOOT (IMMERSION FOOT)

DISCUSSION

Trench foot (immersion foot) results from exposure to cold and wet environments. It can occur in 12 to 24 h and is frequently seen in homeless populations. It is important to note that the clinical presentation is not related to outcome. A seemingly minor case may actually be quite severe or vice versa. The initial phase begins with a vasospastic or ischemic period with alternating vasoconstriction and vasodilation.

SIGNS AND SYMPTOMS

Signs and symptoms include edema, decreased pulse, local pallor, and decreased sensation. The secondary phase begins 12 to 24 h later and consists of a hyperemic or vasodilating phase with bounding pulses which may last between 5 and 10 days.

These patients present with warm or hot, erythematous, edematous, ecchymotic sites, sometimes with blistering and ulceration. They complain of an intense burning or tingling pain. Approximately 2 to 6 weeks later they begin the recovery phase.

TREATMENT

Treatment includes gradual passive rewarming with avoidance of soaking or massage, elevation, avoidance of pressure or further tissue trauma, meticulous local wound care, complete bed rest if a lower extremity is involved, and sometimes hospital admission. Antibiotics are warranted only if infection is present.

COMPLICATIONS

Complications include hypersensitivity to cold with early cyanosis and permanent injury to vessels and nerves. Other more serious sequelae include lymphangitis, cellulitis, thrombophlebitis, and gangrene.

FROSTBITE

DISCUSSION

Frostbite results from excessive cold exposure (−10 to −4°C or 14 to 24.8°F) with actual freezing of tissues and ischemic necrosis secondary to vasoconstriction. It can be classified into two types:

- *Superficial:* Also called first and second degree, reversible injury, or frostnip. Skin and subcutaneous tissue appear white without blanching (no return of color after mild pressure and no capillary refill) and feel soft and rubbery. Patients report decreased sensation, numbness, paresthesia, and pruritus.

- *Deep:* Also called third and fourth degree. This type may involve skin, subcutaneous tissue, muscle, blood vessels, nerves, tendons, and bone. These may appear hard, wooden-like, or edematous. Patients may report mild burning, stinging, numbness, or a feeling of clumsiness in the involved extremity.

Frostbite can be classified into the following grades:

- *First degree:* Partial-thickness skin freezing without blistering, erythema, or edema; skin may peel several days later; hospital admission recommended if extensive; prognosis is excellent.
- *Second degree:* Full-thickness skin freezing with blistering (6 to 24 h) and eschar formation (several days); hospital admission; prognosis is good.
- *Third degree:* Freezing with skin cell death, hemorrhagic blisters, and subcutaneous involvement; hospital admission; prognosis is poor.
- *Fourth degree:* Full-thickness freezing including all tissue to bone; little edema; initially mottled, red, or cyanotic; later dry, black, or mummified; loss of tissue secondary to necrosis and significant deformity; hospital admission; prognosis is extremely poor.

TREATMENT

Initial treatment of frostnip involves application of constant warmth such as gentle pressure with a warm hand (avoid rubbing) or, in the case of a hand or digit, placement into the contralateral axilla. Footwear should be removed from feet and clean, dry socks or a blanket applied. Treatment is aimed at gradual rewarming.

Some authors recommend a rapid rewarming by submersion in a water bath at 40 to 44°C (104 to 108°F) for 15 to 30 min. This can be uncomfortable and require parenteral analgesics secondary to burning pain. Avoid dry heat, such as a stove or open fire, since this is difficult to regulate and burns can develop.

Other contraindications include attempts at rewarming by exercise (e.g., stomping the affected foot on the ground) or by rubbing the body part with snow or immersion in cold water.

To minimize tissue injury, rewarming should be attempted only once; therefore, rewarming should be delayed if a possibility of refreezing exists. Minor involvement may require elevation, meticulous local wound care, and tetanus prophylaxis. Clear fluid blisters can be débrided and covered with aloe vera cream placed every 6 h, or some suggest silver sulfadiazine cream applied every 12 h. If blisters are left in place, many advise aspiration to minimize contact with fluid containing arachidonic acid cascade and then covering the blister with aloe vera cream. Hemorrhagic blisters should be left in place. Avoid tight or occlusive dressings. Immobilization can be utilized if loose, bulky, dry dressings are carefully applied. Some authors prescribe whirlpool treatment at 32.2 to 37.8°C (90 to 100°F) twice daily for 30 min.

Antibiotics are usually given only if indicated (penicillin G, 500,000 U intravenously every 6 h for 2 to 3 days). Ibuprofen, 12 mg/kg per day in divided doses, is helpful even with concurrent narcotic analgesics. The use of low-molecular-weight dextran and anticoagulants have not been consistently documented to be of benefit.

Any serious involvement may require hospital admission and surgical consultation with the possibility of amputation. Last, technetium pyrophosphate technetium 99m scanners may be helpful in predicting viability at 5 to 14 days postexposure.

Smoking is a contraindication since it impairs healing.

BIBLIOGRAPHY

Adler JN et al (eds): *NMS Clinical Manuals: Emergency Medicine.* Baltimore, Lippincott Williams & Wilkins, 1999, pp 643–650.
American Heart Association: *Advanced Cardiac Life Support.* Dallas, American Heart Association, 1997, pp 11.1–11.3.
American Heart Association: *Basic Life Support for Healthcare Providers.* Dallas, American Heart Association, 1994, pp 5.5–5.6.
Auerbach PS (ed): *Wilderness Medicine—Management of Environmental Emergencies,* 3rd ed. St. Louis, Mosby, 1995, pp 51–145.
Cline DM et al: *Emergency Medicine—A Comprehensive Study Guide/Companion Handbook,* 5th ed. New York, McGraw-Hill, 1999, pp 599–604.
Jenkins JL, Braen GR: *Manual of Emergency Medicine,* 4th ed. Philadelphia, Lippincott Williams & Wilkins, 1999, pp 456–460.
Pousada L et al (eds): *Emergency Medicine (House Officer Series),* 2nd ed. Baltimore, Williams & Wilkins, 1996, pp 510–515.
Salyer SW, Bielig L (eds): *Physician Assistant Emergency Handbook.* Philadelphia, W.B. Saunders, 1996, pp 118–121, 135–138.
Tintinalli JE et al (eds): *Emergency Medicine, A Comprehensive Study Guide,* 4th ed. New York, McGraw-Hill, 1996, pp 843–850.

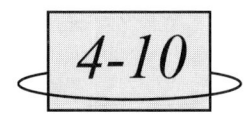

ANAPHYLAXIS
James D. Cannon

DISCUSSION

Anaphylaxis is a dramatic, sudden, adverse systemic response to an injected (bee sting), ingested (food, medicine), or inhaled substance in a previously sensitized person. Rarely, it can result from a topical exposure or even exercise. The immune system becomes hypersensitive, releasing chemical mediators, usually IgE, and in anaphylaxis this can cause cardiovascular collapse and respiratory distress. Table 4-10-1

TABLE 4-10-1. Common Causes of Anaphylactic Reactions

Drugs
Penicillin (including penicillin-contaminated milk)
Cephalosporins (can have cross-reactivity to penicillin because of chemical similarities)
Aspirin
Nonsteroidal anti-inflammatory medications
Sulfa-containing medications
Vancomycin
Radiographic contrast dye
Lidocaine
Vaccines
Blood products

Foods
Milk
Eggs
Shellfish: lobster, clams, shrimp, oysters, scallops
Nuts
Soybeans (including oleic acid, which is in some metered dose inhalers), and soy lecithin. Soy oil in the United States is highly processed and is not a soy allergen
Wheat
Chocolate
Citrus: tomatoes, oranges, lemons, etc.
Food additives: monosodium glutamate (MSG), nitrate and nitrite sulfites, tartrazine dyes
Bee pollen tablets

Environmental Sources
Hymenoptera venom: honey bee, fire ant, and yellowjacket
Insect parts, especially cockroach
Molds
Pollen: trees, grass, plants
Dander: cat (protein in the saliva)
Snake venom

Topical Sources
Spermicidal products
Latex gloves, condoms, etc.
Ophthalmic: fluorescein dye

lists some of the many and varied substances that often cause anaphylaxis.

The true incidence of anaphylaxis is probably underestimated because it is not a reportable disease. One episode of anaphylaxis, related primarily to drug reactions, has been reported for every 2700 hospitalized subjects. Insect stings are probably responsible for at least 50 fatalities per year in the United States. Elevated postmortem tryptase levels have been reported in 12 percent of otherwise healthy adults who died suddenly and in at least 40 percent of victims of sudden infant death syndrome. These elevations in postmortem tryptase level, a highly specific serum marker for mast cell activation, suggest that anaphylaxis was responsible for many of these fatalities.

The most important decision that should be made as it relates to the care of a patient with a possible anaphylactic reaction is the immediate determination of emergent or stable status. Treatment needs to be rapid and aggressive, initiated by office-based, out-of-hospital emergency personnel, and emergency/hospital-based personnel. Always consider 24-h observation in hospital to prevent relapse in the more severe and/or unstable cases. In severe cases, death can come swiftly from intractable bronchospasm, volume depletion, and/or laryngeal edema.

PATHOGENESIS

The chemical mediators that cause anaphylaxis are preformed and released from granules (histamine, tryptase, and others) or are generated from membrane lipids (prostaglandin D_2, leukotrienes, and platelet-activating factor) by the activated mast cell or basophil. These mediators, once active, are released by immunologic mechanisms, and reactions are termed *anaphylactic.* The mediators released by nonimmunologic mechanisms are called *anaphylactoid.* Histamine exerts its pathophysiologic effects via both H_1 and H_2 receptors. Flushing, hypotension, and headache are mediated by both H_1 and H_2 receptors, whereas tachycardia, pruritus, rhinorrhea, and bronchospasm are associated only with H_1 receptors. Increased vascular permeability during anaphylaxis can produce a shift of 50% of intravascular fluid to the extravascular space within 10 minutes. This dramatic shift of effective blood volume causes compensatory catecholamine release and activates the renin–angiotensin–aldosterone system. These internal compensatory responses produce variable effects during anaphylaxis. Some patients experience abnormal elevations in their peripheral vascular resistance, indicating maximal vasoconstriction, whereas others have depressed systemic vascular resistance despite elevated catecholamine levels.

SYMPTOMS

Anaphylaxis can be vague initially, with nasal itching, stuffiness, and a lump in the throat. It can rapidly progress to more serious signs and symptoms (see Table 4-10-2).

OBJECTIVE FINDINGS

The objective findings for anaphylaxis are listed in Table 4-10-3.

DIAGNOSTIC CONSIDERATIONS

Several disorders share the objective features of anaphylaxis. The vasovagal reaction is probably the most common consideration in the differential diagnosis of anaphylaxis. Additional considerations should include those shown in Table 4-10-4.

SPECIAL CONSIDERATIONS

Be mindful of fluid overload in the elderly and people with renal or cardiovascular disease. Because of vascular permeability, pulmonary

TABLE 4-10-2. Signs and Symptoms of Anaphylaxis

Respiratory
Difficulty breathing
Retrosternal pain
Cough
Cardiovascular
Lightheadedness (can be an indicator of vascular collapse)
Palpitations
Loss of consciousness

Cutaneous
Increased warmth of skin
Oropharyngeal swelling (which can be quite painful)
Pruritus

Gastrointestinal
Nausea
Vomiting
Diarrhea
Crampy abdominal pain

edema can develop. Also, a history of heart problems should be elicited before administering epinephrine. However, care cannot be withheld, and the risks versus the benefits need to be assessed.

Individuals on beta-adrenergic antagonists (e.g., metoprolol) may be more likely to experience severe reactions marked by profound hypotension, severe bronchospasm, and paradoxical bradycardia that persists despite treatment with epinephrine. Dosage increases of beta-agonists (e.g., isoproterenol) up to 80-fold are necessary experimentally to overcome beta-receptor blockade.

LABORATORY AND RADIOLOGIC STUDIES

There are no appropriate laboratory and radiologic studies. This is a clinical diagnosis.

TREATMENT

Treatment must be quick and aggressive. A team approach works best. The sequential approach, keeping the ABCs as a high treatment essential, is recommended. A patent airway is the first priority. Oxygen should be administered via facemask or nasal canula. If the airway is obstructed from bronchospasm, laryngospasm, or edema, then the patient needs endotracheal intubation. At least one, and preferably two,

TABLE 4-10-3. Objective Findings in Anaphylaxis

General
Anxiety
Agitation

Respiratory
Wheezing
Tachypnea
Stridor
Use of accessory muscles
Gasping for air
Cough

Cardiovascular
Dysrhythmias
Hypotension
Tachycardia

Cutaneous
Generalized erythema
Edema (orbital, perioral, facial, neck)
Wheals or flares

TABLE 4-10-4. Diagnostic Considerations with Anaphylaxis

Respiratory
Acute asthma
Pulmonary embolism
Airway obstruction

Cardiac
Acute myocardial infarction
Acute congestive heart failure
Cardiac dysrhythmias

Cutaneous
Niacin ingestion
Hereditary angioedema

intravenous lines should be started, with normal saline or Ringer's lactate, wide open, especially if the patient is hypotensive. Vital signs need to be monitored continuously, and the patient should be on a cardiac monitor. Military or medical antishock trousers can be applied if there are sufficient personnel.

Epinephrine is the drug of choice. The condition of the patient determines the route of administration. If there is no evidence of circulatory collapse, then epinephrine, 0.3 to 0.5 mg of a 1:1000 solution, can be given subcutaneously or intramuscularly. (Be sure to draw back on the syringe; inadvertent venous administration can cause severe complications.) This dose can be repeated every 10 to 15 min until the patient improves. If there is no improvement in 30 to 35 min, or if the patient seems to be getting worse, then IV epinephrine is indicated, 0.3 to 0.5 mg of 1:10,000 solution. (If not available, dilute 1 mL of 1:1000 solution epinephrine with 10 mL of normal saline.) It is important to continually assess patient status. If the patient is hypotensive, then a subcutaneous or IM injection of epinephrine is not going to work. If the patient is already in shock and has already been intubated, endotracheal administration is possible, with 5 to 10 mL of 1:10,000 solution followed by four or five rapid ventilations. Hypotension needs to be closely monitored; expect to administer 2 to 4 L of crystalloid solution. However, pulmonary edema can develop due to vascular permeability, especially in the elderly or in patients with cardiovascular or renal disease. Monitor urine output.

Bronchospasm is treated with inhaled bronchodilators. Aerosolized albuterol, 0.5 mL in 3 mL of saline, should be attached to the oxygen tubing. Mild hypotension is sometimes assisted with the use of cimetidine (Tagamet), 300 mg IV, or ranitidine (Zantac), 50 mg IV. Theoretically, it is thought to aid in urticaria also, but this is not an approved indication.

Methylprednisolone (50 to 125 mg) administered by IV push helps prevent recurrent symptoms. The body can respond to allergies for up to 72 h, and corticosteroids control this effectively, as well as the administration of an antihistamine, usually diphenhydramine (Benadryl) 50 mg IM. Supportive measures include hospitalization for 24 h for observation, indicated in moderate to severe reactions. Milder cases that respond quickly in the emergency room can be sent home with corticosteroids, bronchodilators, and antihistamines, after being monitored for up to 8 to 12 h.

Patient Education

Avoid offending substances that cause reactions. The patient will need to carry an emergency epinephrine kit (e.g., EpiPen) if the offending agent could likely recur.

Disposition

Mild cases and stable patients can be discharged home with an oral prednisone taper, diphenhydramine (or other nonsedating branded antihistamine) 25 to 50 mg every 4 to 6 h, cimetidine 400 mg or ranitidine 150 mg twice a day for 1 to 3 days, rest, and if indicated, especially with first episodes, referral to an allergist for further follow-up and care, including skin testing.

ACKNOWLEDGEMENT

The editor would like to acknowledge the significant contribution of Michaela O'Brien-Norton, author of this chapter in the first edition of *Primary Care for Physician Assistants.*

BIBLIOGRAPHY

Austin KF. Diseases of immediate type hypersensitivity. In: Fauci AS, Braunwald E, Isselbacher KJ, et al. *Principles and Practice of Internal Medicine,* 14th ed. New York, McGraw-Hill, 1998, pp. 1860–1864.
Fontanarosa PB, Blanda M. Management of anaphylaxis. *Phys Assist* 18:51–58, 1994.
Kemp SF. Anaphylaxis and serum sickness. In: Rakel, ed. *Conn's Current Therapy* 2000, 52nd ed. New York, Saunders, 2000, pp. 725–729.
Koury SI, Herfel LU. Anaphylaxis and acute allergic reactions. In: Tintinalli et al, eds. *Emergency Medicine: A Comprehensive Study Guide,* 5th ed. New York, McGraw-Hill, 2000, pp. 242–245.
Muelleman RL, Lindzon RD, Silvers WS. Allergy, hypersensitivity, and anaphylaxis. In: Rosen P. *Emergency Medicine: Concepts and Clinical Practice,* 4th ed. St. Louis, Mosby, 1998, pp. 2759–2760.

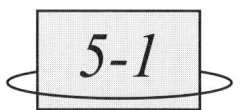

DIABETES MELLITUS
Janice Herbert-Carter

DISCUSSION

Diabetes mellitus, which often is called "sugar diabetes," is a condition in which the pancreas produces insufficient insulin to meet the body's metabolic needs, leading to hyperglycemia (elevated blood glucose). There may be a total lack of insulin production, decreased insulin production, or even hyperinsulinemia, but in all cases the quantity of insulin is insufficient for effective glucose metabolism. About 5 percent of the U.S. population is affected. The disorder involves a spectrum of abnormalities and encompasses variants that primarily affect children and adolescents (type 1), obese middle-aged adults (type 2), and pregnant women (gestational). Also included may be "prediabetic" or "latent" states of impaired glucose tolerance in which the person is not overtly ill but laboratory studies indicate abnormal glucose metabolism.

The etiology of primary diabetes is largely unknown, although hypotheses abound. Viruses, particularly coxsackievirus, may be important in type 1, but heredity plays a part, possibly by making a person susceptible to the effects of the virus. Type 1 diabetes is known to be associated with human leukocyte antigen (HLA) types DR3 and 4, although this is not clinically used in diagnosis or treatment. Heredity clearly is involved in type 2, as evidenced by its occurrence in families and its high incidence in some ethnic groups, but the exact genetics are unclear, probably involving many genes and interactions between genes and the environment. African Americans, Native Americans, Hispanics, Fiji Islanders, and Indians (Asian) are very commonly affected, particularly women.

There are known causes of secondary diabetes. Pancreatic failure with destruction of exocrine and endocrine function as is seen in patients with chronic pancreatitis, pancreatectomy, hemochromatosis, and pancreatic cancer is obvious. Other causes include excess production of hormones that oppose the action of insulin, such as Cushing's syndrome (glucocorticoid excess), glucagonoma, pheochromocytoma (catecholamine excess), and acromegaly (growth hormone excess). Drugs such as thiazide diuretics, synthetic glucocorticoids (prednisone), niacin, and phenytoin (Dilantin) may induce or unmask diabetes. Obesity is a risk factor in gestational and type 2 diabetes, but the risk factors in type 1 diabetes have not been established clearly. Other known risk factors in type 2 diabetes include hypertension, a history of gestational diabetes or delivery of babies over 9 pounds, a previous history of impaired glucose tolerance, family history, and ethnicity.

The pathophysiology of type 1 diabetes (approximately 10 to 20 percent of all diabetic patients) is total failure of insulin production. Autoimmune destruction of beta cells in the pancreatic islets of Langerhans occurs. In type 2 diabetes (approximately 80 to 90 percent of all diabetics), there is typically inadequate insulin production. However, adipose tissue has fewer insulin receptors than do other tissue types, and this contributes to insulin resistance even in the face of hyperinsulinemia. Later in the course of the disorder, the pancreas may no longer be able to maintain the hyperinsulinemic state, and frank insulin deficiency may occur. In gestational diabetes (approximately 4 percent of all pregnancies), the insulin requirement increases but resistance also may increase, leading to inadequate levels and hyperglycemia.

SIGNS AND SYMPTOMS

Signs and symptoms may be divided into acute presenting findings caused by the hyperglycemia and chronic complications resulting from the systemic effects of the disease. Chronic complications are discussed later in this chapter. Two major acute complications—ketoacidosis and hypoglycemia (insulin shock)—are discussed in Chap. 5-7 and 5-8, respectively.

Acute signs and symptoms may be the presenting complaints that lead to a diagnosis or may be indications that an established diabetic patient is out of control. They include thirst (polydipsia), excessive hunger (polyphagia), increased urination (polyuria: large quantities, not simply urinary frequency) and nocturia, blurry vision, fatigue, and weight loss despite increased intake. Many type 2 diabetics may have the disease for years before the diagnosis is made. Therefore, they may present with findings consistent with the long-term systemic effects of diabetes (discussed later in this chapter).

DIAGNOSIS

The hallmark of diabetes mellitus is hyperglycemia. For nonpregnant adults, the following criteria are used to establish the diagnosis:

- Random blood glucose >200 with symptoms as above or
- Fasting blood glucose ≥126 or
- 2-h postprandial glucose ≥200 on an oral glucose tolerance test (GTT)

Any of these criteria must be confirmed by having the same or different criteria repeated on a subsequent day.

Impaired glucose tolerance is defined as an intermediate stage between normal glucose homeostasis and overt diabetes. This is not considered a clinical disorder in and of itself but a risk factor for the development of diabetes and cardiovascular disease. These persons have a fasting plasma glucose ≥110 and <126.

It is important to note that while urine glucose tests may be suggestive, they are never adequate for a diagnosis. Also, GTTs, while diagnostic, are rarely indicated because most patients are easily diagnosed by one of the first two criteria. The exception is that the oral GTT is still used in pregnancy. All pregnant women should be assessed for their level of risk for gestational diabetes at the first prenatal visit. Low-risk women fulfill *all* of the following criteria: <25 years of age, normal body weight, no family history of diabetes, no personal history of abnormal glucose tolerance or poor obstetric outcome, and lack of membership in high-risk ethnic groups. Women at high risk for gestational diabetes should have their glucose checked at the initial prenatal visit, and those who are normal at that time should be rescreened between 24 and 28 weeks. In pregnancy, the patient is given a 50-g glucose load for a 1-h test and a 100-g load for a 3-h test. Nonpregnant patients are given 75 mg of glucose.

LABORATORY TESTS

Elevated blood glucose is assumed in diabetes. Urine glucose is present when the blood glucose is higher than 175. The kidney normally reabsorbs all filtered glucose, but there is a limit. At about 175, the transport maximum (T_{max}) is reached and any excess glucose is spilled into the urine. Unfortunately, there is no direct relationship between urine glucose levels and blood glucose levels above that point. Therefore, urine glucose levels are not reliable gauges of treatment efficacy.

Glycosylated hemoglobin (HbA_{1c}) is used to determine long-term glucose control; it is not used for diagnostic purposes. When blood sugar levels are elevated, hemoglobin irreversibly binds glucose. Thus, the hemoglobin remains glycosylated for the life of the red blood cell (up to 120 days). Patients may have normal glucose at the time of their follow-up visits because they have been careful with diet and medications in the hours or days leading up to phlebotomy but previously may have been out of control for months at a time. Thus, a random or even fasting blood sugar done during a routine office visit may not accurately reflect their level of control over time. The glycosylated hemoglobin level should not be more than 7 percent. If the patient's self-monitoring indicates good control but the HbA_{1c} is elevated, it is wise to check postprandial glucose levels as well. Other laboratory values may be abnormal in certain patients (see Chap. 5-7).

Shorter-term glycemic control may be monitored by using glycosylated serum proteins such as albumin and fructosamine, which may provide evidence of glycemic control over the previous 2 weeks. These tests also may be useful in patients in whom testing HbA_{1c} may be unsatisfactory (i.e., patients with hemolytic anemia).

TREATMENT

The overall goal in diabetes treatment is to maintain normal or nearly normal glucose levels. It is also advisable to attempt to achieve metabolic control of lipids and maintain normal blood pressure. Good control of hyperglycemia has been proven to decrease symptoms and reduce the risk of acute and chronic complications. Metabolic control of lipids and normalization of blood pressure may help reduce cardiovascular and renal complications. Treatment should involve nutritional management, exercise, self-monitoring of glucose, pharmacologic therapy, and continuing patient education and supportive follow-up.

The initial visit once the diagnosis has been established should include a comprehensive history and physical examination. Appropriate laboratory studies (in adults) include fasting lipid profile, HbA_{1c}, serum creatinine, urinalysis, test for microalbuminuria (all type 2 and type 1 if known diagnosis for >5 years), thyroid-stimulating hormone (TSH) in all type 1, and an electrocardiogram. Microalbuminuria may be done as a 24-h urine collection, a spot urine, or a timed sample. There is marked daily variation in the albuminuria levels; therefore, the test should be repeated two or three times over a 3- to 6-month period before a definitive diagnosis of microalbuminuria is made. In a 24-h collection, microalbuminuria is 30 to 300 mg/24. In a spot sample, it is 30 to 300 mg albumin/mg creatinine. Other tests that may be useful include liver function tests to evaluate for fatty liver and establish a baseline of normality before initiating potentially hepatotoxic drugs and a chemistry panel including electrolytes to assess hydration status and the possibility of adverse effects caused by antihypertensive medications (e.g., hyper- or hypokalemia).

Frequent, closely spaced visits may be necessary to bring the disorder under control. Follow-up visits should include smoking cessation assistance if needed, thorough foot examinations yearly or more frequently as warranted, management of dyslipidemia if present, annual screening for microalbuminuria, at least yearly ophthalmologic visits for patients over 30 years old, aggressive management of other cardiovascular risk factors such as hypertension, and dental evaluations. Pneumococcal and influenza vaccines are recommended for diabetic patients regardless of age.

Diet

The goal of medical nutritional therapy is overall health through good nutrition, maintenance of a normal glucose level, provision of adequate nutrients, and prevention of or slowing the progression of complications through glucose control. Nutritional recommendations must be highly individualized. Weight loss is usually helpful but difficult to achieve and maintain in obese type 2 adults. There are no longer specific recommendations for the percentage of calories from protein, carbohydrates, and fats, although it is generally agreed that saturated fats should constitute <10 percent of total calories. Protein restriction may be helpful in slowing the decline of the glomerular filtration rate in patients with established nephropathy but also may contribute to muscle weakness. Fiber intake of 20 to 35 g from a wide variety of food sources (same as for the general population) is recommended. There are no specific recommendations for sodium intake or alcohol. However, alcohol taken without food may lead to hypoglycemia.

Exercise

Exercise is beneficial in type 2 diabetes for promoting glycemic control and decreasing cardiovascular risk. Exercise also may benefit type 1 diabetics, but normal metabolic mechanisms of glucose regulation during exercise are lost in some type 1 diabetes. Excessive production of counterregulatory hormones may induce diabetic ketoacidosis, or, conversely, inadequate food intake in the face of insulin intake and exercise may precipitate hypoglycemia. General recommendations that may help type 1 diabetics include avoiding exercise if the fasting blood sugar is >250 mg/dL. However, carbohydrate should be ingested before exercise if the fasting glucose levels are <100 mg/dL. Type 1 diabetics should be aware of the signs and symptoms of hypoglycemia and have carbohydrate-based foods easily available for as-needed consumption during exercise. It is assumed that all diabetics will have a thorough medical evaluation before undertaking an exercise program. The evaluation should focus especially on cardiovascular risk.

Diabetics with neuropathy must take care not to suffer injuries caused by their inability to sense appropriate painful warning signals. Thus, in patients with loss of protective sensation, treadmills, prolonged walking, jogging, and step exercises are not recommended. Recommended exercises include swimming, cycling, rowing, chair and arm exercises, and other non–weight-bearing exercises. It is important for diabetics to wear properly fitting shoes and check their feet daily for evidence of blisters or infection. Diabetics should never go barefoot, especially if neuropathy is known to be present. In addition, diabetics with retinopathy are prone to retinal detachment and vitreous hemorrhage during strenuous exercise.

Self-Glucose Monitoring

Most patients with type 1 diabetes need to monitor their glucose three to four times daily. Type 2 diabetics on insulin or oral agents should also monitor their glucose, but the optimal frequency has not been established. The goals in both types are not only to maintain optimal whole blood glucose levels (80 to 120 preprandial) but also to prevent and/or detect hypoglycemia. The role of self-glucose monitoring has not been established in stable diet-controlled type 2 diabetics. Patient education about interpretation of the data is crucial if patients are to adjust their diet, exercise, and medication (insulin or oral) regimens on the basis of self-monitoring results. Newer, less painful (compared with fingerstick) methods of glucose self-monitoring may make this task less onerous and achieve more compliance.

Urine glucose testing at home is recommended only for patients who cannot or will not test their blood levels. The limitations of urine glucose testing were discussed above. Urine testing for ketones may, however, be useful in the prevention or early recognition of ketoacidosis. False-positive results may be obtained in patients taking captopril.

Pharmacologic Therapy

Insulin therapy is an absolute requirement for patients with type 1 diabetes and is often necessary in type 2 diabetics. Oral hypoglycemic agents often are used in type 2 diabetics but are *never* appropriate for type 1 diabetics because they work by increasing pancreatic insulin release, which is, of course, totally absent in type 1 patients. Oral hypoglycemic agents also are contraindicated in patients with gestational diabetes. The pregnant pancreas is already producing high levels of insulin, and tighter control with less risk of hypoglycemia is easier to manage in a pregnant patient using insulin than in one using the longer-acting oral agents. It is advisable to convert a type 2 diabetic on oral agents to insulin before conception and to maintain HBA_{1c} levels ≤7 percent.

Most type 1 patients require three to four doses of insulin daily. These doses usually are administered in combinations of an intermediate preparation and a short-acting preparation. Premixed 70/30 N/regular insulin is available but is appropriate only when the ratio has been established, not for initial therapy. Other insulins include 50/50 N/R, lente (intermediate duration of action), ultralente (long duration), Humalog, and 75/25 N/Humalog. Delivery systems include syringes, pumps, and premixed insulin injection pens (especially useful for those with limited vision).

There are now five classes of oral agents available in the United States.

Sulfonylurea drugs are the least expensive and are effective in lowering blood glucose levels. Their most important adverse effect is hypoglycemia, which is particularly significant with the longer-acting agents. Weight gain is a significant drawback to their use but is to be expected because the increased insulin levels they induce stimulate energy storage in adipose tissues. Clinical trials have not demonstrated the superiority of one sulfonylurea over another or of second- over first-generation agents. The most common older sulfonylurea still in use is chlorpropamide (Diabinese). A significant adverse effect with chlorpropamide is hyponatremia. Other first-generations agents include Tolinase and Orinase. Second-generation sulfonylureas include glipizide (Glucotrol)/glyburide (Micronase and DiaBeta), Prandin, Amaryl, and Glucotrol XL.

Metformin (Glucophage) enhances the sensitivity of muscle and liver to insulin, decreasing hepatic gluconeogenesis. It does not increase insulin secretion. It is as effective in reducing blood glucose as are the sulfonylureas but often promotes weight loss and thus may be preferred for initial therapy in obese type 2 diabetics. Metformin has a favorable effect on plasma lipids, lowering low-density lipoprotein (LDL) cholesterol, triglycerides, and free fatty acids. The most common adverse effects are gastrointestinal: abdominal discomfort and diarrhea. Hypoglycemia is rare because metformin does not increase insulin secretion. Unlike its predecessor, phenformin, metformin rarely causes lactic acidosis. The exception is patients with renal insufficiency, in whom metformin is contraindicated. Levels may rise extremely high because the drug is renally excreted. Other contraindications are hepatic failure, respiratory insufficiency/hypoxemia, severe infection, and alcohol abuse. Diabetic patients with symptomatic congestive heart failure may have sufficiently poor renal perfusion to cause metformin retention and thus toxicity. Especially in the elderly, it is advisable to measure creatinine clearance before starting metformin therapy. Diabetics on metformin should avoid radiocontrast dye. If a scan is absolutely necessary, it is best to discontinue the metformin the night before the procedure. After the scan, creatinine should be measured before restarting metformin to ensure that no renal insufficiency has developed.

Acarbose (Precose) and miglitol (Glyset) work by inhibiting small intestinal enzymes that metabolize sugars and starches, thus slowing their absorption. Therefore, they are most effective at decreasing postprandial hyperglycemia by allowing the pancreas more time to respond to a glucose load. Because of their mechanism of action, gastrointestinal adverse effects (e.g., bloating, diarrhea, flatulence) are the most common side effects. Although these drugs themselves do not cause hypoglycemia, they may slow recovery if oral carbohydrates other than glucose are given.

The thiazolidinediones (Actos, Avandia) enhance insulin sensitivity in liver, muscle, and adipose tissue. Their hypoglycemic effect is less than that of sulfonylureas or metformin, but a beneficial effect on plasma lipids often is seen. The thiazolidinediones may take some time to demonstrate their beneficial effect and therefore should not be discontinued before an adequate trial. They may be especially useful in insulin-resistant type 2 patients when used in combination therapy with other oral agents.

Repaglinide stimulates insulin secretion, and its effects (desired and adverse) are similar to those of the sulfonylureas. Repaglinide is given 15 min before meals; the onset of action is rapid, thus controlling postprandial hyperglycemia. This drug is shorter-acting, however, and there may be a lower incidence of hypoglycemia.

Most type 2 diabetics eventually will require combination therapy with two or more oral agents or with oral agents plus insulin. The first step usually is to add a second oral agent, as most patients understandably are reluctant to inject insulin. If this does not achieve glycemic control, either a third oral agent may be added or bedtime dosing of a long-acting type of insulin may be initiated. A mixed-split insulin regimen also may be tried.

COMPLICATIONS

Diabetes affects every organ system. It is the number one cause of blindness in the United States, although with proper eye care, this is often preventable. Diabetic retinopathy may take many forms: proliferative vascular disease, microaneurysms, retinal detachment, infarctions, and exudates. In addition, diabetics have higher rates of cataracts and glaucoma. Blurry vision often is due to acute hyperglycemia but should not be ignored because it may be a sign of a more serious condition. Glasses should not be prescribed routinely, however, until the blood sugar is brought down to normal. Diabetics must see an ophthalmologist at least yearly.

Diabetes is a major risk factor for accelerated atherosclerosis and thus ischemic heart disease and stroke. An important point to remember is that diabetes itself is a cause of endothelial dysfunction, and thus, any elevation of plasma lipids presents a greater risk of atherosclerosis. Any level of hypertension must be treated effectively. Diabetics may have silent ischemia as a result of neuropathy; thus, screening and prevention should be done even in the absence of symptoms. Any signs of ischemia must be addressed promptly.

Diabetes is a major cause of renal failure. The initial sign is microalbuminuria; thus, it is recommended to screen for this problem, which is not apparent on a simple dipstick for proteinuria. Angiotensin-converting enzyme (ACE) inhibitors have been shown to slow the progression of renal disease in patients with microalbuminuria and should be started even in nonhypertensive diabetics. The major contraindication is bilateral renal artery stenosis. In such patient, ACE inhibitors may precipitate acute renal failure. Radiocontrast agents should be avoided if at all possible in order to prevent acute renal failure, especially in patients taking metformin. This drug should be stopped the night before the procedure if the computed tomography (CT) scan is not an emergency procedure. If contrast agents are needed in a diabetic (whether or not the patient is taking metformin), the patient should be well hydrated before, during, and after the procedure.

Neuromuscular disorders in diabetics may take many forms. Autonomic neuropathy may cause gastroparesis with nausea and vomiting, intestinal motility disorders with diarrhea and/or constipation, vasomotor instability with orthostatic hypotension, bladder dysfunction (urinary retention or incontinence), and impotence. Peripheral neuropathy may cause pain, paresthesias, or numbness that can lead to unrecognized trauma, especially of the feet. The result may be prolonged infection and ulcerations with poor wound healing and the eventual need for amputation. Mononeuropathies may cause sensory and/or motor defects such as foot drop, wrist drop, and diplopia.

Skin disorders resulting from diabetes include infections, especially *Candida* vaginitis and balanitis; ulcers; dermopathy; and necrobiosis lipoidica diabeticorum. Type 1 diabetes may be associated with other autoimmune disorders, such as acanthosis nigricans and vitiligo.

Acute complications include ketoacidosis and hypoglycemia, which are discussed in Chapters 5-7 and 5-8, respectively. Infections are also potential severe acute complications. Malignant *Pseudomonas* otitis externa may spread to infect the sinuses and brain. Rhinocerebral mucormycosis may be fatal, beginning with a headache and nasal drainage and ending with coma and death. Other important but less common infections include emphysematous cholecystitis, necrotizing fasciitis, and chronic osteomyelitis.

PEARLS

An important point to remember in caring for diabetic patients is that this disease is more than just hyperglycemia. Normalizing hyperglycemia is crucial but not sufficient. The patient and family need ongoing education and support. The caregiver must be vigilant for complications to provide early diagnosis and treatment and thus prevent more serious complications. A team management approach is best. This disease can have a major lifestyle impact on patients, and the primary care provider should work with a team that includes nurses, social workers, nutritionists, psychologists, and others as needed to prevent morbidity and mortality.

BIBLIOGRAPHY

An excellent reference for more in-depth information is the Clinical Practice Recommendations (updated yearly) published by the American Diabetes Association (ADA) in a supplement to its journal *Diabetes Care*. The full text is available on-line on the ADA Web site at www.diabetes.org.

DeFronzo R: Pharmacologic therapy for type 2 diabetes mellitus. *Ann Intern Med* 131:281–303, 1999.

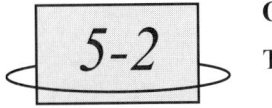

5-2

OSTEOPOROSIS
Timothy C. Evans

DISCUSSION

Osteoporosis is a metabolic disease of bone that is characterized by decreased bone mass; that is, both the mineral component and the organic matrix of bone are decreased. This is in contrast to osteomalacia, in which only mineralization is impaired.

Osteoporosis is a major source of morbidity and mortality. Each year in the United States, osteoporosis results in hundreds of thousands of fractures that have enormous personal and financial costs. The risk of death in the elderly from complications after a hip fracture is 12 to 20 percent.

BONE PHYSIOLOGY

Throughout life, bone is formed and resorbed continuously in a finely regulated process known as *remodeling*. The first step in the process is resorption by cells called *osteoclasts,* which form erosion cavities in bone. Next, *osteoblasts* migrate into the erosion cavities and resynthesize the protein matrix of bone. The matrix is composed primarily of collagen with a number of additional minor protein constituents, most notably osteocalcin. Mineralization of the matrix with a salt of calcium and phosphate called hydroxyapatite occurs over the next several weeks.

The processes of bone formation and resorption are coupled so that neither proceeds without the other. During childhood and adolescence, however, formation is faster than resorption, and so bone density

increases. During the early adult years, bone density is relatively stable. Peak bone density is reached at about age 30 to 35. Thereafter, resorption is faster than formation, and so bone density gradually decreases throughout the rest of life.

Osteoporosis is a clinical disorder in which bone density falls below a threshold at which susceptibility to fracturing increases. An age-related decrease in bone density occurs in all men and women. In women, there is superimposed a period of more rapid loss of bone density for several years around the time of menopause that results from estrogen deficiency. This and the fact that peak bone density is 10 to 15 percent lower in women than in men account for the greater fracture rate from osteoporosis in women.

Although none are completely predictive of symptomatic disease, the factors that have been associated with an increased risk of osteoporosis include female sex, white ancestry, early menopause in women or hypogonadism in men, inactivity, low body weight, low calcium intake during the first 3 decades of life and again after age 60, smoking, and excessive alcohol intake.

CLASSIFICATION

Primary Osteoporosis

Primary osteoporosis is a condition of reduced bone mass and fractures that occurs in postmenopausal women (postmenopausal osteoporosis) and the elderly of both sexes (senile osteoporosis). Two subcategories have been suggested. Type 1 refers to the loss of trabecular bone that occurs in postmenopausal women and frequently is associated with vertebral compression fractures and fractures of the distal wrist. Type 2 refers to the age-related loss of cortical and trabecular bone that occurs in both men and women and is associated with hip fractures. Fractures related to type 1 osteoporosis typically begin to occur in women within about 10 years after menopause, while fractures from type 2 begin about 10 years later.

Secondary Osteoporosis

Secondary osteoporosis refers to decreased bone density resulting from other clinical conditions that affect bone remodeling. Glucocorticoid excess causes increased bone resorption and decreased formation. This deleterious effect may result from endogenous Cushing's syndrome or glucocorticoid administration. Thyrotoxicosis, either endogenous or iatrogenic, causes increased bone resorption. Decreased bone density is a predictable result of long-standing hyperparathyroidism. Certain drugs, such as chronic heparin and anticonvulsants, are associated with osteoporosis. Several malignancies, notably multiple myeloma, may cause diffuse bone density loss.

CLINICAL PRESENTATION

Osteoporosis is asymptomatic, but pain results from its major clinical sequelae: fractures. The fractures most commonly associated with osteoporosis are vertebral compression fractures (primarily of the upper lumbar spine and the middle to lower thoracic spine), Colles' fractures of the distal radius, and fractures of the femoral neck. However, patients with osteoporosis are at increased risk for fractures of all types. Multiple anterior vertebral compression fractures result in the characteristic spine deformity of increased dorsal kyphosis and cervical lordosis known as dowager's hump.

Clinical laboratory tests are typically normal, including calcium, phosphate, and parathyroid hormone. Alkaline phosphatase is usually normal but may be somewhat elevated after a fracture. Abnormalities of blood counts, chemistries, or urine may suggest another underlying disease and should be pursued.

Standard x-rays demonstrate fractures but are insensitive in detecting the loss of bone density (see the material on bone densitometry below).

DIAGNOSIS

In patients with fractures in a typical setting, osteopenia on x-ray, and no other cause of fracture or loss of bone density, the diagnosis of osteoporosis is likely. Establishing bone density loss, however, requires a bone density measurement.

Several techniques are available for bone densitometry, including single- and dual-photon absorptiometry, quantitative computed tomography (CT) scanning, and dual energy x-ray absorptiometry (DEXA). Among these techniques, DEXA is preferred because of its greater precision and lower radiation dose. Bone density determined by DEXA correlates well with the risk of future fractures.

Follow-up and monitoring of osteoporosis are largely clinical, although DEXA performed every 1 to 2 years can show the progression of bone density loss. Several tests are available to measure the rate of bone turnover, including markers of bone resorption such as urinary hydroxyproline and the newer, more specific urinary assays of bone collagen fragments released during resorption. Biochemical serum markers of bone formation include bone-specific alkaline phosphatase and osteocalcin. These indexes of bone turnover are being studied for their potential use in identifying patients at risk for osteoporosis and for monitoring treatment, but there has been insufficient validation of their utility to recommend their routine use.

PREVENTION

Bone density decreases continuously after about age 40. Since most bone density, once lost, cannot be regained, prevention of osteoporosis is much more likely to have a satisfactory clinical result than are attempts to treat established osteoporosis. Prevention begins early in life, when adequate calcium in the diet during the first 3 decades is associated with greater peak bone density and therefore a longer interval of loss later in life before the fracture threshold is reached. This is particularly true for girls, who on average consume significantly less calcium than do boys beginning at puberty. Adequate calcium intake also is particularly important at ages 50 to 60 and should continue thereafter. In general, daily calcium intake for adolescents and adults should be 1200 to 1500 mg.

Regular exercise and the avoidance of smoking and excessive alcohol intake also contribute to maximizing peak bone mass and minimizing the rate of loss in later years.

Among the preventive measures for osteoporosis, none is more effective and applicable to the population at greatest risk than the treatment of hypogonadism in either sex, although numerically this applies mostly to women. Estrogen replacement should be offered to all patients with premature menopause to prevent osteoporosis unless there are contraindications. Similarly, estrogen replacement after natural menopause has been well established in preventing rapid bone loss and decreasing the fracture rate. Estrogen is most effective when used at the time of menopause and the following few years of accelerated bone loss. Since bone loss rapidly resumes when estrogens are discontinued, they should be continued for the long term. When estrogen is given to a woman with an intact uterus, a cyclic or continuous progestogen also should be given to prevent endometrial cancer.

TREATMENT

Once a fracture has occurred, osteoporosis is said to be "established." Several therapies are available for these patients. Intense research efforts are under way to develop this area of pharmacotherapeutics. In all these patients, pain control, avoidance of immobility as much as possible, and safety in ambulation (particularly important in frail elderly persons) should be attended to.

Drug therapy is directed at decreasing bone resorption and increasing bone formation.

Antiresorptive Agents

CALCIUM Dietary calcium supplementation should be provided to ensure 1200 to 1500 mg of elemental calcium intake per day. Several preparations of calcium salts are available. Calcium carbonate is well tolerated and inexpensive.

VITAMIN D The recommended daily allowance of vitamin D of 400 units should be increased to 800 to 1000 units, especially in patients who have limited sun exposure. Calcitriol (active vitamin D, 1,25-dihydroxyvitamin D) also can be used but usually is not necessary and increases the risk of hypercalcemia.

ESTROGEN Estrogen slows the rate of bone resorption, slows bone density loss, and prevents fractures. Conjugated equine estrogen at a dose of 0.625 mg per day or its equivalent provides the beneficial effect on bone. Both oral estrogen and transdermal estrogen are effective. When a patient has an intact uterus, a cyclic or continuous progestogen (for example, medroxyprogesterone 2.5 mg per day) also should be given to prevent endometrial cancer. Selective estrogen receptor modulators (SERMs) have been developed and have beneficial effects on bone density without some of the harmful side effects of estrogen. Ongoing trials are comparing SERMs with estrogen in regard to both benefits, including fracture prevention, and side effects.

CALCITONIN Calcitonin inhibits bone resorption by osteoclasts and has an additional beneficial analgesic effect. It appears to be particularly useful in patients with high-turnover osteoporosis: high urinary hydroxyproline and serum osteocalcin. Both salmon calcitonin and human calcitonin are available, and there is less immunologic resistance to the latter. Although effective, calcitonin is expensive and until recently was administered by subcutaneous injection. An intranasal spray is now available.

BISPHOSPHONATES Bisphosphonates bind to bone mineral, slow osteoclast-mediated resorption, and decrease fracture rates. Several agents have been developed for clinical use in osteoporosis. Newer agents do not impair bone mineralization as did earlier bisphosphonates. Intense clinical research efforts will further define the place of these agents in the prevention and treatment of osteoporosis as adjuncts to and a replacement for estrogen.

Bone-Forming Agents

ANDROGEN Testosterone deficiency in men is a definite cause of osteoporosis and should be treated unless there are contraindications such as prostate cancer. Testosterone treatment increases bone mass, probably by stimulating bone formation. Treatment is with a long-acting testosterone ester (testosterone cypionate or enanthate) 200 mg intramuscularly every 2 weeks. Testosterone also increases bone mass in women, but the virilizing side effects are not acceptable. However, studies are evaluating the potential use in women of testosterone analogues that have less of a virilizing effect while retaining the androgenic effect on bone.

FLUORIDE Fluoride has been known for years to increase bone mass. It has been shown, however, that the increased mass is not associated with decreased fractures and in fact may result in an increased fracture potential, presumably because of an abnormal structure of the bone mineral. Thus, fluoride is not recommended for routine use, but study of its effects continues because it is one of the few agents that increase bone formation.

BIBLIOGRAPHY

Andrews WC: What's new in preventing and treating osteoporosis? *Postgrad Med* 104:89–92, 95–97, 1998.

Fauci AS, Braunwald E, Isselbacher KJ, et al (eds): *Harrison's Principles of Internal Medicine,* 14th ed. New York, McGraw-Hill, 1998.

Liggett NW, Reid DM: Osteoporosis and its management. *Hosp Med* 60:238–242, 1999.

Meunier PJ, Delmas PD, Eastell R, et al: Diagnosis and management of osteoporosis in postmenopausal women: Clinical guidelines: International Committee for Osteoporosis Clinical Guidelines. *Clin Ther* 21:1025–1044, 1999.

Miller PD: Management of osteoporosis. *Adv Intern Med* 44:175–207, 1999.

Miller PD: Management of osteoporosis. *Dis Month* 45:21–54, 1999.

Tierney LM Jr, McPhee SJ, Papadakis MA (eds): *Current Medical Diagnosis and Treatment,* 39th ed. New York, McGraw-Hill, 2000.

Ullom-Minnich P: Prevention of osteoporosis and fractures. *Am Fam Physician* 60:194–202, 1999.

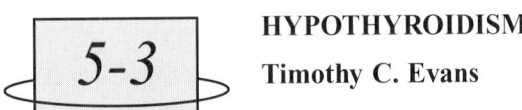

HYPOTHYROIDISM

Timothy C. Evans

DISCUSSION

Thyroid hormone is required by virtually every cell in the body for normal function. It has effects on multiple metabolic processes, including the production and metabolism of other hormones. Thyroid disease may be manifested by low levels of free thyroid hormone (hypothyroidism), increased free thyroid hormone (hyperthyroidism or thyrotoxicosis), or thyroid gland enlargement (goiter; the enlargement of an isolated portion of thyroid tissue is referred to more commonly as a nodule).

There are two forms of thyroid hormone: thyroxine (T_4) and triiodothyronine (T_3). The active form of the hormone is T_3, which contains three iodines and results from monodeiodination of T_4. The conversion of T_4 to T_3 takes place partly in the thyroid gland but primarily in peripheral tissues such as the liver. The thyroid hormones circulate in the blood bound tightly to serum proteins, particularly thyroid-binding globulin (TBG). Much less than 1 percent of the total thyroid hormone is free and available to interact with target cells. Thus, standard measurements of total T_4 and T_3 give an incomplete picture of the thyroid state. Additional tests are used to estimate or measure the amount of free hormone.

Thyroid hormone is secreted by the thyroid gland in response to thyroid-stimulating hormone (TSH) from the pituitary. TSH secretion by the pituitary in turn is stimulated by thyrotropin-releasing hormone from the hypothalamus. The secretory activity of both the pituitary and the hypothalamus is controlled by feedback inhibitory effects of free thyroid hormone in the blood such that increased free thyroid hormone results in decreased pituitary secretion of TSH and decreased free thyroid hormone results in increased TSH secretion.

LABORATORY EVALUATION OF THE THYROID

Thyroid Hormone

Both T_4 and T_3 can be measured accurately by radioimmunoassay. It is important to remember, however, that in each case it is the total circulating hormone concentration that is measured, not the free hormone level, which is the physiologically important fraction. Other tests, therefore, are needed to determine accurately the appropriateness of levels of circulating thyroid hormone. The actual free T_4 or free T_3 can be measured, and this is becoming more readily available in many clinical laboratories.

T_3 Resin Uptake (T_3 Uptake)

In this test, radioactive T_3 is added to the patient's serum to determine the amount of serum protein binding of thyroid hormone. The result, the T_3RU or T_3U, is multiplied by the total T_4 (or T_3) to derive a calculated free T_4 (or T_3) index (FTI), an estimate of the free thyroid hormone.

Thyroid-Stimulating Hormone

TSH assays have been available for some time, and their sensitivity has increased to the point where so-called third-generation assays can accurately distinguish not only between elevated and normal TSH but also between suppressed and normal TSH levels. Since the hypothalamus and the pituitary, like other tissues, respond to free thyroid hormone, TSH is the single most useful thyroid function test. Sensitive assays of TSH have proved invaluable in assessing free thyroid hormone status. An important exception is a patient with hypopituitarism, in whom pituitary function, including TSH secretion, is deficient.

Antithyroid Antibodies

Autoimmune thyroid disease is common, and it is occasionally useful to measure levels of marker antibodies such as antimicrosomal and antithyroglobulin antibodies. Antibodies directed against the thyroid also can cause thyroid disease, as occurs with the thyroid-stimulating antibody of Graves' disease, which is directed against and activates the TSH receptor, resulting in hyperthyroidism. Measurement of this antibody is occasionally useful in Graves' disease patients when the diagnosis is in doubt and in pregnant women when radioiodine uptake and scan cannot be used to diagnose this disease.

Ultrasound

Ultrasound can be useful to define thyroid size and anatomy, determine whether a nodule is solid or cystic, or occasionally guide a needle biopsy of a thyroid nodule.

Radioiodine Uptake and Scan

A tracer dose of radioactive iodine will localize in the thyroid gland within hours of administration. The percentage of the administered radioactivity—the radioiodine uptake—that is detected in the thyroid gives an indication of the relative hormone-producing activity of the gland. Scanning the thyroid to determine the pattern of distribution of radioactivity within the thyroid helps determine whether abnormal function is localized or involves the entire gland.

HYPOTHYROIDISM

Causes of Hypothyroidism

PRIMARY

Autoimmune Thyroiditis   Also called Hashimoto's thyroiditis or lymphocytic thyroiditis, autoimmune thyroiditis results from cell-mediated autoimmune damage of the thyroid and is the most common cause of hypothyroidism. Like other thyroid diseases, it is more common in women than in men and may be associated with other autoimmune diseases. The thyroid is typically modestly enlarged and somewhat firm. Antimicrosomal and antithyroglobulin antibodies are elevated.

Postablative Hypothyroidism   Surgical or radioiodine ablation of the thyroid may result in hypothyroidism, depending on the amount of the gland that is removed or the dose of radioiodine that is administered.

Subclinical Hypothyroidism   Subclinical hypothyroidism is defined as a normal thyroid hormone level in association with increased TSH. Some but not all cases progress to definite hypothyroidism. The degree of TSH elevation is useful in determining the likelihood of progression and the indication for thyroid hormone replacement therapy. In general, subclinical hypothyroidism with TSH higher than 10 mU/L should be treated.

Drug-Induced Hypothyroidism   A number of drugs can interfere with thyroid hormone synthesis or secretion, including high doses of iodine, the iodine-containing antiarrhythmic agent amiodarone, and lithium.

Transient Hypothyroidism   Hypothyroidism lasting for weeks to months and often preceded by a period of hyperthyroidism occurs commonly during the recovery phase of subacute thyroiditis and after about 5 percent of normal pregnancies.

Iodine Deficiency   Hypothyroidism resulting from deficient dietary iodine content is rare in the United States but occurs in isolated inland parts of the world. The chronic underproduction of thyroid hormone results in long-standing TSH excess and often dramatically enlarged thyroid glands, or endemic goiters.

SECONDARY   Hypothyroidism secondary to pituitary or hypothalamic dysfunction is unusual. The deficiency in TSH production may be isolated or may be associated with other pituitary hormone deficiencies.

Clinical Presentation

The most severe forms of hypothyroidism are unusual today. Congenital hypothyroidism (cretinism) is associated with severe mental and motor retardation. In adults, myxedema can progress to include respiratory depression and coma.

More commonly, however, hypothyroidism presents insidiously with nonspecific symptoms such as fatigue and constipation that easily may be overlooked or ascribed to other causes. Characteristic symptoms and signs of hypothyroidism may be absent or may be apparent only after careful reexamination of the patient.

The most common symptoms include fatigue, constipation, cold intolerance, mild weight gain, myalgias and arthralgias, dry skin, dry or brittle hair, menorrhagia, and hoarseness. Intellectual vigor decreases. Carpal tunnel syndrome, obstructive sleep apnea, and pericardial effusions are more common in hypothyroidism.

On physical examination, the patient may appear lethargic with dry skin, nonlustrous hair, and hoarseness. The face may appear puffy, and the lateral half of the eyebrows thin. Mild diastolic hypertension may be present. A delay in the relaxation phase of the deep tendon reflexes is characteristic. Depending on the etiology, the thyroid itself may be nonpalpable or enlarged.

Laboratory Diagnosis

The diagnosis depends on demonstrating low circulating levels of thyroid hormone. Either free T_4 or total FTI, calculated from T_4 along with a T_3RU, should be measured. TSH also should be measured; except for secondary hypothyroidism, this is the most sensitive test for hypothyroidism. Once primary hypothyroidism is established, only TSH is needed to follow the course of the hypothyroidism and its treatment. Serum T_3 is not helpful in the diagnosis of hypothyroidism.

Other laboratory abnormalities include anemia and increased serum cholesterol, creatine kinase, and prolactin.

Treatment

The treatment of hypothyroidism consists of replacement with thyroid hormone. Since the half-life of T_3 is short, replacement is much easier and safer with T_4 (levothyroxine). Administered T_4 is converted naturally in the body to the active form of the hormone, T_3. With few exceptions, therefore, the treatment of hypothyroidism is done with pure synthetic levothyroxine. The average replacement dose for patients with hypothyroidism is 0.1 to 0.125 mg per day given as a single daily dose.

Care should be taken in beginning replacement therapy, especially in frail, elderly patients and those with ischemic heart disease, since thyroid hormone is a cardiac stimulant. In these patients, the starting levothyroxine dose should be 0.0125 to 0.025 mg per day and should be increased slowly over weeks or months. In patients with active ischemic heart disease, treatment of hypothyroidism should be delayed until the coronary occlusive disease has been addressed definitively.

The replacement dose is monitored by following the TSH level. In this way, the pituitary serves as an internal bioassay for the free thyroid hormone level. After starting or changing the dosage level, a 6-week interval should pass before a repeat TSH measurement is done, since it takes time for pituitary TSH production to reach a new steady state. In general, the goal is to normalize but not suppress TSH.

THYROIDITIS

Inflammation of the thyroid occurs in several different settings. All can be associated with hypothyroidism, but none are necessarily associated.

Autoimmune Thyroiditis

As was noted previously, autoimmune thyroiditis, or Hashimoto's thyroiditis, is a result of cell-mediated immune inflammation of the thyroid. Histologic examination of the thyroid shows lymphocytic infiltration. However, the degree of thyroid destruction may not necessarily be sufficient to cause hypothyroidism. If the patient has significant thyroid enlargement or is troubled by the goiter, levothyroxine replacement may be instituted in a euthyroid patient to prevent thyroid growth.

Subacute Thyroiditis

Subacute thyroiditis is a probable viral inflammation of the thyroid associated with fever, myalgias, and a tender enlarged thyroid. The disease is self-limiting but may be associated with thyrotoxicosis in the early stages as a result of leakage of stored thyroid hormone from the inflamed gland and a more prolonged hypothyroid phase that lasts several months during a later phase of recovery. The symptoms of acute thyroid inflammation usually respond to aspirin or nonsteroidal anti-inflammatory drugs. When it occurs, hypothyroidism should be treated, but since the gland usually reverts to normal function eventually, the replacement levothyroxine should be discontinued and TSH should be rechecked after 6 to 12 months of treatment.

Postpartum Thyroiditis

Thyroid dysfunction occurs after about 5 percent of pregnancies. Most patients with this complication have underlying autoimmune thyroiditis. It typically presents with an early mild hyperthyroid phase followed by a more prolonged hypothyroid phase. When hypothyroidism occurs, it should be treated with levothyroxine replacement to normalize TSH. In most patients, the hypothyroidism resolves after 6 to 12 months, but these patients are at risk for the same sequence after subsequent pregnancies.

BIBLIOGRAPHY

Adlin V: Subclinical hypothyroidism: Deciding when to treat. *Am Fam Physician* 57:776–780, 1998.

Benediktsson R, Toft AD: Management of the unexpected result: Compensated hypothyroidism. *Postgrad Med J* 74:729–732, 1998.

Drake WM, Wood DF: Thyroid disease in pregnancy. *Postgrad Med J* 74:583–586, 1998.

Fauci AS, Braunwald E, Isselbacher KJ, et al (eds): *Harrison's Principles of Internal Medicine*, 14th ed. New York, McGraw-Hill, 1998.

Mulder JE: Thyroid disease in women. *Med Clin North Am* 82:103–125, 1998.

Tierney LM Jr, McPhee SJ, Papadakis MA (eds): *Current Medical Diagnosis and Treatment*, 39th ed. New York, McGraw-Hill, 2000.

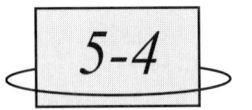

HYPERTHYROIDISM
Timothy C. Evans

DISCUSSION

Thyrotoxicosis is the term applied to any condition in which serum levels of the thyroid hormones thyroxine (T_4) and triiodothyronine (T_3) are excessive. This term often is used interchangeably with *hyperthyroidism,* but strictly speaking, hyperthyroidism applies only to cases in which the excess thyroid hormone comes from the patient's thyroid gland. In almost all forms of thyrotoxicosis, the pituitary secretion of thyroid-stimulating hormone (TSH) is suppressed through feedback inhibition of the pituitary by the increased levels of thyroid hormone.

CAUSES OF THYROTOXICOSIS

The causes of thyrotoxicosis can be subdivided in several ways. A useful distinction can be made by considering the intrinsic activity of the thyroid as shown by the radioiodine uptake (RAIU). In this test, a tracer dose of radioactive iodine is administered to the patient and the radioactivity accumulated in the thyroid is counted 2 to 24 h later. A gland that is metabolically active, producing increased amounts of thyroid hormone, has an increased uptake. When the gland is not actively producing excess hormone, the uptake is low. In cases in which RAIU is increased, a next useful step is to scan the thyroid to demonstrate the pattern of distribution of radioactivity within the gland.

High Radioiodine Uptake

In these diseases, the thyroid is overactive, synthesizing and releasing increased amounts of thyroid hormone. The thyroid activity is autonomous of normal control mechanisms or is stimulated by abnormal activators because pituitary secretion of TSH is appropriately low.

GRAVES' DISEASE By far the most common cause of thyrotoxicosis, Graves' disease is much more common in women than in men. It can be seen at any age but occurs most frequently in the early to midadult years. It is an autoimmune disease and is associated with antimicrosomal and antithyroglobulin antibodies (see Chap. 5-3). It is caused, however, by a unique autoantibody directed against the TSH receptor. When bound to the receptor, this antibody stimulates the thyroid cell just as TSH does when bound to the receptor. The result is diffuse overactivity of the thyroid despite very low levels of TSH. The radioiodine scan shows diffuse increased uptake throughout the gland. There is a familial tendency in Graves's disease, and this disease is associated with an increased incidence of other autoimmune diseases, such as pernicious anemia and myasthenia gravis.

In addition to overactivity of the thyroid gland, Graves' disease is associated with two important clinical manifestations: infiltration of the tissues around the eyes (exophthalmos) and less frequently infiltration of the skin (pretibial myxedema). These manifestations can occur with or without hyperthyroidism and may have a different clinical course than does the thyroid overactivity.

TOXIC MULTINODULAR GOITER Autonomy occasionally develops in long-standing multinodular goiters, with increased thyroid hormone production independent of TSH stimulation. The cause is not understood, but there is no stimulating antibody as there is in Graves' disease. Toxic multinodular goiter occurs primarily in elderly patients. It is not accompanied by eye or skin infiltrative disease and is not associated with other autoimmune phenomena. The thyrotoxicosis is usually not as severe as it is in Graves' disease. The radioiodine scan pattern is patchy, with increased uptake throughout the gland.

AUTONOMOUS THYROID NODULE Also known as a "hot nodule" from its radioiodine scan pattern of a single area of increased uptake surrounded by inactive thyroid tissue, an autonomous thyroid nodule is a variant of toxic multinodular goiter.

Low Radioiodine Uptake

In these cases of thyrotoxicosis, the elevated thyroid hormone levels are not a consequence of increased metabolic synthetic activity of the thyroid. Unlike high-RAIU causes of thyrotoxicosis, these forms of thyrotoxicosis are distinguished by a lack of intrinsic thyroid overactivity, the RAIU is low, and scanning is moot. Since thyroid hormone is increased, however, pituitary TSH secretion is suppressed as it is in high-RAIU thyrotoxicosis.

THYROIDITIS The thyroid contains a large amount of preformed thyroid hormone stored in the colloid space as part of thyroglobulin. In the case of thyroiditis, inflammation in the thyroid gland results in the release of the stored hormone. This occurs most strikingly in the early phase of inflammation of subacute thyroiditis. Mild thyrotoxicosis also occurs occasionally during the course of Hashimoto's thyroiditis, so-called Hashitoxicosis. This occurs commonly after pregnancy and is known as postpartum thyroiditis.

EXOGENOUS THYROID HORMONE The administration of inappropriately large doses of thyroid hormone also causes low-RAIU thyrotoxicosis. This may result from misunderstanding by the patient, failure of the prescriber to adjust the thyroid hormone dose on the basis of the TSH, or occasionally intentional excess dosing by the patient.

Unusual Causes of Thyrotoxicosis

Thyroid tissue contained in ovarian dermoid tumors can function autonomously or in concert with Graves' disease. TSH-secreting pituitary tumors occur rarely and are the only cause of normal or high TSH in association with thyrotoxicosis. High levels of human chorionic gonadotropin (hCG), as are seen in patients with trophoblastic tumors or pregnancy, can cause hyperthyroidism, since hCG is similar in structure to TSH. High levels of iodine, as is seen in patients taking drugs such as amiodarone and iodine-containing radiographic contrast media, can cause hyperthyroidism or hypothyroidism (see Chap. 5-3).

CLINICAL PRESENTATION

Thyrotoxicosis of any cause may cause nervousness, emotional lability, fatigue, heat intolerance, frequent bowel movements, weight loss despite a good appetite, sweating, menstrual irregularities, proximal muscle weakness, dyspnea, and palpitations. The physical findings include stare and lid lag, fine tremor, warm moist skin, tachycardia or atrial fibrillation, and, when thyrotoxicosis is present chronically, osteoporosis. The thyroid gland may or may not be enlarged, depending on the etiology of the thyrotoxicosis; if it is enlarged, it may be either nodular or diffusely enlarged.

Graves' disease has additional specific physical findings. The thyroid gland in patients with Graves' disease is diffusely enlarged and may be so metabolically active that a bruit is heard on thyroid auscultation. In addition to the stare and lid lag of thyrotoxicosis, Graves' ophthalmopathy occurs in 20 to 40 percent of these patients. This may include chemosis, proptosis, and impaired movements of extraocular muscles. When it is severe, exophthalmos can damage vision. Pretibial myxedema occurs in only a small percent of Graves' disease patients and usually is characterized by raised, thickened lesions on the anterior shins.

Occasionally in the elderly, thyrotoxicosis is asymptomatic (so-called apathetic hyperthyroidism) or presents only with atrial fibrillation.

Thyroid storm is an unusual but life-threatening complication of hyperthyroidism that is marked by high fever, tachycardia, vomiting, diarrhea, dehydration, and delirium. The mortality rate is high. It can be precipitated by surgery, a severe medical illness, or radioiodine treatment.

DIAGNOSIS

A number of tests are available to assess thyroid function and anatomy (see Chap. 5-3). The characteristic laboratory abnormalities include increased T_4 and T_3. Since increased serum protein binding [as is seen commonly with estrogen therapy, which increases thyroid-binding globulin (TBG)] results in increased total circulating thyroid hormone but normal free thyroid hormone, it is important to assess the protein binding with a T_3 resin uptake in order to calculate the free thyroid index or measure free T_4 and T_3 directly. T_3 is a more sensitive indicator of hyperthyroidism than is T_4. Occasionally in patients with mild hyperthyroidism, only T_3 is elevated; this is known as T_3 toxicosis. TSH is decreased in all forms of thyrotoxicosis except the rare circumstance of a pituitary tumor that overproduces TSH.

As was noted above, the RAIU and scan can be helpful in distinguishing between the various causes of thyrotoxicosis.

The level of thyroid-stimulating antibody in Graves' disease can be measured, but this is infrequently necessary or helpful except for diagnostic purposes in cases where Graves' eye or skin disease is present without thyrotoxicosis and in Graves' disease during pregnancy. The thyroid-stimulating antibody does cross the placenta and, when present in a significant amount in maternal blood, is predictive of transient neonatal thyrotoxicosis in the newborn.

TREATMENT

The treatment of thyrotoxicosis is based on RAIU. Diseases characterized by increased RAIU respond to antithyroid drugs and radioiodine ablation. Diseases with low RAIU do not.

Treatment Modalities

ANTITHYROID DRUGS The thiourea drugs methimazole and propylthiouracil (PTU) inhibit thyroid hormone synthesis by the thyroid gland. Methimazole is more convenient since it can be taken once a day, but PTU inhibits extrathyroidal conversion of T_4 to T_3 and thus may be somewhat more effective in patients with marked hyperthyroidism. Each medication has side effects, including rashes and hepatitis. The most dangerous side effect is agranulocytosis, which usually resolves when the drug is discontinued. Patients should be advised to watch for fever, other signs of infection, and oral ulcers. Methimazole has been reported to cause the scalp abnormality aplasia cutis in newborns, and so hyperthyroidism in pregnant women is treated with PTU.

RADIOACTIVE IODINE High-RAIU forms of thyrotoxicosis can be treated with doses of radioiodine sufficient to decrease thyroid activity and eliminate excess thyroid hormone production. It typically takes several months after the dose of radioiodine for the thyroid to slow to a new, lower steady state of activity. During the transition period,

antithyroid drugs are continued and the dose is tapered as the thyroid overactivity resolves. A period of pretreatment with antithyroid drugs is also wise in elderly or medically frail patients and those with very overactive thyroids to deplete the gland of stored thyroid hormone before the radioactive damage is inflicted.

THYROID SURGERY Surgery for hyperthyroidism is unusual but occasionally is performed for very large thyroid glands or in the second trimester of pregnancy, when Graves' disease cannot be controlled medically. Pretreatment with antithyroid drugs decreases the chance of thyroid storm.

PROPRANOLOL Propranolol is the beta-adrenergic blocking agent of choice to alleviate the symptoms of tachycardia, nervousness, and sweating. Propranolol does not affect the thyroid itself and can be discontinued when the thyroid overactivity is brought under control. It does decrease peripheral conversion of T_4 to T_3, which is beneficial in the early treatment of symptomatic thyrotoxicosis.

High-RAIU Thyrotoxicosis

Graves' disease usually is treated initially with antithyroid drugs and propranolol if necessary. In young patients with small, modestly overactive glands, there is a significant chance of remission if antithyroid drug suppression is continued for a year and then discontinued. The rate of remission may be increased by adding replacement levothyroxine to the methimazole. Most other patients, as well as those in whom remission is not achieved, are treated with radioiodine ablation. After ablation, some patients become hypothyroid and require thyroid hormone replacement. Over the course of the succeeding years, additional patients eventually become hypothyroid. Long-term follow-up should monitor for this outcome.

Neither multinodular goiter nor toxic adenoma remits with antithyroid drugs. Therefore, after antithyroid drug pretreatment, definitive treatment with radioiodine ablation usually is carried out.

Low-RAIU Thyrotoxicosis

Adrenergic symptoms of thyrotoxicosis can be relieved with propranolol. The hyperthyroidism of thyroiditis is self-limiting and resolves when thyroid inflammation resolves and the store of thyroid hormone in the gland is depleted. No other treatment of the hyperthyroidism is necessary or effective.

In patients overtreated with levothyroxine, the daily dose should be decreased. The patient is followed to determine the dose that normalizes the serum TSH.

BIBLIOGRAPHY

Baker JR Jr: Autoimmune endocrine disease. *JAMA* 278:1931–1937, 1997.
Dabon-Almirante CL, Surks MI: Clinical and laboratory diagnosis of thyrotoxicosis. *Endocrinol Metab Clin North Am* 27:25–35, 1998.
Fauci AS, Braunwald E, Isselbacher KJ, et al (eds): *Harrison's Principles of Internal Medicine,* 14th ed. New York, McGraw-Hill, 1998.
Felz MW, Stein PP: The many "faces" of Graves' disease: Part 1. Eyes, pulse, skin, and neck provide important clues to diagnosis. *Postgrad Med* 106:57–64, 1999.
Felz MW, Stein PP: The many "faces" of Graves' disease: Part 2. Practical diagnostic testing and management options. *Postgrad Med* 106:45–52, 1999.
Haddad G: Is it hyperthyroidism? You can't always tell from the clinical picture. *Postgrad Med* 104:42–44, 53–55, 59, 1998.
Marqusee E, Haden ST, Utiger RD. Subclinical thyrotoxicosis. *Endocrinol Metab Clin North Am* 27:37–49, 1998.
McIver B, Morris JC: The pathogenesis of Graves' disease. *Endocrinol Metab Clin North Am* 27:73–89, 1998.
Mulder JE: Thyroid disease in women. *Med Clin North Am* 82:103–125, 1998.
Tierney LM Jr, McPhee SJ, Papadakis MA (eds): *Current Medical Diagnosis and Treatment,* 39th ed. New York, McGraw-Hill, 2000.

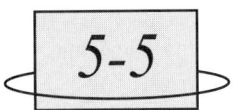

ADRENAL DISORDERS
Timothy C. Evans

DISCUSSION

The adrenal glands are adjacent to the kidneys and are composed of two distinct types of hormone-secreting tissue: the cortex on the outside and the medulla in the center of each gland. The cortex secretes three classes of steroid hormones: glucocorticoids, mineralocorticoids, and androgens. The medulla secretes catecholamines. Diseases of the adrenal generally are suspected because of clinical evidence of a deficiency or excess of these hormones. On other occasions, adrenal masses are found incidentally on abdominal imaging studies performed for unrelated reasons.

ADRENAL CORTEX

Glucocorticoids

The primary glucocorticoid secreted by the adrenal cortex is cortisol. The stimulus for cortisol secretion is adrenocorticotropic hormone (ACTH) from the anterior pituitary. Cortisol is secreted in a diurnal pattern, with the highest levels occurring on awakening and the lowest at bedtime. Physiologic levels of cortisol have modulatory effects on intermediary metabolism, vascular tone, water balance, and inflammation. Cortisol opposes the action of insulin and is secreted briskly in response to stress, both physiologic and psychological.

DEFICIENCY

Clinical Presentation Depending on the rate of development, adrenal insufficiency can present as mild chronic fatigue or fulminant cardiovascular collapse. When the deficiency is only partial, the symptoms may be apparent only in times of stress, such as trauma, surgery, and infection. The classic symptoms include weakness and easy fatigability, hypotension with dehydration and postural drop, and gastrointestinal dysfunction with anorexia, nausea and vomiting, diarrhea, abdominal pain, and weight loss. When the insufficiency is primary, ACTH levels are high and are associated with hyperpigmentation.

Laboratory findings may include hyponatremia, hyperkalemia, hypoglycemia, and hypereosinophilia.

Etiology Adrenal insufficiency may be primary (diseased or absent adrenals) or secondary (insufficient stimulation by ACTH). Primary disease is most commonly an autoimmune phenomenon (Addison's disease), in which case it may be associated with autoimmune disease of the thyroid, gonads, skin (vitiligo), and other tissues. Bilateral adrenal hemorrhage may occur in the setting of anticoagulation or that of critical surgery, trauma, or obstetric illness. Less commonly, disseminated tuberculosis or fungal infections may result in destruction of the adrenal cortices. When the deficiency is primary, mineralocorticoid secretion (see below) as well as glucocorticoid secretion is impaired.

Adrenocortical insufficiency also can be secondary to a lack of ACTH stimulation. By far the most common cause of ACTH deficiency, as well as of adrenal insufficiency overall, is persistent pituitary suppression after the discontinuation of exogenous glucocorticoid administration. It is notable that high-dose glucocorticoid administration for as little as a few weeks can result in prolonged adrenal insufficiency. ACTH deficiency also occurs in the setting of panhypopituitarism, along with deficiencies of other anterior pituitary hormones. In the case of secondary adrenal insufficiency, mineralocorticoid secretion remains relatively normal.

Diagnosis The diagnosis of glucocorticoid insufficiency is suggested by low morning cortisol levels but can be most reliably and reproducibly demonstrated at any time of the day with a cosyntropin stimulation test. In this test, 0.25 mg of cosyntropin is administered intramuscularly or intravenously. The serum cortisol level 30 to 60 min later should be 20 mg/dL or greater. In cases of primary adrenal insufficiency, the ACTH level will be elevated, and in patients with an autoimmune disease, antiadrenal antibodies may be elevated.

Treatment The emergent treatment of patients with cardiovascular collapse from adrenal insufficiency includes immediate intravenous hydrocortisone 100 mg every 6 h and volume repletion with intravenous saline. Treatment is adjusted over hours and days as the clinical picture evolves.

The long-term management of patients with adrenocortical insufficiency requires physiologic levels of glucocorticoid replacement: 30 mg of hydrocortisone or 7.5 mg of prednisone per day in divided doses with two-thirds in the morning and one-third in the evening. Patients with primary insufficiency also may require mineralocorticoid replacement (see below).

The glucocorticoid dose should be increased temporarily for surgery, trauma, or acute illness, and patients should be educated about the risks resulting from discontinuing treatment.

EXCESS

Clinical Presentation Hypercortisolism (Cushing's syndrome) is characterized by central obesity, muscle wasting, thin skin, hypertension, hirsutism, amenorrhea, and osteoporosis. Fatigue and weakness are common, and these patients are subject to infections. Laboratory findings may include hyperglycemia, hypokalemia, and lymphopenia.

Etiology Hypercortisolism most commonly results from prolonged high-dose exogenous glucocorticoid administration, such as for asthma or inflammatory rheumatologic disease. Less commonly, an ACTH-producing pituitary tumor (Cushing's disease) results in hypercortisolism and diffuse adrenal hyperplasia. Infrequently, ACTH excess is due to secretion by other tumors, most commonly small cell bronchogenic lung carcinomas. In the remainder, hypercortisolism results from primary hyperfunction of an adrenal tumor, either an adenoma or a carcinoma.

Diagnosis Iatrogenic glucocorticoid excess is usually apparent from the history. In other patients, the initial diagnosis of hypercortisolism rests on the demonstration of excess, nonsuppressible cortisol production. The best test for this purpose is the 24-h urine free cortisol. More convenient for some patients but less sensitive and specific is the overnight dexamethasone suppression test, in which 1 mg of dexamethasone is taken orally at midnight and a serum cortisol is determined at 8 o'clock the next morning. Normally, the morning cortisol should be suppressed to less than 5 mg/dL. False positives in these tests occur in patients with exogenous obesity, chronic alcoholism, depression, and acute physiologic or psychological stress.

After hypercortisolism has been established, the evaluation turns to the etiology by establishing patterns of cortisol suppressibility with high-dose dexamethasone and assessment of ACTH secretion. Imaging studies of the pituitary, the adrenals, or, for ectopic ACTH, the chest also may be useful.

Treatment The guiding principle of exogenous glucocorticoid administration is to use the minimum dose necessary for the shortest time possible. However, when suppressive doses are necessary, it is important that patients be educated about the risks of discontinuing treatment; if treatment is discontinued, the dose should be tapered gradually to allow the return of endogenous adrenal function.

Treatment of the other causes of hypercortisolism primarily consists of surgical removal of the hyperfunctioning pituitary, adrenal, or ectopic tumor. When hypercortisolism cannot be resolved, ketoconazole can be used to inhibit adrenal cortisol production.

Mineralocorticoids

The primary mineralocorticoid secreted by the adrenal cortex is aldosterone. Aldosterone secretion is stimulated by angiotensin II and hyperkalemia. The renin-angiotensin-aldosterone pathway begins with renin secretion by the kidney in response to low perfusion pressure. Renin converts angiotensinogen from the liver into angiotensin I, and this ultimately results in increased levels of angiotensin II from the action of angiotensin converting enzyme (ACE) on angiotensin I. Aldosterone has its major effect on the renal tubule, where it causes reabsorption of sodium in exchange for potassium and hydrogen ions. In doing this, it helps regulate both volume status and potassium balance.

DEFICIENCY

Clinical Presentation Hypoaldosteronism is seen most commonly in circumstances of primary adrenocortical insufficiency, in which the clinical presentation is dominated by the signs and symptoms of cortisol deficiency. Hypoaldosteronism itself is the major contributor to hyperkalemia, with resultant neuromuscular and cardiac dysfunction manifested by weakness and electrocardiographic (ECG) abnormalities.

Etiology Isolated aldosterone deficiency is unusual and occurs most often in the setting of hyporeninism associated with renal insufficiency and diabetes mellitus. More often, hypoaldosteronism is associated with generalized primary adrenocortical insufficiency (see above).

Diagnosis The specific diagnosis of hypoaldosteronism depends on the demonstration of a deficient aldosterone response (with or without a renin response) to sodium restriction and upright posture. In primary hypoaldosteronism, renin is high but aldosterone is low. In secondary hypoaldosteronism, both renin and aldosterone are low.

Treatment When necessary, mineralocorticoid replacement is accomplished with 0.05 to 0.2 mg oral fludrocortisone daily.

EXCESS

Clinical Presentation Hyperaldosteronism can be primary or secondary to excess renin production by one kidney or both kidneys. Primary hyperaldosteronism results in hypertension, weakness, and polyuria. Hyperaldosteronism accounts for about 1 percent of cases of hypertension. In the absence of other abnormalities, these patients do not have edema. Important laboratory abnormalities include hypokalemia and metabolic alkalosis.

A patient with excess renin from renal artery stenosis that causes unilateral renal underperfusion and hypertensive secondary hyperaldosteronism may have a renal artery bruit.

Etiology In about 70 percent of cases, primary hyperaldosteronism results from a unilateral adrenocortical adenoma (rarely a carcinoma). In most of the remaining cases, the cause is bilateral adrenal hyperplasia. High-renin secondary hyperaldosteronism associated with hypertension results most commonly from renal artery stenosis. Hyperaldosteronism secondary to increased renin secretion also occurs physiologically and without hypertension in other circumstances of renal underperfusion, such as hypovolemia and congestive heart failure.

Diagnosis Hypokalemia in a nonedematous hypertensive patient who is consuming adequate sodium and is not on diuretics is an indication for a diagnostic assessment of hyperaldosteronism. The diagnosis rests on demonstrating nonsuppressibility of aldosterone (and renin in the case of renal artery stenosis) in the presence of a high sodium intake. Ideally, drugs that interfere with the renin-angiotensin-aldosterone system should be discontinued before a definitive evaluation is made.

A useful initial screen for primary hyperaldosteronism is an elevated aldosterone/renin ratio. Confirming tests involve the measurement of aldosterone and renin while patients are on a high-salt diet or after the intravenous infusion of normal saline. In primary hyperaldosteronism, aldosterone is high but renin is low. In secondary hyperaldosteronism, both renin and aldosterone are high. Abdominal computed tomography (CT) or adrenal vein catheterization studies are used to differentiate adenoma from bilateral hyperplasia in primary hyperaldosteronism.

Treatment Unilateral adrenalectomy is used to treat an adenoma or carcinoma. In patients with surgical contraindications or bilateral adrenal hyperplasia, medical management of aldosterone-induced hypertension includes spironolactone, calcium channel blockers, and/or ACE inhibitors. Secondary hyperaldosteronism from renal artery stenosis may be treated with angioplasty or revascularization procedures.

Adrenal Androgens

The adrenal androgens are quite weak compared with testosterone and have little physiologic impact in adults. When present in significant excess, however, they can result in abnormalities. The severity and impact of the abnormalities depend on the age of the patient and the degree of androgen excess. In congenital adrenal hyperplasia (CAH), an enzyme in the biosynthetic pathway of cortisol (and aldosterone) is deficient. In this circumstance, the common precursor accumulates and "spills over" into the adrenal androgen biosynthetic pathway. Adrenal androgens also are secreted in excess by some adrenal carcinomas.

CLINICAL PRESENTATION

In childhood, severe CAH may result in the death of a fetus or infant, sexual ambiguity or a male phenotype in girls, early puberty in boys, accelerated height and bone age, and, depending on the enzyme defect, salt wasting or hypertension. In adult women, a less severe defect of adrenal steroidogenesis can cause hirsutism, oligomenorrhea-amenorrhea, infertility, acne, and temporal balding. In adult women, virilization—clitoromegaly, frontal balding, male-pattern muscularity, and deepening of the voice—suggests adrenal neoplasm.

ETIOLOGY

The most common form of CAH results from a deficiency of 21-hydroxylase. Less commonly, 11β-hydroxylase deficiency occurs. In either case, cortisol production is deficient, and the resultant increased pituitary ACTH drives adrenal steroidogenesis, leading to increased androgen secretion. The aldosterone precursor that accumulates in 11β-hydroxylase deficiency leads to hypertension, while its absence in 21-hydroxylase deficiency leads to salt wasting.

Rarely, adrenal androgen excess results from an adrenocortical carcinoma.

DIAGNOSIS

The diagnosis of CAH depends on the demonstration of an elevation of a precursor to the reaction in the biosynthetic pathway normally catalyzed by the deficient enzymes. The most useful test is serum 17-hydroxyprogesterone. Adrenal androgen excess from hyperplasia or, rarely, from carcinoma is shown by increased levels of dehydroepiandrosterone sulfate (DHEA-S).

TREATMENT

CAH is treated by replacing the critical missing adrenal hormone: cortisol. This results in decreased ACTH levels and resolved overactivity of adrenal steroidogenesis. An adrenal carcinoma requires surgery.

ADRENAL MEDULLA

The adrenal medulla secretes catecholamines—epinephrine and norepinephrine—as part of the sympathetic nervous system in response to various stresses. The catecholamines generally result in increased heart rate and force of cardiac contractility, increased glucose production, and central nervous system excitability. The clinical abnormality of the adrenal medulla is pheochromocytoma, a rare tumor that secretes excess amounts of the catecholamines.

Pheochromocytoma

CLINICAL PRESENTATION   Pheochromocytoma causes less than 1 percent of cases of hypertension. The hypertension may be sustained or paroxysmal. The associated symptoms are variable but classically include paroxysmal headache, palpitations, and diaphoresis in association with acute elevation of blood pressure. There also may be weight loss despite increased appetite and postural hypotension because of volume contraction. Laboratory abnormalities include elevated glucose. Thyroid tests are notably normal.

ETIOLOGY   Most pheochromocytomas are solitary benign tumors. About 10 percent are bilateral, 10 percent are extraadrenal, and 10 percent are malignant. In about 5 percent of cases, the pheochromocytoma is part of familial syndromes as an isolated abnormality or as part of the multiple endocrine neoplasia (MEN) syndrome, types 2a and 2b.

DIAGNOSIS   The diagnosis is established by demonstrating increased excretion of the catecholamines or their metabolites—vanillylmandelic acid (VMA) and metanephrines—in 24-h urine collections. Most pheochromocytomas secrete increased catecholamines continuously, but the sensitivity of testing is increased when it is performed during a hypertensive episode. Localization of the tumor usually is possible with magnetic resonance imaging (MRI) scanning.

TREATMENT   The ultimate treatment of pheochromocytoma is surgical removal. However, correct pre- and intraoperative pharmacologic care is critical and is directed specifically toward catecholamine excess. First, α-blockade is established with phenoxybenzamine and volume expansion is carried out over 7 to 14 days. Only after α-blockade has been established is β-blockade with propranolol introduced. Isolated β-blockade will result in unopposed α-receptor stimulation and dramatic worsening of hypertension.

ADRENAL INCIDENTALOMA

With the widespread availability and use of CT and MRI scanning, an increasing number of adrenal tumors are being discovered incidentally in patients who are scanned for unrelated reasons. Most of these tumors are nonfunctional, and carcinoma is rare in tumors smaller than 5 cm. The finding of an incidental adrenal tumor should prompt a careful history and physical directed toward findings of adrenal hormone excess and a detailed review of the CT or MRI scan, which may suggest the etiology. Laboratory screening for hormone oversecretion may include 24-h urine-free cortisol or an overnight 1-mg dexamethasone suppression test, serum potassium, aldosterone/renin ratio, DHEA-S, and urinary VMA/metanephrines/catecholamines. Functional tumors should be treated appropriately. Tumors 5 cm or larger should be removed. Follow-up CT of smaller nonfunctional tumors should be performed in 6 to 12 months.

BIBLIOGRAPHY

Copeland PM: The incidentally discovered adrenal mass: An update. *The Endocrinologist* 9:415–423, 1999.

Deaton MA, Glorioso JE, McLean DB: Congenital adrenal hyperplasia: Not really a zebra. *Am Fam Physician* 59:1172, 1190–1196, 1999.

Fauci AS, Braunwald E, Isselbacher KJ, et al (eds): *Harrison's Principles of Internal Medicine,* 14th ed. New York, McGraw-Hill, 1998.

Graham DJ, McHenry CR: The adrenal incidentaloma: Guidelines for evaluation and recommendations for management. *Surg Oncol Clin North Am* 7:749–764, 1998.

Hasinski S: Assessment of adrenal glucocorticoid function: Which tests are appropriate for screening? *Postgrad Med* 104:61–64, 69–72, 1998.

Jeffcoate W: Assessment of corticosteroid replacement therapy in adults with adrenal insufficiency. *Ann Clin Biochem* 36:151–157, 1999.

Kleerekoper M, Schiebinger R, Gutai, JP: Steroid therapy for adrenal disorders—getting the dose right. *J Clin Endocrinol Metab* 82:3923–3925, 1997.

Pang S: Congenital adrenal hyperplasia. *Endocrinol Metab Clin North Am* 26:853–891, 1997.

Tierney LM Jr, McPhee SJ, Papadakis MA (eds): *Current Medical Diagnosis and Treatment,* 39th ed. New York, McGraw-Hill, 2000.

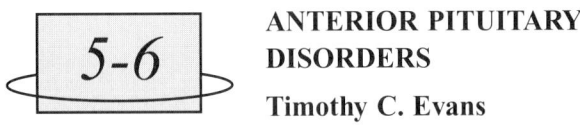

5-6 ANTERIOR PITUITARY DISORDERS

Timothy C. Evans

DISCUSSION

The pituitary gland has anterior and posterior divisions and is located in the sella turcica, a small bony pocket at the base of the cranial vault. The anterior pituitary consists of several different populations of cells that secrete six different peptide hormones: growth hormone (GH), adrenocorticotropic hormone (ACTH), thyroid-stimulating hormone (TSH), luteinizing hormone (LH), follicle-stimulating hormone (FSH), and prolactin. The secretion of these hormones is under the control of the hypothalamus through chemical signals that travel from the hypothalamus to the pituitary via the hypothalamic-pituitary portal circulation. In each case except that of prolactin, the stimulatory signal is a peptide-releasing hormone. Prolactin is unique in that it is under tonic inhibitory control by the hypothalamus. The mediator of this inhibition is dopamine. The posterior pituitary is a direct neuronal extension from the hypothalamus and is discussed in Chap. 5-11.

There are four key anatomic features of the pituitary. The first is its relationship to the hypothalamus, which controls anterior pituitary function through the releasing hormones and dopamine. The second is the location of the pituitary in the sella turcica, which limits the size of the pituitary so that enlargement is generally out of the sella superiorly. The third is the position of the optic chiasm directly above the superior opening into the sella turcica. This means that pituitary enlargement out of the sella results in pressure on or damage to the optic chiasm and characteristic visual field abnormalities. The fourth is the presence of the cavernous sinuses lateral to the sella turcica. Cranial nerves III, IV, and VI pass through the cavernous sinuses, and so lateral extension of a pituitary tumor can result in oculomotor palsies, most frequently of cranial nerve III.

In general, disorders of the pituitary are manifested by the effects of excess secretion of one of the pituitary hormones, a deficiency of one or more pituitary hormones, or pituitary enlargement.

PITUITARY ADENOMAS

Pituitary adenomas are benign pituitary tumors that can be functional or nonfunctional. Functional tumors arise from the cells that secrete pituitary hormones and release excess amounts of the hormone associated with the cells that constitute the tumor. Other tumors are nonfunctional and, like functional tumors, may cause symptoms by compressing the normal pituitary and resulting in decreased secretion of pituitary hormones or through mechanical effects on extrapituitary structures such as the optic chiasm. Small pituitary tumors, less than 1 cm, typically confined to the sella turcica, are termed *microadenomas.* Larger tumors are called *macroadenomas.* When the neurons of the optic chiasm are disrupted, the characteristic visual field defect is bitemporal hemianopsia. Other mass effects include headache and cranial nerve III palsy. The most common functional pituitary tumors secrete prolactin. Next in frequency are GH-secreting tumors, followed by ACTH-secreting tumors. Tumors that secrete excess TSH, LH, or FSH are very unusual. Thirty to 40 percent of pituitary tumors do not secrete excess hormones.

Prolactin

There are many causes of hyperprolactinemia, including physiologic states such as pregnancy and nursing, many drugs, and diseases such as hypothyroidism and pituitary-hypothalamic lesions or tumors that interfere with the delivery of dopamine from the hypothalamus to the pituitary. Another cause is the most common pituitary tumor: a prolactinoma.

CLINICAL PRESENTATION   Prolactin normally stimulates the production of breast milk after childbirth. Excess prolactin also decreases the pituitary gonadotropins, LH and FSH. Consequently, the symptoms of hyperprolactinemia are those of hypogonadism, inappropriate lactation, and infertility. Prolactinomas are more common in women and present with oligo- or amenorrhea and galactorrhea. In men, the symptoms develop gradually and consist of decreased libido and impotence. Because of the menstrual abnormality, prolactinomas tend to be diagnosed in women at an earlier stage than they are in men. In men, the tumors are more likely to be macroadenomas.

DIAGNOSIS   Patients with hypogonadism or galactorrhea should have a prolactin measurement. When prolactin is elevated, the various possibilities in the wide differential diagnosis must be considered. The higher the prolactin level, the more likely the diagnosis of prolactinoma. When there is hyperprolactinemia, a magnetic resonance imaging (MRI) study should be performed to look for a pituitary tumor.

TREATMENT   Prolactinoma is the only pituitary tumor for which the treatment is primarily medical. The dopamine agonist bromocriptine effectively inhibits prolactin secretion and results in a decrease in tumor size. The starting dose is 1.25 mg given at bedtime to minimize the side effects of nausea and postural hypotension. Complete inhibition may require 10 to 15 mg per day in two divided doses. Occasionally, large tumors may require surgery.

Growth Hormone

The second most common functional pituitary tumor secretes GH. This hormone has its primary effect on linear bone growth and has a number of metabolic effects, most notably insulin antagonism. The most characteristic consequence of a GH-secreting tumor is excess growth.

CLINICAL PRESENTATION   In adults, GH excess results in acromegaly, and in children, it results in gigantism. In addition to the increased rate of bone and soft tissue growth, metabolic abnormalities contribute to the clinical picture. It is more common in males than in females.

Children have increased linear bone growth, and adults show enlargement of the hands, feet, and skull. The hands are broad, and the face is characterized by frontal bossing, coarsening of features, oily skin, and the development of spaces between the teeth. The process is so slow that the patient often does not notice the changes; thus, the diagnosis is made only after a long delay. Soft tissue growth results in carpal tunnel syndrome and cardiomegaly with congestive heart failure. Metabolic effects include diabetes mellitus, weight gain, and kidney stones. The tumors have often grown to a large size by the time of diagnosis and are associated with headaches and visual field defects.

DIAGNOSIS   The diagnosis is indicated by the physical findings, diabetes mellitus, or glucose intolerance. Comparison with old photo-

graphs of the patient can be helpful in showing the change in appearance over time. A useful screening test is the measurement of insulin-like growth factor I (IGF-I, also called somatomedin C), which is produced by the liver in response to GH stimulation. Unlike GH, it has a long half-life in serum, and so levels do not vary from minute to minute.

When IGF-I is elevated, serum GH is measured 60 min after 100 g of oral glucose. Since hyperglycemia has the opposite effect on GH that it has on insulin, the GH level should be suppressed to less than 2 ng/mL. Prolactin, which frequently is cosecreted with GH as well as other pituitary hormones, should be measured, since a large tumor may interfere with the normal secretion of other pituitary hormones. After confirmation of GH excess, an MRI is performed to document the anatomy of the pituitary tumor.

TREATMENT   Treatment of GH-secreting pituitary tumors primarily consists of surgical removal. Since these tumors are often macroadenomas, complete removal is often impossible. Other treatment modalities include high-dose bromocriptine, octreotide (an analogue of somatostatin, a natural hormone that inhibits GH secretion), and radiation therapy.

Adrenocorticotropic Hormone

ACTH is the stimulus for cortisol production by the adrenal cortex. Pituitary tumors that secrete excess ACTH constitute Cushing's disease, a form of Cushing's syndrome. Cushing's disease therefore is characterized by the symptoms of hypercortisolism.

CLINICAL PRESENTATION   ACTH-producing tumors are typically microadenomas, and so they usually have no local pituitary mass effects. The symptoms are confined to those of hypercortisolism: centripetal obesity, facial plethora, hypertension, thin skin with easy bruising and abdominal striae, osteoporosis, muscle weakness, and glucose intolerance.

DIAGNOSIS   Hypercortisolism is demonstrated by increased 24-h urine free cortisol or nonsuppression of morning serum cortisol in the 1-mg overnight dexamethasone suppression test or after 2 days of low-dose dexamethasone (0.5 mg every 6 h for eight doses). The next step in the identification of the cause of endogenous hypercortisolism is high-dose dexamethasone suppression test (2 mg dexamethasone every 6 h for eight doses). Classically, ACTH overproduction by a pituitary tumor is suppressed by high-dose dexamethasone, while primary adrenal overproduction and ectopic ACTH-stimulated overproduction are not suppressed.

Since ACTH-producing pituitary tumors are usually small, localization before surgery can be challenging. In addition to MRI, selective catheterization and sampling of ACTH levels in the right and left venous drainage (the petrosal sinuses) of the pituitary gland may help identify the tumor before microsurgery.

HYPOPITUITARISM

Deficient secretion of anterior pituitary hormones can be selective or global: panhypopituitarism. The clinical presentation is determined by the missing hormone or hormones.

Etiology

ISOLATED DEFICIENCIES   An isolated deficiency of anterior pituitary hormones can be congenital or acquired. An acquired deficiency is more common. The most important acquired pituitary hormone functional deficiency is a deficiency of ACTH after prolonged glucocorticoid excess, whether from endogenous hypercortisolism or from exogenous glucocorticoid administration. Likewise, TSH levels may remain suppressed for a time after the resolution of hyperthyroidism. Isolated, reversible gonadotropin deficiency and amenorrhea are seen commonly in women who participate in vigorous athletics or have marked weight loss or a serious physical or psychological illness.

Destructive or space-occupying lesions of the pituitary, such as pituitary tumors, may result in a gradual loss of normal pituitary function. The order of loss is typically GH followed by the gonadotropins, TSH, and ACTH.

A congenital isolated deficiency most often involves GH or the gonadotropins. GH deficiency results in decreased growth velocity and delayed bone development. Gonadotropin deficiency results in delayed puberty and infertility.

PANHYPOPITUITARISM   Complete loss of pituitary function may be a consequence of pituitary tumors, hypothalamic tumors such as craniopharyngiomas, trauma, pituitary or hypothalamic surgery, vascular insufficiency such as postpartum necrosis or pituitary apoplexy, radiation, and infiltrative or granulomatous lesions such as hemochromatosis and sarcoidosis.

Functional loss may be sudden and catastrophic, as in pituitary apoplexy, or gradual, as with pituitary tumor growth. As was noted above, gradual loss usually occurs in the order GH, LH/FSH, TSH, ACTH.

Diagnosis

The diagnosis may involve various measures to visualize the pituitary, such as MRI, or to document other diseases involving the pituitary, such as hemochromatosis and sarcoidosis. Functional testing of the pituitary, however, is the essence of the diagnosis of hypopituitarism.

ADRENOCORTICOTROPIC HORMONE   A deficiency of ACTH is the most critical life-threatening pituitary deficiency. Testing of chronic deficiency, such as that seen after long-term exogenous glucocorticoid administration, may be carried out by measuring the adrenal cortisol response to stimulation by the synthetic ACTH analogue cosyntropin (see Chap. 5-5). This test may be normal, however, in the setting of acute pituitary destruction because the adrenal is still capable of producing cortisol when stimulated. Consequently, a test that stimulates the hypothalamic-pituitary axis occasionally may be required, such as the insulin tolerance test, in which 0.05 to 0.1 unit of regular insulin per kilogram of body weight is administered to lower the blood glucose to less than 40 mg/dL. At this level of hypoglycemia, cortisol should be higher than 19 mg/dL. Pituitary production of GH also can be assessed with this test. The performance of this test requires very close monitoring to avoid dangerous levels of hypoglycemia.

GROWTH HORMONE   The adequacy of GH secretion by the pituitary can be measured simultaneously with ACTH in the insulin tolerance test described above. At the time of significant hypoglycemia, the serum GH level should be higher than 10 ng/mL. Alternative stimuli for GH secretion include levodopa, arginine, clonidine, and exercise.

THYROID-STIMULATING HORMONE   Pituitary TSH production is best tested by measuring serum TSH and free thyroid hormone. Low thyroid hormone with low or inappropriately normal TSH indicates inadequate pituitary TSH secretion. If other pituitary hormones are also deficient, no further thyroid testing is necessary. Before diagnosing isolated TSH deficiency, however, one needs to consider the euthyroid sick syndrome and a deficiency of thyroid-binding globulin.

GONADOTROPINS   Normal menstruation in women and normal testosterone and spermatogenesis in men rule out a gonadotropin deficiency. In patients with amenorrhea, decreased libido, infertility,

impotence, or absent or decreasing secondary sexual characteristics, low LH and FSH in the setting of low estrogen or testosterone confirms a gonadotropin deficiency.

Treatment

In most cases, hormone replacement for pituitary hormone deficiency is done with the missing target organ hormone, except for GH and in the case of the gonadotropins when fertility is desired.

ADRENOCORTICOTROPIC HORMONE   Patients require replacement of cortisol but not aldosterone, since the adrenal glands are intact. Glucocorticoid replacement most often is done with 7.5 mg prednisone or 30 mg hydrocortisone per day, with two-thirds given in the morning and one-third given in the afternoon or evening. The dose is increased temporarily during times of stress such as surgery and acute illness. Patients should be educated carefully about the importance of not discontinuing treatment.

THYROID-STIMULATING HORMONE   Replacement is done with levothyroxine (0.05 to 0.15 mg per day). Since TSH is absent, clinical signs and the free thyroxine level are used to adjust the dose. It is important to note that thyroid hormone accelerates glucocorticoid metabolism so that treatment with levothyroxine before glucocorticoid replacement can worsen adrenal deficiency and precipitate an adrenal crisis. Therefore, glucocorticoid replacement should always precede thyroxine replacement in patients with panhypopituitarism.

GONADOTROPINS   Estrogen-progesterone replacement in women and testosterone replacement in men relieve the symptoms of hypogonadism but do not restore fertility. Ovarian hormone replacement in women can be done with several regimens, such as conjugated estrogens (0.625 mg per day) and medroxyprogesterone (2.5 mg per day). In men, replacement most often is done with testosterone esters given intramuscularly 200 mg every other week. When fertility is desired, ovulation or spermatogenesis stimulation can be attempted with gonadotropin injections over several months.

GROWTH HORMONE   In adults, there is little indication for GH replacement, although research protocols are studying possible benefits on aging, and GH has been approved for use in adults with GH deficiency. In children with isolated GH deficiency or panhypopituitarism whose epiphyses have not closed, growth retardation is treated with synthetic GH injections.

BIBLIOGRAPHY

Fauci AS, Braunwald E, Isselbacher KJ, et al (eds): *Harrison's Principles of Internal Medicine,* 14th ed. New York, McGraw-Hill, 1998.

Lamberts SW, de Herder WW, van der Lely AJ: Pituitary insufficiency. *Lancet* 352:127–134, 1998.

Molitch ME: Pituitary incidentalomas. *Endocrinol Metab Clin North Am* 26:725–740, 1997.

Molitch ME: Pituitary diseases in pregnancy. *Semin Perinatol* 22:457–470, 1998.

Pullan P: Pituitary disease. *Aust Fam Physician* 28:455–461, 1999.

Schmidt DN, Wallace K: How to diagnose hypopituitarism: Learning the features of secondary hormonal deficiencies. *Postgrad Med* 104:77–78, 81–87, 1998.

Shimon I, Melmed S: Management of pituitary tumors. *Ann Intern Med* 129:472–483, 1998.

Tierney LM Jr, McPhee SJ, Papadakis MA (eds): *Current Medical Diagnosis and Treatment,* 39th ed. New York, McGraw-Hill, 2000.

Veznedaroglu E, Armonda RA, Andrews DW: Diagnosis and therapy for pituitary tumors. *Curr Opin Oncol* 11:27–31, 1999.

Yeh PJ, Chen JW: Pituitary tumors: Surgical and medical management. *Surg Oncol* 6:67–92, 1997.

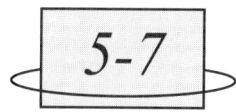

DIABETIC KETOACIDOSIS
Janice Herbert-Carter

DISCUSSION

Diabetic ketoacidosis (DKA) is a very serious acute complication of diabetes mellitus, primarily in type 1 patients. Nondiabetic causes of ketoacidosis include starvation and alcoholism.

PATHOPHYSIOLOGY

Ketoacids (ketones, ketone bodies) are formed by the metabolism of fats. The oxidation of fats does not produce carbon dioxide and water, as is the case with carbohydrates. Instead, fats ultimately produce acetic acid, acetoacetic acid, and B-hydroxybutyric acid, all of which are ketoacids. Under normal conditions, the body produces few of these acids, and their excretion is easily handled. In insulin deficiency states, fat is metabolized preferentially because of the inability to utilize glucose. Thus, excessive amounts of ketones are formed. Their accumulation leads to systemic acidemia, ketoaciduria, and electrolyte imbalance. In addition, some of the problems in diabetic ketoacidosis result from severe hyperglycemia: osmotic diuresis, dehydration, and hyperosmolality.

The precipitating factors are most commonly infection and/or failure to take insulin. Additionally, trauma, emotional stress, or another serious intercurrent illness may initiate DKA. In older diabetics, myocardial infarction or stroke may precipitate this condition.

SIGNS AND SYMPTOMS

The presentation, especially early on, may be nonspecific: abdominal pain, nausea and vomiting, anorexia, malaise, fatigue, thirst, tachycardia, tachypnea, and a fruity odor on the breath. Once the acidosis has progressed, the patient may present obtunded or in a coma. In fact, coma may be the initial presentation of a previously undiagnosed type 1 diabetic patient.

DIFFERENTIAL DIAGNOSIS

A comatose diabetic patient should bring to mind three possibilities: DKA, nonketotic hyperosmolar coma (NKHC), and hypoglycemia. Hypoglycemia is discussed chap. 5-8. NKHC is more common in type 2 diabetics, and acidosis is not present unless it is due to another cause, such as lactic acidosis in septic shock. Severe hyperglycemia, dehydration, osmotic diuresis, and hyperosmolarity are found. The precipitating factors are similar to those in DKA, as is the treatment.

LABORATORY TESTS

Serum ketones are invariably present. Hyperglycemia is also present; it is commonly extreme but sometimes is only moderate. Urine ketones are present but may be erroneously interpreted as negative. The common urine tests for ketones check only for acetoacetate, while the predominant ketone in DKA is β-hydroxybutyrate. Arterial blood gases will demonstrate acidosis (pH < 7.4). Usually, there will also be low pco_2 because tachypnea is a compensatory mechanism for metabolic acidosis. Electrolytes demonstrate an increased anion gap acidosis. Electrolyte abnormalities may be variable, since the degree of dehydration and hyperglycemia affects measured values of sodium, potassium, and phosphate. These electrolytes should be monitored, and adjustments should be made as the dehydration and hyperglycemia are corrected.

TREATMENT

The key to therapy for DKA is regular insulin, ideally given by continuous intravenous infusion in an intensive care setting. If this is not available, periodic bolus intravenous injection is acceptable. The absorption of subcutaneous or intramuscular insulin is unpredictable, and therefore insulin should not be used. Rehydration is as important as is insulin. Vigorous fluid replacement should be given in a diabetic patient with normally functioning cardiovascular and renal systems. Fluid replacement must be attempted more carefully in the face of congestive heart failure or renal failure and in any elderly diabetic. Frequent monitoring of acidosis, electrolytes, vital signs, and hemodynamic status is essential. Insulin therapy should be continued until the acidosis is cleared even if normoglycemia appears first. In such instances, it may be necessary to switch from normal and half-normal saline to dextrose-containing solutions. As acidosis is corrected, potassium and phosphate repletion may be necessary. Bicarbonate therapy is not indicated if the pH is >7.1.

PEARLS

Although DKA has a mortality rate of 5 to 15 percent, it can be managed successfully if it is recognized and treated appropriately. The mainstays of treatment are intravenous regular insulin and fluids. These patients benefit from admission to the intensive care unit because frequent monitoring of hemodynamic status, vital signs, fluid intake and output, electrolytes, and blood gases is important.

ADDITIONAL RESOURCES

Bell DS, Alele J. Diabetic ketoacidosis: why early detection and aggressive treatment are crucial. *Post Grad Med* 101:193–198, 203–204, 1997.
Cefalu WT. Diabetic ketoacidosis. *Critical Care Clin* 7:89, 1991.
Lebovitz HE. Diabetic ketoacidosis. *Lancet* 345:767, 1995.

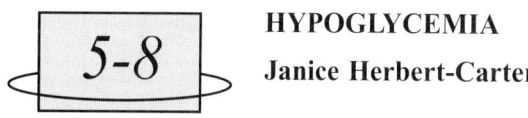

HYPOGLYCEMIA
Janice Herbert-Carter

DISCUSSION

Hypoglycemia is a serious acute disorder in which blood sugar is too low to supply the body's needs, especially the needs of the central nervous system. Any cause of excessive insulin with inadequate glucose intake may produce hypoglycemia. Thus, injection of too much insulin, excessive exercise, ingestion of too much of an oral hypoglycemic agent, failure of hepatic gluconeogenesis, impaired absorption of food from the intestine, and inadequate food intake all may lead to hypoglycemia.

SIGNS AND SYMPTOMS

A hypoglycemic patient may present with sweating, palpitations, hunger, tremor, nervousness, and weakness, all of which result from stimulation of the beta-adrenergic system (epinephrine). These signs may be blunted or absent in a patient taking a beta blocker such as propranolol for hypertension. Additionally, patients may have light-headedness, diplopia, headache, motor incoordination, confusion, obtundation, seizures, and coma as a result of glucose starvation in the central nervous system.

DIFFERENTIAL DIAGNOSIS

The signs and symptoms listed above may be nonspecific, but in a known diabetic patient they should always cause suspicion of hypoglycemia.

In general, it does not hurt to err on the side of caution and give a diabetic patient a dose of glucose. This will almost immediately correct the symptomatology if it is due to hypoglycemia. If it is not, little harm has been done. Hypoglycemia in a nondiabetic has varied causes, including insulinoma; hepatic, renal, pituitary, thyroid, and adrenal diseases; gastrointestinal surgery; severe malnutrition; drugs and poisons (mushroom poisoning, salicylates, alcohol); sepsis; widespread cancer; and surreptitious insulin use. Surreptitious insulin use is seen most often in health care professionals who have knowledge about and access to drugs and syringes. Nevertheless, hypoglycemia in any non-diabetic is a rare finding.

LABORATORY TESTS

The serum glucose must always be low. How low is controversial. In general, most people have symptoms when the serum glucose is less than 50. In known diabetics, further laboratory testing is not needed. If surreptitious insulin injection is suspected, an insulin level together with a peptide C level will be useful. In insulinoma, both insulin and peptide C will be high, indicating excess endogenous insulin production. When hypoglycemia is due to exogenous insulin, the insulin level will be high but the peptide C level will be normal or low.

TREATMENT

Intravenous glucose (dextrose 50% in a water bolus followed by continuous infusion of $D_{10}W$ or D_5W) is the optimal treatment for hypoglycemia. In early stages, an alert patient may notice the signs and symptoms and be able to take oral glucose or a carbohydrate-containing food. Absorption is not certain, however, and the onset of action may be delayed. A comatose patient will awaken quickly if hypoglycemia has not gone on so long that there is permanent brain damage. Even with rapid awakening, a hypoglycemic patient must be monitored carefully. One must remember that the sulfonylureas have long half-lives and that hypoglycemia may recur if glucose infusion is not continued.

ADDITIONAL RESOURCES

Cryer PE, Fisher JN, Shamoon H. Hypoglycemia. *Diabetes Care* 17:734–755, 1994.
Diabetes Control and Complications Trial Research Group, Hypoglycemia in the diabetes control and complications trial. *Diabetes* 46:271–286, 1997.

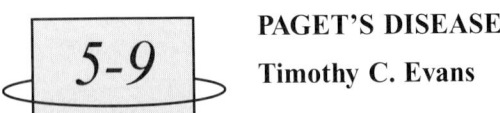

5-9

PAGET'S DISEASE
Timothy C. Evans

ETIOLOGY AND PATHOGENESIS

Paget's disease of bone is a focal bone disease that affects up to 3 percent of individuals over 60 years of age. It is characterized by excess bone lysis followed by replacement initially with vascular fibrous connective tissue and subsequently with bone that has a disorganized structure. Paget's disease resembles a benign bone neoplasm in some respects. Several lines of evidence suggest that Paget's disease may be a consequence of a viral infection.

Paget's disease is initially a localized focal disease and begins with a single site of aggressive bone lysis. After the rapid bone resorption by osteoclasts, fibrous connective tissue is made and bone formation begins, but the osteoblasts are unable to synthesize bone with a normal structure. Instead, the new bone has a disorganized architecture; it is less stable structurally and more liable to fracture.

The process of rapid bone resorption and eventual replacement by abnormal bone may extend from the original focal site, and so the disease may remain localized or extend to involve an entire bone.

In some patients, multiple bones may be involved. During the active phase of resorption and bone re-formation, pagetic bone is extremely vascular. The rapidity of the process and the microscopic structural abnormality of the new bone result in enlargement or deformity of involved bone.

CLINICAL PRESENTATION

Many patients with Paget's disease are asymptomatic, and the diagnosis is made or indicated by incidental x-ray or laboratory findings. In other patients, however, the symptoms include bone pain or deformity, fractures, deafness, and other neurologic deficits.

Pain is the most prominent symptom. The bones of the pelvis are most commonly involved, followed by the femur, skull, tibia, and spine. Pain may be due to the pagetic process and the development of the abnormal microarchitecture and deformity that result. It also may be due to microfractures, especially in weight-bearing bones such as the femur. Gross fractures also occur in pagetic bones and may occur in long bones, vertebrae, and the base of the skull.

Neurologic involvement results from damage to nerves by collapsed or deformed bone. Hearing loss can result from Paget's disease of the bones of the inner ear or from compression of cranial nerve VIII as it passes through the skull. Nerve root or spinal cord compression can result from Paget's disease of the spine.

CLINICAL COMPLICATIONS

In addition to the pain, deformity, fracture, and neurologic consequences of Paget's disease, certain specific complications may arise. When a significant portion of the skeleton is involved, the intense vascularity of pagetic bone during the active phase of resorption and re-formation and the vasodilation in surrounding tissues can result in increased cardiac output. In some elderly patients with cardiac compromise, this can cause high-output cardiac failure.

Osteoarthritis commonly develops in joints adjacent to pagetic bones. Arthritis also can develop secondary to abnormal joint stress caused by deformed or shortened bones.

The hypercalcemia that develops in immobilized patients with Paget's disease can result in kidney stones.

A serious but fortunately uncommon (about 1 percent of patients) complication of Paget's disease is sarcoma of bone. Successful treatment of this malignancy is unusual.

DIAGNOSIS
X-Ray Findings

Radiologic changes in bone are quite specific for Paget's disease. The initial change is the lytic lesion. As bone re-formation follows, there is increased density in the area of new bone. Mixed lesions may show increased thickness, irregular areas of decreased and increased lucency, cortical thickening, and deformity as the bone responds to mechanical stress during remodeling. Fractures may appear as breaks in long bones or as collapsed bone in vertebrae or at the base of the skull.

The early lytic phase may be difficult to detect radiographically. Bone scans are more sensitive and can be used to locate areas of disease or define the extent of bone involvement.

Bone biopsy is seldom necessary, except in cases where primary or metastatic malignant disease is suspected.

Laboratory Tests

Serum calcium, phosphate, and parathyroid hormone (PTH) are typically normal. However, inactivity or bed rest in a patient with Paget's disease can result in hypercalcemia, sometimes of a significant degree. In this circumstance, it is important to eliminate the possibility of primary hyperparathyroidism (by measuring the serum PTH, which will be normal or low in isolated Paget's disease), since coexistent hyper-parathyroidism can increase the rate of progression of Paget's disease.

Several markers of the metabolic activity of bone remodeling can be measured. The most commonly measured, and often the initial indication of the presence of Paget's disease, is alkaline phosphatase. Alkaline phosphatase is elevated, often to very high levels, reflecting the activity of osteoblasts in synthesizing new bone. A newer serum marker of bone formation is osteocalcin, a minor protein constituent of bone that also is elevated in Paget's disease.

Bone resorption markers, which also may be increased, include urine hydroxyproline and newer, more specific indicators of bone degradation: the terminal fragments of bone collagen excreted in the urine.

The differential diagnosis of Paget's disease includes other lytic or destructive diseases of bone, such as multiple myeloma and primary or metastatic malignancy. Blood and tissue diagnostic tests for these diseases should be carried out when appropriate.

TREATMENT

Treatment is usually instituted for pain, neurologic complications, fractures, hypercalcemia, or high cardiac output. Asymptomatic patients require no treatment, although it has been suggested that antiresorptives (see below) be used to prevent more severe disease and its complications. Aspirin or nonsteroidal anti-inflammatory drugs may be used for pain in Paget's disease patients.

Appropriate orthotics should be used, and orthopedic measures should be carried out to maintain the functional geometry of bones, especially the weight-bearing bones of the lower extremities. When orthopedic surgery is necessary, it should be preceded by several weeks of antiresorptive therapy to decrease bleeding from pagetic bone and improve the strength of attachment of prosthetic or stabilizing devices. After surgery of any type, patients should be encouraged to ambulate as soon as medically appropriate to minimize the risk of hypercalcemia.

Medical therapy is directed at decreasing bone resorption by osteoclasts. The primary agents for this purpose are the bisphosphonates and calcitonin. The bisphosphonates have become the treatment of choice for Paget's disease. The newer agents, such as alendronate, pamidronate, residronate, and tiludronate, are more potent than the earlier bisphosphonate etidronate and do not cause the mineralization defect associated with that agent. Oral bisphosphonates are poorly absorbed and so are taken while fasting. The main side effects are gastrointestinal, including esophagitis and esophageal ulcerations.

Both salmon calcitonin and human calcitonin are available and are given by subcutaneous injection. Although used less often than bisphosphonates, calcitonin is available for patients with bisphosphonate intolerance. Antibody formation and insensitivity to salmon calcitonin develop in about 15 percent of these patients, who then can be treated with human calcitonin. Calcitonin administered by nasal spray is now available, but both the injectable and the nasal forms are expensive.

BIBLIOGRAPHY

Fauci AS, Braunwald E, Isselbacher KJ, et al (eds): *Harrison's Principles of Internal Medicine,* 14th ed. New York, McGraw-Hill, 1998.

Hosking DJ: Prediction and assessment of the response of Paget's disease to bisphosphonate treatment. *Bone* 24(Suppl 5):69S–71S, 1999.

Khan SA, Vasikaran S, McCloskey EV, et al: Alendronate in the treatment of Paget's disease of bone. *Bone* 20:263–271, 1997.

Lombardi A: Treatment of Paget's disease of bone with alendronate. *Bone* 24(Suppl 5):59S–61S, 1999.

Reid IR, Nicholson GC, Weinstein RS, et al: Biochemical and radiologic improvement in Paget's disease of bone treated with alendronate: A randomized, placebo-controlled trial. *Am J Med* 101:341–348, 1996 [published erratum appears in *Am J Med* 102:322, 1997].

Siris ES: Goals of treatment for Paget's disease of bone. *J Bone Miner Res* 14(Suppl 2):49–52, 1999.

Tierney LM Jr, McPhee SJ, Papadakis MA (eds): *Current Medical Diagnosis and Treatment,* 39th ed. New York, McGraw-Hill, 2000.

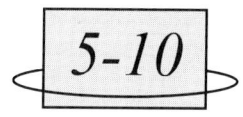

PARATHYROID DISORDERS

Timothy C. Evans

DISCUSSION

The four parathyroid glands are behind and partially in the thyroid gland. The function of the parathyroids is the regulation of serum calcium through the secretion of parathyroid hormone (PTH). Excessive PTH results in hypercalcemia, and insufficient PTH results in hypocalcemia.

CALCIUM METABOLISM

Calcium is a major body constituent, but only about 1 percent of total calcium circulates in the blood; most is in bone. Calcium in the blood is partly bound to protein, with about 55 percent free as ionized calcium. It is the ionized fraction that is required for proper neuromuscular functioning. Consequently, correct interpretation of serum calcium requires that an adjustment of the normal range of total serum calcium be made on the basis of serum albumin because of the protein binding of calcium. When the albumin is low, the normal calcium also is low in a ratio of about 0.8 to 1.0 mg/dL calcium for each gram of albumin (less than 4 g/dL).

The serum calcium level is closely regulated by two hormones—PTH and vitamin D—that act on bone, the kidneys, and the gastrointestinal tract to increase serum calcium. There is no mechanism in humans to lower serum calcium except renal clearance of calcium and the absence of PTH and vitamin D effects.

Parathyroid Hormone

PTH is secreted by the four parathyroid glands in response to hypocalcemia. In turn, PTH raises serum calcium through direct effects on bone and the kidneys and indirect effects on the intestine. PTH stimulates the resorption of bone and decreases the renal clearance of calcium. It also stimulates the renal activation of vitamin D. Each of these mechanisms increases the serum calcium level. When serum-ionized calcium reaches a threshold level, PTH secretion is inhibited.

Vitamin D

The hormone vitamin D is synthesized in the skin and ingested in the diet. With adequate exposure to sunlight, vitamin D is synthesized in adequate amounts and no dietary supplementation is necessary. The critical step in its biosynthesis takes place in the skin under the influence of ultraviolet light. Once it is formed, vitamin D must undergo two hydroxylation steps to become the active agent, 1,25-dihydroxyvitamin D. The first hydroxylation takes place in the liver to form 25-hydroxyvitamin D. The second, rate-limiting hydroxylation to 1,25-dihydroxyvitamin D takes place in the kidney under the influence of PTH. The primary effect of 1,25-dihydroxyvitamin D is increased calcium and phosphate absorption from the intestine.

HYPERCALCEMIA

Hypercalcemia has a wide variety of causes, but 90 percent of cases are caused by primary hyperparathyroidism or malignancy. Other causes include circumstances of high bone turnover such as thyrotoxicosis and immobilization, excess exogenous or endogenous vitamin D, renal disease, and an abnormal upward adjustment of the PTH/calcium set point seen in familial hypocalciuric hypercalcemia (FHH) and lithium therapy.

The PTH in hyperparathyroidism is increased. The PTH in FHH and lithium therapy also may be inappropriately normal or minimally elevated, as is discussed below. All other causes of hypercalcemia are characterized and thus distinguished by appropriately suppressed serum PTH levels. Some malignancies (especially breast cancer) cause hypercalcemia through bony metastasis, others by producing an immunologically distinct protein with PTH-like properties called parathyroid hormone–related protein (PTHrP), and still others by synthesizing vitamin D.

Hypercalcemia of any cause may be associated with symptoms that include anorexia, nausea and vomiting, constipation, weakness, confusion, and polyuria. At higher calcium levels, stupor, coma, and cardiac arrhythmias may occur.

Hyperparathyroidism

Hyperparathyroidism (HPT) is a consequence of excess secretion of PTH. Primary HPT occurs mostly in middle-aged to older adults. It once was thought to be an unusual problem, but an incidence of 0.1 percent has been found in asymptomatic adults since the advent of routine multiphasic serum chemistry analysis. In 80 percent of cases, the cause of primary HPT is a single hyperfunctioning benign parathyroid adenoma. In most of the remaining cases, all four parathyroid glands are hyperplastic and hyperfunctioning, and in a few patients, parathyroid carcinoma is found.

Secondary hyperparathyroidism occurs primarily in the setting of renal disease, in which vitamin D activation is inadequate, leading to decreased intestinal calcium absorption, and phosphate retention impairs bone responsiveness to PTH. In this circumstance, the parathyroids respond with excessive PTH secretion in an attempt to normalize serum calcium from the bone reservoir.

Occasionally, primary HPT is familial as an isolated abnormality or as part of the multiple endocrine neoplasia (MEN) syndrome, types 1 and 2a.

Clinical Findings

The clinical presentation of primary hyperparathyroidism is largely dependent on the level of hypercalcemia. Half or more of patients with primary HPT are asymptomatic and are discovered only when hypercalcemia is found on routine blood testing. In other patients, the symptoms are due to hypercalcemia, calcium deposition in tissues, and the effects of PTH on bone.

Hypercalcemia has a variety of neuromuscular effects. Anorexia, nausea and vomiting, and constipation are common. Neurologic effects, which may be subtle or profound, depending on the calcium level, include fatigue, weakness, confusion, stupor, and coma. Polyuria results from mild renal unresponsiveness to arginine vasopressin. Hypertension is more common in patients with hypercalcemia. Cardiac arrhythmias occur at high calcium levels.

High extracellular calcium can result in the precipitation of calcium salts. This occurs most commonly in the kidney, where about 10 percent of patients with primary HPT present with renal lithiasis. This occurs much less than it did in the past, when hyperparathyroidism went largely undiagnosed until symptoms developed.

Bone pain also occurs in HPT, and in some patients decreased bone density and osteoporosis result from the increased bone turnover. The classic bone disease of HPT, osteitis fibrosa cystica, is now uncommon. This abnormality consists of increased noncalcified space in bones, replacement with fibrous tissue, multiple lytic lesions on x-ray, and subperiosteal resorption that is seen best in the phalanges of the hands. Bone disease is more pronounced in secondary HPT than in primary HPT.

Diagnosis

The diagnosis of HPT begins with a demonstration of hypercalcemia after correction for serum albumin. When there is doubt about the significance of serum protein-binding effects, ionized calcium can be measured, but this is seldom necessary. The distinction of the cause of the hypercalcemia next depends on the serum PTH level.

The advent of hormone radioimmunoassays has made the differential diagnosis of HPT relatively straightforward. With the exceptions discussed below, only the hypercalcemia of HPT is associated with an increased PTH level, and this establishes the diagnosis. In all other cases of hypercalcemia, PTH is appropriately suppressed.

Several assays for PTH are available, but the best is the double antibody immunoradiometric assay (IRMA), which measures the intact PTH molecule. Other assays include the PTH N-terminal and C-terminal assays, which are not as useful. The C-terminal assay in particular is inaccurate in the setting of renal insufficiency, which is a common setting for hypercalcemia.

Clinical evaluation and routine laboratory tests are often sufficient to suggest the correct diagnosis of non–PTH-mediated hypercalcemia, such as malignancy, thyrotoxicosis, and renal disease.

There are two settings in which the cause of hypercalcemia is an abnormal set point of the PTH/calcium threshold. In these patients, the PTH level may not be suppressed in the setting of hypercalcemia and therefore must be distinguished from HPT. These cases are FHH and lithium therapy. In each case, there is an insensitivity of the parathyroid to calcium such that PTH continues to be secreted until the serum calcium level reaches a higher than normal level, at which point PTH secretion is inhibited. The PTH levels are typically normal, which is inappropriate for an increased calcium level, or only slightly increased.

FHH is distinguished from HPT by measuring the urinary excretion of calcium, which is normal to increased in HPT but low in FHH. FHH is a benign condition that does not require treatment and does not respond to parathyroidectomy, and so it is important to exclude it before proceeding to surgery for HPT.

The diagnosis of lithium-induced hypercalcemia is most easily established by demonstrating normalization of laboratory abnormalities when lithium is discontinued.

Treatment

Treatment of significant HPT is surgical. Removal of an adenoma is usually curative. Hyperplasia is treated by removing 3.5 parathyroid glands. Carcinoma is excised with wide margins. Pre- or intraoperative ultrasound can be useful in the localization of a parathyroid adenoma, but other imaging studies are not very helpful in HPT. Although various scanning techniques have been used, none adds much to direct observation carried out by a skilled parathyroid surgeon during neck exploration.

Postoperative hypocalcemia may require large doses of calcium and short-acting vitamin D until the normal function of the remaining parathyroid tissue returns.

Treatment of asymptomatic HPT is more controversial and depends on a number of factors. In general, surgery is recommended for patients less than 50 years old and those with serum calcium more than 1 to 1.5 mg/dL above normal, urinary calcium excretion higher than 400 mg/24 h, renal calcification on x-ray, or bone density more than 2 standard deviations below normal.

Patients who are not operated on should be followed carefully with serum and urinary calcium determinations and periodic radiographic studies.

HYPOCALCEMIA

Like hypercalcemia, hypocalcemia has a wide variety of causes, but it is much less common. Chronic hypocalcemia most often results from hypoparathyroidism, vitamin D insufficiency, or renal disease. Among the many causes of acute or transient hypocalcemia are parathyroidectomy, hypomagnesemia, and pancreatitis.

The symptoms of hypocalcemia include neuromuscular irritability with muscle and abdominal cramps, carpopedal spasm, tingling of the lips and hands, tetany, and convulsions. Chronic hypocalcemia also may be associated with personality changes and cataracts.

The classic physical signs of the neuromuscular irritability of hypocalcemia are Chvostek's sign and Trousseau's sign. Chvostek's sign is a contraction of the facial muscles that is elicited by tapping the facial nerve at its point of entry into the side of the face. Trousseau's sign is a carpal spasm that follows the inflation of a blood pressure cuff on the upper arm.

Hypoparathyroidism

Hypoparathyroidism most often follows parathyroid or thyroid surgery. The deficiency may be transient or permanent. There are also several forms of congenital, familial, and autoimmune hypoparathyroidism. Iron can accumulate in and damage the parathyroids in patients with hemochromatosis or iron overload from multiple transfusions.

Serum calcium corrected for albumin is low, and PTH is low. Serum magnesium should be checked, since magnesium is necessary for PTH secretion and hypomagnesemia will result in reversible hypoparathyroidism.

The goal of treatment is to maintain serum calcium in the low-normal range. Transient hypocalcemia may require only brief supplementation with intravenous or oral calcium, vitamin D, and magnesium if they are deficient. Chronic hypoparathyroidism is treated with calcium 1 to 3 g per day and vitamin D. Several forms of vitamin D are available for use, including vitamin D and 1,25-dihydroxyvitamin D. Vitamin D, ergocalciferol, is given in doses of 25,000 to 200,000 units per day. 1,25-dihydroxyvitamin D, calcitriol, is given in doses of 0.25 to 1.0 mg per day. High doses of vitamin D are required because in the absence of PTH, the 1-hydroxylation step in the kidneys is slow. When they are given along with calcium, however, both forms of vitamin D can result in hypercalcemia, and so careful monitoring is required.

BIBLIOGRAPHY

Beckerman P, Silver J: Vitamin D and the parathyroid. *Am J Med Sci* 317:363–369, 1999.

Fauci AS, Braunwald E, Isselbacher KJ, et al (eds): *Harrison's Principles of Internal Medicine,* 14th ed. New York, McGraw-Hill, 1998.

Grill V, Rankin W, Martin TJ: Parathyroid hormone-related protein (PTHrP) and hypercalcaemia. *Eur J Cancer* 34:222–229, 1998.

Kebebew E, Clark OH: Parathyroid adenoma, hyperplasia, and carcinoma: Localization, technical details of primary neck exploration, and treatment of hypercalcemic crisis. *Surg Oncol Clin North Am* 7:721–748, 1998.

Tierney LM Jr, McPhee SJ, Papadakis MA (eds): *Current Medical Diagnosis and Treatment,* 39th ed. New York, McGraw-Hill, 2000.

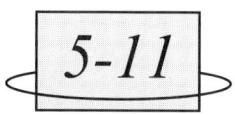

5-11 POSTERIOR PITUITARY DISORDERS

Timothy C. Evans

DISCUSSION

The posterior pituitary is an extension of neurons from specific areas in the hypothalamus through the pituitary stalk to a position posterior to the anterior pituitary in the sella turcica. The hormones secreted by the posterior pituitary are the peptides arginine vasopressin (AVP) [also known as antidiuretic hormone (ADH)] and oxytocin. AVP acts on the renal tubule, primarily at the collecting duct, to cause water reabsorption that results in urinary concentration. The release of AVP is coordinated with activation of the thirst center in the brain, which causes water-seeking behavior. The stimuli for AVP secretion are hemoconcentration and hypovolemia. Osmoreceptors in the hypothalamus are the primary regulators of AVP secretion. Even a small increase in hemoconcentration will result in increased AVP secretion and strikingly increased urine concentration. Hypotension, which is monitored by stretch receptors in the left atrium, carotids, and aorta, is also a potent stimulus for AVP secretion. A number of drugs can stimulate AVP release, and ethanol has a diuretic effect by inhibiting AVP secretion.

Oxytocin is a similar peptide hormone that has its major effects on the uterus and breast, causing uterine contraction and breast milk ejection, respectively, at the time of parturition.

DIABETES INSIPIDUS

Diabetes insipidus (DI) is an uncommon disease characterized by the inappropriate production of large quantities of dilute urine. It is caused by a deficiency of AVP or renal resistance to AVP. It must be distinguished from other causes of diuresis, such as increased water intake, diuretic use, and osmotic diuresis as in diabetes mellitus.

Clinical Presentation

The hallmark of diabetes insipidus is excess urine volume. In its most severe form, urine output may reach 20 L per day. In an otherwise healthy, conscious person, the polyuria is accompanied by intense polydipsia. When free access to water is available, there may be no other symptoms. In less severe forms of DI, with only a partial deficiency of posterior pituitary secretion of AVP, the urine output and thirst are less striking.

When water is not available or the patient is unconscious or unaware of thirst (as in the case of destructive lesions of the thirst center), dehydration, hypotension, and vascular collapse can follow rapidly, depending on the degree of AVP abnormality.

When urine loss is unmatched by water intake, the laboratory abnormalities include hypernatremia and hyperosmolality despite a large-volume hypotonic urine.

Etiology

Diabetes insipidus may be due to insufficient secretion of AVP or an inadequate renal response to AVP. Insufficient posterior pituitary AVP secretion—central DI—has several causes. Neoplastic, either benign or malignant, or infiltrative lesions such as sarcoid granulomas can result in partial or complete loss of AVP secretion. Pituitary or hypothalamic surgery and head trauma can interfere with AVP synthesis or its passage down the pituitary stalk to the posterior pituitary. Idiopathic DI also occurs and can be sporadic or familial. In each of these cases, the abnormality is insufficient secretion of AVP in response to hemoconcentration and hypovolemia.

Inadequate renal sensitivity to AVP is called nephrogenic DI. In this case, AVP is secreted by the posterior pituitary but the urine remains dilute. The causes of nephrogenic DI include intrinsic renal disease, hypokalemia, chronic hypercalcemia, systemic diseases such as sickle cell anemia, and drugs such as lithium and demeclocycline.

Diagnosis

A careful history and physical examination may reveal other causes of polyuria and polydipsia, such as systemic disease, diuretic or other drug use, and excess water intake (oral or intravenous). Serum glucose, potassium, and calcium levels should be checked.

When no other cause is apparent, the essence of DI evaluation is the serum and urine osmolality response to dehydration and AVP administration. Testing should be done under closely monitored conditions. Water intake is withheld, the patient's vital signs are monitored, and serum and urine osmolality are followed frequently. DI is characterized by increasing serum osmolality but persistently low urine osmolality. An injection of AVP (or the synthetic AVP analogue desmopressin) is then administered. Patients with central DI show increased urine concentration, while patients with nephrogenic DI have no response. Serum AVP measured before the administration of exogenous AVP is low in central DI patients and elevated in nephrogenic DI patients.

Treatment

Treatment of central or nephrogenic DI secondary to other central nervous system (CNS), systemic, or renal disease should include attention to the underlying disease. The water metabolism abnormality of central DI is relatively easily and conveniently treated in most patients with desmopressin given as an intranasal spray 0.05 to 0.1 mL once or twice a day. The less common nephrogenic DI is more difficult to treat and may require thiazide diuretics to decrease the glomerular filtration rate and limit renal water loss.

SYNDROME OF INAPPROPRIATE ANTIDIURETIC HORMONE

The syndrome of inappropriate antidiuretic hormone (SIADH) is characterized by euvolemic hyponatremia. By definition, increased AVP (or ADH) is not inappropriate when it is secreted in circumstances of hypovolemia or hyperosmolality. Thus, SIADH is not present in cases of hypovolemic hyponatremia such as mineralocorticoid deficiency, dehydration, or diuretic use with free fluid replacement. Similarly, SIADH is not present in conditions of edematous hypervolemic hyponatremia such as congestive heart failure, the nephrotic syndrome, and renal disease. AVP secretion rates are also high in hypernatremic dehydration without fluid replacement but again are not inappropriate.

Clinical Presentation

Most often SIADH is discovered by the finding of hyponatremia on electrolyte testing. Since SIADH sometimes is associated with other diseases, the symptoms may be limited to those of the underlying disease. In other cases, the hyponatremia itself, if it is severe enough, may cause symptoms that include lethargy, confusion, stupor, and coma. Neuromuscular excitability, muscle twitches, or even seizures can occur if the serum sodium is very low or if the decrease is rapid. Symptoms are unusual if serum sodium is higher than 125 meq/L.

Etiology

Since AVP is synthesized in the hypothalamus, the cause of SIADH is often neurologic. In these cases, which include stroke, meningitis, tumors, and trauma, there is assumed to be an abnormality of neural input to the hypothalamus or of the perception of neural input by the hypothalamus that leads to inappropriate AVP release. In other cases, SIADH results from ectopic overproduction of AVP by tumors, primarily small cell lung carcinomas, and is associated with a variety of other pulmonary diseases, such as infections and asthma. Furthermore, a wide variety of drugs have been associated with SIADH, including hypoglycemic agents such as chlorpropamide, neuroactive drugs such as amitriptyline and carbamazepine, and antineoplastic drugs, among others.

Diagnosis

The diagnosis is suggested by the finding of hyponatremia. Serum uric acid and blood urea nitrogen are frequently low because of increased urinary clearance. The physical examination of volume status is critical in the diagnosis. Dehydration with postural change in pulse and blood pressure and volume overload with edema by definition rule out the diagnosis of SIADH.

Urinary sodium is also helpful in the evaluation of hyponatremia. If urine sodium is low (less than 20 meq/L) and there is evidence of dehydration, total body sodium is depleted and the treatment consists of normal saline. Dehydration and normal or elevated urine sodium suggest renal disease, diuretic use, or adrenocortical insufficiency. The immediate treatment consists of normal saline to replete volume. Expanded volume with low urine sodium suggests inadequate renal perfusion such as that which occurs with congestive heart failure, and the

correct response is to treat the underlying disease. SIADH is characterized by no edema and elevated urinary sodium resulting from increased renal clearance.

Treatment

Just as DI is treated by administering water, SIADH is treated by water restriction and the provision of adequate sodium in the diet. If there are underlying etiologic features that can be treated, such as CNS or pulmonary disease, they obviously should be addressed. The drugs administered to the patient should be reviewed to see if they may be causative and should be modified if possible. Water restriction results in slow, safe correction of hyponatremia. The patient is typically asymptomatic as long as the serum sodium remains above 125 meq/L.

There are circumstances in which more rapid correction of hyponatremia is indicated, but this treatment entails significant risks to the patient. When serum sodium has been chronically low, it is often asymptomatic and can be corrected slowly. When serum sodium is less than 120 meq/L and is associated with symptoms, however, which often occurs when the hyponatremia is very severe or develops rapidly, the correction also should be more rapid. This generally is accomplished by administering hypertonic saline with close monitoring at a rate that leads to a serum sodium increase not exceeding about 0.5 meq/L/h until serum sodium is above 120 meq/L. More rapid correction can lead to brain swelling and a fatal CNS demyelination syndrome called central pontine myelinolysis.

BIBLIOGRAPHY

Fauci AS, Braunwald E, Isselbacher KJ, et al (eds): *Harrison's Principles of Internal Medicine,* 14th ed. New York, McGraw-Hill, 1998.
Miller KL: Diabetes insipidus. *ANNA J* 23:285–292, 1996.
Mitchell DH, Owens B: Replacement therapy: Arginine vasopressin (AVP), growth hormone (GH), cortisol, thyroxine, testosterone and estrogen. *J Neurosci Nurs* 28:140–152, 1996.
Molitch ME: Pituitary diseases in pregnancy. *Semin Perinatol* 22:457–470, 1998.
Naidich MJ, Russell EJ: Current approaches to imaging of the sellar region and pituitary. *Endocrinol Metab Clin North Am* 28:45–79, 1999.
Otsuka F, Kageyama J, Ogura T, Hattori T, Makino H: Sheehan's syndrome of more than 30 years' duration: An endocrine and MRI study of 6 cases. *Endocr J* 45:451–458, 1998.
Tierney LM Jr, McPhee SJ, Papadakis MA (eds): *Current Medical Diagnosis and Treatment,* 39th ed. New York, McGraw-Hill, 2000.

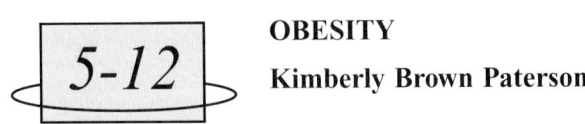

5-12 OBESITY
Kimberly Brown Paterson

DISCUSSION

Obesity is a chronic disease that affects many people and often requires long-term treatment to promote and sustain weight loss. With more than one-third of American adults currently defined as obese [body mass index (BMI) greater than 27 kg/m²], it represents a common and serious health problem. It has been implicated as the cause of many illnesses, including diabetes mellitus, coronary heart disease, hypertension, and several cancers (colon, rectum, prostate, uterus, biliary tract, breast, and ovary).

Studies have shown that diseases associated with obesity, including diabetes, hypertension, and dyslipidemia, can improve after a 10 percent loss in weight.[1] Information from the Third National Health and Nutrition Examination Survey (NHANES III) shows that approximately 33% of men, 36% of women, 14% of children 6 to

11 years of age, and 12% of adolescents 12 to 17 years old are obese. This was a marked increase in the statistics for all the age groups reported in the NHANES II 1976–1980 study.

It is important not only to note weight percentages but also to evaluate weight distribution. Fat distribution patterns are determined by measuring waist and hip circumferences and calculating the waist to hip ratio (WHR).[2]

The android pattern (male-pattern or abdominal obesity) has a WHR higher than 0.85 for females and 0.95 for males. The gynoid pattern (female-pattern or gluteal obesity) has a WHR lower than 0.85 for females and 0.95 for males. Recent data suggest that excess fat around the waist and flank is a greater health hazard than is fat in the thighs and buttocks. Obese patients with a high WHR have a significantly greater risk of diabetes, stroke, coronary artery disease, and early death than do equally obese patients with a lower WHR.[2]

DIAGNOSIS

Until recently, obesity was thought to be related to an excessive intake of calories along with a sedentary lifestyle. However, strong evidence points toward genetic, medical, and environmental factors as influencing the development of obesity. Specific causes of excessive weight are multifactorial. Rare genetic syndromes have been described, as have more common causes, such as insulinoma, hypothalamic disorders, Cushing's syndrome, and the use of corticosteroid drugs. Idiopathic obesity generally is thought to be due to an imbalance between food intake and energy expenditure (including physical activity and metabolic rate).[3]

The diagnosis of obesity is based largely on the history and complete physical examination. Historic information regarding age at onset is particularly important, as prepuberty and young adulthood appear to be sensitive periods for the development of obesity. Family history, eating and exercise behavior, recent weight changes, occupational history, previous weight loss history, and psychosocial factors also should be addressed. Information related to the use of laxatives, hormones, and nutritional supplements should draw attention.

Physical examination should assess the degree and distribution of body fat, overall nutritional status, and, as was noted above, possible secondary causes, including hypothalamic disorders and Cushing's syndrome. Hypothyroidism can cause obesity secondary to diminished energy needs. Cushing's syndrome causes obesity involving centripetal fat stores, the face, and cervical or supraclavicular fat deposits. Insulinoma causes obesity from increased energy intake secondary to recurrent hypoglycemia. The Laurence-Moon-Biedl and Prader-Willi syndromes are rare disorders that are thought to be hypothalamic in origin and feature obesity and hypogonadism.

LABORATORY STUDIES

Further studies to rule out these possible causes should include serum thyroid–stimulating hormone (TSH) determination and dexamethasone suppression testing. Laboratory evaluation of all patients ideally should include cardiac risk factors: serum cholesterol, triglycerides, and glucose.

TREATMENTS

Treatment studies for weight reduction vary widely. The most successful programs include behavior modification and low-fat, low-calorie eating combined with aerobic exercise. The overall goal must be weight maintenance. Most important, the job of the practitioner is to provide long-term follow-up to prevent further weight gain or regain after weight loss. The primary goal of obesity treatment should be to reduce the overall comorbid diseases and improve overall health, not just to make the patient thin. Recent studies show that only 20 percent of patients will lose 20 lb and maintain that loss for over 2 years and

5 percent will maintain a 40-lb weight loss. In light of this information, it can be a difficult task to develop an appropriate program for weight maintenance.

The steps include the following:

1. *Nutritional principles* must apply to obese as well as normal-weight individuals. Low-fat, low-calorie, high-fiber, and complex carbohydrate foods should be the staple of weight loss. Foods that provide large amounts of calories and little nutritional value should be restricted greatly. Special diets that advocate restriction to one or two foods, offer a high protein intake, or limit carbohydrate intake are of little value.
2. *Behavior modification* provides useful techniques. Planning and recording are specific skills that can reveal habits and cues that are emotional and/or situational. They also may provide a source of information that can assist the practitioner in problem solving.
3. *Exercise provides* multiple benefits. An aerobic exercise program most importantly can increase daily energy expenditure. It is also helpful in preventing the decrease in basal energy expenditure seen in low-calorie and low-nutrient diets. Unfortunately, many people believe that no benefit will be gained if they do not participate in vigorous exercise for at least 20 min three or more times week. Revised guidelines from the surgeon general's report on physical activity and health indicate that cardiovascular health can be derived from a routine of 30 min of daily, accumulated activity.[4]
4. *Long-term maintenance* also should be included. Social support can be drawn from a therapist, family members, or peer group involvement to reinforce behavioral change.

Medications, both over the counter and prescriptive, are the most popular obesity treatments. Most often used in the management of obesity are medications known as "appetite suppressants." These medications promote weight loss by decreasing appetite or increasing the feeling of fullness. Appetite suppressants decrease appetite by increasing serotonin or catecholamine, two brain chemicals that affect mood and appetite. Most of the currently available appetite suppressant medications are approved for short-term use only by the U.S. Food and Drug Administration (FDA), meaning a few weeks or months. Sibutramine (Meridia) is the only appetite suppressant approved for longer-term use in significantly obese individuals, although the safety and effectiveness have not been established for use beyond 1 year. A list of prescription appetite-suppressant medications is given in Table 5-12-1.

Because appetite suppressant medications are used to treat a condition that affects millions of people, their potential for side effects is of great concern. Two approved appetite suppressant medications that affect serotonin release and reuptake have been withdrawn from the market (fenfluramine and dexfenfluramine). Medications that affect catecholamine levels (such as phentermine, diethylpropion, and mazindol) may cause symptoms of sleeplessness, nervousness, and euphoria (feeling of well-being). Sibutramine acts on both the serotonin and catecholamine systems, but unlike fenfluramine and dexfenfluramine,

TABLE 5-12-1. Prescription Appetite Suppressant Medications

GENERIC NAME	TRADE NAME
Benzphetamine	Didrex
Dexfenfluramine	Redux (withdrawn)
Diethylpropion	Tenuate, Tenuate Dospan
Fenfluramine	Pondimin (withdrawn)
Mazindol	Sanorex, Mazanor
Phendimetrazine	Bontril, Plegine, Pre-Lu 2, X-Trozine
Phentermine	Adipex-P, Fastin, Ionamin, Obi-trim
Sibutramine	Meridia

it does not cause the release of serotonin from cells. The primary known side effects of sibutramine of concern are elevations in blood pressure and pulse. Patients with poorly controlled high blood pressure, heart disease, irregular heart rhythm, or a history of stroke should not take sibutramine.[6]

Other drugs that may have potential as antiobesity medications include the following:

Orlistat (Xenical): a pancreatic lipase antagonist that prevents absorption of fat in the gastrointestinal (GI) tract
Acarbose (Precose, Prandase): an oral hypoglycemic agent that reduces glucose absorption and may work to reduce weight.[5]

Surgery is usually considered the last resort. More than 100,000 obese patients have opted for vertical-banded gastroplasty or gastric bypass procedures. A BMI above 40—which means about 100 pounds of overweight for men and 80 pounds for women—indicates that a person is severely obese and therefore is a candidate for surgery. This also may be an option for people with a BMI of 35 to 40 who suffer from life-threatening cardiopulmonary problems or diabetes.

The risks for pouch stretching, band erosion, breakdown of staple lines, and leakage of stomach contents into the abdomen are about the same for gastric bypass as they are for vertical-banded gastroplasty. However, because gastric bypass operations cause food to skip the duodenum, where most iron and calcium are absorbed, the risks for nutritional deficiencies are higher in these procedures. Anemia may result from malabsorption of vitamin B_{12} and iron in menstruating women, and decreased absorption of calcium may bring on osteoporosis and metabolic bone disease. Patients may be required to take nutritional supplements that usually prevent these deficiencies.[6]

DISPOSITION

The prevention or avoidance of obesity starts with regular exercise and a reasonable diet, especially in children and young adults. Patient education materials along with excellent advice and answers to tough questions can be obtained from the following sources[6]:

AMERICAN DIETETIC ASSOCIATION
216 West Jackson Boulevard, Suite 700
Chicago, IL 60606-6995
(312) 899-0040
www.eatright.org

AMERICAN HEART ASSOCIATION
7320 Greenville Avenue
Dallas, TX 75231
800-AHA-USA1
www.amhrt.org

LEARN EDUCATION CENTER
P.O. Box 35328
Department 70
Dallas, TX 75235
800-736-7323

LOWFAT LIFELINE
Department 23
P.O. Box 1889
Port Townsend, WA 98368
800-294-9801
lowfat@olympus.net

WEIGHT CONTROL INFORMATION CENTER
1 Win Way
Bethesda, MD 20892
(301) 984-7378
win@info.niddk.nih.gov

REFERENCES

1. Goodrick GK, Foreyt JP: Why treatments for obesity don't last. *J Amer Dietetic Assoc* 91(10):1243–1247, 1991.
2. Schroeder SA: *Current Medical Diagnosis and Treatment*. Norwalk, CT, Appleton & Lange, 1992, pp 950–959.
3. Fauci AS, Braunwald E, Isselbacher KJ, et al (eds): *Harrison's Principles of Internal Medicine,* 14th ed. Companion Handbook. New York, McGraw-Hill, 1998, pp 227–232.
4. Kushner K, Hopson S: Obesity therapy: What works—what doesn't. *Consultant* 38 (3): 511–518, 1998.
5. Paterson KB: *Healthweighs: A Ten Week Comprehensive Weight Management Program.* U.S. Copyright TX 489964, 1991.
6. Ridings H, Rapp D, Boosalis M, Pomeroy C: Primary care management of adult obesity. *Physician Assist* 22(4):35–57, 1998.

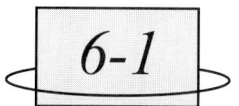

ACUTE GASTROENTERITIS
Anne P. Heinly

DESCRIPTION

Acute gastroenteritis (AGE) is a common diagnosis that is uncommonly hard to define. Some textbooks do not list it as an entity. Alternative names include viral diarrhea, stomach flu, infectious diarrhea, and rotavirus infection. By consensus, it is a self-limiting viral or bacterial inflammation of the stomach and small intestines that produces a characteristic set of symptoms in every human being at some time in his or her life. The colon may be involved with AGE, but these incidents usually are listed independently as colitis (see Chap. 6-4). The vast majority of cases are viral infections (an estimated 40 to 50 percent), and the remainder are probably short-lived food-borne bacterial infections. Infants and young children have on average two episodes of AGE before age 3 and gain immunity to these particular viral pathogens in the process. The majority of adult patients will have two to three episodes of AGE in a lifetime, although environmental factors such as living conditions, widespread food contamination, and travel to developing countries may increase the frequency dramatically.

PATHOGENESIS

Viral infections of the gastrointestinal tract frequently cause nausea and vomiting with a secretory diarrhea. There is an increase in chloride and water secretion with the inhibition of normal intestinal mucosal sodium and water absorption. The result is copious watery diarrhea without pus or blood. Rotavirus infections are more common in children and can cause incredible loss of fluids. The Norwalk virus is more prevalent in school-age children and adults. Both virus and bacteria are found in tainted food and drinking water. They also are spread by the oral-fecal route, which accounts for the majority of community outbreaks. Table 6-1-1 lists the usual causes of acute gastroenteritis. Note the overlap with acute and chronic diarrheal pathogens (see Chap. 6-7).

SYMPTOMS

The classic symptoms of acute gastroenteritis are the sudden onset of watery diarrhea, one stool about every half hour to an hour; nausea and vomiting every 1 or 2 h; and abdominal cramps, malaise (generalized aches and pains), anorexia, fatigue, low-grade fever, dull headache, and chills. These symptoms can appear within 4 h of contamination or as late as 48 h later. The vast majority start resolving in 6 to 24 h. It is not uncommon to see a patient in the office *after* the worst is over.

The very young, the very old, and immunosuppressed patients can become quite ill with this usually self-limiting condition. Infants and toddlers can suffer severe dehydration with a history of decreased tears, less urination, poor feeding, and/or lethargy as key points to explore with the parents. The aged may have a change in mental status or become obtunded secondary to dehydration and electrolyte imbalances. In immunosuppressed persons (HIV, chemotherapy patients, renal disease), these simple infections can be life-threatening with sepsis and prolongation of symptoms. All these groups deserve special attention and close follow-up.

OBJECTIVE

An ill-appearing patient will lie quietly on the examination table, frequently pale and fatigued. Vital signs may reveal a normotensive patient with tachycardia. Orthostatic vital signs may be positive (blood pressure down 10 points, pulse up 20 points), depending on the level of dehydration. Pulses may be diminished with decreased capillary refill. Oral mucosa may be dry with slight halitosis. Check the skin and eyes for evidence of dehydration. Abdominal examination usually reveals a nondistended appearance with hyperactive bowel sounds. Palpation may reveal a soft, diffusely tender abdomen without mass effect or rebound tenderness. The area is usually tympanic, and there is no hepatosplenomegaly. Rectal examination is usually negative for findings, including blood.

DIAGNOSTIC CONSIDERATIONS

The danger of an AGE diagnosis is that so many other disease processes can present with similar symptoms. Clues pointing to AGE include the following: severity of symptoms (AGE is usually mild); peak frequency is in the fall and winter; exposures usually are easily tracked; and the patient should be much improved within 24 to 48 h. However, AGE symptoms can represent anything from early appendicitis to multiple myeloma (see Table 6-1-2). An index of suspicion is required when one sees AGE in a community outbreak. A more serious diagnosis may be lurking, and the young, the elderly, and the immunosuppressed may have a more virulent course.

Raw seafood continues to be a source of AGE, with viral gastroenteritis associated with the consumption of raw shellfish, specifically oysters. Other viral and bacterial pathogens have been identified, including *Vibrio* species, *Salmonella, Campylobacter,* and hepatitis A.

Also consider a different diagnosis when a patient has had several episodes of AGE in a short period. The average adult will have only two to three episodes of AGE in a lifetime. If a patient is having frequent episodes, consider chronic infectious disorders, peptic ulcer disease, irritable bowel syndrome, obstruction disorders, Crohn's disease, and ulcerative colitis.

LABORATORY TESTS

Identification of the specific virus causing an episode of AGE is difficult in common practice. There are laboratories that make the diagnosis with immune electron microscopy and enzyme immunoassays. More commonly, no laboratory studies are done during the first 24 h of a classic acute gastroenteritis. Stool cultures for bacterial causes can be done and are warranted if the patient is very ill, an infant, elderly, or immunosuppressed. Remember, stool culture results can be altered by certain treatments and tests, such as the barium swallow/upper gastrointestinal (UGI) series, D-xylose absorption tests, and antidiarrheal medications. It is advisable to perform cultures first.

Laboratory evaluation should be done if the symptoms have not abated with a clear liquid diet within 24 to 48 h. Laboratory studies should be directed toward the most likely chronic cause of diarrhea, nausea, and vomiting. At the very least, that would include a complete blood count (CBC), chemistry studies, urinalysis (UA) and stool for ova and parasites (O & P), white and red blood cells, and cultures.

TABLE 6-1-1. Acute Gastroenteritis Pathogens

Rotavirus	Virus, usually before age 3 years, partial immunity conferred, community outbreaks in fall and spring, vaccine under development
Norwalk virus	Virus, adults and children, no immunity conferred, food- and water-borne, community outbreaks year-round
Astrovirus	Virus, usually children or immunosuppressed adults, immunity unknown, small community outbreaks year-round
Calcivirus	Same as Norwalk virus
Enteric adenovirus	Same as astrovirus, responsible for up to 10% of community outbreaks
Vibrio species	Bacteria, children and adults, epidemic outbreaks usually in unsanitary conditions (*V. cholerae*), vaccines under development
Cryptosporidium	Coccidian parasite, usually in immunocompromised patients, lasts 1–2 weeks, spread by oral-fecal route
Cyclospora	Coccidian parasite, water-borne transmission, epidemic in unsanitary conditions
Staphylococcus aureus	Bacterial enterotoxin, food-borne from contaminated hands, children and adults, no immunity conferred
Bacillus cereus	Bacterial enterotoxin, cooked rice is most common vector, children and adults, no immunity conferred
Escherichia coli	Bacterial enterotoxin, contaminated undercooked meats, children at greater risk, can be life-threatening, no immunity conferred

RADIOLOGIC (IMAGING) STUDIES

Imaging studies are rarely done for the diagnosis of AGE. One may order a flat and upright plain abdominal radiograph to aid in the differential diagnosis. If symptoms persist, the use of imaging studies increases, depending on what the source is thought to be.

TABLE 6-1-2. Differential Diagnosis for Acute Gastroenteritis

Ulcerative colitis	Diarrhea, blood, pus, LLQ* cramping pain
Crohn's disease	Diarrhea, blood, RLQ* pain

Infectious
  Shigella
  Salmonella
  Campylobacter
  Clostridium difficile
	Diarrhea, usually lasts longer and/or more severe, associated with blood and pus, leukocytosis

Hyperthyroidism	Diarrhea, no blood or pus, no abdominal cramping
Irritable bowel syndrome	Diarrhea, usually associated with stress, no systemic symptoms. Does not wake patient
Medication-induced diarrhea	Magnesium antacids, antibiotics, prokinetic agents, laxative abuse

Acute abdomen
  Appendicitis
  Cholecystitis
  Pancreatitis
  Diverticulitis
	Diarrhea, nausea, vomiting, fever, abdominal pain
	Localization of pain, peritoneal irritation; leukocytosis, chemistry changes

*LLQ = left lower quadrant; RLQ = right lower quadrant.

TREATMENT

The patient will expect an antidiarrheal or antiemetic medication. The real objective in treatment is the replacement of fluids and electrolytes, especially in children and the elderly. Any patient who is unable to tolerate oral fluids will require intravenous fluid replacement. An infant most likely will need hospitalization for rehydration. In children who are able to drink and are not severely ill, oral hydration is recommended. An adult may be able to receive 2 L of fluid in the office setting before being sent home under observation. Table 6-1-3 reviews appropriate clear liquid diets and recommended intravenous (IV) replacement fluids. The patient should sip or drink about 8 oz fluid an hour and can gauge the level of hydration by the frequency of urination.

If the patient is using any medication that may add to dehydration (diuretics), consider stopping it or decreasing the dose during the acute phase of AGE. Antidiarrheals are not recommended (though commonly given) for the vast majority of patients with AGE. Since AGE is a short, self-limiting process and responds well to fluid replacement, medications are not essential. The addition of an antidiarrheal may actually prolong the infectious process. Antibiotics are not appropriate and are ineffective for a viral illness. Antiemetics are not necessary unless the patient is unable to tolerate sipping fluids.

COMPLICATIONS

By far the most common complication is dehydration. Infants can become severely dehydrated very quickly—within hours of the initial symptoms. Signs of dehydration include low urine output, dry mouth and eyelids, orthostatic dizziness, confusion, and change in mentation. In infants, it is important to observe for poor skin turgor and sunken fontanelles as well.

PATIENT EDUCATION

The spread of AGE is primarily by the oral-fecal route. Patients can diminish the spread of the virus in the home by performing good, regular hand washing. Convince patients that they do not need antiemetics and antidiarrheals to deal with simple acute gastroenteritis. Proper education about fluid and electrolyte replacement cannot be stressed enough. Additionally, it is cheaper for the patient to use an electrolyte-rich drink for 24 h than to buy two medications. Another important aspect of education is the admonition to return for follow-up if symptoms persist or increase past 24 to 48 h. The expectation is that the

TABLE 6-1-3. Fluid and Electrolyte Replacement

Oral hydration: water, sodium, potassium, chloride, and citrate
  Pedialyte
  Naturalyte
  Infalyte

WHO/UNICEF oral rehydration salts

Homemade electrolyte solution can be mixed with sugar-free Kool-Aid or similar drink
  Half gallon of water
  4–5 teaspoons of sugar
  1 teaspoon (each) of table salt and baking soda

Intravenous fluids
  Ringer's lactate with 20–40 meq potassium
    Children: 30 mL/kg in first h, then 40 mL/kg in next 2 h
    Adults: 2 L over first 1 1/2 h, then 125 mL/h if needed

Avoid
  Any food should be avoided until hunger pangs begin, usually in 24 h
  Avoid cheese, milk, fried foods, red meat, peanut butter, oils, and foods made of these for at least 24 h, preferably 48 h
  Progress diet with dry crackers, thin soups, bread, and simple fruits

nausea, vomiting, and diarrhea should be gone within 24 h. The fatigue, anorexia, and aches and pain should be gone within 48 h. If symptoms persist, look for exacerbating sources (such as the patient eating an exacerbating meal) or look at the differential diagnoses.

PREVENTION

Prevention comes first. Educate the patient about good hand washing. Also, foods should be kept hot or cold as is appropriate. Refrigerated food should be heated thoroughly to decrease the risk of bacterial food poisoning. A vaccination for rotavirus is under investigation, since that virus is the most common source of AGE in the world and can cause devastating dehydration. Length of immunization is a problem to date. Like the virus itself, the immunity conferred appears to be limited.

PEARLS

After upper respiratory infections, acute gastroenteritis may be the next most common diagnosis. The patient is ill but not writhing in pain. The diarrhea and vomiting usually subside within 6 h. Look for the frequency and timing of diarrhea and vomiting. The average patient will report that he or she woke up and did both about every half hour to an hour. If the patient has been in your office for 1 h and reports that the last stool or vomitus was an hour or more before seeing you, it is likely that this episode is well on the way to resolution. Ensure rehydration and electrolyte replacement and encourage the patient to avoid fatty, greasy, milky foods for at least 24 h. Educate rather than medicate.

BIBLIOGRAPHY

Keepkens MD, Hoekstra JH: Chronic nonspecific diarrhea of childhood: Pathophysiology and management. *Pediatr Clini North Am* 43(2):375–386, 1996.

The management of acute gastroenteritis in young children: American Academy of Pediatrics. *Pediatrics* 97(3): 1996, www.aap.org/policy/gastro.htm.

Rotavirus vaccine for the prevention of rotavirus gastroenteritis among children. *MMWR* 48(RR2):1999.

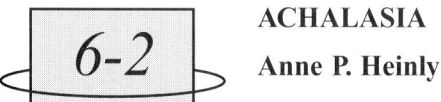

ACHALASIA
Anne P. Heinly

DISCUSSION

Achalasia is the most common motor disorder of the esophagus, affecting 2 to 3 per 10,000 people in a lifetime. The term *achalasia* literally means "failure to relax." It is actually a twofold process: no peristalsis (or very weak peristalsis) and lack of lower esophageal sphincter (LES) relaxation. This combination leads to the retention of ingested food, which progressively dilates the esophageal body. Although the etiology is still unknown, investigations are pursuing a degenerative lesion in the vagus nerve to explain this lack of neuromuscular response. There is equal distribution between men and women, and it is more commonly seen in older individuals.

PATHOGENESIS

The esophagus is basically a conduit for food intake. The upper esophageal sphincter (UES) is constructed entirely of striated muscle and is an important factor in the motor function of the esophagus. The first phase of the swallowing mechanism begins with the oropharyngeal contraction regulated by an intricate neuromuscular reflex, which sends a smooth single peristaltic wave down the entire length of the esophagus. The UES is probably responsible for the sensory input of heartburn and pain arising from a large bolus or tissue irritation. The resting pressure that keeps the UES closed is estimated at 101 mmHg. This is a protective mechanism against regurgitation and can be overcome only by the sudden bursts associated with burping or vomiting.

The body of the esophagus begins as striated muscle and converts to smooth muscle at the distal end. Secondary peristalsis is a normal physiologic response to the presence of a bolus. The spreading contraction aids the continued movement of food to the stomach. The esophagus is lined with squamous epithelium that is easily damaged by pH levels <4. It is the disruption of the squamous epithelium by alcohol, tobacco, chemicals, and the like that predisposes the esophagus to disease.

The final player in achalasia and esophageal disease in general is the LES. Its complex neurohormonal muscular activity defines esophageal emptying. If it is too tight, food cannot exit; if it is too loose, gastric juices can reflux. It can malfunction by pure mechanics, such as obstruction, stricture, ulcer, edema, or varices. It can be affected by neuromuscular diseases, infection, medications, tobacco, and alcohol.

SYMPTOMS

Achalasia classically presents as progressive dysphagia with about one-third of patients complaining of chest pain. These patients develop a cough (especially at night) caused by regurgitation of material trapped in the esophagus traversing the bronchus. Patients may first present with recurrent pneumonia or frequent upper respiratory infections (URIs). With progression of the disease, patients are not able to vomit or belch without great difficulty because they cannot increase intrathoracic pressures sufficiently to overcome the blockage. Weight loss from malnutrition is common late in the disease (food never makes it to the stomach). Halitosis and nocturnal regurgitation are common and can be differentiated from gastroesophageal reflux disease (GERD) regurgitation by the lack of oral ulcers. Patient may describe bizarre postures and maneuvers that literally shake the food down.

OBJECTIVE

The physical examination is usually noncontributory. The most likely finding is evidence of anemia and/or weight loss. Halitosis may be present, and with respiratory complications evidence of pneumonia may be found.

DIAGNOSTIC CONSIDERATIONS

The most common mimickers of achalasia include obstructive diseases. The malignancies and the variant achalasia listed in Table 6-2-1 can confuse the picture until definitive biopsies can be done. Some history clues that favor malignancies include significant weight loss over a short period (6 months or less) and chest pain. While achalasia may cause chest pressure or fullness after meals, carcinomas usually have progressive, steady, deep pain.

LABORATORY TESTS

No specific laboratory studies define achalasia. Standard studies such as complete blood cell count (CBC), chemistries, and *Helicobacter pylori* titers may be helpful in defining anemias and ruling out the differential diagnosis.

RADIOLOGIC (IMAGING) STUDIES

Radiologic studies are the mainstay of diagnosis for achalasia. A simple chest x-ray may reveal a widened mediastinum with air-fluid levels. Barium swallows reveal a distended esophageal body with a

TABLE 6-2-1.   Differential Diagnosis for Achalasia

Vigorous achalasia	Simultaneous, high-amplitude contraction in the distal esophagus with increased LES tone; significant pain and dysphagia, mimics angina
Diffuse esophageal spasm (DES)	Asynchronous, random contractions; chest pain, dysphagia exacerbated by hot or cold foods
Gastric adenocarcinoma	Weight loss, dysphagia, early satiety, pain exacerbated by food, nausea, and vomiting
Squamous cell carcinoma of the esophagus	Progressive dysphagia, weight loss, lymphadenopathy, cough, hoarseness, GI bleeding
Chagas' disease	American trypanosomiasis, megaesophagus, often seen in children, cardiomyopathy, periorbital edema, megacolon, myxedema
Sarcoidosis	Affecting the young, hilar lymphadenopathy (causing achalasia symptoms), pulmonary symptoms with infiltrates, ocular and skin lesions
Scleroderma	80% will have esophageal symptoms, including dysphagia with decreased peristalsis; GERD occurs as well; diffuse fibrosis and vascular changes to the skin, heart, kidneys, etc.
Myasthenia gravis	A pure motor syndrome, it attacks the UES with subsequent dysphagia and cough; ocular symptoms and proximal limb weakness are distinguishing
Angina pectoris	Pressure-like chest pain usually substernal; not usually associated with dysphagia; dyspnea and nausea

beak-like distal LES. The use of amyl nitrite during the barium swallow can help distinguish achalasia from a constricting malignancy; amyl nitrate causes LES relaxation, which will not respond in the presence of achalasia. Esophageal manometry can help differentiate the variant types of achalasia. The archetypical finding reveals no primary peristaltic wave and very low amplitude secondary waves (bolus type). At the LES, resting pressures can be as high as 90 mmHg (normal is 1 to 20 mmHg). The final definitive study is an endoscopic procedure that allows for direct visualization and biopsies. Biopsies may reveal the absence of neural plexus in esophageal muscle layers.

TREATMENT

Calcium channel blockers, nitrates of all varieties, hydralazine, and anticholinergics all have been tried to loosen the LES tone. All have been less than successful. Dilatation of the LES can be accomplished with bougienage (for short-term relief) or pneumatic dilators, which can achieve good results for long periods. The problem with dilatation is that the more often it is performed, the less likely it is to help. An experimental treatment, that appears hopeful is the injection of the LES with botulinum toxin. An intrasphincter injection of toxin provides a strong inhibitor of neuromuscular transmission, causing relaxation for up to 6 weeks in some patients. The most definitive therapy is an esophagomyotomy, incising the anterior LES extending less than 1 cm into the stomach. The myotomy decreases LES pressure, and with a proper procedure the sphincter competency is preserved, although up to 10 percent of patients may develop reflux esophagitis.

COMPLICATIONS

Weight loss, anemia, and pulmonary complications are common in patients with untreated achalasia. During investigation, esophageal rupture can occur. Therapy, however, has its own complications. GERD is the natural consequence of releasing LES tone. The patient may have severe symptoms and require aggressive therapy for control (see Chap. 6-11). The risk of developing esophageal carcinoma from achalasia is unclear. Certainly after myotomy, the risk increases owing to the chronic GERD.

PEARLS

Achalasia and its variants can mimic angina, myocardial infarction, chronic GERD, and other diseases. Esophageal disease warrants careful investigation to rule out malignancies and other systemic diseases. The presentation is quite classic, but it also may present simply as a recurrent URI. Medications are limited, leaving dilatation or surgery as the only option for most patients.

BIBLIOGRAPHY

Gordon JM, Eaker E: Prospective study of esophageal botulinum toxin injections in high-risk achalasia patients. *Am J Gastroenterol* 92(10):1812–1816, 1997.

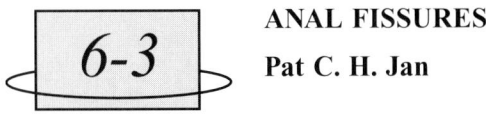

ANAL FISSURES
6-3
Pat C. H. Jan

DISCUSSION

Anal fissures (fissures in ano) are linear tears in the anal mucosa brought on by episodes of diarrhea, constipation, trauma (including anal intercourse), and associated inflammatory bowel disease. Fissures are found in equal numbers in men and women. They commonly are located in the posterior midline and rarely in the anterior midline.

SIGNS AND SYMPTOMS

These patients generally present with complaints of severe anal pain with and after bowel movements. They also may relate episodes of bleeding after each bowel movement. The severity of the pain often leads the patient (especially children) to hold back on future bowel movements. This negative reinforcement leads to the vicious cycle of constipation, pain with defecation, and worsening of the preexisting anal fissure.

OBJECTIVE FINDINGS

Typically the diagnosis can be made by history. In cases of severe pain, it may be difficult to examine the anal canal. Gentle exposure by spreading the buttocks along with verbal reassurance to the patient usually allows sufficient exposure of the anal fissure. Anal fissures generally are located in the posterior midline. Pain occurs when the fissure extends beyond the dentate line. The dentate line is the location of the somatic innervation of the anal canal. In chronic fissures, a hypertrophic papilla that is caused by recurrent episodes of infection can be seen. Distal to the hypertrophic papilla, a sentinel pile is found. Sentinel piles are believed to also be a product of infection of the anal canal. The fissure or anal ulcer lies between these two structures and is the first indication of an anal problem (see Fig. 6-3-1).

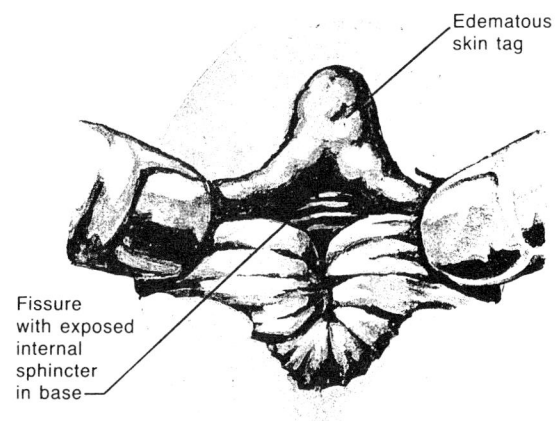

FIGURE 6-3-1. Anal fissure with hypertrophic papilla and sentinel pile. [*From Schwartz SI, Shires GT, Spencer FC (eds): Principles of Surgery, 6th ed. New York, McGraw-Hill, 1994, p 1226. Used with permission of McGraw-Hill, Inc.*]

DIAGNOSTIC CONSIDERATIONS

Anal fissures from constipation, diarrhea, or trauma need to be differentiated from the following disease processes:

• Carcinoma
• Crohn's disease
• Syphilis, primary state
• AIDS colitis

TREATMENT
Medical Management

Medical management generally is used for acute cases. Treatment consists of dietary fiber and/or the use of stool softeners, topical anal anesthetics, and warm sitz baths for 20 min two or three times daily. Botulinum toxin injections and the application of topical nitroglycerin 0.2% are two new treatment options currently under investigation. They work by relaxing the anal sphincter.

Surgical Management

Surgical treatment is reserved for chronic fissures. The patient is taken into the operating room and placed in the jackknife position. Two surgical procedures are available: lateral internal sphincterotomy and anal advancement flap, with the former being the gold standard. The patient is given intravenous sedation along with local anesthesia of 1% lidocaine with epinephrine; 3 to 6 mL of lidocaine is

FIGURE 6-3-2. Lateral internal sphincterotomy, open technique. [*From Schwartz SI, Shires GT, Spencer FC (eds): Principles of Surgery, 6th ed. New York, McGraw-Hill, 1994, p 1227. Used with permission of McGraw-Hill, Inc.*]

used. The internal sphincter is identified and divided by any of the following: cautery, scalpel, or scissors (see Fig. 6-3-2). The external sphincter and fissure are left alone. If any bleeding is encountered, direct pressure to the wound generally stops the blood flow. The wound is left open and allowed to close by secondary intention. The wound generally heals in about 2 to 4 weeks, and the patient usually does not develop a keyhole deformity if the incision is kept lateral and not in the midline. Bupivacaine hydrochloride (Marcaine) 0.25% with epinephrine, which has a longer duration, can be injected into the wound; the patient will have an easier postoperative recovery. The patient is then instructed about perianal hygiene and dietary modifications to prevent constipation. If the patient is unable to adhere to dietary changes, Metamucil or another psyllium-based preparation is suggested as an alternative to produce a large, soft, bulky stool. Patients also are instructed to take two or three sitz baths a day to aid in decreasing inflammation and soothe the wound. An anal advancement flap consists of a rhomboid flap taken at the sentinel pile and placed over the fissure site and sutured in place. The donor site also is sutured closed. Postoperative care instructions consist of good personal hygiene, pain management, a stool softener or fiber, and sitz baths.

Supportive Measures

Patients generally are given a prescription for both oral and topical analgesics. Remember that some oral analgesics can cause constipation, and so a stool softener or fiber also should be used to prevent constipation. A topical analgesic such as dibucaine (Nupercainal) or Hurricane gel can be applied to the wound as needed.

Disposition

Patients are discharged shortly after surgery. They are seen at 1 week, 2 weeks, and 1 month after surgery. Patients are instructed to return earlier if any complications arise.

PATIENT EDUCATION

It is very important for the patient to maintain good perianal hygiene and prevent constipation. Patients are instructed to follow the same postoperative care sheet given to those with hemorrhoidectomies (see Chap. 6-13). If patients do not improve and continue to have pain despite both topical and oral analgesics, they should be reexamined.

COMPLICATIONS

Keyhole deformity and poor wound healing are common complications after a midline sphincterotomy. Lateral internal sphincterotomy is the gold standard for treatment for anal fissures since it does not

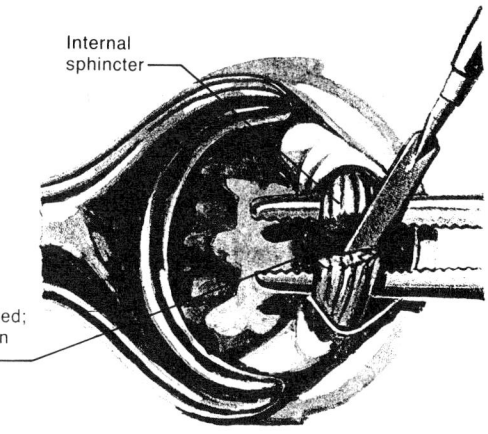

cause these complications. Anal abscesses may develop and require incision and drainage.

NOTES AND PEARLS

Anal fissures are common among pregnant women and usually respond well to conservative treatment consisting of sitz baths, a high-fiber diet, and topical anesthetics. Lateral internal sphincterotomies, if indicated, are delayed until after delivery because of the high probability of anal tears during delivery. Anal intercourse should be considered a possible cause of traumatic or recurrent fissures.

BIBLIOGRAPHY

Beers MH, Berkow R (eds): Anal fissure, in *The Merck Manual,* 17th ed. Whitehouse Station, NJ, Merk, 1999.

Mazier WP: Hemorrhoids, fissures, and pruritus ani (review). *Surg Clin North Am* 74(6):1277–1292, 1995.

Nagle D, Rolandelli RH: Primary care office management of perianal and anal disease. *Primary Care* Sept. 1996, pp 609–614.

Russell TR: Anal fissures, in Way LW (ed): *Current Surgical Diagnosis and Treatment,* 10th ed. Stamford, CT, Appleton & Lange, 1994.

Schwartz SI, Shires GT, Spencer FC (eds): Anal fissures, in *Principles of Surgery,* 7th ed. New York, McGraw-Hill, 1999.

Vogel JD: Comparison of botulinum toxin and nitroglycerin ointment for chronic anal fissure. *N Engl J Med* 341(22):1701. 1999.

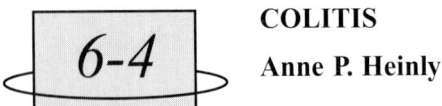

6-4

COLITIS

Anne P. Heinly

COLITIS

DISCUSSION

Colitis is a term that is used easily, but it is difficult to define. The dictionary says that it is "inflammation of the colon," but in general use this can mean anything from acute gastroenteritis to fulminant ulcerative colitis. Most textbooks label an entity *colitis* when there is actual inflammation of the colonic mucosa with structural changes. A brief description of the colon and its anatomy is in order so that clinical practitioners can narrow the differential diagnosis.

The colon (see Fig. 6-4-1) is approximately 1 m in length and frames the intraabdominal contents in an inverted U. Its primary function is the absorption of water and electrolytes, and it finally acts as storage area for feces before evacuation. Considered to have five sections, the colon begins in the right lower quadrant with the cecum, which includes the vermiform appendix and the ileocecal valve. The ascending colon is fairly stationary, having a retroperitoneal attachment, and ends at the hepatic flexure. The transverse colon is quite mobile and can be located from xiphoid to pubis, depending on body habitus and position. The descending colon begins at the splenic flexure and blends into redundancy of the sigmoid colon in the left lower quadrant. The descending colon, like the ascending, is relatively stationary in the retroperitoneum. The sigmoid colon with its excessive tissue is actually the most mobile area. The rectum is part of the colon but often is considered separately, as is the anal area.

The peristaltic motion of the colon is generated from two sets of muscles: an outer longitudinal set (teniae coli) and the inner circular muscle coat. The teniae coli run (as three bands) the entire length of the colon, from cecum to rectum. The teniae coli are just a little shorter than the length of the colon; the ensuing pucker creates the haustra, or outpouching, that are familiar on radiographic examinations of the colon. The presence or absence of the haustra markings can indicate specific disease processes.

Histologically, the colon is fairly simple, with four basic layers. Disease involvement often is measured by the layer or layers affected. The outermost layer is serosa with attached fatty appendixes, an extension of peritoneal fat. The muscle coat is composed of a circular layer forming a spiral effect over the entire length of the colon. The submucosa contains many blood and lymph vessels and dense connective tissue. The innermost layer is the mucosa. It has a special layer of smooth muscle cells called the muscularis mucosae between the submucosa and the mucosa. Unlike the small intestine, the absorption surface is flat with numerous straight tubular crypts. The mucosa is lined with a sheet of columnar epithelial cells. Colitis occurs when the mucosa or underlying structures are inflamed or damaged.

SIGNS AND SYMPTOMS

Because of the many types of colitis, it is important for the clinician to perform a thorough history and physical. History questions should include onset, timing, pattern, radiation, and palliative or exacerbating factors for each presenting symptom. The presenting symptoms may include any of the following: nausea, vomiting, diarrhea (its volume and character), melena, hematochezia, hematemesis, pain, cramping, distention, tenesmus, and constipation. A sexual, travel, and dietary history is essential, since many cases of colitis are infectious. The review of systems should cover extraintestinal symptoms such as joint pain, skin lesions, eye symptoms, and cardiac, pulmonary, hepatic, or renal compromise.

OBJECTIVE FINDINGS

A complete physical examination is a must. Inspect the oral cavity for masses or lesions and the presence or absence of halitosis and examine the neck for lymph node enlargement. An abdominal examination with digital rectal is done for the evaluation of organ enlargement, mass effect, tenderness, and presence of ascites. Do a cardiac and pulmonary examination for evidence of hypovolemia, cardiomyopathies, or pneumonitis. Skin and musculoskeletal examinations may reveal dehydration, malnutrition, or extraintestinal manifestations of disease. Pelvic examinations in women should be done to rule out a gynecologic etiology for the presenting symptoms.

LABORATORY TESTS

Laboratory evaluation includes three to five separate stool samples for ova and parasites (O & P) analysis, culture, and cell counts. Serologic testing should include complete blood cell count (CBC), liver function studies, basic electrolytes, glucose, hepatitis panel, indirect hemagglutination for amebiasis, and screens for sexually transmitted disease such as Venereal Disease Research Laboratories (VDRL), HIV, rapid plasma reagin (RPR), and fluorescent treponemal antibody absorbed (FTA) for syphilis. Antibody titers for cytomegalovirus (CMV), toxoplasma, and herpes simplex virus (HSV) infection may be done. If *Clostridium difficile* is suspected, toxin titers can be done.

RADIOLOGIC (IMAGING) STUDIES

Barium enema may not be indicated in acute situations because of the risk of perforation and should not be done before cultures. Sigmoidoscopy and colonoscopy are the definitive tests because they allow visualization of the tissue and access for biopsy and cultures. See Table 6-4-1 for the pathology associated with each type of colitis.

INTESTINAL AMEBIASIS

Entameba histolytica is the most common form of amebiasis in the United States. It is also found in the tropics and areas with poor

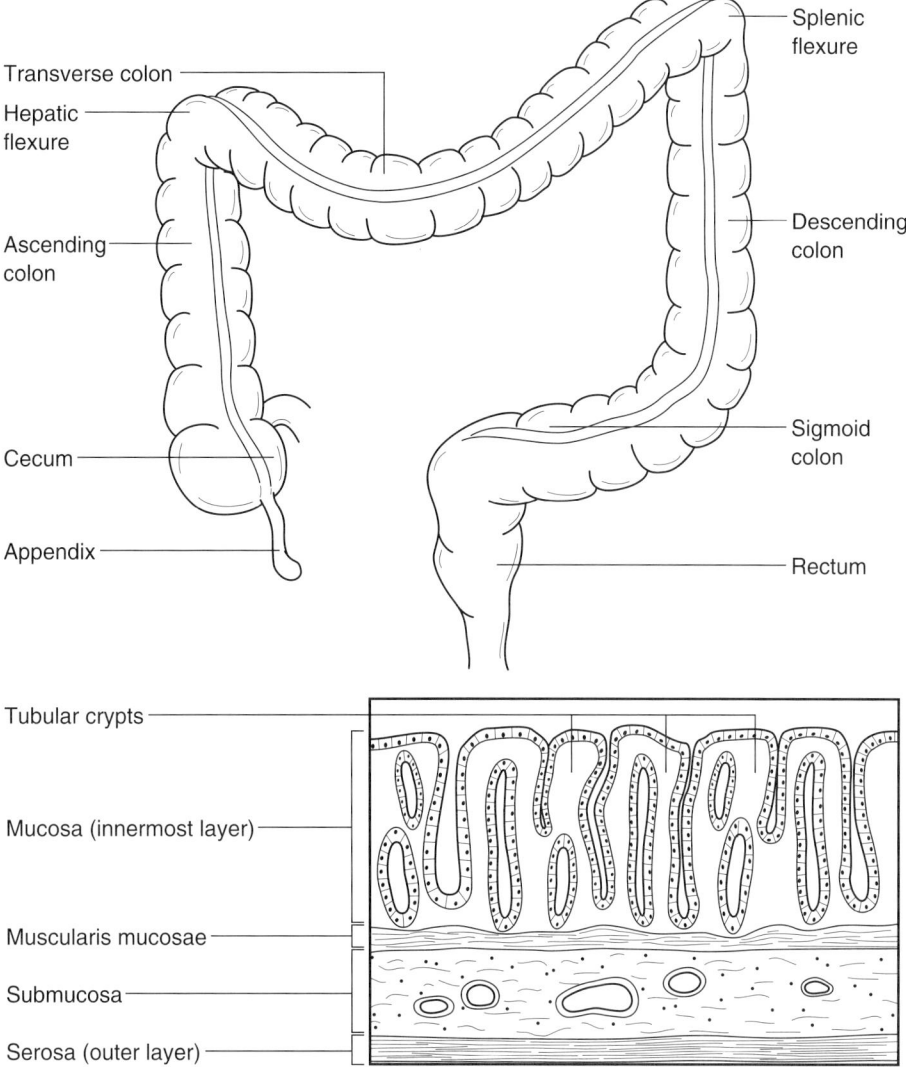

FIGURE 6-4-1. Anatomy of the colon.

sanitation. Symptoms develop 2 to 6 weeks after the ingestion of the infectious cysts. Acutely, these patients have crampy lower abdominal pain and watery, frequent (10 to12 stools daily) small-volume stools that contain scant feces, abundant blood, and mucus. Chronic amebiasis leads to significant malaise and weight loss. Sigmoidoscopy reveals mucosal ulceration, particularly in the cecal and rectal areas. Fulminant disease can form large ulcerative granulomatous masses at the flexures and cecum that may be confused with ulcerative colitis. Stool collection for O & P, cultures, and cell identification is generally diagnostic. Endoscopic findings usually reveal friable mucosa with ulcerations. Treatment includes luminal and tissue amebicides. The luminal drugs iodoquinol, paromomycin, and diloxanide furoate eliminate cysts and trophozoites close to the mucosa. A good tissue amebicide is metronidazole 750 mg tid for 10 days. Several different stools should be checked after therapy to ensure complete eradication.

INFECTIOUS COLITIS

Clostridium perfringens is a common cause of food poisoning in the United States. Rewarmed food is the usual culprit. Like its bacterial cousins, *C. perfringens* is a spore-forming microbe that can germinate during the reheating process. The type A strains can develop 8 to 20 h after ingestion. Enterotoxins are produced in the gastrointestinal (GI) tract, causing hypersecretions, intestinal epithelium damage, and

protein loss into the intestinal lumen. Symptoms include the abrupt onset of watery, profuse diarrhea and epigastric pain. Fever, nausea, and vomiting are infrequent. Mild infections are self-limiting and need supportive treatment. More persistent or fulminant infections may be treated with penicillin G 20 million units a day until the infection is cleared.

Infectious causes of colitis include *Shigella, Salmonella, Campylobacter,* and *Yersinia* species. All these are associated with nausea, abdominal cramps, fever, and diarrhea. *Campylobacter* and *Shigella* are associated with bloody diarrhea. *Campylobacter* may produce liver enlargement. *Shigella, Salmonella,* and *Yersinia* have been associated with Reiter's syndrome, migrating joint pain, and skin lesions. The diagnosis is confirmed by cultures. Sigmoidoscopy will reveal a red, friable, and ulcerated mucosa. Treatment is supportive with correction of dehydration and electrolyte abnormalities. Among these infectious etiologies for colitis, only *Shigella* requires antibiotic therapy, ampicillin 500 mg qid or trimethoprim-sulfamethoxazole bid. The other infections are self-limiting, and in fact, antibiotics given to these patients may tend to lengthen the carrier state of the organism. Diarrhea is a common first symptom for HIV-positive patients. Immunocompromised patients are more susceptible to unusual infectious colitis, including *Candida* spp., *Histoplasma capsulatum,* cytomegalovirus, herpes simplex virus, actinomycosis, and tuberculosis. Symptoms may include fever, abdominal pain, weight loss, anorexia, and diarrhea with or without blood. The elderly, the very young, and cancer patients also may be immunocompromised.

TABLE 6-4-1.   Types of Colitis

TYPES OF COLITIS	SYMPTOMS	STOOL CHARACTER	PATHOLOGY
Amebiasis	Crampy abdominal pain, rarely perforates	Watery, small volume, streaked with blood or mucus	Mucosal ulcerations, rounded, punched-out on x-ray and examination
Clostridium perfringens	Epigastric pain	Watery diarrhea, fecal neutrophils, protein loss	Enterotoxin damages intestinal epithelium
Collagenous	Intermittent abdominal cramping	Chronic, watery, no blood or mucus	Thickened subepithelial layer below colonic mucosa, eosinophilic acellular collagen band
Infectious *Shigella,* *Salmonella,* *Campylobacter,* *Yersinia*	Crampy abdominal pain	Profuse, watery with or without blood and mucus, fecal leukocytes	Inflammation without structural changes
Ischemic	Abdominal pain, hypotension	Rectal bleeding	Submucosal hemorrhage and edema
Pseudomembranous *Clostridium difficile*	Fever, abdominal cramps, pain	Profuse, watery with no blood or mucus	Raised plaques 2–5 mm in diameter interspersed among normal mucosa
Amyloidosis	Diarrhea or constipation	Diarrhea with or without blood	Amyloid deposits
Lymphocytic	Vague colicky pain, chronic course	Watery diarrhea, excessive mucus, no blood	Absence of subepithelial thickening. Lamina propria infiltrated with lymphocytes

COLLAGENOUS COLITIS

The diagnosis of collagenous colitis can be made only by histology. Often dismissed as irritable bowel syndrome (IBS), it is found in middle-aged (fifth to sixth decade) women who have intermittent diarrhea. The diarrhea is chronic and watery without blood, excessive mucus, or cells. The patient may have evidence of arthritis or connective tissue disorders. Barium enema and endoscopy are usually negative. The biopsy, however, reveals a thickened subepithelial layer below the normal-appearing colon mucosa. Treatment with oral sulfasalazine 2 to 3 g daily leads to marked improvement in the majority of patients. Nonsteroidal anti-inflammatory drugs (NSAIDs) should be avoided because they have been associated with intestinal mucosal inflammation. No evidence of severe progression or increased colon cancer risk has been found.

ISCHEMIC COLITIS

Ischemic colitis occurs with the transport of blood away from the intestinal mucosa. This may occur slowly with generalized peripheral vascular disease or acutely with arterial emboli, a dissecting aortic aneurysm, or abdominal surgeries. Radiation therapy to the abdominal or pelvic regions also may trigger an ischemic reaction. The colon receives the majority of its blood supply from the superior and inferior mesenteric arteries. Compromise of the supply or severe hypotension may lead to ischemia. Transient ischemia involves the mucosa or submucosa. Chronic or prolonged ischemia produces damage to the circular muscle layer. Transmural infarction involves all four layers of the colon and usually leads to perforation, gangrene, or even the death of the patient.

Symptoms include severe lower abdominal pain (abdominal angina) and bloody diarrhea, which is quite profuse. The patient often will avoid eating to avoid the pain. When the severity increases, vomiting and hypotension are common. Physical examination reveals an acute abdomen with signs of peritonitis. Barium studies usually reveal the classic "thumbprinting" representing submucosal hemorrhage and edema. Contrast studies may be hazardous, creating the possibility of perforation.

Chronic ischemia may cause stricture formation, ulceration, and granulation tissue. A mesenteric thrombosis is a true life-threatening emergency that calls for early lifesaving therapy and surgical consultation.

PSEUDOMEMBRANOUS COLITIS

Inflammation of the colon associated with the use of antibiotics is the most common cause of pseudomembranous colitis (see Table 6-4-2). It also has been seen with mercury poisoning, intestinal ischemia, and bronchopneumonia. Pseudomembranous colitis is characterized by abscesses in one or several adjacent crypts from which exudative mucus, cellular debris, and leukocytes ooze into the intestinal lumen. In the case of antibiotic use, *C. difficile* is the pathogen that causes the problem. More specifically, *C. difficile* overgrowth results in the release of toxins that in turn cause the symptoms. There are three heat-labile toxins. Toxins A, B, and C cause fluid mobilization. Toxin A causes severe necrosis of the epithelium and bleeding. Toxins A and C cause epithelial cell shedding. The result is a patient with fever, profuse diarrhea, and cramping abdominal pain with leukocytosis. There is seldom excessive mucus, and there may or may not be bleeding. Physical examination may mimic an acute or surgical abdomen. Plain abdominal radiographs may show irregular mucosal outline with blunting of edematous haustra.

TABLE 6-4-2.   Antibiotics Associated with Pseudomembranous Colitis (in Order of Frequency)

Ampicillin/amoxicillin
Cephalosporins
Clindamycin
Sulfamethoxazole-trimethoprim
Other "cillin" drugs
Rarely seen with tetracycline, sulfonamides

TABLE 6-4-3. Differential Diagnosis of Colitis

Neoplasm (carcinoma, adenomatous, polyps)
Diverticula, diverticulitis
Arteriovenous malformations
Behçet's syndrome
Acute gastroenteritis
Bacillary dysentery: salmonella, *Campylobacter*
Herpes simplex virus
Gonorrhea
Lymphogranuloma venereum (LGV)
Irritable bowel syndrome

The diagnosis of pseudomembranous colitis is dependent on the history of antibiotic use within the last 4 to 6 weeks. Most cases of colitis will begin 5 to 7 days after antibiotics are begun, but as many as one-third of cases will not develop symptoms until the antibiotic course is completed. Stool cultures for *C. difficile* are not helpful; it is better to confirm by positive *C. difficile* toxin titer. Toxin B may increase 1000-fold and is considered the hallmark of *C. difficile* infection. Contrast studies should be avoided because of the risk of perforation.

Treatment, of course, includes cessation of the offending antibiotic and the provision of supportive care. Oral metronidazole or intravenous (IV) vancomycin has been used to combat *C. difficile.* The fluoroquinolones appear to be affective in some patients. The patient will show signs of recovery within 24 to 48 h on average. Complications of pseudomembranous colitis include perforation and toxic megacolon, and so rapid therapy is recommended. There is no evidence to suggest that the antibiotic that caused the colitis be avoided in the future, though the colitis can recur with the use of any antibiotic and should be retreated.

PEARLS

With rare exceptions, the many types of colitis have effective treatment options once the type is identified. There is a differential list of processes that may mimic any colitis or contribute to an existing colitis (see Table 6-4-3). Ulcerative colitis and Crohn's disease are covered in Chap. 6-5.

BIBLIOGRAPHY

Cappell MS: Intestinal (mesenteric) vasculopathy: II. Ischemic colitis and chronic mesenteric ischemia. *Gastroenterol Clin* 27(4):827–847, 1998.

Fekety R: Guidelines for the diagnosis and management of *Clostridium difficile*-associated diarrhea and colitis. *Am J Gastroenterol* 92(5):739–749, 1997.

Reed SR: Amebiasis and infections with free-living amebas, in Fauci AS, Braunwald B, Isselbacher KJ, et al: *Harrison's Principles of Internal Medicine,* 14th ed. 1998, pp 1177–1179.

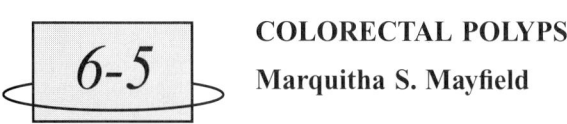

6-5 COLORECTAL POLYPS
Marquitha S. Mayfield

DISCUSSION

Polyps are soft-tissue mucosal lesions that protrude into the lumen of the intestines. They result from excessive proliferation of normal mucosal cells (hyperplastic changes) or neoplastic changes of glandular epithelial cells (adenomatous growths). Polyps can occur anywhere in the intestinal tract. Most occur in the colon and rectum, with 70 to 80 percent of polyps located in the rectosigmoid colon. Polyps may be sessile (broad-based growths) or pedunculated (attached to a stalk), singular or multiple, and vary in size from smaller than 0.5 cm in diameter to larger than 4 cm in diameter. The average polyp is equivalent to 1 cm in diameter. Most polyps are benign; however, some are considered to be premalignant. There is a strong association between adenomatous polyps and the subsequent development of adenocarcinoma of the colon. Dietary factors such as high fat, low fiber, and low calcium may promote malignant transformation. Genetic factors also play a role in the development of colorectal polyps.

The incidence of polyps increases with age. By age 40 years, 20 percent of the adult population will have developed some form of polypoid lesions. Adult males are at greater risk than females (2:1 ratio). There are two primary pathologic groups of polyps, nonneoplastic and neoplastic.

Nonneoplastic Polyps

Nonneoplastic polyps include hyperplastic polyps, hamartomas, inflammatory (pseudopolyps), and juvenile polyps. These benign lesions have no potential for malignant transformation. Hyperplastic polyps are the most common benign tumors. More than 80 percent are located in the rectosigmoid colon, and they are usually less than 4 mm in diameter. Hamartomas are developmental malformations resulting in tumors from the overgrowth of normal tissue. Cells do not reproduce once they reach maturity; therefore the growths are self-limiting and benign. Pseudopolyps are commonly associated with inflammatory changes seen with ulcerative colitis and Crohn's disease. Juvenile polyps are benign colonic growths detected primarily in children and young adults. These polyps are often large, vascular, and attached to long stalks and may bleed or prolapse rectally.

Neoplastic Polyps

Neoplastic polyps include primary adenomatous polyps, which have significant potential for malignant transformation to adenocarcinoma of the colon. Dysplastic changes are slow to develop in adenomatous polyps, and it may take 5 to 10 years for malignant changes to occur. Approximately 25 percent of polyps are found to be adenomatous on histologic report. The prevalence of adenomatous polyps increases with age, with a peak incidence after age 50. Adenomatous polyps may be classified as tubular, tubovillous, or villous adenomas. Malignant potential correlates with the size of the polyp, degree of dysplastic changes, and villous features. Villous adenomas have the greatest potential for malignant transformation (>50 percent), and tubular adenomas, the least potential (20 percent). Tubovillous lesions have a risk for malignant transformation between 20 and 50 percent. Lesions larger than 1 cm in diameter have a 10 percent risk of harboring malignant cells, whereas polyps larger than 2 cm have a 46 percent risk. Sessile adenomas are more likely to harbor malignant changes than pedunculated adenomas. Approximately half the patients with adenomatous polyps have more than one lesion.

SIGNS AND SYMPTOMS

Most patients with colorectal polyps are asymptomatic, with lesions detected on routine endoscopy. Symptoms, when they do occur, consist primarily of intermittent rectal bleeding from ulcerated large polyps. Physical examination findings are uncommon. Digital rectal examination might reveal a palpable rectal mass with large rectal polyps. Gross rectal bleeding may be present. Usually only a positive test for occult bleeding is noted.

DIFFERENTIAL DIAGNOSIS

The differential diagnosis for rectal bleeding includes the following:

• Hemorrhoids
• Upper GI bleeding

- Angiodysplasia
- Diverticular disease
- Infectious diarrhea
- Colorectal cancer
- Ischemic colitis
- Inflammatory bowel disease

SPECIAL CONSIDERATIONS

Familial polyposis is an autosomal-dominant inheritable disorder in which hundreds to thousands of adenomatous polyps form throughout the colon. Lesions often appear during childhood and have a high rate of malignant transformation by age 50. A colectomy is often performed prophylactically. Peutz–Jeghers syndrome is another inherited disorder in which hamartomatous polyps predominate. Lesions are distributed throughout the GI tract, mostly in the small intestine. Although hamartomas are usually benign, patients with Peutz-Jeghers are prone to develop other forms of GI cancer (e.g., gastric, pancreatic, or duodenal malignancies).

Patients with a family history for either of these disorders require enhanced surveillance for early detection of malignant transformation and management of polypoid growths.

LABORATORY AND RADIOLOGIC TESTS

Stool for occult blood is a common screening test used for colorectal cancer. However, it is less sensitive and specific for detecting polyps. Sigmoidoscopy is a better screening test because most colorectal polyps are accessible by the flexible sigmoidoscope. Double-contrast barium enema is also useful and can detect up to 90 percent of polyps larger than 1 cm in diameter. On radiograph, polyps appear as rounded filling defects with sharply defined margins. Colonoscopy is the most reliable method for diagnosing polyps, detecting up to 98 percent of polyps. The entire colon can be visualized and polyps can be removed for histologic evaluation at the same time.

TREATMENT

The mainstay of treatment for colorectal polyps is endoscopic removal. Routine removal of adenomatous polyps significantly reduces the incidence of subsequent development of colorectal cancer. If possible, all colonic polyps should be excised and sent for tissue pathology. A polypectomy using electrocautery techniques can be safely completed through the colonoscope for many sessile and pedunculated lesions. Lesions larger than 3 cm in diameter may require surgical resection. Patients with adenomatous polyps should undergo a repeat colonoscopy within 3 years to detect and remove any additional lesions or residual tissue.

Patients with a family history for inheritable polyposis syndromes may require regular screening sigmoidoscopy beginning at an early age (10 to 20 years).

Supportive Measures

Adopting a diet that is low in saturated fat (<30 percent of total calories), high in fiber (at least three servings daily of fruit and vegetables), as well as limited in the amount of red meat (fewer than three servings per week) and alcohol (fewer than two drinks daily) consumed, may reduce the risk for dysplastic changes of the colorectal mucosa.

Patient Education

The risk for colonic cancer should be explained to all patients with adenomatous polyps. These patients should be encouraged to return for routine follow-up colonoscopy. Instructions on instituting a low-fat, high-fiber diet should also be given.

Disposition

Patients with polyps detected on barium enema or sigmoidoscopy should be referred to a gastroenterologist for diagnostic and therapeutic colonoscopy. Recommendations for repeat "surveillance" colonoscopy vary and are based on pathologic type of the removed polyp and individual risk for cancer. Generally, benign hyperplastic polyps do not require additional follow-up. Patients with adenomatous polyps should have repeat colonoscopy in 3 years. Patients with large polyps, polyps with very dysplastic features, or a strong family history of colon cancer should have repeat colonoscopy sooner.

COMPLICATIONS AND RED FLAGS

Large polyps may precipitate intussusception or cause bowel obstruction. Additionally, polyps may ulcerate and bleed. The major complication, however, is the development of invasive adenocarcinoma of the colon.

OTHER NOTES AND PEARLS

Epidemiologic data from recent studies suggest that the use of NSAIDS (e.g., aspirin and Sulindac) on a daily basis may significantly reduce the incidence of adenomatous polyps and the associated risk for dysplastic changes in some patients.

BIBLIOGRAPHY

Alberts DS, Hixson L, Ahnen D, et al. Do NSAIDS exert their colon cancer chemoprevention activities through the inhibition of mucosal prostaglandin synthetase? *J Cellular Biochem* 22 (suppl):18–23, 1995.

Barker LR, Burton JH, Zieve PD, eds. *Principles of Ambulatory Medicine,* 4th ed. Baltimore, Williams & Wilkins, 1995, pp 472–475.

Ceabert JG. Colorectal cancer: Reducing mortality through early detection and treatment. *Physician Assist* 17:25–42, 1993.

Goroll AH, May LA, Mulley AG Jr, eds. *Primary Care Medicine: Office Evaluation & Management of the Adult Patient,* 4th ed. Philadelphia, Lippincott, 2000, pp. 359, 501, 503–505.

Greenberger NJ. How best to screen for colorectal cancer. *Contemp Nurse Practit* (Clin Focus suppl), summer 1995, pp. 25–31.

Martinez ME, McPherson RS. Aspirin and other nonsteroidal anti-inflammatory drugs and risk of colorectal adenomatous polyps among endoscoped individuals. *Cancer Epidemiol Biomarkers Prev* 4:703–707, 1995.

Neugut AI, Horvath K, Whelan RL, et al. The effect of calcium and vitamin supplements on the incidence and recurrence of colorectal adenomatous polyps. *Cancer* 78:723–728, 1996.

Tierney L, McPhee SJ, Papadakis MA. *Current Medical Diagnosis and Treatment.* New York, McGraw-Hill, 2000, pp. 644–651.

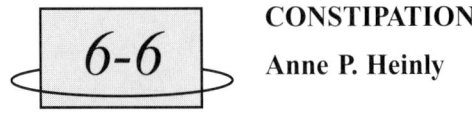

CONSTIPATION

Anne P. Heinly

DISCUSSION

For many people, it is a constitutional right to have at least one bowel movement a day. Failing that, these people will complain of constipation and self-medicate with a laxative. Constipation is a pervasive symptom that affects women more than men and affects the majority of people at least once in their lifetimes. As a symptom, constipation may herald a disease process, but it is not a disease in and of itself. The presence of constipation is highly subjective: A patient may be anxious if the daily routine of three stools a day drops to one; other patients may go several days with no stool evacuation without concern. Constipation is a problem at the extremes of life, affecting infants and toddlers and the elderly most adversely.

PATHOGENESIS

The elimination of stool from the intestinal tract should occur on average three to five times a week and is dependent on multiple elements. The first factor is mobility; slow transit allows the stool to become compact, making it difficult to move. Chronic constipation is usually secondary to slow transit time and redundant colon. Water intake and absorption is another key mechanism. Water and electrolytes normally are reabsorbed from waste product, but if a person has inadequate fluid intake, hard stools develop since the body is conserving fluids. Water also acts as a lubricant. Dietary intake of fiber allows for frequent bulky stools. The average American stool is small and weighs 75 to 150 g, which can be exhausting to move. Fiber adds bulk, increasing the weight (200 to 500 g) and size of the stool. Other elements that slow stool evacuations include prolonged bed rest, lack of exercise, and medication use (see Table 6-6-1). Constipation in the elderly is probably multifactorial, a combination of aging changes, poor diet, lack of exercise, and medication effects.

TABLE 6-6-1. Causes of Constipation

General
  Diet: high fat, low fiber, minimal fruits and vegetables
  Poor bowel habits: ignoring the urge, avoidance of public toilets, avoidance of pain
  Poor exercise habits: sedentary life-style, prolonged bed rest
  Travel: change in schedule or diet, absence of good drinking water

Metabolic
  Hypercalcemia: malignancy, thyrotoxicosis, sarcoidosis, theophylline toxicity
  Hypokalemia: chronic laxative abuse, diuretic therapy, metabolic alkalosis
  Hyponatremia: vomiting, burns, diuretic therapy, cirrhosis, congestive heart failure
  Diabetes: polyuria, thirst, weight loss, ketoacidosis
  Dehydration: excessive heat, lack of thirst mechanism, illness, fever, vomiting

Mechanical
  Redundant, copious bowel
  Pregnancy
  Scarring from radiation therapy
  Surgical adhesions or anastomosis
  Extrinsic or intrinsic tumors/masses

Neuromuscular
  Hirschsprung's disease: congenital aganglionic bowel
  Spinal cord injury
  Paraplegia
  Cerebral vascular accidents
  Muscular dystrophy
  Dementia/Alzheimer's disease
  Parkinsonism
  Depression

Medications
  Smooth muscle relaxants: dicyclomine hydrochloride (Bentyl), verapamil, belladonna
  Antiparkinsonism medications: carbidopa-levodopa (Sinemet), bromocriptine mesylate (Parlodel), amantadine hydrochloride (Symmetrel), Levodopa
  Antidepressants: Tricyclics, chlorpromazine, benzodiazepines
  Calcium- and aluminum-based antacids
  Diuretics: hydrochlorothiazide (HCTZ), furosemide (Lasix), bumetanide (Bumex), spironolactone (Aldactone)
  Iron supplements
  Tranquilizers: chlorpromazine (Thorazine), fluphenazine hydrochloride (Prolixin), haloperidol (Haldol), lithium, trifluoperazine hydrochloride (Stelazine)
  Narcotics and sedatives: morphine, meperidine hydrochloride (Demerol), codeine, chloral hydrate (Noctec), hydroxyzine (Vistaril), zolpidem tartrate (Ambien)

SYMPTOMS

Variable is the key word. Constipation is defined by the patient's perception of what is normal with regard to frequency, consistency (harder than normal), and size. Cramping abdominal pain that comes in wave-like spasms can be described as mild to severe. The pain may be localized or generalized. It is not unusual to have flank pain or pain in the lateral upper quadrants as the stool turns the corner of the hepatic or splenic flexure. With an impaction, a patient may have tenesmus with watery diarrhea escaping around the stool (encopresis). With rare exceptions, the patient does not have systemic symptoms. In addition, there is no weight loss or bleeding. This helps differentiate a constipated patient from one with an acute abdominal event such as appendicitis.

OBJECTIVE

A good history and physical may be sufficient to make the diagnosis. Generally, the patient will present with intermittent pain and normal vital signs. Abdominal examination may reveal a rounded mass effect in the flanks that follows the tract of the colon. Rectal examination is a must. There may be an impaction (see Chap. 6-9). An empty vault does not exclude constipation, as stool may be filling the entire colon but may not have reached the rectal vault. Generally, there is no rebound tenderness or other peritoneal signs.

DIAGNOSTIC CONSIDERATIONS

Risk factors for constipation should be explored: injury, illness, dehydration, a sedentary life-style, and multiple medications (see Table 6-6-2 for the differential diagnosis). In infants, congenital Hirschsprung's disease (small rectal vault, aganglionic colon) presents with constipation, abdominal distention, and vomiting. Toddlers can get into a constipation cycle, delaying defecation because it hurts and then having exceptional difficulty with evacuation, which leads to further avoidance.

The elderly can present with a change in mentation and anorexia. Because of normal physiologic aging changes and/or concomitant illness, an older patient may experience transient blood supply loss to the heart and brain while straining to evacuate stool. Some elderly persons strain so long that rectal prolapse and severe hemorrhoids develop. Urinary retention and fever may complicate the picture in an elderly person.

LABORATORY TESTS

Laboratory testing is necessary only when other disorders are being considered. If laboratory work is ordered, it should include complete blood cell count (CBC) (anemias), electrolytes (hypokalemia, hypercalcemia), thyroid function studies (hypothyroidism), and glucose (diabetes). If the constipation is functional and is due to dehydration, poor diet, or lack of exercise, the laboratory results are usually within normal limits.

TABLE 6-6-2. Differential Diagnosis for Constipation

Irritable bowel syndrome
Hirschsprung's syndrome
Small bowel obstruction
Colon carcinoma
Colonic polyposis
Rectal disease: Crohn's disease, ulcerative colitis, fistulas
Foreign body obstruction
Acute abdomen: appendicitis, diverticulitis

RADIOLOGIC (IMAGING) STUDIES

Plain films of the abdomen are useful in acute constipation. They may reveal gaseous distention of the colon with fecal material throughout the colon. The diagnosis of chronic constipation may be made if 8 or more radiopaque markers are found on plain films 3 days after the ingestion of 20 markers.

A barium enema remains the study of choice in the evaluation of constipation since it can confirm obstructive lesions, redundant colon, megacolon, congenital aberrations, and other problems. Endoscopy is performed to rule out organic lesions, especially in an older patient in whom colon cancer may present with constipation. A full colonoscopy may be beneficial.

TREATMENT

Pharmacologic Management

Medications are separated into classes on the basis of their action in the colon (see Table 6-6-3). Almost all these medications are available over the counter in some form, and so it is critical to find out what the patient has been using for self-medication before recommending a new regimen.

Supportive Measures

Supportive measures include regular exercise, increased fluid intake (preferably water), and the intake of at least 5 to 15 g of dietary fiber daily. Fiber is essential for increasing the bulk of the stool (making it easier to move). Fruits such as dates and prunes, raw or steamed vegetables, and whole grains are considered natural bulking agents. A consultation with a nutritionist is needed in chronic constipation to establish total fiber intake and recommend ways to increase fiber to 30 to 35 g/day. Additional measures include a comfortable and private place for defecation. Children and the elderly are not always afforded the privacy they feel is necessary for comfortable evacuation. Steps should be taken to prevent constipation if a patient is placed on a medication regimen that is likely to cause constipation (narcotics, verapamil).

Complications

Ordinarily, constipation does not produce serious complications. Constipation may be a symptom of a serious problem; therefore, new-onset constipation should be evaluated completely. The most common complication of constipation is hemorrhoids (see Chap. 6-13). Hard stools and extended periods of time on the toilet lead to venous pooling. Hemorrhoids may bleed and/or cause pain. Painful fissures and cracks (see Chap. 6-3) can develop, and rectal prolapse can occur, especially in the elderly. Excessive straining can create poor blood flow to the heart and brain as a result of the prolonged increase in abdominal pressure and may exacerbate cardiac and cerebral vascular disease.

Chronic constipation can lead to laxative abuse. The more often an osmotic or irritant cathartic is used, the more "lazy" the colon will become. Eventually, the intestines become insensitive and fail to work on their own; the result is megacolon with loss of haustration and peristalsis.

PATIENT EDUCATION

Judging from pervasive laxative advertisements, constipation is a common problem. All patients need to be educated about what "normal" bowel habits are and how to avoid constipation. A diet high in fiber and low in fat with adequate fluid intake is the first, best step. Regular exercise, regular times, and a comfortable location for evacuation will help the patient avoid constipation and laxative abuse.

PEARLS

A good history is essential when dealing with constipation. Care should be taken to establish the patient's "normal" bowel habits before his or her perception of the constipation. Investigate the activities of daily living to evaluate mobility, exercise, usual diet, and medication use (over-the-counter and prescription drugs). Encourage the natural fix for constipation—exercise, fiber, and water—before recommending a laxative or a similar intervention. Encourage all patients to respond to the natural urge to defecate as soon as possible; delaying evacuation can exacerbate the situation.

TABLE 6-6-3. Medical Therapy for Constipation

AGENT	MECHANISM OF ACTION	COMMON NAME	DOSE	SIDE EFFECTS
Increased dietary fiber	Natural bulk agents	Fresh fruits, whole grains, vegetables	10–35 g daily	Bloating, flatulence
Bulking Agents Psyllium Methylcellulose Calcium polycarbophil	Add bulk to stool, but increased water intake essential	Metamucil Citrucel FiberCon	1 tbs. 1–3 daily with lots of water	Flatulence, unpalatable, non-compliance
Osmotic agents Magnesium sulfate Milk of magnesia Magnesium citrate Sodium phosphate Lactulose	Draw water into the colonic lumen, inducing peristaltic movement	Chronulac	15 g in water 15–30 mL daily 240 mL on ice 4–8 g in water 15–30 mL daily	Abdominal cramping, watery stools, dehydration, hypermagnesemia
Stimulants Cascara sagrada Calcium salts Senna Castor oil Bisacodyl	Increase intestinal peristalsis by direct action on colon	Senokot Dulcolax	325–650 mg q HS 12–24 mg q HS 2 tablets q HS 15–60 mL q HS 10–15 mg q HS	Cramping, vomiting, malabsorption, dependence, avoid in the elderly
Lubricants Mineral oil	Coat intestinal walls and stool and aid in mobility		5–30 mL at bedtime	Prevents absorption of fat soluble vitamins
Fecal softeners Docusate sodium Docusate calcium Docusate potassium Polaxer	Promote water retention, thereby softening stool (not a laxative)	Colace, Surfak	50–240 mg with water 240 mg daily 100–300 mg daily 480 mg q HS	May increase the systemic absorption of mineral oil.

BIBLIOGRAPHY

Browning SM: Office management of common anorectal problems, constipation, diarrhea and irritable bowel syndrome. *Primary Care Clin Office Pract* 26(1):113–135, 1999.

Talley NJ, Fleming KC, Evans JM, et al: Constipation in an elderly community: A study of prevalence and potential risk. *Am J Gastroenterol* 91(1):19–24, 1996.

Voderholzer WA, Schatke W, Muhldorfer BE, et al: Clinical response to dietary fiber treatment of chronic constipation. *Am J Gastroenterol* 92(1):95–97, 1997.

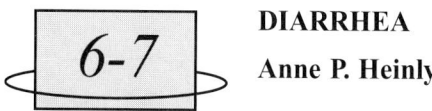

6-7

DIARRHEA
Anne P. Heinly

DESCRIPTION

Diarrhea is one of the most common human symptoms. Caused by a myriad of diseases and medications, it spares no one in any country. The widely held definition of diarrhea is an increase in daily stool weight greater than 250 g with a change in usual bowel habits. Most patients complain of diarrhea when their stool becomes softer, watery, and/or more frequent. Although most sources of diarrhea are acute and self-limiting, other etiologies can be chronic and potentially life-threatening. A logical and knowledgeable approach is required to discern the differences.

PATHOGENESIS

The gastrointestinal tract functions on fluid; on average, a total of 9 L of fluids per day passes through the system from mouth to anus (see Table 6-7-1). The stomach churns ingested food with hydrochloric acid, and the subsequent chyme moves through the pyloric sphincter into the small intestine, where absorption of nutrients, electrolytes, and water takes place. The small intestines have an absorption surface equivalent to the size of an outdoor tennis court. Disease can render it ineffective, reducing the surface to the size of a ping-pong table.

The small intestine has a dynamic flux of absorption and secretions. Approximately 20 ft long, the small intestine includes the C loop of the duodenum, the jejunum, and the ileum. The mucosal layer contains millions of villi whose finger-like projection give the small intestine its incredibly absorptive surface. The microvillous membrane absorbs disaccharides, peptides, and amino acids and is responsible for the cotransport of sodium and D-glucose. Diarrhea represents an interruption of this absorption-secretion cycle in the small intestine and the colon.

Most of the fluid (H_2O) is reabsorbed in the distal ileum and the large intestine, with an average final stool weight of 100 to 150 g containing 60 to 65 percent water. Diarrhea occurs when the water weight increases as a result of decreased absorption or increased fluid secretions. Table 6-7-2 defines the five different mechanisms of diarrhea and their common etiology. Not all causes of diarrhea fit neatly with a mechanism but may involve a combination of factors.

TABLE 6-7-1. Daily Fluid Input to the GI System

Oral intake	2000 mL
Salivary secretions	1500 mL
Gastric juices	2000 mL
Pancreatic juices	2500 mL
Biliary secretions	500 mL
Small intestinal secretions	1000 mL

TABLE 6-7-2. Types of Diarrhea

OSMOTIC

Excess water-soluble molecules in bowel lumen cause water influx into the lumen; watery diarrhea is the consequence. Responds to a clear liquid diet.
- Carbohydrates
- Magnesium products: antacids, food supplements
- Lactose deficiency (milk intolerance)
- Sorbitol use: sugar-free products, diet sodas

SECRETORY

An increase in chloride and water secretion with inhibition of normal active sodium and H_2O absorption and copious watery diarrhea without pus or blood ensues. May or may not respond to fasting or a clear liquid diet.
- Enterotoxins
  - *Vibrio cholerae*
  - Enterotoxigenic *Escherichia coli*
  - *Aeromonas* species
- Hormonal secretagogues
  - Cholecystokinin
  - Substance P
  - Insulin
  - Glucagon
- Gastric hypersecretions
  - Peptic ulcer disease
  - Zollinger-Ellison syndrome
  - Carcinoid syndrome
- Laxatives
  - Bisacodyl
  - Docusate sodium
  - Senna
  - Cascara
  - Phenolphthalein
- Bile salts malabsorption
  - Ileum resection
  - Primary biliary disease
- Fatty acid malabsorption
  - Celiac sprue
  - Bacterial overgrowth

EXUDATIVE

From exudation of protein, mucus, and blood from sites of active inflammation of the bowel wall into the intestinal lumen. There is an abnormal mucosal permeability of the intestinal mucosa.
- Idiopathic
  - Crohn's disease
  - Ulcerative colitis
  - Collagen colitis
  - Whipple's disease
- Infectious
  - *Shigella*
  - *Salmonella*
  - *Campylobacter*
- Ischemic
  - Mesenteric angina or infarction
- Radiation enteritis (a form of ischemic from local radiation therapy)
- Abscess formation (from any source)

ABNORMAL INTESTINAL MOTILITY

Fast transit causes reduced contact; slow transit may cause diarrhea because of bacterial overgrowth.
- Reduced contact with fast transit
  - Hyperthyroidism
  - Postgastrectomy patients or short bowel syndrome
  - Carcinoid syndrome
  - Pheochromocytoma
  - Irritable bowel syndrome
  - Postcholecystectomy
- Decreased motility with slow transit and bacterial overgrowth
  - Diabetes (especially type 1)
  - Hypothyroidism
  - Addison's disease
  - Scleroderma
  - Amyloidosis
  - Postgastrectomy (blind loop syndrome and afferent loop syndrome)

TABLE 6-7-3. Medications and Diarrhea

Diarrhea is a common side effect of numerous medications, including the
following (in no particular order):
- Magnesium antacids
- Sulfa drugs
- Antibiotics: Augmentin, erythromycin
- Antineoplastic: Nolvadex, Adriamycin, Efudex
- Prokinetic agents: Reglan, Propulsid
- Sorbitol: sweetener in many diet foods
- Theophylline products

SYMPTOMS

Evaluating a patient with diarrhea requires a thorough history: a description of the onset, duration, and timing between stools and the color, consistency, and quantity of stool. The presence of blood, mucus, or floating stools provides valuable clues to the etiology:

- Large, watery, soupy, or greasy stools with cramping and periumbilical pain suggest the small bowel.
- Frequent, small quantities of mushy brown stool with mucus or blood, tenesmus, and achy pain suggest the left colon.
- Blood suggests inflammatory, vascular, infectious, or neoplastic etiologies.

The next set of questions should be a good diet history. Does the diarrhea occur before, during, or after meals or at night? Define exposures to other persons with similar symptoms, travel, camping, and HIV risk factors. Then explore medication use (see Table 6-7-3), especially antibiotic use in the last 2 to 6 weeks (see Chap. 6-4). Laxative abuse may cause diarrhea or constipation with a watery diarrhea flowing around an impaction (see Chaps. 6-6 and 6-9).

OBJECTIVES

Because diarrhea can have so many causes, a complete physical examination may be necessary. Every examination should begin with a complete set of orthostatic vital signs and skin inspection for hydration: dry lips, dry eyes, dry oral mucosa, or skin tenting. Severe dehydration may present with a change in mental status: disorientation or altered consciousness. Fever is common with infectious etiologies. The abdominal examination usually reveals mild distention; hyperactive bowel sounds, especially with an infectious etiology; and diffuse, poorly localized tenderness. There is usually no mass effect except with Crohn's disease (right lower quadrant) and diverticulitis (left lower quadrant). Peritoneal signs suggest perforation or toxic megacolon. A digital rectal examination should be done, noting fecal impaction, pain, bleeding, fissures, and fistulas. An occult blood card should be used; the presence or absence of blood helps with the differential diagnosis. Extragastrointestinal symptoms may shed light on the diagnosis as well (see Table 6-7-4).

DIAGNOSTIC CONSIDERATIONS

Complications from diarrhea have two basic mechanisms. The first is water and electrolyte losses and their consequences: dehydration, vascular collapse, and potentially death (i.e., epidemic cholera). The second is malabsorption, which can lead to anemias and weight loss.

Acute Diarrhea

Acute diarrhea is generally secondary to an infection or dietary imprudence. Common viral etiologies are due to the rotavirus and Norwalk virus. Bacterial causes are listed in Table 6-7-5. Parasitic causes include *Giardia lamblia, Cryptosporidium, Cyclospora,* and *Entamoeba histolytica.* The signs and symptoms include loose watery stools, fever, headache, malaise, anorexia, vomiting, myalgia, and

TABLE 6-7-4. Extragastrointestinal Symptoms Associated with Diarrhea

Polyarthritis	Ulcerative colitis, Crohn's disease, Reiter's syndrome, Whipple's disease, AIDS, sarcoidosis
Fever	Amebiasis, lymphoma, tuberculosis, inflammatory bowel disease, carcinoid syndromes
Bruising, purpura	Celiac sprue, tropical sprue, acetaminophen overdose
Conjunctivitis or episcleritis	Crohn's disease, ulcerative colitis, thyroid disease, Reiter's syndrome
Erythema nodosum	Sarcoidosis, acute or chronic pancreatitis, ulcerative colitis, Crohn's disease, radiation therapy, *Campylobacter, Salmonella, Shigella*

abdominal discomfort. Most of these sources of diarrhea are short-lived (24 to 48 h) and require only supportive home care (see Chap. 6-1).

Chronic Diarrhea

Chronic diarrhea is defined as diarrhea that lasts longer than 2 to 3 weeks or that appeared acute, ebbed, and recurred within 2 weeks. Persistent diarrhea requires thorough scrutiny. If the diarrhea contains fat (steatorrhea), malabsorption syndromes should be investigated (see Chap. 6-18). Chronic diarrhea with blood indicates the need to evaluate for inflammatory bowel disease (see Chap. 6-15) or colon cancer (see Chap. 13-5). Watery diarrhea without blood is more likely to be due to a systemic disease such as hyperthyroidism, diabetes, or pheochromocytoma. Recent antibiotic use may provide clues leading to the diagnosis of pseudomembranous colitis (see Chap. 6-4). Complications of any cause for chronic diarrhea include electrolyte and fluid imbalances and malnutrition.

Traveler's Diarrhea

Traveler's diarrhea affects approximately 10 million travelers a year. The vast majority complain of three to four unformed stools daily with classic acute diarrhea symptoms. Anywhere from 50 to 80 percent of cases are caused by dietary ingestion of diarrhea-producing types of bacteria (see Table 6-7-5). The mechanism of traveler's diarrhea is usually secretory and is caused by enterotoxins. *Escherichia coli* and *Salmonella* are relatively common with travel in Asia, Africa, and Latin America. Travelers to Russia and campers in the United States may encounter *Giardia lamblia.* Traveler's diarrhea is a major nuisance on a trip but is rarely life-threatening.

HIV and Diarrhea

Diarrhea may be the presenting symptom of an active HIV infection (see Chap. 9-1). The organisms that cause diarrhea in an immunocompromised patient are commonly the opportunistic type (see Table 6-7-6). Because of the patient's diminished immune system, symptoms may be more severe and recurrent. Bacteremia and sepsis often are seen, and antibiotic therapy is almost always required.

LABORATORY TESTS

Acute diarrhea without blood may not require any laboratory tests. If the acute diarrhea is causing severe symptoms (dehydration) or is bloody, it is evaluated as a chronic diarrhea. Begin with a complete blood cell count (CBC), electrolyte panel, C-reactive protein (CRP), and total protein evaluation. Culture the stool and check for enterotoxins, cells, and ova and parasites (O & P). *Escherichia coli* 0157:H7

TABLE 6-7-5. Bacterial and Viral Sources of Diarrhea

Type/Cause	Characteristics	Remarks
ACUTE DIARRHEA		
Norwalk virus, enterovirus	Watery diarrhea, usually no fever	Supportive hydration, lasts 24–48 h
Vibrio cholerae	Watery diarrhea, usually no fever	Fluid replacement; tetracycline may shorten course
Bacillus cereus	Starts with vomiting, then watery diarrhea, rarely fever	Supportive hydration usually lasts only 24–48 h
Clostridium perfringens	Profuse, watery diarrhea	Supportive hydration lasts 24–98 h
Clostridium difficile	Crampy abdominal pain followed by bloody diarrhea	Cultures not helpful, toxin levels elevated; treat with oral metronidazole (Flagyl) or Vancomycin and fluid replacement
Salmonella spp.	Diarrhea, but usually not profuse, vomiting, low-grade fever	No antibiotics (prolongs carrier stage) useless sepsis is present; fluid replacement
Shigella spp.	Diarrhea with blood and protein, cramps, fever	Severe cases can be treated with sulfa drugs; mild cases are self-limiting; replace fluids
CHRONIC DIARRHEA		
Campylobacter jejuni	Fever, diarrhea, blood, and proteins	Intermittent diarrhea over weeks; treat with erythromycin
Giardia lamblia	Relapsing watery diarrhea, flatulence, bloating, nausea	Can last months; treat with metronidazole
Entamoeba histolytica	Intermittent bloody diarrhea, abdominal pain, weight loss, flatulence	Can be asymptomatic to fulminant; intraluminal: treat with Iodoquinol; systemic: treat with metronidazole
Cyclospora	Relapsing watery diarrhea, weight loss, anorexia	Self-limiting in most patients; life-threatening in AIDS patients

should be sought specifically, as it is implicated in hemolytic uremic syndrome (HUS), which can be life-threatening. *Clostridium difficile* is difficult to culture, and so the toxin levels can be evaluated instead (see Chap. 6-4).

In looking for the cause of chronic diarrhea, the blood count may indicate malabsorption of folate, niacin, or iron. Liver function studies and thyroid studies may be helpful. Hypersecretion states can be associated with elevated gastrin levels. A Sudan black B fat stain can assess malabsorption syndromes (see Chap. 6-18). Check two or three different stools for culture and O & P, since the organisms or their by-products may not be present in every stool. Be sure to obtain all cultures before antibiotic use or barium studies, since both may change the results.

RADIOLOGIC (IMAGING) STUDIES

Plain abdominal films rarely reveal a definitive cause for diarrhea. The one exception is the presence of epigastric calcifications secondary to chronic pancreatitis. Barium studies may reveal the results of exudative diarrhea, neoplasm, diverticulitis, inflammatory bowel disease (IBD), or the spastic colon of irritable bowel syndrome (IBS).

The best study is the sigmoidoscope, which allows direct visualization, cultures, and biopsies. Sigmoidoscopy should be done before barium studies and without the usual hyperosmotic preparation to avoid disturbing the bowel architecture. If no diagnosis is forthcoming, a colonoscope is recommended with multiple biopsies to evaluate the patient for IBD, amebiasis, or amyloidosis. Finally, a computed tomography (CT) scan or magnetic resonance imaging (MRI) study

TABLE 6-7-6. HIV and Diarrhea

Protozoans
Cryptosporidium
Cyclospora
Entamoeba histolytica
Giardia lamblia
Isospora belli
Microsporida
Strongyloides stercoralis
Viruses
Cytomegalovirus
Epstein-Barr
Herpes simplex

may be helpful in defining occult carcinomas, pancreatic pseudocysts, and similar problems.

TREATMENT

The patient comes to a provider because of annoying symptoms, and diarrhea tops the list with most people. Try to treat the underlying source of the diarrhea rather than just the symptom. Since dehydration is a common side effect of diarrhea, rehydration is a fundamental part of treatment. Oral hydration solutions include glucose solution with a combination of essential salts: sodium, potassium, chloride, and citrate. Rehydration formulas are listed in Table 6-1-3. Osmotically induced diarrhea and some secretory diarrhea will diminish or cease completely within 24 h of clear liquids only.

Antidiarrheals such as loperamide (Imodium) 4 mg initial dose followed by 2 mg every 4 to 6 h should be used with care. Loperamide slows the transit time of the intestine and inhibits some intestinal secretions. It does not increase water absorption or change the electrolyte balance. Loperamide should not be used in exudative causes of diarrhea such as ulcerative colitis, pseudomembranous colitis, and acute dysentery because the gut slows down too much and the disease process may be exacerbated.

Diphenoxylate hydrochloride (Lomotil) is very effective in slowing intestinal motility, allowing for increased contact of contents with the mucosal surface. This in turn may increase fluid reabsorption. Like loperamide, diphenoxylate should be used with care and never used in a patient with fever, bloody diarrhea, or the potential of enterotoxin-producing organisms.

Kaolin and pectin are absorbents and gels used in over-the-counter antidiarrhea medications (Kaopectate). For acute diarrhea, these products have not been proved to decrease diarrhea and are not recommended for the treatment of diarrhea of any source.

The use of antidiarrheals is not recommended in children under age 8 or the elderly because of the potential side effects. Treatment of the underlying cause remains the best choice, with adequate fluid and electrolyte replacement regardless of age.

COMPLICATIONS

Acute diarrhea is associated with dehydration with patient complaints of headache, body aches, and anorexia. Electrolyte imbalances may occur with fulminant diarrhea and demand immediate attention to avoid mental status changes or cardiac events. Chronic diarrhea may result in malabsorption of nutrients and vitamins, leading to anemias, muscle atrophy, bone loss, failure to thrive, and so on.

PATIENT EDUCATION

Traveler's diarrhea is preventable if proper care is taken. Travelers should avoid tap water when drinking, brushing teeth, using ice cubes, or rinsing drink ware, fruits, and vegetables. One should try to drink only bottled water or carbonated drinks from containers that are factory-sealed. A traveler should avoid fresh fruits and vegetables unless the traveler peels this food himself or herself. Foods that have been re-warmed, street food, rare meat, raw seafood, doubtfully boiled foods, and food that appears undercooked should not be eaten.

Prophylaxis with antibiotics may be recommended for trips shorter than 2 weeks in certain populations: the elderly and patients with concomitant gastrointestinal (GI) disease, diabetes, renal disease, cancer, or immunosuppression. Currently, trimethoprim-sulfamethoxazole (Bactrim DS) once daily is the recommended prophylaxis. The fluoroquinolones (Cipro, Noroxin) may be used as an alternative.

PEARLS

The most common cause of diarrhea—viruses and bacteria—are easily treated with fluids, bed rest, and time. Encourage the patient to rest and sip fluids all day long, avoid milk products and greasy foods for at least 48 h, and to follow a clear liquid diet for at least 24 h. Do not overprescribe antidiarrheals; they are not innocuous and can be abused. This author never gives a patient more than four tablets for the control of acute diarrhea. This prevents overuse, and if the patient's diarrhea persists, it forces the patient to seek follow-up care and a further workup. Remember that diarrhea is a symptom, not a disease. Look for the underlying cause and treat it appropriately.

BIBLIOGRAPHY

Kneepken CMF, Hoekstra JH: Chronic nonspecific diarrhea in childhood. *Pediatr Clin North Am* 43(2):375–386, 1996.
Kroser JA, Metz DC: Evaluation of the adult patient with diarrhea. *Primary Care Clin Office Pract* 23(3):629–645, 1996.

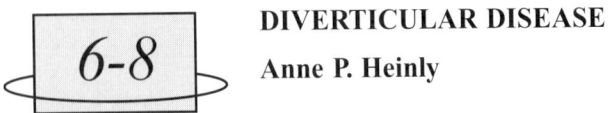

6-8 DIVERTICULAR DISEASE
Anne P. Heinly

DESCRIPTION

Diverticular disease appears to be an unwanted by-product of industrialization, specifically, the milling of whole grains into processed breads and cereals. Virtually unheard of prior to 1900, diverticular disease may be found in up to half of the population in the United States by the age of 70 to 80 years. Diverticular disease has two components: *diverticulosis*, the presence of diverticula, usually asymptomatic, and *diverticulitis*, inflammation of diverticula, usually symptomatic. The development of diverticulosis is unusual before the age of 40, but the risk increases approximately 5 to 10% per decade of life. Of those patients with diverticulosis, perhaps one-fifth will develop diverticulitis, with equal distribution between men and women.

PATHOGENESIS

Diverticula can occur anywhere along the gastrointestinal tract. However, by convention, the term when used independently refers to

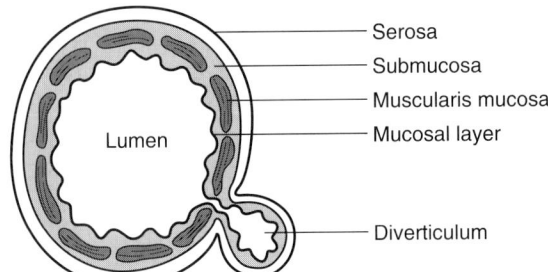

FIGURE 6-8-1. Diverticular disease.

colonic diverticula. The colon has four layers: the serosa (the outer layer), the muscular layer, the submucosa, and the mucosa (the innermost layer). Diverticulum (singular) and diverticula (plural) are actually pseudodiverticula or herniations of the two inner layers through a defect in the muscular band enveloped by the encircling serosa (Fig. 6-8-1). The mechanism of formation appears to be a function of ambient intraluminal pressure in the colon. Because of the low-fiber diet of Americans and persons in other westernized countries, the circular muscles of the colon must contract more forcefully to expel smaller, harder stool products. This leads to an increased intraluminal pressure in segments of the colon, especially the descending and sigmoid colon. Over time, the strength of the colonic connective tissue appears to weaken, and defects in the muscular layer allow for the herniation.

SYMPTOMS

Diverticulosis

More than 80% of patients with diverticulosis will have no symptoms. Diagnosis is made incidentally during other examinations. Those with symptoms may have left lower quadrant (LLQ) crampy abdominal pain, often described as "gripping"—a short, sharp pain followed by 1 to 2 h of dull, achy pain. This is most likely caused by increased intraluminal pressure during colonic peristalsis. With diverticulosis there is no inflammation, so fever, chills, nausea, and peritoneal signs are absent.

The second symptom in patients without inflammation is painless rectal bleeding, which can be quite extensive. The source is usually a single colonic diverticulum in the ascending colon that has enlarged sufficiently to erode or tear the vast arterial supply in the right lower quadrant (RLQ). The blood may be bright red or maroon (seldom black) and may stop spontaneously or continue intermittently for days. Once a bleed has occurred, there is a 50% chance of recurrent bleeds.

Diverticulitis

Diverticulitis is the inflammation of the diverticula. Patients will present with acute abdominal pain, generally persistent and localized to the LLQ. Anorexia, fever, chills, nausea, and vomiting may accompany the pain. A change in bowel habits is common and ranges from sudden onset of constipation to profuse diarrhea. With severe inflammation (multiple microperforations) or frank colonic perforations, peritoneal signs will be present.

OBJECTIVE

With diverticulosis, the patient may have a mass effect in the LLQ. This is most likely the sigmoid colon, which presents as a firm and tender mass. There may be abdominal distention and increased tympany. Diverticulosis seldom presents with peritoneal signs, fever, or vital sign changes.

Diverticulitis, on the other hand, presents with an acute abdomen with quiet or sluggish bowel sounds, distention, rebound tenderness, fever, and vital sign alterations. Peritoneal irritation is often present with positive psoas, obturator, or heel-tap signs. A tender, firm mass effect is common in the LLQ and can be confirmed with pelvic and/or rectal examination. In the elderly, signs may be blunted due to decreased immune response.

DIAGNOSTIC CONSIDERATIONS

A differential diagnosis for symptomatic diverticulosis includes constipation, lactose intolerance, and irritable bowel syndrome. Painless bleeding may be secondary to a variety of sources but it is important to rule out colonic carcinoma, Crohn's disease, and ulcerative colitis, especially in the elderly.

Diverticulitis may mimic any other acute abdominal distress: appendicitis, colitis, acute gastroenteritis, ulcerative colitis, Crohn's disease, and gynecological or urological complaints. The most consistent distinguishing factor is the presence of the mass effect in the LLQ in the majority of diverticulitis episodes.

LABORATORY TESTS

Laboratory findings for diverticulosis will usually be normal. Diverticulitis will commonly reveal an elevated white blood cell count with a left shift (prevalence of polymorphonuclear neutrophil leukocytes). Serum C-reactive protein is elevated, and serum amylase may also climb. In the elderly, the immune response is often blunted so laboratory signs of inflammation may be less dramatic. A urinalysis may reveal hematuria and/or leukocytosis if there has been compromise of the ureters or bladder.

RADIOLOGIC (IMAGING) STUDIES

During acute episodes of diverticulitis, a plain abdominal film may reveal colonic ileus or air fluid levels of a perforation. The best exam to define diverticulosis is a barium enema. Diverticula on a barium enema may appear as solitary lesions or in clumps of pedunculated mushroom-like appendages (Fig. 6-8-2). A barium enema can also demonstrate paracolic abscesses, leaking sacs, fistulas, and strictures caused by the diverticula. The debate still continues on the value of a barium enema during acute diverticulitis. The degree of inflammation may distort the findings and there is risk of perforating a swollen diverticulum or contaminating the peritoneum with contrast medium if a perforation exists.

Computer tomography (CT) scans have been successfully used to diagnosis acute diverticulitis. The benefit is that CT scanning is noninvasive and can detect subtle differences in the colonic walls, fistulas, paracolic abscesses, and perforations. Ultrasound and magnetic resonance imaging may also be used to define the presence of diverticula. Sigmoidoscopy is not recommended during acute episodes and is limited in its ability to diagnosis diverticula. Endoscopy is valuable to rule out the differential diagnosis of cancer, ulcerative colitis, Crohn's disease, or similar disorders. Arteriograms can locate the bleeding source from an asymptomatic diverticulum.

TREATMENT

Conservative treatment for diverticulosis is aimed at decreasing intraluminal pressure. The best therapy for this is a high-fiber diet consisting of whole grains, legumes, fruits, and vegetables. The older recommendation of avoiding foods with small seeds and popcorn has not been shown to affect the disease process. Mild analgesics (acetaminophen) and anticholinergics (Bentyl 10 mg every 6 h) can relieve symptoms of cramping.

Diverticulitis, if mild, can be treated as diverticulosis with the addition of antibiotics (Table 6-8-1). Additionally, the initial diet should be a clear liquid diet to allow for gut rest. After acute symptoms subside, the patient can progress slowly to a high-fiber diet. Many patients can be cared for as outpatients, and elective colon resection is done only for recurrent attacks, fistula formation, or obstruction.

More severely ill patients will require hospitalization and intravenous antibiotics (Table 6-8-1). Surgery is done only for frank perforation, obstruction, or paracolonic abscesses that do not improve with 3 to 7 days of hospital therapy. The optimal situation is to have decreased inflammation prior to surgery to decrease blood loss and surgical risks. There are two surgical approaches: laparotomy with colectomy and resection (when possible) and the newer percutaneous abscess drainage under CT visualization. Obviously, the abscess drainage presents less risk to an acutely ill patient and allows for a delay in the colectomy in 6 to 8 weeks. Delay in colectomy is expedient because it permits the immediate resection (anastomosis) at the time of surgery versus the placement of a colostomy during emergency surgery for perforations. In the elderly, the prospect of one surgery versus two (repair of the colostomy) and the attendant anesthesia risk is an important consideration.

COMPLICATIONS

Diverticular abscess, perforation, fistulas, scarring, obstruction, and bleeding are all complications of diverticular disease. Death occurs rarely but is associated with the infirm elderly and immunocompromised patients. Emergency surgery complications occur in about 10% of patients ranging from cardiac events and pulmonary emboli to sepsis.

PEARLS

A diet high in fiber is probably one of the best things clinicians can recommend for patients. Diverticular disease is a direct result of low fiber in the diet. Colon cancer has been related to low fiber, and constipation is a chronic problem for many Americans. Encourage

TABLE 6-8-1.   Antibiotics for Diverticulitis

Oral

   Metronidazole (Flagyl) 500 mg every 8 h
     with amoxicillin 500 mg every 8 h
   or
   Ciprofloxacin (Cipro) 500 mg bid
   or
   Norfloxacin (Noroxin) 400 mg bid

Intravenous

   Amikacin (Amikin) 15 mg/kg per day divided doses every 8 h
     with metronidazole (Flagyl) 500 mg every 8 h
   or
   Gentamicin (Garamycin) 1 mg/kg every 8 h with clindamycin
     1.5–2.5 mg/kg per day in divided doses every 8 h
   or
   Cefoxitin 1–2 g every 12 h

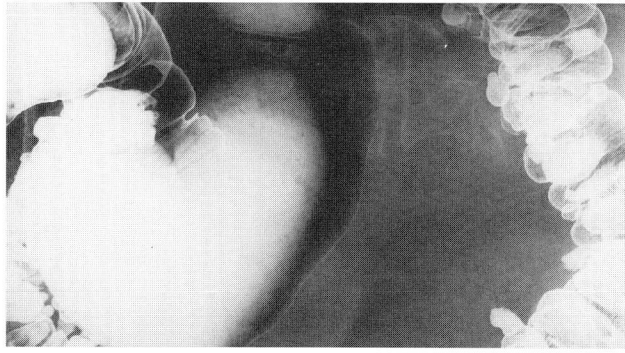

FIGURE 6-8-2. Barium enema demonstrating multiple diverticula.

patients to add 15 to 20 g of high fiber to their daily diet, and diverticular disease may not be the only thing they avoid.

BIBLIOGRAPHY

Sanson TG, Okeefe KP: Gastrointestinal emergencies, part I, evaluation abdominal pain in the elderly. *Emerg Med Clin North Am* 14(3):615–625, 1996.

Practice Parameters for Sigmoid Diverticulitis, Diseases of the Colon and Rectum, 35(2):125–130, Williams & Wilkins, 1995.

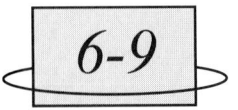

FECAL IMPACTION

Freddi Segal-Gidan

DISCUSSION

Fecal (stool) impaction is a common and often overlooked disorder, particularly among the elderly and immobilized. It has a variable presentation and many potential complications. It generally is thought to be the end result of unrecognized and untreated constipation (see Chap. 6-6). Masses of hard feces accumulate in the rectum, which distends to accommodate an enlarging mass that may back up into the sigmoid colon. It can cause discomfort, pain, delirium, and rarely, in extreme cases, bowel perforation.

Fecal impaction primarily involves the rectum and colon. Changes in the absorption of salt and water from the colon lead to hardening of the stool. Slowing of peristaltic activity causes packing of fecal matter. The rectum is distensible and can accommodate an enlarging fecal mass, but the anal canal has limited distensibility, and therefore the feces become too large to pass.

In hospitalized and immobilized individuals, the common presentation is diarrhea or urinary incontinence. The hard stool of a fecal impaction acts as an irritant against the rectum or colon wall. This causes the production of mucus and fluid, which leak around the mass and cause small amounts of diarrhea, often associated with fecal incontinence. Irritation by the fecal mass also can lead to bleeding.

SYMPTOMS

Impaction usually presents as a subtle and nonspecific finding. Typical symptoms include abdominal pain, anorexia, nausea, and vomiting. Impaction may be associated with complaints of constipation, diarrhea, and incontinence, either urinary or fecal. Often it is the underlying problem in an elderly person who presents with diarrhea or new-onset urinary incontinence, particularly when accompanied by fecal incontinence. Acute confusion (delirium), especially in an elderly or debilitated individual, also may be due to fecal impaction. Elevated temperature, dysrhythmias, and tachycardia caused by impaired motility of the diaphragm from fecal impaction also have been reported.

Whenever the frequency of bowel movements is less than one every other day, a diagnosis of fecal impaction should be considered. There may be a history of no bowel movement for several days or up to a week or more. A history of a prior impaction is also a useful clue.

Medications that delay gastric motility are often a contributing factor (see Table 6-9-1). Depression and psychosis can themselves be associated with constipation. Ironically, the agents used to treat these conditions may worsen the problem and produce impaction as a result of their anticholinergic properties. Fecal impaction occurs at high incidence in association with neurologic conditions that are complicated by immobility, such as stroke, Parkinson's disease, multiple sclerosis (MS), and amyotrophic lateral sclerosis (ALS). Rectal impaction frequently is associated with lumbosacral spinal cord injuries, whereas cervical and thoracic spinal cord injuries tend to cause proximal impactions.

TABLE 6-9-1. Medications That Cause Constipation and Often Contribute to Impaction

Opiate analgesics (codeine)
Tricyclic antidepressants (amitriptyline)
Phenothiazines
Antihypertensives (alpha- and beta-adrenergic blockers, calcium channel blockers)
Diuretics (furosemide, thiazides)
Antacids (aluminum-containing)
Sucralfate
Iron

OBJECTIVE FINDINGS

A digital rectal examination is essential to assess for impaction of the distal bowel. The lack of stool in the rectal ampule or only loose, watery fecal material may be a tip-off to the presence of impaction higher up. Sphincter tone is usually present. The abdominal examination is often completely normal. There may be decreased or few bowel sounds throughout the abdomen, or there may be increased sounds over one region. Fullness may be palpable if a large amount of stool causes distention, especially in thinner individuals. An abdominal mass may be palpated and can be misinterpreted as a tumor or an abdominal aortic aneurysm. Urinary retention may be evident, especially when there is urinary incontinence (usually the overflow type).

DIAGNOSTIC CONSIDERATIONS

Fecal impaction should be considered the underlying cause or a contributing factor in an older adult with diarrhea, urinary incontinence, fecal incontinence, and constipation and in any patient presenting with delirium. Patients with chronic renal failure are predisposed to impaction when there is a disturbance of fluid volume and electrolyte imbalance.

SPECIAL CONSIDERATIONS

The geriatric population is particularly prone to develop fecal impaction as a result of a combination of aging changes in the bowel, low dietary fiber, limited fluid intake, and decreased mobility. Hospitalized and immobilized elderly individuals are especially at risk. Patients with a long history of laxative use (dependency) are also at higher risk for both constipation and fecal impaction.

LABORATORY TESTS

Leukocytosis on a complete blood cell count (CBC) may indicate associated sepsis, usually urinary in origin. Electrolyte abnormalities, particularly hyponatremia and hypokalemia, also may be associated with impaction and/or underlying dehydration. Stool samples should be assessed for occult blood, which may reflect mucosal irritation of an impaction or be a sign of an underlying colon tumor.

RADIOLOGIC STUDIES

A flat-plate x-ray of the abdomen [Kidney, ureter, bladder (KUB)] is useful for the documentation of the presence of an impaction, particularly when it is high in the sigmoid colon. The abdominal x-ray may demonstrate colonic dilatation and an unusual air-fluid level in the small bowel caused by masses of stool or obstruction.

TREATMENT

Disimpaction is essential. It should be initiated manually by rectal examination and stimulation to break up the impaction, followed by an enema (oil retention or Fleet saline). Further manual disimpaction may be necessary. Gentle, progressive dilatation first with one finger and then with two fingers and a scissoring action is used to fragment the impaction and aid its expulsion. Lidocaine jelly for local anesthesia and lubrication may be used. Transvaginal pressure with the other hand in women also may be helpful. Do not use irritant laxatives, as they may irritate the rectal mucosa and cause bleeding. Attempts to remove an impaction from above by catharsis are useless, may worsen the pain, or may contribute to complications.

Normal bowel function should be restored to prevent reimpaction. An essential component of this is a review of the patient's daily food and fluid intake. A diet high in fiber, preferably obtained from fruits, vegetables, and whole grain cereals and with adequate liquids (2 L/day at minimum), is ideal. Dietary fiber can be supplied by Miller's bran added to foods or the use of bulk-producing products (e.g., Metamucil). Stool softeners and lubricants may be required daily in an individual with chronic constipation but pose risks. If there is no stool for 2 days, a glycerine suppository should be administered. If this fails to produce any stool, a saline enema on the third day may be required.

COMPLICATIONS AND RED FLAGS

Fecal incontinence is the most common complication of impaction. Seepage of mucus and stool may lead to decubitus ulceration around the anus. Urinary tract infections also may be caused by fecal contamination from incontinence associated with an impaction. Ulcerations with occult bleeding may result from the pressure and ischemic necrosis on the colon wall that are caused by the fecal mass. Perforation is rare and has a high mortality rate. In a spinal cord–injured patient, autonomic dysreflexia, a potentially life-threatening condition, may be provoked by fecal impaction. Fecalomas may be caused by tumors as well as mimic them.

PEARLS

In the elderly, immobilized, and institutionalized, always keep a high suspicion for underlying fecal impaction. Impaction high in the colon often is associated with an underlying adenocarcinoma.

BIBLIOGRAPHY

Read NW, Celik AF, Katsinelos P: Constipation and incontinence in the elderly. *J Clin Gastroenterol* 20(1):61–70, 1995.
Wrenn K: Fecal impaction. *N Engl J Med* 321(10):658–662, 1989.

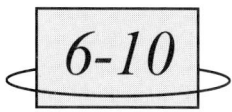

GALLBLADDER DISEASE
Anne P. Heinly

ANATOMY

The gallbladder is a small pear-shaped organ tucked beneath the liver in the right upper quadrant, protected by the anterior rib cage. Its primary function is the storage and subsequent release of bile. Holding approximately 40 mL of bile, the gallbladder releases bile in response to meals, especially fatty meals. The bile is released through the cystic duct into the common bile duct, traveling to the sphincter of Oddi and into the duodenum, and aids in the digestion of fats (see Fig. 6-10-1). Bile is a conglomeration of bile salts (acids), phospholipids, unconjugated bilirubin, and cholesterol held in suspension. Bile acids are detergents that above a critical concentration form aggregates called *micelles*. These micelles are essential for normal intestinal absorption of dietary fats.

CHOLELITHIASIS

DISCUSSION

Between 10 and 20 percent of the general population develops gallstones. Women are twice as likely to develop stones; the acronym "4Fs = female, fat, forty, and fertile" is most likely secondary to the estrogen factor. The likelihood of stone development increases with age. Stones are rare in the Far East and Africa but common among Native Americans and in Chile and Sweden. Although four-fifths remain asymptomatic, found only when abdominal studies are done for other reasons, a small proportion (1 to 4 percent) of patients per year will develop symptoms if stones are present.

PATHOGENESIS

Choleliths, or gallstones, are formed when the concentration of bile salts and cholesterol changes. Eighty percent of all gallstones are cholesterol stones, formed when there is a relative increase in cholesterol biosynthesis and a decrease in bile acid synthesis.[1] A bile acid concentration greater than half will keep cholesterol in solution. Supersaturation of bile with cholesterol, gallbladder hypomotility, and crystal nucleation all promote stone formation. Table 6-10-1 lists risk factors for the formation of cholesterol stones.

Black pigment stones are more common in patients with cirrhosis or chronic hemolytic conditions such as hereditary spherocytosis and sickle cell disease, which are commonly found in the pediatric population. The stones are made up of polymers of bilirubin. Brown pigmented stones are composed of calcium salts of bilirubin and may be associated with infection. *A special note concerning ceftriaxone (Rocephin)*: This drug can cause ceftriaxone-calcium sludge and may present as cholelithiasis. The condition appears to be transient and is reversible with discontinuation of the medication.

SIGNS AND SYMPTOMS

Typical signs and symptoms include biliary colic, which is described as a steady, severe pain that takes several hours to resolve. (Colic is a misnomer because it implies an intermittent process; biliary pain is generally steady.) Pain frequently is located in the right upper quadrant (RUQ) and/or epigastrium and may radiate to the right shoulder, right scapula, or back. Anorexia and nausea with or without vomiting are common. Attacks often are precipitated by a fatty meal, but not always. Bile excretion follows a diurnal pattern, peaking at midnight, and so the patient may awaken with pain. Symptoms often attributed to the presence of gallstones, including belching, bloating, chronic pain, and intolerance of fatty food, are not necessarily exclusive to cholelithiasis.

OBJECTIVE FINDINGS

Right upper quadrant and/or epigastric tenderness without rebound may be noted. The gallbladder may be palpable; Murphy's sign is seen when there is an inspiratory arrest with deep palpation under the midpoint of the right costal margin. Vital signs may show tachycardia with no fever. Rarely, jaundice is seen. Complications of cholelithiasis (see Table 6-10-2) will reveal more physical findings and should be considered with any examination.

DIAGNOSTIC CONSIDERATIONS

It is good to remember that the differential diagnosis can work in reverse: Gallstones may present atypically and manifest as lactose intolerance or gastroesophageal reflux disease. Conversely, the presence of stones may be blamed for symptoms that actually are associated with a totally different disease process. See Table 6-10-3 for the differential diagnosis.

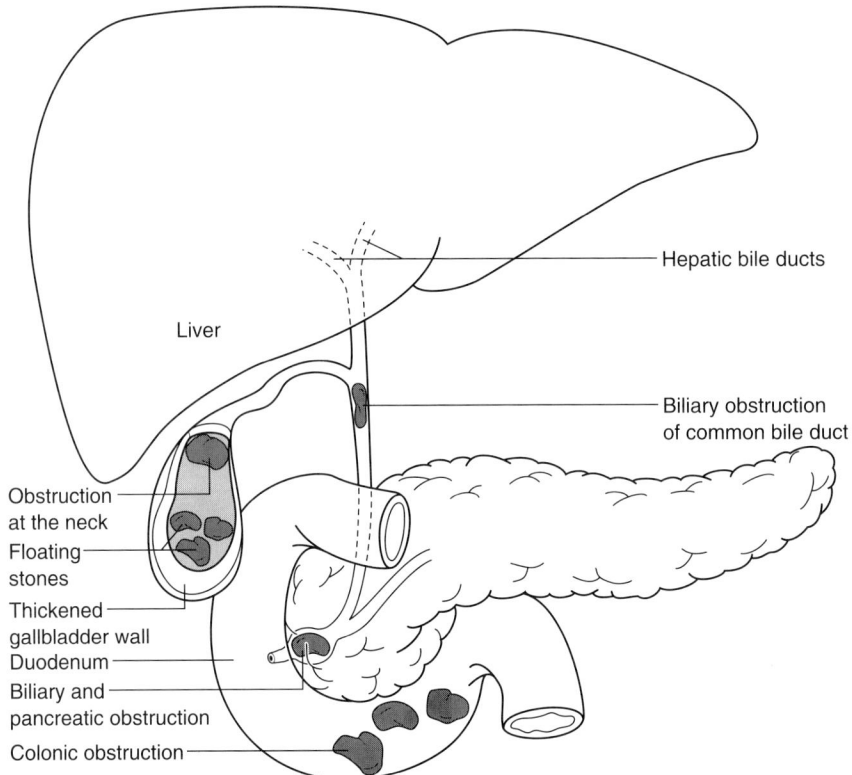

FIGURE 6-10-1. Complications of cholelithiasis.

A special note about gallbladder cancer: The vast majority of patients with gallbladder cancer have choleliths. The choleliths are often solitary and large (3 cm), though no concrete connection has been established between the presence of stones and the development of cancer. It is worthwhile to have a high index of suspicion when one is evaluating a patient with symptoms. Native Americans are at high risk of gallbladder cancer, and with cholelithiasis that risk increases. The take-home point of large stones or a calcified gallbladder wall (porcelain gallbladder) should ring alarm bells for continued evaluation and treatment.

LABORATORY TESTS

Laboratory studies will not diagnose the presence of choleliths but may help differentiate their potential complications. Liver function tests may show an increase in conjugated bilirubin and increased

TABLE 6-10-2. Complications of Cholelithiasis

Cystic duct obstruction
Acute cholecystitis
Cholangitis (sepsis)
Perforation and peritonitis
Fistulization to other abdominal structures
Provoked acute pancreatitis

alkaline phosphatase out of proportion with the mild elevation seen with the other liver enzymes. A serum amylase may be elevated with a common bile duct obstruction, causing acute pancreatitis. A complete blood cell count (CBC) may reveal leukocytosis consistent with inflammation or infection.

RADIOLOGIC (IMAGING) STUDIES

Some choleliths may be radiopaque and easily seen on plain abdominal films. The oral cholecystogram (OCG) has been around for years and has a predictive rate of 90 to 95 percent. However, an OCG may not visualize small stones, takes longer to perform (not good in emergent care), and is contraindicated in pregnant patients and persons with iodinate contrast allergies. The study of choice today is ultrasound.

Gallbladder ultrasound can be done rapidly, accurately identifies stones (even a small one) with a predictive rate of >95 percent, and can give a real-time assessment of gallbladder volume and contractility. Additionally, other abdominal structures are easily visualized and ruled out as a source of pathology. Ultrasound may not be diagnostic in the setting of obesity, ascites, excessive bowel gas, or recent barium studies.

Technetium iminodiacetic acid 99m (IDA) cholescintigraphy (HIDA, DIDA scans) has a predictive value over 95 percent and is especially helpful in revealing a nonfunctional gallbladder with or without stones. This examination generally is done when gallbladder ultrasound has failed to reveal stones but symptoms of gallbladder disease persist. It is not used as the initial diagnostic tool.

TABLE 6-10-1.   Risk Factors for Cholesterol Stones

RISK FACTORS	MECHANISM
Estrogens (childbearing age, OC, HRT)	Reduces synthesis of bile acid, increased cholesterol
Obesity	Increased hepatic secretion of cholesterol
Very low calorie diet	Changes in biliary lipid profile and gallbladder hypomotility
Decreased HDL	HDLs break up cholesterol
Ileal disease (Crohn's)	Decreased bile acid retrieval
Clofibrate (Atromid-S) therapy	Increased hepatic secretion of cholesterol
Hypertriglyceridemia	Change in lipid concentrations
Increasing age	Increased hepatic secretion and decreased bile acids
Type 2 diabetes mellitus	Mechanism not well understood

NOTE: OC = oral contraceptives; HRT = hormone replacement therapy; HDL = high-density lipoprotein.

TABLE 6-10-3. Differential Diagnosis of Cholelithiasis*

DISEASE	HELPFUL LAB DIFFERENTIAL
Pancreatitis	Amylase five times normal, ↑ lipase
Acalculous cholecystitis	Leukocytosis, mild LF abnormalities
Hepatitis (any type)	Elevation of liver enzymes
Peptic ulcer disease	CBC may reveal anemia ± LFS changes
Colon disease	CBC may reveal anemia ± LFS changes
Gastroesophageal reflux disease	CBC may reveal anemia ± LFS changes
Lactose intolerance	No lab changes

Drug-induced cholestasis
   Calcium channel blockers
   Oral hypoglycemics
   Antibiotics
   Tricyclic antidepressants
   Anticonvulsants
   Tranquilizers
	Liver function changes, mild to severe

*Limited list that includes the most common differentials.
NOTE: LF = liver function; CBC = complete blood count; LFS = liver function studies.

TREATMENT

Management of asymptomatic stones is still controversial, but it is generally accepted for the following conditions: nonfunctioning gallbladder, calcified gallbladder wall, history of pancreatitis, and diagnosis of type 2 diabetes mellitus. Studies do not support the presumption that all choleliths require treatment.

There are three treatment choices for symptomatic cholelithiasis: dissolution therapy, laparoscopic cholecystectomy, and open cholecystectomy. Dissolution therapy is a noninvasive medication option that is indicated in approximately one-third of symptomatic patients. The criteria[2] for its use are listed in Table 6-10-4. Ursodiol (ursodeoxycholic acid) increases the bile acid concentration and over 6 months to 2 years can dissolve stones up to 15 mm in size. Complete dissolution occurs in less than half of patients with free-floating stones. The primary adverse effect of the medication is transient diarrhea. Unfortunately, the recurrence of stones is likely, and patients may have complications caused by cystic duct obstruction and inflammation. Smaller stones are still stones and can cause trouble.

Methyl-*tert*-butyl ether (MTBE) has been used as a direct-contact solvent of choleliths. Only one-third of symptomatic patients are candidates for this type of dissolution. The agent is instilled into the gallbladder through a percutaneous catheter placed through the liver [endoscopic retrograde cholangiopancreatography (ERCP)]. Dissolution can occur within 24 h. Cholesterol stones are the only stones affected by this solvent, and recurrence of stones is common. Currently, this procedure is available only at large medical teaching facilities.

Laparoscopic cholecystectomy is the newest procedure. The year 1988 saw the first procedure; since then, the procedure has become commonplace. The most dramatic results of laparoscopic cholecystectomy are a reduction in hospital days, decreased postoperative pain, and a quick return to routine for patients. Patients who should not be considered for laparoscopic surgery include those with widespread peritonitis, severe pancreatitis, septic shock from cholangitis, endstage liver disease, gallbladder cancer, and third-trimester pregnancy.[3]

TABLE 6-10-4. Criteria for Ursodiol (Actigall)

Functional gallbladder
Stones less than 15 mm in diameter
Stones shown to float
Patient is poor candidate for surgery or refuses surgery

Open cholecystectomy remains a safe and effective therapy for symptomatic cholelithiasis. Unlike dissolution therapy, cholecystectomy considerably decreases the recurrence of stones and gallbladder cancer. Additionally, the open approach facilitates bile duct exploration for choledocholithiasis (bile duct stones), which are a potential complication in up to a fourth of these patients. Severe complications of open cholecystectomy are rare, but the cost in hospital days, pain, and time off from work has made this procedure the second choice behind the laparoscopic approach.

Gallstone lithotripsy is being investigated. In countries that use this method of extracorporeal shock wave lithotripsy, stone clearance is as high as 95 percent. Solitary stones up to 20 mm in diameter have been shattered. Complications include transient elevations of liver enzymes, pancreatitis and hematuria. As with dissolution therapy, recurrence is a problem. The U.S. Food and Drug Administration (FDA) has not approved gallbladder lithotripsy in the United States.

Putting prevention into practice is true for cholelithiasis. Several recommendations may help diminish the occurrence of gallstones. Slow weight loss versus drastic weight loss diets may help. Studies found that women who lost 10 kg in a 2-year period had a higher incidence of cholelithiasis then did those who lost 4 to 9 kg.[4] A vegetarian life-style decreases the incidence rate and can be recommended for the prevention of other disease processes as well. Avoidance of medications that are known to precipitate gallstones is a reasonable idea where possible.

SPECIAL CONSIDERATIONS

Three special groups deserve mention in discussing cholelithiasis. The first is North American Indians, who are at high risk for the development of stones and subsequent complications. While "female, fat, forty, and fertile" is generally true, a North American Indian may develop stones in the first or second decade. Additionally, normal-weight women may form gallstones. The rationale for this has been linked to slow intestinal transit time; that is, constipation seems to change the composition of the bile.

Second, children who are incidentally diagnosed with choleliths (often associated with hemolytic anemia, cystic fibrosis, and sickle cell disease) should be considered for prophylactic cholecystectomy because they almost always develop symptoms. Third, the geriatric population frequently is plagued with cholelithiasis. Unfortunately, the normal aging process dulls signs and symptoms as a result of a decrease in immune responses. A geriatric patient with a gangrenous or ruptured gallbladder secondary to stones may not run a fever or reveal a significant leukocytosis. A good history, a physical, and healthy suspicion are required to pick up the source of an acute abdominal event in the elderly.

PEARLS

The majority of people with cholelithiasis never have symptoms, but those who do have pain and nausea. Since pain and nausea are common to many other gastrointestinal disease processes, evaluation for stones or an acalculous nonfunctioning gallbladder is worth the time and effort. Potential complications, especially in the elderly, can be debilitating and life-threatening.

CHOLECYSTITIS

DESCRIPTION

Cholecystitis is inflammation of the gallbladder. It affects more than 15 million people a year, and the vast majority of cases are associated with the presence of choleliths (gallstones). Initially, there may be obstruction to the neck of the gallbladder or the cystic duct by stones (see Fig. 6-10-1). This leads to distention and inflammation. The inflamed gallbladder wall is then colonized by opportunistic bowel flora, and infection ensues. The pathogens most often found include *Escherichia coli, Klebsiella* species, group D streptococci, *Staphylococcus* species,

TABLE 6-10-5. Etiology of Acalculous Cholecystitis

Decreased gallbladder function (↓ motility)

Starvation (very low calorie diets)

Major trauma

Severe burns

Nonbiliary surgery

Prolonged labor

Total parenteral nutrition

Anesthesia induction

Narcotic use

Unusual bacteria
 Leptospira
 Vibrio cholerae
 Salmonella

Parasites: *Isospora bili* found in some AIDS patients

Immunosuppressed patients

Severe atherosclerotic heart disease and peripheral
 vascular disease

TABLE 6-10-6. Differential Diagnosis for Cholecystitis*

Perforated peptic ulcer

Retrocecal appendicitis

Right lower lobe pneumonia

Myocardial infarction

Pancreatitis

Hepatitis

*Partial list—most commonly seen.

LABORATORY TESTS

Laboratory studies should include a CBC that frequently will reveal leukocytosis (10,000 to 15,000) with a left shift. Serum bilirubin may be mildly elevated, as may the alkaline phosphatase.

RADIOLOGIC STUDIES

Gallbladder ultrasound is the diagnostic choice because it is rapid, easily accessed at the bedside, and noninvasive. While the following findings are not exclusive to acute cholecystitis, they help in the diagnosis:

- Gallbladder wall thickening (greater than 4 mm)
- Distention of the gallbladder
- Dependent echogenic bile sludge or stones
- Sonographic Murphy's sign (focal tenderness directly over the visualized gallbladder)

Several ultrasound findings are consistent with an acalculous cholecystitis with gangrene:

- No sonographic Murphy's sign (nerve fibers have been destroyed).
- Inner layer sloughs in the presence of necrosis; may reveal thick mucus within the lumen.
- A frayed or irregular gallbladder wall indicates hemorrhage and microabscesses.

Radionuclide scans (HIDA, DIDA) can diagnose acute cholecystitis or a nonfunctioning gallbladder when bilirubin levels or acute disease precludes the usefulness of other examinations.

COMPLICATIONS

Emphysematous cholecystitis is an acute cholecystitis with ischemia and infection that is caused by a gas-producing organism such as *Clostridium welchii* or *perfringens.* This type is common in elderly men and patients with diabetes. Plain films will reveal gas within the gallbladder lumen and dissection with the gallbladder wall forming a gaseous ring. The mortality rate is high, and surgical intervention is essential.

Cholelithiasis is almost always responsible for chronic cholecystitis. Repeated bouts of subacute cholecystitis lead to a chronic colonization of bacteria in the gallbladder. Surgery is the treatment of choice, with intraoperative and postoperative antibiotic therapy.

Acute cholecystitis when left untreated can lead to gallbladder rupture and gangrene, hepatitis, and pancreatitis. Prompt treatment of this acute abdomen is essential to avoid life-threatening sequelae. Table 6-10-7 lists the complications seen in postcholecystectomy patients.

TREATMENT

Supportive management of acute cholecystitis begins with bed rest and gastrointestinal (GI) tract rest. The patient should be kept NPO (nothing by mouth), or if necessary (to ensure gastric decompression), there may be placement of a nasal gastric tube. Intravenous (IV) therapy for replacement of fluids and electrolytes should be maintained and adjusted to the patient's needs. The elderly can develop CHF and pulmonary edema with fluid overload. Pain relief should not include the use of morphine, which may cause spasms at the sphincter of Oddi. Ketorolac (Toradol) 60 mg IM every 8 h is a good alternative to

and *Clostridium* species.[5] Factors that may predict a serious course include the presence of diabetes, stones more than 2 cm in diameter, a nonpacifying gallbladder, and a calcified gallbladder.

About 20 percent of cases of cholecystitis are caused by an acalculous gallbladder. The incidence is rising, especially in the elderly. Failure to diagnose and treat it early can result in gangrene and perforation of the gallbladder. Reported death rates range from 6 to 67 percent compared with 3 percent for ordinary acute cholecystitis.[6] One possible etiology is decreased blood flow through the cystic artery secondary to congestive heart failure (CHF), arteriosclerosis, diabetes, lymphadenopathy, shock, or metastasis. See Table 6-10-5 for the setting of acute gallbladder inflammation complicating severe underlying illnesses.

SIGNS AND SYMPTOMS

The triad of RUQ pain, fever, and leukocytosis is extremely suggestive of acute cholecystitis. The pain is steady and unremitting, increasing in intensity over 24 h in the RUQ and/or epigastrium. Radiation of pain may be to the right scapula, back, or shoulder. Nausea with vomiting is seen frequently, and the patient may present with evidence of dehydration. A low-grade fever (<103°F) is common. Mild jaundice is present in some patients. The presenting symptoms are the same with calculous and acalculous nonfunctioning gallbladder disease.

OBJECTIVE FINDINGS

Physical examination may show an acutely ill patient, often preferring the fetal position, with fever, mild tachycardia, and shallow respirations. Abdominal examination reveals mild distention, a hypoactive bowel sound, and right upper quadrant tenderness with guarding. Rebound tenderness may occur if there is peritoneal irritation. Murphy's sign is often positive (inspiratory arrest with steady compression of the right costal margin in the midclavicular line). Jaundice and evidence of dehydration may be evident.

DIAGNOSTIC CONSIDERATIONS

The elderly often present differently. As many as half will not have a fever, and a third may have a nontender abdomen. The differential diagnosis can include every "-itis" possible in the abdomen and many pulmonary or cardiac diagnoses as well. Table 6-10-6 lists the most common differentials.

TABLE 6-10-7. Postcholecystectomy Complications

Early complications
    Atelectasis or other pulmonary events
    Subphrenic abscess formation
    Biliary enteric fistula
    Bile leak
    Hemorrhage
    Mechanical obstruction by retained calculi
Late complications
    Biliary strictures
    Retained biliary calculi
    Cystic stump syndrome
    Stenosis of sphincter of Oddi
    Bile-salt-induced diarrhea or gastritis

narcotic use. Improvement generally is seen within 24 h, at which time surgical intervention is considered.

Antibiotic therapy is aimed at gram-negative organisms. One of the commonly used combination antibiotics is ampicillin sodium/sulbactam sodium (Unasyn) 1.5 g every six h by IV piggyback. Single-therapy choices include ampicillin 500 mg qid, cefoperazone (Cefobid) 2–4 g/day in divided doses, and amikacin sulfate (Amikacin) 15 mg/kg/day in divided doses.

Surgical management consists of a cholecystectomy within a few days of the first attack. Early surgery in those without anesthesia risk has limited complications and precludes additional attacks if surgery is delayed for several months. One-fourth of patients who decline surgery will have another significant attack in the future. Seriously ill patients with concomitant disease who have not responded to antibiotics may not be eligible for cholecystectomy. The alternative therapy, done under local anesthesia, is ultrasound-guided percutaneous puncture of the gallbladder.

Laparoscopic cholecystectomy (See "Cholelithiasis," above) is revolutionizing therapy for cholecystitis. An appropriate patient is prepped for surgery. A single trocar needle is inserted through the umbilicus, and the abdomen is distended with CO_2. Once the structures are visualized and judged approachable, two other small incisions are made to essentially triangulate on the gallbladder. With three laparoscopic/trocar devices, the gallbladder is teased away from the liver and the cystic duct is cut and clamped simultaneously. The entire procedure can take as little as 20 min compared to an average of 1.5 h for a standard open cholecystectomy. Only a small number of laparoscopic surgeries are converted to open cholecystectomies intraoperatively.

The expectations for recovery are excellent. Some centers are doing the laparoscopic procedure as day surgery in contrast to open cholecystectomy hospital stays of 2 to 5 days. The patient often goes back to work (without limitations) in 1 week compared to 4 to 6 weeks. The most common complaint among these patients is a feeling of pressure in the abdomen and chest secondary to the CO_2.

PEARLS

Cholecystitis is the most common complication of cholelithiasis and presents with classic symptoms of RUQ pain, fever, and leukocytosis. The pattern of pain is the best clue to the source of this acute abdomen: constant, unremitting and progressive pain in the RUQ. Colonic pain tends to be colicky and pancreatic in the left upper quadrant (LUQ). Additionally, history helps with the common presentation of symptoms in females who are fertile, >40 years old, and obese. Remember the special circumstances of North American Indians, children, and the elderly, in whom a healthy index of suspicion is required to make the diagnosis.

REFERENCES

1. Johnston D, Kaplan M: Pathogenesis and treatment of gallstones. *N Engl J Med* 348(6):412–418, 1993.
2. Shaw M: Current management of symptomatic gallstones. *Postgrad Med* 93(1):183–187, 1993.

3. NIH releases consensus statement on gallstones, bile duct stones and laparoscopic cholecystectomy. *Am Fam Physician* 46(5):1571–1574, 1992.
4. Everhart J: Contributions of obesity and weight loss to gallstone disease. *Ann Intern Med* 119(10):1029–1034, 1993.
5. Greenberger NJ, Isselbacher KJ: Diseases of the gallbladder and bile ducts, in Fauci AS, Braunwald E, Isselbacher KJ (eds): *Harrison's Principles of Internal Medicine*, 14th ed. New York, McGraw-Hill, 1998, chap 302.
6. Chung, SC: Acute acalculous cholecystitis. *Postgrad Med* 98(3): 199–204, 1995.

BIBLIOGRAPHY

Moscati RM: Gatrointestional emergencies: Parts I–II. Cholelithiasis, cholecystitis, and pancreatitis. *Emerg Med Clin North Am* 14(4):719–736, 1996.

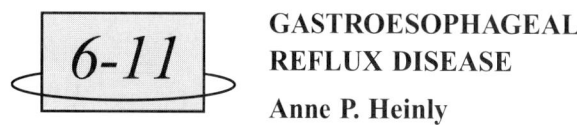

GASTROESOPHAGEAL REFLUX DISEASE
Anne P. Heinly

DISCUSSION

Commercial programming on television provides a hint about the prevalence of gastroesophageal reflux disease (GERD). It is estimated to occur monthly in at least one-third of the adult population, with an equal distribution between men and women. A low estimate of 10 percent of the population has GERD symptoms once a week. Unlike acute illness, GERD tends to be chronic and recurring, with many patients reporting 10 or more years of intermittent symptoms. It is by far the most common esophageal disease process and is known to the public as heartburn, indigestion, or dyspepsia. It often is self-treated with over-the-counter medications for years before patients bring complaints to their health care provider.

PATHOGENESIS

Lined by stratified squamous epithelium, the esophagus acts as a conduit for food transport. The outer longitudinal layer of muscle is primarily striated skeletal muscle, and the inner circular layer is smooth muscle, especially over the distal half of the esophagus. Food is transferred from the mouth to the stomach in three phases: swallowing, esophageal peristalsis, and passage through the lower esophageal sphincter (LES). The main culprit in GERD seems to be a lack of LES tone.

The LES is a physiologic phenomenon functioning at the distal esophagus. The LES relaxes to a pressure of zero in response to the swallowing of a bolus of food, with a combination of muscular attributes and active neural tone regulated by a complex interaction of neural and hormonal factors. LES pressure is easily changed by many different mechanisms (see Table 6-11-1).

Gastroesophageal reflux disease is secondary to a low or absent resting LES pressure, allowing gastric contents to contaminate the esophageal mucosa. The other part of the equation is the gastric contents; the longer hydrochloric acid, bile salts, and pepsin contact the esophageal mucosa, the greater is the chance of injury. Injury to the basal cell layer of the esophagus requires a pH level <4. The body's natural protective mechanism is to replace the injured areas with tissue better suited to low pH levels. Persistent irritation can lead to change of the squamous cell structure to a metaplastic columnar epithelium, a condition called Barrett's esophagitis. Table 6-11-2 lists the protective mechanisms for the esophagus against the elements that cause GERD.

SYMPTOMS

The severity of symptoms does not necessarily translate into the level of tissue injury. The most classic symptom of GERD is heartburn, which is translated variously as burning substernal pain, sternal pressure, an

TABLE 6-11-1. Lower Esophageal Sphincter Tone

LES PRESSURE INCREASED BY = TIGHTER TONE	LES PRESSURE DECREASED BY = LOOSER TONE

Hormones: Tighter tone occurs during gastric churning, preventing reflux
  Gastrin
  Substance P
  Pancreatic polypeptides
  Prostaglandin $F_{2\alpha}$
	Hormones: Loosen tone in response to pyloric antrum chemoactive agents; allow the pyloric sphincter to relax and food to pass to the duodenum; lower LES pressure
	  Secretin
	  Cholecystokinin
	  Glucagon
	  Progesterone
	    Birth control pills
	    Hormone replacement therapy
	  Adenosine

Foods
High-protein foods
	Foods
	  Fats
	  Chocolates
	  Alcohol
	  Peppermint
	  Coffee (caffeine)

Medications and miscellaneous
  Antacids
  Metoclopramide (Reglan)
  Cisapride (Propulsid)
  Histamine
  Raised intraabdominal pressure
	Medication and miscellaneous
	  Beta adrenergics (Alupent, Proventil)
	  Alpha adrenergics (Minipress, Hytrin)
	  Theophyllines
	  Anticholinergic agents
	    Antihistamines
	    Antidepressants
	    Antipsychotics
	  Calcium channel blocking agents
	  Diazepams and barbiturates
	  Dopamine and nitrates
	  Meperidine (Demerol), morphine
	  Smoking
	  Obesity and pregnancy (prolonged increased abdominal pressure)

TABLE 6-11-2. Esophageal Protection and Injury Mechanisms

PROTECTION MECHANISMS	INJURY MECHANISMS

Antireflux barrier: lower esophageal sphincter closes with gastric churning and in response to other stimulants; average resting pressure 20 mmHg.	Weak or incompetent LES: loss of resting tone, pressures as low as 0–10 mmHg
	  Transient LES relaxation secondary to foods, medications, or hormones
	  Disruption of the anatomy—hiatal hernia
	  Loss of neural/hormonal tone—etiology unknown

Luminal clearance: primary and secondary peristaltic waves sweep down the entire esophagus, emptying out the LES each time, leaving limited acidic residue.	Poor luminal clearance: esophagus unable to clear properly
	  Mechanical: strictures, tumors, diverticuli, hiatal hernia, volume of food, poor gastric emptying
	  Tertiary peristalsis: ineffective, random peristalsis of esophagus
	  Neuromuscular disorders: chagas' disease, myasthenia gravis, etc.

Saliva: Salivary bicarbonate neutralizes acid pH; takes 7–10 mL of saliva to neutralize 1 mL of 0.1 N HCl*	Gastric refluxant: HCl, pepsin, bile acids, and trypsin cause mucosal injury or facilitate susceptibility to injury.

Epithelial resistance: mucous layer, unstirred water layer (just adjacent to cell surface with pH 5), and bicarbonate protect the immediate surface	Tobacco use:
	  Decreased mucosal blood flow
	  Decreases LES tone
	  Depresses gastric mucosal prostaglandin synthesis

Tyrosine kinase, an epidermal growth factor, promotes buffering and swift cell replication and replacement.	Interferes with action of H_2 blockers
Rich blood supply and tissue acid-base status allow for waste removal and intact cell-mediated healing factors	
LES/stomach anatomy: acute angle at which esophagus enters stomach creates a type of flap valve	Gastric volume: the fuller the GI tract is, the more likely the acute angle of the LES and stomach will be lost, increasing reflux
Gastric emptying time: along with appropriate esophageal clearance, keeps food on its way	Increased volume from large meals, especially if patient lies down after meal Pyloric obstruction (ulcers, strictures) Obesity, pregnancy, and ascites increase intraabdominal pressure

*Kahrilas P, Hogan P: Physiology of the esophagus, in Sleisenger MH, Fordtran JS: *Gastrointestinal Disease*, 5th ed. Philadelphia, Saunders, 1993, p 384.

uncomfortable chest, or crushing chest pain. The pain may radiate to the neck, back, or left shoulder. Thus, it often confounds a cardiac workup. The pain is ordinarily worse with bending over or lying down, especially after a meal. The pain is improved with antacids, sitting up, or standing. The pain seldom is described as being in the epigastric area.

Associated symptoms include increased belching and regurgitation, which leave a bitter (gastric contents) or salty taste (water brash) in the mouth. Symptoms consistent with complications from GERD include progressive dysphagia (strictures, tumors), chronic cough or recurrent pneumonia (aspiration), exacerbation of asthma (GERD is found in up to 70 percent of asthma patients), and hoarseness and mouth and gingival ulcers (possibly resulting from acidic reflux, especially with nighttime regurgitation). In infants, symptoms include failure to thrive, recurrent upper respiratory infections, and frequent regurgitation. Another unusual indication of possible GERD in children is Sandifer's syndrome, which includes intermittent torticollis and peculiar posturing.

"Red flag" symptoms should prompt rapid evaluation of the patient's disease process. When a patient has red flag symptoms, clinical treatment without investigation is not appropriate. Evaluate GERD as soon as possible when any of the following symptoms are present: progressive dysphagia, recurrent pneumonia, persistent cough, failure to thrive (in children), and evidence of bleeding.

OBJECTIVE FINDINGS

Physical examination is often disappointing. A thorough examination of the mouth, pharynx, lungs, heart, and abdomen is indicated, in addition to a rectal examination. Occasionally, gingival erosion or oral mucosal ulcers are seen. Halitosis may be present. Skin changes such as thickening, Raynaud's phenomenon, sclerodactyly, and telangiectasia may suggest scleroderma, which commonly is associated with esophageal diseases.

Infants and children should be examined for evidence of growth retardation or failure to thrive. Measure height, weight, and head circumference on each visit to track any trends. Stools in both adults and children should be checked for occult blood.

DIAGNOSTIC CONSIDERATIONS

The differential diagnosis includes the skin and all the systems in the chest: respiratory, cardiac, musculoskeletal, gastrointestinal, and

TABLE 6-11-3. Differential Diagnosis of GERD

Achalasia	LES tone too tight, full chest, weight loss, unable to vomit
Defuse esophageal spasm	Strong, random peristalsis: severe stabbing substernal pain, short-lived, exacerbated by hot or cold foods
Infectious esophagitis	Severe, persistent odynophagia, drooling
Chemical ingestion	Severe dysphagia, odynophagia, bleeding
Cardiac pain—MI, angina	Substernal chest pain with radiation to arm or neck, associated with exertion, dyspnea, diaphoresis
Costochondritis	Substernal-sternal chest pain, worse with deep respiration and movement
Pneumonia, pleurisy	Chest pain, generally no radiation pattern, worse with respiration, cough, fever
Biliary tract disease	Epigastric to right upper quadrant pain, radiating to chest, colicky in nature, associated with fat intake
Peptic ulcer disease	Epigastric pain with radiation to chest and back, associated with food intake, stress-induced
Postherpetic syndrome	Dermatome involvement, persistent pain over area, no relation to food intake

neurologic (see Table 6-11-3). Of primary concern is the similarity of cardiac pain to esophageal pain. Angina pectoris and myocardial infarction can mimic GERD, and vice versa. In emergent situations, cardiac sources must be ruled out first. Few people die of acute GERD, but they do die of acute myocardial infarction (MI).

LABORATORY TESTS

No routine laboratory testing defines GERD since it is a structural problem, not a systemic one. Routine laboratory tests, electrocardiography (ECG), and chest x-ray may be done to help rule out the differential diagnosis.

The most definitive test is esophageal pH monitoring. A probe is placed near the LES area, and pH is monitored over a 24-h period. A low esophageal pH is conclusive for GERD. Unfortunately, pH monitoring is not available to all providers and is expensive. The Berstein test can be done readily in most areas. It involves the infusion of a measured amount of hydrochloric acid into the esophagus. It is considered positive if there is reproduction of the patient's symptoms. Esophageal manometry will show decreased LES pressure. Esophagogastroduodenoscopy (EGD) is a useful procedure for direct visualization of lesions, evaluation of strictures and masses, and retrieval of tissue for biopsies.

RADIOLOGIC (IMAGING) STUDIES

The imaging modality of choice for any esophageal disease is a barium swallow. The barium swallow can highlight mucosal injury, ulcerations, strictures, and hiatal hernias. It can help define a relaxed LES or tertiary peristalsis, which may contribute to GERD. A radionuclide scintigraphy uses ^{99m}Tc-sulfur to help indicate esophageal reflux and measure gastric emptying time. Both tests are noninvasive and are readily available to most patients.

TREATMENT

Because many patients treat themselves without a definitive diagnosis, a clinician can make a presumed diagnosis of GERD by history and treat them empirically. The mainstay of therapy is the elimination of precipitating factors. This is best done through good patient

TABLE 6-11-4. General Measures for Control of GERD

THINGS TO DO	THINGS TO AVOID
Small or reasonably sized, well-chewed meals	Lying down within 3 h of a meal Smoking
High-protein diet, low fat	Fatty foods, chocolate, acidic foods
Elevate the head of the bed 3–6 in.	Alcohol, coffee, peppermints Obesity and lack of exercise
Weight control and regular exercise	Medications that cause loss of LES tone

education about life-style changes (see Table 6-11-4). If life-style changes are not enough, medications can be used to decrease acidity, decrease refluxant contact, or tighten LES tone.

Antacids are by far the most common over-the-counter medications used. They neutralize gastric acid and promote healing, but only with frequent dosing. Magnesium-based antacids are the most potent, but 2 tablespoons (30 mL) five times a day may cause diarrhea. Aluminum antacids work well but produce constipation and bind tetracyclines and other medications. Calcium types neutralize acid but can induce rebound hydrochloric acid secretions, creating a vicious cycle. The best antacid is a combination magnesium-aluminum product to get maximum antacid effect with minimal side effects. Many patients like liquid antacids because they relieve symptoms quickly.

Histamine is a potent stimulant of gastric acid. H_2 receptor antagonists (Zantac, Axid, Tagamet, Pepcid) are designed to decrease the acidity of the gastric refluxant by blocking production at the parietal cell. The intermittent use of over-the-counter (OTC) H_2 blockers will diminish symptoms in patients who commit dietary indiscretions such as eating a huge and/or fatty meal or lie down after eating. However, for persistent symptoms, the strength of OTC medications is not sufficient to heal erosive esophagitis.

For more severe GERD, high-dose H_2 blockers or a proton pump inhibitor is recommended (see Table 6-11-5). Omeprazole (Prilosec) inhibits the proton pump within the parietal cell and can create achlorhydria with long-term use. It is an effective therapy for healing esophagitis and has the convenience of a single daily dose. Omeprazole also can be used for maintenance therapy to prevent recurrence of GERD symptoms and sequelae. Yearly follow-up is required when a patient is using omeprazole because persistent achlorhydria can cause pernicious anemia (intrinsic factor, vitamin B_{12} absorption is dependent on parietal cell activity) and may predispose to gastric carcinoma.

Other therapeutic alternatives are the prokinetic agents Reglan and Propulsid. Both tighten LES tone (decreasing reflux contact) and promote rapid gastric emptying. The addition of either one to a regimen of H_2 blockers can be helpful in resistant cases of GERD.

Finally, when all preventive and medication regimens are exhausted, surgery may be done to correct the anatomic defect. Laparoscopic fundoplication is now the procedure of choice for the surgical control of GERD. If Barrett's esophagitis or carcinoma is present, a partial removal of the esophagus may be accomplished. Esophagectomy is the last resort because the sequelae include

TABLE 6-11-5. Medication Regimens for GERD

Mylanta or Maalox, 2 Tbs. 4–5 times a day	Ranitidine (Zantac), 150 mg bid or tid Cimetidine (Tagamet), 300 mg qid
Zantac 75 (OTC), 75 mg bid	Famotidine (Pepcid), 20 mg qd
Tagamet HB (OTC), 150–200 mg qid	Nizatidine (Axid), 150–300 mg qd Omeprazole (Prilosec), 20 mg qd, add if needed
Pepcid AC (OTC), 5 mg bid	Cisapride (Propulsid), 10 mg tid
Axid AR (OTC), 75 mg qd	Metoclopramide (Reglan), 10 mg qid

esophageal clearance problems with regurgitation, weight loss, dumping syndrome, anemia, and other conditions.

COMPLICATIONS

Since most people have episodes of GERD at some time in their lives, it is important to recognize severe symptoms and complications. As a mechanical problem, GERD is recurrent, and so complications can occur at any time and may be exacerbated by age or concomitant disease. The most common complication of GERD is esophagitis with subsequent stricture formation (scarring), which decreases lumen clearance. Perforation, ulceration, hemorrhage, aspiration pneumonia, and obstruction are all possible results of severe GERD.

The most ominous complication of persistent GERD is Barrett's esophagitis. With the presence of Barrett's esophagitis, the risk of adenocarcinoma increases eight- to 11-fold. The squamous cell structure changes to a metaplastic columnar epithelium, which is considered a premalignant state (adenocarcinoma). The intestinal metaplasia progresses slowly up the esophageal mucosa and is associated with ulcerations, bleeding, and stricture formation. An EGD is required for the definitive diagnosis of Barrett's esophagitis, and follow-up includes yearly EGDs for life.

PATIENT EDUCATION

Table 6-11-4 includes all the preventive measures that can be taken to avoid or treat GERD. Patient education should be directed toward these measures. Medications are short-term fixes for the most part and carry their own risk factors with continued use. The commercial media seem to give people permission to eat anything they want, in any quantity, because they can take a pill to solve the subsequent problems. It is better to teach patients good eating habits and avoid medication use completely.

PEARLS

Gastroesophageal reflux disease is a common problem and for the most part is easily resolved with good habits. The trick is to have a high index of suspicion for increasing severity. Unfortunately, severe disease may exhibit limited symptoms, and mild disease may bother a patient tremendously. Any increase or change in symptoms justifies investigation. A patient who seeks medical help has probably tried all the OTC medications, and so evaluation is warranted. In an elderly patient with no previous history of GERD or ulcer disease, evaluation should be done for carcinoma. A common disorder should not lull a diagnostician into a false sense of security.

BIBLIOGRAPHY

Borum ML: Gastrointestinal diseases in women. *Med Clin North Am* 82(1):21–42, 1998.

Lagergren J, Bergstrom R, Lindgren A, et al: Symptomatic gastroesophageal reflux as a risk factor for esophageal adenocarcinoma. *N Engl J Med* 340(11):825–831, 1999.

Wolfe MM, Lichtenstein DR, Singh G: Gastrointestinal toxicity of nonsteroidal antiinflammatory drugs. *N Engl J Med* 340(24):1888–1897, 1999.

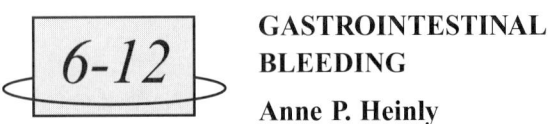

GASTROINTESTINAL BLEEDING

Anne P. Heinly

DESCRIPTION

Between 1 and 2 percent of Americans will be hospitalized for bleeding in the next year, with the vast majority of these bleeds coming from gastrointestinal sources. Blood loss can occur in eight different ways, five of which are common to the gastrointestinal (GI) system. Bloody

vomitus is called *hematemesis;* it may be bright red or have the "coffee-ground" appearance of older, accumulated blood. *Melena* is the presence of 50 to 100 mL of blood in stool, causing black, tarry, and foul-smelling stools. *Hematochezia* denotes rapid bleeding, usually from the lower GI tract, with the presence of bright red or maroon blood from the rectum or mixed with stool. *Occult* bleeding can occur anywhere, but in the GI tract it can be identified with a chemical reagent such as Hemoccult cards. Finally, there is *presumption of bleeding,* in which there are physical findings but no overt or occult bleeding can be identified. This can happen with hemorrhagic pancreatitis.

PATHOGENESIS

The gastrointestinal tract from the mouth to the anus can bleed anywhere at any time. The challenge is to try to define the location, severity, and cause of bleeding. Traditionally, upper GI bleeding comes from any location above the ligament of Treitz and lower GI bleeding originates below that ligament (see Fig. 6-12-1). The GI tract has a complex blood supply with a lot of redundancy to ensure proper digestion and absorption of food. At any given time, up to 25 percent of the blood supply may be involved in digestion. When bleeding occurs as a result of injury or disease, it can be rapid and devastating (chemical ingestion or Boerhaave's syndrome), or it can slowly ooze from a carcinoma or ulceration.

SYMPTOMS

A good history is essential. If bleeding is obvious, questions should include the history of nonsteroidal anti-inflammatory drug (NSAID) use; previous history of bleeding; illnesses that may predispose the patient to bleeding, such as cirrhosis, vitamin deficiency, and malabsorption syndromes; use of medication that might effect coagulation, such as warfarin (Coumadin) or long-term omeprazole use; recent surgeries or instrumentation; use of alcohol or tobacco products; presence of pain or indigestion before bleeding; sexual orientation (HIV syndromes); and family history of bleeding dyscrasias.

Most people can handle a 10 percent volume loss without symptoms. With overt blood loss, a patient may present with sudden fatigue, heart palpitations, increased respiratory rate, dizziness, diaphoresis, nausea, thirst, and/or agitation. As blood volume is lost, the body tries to compensate with an increased pulse in an effort to maintain blood pressure to supply vital organs with needed oxygen and nutrients. In slow, occult blood loss, the patient probably will come to a routine appointment with a history of progressive fatigue, increasing thirst, persistent nausea, inability to maintain the usual physical activities without shortness of breath, or palpitations. In children, failure to thrive may occur. An elderly patient may present with a change in mentation, constipation and/or diarrhea, or loss of appetite.

OBJECTIVE

Quantifying blood loss is quite difficult. Where and what is the source? Is it actively bleeding? If so, how fast? Is there more than one bleeding source or a chronic blood loss overlying an acute bleed? Even today, orthostatic vital signs are still used to judge the effect of blood loss and estimate cardiac reserve. Orthostatic vital signs include blood pressure and pulse determinations from a supine to a sitting to a standing position over a period of 3 to 6 min. Orthostatic vital signs are considered positive when there is a 20-point rise in the pulse rate and a drop in blood pressure of 10 to 15 mmHg from one position to another. Patients with severe blood loss will appear pale or gray, be diaphoretic, and exhibit hypotension, tachycardia, tachypnea, and progressive loss of sensorium.

The obvious bleeding source should not be ignored, but the provider also should do a thorough inspection for other sources or disease processes that may complicate therapy. A complete physical should be done, looking for signs of dehydration (dry mucous membranes), evidence of underlying cirrhosis (jaundice, hepatomegaly), skin lesions (Kaposi's sarcoma), and vascular anomalies (deep vein thrombosis, spider angiomas). Abdominal tenderness with and without peritoneal

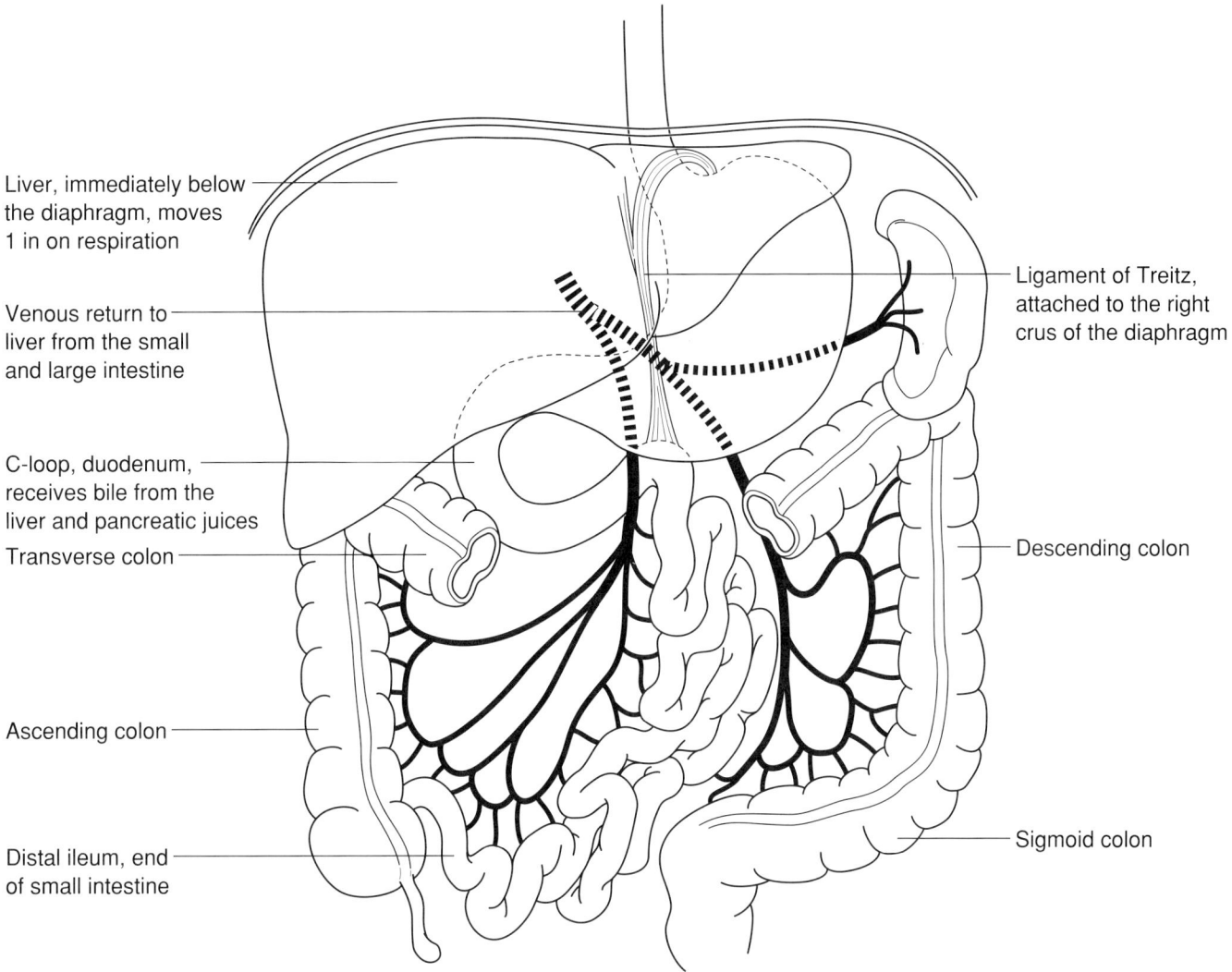

Liver, immediately below the diaphragm, moves 1 in on respiration

Venous return to liver from the small and large intestine

C-loop, duodenum, receives bile from the liver and pancreatic juices

Transverse colon

Ascending colon

Distal ileum, end of small intestine

Ligament of Treitz, attached to the right crus of the diaphragm

Descending colon

Sigmoid colon

FIGURE 6-12-1. GI anatomy in relation to GI bleeding.

signs may indicate ulcer disease or the rupture of a diverticulum. Back pain and tenderness may be secondary to an abdominal aneurysm. Rectal examinations are mandatory with an investigation of GI bleeding to evaluate for blood, hemorrhoids, and polyps.

DIAGNOSTIC CONSIDERATIONS

Upper GI bleeding usually is manifested in two ways. Esophageal and stomach lesions usually cause hematemesis because the blood is an irritant and because of changes in gastric volume. The blood can be bright red, or if it has been accumulating, it may have a dark coffee-ground appearance. Bleeding from ulcer disease, hiatal hernias, or esophageal varices does not necessarily cause hematemesis but may cause melena instead. The blood darkens and mixes with the stool on its 8- to 14-h transit through the small intestine and colon. It is possible to have hematochezia from the upper GI tract, but that usually is associated with massive blood loss (see Table 6-12-1).

Lower GI bleeding can present as melena (slow bleed and transit), which is common with carcinomas, polyps, and diverticular irritation. Inflammatory bowel disease and ischemic bowel disease may cause hematochezia with frank, bright red blood through the rectum. Some researchers attribute maroon-colored stools to lower GI bleeding, estimating that the bleeding location is in the ascending colon because the darker color denotes some transit time but not an extended period in the colon. Occult bleeding can occur from any location, and massive bleeding may produce melena, hematochezia, and hematemesis at the same time (see Table 6-12-2).

LABORATORY TESTS

Fecal occult blood usually is seen on testing cards if the bleeding exceeds 3 to 5 mL a day. Guaiac-based cards (Hemoccult I and II) make use of the pseudoperoxidase function of hemoglobin. These cards have high false-negative and false-positive rates because the location of a bleed, the timing, and diet can affect them. The newer cards (Hemo-Quant) depend on a heme-porphyrin test that can help localize bleeding, but they also have a high false-positive rate. Therefore, fecal occult blood testing remains a simple but nonspecific test.

Blood loss is reflected in hematocrit. With chronic, slow GI bleeding from an ulcer or a similar problem, iron stores are depleted over time and the hematocrit decreases. A complete blood cell count (CBC) will reveal a microcytic, hypochromic anemia. If the anemia is macrocytic, it is most likely secondary to a vitamin deficiency. Rapid blood loss may not register accurately for the first 12 to 72 h because the plasma volume has to return to normal before the hematocrit is valid. It is better to follow orthostatic vital signs, cardiac monitoring, and the clinical picture initially.

The remainder of the laboratory tests are designed to evaluate the organs affected by blood loss. Chemistries should be done to check renal status (uremia can cause GI blood loss) and electrolyte balance. An elevated blood urea nitrogen (BUN) with a normal creatinine indicates blood in the GI tract (BUN is a by-product of hemolysis). Liver enzymes should be done because cirrhosis, portal hypertension, and hypoproteinemia all may be implicated in GI bleeding. Coagulation studies are a must. The bleeding time and prothrombin time with a

TABLE 6-12-1. Sources of Upper Gl Bleeding

DISEASE	SYMPTOMS	TREATMENT OF BLEED

Peptic ulcer disease
  Gastritis or ulcer
  Duodenitis or ulcer
  Zollinger-Ellison
  Gastric antral vascular
    ectasia (GAVE)
	Epigastric pain, worse with empty stomach, usually progressive; occasional patient can have a silent ulcer with bleeding as the first clue	Endoscopic hemostasis most successful with lesion 1–2 cm; surgical removal is considered for severe or numerous bleeding sites; GAVE is associated with systemic sclerosis and recurrent UGI bleeding

Esophageal disease
  Esophagitis (GERD)
  Hiatal hernia
  Varices
  Mallory-Weiss tears
  Boerhaave's syndrome
	GERD presents with substernal pyrosis, increased burping, cough, hoarseness; varices and Mallory-Weiss tears common to alcohol abuse, liver cirrhosis—presents with pain and hematemesis; Boerhaave's is sudden massive bleeding with poor prognosis	Varices may be treated with balloon tamponade, but recurrence is high; more common: variceal sclerotherapy done weekly until varices are obliterated; endoscopic ligation is under investigation as a valid alternative

Carcinomas
  Esophageal
  Gastric
  Duodenal
	Depending on location: progressive dysphagia, early satiety, weight loss, cough, epigastric pain; duodenal may present with jaundice and gallbladder symptoms; bleeding usually occult	Surgical resection is optimal (and hopefully curative) care; palliative therapy may include endoscopic hemostasis

Overdoses
  Warfarin
  Heparin
  Acetaminophen
  Rodent killers
	Widespread bruising, hematuria, hematochezia, hemoptysis, and even joint bleeding; PTT increased within 12–24 h; acetaminophen presents with fine petechiae	Empty stomach by lavage after protecting airway; activated charcoal is recommended; vitamin K 5–10 mg subcutaneously with a unit of fresh frozen plasma for warfarin; watch for relapse

platelet count can help judge the severity of blood loss or the likelihood of more bleeding. A partial thromboplastin time (PTT) double the normal value has a poor prognosis. If circumstances warrant it, look for a drug overdose, especially acetaminophen, warfarin, or heparin, as a possible etiology.

RADIOLOGIC (IMAGING) STUDIES

The decision to be made is: What is the presumed severity of GI bleeding? If bleeding is occult in a young person with limited symptoms, a barium study is acceptable. Depending on the presumed location of the bleeding, a barium swallow for esophageal lesions, an upper gastrointestinal (UGI) series for stomach and duodenal etiologies, a small

bowel follow-through for midgut lesions, or a barium enema for colonic lesions can be recommended.

With massive bleeding, slower bleeding that causes significant symptoms, or bleeding in the very young or elderly, the recommended study is endoscopy. The advantages of an esophagogastroduodenoscopy (EGD) with upper GI bleeding or a colonoscopy, sigmoidoscopy, or anoscopy with lower GI bleeding have increased over the years because of better tools and better-trained practitioners.

A well-trained endoscopist usually can locate the bleeding source and in most cases administer therapeutic modalities. The therapies available with the endoscope are impressive. They include monopolar electrocoagulation, which essentially cauterizes the lesion but does produce a fair amount of tissue damage. Laser therapy, when available,

TABLE 6-12-2. Sources of Lower Gl Bleeding

DISEASE	SYMPTOMS	TREATMENT

Anal disease
  Hemorrhoids
  Anal fissures
  IBD fistulas
  Anal carcinoma
	Hemorrhoids are by far the most common; blood is seen on the stool versus mixed with the stool; usually intermittent; bleeding often painless	Sitz baths and high-fiber diet with stool softeners for hemorrhoids and fissures with topical treatments; surgery only if recurrent. IBD fistulas and carcinoma are surgical referrals

Carcinoma
  Small intestinal CA
  Colonic CA
	Especially in the elderly, a change in bowel habits, weight loss, and occult bleeding may indicate cancer	Resection of the lesion with lymph biopsy and evaluation for metastasis

Inflammatory
  Crohn's disease
  Ulcerative colitis
  Infectious colitis
	Symptoms are disease-specific, but bleeding is usually obvious with lots of diarrhea; especially ulcerative colitis and infectious colitis can bleed briskly	Treatment of all these begins with medical therapy; surgery used as a last resort in most cases

Vascular anomalies
  Bowel ischemia
  Aortoenteric fistula
  Hereditary telangiectasia
  Colonic varices
	Bowel ischemia may be due to obstruction, carcinoma, infection; bleeding is usually brisk with extreme pain; other anomalies may be seen on endoscopy	Bowel resection is done for ischemia and fistula bleeding; sclerotherapy or coagulation by endoscope may contain varices and anomalies

Diverticuli Diverticulitis	May present with LLQ pain, fever, chills, peritoneal signs, and bleeding	Depending on severity and response to medical therapy, colon resection may be done
Solitary ascending diverticulum	May present as abundant, sudden, painless bleeding (hematochezia with bright red or maroon stools)	

NOTE: IBD = inflammatory bowel disease; CA = cancer; LLQ = left lower quadrant.

is the more precise choice for endoscopic hemostasis. Sclerosing therapy uses epinephrine, absolute ethanol, or polidocanol to control bleeding. Epinephrine produces less tissue damage while causing localized vasoconstriction.

The other option for the evaluation of a GI bleed is arteriography. Arteriography is probably still superior to endoscopy when there is massive bleeding because even skilled surgeons cannot see through blood. The arteriogram can localize the bleeding if the blood loss is more than 0.5 mL/min and often can determine the cause of a diverticulum and angiodysplasia. Arteriograms are also better when one is looking for a vascular lesion or anomaly.

Finally, more providers are turning to nuclear scans to localize bleeding. Technetium 99m scintography has a reasonably good record of finding slow bleeding that arteriograms do not pick up. The drawback to nuclear scans, however, is that they are good only for active bleeding sources; they miss intermittent bleeding and are not sufficiently site-specific.

TREATMENT

The first step is to stabilize the patient. Nasogastric tube placement, arteriography, and even endoscopy have to wait for a hemodynamically stable patient. For an orthostatic or shocky patient, two large-bore intravenous lines should be started with rapid fluid resuscitation with either Ringer's solution or normal saline. Replace fluids to compensate for the fluids lost. Monitor the patient's cardiovascular status and urine output.

The next step is blood product replacement. Blood transports oxygen better than intravenous fluid. Blood products should be used to replenish the supply in patients who are down to one-fourth of their normal reserve and patients with evidence of poor tissue perfusion (angina, cyanosis, renal failure, loss of consciousness). Packed red blood cells (PRBC) should be used if improving systemic oxygen delivery is the goal. Fresh frozen plasma or platelets are used to replenish clotting factors and in the presence of severe thrombocytopenia. The rule of thumb is one unit of platelets to every five units of packed RBCs. While evaluating a patient for transfusion, consider whether the bleeding has stopped. Is it likely to recur? Are there other disease processes that may complicate fluid or blood resuscitation [congestive heart failure (CHF), polycythemia]? After the patient's plasma volume is replaced, it will take 12 to 72 h for stabilization. Hematocrit may fluctuate as the volume load settles down. A hematocrit test taken right after a transfusion may underestimate the actual number of RBCs present.

Once fluid and blood replacements are under way, the patient should be evaluated often for vital signs, changes in mentation, blood transfusion reactions, and urine output, and should receive regular electrocardiography (ECG). The use of nasogastric tubes (NGTs) in upper GI bleeding is declining. An NGT may be helpful in washing the upper GI areas before endoscopy, but cold or warm water lavage has not been proved to curtail bleeding.

COMPLICATIONS

Slow or occult bleeding can lead to anemia and fatigue, which may mask or exacerbate other disease processes. Depending on the etiology, the bleeding may be a signal of a more serious problem such as carcinoma. Massive bleeding can cause organ failure because of poor perfusion, which may not be reversible with the resuscitation effort. The ultimate complication is death, which occurs in approximately 14 to 20 percent of those hospitalized with bleeding.

PATIENT EDUCATION

The best way to avoid GI bleeding is to prevent the disease processes that predispose a patient to bleeding. A healthy diet, regular exercise, limited alcohol and NSAID use, and abstention from tobacco go a long way in limiting the possibility of GI bleeding.

PEARLS

Bleeding can occur at any location in the gastrointestinal tract. If the nasogastric lavage is negative for blood, it does not preclude upper GI bleeding. A negative Hemoccult card does not exclude GI bleeding. Sometimes it may seem easier not to notice a low hematocrit on the routine laboratory test, but an investigation may save a life. Be alert for GI bleeders, especially in the elderly. If they progress to massive bleeding, the chances of recovery are quite bleak.

BIBLIOGRAPHY

Peter DJP, Dougherty JM: Evaluation of the patient with gastrointestinal bleeding: An evidence based approach. *Emerg Med Clin North Am* 17(1):239–261, 1999.
Rockey DC: Occult gastrointestinal bleeding. *N Engl J Med* 341(1):38–44, 1999.

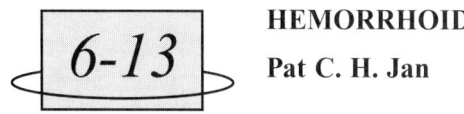

HEMORRHOIDS
Pat C. H. Jan

DISCUSSION

Hemorrhoids, a common anal disease, affect individuals as early as their mid-twenties to as late as their sixties and seventies. Men and women are affected equally. The leading predisposing factor in the formation of both internal and external hemorrhoids is constipation. In addition, many women relate a worsening of existing hemorrhoids after childbirth.

PATHOGENESIS

Hemorrhoids commonly are located in the right anterior, right posterior, and left lateral positions in the anal canal. The anal canal normally has hemorrhoidal tissues, or cushions, that aid in anal continence. Intraluminal pressure caused by straining or pushing from hard stools causes the hemorrhoidal plexus to become engorged and form internal and external hemorrhoids.

SIGNS AND SYMPTOMS

Internal hemorrhoids cause bleeding and prolapse without pain. They can be classified into four types (see Table 6-13-1). External hemorrhoids, by contrast, thrombose and cause pain. They are located below the dentate (pectinate) line. The dentate line has somatic innervation. Thus, structures such as external hemorrhoids located below this line also have sensory innervation.

TABLE 6-13-1. Classification of Internal Hemorrhoids

DEGREE	PHYSICAL FINDINGS
First	Bleeding
Second	Prolapse and spontaneously reducible
Third	Prolapse and requires digital manipulation
Fourth	Prolapse and unable to reduce

OBJECTIVE FINDINGS

Thrombosed external hemorrhoids are tender, hard, and bluish structures located at the anal verge. In an acute thrombosed external hemorrhoid, gentle spreading pressure to the buttocks by the examiner allows enough exposure of the anal verge. Internal hemorrhoids are located above the dentate line in the anal canal. They have a strawberry appearance and can prolapse outside the anal canal. Occasionally, a patient presents with a complex hemorrhoid with both an external component and an internal component. Internal hemorrhoids can be seen easily after the insertion of an anoscope that has been lubricated with petroleum jelly.

DIAGNOSTIC CONSIDERATIONS

When a patient presents with a complaint of rectal bleeding and anal examination does not reveal hemorrhoids, the following should be considered in the differential diagnosis:

- Carcinoma
- Diverticulitis
- Trauma
- Inflammatory bowel disease
- Colon polyps
- Portal hypertension from liver disease

TREATMENT

Medical Management

First-degree and second-degree internal hemorrhoids respond well to conservative treatment with a high-fiber diet or stool softener and decreased time in the bathroom. If patients do not follow the hemorrhoid care protocol, the hemorrhoids may need to be ablated by rubber band ligation or Endo-Lase. Endo-Lase or heat cautery and rubber band ligation can be performed in the office (see Fig. 6-13-1). The tip of the Endo-Lase is applied to the base of the hemorrhoid. Care must be taken to avoid the dentate line to prevent pain to the patient. Several treatments may be required in some patients. Sclerotherapy injections can be used for first-degree and second-degree internal hemorrhoids. Sodium morrhuate, sodium tetradecyl sulfate, or ethanolamine in the amount of 1–2 mL can be injected into the submucosa of each internal hemorrhoid. Unfortunately, there is a higher incidence of recurrence with this method. Rubber band ligation is used for second-degree and sometimes third-degree hemorrhoids (see Fig. 6-13-2). The patient is placed in the right lateral decubitus

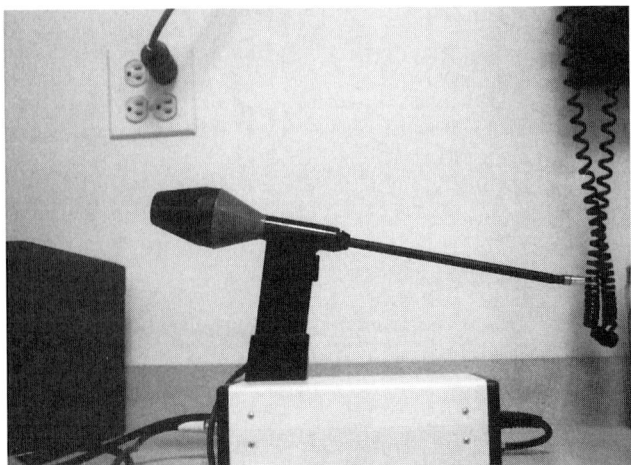

FIGURE 6-13-1. Endo-Lase instrument used for first- and second-degree hemorrhoids.

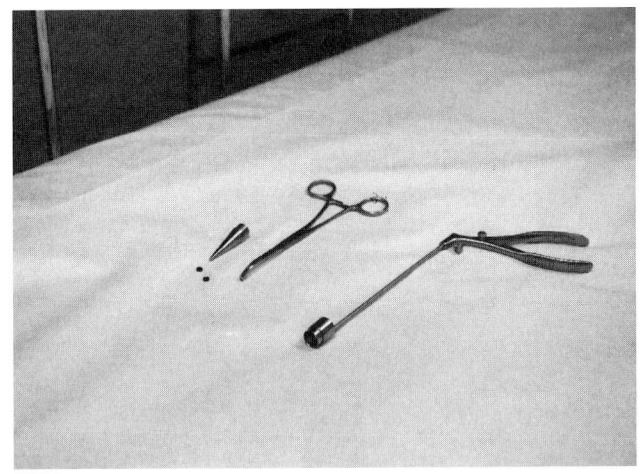

FIGURE 6-13-2. Rubber band ligature used for second- and third-degree hemorrhoids.

position with the legs flexed and the head of the bed bent as in Trendelenburg's position. An anoscope is inserted, and the hemorrhoid is identified. The hemorrhoid is then grasped up and outward as the rubber band ligature is pushed toward the base of the hemorrhoid. The hemorrhoid will atrophy and fall off in about 5 to 7 days. Patients should not feel any pain as long as the rubber band is well above the dentate line. If symptoms continue, excisional hemorrhoidectomy is the next alternative.

Surgical Management

Third- and fourth-degree hemorrhoids require excision. Patients are brought into the operating suite and placed in the jackknife position. The patient is placed under either intravenous sedation with local anesthesia or epidural or general anesthesia. If the patient is placed under intravenous sedation, lidocaine 1% with epinephrine is injected into the base of the hemorrhoids. An elliptical incision is made with a scalpel or cautery. Care is taken to remove the hemorrhoid from the internal sphincter. The sphincter must be identified and preserved. A single surgical gut (chromic) suture is used to approximate the edges. The remaining incision is left open and allowed to heal by secondary intention. The wound is infiltrated with bupivacaine (Marcaine) 0.25% with epinephrine, and dibucaine ointment is applied into the anal canal.

Uncomplicated external thrombosed hemorrhoids can be removed in the office. They are anesthetized with lidocaine 1% with epinephrine. An incision is made with a scalpel, and a hemostat is used to remove all the thrombus, which is purplish. A single inverted suture with either chromic or Vicryl is used to approximate the edges while allowing the remaining incision to heal by secondary intention. Oral analgesics are used for pain management. Patients are given the hemorrhoid care protocol (see Table 6-13-2).

PATIENT EDUCATION

Patients are instructed to increase their dietary intake of both fruits and vegetables. If they are unable to make these dietary modifications, stool softeners and fiber are added to the diet. Patients are reminded not to strain or push during bowel movements and not to spend prolonged time in the bathroom. After each bowel movement, patients should wash the anal area with soap and water. If any tissue prolapses, it should be pushed back gently into the anal canal with the aid of a lubricant such as Anusol or Preparation H. Warm sitz baths are suitable for all postoperative hemorrhoidectomy patients.

TABLE 6-13-2. Hemorrhoid Care Protocol

Keep stool soft
  Eat 3 or more servings of fruits and vegetables each day.
  Drink at least 6 to 8 glasses of fluid per day.
  If feeling constipated, take milk of magnesia (15–30 mL twice daily)
  If difficult to eat enough fruits and vegetables, try to take psyllium
    hydrophilic mucilloid (Metamucil) 1–2 tsp. every day

Limit time on toilet
  Do no spend reading time on toilet
  Go to the toilet when definitely ready; do not sit on toilet and wait
    for bowel movement
  If bowel movement is not coming, do not sit on toilet and strain
  Get up and come back later

Keep anal area clean
  Wash anal area with hand, not washcloth, gently after each bowel
    movement (soap and water)
  Take sitz bath 2–3 times daily for 20 min
  If tissue comes out around the anus, use a product such as Preparation
    H or Anusol to help push tissue back into anal canal with finger

DISPOSITION

Patients are seen 1 week after a medical or surgical procedure. If satisfactory healing has occurred, patients are seen on an as-needed basis. In case of poor wound healing or prolonged pain, patients are seen weekly until postoperative symptoms have subsided.

COMPLICATIONS AND RED FLAGS

The common postoperative complications of Endo-Lase, rubber band ligation, and excisional hemorrhoidectomy are urinary retention, bleeding, infection, anal stenosis, and incontinence. Bleeding can be controlled with adequate coagulation and a pressure dressing. Infections are prevented with a single-dose second-generation cephalosporin, which is given preoperatively. Anal stenosis can be avoided if complex hemorrhoids are removed in stages instead of all at once.

Postoperative edema and excessive excision of the anal derm can lead to stricture. Incontinence is avoided by separating the hemorrhoid off the internal sphincter muscle carefully and limiting the intravenous solution given during the procedure to 400 mL or less.

NOTES AND PEARLS

Since constipation is common among pregnant women, preventive care as well as conservative therapies should be utilized. A high-fiber diet or stool softeners, topical analgesics, and sitz baths should be the recommended therapy until after childbirth. If at that time the hemorrhoids are still painful or bleeding, surgical management is the next step.

Patients who are immunocompromised definitely should receive conservative treatment because surgical procedures performed on this group of patients may lead to sepsis.

BIBLIOGRAPHY

Beers MH, Berkow R: Hemorrhoids, in *The Merck Manual,* 17th ed. Whitehouse Station, NJ, Merck, 1999.
Billingham RP: Hemorrhoids, anal fissure and anorectal abscess and fistula, in Rakel RB (ed): *Conn's Current Therapy.* Philadelphia, Saunders, 1998, p 486.
Hussain JN: Hemorrhoids. *Primary Care,* 26(1):35–51, 1999.
Mazier WP: Hemorrhoids, fissures, and pruritus ani (review). *Surg Clin North Am* 74(6):1277–1292, 1995.
Russell TR: Hemorrhoids, in Way LW (ed): *Current Surgical Diagnosis and Treatment,* 10th ed. Stamford, CT, Appleton & Lange, 1994.
Schwartz, SI, Shires GT, Spencer FC: Hemorrhoids, in *Principles of Surgery,* 7th ed. New York, McGraw-Hill, 1999.

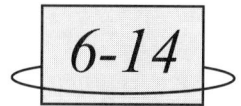

HEPATITIS
JoAnn Deasy

DISCUSSION

Hepatitis is an inflammatory and necrotic disease of liver cells. The hepatitis viruses, which are specific for the liver, can cause acute hepatitis and sometimes chronic hepatitis. Six hepatitis viruses are generally recognized (hepatitis A, B, C, D, E, and G). Chronic hepatitis is defined as elevated liver enzymes for longer than 6 months. Hepatitis B, C, and D viruses can cause chronic disease (see Table 6-14-1).

SYMPTOMS: ACUTE VIRAL HEPATITIS

The clinical course of acute viral hepatitis is variable. It may be asymptomatic, symptomatic but anicteric, or symptomatic and icteric. Rarely, it is very severe and can cause a prolonged illness with a high mortality rate or fulminant disease that may progress to death in a few days or weeks. The onset of symptoms may be gradual or sudden. Early symptoms are usually nonspecific and include anorexia, nausea, vomiting, abdominal discomfort, fatigue, headache, and low-grade fever. The clinician may not be overly suspicious of hepatitis when a patient presents with these symptoms until it is realized that the liver enzymes are elevated. Patients who present with right upper quadrant (RUQ) abdominal pain and jaundice are easier to diagnose. Some patients also have skin rashes, myalgias, arthralgias, diarrhea, and/or itching.

OBJECTIVE FINDINGS

Physical findings may include skin and scleral icterus and mild hepatomegaly with tenderness to percussion and palpation. In a small number of patients, the spleen is palpable. Some patients may have acute arthritis with local pain, redness, and swelling. Joint symptoms and signs usually are associated with hepatitis B and hepatitis E viruses. Dark urine and light stools are also signs of acute viral hepatitis. Clinical signs and symptoms cannot be used to determine the specific virus responsible for hepatitis. Identification of the etiologic virus depends on serologic testing.

LABORATORY FINDINGS

Liver enzymes, specifically alanine aminotransferase (ALT) and aspartate aminotransferase (AST), are released into the blood by damaged liver cells. During acute viral hepatitis, these enzymes may rise to 10 to 20 times their normal values. ALT usually is elevated out of proportion to AST. However, the levels of these enzymes do not correlate with the functional capacity of the liver. The prothrombin time and serum albumin level are used as indicators of hepatic function. Every patient with acute hepatitis needs a prothrombin time done on a same-day basis. Prolongation of the prothrombin time is an ominous sign. Both conjugated and unconjugated bilirubin may become elevated, resulting in jaundice.

HEPATITIS A

Hepatitis A virus (HAV) is an RNA virus that is transmitted via the fecal-oral route or through contaminated water or food, especially shellfish. The virus is resistant to gastric acid and travels from the gastrointestinal tract to hepatocytes, where replication takes place. The virus is shed in bile and excreted in stool. Large amounts of HAV accumulate in stool before symptoms occur, resulting in the spread of the disease unknowingly. In a significant number of persons, HAV infection never becomes clinically apparent. Older adults tend to have worse symptoms than do young adults and children. Diagnosis is made

Table 6-14-1.   The Hepatitis Viruses A through E

	HEPATITIS A	HEPATITIS B	HEPATITIS C	HEPATITIS D	HEPATITIS E
Transmission	Fecal-oral, shellfish	Percutaneous venereal perinatal	Percutaneous venereal	Percutaneous	Fecal-oral
Incubation, days	20–40	60–110	40–60	40	40
Diagnosis	IgM anti-HAV	Acute = HBsAG and HBcAb-IgM Chronic = HBsAg for >6 months	Anti-HCV appears in 5–30 weeks	Anti-HDV	Negative serologies for all hepatitis viruses 1 g Anti-HEV
Course	Acute disease only	Acute and chronic	Acute and chronic	Acute and chronic	Acute disease only
Vaccine	Yes	Yes	No	No	No
Prevention after exposure	Immune globulin + vaccine	HBIG + vaccine	Uncertain	Unknown	Uncertain

by detection of serum IgM anti-HAV, which is present at the onset of symptoms in most patients. IgG anti-HAV reaches a high titer during convalescence and persists indefinitely, conferring immunity. Most cases of hepatitis A resolve over several weeks. In some persons, malaise persists for many months. There is a less than a 1 percent incidence of fulminant hepatitis and death from HAV. There is no progression to chronic hepatitis.

Strategies for the prevention of hepatitis A include hand washing and not eating raw shellfish. HAV is likely to spread when there is close and prolonged contact with infected individuals. Those at risk include household contacts and individuals in settings such as day care centers. Persons who have been exposed to HAV in these settings should be given passive immunoprophylaxis with immune globulin as soon as possible after exposure.

An inactivated hepatitis A vaccine became available in 1995. The vaccine is indicated for persons over age 2 years who are traveling to areas endemic for HAV. The vaccine confers protection 2 weeks after the initial dose; therefore, persons traveling sooner than in 2 weeks should receive a simultaneous injection of immune globulin. In addition to travelers, the vaccine is indicated for men who have sex with men, users of injectable drugs, persons who have chronic liver disease, and persons at occupational risk, such as day care and food service workers. Two injections of hepatitis A vaccine are required: one at time zero and a booster 6 to 12 months after the first.

HEPATITIS E

Hepatitis E is similar to hepatitis A. It is transmitted fecal-orally and has been associated with contaminated food and water. It produces only acute disease, and the clinical course is usually mild and self-limiting. However, in pregnant women hepatitis E causes a high rate (20 percent) of fulminant disease with a high risk of death. Hepatitis E is rare in the United States but is endemic in Southeast Asia, and there have been reported outbreaks in Mexico. The clinician should suspect hepatitis E in a patient with signs and symptoms of hepatitis who has traveled to an endemic area and has negative serologies for hepatitis A, B, and C. There is no commercially available test for hepatitis E at this time; a serologic test is available from the Centers for Disease Control.

HEPATITIS B

Hepatitis B virus (HBV) is a DNA virus that causes both acute and chronic disease. The virus is spread by direct contact with infected blood or body fluids. It is transmitted mainly by sexual contact, both heterosexual and homosexual, and by the sharing of needles among intravenous drug users. It also is transmitted by infected mothers to their babies at birth. In a substantial number of persons, no risk

factor is identified. Ninety to 95 percent of adults infected with HBV recover completely; the other 5 to 10 percent become asymptomatic carriers or develop chronic hepatitis B. Persons with chronic hepatitis B may go on to develop cirrhosis and are at increased risk for developing hepatocellular carcinoma (HCC). The younger a person is when infected with HBV, the greater is that person's likelihood of becoming chronically infected. Fifteen to 20 percent of infected children develop chronic hepatitis B, and more than 90 percent of infected neonates develop chronic infection. The infection becomes chronic if the virus is not eliminated by the immune system during acute disease and continues to replicate. The damage done to the liver in HBV infection is thought to be due to the immunologic response of the host rather than to the cytopathic effect of the virus. Some symptoms, such as rash and arthritis, are more common in hepatitis B than in other types of hepatitis and are thought to be due to the deposition of immune complexes.

The diagnosis of acute hepatitis B can be made with two serologic tests: hepatitis B surface antigen (HBsAg) and IgM hepatitis B core antibody (HBcAb-IgM). If both are positive, the patient has acute hepatitis B. HBsAg is the predominant viral envelope protein. The test for this antigen is the first serologic marker to become positive, appearing as early as 2 to 12 weeks after exposure and preceding the symptoms. HBsAg concentration reaches a peak during acute disease and then usually becomes negative in 3 to 6 months. The persistence of HBsAg beyond 6 months indicates chronic infection. HBcAb-IgM also becomes negative and is replaced by the total hepatitis B core antibody (HBcAb). There is no test for HBcAb-IgG. A positive HBcAb with a negative IgM fraction indicates prior infection. Antibody against HBsAb appears approximately 6 months after the initial infection. The loss of HBsAg and the presence of HBsAb indicate immunity. HBsAb also appears and may persist after hepatitis B vaccination.

Hepatitis B e antigen is another viral antigen. It is released during active viral replication and is associated with infectivity. In acute disease, it appears at approximately the same time as HBsAg and then declines shortly before HBsAg. Persons with chronic hepatitis B should be tested for HBeAg. Hepatitis B DNA (HBV-DNA) is another test of viral replication. Chronic carriers of HBV are positive for HBsAg for longer than 6 months but have undetectable levels of HBeAg and HBV-DNA. The rate of viral replication in these persons is very low, and their infectivity therefore probably is low. These individuals usually show no or minimal evidence of liver damage. Patients who are positive for HBsAg and HBeAg or HBV-DNA have active viral replication and probably high infectivity. Hepatic injury is more likely to occur in these individuals; liver enzymes may or may not be elevated.

To summarize the serologic diagnosis, the presence of HBsAg and HBcAb-IgM indicates acute hepatitis B. HBeAg is also positive in acute hepatitis B. The loss of HBsAg (and HBeAg) and the development of

HBsAb indicate immunity. Chronic hepatitis B (or the carrier state) is diagnosed when the HBsAg is positive for longer than 6 months. The presence of HBeAg or HBV-DNA indicates ongoing viral replication.

Recombinant vaccines against HBV are available and safe and have been incorporated into the childhood immunization schedule. Adolescents should be vaccinated, along with other persons at risk. This includes those who are sexually active with multiple partners, abusers of injectable drugs, and health care workers. All pregnant women should be screened for HBsAg to identify neonates at risk for perinatal infection.

HEPATITIS D (DELTA HEPATITIS)

Hepatitis D virus (HDV) is a defective RNA virus that causes hepatitis only in persons who are already infected with hepatitis B virus. The delta virus is dependent on the continuing presence of hepatitis B surface antigen to replicate. If an individual becomes coinfected with the hepatitis B and hepatitis D viruses at the same time, the risk of fulminant disease is high. Patients with stable chronic hepatitis B who become infected with HDV usually exhibit an exacerbation of their condition with rapid deterioration of liver function. HDV is diagnosed by the serologic test for hepatitis delta antibody. A positive result in a person with HBsAg indicates infection with the delta hepatitis virus. HDV is endemic in Mediterranean countries, the Middle East, and parts of South America. In nonendemic countries, it should be suspected in persons from high-risk groups, such as intravenous drug users and recipients of multiple blood products.

HEPATITIS C

Hepatitis C virus (HCV) has emerged as the major cause of non-A, non-B hepatitis. HCV is an RNA virus that causes both acute and chronic disease. There are at least six HCV genotypes. Although the exact mechanism is not understood, HCV produces disease through cytopathic effects. Until 1986, blood transfusion was responsible for most cases of hepatitis C. Today injectable drug use is the predominant risk factor. Although HCV is spread primarily via the parenteral route, sexual, nonsexual, household contact, and maternal transmission may occur. The transmission of HCV infection through breast milk has not been documented. As with hepatitis B virus, a number of patients with HCV have no identifiable risk factor. The clinical course of acute hepatitis C is generally milder than that of hepatitis A or hepatitis B. A large percentage of these patients are asymptomatic.

The association between HCV, chronic hepatitis, and HCC is well established. It is estimated that approximately 80 percent of persons with hepatitis C infection will go on to develop chronic hepatitis, with persistent or fluctuating ALT elevations that indicate active liver disease occurring in 60 to 70 percent of chronically infected persons. Cirrhosis develops in 10 to 20 percent of persons with chronic hepatitis C over a period of 20 to 30 years, and HCC in 1 to 5 percent. During the time from infection with HCV to the development of cirrhosis, the patient may be asymptomatic.

HCV infection is diagnosed by ordering the hepatitis C antibody test with the second-generation enzyme-linked immunoabsorbent assay (ELISA-2). The time from infection to seroconversion is approximately 6 weeks (range 5 to 30 weeks). HCV antibodies are not neutralizing and offer no protection against current or subsequent infection. Patients with a risk factor for HCV infection and persons with abnormal liver enzymes should be tested for the antibody. The hepatitis C antibody test is associated with false positives in persons with autoimmune disease or any disease that may increase gamma globulins. If a false-positive result is suspected, a confirmatory test for the hepatitis C antibody with the recombinant immunoblot assay second-generation (RIBA-2) method should be done. Serum levels of HCV RNA can be measured by polymerase chain reaction (PCR) or branched-chain DNA assays.

HEPATITIS G

Hepatitis G virus (HGV) has been detected by PCR and is thought to be similar to HCV; it may coexist with hepatitis C. It does not seem to contribute to chronic liver disease.

TREATMENT OF ACUTE VIRAL HEPATITIS AND PATIENT EDUCATION

There is no specific treatment for acute viral hepatitis. Recommended supportive measures include adequate hydration and reduced physical activity. Absolute bed rest is not necessary. A low-fat and high-carbohydrate diet may cause less nausea. Hygiene and stool precautions should be emphasized for patients with hepatitis A and E, and blood and body fluid precautions for those with hepatitis B, C, D, and G. Hepatotoxins, including alcohol and drugs, should be avoided.

INDICATIONS FOR HOSPITALIZATION

Patients with severe nausea and vomiting require hospitalization because of the risk of dehydration and hypoglycemia. Patients with a prolonged prothrombin time or other signs of deteriorating hepatic function should be hospitalized.

TREATMENT OF CHRONIC VIRAL HEPATITIS

Hepatitis B, C, and D can cause chronic disease. The natural history of infection with hepatitis B and C is variable, but both viruses can cause serious liver disease, cirrhosis, and HCC. Chronic hepatitis should be considered in patients with elevated liver enzyme levels that persist for more than 6 months. Interferon alfa-2b is approved for the treatment of chronic hepatitis B and C. Generally, therapy is indicated when chronic infection is present with viral replication occurring and there are histologic changes on liver biopsy. Treatment is limited by the side effects of interferon, including "flu-like" symptoms of headache, fatigue, myalgia, and fever. Psychiatric adverse events also may occur. Patients with chronic hepatitis B or C and replicating virus should be referred to a hepatologist or gastroenterologist for consideration of interferon therapy.

For hepatitis B, interferon alfa is injected subcutaneously at a dose of 5 MU/d or 10 MU three times per week for 16 weeks. Using the HBeAg and HBV-DNA as the end point, there may be up to a 50 percent response rate, depending on patient profile. Recently, antiviral nucleoside analogues such as lamivudine (Epivir) and famciclovir (Famvir) were shown to be effective in the treatment of chronic HBV. These agents suppress viral replication, but typically the virus returns after the cessation of therapy.

Treatment of chronic hepatitis C is recommended for patients with active hepatitis on liver biopsy and HCV RNA in the serum. Studies indicate that interferon treatment in patients with a low pretreatment level of HCV RNA and infection with a genotype other than 1 are more likely to respond. Treatment can be performed with either interferon alfa monotherapy or a combination of interferon and ribavirin, a nucleoside analogue. Patients treated with a combination of ribavirin and interferon have demonstrated sustained response rates of 40 to 50 percent compared with response rates of 15 to 25 percent in patients treated with interferon alone. Combined therapy generally consists of 3 MU of interferon administered three times weekly along with oral ribavirin 1200 mg (depending on the patient's weight) administered in two divided doses daily for 48 weeks. Patients taking ribavirin must be monitored for hemolytic anemia.

DIFFERENTIAL DIAGNOSIS

The differential diagnosis of acute hepatitis includes viral hepatitis, toxic hepatitis (including drug and alcoholic hepatitis), bacterial

Table 6-14-2. Differential Diagnosis of Acute and Chronic Hepatitis

ACUTE HEPATITIS	CHRONIC HEPATITIS
Viral hepatitis	Viral hepatitis
Toxic, drug-induced, alcoholic	Drug-induced and alcoholic
Bacterial hepatitis	Wilson's disease
Biliary obstruction	Hemochromatosis
	Autoimmune hepatitis
	Primary biliary cirrhosis
	Primary sclerosing cholangitis

hepatitis, and biliary obstruction (see Table 6-14-2). Viruses other than the hepatotropic viruses that cause hepatitis include Epstein-Barr virus (infectious mononucleosis), cytomegalovirus, herpes simplex, and less commonly varicella, rubella, mumps, and yellow fever. All medications, prescription and nonprescription, should be considered potential hepatotoxins. An ALT greater than 5000 suggests a toxic hepatitis such as that caused by acetaminophen or other medications. Alcoholic hepatitis is suggested by an AST higher than ALT (ALT is usually <500). Bacteria such as *Salmonella, Campylobacter,* and *Listeria,* can cause hepatitis and should be considered when a patient has acute hepatitis and a fever higher than 101°F. A bilirubin of 10 mg/dL or higher suggests biliary obstruction as the cause of the hepatitis. The differential diagnosis for chronic hepatitis includes viral hepatitis, drug-induced hepatitis, alcoholic hepatitis, Wilson's disease, hemochromatosis, autoimmune hepatitis, primary biliary cirrhosis, and primary sclerosing cholangitis.

BIBLIOGRAPHY

Bowden DS, Moaven LD, Locarnini SA: New hepatitis viruses: Are there enough letters in the alphabet? *Med J Aust* 164(2):87–89, 1996.
Centers for Disease Control: Recommendations for prevention and control of hepatitis C virus (HCV) Infection and HCV-related chronic disease. *MMWR,* 47 (RR-19):1–39, 1999.
Franklin D, Becherer PR, Bacon BR: Hepatitis C virus: What recent studies can tell us. *Postgrad Med* 95(6):121–130, 1994.
Mandell GL, Douglas RG, Bennett JE: *Principles and Practices of Infectious Diseases.* New York, Churchill Livingstone, 1995.

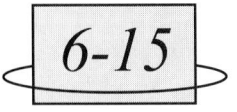 **INFLAMMATORY BOWEL DISEASE**

Anne P. Heinly

DISCUSSION

When inflammatory bowel disease (IBD) is discussed, it is inclusive of two similar but essentially different disease processes: ulcerative colitis and Crohn's disease. Both cause chronic inflammation or ulceration of the intestinal tract. Both are chronic debilitating diseases with systemic manifestations that may have long periods of remission. Both are of unknown etiology. A major distinguishing factor between the two diseases is the underlying tissue pathology: Ulcerative colitis affects the mucosa and submucosa of the colon, whereas Crohn's disease affects all four layers of the colon and/or small intestine (see Table 6-15-1).

PATHOGENESIS

Maintaining a stable environment in the intestinal tract is dependent on several factors: the presence of friendly bacteria, dietary intake, inflammatory triggers, and the host's immune defenses. Inflammatory

TABLE 6-15-1. Comparison of Ulcerative Colitis and Crohn's Disease

ULCERATIVE COLITIS	CROHN'S DISEASE
Symptoms	Symptoms
Acute onset	Insidious onset
LLQ pain	Fatigue
Bloody diarrhea	Weight loss
Fever	Anorexia
Fatigue	RLQ pain
Weight loss	Diarrhea with or without
Anorexia	blood
Rectal tenesmus	Crampy, relieved with defecation
Objective	Objective
Tachycardia	Thin, undernourished
Volume depletion	RLQ tenderness, mass effect
Pale, anemia	Perianal fissures
Fever	Fistula and abscess formation
Abdominal tenderness, peritoneal signs	Pale, anemia
Heme positive	
Systemic manifestations	Systemic manifestations
Inflammatory arthritis	Inflammatory arthritis
Ankylosing spondylitis	Osteoarthritis
Sacroiliitis	Ankylosing spondylitis
Digital clubbing	Sacroiliitis
Episcleritis	Digital clubbing
Pyoderma gangrenosum (common)	Episcleritis
Erythema nodosum (less common)	Erythema nodosum (common)
Aphthous ulcers	Pyoderma gangrenosum (less common)
Cirrhosis (common)	Aphthous ulcers (common)
Pericholangitis (common)	Cirrhosis
Renal stones	Pericholangitis
Growth retardation	Renal stones (common)
	Gallstones (common)
	Growth retardation

bowel disease disrupts this process in an idiopathic manner. There are theories about the cause, but it essentially remains unknown.

Genetics seems to play a role in both branches of IBD. There is a consistent presence of human leukocyte antigen B 27 (HLA-B27) in patients with IBD. Ulcerative colitis is associated with HLA-DR2, and Crohn's disease is associated with HLA-A2.Both are associated with autoimmune disease, autoantibodies, immunoglobulin, and complement deposition. Possible etiologies range from a viral or bacterial trigger of the immune system to abnormal mucosal immunoreactivity, but nothing has been proved. The end point is activation of the inflammatory cells of the gastrointestinal tract, whose products cause varying degrees of tissue damage.

ULCERATIVE COLITIS

DISCUSSION

An estimated 250,000 Americans have ulcerative colitis (UC); it is more common than Crohn's disease. A disease of the young, it is seen from ages 10 to 40 with equal prevalence in men and women. Genetic predisposition may increase the likelihood of developing UC up to 10 times normal. There is a concordance rate for UC in identical twins of 6.3 percent.[1] Ulcerative colitis is more common in the Jewish population and in industrialized countries than in other populations.

PATHOGENESIS

Ulcerative colitis causes the inner lining of the large intestine to die and slough off. Only the mucosal and submucosal layers of the colon are affected, and only rarely is the ileum (distal small intestine) involved. The inflammation predictably starts in the rectum and sigmoid area, which manifests uninterrupted mucosal friability with a propensity to bleed and ulcerate. Ulcerations seldom cause fissures or fistulas. Over time, the chronic mucosal dysplasia deteriorates to adenocarcinoma in many patients.

SYMPTOMS

Typical symptoms include abdominal pain that usually occurs in the left lower quadrant but may be generalized, bloody and/or mucus-containing diarrhea, fever, fatigue, weight loss, and anorexia. Approximately one-fourth of these patients have tenesmus and rectal bleeding. Ulcerative colitis is generally an acute process and can become fulminant over a 24- to 48-h period or present with a slow onset of symptoms that are mistaken for other gastrointestinal (GI) problems. These patients are often quite ill. A small percentage (<10 percent) of patients develop pancolitis with involvement of the entire colon. Among all the possible systemic manifestations, some sort of arthritis is most likely. Twenty percent of these patients will have migratory, inflammatory, or peripheral arthritis with a predilection for the hips, ankles, wrists, and elbows.[2] See Table 6-15-1 for the systemic manifestations of UC.

OBJECTIVE FINDINGS

A patient with UC usually appears quite ill. These patients may be pale, tachycardic, and hypotensive owing to volume depletion and blood loss. Fever frequently is elevated (>103°F), and there may be increased skin turgor. Abdominal examination reveals distention, slow to absent bowel sounds, a firm abdomen (not rigid unless perforation occurs), and tender to light and deep palpation in the left lower quadrant (LLQ) with or without rebound, depending on the level of peritoneal irritation. Rectal examination may reveal exaggerated tenderness and a positive heme check. A complete physical should be done to evaluate for other systemic manifestations.

DIAGNOSTIC CONSIDERATIONS

The differential diagnosis for UC is shown in Table 6-15-2. In sorting out the possibilities, it is helpful to remember pain, bleeding, and age range. These factors help the provider differentiate quickly. Infectious diseases should always be ruled out initially and reconsidered in a patient with known UC. The colon is a warm, dark moist place, and bacteria love to take advantage of it; an exacerbation of UC may have a bacterial trigger.

LABORATORY TESTS

The standard tests for the evaluation of an acute abdomen should be done initially: complete blood cell count (CBC), a chemistry panel for electrolytes, urinalysis, amylase, and plain abdominal films. Stool for ova and parasite (O & P) analysis, fecal leukocytes, and cultures are a must to rule out infectious colitis (see Chap. 6-4). The CBC may reveal a mixed anemia from blood loss and iron deficiency. Liver function studies may be abnormal, and there may be hypoalbuminemia from protein leakage from the ulcerative mucosa. Additional tests may include a sedimentation rate, antinuclear antibodies (ANA), and C-reactive protein.

RADIOLOGIC (IMAGING) STUDIES

A barium enema will reveal the extent and severity of UC. The classic finding of UC on a barium study is loss of haustral markings, giving a "cobblestone" appearance that represents ragged mucosal ulcerations and narrowing of the intestinal lumen. During the acute

TABLE 6-15-2. Differential Diagnosis of Inflammatory Bowel Disease

DISEASE	COMMON SYMPTOMS
Intestinal tuberculosis	Fever, anorexia, nausea, constipation, RLQ pain
Tropical sprue	Profuse frothy diarrhea, anemia, paresthesias, muscle cramps
Amebic colitis	Crampy abdominal pain, watery diarrhea, malaise, weight loss
Infectious colitis *Campylobacter, Shigella, Salmonella, Yersinia*	Bloody diarrhea, generalized abdominal pain, fever, chills
Ischemic colitis	Severe abdominal pain, profuse bloody diarrhea, vomiting, hypotension
Diverticulitis	Elderly, LLQ pain, mass effect, constipation
Whipple's disease	Middle-aged men, steatorrhea, abdominal pain, lymphadenopathy, polyarthritis, GI bleeding
Acute abdomen	Abdominal pain, peritoneal symptoms, fever, tachycardia
Irritable bowel syndrome	Abdominal pain, constipation or diarrhea, ↑ mucus, anxiety component
Colon carcinoma	Altered bowel habits, bloody stools, anemia, sudden weight loss
Pseudomembranous colitis	Profuse watery diarrhea (rarely bloody), tenesmus, antibiotic-related

fulminant phase, the barium enema should be done with great care because the colon is quite friable and perforations are a distinct possibility.

The preferred definitive study is an endoscopic examination with biopsies even during the acute phase. Direct visualization during a sigmoidoscopy or colonoscopy will reveal an irregular mucosal surface with a granular appearance and shallow ulcerations.

TREATMENT

Pharmacologic Management

Pharmacologic management is directed toward the control of symptoms, since there is no definitive cure for ulcerative colitis. Sulfasalazine has been the mainstay of therapy for years. Split by colonic bacterial activity, the effects appear to be topical versus systemic. The active ingredient is mesalamine, with sulfapyridine as the transport mechanism. The probable mechanism of action is an increase in colonic oxidation of glucose.

The pH-dependent 5-amino salicylic acids (5-ASA) are newer oral formulations that deliver mesalamine directly to the colonic tissue. Their advantages are the delivery system and the absence of sulfapyridine, which can cause hypersensitivity and decreased sperm counts in men. Another option is the microsphere formulations, which slowly release medication, beginning in the duodenum and extending to the colon. Rectal 5-ASA preparations have been very successful in controlling UC. Rectal instillation leads to high concentrations in the descending colon (up to the splenic flexure). Efficacy is essentially the same. The side-effect profile and cost determine which medication a patient will tolerate (see Table 6-15-3). Sulfasalazine is used to control mild to moderate disease but is avoided in acute and severe ulcerative colitis since it may cause exacerbation of symptoms.

TABLE 6-15-3. Medical Management of Inflammatory Bowel Disease

MEDICATION	DOSE	SIDE EFFECTS	COMMENTS
Sulfasalazines Delivering drugs, especially helpful in both UC and proctitis	Oral sulfasalazine 2–4 g/d Mesalazine suppositories or enemas 1–4 g/d	Headaches, fever, rash, nausea/vomiting, hepatitis, pancreatitis, pancytopenia, agranulocytosis	Inhibits folic acid ↓ Digoxin ↓ Antibiotic metabolism For left-sided UC, enema or suppositories are excellent
Azathioprine or 6-mercaptopurine (6-MP) Useful in long-term treatment of both UC and Crohn's disease	1.5–2.5 mg/kg/d	Nausea, fever, rash, arthralgias, pancreatitis, hepatitis Potentially bone marrow suppression and/or renal toxicity	May be used in pregnancy; better than cyclosporine or methotrexate in UC
Slow onset of action Cyclosporine used in UC	4 mg/kg/d continuous infusion or orally	Hepatotoxicity, renal failure, hypertension, hyperkalemia	Extensive drug interactions with any drug associated with P450 system
Corticosteroids for immediate control in both UC and Crohn's disease; no proven role in long term therapy	Severe disease Hydrocortisone 300–400 mg/day or Prednisolone 60–80 mg/day or Methylprednisolone 60–80 mg/day or ACTH 120 U/day	Peptic ulcer disease, hypertension, psychiatric disturbances, facial mooning, acne, ecchymosis, cataracts, osteopenia, growth retardation (limited list)	
Metronidazole (Flagyl) for Crohn's disease or ciprofloxacin	750–2000 mg/day in divided doses 500 to 750 mg bid PO	Glossitis, headache, ataxia, vertigo, paresthesias, neutropenia	Alcohol agonist ↑ Warfarin action ↓ Cimetidine clearance ↓ Dilantin clearance

First-line therapy for fulminant UC consists of adrenal steroids. Absorption factors include the level of inflammation, total dosing, and efficiency of delivery. The greater the inflammation, the greater the steroidal absorption. Steroidal systemic side effects thus depend on the level of colonic uptake. The most common dosing is oral prednisone 45 to 60 mg/day. Intravenous prednisolone 40 to 60 mg/day is used if there is a problem with absorption. Improvement is seen in 7 to 10 days, and steroids can be tapered slowly over 4 to 16 weeks.

Cyclosporine inhibits the immune response, which is regulated by T lymphocytes, and is used for refractory UC (notresponsive to steroids). The vast majority of refractory cases will respond to intravenous (IV) therapy of 4 mg/kg/day. Cessation or slowing of rectal bleeding is usually the first clinical sign of improvement.

Azathioprine or its metabolite 6-mercaptopurine has found a role in therapy in patients who have failed sulfasalazine. A potent immunosuppressor, it has the potential to cause remission in up to two-thirds of the selected population. It takes time to work; therapy is usually 2.5 mg/kg/day for at least 12 weeks to prove efficacy. Side effects are common and can be severe, including bone marrow suppression, pancreatitis, fever, rash, and nausea.

Methotrexate also has been used as a major immunosuppressor. It can decrease the use of steroids in patients with severe disease. Treatment consists of intramuscular (IM) injections of 25 mg/week for 6 to 8 weeks. Side effects include hepatic and pulmonary toxicity, nausea, stomatitis, diarrhea, and fatigue.

Additional therapy includes IV fluids and electrolyte replacement. It may be prudent in the acute situation to type and cross-match blood products. Total parenteral nutrition (TPN) is a time-honored treatment for fulminant UC, since it provides complete bowel rest. Patients are given nothing by mouth (NPO) until improvement is seen and then progress to low-roughage meals and elemental diet drinks such as Vivonex, Tolerex, and Vital. Patients who do not respond to any of these therapies are surgical candidates for partial or complete colectomy.

Surgical Management

Approximately one-quarter of patients with UC will require a colectomy at some point in their disease. Surgery is performed for the complications of UC: persistent bleeding, perforations, cancer risks, toxic megacolon, and debilitating illness. Three basic surgeries may be done:

- *Proctocolectomy*: Removal of colon and rectum with ileostomy.
- *Proctocolectomy with continent ileostomy*: A pouch is formed with the ileum inside the abdominal wall. The patient inserts a tube through a small opening in the flank for evacuation of stool.
- *Ileoanal anastomosis*: Called a "pull-through" operation. The ileum is pulled down and secured to the anus for close to normal evacuation of stool. Unfortunately, rectal tone is lost and the patient most likely will have dumping syndrome.

COMPLICATIONS AND RED FLAGS

As many as one-third of ulcerative colitis patients will develop colon cancer. Cancer surveillance is recommended with any exacerbation of UC and 10 years after the diagnosis with or without remission. Colonoscopy with biopsies is recommended once a year to every 2 years. Some gastroenterologists advocate total colectomy as a prophylactic measure against cancer risk. It is best to educate the patient about the risk of cancer and the side effects of a total colectomy.

CROHN'S DISEASE

DISCUSSION

Seen in all countries of the world, Crohn's disease can present at any age. Like UC, it has a peak between ages 10 and 40, but it also has another peak in those age 60 to 80. The idiopathic inflammatory process that can effect any GI mucosa (mouth to anus) has had different names over the years: skip colitis, regional colitis, granulomatous colitis, and transmural colitis.

PATHOGENESIS

Crohn's disease affects all four layers of the intestinal mucosa (transmural), with ulcerations and distinct noncaseating granulomas filling the crypts. Once the process is ingrained, the bowel wall thickens and becomes inflexible and stenotic. Because the disease is transmural, fistulas and perirectal fissures are common and can invade other intraabdominal structures, such as the bladder and ureters. Unlike UC, Crohn's disease is characterized by "skip" lesions; there may be a lesion in the ascending colon and another in the jejunum. Approximately one-third of these patients have small bowel or colon lesions exclusively, but as many as half have lesions in both areas. The vast majority will develop ileal disease at some point, affecting the reabsorption of bile salts.

SYMPTOMS

An insidious onset is characteristic, with vague complaints of fatigue, malaise, weight loss, and low-grade fever. Pain in the right lower quadrant (RLQ) with diarrhea is the most common presentation. The abdominal pain is described as crampy in nature and generally is relieved by defecation. The majority of patients will have watery diarrhea. Mild cases may present with occult bleeding, while more severe cases may have gross GI bleeding. This wide spectrum of disease activity can result in a diagnostic delay. Steatorrhea is possible with small bowel involvement. Perianal disease is prevalent with perianal fistulas, fissures, and abscesses (systemic symptoms are listed in Table 6-15-1). It is important to note that Crohn's disease patients are much more likely to develop gallstones and oxalate kidney stones. Chronic Crohn's disease may present with obstructive symptoms, including nausea and vomiting.

OBJECTIVE

The general appearance of a patient with Crohn's disease is that of a thin and undernourished individual with a low-grade fever. Aphthous ulcerations may be seen in the mouth. A tender mass in the RLQ is common and may be confused with acute appendicitis. A careful rectal examination may reveal perianal scarring, skin tags, fissures, or abscesses. Systemic signs may include erythema nodosum, nail clubbing, and joint inflammation.

DIAGNOSTIC CONSIDERATIONS

The differential diagnosis is essentially the same as that for ulcerative colitis (see Table 6-15-2). The elderly often are misdiagnosed with diverticulosis or ischemic bowel disease.

LABORATORY TESTS

A complete blood count usually reveals a mixed anemia (iron-deficient, vitamin B_{12}–deficient) and an increased white blood cell (WBC) count. An elevated sedimentation rate is common. Chemistries may reveal low albumin, calcium, and sodium. Alkaline phosphatase and gamma globulins usually increase. C-reactive proteins are most closely related to clinical disease activity and are good markers to judge the recovery process.

RADIOLOGIC (IMAGING) STUDIES

Barium studies are essential in the evaluation of Crohn's disease. Since the lesions can occur anywhere, a complete examination includes a barium swallow, an upper gastrointestinal (UGI) series with small bowel follow-through, and a barium enema. Obviously, these procedures should be done in sequence, with the barium enema being the preferred first examination. Radiographic features may include rectal sparing, long longitudinal ulcerations, and mucosal edema that appears as blunting, flattening, thickening, or straightening of the normal bowel patterns. Fibrotic stenosis will cause distortion of landmarks and may appear pipe-like. Fistulization, perforations, and abscess formation also may be seen.

Endoscopy is used as a complement to the barium studies, allowing for biopsies of the strictures, masses, or filling defects. Computed tomography (CT) can demonstrate the transmural thickening and track the fistula formation to the skin, bladder, and retroperitoneum.

TREATMENT

Pharmacologic Management

Medical treatment for Crohn's disease is similar to that for ulcerative colitis with a few differences. Sulfasalazine and its analogues have been quite helpful in controlling inflammation in the colon, but their efficacy in the small bowel is debatable. Corticosteroids have been highly successful in treating Crohn's disease at a dose of 0.25 to 0.75 mg/kg/day. Oral budesonide 9 mg daily can induce remission in patients with ileal disease. Cyclosporine does not improve symptoms or reduce the requirement for other forms of therapy. Another anti-inflammatory that has had some success is methotrexate 12.5 to 15 mg daily. Unfortunately, long-term use may predispose a patient to hepatic fibrosis, pneumonitis, and pulmonary fibrosis.

Metronidazole (Flagyl) 750 to 2000 mg/day has been shown to be at least as effective as sulfasalazines. It reduces or eliminates the need for corticosteroids. Unfortunately, the side-effect profile is not good over the long term, with paresthesias being quite common. Relapse frequency is increased with metronidazole versus sulfasalazine.

Supportive therapy includes good nutrition (a high-protein diet) with the addition of fat-soluble vitamins and vitamin B_{12}. Severe cases of Crohn's disease require total TPN (see Table 6-15-4). Abdominal cramping can be treated with antispasmodics such as dicyclomine (Bentyl) and Donnatal. Diarrhea may be controlled with Imodium 2 to 4 mg every 6 h or Lomotil one or two tablets every 6 h. It is important to rule out ulcerative colitis and bacterial colitis before using either antispasmodics or antidiarrheals, since both can exacerbate these conditions. Bile acid binding resins (Questran or something similar) may be helpful with absorption problems and steatorrhea. Conservative local treatment of perianal disease is recommended, since surgical revisions can lead to worsening fistulas and abscesses.

On the horizon is interleukin-4 (IL-4) gene transfer therapy. Research continues into the connection between calcium-independent nitric oxide synthesis in the colon and the expression of IL-4, a natural anti-inflammatory cytokine. Current research is focusing on how IL-4 can

TABLE 6-15-4. Parenteral Nutrition*

TOTAL PARENTERAL NUTRITION (TPN)†	INGREDIENTS‡
Proteins (amino acids 4.25%)	42.5–50 g
Dextrose (25–50%)	250 (25%) or 125 g (50%)
Calcium	4–5 meq
Magnesium	5–8 meq
Potassium	20–50 meq
Sodium	20–50 meq
Acetate	30–75 meq
Chloride	20–55 meq
Phosphorus	10–20 mM
Multivitamins with biotin, B_{12}, and folic acid	10–15 mL
Heparin: helps prevent venous thrombosis	1000 U

* Daily laboratory tests include full electrolyte set, glucose, CO_2, blood urea nitrogen, weight, and fluid input and output.
† Give through a central line to those who need total bowel rest.
‡ These are recommended starting ranges. They must be adjusted for patient needs by a multidisciplinary team.

inhibit IL-8, thus limiting damage to the colonic mucosa.[1] If this research proves fruitful, it could change therapy for IBD completely.

Surgical Treatment

Surgery is reserved for perforations, abscess drainage, obstructions, intractable disease, and some fistulas. Some fistulas are "innocent," causing no major symptoms or complications. More nuisance fistulas (perianal) are treated with good skin care and topical and/or oral antibiotics. Unfortunately, recurrence of the disease is common after partial intestinal removals, and some patients return to the surgical service on a recurrent basis.

COMPLICATIONS AND RED FLAGS

Cancer Risk

Crohn's disease is recognized for increasing a patient's chances of developing colon cancer fivefold. There also may be an increased risk of small bowel carcinomas. Cancer surveillance should begin about 10 years after the initial diagnosis of Crohn's disease, with routine colonoscopy with biopsies every 1 to 2 years. A sudden change in a patient's usual bowel pattern should prompt an early evaluation. Since colon cancer and Crohn's disease are both possible in the elderly, it is important not to delay the investigation of new symptoms.

Other Inflammatory Bowel Disease Complications

Ulcerative colitis and Crohn's disease predispose patients to electrolyte imbalances and dehydration, especially in hot weather. Hypoalbuminemia may cause varying levels of fluid retention. Weight loss is common to both processes, as is persistent anorexia. One-forth of these children may experience growth retardation (see Table 6-15-5).

SUPPORTIVE MEASURES AND PATIENT EDUCATION

Both ulcerative colitis and Crohn's disease are chronic, often debilitating disease processes that strike patients in the prime of life. The diseases are bad enough in and of themselves, but the therapies used for them can cause at least as much if not more debilitation. Patients with ileostomies must deal with the mechanical needs of emptying an ostomy bag daily, dumping syndrome with malabsorption and dehydration, and psychosexual difficulties, to name a few difficulties. Crohn's disease patients with persistent diarrhea and perianal disease can develop embarrassing rectal incontinence. Rectal or vaginal fistulas can affect sexual activity and complicate birthing in women. Children may suffer growth retardation and vitamin deficiency syndromes. These problems, plus the ever-present risk of colon cancer, make IBD a difficult disease to live with.

Providers must form a trusting relationship with these patients so that they feel free to call when symptoms or concerns overwhelm them. Like the proverbial "headache" patient, chronic disease can test the patience of all concerned. Each new symptom should be approached with the same fervor exhibited in investigating an unknown process. Having IBD does not preclude having a viral acute gastroenteritis (AGE) or appendicitis.

TABLE 6-15-5. Complications of Inflammatory Bowel Disease

Colon cancer: ulcerative colitis > Crohn's
Toxic megacolon: ulcerative colitis > Crohn's
Hemorrhage: ulcerative colitis > Crohn's
Perforation: Crohn's > ulcerative colitis
Fistulas and fissures: Crohn's > ulcerative colitis
Growth retardation: Crohn's > ulcerative colitis
Malabsorption syndromes: Crohn's > ulcerative colitis

It is essential that patients understand the disease process and the expectations concerning the course, progress, chance of remission, and overall prognosis. Good nutrition is key. Both UC and Crohn's disease patients struggle with iron deficiency and low protein, whereas Crohn's disease patients contend with vitamin B_{12} deficiencies. Diet should be high-protein, low-fat (especially after colectomy), and low-residue (avoid raw foods). Ensure that a dietitian follows the patient and tailors a meal plan conducive to individual taste.

Patients may suffer anxiety and/or depressive episodes from the loss of self-image, loss of a job, and marriage difficulties. Psychological needs should be met with appropriate consultation and referral to support groups and professionals.

PEARLS

The diagnosis of IBD usually is not made during the first visit. As with any disease process, the patient should always be instructed to return for care if diarrhea persists more than 24 to 48 h. Past medical history is particularly important in IBD, because the systemic symptoms of IBD may present well ahead of the GI symptoms. Take care in the elderly to keep IBD in the differential, since its treatment is radically different from that for diverticulitis or ischemic bowel disease. The internal medicine department initially cares for the vast majority of these patients, but primary care providers often monitor their follow-up care. Keep the index of suspicion high with changes in disease pattern and remember to do cancer surveillance.

REFERENCES

1. Brown MO: Office management of common anorectal problems, inflammatory bowel disease. *Primary Care Clin Office Pract* 26(1):142–170, 1999.
2. Lugering N, Kucharzik T, Kraft M, et al: Interleukin IL-13 and IL-4 are potent inhibitors of IL-8 secretion by human intestinal epithelial cells. *Dig Dis Sci* 44(3):649–655, 1999.

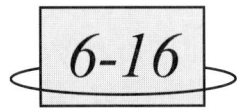

6-16

INTESTINAL OBSTRUCTION
Anne P. Heinly

DESCRIPTION

Intestinal obstruction is simply something inside or outside the intestinal tract that stops or blocks the progress of food or waste. Obstruction is a common phenomenon and accounts for about 20 percent of the emergency surgeries performed each year. *Mechanical obstruction* is something physically in the way or something pressing on the intestine and blocking the path. *Nonmechanical* obstruction (also known as pseudoobstruction) occurs when intestinal peristalsis stops and nothing moves forward or backward. Young people are more likely to have mechanical obstruction in the form of an incarcerated hernia and intussusception (bowel telescoping on itself). The elderly are more likely to have obstruction from carcinomas, volvulus, and diverticulosis. Men and women have an equal chance of having an obstruction, and no age group is safe from the possibility of obstruction.

PATHOGENESIS

Traditionally, intestinal obstruction refers to a partial or complete blockage of the small or large intestine. Esophageal and gastric obstructions are different entities. As described in Chap. 6-18, the small intestine is in charge of digesting and absorbing nutrition and the colon is responsible for continued water and electrolyte retrieval. When obstruction slows or stops this process, harmful things start to happen.

The small intestine, the most common location for obstruction, receives or produces up to 4000 mL of fluid a day. An obstruction allows all that fluid to accumulate, the subsequent pooling causes intestinal wall edema, and vasodilatation ensues, causing even more fluid to pour in. The result is liters of slush backing up with little or no absorption until vomiting is the only way out. Fluid deficits are amassed from intestinal secretions, vomiting, and poor oral intake, and soon there is a dehydrated, hypotensive, ill patient presenting to the emergency department.

Obstruction over time can cause bowel necrosis, which adds the possibility of bleeding, sepsis, electrolyte imbalances, and surgical consequences. Bowel necrosis is more likely to occur when there is a "closed-loop" obstruction or, more simply, an obstruction that blocks two or more points. A volvulus (twisted intestine) is an example, resembling a sausage twisted into a loop, with the stool going nowhere. The result is increasing fluid, increasing pressure, bacterial endotoxins at work, and ultimately bowel wall injury and necrosis.

SYMPTOMS

Small bowel obstruction or proximal obstructions usually present with abdominal pain. The pain usually waxes and wanes as the intestinal peristalsis tries to clear the obstruction. The higher the obstruction is, the faster vomiting occurs, often with bile and partially digested food products. The vomitus is usually copious and has a foul (fecal) smell as a result of bacterial overgrowth. The lower the obstruction is in the tract, the more likely it is that abdominal distention may be a presenting symptom (trapped gas and fluids).

A colonic obstruction more commonly presents with distention, borborygmi, and pain. The pain has a tendency to be dull and steady as opposed to the cramping pain in higher obstructions. It takes longer to get to a vomiting stage because the fluid backup has farther to go and the small intestine can take a fair amount of distention. When the patient does vomit, it is feculent. Patients often complain of constipation or may have "obstipation," which is the passage of stool below the obstruction or watery diarrhea that is able to sneak through. In the elderly, the only symptoms may be distention and constipation because of changes in immune and neurologic status.

OBJECTIVE

Physical findings fluctuate with the location and the duration of the obstruction. An early obstruction or partial obstruction reveals less distention and more bowel sounds such as rushes and gurgles as the bowel tries to clear the obstruction. As the obstruction persists, the abdominal distention can be impressive. The protuberant abdomen can make the patient look 10 months' pregnant. Strangulation, peritonitis secondary to necrosis, sepsis, or complete obstruction can present with absent or very slow bowel sounds and increasing tympany.

A pseudoobstruction patient is less likely to have distention but will have absent bowel sounds because of the lack of peristalsis (adynamic or paralytic ileus). All these patients may have evidence of dehydration: poor turgor, dry oral and eye mucosa, orthostatic vital signs, and/or poor urinary output. A rectal examination is necessary; it may reveal impacted stool, mass, fistula, or blood. Bleeding is not unusual with diverticulitis, carcinoma, ischemia, or intussusception.

DIAGNOSTIC CONSIDERATIONS

Table 6-16-1 reviews the possible causes of obstructions. By far the most common cause is the presence of abdominal adhesions, especially with the small intestine. Colonic obstructions are more likely to be due to carcinoma or diverticuli. Constipation (see Chap. 6-6) sometimes is referred to as the most common type of obstruction. Certainly it is common, but it is generally a temporary condition that seldom causes distention or vomiting.

LABORATORY TESTS

Volume depletion and electrolyte derangement are the most common findings on laboratory evaluation. The complete blood cell count (CBC) may show a high hematocrit owing to volume loss and a mild elevation in white blood cells. The leukocytosis may be more dramatic if necrosis, peritonitis, or sepsis is present. Amylase may be elevated, but like the sedimentation rate, it is nonspecific for the etiology of the obstruction. Urinalysis usually demonstrates the patient's poor fluid status with a high specific gravity. Chemistries may show a metabolic acidosis with rising blood urea nitrogen (BUN) and creatinine. Severity is dependent on the duration of the obstruction, the age of the patient, and concomitant disease processes.

RADIOLOGIC (IMAGING) STUDIES

A plain abdominal film, supine and upright, is usually enough to make the diagnosis of obstruction. Table 6-16-2 reviews possible findings. If the plain films are not sufficient for diagnosis, a barium study is recommended. Barium is preferred to a water-soluble contrast because it does not add to the osmotic fluid confiscation that the obstruction is already causing. The study generally defines the location of the obstruction and often its probable cause. In the case of intussusception or colonic volvulus, the heavy barium may actually help resolve the obstruction.

TREATMENT

Despite the large number of obstruction patients who end up in surgery, the first step is medical management. Correction of electrolyte imbalances and fluid replacement are essential. Stabilization of the cardiac and renal status of the patient is required before any operative therapy. Up to 80 percent of patients with proximal small intestinal obstructions will resolve with early decompression with a nasogastric tube and strict oral fluid restriction (at least for a while). With postoperative paralytic ileus, nasogastric tube (NGT) decompression and fluid restriction may be required for weeks or even months. In these cases, total parenteral nutrition has to be implemented as well. NGT decompression is recommended for all types of obstruction because it puts the intestines at rest and removes secretions.

Surgery is the solution for about 50 percent of obstruction patients. The goal of surgery is to relieve the obstruction with as little disruption of the abdominal contents as possible. Since adhesions frequently cause obstruction, it is important to minimize trauma to the peritoneal tissue during surgery. The second goal is to limit the bowel resection and achieve a clean anastomosis. Laparoscopic abdominal surgery is beginning to reach both goals. Another option for critically ill patients is the placement of metal stents as a temporizing measure. This measure allows for an elective one-stage operation in which the patient is more likely to tolerate the procedure.

The key to therapy for an obstruction is to know when to wait and when to operate. Medical therapy may relieve an obstruction for a time, but recurrence is common. A trial of medical therapy may put the bowel at risk for strangulation, necrosis, and bleeding. Since there is an increased risk of complications, including death with delayed surgery, the decision and timing of surgery can be critical. Serial radiographs, laboratory studies, and physical examinations should be followed carefully to catch subtle progression of the obstruction.

COMPLICATIONS

Before the relief of an obstruction, the complications include volume loss (decreasing cardiac and renal reserves); electrolyte imbalances that can cause acidosis and cardiac arrhythmias; perforation of the bowel at a weak spot (diverticulosis or ulcer), causing a peritonitis, bleeding, shock, or sepsis; and bowel necrosis.

Postsurgical patients are susceptible to wound infection, especially with perforations or in cases of bowel necrosis. In the elderly, the risks

TABLE 6-16-1. Cause of Obstruction

INTRALUMINAL MECHANICAL OBSTRUCTION

Tumors: carcinoma, lymphoma Crohn's disease Diverticulosis, diverticulitis Foreign body: sexual or deviant behavior Gallstones Parasites, worms Intussusception	These occur within the lumen of the intestine, physically blocking the progress of food. In the case of intussusception, the intestine telescopes in on itself, creating an intrinsic blockage.

EXTRALUMINAL MECHANICAL OBSTRUCTION

Volvulus Hernias: inguinal, umbilical, ventral Pregnancy Uterine, ovarian enlargement Adhesions: postsurgical, endometriosis Pseudocysts, abscesses Abdominal aneurysm	Extraluminal obstruction occurs from outside the intestinal lumen. A hernia or volvulus is an extrinsic process caused by the bowel twisting on itself or getting caught in a tight spot. Any enlarged or shifted abdominal structure can compress the bowel, squeezing it closed.

ILEUS OR PSEUDOOBSTRUCTION

Peritoneal insult: trauma, abdominal and nonabdominal surgery, burns, stress Peritonitis: appendicitis, cholecystitis, diverticulitis, ruptured viscous, etc. Electrolyte imbalance, especially potassium, sodium, or magnesium disturbances Ischemia: blood loss from any source, abdominal angina, MI, CVA Renal failure, uremia, liver failure, CHF Renal stones, fractures Infection: sepsis, cellulitis, pneumonia, pancreatitis ulcerative colitis, glomerulonephritis Medications: narcotics, anesthetics, etc.	The intestines are sensitive to multiple stimuli with activity or inactivity triggered by nerves, hormones, or mechanical distention. Ileus occurs because of an insult to the system as a whole, usually affecting the sympathetic nervous system, and the intestinal tract literally stops. Depending on the severity of the stress or insult and the subsequent treatment, the ileus can last only a few hours or for several days.

CHRONIC PSEUDOOBSTRUCTION

Scleroderma Dermatomyositis Amyloidosis Muscular dystrophy Myxedema Diabetes mellitus Parkinson's disease	A chronic problem with slow intestinal transit or propulsion; these patients are prone to develop megacolon. The mechanism seems to be a loss of smooth muscle control, connective tissue loss, and/or neurologic disconnect. The result is relative immobility with chronic constipation, bloating, anorexia, and cramping.

NOTE: MI = myocardial infarction; CVA = cardiovascular accident; CHF = congestive heart failure.

are higher because of decreased organ reserve (they cannot take the hypotension and insult as well) and concomitant diseases. Small intestinal obstructions are less likely to end in death, but as many as 20 percent of colon obstructions result in death despite aggressive therapy and early surgery.

TABLE 6-16-2. Radiologic Findings in Obstruction: Supine and Upright Abdominal Films

FINDINGS	POSSIBLE CAUSE
Multiple air-fluid levels	Small bowel obstruction
Dilated bowel loops folded over on themselves	Small bowel obstruction
Bird's beak appearance	Classic for volvulus
A loop of bowel displacing normal-appearing colonic gas	Closed-loop obstruction
Blurred haustral markings with large loops	May indicate edema and ischemic injury
Evidence of gallstones	Cholelithiasis
Pancreatic calcifications	Possibility of carcinoma
Renal stones	Renal lithiasis
Aortic aneurysm	Aortic aneurysm

PATIENT EDUCATION

Prevention of obstruction is difficult. Adhesions may form even without a history of previous abdominal surgery. Intrinsic problems such as hernias, volvulus, and intussusception are not avoidable. Pancreatic pseudocysts and carcinomas may be preventable with alcohol restriction and a low-fat diet. Postsurgical education should include the likelihood of another obstruction in the future.

PEARLS

An obstruction is a sign of an underlying problem. Stabilize the patient with fluids, decompression, and bowel rest. Look for the underlying cause; an adynamic ileus can be caused by pneumonia or even otitis media in children. Watch for progression of the obstruction and do not delay surgery if there is a risk of strangulation or necrosis.

BIBLIOGRAPHY

Baron TH, Dean PA, Yates MR, et al: Expandable metal stents for treatment of colonic obstruction: Techniques and outcome. *Gastrointest Endosc* 47(3):277–285, 1998.
Lopez-Kostner F, Hool GR, Lavery IC: Management of causes of acute large-bowel obstruction. *Surg Clin North Am* 77(6):1265–1286, 1997.

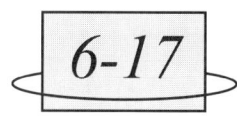

IRRITABLE BOWEL SYNDROME

Anne P. Heinly

DISCUSSION

A common diagnosis that is prevalent among young women, irritable bowel syndrome (IBS) continues to defy definition. A syndrome and not a disease, IBS is a collection of typical symptoms generally associated with aberrant colonic motility, increased visceral sensitivity, and psychopathology. Table 6-17-1 lists the alternative names given to IBS over the years. Although the set of symptoms varies from race to race, there appears to be no specific ethnic predilection for IBS. In making a diagnosis of exclusion, the clinician must first rule out physiologic disease. The reason IBS is not classified as a disease is that its etiology has long eluded researchers. There is no evidence of anatomic or physiologic components that would explain the set of symptoms.

PATHOGENESIS

The primary function of the colon is threefold. The first function is to move waste products out of the system through slow peristaltic movements that for most patients are imperceptible. The second function is the retrieval of essential electrolytes such as potassium, sodium, calcium, and magnesium. The third function is the reabsorption of water. As fecal material is propelled through the gastrointestinal tract, it is condensed, molded, dehydrated, and evacuated by the colon.

The motility of the colon is a mixture of muscle action, hormonal triggers, and nervous system control. Stimulation of the colon may occur with distention, stress, dietary intake, chemical factors, and/or medications. Patients with IBS appear to have a heightened sensitivity to colonic motion and perceive it as crampy abdominal pain. For years, IBS researchers looked for a motility anomaly to explain the set of symptoms. With the availability of small bowel manometry, motor abnormalities have been found in the small bowel and colon. Continuing research is examining "visceral hyperalgesia" (increased sensitivity to pain in an organ). The peripheral nervous system of the gut is composed of multiple nerve terminals. Blocking three (in particular, mu, delta, and kappa) may diminish the neuronal excitability of the colon. Although this information may help with therapeutic modalities, it has not totally accounted for the symptom cycle that IBS patients suffer.

SYMPTOMS

Usually a chronic and recurrent problem, IBS is defined by the three most common symptoms: (1) crampy abdominal pain, (2) associated with gas and bloating, and (3) loose, frequent stools. The pain usually is described as intermittent, mild to moderate, and localized in the lower abdominal quadrants. It is often short-lived (30 min to 1 h) and normally is relieved with defecation. Patients complain of bloating and increased flatulence. Three to four stools will occur in a short period

TABLE 6-17-1. Alternative Names for Irritable Bowel Syndrome

Spastic colon
Spastic colitis
Psychogenic colitis
Irritable colon
Nervous stomach
Mucous colitis
Functional bowel disease

TABLE 6-17-2. Differential Diagnosis for Irritable Bowel Syndrome

Amebic colitis	Crampy abdominal pain, profuse watery diarrhea, malaise, weight loss
Infectious colitis	Bloody diarrhea, generalized abdominal pain, fever and chills, positive laboratory studies
Inflammatory bowel disease (Crohn's disease and ulcerative colitis)	Right or left lower quadrant pain (seldom both), fever, weight loss, diarrhea (with or without blood); peritoneal signs, perianal fissures, biopsy changes
Ischemic colitis	Severe abdominal pain, profuse bloody diarrhea, vomiting and hypotension
Whipple's disease	Middle-aged men, steatorrhea, abdominal pain, polyarthritis and GI bleeding
Acute abdomen Appendicitis Cholecystectomy Diverticulitis Ruptured viscous, etc.	Acute onset, not chronic, steady abdominal pain, fever, tachycardia, peritoneal symptoms, positive laboratory studies
Colon carcinoma	Altered bowel habits, bloody stools, anemia, sudden weight loss; positive endoscopic findings
Lactose intolerance	Abdominal cramping, bloating, and diarrhea 20 to 30 min after a milk or cheese meal; increased flatulence lasting 4 to 6 h; no fever, no systemic symptoms

(2 to 6 h). They are semiformed, brown, and usually nonodorous. Some patients describe stools with mucus. This should not be confused with steatorrhea, in which the stools float and are yellow to gray.

Patients may have the "diarrhea" cycle with alternating constipation. This is manifested by 1 to 2 days of loose stools followed by 5 to 10 days of constipation. Still others have the diarrhea episodes with a persistent sensation of incomplete evacuation. These patients seldom have systemic manifestations such as dehydration, fever, chills, night sweats, nocturnal awakening, and weight loss. Stools are without blood or bacterial overgrowth.

OBJECTIVE

One of the frustrating aspects of this diagnosis is that the physical examination is normal. If the patient is seen during a painful episode, there may be some evidence of abdominal bloating and diffuse, nonspecific abdominal tenderness. The physical should be thorough, with at least a full cardiac, pulmonary, and abdominal examination and a rectal examination.

DIAGNOSTIC CONSIDERATIONS

The differential diagnosis for IBS is enormous. Table 6-17-2 addresses the most likely possibilities. It is vital to rule out anatomic physiologic disease because of the severe consequences associated with some diagnoses. Although it is tempting at times to base a clinical diagnosis on the history and physical alone, that is inappropriate with IBS. A complete workup is required for the diagnosis of IBS to avoid missing a potentially life-threatening disease. Finally, to make the diagnosis of IBS, the patient should have signs and symptoms that are continuous or recurrent for 3 months or more.

LABORATORY TESTS

No laboratory test can define IBS. Laboratory studies are directed toward the differential diagnosis. Standard tests should be done, but additional tests may be necessary to exclude disease. Stool for ova and parasite (O & P) analysis, cell counts, and cultures are the first steps. Complete blood cell count (CBC), sedimentation rates, antinuclear antibodies (ANA), and chemistries are all helpful in finding physiologic disease.

RADIOLOGIC (IMAGING) STUDIES

Radiology studies usually include a full gastrointestinal workup, including an upper gastrointestinal (UGI) series, a small bowel follow-through, and barium enema. The barium studies may reveal an increase in spasticity. Patients also should have, at the very least, a flexible sigmoidoscopy examination to rule out the differential diagnosis. A full colonoscopy may be necessary before a final diagnosis of IBS is made.

TREATMENT

Stress Reduction

Many medical providers can relate to IBS symptoms, remembering a critical test or the moments before an important speech. The colon is responsive to stress. The process is incompletely understood but may be related to cranial nerve X (vagus) stimulation. Anxiety increases blood pressure, pulse, and other functions; the flight-or-fight adrenal surge seems to trigger colonic motility. Thus, IBS patients may benefit from stress reduction. First, map the patient's stress pattern and its relationship to IBS symptoms. If a significant correlation exists, coping mechanisms may be helpful. Be careful not to make this a "psychiatric" diagnosis, since it will not benefit the patient and there is more to IBS than mind control. Biofeedback, exercise, adequate sleep, and stress reduction classes are all recommended if there is an anxiety component.

Diet

Diet is the mainstay of therapy. The cephalic-gastrointestinal (GI) connection has been well established. The mere thought or smell of food can trigger GI secretions and motility. An IBS patient needs to keep a food diary to establish which foods trigger or exacerbate the symptoms. Fats, milk, and the size of the meal are often culprits in an IBS episode and may define its length and severity.

Although it is difficult to make generalized dietary recommendations owing to individual needs, there are two basic goals. The first goal is to regulate (normalize) bowel habits. Regular fiber intake can help achieve this. Increased fiber in the diet will help reabsorb water in a diarrhea-prone patient and add softening bulk in a patient who is prone to constipation. The fiber also keeps the colon slightly distended, decreasing the severity of any spasms that might occur.

Patients can add fiber to their diets with whole grain breads and cereal, legumes, fresh or dried fruits, and vegetables. Whether a patient is adding fiber naturally or with over-the-counter (OTC) bulking agents such as Metamucil, it is important to go slowly. Inform the patient that the initial use of these agents may cause more symptoms for 1 to 2 weeks because gas production will increase. A slow start and small portions will minimize this problem. For those prone to constipation, water intake should be increased to 10 to 12 glasses a day unless there is a medical reason to restrict fluids.

The second goal is small regular meals, avoiding fatty overloads. Large meals, especially fatty ones, can cause cramping and diarrhea because of an osmotic overload. A high-carbohydrate, low-fat diet is suggested with pastas, rice, grainy breads, vegetables, and fruits. Both dietary suggestions come with the recommendation of adequate water intake and regular exercise to promote good bowel habits.

Pharmacologic Management

There is continued research into the etiology of IBS, and treatments are apt to change. Serotonin or 5-hydroxytryptamine (5-HT) has been shown to affect visceral neurotransmitters. Alosetron is a new 5-HT antagonist

TABLE 6-17-3. Medications for Irritable Bowel Syndrome

Bulking agents
  Metamucil
  Citrucel
  FiberCon
	Begin with 1 tbsp/day and increase up to 3 tbsp until regular bowel habit is established	Requires regular use and increased water intake; may cause increased gas and cramping initially

Antispasmodic Bentyl	10–20 mg every 6 h as needed for cramping; may diminish diarrhea as well	May cause mild sedation

Anticholinergic, anxiolytic
  Librax
  Donnatal
	One or two tablets at meals and bedtime; slows the gut and diminishes diarrhea	

Lactose intolerance Lactase supplements	One to two tablets 20–30 min before milk ingestion	Increase gas production and flatulence
Antidepressants Amitriptyline	10–25 mg HS; promotes sleep, slows colon; affects neurotransmitters	Anticholinergic effects
Imipramine	75 mg HS; slows gut; affects neurotransmitters	Anticholinergic effects
Selective Serotonin reuptake inhibitors	Low dose; prokinetic, helpful in constipation; affects neurotransmitters	Usually well tolerated

that affects colonic speed and diminishes contractions, with subsequent pain relief in many patients. Fedotozine is a peripheral kappa agonist that is being investigated for its ability to relieve pain perceptions. Another investigational medication is octreotide, which diminishes perceptions of rectal distention. Table 6-17-3 reviews OTC and prescription medications. It is imperative to remember that these medications may decrease symptoms but do not affect the disease process. Use them judiciously. It is better to use life-style changes such as diet, exercise, and stress relief than to become dependent on medications and risk their side effects.

COMPLICATIONS

Although IBS plagues millions of people a year with an annoying set of symptoms, it has no known major complications. It is not related to inflammatory bowel disease (see Chap. 6-15) or any other type of colitis (see Chap. 6-4). Research has not shown any increase in cancer risk after a diagnosis of IBS.

PEARLS

Patient education is key with IBS. Tell patients what they do not have and reassure them that IBS has no known permanent sequelae. Diet and stress are major components in the vast majority of cases and should be addressed at length with patients. Medications can help but should *not* be relied on for long-term control of symptoms.

Once a diagnosis of IBS has been made, it is dangerous to blame all subsequent GI complaints on IBS. The patient should always be reevaluated. Irritable bowel syndrome is a problem of young women. The very young, the elderly, and men are not likely to have IBS, and so it is important to look for a differential diagnosis. A young woman who has a change in the usual symptoms certainly deserves another look. Providers should not miss disease because of complacency about an ill-defined problem such as IBS.

BIBLIOGRAPHY

Almounajed G, Drossman DA: New aspects of the irritable bowel syndrome. *Primary Care Clin Office Pract* 23(3):477–494, 1996.
Browning SM: Office management of common anorectal problems. *Primary Care Clin Office Pract* 26(1):113–141, 1999.
Quigley EM: Gastric and small intestinal motility in health and disease. *Gastroenterol Clin* 25(1):113–141, 1996.

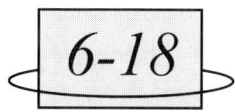

MALABSORPTION
Anne P. Heinly

DESCRIPTION

Malabsorption refers to the body's inability to digest or absorb necessary nutrients from its daily food intake. Numerous disorders can cause a malabsorption syndrome (see Table 6-18-1). Malabsorption to the point of weight loss or vitamin deficiency usually is associated with chronic, long-standing problems. Its prevalence and severity are dependent on the cause. It is best to approach it with a clear understanding of the mechanisms of digestion and nutrient absorption of the gastrointestinal (GI) tract.

PATHOGENESIS

The small intestine, which is located approximately in the middle of the abdominal cavity, is about 15 ft long but has an absorption surface about the size of a basketball court. The duodenum receives digestive enzymes from the pancreas and gallbladder (bile), continuing the breakdown of fats, proteins, and carbohydrates that begins in the stomach. Bile salts produced by the liver are essential for the digestion and absorption of fats. Great detergents, bile salts wash ingested fats and allow the formation of micelles. The micelles then enter the mucosal layer, and the fatty acids and monoglycerides are absorbed by diffusion. The proximal small intestine is responsible for most fat digestion and absorption. The distal ileum is responsible for the reuptake of bile salts, which are returned to the liver in the enteral feedback loop.

The pancreatic enzymes help break down carbohydrates and proteins. Protein polypeptides are disassembled by pancreatic trypsin and chymotrypsin into amino acids that are easily absorbed

TABLE 6-18-1. Causes of Malabsorption

DISEASE	MECHANISM OF MALABSORPTION	SYMPTOMS	TESTS	TREATMENT
Pancreatic insufficiency Chronic pancreatitis Cystic fibrosis Pancreatic cancer Ductal stricture Zollinger-Ellison Syndrome	Loss or destruction of enzyme activity affecting protein and carbohydrate digestion. With ductal strictures the enzymes may be produced but cannot be delivered	Watery diarrhea; may have concomitant IDDM	Low serum albumin; glucose changes	Treat underlying problem. Replace enzymes: 8000 U lipase, 30,000 U protease, 30,000 U amylase before meals and at bedtime
Bile salt insufficiency Liver disease Gallbladder disease Bacterial overgrowth Intestinal obstruction Zollinger-Ellison Crohn's disease with illeum involvement Ileal resection Intestinal vascular disease Intestinal bypass	Absence of or decreased bile acids limit fat digestion and absorption. In the case of vascular disease or postsurgical cases, there is limited contact with available bile salts. Loss of fats and B$_{12}$ ensues in all cases	Steatorrhea, weight loss, anemia, glossitis, neurologic deficits	Low-serum B$_{12}$, macrocytic anemia, positive fecal fat	Cholestyramine can bind colonic bile salts, decreasing diarrhea, not loss of fats. There are no functional bile acid replacements that help with fat digestion. Diet of medium-chain triglycerides recommended
Mucosal defects Amyloidosis Radiation enteritis Celiac sprue Collagenous sprue Tropical sprue Lymphoma Scleroderma Crohn's disease Infectious disease Whipple's disease Samonella Tuberculosis CMV HIV-induced	After digestion, mucosal changes limit absorption of carbohydrate products. Monosaccharides and disaccharides cannot cross the brush border. Severe mucosal disease will affect absorption of all products: fat, proteins, vitamins, carbohydrates, and minerals	Gaseous distention, borborygmi, and osmotic diarrhea are the result Steatorrhea dependent on degree of disease	Mixed anemia acid stools with or without fat; vitamin deficiencies	Correction of underlying disease: e.g., gluten-free diet for celiac sprue, antibiotic therapy for Whipple's disease and tropical sprue
Protein-losing enteropathies Intestinal lymphangiectasis Mechanical blockage of lymphs by extralymph masses Lymphomas	Obstruction of the lymphatics prevents the absorption of the chylomicron and lipoproteins required for production of protein complexes	Edema, ascites, anasarca, steatorrhea, abdominal pain, and fever	Hypoproteinemia, serum albumin decreased	Treat underlying disease

NOTES: IDDM = insulin-dependent diabetes mellitus; CMV = cytomegalovirus.

TABLE 6-18-2.   Vitamin and Mineral Deficiency

VITAMIN OR MINERAL	SYMPTOMS	TESTS	TREATMENT
Vitamin B_{12}	Megaloblastic anemia, weakness, fatigue, glossitis, stomatitis, paresthesias	Decrease serum B_{12} with macrocytic anemia	B_{12} injection 1000 μ monthly
Vitamin B_1 (thiamin)	Anorexia, muscle cramps, paresthesias, loss of reflexes	Decreased serum thiamin	Thiamin injection 100 mg/day for 1 week, then oral dose 5 mg/day
Vitamin B_6 (pyridoxine)	Aphthous ulcers, anemia, glossitis, weakness, neuropathy, and seizures	Decreased pyridoxal phosphate levels	Vitamin B_6 10–20 mg/day
Folic acid	Aphthous ulcers, anemia, glossitis, stomatitis	Normal serum B_{12} with reduced folate level in red blood cells, megaloblastic anemia	Folic acid 1 mg/day
Vitamin A	Night blindness, xerosis, poor wound healing, corneal abrasion, blindness	Serum levels below 30 mg/dL	Vitamin A 30,000 IU for a week
Vitamin D	Rickets osteomalacia, osteoporosis, muscle weakness	Decreased serum calcium and phosphate and vitamin D	Vitamin D 10 mg/day
Vitamin E	Areflexia, disturbances of gait, decreased proprioception and vibrating sensation	Decreased vitamin E (less than 0.5 mg/dL) in relation to lipid profile	Vitamin E 100 IU/day
Vitamin K	Bruising, bleeding	Prothrombin time prolonged	A single dose of subcutaneous vitamin K 15 mg
Calcium	Rickets, osteomalacia, osteoporosis, paresthesias, tetany	Low serum calcium and phosphorus	1200 mg calcium daily
Magnesium	Paresthesia, tetany, weakness, cramps	Low serum magnesium	400 mg magnesium daily
Zinc	Dermatitis, poor wound healing, poor taste	Low serum zinc	15 mg zinc daily

by the proximal and middle jejunum. Amylase breaks down starches and maltose, sucrose, fructose, and lactose. Glucose is readily absorbed by the microvilli of the small intestine, but the other disaccharides have to be split enzymatically before absorption.

The small intestine is also responsible for the absorption of iron; calcium; vitamins A, D, E, and K (see Table 6-18-2); and water. The distal bowel (ileum) absorbs vitamin B_{12} and bile salts. The ability of the small intestine to absorb nutrients is critical to good health. After the absorption process, the final step is into the portal or lymphatic circulation. The portal circulation carries the absorption products to the liver, where protein production, detoxification, and storage take place.

SYMPTOMS

Despite its variety of etiologies, malabsorption almost always presents with one common characteristic: frequent, large, loose, foul-smelling stools. With rare exceptions, fat metabolism is upset, causing an elevation of fecal fat. Additionally, many patients complain of crampy abdominal pain (bloating), and with time, all have weight loss from the loss of calories. Vitamin and mineral deficiencies may be manifested by bone pain, tetany, and weakness (calcium); night blindness and peripheral neuropathies with vitamin A; and purpura and poor clotting with vitamin K.

OBJECTIVE FINDINGS

Physical examination almost always reveals evidence of weight loss and muscle wasting from poor nutrition. Pallor and bruising may be present owing to anemias. Skin dryness, coloration, or texture changes may give clues to specific etiologies such as Crohn's disease, Whipple's disease, and scleroderma. Patients with protein-losing enteropathy may have edema and in the worst cases ascites or anasarca. A complete and thorough physical examination is required to help define the cause of malabsorption.

DIAGNOSTIC CONSIDERATIONS

Simple acute gastroenteritis or diarrhea from any source can cause a mild steatorrhea. The difference between an acute diarrhea state and malabsorption syndrome is time. Most malabsorption etiologies are chronic illnesses that predispose the patient to weight loss and multiple systemic complications. Pancreatic insufficiency can present with watery diarrhea and excessive flatulence just as in irritable bowel syndrome (see Chap. 6-17) but the difference is a persistent intolerance to carbohydrate or lactose meals and weight loss encountered with malabsorption. Chronic diarrhea (a type of malabsorption) may be confused with other malabsorption syndromes. Investigate for infectious origins, especially in patients at risk for immune deficiencies.

LABORATORY TESTS

Among all the areas of the GI system, the small intestines are perhaps the hardest to access. The definition of malabsorption is dependent on laboratory testing. First, the basic laboratory tests should be done to evaluate anemia and vitamin deficiencies: complete blood cell count (CBC), iron studies, vitamin B_{12} level, folate level, calcium level, alkaline phosphatase levels, and protein electrophoresis.

Fecal fat measurement is an unpleasant but necessary mainstay of diagnosis. The average person eliminates 6 g of fat in stools over a 24-h period. The test is conducted with 72 h of stool collection (the unpleasant part) while the patient maintains a high-fat diet (100 g daily); a measurement of more than 15 g of fat in 24 h is considered significant steatorrhea.

Another method is to measure carbohydrate absorption with a D-xylose test. The patient ingests 25 g of D-xylose and then has blood xylose levels checked 2 h after ingestion. If a blood level of 30 mg/dL or more is found, there is normal carbohydrate absorption by the proximal small bowel. If the blood level is low, the urine concentration is examined in 5 h; 4 g or less in the urine indicates mucosal malabsorption.

The Schilling test is used to evaluate vitamin B_{12} deficiency. It has two parts. First the patient ingests a measured dose of radioactive B_{12} and receives an injection of nonlabeled B_{12}. If urinary secretion of the radioactive B_{12} is less than 8 percent of the measured dose, B_{12} malabsorption is confirmed. The next step is to administer intrinsic factor. If the malabsorption rectifies itself, the small bowel is not the problem but an intrinsic factor deficiency exists. The Schilling test is especially helpful in the diagnosis of Crohn's disease (see Chap. 6-15) but may be positive because of bacterial overgrowth and renal failure.

These are the standard first tests when malabsorption is suspected. Borderline tests or tenacious symptoms may warrant further analysis, which may include small intestinal mucosal biopsy (Crohn's disease, celiac disease, Whipple's disease), culturing intestinal aspirate to rule out bacterial overgrowth, and any number of breath tests. Breath tests for glycocholic acid, D-xylose, and glucose hydrogen depend on the metabolic leftovers of absorption-liberating CO_2. The expired breath is examined for radiolabeled CO_2 for each specific test. These tests may be helpful, but their reliability is limited. Gliadin antibodies can help define celiac disease. Protein-losing enteropathies can be confirmed by a fecal alpha$_1$-antitrypsin test.

IMAGING STUDIES

Imaging studies are of limited value. Small bowel barium studies may reveal jejunal dilatation, fold thickening, or segmentation with malabsorption. Sprue typically causes dilatation. Small intestine imaging may reveal jejunal polyps or intestinal pseudoobstruction caused by sclerosis. Imaging for probable causes may be beneficial; for example, a computed tomography (CT) scan for pancreatic pseudocysts, abscesses, or carcinoma may define the malabsorption etiology.

Pancreatic Exocrine Insufficiency

Pancreatic exocrine insufficiency is usually concurrent with a diagnosis of chronic pancreatitis or recurrent episodes of acute pancreatitis. The most common etiology is alcohol abuse, but this condition can occur secondary to trauma, viral infections, and pancreatic carcinoma. With the absence of pancreatic enzymes, the digestion and absorption of fats, proteins, carbohydrates, and fat-soluble vitamins are severely limited. Weight loss, watery diarrhea, and abdominal pain are presenting symptoms. X-ray evaluation may reveal pancreatic calcification in the epigastrium.

Treatment includes an attempt to reduce chronic pancreatitis symptoms. Stop all alcohol ingestion and prescribe pain control, which may require narcotics. Replacement of pancreatic enzymes is essential, though normalization is not achievable. Commercial products such as Viokase and Cotazym S contain enough lipase, protease, and amylase to enhance protein and carbohydrate absorption and alleviate at least some of the steatorrhea. Dosing is generally two or three tablets before each meal and at bedtime.

Bile Acid Insufficiency

Bile acid insufficiency can occur secondary to liver disease, gallbladder disease, faulty ductal delivery, intestinal obstruction, bacterial overgrowth, or disorder of the terminal ileum that interferes with reabsorption. The result in all cases is malabsorption of fat with significant steatorrhea (20 g in 24 h). Protein absorption and carbohydrate absorption usually are maintained. Watery diarrhea because of colonic irritation from bile salts is common.

Treatment is directed at the cause. In the case of bacterial overgrowth, a course of tetracycline or a similar broad-spectrum antibiotic for 10 to 14 days may be successful. In the presence of ileum disease (Crohn's disease), monthly B_{12} injections and cholestyramine 2 g bid are recommended. The cholestyramine helps bind the bile salts, decreasing the diarrhea but not the fat loss.

Celiac Disease

Celiac disease is a disorder of the small bowel mucosa and affects the absorption of fat, protein, carbohydrates, iron, fat-soluble vitamins, and water. The peak incidence is in the first year of life and again in the sixties. It is seen in women more often than in men. In infants and children, the malabsorption can cause failure to thrive, weight loss, infantilism, dwarfism, tetany, mouth ulcers, and angular stomatitis. In adults, there is vertigo, weakness, fatigue, a large appetite with weight loss, explosive flatulence, and diarrhea.

Celiac disease produces a permanent gluten intolerance, with the gliadin fraction of gluten causing the malabsorption of fat. The treatment consists of the elimination of all gluten from the diet. A gluten-free diet includes the removal of all wheat, rye, and barley. In the past, oats were strictly avoided, but extensive testing has revealed that they have no gliadin and the amino acid profile may allow small amounts of oats in the diet. Patients may require calcium and vitamin D supplements. As they reach their teen years, children may be able to resume a regular diet, but they should be counseled about the possible recurrence of symptoms later in life.

Tropical Sprue

Despite the lack of a specific pathogen, tropical sprue appears to be an infection of the small intestinal mucosa. Endemic to most of Asia and some Caribbean islands and parts of South America, epidemics of sprue can last 2 to 10 years. Symptoms may emerge years after one leaves a tropical area. The chief symptom is explosive watery diarrhea followed by pale, frothy foul-smelling greasy stools. Severe malnutrition and water loss cause electrolyte imbalances. Weakness, anemia, paresthesias, glossitis, stomatitis, dry rough skin, flatulence, muscle cramps, night blindness, purpura, and severe weight loss may be seen.

Since megaloblastic anemia is common, vitamin B_{12} 1000 μg intramuscularly is given daily for a week and then monthly for 6 months. Folic acid 5 mg a day and tetracycline 250 mg qid for 1 to 2 months are recommended. Tetracycline dosing may need to be extended for 6 months at half strength (250 mg bid).

Whipple's Disease

Whipple's disease is a rare disorder found in middle-aged men, presumably secondary to an infection of *Trophermyma whippleii*. The onset is insidious, and it can be fatal if not found and treated. These patients have diarrhea with mild steatorrhea, GI bleeding, fever, lymphadenopathy, polyarthritis, edema, and anemia. With progression of the disease, peripheral and finally central neuropathies become evident.

Treatment is with penicillin G 600,000 U intramuscularly bid for 10 days or penicillin VK 250 mg qid for 4 months. About 50 percent of patients may relapse. In relapsing cases, the current recommendation is trimethoprim-sulfamethoxazole or tetracycline for 6 to 12 months. Supplements of vitamin B_{12}, folate, iron, and calcium also are recommended for correction of vitamin deficiencies.

COMPLICATIONS

Certainly the most common complications with any of the malabsorption syndromes are weight loss, electrolyte imbalances, vitamin deficiencies, and dehydration. Without correction, patients, especially young children and the elderly, can suffer permanent damage to vital organs and even death. Celiac disease left untreated leads to marked neurologic deficits that may not be reversible.

PATIENT EDUCATION

Depending on the cause of the malabsorption syndrome, patient education is tailored to the needs of the patient. In the case of bile acid insufficiency or pancreatic exocrine insufficiency, dietary changes are recommended. Generally, a high-protein, low-fat diet is advocated to decrease steatorrhea and diarrhea. A medium-chain triglyceride diet (high in coconut oil) is easier to digest and may help patients tolerate fat intake. Mineral and vitamin supplementation is recommended, including vitamin D (necessary for calcium processing) and magnesium.

PEARLS

Malabsorption may be caused by a variety of diseases that affect the intricate balance of the small intestine. Pancreatic enzymes, bile salts, and intact mucosal surfaces are required to maintain that delicate balance. Identification of these diseases is important to help avoid failure to thrive, weight loss, chronic fatigue, anemia, and systemic manifestations. Virtually all malabsorption syndromes can lead to neurologic deficit and organ failure. It is imperative that a clinician define the cause of recurrent or chronic diarrhea and attempt to ameliorate the symptoms if not the disease.

BIBLIOGRAPHY

Branski D, Lerner A, Lebenthal E: Chronic diarrhea and malabsorption. *Pediatr Clin North Am* 43(2), 1996.
Nehra V: New clinical issues in celiac disease. *Gastroenterol Clin* 27(2), 1998.
O'Duffy JD, Griffing WL, Li CY, et al: Whipple's arthritis. *Arthritis Rheum* 42(4), 1999.

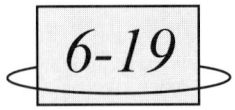

NAUSEA AND VOMITING
Anne P. Heinly

DISCUSSION

Nausea and vomiting often are associated, yet a patient can be nauseated without vomiting and can vomit without first being nauseated. Common to a myriad of diverse conditions, nausea and vomiting are symptoms known to every man, woman, and child at some point in life. Nausea and vomiting can be the early signals of significant disease processes and should be investigated. Nausea is a sensation described variously as queasy, uneasy, churning, gnawing, agitated, or a nervous stomach or abdomen. Nausea may be "anticipatory," caused by an odor, sight, or sound that the patient associates with a bad experience (e.g., chemotherapy). Nausea and vomiting may have mechanical, chemical, or hormonal triggers. There are few diseases or medications that do not have some level of nausea or vomiting associated with them.

PATHOGENESIS

Nausea and vomiting are probably part of the basic regulatory mechanisms of the body, as natural as a pulse or respiration. Nausea may stem from four different locations or a combination of the four. One prime location for nausea is the chemoreceptor trigger zone (CTZ) near the fourth brain ventricle; the vomiting center is on the dorsum of the medulla oblongata. The CTZ seems to be most responsible for the nausea sensation, which is mediated by the second location for nausea production: the vagus nerve (cranial nerve X) and sympathetic pathways. The vagus enervates multiple areas, including the baroreceptors of the heart, aortic arch, and carotid sinuses; the pharynx; the esophagus; and the gastrointestinal (GI) tract to the splenic flexure. The extent of vagus involvement explains why nausea is a symptom in so many processes.

The "vomiting center" has been identified in the medulla near respiratory control; it is affected by histamine and muscarinic cholinergic neurotransmitters. The fourth location for nausea production is in the vestibular apparatus from the labyrinth of the inner ear. Histamine and muscarinic cholinergic neurotransmitters also affect it.

Another association appears to involve vasopressin, a hormone released by the posterior pituitary, which is most sensitive to changes in osmotic pressure (the baroreceptors mentioned above). Research has

shown a marked increase in vasopressin during even brief episodes of nausea. Thus, a disease process that interrupts blood pressure (e.g., infections, medications, motion) can trigger nausea.

Nausea is the sensing side of the equation, and vomiting is the action side. Vomiting is a complex patterned response involving the skeletal muscles and visceral organs of the chest and abdomen. As nausea progresses, at a point of no return the pyloric sphincter loses tone, allowing for bile reflux into the churning stomach. The early retching causes lower esophageal sphincter tone loss, and finally there is a forceful sustained contraction of the diaphragm and abdominal muscles. The force ejects duodenal, gastric, and esophageal contents through the esophagus and out the mouth.

SYMPTOMS: AN APPROACH TO NAUSEA

Given the mechanism of nausea and vomiting and the association with many disease processes, it is important to treat the cause. A thorough history can be quite helpful, especially eliciting the timing and character. If the symptoms have occured over hours or days, consider the following:

- Infectious processes such as acute gastroenteritis (AGE), appendicitis, cholecystitis, otitis media, cellulitis, and streptococcal pharyngitis
- Ingestion of toxins, poisons, or nausea-inducing medications (see Table 6-19-1)
- Pregnancy
- Chronic diseases such as peptic ulcer disease (PUD), myocardial infarction (MI), angina, and Crohn's disease

If the nausea has been present for a week to months, consider partial obstructions, carcinoma, brain tumors, visual or auditory

TABLE 6-19-1. Medications That Cause Nausea (Representative List)

Dopamine agonists	
Dopamine (Levodopa)	Dopamine receptors seem to induce nausea; used for hypotension
Bromocriptine (Parlodel)	Dopamine receptor used in parkinsonism, acromegaly
Narcotics	
Morphine	Reduces gastric motility; used for severe pain control; nausea usually subsides with regular use
Codeine	Reduces gastric motility; nausea worse with increasing doses in most patients
Antibiotics	
Erythromycin	Most likely due to gastric irritation; nausea worse with increasing doses; commonly used antibiotic
Augmentin	Clavulanic acid is probably the culprit; nausea and diarrhea are common
Chemotherapy	
Cisplatin	Most chemotherapy induces some level of nausea, probably from a variety of sources: neurologic toxicity, renal toxicity, and gastric retention Used in the treatment of hormonal tumors; considered the worst for causing nausea
Dacarbazine	Used for the treatment of metastatic melanoma and Hodgkin's disease
Mithracin	Potent antineoplastic used in treatment of testicular cancers
Procarbazine	Used as part of a regimen of vincristine, prednisone, and mustard for treatment of Hodgkin's disease
5-Fluorouracil	Used widely for treatment of colon, rectal, breast, gastric, and pancreatic carcinomas
Methotrexate	An antimetabolite used in the treatment of adult rheumatoid arthritis, severe psoriasis, breast cancer, acute lymphocytic leukemia, osteosarcoma, and small cell carcinomas

sources, motility disorders, and psychogenic causes (anorexia nervosa).

Timing may provide vital clues to the etiology. It is actually unusual to vomit during or immediately after a meal. Psychiatric disorders and esophageal disease are possible culprits. Esophageal diseases such as Zenker's diverticulum, cancer, and strictures are characterized by regurgitation of undigested food, usually without nausea.

Vomiting one or more hours after a meal is associated with infections (any source), gastric outlet obstruction (especially in infants), and decreased gastric motility (illness, chemotherapy). Morning vomiting is associated mostly with pregnancy but occurs with alcohol toxicity, uremia, PUD, and intracranial tumors.

The character of vomit may be telling as well. Old food suggests gastric retention (gastric outlet obstruction, PUD). The presence of bile implies duodenal reflux from cholecystitis, PUD, liver disease, or pancreatitis. Blood may be present as a result of vomiting (Mallory-Weiss tears) or may be the cause of nausea and vomiting (gastric ulcers, PUD, and carcinomas). Fetid breath and emesis may indicate bacterial overgrowth, obstruction, bowel ischemia, or necrosis.

OBJECTIVE FINDINGS

The physical examination should focus on the possible cause of nausea or vomiting. Orthostatic vital signs should be accomplished. Dehydration can cause nausea but seldom vomiting. Infectious disease from any source commonly causes nausea and vomiting. Look for the bottom line with a thorough physical examination, including a rectal or pelvic/prostate examination when indicated.

DIAGNOSTIC CONSIDERATIONS

Table 6-19-2 reviews the differential diagnosis for nausea and vomiting. The commonness of the symptoms defies true classification, and there may be more than one source of the problem. Nausea often is seen with malignancy and may be exacerbated by chemotherapy. Morphine is used for pain control but is well known for its ability to cause nausea. All possible factors should be explored and treated when possible.

TABLE 6-19-2. Causes of Nausea and Vomiting

Infectious origins	
Abdominal	Appendicitis, cholecystitis, ruptured viscous, glomerulonephritis, colitis, diverticulitis, pancreatitis, AGE
Systemic	Especially in infants and children or elderly Otitis media, pneumonia, sinusitis, cellulitis, herpes zoster, PID, prostatitis, epididymitis, meningitis
Hormone-induced	Pregnancy, menses, hypo- or hyperthyroidism, uremia, diabetic ketoacidosis, renal failure, Addison's disease, hypoglycemia
Gastrointestinal sources	Dystonia caused by obstruction, ulcers, strictures, hiatal hernia, volvulus, malignancy, hepatitis, cirrhosis, postsurgical syndromes (afferent loop, dumping), gastric retention, decreased gastric motility from medications
Vascular sources	Acute MI, congestive heart failure, abdominal vascular disease (abdominal angina), headaches, hypotension
Esophageal sources	Zenker's diverticulum, malignancy, GERD, achalasia, strictures, ulcer, candidiasis, CMV
Ear to eye to brain	Ménière's disease, otitis media, labyrinthitis, motion sickness, intracranial pressure from tumors, aneurysms, hydrocephalus, or encephalitis
Medications	See Table 6-19-1

NOTE: AGE = acute gastroenteritis; PID = pelvic inflammatory disease; MI = myocardial infarction; GERD = gastrointestinal reflux disease; CMV = cytomegalovirus.

LABORATORY TESTS

Laboratory assessment is aimed at the presumed cause of the nausea and vomiting and the potential complications. At the very least, an

TABLE 6-19-3. Treatment of Nausea and Vomiting

DRUG	USE	SIDE EFFECTS
Antihistamines Meclizine (Antivert) Hydroxyzine (Vistaril)	Helpful for motion sickness, mild AGE or similar, postoperative nausea. Hydroxyzine good when there is a psychological component to nausea	Sedation, additive effects with other CNS depressives, rare extrapyramidal symptoms
Phenothiazines Prochlorperazine (Compazine) Thiethylperazine (Torecan) Chlorpromazine (Thorazine) Promethazine (Phenergan)	Control of severe nausea, postoperative nausea; used commonly after radiation and chemotherapy	Sedation, interaction with other CNS depressives, extra pyramidal symptoms, blood dyscrasias
Selective 5-HT$_3$ receptor antagonist Ondansetron (Zofran)	Control of severe nausea from chemotherapy and prevention of postoperative nausea	Headache, dizziness, musculoskeletal aches
Butyrophenones Droperidol (Inapsine) Haloperidol (Haldol)	Inapsine is used for pre- and postoperative nausea. Haldol is used for nausea associated with anxiety states	Tardive dyskinesia, neuroleptic malignant syndrome, hypotension
Prokinetics Metoclopramide (Reglan) Cisapride (Propulsid)	Increases lower esophageal sphincter tone and promotes gastric emptying. Used widely for many types of nausea	Extrapyramidal symptoms (Reglan); Arrhythmias (Propulsid)
Benzquinamide (Emete-Con)	Used in patients who do not tolerate the phenothiazines for postsurgical nausea or chemotherapy	Low side-effect profile; drowsiness most common
Treat underlying cause Dehydration Tube decompression for obstruction (NGT or rectal tube) Adrenal crisis—hydrocortisone Drug-induced: reduce or stop drug	Oral or IV fluid replacement with electrolytes	

NOTE: AGE = acute gastroenteritis; NGT = nasogastric tube.

electrolyte survey should be obtained to find evidence of dehydration or electrolyte aberrations.

RADIOLOGIC (IMAGING) STUDIES

Imaging studies, like laboratory studies, are focused on the presumed cause of the nausea and vomiting. It is not wrong to do plain abdominal films to ascertain colonic ileus, free air, renal and gallbladder calculi, or obstructions.

TREATMENT

The key to the treatment of nausea and vomiting is determining the source. Several medications (see Table 6-19-3) are helpful in controlling the symptoms, but they should not be used in place of definitive treatment of the underlying cause of nausea. Two of the most difficult conditions to treat are carcinoma- and chemotherapy-induced nausea and vomiting. Dexamethasone used in conjunction with 5-HT$_3$ agents has been helpful in unresponsive cases. Another medication in trials for difficult nausea is octreotide, which is a somatostatin analogue. It helps control nausea because it inhibits serotonin and most gastric and pancreatic secretions.

COMPLICATIONS

The complications of vomiting can be serious. By far the most common is water and electrolyte loss. Sodium, potassium, hydrogen, and chloride are lost readily, creating a metabolic alkalosis. If diarrhea is present, fluid losses can be impressive and deadly, especially in the elderly and infants. Fluid and electrolyte replacement is essential.

PEARLS

Pay close attention to the timing of the nausea and vomiting. AGE nausea and vomiting occur every 1 to 2 h on average but usually subside within 6 to 8 h and require fluid replacement only. Do not medicate unless necessary. However, if it is known that an essential medication such as chemotherapy or morphine will be used, premedicate with an antiemetic to avoid undue hardship for the patient. Remember to treat the underlying condition.

BIBLIOGRAPHY

Lichter I: Nausea and vomiting in patients with cancer. *Hematol Oncol Clin North Am* 10(1):207–218, 1996.
Murray KR, Christie DL: Vomiting. *Pediatr Revi* 19(10):337–341, 1998.
"Nausea and Vomiting," Health Information (Internet). HTLM<1996, Orbis-AHCN.
"Nausea and Vomiting," National Cancer Institute, No. 208-04466 (Internet). University of Bonn Medical Center, June 1996.

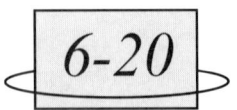

PANCREATIC DISEASE
Anne P. Heinly

ANATOMY

Considered a retroperitoneal organ, the pancreas is about 6 in long and resembles a long, thin chunk of Roquefort cheese. This friable organ is tucked in snugly under the body of the stomach and sits in the curve of the C loop of the duodenum (see Fig. 6-20-1). There is a central duct that connects with the bile duct at the ampulla of Vater, entering the C loop of the duodenum where it dumps its products. Unlike the liver and the spleen, the pancreas does not have an adhesive capsule. The absence of a capsule allows cysts or tumors to grow with relative impunity, at least until they encroach on other abdominal structures.

The importance of the pancreas to normal body function is reflected in its huge blood supply: Branches of the celiac, superior mesenteric, gastroduodenal, and splenic arteries all supply the pancreas. The venous drainage is straight to the portal system as part of the continuous feedback loop between the stomach, liver, and intestines. As with most of the gastrointestinal tract, the vagus nerve (cranial nerve X) innervates the pancreas.

PHYSIOLOGY

The pancreas has one basic function: the excretion of hormones or enzymes that deal with the digestion and absorption of nutrients from daily food intake. The primary endocrine function is located within the islets of Langerhans, which secrete insulin, glucagon, pancreatic polypeptides, and somatostatin, which are essential for glucose utilization (see Chap. 5-1).

The exocrine side of the pancreas is made up of billions of acinar cells that can bud from tiny ductules, which eventually become larger ducts and join to a central duct. The secretory ducts of the acinar cells contain the centroacinar cells. Between the acinar and centroacinar cells, the pancreas secretes 2 to 3 L of digestive enzymes a day. Table 6-20-1 reviews the different enzymes and their functions in regard to digestion and absorption. Because the cells that produce the enzymes also form the transportation system (most other ducts, such as the bile duct, only transport), disease arises when infection, cancer, or medication triggers stimulate autodigestion of the tissues themselves.

The enzyme secretions are dependent on complex feedback loops involving the stomach, liver, and small intestines. Between meals, there is relative pancreatic rest with minimal enzyme secretions that provide for basic cleanup duties. The meal phase is the connection between the brain thinking about food, the nose smelling the food, and the mouth chewing and tasting the food. This "cephalic" phase prepares the bicarbonate brew to be dumped into the duodenum to alkalinize the chyme. The digestion and absorption of food are best done at a pH of 7 to 8.[1] The mediators appear to be cholecystokinin (CCK) and enkephalins in the stomach and liver.

The intestinal phase begins as the chyme is passed into the duodenum. Secretin secretion apparently turns off the gastrin in the stomach and turns on the pancreatic secretions. The amount of secretions is dependent on the fat content of the chyme. The higher the chyme fat content is, the more pancreatic and bile secretions occur. Again, CCK seems to play a major role in this neural and hormonal balancing act. CCK is regulated by the very enzyme it has released: trypsin. Intraluminal trypsin turns the CCK production down or off as needed. Thus, the interaction of secretin, volume, fat, bicarbonate secretions, and finally trypsin operates in an intricate pattern to achieve proper digestion and absorption. Disruption of this balance results in malabsorption at the very least and destruction of the pancreas at worst.

LABORATORY TESTS

The serum amylase test is the most frequently performed test. Care must be taken in interpreting an amylase alone. Amylase is not unique to the pancreas; it is found in the mouth, liver, kidneys, and small intestine and may be produced by a variety of carcinomas. Despite this, a serum amylase level over 300 U is highly indicative of pancreatic disease. To further localize the pancreas, P isoamylase (specific to the pancreas) remains elevated longer, whereas the total amylase is likely to drop rapidly (within 2 to 5 days). Lipase has been relied on increasingly for a clear indication of acute pancreatic disease. Lipase levels rise slowly but are maintained on average for 7 to 14 days. Conditions that can confuse elevated lipase findings are renal failure, bowel obstruction, bowel necrosis, and perforated ulcer disease.

Testing exocrine pancreatic function usually is done to determine the consequence of disease or injury. Persistent nonfunctioning may

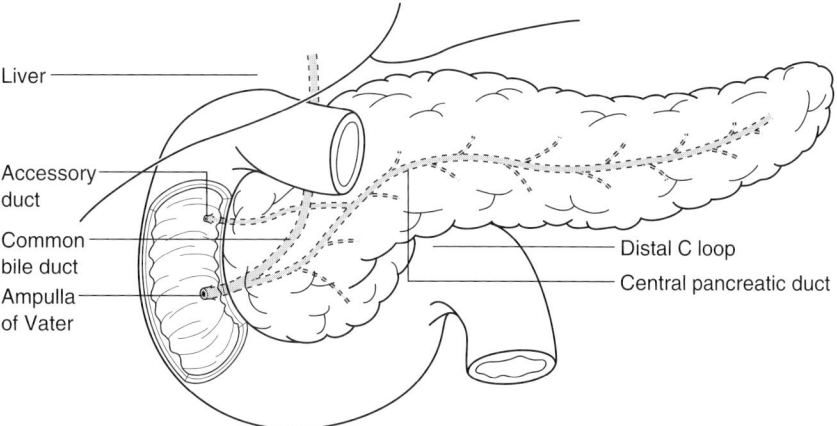

FIGURE 6-20-1. Pancreatic anatomy.

result in a malabsorption syndrome hypertriglyceridemia, vitamin B_{12} loss, hypercalcemia, ascites, or other conditions (see Chap. 6-18). Direct stimulation of the pancreas is the gold standard to determine function. It analyzes the duodenal contents before and after a challenge of secretin and cholecystokinin. This should cause enzyme production;

absence of production indicates widespread, chronic pancreatic disease. See Table 6-20-2 for laboratory findings.

Additional tests include a complete blood cell count (CBC) with possibilities of megaloblastic anemia, chronic blood loss anemia, and/or leukocytosis. Liver function studies and chemistries may reveal hyperglycemia, hypoproteinemia, hypertriglyceridemia, hypocalcemia, increased blood urea nitrogen (BUN), and increased creatinine. Blood gases may show hypoxia.

RADIOLOGIC (IMAGING) STUDIES

Plain abdominal films are valuable about half the time. They may reveal the "sentinel loop," which is a localized ileus involving the jejunum, or a "colon cutoff sign," which is distention of the transverse colon.[2] In a patient with chronic pancreatitis, especially with exocrine insufficiency, the plain film may reveal epigastric calcifications.

Quick, easy, and useful diagnostic information can be gained by using ultrasound, which can delineate edema, pseudocysts, masses, and calcifications. Acute pancreatitis usually presents with enlargement and blunting of the shape owing to edema. Cancer distorts the architecture, and a pseudocyst (common to acute or chronic pancreatitis) is a rounded mass with fluid levels. Ultrasound has drawbacks in that the ileus (bowel gas) can obscure findings, as can obesity, pregnancy, and recent barium studies.

Computer tomograms (CT scans) are helpful in the diagnosis of pancreatic disease. Tumors and pseudocyst show up with contorted structures with or without fluid levels. Endoscopic retrograde cholangiopancreatography (ERCP) utilizes cannulization of the pancreatic duct. This provides definitive information about stenosis, abscesses, tumor size, tumor location, and biopsy potentials.

ACUTE PANCREATITIS

DISCUSSION

Pancreatitis is an inflammatory disease that probably is grossly underdiagnosed. In the past, especially in the United States, most cases of pancreatitis were thought to be due to alcohol abuse. New studies are finding that infections and drugs induce pancreatitis much more commonly than was previously realized. See Table 6-20-3 for the causes of acute pancreatitis. About 1 percent of men and women have at least one episode of acute pancreatitis.

PATHOGENESIS

Although this is still the subject of intense study, the prevailing theory is that the condition of "autodigestion" causes pancreatitis. Trypsin

TABLE 6-20-1. Pancreatic Enzymes

Amylase	Saliva contains amylase, which starts the digestion of starch and glycogen, and the pancreatic amylase continues the job. The small intestinal brush border enzymes convert the final product to glucose
Trypsinogen, proteolytic	Attacks the peptide bonds of protein molecules in the duodenum, resulting in free amino acids, which are then absorbed by the brush border of the jejunum
Chymotrypsinogen, proteolytic	Works with trypsinogen to break catalyzed protein bonds
Proelastase, proteolytic	Cleaves specific protein bonds to liberate amino acids
Procarboxypeptidase A, proteolytic	Continues the protein breakdown at the end of the protein chains, resulting in free amino acids
Procarboxypeptidase B, proteolytic	Continues the protein bond breakdown
Lipase, lipolytic	Breaks down the triglyceride molecule into 2 fatty acids and a monoglyceride; the presence of bile acids and colipase is essential to the process
Prophospholipase A_2, lipolytic	Breaks down the fatty acids, leading to the formation of free fatty acids, which are absorbed to the portal circulation
Carboxylesterase lipase, lipolytic	This enzyme can do a little of everything, cleaving cholesterol ester, lipidsoluble vitamins, triglycerides, monoglycerides, and diglycerides. Bile is required for smooth function
Deoxyribonuclease	Two isozymes that are specific to protein DNA
Ribonuclease	Up to 5 isozymes that are specific to protein RNA
Procolipase	The mediator between lipase and bile acids to aid in triglyceride breakdown
Trypsin inhibitor	A group of 56 amino acids that essentially neutralize trypsin. A protective mechanism from autodigestion

TABLE 6-20-2. Laboratory Findings in Pancreatic Disease

FINDINGS	ACUTE PANCREATITIS	CHRONIC PANCREATITIS	PANCREATIC CANCER
Amylase	>300; elevated 2–12 h after onset; diminishes over 3–5 days	May be normal or only mildly elevated	Rarely elevated
Lipase	>300; elevated 24–72 h after onset; diminishes slowly	May be normal or only mildly elevated	May be normal to mildy elevated
AST	Up to 15 times normal	Mildly elevated	Mildly elevated
ALT	Usually only minimally effected	Usually only minimally effected	Progressive elevation with hepatic metastasis
Bilirubin	Mild elevation	Mild to moderate elevation due to liver congestion	Progressive elevation
Leukocytosis	15,000–20,000 in most cases; may be lower in the elderly	May be normal	Normal
Hyperglycemia	Less insulin production; usually mild	Glucose intolerance or diabetes may occur	Possible occurrence of glucose intolerance or diabetes
Hypocalcemia	Mild; mechanism unknown	Mild to moderate; changes in the parathyroid secretions	
Alkaline phosphatase	Normal	Mildly elevated	>5 times normal in many cases but still not specific

NOTE: AST = aspartate aminotransferase; ALT = alanine aminotransferase.

appears to be stimulated inside the pancreas, allowing the other proteolytic enzymes (chymotrypsin, elastase, carboxypeptidase, and phospholipase) to be activated as well. Since these enzymes are designed to break down cell walls, the enzymatic actions literally "eat the hand that feeds them." The result is edema (inflammatory reaction), vascular injury (hemorrhage), and finally tissue loss and necrosis. Additionally, systemic reactions of bradykinin and histamines cause vasodilation not only in the pancreas but in pulmonary tissue; this accounts for the pulmonary edema seen in fulminant acute pancreatitis.

SYMPTOMS

As with all diseases, there are classic signs (Virchow's triad); with acute pancreatitis, they are midepigastric to left upper quadrant (LUQ) pain, severe nausea and vomiting, and progressive severity. The pain is described as a constant, deep, boring pain, often with radiation to the back. Patients may avoid lying supine because of the increased pain. Patients also may note fever, fatigue, and dizziness. The not so classic symptoms occur in the elderly. In the elderly, the pain may be muted

TABLE 6-20-3. Possible Triggers for Acute Pancreatitis

Gallstones	Bile stasis; bile is essential for lipid breakdown
Alcohol abuse	Mechanism poorly understood, but there is high correlation to disease
Medications Sulfonamides Estrogens NSAIDs ACE inhibitors	Most are dose-related, with mild to severe pancreatitis possible. Certainly rare, the mechanism seems to be an interruption of fat digestion and degeneration of liver function as well
Trauma-surgery	Loss of architecture is secondary to trauma or change in blood supply
Hyperlipidemias	The breakdown of large amounts of triglycerides seems to cause a cytotoxic level of free fatty acids
Pregnancy	Most often associated with concomitant gallstones
Obstruction of ampulla of Vater	Ductal tumor, choledocholithiasis, Crohn's disease, peptic ulcer disease block secretions

NOTE: ACE = angiotensin converting enzyme.

or absent and there is less nausea and vomiting. This presumably is due to the poor immune response of an aging patient. In the elderly, the presenting symptoms may be a change of mentation, shock, and coma.

OBJECTIVE

The physical examination often finds the patient sitting on the table with the knees pulled to the chest, rocking. One of the differentiating signs of severe pancreatitis is that the onset is sudden, and so the abdomen is slightly distended and exquisitely tender without peritoneal signs initially and the stomach is soft and painful. With increasing severity, dehydration and hypotension are evident. With hemorrhagic pancreatitis, bruising or ecchymosis may develop on the flanks (Turner's sign) or periumbilically (Cullen's sign). A quiet abdomen is indicative of an ileus caused by the inflammation. Pulmonary signs may include pneumonitis (crackles), pleural effusion (rhonchi), and frank respiratory distress.

DIAGNOSTIC CONSIDERATIONS

Any source of an acute abdomen is suspect: appendicitis, cholecystitis, perforated ulcer, perforated diverticulitis, severe acute gastroenteritis (AGE), and hepatitis. Another consideration of great importance is an abdominal aortic aneurysm (AAA), which can present with exactly the same symptoms with the addition of a pulsating, expanding mass on examination. Bowel and duct obstruction also can masquerade as acute pancreatitis.

TREATMENT

Monitoring is very important. Progression or abatement of disease should be followed by serial vital signs (dehydration) and frequent blood gases or pulse oxygenation measurements (pulmonary complications). Serial chemistries and possibly electrocardiograms (ECGs) should be monitored for electrolyte changes such as hypocalcemia, hypokalemia, hyperglycemia, and renal functions. With severe pancreatitis, coagulation profiles should be done because disseminated intravascular coagulation (DIC) is a possibility.

There is no definitive treatment for acute pancreatitis. Steroids, H_2 blockers, anticholinergics, glucagon, and antibiotics have been found to be of little or no use in shortening the course of the disease. *Fluid and electrolyte replacement is essential.* Total parenteral nutrition may be an option if the episode lasts more than 5 days and should be accomplished with a multidisciplinary team (see Chap. 6-15, Table 6-15-4). In the past, a nasogastric tube (NGT) was placed to obtain full intestinal rest. If nausea and vomiting are controllable, this is not absolutely necessary, but the patient should be kept strictly NPO (nothing by mouth).

Pain control is the second part of supportive therapy. Traditionally, meperidine (Demerol) has been used, but ketorolac (Toradol) is a great alternative to avoid narcotic loads and side effects. Morphine generally is avoided because it may cause ductal spasm.

Antibiotics may be used if an infectious origin is identified, but the vast majority of acute pancreatitis cases are purely inflammatory; therefore, there is no rationale for the indiscriminate use of antibiotics. Finally, while supporting the patient, look for a treatable etiology such as alcohol abuse, gallstones, choledocholithiasis, and Crohn's disease.

Surgical excision of the pancreas is technically challenging and questionably useful. The drainage of large pseudocysts, persistent pain, hematoma, and abscesses are about the only reasons why most surgeons attempt the process. Postoperative complications are common, and the mortality rate is high.

COMPLICATIONS

Acute pancreatitis is not a benign process; it kills people. Complications include cardiovascular collapse from hypovolemia or hypoproteinemia and even sudden death. Pulmonary complications are usually evident on examination: pleural effusions, pneumonitis, atelectasis, and, in severe disease, adult respiratory distress syndrome. The electrolyte imbalances can cause oliguria and azotemia with progressive renal failure. The pancreatic debris can embolize to the renal artery, brain, or heart. Finally, damage to the pancreas itself can cause diabetes, exocrine insufficiency (with malabsorption), pancreatic pseudocysts, or chronic pancreatitis. Used for years, the Ranson-Imrie criteria for prognosis are quite useful (see Table 6-20-4).

PATIENT EDUCATION

Since alcohol abuse is still the number one trigger for acute pancreatitis, it is a good idea to recommend limited alcohol use to all patients. Other than that, there is really no preventive education available for patients. After acute pancreatitis, the patient should be instructed to avoid all alcohol use. Diet should be tailored to the residual function of the pancreas. Fortunately, a patient can lose up to 90 percent of function before nutrition is severely affected. Most patients do well on a low-fat diet (usually less than 40 g/day) with moderate amounts of carbohydrates and proteins. The diet may need to address diabetic needs as well. Reoccurrence is common, and severity is generally progressive.

TABLE 6-20-4. Ranson-Imrie Criteria

UPON ADMISSION	48 h AFTER ADMISSION	NUMBER CRITERIA
Age over 55 years	Hematocrit drops 10%	0–2 items, 1% mortality rate
White blood count of 16,000	BUN rises >5 mg/dL with adequate hydration	3–4 items, 16% mortality rate
Serum glucose >200 mg/dL	Arterial PO <60 mmHg	5–6 items, 40% mortality rate
Serum LDH >350 IU/L	Serum calcium <8 mg/dL	7–8 items, 100% mortality rate
Serum AST >250 IU/L	Fluid sequestration >4–5 L Serum albumin <3.2 g/dL	

NOTE: LDH = Lactate dehydrogenase; AST = aspartate aminotransferase; BUN = blood urea nitrogen.
SOURCE: Modified from Isselbacher KJ, Braunwald E, Wilson JD, et al: *Harrison's Principles of Internal Medicine,* 14th ed. New York, McGraw-Hill, 1998, p 1743.

PEARLS

Acute pancreatitis is a wait-and-watch process. It is important to be clinically alert to progression of the disease. Pseudocyst can enlarge, hemorrhage can progress, and bacterial infection can ensue. Monitor and support the patient. The average hospital stay for most patients is 7 days, so be patient and vigilant.

CHRONIC PANCREATITIS

DISCUSSION

About 10 percent of patients with acute pancreatitis progress to the chronic phase. It is not clear whether the patient has a series of acute episodes that progressively destroy tissue or whether there is a continuous loss of tissue without significant inflammation. The end result is the same: The incremental loss of pancreatic architecture leads to exocrine insufficiency and diabetes.

SYMPTOMS

Chronic pancreatitis can present as acute but most commonly does not. It often presents with insidious deep pain, steatorrhea (reflecting malabsorption), and insulin-dependent diabetes mellitus. Weight loss owing to malabsorption and jaundice owing to hepatic complications may be evident. Pulmonary symptoms may or may not be present.

OBJECTIVE

Physical examination may reveal a thinning patient with mild jaundice. Mild epigastric or even diffuse abdominal tenderness without distention is the most common finding. Vitamin deficiency anemia is rarely found.

DIAGNOSTIC CONSIDERATIONS

Diagnostic considerations are the same as those for acute pancreatitis.

TREATMENT

Pain and malabsorption are the focus. Pain can be diminished through strict restriction of alcohol products and in some cases a low-fat diet. Some patients may require narcotics for pain control, but this can lead to addiction. Adequate enzyme replacement may diminish the pain syndrome. When all medical therapies are not sufficient to control pain, surgery is considered, but as a surgeon once said, "The pancreas is a skunk you don't want to poke." Surgery is the last resort.

Most chronic pancreatitis patients need enzyme replacement for exocrine dysfunction. Viokase, Cotazym-S, or a similar substance can be used to try to address the malabsorption. Unfortunately, it is difficult to deliver the active enzyme intact to the duodenum at the perfect time. Therefore, the dosing is large and frequent (see Table 6-20-5).

COMPLICATIONS

The long-term life expectancy of a chronic pancreatitis patient is limited; if alcohol is continued, death is likely in 5 to 15 years after the diagnosis. As pancreatic dysfunction progresses, the manifestations and complications of malabsorption become more apparent with weight loss and vitamin deficiencies.

PATIENT EDUCATION

Same as those for acute pancreatitis.

PEARLS

Chronic pancreatitis is also a watching and waiting game. Monitor the nutritional status of the patient. A chemistry profile should be examined

TABLE 6-20-5.   Treatment of Pancreatic Enzyme Deficiency

PREPARATION	LIPASE	TRYPSIN	PROTEOLYTIC ACTIVITY	AMYLASE	DOSE
Cotazym	8000 U	0	30,000	30,000 U	1–3 tablets before each meal or snack
Arco-Lase	25 mg	38 mg	6 g	30 mg	1 tablet with or immediately after meals
Donnazyme	1000 U	0	12,500 U	12,500 U	2 tablets with meals and snacks
Kutrase or Ku-zyme	1200 U	0	6 mg	30 mg	1–2 tablets with meals and snacks
Viokase	8000 U	0	30,000 U	30,000 U	1–2 tablets with meals and snacks or every 2 h after pancreatectomy

for changes in glucose, calcium, magnesium, potassium, and proteins. Adjust diet and supplements to meet the needs of each patient. Involve a multidisciplinary team to ensure maximum results for the patient. With proper care and alcohol abstinence, these patients can live a long life.

PANCREATIC CANCER

DISCUSSION

The prevalence of adenocarcinoma of the pancreas has been on the rise in the last 20 years. Only 5 percent of those patients are likely to survive more than 5 years. Pancreatic cancer is called "the silent cancer" because it seldom is found early. It is recognized as the fourth most common cancer killer in the United States. Black men seem to have the highest risk, but men in general have pancreatic cancer in a 2:1 ratio compared with women.[1] The aged are the most likely to develop cancer, but pancreatic cancer may occur at any age (see Chap. 13-8).

PATHOGENESIS

While adenocarcinoma of the pancreas has no proven etiologies, tobacco abuse (specifically cigarette smoking) has been strongly linked. Tobacco seems to trigger hyperplastic changes in the pancreas that are reversible if a patient stops smoking. Gallbladder disease, alcohol abuse, and acute or chronic pancreatitis do not appear to predispose to pancreatic cancer. The vast majority of cancers arise from the exocrine tissue (ductal system), and symptoms are dictated by the location of the tumor. Periampullary lesions encroach into the common bile duct, duodenum, and liver. Tumors arising in the body or tail of the pancreas usually are found later because encroachment causes less trouble initially. The absence of an adhesive capsule allows the tumors to enlarge unchecked with minimal symptoms. The rich lymphatics and blood supply of the region disseminate the cancer before a patient is aware of the tumor.

SYMPTOMS

A slow and insidious presentation is the norm for pancreatic cancer. Weight loss is common, and a dull aching pain may be noted in the epigastrium or left upper quadrant. The patient may believe it is a muscle pull. With tumors in the body or tail, the nerves of the retroperitoneal areas are invaded and the pain may become much more severe. Patients may complain of a vague nausea and persistent anorexia. With tumors near the ampulla of Vater, painless jaundice may be the presenting symptom with pruritus, nausea, and perhaps vomiting. Though rare in an adult patient, the development of insulin-dependent diabetes mellitus may signal early pancreatic cancer.

OBJECTIVE

The physical examination is usually negative initially. With metastasis of the carcinoma, weight loss with muscle wasting is evident. Jaundice and hepatomegaly are common findings. Evidence of malnutrition may be present: pale (anemia), nail bed changes (vitamin deficiency), and fractures (metastasis and calcium changes).

DIAGNOSTIC CONSIDERATIONS

Pancreatic cancer can masquerade as almost any abdominal complaint. In fact, valuable time often is lost looking for gallstones, ulcers, or malabsorption syndromes in these patients. Worse, most patients may have gallbladder disease or peptic ulcer disease concomitantly, and the clinician may stop investigations after making the presumed diagnosis. The most significant clue is weight loss and malnutrition. Malnutrition syndromes almost always are accompanied by diarrhea with steatorrhea. Significant weight loss indicates cancer until proved otherwise. Gallbladder, Crohn's disease, and similar diseases usually do not involve major weight loss.

LABORATORY TESTS

The most important test is a biopsy. A tissue biopsy can be obtained by ERCP or laparoscopy. The importance comes from the possibilities of nonmalignant ductal tumors and chronic pancreatitis. Both can present as hard masses in the pancreatic area with similar symptoms. Obviously, the treatment and prognosis are quite different. Additionally, the laparoscopic approach allows biopsies of nodes and the surrounding organs; if the laparoscopic findings for metastasis are negative, curative pancreatic resection may be accomplished in up to 20 percent of patients.

IMAGING STUDIES

With improvements in computed tomography (CT) and magnetic resonance imaging (MRI), very good images of the pancreas can be seen. A spiral CT of the abdomen provides high-resolution images without invasive procedures. The odds of resectability by CT estimates compared to surgical findings have reached approximately 75 percent. MRI may be used if patients are unable to tolerate CT contrast material, but it is associated with some false-negative findings.

TREATMENT

Treatment unfortunately is limited to palliative care in the vast majority of patients. However, about 20 percent of patients benefit from pancreaticoduodenectomy. In recent years, pancreatic resection followed by combination radiation and chemotherapy has extended the life span of many patients. There are several factors that bode well for these patients: (1) small tumors measuring <2.5 cm, (2) benign lymph nodes on laparoscopic inspection, and (3) the absence of microvascular invasion (lack of metastasis).[2]

When pancreatic cancer is not resectable, treatment is aimed at quality of life for the approximately 5 months the majority of patients have left. The provider should make every effort to keep the patient comfortable, awake, and functional. As with all terminal diagnoses, the inclusion of a hospice team can be a great help to the patient and family.

Chemotherapy with 5-fluorouracil (5-FU) and radiation therapy can shrink the tumor and provide symptomatic relief of ductal obstruction and jaundice. Morphine or its adjuncts should be titrated to maximum pain relief with minimal sedation effects. The morphine should not be limited for fear of respiratory compromise or addiction. Neither occurs in the vast majority of patients. Patient will need nutritional support and nausea and constipation control as well.

PATIENT EDUCATION

It is important to be honest. Pancreatic cancer (with rare exceptions) is a grave, terminal diagnosis. The patient and family should be educated about expectations and what can be done to make the patient comfortable. One item of specific concern to most families is the ability of the patient to eat. Pancreatic cancer causes profound anorexia. Additionally, as the carcinoma progresses, the ability of the body to process and absorb nutrition slows and eventually stops. Families must be educated about the process so that they will not become petulant with a sick family member for not eating.

PEARLS

The diagnosis of pancreatic cancer is very difficult. It is an index of suspicion that leads to early diagnosis. Once it is diagnosed, be cognizant of the needs of the patient and family. Support and manage symptoms to provide the best quality of life for the patient.

REFERENCES

1. Sleisenger MH, Fordtran JS: *Gastrointestinal Disease.* Philadelphia, Saunders, 1993, vol 2, pp 1585, 1682.
2. Isselbacher KJ, Braunwald E, Wilson JD, et al: *Harrison's Principles of Internal Medicine,* 13th ed. New York, McGraw-Hill, 1994, pp 1519, 1533.

BIBLIOGRAPHY

Banks PA: Practice guidelines in acute pancreatitis. *Am J Gastroenterol* 92(3): 377–385, 1997.
Barkin JS, Goldstein JA: Diagnostic Approach to Pancreatic Cancer. *Gastroenterol Clin* 28(3):709–719, 1999.
Dragonetti GC, Licht H, Rubin W: Pancreatitis, evaluation and treatment. *Primary Care Clin Office Pract* 23(3):525–533, 1996.
Isselbacher KJ, Braunwald E, Wilson JD, et al: *Harrison's Principles of Internal Medicine,* 14th ed. New York, McGraw-Hill, 1998, pp 1741–1751.
McClave SA, Spain DA, Snider HL: Nutritional management in acute and chronic pancreatitis. *Gastroenterol Clin* 27(2):421–431, 1998.

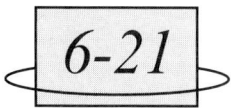

PEPTIC ULCER DISEASE
Anne P. Heinly

DESCRIPTION

Peptic ulcer disease (PUD) encompasses diagnoses of gastritis, duodenitis, and gastric and duodenal ulcers. Zollinger-Ellison (ZE) syndrome is included under the PUD umbrella, although its etiology is quite different from that of the average PUD. It is estimated that 2 of 10 adults have PUD at some point in their lives. PUD is rare before age 6 and becomes apparent in many people in their twenties. In some countries, the estimate is near 100 percent in the elderly. Men are more likely to have episodes of PUD, but it is by no means a sex-specific problem. A previously recurrent disease that was poorly understood, PUD may be well on its way out the door as a chronic illness because of the discovery of *Helicobacter pylori* and its impact on the gastric and duodenal areas of the gastrointestinal (GI) tract.

PATHOGENESIS

Gastric physiology has everything to do with PUD. The stomach has several jobs: mixing and churning foods into chyme; secretion of pepsinogen, which becomes pepsin and initiates protein digestion; secretion of HCl and an intrinsic factor, which are essential for vitamin B_{12} absorption; and secretion of gastrin, which helps regulate stomach, hepatic, and pancreatic enzymes and lowers pyloric, Oddi, and ileocecal sphincter pressures.

The parietal cells of the stomach secrete up to 2 quarts of hydrochloric acid a day. The physiologic triggers are a complex set of chemical, neural, and hormonal factors that participate in feedback loops to turn acid production on and off. The hormone gastrin stimulates the HCl production triggered by thoughts of food, smells, ingestion of food, ingestion of calcium, alcohol use, and medications.

The stomach's defense against excess HCl and the corrosive effect of even normal levels of acid is impressive. A pH level below 1.5 turns HCl production off. Feedback from secretin, cholecystokinin, or glucagon can shut down HCl production. The mucus-producing cells protect the gastric mucosa and prevent back diffusion of HCl. Bicarbonate ions in the "unstirred" water layer, a gel-like line separating parietal cells and mucous cells, provide an alkaline environment perfect for healing. Prostaglandin, which is abundant throughout the gastrium, protects the cells and promotes good blood flow that engenders rapid healing when needed.

In light of all this physiology, providers used to look for exogenous stimulation to upset the natural balance of the gastric environment (see Table 6-21-1). Although all these causes are players, *H. pylori* is the key factor in recurrent ulcer disease [in the absence of nonsteroidal anti-inflammatory drug (NSAID) use or ZE]. *Helicobacter pylori* is an S-shaped bacterium that finds a home between the cells under the stable layer of mucus in the antrum of the stomach. It is estimated that this bacterium is responsible for up to 90 percent of all cases of PUD and is found worldwide. How people are infected with *H. pylori* is debated, but it is thought to be water-borne. To date, reinfection is rare, and so treatment of *H. pylori* is considered curative in the vast majority of patients. *Helicobacter pylori* is thought to cause gastritis or ulcers by producing a urease that causes deterioration of the protective barriers of the mucous layer. Additionally, *H. pylori*

TABLE 6-21-1. Causes of Peptic Ulcer Disease

TRIGGERS FOR PUD	MECHANISM
Helicobacter pylori	Bacterium hidden in the gastric mucosal layer: urease secretion causes chronic inflammation and ulcerations
Medication	
Alcohol	Damages the mucous lining and interferes with healing mechanisms
Aspirin or NSAIDs	Antiprostaglandins; damage to mucous lining and disruption of blood supply occur
Tolazoline	Stimulates gastric secretion and stress ulcers in children treated for pulmonary hypertension
Corticosteroids	Mechanism is poorly understood: probably a feedback interruption
Tobacco	Decreases pancreatic bicarbonate secretion (feedback loop) and mucosal blood flow, hampering healing; inhibits the actions of H_2 blockers
Stress ulcers	
Burns (Curling's ulcer)	Stress ulcers can occur within hours to days of
Intracranial trauma	severe trauma or burns and most likely are
Shock	due to an ischemic phenomenon. As blood
Hypoglycemia	is shunted to damaged area or lost, gastric
Dehydration	protection mechanisms are retarded and
Renal failure	feedback loops are interrupted. Prophylactic
Vasculitis	therapy should be undertaken to avoid complications
Disease	
Cystic fibrosis	Any disease process that changes the feedback
Gastrinoma (ZE)	mechanism of acid secretion, blood supply,
Type 1 MENS	or mucous layer integrity could cause PUD
COPD	
Cirrhosis	
Polycythemia	

NOTE: MENS = multiple endocrine neoplasia syndrome; COPD = chronic obstructive pulmonary disease.

seems to result in unimpeded secretion of gastrin because of a suppressed somatostatin feedback loop.

SYMPTOMS

The classic symptom of PUD is a deep, gnawing, or burning epigastric pain 1 to 3 h after meals (empty stomach) with nocturnal awakenings. Typically, this pain is relieved by food intake and/or antacids. Some patients may not complain of pain, but a careful diet history may reveal that they nibble to the point where the stomach is never empty, providing a buffer to excess acid. The pain may radiate to the back, may go "straight through me," or may be described as an "acid stomach." Many patients self-treat with over-the-counter antacids and H_2 blockers, and so the symptoms may be dulled.

Nausea with or without vomiting is also a common symptom, especially with severe pain. If occult bleeding is occurring with "itis" or ulceration, the patient may present with or without pain in an orthostatic state. Patients complain of dizziness, thirst, syncope, and/or melenic stools. It takes 50 mL of blood to make a melenic stool, and so several stools usually represent a hemoglobin drop of 2 to 4 points.

The symptoms may wax and wane, with several pain episodes over a short period followed by long periods of remission. Patients with PUD often have concomitant histories consistent with gastroesophageal reflux disease (GERD), (see Chap. 6-11) as well. Symptoms of concern, especially in the young and the elderly, include weight loss, anorexia, early satiety, nausea, and vomiting or regurgitation. These symptoms suggest an obstruction caused by stricture formation, gastric outlet syndrome, or carcinoma and merit an immediate workup.

OBJECTIVE

The physical examination may reveal point tenderness in the epigastric to right upper quadrant (RUQ) area in adults. With children, the pain may present periumbilically or be poorly localized. If the patient has eaten recently, this may be muted. Guarding, peritoneal signs, ascites, and percussion changes are not present unless a perforation has occurred. If bleeding has occurred, the patient may have positive orthostatic signs, evidence of dehydration, or, in the worse case, stupor or loss of consciousness. The elderly can present without pain with a change in sensorium or frank shock. A rectal examination with an occult blood examination should be done. Absence of blood in the stool does not preclude PUD or bleeding.

DIAGNOSTIC CONSIDERATIONS

Table 6-21-2 lists the differential diagnosis for PUD. Zollinger-Ellison syndrome is caused by a hypersecretion state in the presence of gastrinomas with a marked increase in severity and recurrence of symptoms. In children, ulcers may present as chronic abdominal pain or gastric outlet syndrome. With outlet syndrome, a gastric succession splash may be found. Congenital pyloric stenosis generally is identified in early infancy as a mass in the RUQ and should not be confused with PUD. Whereas nearly 70 percent of older Americans are likely to have *H. pylori* present, the most common etiology of ulcers is the use of NSAIDs because of their antiprostaglandin effects. In the elderly, as with so many diseases, the symptoms may be muted or absent because of aging changes. Orthostatic changes from blood loss may be the first signal of trouble.

LABORATORY TESTS

There are three ways to identify *H. pylori* in the laboratory. The *H. pylori* serum titer searches for immunoglobulin G and A antibodies to its antigen and is now considered a sensitive test. The second is the breath test for urease response using C-labeled urea. The sensitivity and specificity of the breath test are both in the high 90s. The third laboratory test involves *H. pylori* cultures obtained during endoscopic evaluation. One would think a culture would be the gold standard, but *H. pylori* is a finicky organism and is not easily cultured.

TABLE 6-21-2. Differential Diagnosis of PUD

Gastric carcinoma	Weight loss, early satiety, persistance of pain despite food or medication, anemia
Pancreatitis	Usually associated with alcohol, severe epigastric to LUQ pain, radiating to or from the back, fever, chills, elevated amylase and lipase
Gallbladder disease	Episodic, colicky pain in RUQ to epigastrium with radiation to right shoulder, worse with fatty meals, not relieved with antacids
Abdominal angina (mesenteric in sufficiency)	Severe, debilitating epigastric or umbilical pain 5–15 min after meals. Patient will starve rather suffer the pain. Weight loss, bleeding are common; seen in the elderly
Acute gastroenteritis	Sudden onset of nausea, vomiting, often associated with diarrhea, fever, chills, and aches; short-lived, not recurrent
Corrosive ingestion (accidental in children or suicidal)	Ingestion of strong alkali or acids, sudden onset, burns to lips, mouth, pharynx; epigastric pain with vomiting and hematemesis
Liver disease	Constant deep RUQ and right chest pain, jaundice, ascites; may have evidence of right heart failure

NOTE: LUQ = left upper quadrant; RUQ = right upper quadrant.

Additionally, a complete blood count and chemistries should be run to rule out PUD-induced anemia and other differential diagnoses. Hemoccult cards should be done on three separate occasions to rule out occult bleeding. Since duodenitis or an ulcer may bleed intermittently, stools may not be consistently positive. A negative guaiac does not preclude PUD. When ZE is suspected because of severity or reoccurrence, a serum gastrin level (usually over 500 pg/mL) and secretin stimulation test can be done.

RADIOLOGIC (IMAGING) STUDIES

Certainly a mainstay for years, the upper gastrointestinal (UGI) series with small bowel follow-through can be used to diagnose PUD. The barium study can potentially identify ulcer craters, webs, hiatal hernia, strictures, incompetent sphincters, masses, and contour changes. The distinction between duodenitis or gastritis and ulcer craters is harder to see because GI contour is not affected as drastically. This probably accounts for the almost one-third of false negatives reported with UGIs in the presence of classic symptoms. On the flip side, those who appear to have an identifiable lesion on UGI often have negative endoscopic results because of the mobile and foldable nature of the intestinal tissue itself.

The most definitive diagnosis for PUD and ZE is the endoscopic evaluation. Despite being an invasive test, it does allow direct visualization of all the tissue, permits biopsies and cultures, and provides therapeutic opportunities in case of bleeding. In the presence of severe symptoms that are marginally responsive to medications, endoscopic evaluation may be considered a first-line diagnostic procedure, especially if ZE or cancer is suspected.

TREATMENT

As with all diseases, treatment is tailored to etiology. For a stressed-out smoker, life-style changes may be all that is required. If *H. pylori* is the culprit, a strict medication regimen should be successful. If the PUD is NSAID-induced, medications are used to heal and prevent future ulcers. Table 6-21-3 describes treatment plans in detail. Keep in mind that it may be necessary to address more than one etiology in most patients. In NSAID-induced ulcers, misoprostol, a prostaglandin agonist, helps restore the balance that chronic NSAID use upsets.

TABLE 6-21-3. Treatment Regimens for PUD

REGIMEN	DOSE	SIDE EFFECTS
Life-style changes		
Stop tobacco use	Outstanding recommendations	None known
Stop alcohol use	for any patient	
Low-fat diet		
Avoid stress		
Avoid offending medications		
Helicobacter therapy	Taken concurrently (approximately 90% cure rate)	
Bismuth compound	2 tablets qid for 14 days	Allergies, drug resistance, diarrhea, pseudomembranous colitis,
Metronidazole (Flagyl)	250 mg tid for 14 days	noncompliance
Tetracycline or amoxicillin	500 mg tid for 14 days	
H₂ blocker or omeprazole may be used for control of symptoms		
or	Taken concurrently (approximately 80% cure rate)	As above
Omeprazole	20 mg bid for 14 days	
Clarithromycin	500 mg tid for 14 days	
Relief therapy	To heal an ulcer	Side effects
Antacids (representative)		
Mylanta	2 tbsp qid for 6 weeks	Diarrhea and/or constipation, noncompliance
Maalox	2 tbsp qid for 6 weeks	
Riopan	2 tbsp qid for 6 weeks	
Avoid calcium products, owing to rebound hyperacidity		
H₂ blockers		Cimetidine has the most warnings with drug interactions; may also cause disorientation in the elderly
Ranitidine (Zantac)	150 mg bid for 12 weeks	
Cimetidine (Tagamet)	200 mg qid for 12 weeks	
Famotidine (Pepcid)	20 mg bid for 8 weeks	
Nizatidine (Acid)	150 mg bid for 12 weeks	
Cytoprotective		
Sucralfate (Carafate)	1 g 30 min before meals and at bedtime	Will not work in the presence of concomitant H₂ blockers; needs an acid environment to work; constipation
Misoprostol (Cytotec) (not a first-line medication)	100 μg qid with food to start, may increase to 200 μg as tolerated	Diarrhea, dehydration; use with care in the elderly
Proton pump inhibitor		
Omeprazole (Prilosec)	20 mg qd for 4–8 weeks	Prolong elimination of phenytoin, warfarin, and diazepam; suppression of B₁₂ mechanism; megaloblastic anemia with long-term use

COMPLICATIONS

By far the most common complication of PUD is bleeding. Up to one-fourth of PUD patients have occult blood loss, and about 10 percent have frank bleeding episodes. This can be life-threatening in the very young and the old because of dehydration and organ perfusion problems. Perforation occurs in about 5 percent of patients and presents as a typical acute abdomen with peritoneal signs. Remember, in the elderly, the only "typical" sign may be a change in sensorium; keep that index of suspicion. Duodenal scarring and gastric outlet syndrome may occur, especially with the diagnosis of ZE, which is seen in men more than in women. Finally, chronic gastric irritation can lead to atrophic changes of the gastrium, predisposing the patient to gastric carcinoma. Research is slowly making the link between chronic *H. pylori* infections and gastric cancer, especially in Asia, where gastric carcinomas are quite common. Gastric lymphoma also may be a result of chronic *H. pylori* infection; thus the lesson here is to eradicate *H. pylori* when possible.

PEARLS

Like GERD, peptic ulcer disease is (1) common and (2) self-treated with over-the-counter medications. Inadequate dosing for healing purposes and the likelihood of muted symptoms leading to a chronic problem that goes undetected for years are a concern. The provider's job is to educate patients about ulcer disease and specifically about *H. pylori*. With full treatment many patients will never spend money on antacids again and the serious consequences of undertreated disease

will be eradicated. Life-style changes remain important, so help patients stop smoking, encourage proper diet and exercise, and avoid ulcer-inducing medications when possible.

BIBLIOGRAPHY

Fauci AS, Braunwald E, Isselbacher KJ, et al: Peptic ulcer and gastritis. In *Harrison's Principles of Internal Medicine,* 14th ed. New York, McGraw-Hill, 1998, pp 1596–1605, 1616.
Hunt RH: The management of acid-related disorders: Clinical practice and therapeutic principles. *Am J Gastroenterol,* 92(4):36–40, 1997.

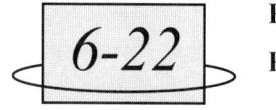 **PILONIDAL DISEASE**
Pat C. H. Jan

DISCUSSION

Epithelial tissues trapped in the natal cleft cause pilonidal disease. It was once thought to have congenital origins but is currently regarded as an acquired lesion. Young adults have the highest incidence of occurrence, with prevalence in males over females and a peak age of 30 years. Patients with a tendency toward hirsutism are predisposed to pilonidal cysts.

PATHOGENESIS

Pilonidal cysts and abscesses are caused by infections of the hair follicles in the natal cleft. The hair, which normally grows at a 90° angle, comes out at a 100° angle instead. The epidermis forms a tunnel-like structure about the hair follicle. There is an increased chance of cyst formation and infection with elongated tunnels. In addition, midline follicles become obstructed by keratin or hair, which leads to a foreign-body reaction. The patient subsequently develops an abscess that can spontaneously drain in the acute case with no further recurrence. Recurrence, however, is extremely common if the hair, which acts as a foreign body, is not removed.

SIGNS AND SYMPTOMS

Patients generally present with pain in the affected areas in acute cases. In chronic states, patients may complain of drainage from the gluteal area. In cases of pilonidal abscess, patients may relate a history of chronic "boils." As mentioned above, the abscess may spontaneously drain.

OBJECTIVE FINDINGS

Physical examination may reveal multiple midline sinuses at the natal cleft with tufts of hair from each sinus (see Fig. 6-22-1). If an abscess is present, the area is generally indurated with mild to severe erythema in the surrounding subcutaneous tissue. There is tenderness to palpation.

DIAGNOSTIC CONSIDERATIONS

Identifying pilonidal disease is straightforward and can be determined by history and physical examination alone. Identification of a pilonidal sinus and tufts of hair can easily rule out gluteal abscess of other origin. Other diseases that may appear similar to pilonidal disease are hidradenitis suppurativa, an infection of the sweat glands; perianal abscess located close to the anus, which should be differentiated from pilonidal abscess; and furuncle, which is an infection of a single hair follicle leading to a pustule and simply requires drainage and antibiotics.

TREATMENT

Medical Management

The most current management of noninfected pilonidal disease is focused on good personal hygiene with weekly shaving of all hairs in the sinus. It is believed that removing the hairs in the sinus tracts can

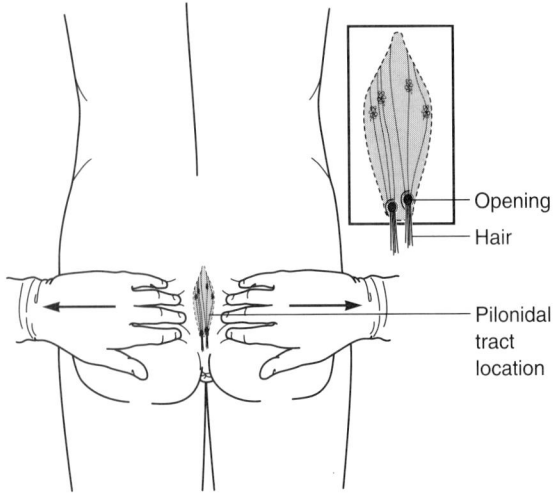

FIGURE 6-22-1. Pilonidal sinus tract.

prevent a foreign-body reaction. In acute pilonidal abscess, incision and drainage are the current mainstays of treatment. Once the infection has subsided, the patient may undergo elective excision of the pilonidal sinus for a more definitive treatment.

Surgical Management

To prevent an acute pilonidal abscess from becoming a chronic infection, excision of the offending sinus needs to be performed. Two treatment options are available. This first technique consists of excision and primary closure of the sinus tract. This is performed under general anesthesia, and the patient is given a broad-spectrum antibiotic. The sinus tract is excised down to the fascia layer. Another technique is to marsupialize the wound. Marsupialization requires excision of the offending tissues down to the epithelized tract of the lowest hair follicle. Skin edges on either side are then sutured to the epithelized tract instead of the fascia. The open area is then cleaned daily. Another technique seldom used today but worth mentioning is healing by secondary intention. The patient requires frequent dressing changes and close monitoring for any signs of potential infection. Good personal hygiene is the key.

PATIENT EDUCATION

Recurrence is common and can be minimized by remembering a few principles:

- Personal hygiene and shaving of all hairs in the gluteal folds helps to decrease the foreign-body reaction caused by the hairs.
- Good postoperative care helps to facilitate wound healing by keeping the wound clean and dry.
- Prevention of constipation decreases straining and decreases pressure to the surgical wound.

DISPOSITION

Postoperative care is extremely important, and patients should be seen weekly until the wound is completely healed. There is always a possibility of poor wound healing and occurrence of drainage, with local infection leading to more sinus tracts. Therefore any drainage or signs of infection (i.e., swelling, erythema, or increased pain) should be reported. Care should be taken to avoid chronic wetness by the overuse of topical ointments.

COMPLICATIONS AND RED FLAGS

The most common complication of pilonidal disease is the development of an abscess with further damage of the surrounding tissue secondary to inflammation. Uncommon but worth mentioning is squamous cell carcinoma arising from recurrent or untreated pilonidal disease. There are approximately 38 cases of such squamous cell carcinoma in the literature. Patients would require both radiation and chemotherapy treatment after excision of the sinus tract. As mentioned, early recognition leads to early treatment with minimal postoperative care, fewer recurrences, and decreased risk of squamous cell cancer.

NOTES AND PEARLS

There is no current universal treatment protocol for pilonidal disease. Recommendations are aimed at good personal hygiene and weekly shaving of hairs in the sinus tract. Marsupialization has the advantage of a rapid postoperative recovery. After multiple recurrences, frustration leads to wide excisions with closure by secondary intention. The drawback of this approach is constant monitoring of the wound for drainage and infection.

BIBLIOGRAPHY

Armstrong JH: Pilonidal sinus disease: The conservative approach. *Arch Surg* 129:914–918, 1994.

Beers MH, Berkow R (eds): Pilonidal disease, in *The Merck Manual,* 17th ed. New Jersey, Whitehouse Station. 1999.

Jones DJ: Pilonidal sinus. *BMJ* 305:410–412, 1992.

Kulaylat MN et al: Multimodality treatment of squamous cell carcinoma complicating pilonidal disease. *Am Surg* 62:922–927, 1996.

Surreal JA: Pilonidal disease. *Surg Clin North Am* 74(6):1309–1315, 1994.

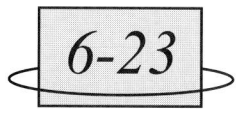

PROCTITIS
Marquitha S. Mayfield

DISCUSSION

Proctitis is a nonspecific term that is used to describe a variety of inflammatory diseases involving the rectal portion of the colon. Most of these diseases have an infectious etiology. Other causes include trauma, radiation therapy for the pelvis, and irritative rectal medications. Ulcerative colitis also can present with strictly rectal involvement in some patients. About 90 percent of these cases never advance beyond an inflammatory proctitis. There is a high incidence of sexually transmitted disease (STD) proctitis, particularly in adult homosexual males with multiple sexual partners. Proctitis may manifest as an acute or chronic inflammatory process and affects 10 to 30 per 100,000 patients in the United States. Adult males are more commonly affected than are females.

SYMPTOMS

Symptoms vary with the etiology and may range from none to severe anorectal pain, bleeding, tenesmus, and/or mucopurulent anal discharge. Common symptoms associated with specific disorders include the following:

- *Gonococcal and chlamydial proctitis*: mucopurulent rectal discharge associated with anal discomfort.
- *Syphilitic proctitis*: mucopurulent discharge initially, tenesmus and transient nontender perianal ulcer(s).
- *Herpes simplex proctitis*: severe rectal pain, tenesmus associated with constipation and draining rectal ulcers. Additionally, if the sacral nerve roots are involved, paresthesias of the buttocks and lower extremities, bladder dysfunction, and impotence may occur.
- *Amebiasis*, Campylobacter, *or* Shigellosis *proctitis:* diarrhea is the hallmark symptom. Fever and abdominal pain also may occur.
- *Inflammatory proctitis*: Bloody diarrhea, tenesmus, and rectal pain occur. Patients with Crohn's disease or ulcerative colitis also may present with fever, malaise, abdominal pain, and weight loss.
- *Radiation proctitis*: rectal pain, tenesmus, diarrhea, and rectal bleeding or discharge.

OBJECTIVE FINDINGS

Physical examination findings vary according to etiology, stage of disease, and severity of the inflammatory response. Unless the anus is involved, few physical examination findings may be noted. Nevertheless, anal skin should be examined for ulcerations, erythema and other inflammatory changes, nodules, vesicular lesions, condylomata, fissures, fistulas, patches of psoriasis with secondary inflammatory bowel disease (IBD), hemorrhoids, and/or discharge. A digital rectal examination may elicit tenderness and/or palpable nodules. Obtain a stool guaiac to detect occult rectal blood.

Classic findings for specific disorders include the following:

- *Herpes proctitis*: perianal vesicular lesions that later ulcerate and become secondarily infected.
- *Inflammatory bowel disease (Crohn's disease) and radiation therapy*: perianal fistulous tracts, perirectal abscesses. Anal skin tags noted on examination have a strong association with Crohn's disease.
- *Gonorrhea and chlamydia*: mucopurulent anal discharge.
- *Syphilis*: mucopurulent anal discharge; nontender, indurated ulcers (chancres).
- *Amebiasis,* Campylobacter, *or* Shigellosis *proctitis*: Possible fever, abdominal tenderness and/or distention, heme-positive stools.

DIFFERENTIAL DIAGNOSIS

Because STDs cause many cases of proctitis, a detailed sexual history should be obtained to help establish a working differential diagnosis. Many cases of proctitis caused by STDs are seen in patients who engage in receptive anal intercourse. Also common in this group is an allergic proctitis caused by chemical irritants in enemas or anal lubricants. The trauma resulting from anal intercourse can result in anorectal tears and/or fissures, which can become secondarily infected. The differential diagnoses for the etiology of proctitis are listed in Table 6-23-1. The most common pathogens isolated by laboratory studies are *Neisseria gonorrhea, Chlamydia* species, and herpes simplex virus.

SPECIAL CONSIDERATIONS

Proctitis in pediatric patients is rare. When it does occur, the disease can have a fulminant course with extension to the sigmoid and more proximal areas of the colon. Consider sexual abuse in any child with STD-related proctitis. Geriatric patients with severe proctitis should be evaluated for ischemic bowel.

LABORATORY AND RADIOLOGIC TESTS

Anoscopy in the office is an effective screening tool. One can visualize the anorectal vault for signs of inflammation and obtain specimens of any discharge. Sigmoidoscopy is indicated in any patient with rectal bleeding, fistulas, fissures, or diarrhea. The rectal mucosa in proctitis appears friable and inflamed, and ulcers may be noted. The architecture of the rectal crypts also may be disrupted. In 15 percent of cases, inflammatory changes may extend beyond the rectal vault to involve the sigmoid colon and/or anus.

TABLE 6-23-1. Differential Diagnoses of Proctitis

Infectious etiology
Sexually transmitted disease
Gonorrhea
Herpes simplex
Chlamydia
Syphilis
Condyloma acuminata
Other
Shigellosis
Campylobacter
Amebiasis
Noninfectious
Inflammatory bowel disease
Ulcerative colitis
Crohn's disease
Other
Trauma
Radiation therapy
Chemical irritants

Additional laboratory studies will help determine the etiology of proctitis and include viral cultures of vesicular lesions to detect herpes simplex, biopsy of anorectal nodules or ulcers to rule out occult malignancy, and tissue histology to confirm the presence of ulcerative colitis or Crohn's disease. Rectal Gram stains for gonorrhea have a low yield. Cultures of the anus are preferred. Also, cultures taken from the rectal wall during anoscopy should be obtained to diagnose chlamydia. Obtain stool cultures to diagnose shigellosis and *Campylobacter.* Serologic studies for syphilis Venereal Disease Research Laboratories (VDRL) or (RPR) and amebiasis (serum antibody testing) may help establish these diagnoses.

TREATMENT

Therapeutic modalities vary with the etiology. The following treatment recommendations are for uncomplicated cases of proctitis. Special considerations and alternative drug regimens are indicated in pregnant or lactating women, children, and patients who are immunocompromised.

Medication

INFLAMMATORY OR RADIATION PROCTITIS Topical steroids (retention enemas or foam) are the treatment of choice for proctitis caused by inflammatory bowel disease or radiation therapy. One applicatorful rectally of Cortifoam (q HS or bid) or Proctofoam-HC (tid or qid) is prescribed for 2 to 3 weeks. A short course of oral steroids (prednisone or Solu-Medrol Dosepak) may be used when the proctitis is unresponsive to these agents. An infectious cause, however, must be ruled out before any steroid therapy is initiated. 5-Aminosalicylic acid agents mesalamine have anti-inflammatory activity and provide an alternative to steroid use. Mesalamine is available as a rectal suspension enema or suppository (Rowasa) for the treatment of active ulcerative proctitis or proctosigmoiditis. Retention enemas usually are given at bedtime and retained for 8 h.

Suppositories are given (one rectally bid and retained for 1 to 3 h). Both require continued treatment for 3 to 6 weeks.

In patients with IBD and more proximal involvement of the colon, oral administration of mesalamine (Asacol and the long-acting form, Pentasa) may be warranted. Doses vary, depending on the agent used. Treatment is continued for 6 to 8 weeks.

CHLAMYDIA PROCTITIS Use azithromycin 1 g orally in a single dose *or* doxycycline 100 mg orally twice a day for 7 days. Alternative regimens include erythromycin 500 mg PO qid for 7 days or ofloxacin 300 mg PO bid for 7 days.

GONORRHEA PROCTITIS Use a single dose of ceftriaxone 125 mg intramuscularly (IM) (drug of choice). Other recommended regimens include cefixime 400 mg or ciprofloxacin 500 mg, both as a single dose orally, *or* ofloxacin 400 mg orally in a single dose plus azithromycin 1 g orally in a single dose, *or* doxycycline 100 mg twice a day orally for 7 days. Alternatively, spectinomycin 2 g IM can be given as a single dose to patients who are unable to take cephalosporins or quinolones. Rectal gonorrhea is difficult to treat, and up to 35 percent of cases may be resistant. Coinfection with *Chlamydia* is often present, and treatment for gonorrhea should provide dual therapy.

HERPES PROCTITIS Use acyclovir (Zovirax) 200 to 400 mg PO five times a day or valacyclovir (Valtrex) 500 mg PO bid. Both are given for 7 to 10 days. Consider chronic suppressive therapy in patients with AIDS or recurrent relapses.

AMEBIASIS Use iodoquinol 650 mg PO tid for 20 days for noninvasive intestinal infections. Use metronidazole (Flagyl) 750 mg PO tid for 5 to 10 days plus iodoquinol (20-day course) for cases of severe invasive proctocolitis.

SHIGELLOSIS/CAMPYLOBACTER Give ciprofloxacin 500 mg PO bid for 5 to 7 days.

Supportive Measures

Patients with anal involvement may benefit from hot sitz baths three to four times a day. Topical anesthetics may help with acute anorectal pain.

PATIENT EDUCATION

Provide instruction on safe sex for STD and HIV prevention. Anal intercourse should be avoided during active treatment.

DISPOSITION

Patients should be reevaluated in 2- to 4-week intervals until completely healed as documented by follow-up sigmoidoscopy. Evaluation and treatment of the sexual partners for all patients being treated for STD-related proctitis also should be completed.

COMPLICATIONS AND RED FLAGS

Rectal abscess, anorectal fistulas, chronic ulcerative colitis, perforation of bowel wall, and treatment failure are the most common complications seen. Suspect these disorders in patients with severe rectal pain, tenesmus, or fever.

BIBLIOGRAPHY

Barker LR, Burton JH, Zieve PD (eds): *Principles of Ambulatory Medicine,* 4th ed. Baltimore, Williams & Wilkins, 1995, pp 1359–1361.

Bassford T: Treatment of common anorectal disorders. *Am Fam Physician* 45(4):1787–1794, 1992.

Centers for Disease Control: 1998 guidelines for treatment of sexually transmitted diseases. *MMWR* 47:1–118, 1998.

Fauci A, Braunwald E, Isselbacher K, et al: *Harrison's Principles of Internal Medicine,* 14th ed. New York, McGraw-Hill, 1998, pp 809, 920, 1085, 1177–1178.

Goroll AH, May LA, Mulley AG Jr (eds): *Primary Care Medicine: Office Evaluation and Management of the Adult Patient,* 4th ed. Philadelphia, Lippincott, 2000, pp 426, 475, 482.

Griffith W, Dambro MR: *5 Minute Clinical Consult.* Philadelphia, Lea & Febinger, 1996, pp 848–850.

Tierney L, McPhee SJ, Papadakis MA: *Current Medical Diagnosis and Treatment,* 39th ed. New York, Lange Medical Books/McGraw-Hill, 2000, pp 652–653.

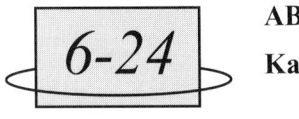

ABDOMINAL HERNIAS

Karen A. Newell

DISCUSSION

Hernia can be defined as the defect through which an organ or part of an organ protrudes from its cavity. Abdominal hernias are the second most common cause of bowel obstruction, trailing postoperative adhesions. This chapter covers primarily those defects located in the abdomen that protrude externally.

Incidence

The incidence of hernia is as follows:

- 75 to 80% groin (direct, indirect, femoral)
- 10% incisional and ventral
- 3 to 8% umbilical

TABLE 6-24-1. Predisposing Factors for Hernias

- Chronic obstructive pulmonary disease
- Obesity
- Pregnancy
- Benign prostatic hypertrophy secondary to chronic urination strain
- Straining during defecation
- Excessive lifting and exercise
- Trauma to transversalis fascia (e.g., from weightlifting)
- Smoking
- Systemic illness
- Ascites
- Aging (related to decreased muscle tone)
- Heredity (connective tissue strength associated with direct inguinal hernia)

Predisposing Factors

Owing to increased intraabdominal pressure and/or decreased muscle strength, a variety of medical problems can cause a hernia (see Table 6-24-1). The layers of the abdomen are shown in Fig. 6-24-1.

TYPES OF HERNIAS

Hernias may be congenital or acquired and consist of these types:

- *Reducible hernia*: Contents return to the abdomen spontaneously with supination or with light manual pressure by the patient or examiner.
- *Incarcerated or irreducible hernia*: Contents are "stuck"; they do not return to the abdomen. If acute, it may be accompanied by crampy abdominal pain, severe localized tenderness, nausea, vomiting (can be feculent), constipation or other change in bowel habits, and fever. This is an impending surgical emergency if the jejunum is involved. This type exhibits more acute symptoms than hernias of the ileum or large bowel do.
- *Strangulated hernia*: The entrapped tissue of the hernia has its blood supply compromised; ischemia and necrosis ensue, bringing about a surgical emergency.

Sliding Hernia

Part of the hernia sac is a portion of an organ (e.g., sigmoid colon or cecum).

Interparietal Hernia

This hernia lies between abdominal wall layers.

Inguinal Hernia

This is the most common site of all hernias, can be direct or indirect, and occurs in males nine times more often than in females; 5% of all males will have an inguinal hernia at some time.

- *Direct inguinal hernia*: Typically affects males over 40 years of age; rare in females. The defect is through the floor of the inguinal canal (Hesselbach's triangle) where the lateral border is the inferior epigastric artery, the inferior border is the inguinal ligament, and the medial border is the lateral edge of the rectus abdominis (see Fig. 6-24-2). These tend not to strangulate as they present as a wide defect visibly noted as a bulge at the external inguinal ring. Usually they are easily reduced and rarely migrate into the scrotum; recurrence after surgical correction is variable, up to about 30%.
- *Indirect inguinal hernia*: This is the most common of the inguinal hernias. They have a tendency to strangulate secondary to narrow defect. Seen often in the first year of life, they are again common between 10 and 30 years of age. Both males and females can be affected, with males affected four times more often than females. These hernias often occur bilaterally. There is a defect in the internal inguinal ring since it is the weakest site of the abdominal wall secondary to the descent of the gonads during embryonic development. The abdominal contents follow a patent processus vaginalis through the spermatic cord (hernia sac lies anteromedial to cord structures) into the scrotum. Therefore, all indirect inguinal hernias are considered congenital: 80% of newborns have a patent processus vaginalis; 40 to 50% of 1-year-olds and 20 to 25% of adults have a patent processus vaginalis.

The processus vaginalis usually closes by 2 to 3 months after birth. Actual herniation occurs in 60% of premature male infants and 1 to 4% of young children, with 45% of these occurring during the first year of life. Since the right gonad is last to migrate and close, 60% occur on the right, 25% on the left, and 15% are bilateral. In children, 10% of those that herniate become incarcerated, and 30% of these go on to strangulate. In girls, the hernia sac can include the ovary, fallopian tube, and/or uterus. Recurrence rate after surgery varies realistically between 5 and 10%.

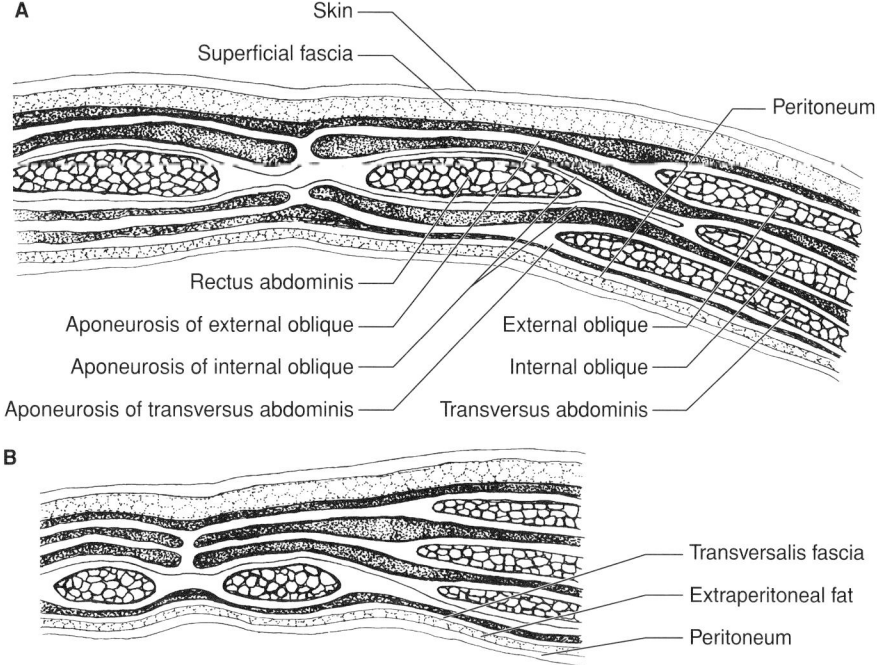

FIGURE 6-24-1. Layers of the abdomen. **A,** Superior to the umbilicus. **B,** Inferior to the umbilicus.

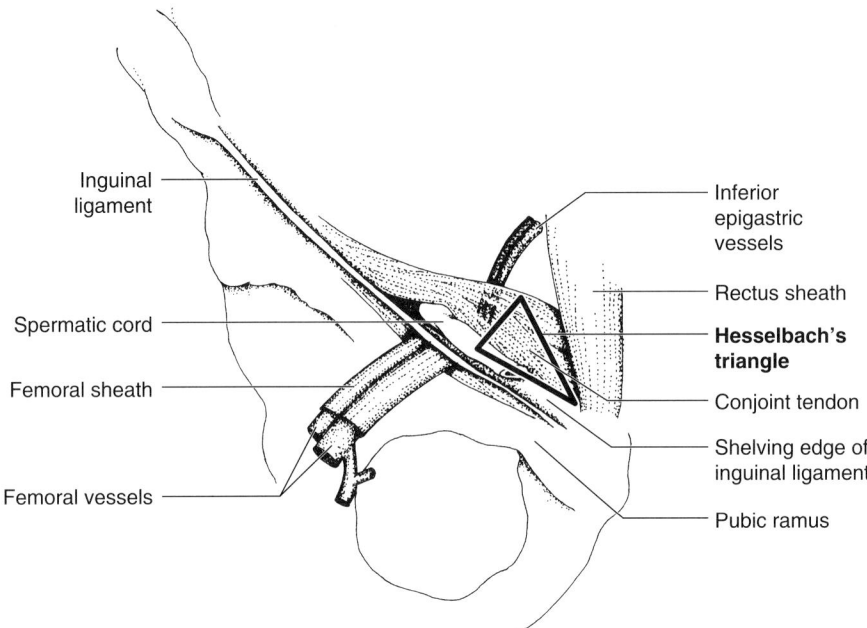

FIGURE 6-24-2. Hesselbach's triangle.

The differential diagnosis of a strangulated inguinal hernia includes the following:

- Testicular torsion of an undescended testicle (absence of a testicle in the scrotum; may have vomiting but not feculent material; see Chap. 18-7)
- Inflamed inguinal lymphadenopathy (usually associated with erythema, edema of the skin and soft tissue, and fever; absence of vomiting and abdominal pain; usually presents with associated genitourinary infection)
- Thrombosis of the spermatic cord (usually presents with marked localized testicular swelling)

Pantaloon Hernia

Combined direct and indirect inguinal hernias are called pantaloon hernias.

Femoral Hernia

These account for 2% of groin hernias in men and one-third of groin hernias in women. Therefore, most are found in females (thought to be associated with a wider pelvis and pregnancy). Right-side hernias are more common than those on the left, may be asymptomatic until incarceration or strangulation, and are located below the inguinal ligament in the femoral triangle (inguinal ligament superiorly), sartorius muscle (laterally), and adductor longus muscle (medially). The highest risk of incarceration or strangulation is secondary to a narrow defect in the transversalis fascia that is usually irreducible. Postsurgical recurrence is about 5 to 10%.

The differential diagnosis of a femoral hernia includes the following:

- Inflamed inguinal lymphadenopathy (absence of vomiting or abdominal pain, more local skin and soft tissue edema, and erythema)
- Thrombosis of a saphenous vein branch (absence of vomiting and abdominal pain; may palpate a thrill when the patient coughs)

Ventral Hernia

Incisional, umbilical, and *epigastric* hernias are all considered ventral hernias, which are identified by protrusion through the abdominal wall,

usually in the midline through the linea alba. These are common after repeated pregnancies or multiple abdominal surgeries that weaken the abdominal musculature; therefore, prevention can be obtained with careful closure of the anterior rectus sheath, since this is the strength of the closure. Usually the small bowel is involved. Patients with incarceration will present with abdominal pain, vomiting, constipation, and localized tenderness.

- *Incisional* hernias are marked by protrusion through a previous incision site by a defect in the fascial closure, a result of 10% of all abdominal surgeries. They are associated with poor surgical technique, increased age, infection, serious systemic illnesses, obesity, smokers or those with chronic obstructive pulmonary disease who cough frequently, and surgical drain tracts. Postsurgical recurrence rates vary depending on the incision size: small, 2 to 5%; medium, 5 to 15%; and large, 25%. Recurrence can be up to 50% in some cases.
- In *umbilical* hernias, the abdominal contents protrude through the umbilicus. The gastrointestinal tract developmentally begins outside of the abdomen and enters the abdomen at 10 weeks in utero through the umbilicus. This remnant passage is usually partially closed at birth but may not be completely sealed until age 4 years (higher incidence seen in those of African descent). This usually closes spontaneously if smaller than 1.5 cm. Surgery is indicated in those with greater than a 2-cm defect or if not completely closed by age 3 to 4 years to prevent incarceration in adulthood. Adult females are more often affected than males. These hernias are associated with marked obesity; therefore, they are often hidden in abdominal fat. Usually the large bowel or omentum is involved, so symptoms are less acute. If the hernia is incarcerated, the patient may present with abdominal pain, vomiting, and localized tenderness with possible palpable swelling.
- *Epigastric* hernias affect 3 to 5% of the population and men more than women. Common ages are 20 to 50 years; 20% are multiple; 80% occur on the midline, located above the umbilicus through the linea alba. They are often found on routine examination. Most are painless but can present with mild tenderness to deep, burning pain, which can radiate to the back; other symptoms may include bloating, nausea, or vomiting. These hernias are exacerbated by large meals and palliated with supination. With an increased incidence of incarceration and strangulation, the postsurgical recurrence rate is 10 to 20%.

Parastomal Hernia

Parastomal hernias are those that develop at a stomal site.

Richter's Hernia

This is an incarcerated antimesenteric portion of the bowel (the side opposite that which is attached to the mesentery); therefore, bowel lumen may remain unaffected and subacute symptoms may occur until perforation and peritonitis develop.

Spigelian Hernia

This is a rare protrusion through the point of intersection of the linea semilunaris and the linea semicircularis. It is usually not visible externally because it is hidden in the abdominal fatty layer.

Perineal Hernia

This is a rare protrusion through the pelvic floor, usually secondary to a previous surgical procedure, such as a prostatectomy.

Lumbar or Dorsal Hernia

This is a protrusion through the lateral abdominal wall at either the inferior lumbar triangle (Petit's; anterior border = external oblique, inferior = iliac crest, and posterior = latissimus dorsi) or superior triangle (Grynfeltt's). Patients describe a "lump" in the flank and a dull, heavy sensation. Incarceration is found in 10%, and the postsurgical recurrence rate is low.

Obturator Hernia

This rare internal hernia follows the obturator vessels and nerve. It is seen in cachectic elderly females who complain of inner thigh pain with radiation to the knee as the obturator nerve is compressed. Crampy abdominal pain with vomiting may accompany the presenting complaint. Rectal examination may reveal a tender, palpable mass in the obturator canal. The mortality rate ranges from 13 to 40% in those who present acutely.

Sciatic Hernia

The least common of all the abdominal hernias, this is an internal hernia that protrudes through the greater sciatic foramen.

Littre's Hernia

This hernia contains a Meckel's diverticulum. It is associated with the inguinal region in 50% of cases; femoral region, 20%; umbilical region, 20%; and other regions, 10%. It is seen more often in males and on the right side.

Diaphragmatic Hernia

This is an internal protrusion through the diaphragm.

Traumatic Hernia

This type of hernia is secondary to direct blunt abdominal trauma.

SIGNS AND SYMPTOMS

Many patients have no symptoms and learn they have a groin hernia only through a routine sports or preemployment physical. Some may experience a gradual onset of discomfort, reported as a dull ache with radiation into the scrotum (if male). If swelling is present, it is typically maximized at the end of the day and disappears with supination. Occasionally a patient will report acute onset of swelling and discomfort after a particularly strenuous straining or lifting episode. In infants who have acutely incarcerated hernias, presentation may consist only of irritability.

Figure 6-24-3 shows the common hernia locations.

PHYSICAL EXAMINATION

A symmetric, circular bulge located just superior to the pubic tubercle can often be seen on inspection in the patient who presents with a direct hernia. A hernia can be visually exacerbated by coughing or by the Valsalva maneuver. Males with a large indirect hernia may present with scrotal enlargement. Otherwise there may not be any visible findings.

The best examination maneuver for detecting an inguinal hernia consists of placing the gloved index finger of the examiner into the external inguinal ring of the patient during standing. Start low by invaginating loose scrotal skin (in the case of the male), aiming superior, and then lateral toward the patient's anterior superior iliac spine (ASIS). Once the examiner's digit is in position, the patient can turn his or her head and cough or perform the Valsalva maneuver. This increase in intraabdominal pressure may force abdominal contents into the inguinal canal secondary to abdominal wall weakness and may allow palpation by the examiner's finger. This is performed bilaterally. When the right index finger is placed in the patient's right inguinal canal and directed at the right ASIS, abdominal contents touching the fingertip may indicate an indirect inguinal hernia and touching the side of the digit suggests a direct hernia. This is not a completely reliable finding, since it may be very difficult to distinguish between the two, but it may be useful in some cases. This procedure is repeated using

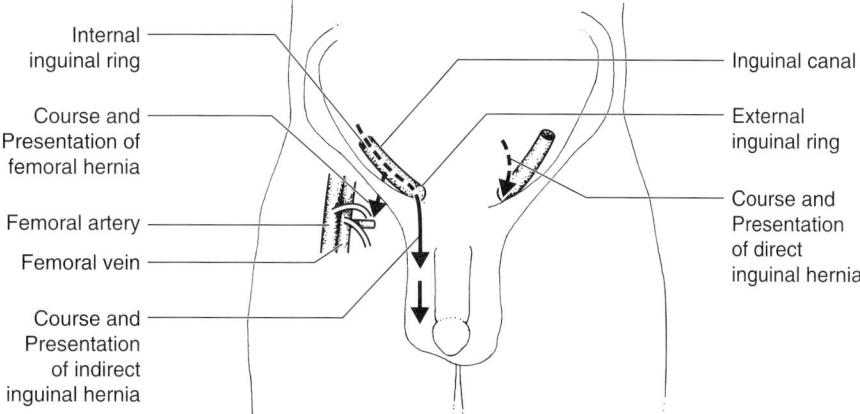

FIGURE 6-24-3. Common hernia locations.

the examiner's left index finger aimed toward the patient's left ASIS within the left inguinal canal. The patient then can be examined in the supine position to determine reducibility. In a male patient suspected of having an incarcerated or strangulated hernia, auscultation of the scrotum can yield bowel sounds if the hernia is detected early. Later, bowel sounds may cease due to further ischemia and necrosis.

Attempting to get fingers above a scrotal mass can help to differentiate between a hernia (cannot get above) and a hydrocele (which one typically can get above). Transillumination of the mass can also help to distinguish between a hydrocele, which typically transilluminates, and a hernia, which does not. Hydroceles are usually described as nontender.

DIAGNOSTIC STUDIES

Vitals signs may demonstrate elevated temperature and slight tachycardia in patients whose hernias are strangulated. Use complete blood cell count for evidence of leukocytosis and left shift in those suspected of strangulation. Electrolytes may be abnormal if strangulation is secondary to dehydration and toxicity. Flat and upright plain films of the chest and abdomen help assess for bowel obstruction and/or perforation. Ultrasound may be helpful in differentiating scrotal masses. Urinalysis may be helpful in differentiating genitourinary involvement. Computed tomography scans are sometimes helpful in difficult cases (internal pelvic and spigelian hernias). Herniography (which consists of intraperitoneal injection of contrast material, then a plain film obtained while the patient performs the Valsalva maneuver) may also be used.

TREATMENT

Some patients benefit from the use of a daytime truss and avoidance of heavy straining or lifting; however, this is temporizing in most and actually contraindicated in those with femoral hernia. Surgical repair (herniorrhaphy or hernioplasty) to reduce the sac and close the defect is the only method of treatment and should be done to prevent the possibility of incarceration or strangulation. This can usually be accomplished electively with local anesthesia and same-day surgery. Most patients can return to a sedentary job within several days or 3 to 6 weeks for those who perform heavy manual labor. Surgical consideration should be given based on the health, activity level, and life-style of the patient. Surgical benefits should outweigh the risks. In acute cases, gentle attempts at manual reduction of the incarceration using the Trendelenburg position can be implemented. However, surgical consultation should be instituted quickly. The patient should be given intravenous fluids and nothing by mouth; a nasogastric tube should be placed. Many types of surgical repair are utilized. It is important to be familiar with the anatomy of the groin (see Fig. 6-24-4). Some of the more common types of surgical repair include:

- *Bassini repair*: This is the most widely used method (originally described in 1887) and involves sewing the conjoined tendon (internal oblique aponeurosis and transversus abdominis aponeurosis, transversalis fascia) to the inguinal ligament, also called Poupart's ligament.
- *Halstead repair*: The external oblique fascia is sutured beneath the spermatic cord; of historical significance only.
- *Lotheissen-McVay repair/Cooper's ligament repair*: This useful indirect hernia repair always requires a relaxing incision in the rectus sheath to relieve tension. It is also effective for femoral hernia repair.
- *Shouldice repair*: This technique involves running a suture closure of the transversalis fascia; the strength in the groin is the transversalis fascia, also known as the shelving margin or iliopubic tract.

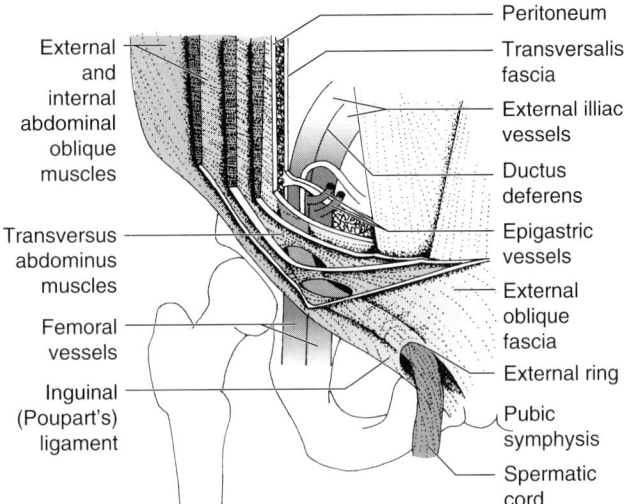

FIGURE 6-24-4. Anatomy of the groin.

- *Lichtenstein repair*: A polypropylene mesh (Marlex) or other synthetic patch is used to repair the transversalis fascial effect.
- *Marcy repair*: The internal ring is surgically tightened.
- *Laparoscopic repair*: This newer closed technique involves stapling and mesh; the long-term results are unknown.

HERNIORRHAPHY AND HERNIOPLASTY COMPLICATIONS

Complications include hemorrhage and severed vas deferens. There can be resection or entrapment of the ilioinguinal nerve, altering skin sensation of the upper thigh, root of the penis, and scrotum (in males) or the mons pubis and labia majora (in females). Entrapment of the genitofemoral nerve can also disrupt skin sensation of the groin and upper thigh. Other possibilities are testicular swelling if ring closure is too tight, recurrence, infection, and failure in diabetic patients secondary to decreased healing and in obese patients secondary to weight. Ischemic orchitis, testicular atrophy, bladder injury, and bowel injury can also occur.

BIBLIOGRAPHY

Adler JN, Planz SH: *NMS Clinical Manuals—Emergency Medicine.* Baltimore, Williams & Wilkins, 1999, pp 159–160.
Bates B: *A Guide to Physical Examination and History Taking.* Philadelphia, Lippincott, 1999, pp 387–403.
Jarrell BE et al: *NMS Clinical Manuals—Surgery,* 4th ed. Philadelphia, Williams & Wilkins, 2000, pp 40–46, 551–554.
Kozol RA et al: *When to Call the Surgeon—Decision-making for Primary Care Providers.* Philadelphia, FA Davis, 1998, pp 167–180.
Lawrence PF et al (eds): *Essentials of General Surgery,* 3d ed. Philadelphia, Lippincott Williams & Wilkins, 2000, pp 195–199.
Niederhuber JE: *Fundamentals of Basic Surgery.* New York, McGraw-Hill, 1998, pp. 390–401.
Schwartz SI et al (eds): *Principles of Surgery,* 6th ed. New York, McGraw-Hill, 1994.
Silen W: *Cope's Early Diagnosis of the Acute Abdomen.* New York, Oxford University Press, 1996, pp 198–205.
Spector SA, Coppola CP: *Surgery—Clinical Companion.* Philadelphia, Lippincott Williams & Wilkins, 1999, pp 245–248.
Tintinalli J et al (eds): *Emergency Medicine: A Comprehensive Study Guide.* New York, McGraw-Hill, 1996, pp 466–468.
Way L (ed): *Current Surgical Diagnosis and Treatment.* Norwall, CT, Appleton and Lange, 1994, pp 712–724.
Zollinger RM Jr, Zollinger RM (eds): *Atlas of Surgical Operations.* New York, McGraw-Hill, 1993, pp 424–447.

ABDOMINAL PAIN
Pat C. H. Jan

DISCUSSION

Abdominal pain is the most common complaint at emergency rooms and outpatient clinics. It is important to identify disease processes involving abdominal pain that require immediate surgical intervention and those which require a complete medical workup.

Common surgical emergencies include small and large bowel obstruction, appendicitis, mesenteric ischemia, cholecystitis, perforated duodenal ulcer, incarcerated inguinal hernia, aortic aneurysm rupture, and ectopic pregnancy.

It is very important to obtain a complete history on each patient. Be sure to ask for the following information: onset (early morning, afternoon, dinner, bedtime), duration (minutes, hours, days), radiation (from left upper quadrant to shoulder, right lower quadrant to lower extremities, epigastric area to back), aggravating factors (types of food or movement that cause the pain to worsen), relieving factors (what makes the pain less or alleviates the pain), quality (sharp, dull, burning, gnawing), bowel habits (diarrhea or constipation), urinary problems (dysuria, hematuria, frequency), and location of pain. Prior medical and surgical history should be obtained along with current medications, vitamins, and herbal products.

SIGNS AND SYMPTOMS
Left Upper Quadrant Pain

Pain in this area can be from a myocardial infarction, duodenal ulcer, splenic injury, or gastroenteritis. The pain can present as sharp, burning, or gnawing. Kehr's sign may be present with splenic injury. It is referred pain to the left shoulder from the splenic area (see Chaps. 6-1 and 6-21).

Left Lower Quadrant Pain

Diverticulitis, inflammatory bowel disease, pelvic inflammatory disease, a kidney stone, endometriosis, ectopic pregnancy, and rupture of an ovarian cyst are common causes of abdominal pain in this area. A careful history of bowel habits, urinary problems, sexually history, and menstruation should be obtained (see Chaps. 6-8, 6-15, 12-8, and 12-9).

Right Upper Quadrant Pain

Palpation of the right upper quadrant for Murphy's sign indicates cholecystitis (see Chap. 6-10). Percuss, palpate the liver, and check the sclera for icterus in case of hepatitis. Also check for chronic alcohol use in patients with pancreatitis and alcoholic liver disease. Retrocecal appendicitis should be ruled out, since it can hide behind the intestine. Pneumonia and pulmonary embolism can cause pain at the costal vertebral angle and should be differentiated from abdominal causes (see Chap. 17-7).

Right Lower Quadrant Pain

Pain may be diffuse, as in early appendicitis, or crampy and nonradiating, as in ectopic pregnancy. Colon obstruction secondary to colon cancer, diverticulitis, and ureterolithiasis are common causes of pain in this area (see Chap. 6-26).

OBJECTIVE FINDINGS
Inspection

Begin with the patient supine with the arms placed at the side. Put the bed in the supine position and look at the abdomen for disten-

tion. If there is dropoff at the costal margins, the abdomen is not distended. Look to see which area of the abdomen is distended. Left upper quadrant distention can be gastric outlet obstruction in a patient with a gastrostomy tube. Right upper quadrant distention can be caused by hepatomegaly. Abdominal distention with bowel sounds may be due to a fecal impaction from prolonged narcotic or laxative abuse leading to constipation. Abdominal distention without bowel sounds is ileus. Bowel obstruction and perforation are common causes.

Auscultation

Hypoactivity to absence of bowel sounds can be heard with ileus. Hyperactive bowel sounds generally are heard in patients with gastroenteritis. High pitch with crescendo-decrescendo is common with bowel obstruction.

Percussion

Percuss over each quadrant for tympany and dullness. Percuss out the borders of the liver. Patients with liver disease may have a distended abdomen filled with ascites. Perform the fluid wave and shifting dullness to determine whether the patient has ascites.

Palpation

Always start from an area of nontenderness and go to the area of pain. Palpate lightly and then deeply to locate the source of the abdominal pain. Locate the abdominal aorta and determine the approximate size, since it can be a source of abdominal pain. Some special maneuvers can be used to help with the diagnosis of abdominal pain. Cutaneous hypersensitivity is caused by pain from gentle squeezing of the skin in the abdominal area between the thumb and the index finger. Deep palpation of one quadrant with peritoneal irritation to the opposite quadrant is a positive Rovsing's sign. A psoas sign is elicited by extension of the right thigh with resistance. It is used as a diagnostic aid in appendicitis. The obturator sign causes pain with flexion and extension of the flexed right thigh. Murphy's sign is tenderness with palpation of the gallbladder with inspiration. A rectal examination should be performed as well.

DIAGNOSTIC CONSIDERATIONS

Common causes of abdominal pain are listed in Table 6-25-1.

Cholecystitis

Cholecystitis presents as right upper quadrant pain that is worse after a fatty meal. The pain is worse with obstruction of the common bile duct by a gallstone. Common risk factors are female, fat, forty, and fertile. Ultrasound is the gold standard. Check liver functions, especially alkaline phosphatase in cases of common bile duct obstruction, cholestasis, hepatitis, or liver abscess (see Chap. 6-10).

Mesenteric (Intestinal) Ischemia

Findings are out of proportion to physical examination with mesenteric ischemia. Patients may present with weight loss and crampy abdominal pain. Utilize angiography to aid in the diagnosis.

Diverticulitis

Diverticulitis presents as left lower quadrant pain. Patients have mild leukocytosis, fever, and chills with perforation. Plain films may illustrate multiple diverticula in the left colon (see Chap. 6-8).

TABLE 6-25-1. Common Causes of Abdominal Pain

DISEASE	SIGNS AND SYMPTOMS	PHYSICAL FINDINGS	X-RAY AND LAB TESTS	TREATMENT	ETIOLOGY
Duodenal ulcers	Epigastric pain; relieved with food; burning sensation	Epigastric tenderness	EGD; (+) CLO; H.pylori	BMT (peptobismol 525 mg tid, flagyl 250 mg tid, amoxicillin 500 mg bid, or tetracycline 500 mg qid) × 14 d or clarithromycin 500 mg tid + omeprazole 40 mg qd × 14 d, then omeprazole 20 mg qd × 14 d	*H. pylori*
Pancreatitis	Initially midepigastric pain; radiating pain to back; nausea and vomiting	Epigastric tenderness; may have abdominal distention; in fetal position; Cullen's sign; Grey Turner's sign	Chem profile (watch glucose, calcium, magnesium); amylase (*p*-isoenzyme); lipase	NPO (allow for pancreas to rest); NG tube (for abdomen distention and nausea, vomiting); pain control (demerol or morphine); delirium tremens (IV w/MVI 10 mL, thiamine 100 mg)	Alcohol; gallstone; drugs
Acute cholecystitis	RUQ pain; nausea, vomiting; fever, chills; pain worse after fatty meal	(+) Murphy's sign; RUQ tenderness	Ultrasound; HIDA scan; plain abdominal x-ray; chemistry profile (watch for increased alkaline phosphatase in obstruction)	Laparotomy; laparoscopic cholecystectomy	Gallstone obstruction; bile stasis (TPN, drugs—rocephin, dehydration)
Small bowel obstruction	Nausea, vomiting; crampy abdomen pain	Abdominal distention; crescendo-decrescendo bowel sound; absent bs; abdomen scar	4 views of abdomen (look for air-fluid levels, dilated loops of bowel)	NG tube; pain control; laparotomy	Previous surgery (adhesions); inflamatory bowel disease (strictures); hernia
Large bowel obstruction	Nausea, vomiting; obstipation; abdomen pain	Abdominal distention; high-pitched bowel sound with rushes	Plain abdominal x-ray (look for dilated loops of bowel); barium enema (stricture)	Laparotomy	Carcinoma; volvulus; diverticular disease
Appendicitis	Periumbilical pain; localized RLQ pain; anorexia; fever/chill	Rebound tenderness; Rosving's sign; psoas sign; obturator sign; heel sign	Plain abdominal x-ray (psoas shadow); barium enema (nonvisualization of appendix); CBC (increased WBC)	Laparotomy; laparoscopic appendectomy	Lymphoid tissue; fecal/fecalith; tumor (carcinoid)
Mesenteric ischemia	Acute abdominal pain; melena	Abdominal distention; shock; minimal PE findings	WBC > 15,000; elevated amylase; elevated CPK; elevated inorganic phosphate; mahogany color peritoneal fluid; ¹³³Xe scan (retained xenon in ischemic bowel); ¹¹¹In scan (infarcted bowel); angiogram	Surgery; heparin administration	Mitral stenosis; connective tissue disease; drugs; trauma
Diverticulitis	LLQ pain; fever, chills; bleeding; crampy abdominal pain	LLQ tenderness; abdomen distention; LLQ mass	Plain film abdominal (mass, obstruction); CT scan (abscess, fistula); barium enema (abscess, stricture, diverticular sac)	Medical treatment (NG tube, IV fluids, pain control, broad-spectrum antibiotic); surgical treatment: primary resection with or without anastomosis	Low dietary fiber; weakness in colon wall
Ectopic pregnancy	Amenorrhea; pelvic pain; sudden nonradiating back pain	Enlarge uterus; adnexal mass; cervical tenderness; abdominal peritoneal signs	Quantitative beta HCG (look for doubling q 48 h); serum progesterone (<30 nm/L); pelvic sonogram (empty gestational sac)	Medical treatment: methotrexate; surgical treatment: salpingectomy, laparoscopic salpingectomy	Pelvic inflammatory disease; IUD use; previous induced abortions
Abdominal aortic aneurysm	Vague abdominal pain	Palpation of abdominal mass	Ultrasound (measure size of aorta); plain film abdominal (calcification); CT scan (size of aorta)	Laparotomy (replace segment of aneurysm wall with graft)	Atherosclerosis

NOTE: EGD = esophagogastroduodenoscopy; CLO = campylobacter-like organism test; BMT = Pepto Bismol + metronidazole + tetracycline; MVI = multivitamin; bs = bowel sound; HIDA = 99m Tc iminodiacetic acid scan; TPN = total pareneteral nutrition; PE = physical examination; CPK = creatine phosphokinase; HCG = human chorionic gonadotrophin; IUD = intrauterine contraceptive device.

Pancreatitis

Epigastric pain with radiation to the back is the typical presentation of pancreatitis. Patients often are found in the fetal position. The abdomen may be distended and tender to palpation. Cullen's sign (peri-umbilical ecchymosis) and Grey Turner's sign (flank ecchymosis) are late findings. Since a history of alcohol abuse is a common cause of pancreatitis, the patient should be placed on delirium tremens (DT) prophylaxis. A drug history should be obtained, since pancreatitis can be drug-induced (see Chap. 6-20).

Duodenal Ulcers

Epigastric pains that are relieved with food denote duodenal ulcers. Perforations are seen on plain abdominal films as free air under the diaphragm. Endoscopic biopsy may reveal *Helicobacter pylori* as the cause of the ulcers (see Chap. 6-21).

Other diseases to keep in mind are ectopic pregnancy, bowel obstruction, endometriosis, inflammatory bowel disease, biliary disease, hernias, and renal disease (see Fig. 6-25-1).

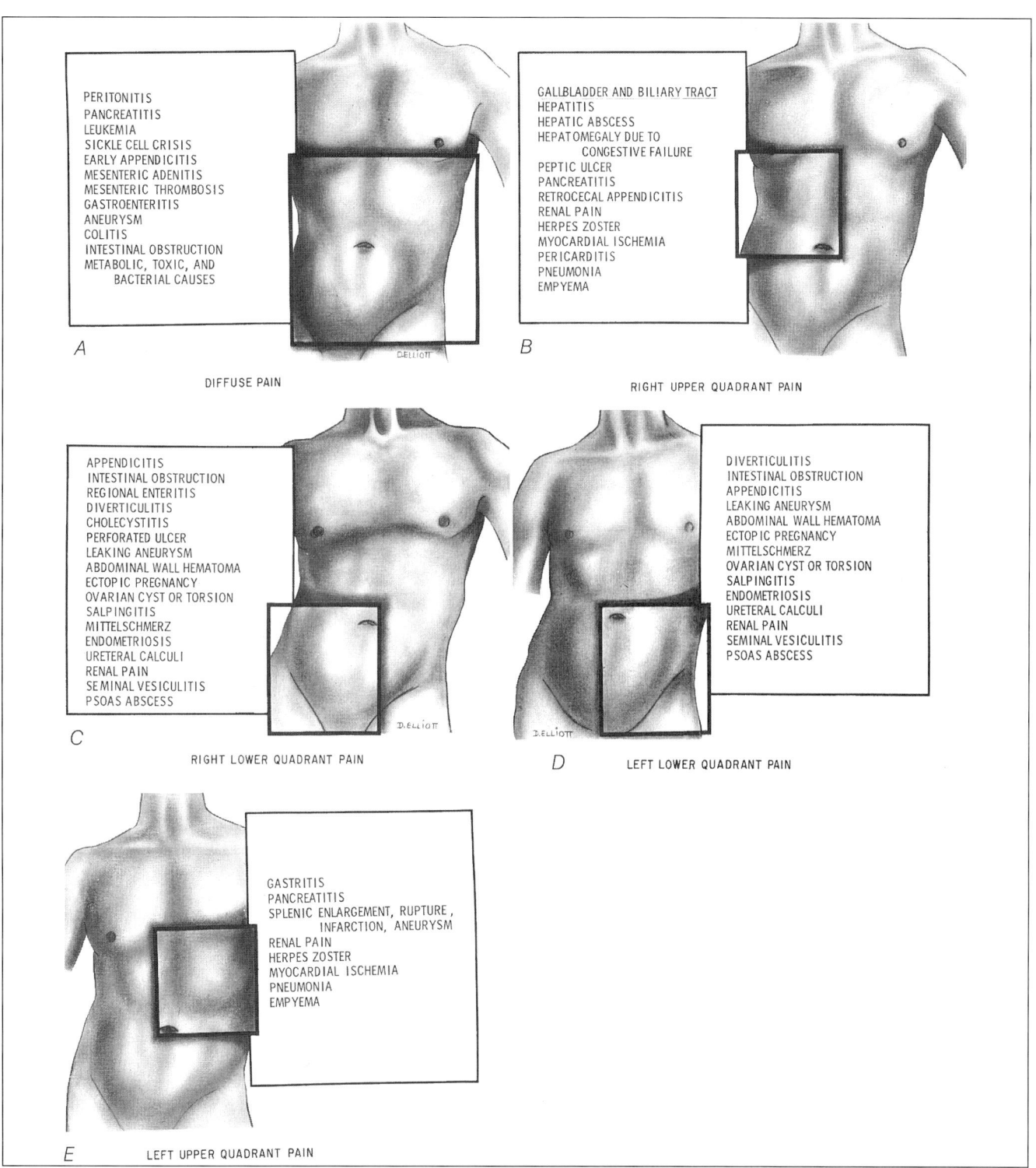

FIGURE 6-25-1. Common causes of abdominal pain. (*From Schwartz SI, Shires GT, Spence FC (eds): Principles of Surgery, 6th ed. New York, McGraw-Hill, 1994, p 1018. Used with permission of McGraw-Hill, Inc.*)

LABORATORY STUDIES

Complete Blood Cell Count

Decreased as well as elevated white blood cell (WBC) count indicates an inflammatory process. This is seen in abdominal abscess formation, perforated viscus, carcinoma, and gynecologic infections. Occasionally, a patient will present with an elevated WBC with no significant findings other than recent surgery or resolution of a recent infection. This is termed a leukemoid reaction. A follow-up WBC will be within the reference range. Steroids also can cause a falsely elevated WBC. If a differential is included in complete blood count (CBC), left shift caused by increased polymorphonuclear leukocytes and increased bands indicate acute bacterial infection. Elevations in lymphocytes can indicate viral infection. Eosinophils can be elevated in a number of disease processes, such as neoplasm, Addison's disease, allergic reaction, collagen vascular disease, and parasitic infections.

Urinalysis

Urinalysis may be useful in demonstrating a urinary tract infection in a female patient presenting with low abdominal pain or hematuria in a patient with renal stones.

Prothrombin Time and Partial Thromboplastin Time

An elevated prothrombin time (PT) and partial thromboplastin time (PTT) will signify worsening liver function. Remember that all coagulation factors are made by the liver except for factor VIII.

Chemistry Profile

Electrolyte abnormalities can be related to small bowel obstruction or gastroenteritis secondary to a bacterial infection. Hyperglycemia may be related to a patient presenting with pancreatitis. Elevations in liver function profile may represent disease processes in the liver or indicate a mesenteric infarction. High levels of alkaline phosphatase are seen in patients with common bile duct obstructions and bone diseases. Amylase and lipase are high in patients with acute pancreatitis. Total bilirubin elevation is associated with liver disease. Creatine phosphokinase (CPK) isoenzymes will help differentiate between cardiac, skeletal muscle, and liver pathology.

RADIOLOGIC STUDIES

Plain Abdominal Films

These films are used to identify perforated viscus by looking for free air under the diaphragm. Small bowel obstruction can be confirmed with visualization of air-fluid levels and distended loops of small bowel (see Figs. 6-25-2 and 6-25-3). Radiopaque gallstones can be seen in the upper right quadrant of the abdominal film. Loss of psoas shadow can indicate appendicitis.

Ultrasonography

Ultrasonography is the gold standard test for gallstones. It is very useful in pelvic pain to identify fibroids, ovarian cysts, empty gestational sacs in ectopic pregnancy, and aortic aneurysms.

Computed Tomography Scan

A computed tomography scan is very useful in identification of abscess formations, diverticular disease, pancreatic cancer, liver cancer, gallstones, and perforated viscus.

Barium and Gastrografin Studies

These studies are useful in locating diverticular disease, fistula formation from inflammatory bowel disease, appendicitis with

FIGURE 6-25-2. Air-fluid levels in left lateral position as seen in small bowel obstruction.

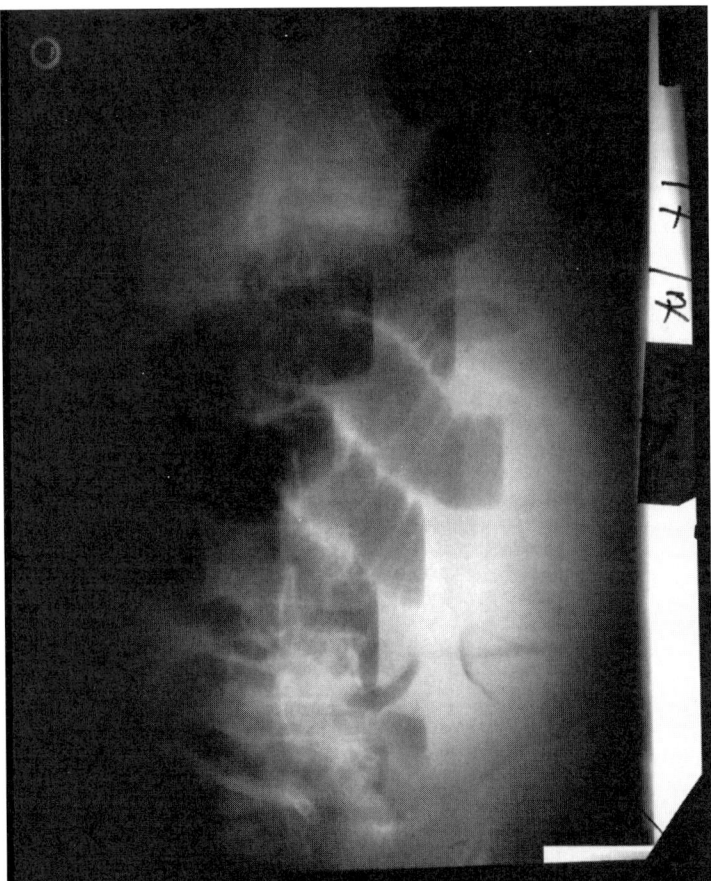

FIGURE 6-25-3. Distended loops of bowel.

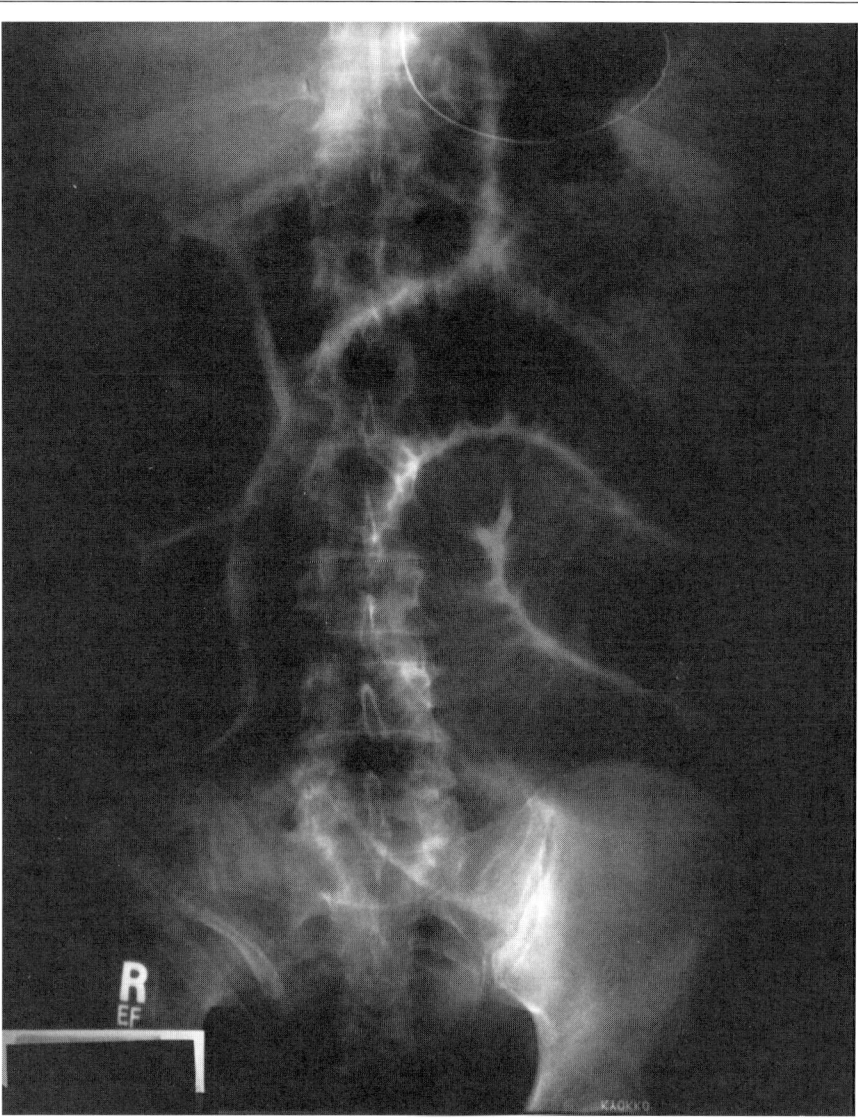

nonfilling appendix, stenosis, and edema at surgical anastomosis sites.

HIDA Scan

Technetium 99 is injected into the patient. Acute cholecystitis or acalcaneous cholecystitis is confirmed when the gallbladder is not visualized.

Angiography

Use an angiogram to demonstrate arterial bleeding, infarction, and stenosis.

NOTES AND PEARLS

Patients with short bowel syndrome secondary to bowel resection from inflammatory bowel disease may present to the emergency room with the complaint of abdominal pain and vomiting. Plain abdominal x-ray films reveal distended loops of small bowel, which are seen in small bowel obstruction. The patient is taken into the operating room, and the abdomen is benign. It is common for the small bowel to become distended in this group of patients because the intestine is adapting. Patients with a history of narcotic abuse may present with a distended abdomen and constipation. Rectal

examination usually reveals fecal impaction, or the patient may have a "lazy bowel" from laxative abuse.

BIBLIOGRAPHY

Nyhus LM: *Abdominal Pain: A Guide to Rapid Diagnosis.* Stamford, CT, Appleton & Lange, 1994.
Schwartz SI, Shires GT, Spencer FC (eds): *Principles of Surgery,* 7th ed. New York, McGraw-Hill, 1999.
Seller R: *Differential Diagnosis of Common Complaints.* Philadelphia, Saunders, 1996.
Zackowski SW: Chronic Recurrent Abdominal Pain. *Emerg Med Clin North Am* 16(4):877–894. 1998.

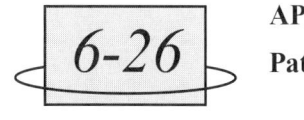

APPENDICITIS

Pat C. H. Jan

DISCUSSION

Acute appendicitis remains a common cause of abdominal pain, often requiring surgical management. Appendicitis occurs equally in males and females until puberty. After puberty, the occurrence rate is higher in males by a ratio of 2:1. Overall, the incidence of appendicitis has decreased since the 1940s. Some authorities say that the decline is attributed to things such as better nutrition and better diagnostic abilities of clinicians.

PATHOGENESIS

Appendicitis is caused by obstruction of the appendiceal lumen. Lymphoid follicle tissue generally appears in the appendix 2 weeks after birth. Hyperplasia of this tissue can be a result of gastrointestinal (GI) infection from bacterial or viral organisms. These follicles can then obstruct the lumen of the appendix. Fecal stasis and fecalith formation are caused by entrapment of small amounts of vegetable fiber in the appendiceal lumen that stimulate mucus secretion. The mucus surrounds the fiber, causing the irritation of the walls of the appendix, which stimulates further mucus secretion, and the appendix becomes obstructed. Foreign bodies and strictures of tumors of the appendix account for a small percentage of appendicitis cases. The common tumor type is carcinoid.

SIGNS AND SYMPTOMS

Patients with acute appendicitis present with abdominal pain as the initial complaint. The abdominal pain starts out as a generalized abdominal discomfort or periumbilical pain that is poorly localized. Patients may complain of crampy abdominal pain or gastroenteritis. As the disease progresses, the pain may shift from the periumbilical area to the right lower quadrant. Before the onset of abdominal pain, the patient may relate a history of decreased appetite or anorexia and general malaise for a few days. Therefore, patients with good appetites are less likely to have appendicitis. Patients may complain of nausea and vomiting as the lumen of the appendix becomes obstructed and distended. An elevated white blood cell count greater than 12,000 and low-grade temperature may or may not be present. Lower back or flank pain may indicate a retrocecal appendix. A pelvic appendix may present as suprapubic pain.

OBJECTIVE FINDINGS

Typically, these patients are found in bed with guarding of the right lower quadrant. They may even have the right leg flexed to prevent irritation and pain. If patients are seen walking about or sitting comfortably in bed, appendicitis is probably unlikely. The first step is to observe the abdomen for distention. This is best accomplished with the bed placed in the supine position and the patient lying flat with the hands at the side. The abdomen is inspected for a dropoff at the costal margins. If the dropoff is seen, the patient is not distended. The costal margin dropoff also can be seen readily in obese patients. Auscultation for bowel sounds is the next step. Hypoactive to absent bowel sounds may be noted with ileus secondary to inflammation of the appendix. Acute appendicitis may present with normoactive bowel sounds. Meanwhile, hyperactive bowel sounds are more common in patients with intestinal obstruction and gastroenteritis.

When performing percussion for tympany or dullness, it is important to start from an area of nontenderness and slowly work toward the place of tenderness. The same principle applies to palpation. If abdominal rigidity is encountered, during palpation, perforation should be suspected. Additional maneuvers, sometimes called special tests, can be utilized in the diagnosis of appendicitis. Cutaneous hypersensitivity is pain caused by gentle squeezing of the skin in the abdominal area between the thumb and index finger. McBurney's point is located approximately one-third of the distance between the anterior superior iliac spine and the umbilicus. This is the point of maximum tenderness. Patients have a positive rebound when they complain of pain after a sudden release from deep palpation at McBurney's point.

There are many ways to elicit peritoneal inflammation; demonstration of pain with any one of these methods will help confirm peritoneal irritation. Rovsing's sign consists of deep palpation of the left lower quadrant of the abdomen to elicit peritoneal irritation in the right lower quadrant. Sometimes the appendix, when inflamed, will cause irritation of the psoas muscle. Resistance with extension of the right thigh elicits the psoas sign. The obturator sign consists of flexion and extension of the flexed right thigh. If it is positive, consider the pelvis as the location of the appendix. In the heel drop test, the patient or child is asked to stand up on the toes and drop down on the heels. This will cause peritoneal irritation. A modified heel drop can be done with the patient in the supine position. In this case, the examiner hits the bottom of the heel and transmits a vibration to the right lower quadrant. Coughing can cause peritoneal irritation in an inflamed appendix. The patient indicates the right lower quadrant as the source of pain and discomfort. Finally, a rectal examination should be performed for tenderness from a suprapubic appendix.

DIAGNOSTIC CONSIDERATIONS

Pain in the right lower quadrant has a myriad of potential etiologies, including but not limited to appendicitis. The following common diseases should be considered in the differential diagnoses.

Enteritis

Patients present with diffuse crampy abdominal pain and episodes of diarrhea. If patients have consumed any food toxins, they may present with fever, chills, and dehydration secondary to diarrhea (see Chap. 6-1).

Pelvic Inflammatory Disease

The patient may relate a worsening of abdominal pain after menstruation. Usually both salpinges are inflamed, and the patient may present with fever, chills, nausea, and vomiting. Physical examination generally demonstrates cervical motion tenderness, and a vaginal discharge may be noted. Sexual history should be ascertained (see Chap. 12-8).

Ectopic Pregnancy

Women of childbearing age, especially those with a past history of pelvic inflammatory disease (PID), may have an ectopic pregnancy. Even in cases where sexual activity is denied (e.g., adolescent females), a pregnancy test should be performed or a pelvic ultrasound ordered (see Chap. 12-6).

Ovarian Cyst

Patients may complain of lower quadrant pain at the start of each month's menstrual cycle. Physical examination can reveal adnexal tenderness. A pelvic sonogram can be used to confirm the diagnosis (see Chap. 12-9).

Mesenteric Adenitis

Patients may present with a history of a recent bout of infection causing enlargement of regional lymph nodes. These patients have diffuse abdominal pain.

Diverticulitis

Although diverticula are more common in the left colon, inflamed right colon diverticula can be difficult to distinguish from appendicitis. Questions should be directed at bowel habits, signs of diarrhea, and blood in the stool (see Chap. 6-8).

Acute Cholecystitis

Acute cholecystitis usually presents with right upper quadrant pain. Pain may be worse after a fatty meal. Signs and symptoms also include fever and chills. Palpation will reveal right upper quadrant tenderness. Ultrasound is the gold standard confirmatory test (see Chap. 6-10).

Ureteral Stones

Sharp, stabbing pains to the right quadrant and back and hematuria are common signs and symptoms of ureteral stones. Intravenous pyelography usually demonstrates kidney stones (see Chap. 18-5).

Other diseases to keep in mind are perforated ulcers, inflammatory bowel disease, and aortic aneurysm.

SPECIAL CONSIDERATIONS

Appendicitis in Children

It is often difficult to get accurate histories from children regarding the onset of abdominal pain and radiation of pain to the right lower quadrant. Parents may unknowingly delay treatment of what they presume is gastroenteritis. Physical examination and special tests may be limited because of fear of the clinician. Children usually present with episodes of diarrhea, fever, chills, and dehydration.

Appendicitis in the Elderly and Mentally Challenged

This is another population of individuals in whom accurate histories may be limited because of poor attention to detail and difficulty with memory retention. These patients often present initially with adverse behavioral changes that may be misinterpreted. Unfortunately, physical examination findings may be unremarkable and diagnostic laboratory findings may be normal or borderline abnormal. Therefore, it is no surprise that many elderly and mentally challenged patients have a perforated appendix when taken into the operating room.

Appendicitis and Pregnancy

Appendicitis is common during the first trimester of pregnancy. Signs and symptoms associated with appendicitis are similar to those found in nonpregnant women. Physical examination findings may not be helpful because the appendix may shift location during pregnancy.

Quite often, there is a delay in surgery because of the concern about inducing premature labor.

LABORATORY TESTS

There may be a mild to moderate elevation of the white blood cell count (WBC) in the range of 10,000 to 17,000. A mild increase in polymorphonuclear cells (a left shift) is also common. A urinalysis may be useful in ruling out a bladder infection or renal stones. Occasionally, if an inflamed appendix rests on the ureter, white blood cells may be seen in the urine.

RADIOLOGIC STUDIES

The following studies can aid in the diagnosis if appendicitis is not apparent from the history and physical examination. They are also useful in identifying other potential causes of abdominal pain. Plain films and/or ultrasound examinations usually are utilized first.

Plain Abdominal Films

Abdominal x-rays may demonstrate distended loops of bowel localized around the site of inflammation, loss of the psoas shadow, or gas in the appendix.

Barium Enema Study

If the appendix is completely filled with the barium, appendicitis is unlikely. However, nonfilling of the appendix can suggest appendicitis (see Figs. 6-26-1 and 6-26-2). Barium studies are not recommended if there is suspicion of a perforated appendix.

FIGURE 6-26-1. Filling of the appendix on barium enema study.

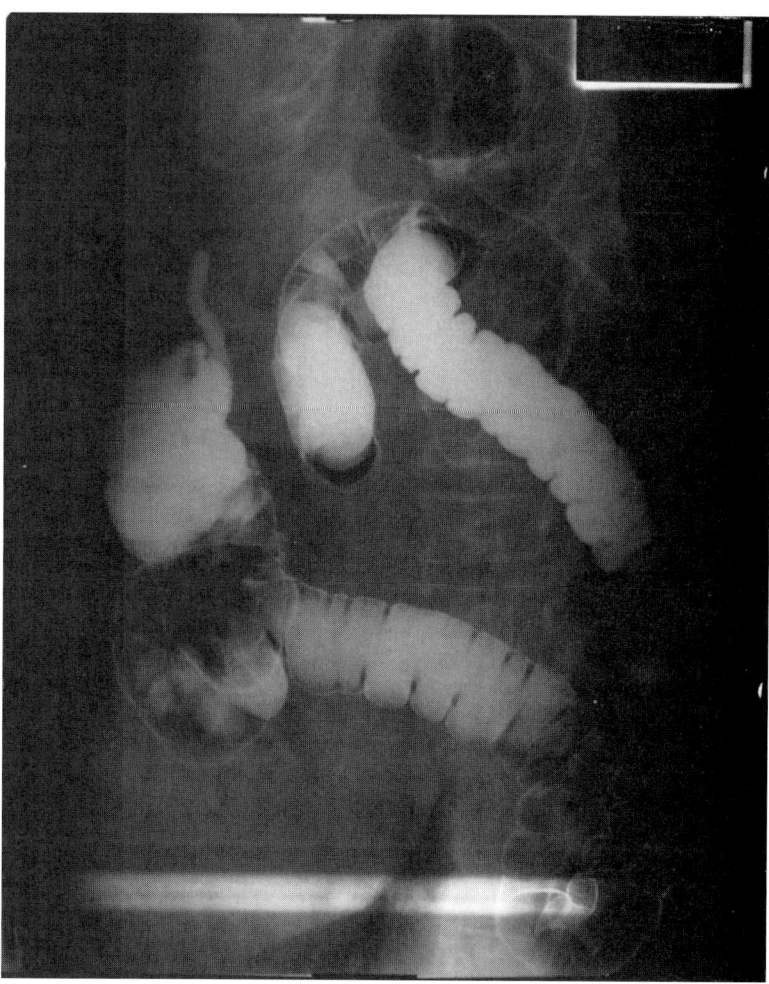

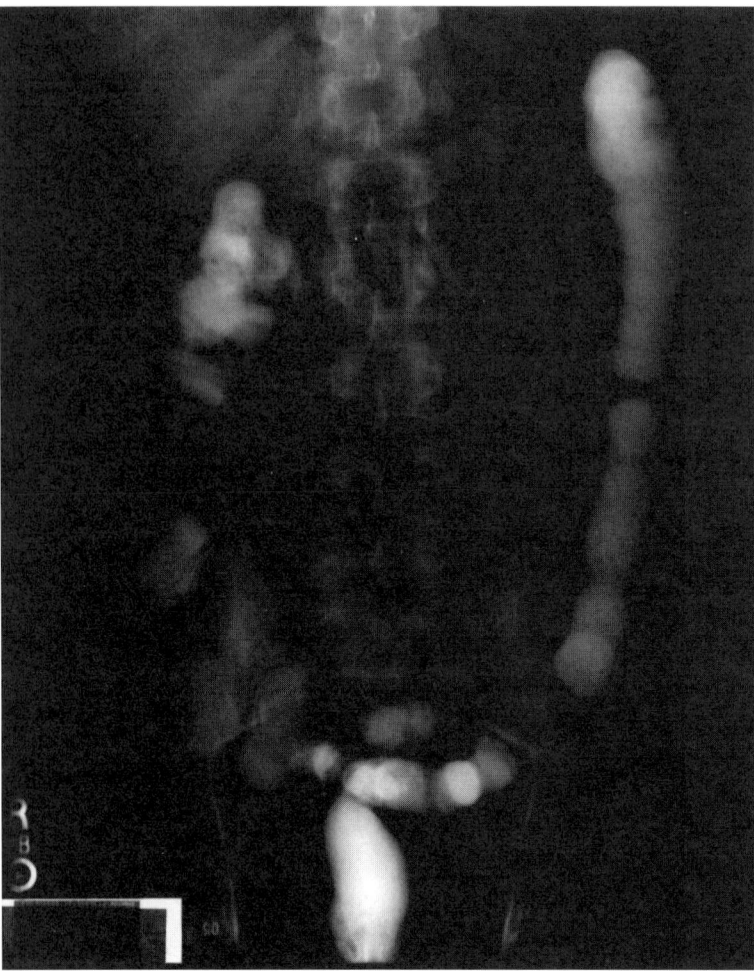

FIGURE 6-26-2. Nonfilling of the appendix on barium enema study.

Ultrasonography

Ultrasonography may demonstrate an inflamed appendix or aid in locating a pelvic mass or abscess.

Computed Tomography Scan

A computed tomography (CT) scan can be useful in finding appendiceal abscess.

TREATMENT

Laparotomy

An incision is made over McBurney's point in patients with classic appendicitis. If there is doubt, a midline incision is used so that other procedures will be feasible if needed (see Fig. 6-26-3). In case of perforation, the subcutaneous layer is left open and allowed to close by secondary intention to minimize infection.

Laproscopic Appendectomy

This procedure can be used when there is doubt from subjective and objective findings. It also can be used to rule out gynecologic pathology. Four ports are inserted into the abdomen, and the appendix artery is divided. The appendix is separated from the cecum and removed from one of the ports. If there is evidence of perforation or purulent drainage, a Jackson-Pratt drain should be placed.

DISPOSITION

Patients initially are followed 1 week after discharge from the hospital and in uncomplicated appendectomy. These patients can be reevaluated in 2 to 3 weeks. In case of perforation or abscess formation, weekly visits are recommended until the abdominal wound is completely healed. Patients are reevaluated in 3 weeks.

COMPLICATIONS AND RED FLAGS

Perforation

Postoperative monitoring for shock and sepsis is required in case of perforation. Patients should be placed on broad-spectrum antibiotics such as clindamycin, plus an aminoglycoside or a second-generation cephalosporin (Mefoxin) or an aminopenicillin (Unasyn) or antipseudomonal penicillin (Timentin) for an additional 5 to 7 days. The subcutaneous layer should be left open to close by secondary intention, and a drain should be left in place.

Appendiceal Abscess

There is some controversy regarding treatment. Some practitioners advocate percutaneous radiologically guided drainage with a scheduled appendectomy at a later date, whereas others recommend immediate appendectomy with evacuation of the abscess. Patients are also placed on broad-spectrum antibiotics for 5 to 7 days postoperatively.

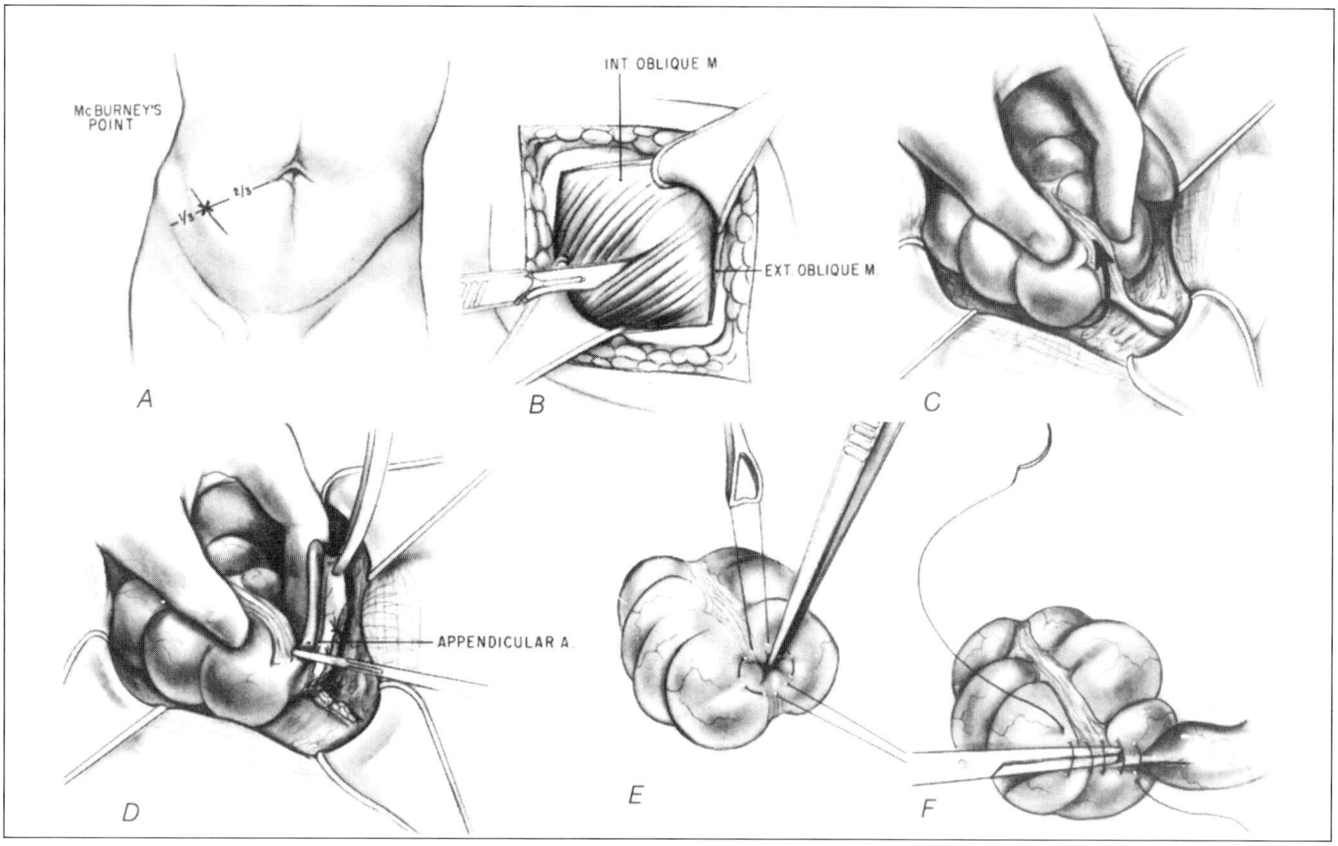

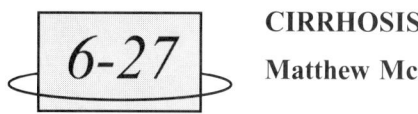

FIGURE 6-26-3. Appendectomy by laparotomy. (*From Schwartz SI, Shires GT, Spencer FC (eds): Principles of Surgery, 6th ed. New York, McGraw-Hill, 1994, p 1315. Used with permission of McGraw-Hill, Inc.*)

Fecal Fistula

A fistula occasionally may occur secondary to loosening of surgical ties and will tend to close spontaneously.

Intestinal Obstruction

This occurs secondary to ileus. A nasogastric tube should be inserted to prevent vomiting and aspiration until normal bowel movements have returned.

PEARLS

The diagnosis of appendicitis is most often a clinical decision. Quite often, the physical examination and laboratory and radiologic studies are inconclusive. Sometimes the clinician has to make the determination of appendicitis by history alone.

BIBLIOGRAPHY

Schwartz SI, Shires GT, Spencer FC (eds): Appendicitis, in *Principles of Surgery,* 7th ed. New York, McGraw-Hill, 1999.

Tierney LM, McPhee SJ, Papadakis, MA (eds): Appendicitis in *Current Medical Diagnosis and Treatment,* 39th ed. Stanford, CT, Lange & McGraw-Hill, 2000, p 625.

Vitello JM: Appendicitis, in Nyhus LM (ed): *Abdominal Pain: A Guide to Rapid Diagnosis.* Stanford, CT, Appleton & Lange, 1995.

Wagner JM, McKinney WP, Carpenter JL: Does this patient have appendicitis? *JAMA* 276:1589, 1996.

6-27

CIRRHOSIS
Matthew McQuillan

DISCUSSION

Cirrhosis is the final common pathway in the course of a variety of chronic, progressive liver diseases that lead to fibrosis and nodular regeneration. Portal hypertension, portosystemic shunting, and impaired excretory and synthetic liver function follow. This irreversible, incurable disease is the eleventh leading cause of death in the United States, with an estimated incidence of 900,000. There are numerous causes of cirrhosis (Table 6-27-1). However, in North America, South America, and Western Europe, most cases can be attributed to alcohol. Worldwide, chronic hepatitis B and C are the major culprits.

SIGNS AND SYMPTOMS

Cirrhosis may be clinically silent and many cases are found incidentally at laparotomy or autopsy. Symptoms (Table 6-27-2) vary depending on the underlying cause, but are most often related to the complications of hepatic dysfunction. It is important to note that up to 40% of patients with cirrhosis are asymptomatic. When symptoms are present, they usually have an insidious onset. A firm, enlarged, nodular liver is an early sign in 70% of cases. Other signs (Table 6-27-3) are usually the complications that accompany longstanding hepatic injury.

TABLE 6-27-1. Etiology of Cirrhosis

Drugs

  Ethanol
  Methotrexate
  Acetaminophen
  Isoniazid
  Methyldopa
  Vitamin A
  Amiodarone

Infections

  Hepatitis B, C, D
  Schistosomiasis
  Brucellosis
  Echinococcosis
  Syphilis

Biliary Obstruction

  Primary biliary cirrhosis
  Secondary biliary obstruction
    Sclerosing cholangitis
    Pancreatic neoplasms
    Bile duct neoplasms
    Iatrogenic or inflammatory biliary stricture
  Cystic fibrosis
  Biliary atresia/neonatal hepatitis
  Congenital biliary cysts

Metabolic Diseases

  Wilson's disease
  Hemochromatosis
  α_1 antitrypsin deficiency
  Carbohydrate disorders
    Fructose intolerance
    Galactosemia
    Glycogen storage diseases
    Lipid disorders, e.g., Wolman's disease, abetalipoproteinemia
  Urea cycle defects
    Ornithine transcarbamylase
  Porphyria
  Amino acid disorders, e.g., tyrosinosis
  Bile acid disorders, e.g., Byler's disease

Vascular Disorders

  Hereditary hemorrhagic telangiectasias
  Right-sided heart failure
  Pericarditis

Autoimmune Disorder

  Autoimmune chronic hepatitis

TABLE 6-27-2. Symptoms of Cirrhosis

Fatigue	Abdominal pain
Weakness	Anorexia
Edema	Fever
Oliguria	Steatorrhea
Azotemia	Osteomalacia
Nausea	Osteoporosis
Vomiting	Melena
Diarrhea	Xerophthalmia
Amenorrhea	Xerostomia
Pruritus	Hematemesis
Impotence	
Arthritis	

DIAGNOSTIC CONSIDERATIONS

Cirrhosis can be comfortably diagnosed based on the subjective and objective findings without the need for an extensive laboratory workup. However, the only definitive diagnosis can be achieved histologically via biopsy, which is considered the gold standard. Traditionally, cirrhosis has been classified based on the presence and size of nodules. The most common system of classification divides cirrhosis into micronodular, macronodular, and mixed forms, all of which can be seen in the same patient simultaneously. It is important to note that this system of classification does not provide any etiologic, functional, or prognostic value. A rare exception is in the cirrhotic patient with a massive "regenerative" nodule, which must be distinguished from a neoplasm.

LABORATORY TESTING

Laboratory abnormalities may be absent or minimal in latent or quiescent cirrhosis. Macrocytic anemia, thrombocytopenia, and coagulopathies are frequent findings. Modest elevations in aspartate aminotransferase (AST) and alkaline phosphates reflect hepatic injury.

RADIOLOGIC AND IMAGING STUDIES

Plain films may reveal hepatic or swelling enlargement. An upper gastrointestinal series may show the presence of esophageal varices. Ultrasonography assists in evaluating liver size and assessing the patency of the splenic, portal, and hepatic veins.

OTHER DIAGNOSTICS

Esophagogastroscopy can confirm the presence and extent of variceal formation.

TREATMENT

Management of the disease is aimed at prevention and treatment of the life-threatening complications such as variceal bleeding and hepatic encephalopathy. It is largely directed toward supportive care. All medications should be used with caution, particularly those metabolized by the liver, which may be severely impaired. Most importantly, patients should be encouraged to abstain from alcohol. Patients who continue to consume alcohol may have a lower threshold of tolerating the toxic effects of acetaminophen. Liver transplantation, the only curative therapy for most causes of cirrhosis, is recommended for worsening functional status, increasing bilirubin, decreasing albumin, worsening coagulopathies, or worsening encephalopathy.

Pharmacologic Management

Prednisone or prednisolone in moderately large doses may be helpful in patients with severe alcoholic hepatitis and encephalopathy; however, glucocorticoids should be avoided in those patients with acute alcoholic hepatitis. Maintenance therapy with colchicine, 0.6 to 1 mg twice daily, has been shown to slow progression in some patients with alcoholic liver disease. It works by inhibiting hepatic fibrogenesis. Spironolactone should be used in patients to increase diuresis, especially if restricted sodium intake is not effective. Begin with 100 mg/d and titrate every 3 to 5 days in increments of 100 mg to a maximum of 400 mg/d.

In patients with chronic hepatitis B, standard treatment is daily interferon α-2b (Intron A) 5 million U subcutaneously daily or 10 million U subcutaneously three times per week for 4 months. For those patients with hepatitis C, transplantation is the only cure.

TABLE 6-27-3. Physical Signs of Cirrhosis

SIGN	COMMENTS
Scleral icterus	Jaundice; present with bilirubin level >3 mg/dL
Kayser-Fleischer rings	Corneal copper deposition seen in Wilson's disease; best diagnosed with slit lamp
Fetor hepaticus	Musty breath odor secondary to accumulation of volatile aromatic substances accumulated in the blood and urine due to defective hepatic metabolism
Gynecomastia	May indicate chronic liver disease in men
Tender hepatomegaly	Congestive hepatomegaly
Small nodular liver	
Courvoisier's sign	Neoplastic extrahepatic biliary obstruction
Palpable spleen	
Venous hum	Auscultate over periumbilical veins; present with portal hypertension
Ascites	Portal hypertension; hypoalbuminemia
Hemorrhoids	Portal hypertension
Guaiac positive stool	Alcoholic gastritis; bleeding esophageal varices; PUD; bleeding hemorrhoids
Testicular atrophy	Chronic liver disease; hemochromatosis
Pedal edema	Hypoalbuminemia; right-sided heart failure
Arthropathy	Hemochromatosis
Asterixis	Flapping tremor; occurs in hepatic encephalopathy
Dysarthria	Spasticity of the muscles used for speaking; seen in Wilson's disease
Choreoathetosis	Abnormal movements of the body
Jaundice	
Palmar erythema	Mottled redness of the thenar and hypothenar eminences
Spider angiomata	
Ecchymoses	Thrombocytopenia or coagulation factor deficiency
Dilated superficial periumbilical veins (caput medusae)	
Increased pigmentation	Hemochromatosis
Xanthomas	Yellow nodule or plaque composed of lipids; due to primary biliary cirrhosis; usually found on the skin
Needle tracks	Viral hepatitis
Terry's nails	Dark red distal nail, pale proximal nail; commonly seen with cirrhosis
Glossitis	Vitamin deficiencies
Cheilosis	Vitamin deficiencies

Primary biliary cirrhosis is treated with daily divided doses of ursodeoxycholic acid, 10 to 15 mg/kg. Hemochromatosis is treated through iron depletion therapy either by way of phlebotomy or iron chelation therapy.

Wilson's disease results in copper accumulation in the liver, central nervous system, and kidneys. D-penicillamine, 1 to 2 g daily in four divided doses, is effective in preventing copper accumulation but does not aid in the regression of the disease.

Diet

Patients should be encouraged to consume 1 g of protein per kilogram of body weight and aim for total caloric intake of 2000 to 3000 kcal per day. A daily multivitamin with 100 mg of thiamine and 1 mg of folic acid is necessary for those patients with Wernicke-Korsakoff disease. Fluid retention necessitates the restriction of sodium. Alcohol is absolutely contraindicated.

Supportive Measures

If ascites and severe edema develop, diagnostic paracentesis is indicated. Ascitic fluid should be analyzed for albumin, cell count, and culture. If the ascites causes respiratory compromise, large-volume paracentesis is effective and can be continued daily.

Patient Education

Alcohol counseling should be strongly encouraged if appropriate.

DISPOSITION

Prognosis for patients with cirrhosis varies according to etiology and clinical stage. However, regardless of etiology, prognosis does correlate with the Child-Turcotte classification (Table 6-27-4). Mean survival times for patients with class A, B, and C cirrhosis are 40, 32, and 8 months, respectively. Most patients with advanced liver disease eventually die as a result of massive variceal hemorrhage and/or profound hepatic encephalopathy. Patients who have had a major complication of cirrhosis and who continue to drink have a 5-year survival of less than 50%. Transplantation is associated with a 5-year survival rate as high as 80%. However, hepatocellular carcinoma, hepatitis B and C, and Budd-Chiari syndrome may recur in the transplanted liver.

COMPLICATIONS AND RED FLAGS

Massive uncontrolled hemorrhage can occur from an upper gastrointestinal bleed via varices, portal hypertensive gastropathy, or a gastroduodenal ulcer. Endoscopic band ligation or sclerotherapy is effective, however, transjugular intrahepatic portosystemic shunts (TIPS) are an alternative to refractory cases of bleeds and ascites. The long-term use of the TIPS method has not been established and therefore it is usually recommended as a short-term alternative until transplantation can be achieved. Vasopressin and intravenous

TABLE 6-27-4. Pugh Modification of the Child-Turcotte Classification of Cirrhosis

FEATURE	SCORE		
	1	2	3
Encephalopathy (stage)	0	1–2	3–4
Ascites	Absent	Slight	Poorly controlled
Bilirubin (mg/dL)	<2.0	2.0–3.0	>3.0
Albumin (g/dL)	>3.5	2.8–3.5	<2.8
Prothrombin time(s)	1.09–4.0	4.0–6.0	>6.0

Each feature is assigned 1, 2, or 3 points.

Class A: 5–6 points

Class B: 7–9 points

Class C: 10–15 points

nitroglycerin can also be used to control bleeding in situations not amenable to other procedures. Propanolol can also lower portal hypertension and prevent the first bleed, but it is ineffective in preventing recurrences.

Spontaneous bacterial peritonitis (SBP), heralded by fever, abdominal pain, ascites, and encephalopathy, can be diagnosed via paracentesis and treated with intravenous antibiotics to cover *Escherichia coli* and pneumococci. Since there is a high mortality rate associated with SBP, survivors are given long-term antibiotics and other patients with cirrhosis are treated prophylactically.

Hepatorenal syndrome is characterized by azotemia, oliguria, hyponatremia, low urinary sodium, and hypotension and occurs in end-stage liver disease. Therapies such as vasopressors do not improve survival. Hepatic encephalopathy results from failure of the liver to metabolize toxic agents, most commonly ammonia. Other causes are alkalosis, hypokalemia, hypovolemia secondary to paracentesis, and hepatic or systemic infections. Treatment can be offered with restricted protein intake and lactulose, 30 mL three to four times daily, which acidifies colonic flora thereby decreasing the uptake of ammonium. The dose should be titrated to produce two or three soft stools per day. Neomycin sulfate is an alternative to lactulose.

NOTES AND PEARLS

To assess the degree of liver injury, look for albumin less than 3 g/dL or an increased prothrombin time of 11 to 16 s. Do not rely on the levels of AST since they do not correlate with the degree of injury. The typical patient with cirrhosis has on a daily basis consumed a pint or more of whiskey, several quarts of wine, or an equivalent amount of beer for at least 10 years.

BIBLIOGRAPHY

Dindzans VJ: Cirrhosis, in *Kochar's Concise Textbook of Medicine,* 3d ed, K Kutty (ed). Baltimore, Williams & Wilkins, 1998, pp 484–489.

Friedman LS; Cirrhosis, in *Current Medical Diagnosis and Treatment,* 39th ed, LM Tierney et al (eds). New York, McGraw-Hill, 2000, pp 671–679.

Friedman LS: Alcoholic liver disease, cirrhosis, and its major sequelae, in *Cecil Textbook of Medicine,* 21st ed, L Goldman, JC Bennett (eds). Philadelphia, W.B. Saunders, 2000, pp 804–816.

Podolsky DK, Isselbacher KJ: Cirrhosis and alcoholic liver disease, in *Harrison's Principles of Internal Medicine,* 14th ed, AS Fauci et al (eds). New York, McGraw-Hill, 1998, pp 1704–1717.

Rosenberg PM, Friedman LS: Cirrhosis, in *Conn's Current Therapy,* RE Rakel (ed). Philadelphia, W.B. Saunders, 1999, pp 460–472.

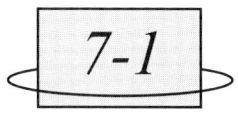

CYSTIC FIBROSIS (MUCOVISCIDOSIS)

William A. Mosier

DISCUSSION

Cystic fibrosis (CF) is the most common debilitating autosomal recessive disease that presents in persons of white European ancestry. It has been estimated that 30,000 Americans are afflicted with this lethal condition. It occurs in over 1 in every 2500 live births. An estimated 4 percent of white people (about 9 million Americans) are carriers of the defective gene. Approximately 1200 new cases of CF are diagnosed annually in the United States. CF usually manifests within the first year of life. The respiratory tract is the organ system that generally determines the prognosis and survival of a CF patient. However, 90 percent of patients with CF also have pancreatic insufficiency and require pancreatic enzyme supplements. Most patients with CF have severe difficulty breathing and maintaining a clear airway. In fact, respiratory tract involvement is responsible for over 90 percent of the morbidity rate of CF. The median survival of patients with CF is only 30 years.

PATHOGENESIS

CF is a genetic-based protein defect. The disease consists of a defect in the protein product of the CF gene called the cystic fibrosis transmembrane conductance regulator (CFTR). The CF gene is a relatively large gene on chromosome 7 that encodes a protein containing 1480 amino acids. The CF gene has 27 subregions (exons) that code for the processed messenger ribonucleic acid (mRNA), which in turn is translated into the protein CFTR. The basic biochemical defect in CF is an abnormality of chloride ion (Cl^-) transport across airway epithelial cells. It has been hypothesized that there is an impaired ability of airway cells to secrete Cl^- through CFTR. CFTR serves as a Cl^- channel in response to cyclic 3′,5′-adenosine monophosphate (cAMP)-mediated secretagogues. An enhanced rate of sodium ion (Na^+) absorption also occurs as a result of increased amiloride-sensitive Na^+ conductance on the luminal membrane and increased Na^+, K^+-ATPase sites on the basolateral membrane. The result is a water imbalance caused by this decreased Cl^- permeability and excessive Na^+ reabsorption. The resulting electrolyte and transport abnormality leads to abnormal airway secretions, impaired mucociliary clearance, and persistent airway infections (predominantly bacterial). Human alveolar macrophage (AM)-derived cytokines are the key to the pathogenesis.

MICROBIOLOGY

The persistent infections that occur with CF cause neutrophils to migrate to the sites of infection. Neutrophils release large amounts of the viscous polyanion deoxyribonucleic acid (DNA) and actin during their routine disintegration. The lysosomal protein elastase also is released at this time. The DNA is present in CF sputum at a concentration of approximately 1 to 15 mg/mL. The DNA, actin, and elastase debris then mix with already present airway secretions. The secretions are retained because of apparently impaired mucociliary clearance in patients with CF. The secretions display increased viscosity and elasticity and decreased pourability. These properties tend to hinder the

upward flow of respiratory tract secretions and inhibit the patient's ability to expectorate sputum. Thus, these secretions are associated with airway obstruction, shortness of breath, and exacerbation of infections. This process also causes an increase in the inflammatory response, which leads to a vicious cycle of further accumulation of leukocyte-derived debris mixing with airway secretions, resulting in more airway obstruction. The retention of these secretions in the airways predisposes CF patients to persistent *Staphylococcus aureus, Pseudomonas aeruginosa,* and *Haemophilus influenzae* infections. Once *P. aeruginosa* becomes established in the lungs of a patient with CF, it is extremely difficult to eradicate. Progressive lung destruction can then result in bronchiectasis, respiratory failure, and eventually premature death. The fungal pathogens found in CF are *Candida* and *Aspergillus* spp. Other gram-negative pathogens occasionally are isolated from CF cultures, including *Escherichia coli,* other *Pseudomonas* spp., and *Klebsiella, Proteus, Enterobacter,* and *Citrobacter* spp. Rarely, *Burkholderia cepacia* may appear. In addition to bacteria, some viruses have been responsible for respiratory tract infections in CF patients, most notably respiratory syncytial virus (RSV) and influenza A virus.

SYMPTOMS

The most common symptoms are chronic cough with sputum production and dyspnea. Symptoms observable in infants include foul-smelling fatty stools, severe constipation in a newborn, weight loss, wheezing, and a salty taste on a baby's skin. The salty taste is due to the blockage of chloride channels, which causes the abnormal sodium balance, resulting in a discharge of excess sodium excreted through the pores. Flatulence also may be a prominent symptom. The typical patient with CF will have 9 days of hospitalization annually related to CF complications from exacerbation of respiratory tract infections.

OBJECTIVE FINDINGS

CF can have varying clinical manifestations. The initial findings in 10 percent of newborns with CF are intestinal obstruction and meconium ileus. The mortality rate among these infants is 20 to 60 percent. Meconium from babies with CF is high in albumin and lactase and is extremely viscous. The first signs are usually a persistent cough and wheezing with a rapid respiratory rate. Gagging, vomiting, and difficulty sleeping as well as recurring respiratory infections are suggestive of CF. Failure to gain weight and the passage of large, frequent bowel movements in association with an excessive appetite are also characteristic features in early childhood (see Table 7-1-1).

DIAGNOSTIC CONSIDERATIONS

Although most cases of CF are diagnosed in childhood, 20 percent of CF patients are not diagnosed until after age 15. Therefore, any young adult who presents with interstitial infiltrates plus chronic sinopulmonary infections with a mucoid variant of *P. aeruginosa,* bronchiectasis, symptoms of asthma, unexplained gastrointestinal complaints, or a family history of similar complaints should receive a sweat chloride test. Rare alternative diagnoses that may be confused with CF on chest radiography include eosinophilic granuloma and lymphangiomyomatosis.

TABLE 7-1-1. Clinical Manifestations of Cystic Fibrosis

Respiratory tract complications
   Viscous secretions causing small duct obstruction
   Bronchitis
   Sinusitis
   Atelectasis
   Emphysema
   Bronchopneumonia
   Bronchiectasis
   Lung abscesses
   Aspergillosis
   Nasal polyposis
   Hemoptysis
   Pneumothorax
   Pulmonary hypertension
   Cor pulmonale
   Respiratory failure

Pancreatic complications
   Steatorrhea
   Deficiencies of vitamins A, D, E, and K
   Diabetes mellitus
   Pancreatic calcifications
   Nutritional and growth failure

Intestinal complications
   Delayed meconium passage at birth
   Peritonitis
   Meconium ileus
   Volvulus
   Ileal atresia
   Rectal prolapse
   Intussusception
   Fecal impaction
   Pneumatosis intestinalis

Hepatobiliary complications
   Mucus hypersecretion
   Cholelithiasis
   Loss of bile salts
   Bile plugging of ductules
   Portal hypertension
   Esophageal varices
   Hypersplenism
   Atrophic gallbladder
   Cirrhosis

Skeletal complications
   Demineralization
   Hypertrophic osteoarthropathy
   Bone retardation

Reproductive system
   Males: sterility and absence of vas deferens, epididymis,
      and seminal vesicles
   Females: decreased fertility, increased viscosity of vaginal secretions

Miscellaneous complications
   Salt depletion
   Heat stroke
   Salivary gland hypertrophy
   Retinal hemorrhage
   Apocrine gland hypertrophy

SPECIAL CONSIDERATIONS

Malabsorption leading to malnutrition is a complication of considerable importance in CF. Because of mucus plugs in the pancreas that block pancreatic enzymes from passing into the small intestine, undigested food passes out of the body in the stool. To control this problem, digestive enzymes must be taken daily as supplements.

LABORATORY TESTS

To confirm the diagnosis of CF, a sweat test with pilocarpine iontophoresis is performed. Sweat chloride concentrations exceeding 60 meq/L are found in 98 percent of patients with CF. A level of 60 meq/L confirms the diagnosis in patients under age 20 years. A value of 80 meq/L is required for the diagnosis in persons age 20 years or older. Gene testing can be used to clarify the diagnosis in equivocal cases or when it is not possible to obtain an adequate sweat collection.

RADIOLOGIC STUDIES

A chest x-ray containing diffusely increased markings with cystic spaces, upper lobe predominance, and hyperinflation is highly characteristic of CF.

OTHER DIAGNOSTICS

Imaging procedures, including magnetic resonance imaging (MRI), computed tomography (CT), and ultrasonography, are useful for identifying pancreatic abnormalities in CF patients. They also can be useful in identifying liver complications.

TREATMENT

The standard of care for CF includes chest physical therapy (CPT), a procedure in which the patient's chest is pounded on to mechanically dislodge lung secretions; enzyme therapy; and antibiotic therapy (see Table 7-1-2).

Medications

Current treatment includes the utilization of medications to hydrolyze extracellular DNA to improve the clearance of airway secretions. Deoxyribonuclease I (DNase) is a naturally occurring enzyme produced by the pancreas and salivary glands that is responsible for this function. Recombinant human DNase I (rhDNase) has been cloned from human pancreatic complementary DNA (cDNA) to be used as a treatment to alter sputum viscoelasticity and improve the clearance of secretions. This medication is referred to commercially as dornase alfa (Pulmozyme). This drug improves forced expiratory volume in 1 second (FEV_1) and helps decrease dyspnea. Its use also has been shown to reduce cough, congestion, and the frequency of respiratory infections. It is available in single-use ampules administered by nebulizer. A typical starting dose is 2.5 mg a day. Possible side effects related to aerosol use include chest pain, dyspepsia, facial edema, laryngitis, pharyngitis, rash, conjunctivitis, and hoarseness. However, these adverse effects are uncommon, mild, and self-limiting.

Another important mainstay of treatment is replacement therapy with pancreatic enzyme preparations, preferably in the form of enteric-coated microspheres. The enzymes are taken with meals and snacks. The enzymes provide only partial relief from maldigestion and

TABLE 7-1-2. Goals of CF Treatment

Improve lung function
Reduce respiratory symptoms
Delay bronchiectasis
Reduce frequency of exacerbations of respiratory tract infections
Reduce use of parenteral antibiotics
Optimize patient's sense of well-being
Minimize number of lost school and/or work days caused by CF-related illness

diarrhea. Doses vary with the age and weight of the patient, the severity of the deficiency, and the contents of a meal. High doses of the enzymes are associated with an increased risk of uricosuria.

Chronic endobronchial infection with *P. aeruginosa* is a major cause of morbidity and mortality in CF patients. Therefore, antibiotic therapy is aimed at controlling its progression. Because *P. aeruginosa* rarely is eradicated once it is established, the chronic production of immune mediators tends to result in a slow progression of the lung disease. For this reason, the efficacy of current antibiotics is limited. Multi-drug-resistant *P. aeruginosa* is a consequence of frequent and prolonged antibiotic therapy. Slowing the emergence of resistance by pairing antibiotics from different classes has been tried with some success. Oral ciprofloxacin plus aerosolized colistin may reduce chronic infection. However, this has not been confirmed in controlled trials. Short-term, high-dose aerosol administration of tobramycin in patients with clinically stable CF has proved to be an efficacious and safe treatment for endobronchial infection with *P. aeruginosa*. Additional drug therapy includes bronchodilators and anti-inflammatory agents such as inhaled corticosteroids, ibuprofen, and antipseudomonal intravenous immunoglobulin (IVIG).

SUPPORTIVE MEASURES

Airway clearance techniques (ACTs), also referred to as CPT, are the primary nonpharmacologic therapies for clearing airway secretions and improving pulmonary function in patients with CF. Although anti-inflammatory agents may aid in reducing inflammation, the physical removal of purulent secretions appears to be more effective in slowing the progression of CF airway disease. Therefore, ACTs are essential for the preservation of pulmonary function in CF patients. However, because traditional CPT can be uncomfortable, alternative ACTs are available, including the following:

* High-frequency chest percussors (such as inflatable vests) that deliver compression pulses to the chest
* Oral oscillators
* Masks used to deliver back pressure to the lungs during expiration

These therapies can combine controlled breathing, autogenic drainage, and a positive expiratory pressure to facilitate airway clearance. Physical exercise is also a valuable adjunct to ACTs in prolonging pulmonary function and improving a patient's quality of life.

Nutritional support and diet therapy are of vital importance in the overall treatment program for CF patients. Because of the malabsorption, the diet should include sufficient calories and protein to provide for normal growth. This usually includes a higher than normal total fat intake to increase the caloric density of the diet. Taking multivitamin and mineral supplements in megadoses, especially the lipid-soluble vitamins such as vitamin E, is usually necessary. Salt supplements during periods of thermal stress or increased sweating also are advised. Great attention must be paid to emotional support issues. CF care centers are available in many communities to implement the specialized care required.

PATIENT EDUCATION

Families should be encouraged to seek a CF support group. These support groups can provide valuable self-help information for both parents and victims of CF. The Cystic Fibrosis Foundation is located at 6931 Arlington Road, Suite 2000, Bethesda, MD 20814, (800) 344-4823. The foundation can be accessed on the Internet at www.cff.org. A wealth of material for families facing this debilitating disease is readily available from the foundation. If there is a family history of CF, couples should be referred for genetic counseling before attempting a pregnancy. Accurate prenatal diagnosis and carrier detection have been available since 1985. Gene testing

can be performed to determine the relationship between genotype and phenotype. Because most patients with CF have digestive problems, nutrition support services must be provided.

DISPOSITION

Diffuse bronchiectasis leading to pulmonary hypertension and its complications are the typical terminal events. The only curative therapy currently available for end-stage bronchiectasis resulting from CF is lung transplantation.

COMPLICATIONS AND RED FLAGS

Two important complications of lower respiratory tract involvement in patients with CF that must be watched for are hemoptysis and pneumothorax. Although antibiotic therapy often is able to eradicate *S. aureus, H. influenzae,* and other bacteria from the respiratory tract, it seldom is able to permanently clear *P. aeruginosa* from the endobronchial space. Because of this resistance, a pulmonary consultation is strongly advised at the first sign of pneumonia.

OTHER NOTES AND PEARLS

In the future, the possibility of recombinant CFTR replacement therapy and recombinant CF gene therapy may allow correction of the basic disease mechanism. Testing is being done using the potassium-sparing diuretic amiloride to block the uptake of sodium ions in airway epithelia. This may suppress the inflammatory milieu in the distal airways of CF patients through its action on AM-derived cytokines, reducing the subsequent injury caused during the release of neutrophil-derived products. Studies are under way using uridine triphosphate (UTP) to induce chloride ion efflux via aerosolized nucleotides. The current strategy in gene therapy for CF is to use recombinant adenoviruses, adeno-associated virus, and liposomes as gene delivery methods. The plasma protein gelsolin, which severs actin filaments, also is being explored as a mucolytic agent. Anti-inflammatory therapy research is under way to study the role of pentoxifylline and antiproteases in the treatment of CF. Investigators also are studying the feasibility of an antipseudomonal vaccine.

BIBLIOGRAPHY

Aitken ML: Cystic fibrosis, in Kelley WN (ed.): *Textbook of Internal Medicine,* 3d ed. Philadelphia, Lippincott-Raven 1997, pp 2002–2007.

Cystic Fibrosis Foundation: Cystic fibrosis—what you should know. Bethesda, MD, Cystic Fibrosis Foundation, 1999.

Hodson ME: Aerosolized dornase alfa (rhDNase) for therapy of cystic fibrosis. *Am J Respir Crit Care Med* 151:S70–S74, 1995.

Knowies MR, Olivier K, Noone P, Boucher RC: Pharmacologic modulation of salt and water in the airway epithelium in cystic fibrosis. *Am J Respir Crit Care Med* 151:S65–S69, 1995.

Schuster A, Fahy JV, Ueki I, Nadel JA: Cystic fibrosis sputum induces a secretory response from airway gland serous cells that can be prevented by neutrophil protease inhibitors. *Eur Respir J* 8:10–14, 1995.

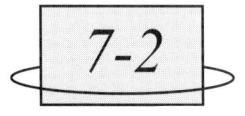

HUMAN GENETIC DISORDERS

Virginia Schneider and Pamela Plotner

DISCUSSION

Investigations into the genetic basis of human disease are on the threshold of revolutionizing the understanding of the pathophysiology and treatment of common and uncommon disorders. Increasingly, knowledge of the basic terms of genetics and the ability to evaluate a

TABLE 7-2-1.   Common Genetic Terms

Malformation	Poor tissue formation and associated defects
Deformation	Normal tissue acted on by mechanical forces
Disruption	Normal tissue acted on by a destructive force
Dysplasia	Lack of normal cellular organization resulting in abnormal tissue formation
Pedigree	A schematic representation of the family history indicating sex, age, and health status of relatives of proband
Genome	All the genes carried by a single gamete, individual, population, or species; the human genome consists of 44 autosomes, 2 sex chromosomes, and the mitochondrial DNA
Karyotype	The chromosomal constitution; also refers to the pictorial arrangement of matched pairs of chromosomes
Genotype	The actual genetic makeup of an individual
Phenotype	External appearance of an individual; produced by genotype interacting with environment
Syndrome	A group of malformations resulting from a single etiology, e.g., chromosomal disorders, single-gene defects, teratogens
Association	A group of malformations frequently found together, e.g., VACTERL, CHARGE, MURCS
Sequence	A group of malformations that arise secondary to initial malformation, e.g., Potter sequence, cleft lip sequence, holoprosencephaly sequence
Multifactorial	More than one factor responsible for the appearance of a trait; genetic and environmental influences acting together
Autosomal dominant	A trait that is produced by one allele regardless of the allele on the homologous chromosome; family histories often show the condition in successive generations, equally expressed in males and females; severity of the condition and/or symptoms may vary considerably even among family members
Autosomal recessive	A trait that is produced only when an allele is present in a homozygous state; the allele has no effect in the presence of a dominant allele (heterozygous state); family histories sometimes show siblings but not parents affected, and patients sometimes have parents who are genetically (blood) related.
Sex-linked trait	A trait carried on the X chromosome; family histories often show multiple affected males related through their mothers or sisters; females usually are not affected
Heterozygous	The occurrence of two different alleles at the same chromosome locus
Homozygous	The occurrence of identical alleles at the same chromosome locus

patient for potential genetic defects are becoming essential to primary care providers. This chapter will familiarize the reader with fundamental concepts and provide references to more complete sources of information about genetic diseases. Genetic disorders generally can be grouped into the categories of chromosomal disorders, monogenic disorders (autosomal dominant, autosomal recessive, and sex-linked disorders), mitochondrial disorders, and multifactorial disorders. The terminology commonly used in genetics is defined in Table 7-2-1.

HISTORY

The features of genetic disease may be obvious or subtle. While often first noted in infancy and childhood, genetic abnormalities may go undiagnosed into adulthood. A family history of genetic disease, a family history of unusual patterns of disability or death, developmental problems, sensory deficits, and abnormalities on physical examination are important clues to the possible presence of a genetic disorder.

A careful history is the place to begin with any patient suspected of having a genetic abnormality. The pregnancy and birth history are most important when the affected individual is an infant or child. The caregiver should be questioned in detail about the course of the pregnancy and any illnesses, complications, or memorable events. These questions generate information about the intrauterine environment and the early physical state of the patient and help differentiate genetic disease from similar findings of nongenetic origin. A wide variety of teratogens (see Table 7-2-2) lead to human malformations.

Vascular accidents and fetal movement may result in disruptions when a strand of amnion becomes wrapped around a limb, causing an intrauterine amputation. Uterine constraints caused by uterine fibroids or a bicornate uterus can result in fetal deformations. Birth trauma may cause anomalies (Erb's palsy) or result from an underlying disorder (hydrocephalus).

A family history is helpful in delineating inheritance patterns. A pedigree is a pictorial outline of the family history (see Table 7-2-3). By displaying the information in the form of a pedigree, one can easily find affected family members and their degree of relatedness. The

TABLE 7-2-2.   Common Teratogens

DRUGS	INFECTIONS	ENVIRONMENT	MATERNAL CONDITIONS
Alcohol	Toxoplasmosis	Radiation	Diabetes
Lithium	Rubella	Lead	Phenylketonuria
Antiepileptic drugs	Cytomegalovirus	Mercury	
Retin A	Herpes	Iodine	
Coumadin	HIV	Carbon monoxide	
Thalidomide	Syphilis		

TABLE 7-2-3.   Pedigree–Common Abbreviations

□	Normal male
○	Normal female
○—□	Normal mating
○=□	Consanguineous mating
■	Individual affected by the trait or disease
◧ ◑	Heterozygote
/	Deceased

TABLE 7-2-4. Family History

Pregnancy and birth
Infections
Drugs
Uterine constraint
Gestational age at delivery
Other family members with similar problem
Consanguinity
Neonatal deaths, stillbirths, miscarriages
Mental retardation, seizures, blindness, deafness
Heart defects, bleeding disorders
Stature, bone defects, musculoskeletal problems

family history should contain at least three generations. Table 7-2-4 outlines important issues in the family history.

PHYSICAL EXAMINATION

Assessment of the patient should include measurement of the height, weight, and frontooccipital circumference and a thorough physical examination for major and minor abnormalities. Major malformations are those which have a significant effect on the patient's life (see Table 7-2-5); minor malformations are more cosmetic defects (see Table 7-2-6).

Identification of a minor malformation should alert the practitioner to examine the patient closely for other malformations; if several minor malformations are found, a search should be made for major malformations (see Fig. 7-2-1).

In addition to specific physical defects, developmental problems and sensory deficits may be significant features of genetic disease. A review of the child's development, social skills, and school history should be made, looking for delays in achieving normal milestones, autism, attention disorders, learning disabilities, and retardation. Major regression from prior abilities is significant. A history of poor growth velocity, failure to thrive, and poor muscle tone also are significant. Hearing loss and early or severe visual problems may be consistent with genetic disease. Sensory, developmental, and intellectual testing may be helpful.

DIAGNOSTICS

You may wish to begin the laboratory assessment or defer this portion of the evaluation to a geneticist, depending on the type of problem

TABLE 7-2-5. Major Malformations

Cataracts
Cleft lip and/or palate
Contractures
Congenital heart defects
Diaphragmatic hernia
Gastroschisis
Genital malformations
Hydrocephalus
Microcephaly
Microphthalmia
Missing digits or limbs
Meningomyelocele
Omphalocele
Renal malformations

TABLE 7-2-6. Minor Malformations

Ear pits and/or tags
Unusually shaped ears
Downslanting eyes
Epicanthal folds
Upslanting eyes
Hypo- or hypertelorism
Facial asymmetry
Hirsutism
White forelock or other hair patch
Abnormal teeth
Smooth philtrum
Micrognathia
Thin upper lip
Hyperextensible joints
Short or tall stature
Syndactyly
Polydactyly
Portwine nevus
Nevi

suspected and the availability of consultants. Typical initial studies to consider include a complete blood count, electrolytes, liver function studies, specific hormone assays (e.g., thyroid function), urinalysis, serum amino acids, urine organic acids, and radiographic tests such as echocardiography, simple radiographs, and ultrasound. Specific genetic tests and their indications are listed in Table 7-2-7.

While the presentation of most genetic diseases is nonemergent, occasionally a quick diagnosis is essential. Particularly keep in mind an infant who presents with symptoms similar to bacterial sepsis after several days of life. This is the typical timing and presentation of genetic metabolic abnormalities such as a urea cycle defect. Abnormal serum ammonia or lactic acid levels will point to the diagnosis quickly.

TABLE 7-2-7. Genetic Testing

1. Karyotype: test a primary care provider is most likely to order during genetic evaluation
   Indications
       Known or suspected chromosome abnormality
       Multiple congenital anomalies, especially when associated with growth and/or mental retardation
       Disorder of sexual differentiation
       Undiagnosed mental retardation
       Selected hematologic malignancies and diseases associated with chromosome instability
       Multiple miscarriages

2. FISH (fluorescence in situ hybridization) analysis
   Fluorescently tagged nucleic acid probes used to identify chromosomes and loci can detect microdeletions, duplications, and chromosome fragments; also can be used for gene mapping

3. Molecular analysis
   Used for detection of known point mutations, small insertions, or deletions; also used for detection of larger insertions, expansions, deletions, or other major structural rearrangements

4. Protein analysis: Chromatography, electrophoresis, Western blots
   Used for detection of known protein abnormalities such as sickle hemoglobin

**Frequency of major malformations versus
number of minor malformations**

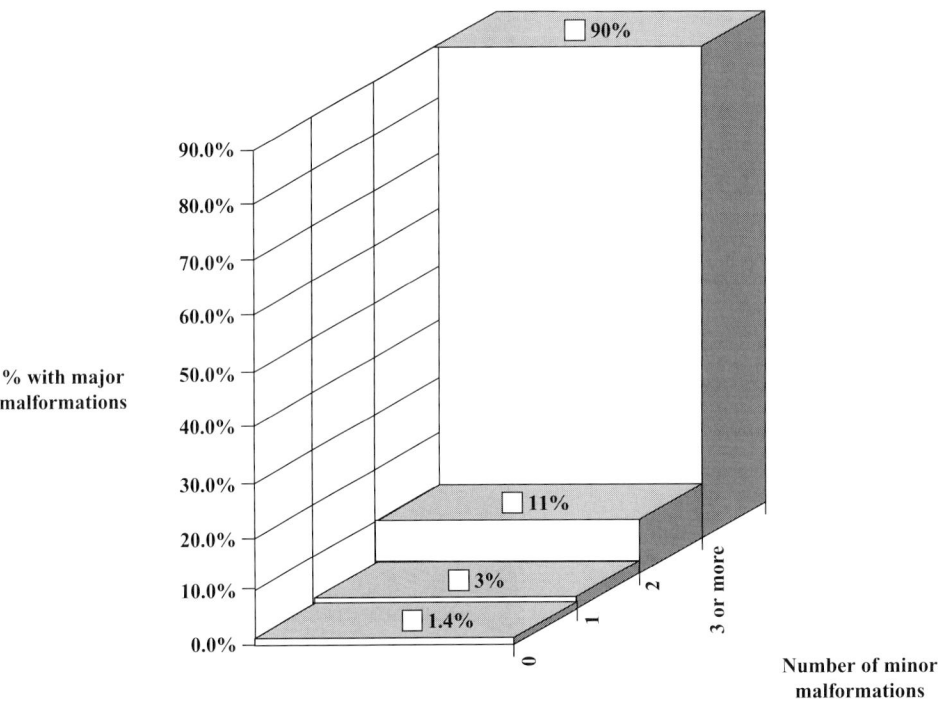

FIGURE 7-2-1. Association between minor and major malformations. (*Adapted from Jones K L: Smith's Recognizable Patterns of Human Malformation, 5th ed. Philadelphia, Saunders, 1988.*)

MAJOR SYNDROMES

The spectrum of known syndromes associated with genetic defects is expanding constantly as new links are identified. A careful history and a physical examination remain the foundation for diagnosis. It is beyond the scope of this chapter to outline all the major genetic defects and their management. Presented here are those most commonly encountered in primary care practice.

Your first job may be to help a family cope with the diagnosis of a genetic disorder in its child. As in dealing with any family whose child has a chronic condition, frequent visits in the beginning lend reassurance and support. Social and family support systems are critical. Support groups and information resources exist for many major and minor genetic syndromes and are invaluable to both parents and practitioners. As the patient grows, resources for education, employment, and adult day care may become an issue about which the practitioner will be asked for guidance.

Chronic care of a patient affected by a genetic disorder is multifactorial. Children with genetic syndromes often grow at rates different from those of their normal counterparts. Special growth charts are available to monitor growth in children with most major syndromes. Besides routine health monitoring, it is important to be aware of the special health problems that are more likely to occur among those with specific syndromes. For example, children with Down syndrome are more likely to develop hypothyroidism and must be monitored for its appearance.

CHROMOSOMAL ABNORMALITIES

Down Syndrome (47 Chromosomes, +21)

The incidence is 1 in 770 births.

COMMON FEATURES

a. Face	b. Eyes	c. Hands and Feet
• Flat occiput	• Upslanting palpebral fissures	• Brachydactyly
• Flat midface	• Epicanthal folds	• Clinodactyly
	• Brushfield spots	• Transverse palmar crease

d. Gastrointestinal	e. Heart Defects	f. Central Nervous System
• Atresias	• Ventricular septal defect	• Hypotonia
	• Tetralogy of Fallot	• Mental retardation
	• Atrioventricular canal	

HEALTH MAINTENANCE ISSUES

a. Increased risk of acute lymphocytic leukemia and hypothyroidism
b. Alantoaxial instability (12 to 20 percent)
c. Mental retardation (IQ usually 25 to 50)
d. Reduced life expectancy

Turner Syndrome (45 Chromosomes, X only)

The incidence is 1 in 2500 liveborn females (2 percent of conceptions, of which >95 percent do not reach term).

COMMON FEATURES

a. Poorly Developed Lymphatics	b. Heart Defects	c. Endocrine
• Lymphedema	• Coarctation	• Short stature
• Cystic hygroma	• Dilated aortic root	• Amenorrhea
• Increased neck folds		• Premature ovarian failure

d. Central Nervous System
- Average IQ
- May have nonverbal difficulties
- May have visual/spatial difficulties

e. Other
- Increased carrying angle of arms
- Broad shield-like chest
- Low posterior hairline

HEALTH MAINTENANCE ISSUES

a. Estrogen for primary amenorrhea and delayed puberty
b. Growth hormone for growth delay
c. Infertility issues and premature menopause
d. Removal of gonadal tissue (increased risk of tumors)
e. Increased incidence of thyroiditis, diabetes, and collagen vascular disease

AUTOSOMAL RECESSIVE DISORDERS

Cystic Fibrosis

a. Most common lethal genetic illness among Caucasians
b. 1 in 25 carrier rate, incidence 1 in 2000 to 2500 births in Caucasians
c. Caused by a defective chloride channel

COMMON FEATURES

a. Pulmonary
- Chronic and/or recurrent upper and lower respiratory infections
- Progressive chronic obstructive lung disease

b. Gastrointestinal
- Pancreatic deficiency
- Malabsorption with failure to thrive
- Meconium ileus

c. Other
- Sweat gland dysfunction

HEALTH MAINTENANCE ISSUES

a. Oral pancreatic enzyme replacement
b. Monitor for type 1 diabetes mellitus
c. Chest physical therapy, routine pulmonary function tests (PFT)
d. Coverage for *Pseudomonas* when ill
e. Influenza immunization
f. Management of associated problems (hyponatremia, rectal prolapse, nasal polyps, sinusitis, ileal obstruction, hemoptysis)

Sickle Cell Anemia

a. A disorder of hemoglobin structure and red blood cell morphology (see Chap. 8-3)
b. 1 in 12 carrier rate in African-Americans; prevalence is 1 in 600.

COMMON FEATURES

a. Anemia and heart failure
b. Sepsis caused by encapsulated bacteria (strep, salmonella)
c. Cerebral infarction in early childhood
d. Septicemia and meningitis in infancy
e. Splenic autoinfarction
f. Pain crisis, dactylitis, priapism
g. Acute chest syndromes

HEALTH MAINTENANCE ISSUES

a. Folic acid, penicillin, pneumococcal vaccine
b. Medic-Alert bracelet
c. Pain management (Tylenol with codeine, morphine)
d. History and physical, complete blood count and reticulocyte count, and education twice a year
e. UA, chemistries, serology, oxygen saturation once a year

f. Baseline hemoglobin typing, electrocardiogram, echocardiogram, and PFT
g. Ophthalmology every 1 to 2 years
h. Gallbladder ultrasound as required

AUTOSOMAL DOMINANT DISORDERS

Marfan Syndrome

a. Disorder of connective tissue (fibrillin gene mutation).
b. Prevalence is 1 in 10,000 in the United States.
c. About 25 percent of cases arise as a new mutation.

COMMON FEATURES

a. Skeletal
- Pectus carinatum or excavatum
- Reduced ratio of upper to lower segments
- Arm span–to–height ratio >1.05
- Wrist and thumb signs
- Scoliosis >20 degrees or spondylolisthesis

b. Ocular
- Ectopia lentis

c. Cardiovascular
- Dilation of ascending aorta
- Mitral valve prolapse

d. Pulmonary
- Spontaneous pneumothorax

HEALTH MAINTENANCE ISSUES

a. Routine review of growth and orthopedic abnormalities
b. Blood pressure monitoring and baseline and routine echocardiograms
c. Beta blockers to slow aortic dilatation and decrease risk of dissection
d. Routine ophthalmologic exams

Neurofibromatosis

a. A neurocutaneous disorder.
b. Prevalence is 1 in 3000.
c. About 50 percent of cases are due to new mutations.

COMMON FEATURES

a. >6 café-au-lait spots of specific size
b. Axillary or inguinal freckling
c. Optic glioma
d. First-degree relative with neurofibromatosis

HEALTH MAINTENANCE ISSUES

a. Routine ophthalmologic, neurologic, developmental, and orthopedic examinations
b. Blood pressure monitoring
c. Monitoring of lesions for malignant changes

SEX-LINKED DISORDERS

Fragile X Syndrome

a. Most common hereditary cause of mental retardation.
b. Prevalence is 1 in 1250 to 2500 males.

COMMON FEATURES

a. Developmental delay or mental retardation (IQ 30 to 65)
b. Abnormal behavioral patterns
c. Large, protuberant, slightly dysmorphic ears
d. Prominent forehead; long, thin face; prominent jaw
e. Mitral valve prolapse
f. Macroorchidism

HEALTH MAINTENANCE ISSUES
a. Routine ophthalmology and cardiac examinations
b. Counseling
c. Developmental intervention
d. Medical treatment of hyperactivity and autistic features

SUMMARY

Whether caring for infants, children, or adults, practitioners must be alert to clues to the presence of genetic disease. A high index of suspicion, a careful history and physical examination, and judicious testing are the keys to diagnosis. Identification of genetic disease is important not only for the individual but in regard to counseling for prevention in future generations. A significant portion of the genetic evaluation can be carried out by the primary care provider, and referral can be made to a genetic specialist for ultimate diagnosis and counseling. Regardless, it is the primary care provider who will be responsible for ongoing care for the special medical and social needs of these patients. The information in this chapter and the resources provided below are intended to help you provide the best possible care for your patients.

ACKNOWLEDGMENT

The author would like to acknowledge Pamela Plotner for her assistance in preparing this chapter.

BIBLIOGRAPHY

Counseling Aids for Geneticists, 3d ed. Greenwood, SC, Greenwood Genetic Center, 1995.
Growth References: Third Trimester to Adulthood. Greenwood, SC, Greenwood Genetic Center, 1998.
Jackson PL, Vessey JA: *Primary Care of the Child with a Chronic Condition,* 2d ed. St. Louis, Mosby Year Book, 1996.
Jones KL: *Smith's Recognizable Patterns of Human Malformation,* 4th ed. Philadelphia, Saunders, 1988.
Scriver CR, Beaudet AL, Sly WS, et al: *The Metabolic and Molecular Bases of Inherited Disease,* vols. I, II, and III, 7th ed. New York, McGraw-Hill, 1995.
Thomas D, Collins FS, Ginsburg D: *Principles of Medical Genetics,* 2d ed. Baltimore, Williams & Wilkins, 1998.
Toomey KE: Medical genetics for the practitioner. *Pediatr Rev* 17(5):163–174, 1996.

Web Sites

NORD (National Organization of Rare Disorders): http://www.rarediseases.org
Online Mendelian Inheritance in Man (OMIM): http://www3.ncbi.nlm.nih.gov/Omim

American Academy of Pediatrics Committee on Genetics Clinical Guidelines

Health supervision for children with achondroplasia. *Pediatrics* 95(3):443–451, 1995.
Health supervision for children with Down syndrome. *Pediatrics* 93(5):855–859, 1994.
Health supervision for children with fragile X syndrome. *Pediatrics* 98(2, part 1), 1996.
Health supervision for children with Marfan syndrome. *Pediatrics* 98(5):978–982, 1996.
Health supervision for children with neurofibromatosis. *Pediatrics* 96(2, part 1):368–372, 1995.
Health supervision for children with sickle cell diseases and their families *Pediatrics* 98(3, part 1):467–472, 1996.
Health supervision for children with Turner syndrome. *Pediatrics* 96(6):1166–1173, 1995.

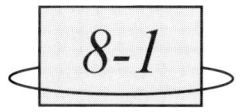

IRON-DEFICIENCY ANEMIA

JoAnn Deasy

DISCUSSION

Iron-deficiency anemia (IDA) occurs when the body's iron supply is inadequate to meet the iron requirement of red blood cells (RBCs) and body tissues. RBCs are responsible for oxygen transport and can be thought of as containers for hemoglobin. The hemoglobin molecule in an RBC releases oxygen to body tissues. The nutritional factors necessary for an RBC to go through proliferation and maturation in bone marrow are iron, folic acid, and vitamin B_{12}. Iron and protoporphyrin form the heme portion of the hemoglobin molecule; globin is the protein portion of the molecule.

The most immature RBC in the bone marrow is the pronormoblast. It divides and matures through various stages, forming the nucleated red blood cell (NRBC) in the bone marrow. The nucleus of this cell disintegrates, forming the immature RBC called the reticulocyte. Some reticulocytes are released into the bloodstream, where after 1 or 2 days they mature into RBCs. The reticulocyte count is an indicator of RBC productivity. An RBC has a life span of approximately 120 days. The spleen removes "old" RBCs.

A state of negative iron balance can first be detected by a low ferritin level that falls as iron stores are depleted. As long as some iron stores remain, other laboratory parameters remain in the normal range, including the serum iron level and transferrin (total iron-binding capacity). At this point, the hemoglobin level is normal and there is no change in red cell morphology. When all the iron stores are completely exhausted, serum iron becomes decreased, total iron-binding capacity rises, and the percent saturation falls. This state, when anemia has not yet developed, can be labeled iron-deficient erythropoiesis. The poor iron supply has an impact on developing RBCs, and finally iron-deficiency anemia develops.

Anemia is clinically defined as a reduction in hemoglobin or hematocrit concentration. Although normal values may vary with different laboratories, anemia is usually present when the hemoglobin is less than 14 g/dL in adult males, less than 12 g/dL in menstruating females, and less than 11 g/dL in pregnant women. In IDA, in addition to a lowered hemoglobin, RBCs become progressively microcytic and hypochromic. Microcytosis is defined as a mean corpuscular volume (MCV) less than 80 femtoliters. Iron-deficiency anemia is the most common cause of microcytic anemia.

PATHOGENESIS

The causes of IDA include blood loss, inadequate dietary intake, and inadequate absorption of iron. In adults, chronic blood loss is the most common cause. This most often results from gastrointestinal bleeding or menstrual loss. A diet deficient in iron is the most common cause in children. In infancy, a diet consisting predominantly of cow's milk may lead to IDA. After age 4 to 6 months, growth requirements are so great that without iron supplementation, iron deficiency is common. Later in childhood, as the caloric intake increases, the diet usually supplies an adequate amount of iron.

SYMPTOMS

The symptoms of IDA and anemias in general depend on the severity of the anemia, the abruptness of onset, age, and the ability of the body to compensate. Until the hemoglobin falls below 10 (hematocrit less than 30 percent), the patient usually does not experience any symptoms. With a hemoglobin level below 10 g/dL, the symptoms of IDA are nonspecific and common to anemia in general. They include fatigue and dyspnea on exertion, faintness, vertigo, palpitations, and a headache with exertion. In obtaining the patient's history, a detailed review of systems (ROS) is essential. The possibility of blood loss may be detected by a careful review of the gastrointestinal system and the menstrual and pregnancy history in females. In the ROS, information regarding frequent blood donations, recurring epistaxis, and toxic exposure also should be ascertained. The patient's nutritional habits, including alcohol intake, merit special attention. Patients with severe IDA may crave ice or, less frequently, have a sore mouth.

OBJECTIVE FINDINGS

Pallor is an indicator of anemia because mucous membranes and skin color reflect hemoglobin levels. In severe anemias, there is an increase in cardiac output, resulting in a rapid pulse and systolic murmur. With iron loss, there is shedding of epithelial cells. Epithelial atrophy results in signs that are specific to IDA: atrophic glossitis, cheilitis, and koilonychia (spooning).

A complete physical examination is necessary. Special attention should be paid to skin color and the color of the mucous membranes. Examinations of the conjunctiva, nail beds, and palmar creases of the hand are usually best for detecting pallor. In patients with severe IDA, the cardiac examination may reveal a forceful apical pulse, hyperactive heart sounds, and a systolic murmur. The abdominal examination and rectal examination with a test of occult blood in the feces are important, as is a pelvic examination in females.

DIFFERENTIAL DIAGNOSES

When microcytic anemia is present, the differential diagnosis includes IDA, thalassemia trait, anemia of chronic disease, sideroblastic anemia, lead poisoning, and copper deficiency (see Table 8-1-1).

DIAGNOSTIC STUDIES

A laboratory diagnosis is necessary to validate the diagnosis of IDA. The most important tests are the complete blood cell count (CBC) using an automated counter, the red cell morphology, and the evaluation of the iron supply by measuring the serum iron, the total iron-binding capacity (TIBC), and the serum ferritin. The CBC and red cell morphology yield a considerable amount of information. If anemia is present based on the hemoglobin level, the RBC indexes should first be examined. If microcytosis is present (MCV <80), IDA is a definite consideration. The mean corpuscular hemoglobin (MCH) usually moves in the same direction as the MCV. Pay attention to the red cell distribution width (RDW). The RDW is a parameter that expresses the degree of variation in cell size (anisocytosis). IDA results in small red blood cells whose size is highly variable; therefore, the RDW is elevated. The RDW discriminates IDA from thalassemia. With thalassemia,

Table 8-1-1. Differential Diagnosis of Microcytic Anemias

ANEMIA	MCV	RBC COUNT	RDW	SERUM FE	TIBC	FERRITIN
IDA	Low	Low	High	Low	High or normal	Low
Thalassemia	Low	Normal or high	Normal	High or normal	Normal	Normal or high
Chronic disease	Normal or low	Normal		Low	Low	Normal or high
Sideroblastic	Normal or low			Normal or high	Normal	High

NOTE: IDA = iron-deficiency anemia; MCV = mean corpuscular volume; RBC = red blood cell; RDW = red cell distribution width; TIBC = total iron-binding capacity.

the red cells are uniformly small and the RDW is normal. The tests needed to evaluate the iron status are serum iron, TIBC, and ferritin. As previously discussed, the serum ferritin, which measures iron stores, is the first measure to fall. This is followed by a decrease in serum iron and an elevation of TIBC. The measurement of serum iron reflects iron bound to serum proteins. Most iron is bound to transferrin. Normally, transferrin is about one-third saturated. Serum total iron-binding capacity represents an approximate estimate of serum transferrin. Bone marrow aspiration is not usually necessary to make the diagnosis of IDA, but if it is done, the bone marrow will reflect diminished iron stores.

Once the diagnosis of IDA is established, a search for the underlying cause must be undertaken. The history may indicate which further tests need to be done. In iron-deficient males and postmenopausal females, there is a strong possibility of occult bleeding from the gastrointestinal (GI) tract; therefore, endoscopic and possibly radiographic investigations of the GI tract should be done.

TREATMENT

Oral Route

This is the preferred treatment. Administer a ferrous iron salt (ferrous gluconate, sulfate, or fumarate or ferrous sulfate syrup) and calculate the dose according to the amount of elemental iron in the salt. For adults, administer 200 mg of elemental iron daily in three divided doses; for children, give 6 mg/kg of elemental iron daily in three divided doses. The maximum dose for children age 1 to 5 years is 45 mg/day, and for those age 6 to 12 years it is 120 mg/day. Most iron tablets contain 60 to 70 mg of elemental iron; thus, three tablets a day provide adequate iron therapy for an adult. Absorption is improved by taking the tablets between meals.

The most common side effect of iron therapy is GI intolerance, particularly heartburn, nausea, and gastric discomfort. If GI intolerance occurs, lower the dose of iron. Iron therapy should be continued until anemia is corrected and then for an additional 6 months to replenish iron stores. During therapy, stools are black.

Parenteral Iron

In situations where oral iron is ineffective because of malabsorption, parental iron can be administered in the form of iron dextran, which can be given by the intramuscular or intravenous (IV) routes. IV is the preferred route. The dosage (in milliliters) is based on the observed hemoglobin, the desired hemoglobin level, and the patient's lean body weight. A dosage chart comes with most product inserts. Anaphylaxis and other hypersensitivity reactions have been reported; therefore, parental iron should be used only when effective oral therapy is clearly impossible. As with oral iron, GI side effects are not uncommon.

Transfusion

Indications for transfusion require individual evaluation of the patient. Generally, persons with hemoglobin less than 6 g/dL require a blood transfusion. Patients with heart disease may require a transfusion at a higher hemoglobin measurement.

PATIENT EDUCATION

Instruct the patient about iron-rich foods. The patient should be informed about the possible causes of the IDA. If the patient is experiencing symptoms such as fatigue and depression, the clinician should tell the patient the extent to which the anemia accounts for the symptoms. In a person without heart disease, it is unlikely that these symptoms can be attributed to anemia unless the hemoglobin is below 10.

DISPOSITION

Unless bleeding is acute, appropriate follow-up consists of seeing the patient in 3 weeks to check on compliance and side effects from the iron therapy and to do a reticulocyte count and CBC. An increased reticulocyte count indicates a response to treatment. At 3 weeks, a 2-g increase in hemoglobin is an adequate response. Failure to respond may indicate continued bleeding, malabsorption of iron, noncompliance, or an incorrect diagnosis. The CBC must be monitored at frequent intervals until the anemia is corrected and then at increasingly longer intervals.

PROGNOSIS

Iron-deficiency anemia caused by dietary factors has an excellent prognosis. When the cause of IDA is bleeding, the prognosis depends on the ability to correct the underlying cause responsible for the bleeding.

BIBLIOGRAPHY

Deasy JA: Clinical interface: Three anemic patients. *Physician Assist* 15(6):58–62, 1991.
Hillman RS, Finch CA: *Red Cell Manual,* 5th ed. Philadelphia, Davis, 1985.
Leiner S, Mays M: Diagnosing microcytic anemia in adults. *Physician Assist* 20(3):24–26, 32–38, 56, 1996.
Ravel R: *Clinical Laboratory Medicine,* 6th ed. St Louis, Mosby, 1995.

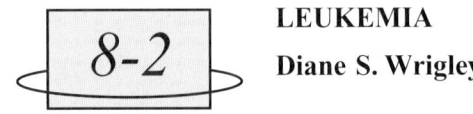

LEUKEMIA
Diane S. Wrigley

DISCUSSION

Discussion of leukemia can be lengthy, confusing, and highly complex. For the purposes of this book and the relevance to practicing physician assistants in clinical medicine, the information presented here is concise and as practical as possible. Leukemia occurs as an acute or a chronic disease. Leukemia is classified by type of blast or blood cell progenitors and according to the course, as follows:

- Acute lymphoblastic leukemia (ALL)
- Acute nonlymphoblastic leukemia (ANLL)
- Chronic myelocytic leukemia (CML)
- Chronic lymphocytic leukemia (CLL)

The yearly incidence is 13.2 in 100,000 in males and 7.7 in 100,000 in females. Seventy percent of leukemias occur in adults, mostly CLL and ANLL, and 30 percent occur in children, mostly ALL. Leukemia is the twentieth most common cause of cancer deaths. The type of leukemia defines the treatment and the prognosis.

With the current cure rate, which is especially good for childhood ALL, estimates are that by the year 2010, 1 in 1000 young adults between 15 and 45 years of age will be a childhood ALL survivor.

PATHOPHYSIOLOGY

Malignant clonal expansion of hematopoietic stem cells leads to an accumulation of abnormal immature blood cell progenitors, or blasts, in bone marrow and other tissues. This process leads to marrow failure. It can be aggressive and rapidly fatal if not treated. The normal differentiation of stem cell maturity is interrupted, and immature cells occur. The systems affected are the heme, lymphatic, and immune systems. Genetics are unknown, but some forms appear to be familial. The precise cause is unknown.

Major factors have been associated with leukemias: Radiation, chemical exposure such as benzene, and the HTLV-1 virus, are contributory or major risk factors. In many cases, exposure to these factors has been high or unusual and the majority exposed have not developed disease; it is presumed that other factors, such as inherited molecular abnormalities, play a role. Latency periods between exposure and the development of disease can vary from 3 to 30 years. Childhood leukemia is being relooked at from an infectious standpoint. Although it is known that leukemia is not contagious, the fact that domestic animals suffer from viral-induced spontaneous leukemias and the role of Epstein-Barr virus in Burkitt's lymphoma lead one to look to infection as a contributory cause. Among the theories considered are that the development of leukemia can arise from a rare response to common infection caused by things such as lack of early exposure to common viruses through decreased breast-feeding and lack of transplacental antibodies secondary to lack of the mother's own exposure. Infection with common microbes at a biologically abnormal time frame for which the immune system is inappropriately programmed is being considered as a possible cause.

SIGNS AND SYMPTOMS

Many of the signs and symptoms are nonspecific, relating to marrow failure or infiltration. There may be fever, bleeding as evidenced by petechiae, easy bruising, oozing, bone pain, pallor, fatigue, lymphadenopathy, hepatosplenomegaly, gingival swelling, and anemia with neutropenia and/or thrombocytopenia.

DIAGNOSTIC CONSIDERATIONS

The considerations here are very broad. All forms of bone marrow failure or invasion must be considered. Often a viral-induced cytopenia with lymphadenopathy and organomegaly can mimic leukemia. Immune and drug-induced cytopenias also must be considered. A large number of patients may have low or normal white blood cell (WBC) counts, and so a thorough examination of the peripheral blood for abnormal cells such as circulating blasts should be done. A careful history should document the onset of symptoms, the date of the last normal blood count, family history, and exposure to chemicals or radiation. Ask whether the patient has had transfusions or a history of disseminated intravascular coagulation (DIC). Assess renal, cardiac, and hepatic function in preparation for possible chemotherapy.

RISK FACTORS

Genetic and chromosomal abnormalities, trisomy 21, and translocations are risk factors for leukemia. Other factors include radiation exposure, immunodeficiency states, chemical and drug exposure such as nitrogen mustard and benzene, preleukemia, and cigarette smoking.

LABORATORY TESTS

A complete blood cell count (CBC) with differential should be done. Look for a reticulocyte count <0.5, an elevated sedimentation rate, elevated lactate dehydrogenase (LDH) or uric acid chemistries, and low immunoglobulins (IgG). The coagulation profile may be abnormal or prolonged. *Caution:* Corticosteroid use may alter laboratory results.

DIAGNOSTIC PROCEDURES

In bone marrow studies, aspirates are stained for cell morphology. This is important for correctly identifying the type of leukemia, since it will have a direct bearing on the treatment and prognosis. Biopsy of the marrow then provides information on cellularity, architecture, and megakaryocytic series. A marrow cell suspension is used for cytochemistries, such as Sudan black, confirming positive myeloblasts. The suspension also can be used for immunophenotyping to differentiate monoclonal versus polyclonal, B lymphocytes versus T lymphocytes, and early versus late. Chromosome studies show ploidy or the presence of a translocation (Philadelphia chromosome), which is of prognostic value.

TREATMENT

Consult with a chemotherapist and use inpatient care for acute leukemia treatment. The overall focus is recognizing and treating signs of infection, bleeding, central nervous system (CNS) involvement, or tissue invasion. Respiratory difficulties, change in vision, and abdominal pain are examples of tissue invasion. Chemotherapy is used to induce a marrow aplasia; if and when it is successful, hematopoiesis from the surviving stem cells leads to repopulation. This stage is called remission and is not to be confused with cure or eradication. Advances in supportive care, indwelling central venous catheters, broad-spectrum antibiotics, antifungals, and blood product support improvements have decreased treatment-related deaths. Immune therapy and vaccination of the body are new and different approaches to leukemia. Efforts to target leukemia cells with radioactive "smart bombs" are showing continued success. Improvements in chemotherapy so that cancer cells can be targeted more specifically are showing promise while decreasing the toxicity side effects.

PATIENT EDUCATION

Patients need an adequately balanced diet and close follow-up on weight checks. There is a need for psychological support for children with leukemia and their families. The emotional reaction of children is age-dependent, but a team approach with providers, nurses, social workers, and psychologists should help with the emotional as well as economic impact on the families.

Platelets and packed red blood cells (RBCs) for transfusion may be given. Isolation may be necessary. It is important to watch for DIC.

Surgical measures include allogeneic bone marrow transplants.

NOTES AND PEARLS

The overall prognosis for childhood leukemias continues to improve, with 80 percent of patients achieving long-term disease-free survival. The following factors have prognostic significance:

- The higher the WBC at diagnosis, the poorer the prognosis.
- Two- to 10-year-olds fare best, adolescents do less well, and infants under 1 year have only a 25 to 30 percent survival rate.
- The presence of CNS disease at diagnosis increases the probability of subsequent relapse.

BIBLIOGRAPHY

Greaves MF: Aetiology of acute leukaemia. *Lancet* 349:344–349, 1997.

Henderson CW: Treatment: New approaches may finally offer hope for leukemia. *Cancer Weekly Plus,* pp 1–2, Oct. 12, 1998.

Hoffman R, Benz EJ, Shattil SJ, et al: *Hematology Principles and Practice.* New York, Churchill Livingstone, 1991, pp 1–2.

Rakel R (ed): *Conn's Current Therapy.* Philadelphia, Saunders, 1995, pp 390–412.

Schrier S, McArthur J: *Hematology.* Seattle, University of Washington School of Medicine, Education Program of the American Society of Hematology, 1993, pp 38–44.

Williams WJ, Beutler E, Erslev AJ, Lichtman MA: *Hematology,* 4th ed. New York, McGraw-Hill, 1990, chap 25.

Wood ME, Bunn PA Jr: *Hematology/Oncology Secrets.* Philadelphia, Hanley & Belfus; St. Louis, Mosby, 1994, chap 27.

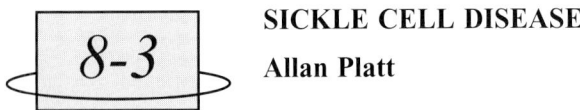

SICKLE CELL DISEASE
8-3
Allan Platt

DISCUSSION

Sickle cell disease is a group of inherited hemoglobin disorders characterized by chronic hemolytic anemia, a heightened susceptibility to infections, end organ damage, and intermittent episodes of vascular occlusion that cause both acute and chronic pain. Sickle cell anemia, the most common variant, results when an individual inherits sickle hemoglobin from both parents. The substitution of valine for the normal glutamic acid in the sixth position of the beta chain alters the hemoglobin molecule so that it crystallizes, elongates, and deforms the red cell into a rigid "sickle" shape when oxygen is released.

It is estimated that 70,000 Americans of different ethnic backgrounds have sickle cell disease. In the United States, sickle cell syndromes are present in 1 in 600 African-Americans. The disease is most common in individuals who are descendants of those from malaria-endemic areas of the world. Inheriting one sickle gene, or sickle cell trait, provides some protection from the red cell parasite malaria. Sickle hemoglobin is found in Africans, Arabs, Turks, Greeks, Italians, Iranians, and Asian Indians. Eight percent of American blacks are carriers of the sickle gene and make less than 50 percent sickle hemoglobin. The carrier state is usually asymptomatic, but hematuria and sickle complications can occur under severe bodily stress such as dehydration, temperature change, or pressure change.

SIGNS AND SYMPTOMS

The clinical manifestations of sickle cell disease are thought to result from increased blood viscosity, changes in red blood cell deformability, fragility, and adherence to vascular walls. The coagulation system also plays a role because markers of increased platelet activation are prevalent in sickle cell patients. Red cell dehydration and deoxygenation enhance deformation into a rigid sickle shape, increasing blood viscosity and capillary plugging.[1] The result is a disruption of blood flow that causes vascular occlusion, hemorrhages, infarctions, and ischemic necrosis. This increased mechanical fragility reduces the red cell survival from a normal 120 days to 15 days, causing a hemolytic

anemia and bone marrow proliferation to keep pace. This marked hemolytic anemia causes increased indirect bilirubin and lactate dehydrogenase (LDH) and a high reticulocyte count.

Intense pain may be caused by the inflammatory response to bone marrow and muscle necrosis, ischemia, or infarction secondary to blood flow obstruction and sludging. Damage can occur to any organ in the body, including the brain, lungs, liver, spleen, kidneys, bones, and eyes.

Management of acute events includes a thorough history, physical examination, laboratory workup, and radiologic examination if necessary. Precipitating causes such as infection, dehydration, hypoxia, and temperature exposure must be identified and corrected. General treatment measures include intravenous (IV) hydration with D_5W, pain medications, and oxygen if the patient is dyspneic or hypoxic. If the patient has evidence of transient ischemic attack (TIA), stroke, chest infarction, multiple organ system failure, or sequestration of red cells in the spleen or liver, phenotypic packed red cell transfusions are indicated. Table 8-3-1 lists the most common signs and symptoms of sickle cell disease. The objective findings, diagnostic considerations, and laboratory, imaging, and treatment options are included.

LABORATORY STUDIES

The definitive test used to diagnose sickle cell syndromes is hemoglobin electrophoresis. Because the HbS and HbC amino acid substitutions change the electrical charge of the protein, the migration pattern of the hemoglobin with electrophoresis or hemoglobin diagnosis using isoelectric focusing (IEF), high-performance liquid chromatography (HPLC), or DNA analysis results in diagnostic patterns with each of the different hemoglobin variants. Diagnosis of Hb S Beta-Thal requires careful evaluation of the red blood cell count and mean corpuscular red cell volume (MCV) and specifically quantification of Hb A, S, A2, and F. A 5-min solubility test named the Sickledex has been used to detect the presence of Hb S in the emergency setting. This test is of little diagnostic value because it does not differentiate sickle syndromes from the benign carrier state (Hb AS). False negatives are also common in newborns and patients with severe anemia.

Most states are performing mandatory hemoglobinopathy testing on all newborns as part of newborn screening programs. Intervention with daily penicillin and parental education about the signs of sickle complications and immunizations, including pneumococcal vaccine, have saved many lives. Other blood tests that should be monitored on a routine basis are a complete blood count (CBC), a reticulocyte count to determine the bone marrow response to the chronic hemolysis, a chemistry profile, and a urinalysis.

PAIN EPISODES

The most common problem for sickle cell patients is the pain episode, a self-limiting and reversible pain in the extremities, back, chest, and abdomen. The severity of pain has been reported to range from mild transient attacks of 5 min to pain lasting days or weeks and requiring hospitalization. The cause of the intense pain is believed to be an inflammatory response to bone marrow necrosis, ischemic muscle, and ischemic bowel resulting from the obstruction and sludging of blood flow produced by sickled erythrocytes. Cumulative ischemic tissue damage and fibrosis can lead to chronic pain. The frequency of pain crisis varies with each individual and depends to some extent on the patient's hemoglobin phenotype, physical condition, and concurrent illness, as well as psychological and social variables.

Pain episodes should be managed as in any other severe, acute pain-producing disease, tailoring the analgesic used and the dose to the level of pain experienced by the patient. Pain intensity should be assessed as a vital sign by using a visual analogue scale or a similar

TABLE 8-3-1. Signs and Symptoms of Sickle Cell Disease

SIGNS AND SYMPTOMS	DIAGNOSTIC TESTS AND DIFFERENTIAL	TREATMENT OPTIONS
Symmetric hand and foot swelling, infant	Hand-foot syndrome	Fluids and pain management
Chills and fever	Sepsis, pneumonia, osteomyelitis; do a CBC, WBC differential (check for elevated bands and total WBC count), blood cultures	Empirically treat with antibiotics until cultures are known; prevent infections with immunization and prophylactic penicillin up to age 6
Headache	Stroke, aneurysm, meningitis; CT scan, MRI-MRA, LP	Treat etiology
Chest pain, dyspnea, cough	Chest syndrome, pneumonia; do a CXR, ABG	Treat empirically with antibiotics and transfusion
Abdominal pain and swelling	Splenic or hepatic sequestration, gallstones; ultrasound or CT, CBC and chemistry profile	Transfusion for sequestration; surgery for gallstones
New weakness, paresthesias, difficulty talking	Stroke; do a CT or MRI-MRA	Transfuse acutely and chronic transfusion program for prevention
Pain in extremities, low back, "typical crisis pain"	Pain crisis; look for precipitating causes such as infection, dehydration, acidosis; do a CBC, reticulocyte count, chemistry profile, and UA	Hydration with oral or IV water; good pain management; Hydrea may prevent crisis
Weakness, lethargy, pallor	Aplastic crisis; do a CBC with reticulocyte count	Transfusion support until bone marrow responds
Acute decline after routine pain crisis: multiple organ failure	Multiple organ system failure evidenced by renal, hepatic failure, ARDS, DIC	Transfusions can be lifesaving
Increasing jaundice	Increased hemolysis or bile duct obstruction; do a CBC, reticulocyte count, and chemistry profile; consider gallbladder ultrasound	Treat etiology; administer folate 1 mg daily to all patients for red cell production demands
Focal bone pain	Consider bone infarction or osteomyelitis; if hip or shoulder pain, consider avascular necrosis (AVN); do a CBC and x-ray the area	For bone infarction and AVN, treat with long-acting NSAIDs and decreased weight bearing

tool at the beginning of treatment and at set intervals to document the response to treatment. A detailed history and a physical examination are important to identify correctable precipitating factors such as infection, dehydration, increased anemia, acidosis from any cause, emotional stress, extreme temperature exposure, and ingestion of other substances, such as alcohol and other recreational drugs. An excellent question to ask the patient is: Is this pain typical of your pain crisis? If the pain is atypical, a search for other causes should be pursued. Headache, chest pain, and abdominal pain should prompt a search for secondary causes and complications. The treatment of pain crisis includes the administration of analgesics including narcotics and nonsteroidal anti-inflammatory drugs (NSAIDs), intracellular hydration with hypotonic oral or intravenous fluids (D_5W), bed rest, treatment of the underlying infection, and treatment of other precipitants.

Oxygen should be administered if a patient has an underlying pulmonary problem and hypoxia is documented by arterial blood gases or pulse oximetry. Pulse oximetry should be monitored as a vital sign, but it becomes less reliable when severe anemia is present. Low oxygen saturation in symptomatic patients must be investigated with arterial blood gases, chest x-rays, and pulmonary testing. When hypoxia is not present, oxygen therapy has been shown to reduce red blood cell production.

Managing acute pain episodes requires controlling pain appropriately, excluding correctable precipitating causes, detecting life-threatening complications, and diagnosing causes of pain unrelated to sickle cell complications. Pain therapy requires choosing agents that are safe and provide rapid analgesia. Pain medication should be administered on a fixed time schedule at an interval that equals the period of adequate analgesia. This will maintain a steady serum drug level, thereby improving control of pain, minimizing complications, and decreasing anxiety in patients. The oral route of administration is the safest. The oral dose needed is always greater than the dose needed with the

parenteral route. Patient-controlled analgesia (PCA) pumps that provide constant low-dose infusion of morphine with defined rescue doses provide excellent pain treatment. The side effects of the narcotic analgesics include itching from histamine release, respiratory depression, nausea, vomiting, hypotension, constipation, increased bladder tone, urinary retention, and a decreased seizure threshold. Synthetic agonist-antagonist agents such as buprenorphine (Buprenex) and nalbuphine (Nubain) are alternative choices for some patients but can cause withdrawal symptoms similar to those of naloxone in patients with very frequent narcotic usage.

Hydration with intravenous hypotonic solutions such as D_5W is a treatment that may slow or stop the sickling process by lowering serum sodium and thus serum osmolality. Reduced serum osmolality moves water into a red blood cell, reducing the concentration of the sickle hemoglobin in the cell. This reverses sickling because the tendency for sickle hemoglobin to polymerize increases with the thirtieth power of the hemoglobin concentration. Fluid should be administered to adults at the rate of 250 mL/h for 8 h and then reduced to 125 mL/h if there are no signs or past history of congestive heart failure, renal failure, or hyponatremia.

OTHER COMPLICATIONS

Bacterial infection is one of the main causes of morbidity and mortality in patients with sickle cell disease. Children less than age 3 are at the greatest risk for fatal sepsis, but patients of any age are at risk for rapid death from sepsis. Splenic function is markedly decreased or absent in patients with sickle cell anemia, leaving the individual at great risk for infection with encapsulated organisms such as *Streptococcus pneumoniae, Haemophilus influenzae,* salmonella, and meningococci, among others. Serious infections such as meningitis, pneumonia, sepsis, and osteomyelitis must be aggressively excluded and treated empirically early to prevent morbidity and mortality. Preventive measures such as pneumococcal and *H. influenzae* vaccine should be administered to all sickle cell patients starting at birth (with Prevnar). Prophylactic daily penicillin should be instituted at birth and should continue until the child is 6 years old.

Splenic sequestration crisis is one of the most serious complications and is second only to infections as a cause of death in infants with sickle cell disease. This event usually occurs between ages 4 months and 3 years but may occur at any age with hemoglobin SC or S-Beta Thal disease. During sequestration episodes, sickle cells are trapped in the spleen, causing a rapid fall in the hemoglobin level and enlargement of the spleen. Sequestration events may be triggered by infection or occur with no apparent antecedent. The onset of signs and symptoms is very rapid and consists of weakness, abdominal pain, fatigue, dyspnea, pending shock, tachycardia, pallor, an enlarging spleen, and a falling hemoglobin hematocrit with a reticulocyte count equal to and usually higher than the patient's baseline. Treatment consists of admission to an intensive care unit (ICU) with aggressive blood transfusions. Emergent splenectomy occasionally is required.

Hepatic sequestration may occur later in life with similar signs and symptoms, including a rapidly enlarging liver and a falling hematocrit. The treatment consists of aggressive simple transfusion or red cell exchange transfusion. Aplastic crisis occurs when the bone marrow slows or stops new red blood cell production. Signs and symptoms are a falling hemoglobin and hematocrit, along with a falling reticulocyte count, weakness, pallor, dyspnea, and dizziness. In sickle cell disease, the absolute reticulocyte count is three to four times the upper limit of normal in compensation for the shortened red blood cell survival. Treatment for aplastic crisis includes immediate hospitalization and blood transfusions to support the hemoglobin level. Sources of the aplastic event, such as infection with parvovirus and folate deficiency, should be sought.

Chest pain, cough, or hypoxia should be evaluated with a chest x-ray. The presence of an infiltrate is the hallmark of acute chest syndrome. Acute chest syndrome (ACS) is an important cause of morbidity and mortality in sickle cell disease. The etiology of ACS includes viruses, atypical bacteria, bone marrow necrosis with fat embolism, and bacteria.[2] Bronchoscopy may be diagnostic and therapeutic. Patients should be treated with transfusions and antibiotics that cover atypical bacteria and pneumococci. Postoperative ACS may be prevented by incentive spirometry.

PREVENTIVE CARE AND PATIENT EDUCATION

The vitamin folic acid or folate should be administered 1 mg daily to most sickle cell patients because dietary intake of folate may not meet the increased requirements for red cell production. Hemoglobin, hematocrit, and reticulocyte counts should be checked periodically to determine a normal baseline for each patient so that significant changes can be identified early. Iron preparations are to be avoided unless serum ferritin, iron, and total iron-binding capacity (TIBC) levels establish a diagnosis of iron deficiency. Iron is recycled in the reticuloendothelial cells and reused for the production of hemoglobin in new red cells. Iron overload may become a problem later in life for sickle cell patients treated with repeated blood transfusion and aggressive oral or parenteral iron supplementation.

Those with sickle cell disease should be evaluated periodically to identify chronic problems, update immunizations, maintain folate acid therapy, and provide patient education and support. Patients and parents should be taught how to read a thermometer and how to seek immediate medical attention when a fever develops or signs of infection appear. Smoking and excessive alcohol intake should be discouraged. Patients should be educated about the importance of drinking 8 to 10 glasses of water or fluid per day. They should avoid extreme temperature changes by dressing properly in hot and cold weather. Excessive physical exertion that repeatedly leads to complications should be

avoided. The patient should be encouraged to find and not exceed his or her personal physical limits in sports and outdoor activities. Educational and vocational goals should be set and actively pursued with positive reinforcement. Overprotectiveness, family and health care overdependence, and chronic illness behavior should be discouraged.

In patients with chronic pain, NSAIDs with renal sparing properties should be administered continuously to maintain analgesic blood levels. Transcutaneous nerve stimulation units, relaxation techniques, and occupational and physical therapy may be used to maintain a functional life-style. Vocational rehabilitation and outside activities are critical in coping with the chronic pain of sickle cell disease. Severe pain can be managed cautiously with long-acting narcotics such as sustained-release oral morphine, sustained-release oxycodone, and methadone.

COMPLICATIONS AND RED FLAGS

All sickle cell patients should be managed with the help of a hematologist skilled in sickle cell care. Generalists can deliver the routine care, but specialists should manage the complications. The best care and consultations are available at several comprehensive sickle cell centers around the United States. Comprehensive sickle cell centers should have facilities to evaluate, treat, and counsel those with any of the complications of the disease. Centers should have support staffs including patient educators, genetic counselors, psychiatric support, vocational rehabilitation, occupational therapy, physical therapy, and health care providers all working together as a multidisciplinary team to solve the complex medical, psychological, and social problems associated with these diseases (visit the Sickle Cell Information Center at http://www.emory.edu/PEDS/SICKLE for clinic locations).

NEW TREATMENTS

Daily administration of oral hydroxyurea (Hydrea) is the first effective pharmacologic intervention documented to provide clinically significantly prevention of complications in sickle cell disease. Treatment with Hydrea has been shown to reduce pain events, hospital admissions, and the need for blood transfusions by 50 percent.[3] It is used in doses starting at 15 to 20 mg/kg/day and increased slowly until a favorable response is obtained or signs of toxicity appear (neutrophil count $<2,000/mm^3$, platelets $<80,000/mm^3$, hemoglobin drop of 2 g/dL, or absolute reticulocyte count $<80,000/mm^3$) or a total dose of 35 mg/kg is reached. When a good clinical response is observed, the patient's fetal hemoglobin increases and total hemoglobin increases an average 1 g/dL. The patient must be monitored with CBCs every 2 weeks for evidence of bone marrow suppression, and only a 2-week supply of Hydrea with no refills should be given to the patient at each visit. Once a stable or maximally tolerated dose is obtained, the patient can be monitored monthly. The long-term benefits of hydroxyurea and its toxicities are unknown. Studies of safety and efficacy are being initiated in children, and this treatment currently is recommended for older children; however, the long-term effects are unknown.

A cooperative study of preoperative transfusion demonstrated that sickle cell patients should have simple transfusions to raise a patient's hemoglobin to 10 g/dL before surgery.[4] These simple transfusions are safer and as effective in preventing postoperative complications as are exchange or aggressive transfusions to decrease the hemoglobin S level below 30 percent. Postoperative complications such as chest syndrome, fever, and alloimmunization with delayed transfusion reactions are common. Alloimmunization can be minimized by giving antigen-matched blood (matched for K, C, E, S, Fy, and Jk antigens). All patients should receive incentive spirometry and be given adequate hydration and oxygenation. Transfusions are still the best acute treatment for life-threatening complications such as stroke, acute chest syndrome, sequestration, and aplastic events. Chronic transfusions are necessary for life to prevent recurrent strokes. Transfusion to hemoglobin levels above 10 may cause hyperviscosity, increased sludging, and complications such as stroke.

New methods for screening for central nervous system (CNS) ischemia, including transcranial Doppler and magnetic resonance imaging and angiography (MRI-MRA), have uncovered a 15 percent incidence of CNS ischemic injury in asymptomatic sickle cell patients. A prospective trial of preventive chronic transfusion therapy in high-risk children demonstrated a 92 percent reduction in strokes.[5] All patients with CNS symptoms should be screened immediately and treated with acute exchange therapy if an infarctive stroke is documented. Strokes and TIAs are associated with a 50 percent or greater recurrence rate unless chronic transfusion therapy is maintained for life. Because of the problems of alloimmunization, blood-borne infection, and chronic iron overload, bone marrow transplantation is considered in young children with strokes. Bone marrow transplantation is an experimental therapy limited to patients who have enough complications from sickle cell disease to warrant the risk of death and long-term complications from the transplantation and who also have a sibling with an identical HLA match. Patients face a 10 percent risk of mortality from the procedure and several months in the hospital in preparation and care after transplantation. Successful transplantation has resulted in the first cures of this genetic disorder.[6] The probability of event-free survival is 84 percent. The problem has been a lack of HLA-matched related donors. Using stem cells from cord blood samples from unrelated donors offers the best promise of meeting this need. Eligible patients can be referred to one of the participating transplant centers across the nation.

On-line guidelines, research updates, and comprehensive clinic locations are available at the Sickle Cell Information Center at http://www.emory.edu/PEDS/SICKLE.

ACKNOWLEDGMENT

The editor would like to acknowledge the significant contribution of Diane Wrigley, the author of this chapter in the first edition of *Primary Care for Physician Assistants.*

REFERENCES

1. Steinberg M: Management of sickle cell disease. *N Engl J Med* 340:1021–1030, 1999.
2. Vichinsky EP, Styles LA, Colangelo LH, Wright EC, Castro O, Nickerson B: Acute chest syndrome in sickle cell disease: Clinical presentation and course: Cooperative Study of Sickle Cell Disease. *Blood* 89(5):1787–1792, 1997.
3. Charache S, Terrin ML, Moore RD, et al: Effect of hydroxyurea on the frequency of painful crisis in sickle cell anemia. *N Engl J Med* 332:1317–1322, 1999.
4. Vichinsky EP, Haberkern CM, Neumayr L, et al: A comparison of conservative and aggressive transfusion regimens in the perioperative management of sickle cell disease: The Preoperative Transfusion in Sickle Cell Disease Study Group. *N Engl J Med* 333(4):206–213, 1995.
5. Adams R, McKie V, Hsu L: Prevention of a first stroke by transfusions in children with sickle cell anemia and abnormal results on transcranial doppler ultrasonography. *N Engl J Med* 339(1):5–11, 1998.
6. Walters MC, Patience M, Leisenring W, Rogers ZR, et al: Collaborative multicenter investigation of marrow transplantation for sickle cell disease: Current results and future directions. *Biol Blood Marrow Transplant* 3(6):310–315, 1997.

Resources: Books and CD-ROMs

Problem Oriented Management of Sickle Cell Syndromes, by James Eckman and Allan Platt. Available at http://www.emory.edu/PEDS/SICKLE.
Stickle Cell Disease: Comprehensive Screening and Management in Newborns and Infants. AHCPR Guidelines 93-0562 and 93-0563.
Acute Pain Management in Infants, Children and Adolescents: Operative and Medical Procedures. AHCPR Guidelines 92-0020, 92-0032, and 92-0019.
Clarice Reid (ed): *Management and Therapy of Sickle Cell Disease.* NIH Publication 95-2117, 3d ed., 1995.

Embury, SH, Hebdel RP, Mohandas N, et al. (eds): *Sickle Cell Disease: Basic Principles and Clinical Practice.* Raven-Lippincott Publishers, Philadelphia, 1994.
Graham Serjeant: *Sickle Cell Disease,* 2d ed. Oxford, UK, Oxford University Press, 1992.
Samir K. Ballas: *Sickle Cell Pain Progress in Pain Research and Management,* vol. 11, 1998.
American Pain Society: *Guideline for the Management of Acute and Chronic Pain in Sickle Cell Disease.* Seattle, WA, 1999.
On-line-Tutorial: The Wellcome Trust Presents: Topics in International Health: Sickle Cell Disease, http://www.wellcome.ac.uk.

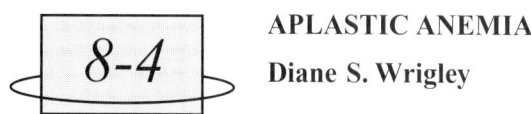

APLASTIC ANEMIA
Diane S. Wrigley

DISCUSSION

In aplastic anemia, the loss of the hematopoietic cells in bone marrow leads to failure to produce adequate numbers of peripheral blood elements. Aplastic anemia also may be referred to as pancytopenia. It can be acquired or genetic. The marrow becomes hypocellular, and hematopoietic cells may occupy as much as 25 percent of the marrow or as little as 0 to 5 percent. The injury to the marrow can be initiated by toxic, radiation, or immunologic etiologies to the erythroid elements. A single blood cell line may be involved at the beginning, followed by a full line of erythroid elements. Although the acquired form can be seen at all ages, two age groups have an increased risk: Young adults 15 to 30 years old and those over age 60 have higher rates than does the general population, which has a rate of 5 to 10 per 1 million. The genetic or constitutional form is limited to children and young adults.

PATHOPHYSIOLOGY

Bone marrow failure results from damage to the hematopoietic stem cells. This can occur because of damage to DNA from exposure to radiation, chemicals such as benzene, and drugs such as chloramphenicol and the cytotoxic drugs used in chemotherapy. Viruses have been known to be cytotoxic to stem precursors; 50 to 75 percent of cases of stem cell damage are idiopathic.

Radiation damage is dependent on the amount of energy absorbed and the radiosensitivity of the tissue. To put this in terms of visualization, doses of radiation are measured in sieverts (Sv). At 0 to 1.0 Sv, there are few if any symptoms. At 100 Sv, there is a 100 percent mortality rate. Cosmic rays give 0.001 Sv compared with a radioactive isotope such as a thyroid scan, which gives 0.0001 Sv.

In this industrialized society, potentially toxic compounds are limitless: insecticides, fertilizers, food additives, and benzene radicals for both household and commercial uses. All hydrocarbons are suspected in the etiology of aplastic anemia, as are insecticides such as pentachlorophenol, lindane, and DDT.

Introduced over 40 years ago, chloramphenicol has an inherent risk of 1 in 20,000 to 30,000 of causing aplastic anemia, but that still is 10 to 20 times the idiopathic risk. The anemia is reversible when the drug is withdrawn. Specifically, chloramphenicol affects the maturation and proliferation of marrow precursor cells and then irreversibly damages the genetic structure of stem cells. Stem cells produced without the influence of the drug return to normal. Other drugs that have been implicated include the nitrobenzene compounds. As many as 75 drugs have been implicated, but the hydantoins, pyrazoles, sulfonamides, and gold have an unusual affinity for this relationship. No specific genetic pattern is detected in acquired aplastic anemia. However, there may be a genetic defect in the ability to handle drug elimination or detoxification, leaving stem cells vulnerable.

Infections such as hepatitis viruses commonly cause up to 5 percent of marrow failures, and Epstein-Barr virus, rubella, parvovirus, and HIV also have been implicated. Paroxysmal nocturnal hemoglobinuria has been associated with pancytopenia.

Immunologic changes such as graft-versus-host disease and other states of immune status change, such as pregnancy, can cause damage to these stem precursors. The presence of antibodies to stem cells is a phenomenon in the immunologic or autoimmune etiology. Suppression of normal stem cell function also can be caused by the action of abnormal stem cells.

Another form of aplastic anemia is inherited. Called Fanconi syndrome or constitutional anemia, it was first described in 1927. There is an autosomal recessive gene in constitutional Fanconi syndrome.

A considerable loss can take place in the marrow before peripheral blood is affected. Pure red cell aplasia is a related syndrome caused by selective failure of the erythroid elements, leaving leukocyte and platelet counts unaffected.

SYMPTOMS

These patients look and feel well. The onset is usually insidious. Symptoms caused by anemia, infections exacerbated by neutropenia, and cutaneous bleeding associated with thrombocytopenia frequently are treated symptomatically until purpura, with its more serious connotations, forces a more complete hematologic evaluation. The less severe form of aplastic anemia is striking in that the symptoms are restricted to the hematologic system. The prognosis is dependent on the degree of anemia. When neutrophil counts are $<500/mm^3$, platelets $<20,000$, and reticulocyte count <1 percent, it is considered severe. In acquired aplastic anemia, bleeding is an early symptom of a severe level, as are fatigue, weakness, shortness of breath (SOB), a pounding sensation in the ears, pallor, and weight loss.

OBJECTIVE FINDINGS

The physical examination may be very unremarkable. Ecchymoses, petechiae, melena, occult stool blood, retinal flame hemorrhage, systolic ejection murmur, menorrhagia, and purpura all may be present. In short, many of the objective findings have to do with hypovolemia and hypoxia from lack of circulating cells. In constitutional anemia, short stature, microcephaly, and renal anomalies prevail.

DIAGNOSTIC CONSIDERATIONS

Beware of other causes of pancytopenia. Lack of peripheral elements can be due to destruction after the marrow has produced them. A bone marrow biopsy will rule this out. A mean corpuscular volume (MCV) greater than 100, indicating a possible megaloblastic anemia from deficiencies that are easily reversible, is a good clue to normal marrow elements. Splenomegaly and lymphadenopathy are conspicuously absent in true aplastic anemia. Other myelodysplastic disorders may be mistaken for aplastic anemia.

SPECIAL CONSIDERATIONS

Persons with early very severe aplastic anemia that is not treated may have a median survival of only 3 to 6 months. Eighty percent of all patients treated with blood transfusions alone die within 18 months to 2 years. Patients undergoing bone marrow transplantation have a 60 to 90 percent chance of being cured. Patient history taking should include careful attention to exposure to drugs and conditions in the workplace and home.

LABORATORY

Do a complete blood cell count (CBC) with evidence of pancytopenia, specifically anemia, leukopenia, neutropenia, and thrombocytopenia but normochromic red blood cells (RBCs). Check for increased bleeding time, a decreased reticulocyte count, normal total iron-binding capacity (TIBC), high MCV (>104), and hematuria. Erythropoietin levels increase up to 500 to 1000 times normal values. Check liver function tests for hepatitis. Check for increased fetal hemoglobin (Fanconi syndrome). Other diagnostic tests include a bone marrow biopsy. Check for increased iron stores, decreased cellularity (<10 percent), and decreased megakaryocytes, myelocytes, and erythroid precursors.

RADIOLOGIC STUDIES

X-ray the radius and thumbs; do a renal ultrasound if constitutional anemia is suspected.

TREATMENT

Admit the patient to a facility with experienced practitioners. The first step in treatment involves discontinuing any exposure to substances that may be causing the disorder. Giving blood transfusions is only a temporary aid and may compromise future successful attempts at bone marrow transplantation. Consider a bone marrow transplant. Eighty percent are done in those under 20 years of age with severe anemia and a human leukocyte antigen (HLA)-compatible donor. If the patient has been transfused, the risk of graft-versus-host reaction increases. For patients older than 40 years and those lacking a suitable marrow donor, give antithymocyte globulin therapy (ATG) at 40 mg/kg/day for 4 days. Hematologic responses equivalent to improving blood counts so that transfusions are no longer required occur in 40 to 50 percent. If cyclosporin is given in conjunction with ATG, response rates increase to 70 to 80 percent with a 5-year survival rate of about 90 percent. Use cyclosporin at 12 mg/kg/day for adults and 15 mg for children. Steroids and cyclophosphamide also are used. Consider androgen therapy. Signs of infection are treated aggressively with parental or broad-spectrum antibiotics. Treatment is empiric. Do not wait for cultures. Ensure scrupulous hand washing. Do platelet transfusions with leukocytes removed for platelet counts under 10,000 because of the risk of an intracranial bleed. Suppress menstruation in females. Avoid aspirin and nonsteroidal anti-inflammatory drugs. For patients who cannot undergo bone marrow transplantation, transfuse with RBCs to get the hemoglobin at 7.0 g or better at 2 U every 2 weeks. If transfusions are to be chronic, an iron chelation, deferoxamine, by the fiftieth unit may be necessary to avoid a secondary hemochromatosis or iron overload.

SUPPORTIVE MEASURES

Give oxygen therapy to help with SOB and lack of hemoglobin transport of O_2. Isolation precautions may be indicated. Encourage a nutritious diet and good oral hygiene.

PATIENT EDUCATION

Avoid likely causative agents and prepare for a search of unrelated donor transplants if other therapies fail.

Further information can be obtained by writing to the Aplastic Anemia Foundation of America, Inc., PO Box 613, Annapolis, MD 21404, (800) 747-2820, http://www.aplastic.org.

BIBLIOGRAPHY

Carson-Dewitt RS: Aplastic anemia, in Oldenerf D, Jeryan C, Boyden K: *Gale Encyclopedia of Medicine,* 1st ed. Gale Research, Farmington Hills, MI, 1999, p 311.

Griffith CJ: Evaluation and management of anemia. *Adv PA* 4(5):33–38, 1996.

Hoffman R, Benz EJ, Shattil SJ, et al: *Hematology Principles and Practice.* New York, Churchill Livingstone, 1991, chap 18.

Williams WJ, Beutler E, Erslev AJ, Lichtman MA: *Hematology,* 4th ed. New York, McGraw-Hill, 1990, chap 18.

Wood ME, Bunn PA Jr: *Hematology/Oncology Secrets.* Philadelphia, Hanley & Belfus; St Louis, Mosby, 1994, pp 43–46.

Young NS: Acquired aplastic anemia. *JAMA* 282:i3–271, 1999.

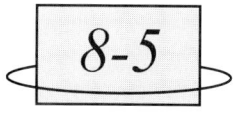

HEMOCHROMATOSIS
Diane S. Wrigley

DISCUSSION

Hemochromatosis, or iron overload disease, is caused by increased iron absorption from the gut. The nature of this defect is unknown. Since the body cannot excrete iron, the excess is stored in organs such as the liver, pancreas, and heart. The condition is genetic, with the homozygote occurring as frequently as 1 in 200 to 1 in 600 persons, with an incidence of clinical disease of 8 to 13 percent of the homozygous population. Normally, two-thirds of the total body iron is found in red blood cells, making up about 2 g of iron. The remaining one-third is found in storage iron that is in the form of iron storage protein, ferritin. The term *hemochromatosis* is used for the state of iron overload with resultant tissue damage.

The heterozygote state occurs in approximately 1 in 10 people, making it the most common abnormal gene in the U.S. population. The clinical disease often is detected between ages 40 and 60, with the ratio of males to females at 8:1. The biggest risk of untreated hemochromatosis is the formation of hepatomas. Once the disease is established, treatment does not affect the clinical outcome of the malignancy. The goal is early identification and treatment to reduce morbidity and mortality.

PATHOPHYSIOLOGY

Iron that is in the reticuloendothelial cells is harmless, but iron stored in parenchymal cells is a noxious agent. The consequences of untreated iron overloading are increased skin pigmentation and hepatomegaly with an increased risk of hepatoma. Iron metabolism appears normal in this disease, but there is a higher level of circulating iron. Iron usually is stored as ferritin, but in this case it can be stored as hemosiderin. Ferritin levels may be as high as 700 and into the thousands. Twenty grams of excess iron is necessary to cause clinical disease.

The signs and symptoms of hemochromatosis are much the same as those of diabetes, arthritis, impotence, and congestive heart failure (CHF). The disease probably is underdiagnosed because the incidence of these diseases is so high.

RISK FACTORS

Loss of blood delays the onset of symptoms, and so menstruating and pregnant women exhibit a lag in time of presentation. Intake of iron in supplement form with not only iron but also vitamin C enhances iron absorption. Increased alcohol consumption enhances iron absorption.

SIGNS AND SYMPTOMS

Look for weakness; abdominal pain; arthralgia, particularly in large joints and the metacarpal phalangeal joint (MCP); loss of libido or sexual potency; amenorrhea; increased skin pigmentation; hepatomegaly; and diabetes mellitus symptoms. Hemochromatosis most often is discovered incidentally or through the evaluation of abdominal pain, joint pain, or weakness.

OBJECTIVE FINDINGS

Hepatomegaly, splenomegaly, jaundice, hepatic tenderness, and increased skin pigmentation can be appreciated on physical examination. Testicular atrophy and gynecomastia, which are found in alcoholism, are often present. A good physical examination with positive confirmation of appropriate laboratory tests exclusively looking for hemochromatosis will result in a proper diagnosis.

DIFFERENTIAL DIAGNOSIS

The differential diagnosis includes repeated transfusions, hereditary anemias with ineffective erythropoiesis, alcoholic cirrhosis, and excessive iron ingestion (rare).

LABORATORY TESTS

Ferritin >300 μg/L for men and >120 for women is diagnostic. If the saturation is >62 percent, the homozygous state can be predicted with 92 percent accuracy. Once it is suspected, a firm diagnosis can be made by liver biopsy, staining specifically for iron and identifying excess iron deposition in hepatocytes. Quantitative iron on the hepatic tissue as well as evidence of cirrhosis also can be checked. Also look for urinary iron; decreased follicle-stimulating hormone (FSH), luteinizing hormone (LH), testosterone, and albumin as indications of hemochromatosis; oral glucose tolerance test to rule out hyperglycemia; and increased serum glutamic-oxaloacetic transaminase (SGOT).

DIAGNOSTICS

Use an echocardiogram to rule out cardiomyopathy. Consider a liver biopsy for iron particles when there is evidence of cirrhosis.

TREATMENT

The best treatment is phlebotomy. One unit of blood contains 250 mg of iron. At least 80 phlebotomies will be necessary to normalize total body iron. Once patients have achieved normal iron levels, only two to four phlebotomies a year will be required for maintenance. Patients with induced (not hereditary) hemochromatosis associated with transfusion therapy should receive treatment with an iron-chelating agent. An iron-free diet is not necessary.

Patients with mild clinical disease have a normal life span. Patients with diabetes mellitus (DM), cardiac damage, or hepatic cirrhosis have decreased survival rates. Phlebotomy at that stage does not decrease the risk of developing a hepatoma.

NOTES AND PEARLS

Hepatic computed tomography and magnetic resonance imaging (MRI) and magnetic susceptibility measurements (MSM) are in the future. The human leukocyte antigen (HLA)–linked iron-loading gene (HFE) associated with the clinical disease known as hereditary hemochromatosis occurs in 10 percent of subjects of European descent. However, current guidelines do not recommend mass genetic testing for this gene. There are many questions to be answered regarding the prevalence and penetration of the gene as well as concerns about the optimal care of asymptomatic people who carry the gene. Gene testing probably will be reserved for screening family members of a diagnosed patient and helping to resolve ambiguous cases. Inclusion of transferrin saturation on routine laboratory screening is being considered.

PATIENT EDUCATION

Teach patients to avoid alcohol and iron-fortified foods. Restrict vitamin C to small doses between meals. Tea chelates iron, and so the patient may drink tea with meals. Once a firm diagnosis of hemochromatosis is made, immediate family members should be screened for the disease. The best treatment is early intervention. Patients may engage in full activity unless there is evidence of significant heart disease.

BIBLIOGRAPHY

Bothwell TH, MacPhail AP: Hereditary hemochromatosis—etiologic, pathologic, and clinical aspects. *Semin Hematol* 35(1):55–71, 1998.

Brandhagen DJ, Fairbanks VF, Batts KP: Update on hereditary hemochromatosis and the HFE gene. *Mayo Clin Proc* 74(9):917–921, 1999.

Williams WJ, Beutler E, Erslev AJ, Lichtman MA: Disorders of iron metabolism, in McCracken A, Jeffers A, Ramos-Englis M, eds.: *Hematology,* 4th ed. New York, McGraw-Hill, 1990, pp 752–758.

Wood ME, Bunn PA Jr: *Hematology/Oncology Secrets.* Philadelphia, Hanley & Belfus; St Louis Mosby, 1994, chap 15.

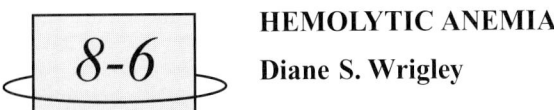

HEMOLYTIC ANEMIA
Diane S. Wrigley

DISCUSSION

Hemolytic anemia can be acquired or inherited. In this disease, red blood cell destruction occurs prematurely as a result of immunologic, physical, or chemical injury. The mechanism of the destruction is the binding of autoantibodies and/or complement to red blood cells. Physical injury may result from cardiac pathology, narrowed heart valves, pathologic shunts, valve prosthesis, and increased tissue temperatures. Chemical causes include exposures to arsenic or copper and inappropriate water exposure. A drop in hemoglobin (Hb) of >1 g/week should be suspicious for excessive blood loss or hemolysis. The congenital form involves intrinsic defects of the red blood cell (RBC) membrane. The clinical manifestations of the acquired and inherited forms are the same. The hereditary form is a common autosomal dominant disease of varying severity.

PATHOGENESIS

Three components of the RBC that are involved in hemolytic anemia are the membrane, the Hb, and the intracellular erythrocyte enzymes that provide adenosine triphosphate (ATP) energy and reducing equivalents. Patients who once had a normal hematocrit and normal reticulocyte count can be diagnosed as having the acquired form as opposed to the inherited form. The mechanism of hemolysis or rupture of the normal RBCs is the same as it is in persons with intrinsic red cell defects. The integrity of the RBC can be overcome when it is exposed to sufficiently severe stress. In hereditary spherocytosis (HS), the RBC intrinsic defect and the intact spleen selection in retaining the abnormal cells contribute to the pathophysiology. In accelerated HS, RBC destruction is a multistep process resulting from dysfunction of the skeletal proteins of the membrane.

RISK FACTORS

Acquired hemolytic anemia is idiopathic in 50 percent of cases. Risk factors include warm and cold antibodies, neoplasias (leukemias, myelomas, lymphomas, thymomas), collagen vascular disease, viral infections, and drugs such as methyldopa, quinidine, penicillin, sulfasalazine, phenazopyridine hydrochloride, and sulfonamides. Additionally, insect venoms, excessive water inhalation in drownings, excessive distilled water in the circulation such as in dialysis or surgical procedures, and increased heat >47°C (extensive burns) may cause hemolysis.

OBJECTIVE FINDINGS

Vital sign findings include increased pulse and change in blood pressure with postural changes. These findings occur with marked blood loss. There is pallor of skin and/or palpebral conjunctival pallor in dark-skinned patients. Splenomegaly and lymphadenopathy also are found.

LABORATORY TESTS

Spherocytes, schistocytes, and helmet cells are found in the peripheral smear in the complete blood cell count (CBC). There is elevation of the mean corpuscular hemoglobin concentration (MCHC) indexes and an elevated reticulocyte count. In looking at automated erythrocyte indexes, an elevated MCHC (35.9 or greater) coupled with an elevated erythrocyte distribution width (greater than 14) is considered an effective screening test for identifying those with HS, showing a specificity of 100 percent. Do an indirect hyperbilirubinemia test and a CBC, noting RBC indexes values and laboratory comments on cells. Also do an osmotic fragility test, which tests the integrity of the RBC membrane. Cells that are susceptible to easy damage will hemolyze at hypertonic saline concentrations. A Coombs' test is positive direct in 90 percent of autoimmune hemolytic anemia patients, since it measures immunoproteins; the indirect Coombs' test measures antibodies that are formed with the glucose-6-phosphate dehydrogenase (G6PD), deficiency. This is an enzyme abnormality that results in the RBC's inability to defend itself against oxidative assaults. The oxidants damage vital cell constituents. Patients lacking the enzyme exhibit signs of hemolysis if exposed to oxidant drugs such as nitrofurantoin or even if they ingest fava beans. Looking at the laboratory's comments and finding "Heinz" bodies should raise the suspicion of G6PD insufficiency. The gene for the G6PD deficiency is on the X chromosome. Look for suspicious drug levels of antimalarials, sulfonamides, nitrofurantoin, chloramphenicol, aspirin, and ascorbic acid, which all may be measured if suspected in a case of hemolytic anemia. Other tests include indirect bilirubin, haptoglobin, IgG and IgM antibodies, and lactate dehydrogenase (LDH).

SYMPTOMS

Symptoms of hemolytic anemia include weakness, fatigue, dyspnea on exertion, dizziness, palpitations, malaise, pallor, splenomegaly and hepatomegaly, anemia, hemoglobinemia, and jaundice.

SUPPORTIVE MEASURES

Ensure rest until the patient is asymptomatic; no special diet or restrictions are required. Check the family history for any hemolytic anemias.

TREATMENT

Give 1 to 1.5 mg/kg/day of prednisone for rapid hemolysis or intravenous (IV) cortisone 400 to 800 mg/day. Consider a splenectomy. Patients having a splenectomy also need to be immunized with pneumococcal vaccine, and pediatric patients may be given daily penicillin prophylaxis because of the high rate of rapidly developing infections in splenectomized populations. Give large amounts of IV gamma globulin 0.5 to 1.0 g/kg infused for 5 days. Prescribe daily chlorambucil

2 to 4 mg orally to decrease the rate of cold agglutinin. Remove offending causes.

PATIENT EDUCATION

Make the patient aware of potentiating factors, if identified, and talk about avoidance in the future. A screening is recommended for the congenital form if one affected relative is identified.

BIBLIOGRAPHY

Griffith CJ: Evaluation and management of anemia. *Adv PA* 4(5):33–38, 1996.
Hoffman R, Benz EJ Jr, Shattil SJ, et al: *Hematology Principles and Practice.* New York, Churchill Livingstone, 1991, chap 37.
Michaels LA, Cohen AR, Zhao H: Screening for hereditary spherocytosis by use of automated erythrocyte indexes. *J Pediatr* 130(6):957–960, 1997.
Williams WJ, Beutler E, Erslev AJ, Lichtman MA: *Hematology,* 4th ed. New York, McGraw-Hill, 1990, chaps 55, 65, 66.

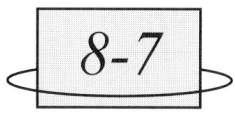

HENOCH-SCHÖNLEIN PURPURA

JoAnn Deasy

DISCUSSION

Henoch-Schönlein purpura (HSP) is a nonthrombocytopenic vasculitis that is more common in childhood but may affect adults. Vasculitis is an inflammatory and often destructive process that affects the arteries and veins. The median age of onset of HSP is 6 years, and males are affected twice as often as are females.[1] The cause of this condition is unknown. An association has been shown with a preceding exposure to an infectious disease agent (particularly viruses causing upper respiratory infections), food, and drugs.

HSP is considered an IgA-mediated vasculitis of small vessels. The most commonly involved organs are the skin, joints, gastrointestinal tract, and kidneys. It has been postulated that there is a trapping of immune complexes in the vessel wall and activation of complement, which results in the production of complement breakdown products that are chemoattractants to polymorphonuclear leukocytes (PMNs). These PMNs accumulate at the site of inflammation and release various enzymes and free radicals, resulting in damage to the vessel wall.[2] Histologically, granulocytes are seen in the walls or perivascular cuff of arterioles or venules.

SIGNS AND SYMPTOMS

The most characteristic manifestation of HSP is the typical rash, which occurs primarily over the buttocks and lower extremities but may involve the entire body. The skin lesions may consist of urticarial wheals, erythematous macules and papules, petechiae, and palpable purpura. New lesions may continue to occur in crops. Arthritis of the large joints and acute abdominal pain may occur. When arthritis occurs before the rash of HSP, the diagnosis can be difficult. The knee and ankle joints are most commonly involved, and the arthralgias may be migratory. When abdominal pain is present, it is usually diffuse and may be severe, presenting as an acute abdomen. The pain often is described as cramp-like and is thought to be due to hemorrhage and the accumulation of fluid primarily in the small intestine. Other gastrointestinal symptoms include bloody or nonbloody diarrhea, nausea, and vomiting. If there is renal involvement, hematuria may be present, but it usually is a later symptom that occurs during the second or third week of the illness.

OBJECTIVE FINDINGS

Petechiae and purpura involve blood that is extravascular; therefore, the color does not blanch with pressure. If swelling of the joints is present, the swelling is often periarticular and not a true joint effusion. The findings on abdominal examination may be inconsistent with the severity of the abdominal pain. The tenderness to palpation is often diffuse, and signs of peritoneal irritation are usually absent. However, intussusception may occur as a complication with associated abdominal distention, and a tubular mass may be palpable.

COMPLICATIONS

Glomerulonephritis and nephrotic syndromes may occur. It is thought that the glomerulonephritis is due to deposition of immune complexes in the glomeruli. Approximately 20 percent of children have renal involvement during on acute attack.[2] Only a small number go on to have persistent renal disease. Death from renal failure has occurred. Intussusception of the small bowel, testicular torsion, and involvement of the central nervous system are other possible complications.

DIAGNOSTIC CONSIDERATIONS

Conditions that may present similarly to HSP include systemic lupus erythematosus, thrombocytopenia purpura, the rash of meningococcemia, subacute bacterial endocarditis, rickettsial diseases, and Waldenström's hyperglobulinemic purpura.

LABORATORY TESTS

A platelet count, platelet function tests, and a bleeding time are ordered. The results should be normal. Urinalysis may show hematuria and proteinuria. Stool occult blood may be positive. IgA may be elevated.

RADIOGRAPHIC STUDIES

If intussusception is suspected, ultrasonography or barium enema should be ordered to confirm this complication.

TREATMENT

There is no specific treatment for HSP. In severe cases, a short course of corticosteroids may provide relief of symptoms but does not alter the course of the disease.

PROGNOSIS AND DISPOSITION

The disease is usually self-limited, and the prognosis for complete recovery is excellent. The illness lasts 4 to 6 weeks in most patients. Attacks may recur in some patients for months to a year after the initial onset. In patients with renal involvement, hematuria and proteinuria may persist and regular periodic follow-up is essential.

REFERENCES

1. Schaller JG, Szer IS: Systemic lupus erythematosus, dermatomyositis, scleroderma, and vasculitis in childhood, in Delley WN, Harris ED Jr, Ruddy S, et al (eds): *Textbook of Rheumatology,* 3d ed. Philadelphia, Saunders, 1989, pp 1340–1341.
2. Athreya BH: Vasculitis in children. *Pediatr Clin North Am* 42(5):1239–1261, 1995.

BIBLIOGRAPHY

Kraft DM, McKee D, Scott C: Henoch-Schönlein purpura: A review. *Am Fam Physician* 58(2):405–408, 1999.
Patrignelli R, Sheikh S, Shaw-Stiffel TA: Henoch-Schönlein purpura. *Postgrad Med* 97(5):123–134, 1995.

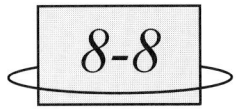

PERNICIOUS ANEMIA
Diane S. Wrigley

DISCUSSION

Pernicious anemia (PA) is a disease of unknown origin in which the basic defect—atrophy of the gastric mucosa (parietal cell)—eventually leads to a lack of intrinsic factor (IF) and hydrochloric acid (HCl) secretion. Vitamin B_{12} (cyanocobalamin) plays an important role in the development of blood cells. It is found in foods such as liver, meats, milk, and legumes. Vitamin B_{12} can be absorbed only when it is attached to intrinsic factor PA and is categorized under the megaloblastic macrocytic anemias: mean corpuscular volume (MCV) >95 percent in the red blood cell (RBC) indexes. The incidence of PA is about 25 cases per 100,000 per year. The average age at onset is 60. The predisposition to developing PA may have a genetic basis, but precise information is lacking. There is a positive family history in up to 30 percent of patients with clinical PA.

PATHOPHYSIOLOGY

Since vitamin B_{12} can be absorbed only by binding to IF, the end result is vitamin B_{12} deficiency. Decreased B_{12} levels affect three systems: the hematopoietic, gastrointestinal, and nervous systems. These macrocytic anemias account for about one-third of anemias because the ability to incorporate B_{12} into new RBC synthesis, impairing DNA synthesis, results in dissociation between the maturation of the nucleus and the cytoplasm in developing cells. An RBC with an immature nucleus has open chromatin and is enlarged or megaloblastic.

There is a significant association of PA with other autoimmune diseases, such as Graves' disease, Hashimoto's thyroiditis, hypoparathyroidism, vitiligo, and adult-onset hypogammaglobulinemia. It is thought that the immune system, which already is out of control with these diseases, becomes indirectly directed against the parietal cells in the gastrointestinal (GI) system.

PA may affect up to 10 percent of the population older than age 70 years. Achlorhydria and partial, subtotal gastrectomies are contributing factors in the elderly, in addition to the loss of pepsin. Total gastrectomy leads to the removal of IF-producing cells. Ninety percent of patients with PA have anti-IF antibodies in the serum or gastric juice. Although a genetic predisposition has been shown, the full expression of pathology, which appears to be autoimmune, may be modified by acquired environmental influences.

RISK FACTORS

Alcoholism with or without liver disease can cause vitamin B_{12} deficiency. Drugs such as ascorbic acid, colchicine, cholestyramine, neomycin, cimetidine, and oral contraceptives have been implicated. Folate deficiency and lack of dietary B_{12} ingestion as well as strict vegetarianism with no dairy products and bacterial overgrowth syndromes in the gut competing for vitamin B_{12} all play a role in macrocytic, megaloblastic anemias. Intestinal worms such as the fish tapeworm may use B_{12}. Conditions affecting the ileum, such as sprue, Whipple's disease, Crohn's disease, tuberculosis, and the Zollinger-Ellison syndrome can cause a vitamin B_{12} deficiency.

LABORATORY TESTS

Look for complete blood cell count (CBC) >95 MCV, decreased reticulocytes, low hemoglobin and hematocrit, and hypersegmented polymorphonuclear sites. Check vitamin B_{12} and folate levels. A Schilling test should be done. Radioactive B_{12} is given orally. The amount excreted in the urine is measured. Patients who lack IF do not absorb B_{12}; therefore, they do not excrete it. Serum methylmalonic acid is increased in >95 percent of B_{12}-deficient patients. Values may be as high as 2,000,000; normal is 70 to 270. B_{12} is essential in mammals as a cofactor in two enzymes. Reduced activity of these critical enzymes leads to an increase in methylmalonic acid.

SYMPTOMS

Symptoms of severe anemia include weight loss, GI symptoms such as bloating and diarrhea, infertility, orthostatic hypotension, loss of proprioception, ataxia, memory loss, abnormal smell or taste, and listlessness or hallucinations. Neurologic symptoms include numbness, tingling, muscle weakness, irritability, confusion, and depression.

OBJECTIVE FINDINGS

Objective findings include glossitis, stomatitis, premature gray hair, neurologic symptoms from paresthesias and dysesthesias of the extremities (particularly the lower extremities), and depression to frank psychosis.

TREATMENT

Give intramuscular or subcutaneous vitamin B_{12} once per week for 8 weeks and then once per month for the rest of the patient's life. Use oral treatment with B_{12} at a dose of 10 mg/day for strict vegetarians.

PATIENT EDUCATION

The response to therapy is the ultimate determination of the existence of a deficiency regardless of the etiology. Symptomatic family members also should be screened. A general family history should be obtained on all patients with PA.

BIBLIOGRAPHY

Carson-Dewitt RS: Pernicious anemia, in Oldenerf D, Jeryan C, Boyden K: *Gale Encyclopedia of Medicine,* 1st ed. Gale Research, Farmington Hills, MI, 1999, p 2224.

Griffith CJ: Evaluation and management of anemia. *Adv PA* 4(5):33–38, 1996.

Wood ME, Bunn PA Jr: *Hematology/Oncology Secrets.* Philadelphia, Hanley & Belfus; St Louis, Mosby, 1994, pp 34–39.

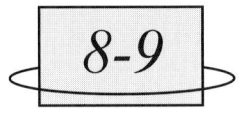

POLYCYTHEMIA VERA
Diane S. Wrigley

DISCUSSION

Polycythemia vera (PV) is one of a group of myeloproliferative disorders with resultant excessive erythroid, myeloid, and megakaryocytic elements in the bone marrow. It is considered a clonal disorder, which means that there is unregulated growth of a malignant cell. Patients with polycythemia have increased numbers of CFU-GEMM (colony-forming units—granulocytes, erythroids, macrophages, megakaryocytes). These units have demonstrated unregulated proliferation in culture in the absence of erythropoietin. The prevalence in the population is 0.5 per 100,000, males slightly outnumber females, and the predominant age is the middle to late years, with the mean being 60 years of age. The incidence seems to increase with age until age 80 years, suggesting that mutational somatic events may play a role in the pathogenesis. Untreated patients have a median survival rate of about 18 months from the diagnosis. Treated patients may live 10 to 15 years.

Individuals with relative or spurious polycythemia have normal red blood cell mass and conditions that reduce the plasma volume, causing hemoconcentration. Real polycythemia or polycythemia vera has an elevated red blood cell (RBC) mass (>36 mL/kg for males and >32 mL/kg for females). Generally, the hematocrit is over 60 percent without any evidence of dehydration. Because of prognostic and treatment differences between PV and a secondary erythrocytosis, a firm diagnosis should be based on determining RBC mass.

PATHOPHYSIOLOGY

The increased blood volume leads to generalized vascular expansion and venous engorgement. The increased blood viscosity is reflected in the characteristic ruddy cyanosis of the skin and mucous membranes. These factors are magnified by the significant decrease in cerebral blood flow that accompanies an elevation of the hematocrit and contributes to the symptoms of headaches, tinnitus, and frequently described feeling of fullness or light-headedness in the head and neck. The consequence is an increase in thrombotic complications, particularly in the cerebrovascular circulation. Epistaxis and upper gastrointestinal (GI) hemorrhage also may occur. The resultant hypervolemia may result in decreased cardiac output, ultimately impairing tissue oxygenation.

The proliferative phase, which is the initial phase, includes ineffective hematopoiesis. A bone marrow biopsy may reveal a trilinear hyperplasia; that is, hemoglobin, platelets, and white blood cell production are increased. The peripheral smear may mirror this. Vascular congestion, splenomegaly, bleeding, and thrombosis are seen in this stage.

The spent phase is seen after about 10 years in a small proportion of patients (5 to 15 percent). Now extensive bone marrow fibrosis and ineffective hematopoiesis are evident. Anemia is due to splenic sequestration, iron deficiency, and excessive bleeding resulting from platelet dysfunction. Between 20 and 50 percent of cases at this stage transform into acute leukemia, which has a poor survival prognosis of 70 percent mortality within 3 years.

DIAGNOSTIC CONSIDERATIONS

Consider secondary polycythemias. Affected individuals have evidence of tissue hypoxia or erythropoietin-secreting tumors. High erythropoietin levels will be detected. This increased level may be appropriate in chronic obstructive pulmonary disease (COPD), sleep apnea, and cardiovascular shunts. Renal disease such as hydronephrosis, cysts, and renal transplants also can account for this level.

LABORATORY TESTS

Do a complete blood cell count (CBC), looking for increased RBC mass and white blood cells (WBCs) greater than 12,000. Check for iron-deficiency anemia [check total iron-binding capacity (TIBC) and percent iron saturation], leukocytosis, elevated leukocyte alkaline phosphatase (LAP) score, increased vitamin B_{12}, increased uric acid and lactate dehydrogenase (LDH), increased platelets higher than 500,000, and a normal erythropoietin level.

OBJECTIVE FINDINGS

In the early stages, there are no objective findings. Then headaches, tinnitus, vertigo, blurred vision, and epistaxis may appear. There is plethora of the hands, face, and feet. There may be arterial and venoocclusive events, sweating, weight loss, splenomegaly or hepatomegaly, bone tenderness and pain, gout, pruritus, and ruddy cyanosis of the complexion. There may be evidence of peripheral vascular disease. However, signs of infection are *not* present.

TREATMENT

Use phlebotomy to reduce hemoglobin to <14 g for males and <12 g for females. Cytoreductive drugs such as hydroxyurea and interferon can be used adjunctively with phlebotomy. ^{32}P and chlorambucil were effective in the past, but the high incidence of leukemia precludes their use except as a last resort.

NOTES AND PEARLS

When a patient shows increased hemoglobin levels, always search for secondary or reversible causes. Consider high altitude, excessive smoking, medications (particularly anabolic steroids and corticosteroids), burns, and stress such as the elusive pheochromocytoma. An iron deficiency may mask an increased RBC volume, as may a folate or vitamin B_{12} deficiency. RBC volumes in obese persons are imprecise. A hypoxic smoker may have polycythemia as well, and so it is important to look for elevated WBCs or an elevated platelet count in these patients. Splenectomy during the proliferative phase of polycythemia vera carries a high thrombolytic risk from the release of a large volume of pooled platelets.

BIBLIOGRAPHY

Dale DC, Federman DD: Hematology. *Sci Am Med* 5:1–10, 1997.
Tefferi A: Diagnosing polycythemia vera—a paradigm shift. *Mayo Clin Proc* 74(2):159–162, 1999.
Williams WJ, Beutler E, Erslev AJ, Lichtman MA: *Hematology,* 4th ed. New York, McGraw-Hill, 1990, chap 21.
Wood ME, Bunn PA Jr: *Hematology/Oncology Secrets.* Philadelphia, Hanley & Belfus; St Louis, Mosby, 1994, pp 50–56.

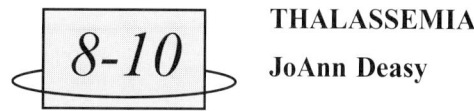

THALASSEMIA
JoAnn Deasy

DISCUSSION

Thalassemias are common hereditary hemoglobinopathies. These patients are classified as having *thalassemia trait (minor), thalassemia intermedia,* or *thalassemia major,* depending on the severity of their anemia. Thalassemia trait is underdiagnosed and frequently misdiagnosed as iron-deficiency anemia. An alert practitioner who recognizes the potential for the prevention of congenital disease and watches for microcytosis on electronic blood counts can identify persons with thalassemia trait. In regard to homozygous thalassemia, an invariably fatal condition can be prevented through the detection and education of heterozygous carriers.

The thalassemias constitute a group of congenital disorders in which there is defective production of the globulin chains, alpha or beta. Alpha thalassemia is due to gene deletion (see Table 8-10-1). Normal individuals inherit two alpha-chain genes from each parent. Deletion of one of the four genes results in a silent carrier state with no hematologic abnormalities. Persons with deletion of two alpha-chain genes have α-thalassemia trait (also referred to as α-thalassemia minor), causing microcytosis with or without anemia. Deletion of three genes causes a compensated hemolytic, microcytic anemia called hemoglobin H disease. Deletion of all four genes (Bart's disease) is incompatible with fetal survival as a result of hydrops fetalis. The diagnosis of homozygous disease is also important because of associated serious obstetric complications in the mother. α-Thalassemia syndromes primarily affect persons from Southeast Asia and China and African-Americans.

The β-thalassemias usually are caused by mutations rather than deletions. Individuals inherit only one beta chain from each parent.

TABLE 8-10-1. Select Gene Combinations in α-Thalassemia

HEMOGLOBIN GENES*	DIAGNOSIS	IMPLICATIONS
$\alpha\alpha/\alpha\alpha + \beta/\beta$	Normal adult hemoglobin	None
$-\alpha/\alpha\alpha + \beta/\beta$	α-Thalassemia silent carrier	None
$-\alpha/-\alpha + \beta/\beta$	α-Thalassemia trait	Moderate microcytic anemia; more common in African-Americans
$--/\alpha\alpha + \beta/\beta$	α-Thalassemia minor	Moderate microcytic anemia; more common in Asians
$--/-\alpha + \beta/\beta$	Hemoglobin H disease	Moderate to severe anemia
$--/-- + \beta/\beta$	α-Thalassemia major (Bart's disease)	Hydrops fetalis, stillbirth, high-risk pregnancy

*Minus sign indicates missing gene.

Therefore, β-thalassemias are heterozygous, homozygous, or compound heterozygous, such as sickle α-thalassemia. The heterozygous state, β-thalassemia trait (β-thalassemia minor), results in a hematologic picture similar to α-thalassemia trait. The homozygous state β-thalassemia major, produces a severe life-threatening anemia sometimes called Cooley's anemia. β-Thalassemia affects persons of Mediterranean origin, African-Americans, and Chinese and other Asians. Thalassemia intermedia patients may have a combined α- and β-thalassemia defect, a milder form of homozygous β-thalassemia, or β-thalassemia with high production levels of hemoglobin F.

SYMPTOMS

Thalassemia trait (minor) is generally asymptomatic, since the degree of anemia is usually mild. Most often thalassemia trait is diagnosed in asymptomatic persons who undergo an evaluation for microcytosis detected on a routine electronic blood count. In differentiating thalassemia trait from iron-deficiency anemia (IDA), the medical history should include questions regarding diet and the possibility of blood loss. Inquiry about the duration of the anemia and previous hemoglobin determinations should be made as well as about racial origin and the presence of anemia in other family members. Persons with thalassemia intermedia and β-thalassemia major have symptoms referable to their anemia: fatigue, dyspnea on exertion, faintness, and palpitations. The presentation of a patient with hemoglobin H disease is clinically that of an α-thalassemia intermedia patient.

OBJECTIVE FINDINGS

No characteristic physical findings are associated with α- or β-thalassemia trait. Hemoglobin H disease can vary in severity. Physical examination of some patients with hemoglobin H disease may reveal pallor and splenomegaly. α-Thalassemia major results in stillbirth. Children affected with β-thalassemia major (Cooley's anemia) develop a severe anemia during the first year of life with numerous subsequent clinical abnormalities. On physical examination, jaundice and hepatosplenomegaly are usually present. There may be sexual and growth retardation and skeletal abnormalities. The findings in thalassemia intermedia vary with the severity of the anemia; hepatosplenomegaly may be present. Transfusion therapy leads to cardiomyopathy and other dysfunctions. Death from cardiac failure generally occurs between ages 20 and 30.

DIFFERENTIAL DIAGNOSIS

The α- and β-thalassemia trait must be differentiated from other causes of microcytosis and frequently is confused with IDA (see Table 8-10-2).

TABLE 8-10-2. Types of Hemoglobin

Adult Hb—Hg A	$\alpha_2\beta_2$	>95% of adult Hb
Fetal Hb—Hb F	$\alpha_2\gamma_2$	70% of Hb at birth <1% of adult Hb
Hb A$_2$	$\alpha_2\delta_2$	<3% of adult Hb

LABORATORY DIAGNOSIS

In persons with uncomplicated α- and β-thalassemia trait, the microcytosis is striking [mean corpuscular volume (MCV) is 60 to 75] and more prominent than the anemia. This is the case because the red blood cell (RBC) count is relatively high, resulting in only a slight decrease in the hemoglobin level or even a normal hemoglobin. This is in contrast to patients with IDA, in whom the anemia is usually more prominent with a lesser degree of microcytosis and with lower RBC counts. The red cell distribution width (RDW) that is generated by an electronic blood count tends to be normal in patients with thalassemia trait because of the uniform microcytosis. IDA produces more anisocytosis (degree of variation in cell size); thus, the RDW tends to be elevated. The peripheral blood smear will reveal microcytic cells with possible hypochromasia and target cells. In patients with β-thalassemia trait, basophilic stippling may be present.

β-Thalassemia trait can be diagnosed by ordering hemoglobin electrophoresis, which will demonstrate an increase in hemoglobin (Hb) A$_2$ (normal <3.5 percent). If IDA and β-thalassemia trait coexist, Hb A$_2$ will not be elevated. Once the IDA is successfully treated, the elevated Hb A$_2$ will be exposed. β-Thalassemia major (Cooley's anemia) is suggested by a severe anemia that becomes evident at 2 to 3 months of age with hypochromic RBCs, target cells, many nucleated RBCs, and a high-risk ethnic origin. The diagnosis is made by demonstrating elevation of Hb F on hemoglobin electrophoresis. In addition, an alkali denaturation test can be done. Hb F is more resistant to denaturation than is Hb A (see Table 8-10-2).

Currently, there is no easy laboratory test that will diagnose α-thalassemia trait. It is usually a diagnosis of exclusion. However, the cord blood of a baby with thalassemia trait or hemoglobin H disease will show the presence of Bart's hemoglobin by electrophoresis in approximate proportion to the severity of the anemia. By age 4 to 6 months, Bart's hemoglobin generally disappears. After that age, globulin chain synthesis studies or the DNA probe technique can be used, but these techniques are available only in research laboratories.

TREATMENT

Usually no treatment is indicated for thalassemia trait. Chronic transfusions are the mainstay of treatment for β-thalassemia major (Cooley's anemia). Iron chelation therapy is used to prevent iron overload. Some individuals with thalassemia intermedia also require transfusions.

PATIENT EDUCATION

Once individuals are diagnosed with thalassemia minor, they should be informed so that they will not be treated with iron unnecessarily in the future. Patient education should include partner screening and preconception counseling.

BIBLIOGRAPHY

Deasy JA: Clinical interface: Three anemic patients. *Physician Assist* 15(6):58–62, 1991.

Hillman RS, Finch CA: *Red Cell Manual,* 5th ed. Philadelphia, Davis, 1985.

Lops VR, Hunter LP, Dixon LR: Anemia in pregnancy. *Am Fam Physician* 51(5):1189–1197, 1995.

Ravel R: *Clinical Laboratory Medicine,* 6th ed. St Louis, Mosby, 1995.

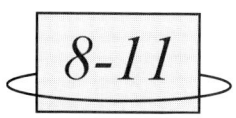

THROMBOCYTOPENIA
Diane S. Wrigley

DISCUSSION

Thrombocytopenia is a decrease in the number of platelets to less than 100,000/mL as a result of platelet destruction, decreased production, sequestration of platelets in the spleen, or a combination of any of these three. It may be a benign incidental finding in an asymptomatic patient or the sign of a potentially life-threatening disorder.

PATHOPHYSIOLOGY

The clinical presentation varies depending on the presence or absence of pancytopenia and the etiology. The hallmark is petechiae, which reflect bleeding at the level of the capillary venule. Usually petechiae develop over the lower extremities because of elevated hydrostatic pressure and constrictive clothing and in the oral mucosa because of the masseter's force on the surface during chewing. Decreased platelets may be due to decreased numbers of megakaryoblasts and replacement of bone marrow by abnormal tissue. Abnormal maturation of megakaryocytes also may contribute. Deficiency of vitamin B_{12} or folate can cause thrombocytopenia resulting from ineffective thrombopoiesis or hematopoietic dysplastic syndromes. Increased destruction of platelets can be secondary to immune disorders such as idiopathic thrombocytopenic purpura (ITP) and systemic lupus erythematosus (SLE); chronic lymphocytic leukemia; infectious diseases such as mononucleosis, cytomegalovirus (CMV), and AIDS; and drugs such as heparin, sulfa, quinidine, acetaminophen, and gold salts. Nonimmune disorders of destruction include disseminated intravascular coagulation (DIC), sepsis, malaria, paroxysmal nocturnal hemoglobinuria (PNH), acute renal transplant rejection, and congenital cyanotic heart disease. Disorders of distribution may occur because of hypersplenism and increased sequestration of platelets.

SYMPTOMS

These patients feel well but may have menorrhagia, easy bruising, petechial rash, excessive bleeding with cuts or dental work, purpura, or splenomegaly.

OBJECTIVE FINDINGS

There are skin and oral mucosal changes. There may be jaundice or petechiae. The lymphatic and hepatosplenic systems must be examined for abnormalities. A complete blood cell count (CBC) peripheral smear establishes the presence of decreased platelets as well as abnormal morphology.

DIAGNOSTIC CONSIDERATIONS

It is necessary to look for the cause. A thorough history should be taken, looking for a previous related illness such as liver disease or connective tissue disease. Consider HIV or hepatitis infections or pregnancy. Ask about a family history of congenital thrombocytopenia. Be suspicious of nutritional causes such as bulimia and anorexia. Correlating the patient's physical examination findings with the results of the CBC and peripheral smear often narrows the search for the underlying cause and eliminates the need for further evaluation or expensive tests.

LABORATORY TESTS

Recommended tests include CBC and reticulocytes, vitamin B_{12} and folate levels, a direct Coombs' test, and a coagulation panel that includes bleeding time. Prothrombin time (PT) and partial thromboplastin time (PTT) are normal.

RADIOLOGIC STUDIES

Use computed tomography (CT) of the head to rule out intracranial bleeding.

OTHER DIAGNOSTICS

Do a bone marrow biopsy if hypoplastic marrow is suspected. A normal marrow with only decreased numbers of megakaryocytes suggests drug ingestion rather than a neoplastic process. A platelet-associated antibody (PA-IgG) test may be useful.

TREATMENT

Remove the offending agent. Replace vitamin B_{12} and folate if indicated. Consider doing a platelet transfusion: One unit equals 10,000 platelets that will circulate approximately 24 h. Give prednisone 20 to 30 mg/day to maintain vascular integrity. Supportive measures include outpatient management unless there is active bleeding. Recommend minimal activity to prevent bruising. Tell the patient to avoid contact or collision sports and not to take aspirin and other platelet-inhibiting drugs.

BIBLIOGRAPHY

Goldstein KH, Abramson N: Efficient diagnosis of thrombocytopenia. *Am Fam Physician* 53(3):555–575, 1996.

Hoffman R, Benz E, Shattil S, et al: *Hematology Principles and Practice.* New York, Churchill Livingstone, 1991, chaps 15, 123, 125.

Wood ME, Bunn PA Jr: *Hematology/Oncology Secrets.* Philadelphia, Hanley & Belfus; St Louis, Mosby, 1994, pp 64–67.

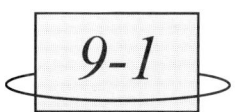

HIV/AIDS
Claire Babcock O'Connell

DISCUSSION

In the early 1980s the first clusters of opportunistic infections and neoplasia in gay men were reported to the Centers for Disease Control and Prevention (CDC). This often fatal syndrome of immune breakdown was designated gay-related immune disease (GRID) and prompted strong public outcry and fear (the "Gay Plague"). In the ensuing years, the number of persons suffering from this acquired immune deficiency state grew exponentially, affecting people from all walks of life around the world. In 1984, after massive epidemiologic analysis and biologic research, the etiology of acquired immunodeficiency syndrome (AIDS) was isolated, and the agent was later named *human immunodeficiency virus* (HIV).

Today, an estimated 40 million people worldwide are believed to have been infected with HIV, two-thirds of whom have met the criteria for the diagnosis of AIDS; over half of these AIDS patients have died. More than half of all cases of HIV infection have occurred in Sub-Saharan Africa; some countries report population infection rates that come close to one in three adults. Asia, China, and India continue to see rapid spread of the virus; transmission rates in North America and Europe have plateaued. Spread of the virus continues in all segments of society despite ongoing public education.

Much has been learned about the biology and clinical spectrum of HIV disease. Treatment options have undergone substantial evolution; reactive treatment against opportunistic infections and neoplasia is being replaced with proactive treatment against the virus. The most recent advances in the treatment of HIV involving triple therapy with reverse transcriptase inhibitors and protease inhibitors have provided the first glimpse at possible cure or at least chronic control of disease progression. However, despite preliminary work on treatment and vaccines, education and public health efforts aimed at controlling the spread of the virus remain the only effective method of halting the epidemic.

Biology of HIV

Current research supports the theory that HIV originated from a mutation of a simian immunodeficiency virus (SIV) in Africa. HIV is a single-stranded RNA virus of the retrovirus family. It is an icosahedron that has a significant ability to mutate. The biology of HIV has been extensively studied; the development of new drugs and vaccines is a direct result of increased understanding of the virus. The virus attaches to the host cell, predominantly the CD4+ (T helper) lymphocytes, fuses with the host cell membrane, and enters the cell. The virion contains reverse transcriptase which is required to produce DNA from RNA, and the DNA then gets integrated into the host nucleus, seizing control of the cell and dictating replication and integration of virus. The infected host cells can no longer function. Loss of functioning T helper cells, to which HIV has the greatest affinity, as well as loss of effective monocytes, macrophages, Langerhans' cells, and other members of the human immune system lead to the profound deficiency state that is characteristic of AIDS.

Transmission

HIV does not survive well outside cells. It quickly dies when exposed to air, heat, or a variety of chemicals. Transmission occurs through bodily fluids: parenteral exposure to blood or blood products (including exchange through contaminated intravenous drug paraphernalia), exchange of sexual fluids through sexual contact, and vertical transmission between an infected mother and her child either perinatally or through breast milk. There has been no documented transmission of HIV through casual contact, tears, saliva, respiratory droplets, or insects. Public health and preventive efforts have highlighted these facts of transmission in attempt to allay public fear and stem the growth of the epidemic. Heterosexual transmission in adolescents and young adults accounts for the majority of new infections throughout the world. Risk factors include multiple sex partners, anal intercourse, prostitution, sex during menses, lack of circumcision, traumatic intercourse, cervical ectopy, and the presence of other sexually transmitted diseases (STDs). Barrier methods using latex condoms are effective against sexual transmission. All blood and blood products since 1985 have been screened for the virus. Occupational risk among health care workers is minimized through the practice of universal precautions. Infected pregnant women receive antiviral treatment in order to reduce the incidence of vertical transmission.

SYMPTOMS

HIV disease should be viewed as a continuum including initial exposure, asymptomatic infection, symptomatic disease, and end-stage AIDS. Progression along the continuum cannot be predicted; the rate of decline varies significantly. Each patient must be evaluated as an individual, and the health care team must make decisions for assessment and treatment throughout the course of the disease.

The Acute HIV Syndrome

More than half of the individuals who contract HIV experience an acute syndrome 3 to 6 weeks after the primary infection. However, many individuals either do not recall symptoms or think the symptoms are a result of other infections or bodily stress. The typical scenario is a constellation of flulike symptoms similar to mononucleosis including fever, pharyngitis, arthralgias and myalgias, headache, lethargy, and anorexia. Patients may also have lymphadenopathy, nausea, vomiting, and diarrhea. The flulike syndrome is associated with the initial dramatic rise in viral count. Less often, patients may experience signs of meningitis, encephalopathy, peripheral neuropathy, or dermatologic conditions.

Unless the clinician maintains a suspicion for HIV infection, the syndrome may be misdiagnosed and the infection will go undetected. Clinicians should be alert for the acute HIV syndrome in any patient presenting with fever and mononucleosis-like symptoms, especially if the patient is sexually active or known to engage in injection drug use. Subsequent disease progression has been linked to the severity of the acute HIV illness, thus making the correct diagnosis at this stage even more important.

The syndrome persists for up to 2 to 3 weeks and gradually wanes. The decline in symptomatology accompanies the immune response. During this time, virologic testing for p24 antigen, HIV RNA, or proviral DNA is positive while antibody testing is negative. In most patients, the immune system begins to produce antibodies to different sections of the virus within 3 weeks of the initial infection. The level of immunity is inversely proportional to the level of virus. Treatment with antiretroviral medications during the acute infection is aimed at eradicating the virus or at least reducing viral load prior to irreversible immune system damage and dissemination of the virus to other tissue.

Clinical Latency

After the acute HIV infection, the virus is sequestered in lymph tissue and the body mounts a response. Viral load declines, antibodies to the virus appear, and molecular changes within the immune system are detectable. Clinically, there is a variable period of freedom from symptoms. This period may last many years (median, 10 years). There are several documented cases of symptom-free periods that are continuing after 2 decades of infection. However, there is no true latent period. It is now known that even in the face of normal immune function and low levels of virus detectable in the blood, the virus continues to multiply. The level of activity and speed of decline in the immune system vary among individuals, ranging from a few weeks to decades, but will occur in all infected patients. Antiretroviral therapy aims to halt this progression. A cure is still not available.

Symptomatic Disease

The onset of clinical symptoms may begin any time after initial infection with HIV. The median length of time between infection and clinical disease is 10 years. The CDC has compiled a list of clinical diseases or states that qualify a patient for a diagnosis of AIDS (Table 9-1-1). This list has been reevaluated and expanded in response to increased epidemiologic and biologic information throughout the history of the HIV epidemic. A diagnosis of AIDS (symptomatic HIV disease) is important for surveillance and gives the patient access to treatment and government-funded community and psychosocial resources.

The most frequent manifestation of HIV disease after the acute syndrome is a generalized lymphadenopathy without another cause. The nodes are multiple, found in more than two locations, larger than 1 cm, smooth, mobile, and persistent. They are caused by a follicular hyperplasia in response to the virus. Biopsy is not indicated unless another separate or confounding pathology is suspected. In general, the lymphadenopathy occurs early in the course of HIV disease, although it may occur after other symptoms of neoplasia or opportunistic infection. Reduction in nodal size or quantity late in HIV disease may be a poor prognostic sign indicating further loss in immune capacity and function.

As the decline in immune function progresses, clinical manifestations become more apparent and frequent. When the CD4+ count falls below 500, patients begin to exhibit clinical signs of oral thrush, herpes simplex or zoster, oral hairy leukoplakia, and declining numbers of platelets, leukocytes, and erythrocytes. Patients may have weight loss, unexplained fevers, dementia, and diarrhea. Below a count of 200, opportunistic infections and neoplasia are very likely to occur. In general, the more common manifestations of advanced HIV disease can be predicted from the CD4+ count (Fig 9-1-1), although exceptions in either direction are possible. Patients can be diagnosed with a disease or condition with higher than predicted CD4+ counts, and there are patients with very low CD4+ counts that do not show any clinical disease.

HIV disease encompasses a myriad of clinical presentations. Clinical syndromes may be due to HIV itself, opportunistic infection, neoplasia, psychosis, or depression (Table 9-1-2). HIV may manifest clinically in any body system or systems. The presentation is widespread and varied. Table 9-1-3 is a list of conditions grouped by system that are typically encountered in HIV disease.

PATIENT HISTORY

The medical history is an important tool for initial evaluation of suspected HIV infection and also for the monitoring of known HIV-positive individuals. Careful attention to behavioral factors is

TABLE 9-1-1. Centers for Disease Control Surveillance Case Definition for AIDS, 1993

A. Indicator diseases diagnosed definitively in the absence of other causes of immunodeficiency and without laboratory evidence of HIV infection
   1. Candidiasis of the esophagus, trachea, bronchi, or lungs
   2. Cryptococcosis, extrapulmonary
   3. Cryptosporidiosis with diarrhea persisting >1 month
   4. Cytomegalovirus disease of any organ excluding liver, spleen, and lymph nodes in a patient >1 month of age
   5. Herpes simplex virus infection causing a mucocutaneous ulcer persisting >1 month, or bronchitis, pneumonia, or esophagitis in a patient >1 month of age
   6. Kaposi's sarcoma in a patient <60 years of age
   7. Lymphoma of the brain (primary) in a patient <60 years of age
   8. Lymphoid interstitial pneumonia and/or pulmonary lymphoid hyperplasia in a child <13 years of age
   9. *Mycobacterium avium* complex or *M. kansasii* disease (disseminated)
   10. *Pneumocystis carinii* pneumonia
   11. Toxoplasmosis of the brain in a patient >1 month of age

B. Indicator diseases diagnosed definitively regardless of the presence of other causes of immunodeficiency and in the presence of laboratory evidence of HIV infection
   1. Any disease listed in section A
   2. Bacterial infections (multiple or recurrent) in children <13 years of age caused by *Haemophilus, Streptococcus,* or other pyogenic bacteria
   3. Coccidioidomycosis, disseminated
   4. HIV encephalopathy
   5. Histoplasmosis, disseminated
   6. Isosporiasis with diarrhea persisting >1 month
   7. Kaposi's sarcoma at any age
   8. Non-Hodgkin's lymphoma of B-cell or unknown phenotype and having the histologic type of small noncleaved lymphoma or immunoblastic sarcoma
   9. Any mycobacterial disease, disseminated, excluding *M. tuberculosis*
   10. *M. tuberculosis,* extrapulmonary
   11. *Salmonella* (nontyphoid) septicemia, recurrent
   12. HIV wasting syndrome

C. Indicator diseases diagnosed presumptively in the presence of laboratory evidence of HIV infection
   1. Candidiasis of the esophagus
   2. Cytomegalovirus retinitis with loss of vision
   3. Kaposi's sarcoma
   4. Lymphoid interstitial pneumonia and/or pulmonary lymphoid hyperplasia in a child <13 years of age
   5. Mycobacterial disease, disseminated
   6. *P. carinii* pneumonia
   7. Toxoplasmosis of the brain in a patient >1 month of age

D. Indicator diseases diagnosed definitively in the absence of other causes of immunodeficiency and in the presence of negative results for HIV infection
   1. *P. carinii* pneumonia
   2. Other indicator diseases listed in section A and CD4+ T lymphocyte count <400/μL

E. The 1993 expanded definition includes
   1. All HIV-infected persons who have CD4+ T lymphocyte counts <200/μL or a CD4+ T lymphocyte percentage of total lymphocytes of <14
   2. Pulmonary tuberculosis
   3. Recurrent pneumonia
   4. Invasive cervical cancer

paramount. A complete sexual history should be performed for all patients with special emphasis on behaviors known to be of high, intermediate, and low risk (Table 9-1-4). The sexual history must be completed free of all judgments and assumptions. Questions should be directed at specific practices; no assumptions should be made during the interview process. A prior history of sexually transmitted diseases,

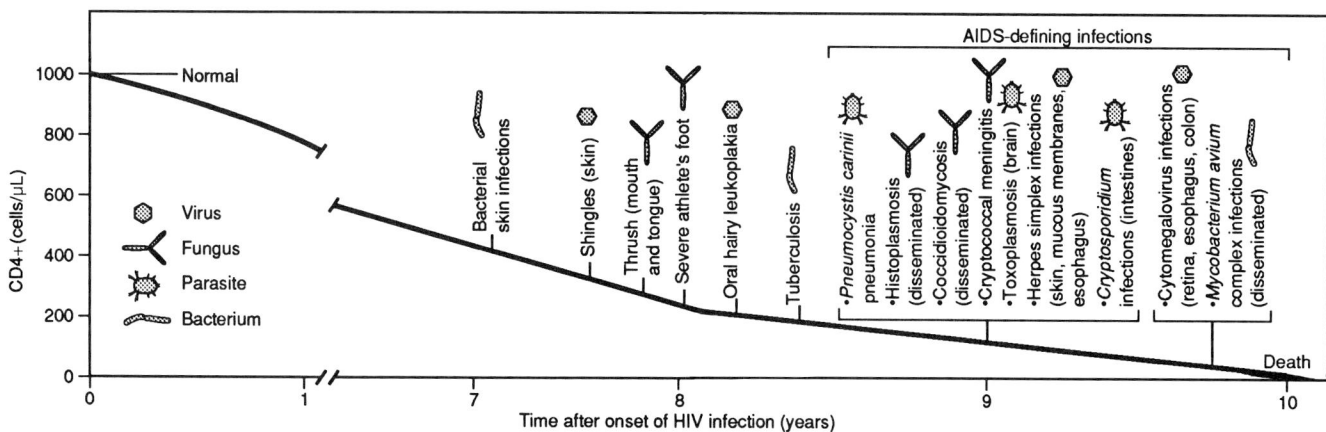

FIGURE 9-1-1. Major opportunistic infections in advanced HIV infection.

hepatitis B, sexual trauma, or prostitution should alert the practitioner to HIV risk. Use of alcohol and recreational drugs must also be assessed; the common correlation with the use of mind-altering substances and unsafe sex is well documented. Sharing needles and

TABLE 9-1-2. Grouping of Common HIV Clinical Conditions by General Etiology

I. HIV Proper

   AIDS dementia
   Aseptic meningitis
   Sensory neuropathy
   AIDS enteropathy
   Renal failure/AIDS nephropathy

II. Opportunistic Infections

   A. Bacterial
      Mycobacterium
      Streptococcus
      Haemophilus
      Staphylococcus
      Pseudomonas
      Neisseria
      Shigella
      Salmonella
      Campylobacter
   B. Fungal
      Cryptococcus
      Coccidioides immitis
      Histoplasma
      Aspergillus
      Microsporida
      Candida
      Isospora
   C. Viral
      Herpes simplex
      Herpes zoster
      Epstein-Barr
      Cytomegalovirus
   D. Protozoan
      Cryptosporidium
      Toxoplasma
      Pneumocystis

III. Neoplasia

   Kaposi's sarcoma
   Non-Hodgkin's lymphoma
   Hodgkin's lymphoma
   Cervical cancer
   Anal cancer

IV. Psychosis and Depression

trading sex for drugs are strong indicators of risk. A patient who is HIV-positive must continue to be counseled regarding behaviors that carry the risks of transmission of HIV to others and contact with potentially fatal pathogens in the face of their own compromised immune system function.

HIV disease can affect virtually any organ or system. A thorough review of systems during each patient encounter is indicated. Constitutional symptoms such as fever, fatigue, and weight loss can be caused by HIV or by infection. Skin changes, respiratory complaints, gastrointestinal or genitourinary symptoms, and changes in mental status may also herald disease progression.

OBJECTIVE FINDINGS

A thorough physical examination is warranted in all patients; specific areas are of particular importance in assessing HIV disease. The respiratory exam and examination of the skin may uncover the first signs of HIV disease; *Pneumocystis carinii* pneumonia and Kaposi's sarcoma remain the most frequent initial conditions in HIV disease. The skin exam may also reveal signs of herpes infection, molluscum contagiosum, syphilis, or *Staphylococcus* infection.

Examination of the oral mucosa may reveal signs of candidiasis, herpes, oral hairy leukoplakia, or Kaposi's sarcoma. Patients with oral candidiasis and dysphagia are presumed to have esophageal candidiasis and do not need to be endoscoped before the initiation of treatment. Lymphadenopathy should be recorded in terms of size, number, location, and tenderness; correlation to HIV disease and/or opportunistic infection is necessary. Biopsy should be reserved for cases in which the nodes are associated with fever or weight loss to assess for lymphoma or mycobacteria.

The genital exam may reveal the lesions or ulcers of sexually transmitted diseases. Pap smears should be performed every 3 months in HIV-positive women to detect cervical dysplasia. The rectum and anus may also exhibit signs of sexually transmitted diseases or cancer.

A complete neurologic exam should be performed on all new HIV-positive patients and in any patient presenting with changing symptoms. Change in mental status may be subtle: caregivers or companions may provide insight into changes in personality or behavior. Motor and sensory examinations and assessment of reflexes will aid in the analysis of neurologic diseases or possible drug side effects such as peripheral neuropathy.

LABORATORY STUDIES

HIV Testing

All testing for HIV should be accompanied by both pre- and posttest counseling regarding past, present, and future risk. The standard test for HIV infection is an enzyme-linked immunosorbent assay (ELISA)

TABLE 9-1-3. Manifestations of HIV Disease by System

Pulmonary
  Pneumocystis carinii pneumonia
  Bacterial pneumonia
  Tuberculosis and other mycobacterial diseases
  Lymphoid interstitial pneumonia
  Disseminated histoplasmosis
  Disseminated coccidioidomycosis
  Aspergillosis
  Cytomegalovirus (CMV)
  Kaposi's sarcoma
  Lymphoma

Gastrointestinal
  Candidiasis (thrush)
  Oral hairy leukoplakia
  Esophagitis
  Acute and chronic diarrhea
    Cryptosporidiosis
    Microsporidiosis
    Mycobacterial
    CMV
    Isosporiasis
    Other bacterial (shigella, shigellosis, campy)
  AIDS enteropathy
  Wasting syndrome
  Lymphoma
  Acalculous cholecystitis

Ophthalmologic
  Retinal disease (cotton wool spots)
  CMV retinitis
  Toxoplasmosis chorioretinitis
  Necrosis (herpes simplex, varicella)
  Optic neuropathy

Hematologic/Oncologic
  Cytopenia
  Thrombocytopenia
  Anemia
  Neutropenia
  Hematopoietic suppression
  Kaposi's sarcoma
  Non-Hodgkin's lymphoma
  Hodgkin's lymphoma
  Cervical cancer
  Anal cancer

Neurologic
  Toxoplasmosis
  Cryptococcal meningitis
  Progressive multifocal leukoencephalopathy
  CMV meningitis
  Syphilis
  Lymphoma
  AIDS dementia
  Aseptic meningitis
  Sensory neuropathy
  Dementia

Renal
  Fluid and electrolyte imbalances
  Acid-base disorders
  Renal failure
  HIV nephropathy

Cardiac
  Ventricular dysfunction
  Myocarditis
  Pericarditis
  Endocarditis
  Arrhythmias

Endocrine
  Adrenal dysfunction
  Hypogonadism
  Hypothyroidism

Rheumatologic
  Arthralgia
  Myopathy
  Reiter's syndrome
  Sjögren's syndrome
  Arthropathy
  Vasculitis

TABLE 9-1-4. Sexual Practices and Risks for HIV/AIDS

Safe
  Massage
  Hugging
  Stroking
  Mutual masturbation (no skin cuts or breakage)
  Self-masturbation
  Dry kissing
  Monogamous relationship between two uninfected partners
  Abstention

Possibly Safe
  French (wet) kissing
  Anal intercourse properly using a latex condom
  Vaginal intercourse properly using a latex condom
  Urine contact (not with mouth, rectum, or any broken or cut skin)

Possibly Unsafe
  Cunnilingus
  Fellatio
  Fellatio without ejaculation
  Sharing of sexual devices

Unsafe
  Receptive anal intercourse without a condom
  Vaginal intercourse without a condom
  Anilingus
  Unprotected anal penetration with the hand
  Anal douching with oral sex
  Multiple sex partners

SOURCE: From PT Cohen: Safe sex, safer sex and prevention of HIV infection, in PT Cohen et al (eds): *The AIDS Knowledge Base.* Waltham, MA, Medical Publishing Group, 1990.

for antibodies to the HIV virus. The HIV test has been available since March 1985. It has a high sensitivity and is relatively inexpensive. False-positive ELISA tests may occur in patients with systemic lupus erythematosus, pregnancy, or in conditions that produce rheumatoid factor or cryoglobulins. False-negative ELISA tests occur in the early "window" period after infection (up to 12 months, average period 3 months) and also in the later stages of symptomatic AIDS. The most frequent cause of false positives or false negatives is lab error. Any positive ELISA test is repeated; if again positive, a confirmatory Western blot (immunoblot) test is performed. If the Western blot is also positive, the patient is diagnosed as HIV-positive. If either of the ELISA tests are positive and the Western blot is negative, or the ELISA is negative but a strong suspicion is held, the patient is retested in 3 months. Meanwhile, all patients should be counseled regarding risk factors and educated to reduce any possible impending risk of transmission to the patient as well as to the patient's contacts. A patient with a negative ELISA or Western blot may indeed be positive for the virus but not as yet mounting an immune response. More recently, the development of recombinant protein ELISA tests have reduced the window period to 20 days; however, this test is not available for general screening, although it is used for screening donated blood.

Laboratory tests are also available for detecting various parts of the virus, such as the p24 antigen and the β_2-microglobulin; other tests measure antibodies to other parts of the virus but are generally confined to the research arena. The p24 antigen is measured to confirm the acute HIV syndrome. Recent scientific advances show potential for some of these testing methods to become part of standard diagnostic protocol. Direct culture of the virus is a very slow process that is performed exclusively in research trials. Several virus particles are undergoing testing in the hopes of developing a vaccine; to date no preventative or therapeutic vaccine is available.

Screening

Risk assessment is an integral component in the fight to eradicate HIV. All patients should be screened for risk factors for HIV exposure and counseled concerning behavioral changes that they may make to reduce their risk of exposure and transmission. Unsafe sexual behavior, substance abuse, history of blood or blood product transfusion, occupational exposure, and tuberculosis should prompt further assessment and encourage HIV testing. All pregnant women should be offered counseling and testing. Patients presenting with generalized lymphadenopathy, unexplained weight loss, chronic diarrhea, fever of unknown origin, recurrent infections, or STDs should alert the practitioner to the possibility of HIV. Any patient requesting HIV testing, regardless of risk, should receive full support of their request without judgment.

Routine Laboratory Analysis

When a patient is known to be HIV-positive, several laboratory tests should be performed on a scheduled basis. Baseline counts of leukocytes, erythrocytes, and platelets are important for prognosis, disease state, and detection of changes resulting from drug therapy. Anemia is very common in HIV disease as is neutropenia, especially if the patient is receiving antiretroviral therapy. Clinicians should monitor cell counts and initiate therapy as is appropriate. Renal function and liver enzymes should also be recorded prior to initiation of any therapy, and, as monitoring tools, serum glucose, protein, and albumin are important in assessing overall health and nutritional status. Changes in liver enzymes may indicate hepatitis or drug toxicity.

Serologic tests for syphilis are recommended; positive screening results should be followed with specific treponemal testing and appropriate antisyphilis therapy. Patients with latent syphilis should have the cerebrospinal fluid (CSF) examined for organisms in light of the high risk of neurologic involvement with syphilis in HIV-positive patients. Skin testing for tuberculosis is mandatory in all HIV-positive patients. Any reaction >5 mm in a patient who is HIV-positive should be treated with a minimum of 1 year of isoniazid. In geographic areas exhibiting higher prevalence of multidrug-resistant tuberculosis, treatment should be adjusted accordingly.

The CD4+ Count

HIV has a particular affinity for CD4+ cells. The virus can attach to the surface of the cells like Velcro, enter the cell, and begin the cycle of viral replication and dysfunction and death of the immune cells. A normal CD4+ count is above 500; most people have above 1000/μL. The CD4+ count was the first widely used method to track HIV disease progression and continues to be valuable when measured in conjunction with viral load. As the disease progresses, the number of CD4+ cells declines, indicating continuing destruction of the immune system. Parameters of CD4+ counts have been established for use in diagnosing HIV disease and in predicting the risk of acquiring opportunistic infection, therefore assisting in the decision for prophy-

laxis (see Fig. 9-1-1). A CD4+ count below 200/μL meets the CDC criteria for AIDS regardless of symptom status. It is also the level that prophylaxis against the most frequent opportunistic infections (*P. carinii* pneumonia, toxoplasmosis) and treatment with retrovirals [zidovudine (Retrovir; AZT)] has generally been recommended, although these recommendations have been controversial over the years and are undergoing renewed analysis in light of the introduction of newer anti-HIV medications.

Viral Load

Quantitative virology is standard in HIV care. It is essential for accurately diagnosing HIV and for staging, monitoring, and directing treatment options. These tests encompass polymerase chain reactions (PCR) to detect viral RNA by augmenting viral replication in the lab and a branched DNA (bDNA) test that detects viral RNA via a light-producing reaction in the lab. The nucleic acid sequence–based amplification (NASBA) is a highly sensitive assay reserved for detecting the virus in patients with very low viral loads. Viral load provides an excellent marker for disease progression. Studies have shown an inverse relationship between viral load and CD4+ count and, therefore, probability of clinical symptoms. As the CD4+ count is a marker of change in the immune system and its ability to function, viral load is a marker of viral progression. Together, the tests are powerful indicators of disease status with or without clinical symptoms. However, it is also widely believed that only about 2% of the virus is circulating in the blood at any time. Therefore, a very low or even negative viral load test does not guarantee a virus-free state even with a high CD4+ count.

Staging

Determination of where a patient lies within the continuum of HIV disease is important in the effort to maximize treatment and improve prognosis. The 1993 CDC AIDS Surveillance Case Definition for Adolescents and Adults is a 3 × 3 matrix that uses CD4+ cell count and clinical status to stage patients (Table 9-1-5). Patients with stage A3, B3, or any C stage (i.e., any AIDS indicator condition or a CD4+ count <200/μL) are considered to have AIDS and must be reported to the local health department in order to assure accurate surveillance and assist in the distribution of federal resources.

TREATMENT

Aggressive treatment against HIV has resulted in significant success in stabilizing patients' immune systems, reducing complications such as opportunistic infections and neoplasias, and prolonging life. In the United States, HIV is no longer a death sentence; proper treatment under the supervision of an expert in HIV management can control the progression of the disease. HIV in developed countries has made the transition from an acutely fatal infection to a chronic disease that requires the expertise of specialized practitioners as the patient ages. In many parts of the world, however, antiretroviral medications are not

TABLE 9-1-5. 1993 AIDS Surveillance Case Definition for Adolescents and Adults

CD4+ CELL CATEGORIES	CLINICAL CATEGORIES		
	A. ASYMPTOMATIC, PGL, OR ACUTE HIV INFECTION	B. SYMPTOMATIC	C. AIDS INDICATOR CONDITION
1. >500/μL (>/=29%)	A1	B1	C1
2. 200–499/μL (14%–28%)	A2	B2	C2
3. <200/μL (<14%)	A3	B3	C3

ABBREVIATION: PGL, Progressive generalized lymphadenopathy.
SOURCE: From Centers for Disease Control and Prevention, Atlanta, GA.

available and HIV continues to be a frequent cause of quick and devastating death.

The goals of treatment in HIV disease are multiple. First and foremost is to identify patients infected with HIV and ensure access to medical treatment and monitoring. Once HIV is identified, a variety of services are needed to manage the complex medical and psychosocial needs of HIV-positive patients. Medical management starts with a full history and physical examination to assess the patient and the present status of the HIV infection as well as any preexisting non-HIV-related diseases or conditions. Control of HIV replication and enhancement of immune function is a constant struggle; the development of new drugs is aimed at balancing this battle. The ultimate goal is to have no HIV units and a fully functional immune system. That goal has not been met, but research is ongoing.

Throughout the course of HIV disease, the prevention, diagnosis, and management of opportunistic infections and malignancies are key to patient survival. Death more commonly is due to overwhelming infection or malignancy than to HIV itself. As patients progress through the stages of HIV disease and end-stage AIDS, simple needs such as housing, transportation, nutritional supplements, emotional counseling, bereavement counseling, legal services, and financial assistance for medical costs and living expenses become important. Health care practitioners must work with other service providers to provide effective and efficient care.

There are four broad areas of treatment: conventional care (prophylaxis and treatment of opportunistic infections, prevention of HIV transmission, and antiretroviral therapy); preventative care and wellness (nutrition, exercise, stress reduction, and elimination of smoking, alcohol excess, and drug abuse); psychological counseling (suicide prevention, management of anxiety and depression, and grief and loss counseling); and nontraditional approaches (hypnosis, biofeedback, physical manipulation, and unorthodox therapies). This chapter will emphasize conventional care.

Antiretroviral therapy is, in general, indicated in patients with the acute HIV syndrome, symptomatic disease, or asymptomatic patients with CD4+ counts below $500/\mu L$ or HIV RNA viral load >10,000 copies/μL by bDNA assay or >20,000 copies/μL by the reverse transcriptase (RT)-PCR assay. Patients who do not fall under these guidelines may defer treatment or opt to begin treatment. The decision should be made in consultation with an HIV specialist and take into account such characteristics as clinical status and history of prior treatment, immune status, risk of disease progression, risk of developing resistance, patient reliability and adherence, risk of medication interaction or side effects, and access to follow-up care. All patients, regardless of clinical or treatment status, should be seen and monitored regularly. Frequency of follow-up and laboratory monitoring will depend on both personal and clinical factors. The patient, in consultation with his or her health care practitioner and HIV specialist, best makes these decisions. Patients need to be informed about treatment options, side effects, and when to notify the practitioner regarding symptoms and changing clinical status.

Table 9-1-6 offers a quick reference guide to the antiretroviral drugs. As of the close of 1999, 14 drugs had been approved for use against HIV. The first antiretroviral available was AZT. AZT is a nucleoside analog reverse transcriptase inhibitor (NRTI). Reverse transcriptase is necessary for the formation of a double-stranded DNA proviral copy of the viral RNA; this class of drugs inhibits this enzyme, thereby blocking further replication by competing with the natural nucleoside triphosphate for binding to reverse transcriptase. Several other NRTIs are available, each with its unique safety profile. NRTIs delay the decline in CD4+ cells, reduce viral load, decrease opportunistic infections, prevent or reduce HIV-associated dementia, and significantly alter the risk of vertical transmission. Side effects include nausea, headache, and fatigue; these symptoms usually abate after the first few weeks of

therapy. Myelosuppression is a serious side effect. The complete blood count (CBC) should be monitored every 3 months. Some patients can survive with seriously low blood cell counts; others may benefit from the addition of granulocyte colony-stimulating factor (G-CSF) or erythropoietin.

Nonnucleoside reverse transcriptase inhibitors (NNRTIs) also inhibit reverse transcriptase activity but do so indirectly by binding to reverse transcriptase at a site remote from the substrate-binding site. There are three NNRTIs available. Resistance is common and, once it emerges, is conferred across the category. They are metabolized by the cytochrome P450 system, and therefore, caution must be used when prescribing other medications if the patient is on an NNRTI.

Protease inhibitors (PIs) block a separate enzyme, protease, which is necessary for the production of mature infectious particles prior to budding of the infected cell. Thus, the replication cycle is broken and HIV is prevented from infecting other cells. PIs are also metabolized by the cytochrome P450 system. When first introduced, PIs resulted in significant reductions in viral load and the first glimpse at cure. However, although highly effective against HIV, especially in combination with other antiretroviral medications, a cure is not in sight yet. PIs were the first antiretroviral associated with abnormal fat distribution (lipodystrophy), but this phenomenon has since been seen in patients without a history of PI therapy.

Current research continues to search for new drugs within the three existing classes and also to develop new classes of drugs with unique mechanisms of action. Preliminary studies have shown promising results with different medications including fusion inhibitors, integrase inhibitors, and nucleocapsid zinc finger inhibitors.

The virus quickly develops resistance to all the retrovirals available when they are used as monotherapy. The virus has a profound ability to mutate. Cross-resistance is frequent. Combination therapy with a minimum of three drugs is standard therapy. Several combinations are possible. Highly active antiretroviral therapy (HAART) has produced significant benefits to patients infected with HIV. There has been a marked decline in mortality and significant reductions in incidence of opportunistic infections, rates of hospitalization, and utilization of home care, skilled facilities, and hospice care. On the forefront in HIV therapy now is the potential for long-term side effects and virologic failure secondary to drug resistance.

Selection of an antiretroviral regimen is guided by the potency of each drug alone and in combination, how well the combination will be tolerated, and the ease with which a patient can adhere to the regimen. Practitioners must be wary of resistance and cross-resistance as they anticipate patient response to a give regimen and allow for future combination possibilities to salvage therapy.

The standard of care for HIV, especially patients naïve to antiretroviral therapy, is a combination of a PI with two NRTIs. When taken correctly, this regimen is highly successful in suppressing viral replication. However, the regimen is complex and side effects are great. Table 9-1-7 lists several other commonly prescribed regimens.

The remarkable ability of HIV to mutate should encourage practitioners to adhere to strict guidelines when treating infected patients. Similar to the management of tuberculosis, optimal dosing of each drug and acute awareness of impending resistance is warranted to provide the best chances of prolonging survival and to avoid the development of virus resistance and cross-resistance between drugs. Noncompliance with recommended dosing regimens, subtherapeutic levels, interactions with other dugs, and the use of monotherapy, intermittent therapy, and sequential therapy may all contribute to the development of resistance. The fear of an emerging multidrug-resistant HIV is very real. It is imperative that practitioners involved in the care of HIV-positive patients remain attuned to the current and evolving knowledge and recommendations regarding treatment with anti-HIV drugs. Patient education is also a crucial element; open communication regarding the need for compliance, the risks of drug–drug interactions, the progression of disease and resistance,

TABLE 9-1-6. Quick Reference Guide to Antiretrovirals*

Nucleoside Analog Reverse Transcriptase Inhibitors (Nucleoside Analogs, NRTIs)

CHEMICAL	GENERIC	BRAND	DOSE	COMMENTS AND COMMON SIDE EFFECTS
AZT	Zidovudine	Retrovir	300 mg twice daily	Initial nausea, headache, fatigue, anemia, neutropenia, neuropathy, myopathy.
3TC	Lamivudine	Epivir	150 mg twice daily	Generally well tolerated. Active against HBV.
AZT + 3TC	Zidovudine Lamivudine	Combivir	1 tablet twice daily	Combination tablet containing 300 mg of AZT and 150 mg of 3TC.
ddI	Didanosine	Videx	200 mg twice daily or 400 mg once daily on empty stomach (>60 kg body weight)	Peripheral neuropathy in 15%, pancreatitis; avoid alcohol. Contains antacid: ok to give at same time as all NRTIs, adefovir, nevirapine, and efavirenz; delavirdine and indinavir must be taken at least 1 h prior to ddI; nelfinavir can be taken 1 h after ddI.
ddC	Zalcitabine	Hivid	0.375–0.75 mg three times daily	Peripheral neuropathy in 17–31% of trial participants; oral ulcers.
d4T	Stavudine	Zerit	20–40 mg twice daily	Peripheral neuropathy (1–4% in early studies; 24% in expanded access patients with CD4+ counts <50).
1592U89	Abacavir	Ziagen	300 mg twice daily	Up to 3% hypersensitivity reaction: fever, malaise, possible rash, GI. Resolves within 2 days after discontinuation. *Do not rechallenge.* Also: rash alone without hypersensitivity.

Nonnucleoside Reverse Transcriptase Inhibitors (NNRTIs)

GENERIC	BRAND	DOSE	COMMENTS AND COMMON SIDE EFFECTS
Nevirapine	Viramune	200 mg (1 tablet) once daily for 2 weeks, then 200 mg twice daily or 400 mg once daily.	Transient rash, hepatitis. P450 3A4 inducer. Once-daily dosing recommendation based on pharmacokinetic data only.
Delavirdine	Rescriptor	400 mg (4 tablets) 3 times daily	Transient rash. P450 3A4 inhibitor.
Efavirenz	Sustiva	600 mg (3 cap) once daily at bedtime	Initial dizziness, insomnia, transient rash, P450 3A4 inducer; avoid clarithromycin.

Protease Inhibitors (PIs)

GENERIC	BRAND	DOSE	COMMENTS AND COMMON SIDE EFFECTS
Saquinavir hard gel cap	Invirase	600 mg (3 cap) 3 times daily with fatty meals	Well tolerated. Limited potency due to poor absorption (4%). In time will be replaced by Fortovase.
Saquinavir soft gel cap	Fortovase	1200 mg (6 cap) 3 times daily with fat-containing food (>28 g)	Improved absorption compared to Invirase. 1600 mg twice daily promising. Store in refrigerator. Stable at room temperature for 3 months.
Ritonavir	Norvir	600 mg (6 cap/7.5 mL) twice daily; start with 300 mg twice daily and increase to full dose over 10 days	Nausea, diarrhea, numb lips for up to 5 weeks or longer; occasional hepatitis. Up to 50% will not tolerate. Currently only available in liquid formulation.
Indinavir	Crixivan	800 mg (2 cap) every 8 hours on empty stomach or with snack containing <2 g of fat. Note: bid dosing ineffective when sole PI	Kidney stones in 6–8%, good hydration essential. Occasional nausea and GI upset. Store in original container which contains dessicant; without this, IDV is stable for only about 3 days.
Nelfinavir	Viracept	750 mg (3 tab) 3 times daily or 1250 mg (5 tab) every 12 hours with food	Diarrhea common, which may respond to Ultrase MT20 enzyme preparations; occasional nausea.
Amprenavir	Agenerase	1200 mg (8 cap) twice daily with or without food	Rash (20%), diarrhea, nausea.

*These tables list all antiretrovirals currently available in U.S. pharmacies and through compassionate use protocols.
SOURCE: From M Schutz: Quick reference guide to antiretrovirals. http://hiv.medscape.com/updates/quickguide.

and the need for thorough follow-up on all recommendations is paramount to maximizing the benefits of treatment.

Supportive Measures

HIV-infected individuals have shown great support of and claim benefit from nontraditional medical approaches to disease. Proper nutrition and nutritional supplements, exercise, stress management, and avoidance of unhealthy habits such as smoking and drug abuse certainly will have a beneficial effect on any disease state. A strong investment in nutritional awareness has been evident in HIV disease; research has shown that proactive nutritional management can prevent or slow the HIV wasting syndrome and reduce the chances of gastrointestinal manifestations of the disease. Optimum healthy living has proved to increase the efficiency of the immune system and thus slows the progression of HIV disease.

TABLE 9-1-7.   Five Regimens for Naïve Patients: Pros and Cons

REGIMEN	ADVANTAGES	DISADVANTAGES
PI + 2 NRTIs	• Standard of care • Well-studied, long-term data • Effective and durable	• PI cross-resistance • Short-term and long-term side effects • Complex regimens
Dual-PI regimens	• More effective? • More durable? • Decreased pill burden/simpler regimens	• Potential for broad cross-resistance • Additive toxicity? • Ritonavir liquid (RTV-containing regimens) • High pill burden (NFV/SQV)
NNRTI + 2 NRTIs	• Allows deferral of PIs • Simple regimens • Well tolerated • Most effective? (EFV)	• Not all NNRTIs equipotent to PIs • Not as effective at high viral loads (NVP, DLV) • NNRTI cross-resistance
NRTI-based regimens (AZT/3TC/ABC) (ddI/d4T/HU)	• Allow deferral of PIs, NNRTIs • Simple regimens • Well tolerated	• Relative potency, durability not established • May be less effective at high viral loads • Blunted CD4+ response with HU • Long-term hydroxyurea toxicity?
PI/NNRTI/NRTI	• Three mechanisms of action • High potency • Induction-maintenance option (high baseline viral loads)	• Drug interactions • Potential for multiclass resistance • Not as well studied

ABBREVIATIONS: 3TC, lamivudine; ABC, abacavir; AZT, zidovudine; d4T, stavudine; ddI, didanosine; DLV, delavirdine; EFV, efavirenz; HU, hydroxyurea; NFV, nelfinavir; NNRTI, nonnucleoside reverse transcriptase inhibitor; NRTI, nucleoside analog reverse transcriptase inhibitor; NVP, nevirapine; PI, protease inhibitor; RTV, ritonavir; SQV, saquinavir.
SOURCE: From Oliva D, Glatt A: HIV infection: Epidemiology, transmission, and screening. *Hospital Medicine* 35(5):31–37, 1999.

HIV advocates have also been on the forefront of other nontraditional or complementary therapies. Hypnosis, biofeedback, acupuncture, imagery, and physical manipulation are just a few of the practices that have been widely used through the years by the general public and have received attention and increased acceptance as a result. Further research is needed before recommendations for alternative or complementary therapies can be made.

SPECIAL CONSIDERATIONS

Women and HIV/AIDS

In the United States, women comprise one of the fastest-growing segments of the HIV epidemic; HIV is the third leading cause of death in women aged 25 to 44 years; one in three new cases of HIV infection occurs in women. Heterosexual transmission and injection drug use account for the vast majority of HIV-infected women. The manifestations of HIV disease in women include all of the opportunistic infections and neoplasias seen in men with the addition of vaginal infections, pelvic inflammatory disease, and cervical dysplasia and cancer. Many of the infections are more aggressive and less responsive to treatment in women, including syphilis, herpes, human papillomavirus, and tuberculosis. In general, infection in women is not detected as early in the course of the disease and treatment is not sought as aggressively as it is in men. Increased public awareness and patient education is needed.

HIV disease and pregnancy is a major concern. The virus can be transmitted in utero, during delivery, or through breast milk. There is no way to predict the chances for vertical transmission in any individual pregnancy. Risk is greatest in mothers with high viral loads, low CD4+ counts, or placental membrane inflammations and/or STD. The results of clinical trials have shown a significant reduction (from 30% to <10%) in the risk of transmission to the fetus with the use of AZT prenatally, at delivery, and in the neonate. Research is ongoing on the role of PIs in pregnancy and the long-term effects of treatment on the infant and the mother. Recent studies have supported the use of routine cesarean section to reduce the risk of infection. The use of artificial rupture of membranes, fetal electrodes, and episiotomies may increase risk and should be avoided. Practitioners need to be aware of the risks of infection and the benefits of treatment. They should counsel all pregnant patients with the recommendation that they be tested for HIV and should never withhold treatment for HIV or its manifestations because of pregnancy.

Pediatric and Adolescent HIV

Children are at risk of HIV through perinatal transmission from an infected mother, through sexual abuse, via contaminated drug-injection equipment, and as recipients of infected blood or blood products. Since the introduction of blood testing in the United States in 1985, the risk through infected blood and blood products has been extremely low. The majority of HIV cases seen in children are through perinatal transmission and can be detected at birth. The expansion of the use of antiretroviral therapy during pregnancy and the neonatal period should result in a reduction of pediatric cases. However, at this time, not all pregnancies and neonates are monitored for HIV infection.

Infants born to infected mothers will be positive for HIV antibodies; continued positivity or positive viral antigen testing confirms infections in the baby. Failure to thrive, continued or recurrent bacterial infections, chronic diarrhea, developmental delay, and persistent thrush, diffuse lung disease, lymphadenopathy, or hepatosplenomegaly constitute the usual manifestation of HIV disease in infants and children.

Lymphoid interstitial pneumonia is the most common AIDS-defining illness in children presenting with nonproductive cough, wheeze, and respiratory distress. Presumptive diagnosis is frequent and there is no specific treatment; symptomatic treatment includes oxygen, bronchodilators, and steroids. Pediatric dosing with antiretroviral medication is recommended.

Occupational Exposure in Health Care Workers

Health care providers are at risk of contamination from bloodborne pathogens such as hepatitis and HIV. HIV is far less likely to be transmitted from such contamination than is hepatitis, but HIV produces greater fear and anxiety. HIV carries a greater degree of social discrimination and ostracism. The fear of contracting HIV through needle-stick injuries, open skin exposure, and splash accidents prompted the development of universal precautions that were formalized by the CDC in the 1980s and have been updated and maintained since. Now known as standard precautions, the main objective is to view each patient encountered as a potential source of contamination and use the same commonsense precautions in every situation. The precautions include wearing gloves and protective equipment whenever exposure to bodily fluids is likely, never recapping needles, and using the proper tools to clean up any spills and dispose of any waste. All health care practitioners should be fully cognizant of and adamantly adhere to all standard precautions.

The risk of transmission of the virus from patient to practitioner when the source patient is known to be HIV-positive is less than 0.3% after a percutaneous exposure (needle-stick injury) and even less so for a mucous membrane or skin exposure. Risk is increased if the source patient has a higher viral load or if the accident involves deep intramuscular penetration or the use of large-gauge hollow needles. Prolonged contact and large volumes of blood or bodily fluids also carry greater risk of transmission (Table 9-1-8). If contamination with bodily fluids does occur, regardless of the status of the source, the first step is to copiously wash the area involved. Hands and other skin surfaces should be washed with soap and water, letting the injury bleed; mucous membranes should be irrigated with water. All such accidents must be reported to the institution at which the accident occurred, and proper counseling and follow-up must be initiated. Baseline HIV testing of the health care worker and the source patient should be performed after consent is obtained. Testing should be repeated 6 weeks, 12 weeks, and 6 months following the incident.

Prophylaxis against HIV following occupational exposure has undergone several changes since the advent of AZT and the development of additional anti-HIV drugs. The current recommendations offer guidance according to the status of the source and the nature of the injury. In all such occupational accidents, the risk of disease must be balanced with the risk and benefits of treatment. For percutaneous injuries, prophylaxis is encouraged for any deep intramuscular puncture and recommended for superficial injuries and accidental skin pricks with a used bloody sharp if the source is in end-stage AIDS. Health care workers who sustain superficial percutaneous injuries associated with an asymptomatic patient can be offered prophylaxis, but it is not recommended or encouraged.

Mucous membrane exposure occurs with accidents such as a splash to the eyes or mouth with bodily fluids or tissue. Prophylaxis is encouraged if the source is in end-stage AIDS and the exposure is large and prolonged; prophylaxis is recommended if the contact is either large or prolonged regardless of source status. Prophylaxis can be offered in the case of small and brief contact, if the recipient strongly desires.

Surface cutaneous exposures are exposures to bodily fluids onto skin that is abraded or chronically chapped, or onto skin that contains a moderate to severe dermatitis without the protection of gloves. Prophylaxis is recommended if the exposure is large and/or prolonged and may be offered for small and brief contact if the exposure occurs onto skin that is nonintact.

Current prophylaxis regimens advise the use of combination drug therapies. AZT should be included in all regimens at the recommended dose of 200 mg orally tid. Addition of another reverse transcriptase inhibitor as well as a PI completes the regimen. Four weeks of full triple regimen is the minimum recommended therapy for serious injuries. HIV testing is done at baseline, 6 weeks (2 weeks after completion of the drug therapy), 12 weeks, and 6 months; all exposed

TABLE 9-1-8. Hierarchy of Infection Risk by Type of Exposure to HIV-Positive Blood

High risk*

- Deep injury (causing bleeding) from a hollow-bore, blood-filled needle
- Direct contact with concentrated virus in a research laboratory

At risk*

- Needle-stick injury or laceration (causing bleeding) from instrument visibly contaminated with blood
- Exposure of an open wound or conjunctivae to blood or to bodily fluid visibly contaminated with blood

Low risk*

- Superficial injury (not causing bleeding)
- Exposure of a closed wound or of mucous membrane other than conjunctivae to blood or to bodily fluid visibly contaminated with blood
- Prolonged blood contact over large areas of skin; skin wound caused by bite

No documented risk

- Contamination of intact skin (small area) by blood
- Injury with instrument not visibly contaminated with blood

*Risk is further increased if source patient is in end-stage AIDS or is in the window period of HIV infection.
SOURCE: From Oliva D, Glatt A: HIV infection: Epidemiology, transmission, and screening. *Hospital Medicine* 35(5):31–37, 1999.

health care workers should receive ongoing counseling, regardless of any treatment option chosen.

BIBLIOGRAPHY

1993 revised classification system for HIV infection and expanded surveillance case definition for AIDS among adolescents and adults, in *Mortality and Morbidity Weekly Report.* Atlanta, GA, Centers for Disease Control and Prevention, 1992.
AMA physician guidelines: HIV blood test counseling, in *AMA Physician Guidelines #511.* American Medical Association Division of Health Science, Atlantic Information Services, 1993.
Daar E: Primary HIV infection. *Medscape HIV/AIDS* Annual Update 5(suppl): 1999.
Gallant J: Antiretroviral strategies and controversies. *Medscape HIV/AIDS* Annual Update 5(suppl), 1999.
Gallant J: The seropositive patient—the initial encounter, in *HIV Clinical Management,* vol 1. Medscape, 2000.
Goldman L, Plum F (eds): *Cecil Textbook of Medicine,* 21st ed. Philadelphia, W. B. Saunders, 2000.
Hammer S: Antiretrovirals: New agents and new targets. *Medscape HIV/AIDS* Annual Update 5(suppl), 1999.
Laurence J: Stopping heterosexual HIV. *AIDS Reader* 9(8):512–513, 518, 1999.
Lewis JE: History of the acquired immunodeficiency syndrome (AIDS) epidemic, in *AIDS and the Allied Health Professions,* JW Hopp, EA Rogers (eds). Philadelphia: F. A. Davis, 1989.
Mayer-Quezada D: Guidelines for occupational exposure. Lecture, New Jersey Academy of Medicine, Mount Laurel, NJ, December 5, 1997.
Muma RD et al: *HIV Manual for Health Care Professionals.* Norwalk, CT, Appleton & Lange, 1994.
Oliva D, Glatt A: HIV infection: Epidemiology, transmission, and screening. *Hospital Medicine* 35(5):31–37; 1999.
Ries K: HIV infection and AIDS: A diagnostic consideration in every patient. *Consultant* 39:3027–3035, 1999.
Shacker T et al: Clinical and epidemiologic features of primary HIV infection. *Ann Intern Med* 125(4):257–264, 1996.
Ungvarski PJ, Flaskerud JH: *HIV/AIDS—A Guide to Primary Care Management,* 4th ed. Philadelphia, Saunders, 1999.
Vanhems P, Toma E: Recognizing primary HIV-1 infection. *Infect Med* 16(2):104–108, 110, 1999.
Weiss W: Lecture: Current guidelines in the diagnosis and treatment of HIV disease. Lecture, Piscataway, NJ, December 9, 1996.

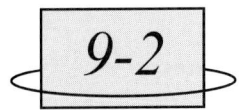

KAPOSI'S SARCOMA

Claire Babcock O'Connell

DISCUSSION

Until the advent of HIV disease, Kaposi's sarcoma (KS) was a malignancy of Mediterranean and Jewish elderly men, certain endemic areas of central Africa, and persons undergoing immunosuppressive therapy after receiving transplants. Since the emergence of HIV disease, KS has become the most frequently encountered neoplasm in infected patients. KS is 20,000 times more common in HIV-positive persons than in the general population of the United States. In the early 1980s, KS was reported in over 40 percent of patients diagnosed as HIV-positive. The frequency has declined in recent years; KS is now seen in 10 to 15 percent of HIV-positive persons. It is 20 times more common in homosexual or bisexual males than in HIV-positive patients without homosexual contact.

The exact cause of KS remains unknown; epidemiologic data point to an infectious cause. KS is believed to be caused by a reactivation process of a herpes virus infection. The newly discovered offending agent had been termed Kaposi's sarcoma–associated herpesvirus (KSHV) and is now known more appropriately as human herpesvirus-8 (HHV-8). Reactivation may be promoted by immunostimulation, immunosuppression, concurrent infections, and genetic, behavioral, and environmental factors. Transmission occurs through human-to-human contact. Research indicates that HHV-8 is a ubiquitous virus, although it is not clinically apparent until a person becomes immunosuppressed.

Histopathologically, KS demonstrates a mixture of different cell types. Lesions predominantly consist of endothelial cells and spindle cells that are enveloped with erythrocytes, altered lymphocytes, and macrophages. The cell of origin is not known, but it is most likely of mesenchymal origin. There are four histologic types of KS: classic KS, endemic KS (equatorial Africa), iatrogenic or posttransplant KS, and AIDS-associated KS.

SYMPTOMS

KS most commonly affects the skin and mucous membranes, although other systems, such as the lungs and the gastrointestinal tract, also may be affected. Lesions usually first appear as small violaceous macules that are not painful or pruritic. The lesions commonly have a surrounding ring of erythema. As the disease progresses, lesions may enlarge and may become nodular and/or confluent. Large plaque-like areas may develop, particularly on the lower legs. The rate of growth and the pattern of progression are highly variable. The most common sites of disease are sun-exposed areas, the hard palate, the posterior pharynx, and the glans penis. The skin over the lesions may break down and necrose; although this is rare, it is very painful.

It is not unusual to find lymphatic involvement in KS presenting as tender lymphadenopathy or painful lymphedema. Pulmonary disease results in respiratory distress and pulmonary effusions; it is commonly mistaken for *Pneumocystis carinii* pneumonia (PCP). KS of the oral cavity is most commonly asymptomatic and must be specifically searched for in any HIV-positive patient. Oral lesions may become painful and interfere with eating. Other lesions along the gastrointestinal (GI) tract may cause malabsorption, bleeding, or diarrhea. In over 40 percent of patients with cutaneous lesions, KS lesions are found in the gut at autopsy.

OBJECTIVE FINDINGS

KS most commonly appears as nonblanching cutaneous lesions that are red to purple in color and painless. They are cosmetically worrisome but do not cause major morbidity. Nodular lesions often are brown in color. Suspicion of visceral involvement necessitates biopsy for confirmation.

DIAGNOSIS

The diagnosis of KS is based on physical findings and patient risk, namely, HIV-infected or otherwise immunocompromised patients. Cutaneous lesions are readily identified, and the diagnosis is not difficult. Punch biopsy findings show a typical mixed pattern. Definitive diagnosis via biopsy is often desired before treatment is initiated. Bacillary angiomatosis is caused by the microbe *Rochalimaea* and may present with similar lesions; the diagnosis is achieved by Warthin-Starry staining of the biopsy, and treatment consists of antibiotics. Oral KS lesions need to be differentiated from lymphoma.

Pulmonary KS and GI KS generally necessitate biopsy for adequate diagnosis. Often bronchoscopy is ordered in a search for PCP, and KS is found. Respiratory distress and pulmonary effusions carry a wide differential; the diagnosis is assisted by patient history and index of suspicion and confirmed by bronchoscopic evidence of submucosal lesions with characteristic biopsy results. Symptoms of GI involvement also present diagnostic difficulty. KS usually is first suspected after other, more common causes of the symptoms (bacterial, parasitic, wasting syndrome) are ruled out; confirmation is done through endoscopy and biopsy.

LABORATORY TESTS

Polymerase chain reactions are available to detect HHV-8 in clinical specimens and disseminated tissues. Other immunologic tests are under investigation. These tests may allow clinicians to detect the risk for KS in both non-HIV-infected patients and those who are infected but are not yet exhibiting signs of KS.

RADIOLOGIC STUDIES

Chest x-rays in pulmonary KS patients show thickened bronchial walls and nodularity. Lesions commonly are found centrally and at major bifurcations. Kerley B lines, pleural effusions, and hilar or mediastinal adenopathy also are seen. Bronchoscopy reveals typical flat red to purple lesions that may appear similar to hemorrhagic lesions produced by bronchoscopic trauma. Intestinal endoscopy reveals typical raised red nodules in KS of the GI tract.

OTHER DIAGNOSTICS

The National Institute of Allergy and Infectious Diseases AIDS Clinical Trials Group has developed a TIS Staging System for Kaposi's sarcoma (see Table 9-2-1). The system is based on tumor (location and extent), immune system (CD4+ T-cell count), and systemic illness. The classification divides patients into two broad categories and is used to predict the prognosis.

TREATMENT

Small, nonpainful lesions that do not involve lymphatics or other organ systems can be simply observed. Excision is possible for small lesions that are cosmetically bothersome. Local radiation, intralesional chemotherapy (vinblastine), and local cryotherapy have been successful, but recurrence is typical. In patients with disseminated disease or extensive cutaneous advancement, systemic combination chemotherapy will provide a 50 percent response rate within the first few weeks. However, the treatment must be continued chronically as the lesions will recur when the chemotherapy is stopped. It is wise to consult an experienced expert when initiating chemotherapy. Severe pulmonary KS also may respond to radiation therapy.

Current research indicates that KS may be treated or even prevented through treatment with the antiviral medications foscarnet and

TABLE 9-2-1. National Institute of Allergy and Infectious Diseases AIDS Clinical Trials Group TIS System for Kaposi's Sarcoma

PARAMETER	GOOD RISK (STAGE 0): ALL OF THE FOLLOWING	POOR RISK (STAGE 1): ANY OF THE FOLLOWING
Tumor (T)	Confined to skin and/or lymph nodes and/or minimal oral disease	Tumor-associated edema or ulceration Extensive oral lesions Gastrointestinal lesions Nonnodal visceral lesions
Immune system (I)	CD4+ T-cell count ≥ 200 cells/μL	CD4+ T-cell count <200 cells/μL
Systemic illness (S)	No B symptoms* Karnofsky performance status >70 No history of opportunistic infection, neurologic disease, lymphoma, or thrush	B symptoms* Karnofsky performance status <70 History of opportunistic infection, neurologic disease, lymphoma, or thrush

*B symptoms = unexplained fever, night sweats, >10 percent involuntary weight loss, or diarrhea persisting for more than 2 weeks.

ganciclovir. Acyclovir has shown no beneficial effects. Aggressive antiretroviral therapy may cause regression of KS if a significant rise in CD4+ cells occurs.

Patient Education

Although KS commonly occurs on sun-exposed areas, there is no evidence that avoidance of sun exposure will help prevent KS. Patients should be made aware of the myriad patterns of development and prognosis. Involvement of the viscera does not imply a poor response to therapy.

COMPLICATIONS

Extensive organ involvement, although rare, can be life-threatening. Extensive pulmonary involvement may be clinically silent for a prolonged period and may occur without cutaneous involvement. Respiratory distress and parenchymal or pleural involvement may cause severe respiratory compromise. Lymphatic involvement may cause severe lymph blockage and the threat of vascular compromise of the extremities or groin.

BIBLIOGRAPHY

Goldman L, Bennett JC (eds.): *Cecil Textbook of Medicine,* 21st ed. Philadelphia, Saunders, 2000.

Lin J-CL. Pathogenesis of Kaposi's sarcoma and human herpesvirus-8. *Infect Med* 5(4):264–272, 1998.

Muma RD, et al: *HIV Manual for Health Care Professionals.* Norwalk, CT, Appleton & Lange, 1994.

Powderly WG: Opportunistic infections. *Medscape HIV/AIDS* 5(Suppl), 1999.

Ungvarski PJ, Flaskerud JH: *HIV/AIDS: A Guide to Primary Care Management.* Philadelphia, Saunders, 1999.

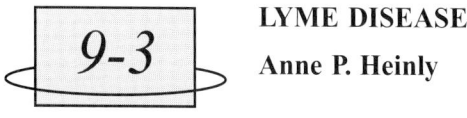

LYME DISEASE

Anne P. Heinly

DISCUSSION

Borrelia burgdorferi is the spirochete that is known to cause Lyme disease. Named for the town of Old Lyme, Connecticut, the disease has been around since the turn of the twentieth century but was not identified as a single infectious disease process until 1975. Well known in the northeastern, midwestern, and Pacific coast areas of the United States, Lyme disease may infect up to 10,000 patients a year. People become a vector for ticks carrying *B. burgdorferi* when hiking through wooded or grassy areas populated by deer. Ticks emerge when the weather warms up, and so infections are most common from May through September, when temperatures are above 2°C (35°F).

PATHOGENESIS

Spirochetes are slender, undulating motile bacteria that form spirals or helixes about 15 mm long. There are three recognized pathologic spirochete classes: *Borrelia* (Lyme disease), *Treponema* (syphilis), and *Leptospira* (leptospirosis). *Borrelia burgdorferi* gains entry to the skin through the bite of an infected deer tick (east and midwest) or a western black-legged tick (Pacific coast). The ixodid tick is very small and populates the growing herds of deer that are spreading throughout the United States. Because the tick lives up to 2 years, there are three distinct growth phases that require a blood meal (biting humans and deer). First, the larvae hatch in the spring and feed on ground hosts (rodents, including mice and rats) and birds that also may act as reservoirs. A year later, the young ticks (the size of a typed period) feed on rodents, and in the fall, they attach to a deer, where they may grow to an impressive 5 mm in size.[1] The small size is important in that most patients never see the tick; the larger pet tick is accused unjustly. *Borrelia burgdorferi* can be transmitted during any blood meal. The spirochete then slowly replicates in the skin and eventually spreads via the lymphatics or bloodstream to other organs. Infection is improbable if the tick is removed within 24 to 36 h of attachment. Lyme disease cannot be transmitted from human to human.

Pregnant women who contract Lyme disease do not appear to have adverse fetal outcomes.

SYMPTOMS

Lyme disease is a continuum. By far the most common initial symptom (stage 1) involves the skin rash (50 percent[2]) erythema migrans (EM). The rash typically appears 10 to 14 days after a bite. The lesion initially appears as a red macule that expands into a red, raised plaque-like round (annular) lesion with central clearing. EM migrates relatively quickly and has no scaling. The rash may appear vesicular or even ulcerative. The final lesion (at 2 to 4 weeks) may be up to 40 cm in size.

Systemic symptoms appear early but may be diagnosed as a viral illness with fever, headache, myalgias, malaise, and vague joint pain. Up to 80 percent of patients with multiple EM lesions have systemic manifestations early.[1]

Stages 2 and 3 can be somewhat blurred. It is accepted that stage 2 symptoms generally occur weeks to months after stage 1, usually involving the skin, central nervous system (CNS), and joints. Stage 3 is the chronic state of untreated Lyme disease, succeeding stage 2 after months or even years. The disseminated phase of the infection tends to be exhibited in three areas.

The joint pain is common (>80 percent[2]) and migratory and almost always includes some neck or back pain. The later stages of the disease involve more arthralgias. There seems to be a predilection for the knees, the temporomandibular joint (TMJ), and large joints. Swelling without heat or erythema is common and usually is not associated with eye symptoms. Polyarticular involvement is seldom seen. In the chronic stage, patients may complain of recurrent bursitis, synovitis, and tendinitis.

With progression of the disease, neurologic symptoms (<15 percent[2]) become evident. Patients may present with meningeal symptoms, facial nerve palsies, peripheral neuropathies, and even radiculopathy.

In stage 2, patients may present with classic viral meningitis symptoms, including headache, stiff neck, and mild photophobia.

Cranial neuropathies are quite prevalent, usually presenting during stage 2. Any patient presenting with a facial palsy (Bell's palsy) should be investigated for Lyme disease. The palsies usually subside in 6 to 8 months. Peripheral neuropathies are manifested by intermittent paresthesias and weakness that may be confused with diseases such as Guillain-Barré. Fortunately, it is rare for a patient to progress to encephalomyelitis (stage 3) or spastic paraparesis. Encephalopathy may cause persistent memory loss, dementia, headache, and difficulty with concentration. Some patients experience chronic fatigue, confusion, depression, mood changes, and sleep changes.

Other symptoms may include cardiac arrhythmias (<5 percent[2]), most frequently heart blocks. The most common heart block is a simple first-degree block. Complete heart block can occur on occasion but rarely remains past 1 to 2 weeks. Third-stage disease rarely includes chronic cardiomyopathy and pericardial effusions. These patients also may present with tachycardia, bradycardia, myocarditis, and pericarditis.

OBJECTIVE FINDINGS

The rash of Lyme disease is the first clue. The erythema usually is red but may be a mottled blue-red with central clearing without scaling. The rash progresses rapidly over days, ranging in size from 20 to 40 cm around. As the lesions become larger, the central clearing may be bright red, ulcerative, or papular (resembling a burn). The rash is typically nontender. A single large lesion is common on the trunk. When there are multiple lesions, EM may be confused with erythema multiforme. A distinguishing feature is that EM typically spares the palms, soles, and mucous membranes. Systemic manifestations may include a low-grade fever, diaphoresis, and mild dehydration.

DIAGNOSTIC CONSIDERATIONS

The differential diagnosis for Lyme disease includes several dermatologic, rheumatologic, and neurologic processes, depending on when the patient is seen (see Table 9-3-1). If the rash is not present on examination, the diagnosis can be hard to establish and a thorough evaluation is essential to rule out major cardiac, neurologic, and arthritic conditions. If a tick-borne disease is considered, one must be sure to rule out Rocky Mountain spotted fever and relapsing fever, as the treatment is quite different. A vital clue is the presence of arthritic symptoms with a normal rheumatoid factor (RF) or antinuclear antibodies (ANA) and the lack of associated symptoms as seen in Reiter's syndrome.

LABORATORY TESTS

Laboratory testing is the mainstay for confirming the diagnosis. A standardized flagellin–enzyme-linked immunosorbent assay (ELISA) serologic test is used in endemic areas. Timing is everything, as testing a day after a presumed bite will yield nothing. The optimal testing time is between 3 and 6 weeks after the bite, when circulating IgM levels are at their peak.[3] An antibody response may take up to 8 weeks to be measurable. False positives may occur because other species of *Borrelia* may contaminate the serologic antigens or react to other spirochetal diseases (e.g., syphilis). If the ELISA is borderline, a Western blot can help detect antibody bands and decrease the number of false-negative and false-positive reports. Because of the imperfections in serologic testing, the final diagnosis is as dependent on the history and clinical presentation as it is on the laboratory findings.

Cultures of the EM skin lesions can yield *B. burgdorferi* but take several days to weeks to incubate. Research continues on ways to isolate the spirochete. Culturing of cerebrospinal fluid (CSF), blood, and synovial fluid has been disappointing as a method of diagnosis. Complete blood count (CBC), rheumatoid factor (RF), antinuclear

TABLE 9-3-1. Differential Diagnosis for Lyme Disease

DISEASE	CHARACTERISTICS
Rocky Mountain spotted fever	*Rickettsia rickettsii*, transmitted by ticks. Sudden onset of fever, headache, and chills for 2–3 weeks. Red rash seen on palms, soles, ankles, and wrists, progressing to a red maculopapular rash on the trunk, buttocks, and axillae. Cough and CNS symptoms occur
Relapsing fever	A *Borrelia* spirochete infection from a louse or tick. Louse-borne is endemic to Africa, China, and Peru; tick-borne is seen worldwide. Characterized by relapsing fever and neurologic symptoms, including deafness, unilateral blindness, and neuropathies
Typhus fever	*Rickettsia typhi*, transmitted by fleas. It causes shaking chills, headache, and fever. Rash begins in the axillae and becomes a dull macular rash involving the entire body eventually. Cough and rales are common. Neurologic effects may include dementia and coma
Juvenile rheumatoid arthritis	Insidious onset of arthralgia (polyarticular), fever, fatigue, myalgia with a fine rash. Sedimentation rate elevated with positive RF in some patients. ANA may be elevated as well
Systemic lupus erythematosus	Insidious onset of myalgia, fever, arthritis symptoms, eye pain and vision changes, and weight loss. Rash is usually erythema nodosum over the legs plus a "butterfly" macular rash over the cheeks and nose. Positive ANA and elevated sedimentation rate
Scleroderma	Insidious onset of joint stiffness, arthralgia, myalgia, and skin changes, including swelling, dryness, and cracking. Dyspnea, weakness, weight loss, and proximal muscle weakness all possible. Increased sedimentation rate and ANA
Tinea corporis	Scaling plaque with well-demarcated annular red rings. Maximum size for most lesions is 5 cm with no central clearing and mild itching. No systemic symptoms
Erythema multiforme	A self-limiting skin sensitivity characterized by sudden onset of rash on palms, soles, and all extensor surfaces. Oral mucosa vesicles and ulcers are common. The lesions may have central clearing and a burning sensation
Encephalitis, viral	Sudden onset of malaise, fever, and neck pain followed by meningeal irritation with stiffness and headache. Myalgias and arthritis symptoms may increase with fever. No rash generally
Meningitis, bacterial	Fever, headache, and neck pain and stiffness, usually after an upper respiratory infection. Rigor, seizures, dementia, loss of concentration, weakness, and photophobia common. A maculopapular rash initially, then petechial with mild pruritus

antibodies (ANA), and other laboratory parameters are usually normal or negative in Lyme disease patients.

RADIOLOGIC (IMAGING) STUDIES

Imaging studies are not generally helpful in diagnosing Lyme disease but may be useful in ruling out various arthritides. In the chronic phase, some joint erosion may be noted, but it is not consistent with the usual joint stiffness and elevated RF or ANA commonly seen with rheumatoid arthritis.

TREATMENT

Lyme disease can be treated at any phase after discovery, with a variable cure rate. Certainly if the history and clinical findings are supported by positive serology, therapy should be started immediately. If the diagnosis is unconfirmed but highly suspected by history and examination, therapy should be started. Table 9-3-2 lists the current therapeutic options. Supportive measures should be tailored to the stage of the disease, the age of the patient, and concomitant diseases. Joint pain may be treated with anti-inflammatories and joint rest. A pacemaker may be necessary for temporary relief of heart blocks. Persistent neuralgias may require antidepressant serotonin reuptake inhibitors therapy.

COMPLICATIONS

As many as 50 percent of patients with untreated Lyme disease may develop recurrent synovitis and migratory arthritis symptoms. The infection may be a trigger for fibromyalgia and/or chronic fatigue syndrome. Peripheral neuropathies and paresthesias are also common complications. Encephalopathies may include memory loss, dementia, poor concentration, and stroke-like symptoms. Some patients treated late in the course of the disease (>60 months) may have permanent damage to the CNS, heart, or joints.

Patient Education

The best treatment is prevention. The recommendations for endemic areas include wearing long sleeves and long pants tucked into the socks. Light-colored clothing is a must, as black ticks then show up better and are more easily removed. A repellent may be helpful (DEET)

TABLE 9-3-2. Treatment of Lyme Disease

SYMPTOM	MEDICATION	TIMING AND CONSIDERATIONS
Erythema migrans (EM)	Doxycycline 100 mg bid or amoxicillin 500 mg tid or cefuroxime 500 mg bid or clarithromycin 500 mg bid Azithromycin 500 mg day 1, then 250 mg × 4 days	Give for 2–3 weeks with the exception of azithromycin: use amoxicillin in children and pregnant or lactating women
Facial palsies CNS disease Cardiac disease Arthritis	Doxycycline 100 mg bid or amoxicillin 500 mg tid or ceftriaxone 2 g/d IV or cefotaxime 2 g/d IV or penicillin G 20–24 million units IV daily	Early symptoms can be treated for 2–3 weeks. Late or severe symptoms should be treated for 3–4 weeks and may require IV therapy

SOURCE: Modified from Sanford J, Gilbert D, Moellering R, et al: *The Ranford Guide to Antimicrobial Therapy.* Vienna, VA, Antimicrobial Therapy, 1997.

but should be used with care in children and the elderly. One should never use repellent near the eyes and should try to avoid thick brush and high grasses, as the ticks do not jump well. After finishing a hike or work, it is necessary to inspect the body for ticks. Removal is accomplished with a tweezer and a gentle but firm tug. One should try not to crush the tick because the body fluids may contaminate the bite area. One must wash the area well, save the tick for inspection, and watch for the development of the rash and/or flu-like symptoms.

In endemic areas, it may be wise to clear the property of ticks, especially for farmers and hunters. Several over-the-counter insecticides are available to treat soil and lawns. All these products should be used with care and according to the manufacturer's instructions. Another measure may include special baits for the field mice and rodents that act as vectors for the ticks. The rodents carry the insecticides into their burrows and kill existing ticks.

PEARLS

On any given day in the spring or summer in an endemic area, parents worry about tick bites. Remember that ticks usually wander over the body for a few hours to find a cozy spot to feed at, and so inspection and brushing off the skin and clothing are the key to prevention. Additionally, the tick needs to be attached for 24 to 36 h before transmission of *B. burgdorferi* occurs. Prophylaxis for even confirmed bites is generally avoided and has not proved effective. Watch for the rash. If you have the rash, systemic symptoms, and the tick, treat it. With today's rapid transit, anyone can present with Lyme disease. If the rash has receded before you see a patient, a high index of suspicion is required to order the serology.

REFERENCES

1. Lyme Disease: Clinical Update for Physicians. American Lyme Disease Foundation, with the CDC of the U.S. Public Health Service, fall 1993.
2. Infectious disease: VII. Leptospirosis. *Sci Am,* 1996, pp 7–15.
3. Recommendations for the use of Lyme disease vaccine. *MMWR* 48(RR-7): 1–25, 1999.

BIBLIOGRAPHY

Berger BW: Current aspects of Lyme disease and other *Borrelia burgdorferi* infections. *Dermatol Clin* 15(2):247–254, 1997.

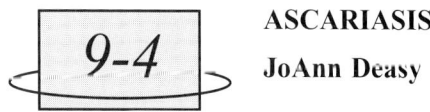

ASCARIASIS
JoAnn Deasy

DISCUSSION

Ascariasis, or roundworm infection, is the most common helminthic infection worldwide. In the United States, approximately 4 million people are infected with *Ascaris lumbricoides,* mostly in the southeast. *Ascaris* eggs reach the soil in feces and in 2 to 3 weeks develop into embryos that are infectious. The eggs can persist for years in the soil. Transmission is usually from hand to mouth. In dry, windy climates, the eggs may become airborne and then be inhaled and swallowed.

The larval worms hatch in the small intestine and migrate through the gut wall into the bloodstream. They are carried through the liver to the alveoli of the lungs. In the course of this migration, the larvae increase in size. By the time they reach the pulmonary capillaries, they are too large to pass through to the left side of the heart. Since their route is blocked, they rupture through the alveolar spaces and are coughed up and swallowed. When they return to the upper intestine, they complete their maturation and mate. The adult worms are white or reddish-yellow and are 15 to 35 cm in length, a little longer than a pencil. Each female produces a daily output of approximately 200,000 ova.

SYMPTOMS

The symptoms are dependent on the intensity of the infection and the organ involved. If the worm load is small, infections may be completely asymptomatic. In the lungs, the worms may cause a pneumonitis known as Löffler's pneumonia. Transient symptoms of fever, cough, substernal burning, wheezing, and shortness of breath are associated with the pneumonia. The presence of adult worms in the intestines may cause vague abdominal discomfort or nausea. Heavier worm loads may result in abdominal pain and malabsorption. Occasionally, a mass of worms may develop and cause intestinal obstruction or an adult worm may migrate to the appendix, bile duct, or pancreatic duct, causing inflammation and obstruction of that organ.

OBJECTIVE FINDINGS

In a patient with pulmonary involvement, wheezes and rales may be heard on auscultation of the lungs. Oxygen desaturation may occur. Occasionally, the collection of worms in the intestine may be large enough to be palpated on abdominal examination. In an asymptomatic individual, the only indication of infection may occur when the adult worms are vomited or passed in the stool.

DIAGNOSTIC CONSIDERATIONS

During the pulmonary stage, ascariasis must be differentiated from asthma and pneumonia caused by bacteria or a virus. The gastrointestinal symptoms must be differentiated from other parasitic infections and other causes of intestinal obstruction.

LABORATORY AND RADIOLOGIC TESTING

To make the diagnosis, a stool examination for ova and parasites should be ordered. Characteristic eggs are seen in the feces. The peripheral blood may exhibit eosinophilia. The pulmonary phase is diagnosed by the finding of larvae and eosinophils in the sputum. Perihilar infiltrates may be seen on chest x-ray.

TREATMENT

The usual treatment consists of mebendazole (Vermox) 100 mg twice daily for 3 days. Albendazole also may be used and has the advantage of being given in a single dose (400 mg). Pyrantel (1 mg/kg, maximum dose 1 g) may be prescribed for pregnant patients. Drug treatment may fail to kill the larvae, and so a follow-up examination of the stool for ova and parasites should be done 2 months after treatment. Ultimately, eradication requires adequate sanitation facilities.

BIBLIOGRAPHY

Juckett G: Common intestinal helminths. *Am Fam Physician* 52(7):2039–2048, 1995.

Mandell GL, Douglas RG, Bennett JE: *Principles and Practice of Infectious Diseases,* 4th ed. New York, Churchill Livingstone, 1995.

Rakel RE: *Conn's Current Therapy 2000.* Philadelphia, Saunders, 2000.

Sherris JC (ed): *Medical Microbiology.* New York, Elsevier, 1990, pp 734–736.

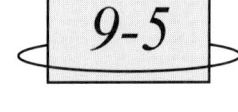

CAT-SCRATCH DISEASE

Katherine Adamson

DESCRIPTION

Anyone who sees children in his or her daily practice will see cat-scratch disease. Cat-scratch disease (CSD) can best be described as a generally benign and self-limiting type of lymphadenitis. CSD most often is encountered in the pediatric population, with an estimated 24,000 cases occurring annually in the United States.[1]

PATHOGENESIS

As one might infer from the name, CSD is transmitted by contact with cats that have picked up the offending organism from the soil. Typically, an immature animal is infected with the causative agent, a small, pleomorphic gram-negative bacillus known as *Bartonella henselae.* The cat remains asymptomatic as it carries the organism in its mouth and paws. CSD most often is transmitted by a scratch or bite, though a lick or even contact with infected secretions has been known to inoculate the disease. Within a few days of contact with an infected cat, the affected individual presents with a small papule that rapidly becomes a vesicle and just as rapidly (two to three days) resolves, leaving a macule that may persist for weeks. This prodromal skin lesion appears at the site of inoculation whether it is a bite, a scratch, or mucous membrane contact with previously broken skin. Days to weeks may go by before the characteristic sign of lymphadenopathy appears.

MICROBIOLOGY

The causative organism of CSD, *B. henselae,* has been isolated from the lymph nodes of affected patients. This organism, formerly known as *Rochalimaea* and briefly called *Afipia felis,* has been associated with bacillary angiomatosis in immunocompromised individuals.[2] An immunocompetent patient generally presents with a limited regional lymphadenopathy that is tender to palpation in the initial stages of the infection. If the lymph tissue is excised in an effort to rule out a more serious etiology, the pathologist will note stellate necrosis and granulomatous inflammation. The bacilli may be demonstrated with silver impregnation stains in approximately one-third of cases.

SYMPTOMS

Typically, a patient with CSD presents to the clinic 2 weeks or so after inoculation. The symptom that prompts parents to bring their children for medical care is invariably a tender enlarged lymph node. The associated symptoms are not unlike those of many infectious disorders: malaise, low-grade fevers [39°C (102°F)], appetite disturbances, and vague generalized aches and pains. Rarely, conjunctival inoculation may lead to an oculoglandular syndrome known as Parinaud's syndrome, which is striking in appearance but has a very good prognosis.

OBJECTIVE FINDINGS

The lymphadenopathy of CSD is proximal to the site of inoculation. Typically, one or two nodes are involved, with disseminated disease reported in patients with an immune deficiency. Since the site of inoculation is most often an upper extremity, the location of the adenopathy probably will be epitrochlear, axillary, or cervical. A small minority of these nodes progress to suppuration, with the vast majority slowly regressing over several weeks. Parinaud's oculoglandular syndrome is notable for preauricular adenopathy, conjunctival granuloma formation, and surprisingly minimal local discomfort and purulent discharge.

DIAGNOSTIC CONSIDERATIONS

Of paramount importance in the diagnosis of CSD is a history of exposure to a cat in the setting of limited lymphadenopathy. Careful questioning will elicit a history of contact with a cat in the vast majority of cases. The clinician should inquire carefully about the presence of the premonitory papule, which may have been forgotten or overlooked. At the same time, the clinician must be aware that this papule is seen in only about one-half of cases of CSD. Other, more devastating etiologies of lymphadenopathy must be included in the differential. This need to rule out malignancy of the lymph node often leads a clinician to search for a definitive diagnosis. Table 9-5-1 includes a partial list of the more common diagnoses that should be included in the differential.

SPECIAL CONSIDERATIONS

The key to preventing CSD lies in limiting opportunities for infected cats to transmit the infection. Parents and children should be warned to avoid stray and unknown animals. Family pets, particularly kittens, should be kept indoors and handled carefully. If a break in the skin occurs, immediate cleansing and wound care will minimize disease transmission. One also must remember that a cat bite or scratch can transmit other organisms. *Pasteurella multocida* presents very differently, with a rapidly developing cellulitis.

LABORATORY TESTS

The diagnosis of CSD is suspected whenever a clinician is confronted with a patient with tender lymphadenopathy of 3 or more weeks' duration and a history of cat exposure. An immunofluorescent antibody (IFA) assay for *B. henselae* is available from the Centers for Disease Control.

RADIOLOGIC STUDIES

Radiographic investigations generally are reserved for investigating other etiologies of lymphadenopathy [i.e., a chest computed tomography (CT)

TABLE 9-5-1. Common Causes of Lymphadenopathy

Infectious
  Viral
    Cytomegalovirus
    Epstein-Barr virus
    Herpes family (varicella, zoster, simplex)
    Human immunodeficiency virus
    Rubella

  Bacterial
    Streptococci
    Staphylococci
    Chlamydia (lymphogranuloma venereum, trachoma)
    Spirochetes (syphilis, leptospirosis)
    Mycobacteria

  Fungal
    Coccidioidomycosis
    Histoplasmosis

Malignancy
  Lymphomas (Hodgkin's and non-Hodgkin's)
  Leukemias
  Metastatic carcinomas (breast, lung, gastrointestinal tract, head, neck)

Hypersensitivity Reactions
  Drug reactions (phenytoin)
  Foreign body (silicone implants)
  Vasculitis (systemic lupus erythematosus, rheumatoid arthritis)

Endocrinopathy
  Hyperthyroidism

Other
  Sarcoid

scan in the workup of lymphoma or a mammogram if axillary adenopathy is due to breast carcinoma].

OTHER DIAGNOSTICS

A skin test for CSD exists, but it is no longer commercially available because of controversy about its safety. The antigen used in the skin test was derived from human lymph node aspirate. This gave rise to concern about viral contaminates that might be present in the antigen.[3] A reasonably reliable diagnosis can be made on the basis of the time-honored methods of a suggestive history and physical findings. The clinical situation of the patient will dictate the clinician's comfort level in choosing between watchful waiting and a more invasive approach (node biopsy). Of course, a tuberculin skin test should be administered to all patients who present with regional lymphadenopathy.

TREATMENT

Medications

Antibiotic therapy is rarely indicated in the treatment of CSD. A variety of antibiotics, including trimethoprim-sulfamethoxazole, rifampin, amoxicillin, ciprofloxacin, and azithromycin, have shown in vitro effectiveness against *B. henselae*. The author is unaware of any controlled clinical trails that demonstrate a clear benefit from using these antibiotics in clinical treatment. Most authors recommend treating only the rare patient who is severely ill.[1] A commonly suggested regimen for an unusually ill patient is combination therapy with a third-generation cephalosporin and an aminoglycoside.

Supportive Measures

Treatment with analgesics is often helpful in controlling the associated symptoms. In addition, the patient should be advised to rest and avoid any activity that may traumatize the involved lymph tissues. In the rare instance where affected nodes painfully suppurate, it can be comforting to aspirate the involved nodes, using sterile technique and a large-bore (16-gauge) needle.

Patient Education

Once the diagnosis has been made, it is important to review the pathogenesis and prognosis with the patient. The patient needs to know that some degree of malaise and activity limitation probably will occur over the recovery period of weeks to a few months.

Disposition

It is vital that all instances of lymphadenopathy be followed at regular intervals until complete resolution has occurred. Early in the course of CSD, this may mean weekly or even twice weekly visits to the office. Once the patient is obviously recovering, it is reasonable to follow the affected nodes every few weeks until they are no longer enlarged.

COMPLICATIONS AND RED FLAGS

In a patient with an intact immune system, complications are fortunately rare. It is possible to see involvement of the central nervous system (encephalitis), liver, spleen, lung, bone, and skin.

NOTES AND PEARLS

It is of the utmost importance that affected lymph nodes be followed sequentially until resolution has occurred. The difficulty of obtaining an accurate node measurement can be minimized through the use of commonly available electrocardiographic (ECG) calipers, measuring the node in both the horizontal and vertical planes.[4]

REFERENCES

1. Spach DH, Koehler JE: *Bartonella*-associated infections. *Infect Dis Clin North Am* 12:137–155, 1998.
2. Tompkins LS: *Bartonella* infections, including cat-scratch disease, in Fauci AS, Braunwald E, Isselbacher KJ, et al (eds): *Harrison's Principles of Internal Medicine,* 14th ed. New York, McGraw-Hill, 1998, pp 983–985.
3. Margileth AM: Cat-scratch disease, in Rakel RE (ed): *Conn's Current Therapy, 1999,* 51st ed. Philadelphia, Saunders, 1999, pp 157–158.
4. Kelly CS, Kelly RE: Lymphadenopathy in children. *Pediatr Clin North Am* 45:881–882, 1998.

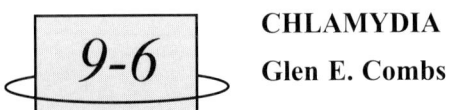

9-6 CHLAMYDIA
Glen E. Combs

DISCUSSION

The etiologic agent of chlamydia is *Chlamydia trachomatis,* an obligate intracellular parasite that causes the currently most common bacterial sexually transmitted disease in the United States. *C. trachomatis* is responsible for more than 4.6 million infections annually in the United States; 20 to 40% of sexually active American women show serologic evidence of exposure. Reported prevalence rates range from 4 to 9% in primary care settings to as high as 30% in sexually transmitted disease (STD) clinics.

Risk factors that have been shown to increase the incidence of infection include multiple sexual partners, a new sexual partner (within the last 2 months), age below 25 years, being unmarried, inconsistent use of barrier contraceptives, and poverty. The incubation period is 7 to 21 days after exposure.

SIGNS, SYMPTOMS, AND OBJECTIVE FINDINGS

Uncomplicated Infections

Studies show that up to 80% of infected women display no apparent signs or symptoms. In symptomatic women, a mucopurulent vaginal discharge and a friable cervix are the most common clinical findings. Dysuria and urinary frequency may occur in women with chlamydial urethritis.

Asymptomatic infection is also common in men (studies show up to 25%). The most common infection sites in men are the urethra and the rectum. Urethritis presenting with a clear or mucopurulent urethral discharge is the most common clinical finding in symptomatic men.

Complicated Infections

In women, a chlamydial infection may migrate into the upper genitourinary tract and present as a bartholinitis, an infection of the Bartholin's ducts; salpingitis; or perihepatitis (infection of the hepatic capsule), also known as the Fitz-Hugh-Curtis syndrome. This syndrome should be suspected in any sexually active woman who presents with right upper quadrant abdominal pain, fever, nausea, and vomiting. A concurrent salpingitis is usually present. Asymptomatic or symptomatic chlamydial infections may persist for months, during which time sexual transmission and complications may occur. Other complications in women include chronic pelvic pain, infertility, and ectopic pregnancy.

In men, complications of a chlamydial infection include epididymitis (presenting as unilateral scrotal pain associated with swelling,

TABLE 9-6-1. Differential Diagnosis of Cervicitis and Urethritis with Chlamydial Infection

Chlamydia trachomatis
Neisseria gonorrhoeae
Trichomonas vaginalis
Ureaplasma urealyticum
Bacterial vaginosis
Candidiasis
Herpes simplex virus
Allergic urethritis/cervicitis (latex)

tenderness, fever, and urethritis; see Chap. 18-4). Additional complications include proctitis (Chap. 6-23), prostatitis (Chap. 18-3), and Reiter's syndrome (urethritis and conjunctivitis occurring at the same time; Chap. 10-9). *Chlamydia* rarely produces systemic infections.

DIAGNOSTIC CONSIDERATIONS

A variety of genital pathogens, many of which are sexually transmitted, may cause urethritis or cervicitis (Table 9-6-1).

SPECIAL CONSIDERATIONS

Management of Sexual Partners

The sexual partners of infected patients must be evaluated and treated. A patient should be instructed to refrain from intercourse until the patient and his or her partner(s) have been adequately treated.

HIV Infection

The treatment regimen of chlamydial infections in HIV-infected patients is no different than the standard treatment regimens for chlamydial infections.

Pregnancy

The prevalence of *C. trachomatis* infection exceeds 5% among all pregnant women. There are specific treatment regimens for associated chlamydial infections in pregnancy.

Chlamydial Infections in Infants

Each year more than 155,000 infants are delivered to mothers infected with *Chlamydia.* Infants exposed to *C. trachomatis* during passage through an infected birth canal may have conjunctivitis (ophthalmia neonatorum) and/or pneumonia. *Chlamydia* is the most common cause of infectious conjunctivitis in infants up to 30 days of age. *Chlamydia* also may produce a subacute pneumonia in infants, commonly presenting up to 90 days of age.

Diagnostic Testing

Serologic testing is not useful in confirming the diagnosis. A laboratory diagnosis of *Chlamydia* relies on culture and nonculture diagnostic testing. Many cases are treated empirically without a laboratory diagnosis.

Cell culture is reliable but expensive. Nonculture tests are DNA probing of secretions and enzyme-linked immunoassay (EIA) (Chlamydiazyme). A number of rapid tests are now available, taking about 10 to 30 min to yield results. The advantages of office testing include ease of processing, rapid results, and increased cost-effectiveness. The main disadvantage of these tests is lower specificity.

TREATMENT

Pharmacologic Management

The recommended regimen is to treat with one of the following:

- Doxycycline 100 mg orally two times per day for 7 days
- Azithromycin 1 g orally in a single dose

Alternative regimens include the following:

- Ofloxacin 300 mg orally two times per day for 7 days
- Erythromycin base 500 mg orally four times per day for 7 days
- Erythromycin ethylsuccinate 800 mg orally four times per day for 7 days
- Sulfisoxazole 500 mg orally four times per day for 10 days (least effective)

The recommended regimen for pregnant women is erythromycin base 500 mg orally four times per day for 7 days. Alternative regimens for pregnant women include:

- Erythromycin base 250 mg orally four times per day for 14 days
- Erythromycin ethylsuccinate 800 mg four times per day for 7 days
- Erythromycin ethylsuccinate 400 mg four times per day for 14 days
- Amoxicillin 500 mg orally three times per day for 7 to 10 days

The recommended regimen for infants with ophthalmia neonatorum or pneumonia caused by *Chlamydia* is erythromycin 50 mg/kg per day orally in divided doses for 10 to 14 days.

PATIENT EDUCATION

Patients must be advised to abstain from sexual activity until they and their partners are cured. Concurrent treatment of partners is essential, even if they are asymptomatic. All sexual partners within the last 60 days should be clinically evaluated and treated. A history of an STD places a patient at increased risk for concurrent and subsequent STDs. When used consistently, condoms are effective in preventing STDs. Patient education in verifying the proper use of condoms should occur during the visit of every patient who has been exposed to STDs.

DISPOSITION

A follow-up test of cure is not mandatory since treatment failures (if medication is taken properly) are uncommon. Retesting should be performed if symptoms persist or reinfection is likely. Owing to higher treatment failure rates with sulfisoxazole and erythromycin, test of cure should be considered. Nonculture (DNA probe) follow-up testing at less than 3 weeks after the completion of therapy may be false positive because of the excretion of dead organisms.

COMPLICATIONS AND RED FLAGS

Many, but not all, states are required to trace and notify the sexual partners of patients with a sexually associated chlamydial infection. All clinicians should be knowledgeable about reporting procedures for communicable diseases in their respective states.

Routine screening for asymptomatic infection in women during the annual pelvic examination is recommended, particularly in high-risk patients. Clinical findings that are suggestive of asymptomatic infection (friable cervix, mucopurulent discharge) should be investigated. Routine screening of asymptomatic infection in men is not cost-effective.

ACKNOWLEDGMENT

The editor would like to acknowledge the significant contribution of Meredith Hansen, author of this chapter in the first edition of *Primary Care for Physician Assistants,* in the preparation of this revised work.

BIBLIOGRAPHY

Centers for Disease Control and Prevention: Recommendations for the prevention and management of *Chlamydia trachomatis* infections: 1993 sexually transmitted diseases treatment guidelines. *MMWR* 42:3–7, 47–56, 1993.
Majeroni BA: Chlamydial cervicitis: Complications and new treatment options. *Am Fam Physician* 49:1825–1828, 1994.
Preventive Services Task Force: *Guide to Clinical Preventive Services,* 2d ed. Alexandria, VA, International Medical Publishing, 1996.
Scholes D et al: Prevention of pelvic inflammatory disease by screening for cervical chlamydial infection. *N Engl J Med* 334:1362–1366, 1996.
Tierney L et al: *Current Medical Diagnosis and Treatment,* 39th ed. Lange Medical Books/McGraw-Hill, 2000, pp 1373–1375.

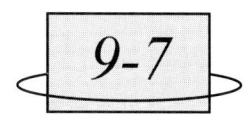

COCCIDIOIDOMYCOSIS
Diane S. Wrigley

DISCUSSION

Coccidioidomycosis (cocci) is a pulmonary fungal infection that is endemic in the southwestern United States. The common names are *cocci* and *valley fever.* Found only in the western hemisphere and in specific areas of Argentina and Central America, coccidioidomycosis is seen largely in the San Joaquin Valley of California and southern Arizona. Coccidioidomycosis is an increasingly important health problem because of the migration of large numbers of persons to endemic areas and increasing numbers of immunocompromised patients. Both the incidence and the severity of fungal infections appear to increase with the progression of HIV disease. From 50,000 to 100,000 people a year develop symptoms of cocci, 35,000 in California alone. Arizona reported a doubling of cases of coccidioidomycosis from 1990 to 1995, with the incidence changing from 7 to 14.9 cases per 100,000. It is the oldest of the major pathologic mycoses. The first case was described in 1892 in an Argentine soldier. A major dust storm in California in 1977 resulted in large amounts of spores being transported to northern and coastal areas several hundred miles away. In 1978, the incidence of cocci had a fourfold increase in the state and a 20-fold increase in the San Joaquin Valley.

PATHOGENESIS

The fungus *Coccidioides immitis* that causes cocci or valley fever is a normal inhabitant of the sandy and saline soil of the lower Sonoran Desert life zone. Infection occurs when liberated spherules are inhaled from disturbed soil through digging, building construction, dust storms, spelunking, archaeological digging, and rodent burrowing. Each spherule of *C. immitis* then releases hundreds of endospores. The infection cannot be transmitted from person to person. After exposure to the spores, with or without symptoms, the body develops immunity. Polymorphonuclear neutrophils (PMNs) in the blood manage to ingest 20 to 30 percent of the circulating endospores. PMNs can digest the outer walls of spherules but may not induce lethal injury. Cell-mediated immunity becomes the key to host defense. Although the lung is the primary site of infection as spores are inhaled, cocci can become progressive and spread hematogenously to involve extrapulmonary sites such as bone, skin, and the central nervous system (CNS). This process is referred to as *dissemination.* It can affect people of all ages without regard to sex, but the very young, the very old, and pregnant women have the worst clinical outcomes. *Coccidioides immitis* is stimulated directly by increased levels of estradiol and progesterone of pregnancy (see Table 9-7-1).

TABLE 9-7-1. Risk Factors for Increased Morbidity of Coccidioidomycosis

- Age group: very young and very old
- Race: Filipino, black, Native American, Hispanic, Asian, white, in order of most to least susceptible
- Negative skin test
- Serum complement fixation >1:64
- Pregnancy: second half and postpartum
- Immunosuppression: HIV, diabetes mellitus, chemotherapy, malignancies

SIGNS AND SYMPTOMS

About 65 percent of these infections are asymptomatic, with no complications. Evidence of exposure to *C. immitis* infection is detected by means of a positive skin test. The cocci spherule antigen is applied in exactly the same manner as a purified protein derivative (PPD) skin test. The results show whether a patient has been exposed to cocci much as a tuberculin skin test shows exposure to mycobacterium. Many symptomatic patients pass the illness off as the "flu" or an uncomplicated upper respiratory infection (URI) (see Table 9-7-2).

The other 35 percent of infections present as a primary pneumonia, often with pleuritic chest pain. Eventually, 95 percent of all cases progress to full resolution without complications. The other 5 percent advance to pulmonary complications such as acute respiratory disease (ARD), a pulmonary nodule or cavity, empyema, and progressive pulmonary involvement with skin lesions, abscesses, arthritis, osteomyelitis, and meningitis. The most common skin manifestations are erythema nodosum and erythema multiforme. The arthritis is experienced mostly in the knees and ankles and is symmetric. It is a result of immune complexes, not dissemination.

OBJECTIVE FINDINGS

Ear, nose, and throat (ENT) examination may reveal minimal to marked congestion with otherwise normal findings. The lungs are clear to auscultation and normal to percussion in asymptomatic and moderately symptomatic individuals. Rales may be heard in those who present with pneumonia. An inspection of the skin that reveals evidence of erythema nodosum or erythema multiforme should increase the suspicion of cocci. Any rash that does not fit a particular pattern in a symptomatic patient should raise the consideration of cocci. Cocci is known as a great "imitator," just as syphilitic rashes are. If a skin test has been administered, any evidence of induration or erythema after 48 h constitutes a "positive." Chest x-rays may range from normal to showing infiltrates that abut fissures and exhibit hilar adenopathy. Paratracheal and superior mediastinal infiltrates or mediastinal widening may signal dissemination.

DIAGNOSTIC CONSIDERATIONS

Cocci is not easily distinguished from other respiratory tract illnesses. The index of suspicion for cocci should increase with the chance of

TABLE 9-7-2. Symptoms of Coccidioidomycosis

SYMPTOM	PREVALENCE, %
Fatigue	77
Fever	46
Cough	64
Headache	22
Arthralgia	22
Chest pain	53
Dyspnea	17
Rash	23

exposure to endemic regions, an erythrocyte sedimentation rate (ESR) <28, signs of erythema nodosum, an absolute lymphocyte count <1.6, and pediatric and adolescent patients with complaints of chest pain.

LABORATORY TESTS

In the complete blood count (CBC), the white blood cell count (WBC) is below 10,000 in 27 percent of cases of eosinophilia. The ESR is elevated above 28. In sputum cultures, *C. immitis* will grow as thin strands of cotton on blood agar plates.

Antibodies Titers or Complement Fixation Titers

Tube precipitin antibodies (TPs) yield IgM or early signs of infection within the first 30 days after exposure to the spores. This is not a prognostic test, but it is useful as a screen for the presence or absence of possible disease. The complement-fixing antigen or IgG is proportional to the disease. These are quantitative antibodies determined by serial dilutions. The titers are reported as <1:2, 1:2, 1:4, 1:8, 1:16, 1:64, 1:132, and 1:264. Titers >1:16 suggest extrapulmonary infections, and titers that increase more than twofold over 2 to 3 weeks increase the suspicion of dissemination. Titers should be followed until the level is <1:2. Often the symptoms disappear as the antibody level drops. Biopsies of lung and skin may have cocci spherules present. A lumbar puncture may show persistent headache, changes in mental status, or neurologic symptoms.

TREATMENT

Most cases resolve without therapy. One must remember that 65 percent of these cases are asymptomatic. Rest and time are the recommended treatment for those who are symptomatic but are not at risk for extrapulmonary disease or dissemination. There is no evidence that treatment can shorten the course of illness or prevent more serious problems.

Immunodeficient patients and those who exhibit signs of extrapulmonary disease or are at risk of dissemination on the basis of x-ray, risk factor, or rising titers may be treated with

- Fluconazole (Diflucan) 400 mg/day
- Itraconazole (Sporanox) 400 mg/day
- Ketoconazole (Nizoral) 400 to 800 mg/day
- Amphotericin B (dose of cumulative therapy to a maximum of 1.0 g intrathecally until improved, followed by ketoconazole at 800 mg/d)

SUPPORTIVE MEASURES

Patients who develop bronchospasm may be treated with β_2-agonists delivered orally or by Medidose inhalers and inhaled corticosteroids. Caution must be exercised in using systemic corticosteroids. Malaise and arthralgias may be treated with nonsteroidal anti-inflammatory drugs (NSAIDs) unless specific contraindications exist.

PATIENT EDUCATION

Patients must limit physically exhausting activities. For the most part, the body's own defense system is the best treatment. One should remove physical education from the school curriculum for students and heavy labor from the work of adults, encouraging bed rest as much as possible until the patient is asymptomatic and/or titers are <1:2. The patient must know the importance of following up on laboratory work for serial titers every 2 to 3 weeks.

Once a person is infected, lifelong immunity should persist. There is no need to repeat skin testing once a positive has been determined.

NOTES AND PEARLS

Medical and indirect costs for the most benign cases are $300 to $5000 per patient. The most severe cases cost $30,000 to $300,000, with physician office visits accounting for 18 percent, lost wages for 12 percent, drugs for 6 percent, and hospitalization for 63 percent of the bill. Kern County in southern California in 1991–1994, a period of an epidemic with unknown specific etiologies, had 8434 cases of cocci at a cost of $66.6 million. The annual cost to the county is $4.8 million.

There is no vaccine available, although many research groups are searching for vaccines for fungal diseases, with *C. immitis* being considered. Genetic vaccination studies carried out in mice showed promise in regard to protection against lethal challenges with *C. immitis.* As well as vaccine research, investigations into the molecular and cellular biology of *C. immitis* and knowledge of the soil ecology supporting the fungus are the goals for future control of the disease. New antifungal drugs are being discovered.

BIBLIOGRAPHY

Dixon DM, Casadevall A, Klein B, Mendoza L: Development of vaccines and their use in the prevention of fungal infections. *Med Mycol* 3b(Suppl1): 57–67, 1998.

Galigiani JN: Coccidioidomycosis: A regional disease of national importance: Rethinking approaches for control. *Ann Intern Med* 16:130(4, Part 1): 293–300, 1999.

Galigiani J: Conferences and reviews. *West J Med,* Aug 1993, pp 153–171.

Jiang C, Magee DM, Quitugua TN: Genetic vaccination against *Coccidioides immitis:* Comparison of vaccine efficacy of recombinant antigen 2 and antigen 2 cDNA. *Infect Immun* 67(2):630–635, 1999.

A Vaccine for Valley Fever. Bakersfield, CA, Rotary America's Valley Fever Research Foundation, 1996.

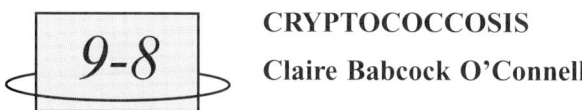

CRYPTOCOCCOSIS

9-8

Claire Babcock O'Connell

DISCUSSION

Cryptococcus neoformans is a common yeast-like fungus that is found in bird droppings and in the soil. The fungus becomes aerosolized and is inhaled by humans; it does not cause disease unless the host is immunocompromised. There is no evidence that cryptococcus is transmitted from human to human or from animal to human. In HIV-positive patients, cryptococcus is the leading cause of fungal meningitis, with an incidence of 6 to 12 percent.

Cryptococcal meningitis is often an indolent process, causing symptoms for weeks or months before being diagnosed. However, it is not uncommon to have a fulminant course of the disease rapidly lead to death. Cryptococcus generally presents in patients with a CD4+ T-cell count below $100/mm^3$. The incidence of cryptococcosis has declined in the HIV-positive patient population with the advent of highly aggressive antiretroviral therapy (HAART).

SIGNS AND SYMPTOMS

The majority of HIV-positive patients with cryptococcal infection present with subacute meningoencephalitis. The symptoms are often subtle and nonspecific. All these patients will have fever. Approximately 40 percent of patients will have nausea and vomiting. One-quarter will complain of changes in mental status (depression, dementia, delirium), headache, and meningeal irritation. Seizures and focal neurologic signs occur but are less common. A few patients with central nervous system infection with cryptococcus will develop cryptococcomas, which show multiple ring-enhancing lesions on magnetic resonance imaging (MRI).

Cryptococcal pulmonary disease occurs in up to 40 percent of HIV-positive patients with cryptococcal infection; more than 90 percent of these patients will have concurrent infection of the central nervous system. Fever, cough, and dyspnea with focal or diffuse interstitial infiltrates aid in the diagnosis of cryptococcal pneumonia.

About half of HIV-positive patients with cryptococcal infection experience fungemia and complain of fatigue and malaise. About 4 to 8 percent may present with fungemia as the only manifestation of cryptococcal infection. Other, less common manifestations of cryptococcal infection are seen more commonly in disseminated, fulminant infection and may include skin lesions, lymph node involvement, oral ulcers, gastroenteritis, hepatitis, splenic dysfunction, arthritis, and prostatitis.

OBJECTIVE FINDINGS

Altered mental status is the most useful physical finding. The Folstein Mini-Mental Status Exam can be used as a screening examination to detect subtle changes in mental status. Subtle changes in personality may be revealed during attentive interviewing. Photophobia and neck stiffness are rare. Manifestations of cryptococcal infection are often subtle and nonspecific. A high index of suspicion and early examination of the cerebrospinal fluid (CSF) are necessary to avoid missing the diagnosis.

DIFFERENTIAL DIAGNOSIS

The differential diagnoses include AIDS dementia complex, toxoplasmosis, progressive multifocal leukoencephalopathy, cytomegalovirus, tuberculosis, syphilis, and lymphoma.

LABORATORY TESTS

Identifying the fungus on India ink stain of the CSF establishes a presumptive diagnosis of cryptococcal meningitis. The diagnosis is further justified if cryptococcal antigen is measured in the CSF or serum. The diagnosis is confirmed by culturing the fungus from the CSF, blood, bone marrow, sputum, or a tissue specimen. Any positive culture, regardless of the site, is considered significant and should prompt treatment against cryptococcus. Treatment, however, should not be delayed while one is waiting for culture results.

In almost all cases of cryptococcal meningitis, CSF antigen testing is positive. In the majority of cases of non-HIV cryptococcal and HIV-positive cryptococcal meningitis, the CSF reveals increased white blood cells (WBC), elevated protein, and a low glucose concentration. In about 20 percent of HIV-positive cases, the antigen is positive but all other CSF findings are normal.

The radiologic findings in cryptococcal meningitis are usually normal. Nonspecific changes such as cortical atrophy, ventricular enlargement, and enhancement of the meninges may be seen on a computed tomography (CT) scan of the head. Mass lesions that may be ring-enhancing on MRI (cryptococcomas) must be differentiated from toxoplasmosis. Pulmonary cryptococcal infection appears as a focal or diffuse interstitial infiltrate but also may cause a lobar or cavitary lesion with pleural effusion and possible hilar or mediastinal adenopathy. A small percentage (<10 percent) of patients present with pulmonary cryptococcal disease without meningitis.

TREATMENT

Medications

Amphotericin B intravenously (IV) at a dose of 0.5 to 0.8 mg/kg/day until the patient shows clinical improvement is the first line of therapy for cryptococcal meningitis. Treatment should be initiated in any patient suspected of having cryptococcal meningitis and continued for a minimum of 2 weeks. Many clinicians add flucytosine (5-FC, Ancobon) at a dose of 100 to 150 mg/kg/day during this 2-week induction period. An alternative therapy is fluconazole (Diflucan) 400 mg PO qd. Fluconazole is not as effective as amphotericin B with or without flucytosine but is better handled by patients and may be chosen as the initial therapy in patients with milder disease. After the 2-week induction period, consolidation therapy with fluconazole (400 mg/day) for 8 weeks is recommended for all patients.

Because of the high recurrence rate (approximately 40 to 60 percent) in successfully treated patients, chronic therapy is recommended for patients with a history of cryptococcal infection. Fluconazole 200 mg/day is the drug of choice for suppression therapy. Itraconazole 200 mg PO qd may be an alternative in patients who are unable to tolerate fluconazole, but its penetration into CSF is not as effective as that of fluconazole.

Amphotericin B is fraught with side effects. Patients complain of headache, fever, chills, nausea, vomiting, hypotension, malaise, muscle and joint pain, and anorexia. It also can cause renal damage. Flucytosine can be very toxic to the bone marrow, causing anemia and neutropenia. Approximately one-half of patients who are started on flucytosine must discontinue the drug because of its toxic effects on bone marrow. Peak serum levels of flucytosine should not rise above 100 μg/mL. Fluconazole often is better tolerated but may cause a rash, gastrointestinal upset including nausea and vomiting, and elevated liver enzymes.

Patient Education

HIV-positive patients and their caretakers should be alert to any changes in mental status or personality. Any subtle changes or reports of headache should prompt a consultation with a health care provider about the possibility of cryptococcal meningitis. Children with HIV disease should avoid areas where bird droppings are common.

Disposition

All patients with CD4+ T-cell counts below 200/mm³ should be monitored for cryptococcal infection. Some clinicians advocate prophylaxis at this level; most clinicians postpone prophylaxis until the CD4+ count drops below 100/mm³. Fluconazole provides effective prophylaxis against cryptococcal infection and *Candida*. Once cryptococcal infection is suspected, treatment is initiated and must be continued indefinitely because of the high recurrence rate. Patients must be monitored for toxic effects of treatment.

COMPLICATIONS AND RED FLAGS

Patients who do not demonstrate a successful response to therapy may develop cryptococcomas within the brain parenchyma and/or spinal cord. In these patients, CSF antigen testing and fungal cultures may be negative; biopsy confirmation is needed. Increased intracranial pressure may lead to papilledema and visual loss or even blindness. Treatment includes shunting. Other possible complications of cryptococcosis include hydrocephalus, encephalitis, brainstem vasculitis, and optic nerve involvement. Regardless of treatment, about one-quarter of patients ill with cryptococcus will die.

BIBLIOGRAPHY

Dobkin JF: Opportunistic infections and AIDS. *Infect Med* 12(Suppl A):58–70, 1995.

Gallant JE: Prophylaxis for opportunistic infections in patients with HIV disease. *Ann Intern Med* 120:932–944, 1994.

Goldman L, Bennett JC (eds): *Cecil Textbook of Medicine,* 21st ed. Philadelphia, Saunders, 2000.

Lane CH (moderator): Recent advances in the management of AIDS-related opportunistic infections. *Ann Intern Med* 120(11):945–954, 1994.

Ungvarski PJ, Flaskerud JH: *HIV/AIDS: A Guide to Primary Care Management.* Philadelphia, Saunders, 1999.

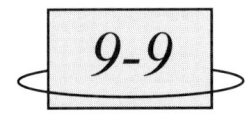

CYTOMEGALOVIRUS INFECTION

Claire Babcock O'Connell

DISCUSSION

Cytomegalovirus (CMV) is a complex double-stranded DNA virus of the herpes family. Infection results in a characteristic enlargement of cells and large intranuclear inclusions with clear halos referred to as "owl's eyes." CMV is found worldwide; it can be detected in urine, feces, saliva, milk, semen, and sexual fluids. CMV is transmitted through intimate or close contact.

Initial contact with the virus causes a mononucleosis-like illness with atypical lymphocytes and T-cell proliferation. Most immunocompetent infected individuals, when first infected, will recover and continue to harbor the virus in multiple tissue sites as a latent infection. Immune compromise, most commonly HIV disease, results in a reactivation of the infection, leading to pneumonia, gastrointestinal disease, sight-threatening retinitis, or disseminated illness. Newly infected neonates display a disseminated cytomegalic inclusion disease that is often fatal. CMV is a very common and problematic posttransfusion infection that accounts for significant morbidity and mortality in the posttransfusion population.

Evidence of infection is apparent in over 90 percent of HIV-positive patients, and clinical disease is apparent in over 40 percent. CMV disease becomes a statistically higher risk in patients with advanced HIV disease when CD4+ T-cell counts drop below 50/mm³. It is rarely the presenting or AIDS-defining infection in HIV-positive patients. CMV also is implicated as a cofactor that furthers immune system compromise and HIV replication with disease progression. The success of highly aggressive antiretroviral therapy (HAART) in recent years has resulted in a decline in the appearance of CMV disease.

SIGNS AND SYMPTOMS

CMV causes many symptoms: colitis, esophagitis, pneumonia, and retinitis are the most common manifestations in HIV-positive patients. Retinitis is the most devastating presentation and the most common cause of blindness in patients with HIV disease. CMV retinitis usually appears with a CD4+ T-cell count of <50/mm³. Patients may present with painless visual loss, blurriness, and visual field defects ("floaters"). One eye usually is affected first, but most cases progress to bilateral infection. Without treatment, the disease can cause complete retinal detachment and permanent blindness. Optic neuritis, uveitis, and conjunctivitis also may develop.

Gastrointestinal (GI) infection with CMV can present anywhere along the GI tract. Difficult and painful swallowing with substernal chest pain is typical of CMV esophagitis. The most common manifestation of CMV in the GI tract is colitis, which presents with diarrhea (with or without melena), crampy abdominal pain, and weight loss. CMV colitis may follow an indolent, prolonged course or, less commonly, a fulminant, abrupt course resulting in perforation and bacteremia.

CMV commonly is isolated from the lungs of HIV-positive patients but is rarely thought to be the primary agent in lung disease. A rare occurrence, CMV pneumonia presents with dyspnea and dry cough. The diagnosis is made when inclusion bodies are found in tissue samples.

CMV also can cause other, less common manifestations, including carditis, pancreatitis, thyroiditis, pyelonephritis, hepatitis, biliary disease, and central nervous system (CNS) involvement, including encephalitis and polyradiculopathy.

OBJECTIVE FINDINGS

Funduscopic changes in retinitis are characteristically white to yellow cheesy retinal exudates with or without hemorrhage. Lesions are found commonly on or near vessels. Involvement of the macula quickly leads to visual loss. Examination of the retina will show inclusion bodies and full-thickness necrosis. All patients with CD4+ counts below 100/mm^3 should be examined and followed by an experienced ophthalmologist.

Early retinal involvement in susceptible patients can be detected through the use of an Amsler Grid. The patient is instructed to stare at the central dot in the middle of a blocked grid. If any part of the grid appears distorted or is missing, the patient is instructed to contact his or her health care practitioner for evaluation.

DIAGNOSTIC STUDIES

A definitive diagnosis of CMV is confirmed by demonstration of CMV inclusion bodies. They can be found in virtually all tissues that may be infected. Viral cultures also can verify the presence of CMV but are not particularly sensitive. Most patients with CD4+ counts less than 100/mm^3 will shed CMV, but this may not necessarily cause a patient's symptoms.

Viral cultures are not highly correlated with patient symptomatology. The demonstration of CMV inclusion bodies (owl's eyes) is a key diagnostic finding. Patients ill with CMV disease will have other laboratory findings, including low CD4+ counts, leukopenia, thrombocytopenia, and abnormal liver enzymes, but these findings could be due to the CMV or other pathologies associated with the immunocompromised state. CMV viral load assays have been developed and may help assess disease severity or progression.

Gastrointestinal endoscopy reveals characteristic multiple shallow ulcers along the mucosa. In the large bowel, it is common to see edema with erythema with erosions and hemorrhage. Biopsy specimens will reveal the inclusion bodies and may confirm the presence of the virus. Multiple biopsies may be required to isolate the virus. Stool cultures are not sensitive; barium enemas are usually normal. Chest x-rays in patients with CMV pneumonia are not well defined; a diffuse interstitial pattern is more common but is not easily distinguished from other causes of interstitial lung disease.

DIFFERENTIAL DIAGNOSIS

CMV retinitis must be differentiated from cotton wool spots, retinal hemorrhages, choroidal granulomas, retinal necrosis syndromes, and retinitis caused by toxoplasmosis or syphilis. An expert should confirm the funduscopic examination.

Esophagitis and colitis caused by CMV can be confused with many other causes of GI inflammation, including *Candida,* other viruses, bacteria, inflammatory bowel diseases, chronic illness, and reaction to medications. Endoscopy findings and inclusion bodies in biopsy specimens are needed for diagnostic certainty. CMV pneumonia is diagnosed only after other causes of the respiratory symptoms are ruled out: *Pneumocystis carinii* pneumonia (PCP), other pathogens, and injury from drugs or radiation.

TREATMENT
Medications

Ganciclovir and foscarnet are the two drugs used in the treatment of CMV. Ganciclovir [dihydroxypropoxymethyl guanine (DHPG)] was the first U.S. Food and Drug Administration (FDA)-approved drug for CMV retinitis and colitis. The dose is 5 mg/kg intravenously (IV) bid for 14 to 21 days. The drug is static to the virus and will halt progression of the disease in 90 percent of patients. The virus is not eradicated; thus, treatment cannot be stopped. The most common and safest route for maintenance therapy is via intraocular implants. Oral ganciclovir (Cytovene) has proved as effective as intravenous ganciclovir for prophylaxis and prevention of recurrence after the disease has been stabilized. The oral dose is 100 mg PO tid.

Foscarnet offers equivalent efficacy against CMV and is useful against ganciclovir-resistant strains. It is given in doses of 60 mg/kg IV tid for 14 to 21 days. Foscarnet therapy also must be continued chronically; maintenance therapy can be either intraocular or intravenous. Clinical trials have indicated that foscarnet therapy may improve survival through its action against HIV and may be the drug of first choice for CMV retinitis in patients with good renal function.

Both drugs have potentially severe side effects. Ganciclovir is toxic to bone marrow, especially when given with zidovudine (AZT), and often is given with granulocyte colony-stimulating factor or granulocyte-macrophage colony-stimulating factor to offset leukopenia. Ganciclovir has caused nausea, vomiting, renal toxicity, and rash. Foscarnet can be toxic to the kidneys; adequate hydration is very important to minimize toxicity. Foscarnet also can cause a rash, fever, and abnormal electrolytes, including calcium, phosphorus, magnesium, and potassium, as well as induce seizures. Hypocalcemia is very likely to occur with foscarnet in the presence of intravenous pentamidine. Recurrent CMV disease in a patient already on maintenance monotherapy is treated with a combination of ganciclovir and foscarnet.

Cidofovir, a nucleotide analogue, can be administered intravenously or intraocularly on a weekly schedule after induction is complete. It is highly effective against CMV but is highly nephrotoxic.

Patient Education

Patients are the most important players in the monitoring of sight. They can be instructed in the use of the Amsler Grid and should be strongly counseled to report to their health care provider if they suspect any change in vision.

Disposition

Close monitoring of blood chemistries and hematologic function is warranted while on treatment. CD4+ levels that start to approach 100/mm^3 or less should alert the practitioner to institute prophylaxis against CMV.

BIBLIOGRAPHY

Dobkin JF: Opportunistic infections and AIDS. *Infect Med* 12(Suppl A):58–70, 1995.

Goldman L, Bennett JC (eds): *Cecil Textbook of Medicine,* 21st ed. Philadelphia, Saunders, 2000.

Lane CH (moderator): Recent advances in the management of AIDS-related opportunistic infections. *Ann Intern Med* 120(11):945–954, 1994.

Muma RD: *HIV Manual for Health Care Professionals.* Norwalk, CT, Appleton & Lange, 1994.

Powderly WG: Opportunistic infections. *Medscape HIV/AIDS* 5(Suppl), 1999.

Sharp V, Ferri S: AIDS update *Clinician Rev* 6(5):115–119, 1996.

Ungvarski PJ, Flaskerud JH: *HIV/AIDS: A Guide to Primary Care Management.* Philadelphia, Saunders, 1999.

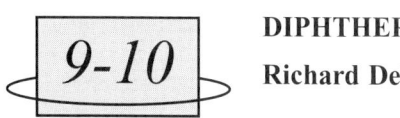

DIPHTHERIA
Richard Dehn

DISCUSSION

Diphtheria is a localized acute infectious disease of the upper respiratory tract mucous membranes or skin caused by the toxin-producing organism *Corynebacterium diphtheriae.* Typically, the primary site of infection is the mucosa of the throat, larynx, or nose; however, in developed countries, cutaneous presentations have become more common. The infection typically is local, and the site of infection is characterized by the formation of a fibrinous pseudomembrane. Serious consequences can result from the pseudomembrane, which can contribute to airway obstruction, and from the production of exotoxin, which can cause myocarditis, neuropathy, and renal failure. In the 1920s, it was discovered that treating diphtheria exotoxin with formaldehyde converts it to a nontoxic substance called diphtheria toxoid and that the vaccination of individuals with diphtheria toxoid results in the production of an antibody known as antitoxin. The antitoxin can neutralize the diphtheria exotoxin but cannot prevent *C. diphtheriae* infection or the carrier state. Immunized individuals tend to have a lower susceptibility to infection by *C. diphtheriae* and, if infected, have a less severe illness.

Before the development of the diphtheria toxoid vaccine in the 1920s, diphtheria was common. In 1921, more than 206,000 cases were reported in the United States, compared with only 22 cases reported from 1980 to 1987. This decrease in incidence in immunized populations has been accompanied by a shift in the age of infected individuals from childhood to adulthood. In unvaccinated populations, diphtheria is primarily a disease of children. Mortality rates of 30 to 50 percent have been reported in patients with untreated disease. Treatment with antitoxin can reduce the mortality rate to 5 to 10 percent.

PATHOGENESIS

Diphtheria is caused by the organism *C. diphtheriae,* a gram-positive slender rod that lacks spores or a capsule. The organism has clubbed ends and has a tendency to branch, producing a cuneiform appearance. In the 1920s, *C. diphtheriae* was classified into the three subtypes—*gravis, intermedius,* and *mitis*—according to the severity of the disease thought at that time to be caused by each subtype. It now is recognized that the severity of clinical diphtheria is dependent on the quantity of exotoxin produced and that all three subtypes of *C. diphtheriae* are capable of producing exotoxin. The ability of the organism to produce exotoxin is conferred by a lysogenic bacteriophage that transmits the gene for toxin production. Infection of a nontoxic strain occurs after the introduction of the bacteriophage, converting the organism to a toxin-producing strain. The toxin produced is a cytotoxic protein that interferes with cell protein synthesis.

Corynebacterium diphtheriae usually is transmitted to the host by intimate contact with an infected patient or carrier. The infection source is often discharges from the nose, throat, or eye or skin lesions of an infected person. Humans are the major reservoir for *C. diphtheriae.* The organism can survive for long periods outside a host and has been known to be transmitted through contaminated food. The incubation period is typically 2 to 3 days but can be up to 1 week. Most commonly the organism colonizes the tonsil or nasopharynx; however, other sites can include the larynx and the skin. The infection tends to remain local; however, toxigenic strains produce exotoxin, which kills adjacent host cells. The destroyed layer of epithelium and the resulting exudate coagulate to form a pseudomembrane containing bacteria, fibrin, leukocytes, and necrotic epithelial cells; the pseudomembrane at first appears yellowish-white but turns gray after about 5 days. The exotoxin is absorbed locally and carried by the blood systemically and can damage cells in distant organ systems. The most common sites of damage are the nervous system and the myocardium, although occasionally the kidneys are affected.

As the disease progresses locally, pharyngeal and laryngeal edema as well as obstruction from the pseudomembrane can contribute to airway compromise. A sudden detachment of the membrane can result in complete airway obstruction. If exotoxin diffuses into the neck tissue, a severe edema known as "bull neck" can result that carries a grave prognosis. If the membrane extends into the bronchi, a virtual cast will result that is almost always fatal. Nasal diphtheria is usually the mildest upper respiratory form of the disease and usually does not produce toxicity. Cutaneous diphtheria generally is not known to be toxin-producing and rarely exhibits a pseudomembrane.

The exotoxin is capable of damaging the heart, nervous system, and kidneys. Clinical myocarditis develops in about 10 percent of patients with diphtheria, usually within the first week of illness. Involvement of the nervous system occurs in 5 to 10 percent of patients with diphtheria. The symptoms vary from an isolated nerve palsy to a Guillain-Barre-appearing syndrome. Nervous system involvement can occur in the first week of the illness but more commonly presents between the second and sixth weeks. Patients who survive diphtheria involving the nervous system do not have residual damage after recovery. A rare but fatal complication of diphtheria is renal failure, which is caused by a toxic nephropathy.

An infection with diphtheria does not necessarily stimulate a patient's natural immunity.

SIGNS AND SYMPTOMS

An infection with *C. diphtheriae* can range from an asymptomatic carrier state, to a single localized lesion without systemic symptoms, to rapidly progressive fatal systemic disease. The severity of the symptoms is a function of the quantity of exotoxin produced, the site and extent of the primary infection, the patient's age, and any preexisting disease. *Corynebacterium diphtheriae* infections of the anterior nasal area, middle ear, and skin rarely produce exotoxins; consequently, these patients usually have no symptoms other than purulent drainage from the involved site. Infections from these sites can become chronic, and the discharge can transmit the organism to others.

Infection of the respiratory tract is usually exotoxin-producing, with the exception of the anterior nasal area. The most common site is tonsillopharyngeal, followed by laryngeal and tracheobronchial. The onset of symptoms is typically insidious, progressing so rapidly that patients seek care within a few days after the start of symptoms. The initial symptom is often a sore throat in adults and nausea and vomiting in children. Half these patients have a moderate fever, and 25 percent have cough, hoarseness, and dysphagia. Other symptoms include chills and rhinorrhea. While patients without toxicity may have only localized symptoms, patients with severe toxicity may be listless and pale and have a tachycardia that can progress quickly to vascular collapse. Diphtheria should be suspected in a patient presenting with tachycardia and a low-grade fever.

The affected local respiratory mucosa initially appears erythematous; this is followed quickly by the appearance of a yellowish-white or gray exudate. These lesions often grow and coalesce within the next 24 h to form a pseudomembrane that progressively thickens, adheres more tightly to the mucosa, and turns a darker gray color. Attempts to dislodge the membrane will cause bleeding. Extensive pseudomembrane formation usually is associated with more severe toxicity.

A particularly malignant form of pharyngeal diphtheria called "bull neck" presents with a rapid onset of extensive pseudomembrane formation, massive edema of the neck, cervical lymphadenopathy, foul-smelling breath, and thick speech. Extension of the pseudomembrane to the larynx or beyond can produce airway obstruction with stridor and cyanosis.

As many as half of at least moderately toxic patients exhibit myocarditis from the direct effect of toxin on myocardial cells. The effect of toxin on neural tissue occurs in 10 to 20 percent of patients and usually presents as a progressive palsy.

Skin lesions rarely produce exotoxin and are found most commonly on the extremities. These infections are usually secondary to a preexisting wound, and the lesions have a "punched-out" well-demarcated ulcerative character with necrotic sloughing of membrane.

DIFFERENTIAL DIAGNOSIS

Corynebacterium diphtheriae justifies the initiation of treatment before the results of cultures are available.

LABORATORY TESTS

Because of the importance of early treatment, therapy often is begun before the diagnosis can be confirmed. The diagnosis of diphtheria is made by culture, and the organisms are evaluated for exotoxin production. The preferred culture medium is Loeffler's medium or tellurite agar, and the laboratory should be informed that diphtheria is suspected. A presumptive diagnosis can be supported by staining exudate with methylene blue, and the presence of deeply staining metachromatic granules is strongly suggestive of infection with *C. diphtheriae.* Beta-hemolytic streptococci are present in 20 to 30 percent of diphtheria infections.

TREATMENT

Hospitalization is advised for symptomatic patients, and those with an infection of the respiratory system should be placed in strict isolation until two cultures from the nose and throat are negative for *C. diphtheriae.* Respiratory, neurologic, cardiac, and renal complications should be monitored carefully. It is important that antitoxin be given as soon as possible to neutralize the toxin that is not yet bound to cells. Antitoxin usually is given as soon as the clinical diagnosis of diphtheria is seriously entertained instead of waiting for the results of cultures.

Since diphtheria antitoxin is derived from horse serum, the patient must be tested for sensitivity before administration. This can be done with a 1:10 antitoxin dilution to the conjunctiva or a 1:100 dilution intradermally. Antitoxin is administered intravenously, with the dose determined by the characteristics of the infection. Suggested doses are 20,000 to 40,000 U for pharyngeal or laryngeal disease that has lasted 48 h, 40,000 to 60,000 U for nasopharyngeal lesions, and 80,000 to 100,000 U for extensive disease lasting more than 3 days or bull neck characteristics. Although antitoxin has no proven value in cutaneous diphtheria, some consultants advise using 20,000 to 40,000 U, since a few cases of toxin-producing cutaneous strains have been reported. Individuals sensitive to antitoxin need to undergo a desensitization procedure before antitoxin administration.

Antimicrobials are required to eradicate the organism and stop further toxin production but should not substitute for antitoxin therapy. Erythromycin 40 to 50 mg/kg/day for 14 days is the drug of choice, and eradication of the organism should be documented after treatment by two negative cultures. Asymptomatic carriers also should receive antibiotics, and eradication of the infection should be documented. A single intramuscular injection of benzathine penicillin 600,000 U for those weighing less than 30 kg and 1,200,000 U for those over 30 kg is an acceptable alternative therapy.

Diphtheria toxoid vaccination will stimulate the host to produce antitoxin for at least 10 years. Most diphtheria cases occur in unvaccinated or inadequately vaccinated individuals. Unvaccinated survivors of diphtheria should begin and complete the immunization series after recovery. Inadequately vaccinated survivors should complete the vaccination regimen. Unvaccinated carriers should begin or complete the immunization series immediately. Close contacts of a suspected patient or carrier should be cultured, receive antimicrobial therapy, and receive a diphtheria toxoid booster if the last vaccination occurred over 5 years earlier. Those with incomplete immunization should immediately resume and complete their immunizations. The administration of antitoxin to unvaccinated close contacts is not recommended.

Vaccination of the population is the key to preventing diphtheria. Children should be vaccinated at 2, 4, and 6 months with a combined diphtheria, tetanus, and acellular pertussis (DTaP) vaccine and again at 18 months and 4 to 6 years of age with a DTaP vaccine. The first three doses should be at least 4 weeks apart, and the fourth dose should follow the third by at least 6 months. A fifth dose is necessary at school entry if the fourth dose was given before age 4. Children under 7 years of age who were not vaccinated in the first year of life should have two vaccinations at least 4 weeks apart, a third vaccination at least

6 months after the second, and a fourth before school entry unless the third dose was given after age 4. It is recommended that only DTaP and not diphtheria (DT), pertussis, tetanus (DPT) be administered to children younger than age 7. Those receiving the vaccination series after age 6 should receive a Td, which has a smaller quantity of diphtheria antitoxin. The first two doses should be administered at least 4 weeks apart, and then a third dose should be administered at least 6 months after the second. Booster vaccinations of Td should be administered every 10 years. DTaP, DTP, DT, and Td vaccinations can be given concurrently with other vaccinations.

Inadequately immunized teenagers and adults are thought to constitute a large pool of individuals susceptible to diphtheria infection. Practitioners should identify all inadequately protected individuals in the population and immunize them.

BIBLIOGRAPHY

Beers MH, Berkow R (eds): *Merck Manual of Diagnosis and Therapy,* 17th ed. Whitehouse Station, NJ, Merck Research Laboratories, 1999, pp 2303–2306.

Chambers HF: Diphtheria, in Tierney LM Jr, McPhee SJ, Papadakis MA (eds): *Current Medical Diagnosis and Treatment,* 39th rev. ed. New York, McGraw-Hill, 2000, pp 1344–1345.

Georges P (ed): Pertussis, in *1997 Red Book: Report of the Committee on Infectious Diseases,* 24th ed., Elk Grove Village, IL, American Academy of Pediatrics, 1997, pp 191–195.

Grossman M: Immunization, in Stites DP, Terr AI, Parslow TG (eds): *Medical Immunology,* 9th ed. Stamford, CT, Appleton & Lange, 1997, pp 772–795.

Holmes RK: Diphtheria, other corynebacterial infections, and anthrax, in Fauci AS, Braunwald E, Isselbacher KJ, et al (eds): *Harrison's Principles of Internal Medicine,* 14th ed. New York, McGraw-Hill, 1998, pp 892–899.

Infections, in Cunningham GF, MacDonald PC, Gant NR, et al (eds): *Williams' Obstetrics,* 20th ed. Norwalk, CT, Appleton & Lange, 1997, pp 1297–1315.

Ogle JW: Infections: bacterial and spirochetal, in Hay WW Jr, Hayward AR, Levin MJ, Sondheimer JM (eds): *Current Pediatric Diagnosis and Treatment,* 14th ed. Stamford, CT, Appleton & Lange, 1999, pp 1027–1028.

Ryan JL: Bacterial diseases, in Stites DP, Terr AI, Parslow TG (eds), *Medical Immunology,* 9th ed. Stamford, CT, Appleton & Lange, 1997, pp 684–693.

Sutter RW: Diphtheria, in Goldman L, Bennett JC (eds): *Cecil Textbook of Medicine,* 21st ed. Philadelphia, Saunders, 2000, pp 1666–1668.

Zimmerman RK: Immunization practices, in Rachel RE (ed): *Conn's Current Therapy,* 2000. Philadelphia, Saunders, 2000, pp 139–145.

Zimmerman RK, Ball, JA: Update on childhood immunizations for the year 2000. *Fam Pract Recert* 22(4):69–80, 1999.

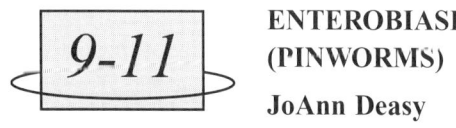

ENTEROBIASIS (PINWORMS)

JoAnn Deasy

DISCUSSION

Pinworms (*Enterobius vermicularis*) are the most common helminthic infection seen by clinicians in the United States. They are intestinal nematodes whose life cycle is confined to humans. The eggs of *E. vermicularis* hatch in the small intestine, where the larvae differentiate into adults and then migrate to the colon. The adult worms are small (about 1 cm in length), whitish in color, and thread-like in appearance. In the colon, mating occurs, and then at night the female worms migrate from the anus to deposit thousands of fertilized eggs on the perianal skin that then may be transferred to clothes, bedding, and the air. Within 6 h, the eggs develop into infectious larvae.

Reinfection can occur when the larvae return to the colon, or eggs can be carried to the mouth on the fingers after anal scratching. Microscopic eggs that have contaminated bedding and other surfaces in the home promote the spread of infection to entire families.

SYMPTOMS

The most common presenting symptoms of pinworms are perianal and perineal pruritus and restless sleep caused by the itching. A heavy infestation with *E. vermicularis* may cause symptoms of vulvovaginitis. Many infections with *E. vermicularis* are asymptomatic.

OBJECTIVE FINDINGS

The physical examination may be entirely normal, or evidence of scratching with excoriations may be present around the anus or the perineal area. Examination of the anus very late at night or early in the morning with a light source may reveal the presence of the glistening adult worms.

DIAGNOSTIC CONSIDERATIONS

The differential diagnosis includes dermatologic problems that may present with localized pruritus, such as contact dermatitis, candidiasis, and inflammation secondary to improper bathroom hygiene.

SPECIAL CONSIDERATIONS

The prevalence of pinworm infections is greatest in children under 12 years of age. Spread in institutionalized settings and to siblings may be quite rapid.

LABORATORY TESTS

The diagnosis is made by recovering the eggs of *E. vermicularis* from perianal skin by using the "Scotch tape" technique and then examining the specimen microscopically. To recover the eggs, a tongue blade covered with a segment of clear cellulose tape is placed sticky side down on the unwashed perianal skin in the morning. The specimen is transferred to a glass slide and then examined microscopically for the colorless eggs, which are flattened on one side. The collection of several specimens on separate mornings increases the detection rate. These eggs are not found in stools, but occasionally the adult worm can be found in feces. Special "pinworm prep kits" are available from some laboratories. Pinworm preparation kits include a plastic paddle with one sticky side to obtain the perianal specimen. The inoculated paddle is then inserted into a plastic test tube for transport and subsequent microscopic examination.

TREATMENT

Pinworm infection is treated with mebendazole (Vermox) in a single oral dose of 100 mg, pyrantel pamoate in a single dose of 11 mg/kg (maximum of 1 g), or albendazole 400 mg once. Pyrantel pamoate is available over the counter. A second dose of medication 10 days later is recommended to ensure effectiveness. Reinfection is very common. The entire family should be treated to ensure eradication.

PATIENT EDUCATION

Clothing and bedding should be washed in hot water. Personal cleanliness is a useful general principle, but there is no good means of preventing pinworm infection.

BIBLIOGRAPHY

Juckett G: Common intestinal helminths. *Am Fam Physician* 52(7):2039–2048, 1995.
Mandell GL, Douglas RG, Bennett JE (eds): *Principles and Practice of Infectious Diseases,* 4th ed. New York, Churchill Livingstone, 1995.
Rakel RE: *Conn's Current Therapy 2000.* Philadelphia, Saunders, 2000.

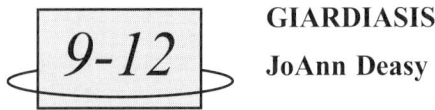

GIARDIASIS

JoAnn Deasy

DISCUSSION

Giardia lamblia is the most clinically significant protozoal pathogen in the United States. *Giardia* has both a trophozoite form and a cyst form. The mature cysts are the infective form of the parasite and generally are transmitted fecally-orally or through the ingestion of contaminated food or water. Sexual transmission, usually homosexual, has been reported. In the duodenum of a new host, the cyst divides into trophozoites. The trophozoites flourish in the duodenum and jejunum, absorbing nutrients from the intestinal tract. Disease manifestations appear to be related to intestinal malabsorption, particularly of fat and carbohydrates. The trophozoites may be carried by the fecal stream to the large intestine, where some trophozoites encyst. The infective cysts are passed in feces and can survive in cold water for more than 2 months; they are resistant to the concentration of chlorine generally used in municipal water systems.

SYMPTOMS

Infection with *Giardia* may result in asymptomatic passage of cysts, an acute case of often self-limited diarrhea, or a chronic syndrome of diarrhea, malabsorption, and weight loss. The presence of symptoms and their severity most likely are related to the number of cysts and the strain of *Giardia* ingested and the individual's immune response to the parasite. The incubation period from the ingestion of the cysts to the development of symptoms is 1 to 2 weeks.

Acute giardiasis is characterized by diarrhea, foul-smelling stools, abdominal cramps and/or pain, bloating, and flatulence. The patient may experience fatigue, nausea, and anorexia. Acute symptoms generally resolve within several weeks. Patients who go on to have chronic symptoms often experience a more profound fatigue and have upper abdominal pain and flatulence. Diarrhea is usually present but may be interrupted by periods of constipation or normal bowel movements. Malabsorption and weight loss may develop.

OBJECTIVE FINDINGS

The physical examination may be entirely unremarkable, or mild epigastric tenderness may be present.

DIAGNOSTIC CONSIDERATIONS

Giardiasis may be confused with diarrhea caused by other parasites or diarrhea caused by viral or bacterial gastroenteritis. Other diseases that should be considered in the differential diagnosis include irritable bowel syndrome, malabsorption syndromes, peptic ulcer disease, lactase deficiency, inflammatory bowel disease, and cholecystitis.

SPECIAL CONSIDERATIONS

All ages and economic groups may become infected with *G. lamblia,* but there is a higher incidence in young children and young adults. Giardiasis is common among non-toilet-trained young children who attend day care centers, and person-to-person transmission to their families may occur. The ingestion of fecally contaminated water accounts for many cases of traveler's diarrhea. Waterborne outbreaks of giardiasis have been reported in the United States. The sources have included untreated stream water, sewage-contaminated municipal water supplies, and chlorinated but inadequately filtered water. It is thought that wild mammals, particularly beavers, have been the reservoir hosts of *Giardia* in some of these outbreaks. Persons with IgA deficiency are more likely to develop symptomatic giardiasis.

LABORATORY TESTS

The diagnosis of giardiasis should be considered in patients who present with prolonged diarrhea, abdominal cramp-like pain, or malabsorption. Recent travel to an endemic area or the presence of children in the home who attend day care centers should raise the index of suspicion. The diagnosis is confirmed by ordering a stool examination for ova and parasites and finding the cyst in semisolid or formed stool specimens or finding the trophozoite in liquid stool. In acutely symptomatic patients, the parasite usually can be demonstrated by examining one to three stool specimens. In chronic cases, passage of the parasite is often intermittent, making confirmation more difficult. Duodenoscopy with biopsy and duodenal fluid sampling for *Giardia* trophozoites are reserved for diagnostically difficult cases. Detection of anti-*Giardia* IgM is compatible with the diagnosis of acute infection. Testing for fecal *Giardia* antigen by enzyme-linked immunosorbent assay (ELISA) has been shown to be sensitive and specific.

TREATMENT

Giardiasis may be treated with metronidazole (Flagyl) 250 mg three times a day for 5 days (pediatric dose, 15 mg/kg/day in three doses). Metronidazole may cause nausea, vomiting, and a metallic taste in the mouth. It also is known to cause a disulfiram-like (Antabuse) reaction with alcohol. As an alternative, furazolidone (Furoxone) 100 mg four times a day for 7 to 10 days for adults or 6 mg/kg/day in four doses for children may be prescribed. Furazolidone comes in a suspension form and therefore is especially useful for treating children under age 5 years. Paromomycin is less effective but may be used during pregnancy in a very symptomatic woman. Although treatment of asymptomatic persons is not clinically required, it should be considered to prevent person-to-person transmission of *Giardia.*

PATIENT EDUCATION

The prevention of giardiasis includes attention to good personal hygiene, particularly hand washing, especially in day care settings. Hikers and travelers should use caution when drinking local water. Adequate disinfection of water can be accomplished by using portable purification systems, available from outdoor supply stores, that filter out *Giardia.*

DISPOSITION

Once a diagnosis of giardiasis is made, consideration should be given to testing other household members. Patients should be reevaluated if their symptoms persist.

BIBLIOGRAPHY

Juckett G: Intestinal protozoa. *Am Fam Physician* 53(8):2507–2516, 1996.
Mandell GL, Douglas RG, Bennett JE (eds): *Principles and Practice of Infectious Diseases,* 4th ed. New York, Churchill Livingstone, 1995.
Sherris JC (ed): *Medical Microbiology.* New York, Elsevier, 1990, pp 734–736.

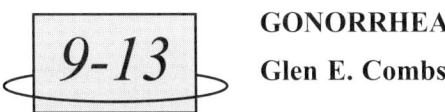

GONORRHEA
Glen E. Combs

DISCUSSION
Etiology

The etiologic agent of gonorrhea is *Neisseria gonorrhoeae,* a gram-negative diplococcus. It may be found intracellularly and extracellularly.

Epidemiology

Gonorrhea is considered the most prevalent sexually transmitted disease (STD) in the United States. It has been estimated that gonorrhea infects more than 2.5 million people annually. Although gonorrhea is reportable in all states, it has been estimated that only 20 to 30% of cases are reported. This alarming statistic underscores the problem for eradication of this STD. Risk factors include multiple sexual partners, young age, early onset of sexual activity, lack of use of barrier contraceptive methods, and a history of a previously diagnosed STD. The average incubation period for the *N. gonorrhoeae* organism is 2 to 5 days.

Multidrug resistance is common with gonococcal infections. Penicillinase-producing *N. gonorrhoeae* (PPNG) has been detected in the United States since 1976. PPNG is currently implicated in 5 to 20% of all gonococcal infections in the United States. Tetracycline- and spectinomycin-resistant gonococcal infections have been documented since the mid-1980s.

SIGNS, SYMPTOMS, AND OBJECTIVE FINDINGS

The clinical syndrome of gonorrhea is broad, ranging from patients who are asymptomatic or superficially symptomatic to patients who have complicated infections at multiple sites or disseminated disease.

Uncomplicated infections remain localized to the site of inoculation. Gonorrhea rarely causes disabling symptoms or sequelae. Of treated cases in the industrial world, 80 to 90% are uncomplicated.

Uncomplicated Infection in Men

Acute urethritis is the most common clinical manifestation of gonorrhea in men. The incubation period ranges from 1 to 14 days, with 2 to 5 days being the average. Symptoms include dysuria, urethral discharge, and meatal erythema. The discharge may be scanty and mucoid or mucopurulent, becoming frankly purulent and profuse within 24 h. Anorectal symptoms include proctalgia, anal pruritus, purulent discharge, and tenesmus. Gonococcal pharyngitis commonly is asymptomatic but may present with a sore throat and an acute tonsillopharyngitis. Pharyngeal infections carry an increased risk of dissemination. Studies have demonstrated that 3 to 7% of men with gonorrhea are asymptomatic.

Complicated Infection in Men

Gonorrhea in men may ascend from the lower genital area to an upper tract site, presenting as an acute epididymitis, an acute or chronic prostatitis, an inguinal lymphadenitis, or urethral stricture formation.

Uncomplicated Infection in Women

Cervicitis is the most common clinical manifestation in women. The incubation period averages 2 to 10 days. Common symptoms include vaginal discharge, dysuria, dyspareunia, dysmenorrhea, and irregular vaginal bleeding. The physical examination may be normal or may show an abnormal cervix with purulent or mucopurulent discharge, erythema, and friability. A high prevalence of coexisting sexually transmitted infections has been demonstrated. Female anorectal and pharyngeal clinical manifestations are identical to the male presentations. Studies have demonstrated that 10 to 20% of women with gonorrhea are asymptomatic.

Complicated Infection in Women

Gonococcal infection in women migrates from the lower genital area and ascends to the fallopian tubes in approximately 15% of infections. This spread may result in endometritis or salpingitis. Chronic salpingitis may lead to scarring in the fallopian tubes, resulting in sterility. Gonorrhea may migrate into the abdomen and create a perihepatitis that also is called the Fitz-Hugh-Curtis syndrome. The symptoms of Fitz-Hugh-Curtis syndrome are right upper quadrant abdominal pain, fever, and nausea. A concurrent salpingitis is common with Fitz-Hugh-Curtis syndrome.

Skene's and Bartholin's glands are commonly infected, resulting in abscess formation. A unilateral Bartholin's abscess may be suggestive of gonorrhea. In pregnancy, the incidence for spontaneous abortion and premature membrane rupture is increased with a concurrent gonococcal infection.

Disseminated Disease

Disseminated gonococcal infections arise from a gonococcal bacteremia, resulting in a triad. It is important to keep in mind that all three presentations of the triad rarely occur at the same time.

1. Skin lesions: papular, pustular, or necrotic
2. Asymmetric arthralgias or septic arthritis
3. Tenosynovitis

Two-thirds of disseminated disease occurs in women. The symptoms of disseminated infection tend to appear immediately after a menstrual cycle. This is thought to occur from sloughing of the endometrium, exposing blood vessels to the infectious organism. Strains of *N. gonorrhoeae* that cause disseminated disease tend to produce mild genitourinary symptoms.

Disseminated gonococcal infections are rarely associated with hepatitis, endocarditis, or meningitis.

DIAGNOSTIC CONSIDERATIONS

A variety of genital pathogens, most of which are sexually transmitted, may cause urethritis or cervicitis. A differential listing is provided in Table 9-13-1.

SPECIAL CONSIDERATIONS

Management of Sexual Partners

The sexual partners of infected patients must be evaluated and treated. Patients should refrain from intercourse until properly treated. Sexual partners of infected patients should also be properly treated prior to resuming sexual activity.

HIV Infection

Treatment of gonorrhea in HIV-infected patients is the same as the standard of care for non-HIV infected patients.

Pregnancy

The standard treatment regimens for gonococcal infections associated with pregnancy are different. Infected women who are pregnant should not be treated with quinolones or tetracyclines.

TABLE 9-13-1. Differential Diagnosis of Cervicitis and Urethritis with Gonococcal Infections

Neisseria gonorrhoeae
Chlamydia trachomatis
Ureaplasma urealyticum
Trichomonas vaginalis
Candidiasis
Bacterial vaginosis
Herpes simplex virus
Allergic urethritis/cervicitis (latex)

Gonococcal Infections in Infants

During delivery, the conjunctiva, pharynx, or rectum of the newborn may become infected. Infants at high risk for gonococcal ophthalmia are those whose mothers did not receive routine prenatal care or have a history of STDs or drug use. Prophylaxis for the prevention of gonococcal ophthalmia has become the standard of care in U.S. hospitals. Topical therapy to the conjunctiva alone is considered inadequate if the infant has a confirmed gonococcal infection. Treatment for gonococcal infections in infants should consist of ceftriaxone 25 to 50 mg/kg intravenously or intramuscularly in a single dose.

LABORATORY TESTING

Isolation of *N. gonorrhoeae* is the diagnostic standard. Gram's stain of exudate (men) represents a presumptive diagnosis when gram-negative diplococci are identified within polymorphonuclear cells. Culture using Thayer-Martin medium is indicated when Gram staining is negative or equivocal. *N. gonorrhoeae* is a fastidious organism that dies quickly. Cultures should be plated immediately and incubated as soon as possible. The existence of coinfection with other STDs is common. All patients with gonococcal infections should be tested for chlamydial infection and syphilis. In addition, infected patients should be counseled about HIV testing.

TREATMENT

Pharmacologic Management

The recommended regimen is ceftriaxone 125 mg intramuscularly in a single dose. Alternative regimens include cefixime 400 mg orally in a single dose, ofloxacin 400 mg orally in a single dose, spectinomycin 2 g given intramuscularly in a single dose, and ciprofloxacin 500 mg orally in a single dose.

Since coinfection with *Chlamydia* is common, these regimens should be followed by a 7-day course of doxycycline or erythromycin. A single 1-g dose of azithromycin is also effective.

The recommended regimen in pregnant women is ceftriaxone 125 mg given intramuscularly in a single dose. This regimen should be followed with a 7-day course of erythromycin.

The recommended regimen for disseminated infection consists of ceftriaxone 1 g intramuscularly or intravenously daily[1] or ceftizoxime 1 g intravenously every 8 h.[2]

Patient Education

Patients must be advised to abstain from sexual activity until they and their partners are cured. Concurrent treatment of all partners is essential even if they are asymptomatic. All sexual partners within the last 30 days should be tested and treated.

A history of an STD places a patient at risk for subsequent STDs. When used consistently, condoms are effective in preventing STDs. Patient education in the proper use of condoms should occur during every patient visit for STDs.

DISPOSITION

A follow-up test of cure is not mandatory, since treatment failures are uncommon. Retesting, including drug sensitivity, should be performed if symptoms persist.

---

[1]This regimen should be given until 24 to 48 h after the resolution of symptoms; then cefixime should be given at 400 mg daily to complete a 7- to 10-day course.

[2]This regimen should be followed with a 7-day course of erythromycin or doxycycline or a single 1-g dose of azithromycin.

COMPLICATIONS AND RED FLAGS

Gonorrhea is a reportable communicable disease in all states. All clinicians who evaluate and treat patients with possible STDs should be knowledgeable about the reporting procedures in their respective states.

Routine screening for asymptomatic infection in women during the annual pelvic examination is recommended, particularly for high-risk patients. Clinical findings that are suggestive of asymptomatic infection include friable cervix, mucopurulent discharge, and chronic pelvic pain. Routine screening for asymptomatic infection in men is not cost-effective.

ACKNOWLEDGMENT

The editor would like to acknowledge the significant contribution of Meredith Hansen, author of this chapter in the first edition of *Primary Care for Physician Assistants,* in the preparation of this revised work.

BIBLIOGRAPHY

Centers for Disease Control and Prevention: 1993 sexually transmitted diseases treatment guidelines. *MMWR* 42(RR-14):3–7, 40–45, 1993.
Centers for Disease Control and Prevention: Gonorrhea—United States, 1998. *MMWR* 49(24):538–542, 2000.
Fauci AS et al (eds): *Harrison's Principles of Internal Medicine,* 14th ed. New York, McGraw-Hill, 1998, pp 915–922.
Preventive Services Task Force: *Guide to Clinical Preventive Services,* 2d ed. Alexandria, VA, International Medical Publishing, 1996.
Tierney L et al (eds): *Current Medical Diagnosis and Treatment,* 39th ed. New York: Lange Medical/McGraw-Hill, 2000, pp 1362–1363.

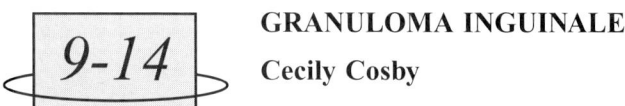

GRANULOMA INGUINALE
Cecily Cosby

DISCUSSION

Granuloma inguinale (GI) is also called donovanosis and is associated with the presence of an intracellular organism known as a Donovan body.[1]

Etiology

The etiologic agent of GI is *Calymmatobacterium granulomatis,* a gram-negative rod. It causes a mildly contagious, chronic, indolent, progressive, autoinoculable, ulcerative disease involving the skin and lymphatics of the genital or perianal areas.[2]

Epidemiology

GI is uncommon in developed countries. The greatest incidence of GI occurs in tropical and subtropical areas, where endemic clusters are found. The reported incidence is 10:1 male:female and is uncommon in Caucasians.[2] Demonstrated HIV coinfection has been found in Africa. The incubation period is broad, falling between 8 and 90 days.

SIGNS, SYMPTOMS, AND OBJECTIVE FINDINGS

The most common initial presentation is a painless granulomatous ulcer at the inoculation site. The lesions are highly vascular, bleed easily on contact, and may become quite disfiguring as the ulcer enlarges.[3] Enlargement of the lesion or lesions occurs by autoinoculation or contiguous spread. Regional lymphadenopathy is uncommon unless there is a secondary bacterial infection.

Dissemination with bony, splenic, or hepatic involvement has been reported. Perianal GI may mimic the condylomata lata of secondary syphilis. Complications of GI include urethral, vaginal, or anal stenosis and lymphatic obstruction that produces a genital edema. A causal relationship involving the development of genital carcinomas secondary to GI has not been proved.

DIAGNOSTIC CONSIDERATIONS

A variety of genital pathogens, most of which are sexually transmitted, cause genital ulcer disease. A differential listing is provided in Table 9-14-1.

SPECIAL CONSIDERATIONS

Management of Sexual Partners

The sexual partners of infected patients must be evaluated and treated. Patients must be told to refrain from intercourse until they are cured. Studies document increased coinfection with HIV and syphilis. Patients must be counseled about HIV testing and tested for syphilis.

HIV Infection

Current studies do not recommend a different treatment regimen for GI when the patient has HIV infection. The addition of a parenteral aminoglycoside should be strongly considered.[3]

Pregnancy

Both pregnant and lactating women should be treated with erythromycin. The addition of a parenteral aminoglycoside should be strongly considered.[3]

LABORATORY TESTING

Serologic testing is not useful in diagnosing GI but is essential in ruling out syphilis and HIV. The most successful method used to identify the Donovan bodies in GI patients is a punch biopsy of the granulation tissue from the border of the lesion or lesions. With the use of Wright-Giemsa staining techniques, the Donovan bodies can be seen within the cytoplasm of large mononuclear cells.

TREATMENT

Pharmacologic Management

Treatment appears to halt progressive destruction of tissue, while prolonged therapy is often required to enable granulation and reepithelialization of the ulcers. Four commonly used antibiotics are effective in the management of GI.[3]

The recommended regimens are trimethoprim-sulfamethoxazole, one double-strength orally twice per day or doxycycline 100 mg orally twice per day. Alternative regimens include ciprofloxacin 750 mg orally twice per day or erythromycin 500 mg orally four times per day. If lesions do not respond within the first few days of therapy, the addition of an aminoglycoside (gentamicin 1 mg/kg intravenously every 8 h) should be considered. Relapse can occur 6 to 18 months later despite

TABLE 9-14-1. Differential Diagnosis of Genital Ulcers (in Order of Relative Frequency in the United States)

Herpes simplex virus
Treponema pallidum (syphilis)
Haemophilus ducreyi (chancroid)
Granuloma inguinale
Lymphogranuloma venereum

effective initial therapy. Therapy is for a minimum of 3 weeks but should be continued until all lesions have healed completely.[3] Other antimicrobials with effectiveness include tetracycline, azithromycin, and ceftriaxone, although no comparative trials have been conducted.[2]

Patient Education

A history of sexually transmitted disease (STD) places a patient at risk for subsequent STDs. Patients should be advised of their increased risk status and counseled on methods to reduce the risk of subsequent STDs. When used consistently, condoms are effective in preventing STDs. Patient education in the proper use of condoms should occur during every patient visit for an STD. Patients need to be advised about sexual abstinence while undergoing treatment for GI.

DISPOSITION

A follow-up test to cure is not necessary in GI. Patients should be followed until signs and symptoms have resolved.[3]

COMPLICATIONS AND RED FLAGS

Because of the uncommon nature of GI in the United States, few states include it in their reportable disease lists. GI should be reported to the appropriate health authorities if required.

ACKNOWLEDGMENT

The editor would like to acknowledge the significant contributions of Meredith Hansen, author of this chapter in the first edition of *Primary Care for Physician Assistants.*

REFERENCES

1. Robinson K: Sexually transmitted infections, in *Pathophysiology: The Biologic Basis for Disease in Adults and Children,* 3d ed, McCance K, Huether S (eds). St. Louis, MO, Mosby, 1998, pp 823–825.
2. Holmes KK: Donovanosis (granuloma inguinale), in *Harrison's Principles of Internal Medicine,* 14th ed, Fauci AS et al (eds). New York, McGraw-Hill, 1998, p 986.
3. Centers for Disease Control and Prevention: 1998 guidelines for treatment of sexually transmitted diseases. *MMWR* 47(RR-1):26–27, 1998.

BIBLIOGRAPHY

Centers for Disease Control and Prevention: 1993 sexually transmitted diseases treatment guidelines. *MMWR* 42(RR-14):4–7, 19–21, 1993.
Goens JL et al: Mucocutaneous manifestations of chancroid, lymphogranuloma venereum and granuloma inguinale. *Am Fam Physician* 49(2):415–425, 1994.
Hoffman I, Schmitz J: Genital ulcer disease. *Postgrad Med* 98(3):67–80, 1995.
Preventive Services Task Force: *Guide to Preventive Clinical Services,* 2d ed. Alexandria, VA, International Medical Publishing, 1996.
Tierney L et al (eds): *Current Medical Diagnosis and Treatment,* 39th ed. New York, Lange/McGraw-Hill, 2000, p 1364.

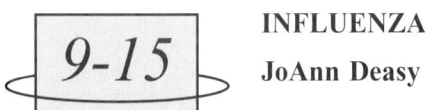

INFLUENZA
JoAnn Deasy

DISCUSSION

Influenza is a common respiratory pathogen of humans caused by RNA viruses of the *Orthomyxoviridae* family. There are three antigenically different groups of influenza viruses, designated as A, B, and C. Influenza A and influenza B are clinically indistinguishable, while in-

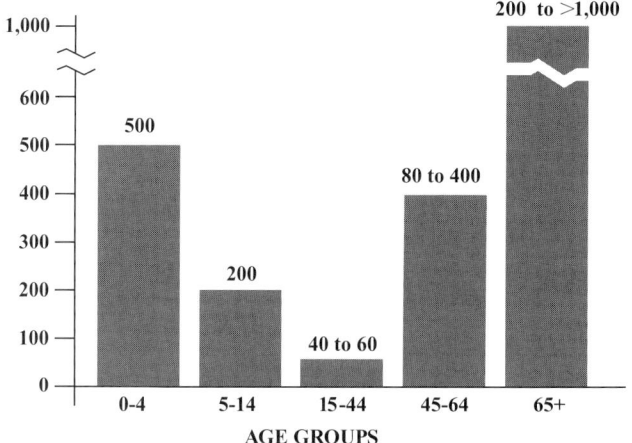

FIGURE 9-15-1. Influenza-related hospitalizations. Hospitalizations per 100,000 U.S. population among people at high risk. (SOURCE: *Centers for Disease Control studies of different influenza epidemics in 1972–1981, 1999.*)

fluenza C causes a milder illness. Influenza is spread by respiratory droplets. The incubation period is 1 to 3 days.

Outbreaks of influenza occur virtually every winter but vary considerably in extent and severity. The major determinants for morbidity and mortality are the virulence of the circulating strain of virus and the preexisting immunity in the population in which the infection occurs. In the United States, 10,000 to 20,000 people die annually from influenza-related illness in nonpandemic years. Influenza virus causes large economic losses from disruption of the workforce and high health care costs. Figure 9-15-1 shows the trend of influenza-related hospitalizations in the United States.

SIGNS AND SYMPTOMS

Influenza is characterized by an abrupt onset of fever [38 to 41°C (101 to 106°F)]; myalgias, especially of the back and thighs; headache; and a nonproductive cough. Coryza and a sore throat are also usually present. Vomiting and diarrhea are rare in adults but common in young children. Influenza can cause severe malaise lasting several days. Physical examination may reveal no signs or minimal signs such as mild pharyngeal infection.

DIFFERENTIAL DIAGNOSIS

In the absence of a community outbreak, influenza can be difficult to diagnose. The differential diagnosis includes other febrile illnesses and other viral respiratory infections.

COMPLICATIONS AND SPECIAL CONSIDERATIONS

Influenza causes damage to the respiratory epithelium that predisposes an individual to a secondary bacterial infection. The most common complications of influenza are acute sinusitis, otitis media, bronchitis, and bacterial pneumonia. Secondary pneumonia most often is caused by *Streptococcus pneumoniae, Haemophilus influenzae,* and *Staphylococcus aureus.* Staphylococcal pneumonia is less common but is the most serious form. A primary pneumonia caused by the influenza virus itself occurs but is rare.

Reye's syndrome can be a hepatic and central nervous system (CNS) complication of influenza and other viral infections (see Chap. 15-4). It occurs almost exclusively in children. Because of the association between Reye's syndrome and aspirin, the administration of aspirin should be avoided. Myocarditis and pericarditis are other rare

TABLE 9-15-1. Antiviral Agents for Influenza

	AMANTADINE	RIMANTADINE	ZANAMIVIR	OSELTAMIVIR
Types of influenza viruses inhibited	Influenza A	Influenza A	Influenza A and B	Influenza A and B
Route of administration	Oral (tablet, capsule, syrup)	Oral (tablet, syrup)	Oral inhalation*	Oral (capsule)
Ages for which treatment is approved	≥1 year	≥14 years	≥12 years	≥18 years
Ages for which prophylaxis is approved	≥1 year	≥1 year	Not approved for prophylaxis	Not approved for prophylaxis

NOTE: Amantadine manufacturers include Endo Pharmaceuticals (Symetrel®—tablet and syrup); Invamed and Rosemont (Amantadine HCL—capsule); and Alpharma, Copley Pharmaceutical, HiTech Pharma, Mikart, Morton Grove, and Pharmaceutical Associates (Amantadine HCL—syrup). Rimantadine is manufactured by Forest Laboratories (Flumadine®—tablet and syrup). Zanamivir is manufactured by Glaxo Wellcome (Relenza®—for inhalation). Oseltamivir is manufactured by Hoffman-La Roche Inc. (Tamiflu®—capsule).
*Zanamivir is administered by using a specially designed plastic oral inhalation device (Diskhaler®). The device and instructions on its use are included in the package with the medication.
SOURCE: Centers for Disease Control and Prevention. *MMWR* 48(RR-14):1–7, 1999.

complications of influenza. In addition to the complications of individual organ systems listed above, elderly and chronically ill persons may experience multisystem deterioration. Persons at high risk for the complications of influenza include those over age 65 and persons with chronic cardiopulmonary or metabolic diseases.

DIAGNOSTICS

A clinical diagnosis of influenza can be made with a high degree of certainty if typical "influenza-like illness" is encountered in the middle of a documented outbreak. The white blood cell (WBC) count may show leukopenia or may be normal. Proteinuria may be present. A chest x-ray will be normal in a patient with uncomplicated influenza. A specific laboratory diagnosis is established by isolating the virus in cell culture from oropharynx or respiratory secretions; however, results take 4 to 5 days. A serologic diagnosis can be made retrospectively by comparing antibody titers in acute and convalescent serums obtained 10 to 14 days apart.

The diagnosis of influenza by office rapid diagnostic tests holds promise for improved disease outcomes and a reduction of inappropriate antibiotic usage. Several rapid tests are available with excellent specificity; however, negative tests cannot be trusted because the sensitivity of these tests ranges from 57% to 81%.

TREATMENT

The treatment of uncomplicated influenza is largely symptomatic and includes antipyretics and analgesics. Aspirin should be avoided because of the risk of Reye's syndrome. Patients should be advised to rest and maintain hydration during acute illness.

Amantadine can be used for the treatment of influenza A but is not effective against influenza B. The administration of amantadine within 48 h of the onset of illness has been shown to reduce the signs and symptoms of influenza by 50%. The usual dose is 200 mg/d in two divided doses for adults. Because the drug is excreted largely by the kidneys, the dose should be reduced in patients with decreased renal function as well as in the elderly (over age 65), for whom the usual dose is 100 mg/d. Amantadine is associated with mild CNS side effects, including jitteriness, anxiety, insomnia, and difficulty concentrating. An increased incidence of seizures has been reported in persons with a history of seizure disorder taking amantadine.

The antiviral rimantadine (200 mg/d in two divided doses) also may be used and is associated with fewer side effects. Rimantadine is preferred in patients with renal failure. It has not been approved for the treatment of influenza in children.

A new class of antiviral medications released in 1999 called *neuramidase inhibitors* are active against both influenza A and influenza B. When administered within 2 days of the onset of symptoms, these agents can reduce by approximately 1 day the duration of symptoms of uncomplicated influenza. At the time of this writing, neuramidase inhibitors are not approved for influenza chemoprophylaxis but are likely to receive that approval in the future. Zanamivir (Relenza) is a neuramidase inhibitor that is available as a dry powder and delivered by oral inhalation. Patients with underlying chronic respiratory diseases may experience bronchoconstriction with administration of zanamivir, and caution is advised. Oseltamivir (Tamiflu) is a neuramidase inhibitor available in capsule form. Dosing should be reduced in persons with renal failure. Nausea and vomiting are the most common adverse effects with oseltamivir. Influenza-specific antiviral agents are adjuncts to vaccine and are not a substitute for vaccination. Table 9-15-1 compares antiviral agents for influenza.

Antibacterial antibiotics should be reserved for bacterial complications only. The persistence of fever beyond 4 days, leukocytosis, or a cough that becomes productive should precipitate a workup to verify or rule out a secondary bacterial infection.

PREVENTION

Prevention may be accomplished by immunoprophylaxis with inactivated (killed-virus) vaccine or chemoprophylaxis with amantadine or rimantadine. Vaccination of persons at high risk each year is the most effective measure for reducing the impact of influenza. Each year's vaccine contains three virus strains (usually two type A and one type B). The vaccine's antigenic formulation changes yearly and is based on the prevalent strains of the preceding year. Influenza vaccine is recommended for any person 6 months of age or older who is at increased risk for influenza-related complications (Table 9-15-2), health care workers and others in close contact with people at high risk for influenza, and individuals who wish to reduce their chances of becoming infected with influenza. Vaccination provides partial immunity (efficacy depends on age, immunocompetence, and how well the vaccine matches circulating influenza strains) for a few months to 1 year. It takes up to 2 weeks for the development of antibodies. Influenza vaccine should be administered in October or November each year. Immunosuppressed individuals may have a decreased antibody response to influenza vaccine but should still be immunized. Two doses 1 month apart may be necessary to achieve a satisfactory antibody response in previously unvaccinated children less than 9 years old.

Influenza vaccine is contraindicated in persons who are known to have anaphylactic hypersensitivity to eggs or other components of the

TABLE 9-15-2. High-Risk Groups in Which Yearly Influenza Vaccine Is Recommended

- Persons 65 years of age or older
- Residents of nursing homes and other chronic care facilities that house persons of any age with chronic medical conditions
- Adults and children with chronic disorders of the pulmonary or cardio-vascular system, including children with asthma
- Adults and children who have required regular medical follow-up or hospital-ization during the preceding year because of chronic metabolic diseases (in-cluding diabetes mellitus), renal dysfunction, hemoglobinopathies, or im-munosuppression (including immunosuppression caused by medications)

SOURCE: From Centers for Disease Control and Prevention 1996.

vaccine. Since influenza vaccine contains only noninfectious viruses or viral antigens, it cannot cause influenza. The most common side effect of vaccination is soreness at the vaccination site. Myalgias and fever occur rarely.

A new live attenuated vaccine delivered intranasally is on the horizon for prevention of influenza A and B; 93% efficacy against culture-confirmed influenza has been demonstrated in trials.

For persons in high-risk groups for whom the influenza vaccine is contraindicated, chemoprophylaxis with amantadine or rimantadine may be indicated throughout the influenza season. The dose is the same as that used for treatment.

PROGNOSIS

The duration of uncomplicated influenza is 1 to 7 days, and the prognosis is excellent. The mortality rate is highest in debilitated persons. In influenza epidemic years in the United States, more than 90% of the deaths attributed to pneumonia and influenza have occurred among persons over 65 years of age.

BIBLIOGRAPHY

Centers for Disease Control and Prevention: Prevention and control of influenza: Recommendations of the Advisory Committee on Immunization Practices. *MMWR* 45(RR-5):1–24, 1996.

Centers for Disease Control and Prevention: Neuraminidase inhibitors for treatment of influenza A and B infections. *MMWR* 48(RR-14):1–7, 1999.

Mandell GL, et al: *Principles and Practice of Infectious Diseases,* 4th ed. New York, Churchill Livingston, 1995.

Rapid diagnostic tests for influenza. *Med Lett Drugs Ther* 41(1068):121–122, 1999.

Small PA Jr: Influenza: Pathogenesis and host defense. *Hosp Pract* 25(11): 51–54, 1990.

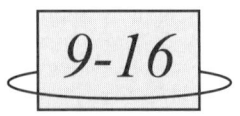

MEASLES/RUBEOLA

Richard Dehn

DISCUSSION

Measles, also known as rubeola and the seven-day measles, is a highly contagious viral illness that is characterized by a prodromal phase consisting of high fevers, cough, malaise, coryza, anorexia, and conjunctivitis. This phase begins 7 to 14 days after exposure, and 2 to 4 days later Koplik's spots appear on the buccal and labial mucosa. A day or two after the appearance of Koplik's spots, the characteristic rash begins, first around the ears and then spreading downward to the trunk and extremities. It begins as irregular macules that rapidly progress to maculopapular lesions. By the time the rash reaches the extremities (usually about 2 days), the earliest lesions have begun to fade to a brownish color, which eventually desquamates.

Before the routine vaccination of American children beginning in 1963, virtually everyone acquired measles, usually before age 10, and this conferred a lifelong immunity. In the prevaccination era, measles epidemics 3 to 4 months long occurred every 2 to 5 years. The justification for vaccination of the nonimmune population is based on the morbidity and mortality rates of the complications that occasionally result from naturally occurring measles infection.

Vaccine products currently in use produce immunity in about 95 percent of the population immunized. After the introduction of widespread immunization in 1963, the annual number of reported cases in the United States decreased from about 500,000 before 1963 to 1497 in 1983. More recently, the annual number of measles cases in the United States increased to more than 27,000, resulting in more than 60 deaths in 1990. The increase in cases has been attributed to populations of nonimmunized preschool children, the immigration of nonimmunized individuals to the United States, and a population of nonimmune but previously vaccinated individuals. The recent rise in measles cases has led to increased efforts to immunize all eligible populations and has resulted in the recommendation that a series of two vaccine doses be used instead of the traditional single-dose protocol. The measles virus is so contagious that cases occur despite high levels of immunity in the population, and so the goal of prevention calls for vaccinating as many individuals in the population as possible. One study demonstrated that an unimmunized individual in the United States has a 35 times greater chance of contracting measles compared with an immunized individual. In the developing world, measles is still a common childhood disease, and it has been estimated that measles causes 1 million to 2 million deaths annually worldwide. In the United States, the mortality rate is 3 in 1000 cases, primarily from respiratory and neurologic complications.

PATHOGENESIS

Measles is caused by a paramyxovirus that is spread by direct contact or by airborne droplets drawn into the host's respiratory tract. It and chickenpox are among the most easily transmitted infectious diseases. After inoculation the virus begins to replicate, and after 2 to 4 days it begins shedding and is communicable to other hosts. The acute infection is characterized by a marked depression of cellular immunity, which is probably a direct viral effect on B and T lymphocytes, and it is during this time that the prodromal symptoms start and progress. The depression of cellular immunity in the prodromal stage commonly produces leukopenia. A few days after upper respiratory symptoms have developed and progressed, the characteristic rash appears, produced by the reemergence of cellular immunity. Patients deficient in cellular immunity do not develop a rash but develop infections that result in death. Half the patients with an underlying malignancy or HIV who contract measles will die. The depression of cellular immunity in the prodromal stage sometimes results in the reactivation of tuberculosis or coccidioidomycosis and is the rationale for the recommendation not to perform skin testing after the administration of a measles vaccination or a case of measles.

In the absence of secondary complications, the appearance of the rash is soon followed by marked improvement in systemic symptoms such as fever as the reinvigorated cellular immunity rapidly reduces the quantity of virus in the host. The end result of a measles infection is a lifelong humoral immunity that is passively transferred to a newborn. Newborns of immune mothers are protected by maternal antibody for the first few months of life.

The depression of cellular immunity also can contribute to the development of infections in other organ systems. Lower respiratory tract infections have been reported in up to 50 percent of measles cases. These infections include primary viral infections such as bronchitis and pneumonia in adults and croup and bronchiolitis in children as well as secondary bacterial infections such as pneumonia, sinusitis, and otitis media. Giant cell pneumonia may develop in immunocompromised patients without the presentation of the characteristic measles rash.

Measles often produces central nervous system symptoms, with a majority of uncomplicated cases exhibiting some transient electroencephalographic (EEG) abnormalities. Between 0.05 and 0.1 percent of cases result in acute encephalitis, with these patients exhibiting fever, seizures, altered sensation, and occasional focal abnormalities. The mortality rate from measles encephalitis is 10 to 20 percent, with more than half these patients having residual neurologic effects. Encephalitis is thought to be due to an immune response directed at myelin structures. Subacute sclerosing panencephalitis (SSPE), a rare condition, can occur years after a measles infection. It is characterized by a progression of mental deterioration, seizures, and myoclonic jerks and is almost always fatal. It rarely occurs in patients whose immunity was conferred by immunization, and so the incidence of SSPE has decreased significantly in developed countries.

Acute measles infection can produce acute viral appendicitis and viral mesenteric adenitis, which can result in abdominal pain. An icteric hepatitis is present in up to 5 percent of adult measles cases. Viral keratitis is common and may progress to corneal ulcerations.

The measles virus poses problems in pregnant women in that maternal infection increases the risk of abortion and low-birth-weight infants. There is no evidence that measles causes birth defects; however, if maternal infection develops shortly before birth, the risk of the neonate developing measles is high. Neonates with measles bear some risk of death, especially if they are born preterm.

Individuals who received the inactivated measles vaccine before 1969 are susceptible to an often severe atypical form of measles. The inactivated vaccine of that era stimulated the production of antibody to only the viral hemagglutinin, not the fusion protein. A natural infection after vaccination with the inactivated vaccine often produced a severe illness with unusual and confusing features such as a noncharacteristic rash, pneumonitis, eosinophilia, coagulopathy, and an elevated erythrocyte sedimentation rate (ESR). The live-virus vaccines administered since 1969 stimulate antibody production to both the viral hemagglutinin and the fusion protein.

SIGNS AND SYMPTOMS

After infection and a 7- to 14-day incubation period, the patient begins to develop a fever, cough, coryza, and conjunctivitis. Fevers can be high and often are accompanied by anorexia, malaise, myalgia, and gastrointestinal symptoms. Within a day or two, an erythematous maculopapular rash develops around and below the ears and quickly spreads downward to affect the trunk and extremities. A few days after the rash appears, the prodromal symptoms often begin to improve, and 5 to 6 days after appearing, the rash begins to turn a brownish color, starting with the earliest-appearing lesions. A generalized lymphadenopathy commonly appears in the prodromal phase and can persist for several weeks. The cough often persists after resolution of the rest of the symptoms.

Two to 4 days after acute symptoms begin, Koplik's spots appear, which are diagnostic for measles. They present as small white to bluish-white specks on a red base. They are typically present on the buccal or labial mucosa opposite the first and second molars.

SPECIAL CONSIDERATIONS

Bacterial infections are the most common complication, and pneumonia and otitis media are the most frequently found secondary infections, with pneumococci and group A streptococci being the most commonly responsible pathogens. Before the development of antibiotics, otitis media secondary to measles resulted in residual hearing loss in as many as 10 percent of cases. Bacterial infections should be suspected when fever recurs or persists and leukocytosis develops. Patients with a compromised immune system are at a much greater risk of secondary infection complications as well as a higher incidence of adverse outcomes from the primary measles virus infection.

DIFFERENTIAL DIAGNOSIS

The diagnosis of measles usually is made through recognition of the pattern of signs and symptoms and is particularly straightforward when Koplik's spots are present. The diagnosis can be difficult when the presentation is atypical, such as in individuals who were immunized with the inactivated measles vaccine, though suspicion should be enhanced if cases have been reported in the local area. Other diagnoses to consider include drug rashes, rubella, scarlet fever, secondary syphilis, Kawasaki disease, and infectious mononucleosis. Several of these diagnoses do not produce a prodrome; however, the diagnosis can be complicated if the patient had an upper respiratory infection before the development of a rash.

LABORATORY TESTS

Measuring acute and convalescent serum antibody titers establishes the definitive diagnosis of measles. The obvious limitation of a diagnosis made by this method is that it is obtained after the patient has recovered and in the process has spread the highly contagious virus to many others. Isolation of the measles virus is difficult, and attempts at virus retrieval are advised only in unusual situations such as atypical measles, encephalitis after vaccination, and pneumonia without a rash in an immunocompromised patient. A complete blood count is helpful, since leukopenia is common in the prodromal phase and when the rash first presents; however, the interpretation may be compromised by the presence of a bacterial infection. A severe leukocytosis with less than 2000 cells/mm^3 is correlated with a poor prognosis.

Measles has been known to produce elevations of liver function tests, and elevations of two to three times the normal values of serum aspartate aminotransferase (AST), lactate dehydrogenase, and creatine phosphokinase are not uncommon. As many as 5 percent of adults with measles exhibit icteric hepatitis with hyperbilirubinemia. One-fifth of these patients have transient electrocardiographic (ECG) changes, though measles-related cardiac complications are rare.

Because measles produces a transient depression of cellular immunity, skin tests that utilize the cellular immune system are inaccurate. These tests include the purified protein derivative (PPD) and other skin tests for tuberculosis, the coccidioidomycosis skin test, the candida control skin test, and skin testing for the identification of allergies. Suppression of immunity sufficient to invalidate these tests results from the measles live-virus vaccine as well as the natural infection, and it is advised that testing be delayed as long as 4 weeks after vaccination or infection.

TREATMENT

Treatment for active measles is generally supportive. Recently, interest in the use of antiviral therapy has increased, as the measles virus is susceptible in vitro to ribavirin. No controlled studies have demonstrated its effectiveness, and ribavirin is not currently U.S. Food and Drug Administration (FDA)-approved for use in measles.

The World Health Organization (WHO) and the United Nations International Children's Emergency Fund (UNICEF) advise the administration of vitamin A to certain populations of children with active measles. It is advised that vitamin A, which is available in the United States as an oral solution containing 50,000 IU/mL, be given to children 6 months to 2 years of age hospitalized with complications and also to patients older than 6 months with immunodeficiency, ophthalmologic evidence of vitamin A deficiency, impaired intestinal absorption, malnutrition including eating disorders, and recent emigration from an area with a measles mortality rate over 1 percent. Vitamin A therapy also is recommended for any population in which the measles mortality rate exceeds 1 percent. The recommended dosage is a single dose of

200,000 IU orally for children 1 year and older and 100,000 IU for children 6 months to 1 year. Children with ophthalmologic evidence of vitamin A deficiency should be re-treated the next day and 4 weeks later. Children taking the 200,000 IU dose may experience a few hours of vomiting and headache.

The most effective treatment is prevention. Most developed countries have devoted resources to the control of measles by promoting mass immunization of the population. The currently available vaccine product is a live attenuated measles virus prepared in chick embryo cell culture. Approximately 95 percent of the recipients reach the desired level of immunity, though it is now known that antibody titers produced by vaccination tend to decrease over time in some individuals, in contrast to naturally acquired immunity, which is lifelong. The decrease in immunity over time in some vaccinated individuals was thought to contribute to the measles epidemics of the 1980s in the United States and led to the recommendation that all individuals born after 1957 receive two vaccinations. The vaccine is available as a single-disease product and in a combination product as measles-mumps-rubella (MMR) vaccine. It generally is advised that the MMR product be administered, since vaccinated individuals are likely to be susceptible to mumps and rubella, unless the cost of the MMR compared with the cost of the measles-only vaccine is prohibitive.

The MMR should be given to susceptible individuals with measles exposure occurring no more than 72 h before vaccination. Vaccination within this time frame can prevent wild virus infection in some cases. This is the treatment most preferred in outbreaks in schools.

Immune globulin (IG) can be given to susceptible individuals up to 6 days after exposure. IG is utilized for the protection of household contacts, contacts 5 to 12 months of age, exposed infants less than 5 months of age if the mother is not immune, exposed immunocompromised individuals, exposed children and adolescents with HIV regardless of MMR status, and exposed pregnant women who are not immune. IG doses should be 0.25 mL/kg intramuscularly (0.5 mL/kg intramuscularly for immunocompromised children), with the maximum dose being 15 mL.

The preferred method of prevention is immunization of the population. All individuals born before 1957 are assumed to be immune to childhood infection from the wild virus; therefore, immunization of this population is unnecessary. MMR should be given to all children at 12 to 15 months of age, and a second dose should be given by 12 years of age. Some schools and public health jurisdictions now require that the second MMR be given for school entry, and this protocol is adequate provided that the first dose was not given before the first birthday. Individuals in the population born after 1956 who received only one MMR or received the inactivated vaccine (before 1969) should be reimmunized.

In areas with a low incidence of measles, the first MMR usually is given at age 15 months. In areas with a high incidence, the first MMR usually is administered at 12 months. During outbreaks, measles vaccine can be administered as early as 6 months; however, since many children immunized at this age do not become immune, those immunized before age 12 months should be reimmunized at 12 to 15 months and then be immunized again before 12 years of age. Immunizations given before the first birthday should not be considered part of the immunization series.

The measles vaccine has been known to produce fever in 5 to 15 percent of nonimmune recipients, usually beginning 7 to 12 days after vaccination and lasting 1 or 2 days but sometimes lasting up to 5 days. Rarely, the vaccine will cause measles or complications of measles, and serious complications occur less frequently than 1 in 1 million. The vaccine is contraindicated during pregnancy, in individuals who have experienced anaphylaxis with egg antigens or neomycin, in individuals with recent administration of IG, and in immunocompromised individuals. Individuals with HIV should be immunized, as should those with inactive tuberculosis. After vaccination, PPD skin testing should be avoided for up to 6 weeks.

BIBLIOGRAPHY

Arruda E, Hayden FG: Paramyxovirus (parainfluenza, mumps, measles, and respiratory syncytial virus), rubella virus, coronavirus, and adenovirus infections, in Stein JH (ed): *Stein Internal Medicine,* 5th ed. Philadelphia, Saunders, 1998, pp 1497–1499.

Beers MH, Berkow R (ed): *Merck Manual of Diagnosis and Therapy,* 17th ed. Whitehouse Station, NJ, Merck Research Laboratories, 1999, pp 2320–2325.

Boickenooghe A, Shandera WX: Infectious diseases: Viral and rickettsial, in Tierney LM Jr, McPhee SJ, Papadakis MA (eds): *Current Medical Diagnosis and Treatment,* 39th rev. ed. New York, McGraw-Hill, 2000, pp 1306–1307.

Brunell PA: Measles, in Goldman L, Bennett JC (eds): *Cecil Textbook of Medicine,* 21st ed. Philadelphia, Saunders, 2000, pp 1802–1804.

Georges P (ed): Pertussis, in *1997 Red Book: Report of the Committee on Infectious Diseases,* 24th ed. Elk Grove Village, IL, American Academy of Pediatrics, 1997, pp 344–457.

Gershon A: Measles, in Fauci AS, Braunwald E, Isselbacher KJ, et al (eds): *Harrison's Principles of Internal Medicine,* 14th ed. New York, McGraw-Hill, 1998, pp 1123–1125.

Grossman M: Immunization, in Stites DP, Terr AI, Parslow TG (eds): *Medical Immunology,* 9th ed. Stamford, CT, Appleton & Lange, 1997, pp 772–795.

Heggie AD: Measles, in Rakel RE (ed): *Conn's Current Therapy, 2000.* Philadelphia, Saunders, 2000, pp 132–134.

Infections, in Cunningham GF, MacDonald PC, Gant NR, et al (eds): *Williams' Obstetrics,* 20th ed. Norwalk, CT, Appleton & Lange, 1997, pp 1297–1315.

Levin MJ: Infections: Viral and rickettsial, in Hay WW Jr, Hayward AR, Levin MJ, Sondheimer JM (eds): *Current Pediatric Diagnosis and Treatment,* 14th ed. Stamford, CT, Appleton & Lange, 1999, pp 969–970.

Mills J: Viral infections, in Stites DP, Terr AI, Parslow TG (eds), *Medical Immunology,* 9th ed. Stamford, CT, Appleton & Lange, 1997, pp 694–705.

Panitch HS, Fishman PS, Bever CT Jr: Demyelinating diseases: Acute disseminated encephalomyelitis, in Stites DP, Terr AI, Parslow TG (eds), *Medical Immunology,* 9th ed. Stamford, CT, Appleton & Lange, 1997, pp 579–590.

Salmon DA, Haber M, Gangarosa EJ, et al: Health consequences of religious and philosophical exemptions from immunization laws: Individual and societal risk of measles. *JAMA* 282(1):47–53, 1999.

Wyde PR, Moore-Poveda DK, De Clercq E, et al: Use of cotton rats to evaluate the efficacy of antivirals in treatment of measles virus infections. *Antimicrob Agents Chemother* 44(5):1146–1152.

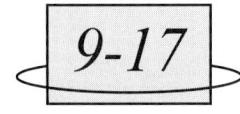

MUMPS

Richard Dehn

DISCUSSION

Mumps is an acute generalized viral infection that characteristically causes painful enlargement of the parotid glands. In most cases, mumps is a benign self-limited illness, especially in the preadolescent age group. After puberty, the severity of the symptoms and complications increases significantly with age.

In unvaccinated populations, mumps is primarily a disease of childhood, and by age 15, over 90 percent of the population will have developed antibodies to mumps. As many as one-third of the cases are asymptomatic, and up to 90 percent of adults without a history of clinical mumps or mumps vaccination will have antibodies to mumps. In the United States, the live attenuated virus vaccine was introduced in 1967 and reduced the incidence of mumps by 98 percent. As a result of the immunization of school-age cohorts, the majority of nonimmune individuals are in the postpubertal age groups. This has contributed to the recent rise of mumps cases in older age groups, which have a higher frequency of complications and more severe symptomatology.

Most patients with clinical mumps have inflammation of the parotid glands. The parotitis of mumps has a characteristic "chipmunk" look, since the swelling lifts the earlobe outward and obscures the angle of the mandible. Often involvement is initially unilateral, followed 2 to 3 days later by contralateral involvement.

PATHOGENESIS

Mumps is caused by a paramyxovirus of which there is only one known serotype, though antigenic differences have been noted with different strains. Humans are the only known host of the mumps virus, although the virus can be introduced into several other mammals. The virus is spread to the host through saliva or secretions from the respiratory system, usually through direct contact or aerosol droplets. The virus is significantly less contagious than measles or chickenpox, though it is contagious enough that epidemics can occur in populations with a small proportion of susceptible individuals. The virus replicates in epithelial cells of the upper respiratory tract and spreads to the regional lymph nodes and then systemically. The virus has a high degree of affinity for glandular and nervous system structures; thus, the clinical manifestations are likely to occur in those organ systems. The incubation period is 7 to 25 days, usually averaging 16 to 18 days. The virus usually is communicable for an average of 7 days, starting 1 to 2 days before parotid involvement and lasting 5 days; however, it has been reported to be communicable as early as 7 days before parotid involvement and to last as long as 9 days after the onset of parotitis. Up to 30 percent of mumps infections are subclinical. Among those who are symptomatic, the most commonly affected single organ is the parotid gland. Most patients with symptomatic mumps experience edema and tenderness of one or more salivary glands.

As many as 15 percent of patients with clinical mumps exhibit symptoms of meningitis, which usually is characterized by headache, lethargy, neck stiffness, and vomiting. The meningitis is thought to be caused by replication of mumps virus in the ependymal cells of the choroid plexus, and virus can be found in the cerebrospinal fluid (CSF). Up to 50 percent of mumps patients symptomatic with parotitis and without meningitis have mild headache and mononuclear pleocytosis of the CSF. Severe encephalitis is rare (1 in 1000 cases) and has a relatively low mortality rate of 0.5 to 2.3 percent, seldom producing residual damage. The mumps virus is known to replicate in the testicles, producing orchitis. Mumps orchitis is an unusual finding in prepubertal males but occurs in up to one-third of postpubertal males. Up to half of cases of mumps orchitis result in testicular atrophy, but sterility is uncommon. Mumps has been noted to cause oophoritis in postpubertal women, though the incidence is only about 5 percent. When the right ovary is involved, the clinical picture can resemble that of acute appendicitis. Premature menopause and infertility have been reported, though both are rare. Occasionally mumps produces mastitis. Several other glandular systems can be infiltrated by the mumps virus and produce clinical symptoms. Pancreatic inflammation can produce the symptoms of acute pancreatitis. Other uncommon presentations of mumps include thyroiditis, myocarditis, arthritis, prostatitis, lacrimal gland involvement, sensorineural deafness, renal function abnormalities, and thrombocytopenia.

There is some evidence that maternal mumps infection in the first trimester of pregnancy may result in an increase in the frequency of spontaneous abortions and may be associated with a greater likelihood of low birthweight, although this evidence is not convincing. No increases in birth defects have been noted in children born to mothers who had clinical mumps during the first trimester. There is no difference in the clinical course of mumps between pregnant patients and nonpregnant patients.

SIGNS AND SYMPTOMS

After the incubation period, the patient experiences a 12- to 24-h prodromal phase characterized by chills, low-grade fever, anorexia, and headache. It is not unusual for the prodrome to be absent. Parotitis then presents as otalgia or jaw tenderness with mastication that worsens over the next 2 or 3 days until the gland reaches its maximum size.

The patient usually experiences pain with chewing or swallowing and finds that the ingestion of acidic liquids causes severe parotid pain. The involved gland is swollen and tender, and the oral outlet ducts of the involved gland appear edematous and inflamed. The parotid gland is most commonly involved, though occasionally the submaxillary gland is involved, producing suprasternal edema. Often the parotid involvement is unilateral, only to be followed by contralateral involvement 2 to 3 days later. Parotid edema peaks on the second or third day and usually resolves within 7 days. Mumps has been known to produce a relapse of symptoms about 2 weeks after resolution, though the incidence of relapse is rare (see Fig. 9-17-1).

Patients with symptomatic mumps commonly have headache and stiff neck. As many as half these patients have a CSF pleocytosis, and up to 15 percent of all symptomatic measles cases progress to symptomatic meningitis. Males are two to three times more likely to have nervous system involvement than are females. Meningitis usually presents 4 to 5 days after the onset of parotitis, though it is not unusual for it to present without parotid involvement. Meningitis symptoms usually resolve within a week but can persist up to 5 weeks.

Encephalitis is an uncommon complication of mumps. The symptoms may develop at the same time as parotid involvement or may present 1 to 2 weeks later. Findings include obtundation, seizures, and high fevers. Unilateral nerve deafness can occur, which is usually temporary. Mumps encephalitis has a low mortality rate, and residual damage is rare.

Orchitis is a common presentation in postpubertal males. The orchitis is usually unilateral, though it can be bilateral in up to one-third of cases. Orchitis typically presents within a week of the onset of parotitis, though it can develop as the only presenting symptom. Orchitis usually presents with severe testicular pain and swelling accompanied by fever, headache, nausea, and vomiting. The acute pain and swelling usually resolve within 7 to 10 days, but the symptoms can persist for several weeks. Up to 50 percent of involved testicles undergo some degree of atrophy after resolution of the infection. Sterility is rare even after bilateral involvement, and the subsequent development of testicular tumors is rare.

Postpubertal females can develop oophoritis and mastitis. Right-sided oophoritis can be confused with acute appendicitis. Pancreatic involvement can present as acute pancreatitis with a clinical picture of nausea, vomiting, severe epigastric pain, fever, and chills. Recovery usually occurs within a week.

Unusual complications include thyroiditis, myocarditis, arthritis, prostatitis, lacrimal gland involvement, sensorineural deafness, renal function abnormalities, and thrombocytopenia.

DIFFERENTIAL DIAGNOSIS

The parotitis of mumps is difficult to differentiate from other possible causes of tender neck masses. The presence of other mumps cases in the area or known exposure to mumps is helpful. Parotitis can be caused by several other viruses, such as influenza A virus, parainfluenza virus, coxsackievirus, and lymphocytic choriomeningitis virus. *Staphylococcus aureus* and streptococcal infections also can cause parotitis as well as diphtheria, typhoid, typhus fever, and infections resulting from poor oral hygiene. Care should be taken not to confuse parotitis with lymphadenopathy. Parotid duct obstruction and tumors should be considered.

Atypical presentations such as mumps meningitis and orchitis are difficult to diagnose. Other causes of orchitis, such as torsion, hematomas, hernias, tumors, epididymitis, and infection with other organisms, should be considered. The diagnosis in these cases probably will rely on laboratory testing.

LABORATORY TESTS

The diagnosis is easy to make from clinical signs in typical cases during an epidemic; however, mumps antibody titer from paired specimens of acute and convalescent sera is diagnostic if a fourfold increase is

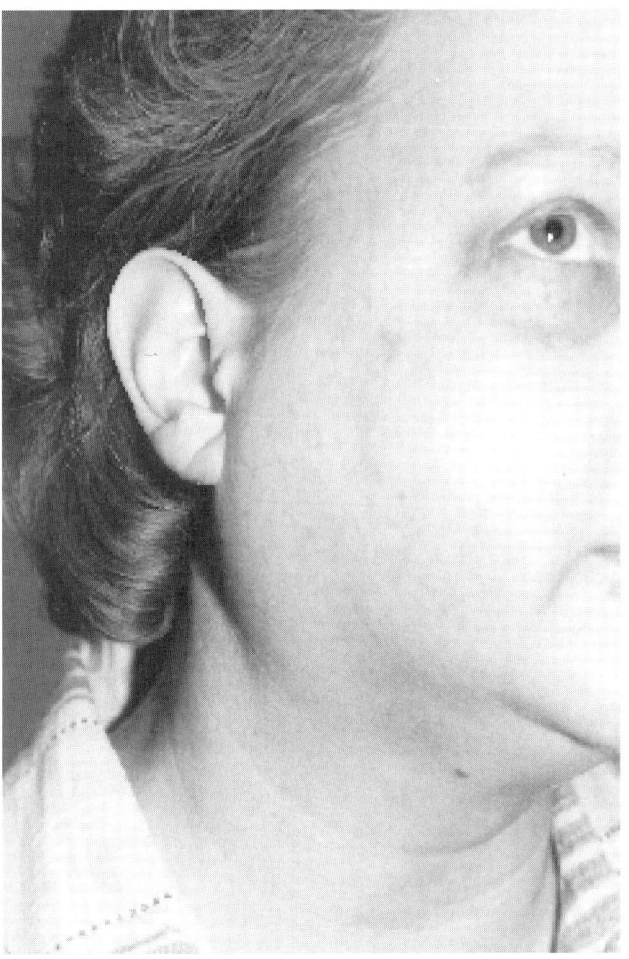

A

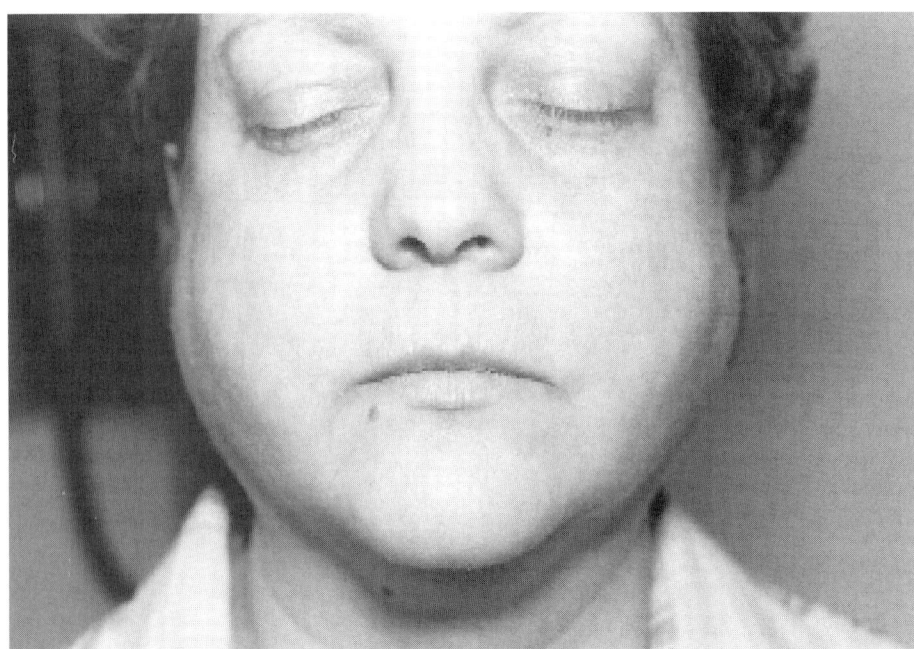

B

FIGURE 9-17-1. Mumps in an adult patient. *A.* Marked parotid swelling characteristic of mumps. *B.* Bilateral parotid swelling in the same patient. (*Photos courtesy of Rodney L. Moser. Used with permission.*)

noted. Mumps virus can be isolated from samples obtained from saliva, urine, and CSF for 4 to 6 days after the onset of parotitis.

The white blood cell count often is unaffected by mumps; however, elevated lymphocytes are not unusual. A white cell count higher than 20,000 with a polymorphonuclear predominance sometimes is found in patients with meningitis or orchitis. Parotid involvement often produces an elevated serum amylase, which complicates the diagnosis of pancreatitis. A normal serum lipase can indicate whether a patient also has pancreatic involvement. Patients with central nervous system (CNS) involvement exhibit abnormalities of the CSF that are consistent with a viral infection.

TREATMENT

Treatment is supportive. Orchitis patients usually are advised to avoid activity, apply cold packs to the affected testicle, and wear appropriate support for the scrotum. Although corticosteroids sometimes are utilized to reduce inflammation of the testicles, there is no evidence that this treatment is beneficial. Isolation from school, child care, and populations of susceptible individuals is appropriate for 9 days after the onset of parotitis. Serious complication such as meningitis, encephalitis, and pancreatitis may require hospitalization.

Mumps immune globulin has been found to be ineffective and has been withdrawn from the market. The administration of mumps live-virus vaccine after exposure is not effective in preventing infection but is not contraindicated.

The prevention of mumps cases through immunization is the preferred treatment. Mumps attenuated live-virus vaccine prepared in chick embryo cell culture was released in 1967 and has produced a 98 percent reduction in the number of cases reported. It produces immunity in 95 percent of those vaccinated, and serologic evidence suggests that immunity obtained from a single dose is long-lasting. It is available as a single-virus vaccine or combined with measles and rubella vaccines (MMR). Since it is known that mumps can transmit through a population that contains only a small proportion of nonimmune individuals, the goal of immunization is the identification and vaccination of all susceptible individuals.

In the United States, all individuals born before 1957 are considered naturally immune and therefore do not need routine immunization. However, immunization in this age group is not contraindicated, as natural immunity will destroy the attenuated live virus of the immunization and those individuals therefore will not have any sort of immunization reaction. Any individual in that age group who is not naturally immune will have immunity conferred by the immunization.

It is recommended that children receive MMR after the first birthday. Generally, this immunization is given at age 15 months. A second MMR is recommended any time from school entry age (4 to 6 years) to the start of puberty. It is advised that the second MMR dose be given before the start of puberty so that individuals who do not receive immunity from the first vaccine will gain protection. Since mumps infection during puberty can involve the testes or ovaries and since the severity of cases increases with age, it is important that immunity be conferred before adolescence. The recent increase in adult mumps cases is indicative of the number of unvaccinated individuals in the population who were born after 1956 and did not receive the vaccine because MMR was not uniformly required for school entry in the 1970s.

Infants have mumps immunity for the first year of life if the mother was immune to mumps. It is this passive immunity that makes it impractical to give the attenuated live-virus vaccine in the first year of life. If an infant receives the mumps vaccine before the first birthday, it should be repeated at 15 months of age and again at school entry or before puberty.

All individuals in the population should be evaluated in regard to mumps immunity status. Individuals not immune by virtue of birth before 1957, not up to date with current immunization recommendations, or not shown by serology testing to be immune should be immunized.

Pregnancy is a contraindication to vaccination. Conception should be avoided for 3 months after vaccination. Inadvertent vaccination during pregnancy poses theoretical risks to the fetus, but there is no evidence that the fetus becomes infected with the virus.

Vaccination should be avoided in individuals who are immunocompromised. The exception to this contraindication is a patient with HIV, who should be immunized with MMR.

Patients who recently have received immune globulin or blood transfusions should avoid vaccination temporarily. The vaccine should be given at least 2 weeks before or 3 months after reception of the immune globulin or blood transfusion. The individual should be protected from mumps during that time by the antibodies in the blood products.

Since the mumps vaccine is derived from chick embryo cell cultures, it should be administered with caution in individuals who are allergic to eggs. Allergic reactions to the vaccine are rare.

The presence of fever is not a contraindication to vaccine administration. Individuals with upper respiratory infections and low-grade fever can be vaccinated; however, individuals who present with a fever suggestive of a more serious illness should have the vaccination withheld until after recovery. In recent studies, no differences were noted in immunity conferred by immunizations given to children with minor illnesses compared with immunizations given to healthy children.

Adverse reactions to mumps vaccination are very rare. Most adverse reactions are time-limited and include neurologic deafness, rash, febrile seizures, parotitis, orchitis, meningitis, encephalitis, pruritus, and purpura. CNS reactions occur at a lower incidence than they do in unvaccinated populations.

BIBLIOGRAPHY

Arruda E, Hayden FG: Paramyxovirus (parainfluenza, mumps, measles, and respiratory syncytial virus), rubella virus, coronavirus, and adenovirus infections, in Stein JH (ed): *Stein Internal Medicine,* 5th ed. Philadelphia, Saunders, 1998, pp 1495–1497.
Beers MH, Berkow R (ed): *Merck Manual of Diagnosis and Therapy,* 17th ed. Whitehouse Station, NJ, Merck Research Laboratories, 1999, pp 2325–2327.
Boickenooghe A, Shandera WX: Infectious diseases: Viral and rickettsial, in Tierney LM Jr, McPhee SJ, Papadakis MA (eds): *Current Medical Diagnosis and Treatment,* 39th rev. ed. New York, McGraw-Hill, 2000, pp 1307–1309.
Georges P (ed): Mumps, in *1997 Red Book: Report of the Committee on Infectious Diseases,* 24th ed. Elk Grove Village, IL, American Academy of Pediatrics, 1997, pp 366–369.
Gnann JW: Mumps, in Goldman L, Bennett JC (eds): *Cecil Textbook of Medicine,* 21st ed. Philadelphia, Saunders, 2000, pp 1808–1810.
Infections, in Cunningham GF, MacDonald PC, Gant NR, et al (eds): *William's Obstetrics,* 20th ed. Norwalk, CT, Appleton & Lange, 1997, pp 1297–1315.
Levin MJ: Infections: Viral and rickettsial, in Hay WW Jr, Hayward AR, Levin MJ, Sondheimer JM (eds): *Current Pediatric Diagnosis and Treatment,* 14th ed. Stamford, CT, Appleton & Lange, 1999, pp 998–999.
Parslow T: Immunogens, antigens, and vaccines, in Parslow T et al (eds): *Medical Immunology,* 10th ed. New York: McGraw-Hill, 2001.
Venglarcik JS: Mumps, in Rakel RE (ed): *Conn's Current Therapy, 2000.* Philadelphia, Saunders, 2000, p 113.

PERTUSSIS
Richard Dehn

DISCUSSION

Pertussis, better known as whooping cough, is a highly communicable bacterial infectious disease with a significant morbidity rate in infants and young children. The illness presents in three distinct stages, the second of which is characterized by a severe paroxysmal cough with a unique inspiratory whoop. Uncomplicated pertussis usually has a 6- to 10-week course, though complications such as pneumonia are not uncommon.

Pertussis is highly contagious, infecting 70 to 100 percent of susceptible individuals. In unvaccinated populations pertussis is endemic, and in undeveloped regions of the world infant and childhood mortality rates are high. Improvements in supportive treatment in the United States at the beginning of the twentieth century and the subsequent development of antibiotics reduced mortality rates from pertussis; however, the incidence did not drop until the early 1950s, when immunization of infants and children became prevalent. Before widespread immunization, the annual incidence in the United States was about 200,000 cases, compared with a recent annual incidence of about 4000 cases. The mortality rate correspondingly dropped from 5000 to 10,000 deaths per year in the prevaccination era to 4 to 11 deaths per year more recently. About three-fourths of the deaths occur in the first year of life. The fatality rate in children less than 6 months of age is 0.5 percent.

The reported incidence of pertussis in the United States increased from 0.54 to 0.95 cases per 100,000 in 1978–1982 to 0.96 to 1.74 cases per 100,000 in 1983–1987. This has been thought to be due primarily to an increase in the proportion of unvaccinated individuals in the very young population. Factors contributing to the increase in the proportion of susceptible infants and young children include a significant number of parents who withhold pertussis vaccine from their children because of the potential side effects, the existence of infant populations not receiving vaccinations, and the immigration of unvaccinated individuals to the United States.

PATHOGENESIS

Pertussis is caused by *Bordetella pertussis,* a nonmotile gram-negative coccobacillus first isolated by Bordet and Gengou in 1906. It usually is transmitted to the host by the inhalation of respiratory secretions from an infected individual. The organisms adhere to ciliated respiratory epithelial cells, where they replicate. *Bordetella pertussis* does not invade farther than the ciliated respiratory epithelial cells. The disease is produced by several bacterial toxins, including the pertussis toxin, which is responsible for lymphocytosis and many of the respiratory symptoms of pertussis. It is felt that the toxins cause tissue damage to specific organs in the respiratory system, since damage and symptoms persist long after the *B. pertussis* organism is no longer present. Further evidence supportive of pertussis being caused by toxins produced by *B. pertussis* is provided by the fact that treating individuals in the incubation period or the early catarrhal stage with antibiotics often ameliorates the disease. In these cases, elimination of *B. pertussis* probably occurs before the production of toxins causes tissue damage. Infection with *B. pertussis* results in the production of antibody for about 5 years, while vaccination with killed whole virus produces about 3 years of immunity. Most older children, adolescents, and adults are susceptible to pertussis, and infections passed to young children by older members of the family are common. A natural infection and the prior completion of immunizations often result in milder subsequent infections. Infections in all individuals other than infants and young children rarely result in serious illness or complications but place susceptible youngsters at risk.

SIGNS AND SYMPTOMS

Pertussis presents in three distinct stages, with the first stage lasting 1 to 2 weeks and the second and third stages usually lasting 2 to 4 weeks. After infection of the host's respiratory tract with *B. pertussis* and a 7- to 10-day incubation period, the first stage, or catarrhal stage, begins. The catarrhal stage is characterized by mild nonspecific upper respiratory symptoms such as rhinorrhea, conjunctival injection, increased lacrimation, sneezing, and a troublesome hacking nocturnal cough that gradually becomes diurnal. Low-grade fever, listlessness, and anorexia are sometimes present; however, a fever higher than 38.3°C

(101.0°F) is suggestive of a bacterial superinfection or a nonpertussis cause of the upper respiratory infection (URI). Pertussis in the catarrhal stage is difficult to distinguish from common URIs and thus often is not recognized at this stage. The host is most infectious to other susceptible individuals during this stage, and so the organism often is passed to others before it is clinically recognized. The catarrhal stage lasts about 2 weeks before the worsening cough becomes paroxysmal.

The second, or paroxysmal, stage is characterized by bouts of 10 to 30 forceful coughs within a span of a few seconds, ending with an inspiratory whoop, though the whoop is not always exhibited in adults and infants. At the peak of the paroxysmal stage, the host may experience as many as 25 paroxysms over a 24-h period, with more occurrences at night than during the day. Paroxysms can be accompanied by cyanosis, sweating, prostration, and exhaustion and often are followed by the expulsion of copious amounts of viscid mucus, which frequently results in vomiting. Cyanosis, neck vein congestion, bulging eyes, and protrusion of the tongue also can be present during attacks, as well as residual petechial hemorrhages, engorged conjunctivae, periorbital edema, and epistaxis. Yawning, sneezing, or eating often provokes attacks. Between attacks, the patient appears normal. Except for a few scattered rhonchi, the chest examination is usually normal. The presence of fever in this stage is suggestive of a secondary infectious process.

After a paroxysmal stage lasting 2 to 4 weeks, the paroxysms gradually decrease in frequency and intensity. Vomiting and other symptoms produced by the intense paroxysms stop. Recovery progresses slowly, usually lasting an additional 3 to 4 weeks; however, this stage can last several months. The paroxysms evolve into a cough that resembles chronic bronchitis, though noxious stimuli and viral URIs can provoke a return of paroxysms.

DIFFERENTIAL DIAGNOSIS

At the onset pertussis is insidious, and in the catarrhal stage it is indistinguishable from a mild viral respiratory infection. Exposure to pertussis may provide a clue to the appropriate diagnosis during the catarrhal stage. The diagnosis of pertussis usually is entertained after the appearance of paroxysms; however, spasmodic coughing is not pathognomonic of pertussis. Bronchiolitis, cystic fibrosis, tuberculosis, foreign bodies, airway compression from lymphadenopathy or malignancy, and chlamydia and viral or mycoplasma pneumonia should be considered. Differentiation usually can be made by careful physical examination, laboratory findings, and the results of a chest x-ray.

COMPLICATIONS

Up to 90 percent of the fatalities caused by pertussis are due to pneumonia, which is the most common serious complication. Interstitial and subcutaneous emphysema and pneumothorax are uncommon consequences of the increased intrathoracic pressure of the paroxysms. This can produce bronchiectasis in debilitated children, resulting in residual emphysema. Mucus plugs can cause atelectases. Severe paroxysms resulting in anoxia can cause hemorrhages into the brain, eyes, skin, and mucous membranes. Cerebral hemorrhage, cerebral edema, and toxic encephalitis may result in severe neurologic disorders. Paroxysms can produce frenulum ulcers as a result of abrasion with the lower incisors, and occasionally they result in rectal prolapse and umbilical herniation. It is not unusual to see convulsions in infants, but they are uncommon in older children. Otitis media is a common complication and should be treated with the appropriate antibiotic.

LABORATORY TESTS

The organism *B. pertussis* can be cultured from nasopharyngeal specimens in the catarrhal and early paroxysmal stages. Unfortunately, the likelihood of obtaining a positive culture starts to decrease at about the time in the course of the illness when the diagnosis of pertussis becomes obvious. A positive culture is considered diagnostic, and false-negative results are common, especially after the fourth week of the illness and in patients who have received antibiotics. Cultures are best plated at the bedside to freshly prepared Bordet-Gengou or charcoal agar medium, using small cotton swabs passed through the nose to the nasopharynx with 28-gauge zinc-coated wire. A direct immunofluorescent assay (DFA) of nasopharyngeal secretions is available at some laboratories but is less sensitive and specific than a culture, sometimes producing false-positive or false-negative results.

No single serologic test is specific or sensitive enough to confirm a diagnosis. Since each individual produces a different antibody response to pertussis infection or vaccination, serologic antibody results are difficult to interpret. Enzyme immunoassays for IgG antibody to pertussis toxin and IgA antibody to *B. pertussis* filamentous hemagglutinin are under investigation as diagnostic tests.

Pertussis often produces lymphocytosis toward the end of the catarrhal stage. White blood cell counts are frequently in the range of 20,000 to 30,000/μL with 60 to 80 percent small lymphocytes, but the counts can be as high as 60,000/μL. The degree of lymphocytosis usually parallels the severity of the cough.

Bronchopneumonia and patchy atelectases often are seen on chest x-ray as thickened bronchi or a "shaggy" heart border.

TREATMENT

Treatment for pertussis once it has reached the paroxysmal stage is primarily supportive. Infants often require hospitalization, and occasionally older individuals may experience complications. Unnecessary manipulation and activity should be discouraged in the acute paroxysmal stage, since any form of stimulation can contribute to increased paroxysms.

Antibiotic therapy can stop the progression of the disease if it is given during the incubation period or the catarrhal stage. Antibiotics also are given to individuals beyond those stages to eradicate the *B. pertussis* organism even though this does not affect the course of the disease, thus preventing transmission of the disease to caretakers and family members. The antibiotic of choice is erythromycin 40 to 50 mg/kg/day in four divided doses, up to 2 g a day, for 14 days. The estolate form of erythromycin (Ilosone) is thought to be more active against *B. pertussis* and is preferred. An alternative to erythromycin is trimethoprim-sulfamethoxazole (Bactrim, Septra), 8 mg/kg/day trimethoprim and 40 mg/kg/day sulfamethoxazole in two divided doses; however, its efficacy has not been well studied. Antibiotic therapy also is recommended for all household contacts and other close contacts irrespective of vaccination status. The host and all contacts should be considered capable of shedding virus until 5 days after the start of antibiotic therapy.

Corticosteroids and albuterol have been used in the paroxysmal stage with variable results. Albuterol is used commonly in Europe, but its effectiveness has not been evaluated carefully. The use of corticosteroids can worsen a complicating infection, though in one study corticosteroid use significantly reduced the frequency of paroxysms. Pertussis immune globulin has been shown to confer no benefit.

Children under 7 years of age should be immunized with pertussis vaccine. A whole-cell killed-virus vaccine developed in the 1940s is available as a single-virus vaccine and as part of a combined vaccine with diphtheria and tetanus toxoids (DTP); however, this vaccine is no longer recommended for children under 7 years of age. The current recommendation for children under 7 years is an acellular pertussis vaccine combined with diphtheria and tetanus toxoids (DTaP). It should be given at 2, 4, and 6 months of age and again at 18 months and at school entry. The pertussis vaccine is associated with increased vaccination reactions with increasing age, and so the pertussis vaccination is not recommended for individuals over 6 years of age. Three doses of whole-cell vaccine are effective in about 80 percent of

recipients, and the immunity persists for about 3 years. The whole-cell pertussis vaccine generally has a higher incidence of adverse reactions than do other vaccines for childhood illnesses. In the United States, media coverage of vaccination reactions has resulted in a significant number of parents refusing to vaccinate their children against pertussis. This population of unvaccinated infants and young children has contributed to the recent increase in the incidence of pertussis.

The most common reactions to the pertussis vaccine are inflammation at the site of injection and fever. As many as half the individuals receiving the whole-cell vaccine experience a local reaction or fever, though the incidence of these side effects is much lower when the acellular vaccine is used. Local reactions can be reduced by the administration of acetaminophen or another appropriate antipyretic at the time of injection and 4 and 8 h after the injection.

Allergic reactions are uncommon, with anaphylaxis occurring in approximately 2 cases per 100,000 injections, though death is extremely rare. The incidence of seizures within 48 h of vaccination with DTP is 1 in 1750 doses. Most of these seizures are thought to be fever-related and are not associated with residual neurologic symptoms or a greater risk of developing epilepsy. Inconsolable crying for more than 3 h occurs in 1 percent of individuals who receive the vaccine and can be seen as long as 48 h after the injection. A hypotonic-hyporesponsive episode presenting as a generalized collapse or shock-like state is seen in 1 in 1750 doses. There is no evidence of residual damage after these episodes. Generally, the incidence of all adverse reactions appears to be lower after the use of acellular vaccine, but large population studies have not been completed on the acellular vaccines.

Many severe reactions to the pertussis vaccine have been alleged but not proved. Severe adverse reactions such as death, encephalopathy, the onset of seizure disorder, developmental delays, and learning disabilities have been temporally related to the administration of the pertussis vaccine. In epidemiologic investigations, the incidence of pertussis vaccine–related severe acute neurologic illness has been estimated to be 1 in 140,000 DTP doses.

Contraindications to pertussis vaccine include an immediate anaphylactic reaction to a prior pertussis vaccination and encephalopathy within 7 days after a prior vaccination. Individuals who experience a convulsion or episodes of inconsolable crying within 3 days of pertussis vaccination, a hypotonic-hyporesponsive episode within 48 h of vaccination, or a fever of 40.5°C (104.9°F) or higher within 48 h of vaccination should consider the risks and benefits of additional vaccinations carefully.

BIBLIOGRAPHY

Beers MH, Berkow R (ed): *Merck Manual of Diagnosis and Therapy,* 17th ed. Whitehouse Station, NJ, Merck Research Laboratories, 1999, pp 2306–2308.

Chambers HF: Infectious diseases: Bacterial and chlamydial, in Tierney LM Jr, McPhee SJ, Papadakis MA (eds): *Current Medical Diagnosis and Treatment,* 39th rev. ed. New York, McGraw-Hill, 2000, pp 1351–1352.

Georges P (ed): Pertussis, in *1997 Red Book: Report of the Committee on Infectious Diseases,* 24th ed. Elk Grove Village, IL, American Academy of Pediatrics, 1997, pp 394–407.

Grossman M: in Stites DP, Terr AI, Parslow TG (eds), *Medical Immunology,* 9th ed. Stamford, CT, Appleton & Lange, 1997, pp 772–795.

Henry NK, Wilson WR, Hendley JO: Infections caused by *Brucella, Francisella tularensis, Pasteurella, Yersinia species,* and *Bordetella pertussis* (whooping cough), in Stein JH (ed): *Stein Internal Medicine,* 5th ed. Philadelphia, Saunders, 1998, pp 1611–1613.

Johnson RB Jr: Whooping cough (pertussis), in Goldman L, Bennett JC (eds): *Cecil Textbook of Medicine,* 21st ed. Philadelphia, Saunders, 2000, pp 1644–1666.

Ogle JW: Infections: Bacterial and spirochetal, in Hay WW Jr, Hayward AR, Levin MJ, Sondheimer JM (eds): *Current Pediatric Diagnosis and Treatment,* 14th ed. Stamford, CT, Appleton & Lange, 1999, pp 1044–1046.

Ogle JW: Pertussis, in Rakel RE (ed): *Conn's Current Therapy,* 2000. Philadelphia, Saunders, 2000, pp 137–139.

Ryan JL: Bacterial diseases, in Stites DP, Terr AI, Parslow TG (eds), *Medical Immunology,* 9th ed. Stamford, CT, Appleton & Lange, 1997, pp 684–693.

Siber GR, Samore MH: Pertussis, in Fauci AS, Braunwald E, Isselbacher KJ, et al (eds): *Harrison's Principles of Internal Medicine,* 14th ed. New York, McGraw-Hill, 1998, pp 933–936.

Zimmerman RK, Ball, JA: Update on childhood immunizations for the year 2000. *Family Pract Recertif* 22(4):69–80, 2000.

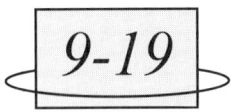

RABIES

Ralph Rice

DISCUSSION

Although rarely seen in the United States, rabies is perhaps the most feared potential consequence of animal bites. However, worldwide, the incidence of rabies is much greater, with the World Health Organization reporting more than 35,000 deaths per year.[1,2] Although rabies previously was considered an endemic disease, mandatory vaccination of dogs and cats and animal control measures enacted in the 1940s and 1950s have resulted in a drop in human rabies in the United States from an average of 55 cases per year in the first half of the twentieth century to less than 1 case per year in 1980.[1,3] Since 1980, a total of 36 cases of human rabies were reported by the Centers for Disease Control and Prevention. The cost of rabies vaccination of pets and postexposure prophylaxis in the United States has been placed at $300 million annually. Each year, between 16,000 and 39,000 people in the United States receive postexposure prophylaxis.[1,4]

Wild animals are the main vector for rabies. The vast majority of rabies infections in humans and domestic animals come from skunks, raccoons, and bats, which account for 83 percent of reported cases. Other wildlife vectors include foxes, bobcats, coyotes, and wolves. Not commonly thought of as carriers of rabies, unvaccinated farm animals accounted for 11 percent of reported domestic animal cases in 1988. Lagomorphs (rabbits and hares) and rodents are uncommon carriers of rabies. Amphibians, fishes, insects, and reptiles are noncarriers.

Rabies is present throughout the United States, with cases having been reported in every state except Hawaii. The prevalence of rabies shows the highest incidence in the following five geographic areas in the 48 contiguous states[2,5,6]:

1. The mid-Atlantic states of Pennsylvania, Maryland, New Jersey, Rhode Island, and West Virginia
2. The southeastern states of Florida, Georgia, Alabama, and South Carolina
3. The south-central states of Texas, Oklahoma, and Arkansas
4. The north-central states of Minnesota, Iowa, and the Dakotas
5. California

New England, the Pacific Northwest, and some Rocky Mountain states, such as Utah, have an incidence of rabies in animals that is below the national average.

PATHOGENESIS

Transmission of the rabies virus most commonly results from inoculation with infected saliva. This may result from a bite, direct contact with mucous membranes, or a break in the skin. Transmission from inhalation has been reported four times: twice in workers in rabies research laboratories and twice after a spelunking exploration in caves inhabited by bats that carried the rabies virus.[3,6,7] Human-to-human transmission of rabies has occurred eight times from corneal transplantation.

Because of the nonspecific early signs and symptoms of rabies, it is important to obtain a history of an animal bite or bat exposure. The type of animal, its behavior, and the circumstances surrounding the injury, along with the location and ownership, if any, of the animal,

TABLE 9-19-1. Factors Influencing Susceptibility to Rabies

Host's genetic background and age
Infecting strain
Size of inoculum
Degree of innervation at site of injury
Proximity to central nervous system

SOURCE: From Baevsky and Bartfield,[1] Fishbein and Robinson.[6]

are important items to obtain in the patient history. Bat bites may be small and go unnoticed, especially during the period of anxiety after an encounter with a bat. The Centers for Disease Control and Prevention (CDC) recommends that in situations in which a bat is physically present and the person cannot reasonably exclude the possibility of a bite exposure and cannot test the bat, exposure to the virus should be considered to have occurred.

A number of variables determine the susceptibility of the host to infection. Table 9-19-1 lists those risk factors.

Initially, the virus replicates within the monocytes near the bite. The virus then enters the peripheral nervous system through unmyelinated terminal sensory and motor neurons. If the initial inoculum is large enough and is in direct contact with peripheral nerves, the virus may enter the nerve immediately. When transmission occurs through inhalation, the virus invades the nervous system through the neuroepithelial cells on the mucosal surface. Once it is in nerve cells, the virus migrates through retrograde axoplasmic flow to the central nervous system (CNS). Symptoms of rabies arise when the virus reaches the CNS. This incubation period, before the onset of symptoms, averages 20 to 90 days[3] but may range from 4 days to 6 years or longer.[1,7,8] In the CNS, the virus replicates almost exclusively in the gray matter, with an ensuing encephalitis. The infection is disseminated through the body along the peripheral nerves and can infect other organs, including the salivary glands, the retinas, and the corneas.

MICROBIOLOGY

The virus that causes rabies is a member of the *Lyssavirus* genus. It is bullet-shaped, measuring 75 by 180 nm and containing a single-stranded RNA genome.

SYMPTOMS AND OBJECTIVE FINDINGS

Rabies infection can be divided into four stages: incubation, prodrome, the neurologic period, and coma.

The incubation stage, described in "Pathogenesis," above, lasts from the time of viral inoculation until the onset of any symptoms. Like the other stages, it is highly variable. During this period, the patient may remain asymptomatic. Most symptoms and signs usually are related to the bite and local wound healing, such as edema and erythema. If the incubation stage is prolonged, the initial injury site may heal. A correct diagnosis during this period is not likely because of the paucity of symptoms.

Progression to the next stage—the prodrome—is associated with a poor outcome. This stage lasts 2 to 10 days. Most patients report pain, pruritus, or paresthesias at the site of the wound or in the entire limb. Itching may be severe to the point of causing significant excoriation. This sensation may be attributed to the proliferation of the virus in the sensory nerves. Fasciculations also may occur at the site of the bite. Other nonspecific constitutional symptoms may include fever, chills, malaise, fatigue, sore throat, headache, nausea, vomiting, anorexia, and a nonproductive cough.

Beginning with the onset of symptoms of CNS involvement and lasting 2 to 10 days, the neurologic stage is marked by progressive deterioration of the patient's mental status. However, there may be periods of normality during this stage. The hallmark symptoms of rabies

TABLE 9-19-2. Nonspecific Findings during the Neurologic Stage of Rabies

Hyperactivity	Hyperreflexia
Hallucinations	Priapism
Muscle spasms	Anisocoria
Opisthotonia	Increased salivation
Lacrimation	Perspiration
Optic neuritis	Diplopia
Facial palsies	Fever to 40.6°C (105°F)

SOURCE: From Baevsky and Bartfield,[1] Doan-Wiggins,[5] Frenia et al.[7]

infection—aerophobia and hydrophobia—usually are seen during this period. Aerophobia, or the fear of moving air, may be elicited by blowing air across a patient's face. This causes spasms of the muscles in the neck and pharynx. A combination of hypersalivation and difficulty swallowing may cause foaming at the mouth. Attempts to drink liquids cause violent, jerky spasms of the diaphragm and in other muscles of inspiration and deglutition, causing hydrophobia. Other nonspecific signs and symptoms during the neurologic stage are listed in Table 9-19-2.

Death during this " furious" phase may result from cardiovascular or respiratory collapse. If the patient does not die or become comatose, a "paralytic" phase may occur. This phase presents similarly to the Guillain-Barré syndrome, with an ascending symmetric or asymmetric paralysis that usually is most pronounced in the bitten extremity. The paralytic phase most commonly is associated with bat bites.

The fourth stage is coma. Death from respiratory arrest, starvation, or dehydration normally occurs within 7 days. Intensive supportive care may prolong survival times, but rabies is almost uniformly fatal. According to the CDC, documented cases of survivors of human rabies in the United States have been limited to a total of four.

DIAGNOSTIC CONSIDERATIONS

During the incubation period, rabies may be misdiagnosed as cellulitis because of a lack of signs other than erythema and edema near the bite area. Presentation during the prodrome stage with nonspecific constitutional symptoms resembling an upper respiratory tract infection or gastroenteritis makes the correct diagnosis of rabies difficult.

More definitive signs and symptoms beginning in the neurologic stage should heighten the suspicion of rabies. The differential diagnosis (see Table 9-19-3) remains extensive.

"Rabies hysteria" also should be considered in symptomatic patients. This occurs in a patient who is knowledgeable about the signs and symptoms of rabies and has a history of an animal bite even though the animal was not rabid.

SPECIAL CONSIDERATIONS

People who are immunocompromised may not develop active immunity and may be predisposed to rabies. Immunosuppressive agents such as steroids should be given during the postexposure period only if they

TABLE 9-19-3. Differential Diagnosis of Rabies during the Neurologic Period

Guillain-Barré syndrome	Tetanus
Brain tumor or abscess	Botulism
Metabolic encephalopathy	Polio
Cerebrovascular accident	Schizophrenia
Drug intoxication or withdrawal	Conversion reaction

SOURCE: From Baevsky and Bartfield,[1] Frenia et al.[7]

are needed to treat other medical conditions. Before immunosuppressive agents are given, vaccination to rabies should have been started and the serum should be tested for antibody production.

A low rabies antibody response has been reported with the administration of human diploid cell vaccine and chloroquine.[7] People traveling to countries with endemic malaria and rabies who are receiving prophylaxis for both should be aware of this interaction.

LABORATORY FINDINGS

A number of limited diagnostic tests are available to confirm rabies. The most common test in the United States is the rapid fluorescent focus inhibition test (RFFIT).[7] In this test, the patient's antibody titer to rabies is compared to a known standard. The results from this test are available within 24 h and have a specificity "approaching 100% with a sensitivity of approximately 90 percent."[1]

Immunofluorescent antibody staining for the viral antigen is another method of diagnosis. Specimens used for this purpose include brain tissue, nerve tissue, neck skin, corneal impressions, serum, cerebrospinal fluid (CSF), and/or saliva. The specimen is exposed to a fluorochrome-labeled antibody or antigen and then examined for fluorescence. Additional tests, often the RFFIT, are recommended to confirm negative results. Antibodies to the rabies virus usually are present in the serum and CSF within 1 week after the development of symptoms.

Mouse inoculation of infected tissue is a technique used to culture the rabies virus and confirm the fluorescent antibody test. If the mouse manifests symptoms of rabies, it is sacrificed and the brain is examined by direct fluorescent antibody testing. It should be noted that in cases of prolonged survival of the patient, mouse inoculation studies along with direct fluorescent antibody staining may be negative.[5,7] This autosterilization phenomenon is "thought to result from a large increase in antirabies antibody."[7]

Sections of brain tissue can be stained with Seller's stain and then examined by microscopy for Negri bodies, which are round or oval inclusion bodies seen in the cytoplasm and the nerve processes. This is the method most commonly used to examine an animal suspected of having rabies.

Standard laboratory tests for the diagnosis of rabies are nonspecific. Blood chemistry studies normally are unaffected by the infection.[1] White blood cell counts may be normal or elevated. A lumbar puncture may show an elevated opening pressure. The CSF may reveal an elevated protein level with a variable leukocytosis. Toxicologic screening of urine or blood is not useful in the diagnosis but can help rule out drug intoxication or withdrawal as a cause of the symptoms.

RADIOLOGIC STUDIES

Although not useful in the diagnosis, computed tomography (CT) of the head may be useful in eliminating a brain tumor or abscess as a cause of the neurologic symptoms.

TREATMENT

As with any animal bite, the first step in proper treatment is to clean the wound and the surrounding area. The incidence of developing rabies may be reduced by up to 90 percent by prompt washing of the area with soap or iodine solution.[1] In the past, quaternary ammonium compounds were recommended for cleaning of the wound. They are now considered not superior to soap.[9]

Pharmacologic Treatment

AFTER EXPOSURE   If a potential rabies exposure has occurred, postexposure prophylaxis should be administered. This consists of two components: passive immunization with immunoglobulin and active immunization with a vaccine.

One dose of human rabies immune globulin (HRIG) is given at the beginning of postexposure immunization, day 0. A dose of 20 IU/kg is given, with half the dose infiltrated around the site of the exposure (if anatomically possible) and the remaining portion given intramuscularly. Only the recommended dose of HRIG should be given, as passive immunization may partially suppress the active production of antibodies.[3,7] If it is not given with the vaccine, HRIG may be given within 7 or 8 days of the first dose of the vaccine. After this time, an antibody response from the active immunization should have occurred. People who have been previously immunized should not receive HRIG.

Active immunization is obtained by administering 1.0 mL of human diploid cell vaccine (HDCV), Rabies Vaccine Absorbed (RVA), or Purified Chick Embryo Cell (PCEC) vaccine intramuscularly into the deltoid or, in children, the anterolateral aspect of the thigh.[4] The vaccine is given on days 0, 3, 7, 14, and 28.[1,6,7] The vaccine should not be mixed in the same syringe as the HRIG or administered at the same site, since neutralization may occur.[7] In cases where the patient has received a previous vaccination, the patient should receive 1.0 mL intramuscularly of the vaccine on days 0 and 3.[1,4,6]

Although there have been no treatment failures reported with the proper postexposure treatment with HRIG and HDCV or RVA in the United States, at least 18 people have contracted rabies outside the United States after receiving the vaccine.[3,6,10] These cases have been associated with improper wound care (inadequate cleaning, inappropriate timing of surgical closure), passive immunization not given or not given around the wound site, or reception of the vaccination in the gluteal region instead of the deltoid.

Treatment should begin as soon as possible after it has been determined that prophylaxis is necessary. Delays up to 5 days after exposure have not affected the success of treatment.[6]

The data involving treatment during pregnancy are limited. No fetal abnormalities have been associated with postexposure prophylaxis,[4,6,7] and pregnancy should not be considered a contraindication to treatment.

The patient's tetanus immunization status should be reviewed. If no booster has been received in the past 5 years or if the patient is unsure of his or her status, tetanus toxoid should be given.[1]

Many animal bites may require antimicrobial therapy (see Chap. 4-4).

BEFORE EXPOSURE For persons with a high risk of rabies exposure, such as veterinarians, animal handlers, laboratory workers, spelunkers, and travelers to areas where rabies is endemic, prophylactic vaccination is recommended.[1,2,4–6] This series should begin at least 30 days before exposure or travel. HDCV, PCEC, or RVA 1.0 mL, should be given intramuscularly in the deltoid on days 0, 7, and 21 or 28. Alternatively, HDCV 0.1 mL of the intradermal formulation may be given intradermally over the deltoid area on days 0, 7, and 21 or 28.[4] The intradermal formulation is only for preexposure vaccination. Booster vaccinations should be given to people who have a continued risk of exposure and a low antibody titer. Preexposure prophylaxis does not eliminate the need for postexposure treatment.

SUPPORTIVE MEASURES

When a case of rabies has progressed through the neurologic phase into the coma phase, intensive cardiovascular and respiratory support is required. As was noted earlier, starvation and dehydration are additional causes of death. All cases are most appropriately managed in an intensive care unit. In addition to supportive measures, some investigators have used antiviral drugs, interferon, and interferon inducers for the treatment of rabies.[11]

PATIENT EDUCATION

People, particularly children, should be warned to avoid contact with wild animals and unfamiliar domestic animals, especially animals that display bizarre, erratic behavior or hypersalivation. Wild animals should not be kept as pets. People with potential rabies exposure and bites of any kind should seek medical attention. People at high risk of exposure should receive prophylactic vaccination. Common sense is the key to prevention.

COMPLICATIONS AND RED FLAGS

Although it is recommended that prophylaxis be started as soon as rabies is suspected, regardless of the time elapsed after exposure, once the virus enters the peripheral nervous system, vaccination can no longer halt the infection.[1,6,7] The body starts to produce antibodies once clinical symptoms occur. There have been three reported cases of neurologic illnesses resembling Guillain-Barré syndrome associated with the vaccine.[4] These cases resolved without sequelae after 12 weeks.

Adverse reactions to rabies prophylaxis are treated in the same manner as are reactions to other vaccines. Local or mild systemic reactions can be treated with anti-inflammatory medications and antipyretics. These minor reactions should not cause discontinuation of treatment. Antihistamines and epinephrine should be readily available in case an anaphylactic reaction occurs. The use of steroids during any reaction should be weighed against the consequence of inhibition of an immune response.

In incidences of anaphylaxis or serious systemic reaction, consideration must be given to the risk of developing rabies before the vaccination series is discontinued. Consultation with a local health department, the CDC, or other qualified experts may help in making this decision.

OTHER NOTES AND PEARLS

Oral vaccines are being tested in an attempt to control rabies in wildlife.[1,6,7,12,13] In parts of Europe, an orally absorbed vaccine distributed by aircraft and by hand has been used to control rabies in foxes. In late 1990, a recombinant rabies vaccine that had been effective in raccoons in the laboratory was distributed on a Virginia coastal island. The results of this and other studies involving skunks have been called "encouraging."[1,6]

Several countries have vaccination schedules that involve fewer doses and fewer clinic visits. One of these schedules, recommended by the World Health Organization, has HDCV given bilaterally intramuscularly on day 0 (two doses) and then one dose given intramuscularly on day 7 and a final intramuscular dose given on day 21.[1,3] This dosing regimen has not been approved in the United States.

Also under investigation are interferon and interferon-inducing agents.[1,7] These agents may have antiviral and immunoregulatory activity, and the results of these studies have been promising.

REFERENCES

1. Baevsky RH, Bartfield JM: Human rabies: A review. *Am J Emerg Med* 11(3):279–286, 1993.
2. Opp D: Rabies in primary care: Evaluating and minimizing risk. *Clin Rev* 9(7):55–68. 1999.
3. Fishbein DB: Rabies. *Infect Dis Clin North Am* 5(1):53–54, 71, 1991.
4. Center for Disease Control: Human rabies prevention—United States, 1999. *MMWR* 48(RR1):1–21, 1999.
5. Doan-Wiggins L: Animal bites and rabies, in Rosen P, Barkin RM, Braen GR, et al (eds): *Emergency Medicine: Concepts and Clinical Practice*. St Louis, Mosby Year Book, 1992, pp 868–875.
6. Fishbein DB, Robinson LE: Rabies. *N Engl J Med* 329(22):1632–1638, 1993.
7. Frenia ML, Lafin SM, Barone JA: Therapy review: Features and treatment of rabies. *Clin Pharm* 11:37–47, 1992.
8. Smith JS, Fishbein DB, Rupprecht CE, Clark K: Unexplained rabies in three immigrants to the United States: A virologic investigation. *N Engl J Med* 324(4):205–211, 1991.
9. American Academy of Pediatrics: Rabies, in Peter G (ed): *2000 Red Book: Report of the Committee on Infectious Diseases*, 25th ed. Elk Grove Village, IL, American Academy of Pediatrics, 1997, pp 476–482.

10. Wilde H, Sirikawin S, Sabcharoen A, et al: Failure of postexposure treatment of rabies in children. *Clin Infect Dis* 22:228–232, 1992.
11. Dutta JK, Dutta TK: Treatment of clinical rabies in man: Drug therapy and other measures. *Clin Pharmacol Ther* 32(11):594–597, 1994.
12. Lawson KF, Chiu H, Crosgrey SJ, et al: Duration of immunity in foxes vaccinated orally with ERA vaccine in bait. *Can J Vet Res* 61(1):39–42, 1997.
13. Fearneyhough MG, Wilson PJ, Clark KA, et al: Results of an oral rabies vaccination program for coyotes. *J Am Vet Med Assoc* 212(4):498–502, 1998.

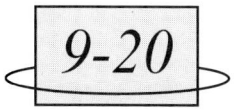

RESPIRATORY SYNCYTIAL VIRUS

Rosslynn S. Byous

DISCUSSION

Respiratory syncytial virus (RSV) is the only viral pathogen that regularly produces an outbreak of infection annually, especially in urban areas. RSV causes acute respiratory manifestations in patients of all ages. RSV is most commonly implicated as the cause of bronchiolitis and pneumonia in infants and young children. RSV is a large enveloped RNA virus that is a member of the Paramyxoviridae family. It has two major strains (A and B), which generally are concurrently present in the host.

Humans are the only infective source of RSV. Transmission is the result of direct or close contact with contaminated secretions. These secretions may be present on fomites or may be contained in droplets. School-age siblings typically infect infants. Viral shedding usually occurs for 3 to 8 days, but this period may be significantly longer in infants, lasting 3 to 4 weeks.

RSV is the most significant cause of lower respiratory tract illnesses in infancy and early childhood, accounting for more than 70 percent of the bronchiolitis cases that are seen and up to 40 percent of the pneumonia cases. Outbreaks typically occur in the fall and winter or the early spring. RSV affects children in the first year of life at a rate as high as 60 percent. Reinfection with RSV is common and manifests itself as a mild respiratory infection and tracheobronchitis in older children or adults. Serious pulmonary infections have been noted in the elderly and in immunocompromised adults.

PATHOPHYSIOLOGY

RSV infects the respiratory epithelial cells, causing the formation of syncytium in the small airways. These airways become obstructed because of an inflammatory response that causes edema and mucus production. As a result of this process, distal atelectasis and hyperexpansion of the lungs occur. These pathologic changes can be attributed to the viral destruction of the epithelium and the local immunologic response.

SYMPTOMS AND OBJECTIVE FINDINGS

The typical child who presents for evaluation will demonstrate the following symptoms: rhinorrhea, pharyngitis, cough, tachypnea, and a low-grade fever. In infants, the only clinical manifestations may be lethargy, poor feeding, and irritability with occasional apneic episodes. As the disease progresses, the child may exhibit wheezing and signs of respiratory distress that include intercostal retraction and tachypnea with or without expiratory wheezing. Tachypnea ranges between 55 and 100/min and may be accompanied by cyanosis and life-threatening respiratory arrest. The hyperinflation of the lungs may produce a "barrel" chest appearance and push the spleen and liver to a palpable position.

In adults, RSV usually presents as the "common cold" with malaise, nasal congestion, and cough for an average of 10 to 14 days. The elderly may present with anything from a simple "cold" to a fatal pneumonia.

TABLE 9-20-1. Differential Diagnosis

Asthma
Foreign body or other airway obstruction
Chlamydial pneumonitis
Cystic fibrosis
Pertussis
Pneumonia

LABORATORY TESTS

Arterial blood gases may reveal an increased level of hypoxemia, and as the infant's condition deteriorates, hypercapnia ensues. Chest roentgenograms may reveal hyperexpansion of the lungs along with a pneumonitis. A nasopharyngeal or pulmonary washing will assist in the confirmation of a diagnosis of RSV. The secretions should be evaluated by the use of rapid diagnostic procedures such as immunofluorescent and enzyme immunoassay techniques. The sensitivity of these assays is in the range of 80 to 90 percent. In addition, serologic testing of acute and convalescent sera may be used to confirm infections. However, the clinician should be aware that infection may not always be accompanied by seroconversion, especially in younger children.

DIFFERENTIAL DIAGNOSIS

In infants, wheezing that is accompanied by a fever and cough may be due to a myriad of sources, including chlamydia and assorted bacterial infections. The clinician also should consider genetic disorders as well as obstructive causes when formulating the list of differentials. Table 9-20-1 reviews the differential diagnoses for an infant or child who presents with a history of wheezing.

COMPLICATIONS

The most commonly seen complication associated with RSV is otitis media. The causative organism typically is a pneumococcus or *Haemophilus influenzae*. With the advent of the sudden exacerbation of fever and leukocytosis, the clinician should suspect that there is a concomitant bacterial infection. Patients with congenital heart disease, pulmonary hypertension, underlying pulmonary pathology, prematurity, or immunodeficiency are at an increased risk of having a severe or fatal RSV infection.

TREATMENT

To adequately manage a patient who has RSV, the clinician must consider the severity of the symptoms, the underlying pathology, and community issues. If there are any signs of respiratory distress, the patient should be hospitalized. The primary goal of managing RSV is the prevention of respiratory distress. Children with severe hypoxia who are incapable of feeding because of respiratory distress should be hospitalized. These patients should receive humidified oxygen and parenteral feeding.

Ribavirin (Virazole) has in vitro antiviral activity that works against RSV. However, because of the cost of the agent and the question of efficacy, ribavirin is used at the discretion of the clinician. Table 9-20-2 lists patient populations that might benefit from its use. The use of antibiotics, decongestants, expectorants, and steroids has not been found to be clinically significant in the treatment of mild cases of RSV.

Immunoprophylaxis against RSV with respiratory syncytial virus immune globulin intravenous (RSV-IGIV) has been approved for use in children less than 24 months of age with bronchopulmonary dysplasia (BPD) or a history of prematurity (<35 weeks' gestation). RSV-IGIV is given once per month just before and during an RSV outbreak. The dose is 15 mL/kg (750 mg/kg). The American Academy of Pediatrics recommends the following immunization guidelines: patients with BPD

TABLE 9-20-2. Ribavirin (Virazole) Treatment Populations

Congenital heart disease

Bronchopulmonary dysplasia

Cystic fibrosis

Previously healthy premature infants (<37 weeks' gestational age)

Immunosuppressed patients

Severely ill children with or without mechanical ventilation

Infant less than 6 weeks of age

Certain neurologic or metabolic illnesses

who are 2 years old or under and are currently receiving oxygen or have received oxygen within the last 6 months before an RSV outbreak and infants with a gestational age under 32 weeks. Premature children with BPD and possible cardiac disease should receive RSV-IGIV. However, children with cardiac disease alone should not receive RSV-IGIV.

To insure adequate prophylaxis, RSV-IGIV should be initiated before the onset of the RSV season (October through December) and terminated at the end (March through May). Children receiving RSV-IGIV should defer their measles-mumps-rubella (MMR) and varicella vaccines for 9 months after the last dose.

PATIENT EDUCATION

In community settings, patient education regarding the necessity of proper hand-washing techniques is paramount. Additionally, clinicians and staff should require all visitors and personnel to follow universal precautions by wearing appropriate gowns and gloves to prevent transmission.

PROGNOSIS

Patients who develop bronchiolitis as a result of RSV rarely have long-term problems; however, 30 to 40 percent of patients who have been hospitalized with this infection will develop postwheezing sequelae in later childhood.

ACKNOWLEDGMENT

The editor would like to acknowledge the significant contributions of Wayne J. van Deusen, the author of this chapter in the first edition of *Primary Care for Physician Assistants.*

BIBLIOGRAPHY

Behrman D, Kliegman R: *Nelson Essentials of Pediatrics,* 3d ed. Philadelphia, Saunders, 1998, p 404.

Hay W, Groothuis J, Hayward A, et al: *Current Pediatric Diagnosis and Treatment,* 13th ed. Stanford, CT, Appleton & Lange, 1997, p 964.

Peter G, Hall B, Haley NA, et al: *1997 Red Book: Report of the Committee on Infectious Diseases,* 24th ed. American Academy of Pediatrics. Elk Grove Village, IL, 1997.

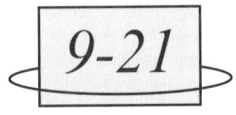

RUBELLA

Richard Dehn

DISCUSSION

Rubella, also known as German measles, is a viral illness that produces relatively mild symptoms. A discrete erythematous maculopapular rash that begins on the face and neck and rapidly spreads to the trunk and extremities characterizes rubella. The rash sometimes is preceded by a low-grade fever and generalized lymphadenopathy, most notably in the suboccipital, postauricular, and posterior cervical nodes. This illness often is called the three-day measles, since the rash usually clears up within 3 to 4 days. Frequently children have subclinical cases or present with only one or two symptoms. Adults are more likely to experience a 1- to 5-day prodrome characterized by low-grade fever, headache, malaise, mild coryza, and conjunctivitis. Up to 50 percent of cases present with a rash, but leukopenia is common. Arthritis, especially in the small joints of the hands, is not an uncommon complication in adults, especially females. Encephalitis is a rare complication.

When rubella occurs in the mother during the first trimester of pregnancy, the fetus has an 80 percent chance of being infected with congenital rubella. Congenital rubella is known to produce a wide range of birth defects, the most common being a triad of malformations affecting the eyes, heart, and nervous system.

Rubella is a relatively benign viral illness in the postnatal population. The ability of rubella to produce serious birth defects when it is contracted by the mother in the first trimester of pregnancy provides justification for an immunization program to control its spread in the general population. In 1969, a live attenuated rubella virus vaccine was released both as a single-virus vaccine and in combination with the measles and mumps vaccines (MMR vaccine), and in the United States recommendations were made for single-dose immunization of susceptible populations. This immunization campaign was directed primarily toward preschool and school-age children so that it would reduce the exposure to pregnant women; it was successful in significantly reducing the incidence of congenital rubella syndrome from 20,000 cases during the 1964 epidemic to 175 cases in 1992. Serology studies have shown that up to 10 percent of the U.S. population is not immune to rubella, and so current immunization strategies have concentrated on immunizing subgroups that are likely to have low immunity, such as teenagers and young adults. Some studies have shown that up to 20 percent of 20-year-old females are not immune to rubella.

PATHOGENESIS

Rubella is caused by a *Rubivirus* that resides only in human reservoirs. Direct contact or aerosol droplets originating from nasopharyngeal secretions transmit the postnatal form of rubella. After an incubation period of 14 to 21 days, symptoms may appear; however, in children, infections are often subclinical and inapparent. It is thought that the virus invades the respiratory tract first and then disseminates to other organ systems. In postnatal cases, the host will spread the virus beginning about a week before the appearance of symptoms and continuing for at least 4 days after the onset of the rash. The illness caused by postnatal rubella is generally benign but is of concern because of the possibility of passing congenital rubella to a first-trimester fetus.

Congenital rubella results from the passing of the virus from an infected mother to her fetus. When a nonimmune mother is infected, the virus replicates in her respiratory system and then disseminates to other organ systems, including the placenta. If the infection presents early in gestation, it will establish a chronic intrauterine infection that will produce endothelial damage to blood vessels, direct cytolysis of cells, and disruption of cellular mitosis. It has been shown that 80 percent of women with rubella infection and a rash during the first 12 gestational weeks have a fetus with congenital infection. At 13 to 14 weeks the incidence of congenital rubella drops to 54 percent, and by the second trimester it drops to 25 percent. The likelihood of congenital infection decreases even further as the pregnancy progresses. One study found birth defects in all infants infected before the eleventh gestational week, in only 35 percent of those infected at 13 to 16 gestational weeks, and in none of those infected after the sixteenth gestational week. These studies do not include several manifestations of congenital rubella that may not be apparent for several years or decades after birth, since the subjects were followed for only 2 years.

SIGNS AND SYMPTOMS

After a 14- to 21-day incubation period, up to 50 percent of children have no signs or symptoms or only a fleeting light rash. A prodromal phase often precedes the appearance of an erythematous maculopapular rash that begins on the face and neck and quickly moves to the trunk and extremities. The prodromal phase often includes low-grade fever, minor upper respiratory symptoms, myalgias, transient polyarthralgias and polyarthritis, and lymphadenopathy that most commonly occur in the suboccipital, postauricular, and posterior cervical nodes. The nodes are usually tender for only a few days but often remain palpable for up to a month. As the age of the host increases, the likelihood of a prodromal phase increases. Most young children do not experience a significant prodromal phase if they experience one at all, while most adults do. Arthralgias and arthritis are most common in adult women. Encephalitis is a rare complication and carries a 20 percent risk of mortality; however, those who recover seldom exhibit permanent damage. Testicular pain is a common complaint in men and may indicate orchitis.

COMPLICATIONS

The major complication of rubella is congenital rubella. Congenital rubella has been associated with a wide range of birth defects. Its effects on the fetus cover a wide range of outcomes from fetal death in utero, to multiple anomalies, to isolated hearing loss. Infants can appear normal at birth only to have anomalies appear later. The most common abnormalities seen in congenital rubella include intrauterine growth retardation, meningoencephalitis, cataracts, glaucoma, retinopathy, hearing loss, patent ductus arteriosus, pulmonary arterial hypoplasia, hepatosplenomegaly, and bone radiolucency. Less commonly seen are thrombocytopenia with purpura, dermal erythropoiesis resulting in bluish-red (blueberry muffin) skin lesions, adenopathy, chromosomal abnormalities, and interstitial pneumonia. Congenital rubella infants require close follow-up, since it is not unusual to later find hearing loss, mental retardation, behavioral disorders, learning disabilities, endocrinopathies, and growth retardation. Infants with congenital rubella commonly continue to shed the virus for several months and sometimes up to a year, placing susceptible individuals at risk. An extended rubella syndrome with progressive panencephalitis and type 1 diabetes may not develop clinically until the second or third decade of life.

DIFFERENTIAL DIAGNOSIS

Because of the nonspecific nature of the signs and symptoms of postnatal rubella, it is difficult to differentiate it from several other common illnesses. Several common viruses, such as echoviruses, parvoviruses, infectious mononucleosis virus, roseola virus, and even measles virus, can produce confusingly similar clinical pictures, as can some bacterial infections, such as streptococcal scarlet fever. It generally is accepted that the diagnosis of postnatal rubella cannot be made solely on the basis of clinical signs and symptoms and that only serologic evidence of infection is diagnostic.

LABORATORY TESTS

The diagnosis of rubella cannot be made reliably from the clinical signs and symptoms because of the nonspecific nature of the illness. The virus sometimes can be detected in throat, blood, and urine samples, but its isolation is time-consuming and expensive.

Most commonly, the diagnosis of rubella infection is made by demonstrating at least a fourfold rise in rubella antibody titers, comparing serum samples from the acute and convalescent stages of the illness. Some laboratories can detect rubella-specific immunoglobulin M (IgM) antibody, which is strongly suggestive of a recent infection. Leukopenia may be present early in the disease course. Other laboratory tests usually are not of much value in the management of postnatal rubella because of the mild nature of the illness.

TREATMENT

Treatment for rubella is supportive and usually is limited to symptomatic treatment for fevers, malaise, arthralgias, and arthritis. Prevention of rubella infections through immunization programs generally is considered the best treatment.

Since 1969, a live attenuated rubella virus vaccine has been available in the United States either as a single-virus vaccine or combined with measles and mumps vaccines (MMR). The current vaccine strain is grown in a human diploid cell line and confers immunity to about 98 percent of those immunized, with minimal side effects. It is thought that a single vaccination confers lifelong immunity to 90 percent of the recipients. Current recommendations call for the immunization of children after 12 months of age with the MMR vaccine and reimmunization at school entry or by 12 years of age. Individuals lacking a second immunization should be reimmunized or demonstrate serologic immunity to rubella. Postexposure immunization is not protective against rubella, but it is not contraindicated since the failure to contract rubella from the exposure will be followed by immunity from the vaccine. Contraindications to vaccination include pregnancy, recent administration of immune globulin (not including Rhogam), and patients with immunosuppression (not including those with HIV). The vaccine should not be given up to 3 months before conception; however, conception less than 3 months after vaccination does not justify terminating the pregnancy, since the maximum theoretical risk for congenital rubella from vaccination is 1.6 percent. Centers for Disease Control and Prevention (CDC) data show that among 226 rubella-susceptible women who accidentally received the rubella vaccine during the first trimester of pregnancy, none of the babies developed congenital defects, although 2 percent had asymptomatic infection. It also is recommended that individuals receiving blood products or Rhogam before vaccine administration have rubella antibodies checked 8 or more weeks after vaccination to assess whether immunity was conferred.

Immune globulin (IG) sometimes is given to pregnant women after rubella exposure, though its use is not advised unless termination of the pregnancy is not an option. Data on this therapy are limited, though a dose of 0.55 mL/kg may prevent or modify the infection in an exposed individual. The data on the effects of IG on the fetus after exposure therapy are even more unclear. Several documented cases have demonstrated the presence of congenital rubella in infants born to mothers treated with IG shortly after exposure.

The most effective treatment for rubella a clinician can provide is to assure that all eligible individuals in the practice are appropriately immunized.

BIBLIOGRAPHY

Arruda E, Hayden FG: Paramyxovirus (parainfluenza, mumps, measles, and respiratory syncytial virus), rubella virus, coronavirus, and adenovirus infections, in Stein JH (ed): *Stein Internal Medicine,* 5th ed. Philadelphia, Saunders, 1998, pp 1500–1502.

Beers MH, Berkow R (ed): *Merck Manual of Diagnosis and Therapy,* 17th ed. Whitehouse Station, NJ, Merck Research Laboratories, 1999, pp 2327–2329.

Boickenooghe A, Shandera WX: Infectious diseases: Viral and rickettsial, in Tierney LM Jr, McPhee SJ, Papadakis MA (eds): *Current Medical Diagnosis and Treatment,* 39th rev. ed. New York, McGraw-Hill, 2000, pp 1310–1312.

Brunell PA: Rubella (German measles), in Goldman L, Bennett JC (eds): *Cecil Textbook of Medicine,* 21st ed. Philadelphia, Saunders, 2000, pp 1805–1806.

Bryant KK, Bratcher DF: Rubella and congenital rubella syndrome, in Rakel RE (ed): *Conn's Current Therapy, 2000.* Philadelphia, Saunders, 2000, pp 130–132.

Cunningham FG, MacDonald PC, Gant NF, et al (eds): *William's Obstetrics,* 20th ed. Stamford, CT, Appleton & Lange, 1997, chap 58.

Georges P (ed): Rubella, in *1997 Red Book: Report of the Committee on Infectious Diseases,* 24th ed. Elk Grove Village, IL, American Academy of Pediatrics, 1997, pp 456–462.

Levin MJ: Infections: Viral and rickettsial, in Hay WW Jr, Hayward AR, Levin MJ, Sondheimer JM (eds): *Current Pediatric Diagnosis and Treatment,* 14th ed. Stamford, CT, Appleton & Lange, 1999, pp 990–992.

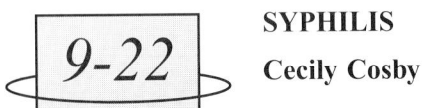

SYPHILIS
Cecily Cosby

DISCUSSION

Etiology

Syphilis is a systemic disease whose etiologic agent is *Treponema pallidum,* a spirochete. Humans are the only host for *T. pallidum.*

Epidemiology

The primary mode of transmission of syphilis is direct contact with infectious exudates from obvious or concealed lesions of the skin, mucous membranes, or body fluids and secretions (semen, saliva, blood, vaginal secretions). Syphilis also may be transmitted transplacentally from the mother to the fetus. Finally, intravenous needle sharing among drug users and blood transfusions can spread the infection. Risk factors known to increase the incidence of infection include multiple sexual partners, intravenous drug use, commercial sex work or sex with a commercial sex worker, young age, and incarceration. The risk of developing syphilis after unprotected sex with an infected partner with early syphilis is approximately 30 to 50 percent. A causal relationship has been established between syphilis and the exchange of sex for "crack" cocaine. The syphilis epidemic peaked in 1990, when 51,060 cases of primary and secondary syphilis and 55,132 cases of early latent syphilis were reported to the Centers for Disease Control and Prevention. Since 1990, the number of reported cases has declined by more than 50 percent. The southern portion of the United States has the highest rates of occurrence. Reported incidence rates are disproportionately higher in blacks and Hispanics.

SIGNS AND SYMPTOMS AND OBJECTIVE FINDINGS

Because of the broad clinical spectrum and diverse treatment regimens, syphilis has been divided into five stages: (1) primary syphilis, (2) secondary syphilis, (3) latent syphilis, (4) tertiary syphilis, and (5) congenital syphilis.

Primary Syphilis

In primary syphilis, the most common clinical manifestation is a painless lesion (chancre) that appears 2 to 6 weeks after exposure. Initially, this lesion appears as a painless papule, but it quickly erodes into an indurated ulcer. Chancres usually are single lesions. The ulcer is generally well marginated. Localized, painless lymphadenopathy usually develops. Because chancres appear at the site of inoculation, they commonly present in the genital area. Chancres also may appear on the tongue, buccal mucosa, and lips. Healing of the chancre is spontaneous.

Secondary Syphilis

Secondary syphilis typically appears 2 to 6 months after primary syphilis. Rarely, there is an overlap of symptoms. In secondary syphilis, the infection has progressed from a regional infection to a systemic one. The most common clinical manifestations of secondary syphilis are skin lesions. Syphilitic skin lesions may imitate a variety of dermatologic conditions (varicella, pityriasis rosea, tinea corporis, seborrheic dermatitis, acne vulgaris, tinea versicolor). These lesions may be transitory or may persist for months. Syphilis should be included in a differential diagnosis if any skin lesions present on the palms of the hands or the soles of the feet. Mucous membrane involvement is common with fused, hypertropic painless papules in intertriginous areas of the body. The lesions present primarily in the genital and rectal areas and are called condylomata lata. Skin and mucous membrane lesions tend to be highly contagious, with the lesion borders teeming with spirochetes. Another common clinical manifestation of secondary syphilis is a generalized alopecia. Common constitutional symptoms include sore throat, fever, chills, headache, weight loss, anorexia, and generalized lymphadenopathy. Uncommon clinical manifestations include arthritis, osteitis, meningitis, iritis, uveitis, and hepatitis. With or without treatment, all the clinical manifestations of secondary syphilis resolve spontaneously.

Latent Syphilis

In latent syphilis, the patient is asymptomatic but diagnostic testing is positive. Latency is divided into two phases. The early latent stage lasts up to 1 year; the late latent stage occurs after 1 year without symptoms. Theoretically, treatment for late latent syphilis requires therapy for a longer duration, because organisms are dividing more slowly; however, the validity of this division and timing is unproved. Latent syphilis often is found incidentally during a routine physical examination or prenatal visit. Unless the patient develops tertiary symptoms, the patient will remain in latent syphilis throughout his or her life.

Tertiary Syphilis

Tertiary syphilis is a chronic inflammatory disease that can affect any organ system. Studies have shown that in patients with tertiary syphilis, cardiovascular syphilis presented in 10 percent, symptomatic neurosyphilis presented in 10 percent, and gummatous syphilis presented in 15 percent. In cardiovascular syphilis, aortitis with aortic insufficiency is the most common complication. Syphilitic aneurysms also may occur. In tertiary neurosyphilis, up to 40 percent of patients may be asymptomatic. In symptomatic neurosyphilis, the clinical manifestations include stroke, seizures, paresis, and tabes dorsalis, which involves destruction of the posterior column of the spinal cord. Neurosyphilis has a broad range of psychiatric and neurologic manifestations (see Table 9-22-1). In gummatous syphilis, the development of gummas may occur on the skin, bone, and respiratory tract. Gummas are slowly enlarging benign granulomatous lesions that are thought to result from a delayed hypersensitivity reaction.

Congenital Syphilis

A dramatic rise in congenital syphilis occurred in the 1990s, particularly in inner cities. Syphilis in pregnancy causes infection in the fetus even if the mother is asymptomatic. Without treatment, 50 percent of the time the infant will die in utero or in the perinatal period. The most common clinical presentation of congenital syphilis is a child who appears healthy at birth but becomes ill weeks to months later. The symptoms include sneezing, rhinitis, and cutaneous lesions. Lymphadenopathy, hematologic abnormalities, and failure to thrive also may be present. Older children may present with interstitial keratitis,

TABLE 9-22-1. Manifestations of Neurosyphilis

Tabes dorsalis
  Ataxia
  Decreased vibratory sensation
  Decreased deep tendon reflexes
  Incontinence
  Cranial nerve palsies
  Argyll Robertson pupils
  Peripheral neuropathies

General paresis
  Tremors
  Personality changes
  Hyperactive reflexes
  Speech disorders

Stroke syndromes

Seizures

Hutchinson's teeth (sharp central incisors), or Clutton's joints (bilateral knee effusions). Making a diagnosis of congenital syphilis requires a high index of suspicion combined with accurate and appropriate testing. When an infant is born to a seropositive mother, the mother and child must be evaluated thoroughly and immediately. This is especially important if there is no record of treatment or if the birth mother was treated less than 1 month before delivery. No infant should leave the hospital without the serologic status of his or her mother having been documented at least once during pregnancy. Serologic testing should be performed at delivery in communities and populations at risk for congenital syphilis.

DIAGNOSTIC CONSIDERATIONS

Syphilis has been recognized as the "great masquerader." A plethora of illnesses mimic syphilis.

Primary Syphilis

Lymphogranuloma venereum, chancroid, herpes simplex, and labial, vaginal, and cervical cancer can mimic a syphilitic chancre. All genital lesions should be considered to be potential syphilis cases.

Secondary Syphilis

Mucocutaneous lesions may imitate a variety of dermatologic disorders. Syphilis should be considered in the diagnostic workup of most dermatologic lesions. Meningitis and hepatitis may be caused by other infectious agents. A patient with alopecia should be tested for syphilis before treatment. Condylomata lata may present as a verrucous lesion, imitating condylomata acuminata (venereal warts). The initial treatment of venereal warts should include a serologic test for syphilis.

Tertiary Syphilis

Tertiary syphilis may affect any organ system. It must be differentiated from a primary neoplasm of the bone, skin, brain, liver, or lungs. Meningitis may be caused by a variety of infectious agents. Syphilis must be included in the differential diagnosis of any patient who presents with a focal neurologic presentation.

SPECIAL CONSIDERATIONS
Management of Sexual Partners

The sexual partners of infected patients must be evaluated and treated. A patient should be instructed to refrain from intercourse until that patient and his or her partners are cured. Persons exposed to a patient

with syphilis in the prior 90 days should be treated regardless of the serologic findings.

HIV Infection

Serologic testing in HIV patients is considered highly accurate. With the exception of neurosyphilis, treatment regimens in HIV-infected patients are identical to those for other patients.

Pregnancy

Pregnant patients should receive the same treatment regimens. If a pregnant patient is allergic to penicillin, she should be hospitalized for desensitization and then treated with penicillin.

DIAGNOSTIC TESTING

Dark-field examination and direct fluorescent antibody testing remain the standard and only definitive methods of diagnosing early syphilis. Considerable skill is required in using this technique. Most hospitals are not equipped to provide these diagnostic tests.

Two types of antibodies are created in response to syphilis: a nontreponemal antibody and a treponemal antibody. Serologic testing has been developed around the two different antibody types. Nontreponemal tests are equally sensitive and are widely used for screening and diagnostic purposes. The two most common nontreponemal tests are the rapid plasma reagin (RPR) and the Venereal Disease Research Laboratories (VDRL). Nontreponemal titers usually correlate with disease activity and may be used as both quantitative and qualitative tests. While both tests are equally sensitive, titers between VDRL and RPR are not interchangeable. In the treatment of patients with primary syphilis, nontreponemal tests become seronegative within 1 year. With secondary syphilis, patients become seronegative within 2 or 3 years after treatment.

The most widely used treponemal test is the fluorescent treponemal antibody absorption (FTA-ABS) test. The two indications for ordering an FTA-ABS test are to confirm a diagnosis of syphilis based on the clinical presentation and to confirm a positive nontreponemal test result. The cost of this test discourages its use for screening purposes. A patient with a reactive treponemal test will have a positive test for his or her lifetime regardless of disease or treatment activity.

False-positive results are a consideration in performing nontreponemal tests for syphilis. The false-positive incidence rate for nontreponemal tests is 5 to 20 percent. Diseases that yield a false-positive result include infectious mononucleosis, herpes simplex, lupus, scleroderma, and various malignancies. False-negatives in nontreponemal tests are uncommon, and false-positive results in treponemal tests are rare. False-negative tests may occur in immunocompromised patients because of a reduced or absent antibody response. Patients tested in the incubating or early primary stages also may have a false-negative reaction, since nonspecific antibodies are not produced until 3 to 4 weeks after spirochete exposure.

No single test can be used for the diagnosis of neurosyphilis in all patients. The diagnosis can be based on various combinations of reactive serologic test results, abnormalities of the cerebrospinal fluid (CSF) cell count, or a reactive VDRL-CSF with or without clinical evidence of disease.

The diagnosis of congenital syphilis requires

- A thorough physical examination
- A quantitative nontreponemal test of the infant's sera, not cord blood
- CSF analysis
- Chest and extremity x-rays
- Complete blood count (CBC)
- Liver function tests
- A pathologic examination of the placenta and amniotic cord

TREATMENT

Since the time of its initial use, penicillin has been the drug of choice for treating all stages of syphilis. There have been reports of rare cases of penicillin resistance.

Pharmacologic Management

For incubating, primary, secondary, and early latent syphilis, benzathine penicillin G is given at 2.4 million units intramuscularly as a single dose. Nonpregnant penicillin-allergic patients who have primary, secondary, or latent syphilis should be treated with one of the following regimens: doxycycline 100 mg orally twice a day for 2 weeks or tetracycline 500 mg orally four times a day for 2 weeks.

For late latent, gummatous, and cardiovascular syphilis, benzathine penicillin G is given at 2.4 million units intramuscularly weekly for 3 weeks. Patients should have a CSF exam to rule out neurosyphilis.

For neurosyphilis, 3 million to 4 million units of aqueous penicillin G is given intravenously every 4 h for 10 to 14 days. Penicillin G is the only documented treatment for neurosyphilis, congenital syphilis, and syphilis in pregnancy. Penicillin-allergic pregnant patients, infants, and patients with neurosyphilis should be treated with penicillin after desensitization. HIV-infected patients should be treated with the same regimens. Penicillin G is the drug of choice for the treatment of syphilis in HIV patients. Desensitization should occur before treatment if the patient is allergic to penicillin.

For congenital syphilis, the patient should receive aqueous penicillin G 50,000 U/kg intravenously every 12 h (first 7 days of life) and then 50,000 U/kg every 8 h for 4 to 7 days or procaine penicillin G 50,000 U/kg intramuscularly daily for 10 to 14 days. Minimal clinical evidence exists regarding the efficacy of alternative treatment regimens.

Patient Education

Patients should be tested for HIV infection and advised to abstain from sexual activity until they and their partners are cured. Concurrent treatment of partners is essential even if they are asymptomatic. A history of a sexually transmitted disease (STD) places a patient at risk for subsequent STDs. When used consistently, condoms are effective in preventing STDs. Patient education in the proper use of condoms should occur during every patient visit for STDs.

DISPOSITION

Treatment failures with penicillin, though uncommon, may occur. Other than serologic retesting, definitive criteria for cure are not available. Patients with early syphilis (incubating, primary, secondary, and early latent) should undergo clinical reassessment and quantitative serologic testing 1, 3, 6, and 12 months after treatment. Patients with a prior history of syphilis will have their test titers decline more slowly than do those of other patients.

Patients with neurosyphilis should have follow-up serologic testing along with CSF examination every 6 months for a minimum of 3 years.

Patients with HIV infection should be assessed clinically and serologically 1, 2, 3, 6, 9, and 12 months after treatment.

Patients who do not have declining serologic titers or remain symptomatic should be assessed for HIV infection, treatment failure, and possible reinfection. All states require notification of syphilis to public health agencies. Physician assistants should be knowledgeable about the reporting procedures for communicable diseases in their states.

COMPLICATIONS AND RED FLAGS

A complication of syphilis treatment is an intense febrile reaction called a Jarisch-Herxheimer reaction; its etiology is unknown. This reaction occurs within 24 h after treatment, is self-limiting, and is common among early syphilis patients. Patients should be counseled about this reaction before the initiation of treatment. Pregnant women who develop a Jarisch-Herxheimer reaction are at increased risk for premature labor or fetal distress. The management of a Jarisch-Herxheimer reaction is limited to supportive care.

BIBLIOGRAPHY

Centers for Disease Control and Prevention: 1998 guidelines for treatment of sexually transmitted diseases. *MMWR* 47(RR-1):28–49 1998.
Hoffman I, Schmitz J: Genital ulcer disease: Management in the HIV era. *Postgrad Med* 98:67–80, 1995.
Isselbacher KJ, Braunwauld E, Wilson JD, et al (eds): *Harrison's Principles of Internal Medicine,* 14th ed. New York, McGraw-Hill, 1994, pp 1023–1033.
Preventive Services Task Force: *Guide to Clinical Preventive Services,* 2d ed. Alexandria, VA, International Medical Publishing, 1996.
Tierney LM Jr, McPhee SJ, Papadakis MA (eds): *Current Medical Diagnosis and Treatment,* 39th ed. New York, McGraw-Hill, 2000, pp 1376–1386.

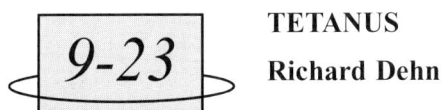

9-23 TETANUS
Richard Dehn

DISCUSSION

Tetanus, also known as lockjaw, is a neurologic disease that is caused by the exotoxin tetanospasmin elaborated by *Clostridium tetani,* a motile, gram-positive, anaerobic spore-forming bacillus. In most cases, the organism is introduced into the host through a contaminated wound, although suitability for infection is not necessarily related to the severity of the wound. The development of clinical tetanus is dependent on contamination of a wound by the organism, tissue characteristics in the area of the wound that are favorable for toxin production, and a susceptible host.

Clostridium tetani spores can be found in 20 to 65 percent of soil samples, with the highest population found in cultivated soil and the lowest in virgin soil. The organism commonly is found in human and animal wastes; thus, areas with poor hygienic practices have more organisms in the soil. As many as 10 percent of humans carry *C. tetani* in the colon. The organism also is found on inanimate objects such as nails and contaminated tools and in household dust. Another source of *C. tetani* is contaminated heroin. In undeveloped countries, the practice of applying contaminated soil or animal feces to an infant's umbilical stump and using contaminated instruments on the stump can cause neonatal tetanus in infants born to unvaccinated mothers.

The exotoxin tetanospasmin is one of the most potent known microbial toxins. The spores can remain viable in the soil for years and are difficult to eradicate. Eradication of the spore requires boiling for a minimum of 4 h or 12 min of autoclaving at 121°C (250°F). When the spores are subjected to an environment with a reduced oxidation-reduction potential, they revert to a vegetative form that produces tetanospasmin. The toxin is absorbed by the peripheral nerves and transported to the spinal neurons at a rate of about 250 mm/day. The toxin also can be carried to the nervous system by blood pathways. The toxin binds irreversibly to the ganglioside membranes of nerve synapses, blocking the release of inhibitory neurotransmitters in the motor neurons. Loss of the inhibitory function results in continuous motor firing, producing a generalized tonic spasticity that usually is superimposed on intermittent tonic convulsions.

Tetanus is not common in the developed world, where a large proportion of the population has been vaccinated. In the United States, 53 cases were reported in 1988, including 1 case of neonatal tetanus.

Almost all tetanus cases occur in unvaccinated or inadequately vaccinated individuals. Most cases occur in older adults, probably as a result of inadequate immunity in older populations. The overall fatality rate is 26 percent; however, 52 percent of patients with tetanus who are over 60 years old die. Although most cases in the United States occur as a result of wounds contaminated by soil, tetanus has occurred after surgery, injections, burns, skin ulcers, and tympanic membrane perforation. Drug addicts appear to be at risk, especially "skin poppers" (those who inject drugs subcutaneously). Heroin that is diluted with quinine lowers oxygen tension at the injection site, creating a favorable environment for the growth of *C. tetani*. Tetanus is common in the undeveloped world, especially in rural areas in warm climates where the soil is cultivated and conditions are unsanitary. It has been estimated that as many as 1 million infants die annually of neonatal tetanus.

PATHOGENESIS

The introduction of *C. tetani* spores into the host usually occurs through a contaminated wound; however, 20 percent of these patients present with no history of trauma or a wound. If the wound is deep, contains necrotic tissue, or contains a foreign body, an anaerobic environment can be established that is favorable for the conversion of the spores to the vegetative form, which produces the exotoxin tetanospasmin. Although the growth of the organism usually is limited to the local wound site, the exotoxin is spread through peripheral nerves and the bloodstream. Eventually the toxin can be disseminated to motor end plates, spinal cord internuncial neurons, and some cranial ganglia, causing a generalized tonic spasticity that usually is superimposed on intermittent tonic convulsions. Peripherally, tetanospasmin can produce neuromuscular blockades, similar to the toxin of botulism, and can have a direct contraction-producing effect on muscles. Clinical symptoms also suggest that tetanospasmin disrupts the sympathetic nervous system. Once the toxin becomes fixed at a binding site, it cannot be reversed; however, patients who survive tetanus have no residual damage. Active infection with *C. tetani* does not produce immunity. Sometimes the effects of the toxin remain local.

SIGNS AND SYMPTOMS

After an incubation period that averages 7 days after the introduction of *C. tetani* spores, neurologic symptoms begin. The most common symptom is jaw stiffness, which often leads to the patient initially presenting to a dentist. Restlessness, irritability, dysphagia, headaches, fevers, sore throat, tonic spasms, and stiffness of the neck, arms, or legs sometimes are seen. Later in the illness, the patient complains of difficulty opening the mouth (trismus); this is why tetanus commonly is called lockjaw. Progression of the muscle spasms involving the facial muscles leads to a characteristic expression with a fixed smile and raised eyebrows called risus sardonicus. Spasms may progress to other muscle groups, including sphincteral spasms, which can cause urinary retention and constipation as well as dysphagia, which can interfere with nutritional intake. The spasms can interfere with respiration, resulting in fatal asphyxia. The spasms often are precipitated by a minor stimulus such as a faint noise or a light touch.

The prognosis is related to the length of incubation and the speed with which the symptoms progress. Severe cases with a poor prognosis present after an incubation period of less than 7 days and have symptoms that evolve over 3 days or less. Moderately severe cases present after an incubation period of less than 10 days, with the symptoms progressing over 3 to 6 days, and mild cases present after 10 or more days, with the symptoms progressing over 4 to 7 days. Tetanus usually lasts 3 to 4 weeks regardless of the severity.

Neonatal tetanus presents in newborns within the first 10 days of life. An infant is susceptible if the mother was not vaccinated. The mortality rate of neonatal tetanus is higher than 70 percent.

DIFFERENTIAL DIAGNOSIS

A patient presenting with spasm or muscle weakness and a history of a wound suggests tetanus. Tetanus can mimic viral or bacterial meningitis or encephalitis, though in tetanus the cerebrospinal fluid (CSF) and the mental status examination are normal. Drugs in the phenothiazine class can produce muscle rigidity similar to that of tetanus. Peritonsillar or retropharyngeal abscesses and other local infections as well as subluxation of the mandible and strychnine poisoning can mimic trismus.

LABORATORY TESTS

Clostridium tetani occasionally can be cultured from the wound; however, the absence of a positive culture does not exclude the diagnosis of tetanus. Laboratory analysis of blood and CSF usually is unaltered by tetanus until the disease produces complicating cardiopulmonary, fluid, and electrolyte problems. The absence of abnormal laboratory and radiologic studies should suggest a diagnosis of tetanus.

TREATMENT

Human tetanus immune globulin (TIG) (Hyper-Tet) should be given as soon as possible at 3000 to 6000 U intramuscularly, avoiding injection in sites where previous tetanus toxoid vaccinations were administered. The purpose of TIG is to neutralize any free tetanospasmin; however, it is not known whether injection directly into the wound site is of any value. Equine tetanus antitoxin can be given if TIG is unavailable, but the patient should first be checked for hypersensitivity to horse serum. Animal serum is far less desirable than TIG because of more rapidly falling antitoxin levels and a considerable risk of serum sickness.

The wound should not be debrided until 3 to 4 h after the administration of immune globulin so that rising antitoxin levels will neutralize the tetanospasmin released during debridement. Thorough debridement is essential to stop the production of tetanospasmin. Metronidazole (Flagyl) is the drug of choice for eradication of the vegetative form of *C. tetani* after debridement. A loading dose of 15 mg/kg is given intravenously over 1 h, followed by 7.5 mg/kg intravenously given over 1 h every 6 h. Procaine penicillin, penicillin G, and cephalosporins are also effective against *C. tetani*.

Additional treatment is supportive while one waits for the slow elimination of the tetanospasmin. Unnecessary stimulation should be avoided. Intravenous fluids and mechanical ventilation may be necessary. Muscle spasms can be controlled with benzodiazepines, chlorpromazine, or short-acting barbiturates. Diazepam (Valium) is the drug of choice, and for mild cases adults can be given 5 to 10 mg orally every 2 to 4 h, though severe cases may require 10 to 20 mg every 3 h by intravenous push. Effective respiration may require the use of a curariform agent.

Tetanus is preventable by vaccination. Under 1 percent of the recently reported tetanus cases in the United States have occurred in adequately vaccinated individuals. A 0.5-mL dose of tetanus toxoid vaccine stimulates active immunity to tetanus, and after completion of the primary series of vaccinations, antitoxin persists for at least 10 years. Additionally, individuals who have completed the primary series of vaccinations can boost their antitoxin levels for another 10 years by receiving an additional tetanus toxoid vaccination.

As a tetanus prevention strategy, it is recommended that all individuals in the population receive tetanus vaccination, preferably the absorbed tetanus toxoid formulation. The vaccination is available as a single agent or in several combinations with vaccines for pertussis [diphtheria-tetanus-pertussis (DTP) or diphtheria–acellular tetanus–pertussis (DTaP)], diphtheria [diphtheria-tetanus (DT) or adult diphtheria-tetanus (Td)], and *Haemophilus influenzae* type b.

Children beginning the initial vaccination series before age 7 should receive a total of five vaccinations. Usually a DTaP is given at 2 months, 4 months, and 6 months of age, followed by a DTaP at 18 months and again before school entry at age 4 to 6 years. If the vaccination schedule is delayed, immunizations should continue with the first three doses given no less than 4 weeks apart, followed by a fourth dose at least 6 months later and a fifth dose at school entry unless the fourth dose was given after the fourth birthday.

Adults and children age 7 years or older beginning the initial vaccination series should receive a first and a second Td injection at least 4 weeks apart and a third Td at least 6 months after the second injection.

After the initial immunization series, a Td vaccination should be administered preventively every 10 years except in individuals who are likely to incur contaminated wounds, who should be vaccinated every 5 years.

Because infection with *C. tetani* does not confer immunity, unvaccinated individuals surviving a case of tetanus who received immune globulin should begin the appropriate vaccination series after recovery from the illness. The vaccinations should be given at a site away from where the immune globulin was given. Individuals surviving a case of tetanus who did not receive immune globulin should begin the vaccination series during convalescence.

Appropriate treatment for individuals sustaining a wound is dependent on whether an individual completed at least three doses of the vaccination series and whether the wound characteristics are favorable for the growth of *C. tetani*. Clean and minor wounds in individuals who have received at least three doses of vaccine do not need revaccination unless the most recent dose was received more than 10 years previously, in which case a Td should be given. Individuals who received fewer than three doses of vaccine and present with a clean and minor wound should begin or continue the immunization series at that time. Individuals who did not receive at least three doses of vaccine and who present with a wound that is not clean or minor should receive a Td if the most recent dose was received more than 5 years earlier. Individuals who did not receive at least three doses of vaccine and who present with a wound that is not clean or minor should receive 250 units of TIG intramuscularly or, after appropriate testing for sensitivity, equine tetanus antitoxin intramuscularly and begin or continue the immunization series at that time. The immunization series always should be administered at a site away from the site of the antitoxin injection. In HIV patients who present with a wound that is not clean or minor, TIG or equine tetanus antitoxin should be given regardless of the immunization history.

Immunizing the mother prenatally can prevent neonatal tetanus. Two doses of vaccine should be administered at least 4 weeks apart so that the second dose is received at least 2 weeks before delivery. Pregnancy is not a contraindication to the administration of a booster dose of tetanus toxoid.

Tetanus is most common in older adults, probably as a result of a lack of immunization compliance in that population. The immunization status of all individuals in the population, including elderly adults, should be assessed periodically and kept current.

The tetanus toxoid vaccination can produce local swelling, redness, and tenderness at the site of injection, especially if antitoxin is present. The administration of Td boosters at intervals shorter than 5 years can produce accentuated side effects. The side effects observed after the administration of combined vaccines often are due to the nontetanus components. Rarely, an individual is allergic to tetanus toxoid, and subsequent injections should be avoided in these individuals.

BIBLIOGRAPHY

Abrutyn E: Tetanus, in Fauci AS, Braunwald E, Isselbacher KJ, et al (eds): *Harrison's Principles of Internal Medicine,* 14th ed. New York, McGraw-Hill, 1998, pp 901–904.

Bartlett JG: Tetanus, in Goldman L, Bennett JC (eds): *Cecil Textbook of Medicine,* 21st ed. Philadelphia, Saunders, 2000, pp 1675–1676.

Beers MH, Berkow R (ed): *Merck Manual of Diagnosis and Therapy,* 17th ed. Whitehouse Station, NJ, Merck Research Laboratories, 1999, pp 1176–1179.

Chambers HF: Infectious diseases: Bacterial and chlamydial, in Tierney LM Jr, McPhee SJ, Papadakis MA (eds): *Current Medical Diagnosis and Treatment,* 39th rev. ed. New York, McGraw-Hill, 2000, pp 1342–1343.

Dressnandt J: Tetanus, in Rakel RE (ed): *Conn's Current Therapy,* 2000. Philadelphia, Saunders, 2000, pp 134–136.

Dworkin R, Leggett J: Gram-positive bacillary infections and clostridial infections, in Stein JH (ed): *Stein Internal Medicine,* 5th ed. Philadelphia, Saunders, 1998, pp 1572–1574.

Georges P (ed): Tetanus, in *1997 Red Book: Report of the Committee on Infectious Diseases,* 24th ed. Elk Grove Village, IL, American Academy of Pediatrics, 1997, pp 518–523.

Ogle JW: Infections: Bacterial and spirochetal, in Hay WW Jr, Hayward AR, Levin MJ, Sondheimer JM (eds): *Current Pediatric Diagnosis and Treatment,* 14th ed. Stamford, CT, Appleton & Lange, 1999, pp 1025–1026.

Zimmerman RK, Ball JA: Update on childhood immunizations for the year 2000. *Fam Pract Recer* 22(4):69–80.

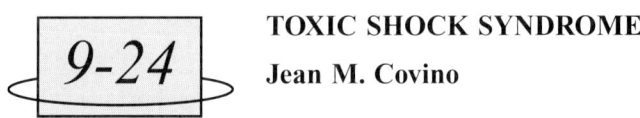

9-24   TOXIC SHOCK SYNDROME
Jean M. Covino

DISCUSSION

Toxic shock syndrome (TSS), a multisystem illness caused by toxin-producing *Staphylococcus aureus,* was first described in 1978. In 1980, TSS was recognized as occurring in epidemic proportions in menstruating women who used tampons.[1] Subsequent research led to the elucidation of the pathophysiology and concentrated efforts targeted at disease control. Those efforts were to some degree successful. From 1980 to 1981, TSS occurred in 6 to 6.2 per 100,000 women. Currently, the prevalence of this disease is 4 per 100,000 women.

PATHOGENESIS

A strong association was found between TSS and the recovery of *S. aureus* from cervical or vaginal cultures obtained from affected women, and a distinct marker toxin, TSST-1, was isolated in up to 90 percent of strains.[2] Staphylococcal enterotoxins B and C1 also may play a role. The pathogenesis involves the establishment of a toxin-producing strain in a nonimmune individual under conditions conducive to toxin production. Presumably, the clinical manifestations of the syndrome are produced when the toxin is absorbed through mucous membranes or from a subcutaneous tissue site of colonization or infection. More recently, group A streptococci infections causing streptococcal toxic shock syndrome have been identified.[3]

EPIDEMIOLOGY

Epidemiologic studies showed a strong association of TSS with the use of tampons. The absorbency of tampons is directly related to the risk for TSS.[4] Public education to limit the duration of use of tampons and the removal of hyperabsorbent tampons from the market have resulted in a decrease in the number of reported cases. Currently, nonmenstrual TSS occurs as frequently as does menstrual TSS. Nonmenstrual TSS has been associated with cutaneous and subcutaneous abscesses, osteomyelitis, postsurgical wound infections, postpartum infection, and gynecologic procedures such as the loop electrosurgical excision procedure (LEEP). TSS also has been reported with the use of diaphragms.

SYMPTOMS AND OBJECTIVE FINDINGS

The onset of menstrual TSS typically occurs on the third or fourth day of menses. In 1980, the Centers for Disease Control and Prevention (CDC) compiled diagnostic criteria:

- Temperature 38.9°C (102°F)
- Rash (diffuse, macular erythroderma that looks like sunburn)

- Hypotension
- Desquamation of palms and soles 1 to 2 weeks after the onset of illness

Streptococcal infection accompanied by hypotension, confusion, or unexplained acute renal insufficiency is a clue to streptococcal TSS. The CDC criteria also include the involvement of three or more of the following organ systems:

- Gastrointestinal (vomiting or diarrhea)
- Muscular (myalgia or elevated creatine phosphokinase twice the upper limit of normal)
- Mucous membranes (hyperemia of vagina, oropharynx, or conjunctivae)
- Renal (blood urea nitrogen or creatinine over twice the upper limit of normal)
- Hematologic (platelet count <100,000/μL)
- Hepatic (total bilirubin, serum glutamic-oxaloacetic transaminase, and serum glutamate pyruvate transaminase over twice the upper limit of normal)
- Neurologic (disorientation or alteration in consciousness without focal neurologic signs)
- Negative tests for Rocky Mountain spotted fever, leptospirosis, and measles
- Negative throat, blood, and cerebrospinal fluid cultures

DIAGNOSTIC CONSIDERATIONS

The differential diagnosis includes any systemic illness associated with fever, rash, hypotension, and multiple organ system involvement, most commonly Kawasaki disease (see Chap. 10-6), Rocky Mountain spotted fever, streptococcal scarlet fever, and bacteremia.

SPECIAL CONSIDERATIONS

Most individuals develop antibodies to TSST-1 by the late teens. Toxic shock occurs predominantly in the population that lacks that antibody because of genetic factors or lack of exposure. It appears that adolescents are at increased risk for TSS.

LABORATORY TESTS

A complete blood count with differential, electrolytes, urinalysis, and renal and hepatic function tests should be done. Gram staining of the vaginal pool, cultures of body cavities (vagina, cervix, oropharynx, anterior nares, and throat), blood, urine, and any lesions and wounds should be done when applicable.

RADIOLOGIC AND OTHER DIAGNOSTIC STUDIES

No radiologic or other diagnostic studies are necessary.

TREATMENT

Therapy is both supportive and specific, with attention to aggressive fluid, electrolyte, and blood product replacement. Tampons and any other foreign bodies should be removed. Identification of the site of infection, drainage, and antibiotic therapy with a β-lactamase-resistant anti-staphylococcal agent such as nafcillin or oxacillin (1 g intravenously every 4 h) should be given. If the patient is penicillin-allergic, vancomycin 500 mg every 6 h is indicated. Antibiotics do not change the course of the illness but may prevent relapses in tampon-associated cases.

Patients should be counseled to

1. Avoid tampon use for at least 8 months
2. Avoid superabsorbent tampons
3. Use tampons only intermittently and use sanitary pads at night
4. Remove the tampon and call a practitioner if vomiting, diarrhea, rash, or fever occurs

Treatment of streptococcal toxic shock syndrome consists of antibiotics and supportive care, with aggressive surgical debridement of soft tissue foci of infection when necessary.

COMPLICATIONS

All suspected patients must be hospitalized. The case fatality ratio of staphylococcal TSS is approximately 3 percent. Up to 30 percent of menstruating women with TSS may have milder recurrences with subsequent menses. The recurrence rate drops to 5 percent if the patient receives β-lactamase-resistant antibiotics early in the disease process. At present, even with aggressive therapy, the mortality rate for streptococcal TSS can exceed 50 percent.

OTHER NOTES AND PEARLS

TSS may be present in a milder version, and so a high index of suspicion must be maintained. More severe cases most likely will present to the emergency room. Although TSS is not currently a common illness, the risk of TSS can be further reduced by counseling all menstruating female patients to use tampons intermittently, alternating with sanitary pads, and to use the least absorbent tampon that is necessary.

REFERENCES

1. Shands KN, Schmid GP, Dan BB: Toxic-shock syndrome in menstruating women: Association with tampon use and *Staphylococcus aureus* and clinical features in 52 cases. *N Engl J Med* 303:1436–1442, 1980.
2. Bohach GA, Fast DJ, Nelson RD: Staphylococcal and streptococcal pyrogenic toxins involved in toxic shock syndrome and related illnesses. *Crit Rev Microbiol* 17:251–272, 1990.
3. Hauser AR: Another toxic shock syndrome: Streptococcal infection is even more dangerous than the staphylococcal form. *Postgrad Med* 104(6):31–34, 43–44 1998.
4. Berkley SF, Hightower AW, Broome CV, et al: The relationship of tampon characteristics to menstrual toxic syndrome. *JAMA* 258:917–920, 1987.

BIBLIOGRAPHY

DeCherney AH, Pernoll ML (eds): *Current Obstetric and Gynecology Diagnosis and Treatment,* 8th ed. Norwalk, CT, Appleton & Lange, 1994.
Ryan KJ, Berkowitz RS, Barbieri RL: *Kistner's Gynecology,* 6th ed. St. Louis, Mosby Year Book, 1995.

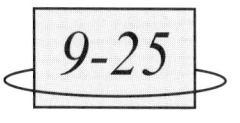

TOXOPLASMOSIS
Dana Gallagher

DISCUSSION

Toxoplasmosis is a disease caused by the protozoan parasite *Toxoplasma gondii.* Transmission of the parasite can occur either congenitally or in adulthood.

Congenital acquisition occurs when nonimmune women are infected during pregnancy. Although maternal infection is typically mild, it can be devastating to the fetus. The severity of fetal sequelae is inversely proportional to gestational age at the time of the mother's infection.[1] Up to 50 percent of newly infected pregnant women pass the infection to their fetuses[2]; the risk of infection in the United States is about 1 in 1000 live births.[1]

Adult acquisition is usually a clinical "nonevent" in an immunocompetent adult, as these infections are asymptomatic. However, new or recrudescent infection with *T. gondii* can be a serious problem in immunosuppressed individuals, especially those with AIDS. In a pregnant AIDS patient, toxoplasmosis infection may reactivate and rarely cause congenital infection.[3,4]

PATHOGENESIS

With the exception of vertical transmission from an infected woman to her fetus, *T. gondii* is not transmitted from person to person. Cats are the definitive host of the parasite; oocysts pass through the feline gut lumen and out into the feces.[5] In children and adults, transmission can result from contact with litter boxes, sandboxes, and playgrounds in which cats have defecated.

Because the intermediate hosts of viable cysts include cattle, goats, and poultry, infections also may occur after the eating of raw or undercooked meat or the drinking of contaminated milk. *Toxoplasma gondii* also can be transmitted by transfusion or organ transplantation.

SYMPTOMS

Acquiring toxoplasmosis congenitally can result in microcephalus or hydrocephalus at birth and a variety of conditions later in childhood, including chorioretinitis, thrombocytopenia, mental retardation, hepatosplenomegaly, jaundice, cerebral calcifications, and abnormal findings in cerebrospinal fluid (elevated protein, pleocytosis).[6] Congenital toxoplasmosis also causes stillbirth.

In pregnant women, toxoplasmosis may be asymptomatic or may present with flu-like symptoms of fever, malaise, and generalized lymphadenopathy.

The most common manifestation of toxoplasmosis in AIDS patients is encephalitis presenting with focal neurologic findings such as altered mental status, seizures, and/or hemiparesis with or without headache and fever. However, *T. gondii* should be an etiologic suspect in pneumonitis and any unexplained disorder of the ocular, integumentary, cardiac, gastrointestinal, and/or genitourinary systems of AIDS patients.[7] Infection with *T. gondii* is asymptomatic in immunocompetent adults.

LABORATORY TESTS

Infection with *T. gondii* causes antibody reactions that are identifiable in blood; approximately 55 percent of all Americans[8] have been infected. However, it has been estimated that 80 percent of American women are uninfected and susceptible.[1] Therefore, prevention of congenital transmission is a critical issue.

A toxoplasmosis titer (the T in the TORCH obstetric panel) should be drawn at the first prenatal visit. The presence of IgM antibody indicates current infection.[9] This result should prompt a referral for genetics counseling.

A toxoplasmosis titer also is drawn at the initial evaluation of an HIV-positive patient. The purpose of the titer is to document the presence of IgG or IgM antibody and, if the titer is positive, to consider toxoplasmosis in any future presentation of neurologic symptoms. Toxoplasmosis typically does not reactivate until the CD count is $100/\mu L$. The prophylaxis for *Pneumocystis carinii* pneumonia (Bactrim DS one tablet orally every day), which usually is instituted when CD4 counts are $200/\mu L$, prevents toxoplasmosis as well[10] (see Chap. 17-6).

RADIOLOGIC STUDIES

If diagnosed with toxoplasmosis in the primary care setting, AIDS patients and those infected congenitally should be referred for specialty care. They probably will undergo computed tomography (CT) brain scanning to ascertain the extent of infection and the response to treatment.

TREATMENT

Congenital Infection

PHARMACOLOGIC MANAGEMENT Because of the potential for drug toxicity to the fetus, a specialist should be consulted to institute treatment during pregnancy. An infectious disease specialist or another specialist should manage chemoprophylaxis and treatment in newborns and young children.

PATIENT EDUCATION To avoid infection, pregnant women should be advised not to clean cat litter boxes. They need not, however, avoid ordinary household contact with their pets.

An infected pregnant woman should be referred to a genetics counselor for a complete case-specific review of potential fetal effects and treatment options. Referrals for pregnancy termination should be made at the patient's request.

AIDS

PHARMACOLOGIC MANAGEMENT AIDS patients with toxoplasmosis usually are hospitalized acutely for a multidrug treatment regimen[11] and then receive suppressive therapy for the rest of their lives. An infectious diseases or AIDS specialist should handle the ongoing management of AIDS patients (see Chap. 9-1).

Patient Education

Patients with HIV should be advised not to clean cat litter boxes and, if it is necessary to do so, be gloved and masked. Patients should not be advised to give away their cats, because the companionship of pets improves the quality of life.

COMPLICATIONS AND RED FLAGS

Immunocompromised individuals with toxoplasmosis need immediate referral to a specialist for further diagnostics and treatment.

NOTES AND PEARLS

With regard to treatment, national collaborative U.S. studies are continuing to determine the best therapeutic regimens for the treatment of congenital toxoplasmosis and toxoplasmosis in AIDS patients.

REFERENCES

1. Stamos JK, Rowley AH: Timely diagnosis of congenital infections. *Pediatr Clin North Am* 41:1020, 1994.
2. Holliman RE: Congenital toxoplasmosis: Prevention, screening and treatment. *J Hosp Infect* 30(Suppl):180, 1995.
3. Benenson AS (ed): Toxoplasmosis, congenital toxoplasmosis, in *Control of Communicable Diseases Manual,* 16th ed. Washington, DC, American Public Health Association, 1995, p 468.
4. Biedermann K, Flepp M, Fierz W, et al: Pregnancy, immunosuppression and reactivation of latent toxoplasmosis. *J Perinat Med* 23:191–203, 1995.
5. Cano RJ, Colome JS: Diseases of the blood, lymph, muscle, and internal organs, in *Essentials of Microbiology.* St. Paul, MN, West, 1994, p 534.
6. Hensyl WR (ed): *Stedman's Medical Dictionary,* 25th ed. Baltimore, Williams & Wilkins, 1991, p 1614.
7. Israelski DM, Remington JS: AIDS-associated toxoplasmosis, in Sawde MA, Volberdine PA (eds), *The Medical Management of AIDS,* 3d ed. Philadelphia, Saunders, 1992, pp 320–321.
8. Goldsmith RS: Toxoplasmosis, in Tierney LM Jr, McPhee SJ, Papadakis MA (eds), *Current Medical Diagnosis and Treatment,* 38th ed. New York, McGraw-Hill, 2000, pp 1427–1429.
9. Jancin B: Toxoplasmosis testing urged before pregnancy. *Obstet Gynecol News,* April 1, 1996, p 12.
10. Amin NM: What's wrong with this picture? *Consultant,* June 1999, p. 1696.
11. Sanford JP, Sande MA, Gilbert DN: *The Sanford Guide to HIV/AIDS Therapy.* Vienna, VA, Antimicrobial Therapy, 1995, p 81.

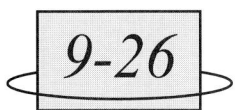

9-26

VARICELLA (CHICKENPOX)
William H. Fenn

DISCUSSION

Varicella (chickenpox) is one of the most common exanthems of childhood. Over 90 percent of cases occur before age 10, with only 5 percent occurring in persons over 15 years of age. In the United States, acquisition of this disorder is almost universal, with more than 3 million cases annually. It is a major cause of lost time from school (morbidity), but in healthy children it has a low mortality rate (2 to 3 deaths per 100,000 cases). The peak incidence occurs in late winter and spring.

PATHOPHYSIOLOGY

Varicella is caused by the varicella-zoster virus (VZV), a herpesvirus whose only known reservoir is humans. The disease is highly contagious (70 to 90 percent rate) via airborne droplets and direct transmission. Initial entry occurs in the nasopharynx, with a secondary viremia leading to the characteristic cutaneous eruption after an incubation period of 10 days to 2 weeks. Because colonization and initial replication in the nasopharynx occur before the rash, patients generally are contagious 1 to 4 days before the rash appears. Generally, the eruption lasts 4 to 5 days. As the lesions resolve, becoming noncontagious by crusting, VZV recedes to the secondary ganglia in a latent phase. One episode generally confers permanent immunity, although documented cases of second infections have occurred and subsequent reactivation of the virus is common (see Chap. 2-17).

SIGNS AND SYMPTOMS

Adult patients especially may complain of a mild prodrome of myalgias, fever, malaise, and headaches, but children frequently have no prodromal symptoms. The presentation is usually a pruritic vesicular rash that generally is accompanied by fever, malaise, anorexia, and a nonproductive cough. The rash generally starts on the face, with rapid spread to the trunk, where it predominates. The patient or parents may describe the rapid appearance of multiple "crops" of lesions over the course of a day.

OBJECTIVE FINDINGS

The characteristic varicella lesion is described as a "dewdrop on a rose petal" and occurs singly and in groups. The generalized exanthem starts as a rose-colored macule, evolving quickly into a papule, followed by the classic vesicles and pustules, which rapidly rupture and crust. At any given time, all lesion types occur simultaneously [see Figs. 9-26-1 (Plate 32) and 9-26-2 (Plate 33)]. This was a clinical observation in the past that was useful in distinguishing VZV from smallpox infections. The lesions are more numerous on the trunk but occur on all areas of the skin and may involve the mucous membranes as well. A low-grade fever is usually present. Lymphadenopathy also may be present.

DIAGNOSTIC CONSIDERATIONS

A diagnosis of varicella is usually not difficult to establish. Disseminated herpes simplex virus (HSV) infection or disseminated vaccinia should be considered in immunocompromised populations.

SPECIAL CONSIDERATIONS

The course of the disease is generally more disabling in adults. Immunocompromised patients also have a more serious course with a

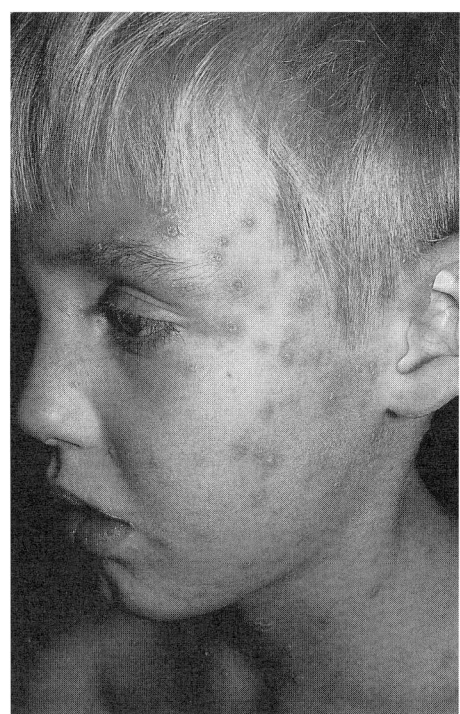

FIGURE 9-26-1. (Plate 32). Pediatric varicella with multiple vesicles and crusting. (*Photo courtesy of Rodney L. Moser. Used with permission.*)

high potential for complications and merit consideration for aggressive treatment.

LABORATORY TESTS

Although the diagnosis of varicella is usually obvious, Tzanck smears (see Chap. 2-16) occasionally may be useful. Viral cultures are possible, although the yield is low; therefore, they are of little clinical use. Immunofluorescence staining of vesicle smears allows for direct identification when needed. Serologic studies are useful only retrospectively.

RADIOLOGIC AND OTHER DIAGNOSTIC STUDIES

No radiologic or diagnostic studies are necessary.

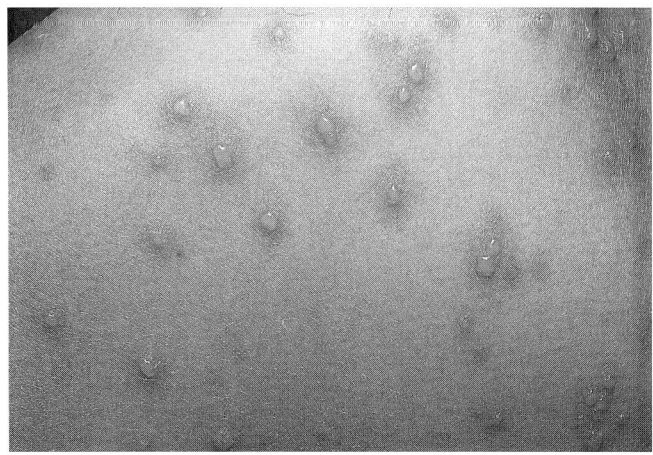

FIGURE 9-26-2. (Plate 33). Close-up of varicella vesicles showing the characteristic "dewdrop on a rose petal" appearance. (*Photo courtesy of Rodney L. Moser. Used with permission.*)

TREATMENT

Pharmacologic Management

Pharmacologic management remains somewhat controversial. Generally, systemic antihistamines are all that is necessary for relief of symptoms. Acyclovir (Zovirax), an antiviral agent, has been approved for the treatment of varicella, and reductions in lesion count and healing time have been documented when treatment is begun within the first 24 h of the disease. Acyclovir is clearly indicated in high-risk populations and adults, but whether its routine use in otherwise healthy children is indicated is a matter of considerable debate. Most authorities do not recommend the routine use of acyclovir. When acyclovir is used in varicella, a regimen of 80 mg/kg/day in four divided doses is used for children and 800 mg four times daily is used for adults. Treatment duration is 5 to 10 days. Antipyretics may be used; however, aspirin must be avoided because of its high degree of association with Reye's syndrome.

Supportive Measures

Measures to reduce scratching and thus reduce the well-known "pock" marking are helpful. Cool baths and compresses, oatmeal baths (Aveeno), and calamine lotion may be employed. Having children wear gloves or socks on their hands when they go to bed may reduce nocturnal scratching. Isolation of the patient while contagious generally is recommended, but as a result of the high rate of contagion and preclinical communicability, this is of limited practical effect. Most school districts require either a provider's statement of noncommunicability or the complete resolution of all lesions before readmitting a child to school after a varicella infection.

Patient Education

Patients and their parents should be educated about the expected course of the disease and the pros and cons of any specific treatment. One must ensure that the parents are well aware of the need to avoid aspirin. They should be advised that patients are no longer contagious when all lesions have crusted and no new lesions are appearing. The practitioner should inquire about nonimmune household contacts and advise the parents about the high degree of likelihood that those contacts subsequently will display symptoms.

Prevention

The introduction into the United States in 1995 of an approved VZV vaccine promises to reduce the morbidity rate of varicella greatly. Current recommendations of the Centers for Disease Control and Prevention's Advisory Committee on Immunization Practices call for children to receive a single vaccine dose between 12 and 18 months of age, along with teenagers who lack a reliable history or serologic markers of the disease. Additional newer recommendations include the routine vaccination of nonimmune teachers, day care workers, college students, prison inmates, military personnel, nonpregnant females of childbearing age, international travelers, and health care workers—in short, almost everyone. Special consideration must be given to HIV-positive individuals, in whom the vaccine may be contraindicated. Reduction in disease occurrence also can be obtained by vaccinating nonimmune individuals within 3 to 5 days of confirmed exposure. Differing rates of efficacy have been reported in different study models, but the long-term results of mass immunizations are not yet evident.

High-risk nonimmune patients who have been exposed to varicella should receive varicella-zoster immune globulin (VZIG).

Disposition

Follow-up evaluation is not necessary in uncomplicated cases.

COMPLICATIONS AND RED FLAGS

Secondary bacterial infection of skin lesions is common and can lead to scarring. Progressive cough and fever, particularly in adults and very young children, should raise the suspicion of varicella pneumonia. Meningeal signs may suggest varicella encephalitis.

OTHER NOTES AND PEARLS

Many providers accept a parent's phone diagnosis and direct treatment without examining the patient. It is important to recognize the pitfalls of this practice in an era of risk management. However, it would be irresponsible to simply ask that a potentially infected child be brought into a crowded waiting room. Strategies such as bringing suspect patients in through an alternative entrance at the end of a clinical day can obviate these concerns.

BIBLIOGRAPHY

Fitzpatrick TB, Eisen AZ, Wolff K, et al (eds): *Dermatology in General Medicine,* 4th ed. New York, McGraw-Hill, 1993, pp 2543–2567.
Holmes SJ: Review of recommendations of the Advisory Committee on Immunization Practices, Centers for Disease Control and Prevention, on varicella vaccine. *J Infect Dis* 174(Suppl 3):S342–S344, 1996.
Lookingbill DP, Marks JG: *Principles of Dermatology,* 2d ed. Philadelphia, Saunders, 1993, pp 167–168.

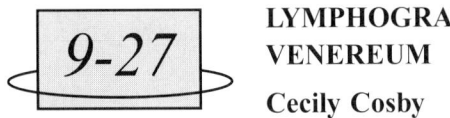

LYMPHOGRANULOMA VENEREUM

Cecily Cosby

DISCUSSION

Etiology

The etiologic agent of lymphogranuloma venereum (LGV) is *Chlamydia trachomatis,* invasive serotypes L1, L2, and L3.[1] LGV is a sexually acquired chlamydial infection. These chlamydial serotypes are different from those that cause urethritis and cervicitis.

Epidemiology

While LGV is endemic in tropical regions, it is uncommon in the United States. Reported cases number less than 500 per year.[2] Risk factors include sexual contact with partners from endemic regions; infection is acquired through contact with contaminated exudates from active lesions. The frequency of infection following exposure is believed to be lower than that for gonorrhea and syphilis, with a male:female ratio of cases in the United States of 3.4:1.[2] The incubation period is 1 to 4 weeks after exposure.[1] Occult infections are common.

SIGNS, SYMPTOMS, AND OBJECTIVE FINDINGS

Lymphogranuloma venereum can be divided into three clinical stages.[1] Stage I presents as a painless papule that ulcerates, as urethritis, or as multiple lesions (usually pustules) that quickly ulcerate. These lesions resolve without treatment. Frequently, they go unnoticed by the patient.

In stage II, after the lesions disappear, the infection migrates to the pelvic and rectal lymphatic chains. The most common clinical presentation of LGV is tender, unilateral inguinal lymphadenopathy. The lymphadenopathy may progress to bubo formation, an accumulation of tender lymph nodes that may undergo suppuration. Buboes may become fluctuant and rupture. Sinus formation commonly results from spontaneous rupture. Anorectal presentations include proctitis and

TABLE 9-27-1. Differential Diagnosis of Genital Ulcers (in Order of Relative Frequency in the United States)

Herpes simplex virus
Treponema pallidum (syphilis)
Haemophilus ducreyi (chancroid)
Granuloma inguinale
Lymphogranuloma venereum

rectovaginal and perianal fistula formation. In women, inguinal nodes are less commonly affected and involvement is mainly of the pelvic nodes with extension into the rectum. Disseminated disease occurs infrequently, resulting in fever, nausea, arthritis, and meningismus.

In stage III, regional lymphadenopathy resolves in 2 to 3 months with or without treatment. Scrotal and penile elephantiasis has been reported sporadically in endemic areas.

The most frequent clinical manifestation of LGV among heterosexual men is tender inguinal and/or femoral lymphadenopathy that is usually unilateral. Women and homosexually active men might have proctocolitis or inflammatory involvement of perirectal or perianal lymphatic tissues that can result in fistulas and strictures.[3]

DIAGNOSTIC CONSIDERATIONS

Ideally, the sexually transmitted disease (STD) workup of a patient with genital ulcers includes serologic testing for syphilis, culture for *Haemophilus ducreyi* (chancroid), and viral culture for herpes simplex virus (HSV). In the United States, the most common causes of genital ulcers are HSV, primary syphilis, and chancroid.[3] The relative frequency of each differs by geographic area and patient population.[3] Studies have shown that coinfection with multiple diseases is present in 3 to 10% of patients with genital ulcers. A differential listing is given in Table 9-27-1.

SPECIAL CONSIDERATIONS

HIV Infection

Treatment of LGV infection in HIV-infected patients is identical to the treatment regimens listed under "Treatment," below. Anecdotal evidence suggests it may require prolonged therapy and that resolution might be delayed.[3]

Pregnancy

The treatment regimen for pregnant patients is the erythromycin regimen listed under "Treatment," below.

DIAGNOSTIC TESTS

The diagnosis is made by culture of the bubo aspirate or a serologic complement fixation test. These tests are expensive and not commonly available. A complement fixation test result higher than 1:32 is indicative of active disease. Occasionally, the diagnosis is made by excluding syphilis, chancroid, or HSV.

TREATMENT

Pharmacologic Management

The recommended regimen is doxycycline 100 mg orally two times per day for 21 days. An alternative regimen is erythromycin base 500 mg orally four times per day for 21 days.[3]

The activity of azithromycin suggests that it may be effective in multiple doses over 2 to 3 weeks, but clinical data are lacking.[3]

Surgical Management

Aspiration of fluctuant lymph nodes or buboes through intact tissue may prevent spontaneous rupture and subsequent fistula formation.

Patient Education

Genital lesions significantly increase the risk of acquiring HIV infection. HIV testing should be considered and offered to patients with genital ulcers. These patients must be advised to refrain from sexual activity until they and their partners are cured. Any sexual partner in the past 30 days should be examined and treated.

When used consistently, condoms are effective in the prevention of STDs. Patient education in the proper use of condoms should occur during every STD patient visit.

Disposition

A follow-up test to cure is not required. The disease course may be long and potentially disfiguring. The therapeutic response is monitored by resolution of the symptoms. Longer-term pharmacologic treatment than the regimen listed above may be indicated.

COMPLICATIONS AND RED FLAGS

Few states require partner contact tracing and notification for LGV infections. Physician assistants should be knowledgeable about the reporting procedures for communicable diseases in their states.

ACKNOWLEDGMENT

The editor would like to acknowledge the significant contributions of Meredith Hansen, author of this chapter in the first edition of *Primary Care for Physician Assistants.*

REFERENCES

1. Robinson K: Sexually transmitted infections, in *Pathophysiology: The Biologic Basis for Disease in Adults and Children,* 3rd ed, K McCance, S Huether (eds). St. Louis, MO, Mosby, 1998, pp 829–830.
2. Stamm WE: Chlamydial infections, in *Harrison's Principles of Internal Medicine,* 14th ed, AS Fauci et al (eds). New York, McGraw-Hill, 1998 p 1058.
3. Centers for Disease Control and Prevention: 1998 guidelines for treatment of sexually transmitted diseases. *MMWR* 47(RR-1):27–28, 1998.

BIBLIOGRAPHY

Centers for Disease Control and Prevention: 1993 sexually transmitted diseases treatment guidelines. *MMWR* 42(RR-14):3–7, 47–56, 1993.
Goens JL et al: Mucocutaneous manifestations of chancroid, lymphogranuloma venereum and granuloma inguinale. *Am Fam Physician* 49:415–423, 1994
Preventive Services Task Force: *Guide to Clinical Preventive Services,* 2d ed. Alexandria, VA, International Medical Publishing, 1996.
Tierney L et al: *Current Medical Diagnosis and Treatment,* 39th ed. New York Lange/McGraw-Hill, 2000, p 1373.

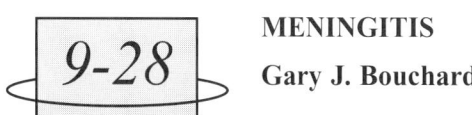

MENINGITIS
Gary J. Bouchard

DISCUSSION

Meningitis is a central nervous system inflammation of the arachnoid and the pia mater that usually is caused by an infection of the cerebrospinal fluid, which flows between them. The inflammation also may extend to the ventricles. Infectious etiologies are the most common.

While bacterial and viral infections are encountered commonly, fungal and parasitic infections also may be seen. Noninfectious causes such as neoplasm, drugs, and systemic diseases also may lead to meningeal inflammation.

Meningitis traditionally has been classified as either bacterial meningitis or aseptic meningitis, with the latter referring to cases in which an infectious etiology is not immediately apparent by standard testing of the cerebrospinal fluid. This nomenclature is somewhat misleading, since describing a case of meningitis as aseptic gives the false impression of a noninfectious etiology. In fact, a viral infection is the leading cause of "aseptic" meningitis. Despite the possible confusion resulting from this nomenclature, it is still clinically useful to distinguish bacterial from nonbacterial etiologies. The distinction is not merely a semantic one; bacterial and "aseptic" meningitis vary with regard to both treatment and prognosis.

Bacterial Etiologies

Haemophilus influenzae type b (Hib) had long been the most common cause of meningitis in children under age 5. However, Hib infections in general and *Haemophilus* meningitis in particular have been declining since the Hib vaccine was introduced in the United States in 1988. Since that time, *Streptococcus pneumoniae* has supplanted Hib as the most common etiologic agent of meningitis in children under age 5. *Neisseria meningitidis* also appears with greater frequency than does Hib in recent studies of pediatric populations.

In adults with community-acquired meningitis, the most frequently encountered bacterial etiologies are *S. pneumoniae, N. meningitidis,* and *Listeria monocytogenes.* The epidemiologic picture will differ in a tertiary care setting. Hospital-acquired bacterial meningitis accounts for a growing percentage of total cases of adult meningitis. Nosocomial meningitis often is attributed to recent neurosurgery or immunocompromise. The most frequently seen etiologies in such cases are gram-negative bacilli such as *Escherichia coli* and *Klebsiella, Staphylococcus aureus,* and coagulase-negative staphylococci.

Nonbacterial Infectious Etiologies

Approximately 10,000 cases of "aseptic" meningitis are reported annually in the United States. Approximately 80 percent of "aseptic" cases attributable to an identified pathogen are caused by enteroviruses such as echovirus and coxsackievirus. Less often, herpesvirus, mumps virus, arbovirus, and HIV are implicated. Of the remaining causes of aseptic meningitis, the most important diagnostic consideration is an extrameningeal infectious focus of bacterial infection or incompletely treated bacterial meningitis. In these cases, patients with negative cerebrospinal fluid (CSF) cultures still require antibiotic therapy.

Noninfectious Causes

Noninfectious causes include meningeal tumors, vasculitis, systemic lupus erythematosus, sarcoidosis, and chemical irritation by drugs such as trimethoprim-sulfamethoxazole and nonsteroidal anti-inflammatory drugs.

SYMPTOMS AND OBJECTIVE FINDINGS

Most patients with meningitis can identify a localized predisposing infectious process that preceded the neurologic symptoms. These processes can include upper respiratory infections, mastoiditis, sinusitis, pneumonia, and a nonspecific febrile illness. The development of symptoms over time may help differentiate among infectious etiologies. Viral meningitis is variable in its course. Patients may become symptomatic within several hours, or symptoms may develop over several days. Bacterial meningitis is most often abrupt in onset, with symptoms developing within hours up to 1 day. Fungal and tuberculous meningitis may take as long as 2 weeks to develop symptoms.

Clinical findings of meningitis include fever, generalized convulsions, severe headache, vomiting, and neck stiffness. Muscle aches, backache, and generalized weakness also may be seen. The physical examination may reveal tachycardia, hypotension, and positive Kernig's and Brudzinski's signs. There also may be meningismus, or resistance to passive forward flexion of the neck. A generalized petechial rash may be seen, and when it is present, a diagnosis of *N. meningitidis* infection is favored. A complete examination of the head and neck may reveal a causative infectious focus. The examiner should assess the patient for papilledema, which indicates increased intracranial pressure that can complicate a lumbar puncture. A complete neurologic exam also should be performed, and the patient's status should be monitored with periodic neurologic checks. As the disease progresses, focal neurologic signs may develop. The level of consciousness may deteriorate from confusion to obtundation or coma.

DIAGNOSTIC CONSIDERATIONS

Parameningeal infections of the central nervous system such as brain abscess, epidural abscess, subdural empyema, and encephalitis are major considerations in the differential diagnosis. Focal neurologic findings should alert the practitioner to the possibility of a space-occupying infection. Other considerations in the differential diagnosis of meningitis include malaria, tuberculosis and fungal infections, subarachnoid hemorrhage, neoplasms, and toxic shock syndrome.

SPECIAL CONSIDERATIONS

Infants may lack the classic clinical findings of meningeal irritation. A high index of suspicion should be maintained in evaluating vague signs such as poor feeding, irritability, and lethargy in these populations. Early evaluation of the CSF should be performed even in the absence of meningeal signs. The elderly may also lack the classic clinical findings of meningeal irritation. Lethargy may be the only presenting condition in this population. A full septic workup including evaluation of the CSF should be performed.

LABORATORY STUDIES

In bacterial meningitis, the most valuable diagnostic test is CSF analysis. The CSF will show moderately increased opening pressure, large numbers of bacteria on Gram stain, neutrophilia and a leukocyte count greater than $1000/\text{mm}^3$, elevated protein levels above 150 mg/dL, and glucose levels decreased to below 40 mg/dL. Cultures of the CSF are positive in 80 percent of cases. In patients with viral meningitis, there is a predominance of lymphocytes in the CSF, with protein mildly elevated and normal glucose. Blood tests provide little conclusive information about the meningitis. Positive findings may include an elevated white blood cell count and an elevated erythrocyte sedimentation rate. Blood cultures may be positive. Serum blood urea nitrogen, creatinine, and electrolytes should be documented to assess secondary abnormalities such as syndrome of inappropriate antidiuretic hormone (SIADH) and to monitor for adverse effects of pharmacologic therapy.

RADIOLOGIC STUDIES

A chest x-ray helps demonstrate pneumonia or an abscess as a source of infection. Similarly, sinus and skull films were used in the past to demonstrate infectious foci. Computed tomography and magnetic resonance imaging now provide better visualization of structures and masses in the central nervous system.

COMPLICATIONS

If SIADH secretion occurs, fluid limitation may be necessary. Shock and coagulopathies (from mild thrombocytopenia to disseminated intravascular coagulation) are usually a result of bacteremia, not a consequence of the meningitis per se. Adrenocortical hemorrhages (Waterhouse-Friderichsen syndrome) may occur in meningococcemia with or without meningitis. The incidence of septic complications such as endocarditis and septic arthritis has been reduced greatly by early recognition and treatment of meningitis.

TREATMENT

Appropriate, timely antibiotic therapy is the standard of care for bacterial meningitis. It is important to begin empirical antibiotic therapy as soon as possible. Therapy should be adjusted as a definitive diagnosis is made and as drug sensitivities are established. In neonates, combination therapy with ampicillin plus cefotaxime is recommended. In children and adults, monotherapy with a third-generation cephalosporin such as cefotaxime or ceftriaxone provides good coverage against the most likely organisms. Ampicillin is added to the regimen if *Listeria* coverage is warranted. Chloramphenicol is a good alternative for penicillin- and cephalosporin-allergic patients. Trimethoprim-sulfamethoxazole provides *Listeria* coverage in penicillin-allergic patients.

There has been a growing incidence of meningitis caused by penicillin-resistant strains. Information from the Centers for Disease Control and Prevention (CDC) and local health agencies is helpful in determining the likelihood of resistance in a specific patient population. Vancomycin or rifampin is added to the regimen if penicillin resistance is likely. Antibiotics should be administered in full doses parenterally for 10 to 14 days of treatment.

Most viral etiologies cause meningitis that is relatively benign and self-limited. Symptomatic treatment is needed. Rest, fluids, analgesics, and antipyretics will enhance patient comfort as the infection resolves. Care should be taken to ensure no other urgent condition is causing the "aseptic" meningitis, such as neoplasia, HIV, tuberculosis, cryptococcus, syphilis, or a bacterial meningitis that has been initially misdiagnosed or inadequately treated. Repeat lumbar punctures may be required.

Many of the neurologic sequelae of meningitis are due to uncontrolled cerebral edema during the acute illness. Mannitol or dexamethasone may be used to manage the increased intracranial pressure caused by brain swelling. Routine use of intravenous dexamethasone without clinical evidence of edema has been shown to be useful in reducing neurologic sequelae in children with bacterial meningitis. It is especially useful in preventing sensorineural hearing loss. Similar benefits of routine dexamethasone use have not been established in adults.

PATIENT EDUCATION

Prophylactic treatment of household contacts may be indicated. A daily dose of rifampin given for 4 days is used. Observation of contacts should continue for a full week. No prophylaxis is indicated if more than 2 weeks has passed since the discovery of the initial case.

Infant immunization against *H. influenzae* has greatly reduced the incidence of bacterial meningitis, and parents should be encouraged to immunize their children according to pediatric immunization guidelines. The immunization of adult populations at high risk for meningococcal and pneumococcal infections also is warranted.

ACKNOWLEDGMENT

The editor would like to acknowledge the significant contributions of Michaela O'Brien-Norton, the author of this chapter in the first edition of *Primary Care for Physician Assistants.*

BIBLIOGRAPHY

Adams RD, Victor M, Ropper AH: Acute bacterial meningitis, in Adams RD, Victor M, Ropper AH (eds): *Principles of Neurology,* 6th ed. New York, McGraw-Hill, 1997, pp. 696–749.

Davis LE: Central nervous system infections, in Weiner WJ, Goetz CG (eds.): *Neurology for the Non-Neurologist,* 4th ed. Philadelphia, Lippincott Williams & Wilkins, 1999, pp. 397–406.

Phillips EJ, Simor AE: Bacterial meningitis in children and adults: Changes in community-acquired disease may affect patient care. *Postgrad Med* 103(3):102–117, 1998.

Swartz MN: Bacterial meningitis, in Goldman L, Bennett JC (eds.): *Cecil Textbook of Medicine,* 21st ed. Philadelphia, Saunders, 2000, pp. 1645–1654.

Townsend GC, Scheld WM: Infections of the central nervous system. *Adv Intern Med* 43:403–437, 1998.

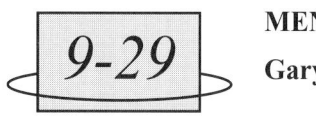

MENINGOCOCCEMIA
Gary J. Bouchard

DISCUSSION

Meningococcal septicemia is characterized by rapidly progressive systemic illness that may take a patient from appearing well to being in a critical condition within hours. The incidence of meningococcal infection is 1 to 2 cases per year per 100,000 population in the United States.

Neisseria meningitides is an aerobic gram-negative diplococcus that primarily colonizes the nasopharynx after droplet transmission. Once the nasopharynx has been colonized, the organism may cause pharyngitis, but more often it remains in an asymptomatic carrier state. In certain colonized patients, for reasons that are not understood, the organism invades the bloodstream within hours or days of colonization. The resulting meningococcemia can be mild and transient or fulminant in its clinical course. The factors that determine the course of the disease are poorly understood, but host factors such as immune globulin and complement deficiencies have been implicated in fulminant meningococcemia.

SYMPTOMS AND OBJECTIVE FINDINGS

The upper respiratory infection caused by *N. meningitides* presents with cough, headache, sore throat, and malaise. As the organism enters the bloodstream, symptoms and signs vary along a continuum of severity. The most benign form is a mild transient bacteremia that causes a febrile illness and few (if any) petechial skin lesions.

A more severe acute meningococcemia may occur, most typically after several days of upper respiratory symptoms. This phase is marked by the abrupt appearance of high fever, shaking chills, and worsening malaise. Generalized weakness, myalgias, arthralgias, nausea, vomiting, difficulty concentrating, and headache may be seen with an abrupt onset. Petechial skin lesions appearing in crops are characteristic of meningococcemia. The lesions usually are located on the ankles, wrists, and axillae. The palms, soles, and head usually are spared.

In advanced disease, the rash may be seen over the entire body. In rare cases, tachycardia and hypotension progress to vascular collapse. Meningeal signs may or may not be present; meningococcemia occurs with or without meningococcal meningitis. Seizures often accompany changes in mental status, which may deteriorate from confusion and delirium to coma

DIAGNOSTIC CONSIDERATIONS

Bacteremia of a different etiology should be considered, including *Streptococcus pneumoniae, Haemophilus influenzae,* and *N. gonorrhoeae.*

A questionable etiology should not delay treatment with broad-spectrum antibiotics covering the presumptive organisms.

Other considerations in the differential diagnosis include

- Viral exanthems
- Rocky Mountain spotted fever
- Typhus
- Typhoid fever
- Subacute bacterial endocarditis
- Vasculitis syndromes (polyarteritis nodosa, Henoch-Schönlein purpura)
- Toxic shock syndrome
- Acute rheumatic fever

SPECIAL CONSIDERATIONS

In children, it is often difficult to distinguish meningococcal bacteremia from other benign febrile illnesses, especially if the classic skin lesions are not present. Otitis media, a viral upper respiratory infection (URI), and gastroenteritis are common erroneous initial diagnoses that later are proved by culture to be caused by *N. meningitides.*

LABORATORY TESTS

The diagnosis of a systemic *N. meningitides* infection is made by isolating the organism from blood or cerebrospinal fluid or with a punch biopsy or needle aspiration of skin lesions. Cultures should be taken from these sites. Specimens may also be Gram stained for the presence of gram-negative diplococci. The Gram stain may be more reliable than cultures if antibiotics were begun before specimens were obtained. Nasopharyngeal cultures are not helpful because of the common carrier state.

Other helpful laboratory studies include a complete blood count with platelet count, coagulation studies, and creatine kinase. These studies aid in determining the prognosis and monitoring the patient for complications such as disseminated intravascular coagulation and myocardial dysfunction.

TREATMENT

Treatment with penicillin G has been effective for years and remains the treatment of choice. Initially, adults should be given 24 million U/day intravenously in divided doses every 2 to 4 h. Infants and children should be given 250,000 U/kg/day intravenously in divided doses every 4 h. The treatment duration is usually 10 to 14 days. Chloramphenicol is used in penicillin-allergic patients. The dosage of chloramphenicol is 75 to 100 mg/kg per day intravenously in divided doses every 6 h. The dosage of chloramphenicol should not exceed 4 g/day.

Hospitalization and isolation are necessary during the acute phase of the illness. Intensive care may be needed in cases of fulminant meningococcemia. Nutritional status, fluid balance, and renal and cardiac function must be monitored closely to achieve the most favorable outcome. A consultation with an infectious disease specialist may be an invaluable resource in the management of these patients.

COMPLICATIONS AND RED FLAGS

Waterhouse-Friderichsen syndrome or purpura fulminans occurs in 5 to 10 percent of cases. This complication is marked by a rapid progression of apprehension, restlessness, and delirium. The skin lesions often spread and become ecchymotic, a sign of extensive intracutaneous hemorrhage. Vasomotor collapse and shock occur. Intravascular coagulation is common, and renal failure or bilateral adrenal hemorrhage may occur. Mortality is high even with appropriate antimicrobial therapy.

Cranial nerve damage may occur acutely, with a residual deficit in some cases. This usually is related to the brain swelling associated with concomitant meningococcal meningitis.

PATIENT EDUCATION

In some cases, prophylactic treatment of household contacts is indicated. A daily dose of rifampin 20 mg/kg for 4 days is used. No prophylaxis is indicated if more than 2 weeks has passed since the discovery of the initial case. There is no immunogenic effect of the vaccine in patients less than 2 years of age. Observation of contacts should continue for at least a full week.

Populations at high risk for meningococcal infections should receive vaccinations. These groups include military recruits, health care workers with close patient contact, patients with asplenia or terminal complement deficiency, and travelers to regions where there are epidemic levels of meningococcal disease.

ACKNOWLEDGMENT

The editor would like to acknowledge the significant contributions of Michaela O'Brien-Norton, the author of this chapter in the first edition of *Primary Care for Physician Assistants.*

BIBLIOGRAPHY

Apicella MA: Meningococcal infections, in Goldman L, Bennett JC (eds.): *Cecil Textbook of Medicine,* 21st ed. Philadelphia, Saunders, 2000, pp. 1655–1659.

Boslego JW, Tramont EC: *Neisseria meningitidis,* in Gorbach SL, Bartlett JG, Blacklow NR (eds.): *Infectious Disease.* Philadelphia, Saunders, 1998, pp 1769–1774.

Turbiak TW, Reich JJ: Bacterial infections, in Rosen P, Barkin R (eds.): *Emergency Medicine: Concepts and Clinical Practice.* St. Louis, Mosby, 1999, pp. 2519–2523.

9-30

FOOD-BORNE DISEASES

Rick Davis

DISCUSSION

Food-borne illness is a significant health problem in the United States and worldwide. Approximately 10 percent of the populations of industrialized countries experiences food-borne diseases annually.[1] The incidence is greatly affected by temperature and biological contamination of areas where food is produced and processed. The estimated incidence in the United States of food-borne diseases is 76 million, with 325,000 hospitalizations and 5000 deaths annually.[2] However, many cases are not reported. Transmission of the illness usually occurs through ingestion of contaminated food and person-to-person spread by the oral-fecal route. Young children, the elderly, and immunocompromised patients are especially at risk of developing serious illness and death from food-borne disease. Several factors have contributed recently to the changing epidemiology of food-borne disease, including greater consumption of raw or undercooked shellfish, vegetables, and meats; increased consumption of commercially prepared foods; new methods of mass food production; and microbial adaptation.[1,3]

Food-borne disease can be categorized by the offending agents, such as bacteria, viruses, parasites, and chemical toxins, or by the predominant symptoms, incubation period, and duration of illness. This chapter covers four of the most common bacterial pathogens: *Salmonella, Shigella, Campylobacter jejuni,* and *Escherichia coli* 0157:H7.

SHIGELLOSIS

DISCUSSION

The "Shiga bacillus" was first described in 1898 by Kiyoshi Shiga and later was called *Shiga dysenteriae*. The term *dysentery* refers to a diarrheal stool that contains pus (polymorphonuclear leukocytes) and blood.

Epidemiology

Between 15,000 and 18,000 cases of shigellosis are reported annually in the United States. Isolates of *Shigella sonnei* account for 77 percent, and *S. flexneri* accounts for 16 percent of cases in the industrialized world, while *S. flexneri* is the predominant isolate (60 percent) in developing countries. Humans and primates are the only reservoirs for *S. sonnei*. As few as 10 to 100 organisms can cause infection. This is in contrast to *Salmonella*, which may require $>10^7$ organisms to cause infection. Transmission is predominantly through the fecal-oral route by close personal contact, as in day care centers, or ingestion of contaminated food or water. Shigellosis is endemic in Mexico, Central America, India, and southeastern Asia.[4]

Microbiology

Shigella spp. are members of the family Enterobacteriaceae and are closely related to *Escherichia* spp. They are aerobic nonmotile gram-negative rods, of which there are four major subgroups: *S. dysenteriae* (subgroup A), *S. flexneri* (subgroup B), *S. boydii* (subgroup C), and *S. sonnei* (subgroup D). *Shigella* spp. can develop resistance to gastric acid and ultimately invade the colonic epithelium and produce an enterotoxin (Shiga toxin).[5]

SIGNS AND SYMPTOMS

The classic clinical presentation of bacillary dysentery is cramping lower abdominal pain, fever, tenesmus (a painful urge to defecate with little or no evacuation), and multiple low-volume stools with bloody mucus. The symptoms usually begin within 24 to 72 h of ingestion and last for 5 to 7 days in adults and 2 to 3 days in children. The volume of diarrhea is usually less than 1 L per day. Malnourished children and debilitated adults are at risk of a more severe clinical course.

DIAGNOSTIC STUDIES

The clinical suspicion of shigellosis should be made in any patient with acute bloody diarrhea, abdominal cramps, and fever. Stool examination for fecal leukocytes and blood supports a diagnosis of dysentery. However, this cannot be differentiated from an acute presentation of ulcerative colitis (see Chap. 6-4) or other dysentery-producing pathogens, such as *Campylobacter* spp., *E. coli* 0157:H7, and *Salmonella* spp.

A stool culture should be performed to confirm the diagnosis and antibiotic sensitivity. Sigmoidoscopy is usually not necessary within the initial 4 or 5 days of symptoms. If the symptoms continue after treatment or last more than 6 weeks, sigmoidoscopy with biopsy is indicated. If patients recently have been treated with antibiotics before the onset of diarrhea, a stool specimen for a *Clostridium difficile* assay should be obtained.

TREATMENT

Many patients with mild symptoms clear the infection without antibiotic therapy. Oral rehydration therapy is indicated for patients with mild disease. However, moderate to severe diarrhea may require intravenous fluid hydration. Traditionally, hypomotility agents are avoided in patients with dysentery to prevent the possible complication of toxic megacolon. However, some authors recommend the use of a hypomotility agent such as loperamide in patients with mild symptoms but no fever. A primary regimen for adults consists of a fluoroquinolone such as ciprofloxacin 500 mg or norfloxacin 400 mg orally bid for 3 days. An alternative regimen is trimethoprim-sulfamethoxazole (TMP-SMX, Septra DS) bid orally for 3 days. Resistance to trimethoprim-sulfamethoxazole is high, especially in the tropics. It has been suggested that shigellosis that is inadequately treated with TMP-SMX may increase the risk of developing the hemolytic-uremic syndrome.[6] Since shigellosis is a highly contagious disease, careful hand washing by the patient, family members, and the health care delivery team should be strongly encouraged. Shigellosis is a reportable disease in many areas. One can refer to the local health department for reporting requirements.

SALMONELLOSIS

DISCUSSION

Nontyphoidal Salmonellosis

Infections caused by any *Salmonella* sp. other than *Salmonella typhi* and *S. paratyphi* are termed nontyphoidal salmonellosis. These species are the most common causes of bacterial food-borne illness in the United States. The infections are divided into several clinical conditions, which include typhoid fever. Gastroenteritis with dysentery and dehydration is common, but bacteremia is less common in immunocompetent individuals. Complications of salmonella infection include endocarditis, arthritis, and meningitis. An asymptomatic chronic carrier state occurs in less than 1 percent of patients.[5]

Microbiology

The genus *Salmonella* includes a large group of gram-negative bacilli with over 2000 serotypes. They are primarily intestinal parasites but may be found in contaminated water and sewage. *Salmonella enteritidis* has become the most common source of salmonella infection in the United States. It is found in undercooked eggs, homemade and unpasteurized ice cream, poultry, and livestock. The bacteria invade the ileal mucosa and to a lesser extent the colonic epithelium after oral ingestion. They also may produce an enterotoxin that plays a role in the initial diarrhea. The development of infection is dependent on the age and health of the host as well as the number of organisms ingested (10^4 to 10^8).

Epidemiology

Salmonella spp. are a leading cause of food-borne illness in the world and the United States. The most common serotypes are *S. enteritidis*, *S. typhimurium*, *S. heidelberg*, and *S. newport*. The incidence of laboratory-confirmed salmonella infection in the United States has been estimated at 13.9 cases per 100,000 population, second to *Campylobacter* infection.[7] However, over 1 million cases of salmonellosis are suspected each year, since the disease is underreported.

Signs and Symptoms

Symptoms from salmonella gastroenteritis usually occur 6 to 48 h after ingestion but may be delayed for 7 to 12 days. The initial symptoms may be as mild as a few loose stools or as serious as severe watery diarrhea. A dysentery syndrome can occur, with colonic infection with frequent bloody mucoid stools of small volume, lower abdominal cramping, fever [usually $<38.9°C$, ($102°F$)], malaise, nausea, and vomiting that may last from 1 week to 2 or 3 months. The more common mild form of gastroenteritis usually lasts <5 days. Young children, the elderly, and immunocompromised patients are more likely to have a more severe course and a greater chance of complications.

Conditions that predispose patients to salmonella infection include hemolytic anemia, immunosuppression, achlorhydria, malignancy, and inflammatory bowel disease.

DIAGNOSTIC STUDIES

The diagnosis is made by means of a strong clinical suspicion and a stool culture. Sigmoidoscopy and biopsy usually are not indicated unless the diarrhea becomes chronic (>6 weeks), and inflammatory bowel disease should be excluded.

TREATMENT

Supportive treatment with oral rehydration is indicated in patients with mild to moderate disease. Antibiotic therapy should be avoided in this group because of the risk of prolonging a chronic carrier state (>1 year). However, patients with severe disease and patients at risk for complications from salmonella infection (malignancy, immunosuppression, prosthetic valves, hemolytic anemias, and sepsis) should be treated judiciously.

The primary therapy for adults is ciprofloxacin 500 mg or norfloxacin 400 mg orally bid for 3 days. Alternative therapies include TMX-SMP-DS or Septra-DS orally bid for 3 to 5 days, but antibiotic resistance is high, especially in the tropics.[6]

TYPHOID FEVER

DISCUSSION

Typhoid, or enteric fever, usually is caused by *S. typhi* but also can be caused by *S. paratyphi. Salmonella typhi* is found in humans who are chronic carriers and in contaminated food and water systems. Flooding of a community sewage system with subsequent contamination of the drinking water supply is a common source.

SIGNS AND SYMPTOMS

Clinically, these patients gradually develop fevers to 40 to 41°C (104 to 105.8°F) during the first week with an associated malaise, headache, and chills. Typically, the pulse rate is not elevated as it is in other febrile conditions. If untreated, the fever may last from 4 to 8 weeks. Splenomegaly may be seen, and during the first week of illness "rose spots" may be observed on the chest and abdomen; these are small erythematous macules and papules that blanch. Constipation may occur early, followed by a mild diarrheal illness.

Complications are rare but carry a high mortality rate when they occur. Intestinal perforation and peritonitis are the most common, followed by biliary tract disease, septic shock, meningitis, and septic arthritis.

DIAGNOSTIC STUDIES

The diagnosis is made by isolation of the organism, usually by blood culture. Stool cultures may be positive by the second to third week of infection. Antibiotic sensitivity should be tested, as there is a high rate of drug resistance.

TREATMENT

The recommended therapy is ciprofloxacin 500 mg orally bid for 10 days or ceftriaxone 2.0 g a day intravenously for 5 days. If a patient is in shock or has declining mental status, consider the administration of dexamethasone just before antibiotic administration.

An alternative treatment is chloramphenicol 500 mg qid orally or intravenously for 14 days.[6]

Campylobacter INFECTION

DISCUSSION

Campylobacter spp. are present in several human infections, but *Campylobacter jejuni* is a major cause of acute dysentery in the United States, with estimates of 2.1 million to 2.4 million cases. However, most cases are underreported or unconfirmed. The Centers for Disease Control and Prevention estimate the incidence of laboratory-confirmed cases of *C. jejuni*–induced food-borne illness at 19.7 per 100,000 population, exceeding salmonellosis at 13.9 and shigellosis at 7.2 per 100,000.[7]

Campylobacter jejuni is a motile gram-negative rod or spiral. Transmission occurs by the fecal-oral route and is associated with the ingestion of poultry, eggs, and raw milk and with sick pets (e.g., puppies). The pathophysiology is not well understood. However, the infectious dose is low, with as little as 500 organisms necessary to cause clinical symptoms. The pathogenesis may be via intestinal mucosal invasion and toxin production. It is commonly a disease of children under 5 years of age, especially in day care settings, and young adults. The incubation period is between 1 and 6 days, while the clinical symptoms usually last less than 1 week. Complications of *C. jejuni* infection include toxic megacolon, Reiter's syndrome (see Chap. 10-9), Guillain-Barré syndrome, and hemolytic-uremic syndrome (HUS).[8]

SIGNS AND SYMPTOMS

The clinical features include an initial fatigue and myalgia followed by nausea, anorexia, lower abdominal cramping pain, and watery or bloody diarrhea (commonly more than 10 stools per day). Stool examination is frequently positive for fecal leukocytes and blood.

DIAGNOSTIC STUDIES

The diagnosis usually is made by isolating the organism from stool or blood samples. Stool specimens should be fresh (less than 2 h after collection) as the characteristic "darting motility" of the spiral or comma-shaped organisms can be seen on dark-field microscopic examination.[8]

TREATMENT

The infection is usually self-limiting, but moderately severe cases may benefit from antibiotic therapy. The primary treatment regimen in adults consists of ciprofloxacin 500 mg or norfloxacin 400 mg orally bid for 5 days. *Campylobacter jejuni* resistance to quinolone treatment is markedly increasing in Southeast Asia, northern Africa, Spain, and Mexico. An alternative therapy would be azithromycin 500 mg orally qid for 3 days or erythromycin 500 mg orally qid for 5 days.[6]

ENTEROHEMORRHAGIC *Escherichia coli*

DISCUSSION

Escherichia coli 0157:H7 is an emerging food-borne pathogen in the United States and is associated with significant morbidity and HUS. Infection causes a bloody diarrhea that often is associated with the consumption of unpasteurized milk or contaminated beef, especially undercooked hamburger. The organism is present in the intestinal tract of cows. The beef often becomes contaminated during processing, at the time of slaughter. Grinding of hamburger transfers the pathogens to the interior of the meat, where they may survive inadequate cooking temperatures (<155°F). The pathophysiology is incompletely understood, but the organism is believed to adhere to the intestinal mucosal surface and produce enterotoxins similar to Shiga toxin.

SIGNS AND SYMPTOMS

The clinical features vary from watery, nonbloody diarrhea and abdominal cramps to bloody diarrhea, fever, nausea, and vomiting. Children less than 5 years old and the elderly are susceptible to a more severe clinical course. Most cases of HUS occur in patients with bloody diarrhea.

DIAGNOSTIC STUDIES

Stools are usually positive for blood and fecal leukocytes. The organism can be cultured from the stool on a special agar from which the 0157 antigen can be assayed. It is recommended that all diarrheal bloody stool specimens be cultured for *E. coli* 0157:H7.

TREATMENT

Currently, no antibiotic treatment is recommended. Conflicting data suggest that antibiotic treatment early in the course of the illness will prevent the development of HUS, while other investigators suggest that antimicrobial therapy may be a cofactor in the development of HUS.[9] One week after the onset of diarrhea, all patients should be monitored for the signs and symptoms of HUS, such as decreased urinary output and pallor. Management is supportive and includes adequate maintenance of fluid and electrolyte balance and frequently dialysis.

PREVENTION

Changes in the production, processing, and marketing of the food supply have contributed to new food-borne pathogens and changes in the epidemiology of food-borne disease. Improved sanitation in food animal production, prevention of contamination, and education of food handlers and consumers (careful hand washing, cooking meat to the proper temperature, etc.) are necessary to reduce the risk of food-borne disease.

REFERENCES

1. Kaferstein F, Abdussalam M: Food safety in the 21st century. *Bull World Health Org* 77:347–351, 1999.
2. Mead PS, Slutsker L, Dietz V, et al: Food-related illness and death in the United States. *Emerg Infect Dis* 5:607–625, 1999.
3. Altekruse SF, Swerdlow DL: The changing epidemiology of food-borne diseases. *Am J Med Sci* 311:23–29, 1996.
4. Kotloff KL, Winickoff JP, Ivanoff B, et al: Global burden of *Shigella* infections: Implication for vaccine development and implementation of control strategies. *Bull World Health Org* 77:651–665, 1999.
5. Edwards BH: *Salmonella* and *Shigella* species. *Clin Lab Med* 19:469–487, 1999.
6. Gilbert DN, Moellering RD, Sande MA: *Guide to Antimicrobial Therapy*, 29th ed. Hyde Park, VT, Anitmicrobial Therapy, 1999, pp 12–13.
7. Centers for Disease Control: Incidence of foodborne illnesses: Preliminary data from the Foodborne Diseases Active Surveillance Network (FoodNet) United States, 1998. *MMWR* 48:189–194, 1999.
8. Fields PI, Swerdlow DL: *Campylobacter jejuni*. *Clin Lab Med* 19:489–503, 1999.
9. Mead PS, Griffin PM: *Escherichia coli* 0157:H7. *Lancet* 352:1207–1212, 1998.

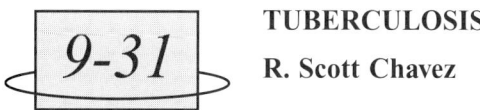

TUBERCULOSIS

R. Scott Chavez

DISCUSSION

Tuberculosis (TB) is caused by an aerobic tubercle bacillus of the genus *Mycobacterium*. Most mycobacteria can be isolated easily from environmental sources and are not pathogenic for humans. However, *Mycobacterium tuberculosis* is transmitted from person to person through the respiratory route and is highly communicable. If left unchecked, pulmonary tuberculosis has a morbidity rate of 33 percent and a mortality rate of 60 percent. On average, TB patients have a 22-year course of disease progression.

In 1985, the United States began tracking annual TB increases, with a 20.1 percent net gain in that year. In 1992, the United States reported a rate of 10.5 cases per 100,000 population. Owing to aggressive public health measures, the overall incidence of TB infection in the United States in 1997 declined to a rate of 7.4 cases per 100,000 general population, an all-time low.[1] While the United States is experiencing low rates of TB infection overall, a number of groups continue to be at high risk for TB infection. High-risk groups include persons infected with human immunodeficiency virus (HIV), illicit drug users, residents and employees in high-risk settings (nursing homes, correctional institutions, homeless shelters, and institutions for the mentally ill), foreign-born persons, some low-income and medically underserved persons, and health care workers who serve high-risk patients.

TB outside the United States is a major public health problem. It is estimated that 95 percent of the TB burden worldwide exists in middle-income and low-income countries. Multidrug-resistant strains are on the rise in third world countries, leading to failure of standardized short-course chemotherapy. More important, many countries do not have access to second-line drugs to manage multidrug-resistant tuberculosis (MDRTB), and this furthers the dissemination of MDRTB worldwide.[2] The World Health Organization (WHO) has reported that the incidence of TB has risen 6 percent in foreign-born persons living in the United States. Foreign-born Hispanic persons accounted for 10 percent of the 20,973 U.S. TB cases in 1996, and of all foreign-born Hispanic TB patients, 83 percent live in the four states bordering Mexico.[3]

Other high-risk groups are the young and the poor. These persons are more at risk for exposure to TB because of the fact that they live and work where the infection is most often found. Malnutrition, stress, and a compromised immune status are risk factors for promoting TB exposure. TB cases among nonwhites tend to be twice those among whites. Of special concern are blacks, Hispanics, Haitians, and Southeast Asian minorities. Individuals who are at high risk for TB are listed in Table 9-31-1.

PATHOGENESIS

Tuberculosis, a chronic bacterial infection, is caused by *M. tuberculosis*, which can affect multiple organs but usually manifests in the lungs. *Mycobacterium tuberculosis* is transmitted primarily through the respiratory route, although it can be transmitted through other routes. As an aerobic tubercle bacilli, *M. tuberculosis* is carried in respiratory secretions by forming nuclei that are carried on liquid droplets that are transported during sneezing, spitting, coughing, or even speaking. What makes *M. tuberculosis* most troublesome is that it remains airborne for a considerable time after the liquid droplets have evaporated. Inhalation of just a few of the bacilli is needed for a person to become infected. The contagiousness of TB is dependent on the frequency and force of a host's cough, the number of bacilli in the expectorate, and the virulence of the infection. Patients who have extensive cavitary pulmonary TB, laryngeal TB, and endobronchial disease are highly contagious and should be handled with caution.

In spite of its contagiousness, three factors aid in the control of TB:

1. Mycobacteria bacilli are susceptible to ultraviolet radiation.
2. Most TB-infected patients do not excrete large amounts of *M. tuberculosis*.
3. Most TB patients become noninfectious within 2 weeks after being placed on chemotherapy.

A good TB intervention program is predicated on providing adequate ventilation, cough suppression, and appropriate antibiotic chemotherapy.

TABLE 9-31-1. Individuals at High Risk for Tuberculosis

Individuals at high risk for tuberculosis infection are those who

Have within the past 2 years a history of *Mycobacterium tuberculosis* infection or a history of inadequately treated tuberculosis

Share household or other enclosed environments with persons known or suspected to have tuberculosis

Are infected with the human immunodeficiency virus

Use high-risk substances (e.g., crack cocaine) or inject illicit drugs

Reside or work in settings where TB-infected individuals are aggregated (e.g., correctional institutions, nursing homes, mental institutions, shelters for the homeless)

Are health care workers who provide care to high-risk clients

Are foreign-born and have arrived within 5 years from countries that have a high incidence or prevalence of tuberculosis (e.g., countries in Africa, Asia, and Latin America)

Have been locally identified as high-risk racial or ethnic minority populations and as being medically underserved or low-income populations

Are elderly

Are less than 4 years of age or are infants, children, and adolescents who have been exposed to adults in high-risk categories

Have chest radiographic findings suggestive of previous tuberculosis

Received inadequate treatment or no treatment

Have diabetes mellitus

Have silicosis

Have had an organ transplantation

Have had prolonged corticosteroid therapy (e.g., prednisone in a dose of 15 mg or more per day for 1 month or more) or other immunosuppressive therapy

Have a history of cancer of the head and neck

Have a history of hematologic and reticuloendothelial diseases (e.g., leukemia and lymphoma)

Have a history of end-stage renal disease

Have had intestinal bypass or gastrectomy

Have had a chronic malabsorption syndrome

Weigh 10 percent or more below ideal body weight

Microbiology

When the tiny (1 to 5 μ in diameter) airborne droplet nuclei of *M. tuberculosis* are inhaled, they become established in the pulmonary tissues and in some susceptible individuals may manifest throughout the body. In the initial 8 weeks of an *M. tuberculosis* infection, the tubercle bacilli multiply in an intracellular environment. Lymphocytes and monocytes begin to interact with the bacilli and create a cell-mediated hypersensitivity. *Mycobacterium tuberculosis* affects monocytes and transforms them into specialized histiocytic cells that form into granulomas. It is known that mycobacteria can remain dormant in microphages for many years, forming granulomas that become calcified and eventually are detectable on a chest radiograph.

Macrophages transport the bacilli to regional lymph nodes that may calcify in the node, providing access for systemic infection. A patient with both a calcified hilar lymph node and a calcified peripheral lung granuloma has a Ghon complex. The initial TB infection may remain dormant for months, years, or even decades; however, it eventually progresses to full reactivation tubercular disease.

SYMPTOMS

Generally, patients with primary TB are asymptomatic. Usually, the onset of pulmonary TB is insidious and deteriorates the host through a chronic and progressive course. Primary TB may not progress to clinical symptomatology until long after the initial infection. Some patients may present with only an inferior or midlung pneumonia that is nonspecific and resolves without complications. However, primary TB may fulminate into full clinical tubercular disease shortly after the initial infection. The point to remember about TB is that it is a chronic wasting disease that varies in its presentation. TB is known as the "great masquerader." There may be minimal infiltration that produces

no clinical illness, or there may be extensive bacterial involvement that produces significant symptomatology. A patient can complain of fatigue, exhaustion, muscle weakness, weight loss, low-grade fever, and drenching night sweats as constitutional symptoms of reactivated pulmonary tuberculosis.

The primary respiratory symptom of TB is a chronic nonproductive cough. When sputum is produced, it is usually scanty and nonpurulent. If there is any hemoptysis, it usually is confined to blood streaking of the sputum. TB patients rarely have massive life-threatening hemoptysis.

OBJECTIVE FINDINGS

Generally, there are few physical examination findings in patients with pulmonary TB. Inspection of the chest cavity yields little information about the disease unless there is extensive wasting and the accessory respiratory muscles are pronounced as a result of the labored breathing or cough. Percussion along the isthmus and clavicles may reveal dullness, but only in patients with extensive tubercular apical disease. Auscultation may reveal little information except when there is apical disease (wheeze) or extensive cavitation (amphoric breath sounds).

DIAGNOSTIC SCREENING

The tuberculin skin test is the standard method of screening for *M. tuberculosis* infection. The tuberculin purified protein derivative (PPD) is the preferred antigen. It should be applied in the intermediate-strength dose through the intracutaneous Mantoux test. Using a tuberculin disposable syringe with a 26- or 27-gauge needle, 0.1 mL of PPD tuberculin containing 5 tuberculin units (TUs) or intermediate-strength tuberculin should be injected by the Mantoux method (intradermally into the volar surface of the forearm, approximately 1 to 2 in below the antecubital fossa). The Mantoux injection is made just under the surface of the skin with the needle bevel facing upward. A 6- to 10-mm-diameter wheal is formed from the injection.

Within 48 to 72 h, the patient's sensitivity reaction to the PPD injection should be measured. The tuberculin skin test must be measured crosswise to the axis of the forearm. Measurement of the transverse diameter of the induration provides an assessment of current or past mycobacterial infection in the patient. Care should be taken to measure only the induration, not the erythema around the site.

The standard recording of a PPD measurement is made in millimeters, not in terms of one's observation of "positive" or "negative." A nonreactive PPD test is recorded as 00 mm when there is erythema with no induration. PPDs can be measured accurately up to 1 week after application. However, if the PPD reading is taken after 3 days beyond its implantation and the results appear negative, the standard of care requires a repeat Mantoux test. Table 9-31-2 describes the guidelines for interpreting positive skin reactions. A recent tuberculin skin test conversion is defined as an increase in induration of 10 mm or more within a 2-year period, regardless of age.

TABLE 9-31-2. Population Group and PPD Reaction Size

POPULATION GROUP	POSITIVE PPD REACTION, mm
Patients with close contacts who have active TB	5 mm
HIV-infected persons	5 mm
Patients with chest radiographs with fibrosis (healed TB)	5 mm
Population groups at high risk of tuberculosis	10 mm
Health care workers who provide care to TB patients and who have no other risk factors	10 mm
Persons who do not meet any of the above criteria	15 mm
Other risk factors	15 mm

It is important to remember that the larger the tuberculin reaction is, the more specific it is for *M. tuberculosis;* in general, a confidence level of 100 percent specificity is reached when PPD reactions of 15 mm are approached. However, caution should be exercised in interpreting PPD readings. The presence or absence of TB is not directly correlated to the size of the PPD skin reaction. Studies have demonstrated that noninfected, asymptomatic populations can have tuberculin skin reaction distributions identical to those of patients with known tuberculosis.

False positives may result when a patient has been exposed to nonpathogenic environmental mycobacteria. The environmental climate greatly influences false positives. For example, in northern climates false reactions to tuberculin reactivity are rather rare, while in the southeast coastal area of the United States nonspecific tuberculin reactivity is found commonly. Generally, reactions smaller than 10 mm are read as cross-reactions to environmental mycobacterial antigens and are not significant. Other causes of false positives include error in administration of the test, previous bacille Calmette-Guérin (BCG) vaccination, and the booster phenomenon.[4]

False negatives can occur for a variety of reasons, such as acute infections, live-virus vaccines, poor nutritional status, metabolic derangements, immunosuppressive therapy, patients 45 years or older, alcoholism, renal failure, corticosteroid use, zinc deficiency, lymphoid disease, and inaccurate reading of the induration. False negatives often occur in the elderly, who frequently fail to react to initial testing. A repeat PPD test should be applied 7 to 10 days after the initial test. It is significant if a reaction occurs on the second PPD application in the elderly.

False-negative results also may be obtained through technical errors such as the use of outdated materials or storage, dilution, contamination, and adsorption of tuberculin antigen material. Injecting subcutaneously, keeping PPD in syringes too long before use, and reading or recording errors by inexperienced readers are other causes of false negatives.

Extreme tuberculin skin reactions are rare. However, if a patient complains of intense itching or a severe reaction 3 days after the administration of PPD, relief can be sought through the application of a strong topical steroid (e.g., triamcinolone ointment 0.1%).

Of greatest concern in tuberculosis surveillance is anergy. Anergy is the absence of a tuberculin skin reaction in infected persons and should not be confused with false negatives. Tuberculin skin testing fails in a number of cases: 15 percent of patients with newly acquired TB, approximately 50 percent of miliary TB patients and 33 percent of tuberculous pleurisy patients, and any individual who is immunosuppressed. Studies have demonstrated that 17 to 24 percent of hospitalized TB patients and 5 percent of ambulatory TB patients have a negative tuberculin skin test at the time of diagnosis. A study of men admitted to New York jails and detoxification centers demonstrated that poor nutritional status, weight loss, and needle sharing result in anergy. Generally, a positive skin test will occur 2 weeks after the initial therapy and some weight gain.

Caution should be followed in repeating PPD skin tests. In a person infected with *M. tuberculosis* as well as in an uninfected person, repeated PPD testing may cause hypersensitivity and result in a boosted reaction size. This reaction, whether it is due to nonspecific reactivity or to TB, should be read and judged with caution. Any small increase should be looked at with suspicion. It is best to think of the booster phenomenon as a "recall of waned immunity." The American Thoracic Society (ATS) and the Centers for Disease Control (CDC) define boosting as "an increase of more than 6 mm of induration from an initial negative test result to one that is positive." The concept of boosting is important in serial tuberculin testing because it may lead to an error in interpretation and unnecessary therapy. The boosting phenomenon, which was first observed in 1934, became more prevalent in the 1970s, when reports of TB

TABLE 9-31-3. Diagnostic Standards and Classification of Tuberculosis in Adults and Children

CLASS O

No tuberculosis exposure, not infected. No history of exposure to TB and, if tested, a negative PPD

CLASS I

Tuberculosis exposure, no evidence of infection. A positive history of TB exposure; however, a negative PPD. Treatment depends on degree of exposure to *M. tuberculosis* and patient's immune status. At minimum, a repeat PPD should be obtained 10 weeks after exposure and treatment for latent TB should be considered. Children under age 15 and HIV-positive patients should be treated for latent TB

CLASS II

Latent tuberculosis infection, no disease. Patients in this class have a positive PPD test and no clinical, bacteriologic, or radiographic evidence of active disease. Clinicians should consider treatment of latent TB infection for high-risk groups.

CLASS III

Tuberculosis, clinically active. To be placed in this class, a patient must have all studies completed. There must be clinical, bacteriologic, or radiographic evidence. The isolation of *M. tuberculosis* is necessary for a patient to be classified in this group. The patient should remain in this class until all treatment is completed for the current infection

CLASS IV

Tuberculosis, not clinically active. To be classified in this group, a patient must have a past history of a positive PPD, a previous episode of TB, or abnormal radiographic findings that were stable. Patients in this class must have negative bacteriologic studies and no clinical radiographic evidence of current disease. If current clinically active disease has not been ruled out, the patient should be classified as tuberculosis-suspect (class V)

CLASS V

Tuberculosis suspect (diagnosis pending). This classification is used when a diagnosis of TB is being considered, whether the patient is being treated or not. An individual should not be in this class for more than 3 months and should be reclassified as soon as possible

SOURCE: Adapted from American Thoracic Society and Centers for Disease Control and Prevention.

conversion in hospital employees increased 10 percent. Boosting rarely occurs before 1 week after the initial testing. Boosting occurs in any age group but is encountered more frequently after 55 years of age. To account for the boosting phenomenon, a two-step tuberculin skin testing protocol is recommended for persons with a high degree of suspicion for TB. The first test in a serial tuberculin skin test is read 7 days after application, and if there is less than 10 mm of induration, a second test is applied immediately and read 2 to 3 days later.

In 1999, the ATS and the CDC recommended targeted testing, classification, and treatment for latent and active TB (see Table 9-31-3). Patients with tuberculosis infection but no evidence of active disease are described as having latent TB. Ruling out active disease becomes very important. A negative PPD test in a person who has close contact with an individual who has active TB is said to indicate a latent TB infection. A repeat PPD test should be done at the 3-month interval. If it is negative, treatment can be stopped. If it is positive, a chest radiograph should be obtained and the patient should be worked up for active tuberculosis.

LABORATORY STUDIES

The diagnosis of TB is confirmed through bacteriologic examination of the sputum, urine, body fluids, or tissues of the patient. Patients with pulmonary TB most likely will have tubercle bacilli in their sputum. Most mycobacteria are acid-fast organisms that retain certain dyes after being washed in an acid solution. When a report indicates that acid-fast bacilli

(AFB) are present on a stained sputum smear, one should suspect a diagnosis of TB. However, TB can be confirmed only after a culture has been grown and identified as *M. tuberculosis*. It takes approximately 4 to 8 weeks to obtain a primary isolation on classic media.

RADIOLOGIC STUDIES

The chest radiograph remains the essential tool for the diagnosis and evaluation of TB. The most typical lesion of pulmonary TB is multinodular infiltration in the apical posterior segments of the upper lobes and the superior segments of the lower lobes. Pulmonary TB patients frequently have cavitation with substantial amounts of infiltration in the same pulmonary segments. The standard views are posterior-anterior (PA) and lateral; however, on occasion lordotic views can obtain views of pulmonary tissue obscured by the intersection of the third and fourth posterior ribs, the second anterior rib, and the clavicle. Serial films are important in judging the progression and activity of tuberculosis. In time, as the tuberculosis becomes inactive or heals, there will be fibrotic scarring. Healed primary lesions may calcify with the passing of years.

OTHER DIAGNOSTICS

Peripheral blood studies may demonstrate monocytes in the range of 8 to 10 percent, an elevated erythrocyte sedimentation rate, and modest anemia. Otherwise, blood and chemical studies do not help in the diagnosis of pulmonary TB.

TREATMENT

Pharmacologic Management

The ATS-CDC recommendations specify the treatment of latent tuberculosis infection (formerly known as preventive therapy or chemoprophylaxis) for a 9-month regimen of isoniazid (INH) 5 mg/kg/day to a maximum of 300 mg/day. The ATS-CDC recognizes that a 6-month course of treatment "may provide a more favorable outcome from a cost-effectiveness standpoint." It is recommended that health care providers consider patient adherence to treatment and local health department recommendations when considering the length of treatment. A patient with latent TB infection should be assessed monthly for hepatotoxicity, anemia, and neurotoxicity. Patients with latent TB infection who are exposed to MDRTB should be treated with two drugs.

Adult patients with active tuberculosis (positive PPD test, positive findings on chest radiography, and a positive AFB) should be treated with a four-drug regimen (see Table 9-31-4). After 2 months of

administration of the four-drug regimen and negative repeat sputum cultures, patients can be placed on an INH and rifampin combination therapy for another 4 months. Monthly sputum smears and cultures should be performed.

If patients are compliant and take effective drugs, symptomatic improvement occurs within the first 2 to 3 weeks. Most patients will convert to negative AFB sputum within the first 2 months. Radiographic evidence of clearing of infiltrates may occur within the first month but usually is recognized between the second and fourth months. Serial chest films between 3 and 6 months demonstrate radiologic stability. Drug therapy should be continued 6 months beyond the time when the patient reaches radiographic stability.

Nonpharmacologic Management

Lack of patient adherence to treatment contributes to the emergence and transmission of drug-resistant organisms. Most patient defaults occur within the first 6 months of a treatment program. Directly observed therapy (DOT) is used to maintain patient compliance and is the single most effective public health strategy against TB. An on-site DOT program; a comprehensive coordination of medical, nursing, and social services; and motivated patients can ensure an effective public health strategy to combat TB.

Supportive Measures

Patients' activity and diet can be regular and as tolerated. TB patients are not contagious after a few days of treatment. Children, elderly patients, and pregnant patients require additional supportive measures. Bacille Calmette-Guérin (BCG) should be given to uninfected children who are at high risk or when INH is not feasible. Elderly patients generally experience more pronounced side effects of INH. Pregnant patients should be given pyridoxine.

Patient Education

Patients should be instructed about the pathogenesis of their disease and the importance of completing the full course of prescribed therapy. They also should be instructed that rifampin colors tears, secretions, and urine orange. Patients with contact lens should be informed that rifampin may stain their lenses permanently. A well-educated patient and an alert provider are the principal safeguards against drug hepatitis. Generally, there are few complications, and if the patient is compliant with the medication regimen, full resolution of the disease can be expected. Patients should be followed every 2 to 3 months with chest radiographs. Children should be seen every 2 to 4 weeks.

TABLE 9-31-4. First-Line Drugs for Active Tuberculosis

DRUG	DAILY DOSING (GIVEN BY DIRECTLY OBSERVED THERAPY ONLY)	ADVERSE REACTION
Isoniazid	Children: 10 mg/kg orally or IM Adults: 300 mg orally or IM Maximum 300 mg	Elevation of hepatic enzyme levels, hepatitis, neuropathy, central nervous system effects
Rifampin (Rifadin)	Children: 10 to 20 mg/kg orally or IV Adults: 10 mg/kg to maximum of 600 mg	Orange discoloration of secretions and urine, gastrointestinal tract upset, hepatitis, bleeding problems, flu-like symptoms, drug interactions, rash
Pyrazinamide	Children: 20 to 30 mg/kg orally Adults: 25 mg/kg orally Maximum 2 g	Gastrointestinal tract upset, hepatitis, hyperuricemia, arthralgias
Ethambutol (Myambutol)	Children and adults: 15 to 25 mg/kg orally	Optic neuritis

COMPLICATIONS AND RED FLAGS

MDRTB is tuberculosis disease that is resistant to at least isoniazid and rifampin. MDRTB is a growing problem in the treatment and management of TB. There is a high prevalence rate of MDRTB in the former Soviet Union, Asia, the Dominican Republic, and Argentina. At-risk populations for MDRTB include HIV-positive individuals; intravenous drug abusers; homeless people; people working or living in correctional institutions, nursing homes, and mental institutions; people exposed to patients with active TB; and health care workers. A high degree of suspicion for primary drug resistance should be raised when a patient has been exposed to noncompliant TB patients or MDRTB patients. Treatment, which must be individualized and based on susceptibility studies, should be initiated only in consultation with local experts or public health authorities. Some public health authorities add a fluoroquinolone to the initial protocol, with final decisions on therapy made after drug resistance studies have been completed. A fifth drug such as streptomycin, cycloserine, or ethionamide may be added.

Drug toxicity is always a concern in multiple-drug therapy. Since there are multiple-drug regimens for TB, toxicity is a factor in the choice of therapy. The toxicity of greatest concern is hepatitis. Approximately 3 to 5 percent of patients taking isoniazid and rifampin have a level of toxicity that requires a change in the regimen. Another 1.5 percent of patients taking isoniazid and ethambutol develop toxicities that require a regimen change. Approximately 30 percent of Asian groups and 2 to 5 percent of other populations have toxicity from isoniazid and thiacetazone. Generally, 25 percent of HIV-infected persons develop toxicity from anti-TB drugs as well. To prevent toxicity side effects, the elderly, diabetic patients, alcoholic patients, and malnourished patients should be given pyridoxine (50 mg/day) concomitantly with isoniazid. Finally, there is little to gain from monitoring liver function serum enzymes, since normal values do not predict the absence or presence of toxicity, and isoniazid may cause a transient rise to three times the normal value.

NOTES AND PEARLS

The recent use of nucleic acid amplification techniques has allowed researchers to isolate and identify *M. tuberculosis.* This technique is evolving rapidly and will make laboratory diagnosis more effective and efficient, enhancing diagnostic certainty. Facing worldwide escalating TB rates, public health officials and clinicians must focus on the efficacy and efficiency of control measures to improve existing programs and determine how TB is increasing in developing and underdeveloped countries.

PATIENT RESOURCES

Facts about the TB Skin Test and *Facts about Tuberculosis.* American Lung Association, 1740 Broadway, New York, NY 10019-4373, (212) 315-8700.
TB: Get the Facts and *Tuberculosis: Connection between TB and HIV.* Centers for Disease Control and Prevention, Information Services Office, 1600 Clifton Road NE, Atlanta, GA 30333, (800) 311-3435, http://www.cdc.gov.
The American Academy of Family Physicians Web site has patient information on TB and other health topics: http://www.familydoctor.org.
National Jewish Medical and Research Center, 1400 Jackson Street, Denver CO 80206, (800) 222-5864, http://www.njc.org.
TB Care Guide: Highlights from Core Curriculum on Tuberculosis. Atlanta, U.S. Department of Health and Human Services, Public Health Services, Centers for Disease Control and Prevention, National Center for Prevention Services, Division of Tuberculosis Elimination, 1994; pp 19–26.

PROVIDER RESOURCES

Core Curriculum on Tuberculosis. American Thoracic Society/Centers for Disease Control, Division of Tuberculosis Elimination, National Center for Prevention Services, Centers for Disease Control and Prevention, 1600 Clifton Road, Mailstop E-10, Atlanta, GA 30333, (404) 639-2508.

Initial Therapy for TB in the Era of Multiple Drug Resistance and Mantoux Tuberculin Skin Testing (videotape). Centers for Disease Control and Prevention, Information Services, 1600 Clifton Road NE, Atlanta, GA 30333, (404) 639-1819.
The Georgia TB Reference Guide. Atlanta Tuberculosis Prevention Coalition, http://www.ph.dhr.state.ga.us/epi/manuals/pdf/tbguide99.pdf.
The American Thoracic Society. *Diagnostic Standards and Classification of Tuberculosis in Adults and Children,* http://www.cdc.gov/nchstp/tb/pubs/1376.pdf.

REFERENCES

1. Centers for Disease Control and Prevention: Tuberculosis morbidity—United States, 1997. *MMWR* 47:253–256, 1998.
2. Espinal MA, Kim SJ, Suarez PG, et al: Standard short-course chemotherapy for drug-resistant tuberculosis: Treatment outcomes in 6 countries. *JAMA* 283(19):2437–2545, 2000.
3. Wells CD, Ocana M, Moser K, et al: A study of tuberculosis among foreign-born Hispanic persons in the U.S. states bordering Mexico. *Am J Respir Crit Care Med* 159(3):834–837, 1999.
4. Hoft DF, Tennant JM: Persistence and boosting of bacille Calmette-Guérin-induced delayed-type hypersensitivity. *Ann Intern Med* 131(1):32–36, 1999.

BIBLIOGRAPHY

Bradford WZ, Daley CL: Multiple drug-resistant tuberculosis. *Infect Dis Clin North Am* 12:157–172, 1998.
Essential components of a tuberculosis prevention and control program: Recommendations of the Advisory Council for the Elimination of Tuberculosis. *MMWR* 44:1–16, 1995.
Guidelines for preventing the transmission of *Mycobacterium tuberculosis* in health-care facilities, 1994. *MMWR* 43:1–132, 1994.
Kendig EL, Kirkpatrick BV, Carter WH, et al: Underreading of the tuberculin skin test reaction. *Chest* 113:1175–1177, 1998.
LoBue PA, Catanzaro A, Dutt AK, Stead W: Tuberculosis: Part 2. *Dis Month* 43:181–274, 1997.
McCollister P, Neff NE: Outpatient management of tuberculosis. *Am Fam Physician* 53:1579–1594, 1996.
McDermott U, Glassroth J, Mehta JB, Dutt AK: Tuberculosis: Part 1. *Dis Month* 43:113–180, 1997.
Prevention and treatment of tuberculosis among patients infected with human immunodeficiency virus: Principles of therapy and revised recommendations. *MMWR* 47:1–58, 1998.
Sumarlojo E, Geiter L, Miller B, Hale B: Can physicians treat tuberculosis? Report on a national survey of physician practices. *Am J Public Health* 87:2008–2011, 1997.
Zuber PL, McKenna MT, Binkin NJ, et al: Long-term risk of tuberculosis among foreign-born persons in the United States. *JAMA* 278:304–307, 1997.

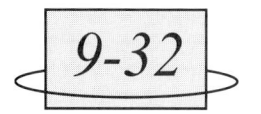

HISTOPLASMOSIS
Kathryn Frake

DISCUSSION

Histoplasma capsulatum is a dimorphic fungus that is present in soil, particularly soil contaminated with the fecal material of blackbirds, pigeons, and chickens. Birds themselves are not carriers of *H. capsulatum;* however, the fungus grows well in soil that is nitrogen-enriched from bird droppings. Bats can be infected with the fungus, and *H. capsulatum* is excreted in their feces. Inhalation of spores from disturbed soil causes human infection and may result in a variety of clinical manifestations, depending on the amount of inoculum inhaled, the nature of the infecting aerosol, and the host's immunity.

H. capsulatum is present in temperate climates worldwide and is endemic in the United States along the Ohio and Mississippi river valleys. The endemic area also includes parts of Texas, Virginia, Delaware, and Maryland. Among individuals living in endemic areas, nearly 100% have positive *Histoplasma* skin test reactivity. Isolated outbreaks have occurred in other areas. In New York City, for example, cases have been seen among people who have lived in Puerto Rico, the Dominican Republic, and Colombia. Other outbreaks have been described in San Francisco, Los Angeles, Minnesota, Iowa, and Florida, suggesting that there may be areas of *H. capsulatum*–contaminated soils outside the endemic region. Historically, most outbreaks result from massive exposure to *H. capsulatum* spores from large soil disturbances at the fringes of endemic areas, where the population lacks natural immunity, or in large cities where a proportion of the population is immunodeficient from HIV infection.

There are approximately 500,000 new *H. capsulatum* infections per year; however, in endemic areas very few individuals develop active disease. Among AIDS patients, the overall rate of histoplasmosis is 2 to 5% in the endemic areas of the United States and up to 25% in certain cities, such as Indianapolis, Kansas City, and Memphis.

PATHOGENESIS

After inhalation of *H. capsulatum* into the alveoli of the lungs, dissemination occurs via the blood and lymphatics. Circulating organisms are removed by the cells of the reticuloendothelial system (spleen, liver, bone marrow), but the fungus is not destroyed until 2 to 3 weeks later, when cell-mediated immunity develops. This immune response causes intense inflammation at sites of infection, and necrosis and calcification may occur. The results of this immune response may be noted as an incidental finding on a chest radiograph that demonstrates numerous small calcifications of uniform size.

In those with deficient cell-mediated immunity (AIDS patients, individuals receiving chronic glucocorticoids, patients on chemotherapy, and those with certain hematologic malignancies), a progressive form of primary infection may develop. Rarely, a progressive primary infection is seen in patients with normal immune systems. It is suspected that an unknown immune deficit exists in these so-called normal hosts. Additionally, a progressive primary infection of the lung that mimics tuberculosis can be seen in smokers with underlying chronic obstructive pulmonary disease (COPD).

SIGNS AND SYMPTOMS

Acute Primary Histoplasmosis

Sixty to ninety percent of primary histoplasmosis infections are asymptomatic. Clinically apparent infections are mild to moderate in severity with nonspecific presentations. Infants and young children are more likely to develop symptoms than are immune-competent adults, and immune-deficient patients are more likely to progress to serious complications from primary infection.

The incubation period of primary infection is 3 to 21 days. In those who do have symptoms, fever, headache, malaise, a nonproductive cough, and substernal chest pain with inspiration are common. Pericarditis, which resolves in 1 to 3 months without treatment, may be present in up to 5%. Rarely, acute respiratory distress syndrome (ARDS) develops after extremely heavy exposures. Most ARDS patients improve after 2 to 6 weeks if they survive the initial critical care management. Females who are symptomatic are at greater risk of developing rheumatologic manifestations such as arthralgias, erythema multiforme, and erythema nodosum.

The lung examination is usually normal. Hepatosplenomegaly may be appreciated, particularly in children. Routine laboratory studies are nondiagnostic or may reveal mild anemia and elevated alkaline phosphatase in more severe cases. Chest radiography in asymptomatic patients is normal. In symptomatic patients, typical findings include patchy infiltrates with hilar and mediastinal adenopathy. Sputum may be cultured and is positive in 10 to 15% of patients with symptoms.

Influenza (see Chap. 9-15) is the most common misdiagnosis; however, the sore throat and coryza typical of influenza are uncommon. Hilar adenopathy on chest radiography also may be seen in sarcoidosis and lymphoma patients, and the histopathology of sarcoidosis and histoplasmosis may be indistinguishable. Elevated serum angiotensin converting enzyme (ACE) levels, which are often seen in sarcoidosis, may be seen in histoplasmosis as well, further confusing the diagnosis. Since most patients improve without treatment, the diagnosis is missed in the vast majority.

Chronic Pulmonary Histoplasmosis

Chronic pulmonary histoplasmosis (CPH) primarily affects males >50 years old with underlying COPD. CPH localizes to the apical regions of the lungs and causes chronic cough, weight loss, low-grade fever, and fatigue. Night sweats are not common. Twenty percent of these patients develop cavitary lesions. The result of CPH is progressive worsening of the underlying COPD. If untreated, these cases sometimes resolve spontaneously. In most, however, insidious progression occurs.

Progressive Disseminated Histoplasmosis

Progressive disseminated histoplasmosis (PDH) occurs in 1 in 2000 healthy adults. It is more common in immunosuppressed patients, infants, and small children. Those with AIDS who reside in endemic areas are particularly susceptible. The clinical manifestations of PDH include:

- *Chronic PDH:* waxing and waning symptomatology
- *Subacute PDH:* waxing and waning but relentless course
- *Acute PDH:* fulminant, rapidly fatal course

Chronic PDH

Skin lesions are the most common clinically apparent manifestation of chronic PDH. Mouth ulcers are the cutaneous lesions that are most frequently seen. The ulcers are usually painful with heaped-up borders and may be mistaken for a malignancy. Hepatosplenomegaly is present in 30% of cases. Chest radiography is negative, and laboratory studies are not usually helpful but may demonstrate mild anemia, leukopenia, and thrombocytopenia. Gradual weight loss, fatigue, and low-grade fevers occur in approximately 30% of these patients. The course is very protracted with asymptomatic periods, making the diagnosis extremely difficult.

Subacute PDH

Fever, weight loss, and malaise are consistent findings. Hepatosplenomegaly is more common, as are oral ulcers. Half these patients have anemia, leukopenia, and thrombocytopenia. The adrenal glands are commonly affected, and 5 to 10% of these patients develop adrenal insufficiency. Gastrointestinal masses and fistulations, endocarditis, chronic meningitis, and cerebral mass lesions may occur. Subacute PDH progresses to death in 2 to 24 months if left untreated.

Acute PDH

The incidence of acute PDH is rising along with the AIDS epidemic. Other susceptible individuals include the very young and those with lymphoblastic leukemia and Hodgkin's disease. In AIDS patients, acute PDH is often the AIDS-defining illness. CD4+ counts are usually <200 cells/μL. Fever, weight loss, fatigue, cough, and dyspnea are common. Hepatosplenomegaly and lymphadenopathy may be seen. The appearance of skin lesions varies considerably, with the most common presentation being diffuse, erythematous maculopapular eruptions. Purpuric lesions, skin ulcers, and vegetative lesions also may be seen. Mouth ulcers are less common, and the overall incidence of skin lesions (approximately 10%) is lower than that of chronic PDH. Anemia, thrombocytopenia, and leukopenia are very common. Chest radiography may demonstrate infiltrates or may be normal. CNS involvement is seen in 5 to 20% of cases. If untreated, acute PDH is always fatal, usually within a few weeks.

DIAGNOSTIC STUDIES

Culture and Tissue Staining

The diagnosis requires growth of the fungus from body tissues or fluid samples or staining for yeast forms in tissue sections. Cultures may require 4 to 6 weeks for growth; however, a DNA probe specific for *Histoplasma* permits the identification of an isolate in 1 to 3 weeks. Success rates for culture vary from laboratory to laboratory, depending on experience. Sputum is positive in only 10 to 15% of those with acute pulmonary disease; however, sputum from patients with chronic histoplasmosis or cavitary lesions is more likely to be positive. In AIDS patients with acute PDH and abnormal chest radiographs, bronchial aspirates are positive in 80 to 90%. Blood and bone marrow are rarely positive in those with chronic PDH, but biopsy of oral lesions is usually diagnostic.

Serologic Tests

Tests for complement fixation antibodies are the most widely used. In endemic areas, 2 to 12% of the population will have chronically positive cultures. As a result, the lowest titer considered to be positive is 1:8. A single test of 1:32 or higher is more suggestive of histoplasmosis, while titers of 1:8 or 1:16 are less compelling but should be considered suspicious in the right clinical setting. Antibodies are detected in 5 to 15% of cases approximately 3 weeks after exposure and in 75 to 95% after 6 weeks; 30 to 50% of immunodeficient hosts, however, fail to develop antibodies at sufficient titers for diagnosis.

Antigen Detection

The antigen detection technique is useful in patients who are immunodeficient when serologic titers are unreliable. *Histoplasma* antigen may be detected in the urine or serum by radioimmune assay (RIA). RIA can detect antigen in the serum of 50% of AIDS patients with acute PDH and in 90% of urine samples. It is less useful in those with self-limiting pulmonary histoplasmosis or cavitary disease.

The monitoring of urinary antigen may be used to determine the initial response to therapy and to detect relapses in AIDS patients who are on chronic suppressive therapy.

Skin Testing

Skin testing is of value only epidemiologically for mapping the distribution of the fungus. It is of little use for diagnosis.

TREATMENT

Acute Primary Histoplasmosis

No treatment is necessary unless the patient is severely ill. Ketoconazole 400 mg/d or itraconazole 200 mg/d for 4 to 6 weeks may be used. Amphotericin B may be used at 0.7 mg/kg per day for 2 to 3 weeks if an azole is contraindicated.

Chronic Pulmonary Histoplasmosis

Asymptomatic patients with thin-walled cavities and areas of interstitial pneumonitis may be followed radiographically over 2 to 4 months if they are not immunocompromised. Those with worsening or persistent radiographic pictures should be treated, along with symptomatic patients and those with thick-walled cavities.

Amphotericin B may be used at 0.7 mg/kg per day to a total dose of at least 35 mg/kg. The relapse rate is high (20%), and surgical resection may be required in patients with relapse or progressive disease despite treatment. Ketoconazole and itraconazole may also be used at 400 mg/d and 200 mg/d, respectively, for 6 to 12 months. Efficacy is similar between the azoles and amphotericin B.

Chronic and Subacute PDH

Amphotericin B or the azoles at the same doses as those listed above may be used. Amphotericin B is the drug of choice if the patient is immunocompromised.

Acute PDH (Including Immune-Compromised Hosts)

Emergent treatment with amphotericin B is needed. A 1-mg test dose is not advised, as this can cause a considerable delay in treatment. A dose of 25 to 30 mg given intravenously is administered immediately over several hours, followed by 0.7 to 1 mg/kg per day to a total dose of 35 mg/kg or 2.5 g.

Fifty percent or more of AIDS patients relapse after therapy; therefore, chronic suppression treatment is required with itraconazole at 200 mg/d. Urinary antigen should be monitored at the beginning and end of induction and every few months thereafter. Any increase in urinary antigen of at least 2 units should prompt additional studies, as this may indicate relapse.

BIBLIOGRAPHY

Deepe G: *Histoplasma capsulatum,* in *Principles and Practice of Infectious Diseases,* 5th ed, GL Mandell et al (eds). New York, Churchill Livingstone, 2000.

Johnson PC, Sarusi GA: Infections caused by dimorphic fungi, in *Principles and Practice of Infectious Diseases,* 4th ed, GL Mandell et al (eds). New York, Churchill Livingstone, 1995.

Wheat J: Endemic mycosis in AIDS: A clinical review. *Clin Microbiol Rev* 8(1):146–159, 1995.

Wheat J, et al: Itraconazole treatment of disseminated histoplasmosis in patients with the acquired immunodeficiency syndrome. AIDS Clinical Trial Group. *Am J Med* 98(4):336–342, 1995.

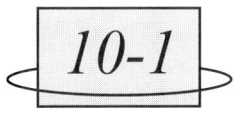

COMMON COMPLAINTS OF THE WRIST, ELBOW, SHOULDER, AND ANKLE

Gloria Stewart

TENDINITIS

DISCUSSION

The tendon transfers the force of the muscle contraction to the bone, which in turn produces movement of the joint. Tendons can withstand large forces, with a breaking point that is said to be similar to steel. As a person ages, the strength of tendons is reduced, fibers shrink and stiffen, frequently resulting in tears from overuse. Tendons appear white because they are relatively avascular, consisting of approximately 30% closely packed collagen fibers, 2% elastin, and 68% water. The muscle-tendon unit can be divided into three areas of concern. Region one is the insertion of the muscle into the tendon. An inflammatory response to injury located in this area would be referred to this as *peritendinitis,* whereas an inflammatory response to injury in region three, at the insertion of the tendon into the bone, is referred to as *tendinitis* (tendinosis). Tendinitis is considered to be an overuse syndrome, which involves a chronic inflammation process. An inflammatory response that occurs in the synovial sheath surrounding the tendon in the middle section of the muscle-tendon unit, region two, is referred to as *tenosynovitis.* Tenosynovitis of the tendon sheath may be due to strain from overuse, a direct blow, or an infection.

Trauma initiates an increase in blood supply, the invasion of inflammatory cells, oversecretion of synovial fluid, and an increase in fibronectin content, which cause adhesions between the tendon and its surroundings. Usually, the sites of tendon injury are located where the muscle-tendon units cross more than one joint, where repetitive high eccentric work loads generally occur. This process is time dependent, characterized by tissue repair, regeneration, or scar formation from repeated microtraumas, or the destruction of a small number of cells. Inflammation is a necessary response to trauma. Macrotrauma, which is acute tissue destruction, is characterized by a defined time of onset, such as a sudden traumatic episode, like a spontaneous disruption of the tendon. Microtraumatic tendon injury is the chronic abusive load or overuse of the tendon, which results in an inflammatory response and is often found in patients who engage in repetitive overhand motions.

An accurate history and physical examination of the area of complaint should be explored for the various reasons that could cause tendinitis. Factors that lead to tendinitis may be best understood by grouping them as either intrinsic or extrinsic. Intrinsic factors include malalignment, excessive pronation, femoral neck anteversion, limb length discrepancy, muscular imbalance, and muscular insufficiency. Extrinsic factors include training errors, excessive distance running, excessive intensity, hill work, improper technique, fatigue, running on hard or uneven surfaces, environmental conditions, and inadequate footwear and equipment.

SYMPTOMS

Typically the patient will present with a history of a gradual onset of localized pain and tenderness over the insertion of the tendon. *Celsius*

(first century A.D.) defines the four cardinal signs of inflammatory response as "rubor et tumor cum calore et dolore": redness and swelling with heat and pain that can be reproduced as the patient moves the tendon. Tenosynovitis in its acute state will present with pain on function, which progresses to pain at rest and diffuse swelling. Crepitation may also be felt by placing one's fingers over the involved tendon while it slides up and down. In a patient with chronic tenosynovitis the tendons may become thickened.

DIAGNOSTIC TESTS

Conventional radiographs, ultrasound, and computed tomography (CT) have a limited role in the diagnosis of injuries of tendons and muscles. Arthrography has been useful for evaluating injury to the rotator cuff, but the most useful diagnostic tool for the evaluation of an injured tendon is magnetic resonance imaging (MRI). The use of MRI with high intrinsic tissue contrast can separate normal from abnormal tendons. In an MRI the normal tendons appear dark while fat appears bright, and muscle will have an intermediate contrast.

TREATMENT

Rest

The initial treatment of tendinitis should include rest. The practitioner should have the patient avoid weight-bearing for the first 24 hours and then slowly increase the motion and load to the area as tolerated. The key to any treatment is gradual progressive challenges in intensity and load. There is evidence that the repetitive motion may create positive signals for postinjury repair, and a modified load has been shown to be important to a successful return to prior performance levels.

Cold Modalities

The use of cold as a treatment modality produces an initial circulatory response of vasoconstriction resulting in reduced edema. There is a secondary circulatory response that is called *cold-induced vasodilation.* This secondary response occurs mainly in the periphery following cold immersion. Cold exposure blocks sensory transmission of the pain impulse, which in turn helps to decrease muscle spasm and thus helps the patient control the pain. The use of cold exposure for an acute injury helps in the prevention of hemorrhage, inflammation, edema, muscle spasm, and pain. The use of cold exposure for a chronic complaint will help the patient by preventing additional inflammation that occurs as a result of the rehabilitation process. Conventional cold therapy includes ice packs, ice-cup massage, and ice immersion baths. There are also commercially prepared products, including gel refrigerant packs, chemical packs, and coolant sprays. Commercially prepared products should have a warning that potential package breakage could result in chemical burns and injuries. Contraindications to using cold therapy are Raynaud's phenomenon, cardiovascular disease, cryoglobulinemia, and paroxysmal cold hemoglobinuria. Other problems with cold therapy are allergy, anesthetic skin, and arthritic conditions.

Heat Modalities

Heat has always been an accepted method of treatment. The use of heat produces vascular changes by causing vasodilation, which produces an analgesic effect and also helps move nutrients and oxygen into the affected area and remove waste products. It has been suggested that for each 10°C (18°F) rise in temperature, the cell's chemical activity and the metabolic rate will increase two to three times.

Various methods of heat modality include warm whirlpool baths, paraffin wax, moist heat packs, infrared heat, and therapeutic ultrasound. Each of these modalities helps to raise the temperature and, therefore, increase vasodilation. Warm whirlpools are usually taken at a temperature of 39 to 41°C (102 to 106°F) for 15 to 20 minutes, depending on the body area. During the treatment the patient should actively move the body part in the whirlpool within his or her pain tolerance. Paraffin wax is used mainly for the smaller joints of the body, such as fingers, hands, and wrists. Heat modalities are used in 20- to 30-minute increments.

Cold and Heat Combined

The combination of cold and heat therapies, called *contrast baths,* is another modality for treatment of tendinitis. The heat therapy should be from 39 to 41°C (102 to 106°F) and the cold therapy from 10 to 15.5°C (50 to 60°F). Suggested time for each modality varies according to each practitioner's preference. Some sources suggest 5 minutes for heat and 1 to 2 minutes for cold, alternating for 30 minutes, while others suggest 1 minute heat and 30 seconds cold or 30 seconds heat with 1 minute cold. The treatment should always end with cold treatment. Theoretically, this method produces a maximum increase in blood flow to the involved area, which should increase the healing process.

PHARMACOLOGIC TREATMENT

The use of nonsteroidal anti-inflammatory drugs (NSAIDs) can be controversial. The suggested uses for NSAIDs are to control pain, to act as an anti-inflammatory agent that would presumably allow early activity, and to decrease inflammation, presumably resulting in faster healing. However, it is necessary to remember that inflammation is a natural and necessary process for response to trauma. There have been studies that suggest that NSAIDs do not seriously delay the healing process and that the person can return to activity more quickly with NSAIDs being part of the treatment. Another part of the controversy involves the adverse effects of gastrointestinal (GI) upset, nausea, dyspepsia (one in three patients), ulcers (1 to 2%), and skin eruptions of pruritus and urticaria. It is said that approximately 50% of all patients will have an adverse reaction and that of this group, 1 to 2% of these reactions could be serious. The practitioner must remember the "triad syndrome"—a patient with asthma, nasal polyps, and aspirin intolerance could have fatal reactions to NSAIDs.

REHABILITATION

There are three phases of tendon healing:

1. Cellular reaction to injury
2. Fibrous protein and collagen synthesis
3. Scar remodeling

This inflammatory process lasts approximately 5 to 7 days with the second phase of collagen synthesis starting 3 days after injury. It is necessary to consider the duration of injury vulnerability, always remembering that vulnerability to reinjury is proportional to the original severity of the tendon damage, the person's rate of healing, and the demand upon the tendon. Injured connective tissue may only have 70 to 80% of its original structural and biomechanical integrity up to and beyond 12 months after injury. Immobilization is detrimental to the outcome strength of the repaired tendon, adding a longer recovery time once immobilization is discontinued. Therefore, the practitioner must weigh the benefits versus the risks of each component of the treatment prescribed.

Most of the common types of tendinitis respond to a program of stretching and strengthening. The program should be progressive in both intensity and the amount of load on the tendon. It is important for a patient to hold each for a minimum of 10 to 30 seconds and to perform a minimum of 3 sets of 10 repetitions each day. It is critical to remember that all rehabilitation programs should begin with a program of ice prior to stretching and strengthening, and each session should conclude with the application of ice for an additional 20 minutes. An example of such a program would be:

• Ice for 10 to 15 minutes
• Warm up the area for 10 minutes with passive or active range-of-motion activities
• Perform stretching and strengthening exercises in a progressive program
• Ice for 20 minutes

BURSITIS

DISCUSSION

The bursa is the fluid-filled sac formed by two layers of synovial tissue; it contains a thin layer of joint fluid. The bursa is located in places where friction would occur within the body tissues, such as between tendon and bone or between skin and bone. Acute bursitis occurs because of sudden direct trauma to areas such as the prepatellar (between the patella and the skin) and the olecranon (between the olecranon process of the ulna and the skin). Overuse or repetitive trauma of muscles or tendons, constant external compression, or trauma (healing) causes chronic bursitis. In both acute and chronic bursitis the inflammatory reaction occurs within the bursa.

SYMPTOMS

Swelling, pain, some loss of function, and an increase in fluid in the bursa occurs. Chronic bursitis may result in the walls of the bursa thickening, possibly leading to calcific deposits and degeneration of the internal lining of the bursa.

TREATMENT

Use rest, compression, heat, and NSAIDs, and protect from further injury.

PAINFUL WRIST

Common complaints of a painful wrist include wrist tendinitis (see "Tendinitis," above), deQuervain tenosynovitis, carpometacarpal osteoarthritis, and ganglion cysts.

DeQuervain Tenosynovitis

DISCUSSION

DeQuervain tenosynovitis is an inflammation of the extensor pollicis brevis and abductor pollicis longus tendons of the thumb caused by overuse or repetitive gripping. This leads to the irritation of the tendons and the tendon sheath, resulting in a stenosing tenosynovitis (see Fig. 10-1-1).

SYMPTOMS

The patient will complain of pain, sharp or aching, which may radiate into the hand or forearm, and the inability to grip. There is local point

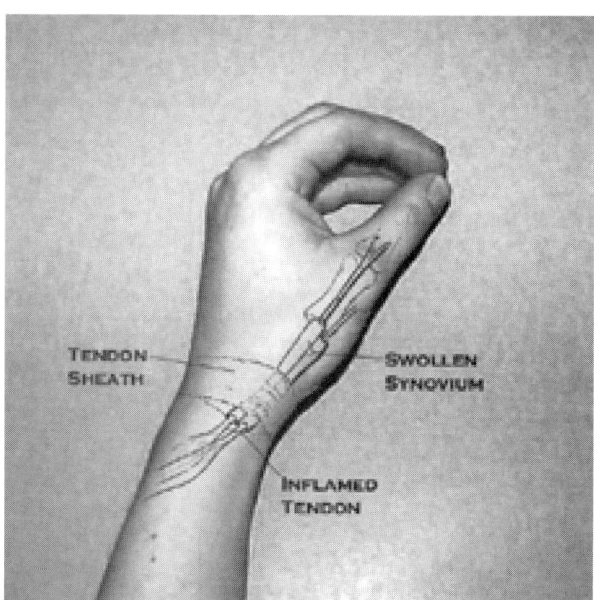

FIGURE 10-1-1. Stenosing tenosinovitis.

tenderness over the radial styloid process and weakness during thumb extension and abduction. Isometric or resistive extension or abduction of the thumb aggravates the pain. Patients may have a positive Finkelstein test. (Have the patient place his or her thumb into opposition (Fig. 10-1-2) and then curl the fingers over the thumb, that is, make a fist with the thumb inside.) Then ask the patient to put the wrist into ulnar deviation, causing a stretching of the tendon (Fig. 10-1-3). Pain in the extensor pollicis longus, extensor pollicis brevis, and abductor pollicis longus thumb tendons indicates a positive Finkelstein test result.

DIAGNOSTIC TESTS

X-rays of the wrist and thumb are usually normal but would be appropriate to rule out other differential diagnoses. The standard views include anteroposterior (AP), lateral, and pronation oblique and axial.

TREATMENT

The initial treatment consists of rest, ice, NSAIDs, and possibly phonophoresis. After the acute signs have resolved, ice treatment before and after passive stretching will help prevent a recurrence. Treatment is effective for 25 to 75% of those patients who receive only rest and immobilization. If conservative treatment fails, then a local injection of steroids or surgical decompression can be considered.

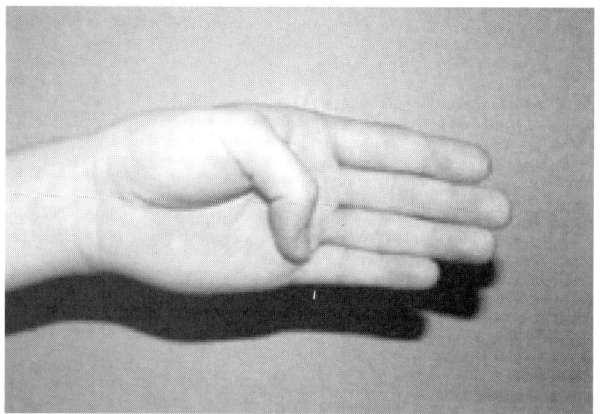

FIGURE 10-1-2. The first part of a Finkelstein test: the patient places the thumb into opposition.

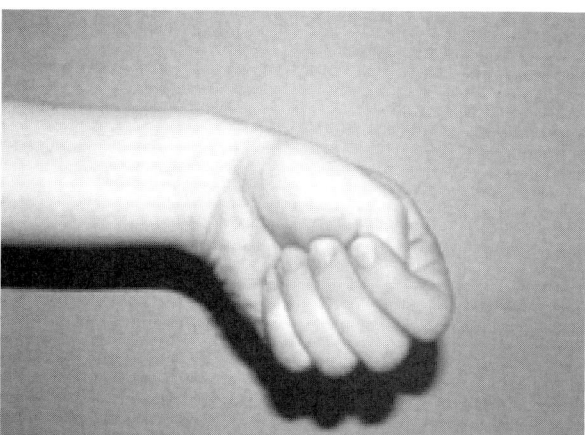

FIGURE 10-1-3. Finkelstein test (continued): the patient curls the fingers over the thumb and puts the wrist into ulnar deviation.

Carpometacarpal Osteoarthritis

DISCUSSION

The carpometacarpal (CMC) area is one of the more common sites for osteoarthritis. Patients who do repetitive gripping and grasping or who work with machinery that involves excessive vibration will often complain of pain at the base of the thumb (see Fig. 10-1-4).

SYMPTOMS

The patient may experience some joint crepitation with circumduction. Generally, there will be swelling, inflammation, and pain when the joint is moved to its extremes, and local tenderness over the volar and radial aspects of the joint. If this condition continues for several years, there will be bone enlargement at the base of the thumb, which may cause a bony deformity (shelf sign) and loss of motion. The patient may also experience subluxation of the joint.

DIAGNOSTIC TESTS

The x-ray of the thumb and wrist will usually show joint narrowing, spur formation, and some varying degree of bony sclerosis.

TREATMENT

Conservative treatment for this condition is initially rest, restriction of gripping and grasping motions, and administration of NSAIDs. If the condition does not improve, referral of the patient to a hand surgeon

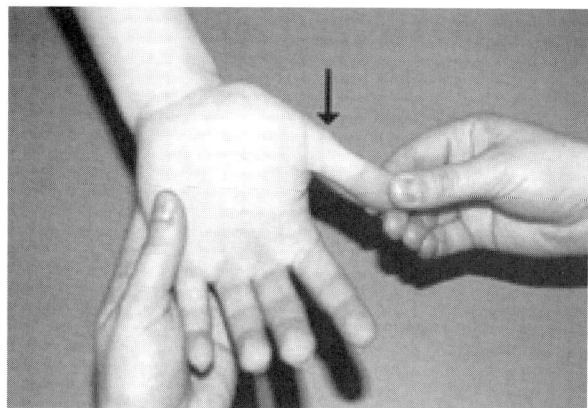

FIGURE 10-1-4. The carpometacarpal area at the base of the thumb.

is appropriate for possible local injection of steroids, implant arthroplasty, or tendon graft interposition.

Ganglion Cysts

DISCUSSION

A wrist ganglion is the herniation of the joint capsule or of the synovial sheath of a tendon. The cyst, containing a mucinous colorless fluid and a benign palpable mobile mass with minimal tenderness to pressure, usually appears slowly on the dorsal or volar radial aspect of the wrist (see Chap. 10-22).

TREATMENT

The general procedure for treatment of a ganglion cyst is aspiration with chemical cauterization and application of a compression bandage. If the cyst returns, than the next appropriate measure is to refer for surgical removal. This does not mean that a new cyst will not form; there is a recurrence rate of 5 to 10% with surgical excision (see Figs. 10-1-5 and 10-1-6).

DIFFERENTIAL DIAGNOSIS

The differential diagnosis for wrist ganglion includes carpal scaphoid fracture, base of the second and third metacarpal fracture, hamate hook fracture, Colles' fracture, carpal tunnel syndrome, dislocation of the lunate, bone tumor, and soft tissue tumor (benign or malignant).

PAINFUL ELBOW

Lateral and Medial Epicondylitis

DISCUSSION

Lateral epicondylitis (tennis elbow) is an inflammatory response to overuse of the extensor-supinator muscles attached to the lateral epicondyle from forced extension of the wrist, causing microtearing of

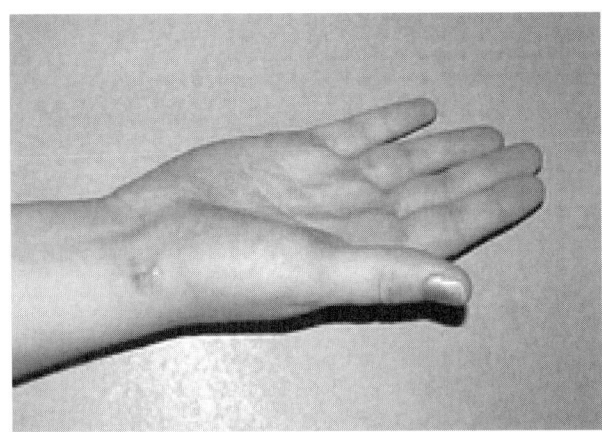

FIGURE 10-1-6. Ganglion cyst at the base of the thumb.

the extensor carpi radialis and the extensor carpi ulnaris, resulting in soft tissue failure. Medial epicondylitis (Little League elbow, golfer's elbow) is the inflammatory response to overuse of the flexor-pronator muscles attached to the medial epicondyle of the humerus.

SYMPTOMS

The patient will experience pain and weakness of the arm, with positive point tenderness over the lateral or medial epicondyle, and with pain that may radiate down the forearm or up into the brachial radialis in the case of lateral epicondylitis. This localized area is usually between the radial head and the lateral epicondyle. Pain is aggravated by resistive wrist extension/flexion and a strong gripping motion. Generally, there will be full range of motion, but in some cases there will be an inability to fully extend the elbow. Swelling of the epicondyle may or may not always be present. To test the elbow, apply resistance to the patient's extended hand with the elbow flexed from 45 to 90° while palpating either the lateral or medial epicondyle at the point of local tenderness. This maneuver will result in moderate to severe pain over the epicondyle (see Figs. 10-1-7 and 10-1-8).

DIAGNOSTIC TESTS

X-rays and laboratory tests are not necessary in the diagnosis of epicondylitis. However, x-rays would be used to distinguish a fracture or dislocation. The standard x-rays could include AP, lateral, and internal and external oblique; a reverse axial view may also be helpful. MRI is now used to diagnose any change in the tendons and ligaments.

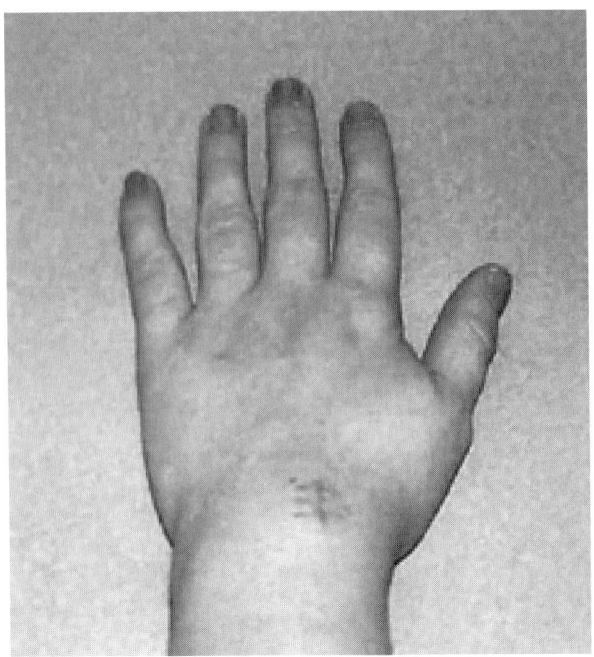

FIGURE 10-1-5. Ganglion cyst on the back of the hand.

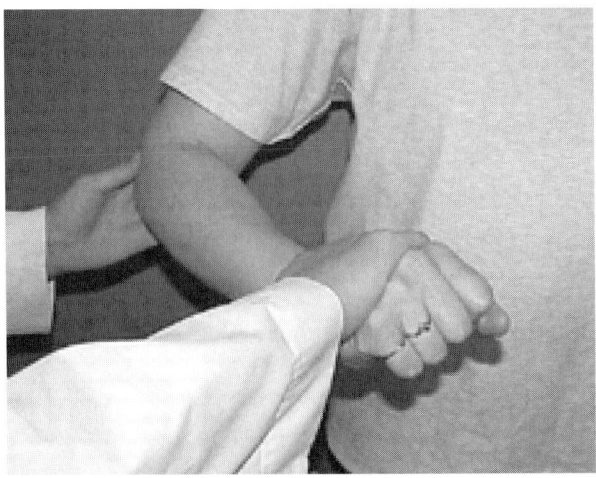

FIGURE 10-1-7. Testing the elbow for lateral epicondylitis.

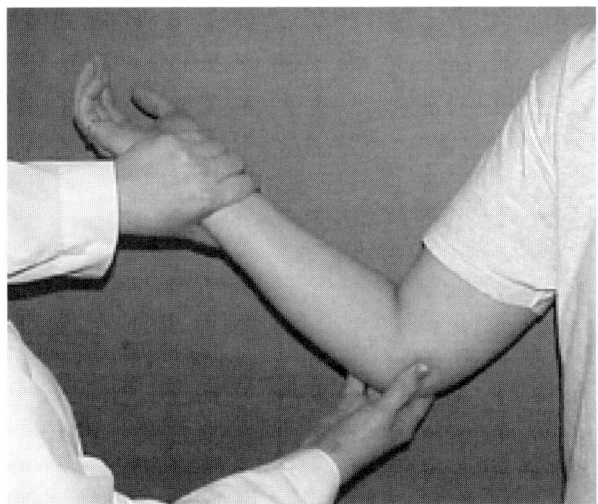

FIGURE 10-1-8. Testing the elbow for medial epicondylitis.

TREATMENT

Treatment of either lateral or medial epicondylitis includes rest, ice, phonophoresis, curvilinear bend, NSAIDs, and strengthening and stretching exercises. The key in treating epicondylitis is to have the patient begin a program of ice massage and stretching. The patient should stretch the arm so as to feel the stretch on either the lateral or medial epicondyle. The patient should hold the stretch position from 10 to 30 seconds for 10 repetitions, three times daily. Ideally, the patient would then progress to isotonic exercises that would strengthen the extensor or flexion muscles, always remembering the patient should begin with low weight (1 lb) and increase only after experiencing no pain or discomfort after the strengthening exercises. If conservative measures do not result in recovery, then the use of steroid injections would be appropriate. After a steroid injection the patient should rest the affected area for several weeks to ensure the healing process and to prevent any spontaneous rupture of the tendon.

DIFFERENTIAL DIAGNOSIS

The differential diagnosis for epicondylitis includes sprain of the collateral ligaments of the elbow, strain of the musculotendinous units of the upper extremity, fractures of the ulnar or radius, osteochondritis dissecans, and dislocation of the radial head. Dislocation of the radial head in association with an ulnar fracture is called a *Monteggia fracture.* Dislocation of the ulna with a fractured radius is called a *Galeazzi fracture.* Other problems to consider include dislocation of the olecranon process, referred pain of carpal tunnel syndrome, cervical radiculopathy, and rotator cuff tendinitis.

Olecranon Bursitis

DISCUSSION

Olecranon bursitis is the inflammation of the bursa located between the olecranon process of the ulna and the overlying skin. This inflammation can be caused by gradual (chronic) multiple small blows (draftsman's elbow, student's elbow), a single traumatic blow, repetitive flexion and extension of the elbow, or infection.

SYMPTOMS

The most common symptoms include stiffness and swelling posteriorly and tenderness. If there is pain, malaise, fever, and erythema, then infectious bursitis must be considered. If the bursitis becomes a chronic condition, there is the possibility of thickening of the bursal sac in 10 to 20% of patients.

DIAGNOSTIC TESTS

X-rays are considered to be unnecessary for the diagnosis, unless there is a question of a possible fracture or dislocation. If infectious bursitis is being considered, the practitioner should aspirate the elbow and get the following laboratory values to evaluate the fluid: cell count, gram stain, crystal analysis, and hematocrit.

TREATMENT

Conservative treatment includes rest, ice, NSAIDs or other analgesics for pain, and compression. Remember that with an elbow that has marked swelling, heat, and erythema, the fluid will have to be aspirated to rule out sepsis. If conservative treatment does not produce results, the practitioner can refer for aspiration and steroid injections. With chronic olecranon bursitis, the patient should be referred for possible surgical excision.

DIFFERENTIAL DIAGNOSIS

The differential diagnosis for olecranon bursitis includes gout, infection, and fracture of the olecranon process of the ulna.

PAINFUL SHOULDER

Common complaints of a painful shoulder include acromioclavicular (AC) separations and sprains, bicipital tendinitis, rotator cuff tears, and adhesive capsulitis.

Acromioclavicular Joint: Separations and Sprains

DISCUSSION

The AC joint and ligaments are susceptible to injury from trauma and from overuse syndromes. The joint comprises three important ligaments that hold the acromion, clavicle, and coracoid process together. They are the AC ligament, the coracoclavicular AC ligament, and the coracoacromial ligament. During trauma the ligaments can experience varying degrees of tearing. A first-degree sprain of any of the ligaments is a stretching or partial disruption of the ligament. A second-degree sprain and/or separation is partial tearing of the superior and inferior AC ligament. A third-degree sprain and/or separation is a complete tearing of the superior and inferior AC and the coracoclavicular ligaments, and when the AC ligament and the coracoclavicular ligament are both completely torn, then this is often referred to as a third-degree sprain or separation.

SYMPTOMS

The patient presents with the arm held close to the side and complains of pain and tenderness to palpation, and there may be swelling and deformity. Pain is also produced with downward traction or possible adduction across the chest. A second- or third-degree separation or sprain may include joint widening when traction is applied. A first-degree sprain presents with point tenderness, pain during range of motion (ROM), and no deformity. A second-degree sprain or separation also has point tenderness, decreased ROM in abduction, and slight deformity. A third-degree sprain or separation will have point tenderness, decreased ROM, and increased deformity.

DIAGNOSTIC TESTS

Suggested x-ray views include AP, lateral, axillary, and internal and external AP views. The use of weighted x-ray views of the shoulder may show widening between the clavicle and the acromial process. If this demonstrates a >5-mm separation, then this is an indication of a separation.

TREATMENT

The initial treatment is to limit the ROM of the arm. This can be accomplished by the use of a shoulder immobilizer for 2 to 4 weeks or until the patient does not experience pain. The shoulder should be treated with ice for the first 48 to 72 hours. The patient should not be allowed to lift objects that weigh more than 10 to 20 lb and may return to activity only after full ROM without pain is present.

Bicipital Tendinitis

DISCUSSION

The tendon of the long head of the biceps can become inflamed as it passes through the bicipital (intertubercular) groove of the anterior head of the humerus. This tendon extends intra-articularly under the acromial process through the rotator cuff to its insertion at the top of the glenoid. Repeated irritation of this tendon leads to microtearing and degenerative changes. This process could lead to spontaneous rupture and also subluxation of the tendon out of its groove, which generally occurs when the transverse ligament is ruptured.

SYMPTOMS

Pain aggravated by lifting or overhead pushing and pulling that is localized to the proximal humerus and anterior shoulder joint is diagnostic. There will be localized tenderness approximately 1 inch below the anterolateral tip of the acromion, when the practitioner palpates the passively moving arm during internal and external rotation. Resistive supination of the forearm with elbow flexion aggravates the pain. A positive Yergason test is used to measure instability and produces pain in the bicipital groove as the patient flexes the elbow at a 90° angle with the wrist supinated against resistance. (see Fig. 10-1-9). A bicipital

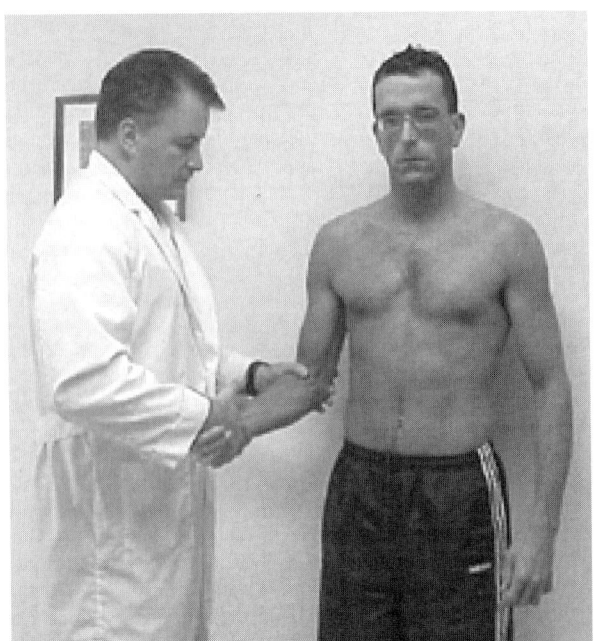

FIGURE 10-1-9. Yergason test for bicipital tendinitis.

tendon that has ruptured presents as a bulge several inches above the antecubital fossa. The patient experiences a popping or snapping sensation as the tendon ruptures.

DIAGNOSTIC TESTS

X-rays do not show tendinitis but help in the evaluation of possible calcification in the bicipital groove.

TREATMENT

Rest, ice, phonophoresis, high-voltage electric stimulation, and NSAIDs are all appropriate modalities of treatment. After the first 24 to 48 hours, the patient should begin with pendulum stretch exercises, progressing to isotonic exercises to help strengthen the tendon's internal and external rotators and avoiding horizontal abduction during the early stages of rehabilitation. If after 6 months conservative treatment is unsuccessful, then the patient should be considered a candidate for surgical intervention. Ten percent of cases progress to spontaneous rupture. Surgical repair of a biceps tendon rupture is not usually suggested for noncompetitive patients.

Rotator Cuff Tears

DISCUSSION

The rotator cuff muscles of the shoulder include the supraspinatus, infraspinatus, teres minor, and subscapularis (SITS). The mechanism of injury (MOI) of rotator cuff injuries is the loss of normal integrity of the tendons from repetitive overhead activities, such as pitching, swimming, and serving in tennis, all of which cause microtrauma. The most likely tendon to be injured is that of the supraspinatus and then the infraspinatus muscles. As a patient engages in repetitive overuse activities, the rotator cuff may impinge on the acromion and the overlying coracoacromial ligament, causing microtrauma to the cuff and resulting in local inflammation, edema, cuff softening, pain, and poor function of the cuff. The poor blood supply to the tendon is suggested as one cause of early degeneration. Other MOIs that cause rotator cuff tears would be those of an acute injury, such as a fall on an outstretched arm or directly onto the outer shoulder that causes the humeral head to impact against the acromion, which could cause a tear to the cuff.

SYMPTOMS

The patient experiences pain and weakness on external rotation and abduction. This position is commonly called the "empty can" position: the arm is in 90° ≠ of horizontal abduction, 30° ≠ of forward flexion, and internally rotated (see Fig. 10-1-10). When the patient has a partial tear, the motion of reaching overhead is not smooth. A patient who has a complete tear is unable to reach overhead, migrate anteriorly and superiorly, and may have the drop arm sign (see Fig. 10-1-11). The patient has decreased ROM, muscle atrophy, muscle weakness, and crepitus in the supraspinatus. There may also be swelling of the subacromial bursa and the glenohumeral joint with large rotator cuff tears.

DIAGNOSTIC TESTS

The use of routine x-rays does not help in the diagnosis of rotator cuff tears but may show rotator cuff tendon calcification in approximately 30% of cases. The standard views for the shoulder are transaxillary lateral, AP internal, and AP external. MRI is now used to show large transverse tears, but it may not be able to differentiate partial tears. MRI has been shown to be 95 to 100% accurate for full thickness tears and approximately 80% accurate for partial thickness tears. The use of arthrography has been beneficial to the diagnosis of tears of the rotator cuff. Other diagnostic tests used for differential diagnoses could

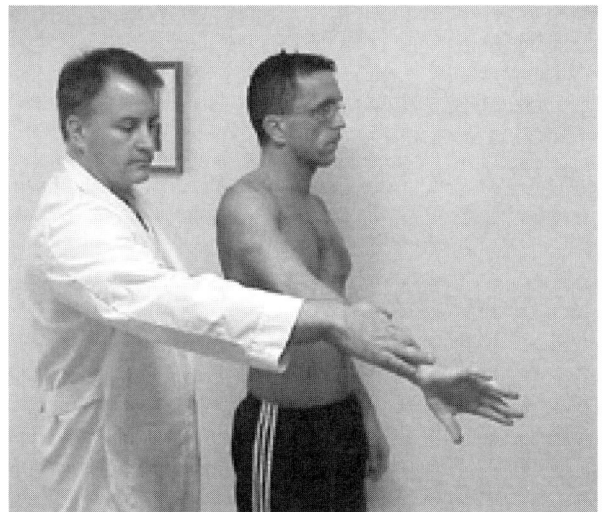

FIGURE 10-1-10. The "empty can" position.

include erythrocyte sedimentation rate, a complete blood count, and a rheumatoid factor.

TREATMENT

If the underlying problem is tendinitis, treatment is the same as for most tendinitis injuries. This includes rest, restriction of overhead motion, cold or heat, iontophoresis or phonophoresis, microelectric nerve stimulation, NSAIDs, and stretching and strengthening programs (ice prior to and after exercise program). A patient who does not respond to conservative treatments should be referred for possible steroid injection or surgery. Steroids must be used with caution because of the degeneration of the tendon and softening of the cuff during the early stages following injection. Surgery should be a consideration after 6 months to 1 year of conservative treatment with the understanding that there is a 95% success rate with conservative treatment.

Adhesive Capsulitis: Frozen Shoulder

DISCUSSION

When the patient complains of shoulder pain with significant loss of shoulder ROM, consider the diagnosis of adhesive capsulitis. Whenever a patient experiences any type of inflammatory process, such as

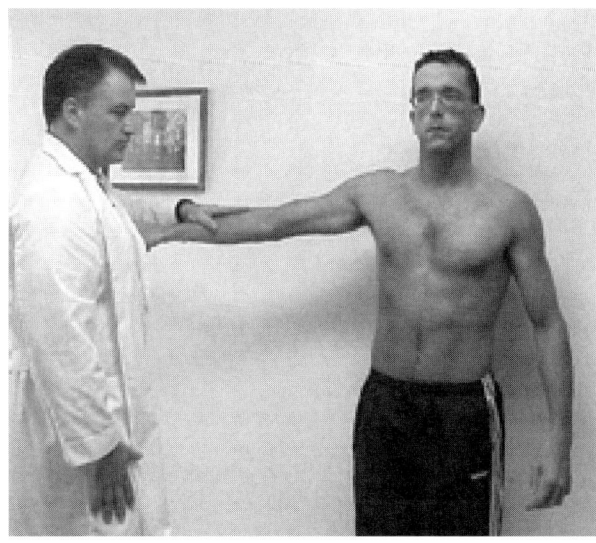

FIGURE 10-1-11. The drop arm sign.

rotator cuff tendinitis, acute subacromial bursitis, or fractures that occur at the head or neck of the humerus, it could lead to progressive limitation in the ROM. Adhesions often form between the joint capsule and the humeral head. This condition can also be caused by the lack of complete ROM over a long period of time. Commonly, this is associated with older adults who do not raise their arms over their head on a daily basis and is often referred to as a frozen shoulder.

SYMPTOMS

The patient may complain of shoulder pain or discomfort, occurring primarily at night, with decreased ROM (external rotation and abduction). As the condition progresses, the pain diminishes, and the ROM becomes progressively less. Common findings in a patient include an inability to raise the arms above the head and a decrease in passive ROM. Normal external rotation is 90°, and normal abduction is from 90 to 120°. The patient is unable to perform the Apley scratch test, which requires patients to reach the midback at the T8 to T10 ventral level with one hand.

DIAGNOSTIC TESTS

Routine shoulder x-rays can be used to help differentiate the diagnosis. Another radiology test that is used is arthrography, in which a normal glenohumeral joint fills with 7 or 8 mL of the contrast agent, as compared with a joint in an advanced case of adhesive capsulitis that will only accept 4 to 5 mL of contrast agent.

TREATMENT

Conservative treatment involves the slow program of heat application prior to stretching with weighted pendulum exercises and passive stretch exercises.

DIFFERENTIAL DIAGNOSIS

The differential diagnosis for adhesive capsulitis includes sternoclavicular dislocation, clavicular fractures, cervical disk disease, brachial plexus (thoracic outlet syndrome), and referred pain of spleen and gallbladder.

PAINFUL ANKLE

Common complaints of a painful ankle include lateral and medial ankle ligament sprains, peroneal tendon injury, and Achilles tendinitis.

Lateral Ankle Ligament Sprains

DISCUSSION

The ankle is one of the most commonly injured joints of patients involved in sports and everyday activities. The three bony structures that make up the ankle joint (hinge joint) are the talus, distal fibula, and distal tibia. There are also three ligamentous complexes that help to stabilize the joint: the lateral complex, medial complex, and interosseous complex (syndesmotic ligaments). Lateral ankle sprains account for 85 to 95% of all ankle sprains and involve the lateral ligamentous complex of the anterior talofibular ligament, the calcaneofibular ligament, and the posterior talofibular ligament (see Fig. 10-1-12). An ankle placed in a plantar flexed position has increased instability because of the position of the talus in the mortise. This position also causes the anterior talofibular ligament to be taut and at risk for injury, since the medial malleolus may act as a fulcrum, predisposing the ankle to lateral or inversion sprains. The MOI is usually a cutting action or landing on an uneven surface, such as another person's foot.

A lateral inversion sprain of the ankle most commonly occurs from the anterior ligament to the posterior ligament, with the most frequent

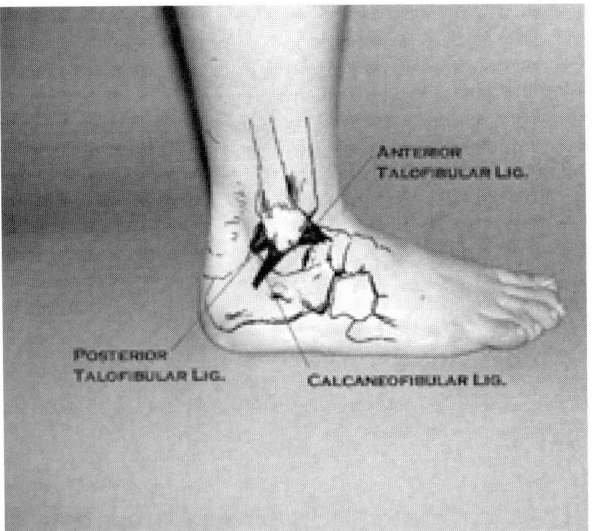

FIGURE 10-1-12. Affected areas of lateral ankle ligament sprains.

being an anterior talofibular ligament sprain. Sprains are classified as first, second, and third degree. A first-degree sprain has minor tearing of the ligament, usually of the ankle. A second-degree sprain is a partial tear of the anterior talofibular ligament with a minimal tear of the calcaneofibular ligament, resulting in ankle instability. A third-degree lateral sprain is a complete tear of the ligament with gross instability of the ankle joint.

SYMPTOMS

The patient complains of pain and joint tenderness over the injured ligament, localized swelling, decreased ROM, and ecchymosis, and may even have a palpable gap in the ligament. To differentiate further the degree of injury: with a first-degree lateral ankle sprain there is point tenderness over the anterior talofibular ligament, with little or no instability, a negative anterior drawer sign, and negative stress x-ray; with a second-degree ankle sprain there is also a moderate anterior drawer sign, with normal stress x-rays or minimal talar tilt with moderate instability; and with a third-degree ankle sprain there is both a positive anterior drawer sign and positive stress films.

To perform an anterior drawer test, grasp the patient's heel by cupping it firmly in one hand. While pulling the foot forward, push posteriorly on the anterior aspect of the distal tibia with the other hand (Fig. 10-1-13). To complete the evaluation of the ankle, a compression

test and/or heel tap should be performed (Figs. 10-1-14 and 10-1-15). A positive compression test and/or heel tap is usually associated with a fracture.

DIAGNOSTIC TESTS

Routine x-rays of all ankle injuries include AP, lateral, mortise (AP with external rotation of 15 to 20% of the foot), oblique, and inversion stress. These help differentiate the type of ankle injury, for example, sprain or fracture. If the x-ray indicates 15 to 30° of tilt of the talus within the mortise, then the anterior talofibular ligament and the calcaneofibular ligament are torn.

TREATMENT

The initial treatment for an acute ankle sprain includes rest, ice, compression, and elevation (RICE) and the use of NSAIDs. Rest requires non–weight-bearing for the first 24 hours. Ice should be applied 20 minutes on and 20 minutes off while awake during the first 24 hours. Compression can be accomplished by the use of an elastic wrap, with care given to proper circulation. A more successful procedure for compression is to apply an open-basket taping procedure or an Unna boot (see Figs. 10-1-16 and 10-1-17). The open-basket taping allows for swelling to form on the dorsal surface not in the ankle mortise. All the procedures for compression should be applied with the ankle in neutral position, so that the ankle mortise is closed. This helps prevent further swelling within the mortise and reduces the recovery time of the patient. Finally, elevation of the ankle should be above the heart to help reduce the dependent swelling. A second-degree sprain requires more rehabilitation time, whereas treatment for a third-degree sprain may include surgical repair of the ligament. The use of cold whirlpools for 15 to 20 minutes two to three times daily helps speed recovery. The use of cold helps to produce a local anesthesia, which decreases tissue metabolism and ultimately causes vasodilation, which assists in the reduction of swelling and removal of hematoma. During the whirlpool treatment, the patient should be asked to move the ankle in flexion and extension because it has been shown that early progressive weight-bearing and movement encourages early healing and return to normal function. Refer back to the discussion on tendinitis for further explanation. Any rehabilitation program should begin with a cold whirlpool, progress to resistive exercises including heel cord stretching, continue with application of cold for 20 minutes, and conclude with taping or putting an air cast on the ankle until no pain occurs and

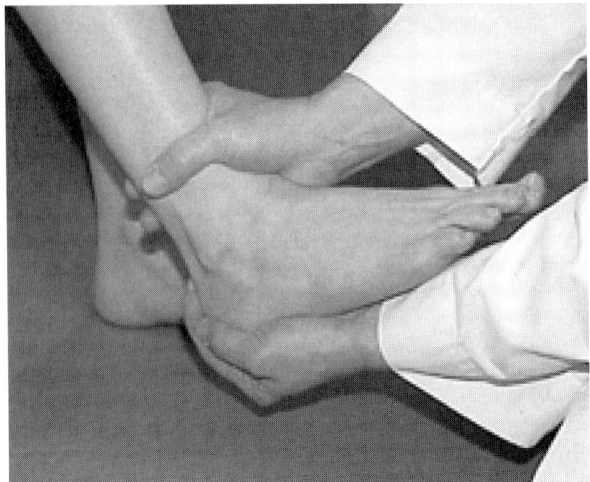

FIGURE 10-1-13. Anterior drawer test.

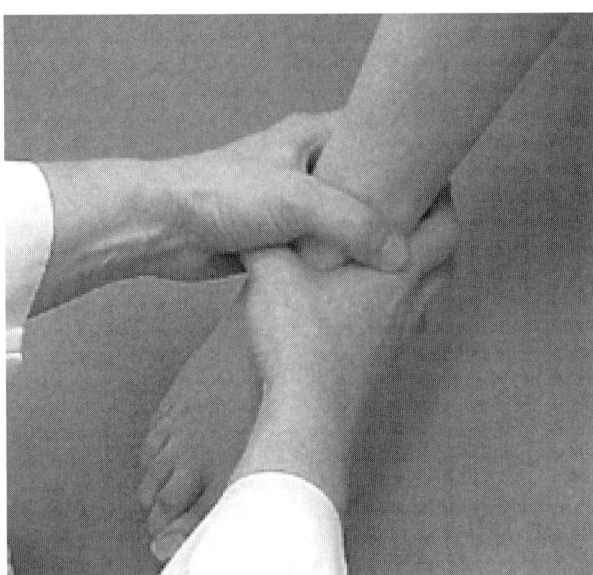

FIGURE 10-1-14. Compression test.

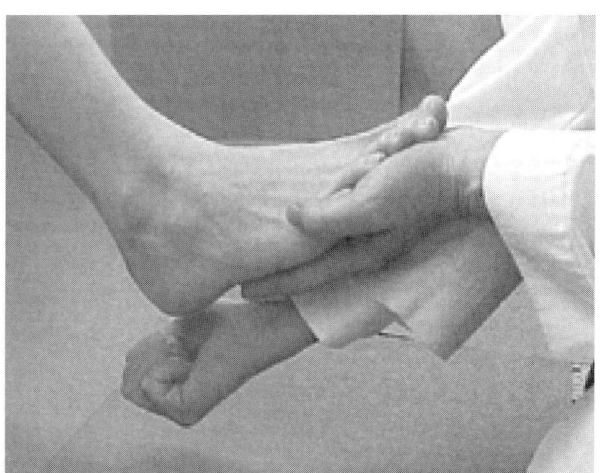

FIGURE 10-1-15. Heel tap.

stability returns. The patient should work on strengthening the ankle, with particular attention to restoring full strength to the peroneal muscles.

MEDIAL ANKLE LIGAMENT SPRAINS

DISCUSSION

The ligament of the medial complex of the ankle is called the *deltoid ligament.* It consists of both superficial and deep fibers and serves as the primary resistance to foot eversion. The medial ligament sprain or eversion sprain occurs less frequently and is often associated with a fracture of the lateral malleolus and/or rupture of the syndesmosis. The most common MOI is any action similar to stepping into a hole.

SYMPTOMS

The patient complains of pain, point tenderness, swelling, decreased ROM, and ecchymosis with increased instability.

DIAGNOSTIC TESTS

Routine x-rays of all ankle injuries include AP, lateral, and oblique. These help differentiate the type of ankle injury, that is, sprain or fracture.

TREATMENT

The initial treatment should be RICE and NSAIDs. (see "Lateral Ankle Ligament Sprains," above.)

Peroneal Tendon Injuries

The peroneal tendons act as the primary lateral dynamic stabilizers of the ankle joint, and injury to these tendons occurs during forced plantar flexion and valgus of the foot. This occurs during maximal eccentric contraction when a load is applied. Injuries to these tendons include tendinitis, subluxation, and rupture.

Peroneal Tendinitis

DISCUSSION

Tendinitis occurs because of the placement of tendons around the lateral malleolus (see Fig. 10-1-18). Because of the pulley action around the tendon, the results can be decreased vascularity, inflammation, and degenerative changes.

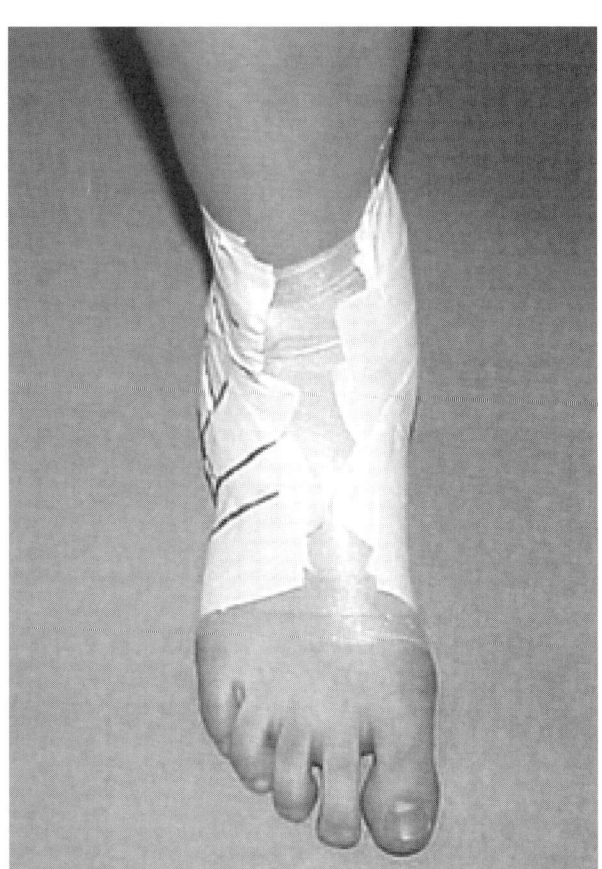

FIGURE 10-1-16. Elastic wrap.

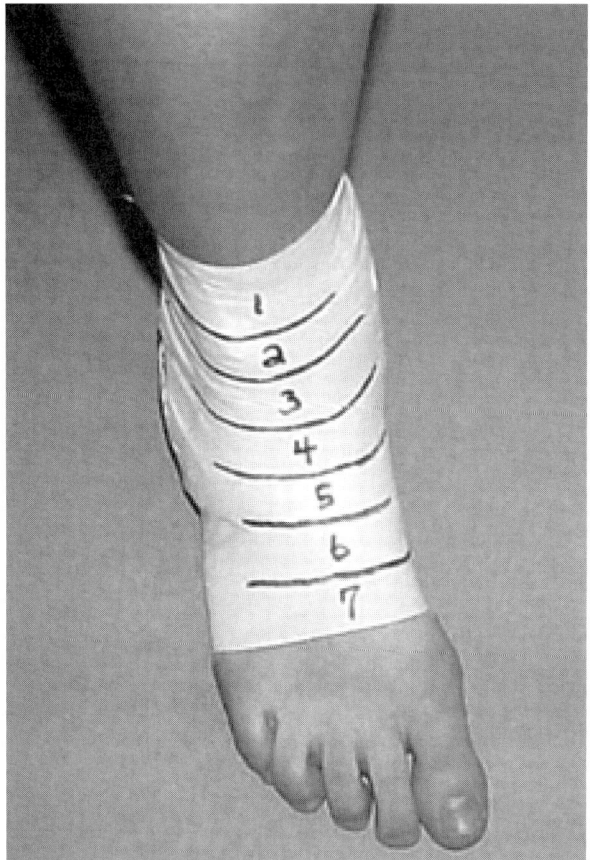

FIGURE 10-1-17. Open-basket taping procedure.

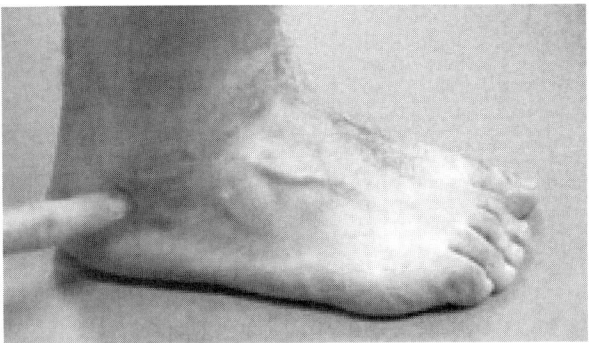

FIGURE 10-1-18. Placement of tendons around the lateral maleolus.

SYMPTOMS

The patient complains of pain and point tenderness over the lateral malleolus, swelling, ecchymosis, and increased pain with active eversion.

DIAGNOSTIC TESTS

Standard lower leg and ankle x-rays are appropriate, but MRI provides more information in determining the degree of injury to the tendon. (See "Tendinitis" above for further information about the use of MRI.)

TREATMENT

The initial treatment should be RICE and NSAIDs. (See "Lateral Ankle Ligament Sprains," above.) It is important to remember that the inflammatory response lasts approximately 48 hours and is vital to the healing phase. Since collagen protein is produced 3 to 4 days following injury, it is necessary to limit inflammation by the use of NSAIDs and cryotherapy. (See "Tendinitis," above.)

Peroneal Subluxation

DISCUSSION

The MOI is a forceful dorsiflexion with inversion and contracture of the peroneal tendons, which causes the retinaculum of the joint to rupture and the tendons to subluxate in front of the distal fibula.

SYMPTOMS

The patient complains of swelling and point tenderness with possible subluxation (snapping) of the tendons.

DIAGNOSTIC TESTS

Standard lower leg and ankle x-rays are appropriate, but MRI provides more information in determining the degree of injury to the tendon. (See "Tendinitis" above for further information about the use of MRI.)

TREATMENT

The initial treatment should be RICE and NSAIDs, then non–weight-bearing for 4 weeks in a cast or surgery.

Peroneal Rupture

This is rare and would require surgery.

Achilles Tendinitis

DISCUSSION

The Achilles tendon is the largest tendon in the body. An inflammatory response to overload triggered by microscopic tearing of the collagen fibers is a complaint of the lower leg. This could occur because of both intrinsic and extrinsic conditions. The intrinsic conditions include malalignment, tight hamstrings or calf muscles, cavus feet, heel or forefoot varus deformity, excessive supination and hyperpronation in midstance, and tight heel cord. The extrinsic conditions are often the result of training errors, such as increased mileage, increased intensity of the sessions, repetitive hill running, progressing too quickly, running on uneven surfaces, and poor shoes.

SYMPTOMS

The patient complains of pain, swelling, crepitation, heat, erythema, weakness secondary to pain, decreased motion, and tenderness to palpation. Chronic symptoms include increased vascularity, thickening of tissue (tenosynovitis), and possibly nodules.

DIAGNOSTIC TESTS

Standard lower leg and ankle x-rays are appropriate, but MRI provides more information in determining the degree of injury to the tendon. (See "Tendinitis" above for further information about the use of MRI.)

TREATMENT

The initial treatment should be RICE, NSAIDs, gentle stretching, ultrasound, and orthotics, which may include the use of a heel lift (0.5 to 0.75 inches). The nodules can be surgically removed. Steroid injections should be avoided because they weaken the tendon, which could result in rupture.

Achilles Rupture

DISCUSSION

Achilles rupture usually occurs as a result of a rapid push-off with the knee extended or landing with the foot in dorsiflexion. The rupture occurs more often 1 to 2 inches above the insertion on the calcaneus, with patients describing the injury as if someone had kicked them in the back of the leg.

SYMPTOMS

Patients initially complain that they feel as if someone kicked the back of their leg. They present with pain, swelling, possibly a palpable gap, weak or absent plantar flexion of the foot, inability to walk on the toes, and possibly a positive Thompson test. The Thompson test is performed by squeezing the muscle belly of the gastrocnemius-soleus muscle while the patient is either in the prone position or on the knees in a chair. Squeezing the muscle will normally cause the ankle to plantar flex (see Fig. 10-1-19).

DIAGNOSTIC TESTS

Standard lower leg and ankle x-rays are appropriate, but MRI provides more information in determining the degree of injury to the tendon. (See "Tendinitis" above for further information about the use of MRI.)

TREATMENT

The initial treatment should be RICE and NSAIDs. Following this, conservative treatment includes casting the lower leg in slight plantar

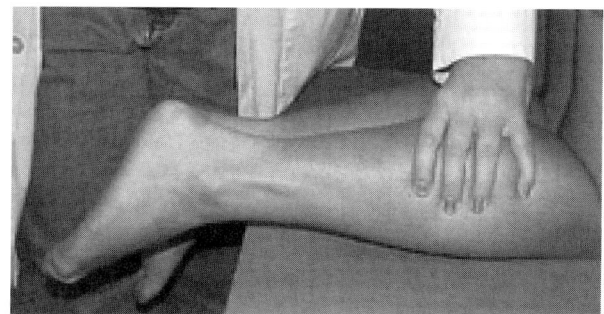

FIGURE 10-1-19. The Thompson test.

flexion for 3 to 6 weeks. This is the procedure often followed for older or nonactive patients and for partial tears of the Achilles tendon. For a complete tear of the tendon, and for athletes, the surgical approach is preferred. Surgery restores 75% to 90% of original function and requires an aggressive rehabilitation program of 3 to 4 months.

DIFFERENTIAL DIAGNOSIS OF COMMON ANKLE PAIN

The differential diagnosis should include undisplaced spiral fracture of the fibula, avulsion fracture of the distal tip of the fibula, fracture of the fifth metatarsal, posterior tibial tendinitis, and stress fracture.

BIBLIOGRAPHY

Anderson B: *Office Orthopedics for Primary Care Diagnosis and Treatment.* Philadelphia, Saunders, 1995.
Anderson M, Hall S: *Sports Injury Management.* Baltimore, Williams & Wilkins, 1995.
Donnelly R: Recognizing and managing Achilles tendon rupture. *JAAPA* 7:406–414, 1994.
Kahler D, McCue F III: Metacarpophalangeal and proximal interphalangeal joint injuries of the hand, including the thumb—Injuries of the hand and wrist. *Clin Sports Med* 11:57–76, 1992.
Kiefhaber T, Stern P: Upper extremity tendinitis and overuse syndromes in the athlete—Injuries of the hand and wrist. *Clin Sports Med* 11:39–56, 1992.
Mirabetio S et al: The wrist: Field evaluation and treatment—Injuries of the hand and wrist. *Clin Sports Med* 11:1–26, 1992.
O'Brien M: Functional anatomy and physiology of tendons—Tendinitis I. Basic concepts. *Clin Sports Med* 11:505–520, 1992.
Snider RK (ed.): *The Essentials of Musculoskeletal Care.* Rosemont, IL, American Academy of Orthopaedic Surgeons, 1997.

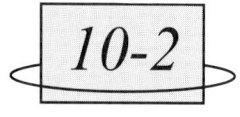

COMMON FRACTURES AND DISLOCATIONS

Karen A. Newell

DISCUSSION

The intent of this chapter is to review pertinent anatomy and basic orthopedic principles involved in the identification, management, and treatment of common fractures and dislocations. The various types of fractures are listed in Table 10-2-1 and Fig. 10-2-1. The various types of reductions and a listing of abnormal healing definitions are found in Table 10-2-2.

It is imperative that accurate terminology and description be used when discussing specific fractures. Fractures are always discussed with the location of the distal fragments in relation to the proximal fragment. *Displacement* refers to an amount of lateral movement of the distal fragment with relationship to the more proximal fragment while

TABLE 10-2-1. Types of Fractures and Dislocations

Open or compound fracture	
Fracture communicates with the outside environment through skin that is broken (may be subtle). (See Table 10-2-3 for the Gustilo-Anderson classification.)	
Closed or simple fracture	
Fracture has no potential for communication with the outside environment. Skin is intact.	
Complete fracture	
Both cortices are broken.	
Incomplete fracture	
One cortex is broken. Example: greenstick, buckle, or torus (common in children), where force applied bows the bone in such a way that only one side fractures.	
Transverse fracture	
Fracture line is perpendicular to the long axis of the bone.	
Oblique fracture	
Fracture line runs oblique to the long axis of the bone.	
Spiral fracture	
Fracture is associated with rotational forces that spiral down the long axis of the bone.	
Comminuted fracture	
Fracture produces two or more fragments.	
Segmental fracture	
This type of comminuted fracture involves a free central fragment between two main sections of bone.	
Articular fracture	
Fracture extends into or involves the articulating surface of a joint.	
Pathologic fracture	
Fracture occurs secondary to diseased or abnormal bone.	
Stress fracture	
Repetitive forces can weaken bone.	
Avulsion fracture	
Ligaments or tendons have pulled off a bony fragment ("chip").	
Depressed fracture	
Fracture fragment is depressed below the bone surface.	
Impaction	
This crush injury occurs when bone is forced into bone. A compression of bone.	
Dislocation	
The articular surfaces of bones that usually form a joint are completely out of contact with one another; usually associated with damage to the joint capsule and surrounding soft tissue structures.	
Subluxation	
Incomplete dislocations in which the articular surfaces of bones that usually form a joint are partially out of contact with one another.	

maintaining alignment with the long axis of the bone (e.g., 50% displaced means half the bone width is displaced laterally between the distal and proximal fragments).

Nondisplaced fractures (without lateral movement of the distal fragment) maintain alignment with the long axis of the bone on both anteroposterior and lateral x-ray views. *Separation* refers to the distance in millimeters the two fragments are from each other

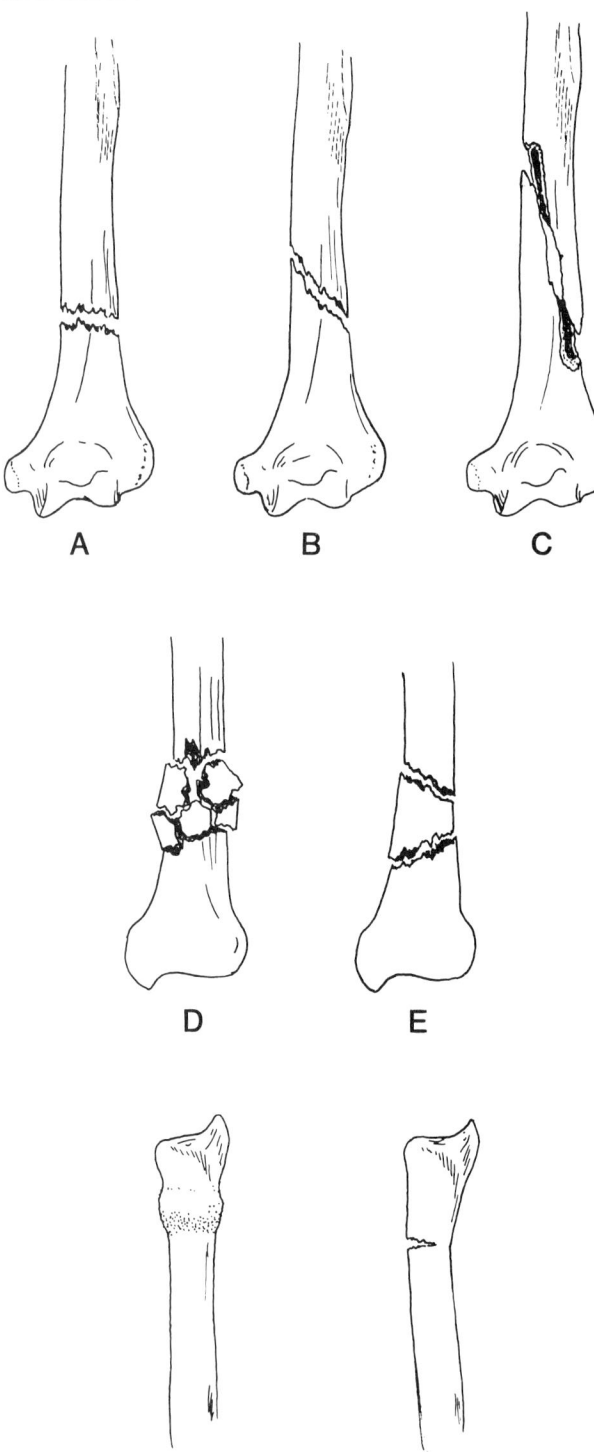

FIGURE 10-2-1. Fracture line orientation. (A) Transverse. (B) Oblique. (C) Spiral. (D) Comminuted. (E) Segmental. (F) Torus. (G) Greenstick. (*SOURCE: From Tintinalli et al. Used with permission from 5th ed. p. 1743 old Fig. 259-1.*)

(see Fig. 10-2-2). The distal fragment long axis and the proximal fragment long axis are at an angle that can be measured in degrees and described with the distal fragment location with respect to the proximal fragment; this measurement is called *angulation.*

RED FLAGS

Any open fracture or joint requires immediate consultation with an orthopedic service and typically is surgically irrigated in the operating

TABLE 10-2-2. Types of Reductions and Abnormal Healing Definitions

CLOSED REDUCTION
Correction of the fracture from external manipulation, considered conservative management
Open reduction internal fixation (ORIF)
Correction of the fracture by surgical repair usually requiring placement of hardware (e.g., plates, screws)

DELAYED UNION
Slow bone healing (usually considered delayed if not fully healed by 6 months)
Nonunion
Failure of fragments of bone to demonstrate radiologic evidence of healing by 4 to 6 months
Malunion
Fracture that has healed in an unacceptable position (usually angulated, rotated, or shortened)

room. On initial presentation give consideration to obtaining wound cultures, keeping the patient off foods and liquids, initiating intravenous prophylactic antibiotics such as 1 g cefazolin or 1 g ceftriaxone, and considering tetanus prophylaxis. The wound should be dressed with sterile gauze soaked in normal saline covering any exposed bone. It is important to note whether the fracture extends into the joint line or articulating surface (intra-articular). These often require special consideration by an orthopedic service (See Table 10-2-3.)

Fractures in children that involve the epiphyseal plate, which is the location for bone growth, are particularly important and should include consultation with an orthopedic service, particularly if they are displaced (see Fig. 10-2-3).

HISTORY

A detailed mechanism of injury is invaluable information obtained from the patient or any witnesses in orthopedic trauma. The specific location of the pain and what type of motion exacerbates or relieves the pain is also helpful information. Check for any areas of anesthesia or paresthesia. Get previous medical and surgical history, including current medications and allergies. Knowledge of the patient's dominant hand, occupation, and serious hobbies are important for clinical decision-making. Carefully document, including any previous musculoskeletal injury and baseline status prior to new injury. Obtaining past medical history of conditions such as diabetes mellitus, peripheral vascular disease, smoking, and chronic steroid use is important, as these factors may impair healing.

PHYSICAL EXAMINATION

Carefully inspect the skin for associated laceration, abrasion, or communication with the underlying fracture or joint. Note any swelling,

TABLE 10-2-3. Gustilo-Anderson Open Fracture Classification

TYPE	DESCRIPTION
I	Low-energy wound that is usually less than 1 cm, often caused by bone piercing the skin
II	Wound greater than 1 cm in length with moderate soft tissue damage secondary to higher-energy trauma
III	High-energy wound that is usually greater than 10 cm with extensive soft tissue damage (other injuries considered type III include high-velocity gunshot wound, segmental fracture, coexisting vascular injury, significant diaphyseal bone loss, fracture sustained in agricultural environment, and crush injury from a moving vehicle)

SOURCE: From Kozin and Berlet. Handbook of Common Orthopaedic Fractures, *2nd ed, p. 162.*

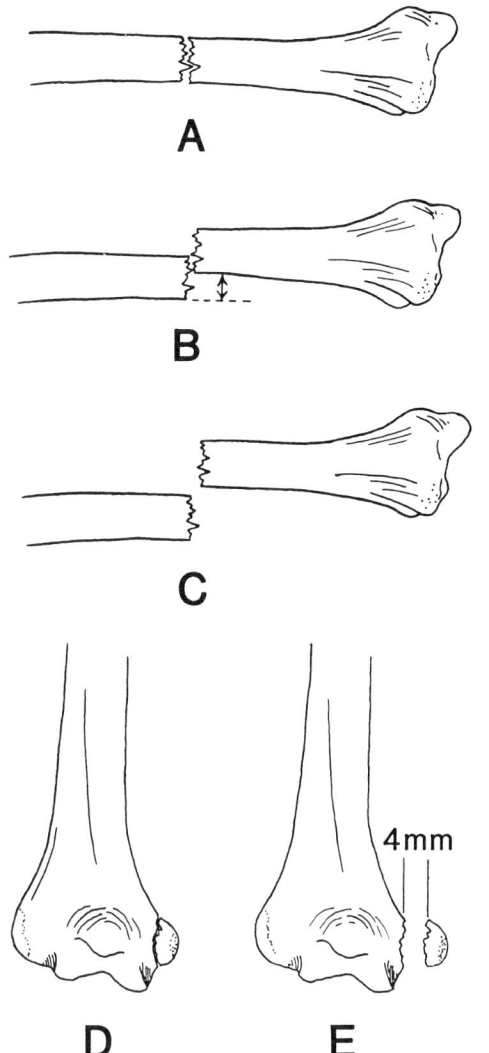

FIGURE 10-2-2. Fracture displacement and separation: **(A)** No displacement, slight separation; **(B)** 50% dorsal displacement; **(C)** Complete dorsal displacement; **(D)** Nondisplaced, no separation; **(E)** 4 mm separation. (*SOURCE: From Tintinalli et al, p 1209. Used with permission.*)

discoloration, or deformity of the site. Thoroughly palpate, including all bones and joints, especially the joint above and the joint below the injury site. Perform a meticulous neurovascular examination, including range of motion, motor, and sensory functions, all pulses, and capillary refill distal to the affected extremity. It may be helpful to compare with the contralateral side. Do not administer local anesthetics until after the sensory examination. All jewelry on the affected extremity should be removed. A ring cutter may be necessary in some cases.

RADIOLOGIC STUDIES

Consider obtaining films of the joint above and the joint below the injury site. Possible films of the uninvolved side for comparison are especially helpful in children with physis injury. Typical views include anteroposterior (AP), lateral, and sometimes oblique. Many special views are available and consultation with the radiologist may be helpful. Providing a succinct yet careful description of the mechanism of injury and notation of any point tenderness may prompt the radiologist to consider obtaining special views.

GENERAL TREATMENT

Emergent treatment of the multitrauma patient includes ABCs (airway, breathing, and circulation) for those injuries that may be life threat-

ening. Once serious injuries of the head, chest, and abdomen have been addressed and the patient is stable, attention can be turned toward the orthopedic injuries.

In general, measures include

• Elevation of the affected extremity
• Cold compresses to minimize swelling
• Immobilization (often splinting) of the joints above and below the injury
• Analgesics
• Reduction consideration, postreduction immobilization, postreduction films
• Disposition (admission vs. home) and follow-up arrangements

Communication

In addition to thoroughly examining an injury, one of the most important skills a clinician can possess is the ability to accurately describe and document the findings (both anatomically and radiologically). Correctly conveying this information to colleagues and consultants ensures optimal treatment; it is at this step that mistakes can occur with misinterpretation regarding a specific injury. An organized systematic description is best and should include specifically which bone is involved; the location of the fracture on the bone itself; whether it is open or closed, displaced or nondisplaced; whether it involves the joint articular surfaces; and any rotational or angular component. A complete description might be: "closed right third transverse midshaft proximal phalangeal fracture that is nondisplaced, and separated 2 mm; the distal fragment is angulated in the dorsal direction by 10 degrees."

COMMON FRACTURES AND DISLOCATIONS OF THE UPPER EXTREMITIES

Shoulder Anterior Dislocations

In shoulder dislocations, 90% to 95% are anterior, the most common major joint dislocation. This injury often recurs. The mechanism is usually abduction and external rotation of the arm. The presentation is usually severe pain and immobility of the shoulder. A visible deformity will be noted since the acromion will appear prominent, with a "squared-off" appearance of the normal shoulder curvature. Usually, the patient is holding the affected arm with the contralateral hand in slight abduction. During physical examination, pay particular attention to the sensation of the lateral shoulder, since there may be axillary nerve damage. On x-ray, it is important to look for an associated fracture of the humeral tuberosities; often a Hill-Sachs lesion is noted (compression divot on humeral head).

Successful reduction can be done in the emergency department after ruling out coexistence of other upper extremity fractures by using one of three methods described below.

STIMSON TECHNIQUE   Attempt passive reduction with a 10- to 15-lb weight secured to the affected wrist with the patient lying prone on a stretcher for 20 to 30 minutes. An analgesia such as morphine, 3 to 5 mg intravenously every 10 to 15 minutes, can be utilized to help relax musculature. Naloxone, 0.4 to 2 mg intravenously every few minutes, may be required for reversal in some cases. Occasionally slight internal and external rotation by the clinician while in this position may be enough to complete the reduction (see Fig. 10-2-4).

MILCH TECHNIQUE   The clinician slowly abducts and externally rotates the arm to an overhead position with the elbow extended while the patient is supine. Gentle traction can be applied (see Fig. 10-2-5).

TRACTION-COUNTERTRACTION TECHNIQUE   Sustained traction is applied to the humerus toward the elbow by one person, while counter traction is applied to the thorax with a sheet wrapped around the patient's chest by another individual (see Fig. 10-2-6).

Class I
Fracture through the growth plate.
Treatment is closed reduction.

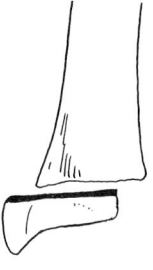

I

Class II
Fracture through the growth plate and
metaphysis. Treatment is closed reduction.

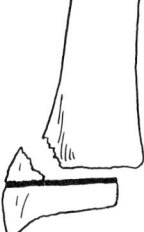

II

Class III
Fracture through the growth plate and epiphysis.
Treatment is either open or closed reduction.

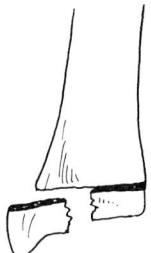

III

Class IV
Fracture through the metaphysis, growth plate, and
epiphysis. Treatment is usually open reduction.

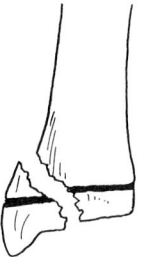

IV

Class V
Growth plate crushed; may not be evident on
X-rays. Often associated with growth disturbances.

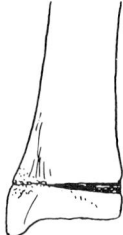

V

FIGURE 10-2-3. Salter-Harris classification of epiphyseal fractures. (*SOURCE: From Tintinalli et al, p 1745. Used with permission.*)

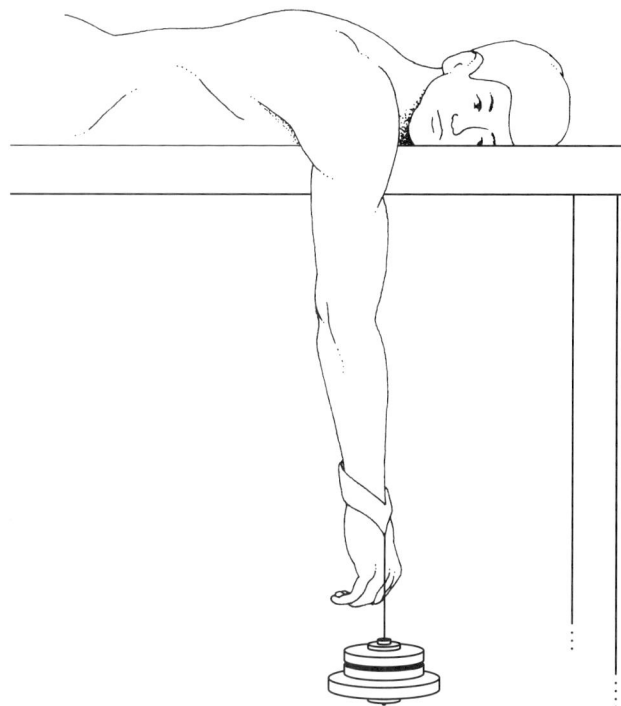

FIGURE 10-2-4. Stimson technique for reduction of anterior dislocations.

Post-reduction films should confirm reduction. Neurovascular reassessment is required following reduction. The patient should be instructed to wear a sling (with frequent removal for range of motion exercises, avoiding abduction and external rotation) and to use analgesics. An orthopedic follow-up should be scheduled in 3 to 5 days.

Shoulder Posterior Dislocations

While rare, the mechanism of injury occurs with direct trauma to the front of the shoulder (as from landing on an outstretched hand during a fall). It can occur during seizure, as the posterior muscles are stronger than the anterior, resulting in forceful muscle contraction that pulls the humeral head out of the glenoid fossa. The injury presents with severe discomfort; visible prominence may be noted posteriorly with

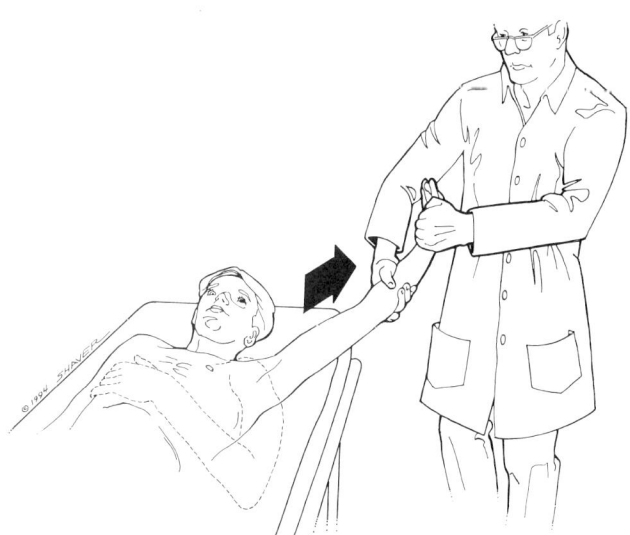

FIGURE 10-2-5. Milch technique. (*source: Tintinalli et al, p 1241. Used with permission.*)

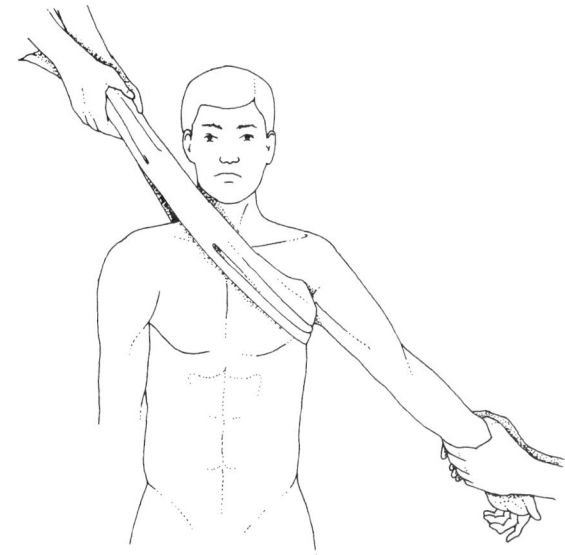

FIGURE 10-2-6. Traction-counteraction technique for reducing anterior shoulder dislocations.

relatively shallow anterior shoulder appearance. The arm may be held adducted against the chest and internally rotated. During physical examination the patient resists movement, especially abduction, and is unable to externally rotate past neutral. This dislocation is often missed on x-rays (estimated up to 50%); therefore, always order AP *and* lateral views (i.e., two views). Axillary views (scapular Y) may be helpful in those read as negative if a high clinical index of suspicion exists; however, they may be difficult to obtain secondary to the patient's inability to abduct.

Reduction may require sedation or general anesthesia. Postreduction films should confirm reduction, neurovascular reassessment (especially axillary nerve), sling and swathe with frequent removal for range of motion exercises (avoiding abduction and external rotation), analgesics, and orthopedic follow-up in 3 to 5 days.

Clavicle Fractures

The most common fracture in children, clavicle fractures usually result from a blow to the shoulder or a fall onto an outstretched hand. They present with localized tenderness, edema, and deformity. During physical examination consider the possibility of great vessel injury. Plain x-ray views may miss this fracture; a computed tomography (CT) scan may be required. Treatment includes figure-of-eight dressing for fractures involving the medial two-thirds of the clavicle for 4 to 6 weeks or a sling for nondisplaced fractures of the lateral one-third (those at the lateral one-third that are displaced by 50% require orthopedic referral). Dressings and slings should be removed each day for gentle range-of-motion exercises. Severe cases should leave the figure of eight dressing in place for the first several days.

Acromioclavicular Joint Injuries (Shoulder Separation)

There are three types of acromioclavicular (AC) joint injuries:

- Type I: Minor ligamentous sprain; tender over AC joint
- Type II: Widened AC joint secondary to partial ligament rupture; may have obvious deformity
- Type III: Complete rupture of the AC ligaments with significant joint widening and deformity; sometimes warrants open reduction internal fixation (ORIF)

Stress or weight-bearing view x-rays should be considered. Treatment consists of rest, ice, analgesics, and immobilization with a figure-of-eight bandage or upper extremity sling with early rehabilitation.

Proximal Humeral Fractures

These fractures usually occur in the elderly, secondary to a fall on an outstretched hand, and present with pain, tenderness, deformity, edema, and ecchymosis. During physical examination, assess the axillary nerve (by testing lateral shoulder sensation) as well as other nerves and arteries. X-rays should include the AP, lateral, and axillary views. Treatment of uncomplicated, minimally displaced fractures requires sling and swathe, analgesia, and orthopedic referral. Other cases require orthopedic consultation for operative consideration. Potential complications include adhesive capsulitis (frozen shoulder), which can be prevented with early rehabilitation.

Humeral Shaft Fractures

Occurring in healthy active adults, this fracture occurs in the middle third of the humerus. A blow to the shoulder, a fall onto an outstretched hand, a motor vehicle accident, or a gunshot wound is often the cause. Patients present with pain, tenderness, deformity, edema, and ecchymosis. During the physical examination, carefully assess the radial nerve, as it is often an associated injury (assess wrist extension). Obtain AP and tangential scapular lateral views of the humerus.

Treatment of uncomplicated fractures consists of coaptation U splint/sugar tong splint of the upper arm, sling and swathe, appropriate analgesics, and an orthopedic referral in 3 to 5 days.

Distal Humeral Fractures

These fractures are often supracondylar in children and intra-articular in adults. X-rays may have a posterior fat pad sign (radiolucent area suggestive of intra-articular bleeding) on lateral view. Treatment is usually ORIF with close neurovascular follow-up. Complications may involve injury to the median, ulnar, or radial nerves secondary to swelling. This fracture may also involve brachial artery injury.

Radial Head Subluxations (Nursemaid's Elbow)

Subluxation of the radial head is common in children from 1 to 4 years of age since the radial head is the same size as the neck; after age 7 occurrence is rare since the radial head enlarges and is more difficult to subluxate. The mechanism of injury is usually a sudden jerk of the hand while the forearm is extended and pronated.

The child avoids use of the affected arm but does not appear in great distress; the forearm is held in slight flexion and pronation and resists supination. There is usually no edema. X-rays are not indicated unless history warrants it.

Reduction is accomplished when the clinician places his or her thumb over the radial head, while the other hand placed at the wrist initiates full supination; a palpable "click" should be felt. If not, fully flex the arm at the elbow or fully extend and reattempt this maneuver. It may require repeated attempts. No immobilization is required unless multiple episodes occur, which warrant a sling or long arm cast and orthopedic follow-up.

Radial Head and Neck Fractures

Trivial trauma will cause radial head and neck fractures presenting with vague discomfort noted over the proximal forearm. X-ray is often normal despite fracture; occasionally a positive fat pad sign (radiolucent area noted on lateral view just posterior to the distal humerus, suggestive of intra-articular bleeding) will be seen. Physical examination reveals exacerbation of pain with rotation of the forearm and hyperflexion and hyperextension at the elbow. Treatment for uncomplicated cases includes sling (remove completely at night and several times during the day for gentle range of motion if tolerated), analgesics, ice compresses, and orthopedic follow-up in 10 to 12 days. Films repeated at this time may show a fracture line.

Elbow Dislocations

Most elbow dislocations are posterior due to falls onto an outstretched hand. The elbow is usually held at 45° of flexion and may develop marked edema. Careful neurovascular assessment with attention to the brachial artery and the ulnar, radial, and median nerves is critical. Lateral view demonstrates posterior displacement of both the radius and ulna; AP view may show either medial or lateral displacement with the radius and ulna normally aligned with relationship to each other; this may be associated with other injuries. After appropriate sedation, these dislocations can be reduced by gentle wrist and forearm traction applied by one clinician, while another clinician provides countertraction on the upper arm. Next, downward pressure is applied to the proximal forearm to disengage the coronoid process, and the elbow is flexed. A palpable "clunk" can be felt: full range of motion should be possible. If not, entrapment might have occurred. Splint the patient at 90° flexion from the axilla to the base of the digits.

Nightstick Fractures

Trauma to the ulna results when a person attempts to protect him- or herself by blocking blows during an altercation (see Fig. 10-2-7). Patients often present with pain and edema over the ulnar aspect of the forearm. Nightstick fractures are treated by reduction followed by a long arm splint. ORIF may be necessary if conservative reduction fails.

Colles' and Smith's Fractures

The common fractures of the distal radius due to falls onto an outstretched hand present with pain, swelling, tenderness, "dinner fork" deformity (Colles' fracture), and limited range of motion. It is important to pay attention to the radioulnar joint and median nerve assessment.

Colles' fracture is just proximal to the distal radius and dorsal displacement of the distal radius and angulation of the distal fragment in the dorsal direction (also known as volar apex angulation since the apex of the angle points volar; see Fig. 10-2-8). Treatment includes a volar wrist splint, elevation, analgesics, and orthopedic follow-up in 3 to 5 days (for Colles' fracture).

Smith's fracture (reverse Colles' fracture) involves volar displacement of the distal radius and a reverse angle. Orthopedic consultation is required, as these fractures are considered unstable.

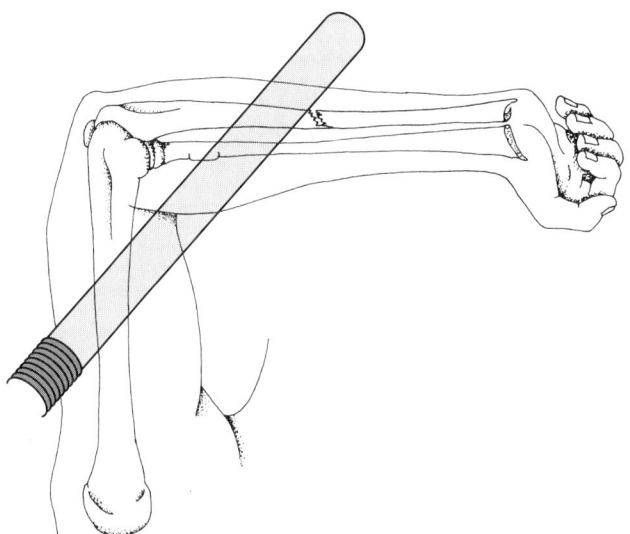

FIGURE 10-2-7. Nightstick fracture. *source: Kozin SH, Berlet AC: Handbook of Common Orthopaedic Fractures, 4th ed., Medical Surveillance, 2000. Used with permission.*

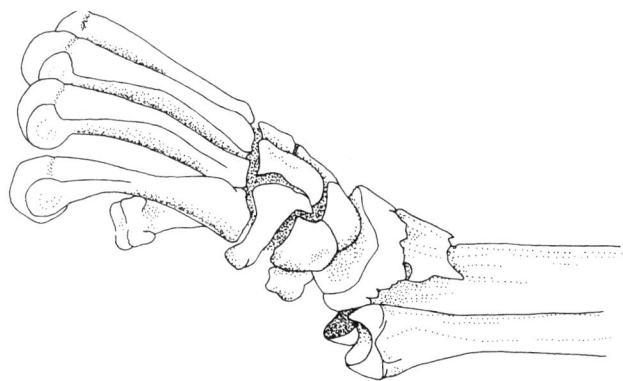

FIGURE 10-2-8. Colle's fracture. *SOURCE: Kozin SH, Berlet AC:* Handbook of Common Orthopaedic Fractures, *4th ed., Medical Surveillance, 2000. Used with permission.*

Monteggia's Fractures and Dislocations

This ulna fracture usually occurs in the proximal third with radial head dislocation because of forced pronation of the forearm or a direct blow over the posterior aspect of the ulna (see Fig. 10-2-9). Clinical presentation includes pain at the elbow, resistance to flexion and extension, and a shortened forearm with palpable radial head in the antecubital fossa. Be sure to assess for radial nerve involvement. Treatment is an orthopedic referral, since these are often operatively corrected.

Galeazzi's Fractures

Galeazzi's fracture is a radius fracture usually located at the junction of the middle and distal thirds with subluxation of the inferior radioulnar joint due to a direct blow on the dorsolateral wrist or from a fall (see Fig. 10-2-10). The ulna head may be prominent on examination. X-ray reveals a widened space between the distal radius and ulna on AP films. Treatment is an open reduction internal fixation (ORIF).

Scaphoid and Navicular Fractures

A fall on an outstretched hand can cause a fracture that presents with point tenderness localized to the anatomical snuffbox; there may be swelling but many look normal. X-rays are often read as negative since the fracture may not show initially (repeat films at 10 to 14 days may demonstrate the fracture line due to bone resorption). If the patient has pain with snuffbox pressure despite normal films (including a scaphoid view), treat in a thumb spica splint for 4 to 6 weeks. These fractures are often missed and because of the blood supply, which may be interrupted, they may subject a patient to avascular necrosis.

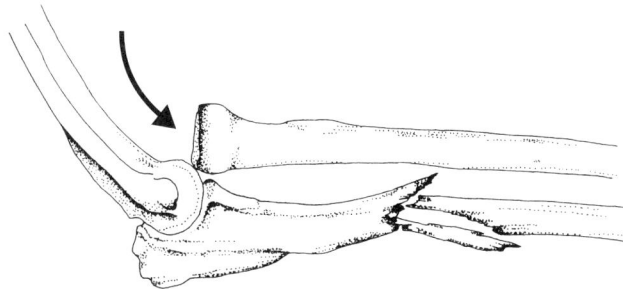

FIGURE 10-2-9. Monteggia's fracture. *SOURCE: Kozin SH, Berlet AC:* Handbook of Common Orthopaedic Fractures, *4th ed., Medical Surveillance, 2000. Used with permission.*

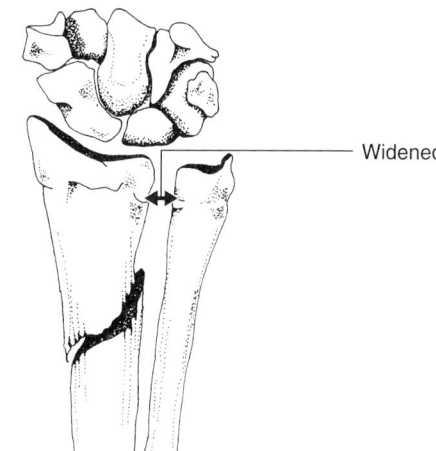

Widened

FIGURE 10-2-10. Galeazzi's fracture. *SOURCE: Kozin SH, Berlet AC:* Handbook of Common Orthopaedic Fractures, *4th ed., Medical Surveillance, 2000. Used with permission.*

Bennett's Fractures

A fracture of the base of the first metacarpal occurs from axial loading to the thumb. Bennett's fracture often requires surgical repair (see Fig. 10-2-11).

Rolando's Fractures

Fractures of the base of the first metacarpal occur due to axial loading to the thumb. Treatment often requires surgical repair (see Fig. 10-2-12).

Metacarpal Shaft Fractures

Nondisplaced fractures can be treated in a gutter splint with orthopedic follow-up. Those with any displacement, angulation, or rotation require prompt orthopedic referral.

Metacarpal Neck Fractures

Fractures of the metacarpal neck are commonly seen in the fourth and fifth digits. Boxer's fracture (fifth digit) results from striking an object with the closed fist. Usually the distal fracture fragment appears angulated

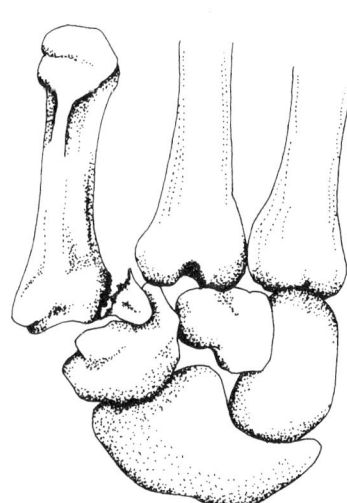

FIGURE 10-2-11. Bennett's fracture. *SOURCE: Kozin SH, Berlet AC:* Handbook of Common Orthopaedic Fractures, *4th ed., Medical Surveillance, 2000. Used with permission.*

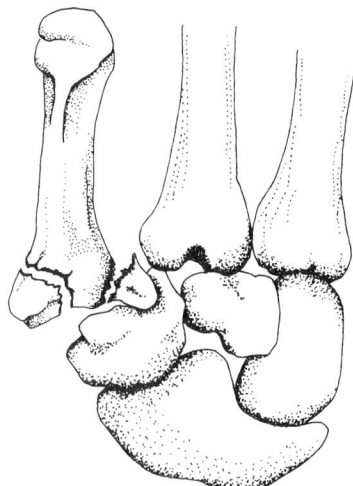

FIGURE 10-2-12. Rolando's fracture. *SOURCE: Kozin SH, Berlet AC: Handbook of Common Orthopaedic Fractures, 4th ed., Medical Surveillance, 2000. Used with permission.*

in the volar direction on x-ray (dorsal apex angulation). It presents with localized tenderness and edema, and there may be a loss of knuckle prominence while making a fist. Obtain AP, lateral, and oblique views. The fourth digit can accept up to 20° of distal fragment volar angulation and the fifth up to 40° of distal fragment volar angulation to be considered acceptable without functional compromise, provided no rotational component is present. (Have patient make a fist; look at fingernails for rotational asymmetry.) If greater than the accepted angles are noted on x-ray, a hematoma block is placed, which involves injecting 3 to 5 mL of 1% plain lidocaine into the fracture site by an experienced clinician (expiration of dark blood confirms location). After waiting 15 minutes for the optimal anesthetic effect, an attempt at closed reduction is performed to obtain a more acceptable angle. Splint in an ulnar gutter splint with the fourth and fifth metacarpophalangeal joints at 90°, the fourth and fifth interphalangeal joints fully extended, and the wrist in 15° of extension. Analgesics, such as ibuprofen, 400 mg orally with food every 6 hours, and elevation are recommended. An orthopedic follow-up in 5 to 7 days completes the treatment.

PITFALLS Careful examination of the skin overlying the metacarpophalangeal joint is imperative if history suggests striking another person in the mouth (clenched fist injury) since human oral contaminants may have been introduced into the joint space. These are treated aggressively as a human bite to prevent severe infection. They often present with severe soft tissue hand infection 3 to 5 days after injury with little external sign of laceration from tooth and no recollection of previous trauma these often require operative irrigation. Second and third metacarpal neck fractures require almost perfect reduction to maintain normal hand function and are best referred for orthopedic consultation.

Proximal and Middle Phalanx Fractures

Often referred to an orthopedic service for operative repair, proximal and middle phalanx fractures usually involve articular surfaces, displacement, or rotation.

Interphalangeal Dislocations

These dislocations are very common and may be associated with ligamentous injury. Check and document neurovascular functioning. Often the distal fragment resides dorsally. Use x-ray to rule out associated fracture. Reduction may be accomplished with 1% plain lidocaine digital block but is not mandatory. While stabilizing the proximal segment, the distal segment is pulled longitudinally and is flexed at the proximal interphalangeal joint (PIP), reducing the dislocation. Perform the

postreduction assessment to determine whether collateral ligaments are intact and note full restoration of motor function. Discharge with a volar splint with the PIP segment flexed at 15 to 20° and recommend early orthopedic follow-up in 3 to 5 days. If reduction is not easy, then refer to an orthopedic specialist, since it may require open reduction secondary to soft tissue entrapment.

Mallet Avulsion Fractures

The extensor tendon pulls off a segment of bone in these fractures. Surgical treatment should be considered if the segment is greater than 25% of the articular surface, as it may require operative pinning. If the segment is less than 25%, it may be treated in an extension splint of the distal interphalangeal joint (DIP) where the PIP is free. This can result in a permanent mallet finger deformity if not monitored carefully.

Distal Phalanx Fracture: Tuft Fractures

The mechanism of injury usually involves smashing a fingertip in a door or trauma from dropped objects. Take care to rule out open fracture that is often associated with nail bed injury; this may require careful repair. Evacuation of subungual hematoma (use portable electrocautery rather than paper clip or 18G-needle method) may be required if the injury is less than 72 hours old and the patient is symptomatic. Caution: do not iatrogenically turn a closed fracture into an open one. Consultation for cases involving displacement, articular surface, or significant soft tissue involvement is recommended. Uncomplicated cases can be treated with a DIP splint with the PIP free. Analgesics are often helpful as these fractures are very painful.

FRACTURES AND DISLOCATIONS OF THE LOWER EXTREMITIES

Pelvic Fractures

The mechanism of injury is usually due to high-energy trauma (motor vehicle accident, fall from height). It is the second most common cause of death associated with trauma (head injury is first); 50% have other fractures or major injuries. Pelvic fractures are commonly associated with bladder rupture, urethral tear, and sacral root damage and usually associated with multiple life-threatening injuries, hemorrhagic shock, pelvic or perineal edema, ecchymosis, and hematoma. After attention to head, thoracic, abdominal, and genitourinary injuries, perform a urethral, pelvic, and rectal examination looking for a high-riding prostate, decreased or absent sphincter tone, blood at the urethral meatus, vaginal or rectal laceration, or hematoma. Perform a complete neurovascular assessment. Attempt to rock the pelvis by exerting bimedial pressure and anterior to posterior pressure to each anterior superior iliac spine and anterior to posterior pressure over the pubic rami. X-ray may include a variety of views such as AP, lateral, internal and external oblique (Judet views), and inlet and outlet plain films. Look for a widened sacroiliac joint or symphysis pubis and disruption of the pelvic ring; this often requires CT scans or other special vascular or urologic studies. Treatment consists of close cardiovascular monitoring for hemorrhagic shock, orthopedic consultation, and admission.

Hip Dislocations

Most hip dislocations occur posteriorly as a result of a motor vehicle accident in which the flexed knees strike the dashboard, causing the hip to dislocate posteriorly. They present with severe discomfort of the hip and inability to ambulate. Physical examination reveals a shortened, slightly flexed, adducted, and internally rotated lower extremity. This can coexist with associated fractures of the femur or acetabulum. Prompt reduction by an orthopedic service within 6 hours minimizes the chances of avascular necrosis from interrupted blood supply to the femoral head.

Slipped Capital Femoral Epiphysis

Occurring in children or adolescents with minor or unrecalled trauma, this injury may occur bilaterally. It presents with groin pain after activity, hip or knee pain, and limp. Physical examination reveals pain is exacerbated with internal rotation of the hip. AP, lateral, and frog leg (hips flexed to 90° and abducted 45°) x-rays demonstrate posterior and inferior displaced femoral epiphysis. Treatment includes crutches and orthopedic consultation. Late complications include avascular necrosis of the femoral head and premature closure of the epiphyseal plate.

Femoral Shaft Fractures

Femoral shaft fractures are caused by direct blow, twisting of the leg, or gunshot wounds, and are usually associated with high-energy trauma. There may be multiple injuries (e.g., pelvis and knee) and significant blood loss. The limb may appear shortened or angulated. Careful skin and neurovascular examination should be done to rule out open fracture and involvement of the femoral artery or sciatic nerve. Treatment includes intravenous fluids, monitoring for hemorrhagic shock, traction splint, orthopedic referral for surgical intervention, and admission.

Patellar Dislocations

Caused by a twisting force on an extended knee, patellar dislocation often recurs because the medial joint capsule is damaged. The patella may be found laterally with severe pain and deformity noted. It often spontaneously reduces itself. If reduction is necessary, this is accomplished with hyperextension of the knee, flexion at the hip, and manual manipulation of patella back into place. Postreduction x-ray should be done to rule out associated fracture. Immobilization for 2 to 3 weeks in a Jones splint or straight-leg knee immobilizer that does not incorporate the ankle is recommended. Later physical therapy can be utilized to strengthen the vastus medialis to prevent recurrence.

Tibial Shaft Fractures

The tibiae are the most frequently fractured long bones. Often an open fracture is associated with a fibular fracture from direct blow, twisting forces, or gunshot wound. Be sure to carefully examine the skin because the anterior bone surface is very close to the skin. Also be sure to carefully check for neurovascular compromise. Be watchful of compartment syndrome; beware as it can exist in the presence of normal skin color and pulses. Serial checks will be necessary. Treatment includes repeated evaluation analgesics, traction splint, orthopedic referral, and admission.

Maisonneuve Fractures

These fractures involve a ruptured deltoid ligament with a high fibular fracture with pain over lateral proximal leg over proximal fibula

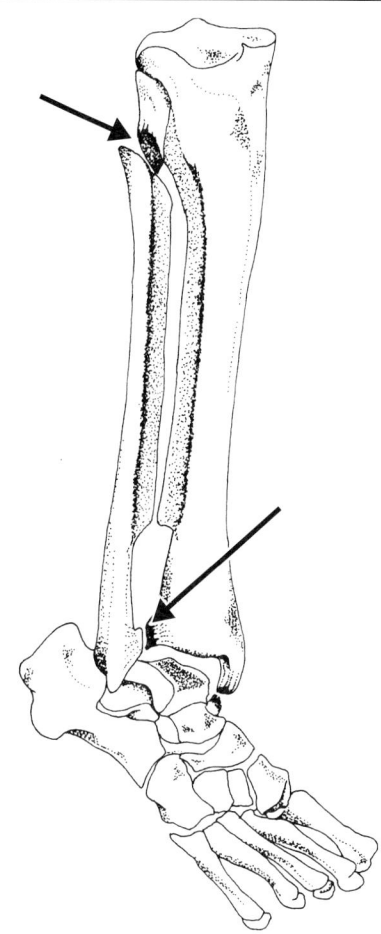

FIGURE 10-2-13. Maisonneuve's fracture. *SOURCE: Kozin SH, Berlet AC: Handbook of Common Orthopaedic Fractures, 4th ed., Medical Surveillance, 2000. Used with permission.*

(see Fig. 10-2-13). A wide mortise despite negative leg and ankle films will be seen on x-ray. Treatment is usually operative to restore joint articular surfaces and syndesmosis.

Ankle Fractures

This very common injury is due to plantar flexion and inversion injury—the "twisted ankle." It presents with pain and often swelling over the lateral ankle. Determine areas of point tenderness and assess neurovascular status and areas of weakness. Check the base of the fifth metatarsal and if involved obtain foot films in addition to ankle films. X ray includes the AP, lateral, and mortise views of the ankle. Figure 10-2-14 shows the Weber classification of fibular fractures.

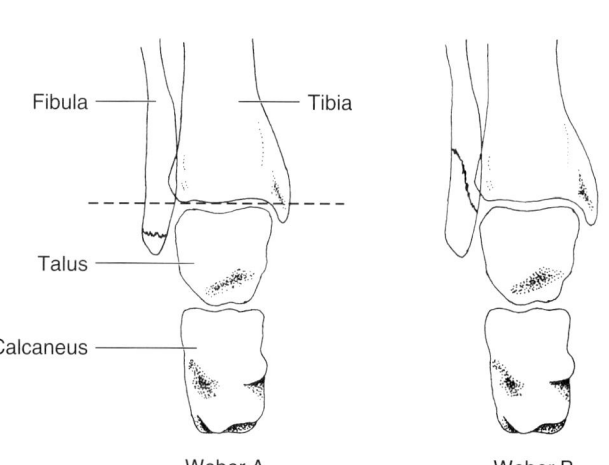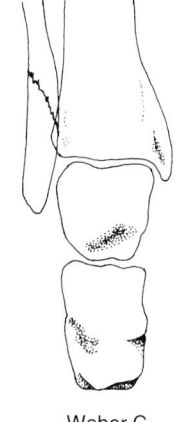

FIGURE 10-2-14. Weber classification.
Type A fibula fracture is avulsed distal to the joint line. Conservative treatment.
Type B fibula fracture is spiral pattern beginning at the level of the joint line and extending proximal. If stable, conservative treatment.
Type C fibula fracture occurs proximal to the joint line associated with syndesmotic interruption. Often, ORIF.

Fibula — Tibia
Talus
Calcaneus

Weber A   Weber B   Weber C

Calcaneal Fractures

These are the most common fracture of the tarsal bones, typically due to a fall or jump with an unstable landing. Presenting with pain, swelling, and tenderness over the medial or lateral heel, they may have from full range of motion at the ankle but extreme dorsiflexion produces pain.

On x-ray, one should obtain AP, lateral, and axial x-ray views. There may be associated injuries, often involving the spine and bilateral lower extremities.

Treatment of medial or lateral calcaneal tuberosity fracture (nondisplaced) includes ice, elevation, non–weight-bearing (crutches) for 1 to 2 weeks, and then a well-molded walking cast with initiation of partial weight-bearing for 8 weeks. For a displaced fracture an orthopedic referral for closed manipulation or ORIF is recommended.

Calcaneal Posterior Tuberosity Fractures

Nondisplaced fractures are treated with a non–weight-bearing cast with the foot in equinus for 6 to 8 weeks, followed by an orthopedic follow-up. Complications include arthritis, stiffness, chronic pain, spur formation, and nerve entrapment.

Talar Fractures

These are the second most common fracture of the tarsal bones. Anterior and posterior talar avulsion fractures are caused by twist injury and are often associated with an audible "pop." They present with tenderness, edema, and pain exacerbated by motion. X-ray is often confused with os trigonum (a normal variant that has smooth, round, bilateral, sclerotic margins). Treatment includes ice, elevation, immobilization (a short walking cast with the ankle in neutral position or a cast in 15° of equinus if treating a posterior avulsion fracture). If the fracture fragment is greater than 0.5 cm it may require surgical manipulation. Because talar head, neck, and body fractures or dislocations often have peroneal tendon involvement, they are prone to development of avascular necrosis and can result in delayed union; therefore these injuries should get prompt orthopedic referral.

Lisfranc's Fractures (Tarsometatarsal Dislocations)

Fracture or dislocation at the base of the second metatarsal resulting in tarsometatarsal joint disruption is usually caused by falls or motor vehicle accidents, often with a rotational component.

This type of fracture usually presents with severe pain and edema. Conduct a careful sensory exam since these fractures are often associated with nerve or blood supply compromise. Order AP, lateral, and oblique films. It may require comparison films or stress views. Greater then 2-mm displacement requires ORIF. Treatment includes analgesics, ice, elevation, and orthopedic referral. Complications include chronic foot pain and swelling, deformity, degenerative arthritis, and circulatory abnormalities. Complications are particularly common in persons with diabetes.

Fifth Metatarsal Fractures

It is important to distinguish between avulsion (ballerina) fractures and Jones (transverse) fractures (see Fig. 10-2-15). The mechanism of injury is often plantar flexion and inversion injury (ballerina) versus forceful planting of the foot as in motor vehicle accidents or dropped objects on the foot (transverse). Both may have point tenderness over the base of the fifth metatarsal; there may be edema and ecchymosis. Treatment includes a hard-soled shoe for ballerina fractures versus a short leg splint for transverse fractures. In all ankle injuries be sure to assess the base of the fifth metatarsal because it is often missed. X-ray views should be based on where point tenderness exists. Many patients with fifth metatarsal fractures have had ankle films but no radiologic assessment of the foot. Jones fractures are notorious for

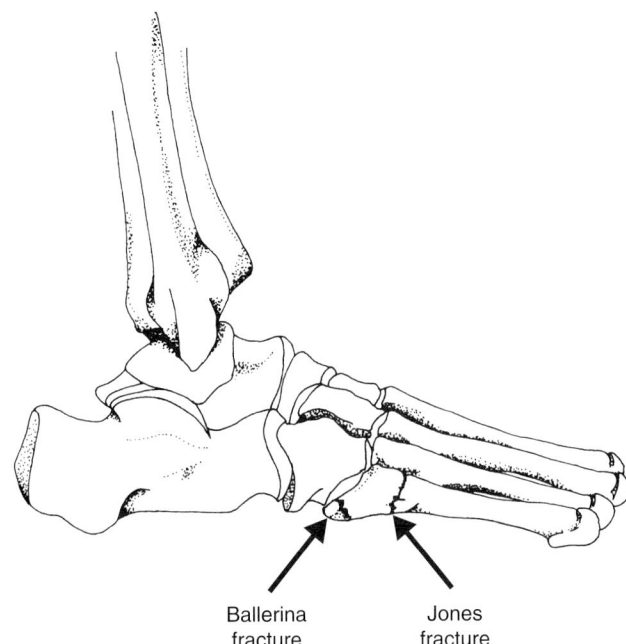

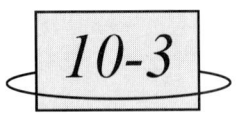

Ballerina Jones
fracture fracture

FIGURE 10-2-15. Ballerina and Jones fractures. *SOURCE: Kozin SH, Berlet AC:* Handbook of Common Orthopaedic Fractures, *4th ed., Medical Surveillance, 2000. Used with permission.*

developing nonunion or delayed union, so they require close follow-up and orthopedic consultation.

BIBLIOGRAPHY

Cline DM et al: *Emergency Medicine: A Comprehensive Study Guide—Companion Handbook,* 5th ed, New York, McGraw-Hill, 2000, pp 871–903.

Jenkins JL, Braen GR: *Manual of Emergency Medicine,* 4th ed, Philadelphia, Lippincott Williams & Wilkins, 2000, pp 82–112.

Kozin SH, Berlet AC: *Handbook of Common Orthopaedic Fractures,* 2nd ed, West Chester, PA, Medical Surveillance, 1992.

Plantz SH, Adler JN: *NMS Emergency Medicine.* Baltimore, Williams & Wilkins, 1998, pp 565–579.

Simon RR, Koeningsknecht SJ: *Emergency Orthopedics/The Extremities,* 3rd ed, Norwalk, CT, Appleton and Lange, 1996.

Skinner HB (ed): *Current Diagnosis and Treatment in Orthopedics.* New York, McGraw-Hill, 1998, pp 51–115.

Tintinalli JE et al: *Emergency Medicine: A Comprehensive Guide,* 4th ed, New York, McGraw-Hill, 1996.

10-3 RHEUMATOID ARTHRITIS

Pamela Moyers Scott

DISCUSSION

Rheumatoid arthritis (RA) is a chronic, systemic disease characterized by symmetric synovial inflammation of the peripheral joints, especially the proximal interphalangeal and metacarpophalangeal joints of the hands, wrists, elbows, knees, ankles, and subtalar joints of the feet. Its etiology is unknown.

Rheumatoid arthritis affects approximately 0.8% of the U.S. population[1] and is more common in women than men. There appears to be a genetic predisposition to developing RA. Onset of symptoms is generally in the fourth or fifth decade of life. Advancing age is a risk factor for developing RA. Symptoms can vary from intermittent arthralgias to severe, debilitating deformities and extra-articular manifestations.

SIGNS AND SYMPTOMS

Generally the presenting complaint in a patient with RA is pain, swelling, and stiffness of the aforementioned joints. The pain is usually bilateral and aggravated by movement. Morning stiffness, or that occurring after periods of inactivity, often lasts more than 1 hour.

Constitutional symptoms are also common. They include low-grade fever, early afternoon fatigue, malaise, weakness, anorexia, and weight loss.

OBJECTIVE FINDINGS

On physical examination, the affected joints reveal swelling, tenderness, decreased range of motion, and warmth secondary to the synovial inflammation. Erythema is generally not present. If the inflammation is not controlled, several characteristic deformities can occur:

• *Z deformity,* caused by radial deviation of the wrist and ulnar deviation of the fingers
• *Swan-neck deformity,* due to hyperextension of the proximal interphalangeal joints (PIPs) and flexion of the distal interphalangeal joints (DIPs)
• *Boutonniere deformity,* defined as flexion deformity of the PIPs with extension of the DIPs

Extra-articular manifestations consist of dermatologic complications such as vasculitis and rheumatoid nodules. Rheumatoid nodules are subcutaneous nodules of varying sizes that occur on the extensor surfaces of the periarticular structures, especially the elbows, sacrum, and occiput. The presence of rheumatoid nodules or vasculitis indicates a more aggressive form of RA. On physical examination, the affected joints reveal swelling, tenderness, decreased range of motion, and warmth secondary to the synovial inflammation. Erythema is generally not present.

Cardiac and pulmonary manifestations are also seen. Most cardiac disease is asymptomatic; it can consist of pericarditis and inflammatory lesions similar to rheumatoid nodules forming in the myocardium and heart valves.[2]

Pulmonary complications can be asymptomatic, such as rheumatoid pleural disease, or life threatening when pleural nodule-like lesions become infected and cavitate or rupture into the pleural space, causing a pneumothorax.[2] Chronic obstructive pulmonary disease can occur, consisting of dyspnea, chronic cough, interstitial fibrosis, and/or bronchiectasis.

Central nervous system involvement is rare; however, rheumatoid vasculitis and rheumatoid nodule-like granulomas occasionally develop in the meninges.[2] Extracranial rheumatoid vasculitis is rarely associated with a mononeuritis multiplex syndrome, and proliferating synovium can compress nerve roots, producing neurologic symptoms.

Ophthalmologic complications can include Sjögren's syndrome, episcleritis, scleritis, and scleromalacia perforans.[2]

DIAGNOSTIC CONSIDERATIONS

The diagnostic criteria for RA appear in Table 10-3-1. Other collagen vascular diseases (e.g., lupus, polyarteritis, progressive systemic sclerosis) must be considered in the differential. Systemic diseases with joint manifestations, such as acute rheumatic fever, sarcoidosis, and amyloidosis, must also be considered. Infectious joint disease (e.g., gonococcal arthritis, viral arthritis, Lyme disease) and other forms of arthritis (e.g., osteoarthritis, ankylosing spondylitis, gouty arthritis, psoriatic arthritis) are other considerations.

SPECIAL CONSIDERATIONS

Juvenile arthritis (JA), previously termed juvenile rheumatoid arthritis (JRA), is estimated to affect approximately 0.05 to 0.1% of children in the United States.[3] It is characterized by the objective findings of chronic inflammation in one or more joints for at least 6 weeks dura-

TABLE 10-3-1. Criteria for the Diagnosis of Rheumatoid Arthritis

At least four of the following criteria must be present to establish the diagnosis of rheumatoid arthritis (RA):

1. Morning stiffness of >1 h for at least 6 weeks
2. Arthritis (diagnosed by a health care provider) simultaneously present in >3 peripheral joints, for a minimum of 6 weeks duration
3. Arthritis of the wrists or metacarpophalangeal or proximal interphalangeal joints of the hands (diagnosed by a health care provider) and present for a minimum of 6 weeks
4. Peripheral joint arthritis that is symmetric, observed by a health care provider, and present for a minimum of 6 weeks
5. Rheumatoid nodules diagnosed by a health care provider
6. Positive serum rheumatoid factor done by a method that has a false-positive rate <5% in unaffected control subjects
7. Radiographic changes that are characteristic for RA—hand x-rays revealing erosions or unequivocal bony decalcification

SOURCE: Modified from Lipsky.[1]

tion in someone <16 years old. As with RA, there are no specific diagnostic tests and the etiology remains unknown.

LABORATORY TESTS

There are no specific tests to establish or exclude the diagnosis of RA. The rheumatoid factor (RF) is present in approximately 85% of all patients with rheumatoid arthritis.[4] However, it is also present in approximately 5% of the general population and 10 to 20% of individuals >65 years old.[1] RF can also be seen with other connective tissue diseases and various infectious processes (e.g., syphilis, hepatitis, rubella, influenza, mononucleosis, malaria). Although RF is nondiagnostic, it has some prognostic value for patients with RA. Higher titers are associated with more severe forms of the disease and more extra-articular manifestations. Additionally, RF-negative patients who become RF-positive later in the course of their disease have the same prognosis and complications as patients who have been RF-positive from the onset.[4]

The erythrocyte sedimentation rate (ESR) and the C-reactive protein (CRP), both measurements of inflammation, are generally elevated in individuals with RA. However, there is a small subset of patients with active inflammation who have normal ESRs.[4] A normocytic, normochromic anemia can also be present. Other laboratory abnormalities can include thrombocytosis, eosinophilia, hypergammaglobulinemia, and hypocomplementemia.[4]

RADIOGRAPHIC STUDIES

Since the earliest signs of erosions are not evident on x-ray studies for 6 months,[5] routine baseline radiographic studies are not indicated. Roentgenograms are indicated when there is clinical evidence of disease progression despite therapy, concern for joint erosion, or need for corroborating evidence of the clinical impression.[6]

OTHER DIAGNOSTICS

Synovial fluid analysis will confirm the presence of an inflammatory arthritis; however, it is not specific or necessary for the diagnosis of RA.[1]

TREATMENT

The goals of treatment of rheumatoid arthritis are to relieve pain and inflammation, prevent deformity and disability, and educate the patient regarding the disease process.

Pharmacologic Management

All patients with RA should be placed on a nonsteroidal anti-inflammatory drug (NSAID). None of the currently available NSAIDs appear to be superior to another in the treatment of RA. When choosing an NSAID, one must consider the impact of side effects, costs, dosing convenience, and compliance for each individual patient.

The risk of gastrointestinal (GI) toxicity, especially hemorrhage, is a serious complication of NSAID therapy. Cytoprotective agents, such as misoprostol (Cytotec), should be considered in all patients receiving an NSAID. Risk factors that increase the likelihood of an adverse GI complication include a previous GI bleed, history of peptic ulcer disease, advancing age, smoking, and oral corticosteroid therapy. Misoprostol is currently the only agent with FDA approval for this purpose. For ease of administration, it is now available in combination with diclofenac sodium (Arthrotec) as a single pill. Although not FDA approved, omeprazole (Prilosec) and famotidine (Pepcid) have also been successfully used to decrease the risk of GI toxicity from an NSAID.[7] The newer cyclooxygenase enzyme-2 (COX-2) inhibitors, such as celecoxib (Celebrex) and rofecoxib (Vioxx), lessen the likelihood of a GI bleed; however, they do not eliminate it because they still affect gastric prostaglandin E2.[8]

NSAIDs are also associated with renal and hepatotoxicity. The greatest risk for renal complications occur in the elderly, diabetics, hypertensives, individuals with preexisting renal disease, and patients on diuretic therapy. Patients who consume large amounts of alcohol are probably at the greatest risk of hepatic complications.

Before instituting NSAID therapy, obtain baseline liver functions, renal functions, potassium, and complete blood count (CBC). CBC, creatinine, and potassium tests should be repeated in 1 month and again every 6 months thereafter.[7] If the initial liver function testing is normal, then additional testing is usually unnecessary.[7]

If the patient is intolerant of NSAIDs or has an aspirin allergy, the nonacetylated salicylates such as salsalate (Salflex, Disalcid) and choline magnesium trisalicylate (Trilisate) may be effective. These drugs are associated with less renal and GI toxicity than the other NSAIDs; however, they are usually not as effective.

If the patient does not respond to a 12-week course of therapy, or if the patient has poor prognostic features (defined as RF-positive, family history of severe RA, severe synovitis especially with functional limitations, joint erosions, and extra-articular manifestations[9]), he or she needs to be on a disease-modifying antirheumatic drug (DMARD). Most experts now recommend a consultation with a rheumatologist before starting or shortly after beginning therapy with a DMARD.[6,10] In fact, treatment outcomes appear to be better if the patient sees a rheumatologist early in the course of the disease.[5]

Those individuals with mild disease and no poor prognostic features who fail to get relief from NSAID therapy alone should be started on hydroxychloroquine (Plaquenil), sulfasalazine (Azulfidine), or oral gold, auranofin (Ridaura).[9] The hydroxychloroquine dose is 400 to 600 mg a day. No additional laboratory monitoring is required with this drug; however, the patient should have a baseline and regular (every 3 months) complete ophthalmologic examinations to evaluate for signs of retinal toxicity.[11]

The starting dose of auranofin is 6 mg/d.[12] Before initiating therapy, a CBC with differential and platelets, a urinalysis (U/A), and tests of renal and hepatic functions should be performed. The CBC and U/A should be repeated monthly to evaluate for the side effects of leukopenia, granulocytopenia, proteinuria, and hematuria; the hepatic and renal functions should be repeated as appropriate.[12]

For individuals with moderately severe disease or poor prognostic indicators, DMARD choices include injectable gold (Myochrysine), gold sodium thiomalate, oral gold (Ridaura), auranofin, or methotrexate (Rheumatrex).[9] A 3- to 5-day course of oral corticosteroids is also indicated.[9]

For individuals with severe disease and poor prognostic indicators, DMARD first-line choices include oral gold, parenteral gold, or methotrexate.[9] Second-line agents include azathioprine (Imuran) and penicillamine (Cuprimine).[9] Corticosteroids are also indicated; dosing depends on the patient's clinical condition.[9]

Combinations of DMARDs are now being utilized with increased effectiveness but no increased toxicity.[13–15] Etanercept (Enbrel) represents a new class of medications available for the treatment of RA, anti-TNF (tumor necrosis factor) agents. It is indicated when DMARD therapy does not produce an adequate response.[14] Alone or in combination with methotrexate, preliminary studies indicate that etanercept is very effective.[14,16] The human tumor necrosis factor-alpha, infliximab (Remicade) was recently approved for the treatment of RA in combination with methotrexate in patients with an inadequate response to methotrexate therapy. The recommended dose is 3 mg/kg as an intravenous infusion on days 1, 14, and 42 and then 9 mg/kg 8 weeks thereafter.[17] At least half of all patients on this combination experienced a reduction in their symptoms.[18] It should be used with caution in patients with chronic infections, recurrent infections, or immunosupression.[17]

Leflunomide (Arava), representing a new class of DMARDs, was also recently released for use in RA. It appears equal in treatment effectiveness and toxicity to methotrexate.[14,16]

Other effective therapies for pain control include opioids and intra-articular corticosteroids. Long-acting, controlled-release morphine or oxycodone, taken at regular intervals, are preferred over short-acting, as-needed preparations.[15] Intra-articular corticosteroid injections should not be given more frequently than at 3- to 4-month intervals.

Surgical Management

Earlier surgical intervention is now indicated. Patients tend to have better results if the surgery is performed before advanced deformities, joint disabilities, contractures, and/or muscle atrophy occurs.[19] Possible surgical interventions include tendon repair or reconstruction, tenosynovectomy, synovectomy, osteotomy, soft tissue arthroplasty, resection arthroplasty, fusion, joint debridement, and joint replacement.[19]

Supportive Measures

Daily exercise with the goal of maintaining or increasing joint mobility and muscle strength is an important component of the treatment plan. Adequate rest, including naps, is essential. Splints, orthotic devices, and physical therapy are also useful modalities.

PATIENT EDUCATION

The patient and family have to be educated on the disease process itself, the purpose of each intervention (including physical therapy, medications, laboratory monitoring, and exercise), and potential complications from medications. They can obtain more information by contacting the Arthritis Foundation at 1-800-283-7800 or at http://www.arthritis.org.

DISPOSITION

The severity of the symptoms and the medications used to treat the patient determine the frequency for follow-up. At each visit, the activity level of the disease should be assessed. At a minimum this should consist of an ESR; questions regarding pain status, presence of swelling, changes in morning stiffness, and amount of fatigue; and a physical examination of the affected joints. Other laboratory studies are indicated based on the patient's complaints and current medications.

COMPLICATIONS

The patient should be referred to a rheumatologist if he or she is being considered for a DMARD, not responding to therapy, has significant disease, or has extra-articular complications.

OTHER NOTES AND PEARLS

Other medications being explored for their use in RA include mycophenolate mofetil, an antirejection drug for cardiac and renal allograft rejection,[14] and minocycline, the antibiotic that is also a metalloproteinase inhibitor.[6] Cytokine inhibitors and other biologic agents are currently being evaluated also.[6,20]

REFERENCES

1. Lipsky PE: Rheumatoid arthritis, in *Harrison's Principles of Internal Medicine,* 14th ed, AS Fauci et al (eds). New York, McGraw-Hill, 1998, pp 1880–1888.
2. Hess E: Rheumatoid arthritis—Epidemiology, etiology, rheumatoid factor, pathology, pathogenesis, in *Primer on the Rheumatic Diseases,* 9th ed, RH Schumacher (ed). Atlanta, GA, Arthritis Foundation, 1988, pp 83–96.
3. Gewanter HL: Juvenile rheumatoid, in *Primary Pediatric Care,* 3d ed, RA Hoekelman (ed). St. Louis, MO, Mosby, 1997, pp 1382–1389.
4. Anderson RJ: Rheumatoid arthritis—Clinical and laboratory features, in *Primer on the Rheumatic Diseases,* 11th ed, JH Klippel (ed). Atlanta, GA, Arthritis Foundation, 1997, pp 161–167.
5. Haque NU et al: Early rheumatoid arthritis: Detection and risk stratification. *Journal of Musculoskeletal Medicine* April:58–67, 1998.
6. Hunder GG et al: Rheumatoid arthritis: Progress in research and clinical management. *Journal of Musculoskeletal Medicine* November:22–35,1998.
7. Clough J et al: The new thinking on osteoarthritis. *Patient Care* 30:110–137, 1996.
8. Cryer B, Feldman M: Cyclooxygenase-1 and cyclooxygenase-2 selectivity of widely used nonsteroidal anti-inflammatory drugs. *Am J Med* 104:413–421, 1998.
9. Paget SA: Rheumatoid arthritis—Treatment, in JH Klippel (ed) *Primer on the Rheumatic Diseases,* 11th ed, Atlanta, GA, Arthritis Foundation, 1997, pp 168–174.
10. Klippel JH (ed): Appendix II, in *Primer on the Rheumatic Diseases,* 11th ed, JH Klippel. Atlanta, GA, Arthritis Foundation, 1997, pp 465–472.
11. Sanofi-Synthelabo: Plaquenil, in *Physicians' Desk Reference,* 55th ed, Montvale, NJ, 2001, pp. 2860–2862.
12. Connitics Corporation: Ridaura, in *Physicians' Desk Reference,* Montvale, NJ, R Arky (ed). 1999, pp 903–904.
13. O'Dell JR et al: Treatment of rheumatoid arthritis with methotrexate alone, sulfasalazine, and hydroxychloroquine, or a combination of all three medications. *N Engl J Med* 334:1287–1291, 1996.
14. Klahr PD et al: New treatments for osteoarthritis and rheumatoid arthritis. *Emerg Med* May:28–44, 1999.
15. Lipman AG: Rheumatoid arthritis: Newest strategies to control the pain. *Consultant* April:1228–1244, 1999.
16. Clinical update: New treatments for RA: Highlights from the ACR meeting. *Women's Health in Primary Care* 2:101–102, 1999.
17. Centocor Inc: Remicaid, in *Physicians' Desk Reference* (PDR), 55th ed, Montvale, NJ, Medical Economics Company, Inc., 2001, pp 1083–1088.
18. Maini RN, et al: Therapeutic efficacy of multiple intravenous infusions of anti-tumor necrosis factor-alpha monoclonal antibody combined with low-dose weekly methotrexate in rheumatoid arthritis. *Arthritis Rheum* 41(9):1552–1563, 1998.
19. Ballard WT, Buckwalter JB: Operative treatment of rheumatic disease, in *Primer on the Rheumatic Diseases,* 11th ed, JH Klippel (ed). Atlanta, GA, Arthritis Foundation, 1997, pp 443–449.
20. Moreland L, Koopman W: Biologic agents as potential new therapies for rheumatoid disease, in *Primer on the Rheumatic Diseases,* 11th ed, JH Klippel (ed). Atlanta, GA, Arthritis Foundation, 1997, pp 437–442.

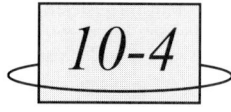

ANKYLOSING SPONDYLITIS
Pamela Moyers Scott

DISCUSSION

Ankylosing spondylitis (AS), also known as Marie-Strümpell disease and Bechterew's disease, is an inflammatory arthritis that primarily affects the axial skeleton and occasionally the large peripheral joints. Although AS is considered a rheumatoid disease, its main pathologic changes are concentrated around the enthesis, not the synovium as seen in rheumatoid arthritis. For purposes of classification, it is considered to be one of the seronegative spondyloarthropathies. The pathogenesis is uncertain; most consider it to be an immune-mediated disease.

Patients begin noticing symptoms in late adolescence or early twenties. Onset of symptoms after the age of 40 years is rare. There appears to be familial clustering of the disease. AS affects more men than women. The course of the disease ranges from mild stiffness to a completely fused spine with severe peripheral joint arthritis and extra-articular complications.

SIGNS AND SYMPTOMS

The presenting symptom of AS is generally an aching low back pain. It is associated with morning stiffness and stiffness following inactivity that can last up to several hours; however, these symptoms decrease with exercise and activity. Nocturnal exacerbations of pain can occur. In later stages of the disease, pain can be constant. However, most patients have episodes of pain-free periods followed by acute exacerbations.

Occasionally, other structures will be the site of the presenting symptom of AS. Most commonly these sites include the costosternal junctions, spinous processes, iliac crests, greater trochanters, ischial tuberosities, tibial tubercles, and heels.[1]

Constitutional symptoms (i.e., low-grade fever, fatigue, weight loss, anorexia, and night sweats) are sometimes the presenting complaint. This is especially true in adolescents.[1]

Although extra-articular involvement does occur, it is rarely the presenting symptom. The most common is acute anterior uveitis. Other such involvement includes neurogenic conditions, such as sciatica, cauda equina syndrome, and complications resulting from spinal fractures; cardiac conditions, including aortic insufficiency, conduction defects, and cardiomegaly; and pulmonary conditions, manifesting as pulmonary fibrosis, cyst formation, and *Aspergillus* infections.[1]

OBJECTIVE FINDINGS

Limited spinal motion is always present in AS. The Schober test is probably the simplest and quickest method for obtaining an objective assessment. To perform this maneuver, find the patient's iliac crests, visually make a line connecting the two, and mark where this line intersects with the spine. Then make an "X" 5 cm above and 10 cm below this mark. Have the patient flex forward as much as possible, then remeasure the distance between the two marks. An increase of ≥5 cm between the two measurements is considered normal. However, some experts feel the distraction is age dependent and should be greater than this in younger individuals.[2]

Limited chest expansion is also a characteristic finding. It is quantitatively evaluated by measuring the difference between maximum inspiration and maximum forced expiration around the chest at the nipple line in men and just below the breasts in women. Normal chest expansion is considered to be ≥5 cm. Bony tenderness and/or muscle spasms may or may not be present. Loss of lumbar lordosis, accentuation of thoracic kyphosis, and cervical forward flexion are sometimes evident on physical examination. In severe disease, flexure contractures of the hip and knee are evident.

TABLE 10-4-1. Diagnostic Criteria for Ankylosing Spondylitis

According to the modified New York criteria, the presence of radiographic-confirmed sacroiliitis plus one of the following criteria is diagnostic for ankylosing spondylitis.

- History of inflammatory back pain consisting of an insidious onset before 40 years of age and morning stiffness with resolution by exercise or activity, present for >3 months before seeking treatment.
- Decreased range of motion of the lumbar spine as defined by the Schober test.
- Limited chest expansion.

SOURCE: *Adapted from Taurog and Lipsky.[1]*

If involved, physical findings related to the aforementioned extra-articular complications will be present.

DIAGNOSTIC CONSIDERATIONS

The modified New York criteria for diagnosing ankylosing spondylitis are outlined in Table 10-4-1. AS must be distinguished from the other seronegative spondyloarthropathies such as Reiter's syndrome (characterized by a more sudden onset, mucous membrane involvement, conjunctivitis, and urethritis), psoriatic arthropathy (characterized by psoriatic dermatological involvement), intestinal arthropathy (characterized by gastrointestinal involvement and a sudden onset if affecting peripheral joints), and reactive arthropathy (a nonspecific form of seronegative spondyloarthropathy with a sudden onset).

Other conditions in the differential include rheumatoid arthritis, osteoarthritis, herniated intervertebral disc, and diffuse idiopathic skeletal hyperostosis (DISH) syndrome.

SPECIAL CONSIDERATIONS

Onset of AS during adolescence is generally associated with a more severe form of the disease and a poorer prognosis. AS in women tends to progress less frequently to total ankylosis. Women often have more peripheral arthritis and incidence of isolated cervical ankylosis.[1]

LABORATORY TESTS

There are no laboratory tests specific for AS. The HLA-B27 antigen is present in approximately 90% of patients with AS of most ethnic groups; however, it is present in only approximately 50% of African Americans with AS.[1] Additionally, the antigen occurs in 4 to 8% of all Caucasians and 2 to 4% of all blacks.[2] Therefore, a negative result is more useful in excluding the diagnosis than a positive result is in confirming the diagnosis.

The erythrocyte sedimentation rate (ESR) is mildly elevated in individuals with active disease. C-reactive protein and IgA levels are often elevated. Rheumatoid factors and antinuclear antibodies are negative unless AS is accompanied by another rheumatoid disease. Occasionally, a mild normocytic, normochromic anemia may be seen. The alkaline phosphatase is increased in severe disease.

RADIOGRAPHIC STUDIES

Lumbar spine x-rays initially reveal findings consistent with bilateral sacroiliitis (blurring of the cortical margins of the sacroiliac joints, followed by erosions, sclerosis, and pseudo-widening of the joint space). Early changes seen in the spine itself consist of diffuse vertebral squaring, osteoporosis, spotty ligament calcifications, and early syndesmophytes (a bony formation that occurs as the outer annular fibers erode). As the syndesmophytes continue to grow and the ligamentous calcifications become diffuse, the vertebral bodies become fused. This represents the classic bamboo spine of AS; however, this finding is seen only in a minority of the patients with severe disease.

OTHER DIAGNOSTICS

Other diagnostic procedures are unnecessary unless the patient is experiencing extra-articular symptoms.

TREATMENT

The goals of treatment are to alleviate pain and prevent, delay, or correct deformities.

Pharmacologic Management

Nonsteroidal anti-inflammatory drugs (NSAIDs) are currently the drugs of choice. Indomethacin (Indocin) is often considered by many authorities to be the most effective NSAID for the treatment of AS.[1,2] However, others have been utilized effectively. When choosing an NSAID, one must consider the impact of side effects, costs, dosing convenience, and compliance for each individual patient.

The risk of gastrointestinal (GI) toxicity, especially hemorrhage, is a serious complication of NSAID therapy. Cytoprotective agents, such as misoprostol (Cytotec), should be considered in all patients receiving an NSAID. Risk factors that increase the likelihood of an adverse GI complication include a previous GI bleed, history of peptic ulcer disease, advancing age, smoking, and oral corticosteroid therapy. Misoprostol is currently the only agent with FDA approval for this purpose. For ease of administration, it is now available in combination with diclofenac sodium (Arthrotec) as a single pill. Although not FDA approved, omeprazole (Prilosec) and famotidine (Pepcid) have also been successfully used to decrease the risk of GI toxicity from NSAIDs.[3] The newer cyclooxygenase enzyme-2 (COX-2) inhibitors, such as celecoxib (Celebrex) and rofecoxib (Vioxx), lessen the likelihood of a GI bleed; however, they do not eliminate it because they still affect gastric prostaglandin E2.[4]

NSAIDs are also associated with renal and hepatotoxicity. The greatest risk for renal complications occurs in the elderly, diabetics, hypertensives, individuals with preexisting renal disease, and patients on diuretic therapy. Patients who consume large amounts of alcohol are probably at the greatest risk of hepatic complications.

Before instituting NSAID therapy, obtain baseline liver functions, renal functions, potassium, and a complete blood count (CBC). A CBC and tests for creatinine and potassium should be repeated in 1 month and again every 6 months thereafter.[3] If the initial liver function testing is normal, then additional testing is usually unnecessary.[3]

Sulfasalazine (Azulfidine), which is indicated for the treatment of ulcerative colitis, has been proven to be effective in reducing the pain and inflammation associated with AS.[1,5] The dosage is 2 to 3 g/d.[1]

Narcotics and muscle relaxants should be used only for limited periods of time for acute exacerbations. Oral corticosteroids do not have a role in the treatment of AS. Intra-articular corticosteroids may be beneficial when peripheral joint pain is the main concern. They should not be given any more frequently than once every 3 to 4 months.

Surgical Management

Total hip arthroplasty is indicated in a patient with severe hip joint arthritis. Other surgical procedures that may benefit patients with AS are correction of extreme flexion of the spine or of atlantoaxial subluxation.[1]

SUPPORTIVE MEASURES

Daily exercise is essential in the treatment of the patient with AS. Stretching and strengthening exercises have to be an integral component of these programs in order to maintain and/or improve range of motion and to prevent contractures and deformities. Postural training, including sleep positions, is also required. A competent physical therapist, with experience in treating AS patients, will be able to assist in devising individualized exercise programs.

PATIENT EDUCATION

Patient and family education regarding AS and its potential complications is essential. The expectations of therapy, including the importance of regular exercise, regular follow-up, and potential adverse reactions from their medications, also need to be discussed. Additionally, the patient needs to be informed that there is a 10 to 20% risk of their children having the disease.[7]

DISPOSITION

At a minimum, the patient should be seen at 3- to 6-month intervals. Each visit should include measurements of the patient's height, chest expansion, lumbar flexion (Schober test), and occiput-to-wall distance with the thoracic spine held against the wall. The patient should also be monitored for problems and potential adverse reactions to medications. Obviously, if the patient has a more severe form of the disease or extra-articular complications, more frequent follow-up will probably be required.

COMPLICATIONS

Patients should be referred to a rheumatologist if they not responding to therapy or have complex extra-articular manifestations.

OTHER NOTES AND PEARLS

There are some theories that exist that implicate infective agents as the precipitating factor for acute flares; the two most implicated organisms are *Klebsiella* and *Mycoplasma*.[7]

REFERENCES

1. Taurog JD, Lipsky PE: Ankylosing spondylitis, reactive arthritis, and undifferentiated spondyloarthropathy, in *Harrison's Principles of Internal Medicine,* 14th ed, AS Fauci et al (eds). New York, McGraw-Hill, 1998, pp 1904–1909.
2. Hellmann DB: Ankylosing spondylitis: Why the morning stiffness in a younger patient? *Consultant* 36:2169–2172, 1996.
3. Clough J et al: The new thinking on osteoarthritis. *Patient Care* 30:110–137, 1996.
4. Cryer B, Feldman M: Cyclooxygenase-1 and cyclooxygenase-2 selectivity of widely used nonsteroidal anti-inflammatory drugs. *Am J Med* 104:413–421, 1998.
5. Dougados M et al: Sulfasalazine in the treatment of spondyloarthropathy: A randomized, multicenter, double blind, placebo-controlled study. *Arthritis Rheum* 38:618–627, 1995.
6. Khan MA: Ankylosing spondylitis, in *Primer on the Rheumatic Diseases,* 11th ed, JH Klippel. Atlanta, GA, Arthritis Foundation, 1997, pp 189–193.
7. Calin A: Ankylosing spondylitis and the spondyloarthropathies, in *Primer on the Rheumatic Diseases,* 9th ed, HR Schumacher (ed). Atlanta, GA, Arthritis Foundation, 1988, pp 142–147.

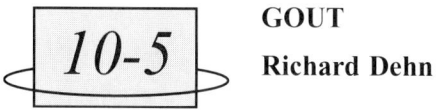

GOUT
Richard Dehn

DISCUSSION

Gout is a unique form of recurrent acute arthritis caused by the precipitation of monosodium urate crystals into the synovial fluid of the joints. It most often is characterized by the abrupt onset of a monoarticular arthritis that starts as an agonizing, pulsating pain followed by a quick progression of excruciatingly tender erythematous edema known as pseudocellulitis.

Gout most frequently presents in middle-aged males, with a peak age at onset of 45. The overall incidence is 1%, though prevalence increases with age, approaching 5% in men over 65. The initial arthritic attack is almost always in a lower extremity, most often affects a single joint, and over half the time is in the metatarsophalangeal joint of the great toe. Other joints are less frequently involved in early attacks and include the joints of the foot, ankle, and knee. The first attack often occurs at night, with the patient reporting no symptoms or a slight tingling sensation upon retiring. The attack rapidly progresses to a point where the joint is so inflamed and tender that the patient cannot tolerate the weight of bedcovers on it. On examination, the joint inflammation may be so intense that it suggests a septic joint or cellulitis.

Attacks often follow a minor trauma, an emotionally stressful experience, surgery, the stress of a medical illness, fatigue, or overindulgence in food or alcohol. The first attack may be quite short, and a second attack may not occur for several years. Without treatment, attacks become more frequent and last longer, and continued progression leads to the development of destructive tophi and renal involvement.

PATHOGENESIS

Gout is caused by the deposition of urates in various locations in the body, producing secondary problems. The urates are deposited as a result of chronically high concentrations of serum uric acid. The urate precipitants are found as urate crystals in the joint synovial fluid, encapsulated lesions containing urate crystals known as tophi that usually are located near joints, urate crystals deposited interstitially in the kidney, and uric acid stones in the urinary system. The presence of urate crystals in body structures initiates an inflammatory response that leads to the symptoms. When the urate crystals in the synovial fluid elicit an inflammatory response, the presentation is that of acute gouty arthritis. The tophaceous urate crystal deposits stimulate a chronic low-grade inflammatory response, with the chemical mediators of the inflammation producing the destruction of nearby tissues, usually bone or cartilage. Similarly, urate crystal deposits in the kidney stimulate an inflammatory response that over time decreases renal function. Additionally, uric acid urolithiasis can cause obstructive renal disease.

The extravascular deposition of urate crystals is a response to chronically high concentrations of uric acid in the serum. If uric acid concentrations in the serum are lowered, the extravascular deposits dissolve and the urates return to the serum. If serum concentrations are kept low over a long period, extravascular deposits disappear.

High serum levels of uric acid are caused by a metabolic overproduction of uric acid, urinary underexcretion of uric acid, or a combination of both mechanisms. It is believed that most cases of gout are caused by decreased renal clearance of urate. This may be a primary idiopathic abnormality, may be secondary to pharmacologic agents, or may be secondary to renal disease. Overproduction most often is caused by a genetically transmitted mechanism; however, it also can be secondary to any condition that exhibits increased rates of cell proliferation and cell death, such as leukemia or psoriasis. Only about 1 in 10 cases of gout is due to overproduction, which is defined as the urinary excretion of more than 1 g of uric acid over a 24-h period.

Gout is associated with increased body mass, hypertension, and hypertriglyceridemia. Although diet is a factor in the overproduction of urates, restrictions of the consumption of high-purine foods is only of marginal value, with the possible exception of organ meats and beer.

Many commonly used pharmacologic agents reduce renal uric acid excretion. Thiazide diuretics, furosemide, pyrazinamide, ethambutol, and cyclosporine can all increase serum uric acid concentrations through this mechanism. Aspirin also decreases renal urate excretion when used in higher doses and therefore should be avoided by patients predisposed to gout.

LABORATORY TESTING

Virtually all patients with gout have above-average serum uric acid levels, and a majority have elevated levels. A normal serum uric acid level at the time of an acute attack probably is due to a stress-induced uricosuric process; however, most patients present with an elevated or high-normal level.

The gold standard in the diagnosis of gout is identification of urate crystals in synovial fluid from the inflamed joint. The crystals are visible inside polymorphonuclear leukocytes. Aspirating the joint for evidence of urate crystals is essential to differentiate gout from pseudogout, which usually is caused by deposition of calcium pyrophosphate dihydrate crystals. Joint aspiration also rules out a septic joint process.

A measurement of uric acid renal clearance can be calculated by a 24-h urine collection. In the typical middle-aged male patient, this is not particularly useful, but in identifying a patient in whom gout is secondary to overproduction from a disease state or underexcretion is secondary to renal failure, 24-h urine studies are valuable. A spot estimate can be calculated to make a rough estimate of whether the patient's hyperuricemia is a result of overproduction or underexcretion by obtaining a random urine uric acid and multiplying the value by the serum creatinine value. This product then should be divided by the random urine creatinine. A result <0.6 is likely to point to underexcretion; if it is >0.6, overproduction should be suspected; and if it is approximately 0.6, a mixed cause should be considered.

DIAGNOSTIC CONSIDERATIONS

In acute attacks of arthritis, despite the characteristic history and physical findings suggestive of gout, several other diagnoses should be considered. Pseudogout can be confused easily with gout; however, pseudogout usually is found in larger joints. Both gout and pseudogout will respond to anti-inflammatory acute treatments; however, pseudogout will not respond to uric acid reduction therapies. The only definitive diagnostic test for accurately discriminating gout from pseudogout is synovial fluid aspiration analysis. A septic joint process also should be entertained and ruled out.

In an acute gouty arthritis patient, one should consider the possibility that the urate hyperproduction could be secondary to a malignancy or hyperthyroidism or that the urate underexcretion could be secondary to renal disease. Additionally, patients with gout should be evaluated for treatable associated signs and symptoms such as obesity, hypertension, hyperlipidemias, and diabetes mellitus.

TREATMENT

Pharmacologic Management

Treatment of gout is determined by whether the patient is in the acute stage or the asymptomatic stage. In the acute stage, treatment is aimed at stopping the inflammatory process in the affected joint. This typically is done by giving high doses of a short-half-life nonsteroidal anti-inflammatory drug (NSAID) such as ibuprofen 800 mg qid or indomethacin with a 100-mg loading dose followed by 50 mg qid. These regimens are continued until the joint improves dramatically, usually in a few days, and then are reduced to 600 mg tid for ibuprofen and 50 mg tid for indomethacin.

Colchicine also can be used, one tablet (0.6 mg) every 1 to 2 h until the symptoms improve, gastrointestinal (GI) toxicity occurs, or a maximum of 7 g has been taken in 48 h. If the symptoms improve, the dose should be reduced to 0.6 mg two times daily. The use of colchicine should be monitored carefully owing to its potential toxicity.

Corticosteroids can be used in either parenteral or oral formulations. A course of oral prednisone 40 to 60 mg daily for 1 week with a tapered withdrawal or a single intramuscular injection of a sustained-released corticosteroid such as triamcinolone (Kenalog) 40 to 60 mg can be used if NSAIDs are contraindicated. Injection of corticosteroids into the joint is also effective; however, it is important that the volume injected by kept to a minimum since large volumes increase the symptoms. Injection of the joint requires starting an additional anti-inflammatory agent to prevent resumption of the gout symptoms in a few days.

Adrenocorticotropic hormone (ACTH) is effective and is appropriate in patients who are unable to use NSAIDs or corticosteroids. It has a faster onset of action than do other agents but must be given intramuscularly, intravenously, or subcutaneously. It also has a rebound effect, requiring the addition of another agent after the symptoms have improved.

Additionally, patients with acute gout should be advised to avoid dehydration to enhance uric acid renal clearance and prevent the accumulation of urate crystals in the kidneys.

Supportive Measures

The goal of the treatment of symptomatic gout is to prevent future attacks. Overweight patients should be advised to reduce their body mass to reduce uric acid production, and excesses of food and alcohol consumption should be avoided. A significant number of first-attack patients will not experience another attack and many others will not have the second attack for several years, and so it is not unreasonable to stop treating these asymptomatic gout patients after 2 weeks of anti-inflammatory medications. Patients experiencing more than two attacks a year are candidates for prophylactic NSAID or colchicine therapy or may elect to use an agent to lower serum uric acid. Patients who exhibit tophi or renal involvement also should be placed on an agent that lowers serum uric acid.

Pharmacologic agents that reduce uric acid synthesis or increase renal excretion of uric acid can reduce serum uric acid. Allopurinol is effective in inhibiting the production of uric acid, and once-a-day dosing makes it convenient to take. It should be started at 100 mg daily and increased until serum uric acid levels off in the range of 5 to 6 mg/dL. Serious toxic side effects such as rashes, interstitial nephritis, liver damage, fever, leukocytosis, and bone marrow suppression usually present early in treatment, and so it is important to begin with a low dose.

Uricosuric agents also can be used to increase the renal excretion of uric acid. Probenecid (Benemid) 250 mg twice daily can be given and titrated up to 2 g daily in divided doses until serum uric acid levels off at the range of 5 to 6 mg/dL. Sulfinpyrazone (Anturane) can be started at 100 mg twice daily and titrated up to 800 mg/day until the desired serum uric acid level is attained.

Because allopurinol is more convenient to take and has fewer interactions with other medications, it is used most commonly for serum acid reduction despite the fact that most gout patients are underexcreters, it is more expensive than uricosuric agents, and it can produce more serious side effects than do the uricosuric agents.

One must remember that when starting an agent that lowers uric acid, sudden changes in serum uric acid levels are likely to trigger an acute gout attack. When one is starting a patient on allopurinol or a uricosuric agent, an anti-inflammatory agent also should be started, such as an NSAID or low-dose colchicine 0.6 mg twice daily. This should be continued until the serum uric acid levels have reached the desired therapeutic range.

BIBLIOGRAPHY

Beers MH, Berkow R (eds): *Merck Manual of Diagnosis and Therapy,* 17th ed, Whitehouse Station, NJ, Merck Research Laboratories, 1999, pp 460–464.

Brasington RD: Hyperuricemia and gout, in Rakel RE (ed): *Conn's Current Therapy 2000.* Philadelphia, Saunders, 2000, pp 576–578.

Hellmann DB, Stone JH: Arthritis and musculoskeletal disorders, in Tierney LM Jr, McPhee SJ, Papadakis MA (eds): *Current Medical Diagnosis and Treatment,* 39th rev. ed, New York, McGraw-Hill, 2000, pp 810–814.

Hershfield MS: Gout and uric acid metabolism, in Goldman L, Bennett JC (eds): *Cecil Textbook of Medicine,* 21st ed, Philadelphia, Saunders, 2000, pp 1541–1548.

Terkeltaub RA: Gout and hyperuricemia, in Stein JH (ed): *Stein Internal Medicine,* 5th ed, Philadelphia, Saunders, 1998, pp 1268–1276.

Wortmann RL: Gout and other disorders of purine metabolism, in Fauci AS, Braunwald E, Isselbacher KJ, et al (eds): *Harrison's Principles of Internal Medicine,* 14th ed, New York, McGraw-Hill, 1998, pp 2158–2166.

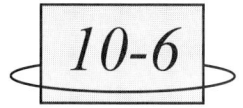

KAWASAKI DISEASE
Ricky Kortyna and Deborah Kortyna

DISCUSSION

In 1967 Tomisaku Kawasaki reported on 50 Japanese children with a new constellation of symptoms, which he termed the *mucocutaneous lymph node syndrome.* Since his original paper the eponym *Kawasaki disease* has replaced mucocutaneous lymph node syndrome. There have been an additional 140,000 cases in Japan since the original report.[1] The disease has been described throughout the world but remains six times more common in children who are of Asian descent than in Caucasians and three times more common in Asians than in African Americans. It is the leading cause of acquired heart disease in children in the United States.[2,3]

Kawasaki disease is almost never seen in adults and is most often observed in children under the age of 5 years with a peak between the ages of 1 and 3 years. The male:female ratio is 1.5:1 and the disease is five times more likely to be fatal in males.[4] In the United States the occurrence in children under the age of 5 years is 9 per 100,000. The incidence is higher during the winter and spring. Person-to-person transmission is rare, only around 2% of cases, yet there were several epidemics reported in the 1980s.[4]

Kawasaki disease is an arteritis involving the small, medium, and large arteries with frequent involvement of the coronary arteries. The etiology of this disease remains unknown but it is thought that a virus, perhaps a lymphotropic retrovirus[5] or parvovirus B19,[6] may start the chain of events leading to vasculitis. Other infectious agents including Rickettsia, *Streptococcus viridans, Staphylococcus, Propionibacterium,* and *Candida* have been proposed.[7,8] The clinical findings mimic those of toxin-producing diseases, and reports of effective treatment with intravenous immune globulin (IVIG) are also similar to the observations noted with toxin-producing diseases.[4] Other explanations have included exposures to varied environmental substances such as heavy metals, pollutants, and rug shampoo.[5,9] Whatever the etiology turns out to be, it is known that the immune system is involved during the acute stage of the disease.[7]

Pathology

The vasculitis of Kawasaki disease resembles that of polyarteritis nodosa. The entire vessel wall demonstrates inflammation and necrosis. Of particular clinical importance is the damage potentially done to the coronary arteries, which ranges from mild changes with only intimal involvement to severe destruction of the entire vessel with skip or segmental necrosis. When the acute phase of the disease begins to subside the patient is at risk for the development of coronary artery aneurysms and possibly thrombosis with myocardial infarction.[2]

CLINICAL MANIFESTATIONS

There is no specific laboratory test for Kawasaki disease as the cause remains unknown; the diagnosis is based on clinical findings.[1] The clinical features are shown in Table 10-6-1.

TABLE 10-6-1. Clinical Features of Kawasaki Disease

Fever of >40°C of at least 5 days duration, unresponsive to antibiotics, and four of the following:
- Extremity changes such as desquamation of hands/feet, palmar/plantar erythema, Beau's lines
- Polymorphous exanthem
- Lymphadenopathy: unilateral cervical
- Mucosal changes such as strawberry tongue, dry cracked lips, and erythema of the oral mucosa
- Conjunctival injection: bilateral, painless, with limbal sparing

Kawasaki disease has three distinct phases. The first or acute phase is marked by the onset of a fever, unresponsive to antipyretics, which exceeds 40.6°C (105°F) in 40% of cases. Affected children are highly irritable. Bilateral anterior triangle cervical lymphadenopathy occurs but disappears rapidly. Bilateral conjunctival injection may also appear. Within several days a polymorphous truncal rash emerges which resembles the rashes of scarlatina, measles, Rocky Mountain spotted fever, and erythema multiforme, all of which are diseases included in the differential for Kawasaki disease.

Cardiac manifestations during this phase include tachycardia out of proportion to the fever, electrocardiogram (ECG) changes as discussed below, congestive heart failure, gallop rhythms, and pericardial effusions as demonstrated on echocardiograms. Aneurysm development can occur in other major vessels such as the aorta and iliac arteries.[8] The hands and feet become edematous and the palms and soles redden. Children may refuse to hold objects.[1] This phase lasts from 7 to 10 days with parents usually consulting a health care provider within the first 3 to 4 days.

The second or subacute phase occurs after 7 to 10 days and is characterized by the continuation of a high fever unresponsive to antibiotics or antipyretics. The fever may last up to 12 days if the underlying disease is not treated. At this stage the child appears ill, the conjunctivitis worsens, and subconjunctival hemorrhages occur. The lips and oral mucosal membranes become hyperemic, the lips also become dry and cracked, and the tongue takes on a strawberry appearance.

Gastrointestinal manifestations include hepatomegaly that resolves quickly, diarrhea, vomiting, abdominal pain, and paralytic ileus. An enlarged, tender liver should make one suspect acalculous cholecystitis, which is confirmed via ultrasound.

Arthritis usually occurs during this phase as does desquamation of the palms and soles. The desquamation begins at the fingertips and later involves the hands and feet.

Because of the fever and irritability, about 25% of patients are suspected of having meningitis and have a lumbar puncture done. The cerebrospinal fluid is consistent with aseptic meningitis.[7] Other neurological sequelae such as facial nerve palsies, seizures, ataxia, and hemiplegia have been reported.[10,11]

Rare findings may include testicular swelling and gangrene of the extremities.[7,8]

The third or convalescence phase lasts from 6 to 8 weeks. The arthritis may persist. Both myocardial infarctions and coronary artery aneurysm rupture may occur at this phase. Beau's lines, which are transverse ridges of the nails, occur several months after the acute illness.[1,8]

Complications

The most notorious complication is that of coronary artery aneurysm formation, which occurs in up to 20% of all patients. Half of the aneurysm abnormalities spontaneously resolve within 18 months; however, there is still a 1 to 2% overall mortality rate with about 70% of all deaths occurring within 45 days of the onset of fever.[5,7] The left coronary artery is involved four times more often than the right.[11] Myocardial infarction secondary to thrombosis of an aneurysm can lead to death. Those patients with the largest aneurysms are at the largest risk for infarction.[3]

DIFFERENTIAL DIAGNOSIS

The differential for Kawasaki disease can be rather broad. The rash may be confused with scarlatina, Rocky Mountain spotted fever, measles, erythema multiforme, staphylococcal scalded skin syndrome, toxic shock syndrome, leptospirosis, and drug reactions (especially to sulfonamides).[5,12]

The arthritis of Kawasaki disease may be confused with that of juvenile rheumatoid arthritis or systemic lupus erythematosus.

TABLE 10-6-2. Laboratory Test Results in Kawasaki Disease

TESTS	RESULTS
CBC and differential	Moderate leukocytosis of 20,000–30,000 cells with a left shift initially and later a lymphocytosis. The counts generally peak at the end of the second week. Additionally there is a drop in the hematocrit most prevalent at the end of the second week.
Thrombocytosis	Occurs in about 80% of all patients and may reach a level of 1,000,000. It peaks at the third week of illness.[8]
ESR	Becomes elevated to around 55 mm/h and returns to normal at about 8 weeks.
C-reactive protein	Elevated, then returns to normal in 8 weeks.
α_1 antitrypsin	Elevated, then returns to normal in 8 weeks.
Cerebrospinal fluid	Elevation of mononuclear cells with a normal protein and glucose.
Liver function studies	Elevation of the serum alanine aminotransferase and occasionally of bilirubin.
Urinalysis	Sterile pyuria with mononuclear cells is found if a clean catch is done. This finding is missed on a bladder tap. Proteinuria may be present.
Joint aspiration	Increase in the WBCs, especially neutrophils, in those with arthritis.
Cardiac troponin 1	This biological marker helps with the diagnosis of myocarditis early in the course of the disease and may also be used to follow the efficacy of IVIG.[13]
Cytokines	Although not routinely ordered, there have been reports of elevation of serum interleukin 1, 2, 4, 6, 8, and 10, tumor necrosis factor α, CD14+ T cells, and plasma endothelin-1.[5,8,14]

ABBREVIATIONS: CBC, complete blood count; ESR, erythrocyte sedimentation rate; IVIG, intravenous immune globulin; WBCs, white blood cells.

LABORATORY STUDIES

Laboratory studies and the results commonly seen in Kawasaki disease are shown in Table 10-6-2.

RADIOGRAPHIC AND OTHER TESTS

Echocardiograms are essential to determine the presence and degree of aneurysm formation.

Gallium 67 citrate scanning may help in determining myocardial inflammation.

Coronary arteriography, although invasive, is the gold standard for the evaluation of coronary aneurysms. This should be done in those patients with echocardiographically proven coronary aneurysms.[15]

ECG findings are nonspecific with mild PR-interval prolongation, T-wave flattening or inversion, and nonspecific ST-T segment changes.[4]

TREATMENT

The acute phase should be treated with IVIG, 2 g/kg as a single dose over 12 hours. A repeat dose is given if the fever reoccurs within 72 hours. Those requiring a second dose of IVIG have a higher rate of complications than those who require only one dose.[4] IVIG has reduced the rate of coronary artery aneurysm formation by half if given with the first 10 days of the disease.[3]

High-dose aspirin is administered at 20 mg/kg per dose every 6 hours from the start of the diagnosis until day 14 of the disease. If the echocardiogram is normal, a lower dose of 3 to 5 mg/kg per day for 2 to 3 months is given.[15] Aspirin can be discontinued once the thrombocytosis is corrected and the erythrocyte sedimentation rate and C-reactive protein are normalized. Aspirin is continued indefinitely in those with coronary artery aneurysms.[9]

Corticosteroid therapy is contraindicated as it may lead to the development of further coronary artery aneurysms.[7]

DISPOSITION

Once the diagnosis of Kawasaki disease is suspected, the patient should be admitted to the hospital for observation and stabilization. Serial echocardiograms may be indicated. Those patients with proven coronary artery aneurysm are followed as outpatients with serial echocardiograms.

COMPLICATIONS AND RED FLAGS

The difficulty with making the diagnosis of Kawasaki disease is that it does not have a typical pattern and the symptoms mimic those of so many other diseases.

If the patient is on aspirin for a prolonged period of time, a salicylate level should be drawn, especially if signs of toxicity such as nausea, lethargy, or hypercapnia occur.[4]

Children with Kawasaki disease should not be given live virus vaccines for at least 11 months after receiving IVIG since the preparation may neutralize the vaccine.[1,8]

ACKNOWLEDGMENT

The editor would like to acknowledge the significant contribution of Wayne van Deusen, author of this chapter in the first edition of *Primary Care for Physician Assistants.*

REFERENCES

1. Rowley AH, Shulman ST: Kawasaki syndrome. *Pediatr Clin North Am* 46(2):313–329, 1999.
2. Schoen FJ, Cotran RS: Blood vessels: Kawasaki syndrome (mucocutaneous lymph node syndrome), in *Robbins Pathologic Basis of Disease,* RS Cotran et al (eds). Philadelphia, Saunders, 1999, p 521.
3. Pahl E: Kawasaki disease: Cardiac sequelae and management. *Pediatr Ann* 26(2):112–115, 1997.
4. Bradley DJ, Glode MP: Kawasaki disease: The mystery continues. *West J Med* 168:23–29, 1998.
5. Barkin RM, Rosen P: Infectious disorders: Kawasaki syndrome, in *Emergency Pediatrics: A Guide to Ambulatory Care,* RM Barkin, P Rosen (eds). St. Louis, Mosby, 1999, pp 707–709.
6. Gotlieb AI et al: Blood vessels: Kawasaki disease (mucocutaneous lymph node syndrome), in *Pathology,* E Rubin, JL Farber (eds). Philadelphia, Lippincott-Raven, 1999, 518–519.
7. Taubert KA, Shulman ST: Kawasaki disease. *Am Fam Physician* 59(11): 3093–3101, 1999.
8. Barron KS: Kawasaki disease in children. *Curr Opin Rheumatol* 10:29–37, 1998.
9. Eichenfield A: Rheumatic diseases: Kawasaki disease, in *Rudolph's Fundamentals of Pediatrics,* AM Rudolph, RK Kamei (eds). Stamford, CT, Appleton and Lange, 1998, p 231.
10. Chung CJ, Stein L: Kawasaki disease: A review. *Radiology* 208:25–33, 1998.
11. McDonald D et al: Neurological complications of kawasaki disease. *Arch Dis Child* 75(2):200, 1998.
12. Fitzpatrick TB et al: Kawasaki's disease, in *Color Atlas and Synopsis of Clinical Dermatology: Common and Serious Diseases.* New York, McGraw-Hill, 1997.
13. Kim M, Kim KK: Changes in cardiac troponin I in Kawasaki disease before and after treatment in intravenous gammaglobin. *Jpn Circ J* 62:479–482, 1998.
14. Wallach J: *Interpretation of Diagnostic Tests,* 6th ed, Boston, Little, Brown, 1996.
15. Wolfe RR: Cardiovascular diseases, in *Current Pediatric Diagnosis and Treatment,* WW Hay (ed). Stamford, CT, Appleton and Lange, 1997, p 524.

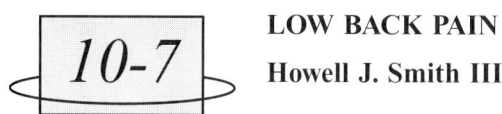

LOW BACK PAIN

Howell J. Smith III

DISCUSSION

Low back pain (LBP) produces a short-term impairment in at least 80% of the U.S. population at some time in each person's life. Causes for LBP are numerous. Mechanical pain resulting from injuries to muscles, tendons, ligaments, deep fascia, disks, or bones accounts for most cases of back pain. The remaining sources include cauda equina syndrome, infection, aortic aneurysm, and neoplasms. These conditions require immediate intervention to prevent further neurologic deficits, massive blood loss, shock, or subsequent death. Low back problems are one of the most common reasons patients seek medical care. It is essential that health care providers obtain a careful medical history and then perform a thorough physical examination that is guided by the symptoms. Using the history and physical examination, a treatment plan is then developed using the flow chart shown in Fig. 10-7-1. Referral to appropriate specialists should occur when primary care providers believe the condition exceeds their expertise. Additionally, consultation is indicated when the patient's condition deteriorates, if the neurologic deficit progresses, or if a secondary cause of back pain is identified that requires skills beyond those of a primary care provider.

MECHANICAL LOW BACK PAIN

This condition most commonly occurs during the productive years, between ages 30 and 60 years. Even though this is by far the most common cause of LBP, it should be a diagnosis of exclusion after other causes have been ruled out. At increased risk for LBP are individuals with poor conditioning, poor abdominal musculature, poor posture, poor body mechanics, or those who are pregnant or obese. Additionally, those working in occupations with heavy exertional activities or those who are exposed to vibrations by vehicles or heavy machinery are more prone to LBP. Underlying psychological etiologies are common and may include manipulation, boredom, dissatisfaction with jobs or personal lives, drug and alcohol addiction, and clinical depression. Secondary gain, whether it be workers' compensation, a settlement from a lawsuit, or attention, is frequently associated with chronic LBP patients.

SYMPTOMS

The symptom that is most indicative of mechanical low back is intermittent pain that correlates with certain body postures or positions. The pain and discomfort are apt to be acute in onset. Many patients may be able to relate an identifiable cause for their pain, like moving or unusual weekend athletic activity. Symptoms are usually aggravated with activities and are improved with rest. Between 30 and 60% of patients report a prior history of back pain. The natural progression of those presenting with mechanical LBP has been demonstrated to be that 50% of patients will recover within 2 weeks and 90% recover by 4 weeks. Acute exacerbations generally last less than 3 months, and chronic exacerbations last 3 months or longer. Fortunately, less than 5% of patients will develop a chronic low back syndrome.

OBJECTIVE FINDINGS

Most patients who present with lumbosacral strain have a diffuse area of tenderness on the affected side. Range of motion of the spine, hips, or lower extremities may be restricted by pain. The examination is unremarkable for neurologic findings. Motor strength, sensation, and deep tendon reflexes are intact. The Babinski test is negative. Rectal tone is good. The straight-leg raising (SLR) test is negative. Although not very specific, the SLR test is a sensitive indicator for disk herniations at the L4-L5 and L5-S1 levels. Leg length discrepancy as well as hamstring tightness are commonly overlooked as sources for LBP.

RADIOLOGIC STUDIES

Anteroposterior and lateral x-rays, when indicated, are standard views for the initial evaluation of uncomplicated LBP.

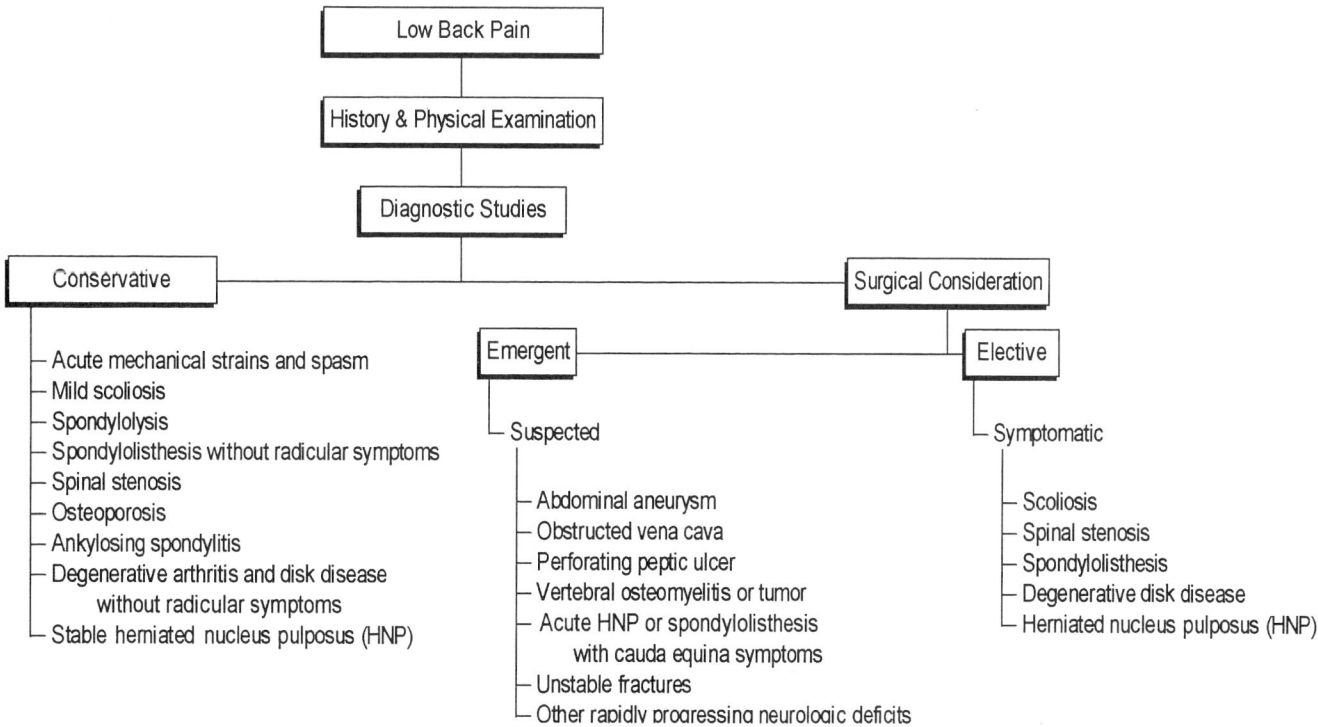

FIGURE 10-7-1. Low back pain algorithm.

TREATMENT

Pharmacologic Management

Acetaminophen can be used for mild to moderate cases. Unless contraindicated, nonsteroidal anti-inflammatory drugs (NSAIDs) are prescribed for moderate to severe cases. Patients who have self-medicated with over-the-counter NSAIDs prior to presentation are usually not taking full therapeutic dosages. If a patient's response to the first prescribed NSAID is inadequate, changing medications is often helpful. Muscle relaxants should be reserved for those patients with muscle spasm, since most cause sedation. This may interfere with the patient returning to work and mobilizing early. Narcotic agents should be used only if the previous treatment fails. If prescribed at all, they should be for no longer than 3 weeks to avoid addiction. Narcotic use should be carefully monitored in patients with chronic pain syndromes. Tricyclic antidepressants may be an appropriate adjunct for patients with chronic LBP.

Supportive Measures

Modalities such as ice, heat, and ultrasound are often helpful. Traction and lumbosacral corsets have not proved effective in the treatment of acute low back symptoms. During the past 5 years, the treatment strategy has changed from prolonged bed rest to encouraging early mobility. New studies indicate that no bed rest and performing normal activities as pain allows is superior to placing the patient on bed rest. Bed rest is utilized for patients with severe acute LBP and should be kept to a minimum. Two days have been shown to be as effective as 7 days. Patients placed on bed rest should be instructed to avoid sitting while in bed.

PATIENT EDUCATION

Patients should be instructed on use of proper body mechanics when lifting and advised to use good postural positions. Enrollment in "low back school" or a referral to physical therapy has proved beneficial to reduce recurrence of symptoms. Abdominal strengthening exercises can begin when pain subsides.

HERNIATED LUMBAR DISK

Lumbar disk herniation is found most commonly in individuals between the ages of 20 and 50 years. Disks can protrude, extrude, or be free fragments in the canal. Individuals at increased risk are those in occupations that require prolonged sitting and repetitive lifting. Disk herniations most commonly occur at the L4-L5 and L5-S1 levels. Most herniations are posterolateral because the posterior longitudinal ligament is the weakest. In acute injuries, the pain is usually severe and is commonly associated with a flexion strain or other traumatic event.

Sciatica and radicular symptoms may be present, and the patient may report pain relief with rest. Cauda equina compression syndrome involves an acute massive central disk prolapse and presents with paresthesias and pain in the posterior thighs and legs. There are varying degrees of motor function loss in the legs and feet, and possible bowel and bladder dysfunction. This is truly an emergency that requires immediate referral to an orthopedic spine surgeon or neurosurgeon. An immediate magnetic resonance imaging (MRI) scan and surgery (as directed by MRI findings) are necessary to arrest progression of neurologic loss.

Individuals with chronic disk herniation report a wide range of symptoms. With aging, degenerative disk changes include loss of water content and annular tears, which predisposes to herniation of nuclear material. Most individuals with this condition have symptoms that progress gradually and intensify. The pain may be dull to severe and may not necessarily be present in the back. The hallmark complaint is lower extremity pain that radiates from the buttocks to the posterolateral thigh and calf and frequently into the foot. Valsalva

and other straining maneuvers that may further compress the involved neurologic structure frequently intensify the symptoms. Clinically, on physical examination, the amount of sensory and motor changes directly correlates with the degree of compression. Conservative treatment methods previously mentioned are generally attempted for mild and transient conditions. Unresolved conditions and those that progressively worsen are considered surgical candidates, based on MRI, electromyogram (EMG), and nerve conduction velocity (NCV) studies.

VERTEBRAL ETIOLOGIES

SCOLIOSIS

Most severe cases of scoliosis are identified in adolescence. Surgical intervention is indicated for severe and unstable cases. Mild scoliosis, which is often detected when evaluating adults with LBP, is generally treated like mechanical LBP.

SPONDYLOLYSIS

A defect in the pars interarticularis is the most common cause of LBP in children and adolescents. The defect is thought to be a fatigue fracture from repetitive hyperextension stresses. It is commonly found in gymnasts, divers, football linemen, and weightlifters.

Although spondylolysis can be seen on some lateral studies, an oblique view best visualizes the defect. When present, the pars defect appears as a defect or break in the "Scottie dog's neck." Defining acute versus chronic etiologies can become an issue, especially in workers' compensation cases. A nuclear scan with an increased uptake is consistent with an active lesion or fracture. Treatment of acute injuries should include avoidance of heavy lifting and hyperextension activities. Symptomatic relief measures should include rest and NSAIDs.

SPONDYLOLISTHESIS

Spondylolisthesis is the anterior displacement of one vertebra on another. It most commonly occurs at L4-L5 or L5-S1. The slippage is usually due to a pars interarticularis defect (see Fig. 10-7-2).

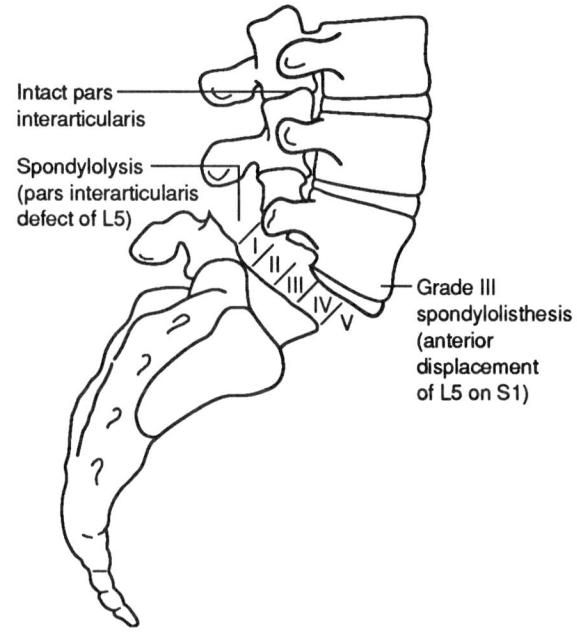

Intact pars interarticularis

Spondylolysis (pars interarticularis defect of L5)

Grade III spondylolisthesis (anterior displacement of L5 on S1)

FIGURE 10-7-2. Spondylolysis and spondylolisthesis.

The severity of the slip is based on the amount of displacement or degree of the spinal column compared with S1 on the lateral x-ray:

Grade I = 0 to 25%
Grade II = 25 to 50%
Grade III = 50 to 75%
Grade IV = 75 to 100%
Grade V = >100%

More than 100% displacement is called *spondyloptosis.*

Patients with less than 50% displacement (grades I and II) usually can be asymptomatic or have minimal mechanical LBP symptoms. Patients with slippages of greater than 50% (grades III, IV, and V) usually experience moderate to severe pain and sciatica and may complain of a variety of lower extremity neurologic symptoms. The degree of neurologic involvement runs from rare to the possibility of a full-blown cauda equina syndrome in high-degree slips. The treatment for asymptomatic spondylolysis and a minimal spondylolisthesis is observation with no restrictions. There is a 60% success rate of treating symptomatic grades I and II spondylolisthesis patients with conservative treatment. Spinal fusion is often necessary to stabilize patients with grades III, IV, and V slippages. Most neurologic deficits are L5 radiculopathy associated with L5-S1 spondylolisthesis. Cauda equina symptoms are associated with grades III, IV, or V slips. Fortunately, this amount of neurologic loss is rare. Suspicion of cauda equina involvement is an emergency that needs immediate attention by either an orthopedic spine surgeon or a neurosurgeon.

SPINAL STENOSIS

Spinal stenosis is a three-joint complex (disk and facet joints) condition that narrows the neural foramen, creating compression on the spinal cord. Most cases of stenosis are from the degenerative changes of a collapsing disk and subsequent facet arthritis. The average age of a patient with stenosis is 60 years. Stenosis is the most common cause for neurologic leg pain in the elderly. Patients with stenosis have a narrowing of the central canal and the lateral recesses where the nerve roots are contained (see Fig. 10-7-3). This can create a lumbosacral radiculopathy and neurogenic claudication. Most patients complain that the pain worsens during the day. A common description is low back and bilateral extremity pain in the buttocks, legs, and thighs after ambulating or standing. Patients also relate that downhill walking makes the pain worse. Neurogenic claudication pain is relieved by 15 to 30 min in a supine position with a pillow under the knees. Patients also report relief of their symptoms by leaning forward while standing, which has been termed the "shopping cart" position. The physical examination may be normal. Increased discomfort with spinal extension suggests stenosis. Neurologic findings vary and, when present, impairment at several spinal levels is often noted.

Radiographs usually demonstrate extensive vertebral osteophytes and degenerative disk disease. MRI and computed tomography (CT) studies are used to evaluate the severity of the condition and for preoperative planning. Conservative treatment consists of NSAIDs and avoidance of aggravating activities such as walking. Bicycling may be recommended as an alternative aerobic activity. Epidural steroid injections may provide short-term relief. Surgical decompression is needed for long-term resolution for those with significant discomfort and neurologic compression.

OSTEOPOROSIS

This is the most common cause of metabolic bone disease in the United States. This age-related decrease in bone mass, most commonly seen in postmenopausal women, is usually associated with the loss of estrogen. Osteoporosis is a contributing cause of 1 million fractures per year. This process primarily affects the cancellous bone. The spine, hip, and pelvis are the most commonly affected areas. Most vertebral fractures secondary to osteoporosis occur between T11 and L1. Individuals affected may be completely asymptomatic or may suffer from severe back pain (see Chap. 5-2).

ANKYLOSING SPONDYLITIS

This chronic systemic inflammatory disease of the joints and the axial skeleton commonly has an onset in the late teens or early twenties and usually occurs before age 40. This disorder affects three times more men than women. The onset is gradual with intermittent exacerbations and back pain radiating down the leg(s) posteriorly. Complaints of progressive morning stiffness over several months that is relieved with exercise are common. Physical examination findings may include painful sacroiliac joints, reduced mobility of the spine, and possible uveitis. Studies indicate that 85% of patients with ankylosing spondylitis (AS) have an elevated erythrocyte sedimentation rate (ESR), the rheumatoid factor is generally negative, and HLA-B27 antigen is present in 90% of cases. The earliest x-ray changes are widening and sclerosis of both sacroiliac joints, which are best visualized on the anteroposterior pelvis view. As the disease progresses, x-ray changes may include what has been labeled the "bamboo" spine. This appearance is a combination of calcification of the anterior spinal ligament and bony bridging of the vertebral bodies. Treatment consists of stressing the importance of postural breathing, NSAIDs, and physical therapy (see Chap. 10-4).

SPINAL TUMORS

Primary spinal tumors are rare, accounting for less than 10% of all bone tumors. Tumors in individuals younger than 21 years are usually benign. More than 70% of primary spinal tumors in individuals older

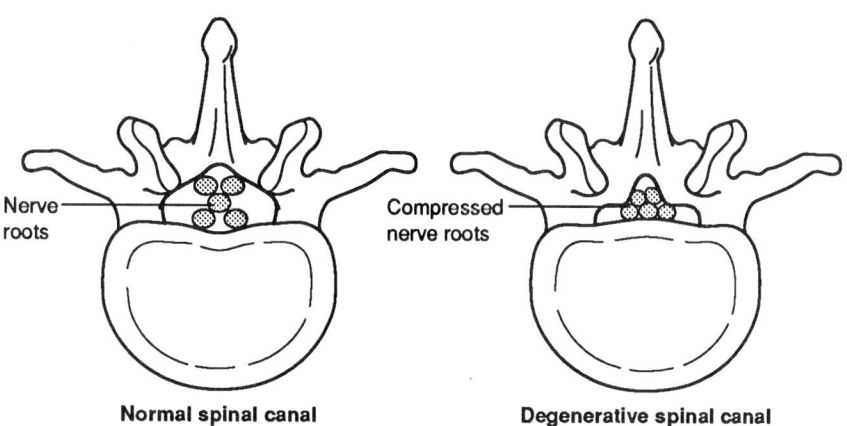

FIGURE 10-7-3. Spinal stenosis.

than 21 years are malignant. Multiple myeloma (see Chap. 13-12) is the most common primary bone tumor. Metastatic tumors are common. Between 50 and 70% of individuals with terminal cancer have vertebral metastasis. More than 75% of tumors in the vertebral body are malignant. Known malignancy and a tender spinous process, with or without back pain, is extremely suspicious for a vertebral or epidural metabolic disease. Night pain that is slow, progressive, persistent, dull, and made worse by recumbency should also be aggressively investigated. Neurologic deficits are common at the time of presentation. X-rays may identify only as little as 30% of spine lesions associated with pain. Nuclear imaging demonstrates increased uptake in areas of activity. CT scan is utilized to evaluate the extent of the tumor. Treatment consists of a biopsy, radiation therapy and chemotherapy, or, in selected cases, surgical excision with spine stabilization.

SPINAL INFECTIONS

Infections of the vertebrae (osteomyelitis; see Chap. 10-17) and of the soft tissues surrounding the spine are rare and are commonly associated with a postoperative surgical procedure or injection. Other causes may include tuberculosis, primary or metastatic tumors of the spine and spinal cord, or infections secondary to myelograms. The most common organisms cultured are *Staphylococcus aureus, Pseudomonas,* and *Escherichia coli.* Individuals with increased risks include drug abusers, those with diabetes mellitus, and those who are immunologically suppressed. Back pain, malaise, fever, sepsis, wound drainage, and an elevated ESR are classic at presentation. The neurologic examination may be normal to a complete cauda equina compression, which is a frequent presentation with spinal tumors. Conditions with acute neurologic changes that are progressing to cauda equina compression need immediate surgical intervention. Other infectious processes require a combination of wound management techniques that include incision and drainage and intravenous antibiotics.

REFERRED PAIN

The causes for referred pain to the back are numerous, many of which can be life-threatening. Etiologies may include herpes zoster, renal calculi, urinary tract infection, peptic ulcer disease, carcinoma of the pancreas, prostatitis, prostatic carcinoma, inferior vena cava obstruction, and abdominal aortic aneurysm. Pain may be intermittent or acute and excruciating. Patients will normally present with the expected signs and symptoms for the particular condition. Treatment is directed by the severity of the condition at the time the patient presents.

DIAGNOSTIC STUDIES

It is important to carefully choose the diagnostic studies ordered and then place them into a proper perspective when evaluating LBP. Some studies are costly, and all can be misleading, which can confuse the treatment plan.

Radiologic Studies

Anteroposterior and lateral x-rays are baseline studies. Additional views may include a "coned down" (spot) view of the lumbar and sacral spine. Oblique, flexion, and extension views are taken to more clearly define and evaluate specific etiologic pathologies. Lumbosacral x-rays in general have a very low specificity. Degenerative changes in patients older than 40 years are not uncommon. For this reason, some clinicians may not order x-rays while initially evaluating apparent simple mechanical strains. X-rays should be obtained when a fracture, metastatic bone disease, infection, chronic inflammatory disease, or a congenital or developmental anomaly is suspected. Spinal radiographs may be required for medicolegal documentation by workers' compensation protocols to assess for pre-existing conditions.

Specialized Studies

Specialized studies may be required to assess for a more definitive diagnosis. MRI is best utilized to evaluate soft tissue structures and neural compression. Research investigation conducted on asymptomatic individuals demonstrated that more than 33% had a substantial abnormality. CT is best utilized to evaluate osseous structures. It should be noted that CT imaging, like MRI, is expensive and has shown a large number of asymptomatic individuals with abnormalities. EMG and NCV are usually reserved for individuals with neurologic changes to assess the physiologic integrity and level of nerve root involvement. Nuclear imaging is helpful to diagnose acute subtle fractures, as well as neoplastic and infectious lesions.

Serum Tests

A complete blood cell count (CBC) and ESR are relatively inexpensive and should be performed when assessing the patient for possible infection, inflammatory processes, and blood loss. A decreased hemoglobin and hematocrit are diagnostic for anemias with various pathologies. The white blood cell count is generally elevated in infectious processes, and the ESR is the most sensitive and early indicator for an inflammatory response. Additional serum tests may be ordered as appropriate, including serum calcium, alkaline phosphatase, serum protein electrophoresis, rheumatoid factor, antinuclear antibodies, and HLA-B27.

RED FLAGS

Individuals with recent trauma, as from a motor vehicle accident, fall, or strenuous lifting activity, are at an increased risk for fracture, disk herniation, and spinal cord compression. Patients older than 50 years of age are at an increased risk for carcinomas and infections. The history, physical examination, and diagnostic studies should be ordered with these considerations in mind.

CONCLUSIONS AND OUTLOOK

Back and spine disorders are the most frequent and most costly musculoskeletal conditions causing limited activity during the working years. Back impairment is the most common chronic impairment for individuals under the age of 45 years and ranks third behind arthritis and heart disease for individuals in the 45- to 64-year-old age group. Low back pain is a major cause of time and productivity loss at work. More than 400,000 U.S. workers are disabled annually by back pain. Medical care costs for LBP are more than $13 billion annually. Primary care providers must be comfortable in evaluating and treating patients with LBP. Recently there has been an acute interest and awareness in fitness and health that will hopefully decrease the morbidity associated with chronic lower back disability. Many large corporations have installed fitness gyms and other incentives in an attempt to reduce stress and improve employee fitness and health, thus reducing time lost from the workplace.

BIBLIOGRAPHY

Frymoyer JW: Lumbar spine, in *Orthopaedic Knowledge,* Update 4. Rosemont, IL, American Academy of Orthopaedic Surgeons, 1993, pp 491–498.

Hellmann DB: Arthritis and musculoskeletal disorders, in *Current Medical Diagnosis and Treatment,* LM Tierney Jr et al (eds). New York, Lange Medical/McGraw-Hill, 2000, pp 817–819, 1009–1012.

U.S. Department of Health and Human Services: *Acute Low Back Problems in Adults: Assessment and Treatment,* AHCPR Publication 95-06343, 1994.

Way LW: Orthopedics, in *Current Surgical Diagnosis and Treatment.* East Norwalk, CT, McGraw-Hill, 1994, pp 1101–1104.

Winter RB: Tumors and infections of the spine, in *American Academy of Orthopaedic Surgeons, Eleventh Annual Comprehensive Review Course.* Chicago, 1995.

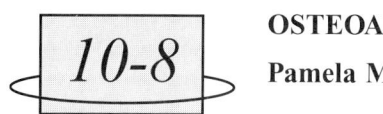

OSTEOARTHRITIS
Pamela Moyers Scott

DISCUSSION

Osteoarthritis (OA), or degenerative joint disease (DJD), is the most common form of arthritis. It is characterized by a progressive loss of articular cartilage and new bone formation consisting of osteophytes (at the joint margins) and sclerosis (subchondral). OA is estimated to affect approximately 16 million Americans.[1] By age 75 years, essentially everyone has radiographic evidence of OA in at least one joint.[2] Until age 55 years, men and women are equally affected; after age 55, women are affected with much greater frequency.[2]

Other risk factors for OA include obesity, repetitive joint usage (either occupational or recreational), significant joint trauma, coexisting inflammatory joint diseases, metabolic disorders, endocrine abnormalities, congenital defects, and a genetic predisposition. Racial differences also exist; however, it is unclear whether they are related to genetics or lifestyle.[3]

SIGNS AND SYMPTOMS

The predominant symptom of osteoarthritis is pain. It is generally aggravated by activity and alleviated by rest. In the more advanced stages of the disease, the pain can be constant. It is most often defined as a deep ache and confined to one or a few joints. It is generally unilateral, although bilateral disease involvement is possible. Onset is usually insidious. The most commonly affected joints are the knees, hips, spine, metacarpophalangeal joints of the thumbs, and distal interphalangeal joints of the hands.

OA may be associated with stiffness following a period of inactivity, including sleeping at night. However, the stiffness is usually completely resolved within 30 minutes. Unless another condition is associated with OA, systemic symptoms and inflammation are generally absent.

OBJECTIVE FINDINGS

The findings on physical examination depend on the joint involved and the extent of the involvement. Varying degrees of tenderness to palpation and limitations in range of motion are present. Instability, bony enlargement, crepitus, synovial effusions, and synovitis may be present. As the disease progresses, these findings become more prominent and can lead to gross deformities of the affected joints.

The presence of bony enlargement of the distal interphalangeal joints (Heberden's nodes) and the proximal interphalangeal joints (Bouchard's nodes) are pathognomonic for OA.

DIAGNOSTIC CONSIDERATIONS

The diagnosis of OA can usually be made on the basis of history and physical examination alone. However, other forms of arthritis should be considered in the differential, including rheumatoid, gouty, psoriatic, erosive inflammatory, and spondyloarthropathic. Bursitis and tendinitis can sometimes mimic OA.

SPECIAL CONSIDERATIONS

OA frequently occurs as a result of an associated disease state and/or causative factor. These conditions include acute and repetitive trauma; inflammatory arthritis; bone diseases, such as Paget's disease and osteoporosis; metabolic and endocrine disorders including diabetes mellitus, hypothyroidism, hyperparathyroidism, acromegaly, hemochromatosis, gout, and ochronosis; congenital and developmental diseases, like Legg-Calvé-Perthes disease, slipped epiphysis, and bone dysplasias;

Charcot's joints; and frostbite.[3] When this occurs, OA is classified as secondary OA. OA without a causative factor or associated disease state is termed primary (or idiopathic).

LABORATORY TESTS

Laboratory studies in the evaluation of OA, are indicated only to rule out other etiologies or secondary causes. In OA, the erythrocyte sedimentation rate (ESR) is normal to slightly elevated.

RADIOGRAPHIC STUDIES

Plain films of the affected joint may confirm the diagnosis. Very early in the course of the disease, however, the x-ray may be normal. Typical radiographic findings of OA include joint space narrowing, osteophytes, sclerosis, and possibly bony cyst formation. When interpreting these radiographic results in the evaluation of a patient with joint pain, it is important to remember that the severity of the disease on x-ray does not necessarily correlate with the severity of symptoms.

OTHER DIAGNOSTICS

Other diagnostic studies are not necessary to make the diagnosis of OA. However, they may be required to determine the etiology of secondary OA.

TREATMENT

Since a cure does not exist for OA, therapy is aimed at reducing pain, maintaining or improving function, minimizing physical disability, and avoiding medication side effects.[4]

Pharmacologic Management

The first-line medication of OA is acetaminophen in a fixed or as-needed dose up to a maximum of 4 g/d. Although long-term acetaminophen usage has been associated with liver toxicity, it most often occurs in association with heavy alcohol consumption.[5] Patients should be counseled accordingly. Long-term acetaminophen usage has also been associated with renal failure; however, the incidence appears to be less than that seen with long-term nonsteroidal anti-inflammatory drug (NSAID) usage.[5]

In patients who do not respond to maximum acetaminophen therapy and nonpharmacologic approaches, an NSAID is then the drug of choice. None of the currently available NSAIDs appear to be superior to another in the treatment of OA.[3] When choosing an NSAID, one must consider the impact of side effects, costs, dosing convenience, and compliance for each individual patient.

The risk of gastrointestinal (GI) toxicity, especially hemorrhage, is a serious complication of NSAID therapy. Cytoprotective agents, such as misoprostol (Cytotec), should be considered in all patients receiving an NSAID. Risk factors that increase the likelihood of an adverse GI complication include a previous GI bleed, history of peptic ulcer disease, advancing age, smoking, and oral corticosteroid therapy. Misoprostol is currently the only agent with FDA approval for this purpose. For ease of administration, it is now available in combination with diclofenac sodium (Arthrotec) as a single pill. Although not FDA approved, omeprazole (Prilosec) and famotidine (Pepcid) have also been successfully used to decrease the risk of GI toxicity from an NSAID.[5] The newer cyclooxygenase enzyme-2 (COX-2) inhibitors, such as celecoxib (Celebrex) and rofecoxib (Vioxx), lessen the likelihood of a GI bleed; however, they do not eliminate it because they still affect gastric prostaglandin E2.[6]

NSAIDs are also associated with renal and hepatotoxicity. The greatest risk for renal complications occurs in the elderly, diabetics, hypertensives, individuals with preexisting renal disease, and patients on diuretic therapy. Patients who consume large amounts of alcohol are probably at the greatest risk of hepatic complications.

Before instituting NSAID therapy, obtain baseline liver functions, renal functions, potassium, and a complete blood count (CBC). A CBC and tests for creatinine and potassium should be repeated in 1 month and again every 6 months thereafter.[5] If the initial liver function testing is normal, then additional testing is usually unnecessary.[5]

If the NSAID alone does not control the patient's symptoms, consider adding acetaminophen on an as-needed basis. If the patient is intolerant of NSAIDs or has an aspirin allergy, the nonacetylated salicylates such as salsalate (Salflex, Disalcid) and choline magnesium trisalicylate (Trilisate) may be effective. These drugs are associated with less renal and GI toxicity than the other NSAIDs; however, they are usually not as effective.

Opiates are also utilized in the treatment of OA. Their primary role is in providing immediate relief in acute flares of symptoms. However, they are being used long term in the management of OA in individuals who are poor surgical candidates and in whom other treatments fail to provide relief, in patients who cannot tolerate any of the other oral regimens, and in individuals for whom the risks of NSAID complications outweigh the hazards of long-term opioid therapy (i.e., addiction and impairment).

The dietary supplements glucosamine sulfate and chondroitin sulfate have been shown superior to placebo in reducing the symptoms of OA in short-term U.S. and European studies.[7–10] However, they have not stood up to the ACR's (American College of Rheumatology) review[11] and offer no convincing data to support claims that they prevent cartilage erosion, stimulate glycosaminoglycan production, and have anti-inflammatory properties.[7] Nevertheless, because of their excellent safety profile, some are recommending their use, along with nonpharmacologic therapies in the treatment of mild to moderate OA.[9,10]

Intra-articular hylan G-F 20 (Synvisc) and sodium hyaluronate (Hyalgan) are options for individuals who are not responding to conservative therapy. They consist of a series of weekly intra-articular injections for 3 and 5 weeks, respectively. They should be used in caution, if not avoided, in individuals allergic to eggs, feathers, and avian products.[7] Although several studies have shown them to be equally as effective as NSAIDs in reducing the pain of OA,[7,8,11] they do not affect the progression of the disease or improve joint functioning.[7]

Intra- or periarticular injections of corticosteroid may provide the patient with relief. They should not be used in anyone contemplating arthroplasty in the near future because they could cause a residual infection of the joint leading to an infected prosthesis. They should not be given any more frequently than every 3 to 4 months because they might increase the rate of cartilage breakdown.

Injectable and oral corticosteroids have no role in the treatment of OA. Tricyclic antidepressants (TCAs) and centrally acting antispasmodics have also been utilized with success.[12]

Nonpharmacologic Management

Exercise is essential in the treatment plan for patients with osteoarthritis. Low-impact exercise such as aerobics, water aerobics, swimming, and recumbent bicycling are preferred. Also, exercises to strengthen the muscles around the affected joint are essential. Any activity that causes pain that persists for greater than 2 hours should be avoided. Additionally, if the joint becomes painful during exercise, the patient must take a break. Persistent pain associated with activity should be treated with ice and rest and a modification of the exercise regimen may be necessary. Weight loss is essential because obesity can cause an accelerated rate of destruction of the weight-bearing joints, especially the knees. Even modest weight loss can result in a significant reduction of symptoms in OA.

Some patients respond to the topical application of heat, some cold, and others alternating heat and cold (known as contrast baths). Another topical therapy that many patents respond to is capsaicin cream (Zostrix), 0.025% to 0.25%, several times per day. Rubefacients containing methyl salicylate (e.g., Thera-Gesic) and various sports creams have also been effective in reducing the pain for some patients.

Surgical Management

Total joint arthroplasty (TJA) is the ultimate solution in the treatment of OA. However, because of the risks associated with surgery, the risk of mechanical failure, and the possibility of repeat procedures, TJA is indicated only when all other treatment options have been unsuccessful. Other surgical options include arthroscopic joint washout tidal lavage, osteotomy, chondroplasty, and laminectomy.

SUPPORTIVE MEASURES

In addition to the nonpharmacologic approaches previously mentioned, physical therapy often increases function and decreases pain in osteoarthritic joints.

PATIENT EDUCATION

The patient must be made aware that treatment will control but not cure the disease. Advise the patient that OA is usually a progressive disease process that often requires increased medical management, including the possibility of surgery. The importance of the nonpharmacologic modalities must be stressed. Finally, the patient needs to be aware of the potential complications from the drug therapies. Patients may obtain additional information and resources by contacting the Arthritis Foundation at 1-800-283-7800 or http://www.arthritis.org.

FUTURE MANAGEMENT

Preliminary research is being done on disease-modifying medications for OA. They include tetracyclines, glycosaminoglycan polysulfuric acid, glycosaminoglycan-peptide complex, pentosan polysulfate, and metalloproteinase-inhibiting peptides.[8] The roles of vitamins D, C, and E are also being explored.[11] Investigations are underway working with growth factor and cytokine manipulation as well as genetic therapy.[8]

Research is also being conducted on techniques to diagnose OA based on serology testing for the macromolecules being released from degenerating bone and cartilage (e.g., glycosaminoglycans).[3]

COMPLICATIONS AND RED FLAGS

Patients who are not adequately responding to conservative treatment should be referred to an orthopedic surgeon.

OTHER NOTES AND PEARLS

Articular cartilage is essentially aneural. Therefore, the pain associated with OA has an etiology in other intra- and/or periarticular structures.

REFERENCES

1. Primary care update. New management guidelines in osteoarthritis of the hip. *Consultant* 2:314–343, 1996.
2. Fife R: Osteoarthritis, epidemiology, pathology, and pathogenesis, in *Primer on the Rheumatic Diseases,* 11th ed, JH Klippel (ed). Atlanta, GA, Arthritis Foundation, 1997, pp 216–218.
3. Brandt K: Osteoarthritis, in *Harrison's Principles of Internal Medicine,* 14th ed, AS Fauci et al (eds). New York, McGraw-Hill, 1998, pp 1935–1941.

4. Hochberg MC: Osteoarthritis, clinical features and treatment, in *Primer on the Rheumatic Diseases,* 11th ed, JH Klippel (ed). Atlanta, GA, Arthritis Foundation, 1997, pp 218–221.

5. Clough J et al: The new thinking on osteoarthritis. *Patient Care* 30:110–137, 1996.

6. Cryer B, Feldman M: Cyclooxygenase-1 and cyclooxygenase-2 selectivity of widely used nonsteroidal anti-inflammatory drugs. *Am J Med* 104:413–421, 1998.

7. Klahr PD et al: New treatments for osteoarthritis and rheumatoid arthritis. *Emerg Med* May:28–44, 1999.

8. Lozada CJ, Altman RD: New drug therapies for osteoarthritis. *J Musculoskeletal Med* Oct:35–40, 1998.

9. Hungerford DS: Treating osteoarthritis with chondroprotective agents. *Orthopedic Special Edition: A Compendium of Educational Reviews* 4:1–4, 1998.

10. Schiedermayer D: Glucosamine sulfate for the treatment of osteoarthritis. *Alternative Medicine Alert* 1:121–124, 1998.

11. Hunder GG et al: Primary care, rheumatology, and osteoarthritis now and tomorrow. *J Musculoskeletal Med* Sept:7–22, 1998.

12. Lozada CJ, Altman RD: Osteoarthritis: A comprehensive approach to management. *J Musculoskeletal Med* Nov:26–38, 1998.

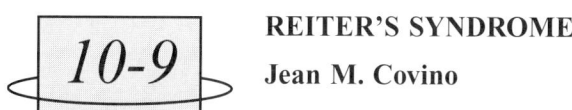

REITER'S SYNDROME
Jean M. Covino

DISCUSSION

Reiter's syndrome is a form of reactive arthritis (ReA) that refers to an acute, nonsuppurative sterile inflammatory condition that occurs in response to an infectious process (usually enteric or urogenital) elsewhere in the body. Reiter's syndrome is the most common form of ReA and consists of mucocutaneous, urogenital, and ocular manifestations.

PATHOGENESIS

Reiter's syndrome occurs predominantly in individuals with the histocompatibility locus A B27 (HLA-B27) haplotype. The pathogenesis of Reiter's syndrome is poorly understood and a topic of ongoing research. Most investigators postulate that a preceding infection serves as a trigger in a genetically predisposed host and that the disease may then persist or recur despite eradication of the infection.[1] The mechanism by which inflammation or infection of a mucosal surface may initiate a sustained systemic illness or the way in which the organisms reach the affected joints is unknown. What is known is that initial manifestations of Reiter's syndrome tend to be more severe and that the natural course is more aggressive in persons with the HLA-B27 haplotype than in those without it.[1] The HLA-B27 haplotype is found in 70 to 80% of white patients with Reiter's syndrome, compared with 6 to 8% of whites in the general population; in blacks with Reiter's syndrome, the reported prevalence of HLA-B27 has varied from 15 to 75%, compared with about 2% among blacks in the general population.[2]

Incidence and Epidemiology

Although cases of Reiter's syndrome have been reported worldwide, the incidence and prevalence of this disease are uncertain and may vary geographically.[1] Epidemiologically, it is characterized by both an endemic or venereal form that usually is sexually acquired and a less common epidemic or dysenteric form that most often is associated with enteric infections. Although postdysenteric Reiter's syndrome occurs in children, most of these patients are adults. The peak onset of Reiter's syndrome occurs during the third decade of life.[1] Postvenereal Reiter's syndrome affects men more than women; male-female ratios ranging from 9:1 to 5:1 have been reported.[2] The ratio was once thought to be 20:1, but this was most likely the result of underreporting of cases in women, who often have less severe disease. The dysenteric form of Reiter's syndrome affects equal numbers in both sexes.[2]

Microbiology

Chlamydia trachomatis (serotypes D through K) is the infectious organism found most frequently in patients with Reiter's syndrome. It has been documented in approximately 50% of men with sexually acquired Reiter's syndrome.[1,2] At least 50% of all patients with Reiter's syndrome have high antichlamydial antibodies suggestive of a recent infection.[2,3] *Ureaplasma urealyticum* is another possible candidate. Enteric pathogens implicated in Reiter's syndrome include *Campylobacter, Shigella, Salmonella, Yersinia,* and possibly *Cryptosporidium* and *Giardia* species.

SIGNS AND SYMPTOMS

The diagnosis is straightforward in patients with arthritis, conjunctivitis, and urethritis. However, fewer than one-third of patients with Reiter's syndrome present with all three clinical findings.[2]

Urogenital findings include urethritis, dysuria, and prostatitis in males. Urethritis is an early symptom and can occur 2 to 4 weeks after sexual exposure or the cessation of a gastrointestinal illness. Women may present with cervicitis or vaginitis. However, a clear spectrum of urogenital symptoms in women with Reiter's syndrome still needs to be described.

Ocular manifestations occur in up to 50% of patients with the sexually acquired form of the disease and up to 90% of cases after the epidemic form of the disease. As with other symptoms, the ocular manifestations may be recurrent. Conjunctivitis, often mild enough to go unnoticed, is the most common ocular manifestation. Although uncommon at initial presentation, keratitis, iritis, and uveitis are other possible symptoms.

Arthritic manifestation is the last clinical feature of the triad to occur. Asymmetric polyarticular synovitis-tendinitis can be seen initially, followed by persistence in one or two joints. Any joint can be involved, but the knees, ankles, and toes are the most commonly affected. Later involvement may include the fingers and the wrists. Tendon insertion sites (entheses) are common points of inflammation, and these areas include the insertion of the Achilles tendon and the plantar fascia. A classic enthesitic feature is dactylitis, which causes "sausage-shaped" fingers or toes. This clinical finding occurs only in Reiter's syndrome and psoriatic arthritis. Sacroiliitis occurs in up to 10% of cases acutely and more commonly in those with chronic Reiter's syndrome.

Dermatologic manifestations often include mucocutaneous lesions, which occur in about 50% of patients. Circinate balanitis is the most common cutaneous manifestation, occurring in approximately 20 to 40% and up to 85% of men with the sexually acquired form of the syndrome. These lesions start as vesicles that quickly rupture to form painless superficial erosions, which in circumcised individuals can form crusts similar to the lesions of keratodermia blennorrhagica. Lesions of keratoderma blennorrhagica begin as erythematous macules that gradually enlarge to form hyperkeratotic papules, sometimes with red halos and occasionally with central clearing. The lesions most commonly appear on the plantar surfaces of the feet but may occur anywhere. They resemble psoriasis both grossly and histologically. In as many as 20% of patients with Reiter's syndrome, especially those with the sexually acquired form, painless shallow ulcers can occur on the tongue, palate, buccal mucosa, tonsillar pillars, or pharynx. Nail involvement occurs in as many as 19% of patients, manifested by thickening and brown-yellow discoloration.

Other systemic manifestations include malaise, fever, anorexia, and weight loss. Transient and usually benign electrocardiographic abnormalities, including atrioventricular conduction disturbances, ST-segment elevation or depression, and nonspecific T-wave changes, can occur.

DIAGNOSTIC CONSIDERATIONS

Other arthritic conditions that should be considered in the differential diagnosis of Reiter's syndrome include ankylosing spondylitis, colitic arthritis, gonococcal arthritis, systemic lupus erythematosus, Lyme disease, psoriatic arthritis, rheumatic fever, rheumatoid arthritis, and gouty arthritis (see Chap. 10-5).

SPECIAL CONSIDERATIONS

Reactive arthritis may occur in HIV-infected patients and is sometimes the initial manifestation of the disease.[4] The diagnosis of reactive arthritis should be considered in any patient with an asymmetric oligoarticular polyarthritis. Conversely, HIV infection should be considered in any new case of reactive arthritis in which the etiology is at all unclear. In these patients, arthritis may be severe and may progress more rapidly.[5,6]

LABORATORY TESTS

Laboratory findings are nonspecific and do not help establish a diagnosis. The erythrocyte sedimentation rate (ESR) and C-reactive protein levels usually are elevated but do not correlate with disease activity. Mild anemia and leukocytosis may occur.

RADIOLOGIC STUDIES

In early disease, there are usually no significant radiographic findings or evidence of soft tissue swelling. With persistent disease, there may be radiographic evidence of joint space erosion, periostitis with reactive new bone formation, or spurs at the insertion of the plantar fascia. About 50% of these patients have evidence of sacroiliitis.

OTHER DIAGNOSTICS

Synovial fluid analysis is rarely specific and resembles septic arthritis. It may show a white blood cell count of 500 to 50,000 cells/μL, predominantly neutrophils, elevated protein and complement levels, and normal glucose levels. A Gram stain should be negative for any organisms. Microbiological identification of specific organisms is helpful but usually is not successful. Attempts to culture the infectious agent from the urethra, cervix, or stool should be made if possible. Antichlamydia antibody tests for IgG and IgM may prove the presence of infection but are not necessary for the diagnosis and are lengthy and costly.

TREATMENT

Although there is no cure for Reiter's syndrome, antibiotic therapy is indicated when *Chlamydia* is the suspected causative agent. Some data suggest that recurrent arthritis is much lower in patients treated with antibiotics for chlamydial urethritis.[7] Most authorities currently recommend doxycycline 100 mg two times daily for up to 3 months based on the patient's clinical response. Whether antibiotics are indicated for patients with postdysenteric Reiter's syndrome is unknown because few clinical studies are available in this subgroup.

Treatment with nonsteroidal anti-inflammatory drugs (NSAIDs) such as indomethacin (Indocin) (75 to 150 mg/day in divided doses) may help alleviate some of the arthritic symptoms. Other NSAIDs also may be effective. Corticosteroid therapy given orally is not effective, but intraarticular steroids injected in patients with large knee effusions can be helpful. Sulfasalazine (Azulfidine), methotrexate (Rheumatrex), azathioprine (Imuran), and bromocriptine mesylate (Parlodel) may help patients with persistent debilitating disease that is refractory to NSAIDs.

Physical therapy also may help alleviate some symptoms.

COMPLICATIONS AND RED FLAGS

The overall prognosis of Reiter's syndrome is good. Most patients are symptom-free 2 months to 1 year after the diagnosis is made. The acute syndrome may recur in about 15% of patients and may manifest as back pain, heel pain, arthritis, or any of the initial symptoms. Twenty percent of patients may develop chronic arthritic symptoms with the potential for degenerative changes. Other documented long-term sequelae, especially in sexually acquired cases, include complete heart block, myocarditis, pericarditis, acute aortitis with aortic valve incompetence, and congestive heart failure. Testing for HIV infection is warranted in all patients with persistent symptoms. Death from Reiter's syndrome is rare.

NOTES AND PEARLS

Since Reiter's syndrome is a clinical diagnosis with no definitive laboratory test, a high index of suspicion must be maintained. Always consider this diagnosis in a patient with asymmetric inflammatory arthritis or tendinitis. A careful history may elicit genitourinary or ocular symptoms 1 to 4 weeks before the reactive disease. Careful inspection of the glans penis, including retraction of the foreskin, and the oral mucosa in all male patients presenting with acute arthritic symptoms is essential.

REFERENCES

1. Keat A: Reiter's syndrome and reactive arthritis in perspective. *N Engl J Med* 309:1606, 1983.
2. Cush JJ, Lipsky PE: Reiter's syndrome and reactive arthritis, in McCarty DJ, Koopman WJ (eds): *Arthritis and Allied Conditions,* 12th ed, Philadelphia, Lea & Febiger, 1993.
3. Handsfield HH, Pollock PS: Arthritis associated with sexually transmitted diseases, in Holmes KK, Mardh PA (eds): *Sexually Transmitted Diseases,* 2d ed, New York, McGraw-Hill, 1990.
4. Winchester R, Bernstein DH, Fisher HD, et al: The co-occurrence of Reiter's syndrome and acquired immunodeficiency. *Ann Intern Med* 106(1):19–26, 1987.
5. Barth WF, Segal K: Reactive arthritis (Reiter's syndrome). *Am Fam Physician* 60:499–503, 1999.
6. Clark MR, Solinger AM, Hochberg MC: Human immunodeficiency virus infection is not associated with Reiter's syndrome: Data from three large cohort studies. *Rheum Dis Clin North Am* 128(1):267–276, 1992.
7. Bardin T, Enel C, Cornelis F, et al: Antibiotic treatment of venereal disease and Reiter's syndrome in a Greenland population. *Arthritis Rheum* 35(2):190–194, 1992.

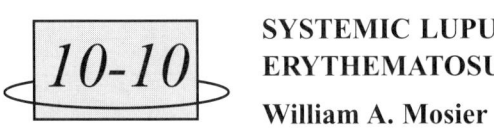

10-10 SYSTEMIC LUPUS ERYTHEMATOSUS
William A. Mosier

DISCUSSION

Systemic lupus erythematosus (SLE) is a chronic multisystemic inflammatory disease. Its chief characteristic is the development of abnormal immune system products that the body fails to suppress. SLE is named for the erythematous rash that appears on the face in about 50% of cases. In fact, the term *lupus* (Latin for "wolf") was first applied to the disease in 1230 A.D. because of the rash, which resembles the mask appearance over the malar eminence of a wolf's face. SLE can vary greatly in its presenting symptoms, clinical manifestation, and course.

A hallmark of SLE is the presence of antibodies to nuclear components found in the blood. The typical case of SLE progresses in a chronic, irregular manner. Episodes of active disease are interspersed with long periods of seemingly complete or nearly complete remission. SLE may present in a mild form. Although it is not typical, SLE can have a fulminating presentation that is rapidly fatal. Infection is a major cause of morbidity and mortality rates in patients with SLE. Some patients die from vascular lesions affecting the central nervous system (CNS), the heart, or the kidneys, whereas others die from the complications of secondary infection. There is no known cure.

Almost 90% of all cases occur in women. Overall, SLE affects women eight times more often than it does men. At age 30 years, the ratio of women to men is 10:1. The ratio in juveniles is closer to 2:1 and in persons over age 65 years the ratio appears to be about 3:1. The prevalence rate among women between ages 15 and 64 years is 1 in 700 women. Symptoms usually appear between ages 15 and 25 years. The prevalence in the general population is about 1 in 1000.

Although SLE affects all ethnic groups, in the United States the prevalence is three times higher among African Americans than Caucasians. It may be slightly more common in the Native American population than in Caucasians. Data are unclear as to its actual prevalence in the Asian population.

PATHOGENESIS

SLE is a disease of unknown etiology. It may actually represent several different disease entities that manifest a clinical expression through a common pathway. It is a disease of immunologic malfunctioning. This malfunctioning results in autoimmune reactions against host antigens that lead to inflammation and tissue damage resulting in cellular and organ dysfunction. Both environmental and genetic factors play an important role in the cause and pathogenesis of SLE. A hereditary complement deficiency has been identified at C2 and C4. The resulting malfunction produces an autoimmune reaction against host antigens that leads to inflammation and tissue damage causing cellular and organ dysfunction. Identified genetic markers for SLE include HLA-B8, HLA-DR2, and HLA-DR3. The serum of patients with SLE contains antibodies to nuclear antigens (see "Laboratory Tests," below). The apparent diversity of antibodies in SLE may be explained by the common chemical features among the antigens, rather than by any diversity of antibody specificities. The antibodies to nuclear antigens (ANA) participate in the pathogenesis of SLE by forming antigen–antibody complexes with their specific antigens. Bacterial, chemical, or viral antigens in genetically predisposed individuals may trigger SLE. Drugs, such as hydralazine and procainamide, can induce a disease state that appears identical with SLE (see Table 10-10-1). A genetic predisposition for SLE is suggested by the increased rate of subclinical abnormalities discovered in relatives of patients with SLE and by the increased occurrence of SLE in the second twin in monozygotic twins. Most cases of SLE are idiopathic. Drug-induced lupus is clinically different from idiopathic SLE (see Table 10-10-2).

SYMPTOMS

A young female patient presenting with a fever, rash, and arthritic pain should be evaluated for SLE. About 90% of all patients with SLE experience nondeforming arthritis. Morning stiffness, usually due to arthralgia, with swelling and effusion is common. About 50% of patients with SLE are photosensitive. Those with photosensitivity may experience a worsening of symptoms after sun exposure.

Alopecia may often occur; however, it is usually reversible. Ulcerations of the mouth and lips may also occur. The two principal affec-

TABLE 10-10-1. Medications That Can Induce Symptoms of SLE

Acebutolol	Ethosuximide
Atenolol	Hydralazine
Carbamazepine	Isoniazid
Chlorpromazine	Labetalol
Clonidine	Methyldopa
D-penicillamine	Procainamide

TABLE 10-10-2. American College of Rheumatology Criteria for the Classification of SLE

Malar rash
Discoid rash
Photosensitivity
Oral or nasopharyngeal ulcers
Nonerosive arthritis
Pleuritis
Pericarditis
Proteinuria (>500 mg/dL)
Cast cells
Psychosis
Seizures
Hemolytic anemia
Leukopenia (<4000/mL)
Lymphopenia (<1500/mL)
Thrombocytopenia (<100,000/mL)
Antinuclear antibodies
Anti-dsDNA
Anti-Smith antigen
False-positive Venereal Disease Research Laboratories test for syphilis
Positive lupus erythematosus cell preparation

SOURCE: *American College of Rheumatology, www.rheumatology.org*

tive symptoms encountered in SLE are anxiety and depressed mood. Headaches are also a common complaint.

OBJECTIVE FINDINGS

Because the severity of symptoms can vary so greatly and because they may appear slowly over many years, diagnosis may also be delayed for many years. The three most common clinical findings are fever, rash, and arthritic pain. Other findings may include cardiac abnormalities, hemolytic anemia, neurologic abnormalities, polyarthralgia, polyserositis (such as pleurisy and pericarditis), renal abnormalities, and thrombocytopenia purpura.

After an acute attack of SLE, remission usually occurs. There can typically be an interval of several symptom-free years. However, an eventual reoccurrence is likely. In any case the course is unpredictable and may recur without apparent cause. Factors that can precipitate exacerbation are certain medications, emotional or physical stress, infection, sunlight, and the trauma of surgery.

Fever Involvement

A low-grade fever occurs in the majority of patients with SLE. Less frequently, a high-grade fever may manifest in isolation or may accompany multisystemic involvement. Caution must be taken to differentiate a fever caused by SLE from one caused by a secondary infection.

Musculoskeletal Involvement

An acute attack of SLE may consist of symmetric and polyarticular arthritis. The hands, wrists, elbows, knees, and ankles are commonly involved. The inflammatory appearance of the joints may or may not be notable. Myalgia and muscle weakness are common. Symptoms of fibromyalgia are also common in SLE.

Skin Involvement

Skin lesions can be an important diagnostic clue to SLE. A patient with SLE may present with subacute, acute, or chronic skin involvement. Although acute cutaneous lupus typically presents as an erythematous rash with a butterfly shape extending from the bridge of the nose to the malar areas; it may occur in other sun-exposed areas. The subacute cutaneous lupus typically consists of an erythematous, papulosquamous eruption. The eruptions may appear annular. These discoid lesions may be found on the face, neck, or scalp. In chronic cutaneous lupus, there are patches of atrophic skin, depigmented at the center with increasing degrees of pigmentation toward the edges. Telangiectasia, scaling, periungual erythema, and palmar erythema may also be present. Alopecia is a typical finding. However, this plugging of hair follicles often resolves during periods of remission.

Renal Involvement

Lupus nephritis may be present in most cases of SLE. It is a benign focal proliferative lesion that usually resolves spontaneously. A remitting and relapsing membranous glomerulonephritis may produce a nephrotic syndrome. A progressive renal failure may develop. Renal insufficiency and renal hypertension may result from a diffuse proliferative glomerulonephritis. In more than 50% of lupus patients with renal disease, the pathology changes over time.

Nervous System Involvement

CNS involvement occurs in about 50% of patients with SLE. Reactive depression is the most common presentation. About 20% of patients with SLE have an organic brain syndrome involving varying degrees of disorientation, intellectual deterioration, and memory impairment. Approximately 10% of patients with SLE may manifest psychosis. Patients who develop psychosis may show evidence of seizure activity. The cranial nerves may be affected, causing facial weakness, ptosis, or diplopia. The CNS manifestations are usually transient. Even the psychosis may be episodic and will often clear dramatically. Cranial or peripheral neuropathies, headaches, chorea, ataxia, impaired work capacity, and impaired social functioning may also be present.

Cardiac Involvement

The most common cardiac manifestation is pericarditis. Pericardial effusion may be present. A friction rub is often identifiable on auscultation. Raynaud's phenomenon (cold- or stress-induced vasospasms of the hands and feet) can be observed in 30% of SLE patients. About 15% of patients with SLE may have cardiac valvular disease. Atherosclerotic coronary artery disease may account for as many as 30% of SLE deaths.

Pulmonary Involvement

A possible cause of an audible friction rub could be pleural effusion. Acute or chronic parenchymal pulmonary involvement may be present in SLE, as may acute lupus pneumonitis. The latter is characterized by a sudden onset of fever and dyspnea with pulmonary infiltrates. Alveolar hemorrhage is the second most prevalent syndrome. It manifests, as the name implies, with bleeding in the lungs and an inevitable decrease in hematocrit. If not treated promptly, both syndromes can quickly progress to respiratory failure. An interstitial lung disease may develop and manifest as either inflammatory alveolitis or interstitial fibrosis. Inflammatory alveolitis responds to immunosuppressive therapy, whereas interstitial fibrosis does not. The pulmonary hypertension that can manifest in SLE presents with dyspnea on exertion. The pulmonary involvement can resemble primary pulmonary hypertension.

DIAGNOSTIC CONSIDERATIONS

SLE can mimic many conditions, especially those involving an inflammatory process. The differential diagnosis includes rheumatoid arthritis, scleroderma, mixed connective tissue disease (MCTD), metastatic malignancy, thyroid disease, primary fibromyalgia, Lyme disease, and various cutaneous rashes. It can also be misdiagnosed as a simple fever of unknown origin.

SPECIAL CONSIDERATIONS

It is imperative to remember that patients with active SLE are predisposed to opportunistic infections. Another important consideration is the emotional state of patients with SLE because their psychological condition will influence their perception of pain, their physical functioning, the successfulness of rehabilitation, and their quality of life.

SLE does not affect fertility, and pregnancy is not necessarily contraindicated. A patient with active SLE may experience flare-ups during pregnancy. However, there is no increased risk of flare-ups as a result of pregnancy.

LABORATORY TESTS

The diagnosis of SLE is confirmed by the finding of abnormal ANA levels (titers of 1:80 or higher). The most specific finding in active SLE is a high titer of double-stranded deoxyribonucleic acid antibodies (anti-dsDNA). Other antigen specificities that may be found in SLE are anti-DNP (deoxyribonucleoprotein), anti-RNA (ribonucleic acid), anti-histones, anti-Sm (Smith), anti-nRNP (non-histone ribonucleoprotein), anti-PCNA (proliferating cell nuclear antigen), antinuclear matrix, anti-Golgi, and/or antiribosomes.

Elevated serum levels of autoantibodies to ribosomal P proteins are specific for SLE when psychiatric symptoms are present. Antineuronal antibodies are found in as many as three-fourths of patients with neuropsychiatric symptoms of SLE. High titers to anti-dsDNA are encountered in roughly 50% of patients with SLE. Anti-Sm antibodies are highly specific for SLE. However, they occur in only 50% of cases.

Antibodies to DNA can be determined by indirect immunofluorescence, immunodiffusion, counterimmunoelectrophoresis (CIE), hemagglutination, radioimmunosorbent assay (RIA), and enzyme-linked immunosorbent assay (ELISA).

LE cells (live neutrophils that engulf the nucleus of dead, fragmented neutrophils after being bound by ANA and complement) are found in the joint fluid, bone marrow, and pleural and pericardial effusion of more than 85% of patients with SLE.

Humoral immune phenomena may be uncovered by studying the immunoglobulins. Serum protein electrophoresis may demonstrate elevated gamma globulin. Lupus anticoagulants, which are sometimes seen in SLE, are immunoglobulins of IgG or IgM class that bind to phospholipids. They are present in 10% of patients with SLE. Both congenital and acquired IgA deficiency has been associated with SLE.

Cellular immune phenomena may be demonstrated with major histocompatibility complex (MHC) of the DR3 type in more than 50% of cases. Complement components C3, C4, and CH_{50} (hemolytic complement) may demonstrate an alternate pattern in SLE. C3 may be normal in acute SLE but low in active or chronic SLE. C4 may appear normal in chronic SLE but low in the acute, active state. Low CH_{50} can be associated with active SLE whether acute or chronic. Measurement of static and functional complement levels may be a useful guide to the activity of SLE in a specific patient.

The lupus band test is a skin biopsy that is positive for IgG or IgM in more than 90% of specimens taken from patients with SLE. Biopsies from sun-exposed skin of the dorsum of the forearm are positive more than 80% of the time. However, a positive test is not specific only to SLE.

Hematologic findings may demonstrate a hemolytic anemia, leukopenia (<4000/mL), lymphopenia (<1500/mL), or thrombocytopenia (platelets <100,000/μL). A false-positive result on the Venereal Disease Research Laboratories (VDRL) serologic test for syphilis is a common finding in patients with SLE.

Urinalysis may uncover proteinuria (>500 mg/24 h), pyuria, hematuria, and granular or red cell casts.

RADIOLOGIC STUDIES

When pulmonary involvement is suspected, a chest radiograph may indicate patchy alveolar infiltrates, which can be indicative of acute lupus pneumonitis.

OTHER DIAGNOSTICS

Analysis of synovial fluid may evidence only mild inflammation. Leukocytes are typically lower than the count found in rheumatoid arthritis. Histologic synovial tissue study may reveal significantly less inflammatory response than is seen in rheumatoid arthritis. A limited joint infiltration of lymphocytes and plasma cells with marginal evidence of edema and some fibrinoid necrosis are often the only histologic synovial findings.

Magnetic resonance imaging (MRI) may be useful for revealing abnormalities associated with the neuropsychiatric manifestations of SLE. Symmetrically distributed areas of increased signal intensity in the subcortical white matter may be present in patients with cognitive dysfunction, generalized seizures, or psychosis. These abnormalities are not present when the patient is in remission.

TREATMENT

Treatment for the various presentations of SLE is controversial. Response to treatment is difficult to evaluate because the symptom patterns and course vary so greatly from patient to patient. However, appropriate health care management would include routine monitoring of symptoms on an outpatient basis.

Pharmacologic Management

The usual treatment is with immunosuppressive drugs, such as prednisone (5 to 15/mg/d). In the majority of patients, the cutaneous lesions of SLE respond to antimalarial drugs such as chloroquine and hydroxychloroquine. In some instances arthritis and arthralgia also respond to these drugs. Maintenance therapy with hydroxychloroquine may even reduce the frequency of flare-ups. Patients found to be resistant to antimalarial medication may respond to azathioprine, dapsone, or the retinoids. Nonsteroidal anti-inflammatory medications can be useful for many patients suffering from active SLE. However, care must be taken to avoid the typical gastrointestinal side effects as well as an aspirin-induced hepatitis that may present in patients with active SLE. Salicylates must be avoided in cases of severe thrombocytopenia and when renal disease is present. The treatment of depression and fibromyalgia secondary to SLE may respond to tricyclic antidepressants and selective serotonin reuptake inhibitors.

Supportive Measures

Bed rest is indicated for patients with active SLE. Because emotional and physical stress can have a negative impact on the immune system, patients should be encouraged to avoid high-pressure situations.

PATIENT EDUCATION

Because all SLE-related skin lesions are either precipitated or exacerbated by sun exposure, patients should be cautioned against exposure without sun block. Patients must be taught that sunlight exposure can also cause flare-ups in other organ systems, not only the skin. When exposure to sunlight cannot be avoided, patients should be instructed to use sunscreens that contain para-aminobenzoic acid (PABA) and also have a high sun protection factor (SPF) rating of at least 30. Patients with SLE should be encouraged to remain as physically active as possible. Patients should be taught that active exercise may strengthen the immune system, but that too much exercise will produce unhealthy stress. Patients should also be taught relaxation techniques to use during periods of stress. Patient and family education are critical. Many symptoms of SLE improve with the proper balance of exercise, rest, and adequate stress management. It is also important for patients to understand the need for early intervention when infections occur. Patients should be encouraged to consult with their health care provider when symptoms of an infection first become noticeable.

DISPOSITION

Follow-up and management depend on whether the patient is in a period of remission or exacerbation of symptoms. The prognosis for patients with SLE is difficult to determine. The most frequent cause of death is active renal disease often accompanied by complications in other organ systems as well as a superimposed infection. Any follow-up activity must be planned so as to ensure a timely intervention of management that will assist the patient in maintaining a satisfactory quality of life.

COMPLICATIONS AND RED FLAGS

Because the toxicity from corticosteroids is predictable and cumulative over time, extreme care must be taken when treating with these preparations. The incidence of herpes zoster occurring because a patient is being treated with immunosuppressive drugs can be as high as 20%. Steroid-induced psychosis is also a serious complication. Controversy exists over the use of postmenopausal estrogen replacement therapy in women diagnosed with SLE. There is evidence that postmenopausal estrogen is associated with an increased risk of developing SLE.

OTHER NOTES AND PEARLS

Elevated serum levels of autoantibodies to ribosomal P proteins are not associated with nonpsychiatric manifestations of SLE. They are a useful measure because they are specific for SLE only when there is severe depression or psychosis. Although most patients with SLE follow a course of exacerbation and remission of symptoms, some will experience a spontaneous and permanent remission. Patients with drug-induced lupus will experience a gradual decrease in symptoms upon discontinuation of the offending agent. The Lupus Foundation of America is a useful resource for both health care providers and patients for material about SLE. The foundation's address is 1717 Massachusetts Avenue NW, Suite 203, Washington, DC 20036. The phone number is 1-800-558-0121.

BIBLIOGRAPHY

Gremillion RB: Update on systemic lupus erythematosus. *Clinical Advisor* Feb 74–84, 2000.
Kelley WN (ed): *Textbook of Rheumatology.* Philadelphia, Saunders, 1997, pp 1015–1054.
McGuire JL, Lambert RE: Systemic lupus erythematosus and overlap syndromes, in *Textbook of Internal Medicine,* 3d ed, WN Kelley et al (eds). Philadelphia, Lippincott-Raven, 1997.
Robinson DR: Systemic lupus erythematosus. Rheumatology, in *Scientific American Medicine,* Dare DC, Federman DD (eds). New York, Scientific American, 1996.
Sanchet-Guerrero J et al: Postmenopausal estrogen therapy and the risk for developing systemic lupus erythematosus. *Ann Intern Med* 122:430, 1995.

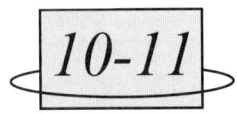

CARPAL TUNNEL SYNDROME

David Zinsmeister

DISCUSSION

Carpal tunnel syndrome is the most common peripheral nerve entrapment. Due to the anatomy of the wrist, the median nerve is subject to compression and perhaps ischemia in the confined space formed by the carpal bones and transverse carpal ligament. It commonly occurs alone due to repetitive overuse; however, it may be present in association with local or systemic conditions that alter the space of the carpal tunnel. The disorder is three times more common in women then in men and occurs most often in middle age. The dominant hand is usually the first to be involved but symptoms are frequently bilateral by the time the patient presents. Numerous studies have linked carpal tunnel syndrome to the workplace with some reporting as high as 56% of all cases directly attributed to occupational activities.

PATHOGENESIS

The carpal tunnel is formed by the bones of the carpus on the dorsal aspect of the wrist and the transverse carpal ligament (flexor retinaculum) on the volar aspect. Within the tunnel lie the median nerve, the flexor digitorum superficialis and profundus tendons, the flexor pollicis longus tendon, and synovial sheaths (Fig. 10-11-1). Compression of the median nerve within this fibro-osseous canal can arise from any condition that causes an alteration in the volume of the tunnel.

Repetitive overuse is the most common cause of median nerve compression at the wrist. Actions performed repetitively in the workplace or during leisure activities may result in swelling of the synovium or thickening of the transverse carpal ligament, causing compression of the nerve. Other common local causes include osseous changes due to fractures, dislocations, or arthritic changes in the bone that compromise the space within the tunnel. A variety of systemic conditions can cause carpal tunnel syndrome; a complete listing can be found in Table 10-11-1. Rarely, carpal tunnel syndrome can be of familial origin.

Regardless of the cause of reduced space within the tunnel, the median nerve, which can be likened to the consistency of overcooked spaghetti, is compressed by the unyielding fibrous and osseous structures that form the tunnel or occupy it with the nerve. At the microscopic level, compression impedes the venous return of the nerve, which impairs the intrafunicular circulation. This results in increased pressure that leads to ischemia, anoxia, and impaired nutrition of the nerve. Edema occurs and protein leakage into the surrounding tissue promotes the proliferation of fibroblasts that form constrictive endoneural tissue. Finally, wallerian degeneration occurs with loss of axons, and the few surviving nerve fibers become encased in a dense, avascular epineurium.

TABLE 10-11-1. Causes of Carpal Tunnel Syndrome

Local	Connective Tissue Disorders
Repetitive overuse	Rheumatoid arthritis
Flexor tenosynovitis	Scleroderma
Wrist fractures and dislocations	Polymyalgia rheumatica
Hematomas	Systemic lupus erythematosus
Infections	Gout
Carpal tunnel stenosis	Chondrocalcinosis (pseudogout)
Exostosis/osteophytes	Amyloidosis
Ganglion cyst	
Anomalous muscles and tendons	

Endocrine Disorders	Other
Diabetes mellitus	Pregnancy
Hypothyroidism	Long-term renal failure
Hyperthyroidism	Multiple myeloma
Acromegaly	Familial carpal tunnel syndrome
Calcium abnormalities	Other polyneuropathies
	Estrogen/progesterone
	Snake bite
	Vitamin B_6 deficiency (?)
	Idiopathic causes

Variations in the sensory and motor distribution of the median nerve must be kept in mind when evaluating a patient with suspected carpal tunnel syndrome. The palmar cutaneous branch that supplies the proximal palm exits the median nerve radially before entering the carpal tunnel. Due to overlapping innervation from the ulnar, radial, and lateral cutaneous nerves, compression of this branch rarely causes a discernible loss of sensation in the proximal palm in carpal tunnel syndrome.

As the median nerve exits the carpal tunnel, its sensory fibers divide into common digital nerves, which supply the distal palm and further subdivide near the web space into the proper digital nerves, which supply the thumb and fingers. The typical sensory innervation pattern of the thumb and fingers by the median nerve includes the palmar aspect of the thumb, index finger, and long finger and the radial aspect of the ring finger. The nerves supply the tips of the digits and extend dorsally to the distal interphalangeal joint of the fingers and the interphalangeal joint of the thumb (Fig. 10-11-2). Common variations of this pattern include innervation of the ulnar side of the

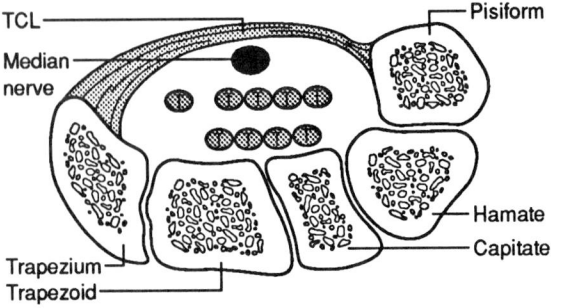

FIGURE 10-11-1. The carpal tunnel and its contents. TCL= transverse carpal ligament.

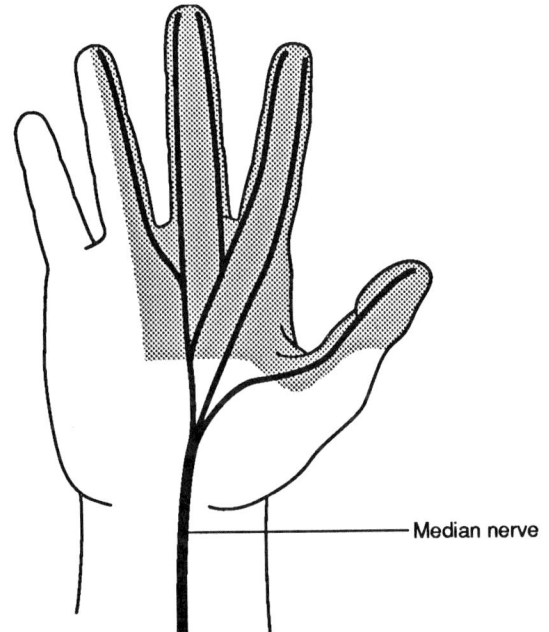

FIGURE 10-11-2. The normal pattern of the sensory distribution of the median nerve in the hand.

ring finger by the median nerve and ulnar nerve innervation that extends to the ulnar aspect of the long finger. Cadaver studies have shown that in 80% of the specimens dissected, the ulnar aspect of the ring finger was innervated by both the radial and ulnar nerves.

Distal to the transverse carpal ligament, the recurrent motor branch supplies the muscles of the thenar eminence. The typical pattern includes the abductor pollicis brevis, opponens pollicis, and flexor pollicis brevis. This pattern, however, is present in only one-third of the population. Variations include ulnar innervation to one or all of the thenar muscles or combinations of innervation by both the median and ulnar nerves to the individual muscles. The terminal motor branches of the median nerve usually supply the lumbricals of the index and long fingers. The most common variation of this pattern is partial innervation of the long finger lumbrical by the median nerve.

The median nerve also carries sympathetic fibers that supply the skin, blood vessels, and sweat glands. When compression affects the pseudomotor and vasomotor fibers in carpal tunnel syndrome, trophic changes in the skin and coolness and dryness of the palm and digits occur.

SYMPTOMS

When evaluating a patient with suspected carpal tunnel syndrome one must keep in mind the seemingly endless variety of terms that a patient may use to describe the symptoms. While terms such as paresthesia (tingling), dysesthesia (an unpleasant perception to a normal stimulus), and hyperesthesia (an elevated threshold to stimulus perception) have very specific implications, patients speak in terms of numbness, "crawling bugs," and burning pain. Further affecting the patients' inability to communicate their experience is the anatomic and physiologic differences between the A delta and C fibers that are responsible for nociception.

A delta fibers are responsible for the ability to sense acute pain. They are dense and myelinated, and they have the ability to transmit rapidly via direct pathways to specific areas of the cortex. C fibers, which are responsible for sensation in chronic conditions, are sparse and unmyelinated but transmit slowly and are integrated with several other pathways before they reach a wide area of the cortex. Since carpal tunnel syndrome is a chronic compression neuropathy, transmission of the patient's sensations occurs primarily through C fiber pathways. This results in the inability to precisely describe the sensation felt or define its exact location.

At the onset, the symptoms of carpal tunnel syndrome are usually preceded by activities such as typing, use of vibrating tools, or fine detail work that requires wrist flexion. Early in the course of the process the pain is intermittent and described as a dull ache at the wrist during or shortly after use. As time progresses, the patient classically complains of burning pain, numbness, and tingling in the areas of the hand supplied by the median nerve. As compression of the nerve continues, the symptoms become constant and more severe. The pain may begin to radiate up the arm and can be felt as high as the shoulder. A pattern may develop in which the patient wakes up 2 to 3 hours after retiring because of pain and numbness in the hand. This is due to the loss of conscious control of the wrist extensors while sleeping, which causes the wrist to flex, thus narrowing the carpal tunnel.

Clumsiness and weakness are common complaints with carpal tunnel syndrome and can be attributed to both altered sensation and muscle weakness. Patients may report dropping objects and the inability to perform fine motor skills that require the use of the thumb and index finger. These symptoms suggest involvement of the recurrent motor branch of the median nerve that innervates the muscles of the thenar eminence and the terminal motor branch that supplies the lumbricals.

When asked to demonstrate what they do to relieve their symptoms, most patients will shake their wrist. This is known as the "flick" sign and is common in patients with carpal tunnel syndrome.

OBJECTIVE FINDINGS

Upon inspection of the hand and wrist the examiner should make note of the color, temperature, and texture of the skin and the presence or absence of thenar muscle atrophy. With the exception of advanced cases of carpal tunnel syndrome with severe compression of the median nerve, the inspection portion of the examination should be normal. At the end stages of long-standing compression, the tips of the thumb, index finger, long finger, and ring finger become smooth, cool, and dry due to trophic changes of sensory and autonomic impairment. Atrophy of the thenar muscles is a late finding and when present indicates that sensory involvement and weakness are advanced.

The sensory examination should begin by asking the patient to outline the area of sensory abnormality. Once this is defined, testing light touch is frequently all that is required to confirm the involved area. If results are negative, gentle pinprick is useful to reveal the deficit. Two-point discrimination is often a late finding and if affected will typically be 1 cm or greater. In the normal, uncallused hand two-point discrimination is 5 to 6 mm. In order to obtain a baseline, the unaffected hand and the ulnar distribution of the affected hand should be tested first since a 1-to-2-mm variance in two-point discrimination among individuals can be expected. Testing of vibratory sense with a tuning fork is useful when evaluating polyneuropathies but is of limited value in compression neuropathies such as carpal tunnel syndrome.

Phalen's test is a provocative method of eliciting symptoms in patients without objective neurologic deficits and has been found in 76% of patients with carpal tunnel syndrome. This test can easily reproduce the symptoms by having the patient markedly flex the wrist for 1 minute. After 1 minute has elapsed, paresthesias or numbness in the distribution of the median nerve occur if compression is present. Even if paresthesias do not develop, sensory examination will typically reveal areas of hyperesthesia within the sensory distribution of the median nerve. It must be noted that paresthesias will develop in normal persons if wrist flexion is sustained long enough and will result in a false-positive Phalen's sign.

Tinel's sign can be elicited by tapping along the course of the nerve as it passes under the transverse carpal ligament. A positive Tinel's sign is present when paresthesias are reproduced by the tapping. Pain at the wrist without paresthesias should be considered percussion tenderness and does not constitute a positive Tinel's sign. The symptoms produced by Phalen's and Tinel's tests may not be present equally in the sensory distribution of the median nerve. This is due to the arrangement of the nerve fibers with those supplying the long finger being closest to the transverse carpal ligament.

The motor examination is usually normal except in advanced cases of carpal tunnel syndrome. When motor deficits are noted, severe compression of the median nerve is present. Motor testing is normally limited to the abductor pollicis brevis since it is the least likely of the thenar muscles to receive innervation from the ulnar nerve and the easiest to isolate. The abductor pollicis brevis is tested for strength by having the patient abduct the thumb away from the palm against resistance. It is important to ensure that the thumb is in a plane perpendicular to the palm when conducting this test, otherwise the extensor muscles will assist with the movement.

DIFFERENTIAL DIAGNOSIS

Table 10-11-1 provides a list of local and systemic conditions associated with carpal tunnel syndrome. These processes can be eliminated in the differential by the absence of other symptoms and signs noted during the general history and physical examination. Of prime importance is to exclude entrapment of the median nerve at other levels or nerve root involvement (Fig. 10-11-3).

Entrapment of C6 or C7 spinal nerve roots can also cause pain and paresthesias in the fingers innervated by the median nerve along with pain in the forearm and shoulder. Nerve root involvement, however,

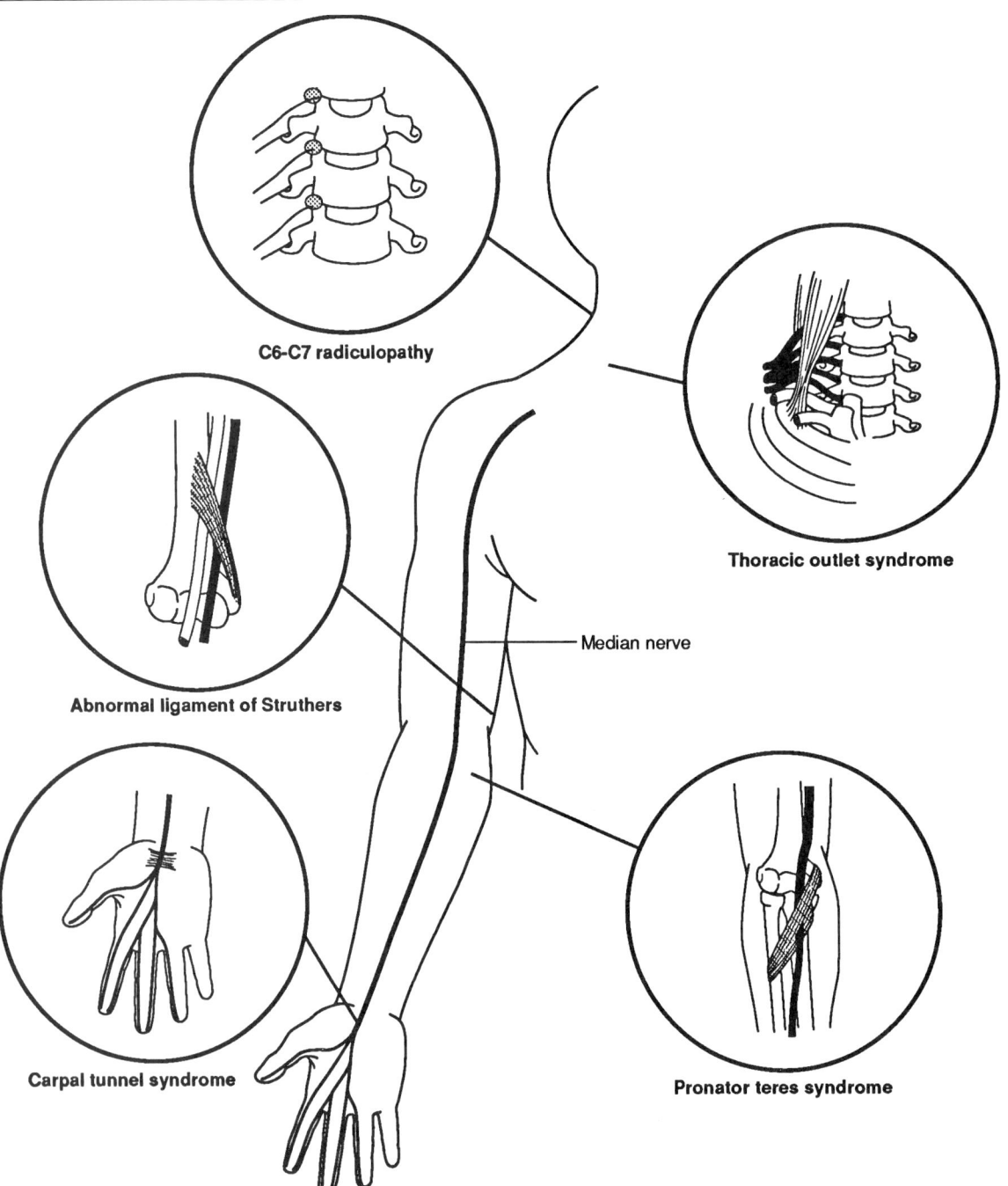

FIGURE 10-11-3. Sites of entrapment of the median nerve and its origins.

is usually accompanied by pain and stiffness in the neck and rarely is bilateral or develops the pattern of night pain. In addition, nerve root entrapment at these levels will cause pain and paresthesias in the dorsal aspect of the hand and will involve the reflexes and motor strength at higher levels in the upper extremity.

Thoracic outlet syndrome may mimic carpal tunnel syndrome in that thenar atrophy may present. The sensory abnormalities in thoracic outlet syndrome will differ and present in the dermatomes of C8 and T1, involving the ring and little fingers and the medial aspect of the forearm.

In 2% of the population a spur occurs at the medial supracondylar region of the distal humerus. When the spur is present the ligament of Struthers may be abnormally attached to it and form a canal through which the median nerve and brachial artery pass. Compression may occur with repetitive flexion of the elbow and resemble carpal tunnel syndrome. In addition to the picture of median nerve compression, the

classic presentation of pain, pallor, pulselessness, paresthesias, and paralysis that indicate arterial occlusion will occur in the regions distal to the elbow that are supplied by the brachial artery.

Compression of the median nerve can occur at the proximal forearm where the nerve passes between the two heads of the pronator teres. The symptoms associated with pronator teres syndrome are an aching pain in the anterior aspect of the forearm that is worsened by activities that involve repeated pronation and pain and paresthesias in the median nerve distribution in the hand. Physical exam findings include a hard, tender pronator teres and a Tinel's sign over the muscle.

A small number of patients may have carpal tunnel syndrome and another coexisting neuropathy that contributes to their symptoms. Most commonly a cervical radiculopathy is the other process involved. When this occurs the term *double crush syndrome* is applied. Although no evidence exists to establish whether there is a pathologic connection or the conditions coexist purely by chance, double crush syndrome should be suspected in the patient with profound symptoms or an atypical presentation of carpal tunnel syndrome.

DIAGNOSTIC STUDIES (NERVE TESTING)

Nerve conduction velocity (NCV) and electromyogram (EMG) are valuable studies that can be readily obtained to aid in the diagnosis of carpal tunnel syndrome. NCV tests can be performed on both motor and sensory nerves. To test the motor portion of the median nerve in carpal tunnel syndrome, electrodes are placed at various points along the nerve to stimulate the abductor pollicis brevis. The latency, which is the time from the onset of the stimulus until the muscle responds, is then measured. From this conduction velocity, amplitude, and duration can be obtained. If a sensory portion of the median nerve is being tested, an electrode is placed proximal to the transverse carpal ligament and a recording of the potential is obtained distally. As with motor testing, sensory responses are calculated and reported in terms of conduction velocity, amplitude, and duration.

Conduction velocity is a direct measurement of the latency and records the time from stimulus to response. In carpal tunnel syndrome NCV will be delayed due to the demyelination of median nerve fibers. Amplitude, which represents the number of functioning myelinated fibers that can carry the stimuli, is reduced in carpal tunnel syndrome. Duration indicates the uniformity of the conduction velocity of the axons and will be increased (dispersed) if carpal tunnel syndrome is present.

Electromyographic examination of suspected carpal tunnel syndrome consists of inserting a needle electrode into the abductor pollicis brevis and measuring the electrical activity when the muscle is relaxed and again when it is fully contracted. During full relaxation the electrical activity of the abductor pollicis brevis will be silent if the muscle is normal. If carpal tunnel syndrome is present, wallerian degeneration has occurred, and the axons are disrupted, the denerved muscle will spontaneously fire during relaxation and produce fibrillation potentials and positive sharp waves. Fibrillation potentials on the EMG resemble the pattern of atrial fibrillation on electrocardiograms (ECGs) and positive sharp waves look very similar to a pathologic Q wave found in myocardial infarction. Fibrillation potentials and positive sharp waves can be found in a variety of muscle disorders and should therefore not be considered diagnostic of carpal tunnel syndrome.

RADIOLOGIC (IMAGING) STUDIES

Radiographs of the wrist may reveal an osseous cause for median nerve compression at the wrist. Malunion of old fractures of the radius, ulna, and carpal bones along with arthritic spurs may extend into the tunnel and reduce its space. Posteroanterior, lateral, oblique, and carpal tunnel views are routinely used to evaluate the wrist. Computed tomography (CT) has been used to evaluate the size of the carpal tunnel in research but has yet to provide a direct correlation to the clinical syndrome and is not routinely used. Magnetic resonance imaging (MRI) has provided a means to view the median nerve, tendons, sheaths, and transverse carpal ligament but, as with CT, the clinical relevance of MRI findings is lacking.

TREATMENT

Conservative treatment of carpal tunnel syndrome consists of splinting the wrist in the neutral position and avoiding repetitive activities of the hand and wrist. Anti-inflammatory agents are prescribed to reduce the inflammation and swelling of the synovial tissues. Corticosteroid injections into the carpal tunnel are useful adjuncts in treating carpal tunnel syndrome. If injections are utilized the median nerve should be avoided. The purpose of the steroid is not to treat the nerve directly but to reduce the inflammation and swelling of the surrounding synovium. Referral to a therapist for tendon gliding exercises and custom splinting is also

helpful in conservative management. These modalities reduce or eliminate the symptoms in about two-thirds of the patients with mild to moderate compression neuropathy.

Patients who fail to respond to conservative therapy or who have marked symptoms such as sensory loss, weakness, or atrophy at the time of presentation are candidates for surgery. In most cases the procedure simply consists of releasing the transverse carpal ligament through an incision in the palm. If indicated, some patients may require a synovectomy or neurolysis. Endoscopic release is frequently employed and facilitates early hand mobilization. Compression dressing and splinting are continued for several weeks postoperatively followed by supervised therapy. Most patients report resolution of pain, paresthesias, and nocturnal symptoms once the incisional pain has dissipated. Return of full sensation and strength may take several months after the surgery. If thenar atrophy is present preoperatively, the recovery period can be prolonged.

COMPLICATIONS

Complications most commonly reported include wound infection, incomplete relief of symptoms, prolonged scar pain, and return of the syndrome after initial surgical success. In rare instances reflex sympathetic dystrophy, bowstringing of the flexor tendons, and joint contractures occur.

BIBLIOGRAPHY

Goldner RD, Goldner JL: Compression neuropathies of the hand and forearm, in *Textbook of Surgery,* 15th ed, Philadelphia, Sabiston DC (ed). Saunders, 1997, pp 1479–1486.

Griffin JW: Peripheral neuropathies, in *The Principles and Practice of Medicine,* 23d ed, Stobo JD (ed). Stamford, CT, Appleton & Lange, 1996, pp 881–889.

McCue FC: Median nerve entrapment at the elbow in athletes. *Operative Techniques in Sports Medicine* 4(1):21–27, 1996.

Palmar D: Carpal tunnel syndrome in athletes. *Operative Techniques in Sports Medicine* 4(1):33–39, 1996.

Stewart JD: *Focal Peripheral Neuropathies,* 2d ed, New York, Raven, 1993.

Venna N: Peripheral neuropathies, in *Textbook of Primary Care Medicine,* 2d ed, Noble J (ed). St. Louis, Mosby, 1996, pp 1408–1431.

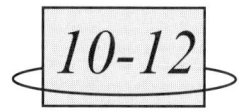

CERVICAL STRAIN AND SPRAIN

Stephen M. Cohen

DISCUSSION

The neck injury termed *whiplash* was first described by an American orthopedist in 1928. Cervical strain (muscle-tendon injury) and/or sprain (ligamentous injury) primarily involve damage to the soft tissues of both the anterior and the posterior neck. Although most episodes result from hyperextension forces, hyperflexion and rotational forces also may cause injury to soft tissue. This injury primarily affects adults. Motor vehicle collisions, diving accidents, and falls account for the primary mechanisms in this injury.

The damage to soft tissue is directly proportional to the forces applied and creates a continuous scale of injury from minimal to severe. Any structure in the neck can be damaged by the forces of extreme or rapid flexion, extension, or rotation. Muscle, tendons, ligaments, the esophagus, the trachea, nerve roots, the sympathetic chain, and fascia all may be damaged. The resulting tissue swelling and inflammation can compound the initial damage.

Often overlooked in neck injury is the risk of cerebral concussion and contusion. When the head is thrown forward, rapid deceleration occurs as the neck flexes to the full forward position. However, the brain continues its forward movement (as a result of inertia) and strikes the frontal cranial vault. A similar injury can occur posteriorly as the head decelerates when the neck goes into full extension. This phenomenon may explain much of the brain damage noted in "shaken baby syndrome." As a result of the brain injury, many patients who experience a cervical strain or sprain injury have abnormal electroencephalograms (EEGs) and associated complaints. This underappreciated phenomenon may account for many of the psychiatric and cognitive symptoms in patients with chronic complaints after neck injury.

SIGNS AND SYMPTOMS

The most common symptoms reported at presentation are acute, delayed, or chronic headache; dizziness; hearing loss; visual disturbances; alterations in smell or taste; and difficulty in cognitive function (primarily word differentiation, concentration, and short-term memory).

Symptoms are extremely variable, depending on forces applied, the mechanism and degree of injury, and the chronology of presentation. Headache is often described as tension-like, starting at the base of the skull near the suboccipital triangle or occiput, shoulders, or midback. The common occurrence of muscle spasm can affect thoracic back, neck, shoulder, and facial muscles.

Aggravation or acute onset of temporal mandibular joint dysfunction and pain has been reported. In a delayed or chronic presentation, the pain of the original injury can be re-created by triggers such as posture and stress days, weeks, or months after the injury.

OBJECTIVE FINDINGS

Often there are delayed symptoms with cervical strain or sprain. As soft tissue swelling progresses, the neck musculature becomes stiff and may progress to painful spasm. Neck range of motion often becomes decreased. Pain often centers around the neck and suboccipital region, although symptoms may include upper back and shoulder pain if spasm persists and spreads caudally.

The mechanics of neck injury may cause symptoms to begin from any previous injured disk herniation or musculoskeletal condition. Underlying and preexisting disease processes in the neck that may precipitate pain in flexion or extension injuries include arthritis, disk annulus fracture, microtears and herniation, and spondylosis. The pain from underlying neck entities is often of a magnitude that exceeds what might be expected with a given mechanism of injury. Additionally, the mechanics of injury may facilitate new fracturing of the disk annulus or facet joint surfaces.

Neurologic examinations most often are normal or without significant findings. Severe mechanical injury may stretch nerve roots and the sympathetic nerve chain, causing symptoms of blurred vision, tinnitus, nausea, vomiting, and occasional dizziness. Pronounced neck and upper back spasm can present with numbness and tingling sensations superficially but rarely will be confused with peripheral nerve or radicular injury. If unilateral sternocleidomastoid muscle damage and swelling occurs, torticollis of varying degrees may occur acutely.

DIAGNOSTIC CONSIDERATIONS

Diagnosis and proper evaluation begin with a complete history and physical examination with concentration on the musculoskeletal and neurologic components of the head, neck, upper torso, and extremities. A careful examination should focus on the discovery of underlying and preexisting conditions separate from the often obvious soft tissue injury.

SPECIAL CONSIDERATIONS

Many cervical injuries, especially from motor vehicle accidents, present "packaged" by emergency medical personnel to the emergency department. The use of a rigid collar and backboard in these cases demands attention to neurologic evaluation and the consideration of more severe injury. Proper evaluation and judgment are necessary to guide the removal of these appliances. At a minimum, a full lateral roentgenogram (visualizing completely to the C7–T1 disk space) should be accomplished before the removal of any pre–hospital-applied collars.

LABORATORY STUDIES

With injury secondary to forceful trauma of unknown cause, a blood alcohol, drug screen, glucose, and complete blood cell count (CBC) may be warranted. Laboratory examination to evaluate the extent of cervical soft tissue injury is not necessary or helpful apart from determining the medical cause of the injury or contributing factors leading to the mechanism of the injury.

RADIOLOGIC STUDIES

Radiographic evaluation in sprain or strain injury most often is normal. Progression of symptoms, muscle spasm, and increased chronicity can cause reversal of the normal curvature on lateral neck films. This presentation often is noted on chiropractic examination but is insignificant on initial presentation unless it is accompanied by degenerative changes or segmental collapse. Correlation with long-term structural changes has not been shown.

Although only 80 to 85 percent accurate at detecting abnormality, anterior-posterior (AP) roentgenograms and lateral plain roentgenograms of the cervical spine are considered the minimal examination to rule out structural abnormality. Serious bony injuries have been detected in "minor" presentations of neck pain and stiffness after low-velocity events. Although this is uncommon, a high index of suspicion should be present in the evaluation of all neck injury.

The essence of radiologic examination is to rule out a subluxation or fracture associated with a soft tissue injury. A concerted effort must be made to clearly visualize C1–C7 with preference for seeing the top of T1 if possible. A "swimmer's" view of C7 may be necessary if this cannot be accomplished. Lateral examinations often can be utilized to assess the severity of prevertebral soft tissue swelling. Attention must be directed to the alignment of spinous processes on AP views of the cervical spine to detect malrotation defects and ligamentous rupture in the rotational plane.

In addition to AP and lateral radiographs, flexion and extension views can be very helpful, some say essential, in delineating and defining ligamentous injury in patients with whiplash. The practitioner should remember the significant role the ligamentous structures play in stabilization. The degrees of "kinking," or kyphosis, and "fanning," or spread of spinous processes, are useful observations to separate minor soft tissue injury from more significant ligamentous tears. Wide-spaced spinous processes on lateral radiographs may indicate complete disruption of ligamentous structures.

OTHER DIAGNOSTICS

Computed tomography (CT) and magnetic resonance imaging (MRI) may be indicated to evaluate the extent of swelling and damage. These examinations also may be utilized to delineate small or occult fractures associated with the injury. Bone scans generally are not indicated, since most will be "hot" throughout the area because of acute inflammation and swelling. Tomograms may assist in the visualization of occult or suspected fractures but are not helpful in acute presentations.

TREATMENT

Pharmacologic Management

Nonsteroidal anti-inflammatory drugs (NSAIDs) in combination with analgesics given in the amounts necessary to relieve pain in the acute phases are essential. A muscle relaxant medication such as metaxalone or methocarbamol in combination with salicylate or anti-inflammatory medication for acute spasm is well tolerated and assists in treating the most common cause of acute pain.

Rarely is diazepam (Valium) or a narcotic necessary in either the acute or the chronic stage, and both should be avoided if possible. Regardless of the medication, care must be taken to ensure proper instruction, patient use, and follow-up. These medications are not intended for use in children, and caution must be used in adolescents. The most common musculoskeletal pain and spasm medications are noted (see Table 10-12-1).

Vitamin C in doses of 500 to 1500 mg orally per day may assist in the healing of soft tissue and is a useful adjunct in the treatment of suspected soft tissue damage in the cervical spine region. Commercially available over-the-counter (OTC) preparations are sufficient and cost-effective for this purpose.

In severe cases with suspected transient cord compression, methylprednisolone given within 8 h of injury may be helpful in preventing more permanent cellular changes in the soft tissue zone of injury, especially if nerve tissue is involved centrally or peripherally. These patients require hospitalization and MRI or CT evaluation of the spinal cord and column.

Supportive Measures

Aggressive applications of conservative treatment modalities are essential in whiplash injury. Rest with 48 to 72 h (primary inflammatory period) of cold-pack therapy is beneficial in reducing inflammation and acute pain. Treatment in an acute injury should then be followed by physical examination to reassess the symptoms. Moist hot packs, manual muscle therapy, trigger point manual therapy, electrical stimulation, and other modalities can relieve the pain and spasm associated with injury once the primary inflammatory period has passed.

Although many clinicians recommend a soft foam collar for support in the early phases of injury, there is no proven stabilization with their use. Soft collars appear not to alter the degree of persistent pain in patients who develop chronic syndromes. The use of soft collars may lead the patient to long-term psychological dependency on such appliances and is not recommended.

Once the acute inflammatory phase has passed, range of motion (ROM) must be performed with slow and controlled movement. Once motion becomes stiff and reduced from the full range, it may be difficult to recover full motion as time progresses. Gentle ROM exercise in

a warm shower twice daily is very beneficial to facilitate early motion of a stiff neck. This may be begun as early as 4 to 7 days after injury, depending on the severity and the results of follow-up examination.

Aerobic exercise is recommended to ensure circulatory enhancement in the area of injury. Walking, bike riding, swimming, and easy jogging are best to avoid jarring from high-impact exercise. Recommend a program of three to four sessions of exercise per week for 20 to 40 min/day. The usual precautions in prescribing aerobic exercise to any patient should be employed, including evaluation of other anatomic and physiologic subsystems.

PATIENT EDUCATION

Patient education and support are vital in the acute injury and the chronic syndrome. The emotional impact of this injury can be disabling and severe. Many patients describe not being "believed" and being treated indifferently by practitioners, which causes great anxiety in a patient with chronic or reoccurring symptoms. Depression is also an extremely common diagnosis in chronic pain syndromes of the neck. Support and complete patient education throughout the process of therapy, which may last for months or years, is vital to a positive outcome. "Learn to live with it" instruction often is unjustified, since improvement is possible with attention and persistent conservative treatment.

The regularly prescribed use of muscle relaxant and anti-inflammatory medication cannot be stressed enough in the acute phase of this injury (24 to 72 hours). The patient must clearly understand that waiting until symptoms begin or get worse is often "too late." PRN (as needed) instruction has no place in the treatment of the acute phase of whiplash injury.

DISPOSITION

Most patients recuperate from this type of injury in 30 to 60 days with conservative care. The remaining 35% continue to have varying degrees of symptoms from months to years. Approximately 18% have persistent symptoms that they attribute to the primary traumatic event after 2 years. Most members of this group have identifiable preexisting conditions before injury. Relapse and setback in treatment commonly cause the patient to become frustrated with therapy. This is to be expected and is a normal course for strain or sprain injury to the cervical spine. The practitioner should be patient and attentive to these concerns.

As the patient begins to heal, triggering events may cause setback, pain, and spasm. Posture (work, sleep, and recreation), stress, recreational activity, and other environmental factors can stimulate muscle spasm and

TABLE 10-12-1. Muscle Relaxant Medications

Metaxalone 400 mg (Skelexin)	800 mg 3–4 times daily for 7–10 days	For muscle spasm pain, not in renal or hepatic deficiency. Watch for drug-induced anemia. Must take regularly to gain blood levels
Cyclobezaprine 10-mg tabs (Flexeril)	10 mg, 3 tid for muscle spasm; 60 mg maximum; no longer than 3 weeks	Danger in cardiac disease, thyroid disease, or with MAOIs. May cause drowsiness, dizziness, GI upset, HA
Orphenadrin citrate 100 mg (Norflex), sustained release	100 mg bid for painful muscle spasm	Contains sulfites. Precautions: coronary disease, arrhythmia, asthma. Interacts with anticholinergic, ETOH, and CNS depressants. May cause tachycardia, dizziness, GI upset, urinary retention
Chlorzoxazone (Parafon Forte)	500 mg qid; 750 mg max qid	Potentiation hazard with CNS depressants and alcohol. GI upset not uncommon. Hepatocellular toxicity (rare)
Methocarbamal (Robaxin)	1.5 g 4 times daily for 48–72 h, then 4 g daily (divided)	May potentiate CNS depressants. Drowsiness, dizziness, GI disturbance, blurred vision, HA reported
Carisoprodol (Soma)	350 mg 4 times daily	Contraindicated in porphyria. Potentiates CNS depressants; may cause orthostatic hypotension, rash, tachycardia, epigastric distress

NOTE: MAOI = monoamine oxidase inhibitor; HA = headache; ETOH = ethyl alcohol.

acute pain attacks. Psychological support and therapy modalities should be utilized to break spasm cycles, gain patient confidence, and facilitate long-term healing and dealing with the injury. This may involve months or years.

Permanent laxity of supporting structures may be identified after the conversion to a chronic pain syndrome. Chronic pain presentations after injury demand regular evaluation for instability and structural changes. This is especially true in any new or progressive radiculopathy after a strain or sprain injury.

COMPLICATIONS AND RED FLAGS

Immediate attention should be directed toward any neurologic deficit (paresthesia, muscle weakness, loss of reflexes, sensory loss, or radiculopathy) or radiographic evidence of more severe bony injury. Any deficit in the acute presentation should be considered for additional studies such as MRI and immediate stabilization with a rigid collar system and a neurologic consultation.

Any difficulty swallowing or talking should alert the evaluator to the possibility of significant soft tissue swelling in the neck. Airway support may be indicated in severe injuries and should be available. Facial or chest injury alerts the examiner to the strong possibility of more severe underlying bony injury in the head, face, and/or spine.

The examiner should remain alert to signs and symptoms that indicate more severe injury or complications. Epidural hematoma, internal carotid artery occlusion, abducens nerve palsy, and retropharyngeal hematoma have been reported in whiplash injury. Additionally, any transient ischemic attacks, dizziness, or similar events within 3 months of a whiplash injury should alert the practitioner to the possibility of circulatory injury, especially in the posterior cerebral system.

NOTES AND PEARLS

Any acute strain or sprain injury of the cervical spine can aggravate preexisting cervical inflammatory or degenerative processes. Old radiographic studies should be obtained for comparison when possible, because this vital information can be helpful in evaluating pain syndromes. Additionally, facet arthritides cannot be ignored. Degenerative facet joint surfaces, when aggravated by acute strain or sprain injuries, can manifest with severe spasm and a chronic course.

Patients with small vertebral canal architecture (congenital small diameter) appear to have a more chronic course and a worse prognosis. In such cases, the stretch and microtears of superficial neural structures adjacent to and including the cord may inhibit expeditious recovery.

Patient support and rigorous patient education about the use of medication, modalities, ROM, heat or cold therapy, and support systems often make the difference between patient satisfaction and treatment failure. Rapid and aggressive management of the acute trauma may prevent or substantially reduce chronic pain syndromes after neck injury.

BIBLIOGRAPHY

Bogduk N, Teasell R: Whiplash—the evidence for an organic etiology. *Arch Neurol* 57(4):590–591, 2000.

Griffiths HJ, Olson PN, Everson LI, et al: Hyperextension strain or "whiplash" injuries to the cervical spine. *Skeletal Radiol* 24(4):263–266, 1995.

Helliwell PS, Evans PF, Wright V: The straight cervical spine: Does it indicate muscle spasm? *J Bone Joint Surg* 76:103–106, 1994.

Mercier LR: *Practical Orthopedics.* St Louis, Mosby, 1995.

Pennie BH, Agambar LJ: Whiplash injuries. *J Bone Joint Surg* 72:277, 1990.

Praemer A, Furner S: *Musculoskeletal Conditions in the United States.* Park Ridge, IL, American Academy of Orthopedic Surgeons, 1992.

Radanov BP, Sturenegger M, DiStefano G: Long-term outcome after whiplash injury: A 2-year follow-up considering features of injury mechanism and somatic, radiologic, and psychosocial findings. *Medicine (Baltimore)* 74(5):281–297, 1995.

Viktrup L, Knudsen GM, Hansen SH: Delayed onset of fatal basilar thrombotic embolus after whiplash. *Stroke* 26(11):2194–2196, 1995.

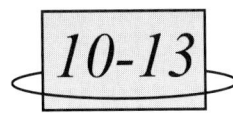

HIP FRACTURES
David Zinsmeister

DESCRIPTION

The term *hip fracture* by convention applies to fractures of the proximal femur. Common locations for fracture are the femoral neck, the intertrochanteric region, and the subtrochanteric region, with isolated fractures of the greater and lesser trochanter occurring less frequently. Stress fractures of the hip are becoming more prevalent, and the hip is a relatively common site of pathologic fracture. Fractures of the femoral head occur with dislocation of the hip and fracture of the acetabulum and generally are not considered hip fractures.

Femoral neck fractures occur at the subcapital, neck, and basicervical regions. Intertrochanteric fractures are defined as the primary fracture line extending between the greater and lesser trochanters, and subtrochanteric fractures are those with the primary fracture between the lesser trochanter and a point 5 cm distal. Each type of fracture has variants that significantly alter treatment and prognosis, based on the anatomic and biomechanical influences at the fracture site (see Boxes 10-13-1 and 10-13-2).

PATHOGENESIS

As the average age of the population has increased, the incidence of hip fractures also has climbed dramatically; between 1965 and 1981, the number of hip fractures almost tripled. Currently, more than 275,000 hip fractures occur each year in the United States, with the estimated cost of treatment exceeding $6 billion. By the year 2040, the incidence of hip fracture is projected to be 500,000 per year. Among Medicare patients, the rate of fracture was highest in the South and the lowest in the Northeast.

Age, sex, and race place certain individuals at a higher risk for hip fracture. More than 85% of all hip fractures occur in individuals over 65 years old. By age 80, 93% of all women will have sustained at least one fracture, and in approximately 33% of cases, that will be a hip fracture. White women are at twice the risk for hip fractures as are blacks and Hispanics and at 2.7 times the risk as are white men.

The relationship of osteoporosis and osteomalacia to hip fracture has been studied extensively. They are contributing factors to the frequency of hip fractures. Osteoporosis (decreased density with normal mineralization) and osteomalacia (decreased mineralization) result in a density or mineralization level below what is required for mechanical support. It has been reported that by age 65, 50% of all women have a bone density or mineral content below the threshold required for sustaining a fracture and that by age 85, 100% of women are below this threshold. Other risk factors include the use of psychotropic drugs, Alzheimer's disease, excessive alcohol intake, and a prior history of hip fracture. Radiographically, osteoporosis and osteomalacia are indistinguishable. Clinical manifestations, laboratory studies, and noninvasive methods to determine bone density help differentiate between the two processes, but bone biopsy is required for a definitive diagnosis.

Mortality rates within the first year after injury vary from 14 to 21%. Patients with significant medical problems had a 1-year mortality rate of 49.4% compared with 8.0% for healthier patients (American Society of Anesthesiologists III/IV). Patients are at the greatest risk of death within the first year after injury, and the mortality rate 1-year after a fracture is comparable to that of the age- and sex-matched population that has not sustained a hip fracture.

BOX 10-13-1

SKELETAL AND VASCULAR ANATOMY

Cortical bone is thinnest at the femoral neck and contributes to the higher incidence of fractures in this area. The metaphyseal region is largely trabecular bone and contains the calcar femorale, a dense plate of cortical bone that serves as a posteromedial buttress. Intertrochanteric and subtrochanteric fractures involving this buttress create instability in this region and increase the risk of malunion and nonunion. The proximal femoral diaphysis consists largely of cortical bone, and when subtrochanteric fractures occur, there is less surface area for healing; this may lead to delayed union, nonunion, and malunion.

The proximal femur receives its blood supply from branches of the femoral artery and the foveal artery (see Fig. 10-13-A). The retinacular arteries supply the neck and most of the femoral head. Although the foveal artery provides blood to the femoral head, its contribution alone is sufficient to sustain viability. Therefore, disruption of the retinacular vessels in femoral neck fractures increases the likelihood of osteonecrosis of the head and nonunion.

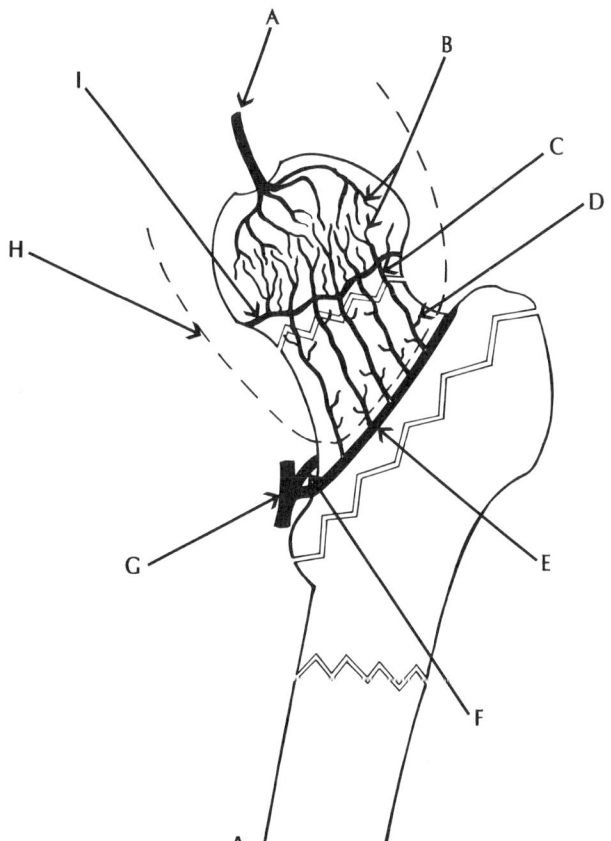

FIGURE 10-13-A. Vascular anatomy of the proximal femur. *A.* Foveal artery. *B.* Epiphyseal arteries. *C.* Retinacular arteries. *D.* Metaphyseal arteries; extracapsular arterial ring. *E.* Lateral femoral circumflex. *F.* Medial femoral circumflex. *G.* Femoral artery. *H.* Capsule. *I.* Intracapsular arterial ring.

BOX 10-13-2

BIOMECHANICS

Forces applied across the hip from body weight and muscle can amount to three times body weight in a single-limb stance. In the early 1900s, Koch,[1] using theoretical analysis, calculated that compression stress at the medial cortex of the subtrochanteric region exceeds 1200 pounds per square inch. This was confirmed over 50 years later using strain gauge measurements.

Ward in 1838 was the first to describe the trabecular orientation of the proximal femur that represents the bone's response to stress that is known as Wolff's law. He identified five trabecular groups that result from bone formation in response to compression, tension, and muscle counterbalance.

In 1976, Singh[2] devised a grading system for osteoporosis that is based on the disappearance pattern of these trabecular groups, as determined by x-ray films. The trabeculae in Ward's triangle are the first to disappear, followed by the secondary compressive, secondary tensile, primary tensile, and eventually primary compressive groups. The disappearance pattern is a useful guide to estimating the degree of osteopenia present (see Fig. 10-13-B).

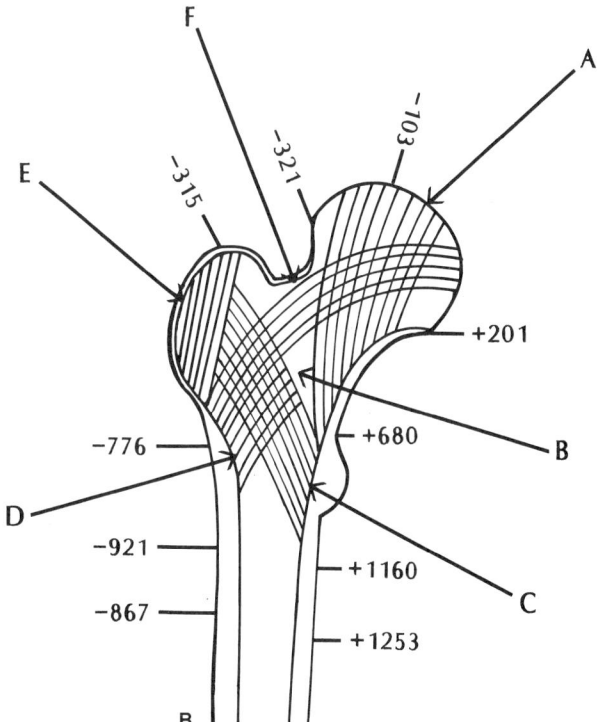

FIGURE 10-13-B. The bone's response to forces across the hip. Trabecular group patterns as described by Ward. *A.* Primary compressive. *B.* Ward's triangle. *C.* Secondary compressive. *D.* Secondary tensile. *E.* Greater trochanter. *F.* Primary tensile. Numbers on periphery indicate pounds per square inch as calculated by Koch. Positive numbers represent compressive stress; negative numbers indicate tension stress.

HISTORY

Hip fractures in young adults usually result from high-energy trauma such as a motor vehicle accident or a fall from a great height. In the absence of a history of either of these injuries, inquiry should be made about alcohol use, current medications, and medical conditions that may have predisposed a patient to fracture from a simple fall. A history of insidious groin pain that occurs with increased activity in a young, active adult may indicate stress fracture.

In the elderly, hip fracture occurs with minor trauma such as falls in the home, missteps, and twisting injuries. Preexisting medical conditions such as diabetes mellitus, cardiac arrhythmias, disorders of equilibrium, cancer, arthritis, and neurologic conditions that result in muscular paresis, weakness, and instability are common and may increase the risk of falls. Current medications should be assessed as possible contributing factors. In patients over age 75, the fall is more likely to be caused by organ failure than by an accident.

OBJECTIVE FINDINGS

In young adults with a hip fracture, concomitant injuries resulting from high-velocity trauma are common and should be sought aggressively. Common coexisting injuries include those of the chest, abdomen, and spine and head injury of a life-threatening nature that requires emergency treatment. Once life-threatening injuries are stabilized, obvious injuries of the extremity should not become the total focus of attention and preclude a complete orthopedic examination. Subtle hip fractures occasionally are missed because of a more dramatic fracture of the ipsilateral femoral shaft (see Fig. 10-13-1).

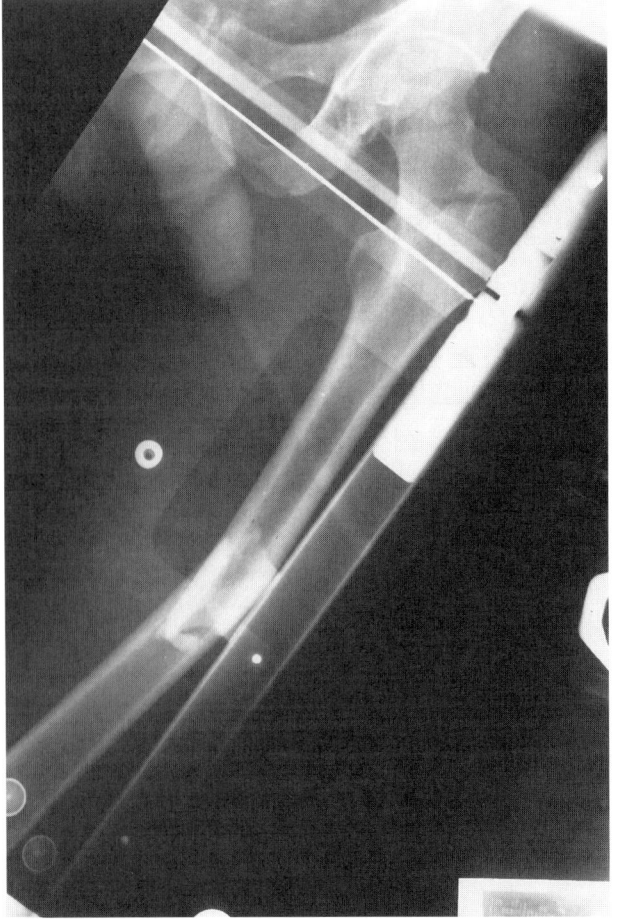

FIGURE 10-13-1. Fracture of the femoral shaft and ipsilateral basicervical fracture of the proximal femur in a polytrauma patient.

In contrast, hip fractures in the elderly are usually isolated injuries. The physical examination should be complete and ensure that medical conditions are stabilized before surgery and that previously unrecognized conditions are identified and treated.

Physical findings on examination of the hip vary, depending on the location of the fracture and the degree of displacement. In a stress fracture of the femoral neck, the patient may be ambulatory with an antalgic gait. Range of motion is usually normal, and tenderness may be elicited over Scarpa's triangle. Displaced femoral neck fractures present with the classic findings of shortening, abduction, and external rotation of the injured extremity. Any attempt at motion will elicit extreme pain. In the case of an impacted or nondisplaced femoral neck fracture, the patient may remain ambulatory for several days before presentation, with physical findings similar to those of a femoral neck stress fracture.

Intertrochanteric fractures have the features of the displaced femoral neck fracture except that a greater degree of external rotation and generalized hip tenderness with swelling exists. Subtrochanteric fractures result in varus angulation distal to the greater trochanter. This physical finding is caused by the pull of the hip abductors and flexors on the proximal fragment and the hip adductors on the distal fragment. Hip examination findings vary with pathologic fractures, depending on the type of tumor, its location, and the extent of cortical involvement.

IMAGING STUDIES

Good-quality anterior-posterior radiographs of the pelvis and anterior-posterior and true lateral films of the hip are the mainstays in the diagnosis of hip fracture. If hemiarthroplasty or total hip arthroplasty is being considered, a low anterior-posterior view of the pelvis should be obtained for component measurement. Tomograms are helpful in detecting discrete, nondisplaced femoral neck fractures. Technetium 99m scanning assists in the diagnosis of nondisplaced and stress fractures of the femoral neck and aids in tumor evaluation. Currently, computed tomography and magnetic resonance imaging play a limited role in traumatic fractures of the hip but help in the evaluation of the cortex and medullary canal in patients with pathologic fractures.

TREATMENT

Femoral Neck Fractures

The classification of femoral neck fractures by Garden[3] consists of four types based on the amount of displacement shown on prereduction radiographs (see Fig. 10-13-2). Type I is an incomplete or complete fracture impacted with valgus angulation of the head, type II is a complete fracture without displacement, type III is a complete fracture with partial displacement, and type IV is a complete fracture with total displacement.

Type I and type II fractures are considered stable because of preservation of the retinacular vessels and carry the best prognosis. Displaced type III and type IV fractures are comminuted posteriorly, which renders the fracture unstable and results in a higher incidence of nonunion and osteonecrosis resulting from vascular insufficiency to the femoral head.

General agreement exists that in a young, active adult, the femoral head should be preserved and the fracture should be internally fixed with multiple pins or screws. In treating an elderly patient, most authors advocate pin or screw fixation in type I (see Fig. 10-13-3) and type II fractures and hemiarthroplasty or total hip arthroplasty for type III and type IV (see Fig. 10-13-4) fractures under certain conditions. Relative indications for selecting arthroplasty over internal fixation include physiologic age over 70, failure to achieve adequate reduction, advanced arthritis, osteogenic bone stock, Parkinson's disease, spastic hemiplegia, and pathologic fracture. Both internal fixation and arthroplasty have been reported as acceptable forms of treatment for displaced femoral neck fractures in the elderly, but a consensus on optimal treatment has not been reached.

FEMORAL NECK FRACTURES

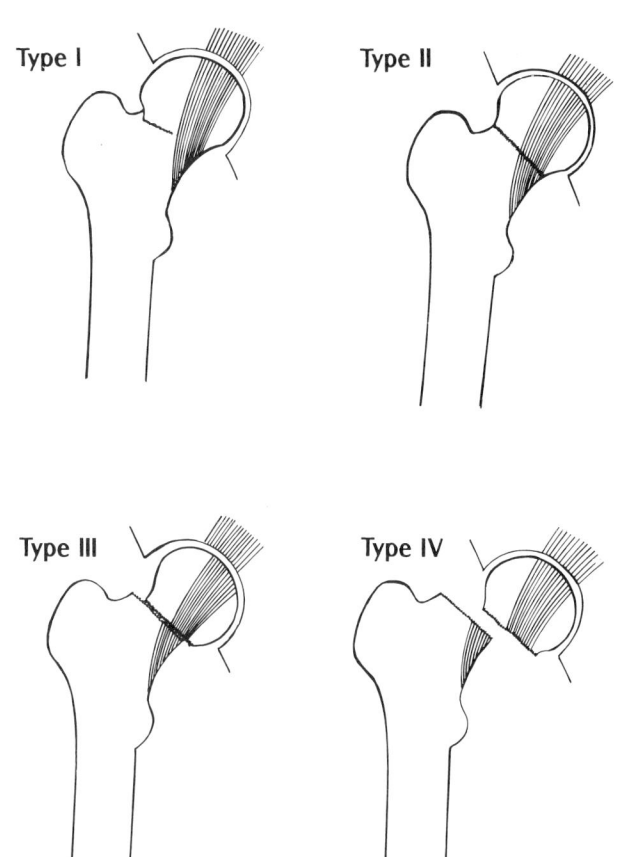

FIGURE 10-13-2. Garden's classification of femoral neck fractures. (*From Garden*[3] *with permission.*)

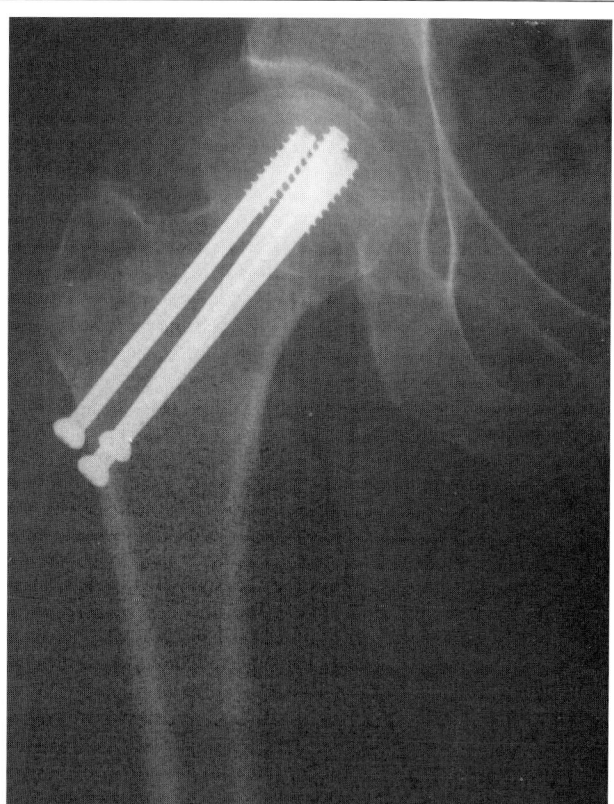

FIGURE 10-13-3. Type I femoral neck fracture in an elderly woman. The fracture is internally fixed with cannulated screws.

Intertrochanteric Fractures

The integrity of the posteromedial buttress is of prime importance in intertrochanteric fractures. Posteromedial comminution and fracture extension result in loss of stability and varus collapse. Kyle and Gustilo's modification[4] of Boyd's classification of intertrochanteric fractures recognizes four basic types of fractures based on the location and degree of comminution that affects stability (see Fig. 10-13-5). Type I is a stable, nondisplaced intertrochanteric fracture, whereas type II is a stable, displaced intertrochanteric fracture with fracture of the lesser trochanter and varus deformity. Type III is an unstable, displaced intertrochanteric fracture with fracture of the greater trochanter, posteromedial comminution, and varus deformity, and type IV is an unstable, displaced intertrochanteric fracture with subtrochanteric extension, posteromedial comminution, fracture of the greater trochanter, and varus deformity.

Internal fixation of intertrochanteric fractures centers on correcting the varus deformity and regaining and maintaining stability. The sliding compression screw and side plate device usually is used to treat stable and unstable fractures. It allows controlled impaction of the fracture and resists deforming forces (see Fig. 10-13-6).

Subtrochanteric Fractures

Russell and Taylor's classification system[5] for subtrochanteric fractures incorporates extension of the fracture into the piriformis fossa and posteromedial cortex, a process that alters treatment and prognosis (see Fig. 10-13-7). Within this classification system, type I fractures do not extend into the piriformis fossa with type II involving

the fossa, "A" indicates sparing of the posteromedial cortex, and "B" indicates comminution and inadequate posteromedial support. This combination results in four fracture types—IA, IB, IIA, and IIB—with IA having the best prognosis and IIB having the worst.

With the piriformis fossa and lesser trochanter intact, type IA fractures are treated with standard intramedullary nailing that locks into the calcar femorale. Type IB fractures that are comminuted posteromedially, thus preventing locking in this region, are internally fixed with a reconstruction nail that locks in the femoral head (see Fig. 10-13-8). Type II fractures that involve the fossa and prevent nail introduction are treated with a compression screw and side plate device that stabilizes the fracture. Indirect reduction techniques and bone grafting are helpful adjunctive methods in these difficult cases.

Stress Fractures of the Femoral Neck

A recent prospective study of 1049 stress fractures identified 54 femoral neck stress fractures in 49 patients. Numerous classification systems for this type of fracture exist, and all center on the involvement of the compression and tension cortices. If only the compression side is involved (see Fig. 10–13-9), treatment consists of rest and restricted weight bearing. In the case of tension side fracture, disruption of both cortices, or displacement, the fracture is internally fixed with multiple parallel pins or screws. Callus, sclerosis, and fracture may not be apparent radiographically for several weeks after the onset of pain, and scintigraphy is required for early diagnosis and assessment of the tension side.

Pathologic Fractures

Metastatic neoplasms are the most common malignant bone tumor, with the femur being fourth in the frequency of osseous sites for metastasis. Primary tumors that frequently metastasize to bone are breast,

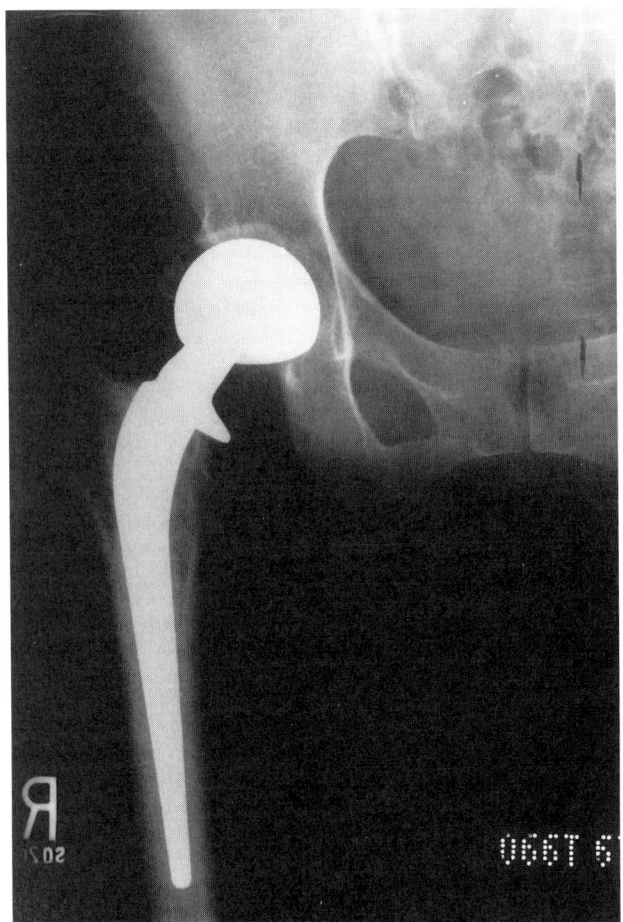

FIGURE 10-13-4. Postoperative radiograph of a patient with a type IV femoral neck fracture treated with cemented bipolar hemiarthroplasty.

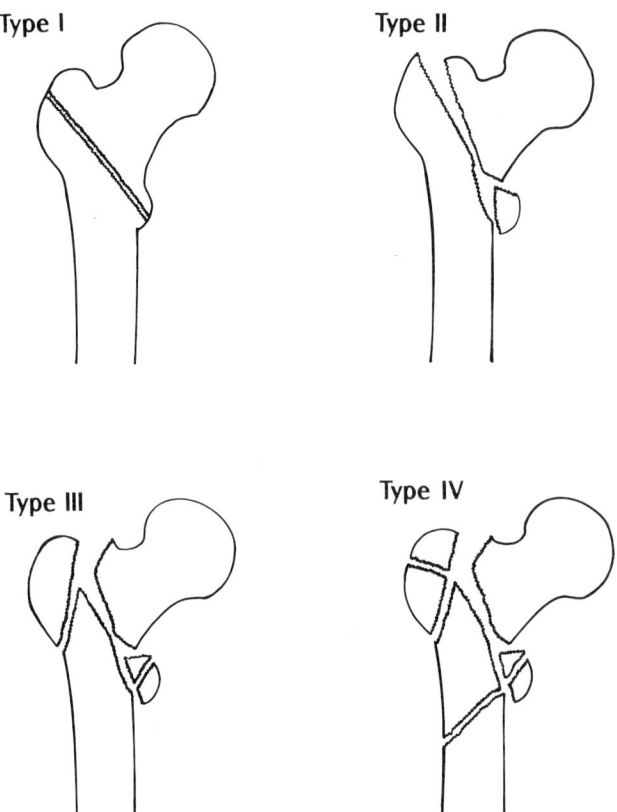

FIGURE 10-13-5. Kyle and Gustilo's modification of Boyd's classification of intertrochanteric fractures. (*From Kyle et al[4] with permission.*)

lung, thyroid, kidney, and prostate tumors, with hematogenous spread being the usual route. Radiation therapy is the principal treatment modality for bony metastasis, and the goals of internal fixation are pain relief, restoration of function, and early mobilization, thus enhancing quality of life and facilitating the provision of care.

Indications for internal fixation of impending pathologic fractures are a painful lesion more than 2.5 cm in diameter and destruction of more than 50% of the cortex. In addition to sparing the patient the painful experience of acute fracture, fixation of impending pathologic fractures results in lower surgical mortality and fewer complications.

SPECIAL CONSIDERATIONS

Indications for the nonoperative treatment of hip fractures are rare. Operative fixation generally is considered the conservative option, with relative contraindications limited to nonambulatory, severely demented patients in little pain and those with life-threatening conditions who are at a high risk of death from anesthesia. However, patients with severe traumatic brain injury can experience spontaneous and often dramatic recovery. Therefore, if otherwise indicated, operative fixation of the fracture should be accomplished under the optimistic assumption that the patient will achieve normal ambulatory status.

AFTERCARE

The principal goals of aftercare of all hip fractures are early mobilization and prevention of complications. The patient should sit upright within the first 24 hours after surgery and begin assisted touchdown weight bearing as soon as it can be tolerated. Progression to full weight bearing with a cane or walker is advanced during the next 6 to 12 weeks, depending on the fracture type. Hip and knee range-of-motion exercises are initiated and advanced during the process of fracture healing.

Various methods exist for using prophylactic anticoagulants in hip fracture patients. The goals of therapy are to provide adequate protection against thromboembolic disease and decrease the risk of bleeding. Support stockings, foot pumps, and elevation of the extremity also help venous return. Prophylactic cephalosporin antibiotics are used and continued for 24 to 72 hours postoperatively. Discharge planning for the elderly should include an evaluation of the home environment and often requires the assistance of social service and home nursing agencies.

COMPLICATIONS AND RED FLAGS

Early significant complications are wound infection and thromboembolic disease. Elderly patients are more susceptible to cardiac failure, pulmonary insufficiency, and genitourinary infections, especially if immobilization is prolonged. A polytrauma patient is at increased risk for adult respiratory distress syndrome, shock, and disseminated intravascular coagulation.

Osteonecrosis and nonunion continue to be the main complications of displaced femoral neck fractures in young adults treated with pins or screws. The incidence of nonunion and osteonecrosis ranges from 5.5% to 14% and 19% to 33%, respectively. Complications for elderly patients treated with arthroplasty include component loosening, acetabular erosion, and heterotopic ossification. Reoperation rates for component loosening and acetabular erosion have been reported as 13.7% for fixed femoral head devices and 7.2% for cemented bipolar prosthesis. Heterotopic bone formation of significance occurs in 1% to 2% of arthroplasty patients.

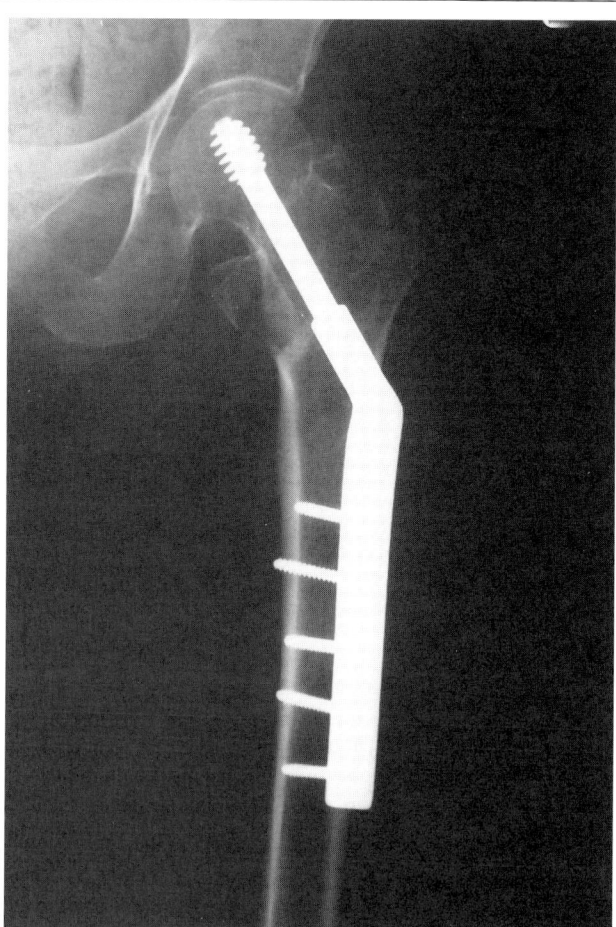

FIGURE 10-13-6. Type III intertrochanteric fracture after internal fixation with a sliding compression screw and side plate device.

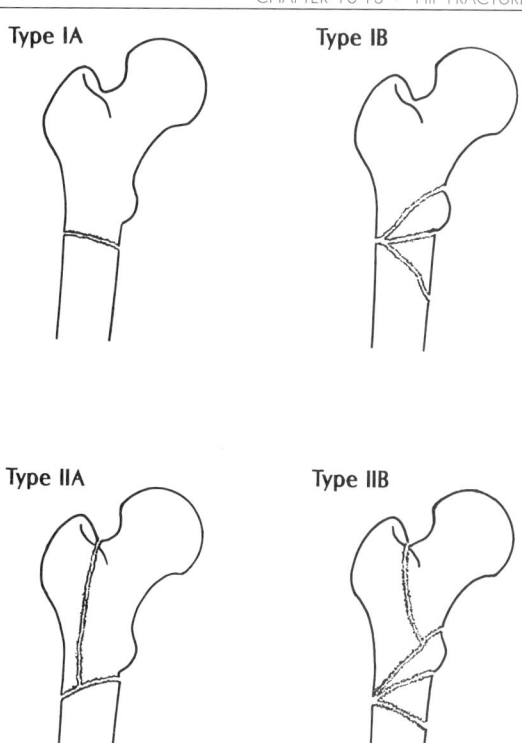

Type IA   Type IB

Type IIA   Type IIB

FIGURE 10-13-7. Russell and Taylor's classification of subtrochanteric fractures. (*From Russell[5] with permission.*)

Complications of intertrochanteric and subtrochanteric fractures treated with a sliding compression screw and side plate device are penetration of the femoral head and neck and device failure resulting in nonunion and malunion. Failure rates vary, depending on fracture stability, from 4.8% to 11.5% in intertrochanteric fractures and a reported nonunion rate of 5% in a variety of subtrochanteric fractures. In a series of 22 subtrochanteric fractures treated with interlocking medullary nailing, one delayed union and one nonunion were reported.

NOTES AND PEARLS

The incidence of hip fracture can be expected to increase as the average life expectancy for Americans becomes longer. In the elderly population, white women with type I osteoporosis are at the greatest risk for hip fracture from minor trauma. High-energy trauma is the predominant cause for hip fracture in young adults, who frequently sustain concomitant life-threatening injuries.

The primary diagnostic tool in the evaluation of hip fractures is fracture classifications based on plain radiographs. To be useful, a classification system must guide appropriate treatment and indicate prognosis. Numerous classifications exist, and the practitioner should consider the strengths and weaknesses of each when selecting a classification system for use.

Surgery is the treatment of choice for fracture of the hip with few contraindications. Femoral neck, intertrochanteric, and subtrochanteric fracture are the types usually encountered, each with its own variants that alter the treatment and prognosis. Aftercare of a patient with fracture of the hip is individualized on the basis of the patient's needs,

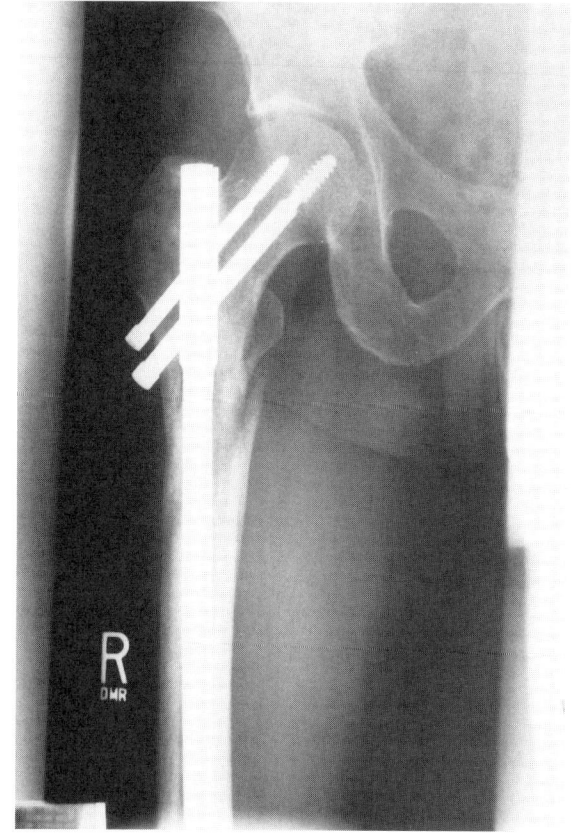

FIGURE 10-13-8. Type IB subtrochanteric fracture after fixation with an interlocking reconstruction nail introduced into the piriformis fossa.

Russell TA: Fractures of the hip and pelvis, in Crenshaw AH (ed): *Campbell's Operative Orthopaedics,* 8th ed, St. Louis, Mosby Year Book, 1992, pp 895–987.

Zinsmeister DE: The diagnosis and treatment of hip fractures. *J Am Acad Physician Assist* 8(6):542–551, 1993.

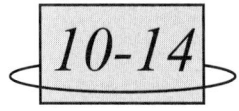

TRAUMATIC KNEE PAIN
David Zinsmeister
Howell J. Smith III

DISCUSSION

Pain, to a greater or lesser extent, is a feature of any traumatic process involving the knee. When eliciting a history of traumatic knee pain it is useful to develop an all-inclusive, systematic approach in order to avoid the pitfall of focusing on the pain rather than the associated symptoms and signs that will be of significance in establishing the diagnosis.

Pain related to trauma is rapid in onset and the patient is evaluated at an early point in the process, usually within hours or days. A key feature in evaluating pain due to trauma is the mechanism of injury. With an understanding of the anatomy of the knee and the biomechanical forces that act upon the knee, the physician assistant can, in the interview process, identify the structures involved, question the patient on related symptoms, and confirm the diagnosis with a systematic approach to the physical exam (see Fig. 10-14-1).

Mechanism of Injury

A sudden twisting of the knee with the foot planted, the knee flexed, and the tibia internally rotated may tear the anterior cruciate ligament (ACL), the medial collateral ligament (MCL), or the medial meniscus. With the knee in this position, the ACL is taut. If enough force is applied through either forward momentum or a blow from behind (a clipping injury) the ligament stretches beyond its elastic limits and tears. As the ligament tears, the tibia translates anteriomedially and can shear the medial meniscus. If enough valgus stress is applied during a clipping injury, fibers of the MCL may also be torn.

When a pure varus or valgus stress is applied to the knee the primary and secondary stabilizers can be involved. The primary stabilizer for the medial aspect of the knee is the MCL with the secondary stabilizers being the anterior and posterior cruciate ligaments. The lateral collateral ligament (LCL) primarily stabilizes the lateral aspect of the knee; the anterior and posterior cruciate ligaments provide secondary support.

A history of a major force applied just below the knee joint that forces the tibia posteriorly or a sudden stop, such as stepping in a shallow hole, that forces the femur anteriorly can cause an isolated tear of the posterior cruciate ligament (PCL) or posteriorly dislocate the knee and damage the popliteal artery.

A direct fall on the knee will involve the anterior structures of the knee. Commonly injured are the bursae, patella, and the articular surface of the femur. Fracture of the patella may result as well as osteochondral fracture of the articular cartilage of the patella or femur. Due to its unprotected location the prepatellar bursa is usually involved to some degree in any injury, however minor, to the anterior surface of the knee from blunt trauma.

Knee pain originating from trauma of the extensor mechanism requires violent contraction of the quadriceps against resistance. This is commonly seen in basketball players during a rebound play when an attempt is made to extend the weight-bearing leg against the downward

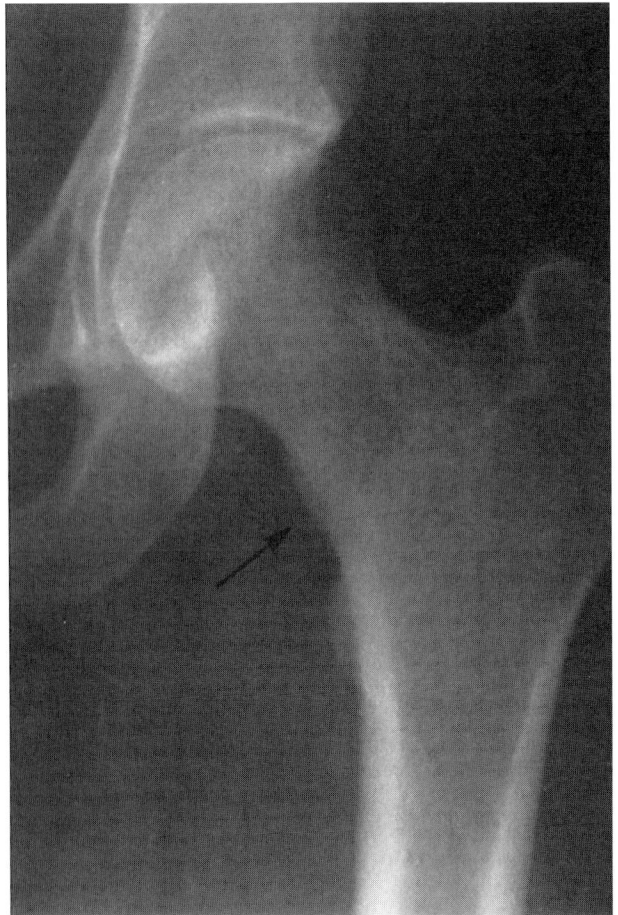

FIGURE 10-13-9. Callus formation (*arrow*) indicating stress fracture of the compression cortex.

with early mobilization and the prevention of complications being common goals in the treatment of all hip fractures.

REFERENCES

1. Koch JC: The laws of bone architecture. *Am J Anat* 21:177, 1917.
2. Singh M, Nagrath AR, Manini PS: Changes in the trabecular pattern of the upper end of the femur as an index of osteoporosis. *J Bone Joint Surg* 52A:457–467, 1976.
3. Garden RS: Low angle fixation in fractures of the femoral neck. *J Bone Joint Surg* 438:647, 1961.
4. Kyle RF, Gustilo RB, Premer RF: Analysis of 622 intertrochanteric hip fractures: A retrospective and prospective study. *J Bone Joint Surg* 61A:216–221, 1979.
5. Russell TA: Fractures of the hip and pelvis, in Crenshaw AH (ed): *Campbell's Operative Orthopaedics,* 8th ed, St Louis, Mosby Year Book, 1992, vol 2, pp 895–987.

BIBLIOGRAPHY

DeLee JC: Fractures and dislocations of the hip, in Rockwood CA, Green DP (eds): *Fractures in Adults,* 3d ed, Philadelphia, Lippincott, 1996, pp 1659–1826.

Laros GS: Intertrochanteric fractures, in Evarts CM (ed): *Surgery of the Musculoskeletal System,* 2d ed, New York, Churchill Livingstone, 1990, pp 2613–2639.

Lhowe DW: Intracapsular fractures of the femoral neck, in Evarts CM (ed): *Surgery of the Musculoskeletal System,* 2d ed, New York, Churchill Livingstone, 1990, pp 2549–2592.

Michelson JD, Cowen EL, Morris MT: Epidemiology of hip fractures among the elderly. *Clin Orthop* 311:129–135, 1995.

ACUTELY INJURED KNEE

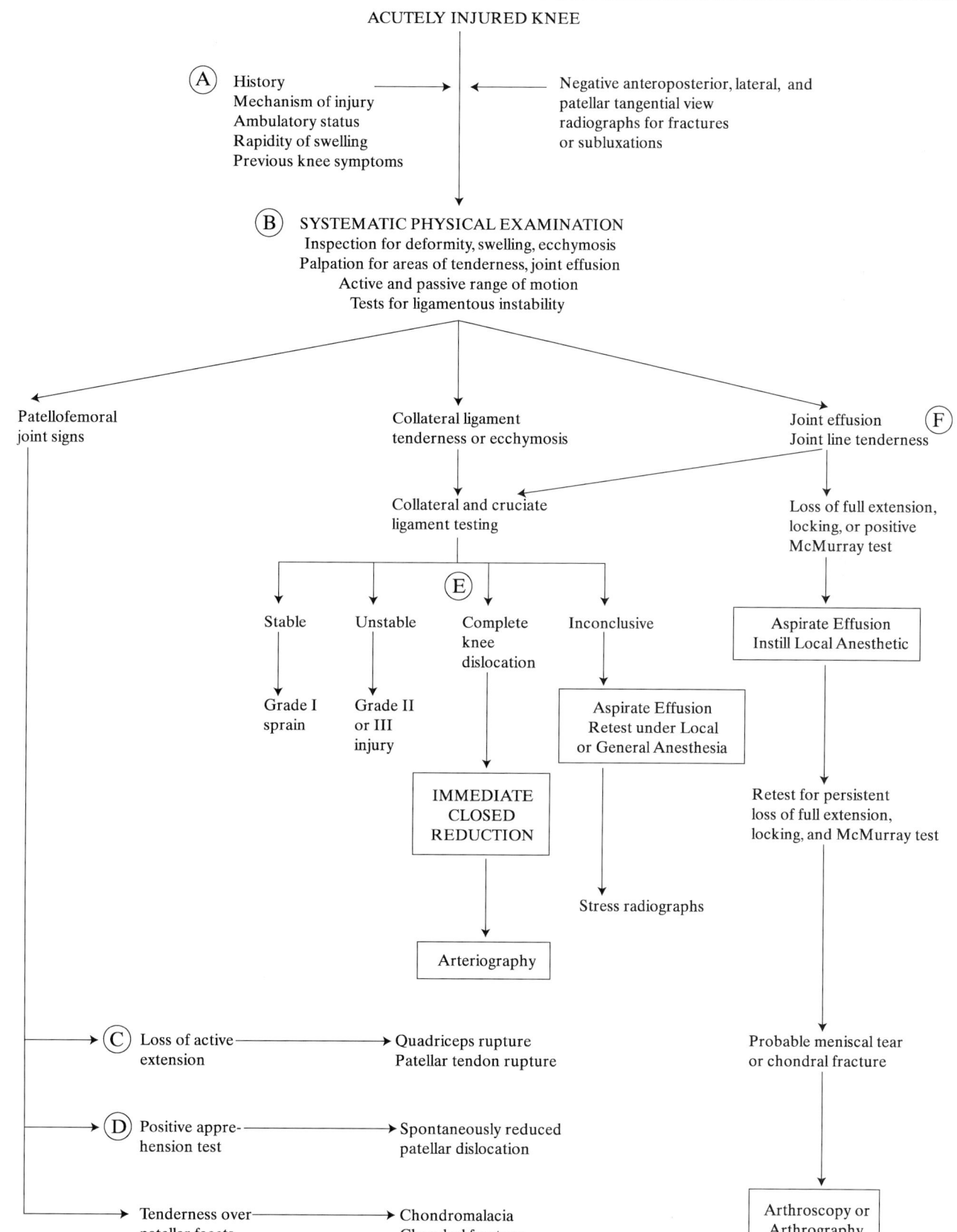

FIGURE 10-14-1. Algorithm for the evaluation of traumatic knee pain. (*Published with permission from RW Buchholz, FG Lippert, DR Wenger (eds): Orthopaedic Decision Making. Toronto, Decker, 1984, pp 46–47.*)

force of the body. When this occurs the extensor mechanism can sustain four types of injury:

1. A tear of the quadriceps tendon
2. A transverse fracture of the patella
3. A tear of the patella tendon
4. An avulsion of the tibial tubercle

Patella dislocation can occur due to virtually any rotational force on the knee. Because of the alignment of the proximal and distal tendinous attachments and the pull of the vastus lateralis, the patella will dislocate laterally and in the process tear the medial retinaculum. The patient will usually give a history of a twisting injury to the knee and a deformity that followed. Since most patella dislocations will spontaneously reduce, the deformity usually will not be present when the patient presents.

Effusion

Effusion is the presence of free fluid within the joint. The two primary sources of effusion in the acutely injured knee are blood and inflammatory fluid. The onset of the effusion in relationship to the injury is a key differentiating point for establishing clinically whether the effusion is secondary to bleeding or from the accumulation of inflammatory fluid. Bleeding within the knee can come from four sources:

1. A torn ligament
2. A torn tendon
3. A fracture
4. A torn meniscus

The tibial intracondylar artery lies on the anterior surface of the ACL and is covered by the ligamentum mucosa. When the ACL is stretched or torn the artery is damaged and the joint fills with blood. Since this is arterial bleeding, the effusion is rapid and the artery will continue to bleed until enough blood accumulates within the knee to tamponade the bleeding. The typical history obtained when an ACL is torn is that of an inversion injury to the knee followed by a massive, rapid effusion that is present within 5 to 10 minutes following the injury.

The vascular supply to the meniscus is limited to the outer one-third, with the central two-thirds being avascular. This has led to the terminology of the *red zone* (vascular) and the *white zone* (avascular) being applied to meniscal tears. The terms are more than descriptive since treatment and prognosis also depend on the zone of injury. When a meniscus is torn within the red zone, bleeding occurs but at a much slower rate than when the ACL is torn. Effusion in a meniscal tear follows the pattern of what appears to be minor swelling at the time of injury but pronounced effusion upon arising the next day. This is due not only to the accumulation of blood within the knee but also to inflammation of the synovium secondary to bleeding, which causes the production of inflammatory fluid within 6 to 8 hours. If a meniscal tear occurs within the white zone, inflammatory fluid will form but usually at a slower rate.

Locking

True locking occurs when the knee cannot be fully extended due to a mechanical obstruction. When trying to elicit this symptom during the history one must be careful in questioning the patient. When carefully questioned, most patients who think locking is present will actually describe stiffness. When true locking occurs it is usually unexpected and the patient is unable to extend the knee past a given point. The endpoint of extension is usually the point of maximum pain and in order to fully extend the knee past the obstructed end point some type of manipulation is required, a pop is felt, and the knee will freely move again.

The most common cause of knee locking is a torn meniscus. Locking, however, will occur only if the torn portion is detached from the central body of the meniscus to the point that it freely extends into the joint and impinges between the femur and tibia. Other causes of locking include an osteochondral fracture that is detached and free to migrate within the joint (joint mouse) and a large tibial remnant of a torn ACL.

Instability

A patient usually describes instability as "giving way" and, when present, it indicates injury to the primary or secondary ligamentous stabilizers of the knee. Isolated tears of the MCL and LCL rarely produce symptoms of instability. In contrast, tears of the ACL and PCL typically cause pronounced symptoms. ACL tears are noted by most patients to be symptomatic when pivoting is attempted; however, some may experience marked "giving way" in straight-line walking.

PHYSICAL EXAMINATION

General

The patient should be dressed in a way that allows full exposure of both lower extremities from the feet to the upper thighs. For ambulatory patients the knee examination begins by assessing gait. A gross assessment can be performed by observing the patient as he or she walks into the examination room. Both lower extremities should be inspected for symmetry (quadriceps atrophy, gross effusion), the general condition of the skin (erythema, ecchymosis, abrasions, wounds), and range of motion. The examiner should then carefully palpate the bony structures, joint lines, muscles, ligaments, tendons, bursae, and popliteal area, noting areas of tenderness or edema. Generally, range-of-motion and other specialized tests are performed on the uninjured knee first. This gives the examiner a baseline for comparison and demonstrates to the patient the maneuvers that will be performed on the injured knee.

Palpation

A careful and systematic palpation of the bony and soft tissue structures of the knee can provide the examiner with a considerable amount of information as to which structures may be involved in the injured knee. Palpable tenderness in the acutely injured knee is typically pinpoint and is a key diagnostic indicator as compared with the generalized tenderness found in chronic knee pain. Since many of the knee's contours disappear when the knee is fully extended, more accurate information can be obtained when the knee is palpated in a flexed position. One of the easiest positions for both the patient and examiner is to have the patient sit on an exam table with the examiner sitting on a stool facing the patient. An alternative position is to place the patient supine and flex the knee. Both of these non–weight-bearing positions relax the muscles, tendons, and ligaments surrounding the knee joint.

Palpation of the anterior aspect of the knee should begin with the extensor mechanism and proceed from proximal to distal to include the quadriceps tendon, patella, patellar tendon, and tibial tubercle. Any tenderness or defects in these structures can indicate injury to the mechanism. The medial retinaculum should also be examined. Tenderness along the medial retinaculum, with or without a palpable defect, may be the only indication of a patella dislocation that has spontaneously reduced. The examination should then proceed to the femoral condyles. Tenderness along the condyles may indicate the presence of an osteochondral fracture.

There are four bursae located around the anterior aspect of the knee that can cause pain in the traumatized knee:

1. The prepatellar bursa
2. The superficial infrapatellar bursa
3. The deep infrapatellar bursa
4. The pes anserinus bursa

The prepatellar bursa overlies the patella, the superficial and deep infrapatellar bursae are anterior and posterior to the patellar tendon, and the pes anserinus bursa is located at the flare of the medial tibial plateau, just medial to the tibial tubercle. When palpating the bursae, swelling, crepitus, and tenderness are key signs that indicate traumatic inflammation, which may be the source of pain.

The medial and lateral joint lines should then be palpated for defects and tenderness. Since several overlying structures are present at the joint lines, palpation must continue beyond the joint lines to isolate the structures involved. When palpating for the medial meniscus, the tibia should be internally rotated. In this position the medial meniscus becomes more prominent along the upper medial tibial plateau both anteriorly and posteriorly. The lateral joint line should be examined in a similar manner to detect any tenderness that may indicate a lateral meniscal tear. Palpation of the joint lines should extend to the posterior aspect of the knee since the posterior horn of the meniscus is a common location for tears. Tenderness in this region may be the only finding to indicate meniscal pathology.

In addition to meniscal tears, central joint line tenderness may indicate damage to the MCL or LCL. When central tenderness is noted at the medial joint line, palpation should continue proximally to the medial epicondyle of the femur and distally to the medial tibial plateau. If central tenderness is noted at the lateral joint line the central area should be palpated from the lateral epicondyle of the femur to the head of the fibula. Any tenderness extending into the regions described above will help the examiner to differentiate a ligament injury from meniscal pathology.

The posterior area of the knee should be palpated for the pulse of the popliteal artery, which lies deep to the fascia, posterior tibial nerve, and popliteal vein. Since the artery is well protected it is rarely injured except in posterior dislocations of the knee. However, the artery should be palpated in all cases of traumatic knee pain to exclude vascular compromise due to swelling.

Measuring Range of Motion

Range of motion is measured with the patient lying supine. The patient is then instructed to raise the entire lower extremity with the knee fully extended as high as he or she can off the table and hold it at the end-point. This motion is actually due to contraction of the iliopsoas muscle but is critical to ensure that the leg has adequate clearance off the exam table. The patient is then instructed to flex the knee as far as he or she can (try to touch the posterior thigh with the heel of the foot) and a measurement of flexion is taken with a goniometer. The patient is then asked to extend the knee as far as he or she can and a measurement of extension is recorded. In the normal knee, the range of motion arc is from 0° of extension to 135° of flexion.

In the event of a disruption of the extensor mechanism, the leg cannot be extended actively despite the patient's best efforts and will have to be supported against gravity. If a large tear of the meniscus is present and displaced into the joint the patient will be able to fully flex the knee; however, extension will block at a given point (locked knee). This can be confirmed by the examiner while attempting to passively extend the knee. If the examiner cannot passively extend the knee past the same point then mechanical obstruction of extension is confirmed. Comparison of active and passive knee extension is also useful to help differentiate extension lag from flexion contracture in the patient with chronic knee pain.

Measuring Quadriceps Atrophy

Appreciable quadriceps atrophy is most commonly the result of a chronic knee problem and typically involves the vastus medialis. This muscle is responsible for the last 30° of extension and is the first to atrophy if a condition is present that prevents the patient from achieving full extension. An acute injury may present with atrophy but should prompt the examiner to inquire about previous injuries. Quadriceps atrophy, if noted visually, should be confirmed and quantified by

measuring the circumference of both quadriceps muscle groups at a specified point proximal to the superior pole of the patella. The measurements should then be documented, comparing the right and left circumferences in centimeters and the distance from the superior pole of the patella at which each measurement was obtained. An example of documenting the finding would be, "Circumferential quadriceps measurements obtained 10 cm proximal to the superior pole of the patella: right 45 cm, left 43 cm."

Tests for Joint Effusion

Two tests commonly used to detect the presence of an effusion are the bulge test and the patella ballottement test.

- The bulge test is performed with the patient in the supine position with the knees fully extended and relaxed. The suprapatellar pouch is then massaged or "milked" distally while the examiner inspects for a bulge at the medial sulcus, which, if present, indicates effusion.
- The patella ballottement test is performed with the knee in the same position as described above. When performing this test the examiner applies downward pressure to the patella, compressing it against the femoral condyle. If an effusion is present, the examiner will appreciate a click when the downward pressure is applied.

Tests for Meniscal Pathology

Two tests can be used to detect meniscal pathology.

- The McMurray test is the maneuver most commonly used to detect tears in either the medial or lateral meniscus. To perform the test the patient is placed is the supine position and the knee is passively flexed. To test the medial meniscus the leg is internally rotated by grasping the ankle with one hand and applying a slight valgus stress to the knee with the other and then slowly bringing the knee to full extension. To test the lateral meniscus the leg is externally rotated and varus stress is applied. A palpable or audible click, which occurs at the joint line when the knee approaches full extension, suggests a meniscal tear. In order to determine that the click originates from the joint line the examiner should place the palm of the hand used to apply the varus or valgus stress over the patella and the thumb and index finger at the joint lines since clicks can come from other structures within the knee. One must keep in mind that a meniscal tear may be present even if the McMurray test fails to elicit a click at the joint line. The stress and rotation maneuvers applied to the knee while performing the test force the femoral condyle to glide over the torn portion of the meniscus and to displace it; the click is produced when the femoral condyle slips off the torn portion. If the tear is too small for the condyle to displace no click will occur but the patient will usually still experience pain or discomfort.
- The Apley compression/distraction test is another method used for detection of meniscal pathology and is helpful in differentiating the source of medial and lateral joint line pain. The test is performed with the patient in the prone position with the knee flexed to 90°. The examiner then exerts downward pressure on the foot. By applying downward pressure the meniscus is compressed between the femoral condyles and the tibial plateau and, if a tear is present, pain can be elicited at either the medial and lateral joint lines. If the patient does not experience pain on compression the examiner then stabilizes the thigh with one hand and pulls upward on the leg with the other. If the joint line pain is due to an injury of the medial or lateral collateral ligaments pain will be elicited upon distraction.

Tests for Ligamentous Stability

Due to the wide variation of ligamentous laxity among individuals the uninjured knee should be examined first in order to establish a baseline.

Some patients will have extremely tight knees while others will have loose knees. The variance is so great that the uninjured knee in a patient with a significant degree of ligamentous laxity will resemble a complete ligament tear in a patient with normally tight knees.

The MCL and LCL are tested by applying varus and valgus stress to the knee. To perform these tests the patient is placed in the supine or sitting position and the examiner supports the lower extremity with the knee fully extended to facilitate complete relaxation of the quadriceps and hamstring muscles. To test the MCL valgus stress is applied by pressing on the lateral aspect of the knee while at the same time distracting the leg laterally. To test the LCL varus stress is applied by pressing on the medial aspect of the knee and simultaneously distracting the leg medially.

The knee should be examined for joint laxity by applying valgus and varus stress with the knee in full extension and flexed to 30°. With the knee in full extension the ACL and PCL act as secondary stabilizers and may prevent the examiner from appreciating the full extent of injury sustained by the MCL or LCL. With the knee flexed to 30° the ACL and PCL are relaxed and the joint line will open significantly if a complete disruption (3° sprain) of the ligament has occurred. If a 1° sprain (stretching) or 2° sprain (partial disruption) is present the patient will experience pain when the MCL or LCL is stressed but the joint line will not open.

The integrity of the ACL is best assessed by the Lachman test and is well tolerated, if performed correctly, by patients with acute ACL tears. To perform the test the patient is placed in the supine position on the examination table and the examiner stands next to the injured knee. The patient is then instructed to relax all muscles and to remain supine during the examination. (Most patients will attempt to partially sit up to view the test; however, this will cause the quadriceps and hamstrings to contract, which will produce a false-negative test.) The examiner then stabilizes the distal femur just above the knee with one hand and passively flexes the knee to 15° with slight external rotation. The tibia is then grasped with the other hand just below the knee and a downward motion is applied to the femur while an upward motion is applied to the tibia. If the ACL is intact, the degree of tibial translation in relationship to the femur should be equal to the uninjured knee. If the extent of tibial translation is greater but has a soft end-point, the ACL is partially torn. If the tibia freely translates anteriorly from the femur the ACL is completely torn.

The integrity of the ACL can also be determined by the anterior drawer test. This test is performed in the supine position with the hip and knee flexed and the patient's foot flat on the table. The examiner stabilizes the extremity by lightly sitting on the foot from the side of the examination table. The hands of the examiner are then "cupped" around the proximal tibia into the popliteal fossa and the examiner gently pulls the proximal tibia forward to assess the amount of anterior tibial translation in relationship to the femoral condyles. To perform the posterior drawer test in order to assess the integrity of the PCL, the examiner simply pushes the proximal tibia posteriorly to determine the amount of posterior tibial translation in relationship to the femoral condyles.

NOTES AND PEARLS

The acutely injured knee should be examined as soon as possible since edema, point tenderness, and discoloration will initially be localized over the injured structures. Over time, as the edema, ecchymosis, and tenderness become more diffuse, isolating the specifically injured structures becomes more difficult. A careful neurovascular exam should be performed, especially with an edematous knee, since the popliteal vessels are frequently injured with posterior knee dislocations. The inability to bear weight, guarding to prevent movement of the knee joint, and marked edema or ecchymosis are signs that are highly suggestive of a severe injury.

BIBLIOGRAPHY

Bradford DS et al: Orthopedics, in *Current Surgical Diagnosis and Treatment,* 10th ed, Way LW (ed). Norwalk, CT, Appleton & Lange, 1994, pp 1011–1129.

Buchholz RW et al (eds): *Orthopedic Decision Making.* Toronto, Decker, 1984, pp 46–47.

Caldwell GL et al: Functional anatomy and biomechanics of the meniscus, in *Operative Techniques in Sports Medicine,* vol 2, number 3. Philadelphia, Saunders, 1994, pp 152–163.

Giles RS et al: Injuries of the knee, in *Fractures in Adults,* vol 2, 4th ed, Rockwood CA, Green DP (eds). Philadelphia, Lippincott, 1996, pp 2001–2126.

Greenleaf JE: Physical diagnosis of collateral ligament and combined ligament injuries, in *Operative Techniques in Sports Medicine,* vol 4, number 3, Philadelphia, Saunders, 1996, pp 148–157.

Seidel HM et al (eds): *Mosby's Guide to Physical Examination,* 3d ed, St. Louis, Mosby, 1995, pp 644–711.

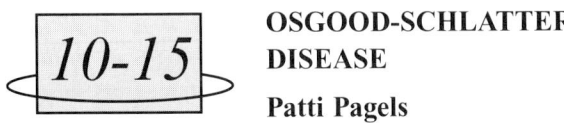

OSGOOD-SCHLATTER DISEASE
Patti Pagels

DISCUSSION

Osgood-Schlatter disease is an overuse syndrome that occurs exclusively in young people (age 8 to 18) causing pain, swelling, and erythema of the anterior tibial tubercle (see Fig. 10-15-1). It is commonly referred to as *traction apophysitis.* The apophysis (unique to the immature skeleton) is a growing layer of bone that attaches the infrapatellar tendon of the quadriceps to the anterior tibial tubercle. During the growth spurt, an imbalance develops between the apophysis and the quadriceps. Traction is placed on the loosely attached apophysis by the somewhat inflexible quadriceps, making it susceptible to injury. Forceful, repetitive contraction of the quadriceps during activities involving running, jumping, and pivoting can avulse the apophysis completely or partially from the tibial tubercle. Continued activity after apophyseal injury leads to inflammation. If athletic activities are not

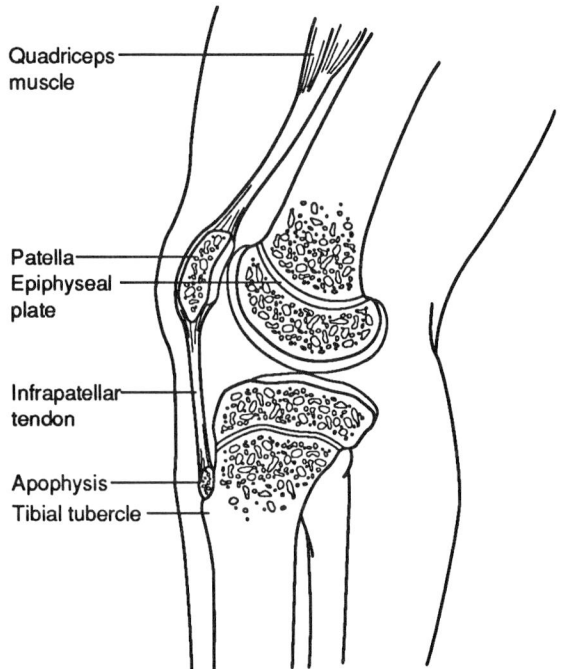

FIGURE 10-15-1. Lateral view of tibial tubercle, apophysis, and quadriceps muscle.

modified, swelling and erythema may result from a painful nonunion between the apophysis and the tibial tubercle.[1] Since the apophysis is not contiguous with the physis (growth plate), this condition is rarely serious. Conservative measures and skeletal maturity bring resolution to the vast majority of cases. The prevalence and incidence of traction apophysitis are unknown. Approximately 20 to 25 percent of patients present with a bilateral condition.[2] Subsets of patients at the greatest risk for developing this condition are ages 11 to 15, males more often than females, those at the peak of the growth spurt, and especially young athletes who participate in a single sport year-round.[1]

SIGNS AND SYMPTOMS

The most common signs include pain, swelling, and erythema of the anterior tibial tubercle, often resulting in a painful limp. Symptoms are insidious in onset and may involve a mild ache to severe pain. Pain usually is accentuated by patellar function.

Examination of an adolescent with painful limp should focus initially on the musculoskeletal system. It is important to exclude systemic conditions that could manifest as joint or bone pain. Since hip pain often is referred to the knee, a thorough examination of both hips and knees is indicated. Osgood-Schlatter disease is a diagnosis made by history and direct physical examination of the knee. It is considered good practice to follow up the physical assessment with a radiograph of both knees to rule out other, more serious conditions (see "Radiologic Studies," below).

Typical and atypical physical examination findings are listed in Table 10-15-1. Atypical findings warrant a search for other causes.

DIAGNOSTIC CONSIDERATIONS

A painful limp in an adolescent can result from other causes. In evaluating suspected Osgood-Schlatter disease, it is important to consider both common and uncommon differentials (see Table 10-15-2).

SPECIAL CONSIDERATIONS

Other factors that may contribute to overuse injuries are malalignment of extremities and physiologic deficits. Evaluate the patient for pes planus, Q-angle derangement, antagonist-agonist muscle strength imbalances, differences in leg length, and inflexibility. The history also should focus on the overall training environment, training techniques, whether proper equipment is employed, the type of footwear used during practice, and training schedules (frequency, intensity, and duration). One or a combination of these factors may be responsible for the overuse syndrome or the exacerbation of the current problem.[3]

The sports notorious for producing this overuse syndrome are long-distance running, jumping, basketball, and soccer. Adolescents may

TABLE 10-15-1. Physical Examination Findings in Osgood-Schlatter Disease

Typical findings
  Localized pain, swelling, and erythema over the anterior tibial tubercle
  Increased knee pain with squatting, crouching, or jumping
  Pain increasing with resisted extension of the knee at 90°
  No pain with straight leg raise
  Bilateral in 25% of patients

Atypical findings
  Acute onset
  Medial or lateral knee tenderness
  Ballottable patella or effusion
  Cruciate or collateral ligament laxity
  Joint warmth
  Popping, clicking, or crepitus
  Hip pain
  Fever or multiple joints with tenderness, erythema, or swelling

TABLE 10-15-2. Differential Diagnosis of Osgood-Schlatter Disease

Common differentials
  Sindig-Larsen-Johansson syndrome
  Trauma
  Tibial stress or plateau fractures
  Patellofemoral stress syndrome
  Patellar tendinitis
  Shin splints

Uncommon differentials
  Slipped capital femoral epiphysis
  Juvenile rheumatoid arthritis
  Neoplasia
  Sickle cell pain crisis
  Legg-Calvé-Perthes disease
  Septic arthritis or osteomyelitis
  Disseminated gonococcal infection

experience pain and discomfort at the knee for up to 2 years, particularly if they remain physically active. The swelling at the anterior tibial tuberosity may persist into adulthood.

LABORATORY STUDIES

Laboratory testing is not required unless a systemic condition or a septic joint is suspected. Tests to rule out these conditions may be appropriate in the primary care setting.

RADIOLOGIC STUDIES

A simple anterior-posterior (AP) and lateral view of both knees for comparison, with attention to the proximal tibia, can rule out other lesions and confirm the diagnosis of Osgood-Schlatter disease. Expected findings are an ill-defined patellar tendon, an edematous intrapatellar fat pad, and excavation of the anterior aspect of the ossification center of the tibial tubercle. An early diagnosis can be made from soft tissue signs alone. Apophysis fragmentation and displacement are not essential for the diagnosis.[4]

Small spicules of bone within the patellar tendon sometimes are seen. These avulsions usually reunite over time. A very small number of patients complain of persistent pain and may require surgical excision of the unattached fragment or fragments.

TREATMENT

Treatment is conservative and focuses on pain control. A trial of nonsteroidal anti-inflammatory drugs (NSAIDs)[1] taken with meals may bring relief. A short course of analgesics may be considered when pain is severe. Activity should be restricted during analgesic use.

Local steroid injections are not recommended, since they weaken tendons.

SUPPORTIVE MEASURES

The mainstays of treatment are rest, ice, compression, and elevation (RICE) and modified activity. Pads to protect the knee from direct pressure may be beneficial in some patients. If pain is pronounced, a trial of crutches or a knee immobilizer in extension for 2 to 3 weeks may bring relief.[1] If indicated, modify the training environment and correct physiologic and anatomic defects when possible. Plaster casting is no longer a recommended treatment.

PATIENT EDUCATION

Education should include the parents in an effort to reduce the number of visits for the same problem and costly trips to specialists.

To prevent symptom flare-ups, the following steps are recommended:

1. Ice the affected knee immediately after activity. Frozen bags of peas work well.
2. Have the patient do quadriceps strengthening and stretching[1] with 30 daily repetitions of straight leg rises for 2 to 3 weeks, followed by another 2 to 3 weeks with 5- or 10-lb weights added to the ankles.
3. Activity should be stopped at the onset of pain to prevent extension of the inflammatory cycle.
4. Use protective padding against direct trauma to the tubercle during athletic activities.
5. Activities that aggravate the symptoms may have to be eliminated until skeletal maturity has been achieved.
6. Check footwear and other gear for proper fit.

DISPOSITION

Conservative measures can be employed safely for up to 2 years or until skeletal maturity is complete.

COMPLICATIONS

Seek consultation for prolonged disability that does not respond to conservative measures or symptoms that persist beyond age 18 or longer than 2 years. In rare cases, surgical excision of ossicles embedded in the infrapatellar tendon may be indicated to relieve pain. The lesion may heal, but the tibial tuberosity may remain enlarged and prominent.

PEARLS

Osgood-Schlatter disease in a pubescent athlete probably originates from mechanical, growth, or traumatic factors or a combination of these factors.[5]

Osgood-Schlatter disease sounds ominous. Take the time to educate and assure the child's family that this is a self-limited condition with a very low risk for surgery or permanent disability.

The American Academy of Family Physicians provides a patient information sheet on Osgood-Schlatter disease. It is an excellent resource for patients and families that may be reproduced for nonprofit educational purposes.

REFERENCES

1. Peck DM: Apophyseal injuries in the young athlete. *Am Fam Physician* 51(8):1891–1895, 1897–1898, 1995.
2. Behrman RE, Kleigman RM, Nelson WE, Vaughan VC III: *Nelson Textbook of Pediatrics,* 14th ed, Philadelphia, Saunders, 1992, p 1705.
3. Shell D, Miller K: Managing overuse injuries in young athletes. *The Challenge of Pain,* 1998, pp 22–27.
4. Keats TE: The emergency x-ray. *Emerg Med* 149–150, Feb 1998.
5. Aparicio G, Abril JC, Calvo E, Alvarez L: Radiological study of patellar height in Osgood-Schlatter disease. *J Pediatr Orthop* 17:63–66, 1997.

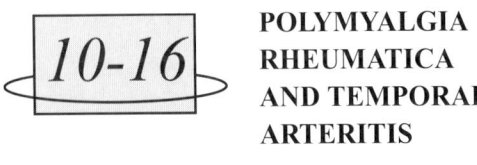

POLYMYALGIA RHEUMATICA AND TEMPORAL ARTERITIS

Daniel P. Radawski

DISCUSSION

Polymyalgia rheumatica (PMR) is a disease characterized by aching and stiffness primarily in the proximal muscles and synovial joints of the shoulder and hip girdle of patients age 50 years and older. The chief pathologic finding in PMR is lymphocytic synovitis in these joints. The etiology of PMR is poorly understood, but genetic, immunologic, and environmental factors are thought to play a role. The prevalence of PMR is approximately 1 in 200 persons older than 50 years with an incidence rate of 50 per 100,000 persons over age 50. PMR tends to be self-limited with symptoms of several months' to several years' duration.

Temporal arteritis (TA) is also known as giant cell, cranial, or granulomatous arteritis. TA is a vasculitis that also occurs in patients older than 50 years and most often affects the temporal artery, but it may affect any branch of the cranial arteries originating from the arch of the aorta. A subtle, more generalized vasculitis may accompany TA. Biopsies of an affected artery demonstrate granulomatous inflammatory infiltrates. The inflammation is often segmental or patchy with histiocytes, monocytes, lymphocytes, and giant and other cells infiltrating the vessel walls. However, the biopsies may be negative in up to 50% of cases.

The etiology of TA is unknown, but environmental factors such as infectious agents, exposure to sunlight, and contact with birds may be involved along with genetic and immunologic factors. Human parvovirus B19 has recently been identified in temporal artery tissues in TA patients. The recent observation in Minnesota of a regular cyclic pattern in incidence rates over time may also support the hypothesis of an infectious cause for TA. The prevalence of TA is about 1 in 500 persons older than 50 years with an average annual incidence of approximately 20 per 100,000 persons over age 50. TA may lead to irreversible blindness or stroke if untreated.

Both PMR and TA occur more frequently in patients of central and northern European ethnic backgrounds. The incidence is less frequent in Asian and African American groups and southern Europeans. They occur in women twice as frequently as in men. Of patients who have PMR, 50% are also found to have TA. Patients with TA are also found to have PMR in a range from 18 to 78%.

SIGNS AND SYMPTOMS

PMR is characterized by aching and stiffness of the shoulder and pelvic girdle muscles and may be of abrupt or gradual onset. These symptoms most often occur in the morning on arising and should, for diagnostic consideration, last for at least 1 hour or more and be present for 1 month or longer. Aching and stiffness also follow other periods of inactivity. This pain and stiffness may begin in one location but soon becomes symmetric and may involve other areas including the buttocks and neck. The distal upper and lower extremities may also be involved. The discomfort may become severe enough to interfere with usual activities and may be associated with systematic constitutional symptoms such as fatigue, loss of sleep and/or weight, or low-grade fever. The symptoms are generally unremitting.

Headache is the most common symptom of TA. The headache may be mild or severe and, as mentioned, is most often present in the region of the temporal artery but infrequently may present in other areas of the head including frontal and occipital areas, depending on the cranial artery affected. Jaw claudication is the next most frequently encountered symptom, occurring in approximately 50% of patients. Jaw claudication is more likely to occur with increased use of the muscles of mastication during prolonged chewing of foods such as meat. Visual disturbances occur in approximately 30% of patients and may include diplopia, blurred vision, transient visual loss (amaurosis fugax), and partial or complete, irreversible blindness. Mononeuritis multiplex or polyneuropathy may also be present. Patients with TA may have transient ischemic attacks or strokes that are preventable or treatable with prompt administration of sufficient doses of parenteral corticosteroids. Constitutional symptoms such as fever, malaise, or fatigue may be present.

OBJECTIVE FINDINGS

Objective findings in PMR are minimal. PMR is a diagnosis of exclusion with objective findings often being related to other diseases. Muscle tenderness may be present, but in objective testing muscle weakness is most often nonexistent or minimal and must be differentiated from hesitancy to perform strength testing because of pain and/or tenderness. Painful areas are less tender to examination than would be expected by the history of disability and pain. Synovial thickening may occur and is most often present in the wrist or knees but is usually mild. Swelling has been noted in the hands and feet in some instances along with pitting edema.

The objective findings in TA may be enlargement, tenderness, and/or erythema over the affected temporal, occipital, or other scalp artery. Bruits or pulse deficits may be present over the carotid, subclavian, or brachial arteries. Large artery and aortic arch involvement may be present initially or later as part of the disease. Funduscopic examination in patients with visual symptoms may include papilledema, hemorrhage, and/or exudates. Optic nerve atrophy may appear later.

DIAGNOSTIC CONSIDERATIONS

Because of the overlap of PMR and TA, signs and/or symptoms and objective findings of PMR may be present in TA. Conversely, history and physical examination of patients with PMR necessitates evaluation for possible symptoms and signs of TA. At present, temporal artery biopsy is not generally recommended in patients with PMR who are asymptomatic for TA. The diagnosis of PMR to a significant degree is a diagnosis of clinical exclusion of other diseases. The differential diagnosis for PMR includes late-onset rheumatoid arthritis (RA) and other rheumatic diseases, including polymyositis, systemic lupus erythematosus, and granulomatous vasculitis. Fibromyalgia, bacterial endocarditis, hypothyroidism, amyloidosis, and paraneoplastic syndromes secondary to malignant neoplasms may also be considered. It may be difficult to distinguish PMR from RA. The absence of rheumatoid factor, a more benign course, constitutional symptoms, and large joint involvement with abrupt onset indicate PMR. Polymyositis and systemic lupus erythematosus can be identified with associated symptoms and signs and by screening with creatine kinase and antinuclear-antibody testing, respectively. Patients with fibromyalgia should meet the criteria of 11 of 18 specific tender points on digital palpation as determined by the American College of Rheumatology. (The locations of these specific tender points are diagrammed in many textbooks, including *The Arthritis Foundation Primer on the Rheumatic Diseases,* Chap. 41.) These patients also have a history of widespread pain and other associated symptoms. Patients with bacterial endocarditis include a subset of patients whose bacterial endocarditis is accompanied by prominent musculoskeletal symptoms early in the course of the disease. These patients also display various stigmata of bacterial endocarditis. Patients with hypothyroid myopathy should have other signs and symptoms of hypothyroidism with concomitant abnormalities in a third-generation test for thyroid-stimulating hormone. Amyloidosis may be considered if there is typical skin, renal, and/or cardiac system involvement. If amyloidosis is considered appropriate, biopsy specimens should be obtained from subcutaneous fat, skin, kidney, or rectum and should be positive when stained with Congo red. Associated symptoms, signs, and tests that indicate malignancy usually identify patients with muscle tenderness from paraneoplastic PMR syndrome. The malignant neoplasms associated with paraneoplastic PMR syndrome include many hematopoietic and nonhematopoietic cancers.

The differential diagnostic considerations for TA include the following: tension vascular headaches, temporal mandibular joint dysfunction, systemic infections, amyloidosis or autoimmune diseases with prominent vascular involvement, neoplasms, and atherosclerotic vascular disease. Tension vascular headaches may be similar in location to TA with tenderness of the muscles. However, there should be no enlargement of vessels or unexplained erythema, elevated sedimentation rate increases, or vision or central nervous system changes. Temporal mandibular joint dysfunction should be discernible on history and physical examination. The other conditions should be differentiated on the basis of associated findings.

LABORATORY STUDIES

In both PMR and TA the erythrocyte sedimentation rate (ESR) as determined by the Westergren method is usually elevated. With PMR, the average ESR is 40 mm/h as minimal criterion for the diagnosis. With TA, the average ESR is 80 to 100 mm/h. However, the ESR may be normal and a normal ESR does not rule out PMR or TA. Elevated C-reactive proteins and anticardiolipin antibodies; a normochromic, normocytic anemia; leukocytosis; thrombocytosis; a mild elevation in hepatic enzymes; and an inflammatory response pattern of serum protein electrophoresis may be seen in both PMR and TA. Radiologic studies including ultrasound are not usually performed in PMR and are infrequently performed in TA. PMR does not usually require other diagnostic tests. A biopsy on a 3- to 5-cm segment of clinically abnormal artery should be performed in suspected TA. This biopsy should be obtained prior to initiating therapy when possible, since corticosteroids rapidly suppress the inflammatory findings. However, histologic features remain normal up to 2 weeks or more after the initiation of corticosteroid therapy in TA. Multiple thin sections of biopsy specimens should be examined after appropriate staining. The specimens should be examined for the stigmata of chronic vasculitis.

TREATMENT

Corticosteroids are the treatment of choice for both PMR and TA. With PMR, 10 to 20 mg of prednisone is given in a single or divided daily dose. This should bring prompt relief of the symptoms within 24 to 48 hours. Rapid resolution of pain and stiffness suggests the diagnosis of PMR. Slow tapering of the corticosteroids over months to minimize symptomatic flare-ups is usually indicated. From 15% to 70% of patients still require corticosteroids after 2 years, and 25% to 50% experience relapse after termination of corticosteroids. The route of corticosteroid treatment in TA is determined by symptomatology. If visual or stroke-like symptoms are imminent or present, aggressive and immediate therapy with significant doses of intravenous steroids is indicated. Otherwise, TA is treated with 40 to 60 mg of prednisone daily given in a single or divided dose. Once the clinical symptoms and laboratory tests have normalized, the steroid dose may be decreased by approximately 10% of the total dose per week. At levels below 10 mg/d, the reduction should be spaced at wider intervals. Nonsteroidal anti-inflammatory drugs may be helpful in low-grade PMR.

In both PMR and TA, patients should be followed at regular intervals. In PMR, the improvement or increase of muscle aching and stiffness should be closely followed with appropriate adjustment of steroids. In TA the patient should be seen on a more frequent basis not only to assess the course of the disease but also to determine the absence or presence of visual or central nervous system symptoms. Relapses of PMR or TA may occur after reduction of doses or cessation of therapy and require increases in doses and reevaluation of the tapering schedule.

SPECIAL CONSIDERATIONS

Patients on long-term corticosteroids for PMR or TA should be evaluated and educated about the gastrointestinal and osteoporotic effects of the drugs. Female, elderly male, and other patients at risk for osteoporosis should receive initial and subsequent bone mineral density studies. All patients should receive appropriate drugs to prevent and/or treat osteoporosis. Thoracic arch aneurysm may be a late manifestation of TA occurring 5 to 7 years after the initial diagnosis. These aneurysms may rupture. Evaluation for this complication should be considered.

PATIENT EDUCATION

Patients with PMR and TA should be educated regarding the course and potential complications of their illness. Teach patients with PMR the signs and symptoms of TA, and also teach patients with TA the signs and symptoms of PMR. Patients should know to seek immediate medical attention if visual or central nervous system symptoms occur. Patients should also be educated about the side effects of corticosteroid and other drugs that may be used in treatment. These patients should understand the course of their illness and central nervous system complications including diplopia, blindness, blurring, partial vision loss, transient ischemic attacks, and stroke.

OTHER NOTES AND PEARLS

PMR should be considered in patients 50 years or older with persistent, bilateral proximal shoulder and/or hip girdle pain and stiffness of greater than 1 month in duration lasting for more than 1 hour following periods of inactivity. Consider the diagnosis of TA in patients who are 50 years old or older with new-onset headaches that involve the region of the superficial temporal artery. Observe the temporal artery for signs of disease, including enlargement, erythema, or tenderness. Include TA in the differential diagnosis of older patients who have new-onset frontal or occipital headaches.

ACKNOWLEDGMENT

The editor would like to acknowledge the contribution of Laura Capozzi, coauthor of this chapter in the first edition of *Primary Care for Physician Assistants.*

BIBLIOGRAPHY

Bennett J, Plum F: *Cecil Textbook of Medicine,* 20th ed, Philadelphia, Saunders, 1996.

Brooks RC, McGee SR: Diagnostic dilemmas in polymyalgia rheumatica. *Arch Intern Med* 157:162–168, 1997.

Fauci AS, et al (eds): *Harrison's Principles of Internal Medicine,* 15th ed, New York, McGraw-Hill, 2000.

Guerrero E, Fang M: Polymyalgia rheumatica and the elderly patient. *Clin Geriatr* 7(6):5054, 1999.

Hunder G: Polymyalgia rheumatica/giant cell arteritis. Mayo Clinic, 18th Annual Practice of Internal Medicine. Rochester, MN, May 1997.

Hurst J: *Medicine for the Practicing Physician,* 4th ed, Stamford, CT, Appleton & Lange, 1996.

Salvarani C, et al: The incidence of giant cell arteritis in Olmstead County, Minnesota: Apparent fluctuations in a cyclic pattern. *Ann Intern Med* 123(3):192–194, 1995.

Weylan OM et al: *Primer on the Rheumatic Diseases: An Official Publication of the Arthritis Foundation,* 11th ed, 1998.

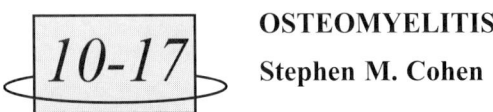

OSTEOMYELITIS

Stephen M. Cohen

DISCUSSION

The term *osteomyelitis* customarily describes an inflammatory process of the bone and attached structures, including joint and muscle attachments. The term most often suggests an acute or chronic inflammation caused by a microorganism. The terminology is most commonly applied to bacterial infection, but any microorganism can cause an inflammatory reaction. Fungal and viral infections also have been found to be causative agents in osteomyelitis.

Generally, osteomyelitis is categorized by the pathway of infection and host vascularity. Hematogenous osteomyelitis occurs when spread of infection occurs through the bloodstream from distant infection foci. Contiguous osteomyelitis, the most common type, occurs secondary to infection of tissue close to the bone, resulting in direct spread of the contaminant. When vascular insufficiency is present, as in diabetes and aging, infection is most often contiguous, and the diminished vascular status can accelerate the local effects of the infection. Whether hematogenous or contiguous with or without vascular insufficiency, bone infection requires prompt and deliberate attention to limit the morbidity rate, structural damage, and deformity.

SIGNS AND SYMPTOMS

Osteomyelitis may present with local and/or systemic signs of infection. Systemically, the patient may present with malaise, fever, chills, night sweats, anorexia, and/or irritability as in any generalized infective process. Local signs and symptoms may help identify anatomic involvement. Local signs and symptoms may include limitation of motion around the infection, erythema, drainage through sinus tracts, nonhealing wounds or ulcers, local swelling, pain, warmth, and discomfort. Joint dysfunction, pain, and limited motion may occur if the joint is involved or is in close proximity to the bone infection. Presenting features may be chronic or acute, depending on the duration and onset.

DIAGNOSTIC CONSIDERATIONS

Diagnosis and proper evaluation begin with a complete history and physical examination with a keen focus on the history of the present illness. The chronology of symptoms related to causative events is often the key to the proper diagnosis. Risk factors should be noted and may include neuropathies, fractures, intravenous drug use and abuse, renal failure and hemodialysis, internal fixation, and vascular insufficiency, as in peripheral vascular disease or diabetes. The history also should include an inquiry about recent pharyngitis, cellulitis, abscesses, respiratory infection, animal bites, diabetes, and puncture wounds. The detailed history also should include prior antibiotic treatment and use for the bone presentation and other subsystems. Host immunologic status always must be considered, especially in vertebral bone infection.

Etiologic Considerations

Most often hematogenous osteomyelitis is of bacterial origin, most commonly *Staphylococcus aureus.* After *S. aureus,* the common etiologic bacteria vary with the age at presentation. In neonates, group B streptococci and *Escherichia coli* are the most common after *S. aureus.* In the age group from 1 month to 16 years, *Haemophilus influenzae* and group A streptococci are common along with *S. aureus.*

In an adult over age 16 years, the clinician must consider gram-negative bacilli and anaerobes in addition to streptococci and *S. aureus.* Gram-negative bacteria such as *Pseudomonas* and *Klebsiella* are common in immunosuppression, nosocomial infection, and intravenous drug abuse. *Escherichia coli* is usually the cause of spinal osteomyelitis after urinary tract infection or instrumentation. In patients with sickle cell disease, infections with *S. aureus* and *Salmonella* are not uncommon.

Differential Diagnosis

Other disease states that may present concurrently or in a similar manner to osteomyelitis include osteoarthritis, rheumatoid and crystalline arthritis, stress fractures, neuropathic joint syndromes, bone and joint tumors, aseptic bone infarction, and other systemic infections.

LABORATORY STUDIES

Optimally, a sample of fluid or a tissue sample from the infected area is required for accurate and precise diagnosis. Culture and antibiotic sensitivity of these samples or histologic examination provide the best demonstration of diagnostic features. Blood cultures are unpredictable and may show up to 50% false negatives in hematogenous osteomyelitis.

The white blood cell (WBC) count can be variable in chronic osteomyelitis but often is elevated in acute disease. The erythrocyte sedimentation rate (ESR) is nonspecific and often is elevated. Caution must be applied to the evaluation of patients who have had prior treatment with surgery or antibiotics, since presentation features may make the diagnosis difficult. This is especially true in a chronic presentation.

RADIOLOGIC STUDIES

Although findings may not appear until later in the infection course, plain radiographs of painful or locally inflamed areas can be diagnostic. On plain film, acute osteomyelitis may produce soft tissue swelling, periosteal reaction, cortical irregularities, and/or demineralization. Fewer than one-third of cases have plain film evidence of osteomyelitis at 7 to 10 days. Most cases do not manifest radiographic evidence of infection until 3 to 4 weeks.

Computed tomography (CT) scan may show increased density within the marrow, but this may be difficult to visualize early in the disease course.

Magnetic resonance imaging (MRI) may show replacement of marrow fat with edema (water) and exudate, resulting in a decreased signal on T1 and an increased signal on T2 images. This finding is not specific for osteomyelitis, however, and also can be found in tumor, acute infarction, or fracture. The sensitivity and specificity of MRI for the detection of acute osteomyelitis are about 95%. MRI may be particularly useful in the evaluation of spine osteomyelitis, showing a characteristic pattern of confluent vertebral body and disk involvement.

Indium 111 WBC imaging has shown promise in the imaging of adult osteomyelitis. In this technique, 60 mL of the patient's blood is removed, spun down to obtain WBCs for labeling, and then reinjected. Images are performed 24 hours after injection. Uptake occurs at the site of any infection or inflammation with WBC aggregation. Infections that do not generate a significant leukocyte response tie (chronic, parasitic, or fungal infection) may best be evaluated with other techniques. Indium 111 WBC imaging is not performed commonly in children because of the high radiation exposure and the potential for more mutagenic effects on lymphocytes in light of the expected longer life span of a child.

Technetium-99m-methylene diphosphonate (MDP) bone scan is highly sensitive but not very specific for osteomyelitis. Any insult to bone may produce an abnormality. The three-phase bone scan has a reported sensitivity of 95% and a specificity of 78% for the identification of osteomyelitis in nontraumatized bone. The specificity drops to about 35% in patients with complicating bone conditions such as recent surgery and hardware. In an adult, a negative result on a bone scan essentially rules out infection. Bone scans may remain positive on delayed images for up to 1 to 2 years after successful treatment of osteomyelitis because of continued remodeling. Gallium imaging is better in assessing the response to treatment.

The addition of gallium 67 imaging to conventional radiologic studies of bone has been reported to increase specificity and provide a slight improvement in sensitivity. The gallium scan can be positive as early as 4 hours after the onset of infection and is usually positive by 24 hours. Gallium imaging is hindered by the same lack of specificity as conventional bone scintigraphy because gallium localizes to bone

as a calcium-like material. In osteomyelitis, gallium uptake should be either equal to or greater in intensity than the uptake on the bone scan. The normal limb is used to determine the degree of intensity of the abnormality. A normal gallium scan virtually excludes the diagnosis of acute osteomyelitis with a high degree of certainty.

Gallium is also effective in identifying osteomyelitis in neonates and children owing to better identification of lesions adjacent to the growth plates. In this setting, a gallium examination should be used when the bone scan is inconclusive or shows a cold defect. After treatment, uptake of gallium should decrease even if the bone scan remains abnormal. Gallium activity frequently does not return completely to normal, but this should not be considered indicative of chronic osteomyelitis. If the gallium scan does return to normal, a cure can be predicted with high reliability.

Bone marrow scintigraphy in acute osteomyelitis may show a marrow defect in approximately 5 days. This can be useful in the differentiation of bone infarction from infection in sickle cell disease patients who present with acute symptoms.

OTHER DIAGNOSTICS

When fluid aspiration is not possible or is unobtainable, a needle biopsy (open or closed) may be necessary to obtain tissue suitable for histologic study and culture.

CLASSIFICATION

The Cierny (University of Texas) classification system uses the following categories for osteomyelitis:

1. *Type I. Medullary:* The primary lesion is endosteal, the etiology is variable, the nidus is constant, there is an ischemic scan, chronic granulations are present, and the trabeculae are sequestered.
2. *Type II. Superficial:* The outer surface of bone is affected, and there is a compromised soft tissue envelope surrounding the bone.
3. *Type III. Localized:* There is full-thickness cortical involvement, and infection usually begins after trauma. The entire lesion can be excised completely and covered with a cuff made of viable tissue while preserving bone.
4. *Type IV. Diffuse:* There is circumferential complete bone involvement where an intercalary segment of skeleton must be removed to effect treatment and cure. There may be an infected nonunion and/or an end-stage septic joint present with obvious destruction.

The Time Element Classification has the following types:

1. *Acute.* Acute inflammation, inflammation of periosteum
2. *Chronic.* Long-term with soft and bone tissue changes
3. *Subacute.* Without signs and symptoms; silent infection

TREATMENT

Successful treatment is proportional to the virulence of disease, suitable antibiotic use, the bone involved, the status of the blood supply, and treatment duration. The overall goals of therapy are to stop continued infection and spread, stop sepsis and death, reduce signs and symptoms, and prevent the complications of infection, including bone and tissue loss and disability. With prudent and timely treatment, the morbidity rate can be reduced and limb salvage can be accomplished. Beginning treatment immediately in adult chronic osteomyelitis is less important than it is in acute or subacute processes.

Pharmacologic Management

As in all infectious disease therapy, antimicrobial agent therapy should be based on susceptibility testing (sensitivity) and organism identification by a sample of fluid or tissue taken before the start of therapy.

TABLE 10-17-1. Empirical Intravenous Therapy Guidelines

ORGANISM OR CIRCUMSTANCES	MEDICATION AND DOSING
Staphylococcus aureus and coagulase-negative *Staphylococcus*	Nafcillin* or cloxacillin 2 g IV q 4–6 h
Penicillin allergy	Clindamycin† 600 mg IV q 8 h
Methicillin-resistant	Vancomycin‡ 1 g IV q 12 h
Staphylococcus or empirical when infection involves prosthetic joint	
Coagulase-negative *Staphylococcus*	Nafcillin 2 g IV q 4–6 h
Streptococcus	Penicillin G 2–4 million units IV q 4 h or cefazolin 1 g IV q 8 h
Enteric gram-negative bacilli or *Pseudomonas*	Piperacillin 4 g IV q 4–6 h plus aminoglycoside
Mixed aerobic and anaerobic organisms (diabetes or animal or human bite wound)	β-lactamase inhibitor combination therapy (e.g., ticarcillin = clavulanate 3.1 g q 6 h IV)
Mixed gram-positive and anaerobic organisms	Clindamycin 600 mg IV q 8 h
High-risk patient (e.g., IV drug abuse and hemodialysis patients)	Cloxacillin or nafcillin with gentamicin (gentamicin =1.5 mg/kg IV q 8 h)
High-risk patient with penicillin allergy (when aminoglycoside is contraindicated)	Clindamycin with gentamicin or clindamycin with ceftriaxone or cefotaxime or ciprofloxacin

*Adding metronidazole to either nafcillin or cloxacillin has the same spectrum of activity as clindamycin alone.
†Watch for diarrhea with and without *Clostridium difficile* infection with clindamycin.
‡Watch for ototoxicity with extended therapy.

Initial therapy begins immediately with intravenous antimicrobial agents on diagnosis and continues for 2 to 3 days (see Table 10-17-1).

Further treatment of acute osteomyelitis is based on reassessment of the patient, but it should continue for 4 to 6 weeks at a minimum on an outpatient basis. Chronic osteomyelitis may require longer therapy. Oral antibiotics are used only after intravenous therapy is complete, an organism is identified, and patient compliance is assured (see Table 10-17-2).

Antimicrobial therapy also may be administered locally in the form of antimicrobial-impregnated polymethylmethacrylate (PMMA) beads implanted at the time of surgery.

Surgery

Most cases of chronic osteomyelitis require debridement surgery in addition to antibiotic therapy. Surgery is the treatment of choice in chronic osteomyelitis and should be considered strongly in initial, acute infection. Infective tissue has the ability to lie dormant, and wide surgical excision of all subacute infected tissue is mandatory for cure. Current understanding of osteomyelitis requires clinicians to understand that incomplete excision represents wasted effort. The principles of surgery include adequate drainage; thorough debridement of granulation, scar,

TABLE 10-17-2. Commonly Used Oral Therapy in Osteomyelitis (After Intravenous Therapy)

Medication	Dose
Cloxacillin	1 g PO q 6 h
Ciprofloxacin	750 mg PO bid
Clindamycin	300 mg PO q 6 h

and dead bone; obliteration of dead space; and directed, specific antibiotic therapy. This surgical process often entails creating wide margins of excision with large tissue defects. Defect management is accomplished with cancellous bone graft, simple approximation, transposition of local tissues, and vascularized tissue flaps. Secondary intent healing is not recommended because it leaves an avascular scar.

The surgeon may consider the temporary implantation of antibiotic-impregnated PMMA (bone cement) beads into the surgical wound. Methylmethacrylate beads impregnated with antibiotic have been utilized by some surgeons to increase the level of antibiosis at the wound site in patients with chronic osteomyelitis. There is a risk that the presence of these beads may inhibit the obliteration of dead space after surgery. Positive results with beads appear to be directly related to the extent and success of debridement and the adequacy of wound coverage.

Surgical intervention is accomplished for debridement, to remove inflammatory tissue, to reduce the bacterial load factor, and to establish an environment in which antibiotics work more efficiently. Free tissue transfer flaps and bone grafting to fill tissue voids left by surgical excision currently appear to offer the best chance for the successful treatment of osteomyelitis by helping to increase circulation to the area.

PATIENT EDUCATION

Patients must be included in all decisions about treatment so that they may understand the potentially chronic nature of this disease. Cure of osteomyelitis with medical treatment alone or inadequate surgical debridement is unpredictable and uncertain. Most patients underestimate the commitment to the treatment course once it has begun. Additionally, weight bearing or mechanical stress on the infected bone can reduce healing potential and potentiate infection. Patients must be instructed to remain non–weight-bearing.

DISPOSITION

Medical treatment is extremely unpredictable when it is utilized without surgical debridement. Because cure rates are low in the long bones without surgery, recurrence can be assumed with antibiotic treatment only. If hematogenous spread can be verified, the rate of cure with antibiotics alone increases. Antibiotic compliance and correct dosing for 6 weeks or longer are mandatory for cure. The patient may be monitored in the treatment period with antimicrobial blood levels, antibacterial titer, and ESR.

COMPLICATIONS AND RED FLAGS

Complications of acute osteomyelitis include death, chronic osteomyelitis, growth disturbance, physeal damage, involvement of the adjacent joint, local extension into soft tissues and abscess formation, pathologic fracture, bacteremia, and prosthetic loosening (if involved).

Chronic recurrent multifocal osteomyelitis (CRMO) is a complication that was first described in 1972. It is a subacute form of osteomyelitis that is characterized by symmetric bone lesions and associated with palmoplantar pustulosis. The etiology of CRMO has been hypothesized to be immune or viral. CRMO occurs most often in older children, and blood cultures are often negative. Slow resolution followed by recurrence months to years later is the course.

PEDIATRIC CONSIDERATIONS

Any child who has sustained minor trauma and has not recovered appropriately should be considered for osteomyelitis. In children, osteomyelitis develops mostly in males between 8 and 12 years old. Pediatric bone infection most commonly occurs in the metaphyseal region of the long bones, where turbulent, slowed blood flow near the growth plate and decreased phagocytic activity may favor bacterial deposition. Transient bacteremia, considered a probable cause, is common in pediatrics and may be initiated by toothbrushing, pharyngitis, ear infection, or similar minor events. Recent varicella infection may predispose to streptococcal osteomyelitis. *Salmonella* osteomyelitis has been noted in pediatric patients with sickle cell disease.

Epiphyseal and joint involvement is common in children under 18 months of age because of the presence of transphyseal vessels. In older children, the growth plate prevents the spread of infection into the epiphysis. In neonates with osteomyelitis, systemic disturbances may be mild or absent. Detection therefore is frequently delayed, and involvement can be multicentric. Differential diagnosis must include juvenile rheumatoid arthritis and tumors such as Ewing's sarcoma. Radiographic signs may take 7 to 10 days to become evident. Culture of aspirate material is more reliable than Gram stain and blood cultures.

OTHER NOTES AND PEARLS

Hematogenous vertebral osteomyelitis is almost always a monomicrobial infection that affects the older population. *Staphylococcus aureus* is the most common microorganism isolated in this group. Gram-negative bacilli may be seen in elderly males with urinary tract infections. Hematogenous vertebral osteomyelitis is treated primarily by conservative care in the form of immobilization and parenteral antibiotics. Indications for surgery are rare, and surgery should be reserved for patients resistant to treatment or with septic course, abscess formation, or neurologic deficits.

BIBLIOGRAPHY

Anthony JP, Mathes SJ: Update on chronic osteomyelitis. *Clin Plast Surg* 18:515–523, 1991.

Anthony JP, Mathes SJ, Alpert BS: The muscle flap in the treatment of chronic lower extremity osteomyelitis: Results in patients over 5 years after treatment. *Plast Reconstr Surg* 88:311–318, 1991.

Dirschl DR, Almekinder LC: Osteomyelitis—common causes and treatment recommendations. *Drugs* 45:29–43, 1993.

Job ML, Matthews HW: Bone and joint infection, in Herfindal E, Gourley D (eds): *Textbook of Therapeutics.* Baltimore, Williams & Wilkins, 1996.

MacDougall CA, McCormack J: Drug therapy in osteomyelitis, in McCormack J, Brown G, Levine M, et al (eds): *Drug Therapy Decision Making Guide* Philadelphia, Saunders, 1996.

Mader JT, Shirtliff ME, Bergquist SC, Calhoun J: Antimicrobial treatment of chronic osteomyelitis. *Clin Orthop* 360:47–65, 1999.

Mandell GL, Douglas RG Jr, Bennett JE (eds): *Principles and Practice of Infectious Diseases,* 3d ed, Toronto, Little, Brown, 1991.

Mercier LR: *Practical Orthopedics* St Louis, Mosby, 1995.

Steffanovski N, Van Voris LP: Pyogenic vertebral osteomyelitis. *Contemp Orthop* 31:159–164, 1995.

Tetsworth K, Cierny G: Osteomyelitis debridement techniques. *Clin Orthop* 360:87–96, 1999.

Vibhagool A, Calhoun J, Mader J, et al: Therapy of bone and joint infection. *Hosp Forum* 28:63–85, 1993.

Wladvogel FA: Osteomyelitis, in Gorbach S, Bartlett J, Blacklow N (eds): *Infectious Diseases* Philadelphia, Saunders, 1992.

Wirganowicz PZ: Aggressive surgical management of chronic osteomyelitis. *University of Pennsylvania Orthopedics J,* vol 12, 1999, http://health.upenn.edu/ortho/oj/1999/html/oj12sp99p7.html.

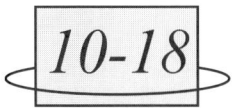

HEEL PAIN AND PLANTAR FASCIITIS

Sandra Martin

DISCUSSION

Heel and arch pain account for a large percentage of foot symptoms with which patients present to the medical office. It is important to first identify where the heel pain is located. It may be plantar or posterior heel pain, and there are multiple causes of both types.

Some of the more common differential diagnoses of plantar heel pain are:

• Insertional plantar fasciitis (proximal plantar fasciitis, heel spur syndrome)
• Plantar fat pad atrophy
• Stress fracture of the calcaneus
• Tumor of the calcaneus
• Irritation of the first (calcaneal) branch of the lateral plantar nerve
• Systemic diseases

Differential diagnoses of posterior heel pain include:

• Insertional Achilles tendinitis
• Achilles tendon rupture
• Calcaneal apophysitis (Sever's disease)
• Fracture of the calcaneus
• Retrocalcaneal bursitis (with or without Haglund's deformity)

SUBJECTIVE AND OBJECTIVE FINDINGS

A detailed history of the symptoms should include information relating to the onset, location, duration, aggravating factors, alleviating factors, and nature of the pain. Information regarding the relationship of the symptoms to activities both at work and during leisure time is also important. A history of recent trauma or change in activities should be considered. A general medical history including rheumatologic history is also important.

Insertional Plantar Fasciitis (Proximal Plantar Fasciitis)

Symptoms are usually greatest with first weight-bearing in the morning or weight-bearing after resting. The initial morning symptoms usually resolve only to resurface later in the day. Symptoms are decreased by wearing either shoes that elevate the heel at least 1 inch above the ball of the foot or athletic shoes with good arch support. Conversely, symptoms are worse when barefoot or wearing flat or negative-heeled shoes. There is tenderness to palpation of the plantar medial aspect of the heel in the area of the insertion of the medial slip of the plantar fascia. There may be a history of recent increase in weight or weight-bearing activity level.

The presence or absence of a plantar calcaneal spur does not correlate with the presence or absence of symptoms. Symptoms are an inflammatory response of the pull of the plantar fascia on the periosteum at its insertion in the calcaneus. Sometimes, a heel spur results as subperiosteal traction causes new bone formation. However, this does not contribute to the symptoms. There is frequently a misconception by both the physician and the patient that the bone spur itself has to be alleviated for the symptoms to resolve.

Plantar Fat Pad Atrophy

This condition frequently occurs in elderly patients. Symptoms are usually not present first thing in the morning or with weight-bearing after resting. The symptoms increase with increased activity and are worse on hard surfaces or with hard-soled shoes; symptoms decrease with decreased activity and padding of the heel area. The plantar aspect of the calcaneus is easily palpable. The plantar fascia is usually not tender.

Stress Fracture of the Calcaneus

Symptoms frequently follow a fall or an activity requiring the patient to repeatedly land on his or her heel or prolonged activity on hard surfaces. Symptoms may be gradual or acute in nature. Pain is diffuse in the heel. Compression of the heel (medial and lateral) usually reproduces the pain. The plantar aspect of the heel is not necessarily tender. The fracture may be seen on a lateral x-ray as a sclerotic band.

Tumor of the Calcaneus

This can present in many ways. Symptoms are usually gradual in onset and not related to weight-bearing or activity level. Radiographs and other imaging studies help to make the diagnosis.

Irritation of the First Branch of the Lateral Plantar Nerve

This is a frequently missed diagnosis. There is usually a history of prolonged activity on the toes of the foot (e.g., ballet dancers, sprinters). The nerve supplies the periosteum of the plantar medial calcaneal tuberosity, and entrapment can occur in a few different sites along its path. The diagnosis is a clinical one. Pain is generally greatest after prolonged weight-bearing or at the end of the day. Tenderness can be elicited by palpation over the medial calcaneal tuberosity, more medial than plantar. There may be some discomfort with percussion of the area.

Systemic Diseases

Symptoms are usually bilateral and not directly related to weight-bearing activity. This is frequently associated with the seronegative arthropathies and screening tests should include HLA-B27 and sedimentation rate. It is very important to obtain a detailed history relating to other areas of symptoms.

Insertional Achilles Tendinitis

Tenderness is usually at the insertion of the Achilles tendon in the middle third of the posterior calcaneus. Dorsiflexion of the ankle may produce symptoms. The patient may have either a tight Achilles tendon (equinus) with limited dorsiflexion of the ankle or other mechanical factors that require an extra stretching of the tendon. A common cause of insertional Achilles tendinitis in women is switching from high-heeled shoes to flat shoes or barefoot. Lateral x-ray may reveal spurring of the calcaneus at the site of the insertion of the tendon. However, symptoms are usually related to an inflammation in that area and not the spurring unless it shows signs of fracture.

Achilles Tendon Rupture

Frequently found in middle-aged athletes but also seen in younger ones, Achilles tendon rupture often occurs with an acute, painful popping or tearing sensation after jumping, running, or landing. Pain quickly resolves, but there is difficulty walking. There may be a palpable void in the tendon. The most reliable test is Thompson's test, which is performed with the patient prone and the feet hanging off the examination table. The test is positive when there is no plantar flexion at the ankle when the calf is squeezed. The test is less reliable as the time since injury increases. Magnetic resonance imaging may be necessary to confirm the diagnosis.

Calcaneal Apophysitis (Sever's Disease)

There is a secondary growth plate, apophysis, that occurs in the lateral aspect of the calcaneus in response to the pull of the Achilles tendon. This area is frequently inflamed, especially during a period of active growth or increased physical activity. This inflammation is known as Sever's disease or as calcaneal apophysitis, and is common in the active 9- to 11-year-old athlete.

The posterior calcaneus is tender to medial-lateral pressure, and there is usually minimal or no tenderness at the insertion of the Achilles tendon or medial slip of the plantar fascia. The Achilles tendon may be tight, and excessive pronation is usually present. The calcaneal apophysis usually opens between 4 and 8 years in females and 7 to 11 years in males. This condition has recently increased in avid young soccer players because of the mechanical factors associated with soccer shoes

and playing on grass, in addition to the frequency with which many youth are playing the sport. Radiographs are useful only to show whether the apophysis is open and to rule out tumors. The appearance of the apophysis is normally irregular and does not have any changes that are diagnostic for Sever's disease.

Retrocalcaneal Bursitis and Haglund's Deformity

This condition is palpated deep to the Achilles tendon and presents as a tender swelling with irregular borders. Radiographs may show a soft tissue enlargement in this area, sometimes with increased density. A Haglund's deformity, osseous enlargement of the calcaneus (usually posterolaterally), is frequently seen in association with a bursa. Both the bursa and the osseous deformity are thought to be mechanical in etiology.

TREATMENT

The goal of treatment of heel pain should be to treat the symptoms and alleviate the causative factors.

Insertional Plantar Fasciitis

Insertional plantar fasciitis (heel spur syndrome, proximal plantar fasciitis) should be treated conservatively. More than 90% of the symptoms usually resolve without surgical intervention. There is no consensus as to the order in which the various therapies should be utilized. Stretching of both the Achilles tendon and the plantar fascia, not only before and after activity but also throughout the day, can help relieve symptoms. A night splint to be worn during sleep will help prevent contracture of the plantar fascia with plantar flexion of the ankle. Custom functional orthotics can help modify foot function and alleviate the stresses on the plantar fascia. Modification of activities that aggravate the symptoms is necessary. Nonsteroidal anti-inflammatory drugs (NSAIDs) may be used. Steroid injections for insertional plantar fasciitis should be targeted toward the point of maximum tenderness, which is usually around the insertion of the medial aspect of the plantar fascia into the plantar medial aspect of the calcaneus. A medial approach to the injection is frequently less painful than a plantar approach. Casting in the neutral ankle and subtalar joint positions allows the soft tissues to remain stretched out and alleviates the recurrent inflammation.

Plantar Fat Pad Atrophy

A cushioning pad or a heel cup to contain the existing soft tissue beneath the calcaneus is used in most cases. Shoes can be modified to have additional padding.

Stress Fracture of the Calcaneus

Treatment is dependent upon the site of the fracture and whether it involves the subtalar joint. Casting is frequently used, both non–weight-bearing and weight-bearing. If the subtalar joint is involved, the patient should be referred to a foot surgeon for further evaluation.

Tumor of the Calcaneus

These cases should be referred to the appropriate specialist for evaluation and treatment. Many tumors are benign but, due to the fragile nature of the calcaneus, frequently should be surgically curetted and packed with bone.

Irritation of the First Branch of the Lateral Plantar Nerve

This usually has a mechanical etiology. It can be treated mechanically with orthotics or supports available over the counter. It can also be treated with local steroid injection to decrease the inflammation of the nerve.

Systemic Diseases

The underlying disease should be investigated and treated.

Insertional Achilles Tendinitis

Avoid injecting steroids into the area of the insertion of the Achilles tendon into the calcaneus. This can cause rupture of the insertion and require surgical repair. It can also cause fibrosis and changes within the substance of the tendon that will require surgical debridement. Treatment is mechanical to alleviate the excessive stress on the tendon and allow the inflammation to resolve. Heel lifts, night splints, heeled shoes, orthotics to prevent excessive pronation, and NSAIDs all frequently help. It may be necessary to place the patient in a weight-bearing cast slightly plantar flexed and then progress to a neutral cast.

Achilles Tendon Rupture

Controversy exists as to the treatment of a ruptured Achilles tendon. It should either be primarily repaired by surgery or treated with cast immobilization.

Calcaneal Apophysitis (Sever's Disease)

Achilles stretching, heel lifts, and rest from aggravating factors frequently alleviate all of the symptoms. However, if symptoms persist, functional orthotics or cast immobilization may be necessary. This is usually a self-limiting problem.

Retrocalcaneal Bursitis and Haglund's Deformity

Identifying the aggravating factors, changing shoes, and avoiding aggravating activities best treat this form of bursitis. Rest, ice, and NSAIDs may also be beneficial. If symptoms persist, mechanical control of the heel in the shoe with a functional orthotic may be necessary. Occasionally, surgical excision of the osseous or soft tissue abnormality is required.

BIBLIOGRAPHY

Mandracchia VJ (ed): *Clinics in Podiatric Medicine and Surger* Saunders, 1999.
Myerson MS (ed): *Foot and Ankle Clinics* Saunders, 1998.
————: *Foot and Ankle Clinics* Saunders, 1999.
————: *Foot and Ankle Disorders,* vol 2 Saunders, 2000.
Ross JA (ed): *Clinics in Podiatric Medicine and Surgery* 1997.
Scurran BL (ed): *Foot and Ankle Trauma* Churchill Livingstone, 1989.
Torg JS (ed): *Clinics in Sports Medicine* Saunders, 1982.

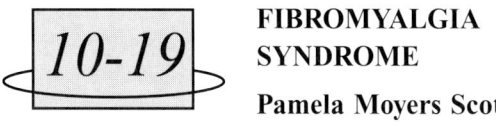

FIBROMYALGIA SYNDROME

Pamela Moyers Scott

DISCUSSION

Fibromyalgia syndrome (FMS) is a frequently encountered condition characterized by widespread musculoskeletal pain, stiffness, fatigue, and multiple tender points in specific areas upon physical examination. Because of its lack of specific laboratory abnormalities, until recently it was considered to be a "psychological" disease. The cause is unknown.

There is a strong female preponderance (greater than 75% in most studies).[1] Peak incidence is between 20 and 60 years of age.[1] However, it has been diagnosed in children.[2]

SIGNS AND SYMPTOMS

Diffuse muscle pain is often the presenting complaint. It is generally concentrated in axial locations. The majority of patients with FMS describe the pain as aching. However, other pain characteristics include shooting, burning, penetrating, and throbbing.[3]

The pain is usually accompanied by general stiffness, often worse in the morning. Severe fatigue is also present, and occasionally it is the presenting symptom. Sleep tends to be nonrestorative.

Other symptoms include subjective soft tissue swelling, usually in the extremities (articular and nonarticular forms have been reported); reticular skin discoloration; and features of connective tissue disease such as Raynaud's phenomenon and xerostomia.[3] Associated conditions include irritable bowel syndrome, primary dysmenorrhea, female urethral syndrome, anxiety, depression, tension headaches, migraine headaches, temporomandibular joint syndrome, restless legs syndrome, esophageal dysmotility, "allergic" symptoms, sensorineural hearing loss, ocular dysmotility, and vestibular abnormalities.[1,3,4] Symptoms tend to be exacerbated by physical activity, inactivity, emotional stress, poor or inadequate sleep, and humid weather.[1]

OBJECTIVE FINDINGS

On physical examination, the patient will experience some degree of pain with palpation of specific tender points (see Fig. 10-19-1) using approximately 4 kg of pressure. Digital palpation appears to be equally accurate as dolorimetry in establishing the diagnosis of FMS.[5] Control sites, e.g., forehead, thumbnail, and anterior thigh, should be nontender to palpation.

DIAGNOSTIC CONSIDERATIONS

The American College of Rheumatology has established criteria for the diagnosis of FMS. Widespread pain (defined as pain on both sides of the body and above and below the waist) and axial pain (defined as pain in the cervical or thoracic spine, anterior chest, or low back) of at least 3 months' duration along with 11 of the 18 tender points (see Fig. 10-19-1) must be present.[6]

SPECIAL CONSIDERATIONS

Individuals who are experiencing the predominate symptoms of FMS but have less that 11 tender points could still have FMS.[1]

LABORATORY TESTS

There are no laboratory tests to confirm the diagnosis of FMS. However, the diagnostic evaluation should include a complete blood count, chemistry panel, erythrocyte sedimentation rate, thyroid-stimulating hormone test, and a urinalysis. Unless there is an underlying disease, all of these studies should be normal.

RADIOGRAPHIC AND IMAGING STUDIES

Unless there is an underlying abnormality, radiographic and imaging studies are normal in a patient with FMS.

OTHER DIAGNOSTICS

Although not necessary to confirm the diagnosis of FMS, elevated levels of substance P have been consistently identified in the cerebrospinal fluid, and decreased plasma levels of serotonin have been found in patients with FMS.[1,3] Sleep electroencephalogram studies generally will reveal a non–rapid eye movement anomaly.[1,3,5] Muscle biopsies reveal no distinct histopathologic abnormalities.[1,3,5]

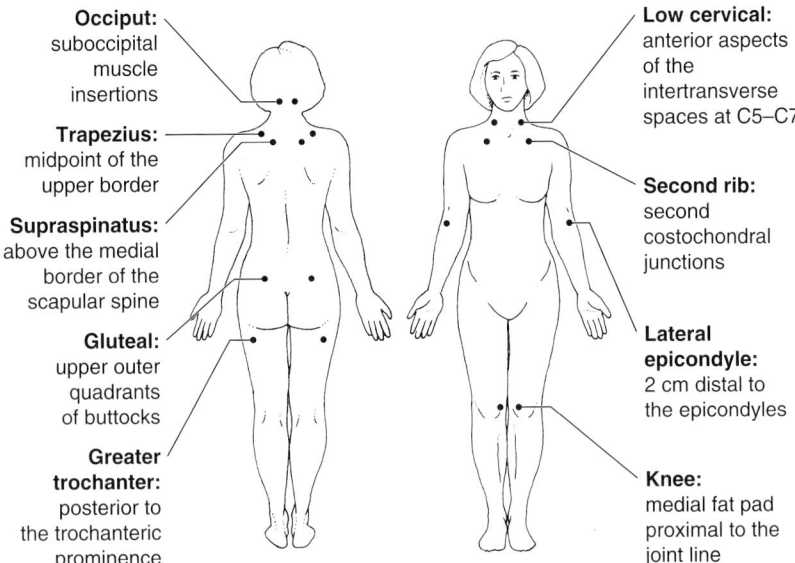

FIGURE 10-19-1 Location of tender points in fibromyalgia. *SOURCE: From the* Primer on Rheumatic Diseases, *11th ed, copyright 1997. Used by permission of the Arthritis Foundation. For more information, please call the Arthritis Foundation's information line at 1-800-283-7800.*

TREATMENT

Patient education, reassurance, and lifestyle modifications are the cornerstone of therapy for FMS.

MEDICATIONS

Low-dose tricyclic antidepressants are considered the drug of choice for FMS. The most commonly used are amitriptyline (Elavil) 10 to 25 mg or doxepin (Sinequan) 10 to 25 mg each given approximately 1 to 2 hours before going to bed. It is theorized that their effectiveness is due to their ability to provide restorative sleep. Other medications utilized to improve sleep are cyclobenzaprine (Flexeril) 10 to 20 mg[5] and alprazolam (Xanax)[1] 0.5 to 2 mg, also given 1 to 2 hours before bedtime.

Selective serotonin reuptake inhibitors have been utilized with success in some patients, especially if there is a coexisting depression.[7–9] Nonsteroidal anti-inflammatory drugs offer little if any improvement of symptoms.[1,5] Their benefit may be enhanced by combining them with the above agents.[1] Glucocorticosteroids offer no benefit and should not be used.[1,5] Most experts advise against using narcotic analgesics in patients with FMS.[1,5,9] Carbidopa/levodopa (Sinemet), capsaicin cream, topical lidocaine, tramadol (Ultram), 5-hydroxytryptophan, and a proprietary combination of malic acid and magnesium have been proven effective in alleviating the symptoms of FMS.[9]

SUPPORTIVE MEASURES

Stretching and low-impact aerobic exercises seem to be beneficial. The patient needs to start slow and gradually work up to 20 to 30 minutes three to four times a week.[5] Trigger point injections with local anesthetics and corticosteroids are often beneficial. Physical therapy, including ultrasound, whirlpool, and electrical stimulation treatments, also seems to provide temporary relief. Adequate sleep is essential. Biofeedback, meditation, acupuncture, and massage may reduce symptoms.[1] Associated stress, anxiety, and depression must be addressed and treated. FMS support groups are often helpful. (Local organizations can be identified by contacting the Fibromyalgia Alliance of America, PO Box 21990, Columbus, OH 43221-0990.)

Activity level and occupational requirements may have to be modified. Studies indicate that 10 to 25% of patients with FMS are not able to work in any capacity.[5] Unfortunately, most governmental agencies do not provide disability payments for the diagnosis of FMS.[3]

PATIENT EDUCATION

Patients need to be advised of the diagnosis and reassured that nothing life-threatening is occurring. Furthermore, they must be reassured that they do have a physical, not a psychological, condition. Lifestyle modifications are the cornerstone of therapy.

DISPOSITION

While changes are being made in the treatment, patients should be seen on a monthly basis. Once their condition stabilizes, the frequency can be decreased to every 3 months.

COMPLICATIONS AND RED FLAGS

Patients with FMS should be referred to a specialist if they fail to respond after several months of treatment. If narcotics are required to manage their pain, they should be immediately referred to a pain management clinic. If initial evaluation reveals tender control trigger points, the patient should be referred for a psychological evaluation. Additionally, if the diagnosis is uncertain, a consultation should be done.

OTHER NOTES AND PEARLS

Treatment is aimed at reducing and controlling symptoms. Unfortunately, total resolution of symptoms occurs in the minority. Patients who respond to therapy still report persistent, but milder and tolerable, pain.[3] A 1994 study revealed that 25% of patients with FMS were in remission at 2 years after diagnosis.[10] Better outcomes are associated with younger age and less severe symptoms at presentation.[1]

REFERENCES

1. Freundlich B, Leventhal L: Diffuse pain syndromes, in *Primer on the Rheumatic Diseases,* 11th ed, J Klippel (ed). Atlanta, GA, Arthritis Foundation, 1997, pp 123–127.
2. Miller M: Musculoskeletal pain syndromes, in *Nelson Textbook of Pediatrics,* 16th ed, Behrman R, Kliegman R, Jenson J (eds). Philadelphia, Saunders, 2000, pp 732–733.
3. Yunus M, Masi A: Fibromyalgia, restless legs syndrome, periodic limb movement disorder, and psychogenic pain, in *Arthritis and Allied Conditions: A Textbook of Rheumatology,* 12th ed, McCarty D, Koopman W (eds). Philadelphia, Lea and Febiger, 1993, pp 1383–1405.

4. Clauw D: Fibromyalgia: More that just a musculoskeletal disease. *Am Fam Physician* 52:843–851, 1995.

5. Gilliland B: Relapsing polychondritis and other arthritides, in *Harrison's Principles of Internal Medicine,* 14th ed, Fauci A et al (eds). New York, McGraw-Hill, 1998, pp 1955–1957.

6. Wolfe F et al: The American College of Rheumatology 1990 criteria for the classification of fibromylagia: Report of the multicenter criteria committee. *Arthritis Rheum* 33:160–172, 1990.

7. Yunus M: Fibromyalgia syndrome: Is there any effective therapy. *Consultant* June:1279–1285, 1996.

8. Silverman S: Using drugs effectively in the treatment of fibromyalgia. *Journal of Musculoskeletal Medicine* December:29–34, 1994.

9. Russlee IJ: Fibromyalgia syndrome: Formulating a strategy for relief. *Journal of Musculoskeletal Medicine* November:4–20, 1998.

10. Granges G et al: Fibromyalgia syndrome: Assessment of the severity of the condition 2 years after diagnosis. *J Rheumatol* 21:523–529, 1994.

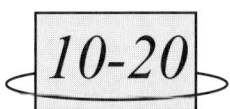

SCLERODERMA (SYSTEMIC SCLEROSIS)

Theresa Horvath

DISCUSSION

Systemic sclerosis, also known as *scleroderma,* is a progressive fibrotic condition of unknown origin. Once thought to be an autoimmune disorder, it is a heterogeneous, complex disease that disturbs humoral and cellular immunity. The exact pathogenesis is unknown, although endothelial cell injury, disruption of collagen synthesis, and abnormal immune states have been implicated.

There are two main variants of the disease, *localized scleroderma* and *systemic sclerosis.* The terms are often interchanged, but localized scleroderma refers to a more constrained set of symptoms involving the skin, primarily, and is also called *limited disease.* Systemic sclerosis is most often progressive and affects the internal organs, and is also called *diffuse disease.*

Systemic sclerosis is relatively rare, affecting from 14 to 19 per 1 million people (Michet, 1998). Women are affected with greater frequency than men, and African-American women are at greatest risk. Onset of the disease is usually between 45 and 55 years of age, although African-American women tend to develop the disease 10 years earlier than others. Furthermore, the Amerindian HLA haplotype HLA DRB1*1602, found among full-blooded Choctaw Indians, is the most strongly predictive genetic factor for scleroderma (Michet, 1998).

Viral and environmental factors have been implicated in the occurrence of systemic sclerosis. Retrovirus and cytomegalovirus may play a role in causing systemic sclerosis, as might exposure to vinyl chloride, trichloroethylene, Spanish rapeseed oil, and products containing tryptophan, bleomycin, or silica (Artlett et al, 1999).

SIGNS AND SYMPTOMS

The most classic symptom of both scleroderma and systemic sclerosis is sclerodactyly. Skin thickening always begins in the fingers and is usually preceded by puffiness. Puffy fingers may be the only presenting sign for years in a patient with limited disease. In diffuse disease, the puffiness may extend to the whole hand, foot, and ankle. Skin thickening may continue for 3 or 4 years and spread from the fingers to the extremities or trunk. The extent and severity of skin thickening is unpredictable. Other dermatologic changes include pigmentation, dryness, pruritus, hair loss, and telangiectasia.

Most all patients have Raynaud's phenomenon. In limited disease, Raynaud's phenomenon may precede all other symptoms for as much as 10 or 20 years. In diffuse disease, systemic disease or significant swelling may occur soon after the onset of Raynaud's. The Raynaud's may progress to pitting scars or ulcers of the fingers, or nailfold

infarcts, except in those with localized scleroderma, who will not experience capillary damage.

Morning stiffness and polyarthralgias are common. In diffuse disease, significant polyarthralgias occur early, placing these patients at risk for contracture, especially if hand swelling and skin tightening accompany joint pain. Flexion contractures may progress to clawlike hand deformity, resulting in serious disability. Carpal tunnel syndrome is a frequent sign of early diffuse disease. Tendon friction rubs of the extensor and flexor aspects of the fingers, forearms, and ankles can be palpated during active motion.

Proximal muscle weakness may occur in one of two forms. The mild variant is far more common, and the weakness, pain, or atrophy can be nonprogressive, noninflammatory, and mild, and treated easily, often just with exercise. The severe variant is an inflammatory myositis, similar to that of polymyositis, and requires treatment with either steroids or immunosuppressive agents (Steen, 1998).

Calcinosis along the fingers, olecranon, and prepatellar bursae is common in limited disease. It can also occur in the buttocks and along the spinal cord, leading to infection should the calcium crystals extrude.

End-Organ Damage

Among the serious manifestations of systemic sclerosis resulting in irreversible damage, esophageal hypomobility caused by weakness of esophageal smooth muscle is by far the most common. Smooth muscle dysfunction can also occur in the small intestine, leading to abdominal pain, bloating, and vomiting. Smooth muscle abnormalities in the colon and rectum may lead to obstipation, incontinence, or rectal prolapse.

Pulmonary disease is the second most common end-organ damage. Interstitial fibrosis is a severe and possibly fatal complication. There are often no pulmonary symptoms during the first 5 years of disease, when damage to the lungs is the greatest. New-onset dyspnea or a decreasing FVC may be the only signs or symptoms of warning. Although pleural thickening, effusions, and rubs, and pneumothorax, are possible complications, pulmonary hypertension is the most dangerous manifestation of systemic sclerosis. It is suspected when severe dyspnea does not correlate with the degree of fibrosis on chest x-ray, or level of FEV. Although pulmonary interstitial fibrosis is the most common cause of death, pulmonary hypertension has the worst prognosis, with most patients living less than 2 years after diagnosis.

Cardiac involvement is seen mostly in patients with diffuse disease. Congestive heart failure is the most common, although pericarditis and conduction problems leading to complete heart block are also seen. Acute renal crisis develops suddenly as a result of malignant arterial hypertension. Angiotensin-converting enzyme inhibitors have greatly reduced the potential of this complication, and what was once a severe and feared manifestation of systemic sclerosis is now rarely seen. A Sjögren's-like syndrome of dry eyes and mouth occurs as well as hypothyroidism and parotid gland enlargement.

Impotence is very common among men with scleroderma. Depression similar to that suffered by patients with any chronic illness is a risk in systemic sclerosis.

OBJECTIVE FINDINGS

Localized scleroderma is composed of three subtypes: morphea, generalized morphea, and linear scleroderma. Morphea is characterized by dermal or subcutaneous dermal plaques. This type of scleroderma occurs most frequently in young women. There are scleroderma-like conditions, such as lichen sclerosus et atrophicus, that present with morphea as well. Generalized morphea describes the minority of cases in which the dermal plaques are more numerous, larger, and coalesce. Linear scleroderma usually consists of a singular linear sclerotic lesion, often on an extremity or the forehead.

Systemic sclerosis is a progressive condition characterized by fibrosis involving the skin as well as internal organs and is composed of two subtypes, limited disease or diffuse disease. Limited disease affects acral skin such as the hands, forearms, legs, and face, and has the better prognosis. Cutaneous findings such as digit or hand edema, or discrete lesions or skin thickening, are often the presenting signs in patients with limited disease. Almost all patients with limited disease will have a long history of Raynaud's phenomenon. New symptoms appear slowly within this group. Diffuse disease involves the proximal extremities and truncal areas.

Limited systemic sclerosis was characterized in the past by the acronym CREST, which signified Calcinosis, Raynaud's, Esophageal dysmotility, Sclerodactyly, and Telangiectasia. CREST did not adequately describe the disease, which has been found to be more variable than the presence of the five conditions would suggest, and has been replaced by the new classification system.

Rapid progression of symptoms is the chief distinguishing factor of the diffuse disease from the limited variant. Organ damage is more common and more severe in diffuse disease, although either group may be initially diagnosed on the basis of a life-threatening condition such as pulmonary hypertension. Localized scleroderma infrequently manifests in systemic disease, and rarely develops into systemic sclerosis, whereas both types of systemic sclerosis involve systemic complications. Esophageal or gastrointestinal dysmotility, or pulmonary diseases such as pulmonary fibrosis or pulmonary hypertension, are the most common. Renal disease is uncommon, but a grave prognostic indicator.

A third type of this disorder is the *overlap syndromes,* which include polymyositis, Sjögren's syndrome, or lupus erythematosus or other mixed connective tissue diseases where the patient has features of both diseases. *Sclerodermoid disorders* are groups of disease, often among selected patient groups, that have features of scleroderma due to a primary disease or risk factor. Scleroderma diabeticorum (cutaneous indurations among poorly controlled insulin-dependent diabetics), scleromyxedema, sclerodermiform chronic graft-versus-host disease, and scleroderma-like changes of porphyria are all examples of this form of the disease.

DIAGNOSTIC CONSIDERATIONS

There are three situations in which the inclusion or exclusion of scleroderma or systemic sclerosis should be considered. The first is in the overlap syndromes. Although there many diseases that coexist with systemic sclerosis, extracting a scleroderma component is important only if it impacts treatment. This is especially important in the scleroderma-like conditions, which are secondary to a primary illness, necessitating treatment for the primary condition.

The second situation involves conditions that mimic scleroderma. Eosinophilic fasciitis and eosinophilia myalgia syndrome are two examples of idiopathic scleroderma-like conditions. Eosinophilic fasciitis lacks the hallmark sign of scleroderma. Although this disorder presents with skin thickening, it involves the extremities and trunk but not the fingers, which is essential for a diagnosis of scleroderma.

Finally, scleroderma and systemic sclerosis should be considered in patients with either new-onset or long-standing Raynaud's phenomenon. As new-onset Raynaud's is more likely to present with diffuse systemic sclerosis, screening tests should be performed for pulmonary, renal, gastrointestinal, or cardiac damage.

LABORATORY AND RADIOLOGIC STUDIES

As in many rheumatologic diseases, serologic testing plays a role, although a definitive marker has not yet been found. Antinuclear antibodies are positive in nearly all patients in a speckled, centromere, and nucleolar pattern. More specifically, anticentromere antibodies and antitopoisomerase (formerly anti-Scl 70 or Scl 96) markers play a role in the diagnosis and prognosis of systemic sclerosis. Anticentromere antibodies are present in 50% to 80% of patients with limited-type disease, and their presence is associated with a favorable prognosis. They are not as specific as antitopoisomerase antibodies, however, which in high titers are extremely reliable to diagnosis diffuse systemic sclerosis. There are patients who are seronegative to both of these tests, and there is a group of new tests, not yet widely accessible, that can be used to diagnose these patients.

Chest radiographs are helpful in diagnosing pulmonary disease, especially when bibasilar fibrosis is shown. Pulmonary function tests show a restrictive pattern with a decreased vital force capacity in fibrosis. For screening purposes, ventilation perfusion scans should be included when a diagnosis of systemic sclerosis is made. Electrocardiogram, echocardiography, and nuclear cardiac studies will diagnose asymptomatic conduction defects, arrhythmias, and pericarditis. X-rays of the extremities are important when erosive arthropathy is suspected.

TREATMENT

No pharmacologic or other therapy has been found to treat systemic sclerosis. Prompt and accurate diagnosis of organ complications is the key to good management of this disease. Patients may experience episodic remissions. Cutaneous symptoms, especially skin tightening, may improve over time, while damage to internal organs generally does not. Raynaud's phenomenon may be treated with calcium channel blockers, prostacyclin analogues or topical nitroglycerin. D-penicillamine has been shown effective for cutaneous lesions. Judicious skin hygiene and care should be stressed.

Angiotensin-converting enzyme inhibitors have greatly reduced renal morbidity. Proton-pump inhibitors, histamine agonists, and metoclopramide or cisapride may help increase lower esophageal sphincter tone. Oral prednisone is indicated for patients with myopathy. Local injections of corticosteroids, nonsteroidal anti-inflammatory agents, physical therapy, stretching exercises and local heat applications may decrease arthralgias. Range-of-motion exercises can prevent contracture.

Referrals to physical therapy and gastroenterology may be helpful early in the disease course, omitting sufficient trials of conservative therapy. Good behavioral medicine can ease the psychosocial effects of the disease as well.

BIBLIOGRAPHY

Artlett CM, Smith JB, Jimenez SA. New perspectives on the etiology of systemic sclerosis. *Mol Med Today* 5:72–78, 1999.

Callen JP. Collagen vascular diseases. *Med Clin North Am* 82:1217–1237, 1998.

Kerin K, Yost JH. Advances in the diagnosis and management of scleroderma-related vascular complications. *Compr Ther* 24:574–58, 1998.

Meyer O. How useful are serum autoantibodies in the diagnosis and prognosis of systemic sclerosis? *Clin Rheumatol* 17:179–180, 1998.

Michet C. Update in the epidemiology of the rheumatic diseases. *Curr Opin Rheumatol* 10:129–135, 1998.

Steen VD. Clinical manifestations of systemic sclerosis. *Semin Cutan Med Surg* 17:48–54, 1998.

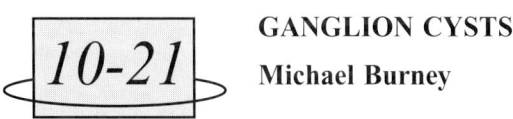

GANGLION CYSTS
Michael Burney

DISCUSSION

Ganglion cysts are structures filled with mucinous fluid, most commonly located in the wrist. Most cysts come from an adjacent joint or tendon sheath. The most common sites include the dorsal wrist, palmar wrist, and flexor sheath of the fingers.[1,2] The etiology is unclear, but trauma is thought to be a causative factor.[3,4] Ganglion cysts are more common with people who engage in repetitive motion activities.[1]

SIGNS AND SYMPTOMS

Ganglia are generally painless except for local swelling. Dorsal ganglia are prone to cause a dull ache.[10] Ganglia located in the fingers may cause tenderness with grasping activities.[2,3] Rarely, compressive symptoms may accompany a cyst that pushes on the median or ulnar nerve, causing numbness and/or weakness of the intrinsic muscles of the hand.[2,5]

OBJECTIVE FINDINGS

The examiner finds a palpable mass on the dorsal or palmar aspect of the wrist or the flexor sheath of the fingers. Normal wrist range of motion is usually the finding. Flexion of the wrist usually accentuates a dorsal wrist ganglion. Tenderness is usually noted with gentle pressure to the cyst.[1,2]

DIAGNOSTIC CONSIDERATIONS

Aspiration of thick mucinous fluid confirms the diagnosis of ganglion cyst.[6]

The differential diagnosis for a finger mass over the DIP joint includes Heberden's nodes of osteoarthritis, gouty tophus, giant cell tumor of the tendon sheath, or a large callous from writing.[3]

Palmar digital masses require the differential diagnosis of epidermal inclusion cyst, foreign body, giant cell tumor, lipoma, and neurilemoma.[3]

LABORATORY TESTS

There are no laboratory tests that assist in diagnosing ganglion cysts.

RADIOLOGIC AND IMAGING STUDIES

Obtain plain posteroanterior and lateral wrist films to rule out osteogenic pathology, such as intraosseous ganglion, Kienböck disease, arthritis, bone tumor (benign or malignant), or fractures. Findings of plain films are negative.[2] Table 10-21-1 lists the common radiographic findings for differential diagnosis of a wrist mass.

TREATMENT

Supportive measures (diet, rest, and exercise) form the basis of treatment. Reassurance that the diagnosis of ganglion cyst is not a serious problem should be reinforced with the patient.[2,6] The natural history of ganglion cysts shows a resolution rate of 28 to 58%.

Immobilization of the wrist with a Velcro splint may help to decrease the size of the cyst after a period of rest, along with a decrease in repetitive motion activities.[1,2,6] Immobilization of wrist ganglions

TABLE 10-21-1. Radiographic Findings for Differential Diagnosis of Wrist Masses

DIAGNOSTIC CONSIDERATIONS	RADIOGRAPHIC FINDINGS
Arthritis	Positive
Bone tumor	Positive
Intraosseous ganglion (evident on radiographs)	Positive
Kienböck disease (avascular necrosis of the lunate)	Positive
Soft tissue tumor, benign or malignant	Negative
Fractures (scaphoid, hamate, distal radius, metacarpals)	Positive

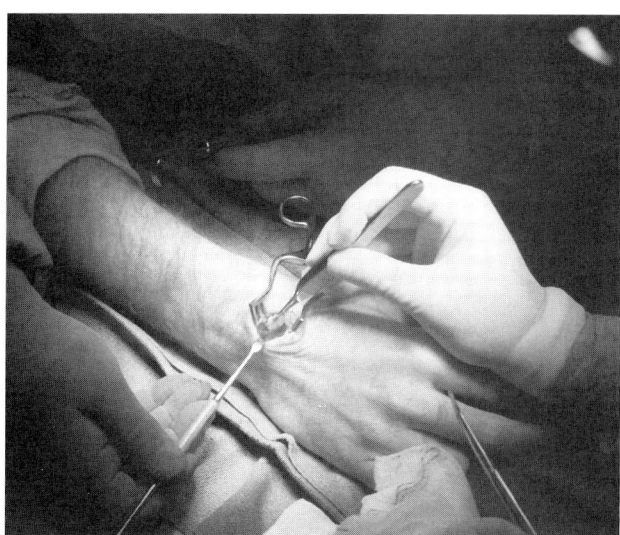

FIGURE 10-21-1. Surgical view of the dorsal ganglion cyst of the author.

does not improve the treatment of ganglions over perforation and aspiration alone.[8]

Pharmacologic Management

Patients whose ganglia fail to resolve after supportive measures may need to have the ganglion aspirated by a large-bore needle, followed by a compressive dressing. Injection of a corticosteroid is used when aspiration alone fails to improve the symptoms.[7] Infrequent complications of corticosteroid and lidocaine injections include subcutaneous atrophy, skin depigmentation, and tendon rupture.[3] Patients should avoid repetitive activity of the injected cystic area for 3 to 4 weeks. Icing for 10 minutes three to four times a day for 3 days after aspiration and injection is recommended.[2]

DISPOSITION/INDICATIONS FOR SURGICAL REFERRAL

Patients who fail conservative treatment, aspiration, and/or injection of a corticosteroid should be referred to a hand surgeon for consultation after a 12-week period.[6] Any mass that does not appear to be a ganglion should be evaluated and referred to a hand surgeon for further evaluation.

Figures 10-21-1 and 10-21-2 shows the author's own dorsal ganglion cyst, including an intraoperative view.

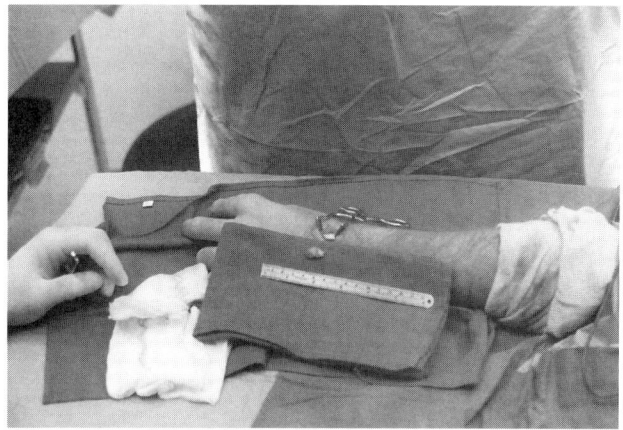

FIGURE 10-21-2. Intraoperative view of the author's dorsal ganglion cyst.

COMPLICATIONS AND RED FLAGS

Radial artery injury can occur following aspiration of volar wrist ganglions.[2]

Rarely, surgical complications from ganglionectomy include recurrence of the ganglion, superficial infection, tendinitis, and pain dystrophy.[9] Needle rupture of digital flexor sheath ganglia may cause digital nerve injury if the cyst is located near a neurovascular bundle of a finger.[3] Recurrence of ganglia in patients following ganglionectomy is between 5 and 10%.[2]

OTHER NOTES AND PEARLS

Clinicians who do not feel comfortable aspirating and injecting ganglion cysts in any anatomic location should refer patients to a hand surgeon for treatment. Patients suffering from wrist pain of unknown etiology may have an occult wrist ganglion and should be referred to a hand specialist for further workup and treatment.

REFERENCES

1. Crowther C: *Primary Orthopedic Care.* St. Louis, Mosby, 1999.
2. Snider R: *Essentials of Musculoskeletal Care.* Rosemont, IL, American Academy of Orthopedic Surgeons, 1997.
3. Peimer C: *Surgery of the Hand and Upper Extremity.* New York, McGraw-Hill, 1996.
4. Klippel J: *Primer on Rheumatic Diseases,* 11th ed. Atlanta, GA, Arthritis Foundation, 1997.
5. Boyles J: *Bunnell's Surgery of the Hand,* 5th ed. Philadelphia, Lippincott, 1970.
6. Anderson B: *Office Orthopedics for Primary Care,* 2nd ed. Philadelphia, Saunders, 1999.
7. Vo P et al: Evaluating dorsal wrist pain: MRI diagnosis of occult dorsal wrist ganglion. *J Hand Surg* 20A:667–670, 1995.
8. Korman J et al: Efficacy of immobilization following aspiration of carpal and digital ganglions. *J Hand Surg* 17A:1097–1099, 1992.
9. Wright T et al: Anterior wrist ganglion. *J Hand Surg* 19A:954–958, 1994.
10. Osterman A, Raphael J: Arthroscopic resection of dorsal ganglion of the wrist, in *Hand Clinics,* Philadelphia, 1995.

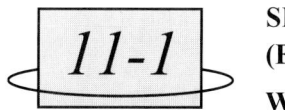

SEIZURE DISORDERS (EPILEPSY)

William A. Mosier

DISCUSSION

A seizure disorder (epilepsy) is best described as a symptom of brain dysfunction involving a paroxysmal and disorganized depolarization of neurons in the brain and the spread of the resulting discharge. The word *epilepsy* is derived from the Greek *epilepsia,* "a seizing." It refers to the many varying types of recurrent seizures produced by sudden, excessive neuronal discharges in the brain. A seizure is an uncontrolled synchronous firing of a group of cerebral neurons. The spread of a seizure involves the progression of surges of disorganized electrical impulses in the brain to surrounding or closely interconnected groups of neurons, engaging them in similar activity. Many abnormal depolarizations have no clinical manifestations; however, when manifestations are present, the result is seizure activity. The term *epilepsy* encompasses convulsive "disorders" with loss of consciousness as well as nonconvulsive seizures with only a slight change in conscious awareness. Generally, the term *epilepsy* is reserved for patients who have experienced at least two and usually three recurrent seizures without clear precipitating factors. Seizures produced by cerebral ischemia, hypoxia, hypoglycemia, cocaine abuse, and withdrawal from alcohol, barbiturates, or benzodiazepines should not be referred to as epilepsy.

The prevalence of seizure disorders is roughly 6 in 1000 in the general population. In the United States, about 1% of the population, approximately 2 million people, has active epilepsy. Another 7 million persons have had at least one seizure at some point during their lifetimes. This represents 1 in every 11 persons. It has been estimated that 200,000 persons experience seizures more than once a month.

It also has been estimated that one-fourth of all patients with seizure disorders continue to experience seizure activity despite receiving treatment. Although seizures can develop at any time in life, 75 percent of new cases present in childhood. Seizure disorders are slightly more prevalent in males and in persons in lower socioeconomic groups.

The two most widely accepted ways of classifying seizures are the International Classification of Epileptic Seizures (ICES) and the International Classification of Epilepsies (ICE). In these systems, seizures are divided into two broad categories: (1) generalized seizures and (2) localization-related (partial, focal) seizures.

Generalized seizures are most often genetic in origin and begin from both sides of the brain simultaneously. Localization-related seizures usually are restricted to specific regions of the brain and most often are acquired. These so-called local seizures can be separated further into simple and complex seizures. The most common idiopathic localization-related seizure disorder is benign childhood epilepsy with centrotemporal spikes (benign rolandic epilepsy). It occurs most frequently between ages 3 and 13. It presents with simple partial seizures manifesting sensorimotor symptoms that affect predominantly the face, particularly the mouth.

Seizures also can be divided into two types: convulsive and nonconvulsive. The most familiar expression of convulsive seizures is the generalized tonic-clonic form often referred to as grand mal seizures. They commonly begin in late adolescence. The most familiar expression of nonconvulsive seizures is called an absence seizure (petit mal). These seizures usually begin in early childhood (see Table 11-1-1).

PATHOGENESIS

The causes of seizures are as varied as the possible clinical manifestations. Seizures may result from idiopathic factors or may be produced by disease processes or brain trauma. Given the appropriate chemical and electrical stimuli, seizure activity can occur even in a "normal" brain. Certain regions of the brain are particularly sensitive to seizure activity, especially the motor cortex and the limbic system. The temporal lobe, the amygdala, and the hippocampus are all especially susceptible to biochemical disturbances. Age and developmental factors are significant influences in the genesis of seizure disorders (see Table 11-1-2).

SIGNS AND SYMPTOMS

One of every five individuals diagnosed with a seizure disorder (epilepsy) may not actually have epilepsy. The most important factor in seeking a diagnosis is taking a thorough history of the initial seizure and any subsequent presumed seizures as well as a detailed family history. The history frequently uncovers the seizure type. The interview must include questioning about a history of early-morning seizure activity or jerking behavior and establishing whether the patient felt tired after a seizure. Evidence of feeling fatigue during the postictal state can rule out absence seizures, which are marked by a rapid return to feeling normal.

Seizure disorders are classified according to their presenting clinical features and the patterns that are observed on the electroencephalogram. Because an accurate diagnosis of a seizure disorder involves so many factors, the following diagnostic considerations should apply in assessing a patient. A determination must be made of

1. Whether seizure activity actually occurred
2. Whether the seizures are localized or generalized in nature
3. Whether consciousness was impaired
4. Whether convulsions occurred

Generalized seizures of the tonic-clonic type are characterized by an aura (a rising or sinking sensation) followed by a sudden loss of consciousness. During the period of unconsciousness, the body develops a tonic (stiffening) response that usually lasts less than a minute. Then the body undergoes a series of muscle contractions that represent the clonic phase. The entire seizure typically may last 3 minutes.

Generalized absence seizures usually present as brief, mild episodes lasting only 5 to 30 seconds. They tend to cause no dramatic physical changes and may go unnoticed. An absence seizure is characterized by a sudden stop in activity and a blank, vacant stare that lasts only seconds. The individual may then immediately resume activity, completely unaware that he or she just experienced a seizure.

Partial seizures can be classified as complex or simple. A partial seizure with impaired consciousness is referred to as a complex partial seizure. A partial seizure without compromised consciousness is called a simple partial seizure. When a seizure persists for an extended period, more than 30 minutes, or occurs so frequently that there is no recovery between attacks, this is referred to as status epilepticus (see "Complications and Red Flags," below).

TABLE 11-1-1. Classification of the More Common Seizures

TYPE	CHARACTERISTICS	LOCATION
LOCALIZATION-RELATED SEIZURES (FOCAL, LOCAL, PARTIAL)		
Motor	Aura	Cortical foci of spikes and slow waves seen on EEG
Sensory Somatosensory	Tingling, numbness	Parietal lobe
Visual	Flashing lights and color	Occipital lobe
Temporal lobe Complex partial (psychomotor)	Lip smacking, chewing	Anterior temporal lobe foci
GENERALIZED SEIZURES		
Tonic-clonic (grand mal)	Aura, unconsciousness, tonic-clonic movements, postictal drowsiness	Single or multiple cortical foci of spikes seen on EEG; can be in any area of cortex
Absence (petit mal)	Staring, speech arrest (brief spells)	Synchronous, symmetric, 3/s spike-and-wave discharges with no cortical localization seen on EEG
Myoclonic	Quick repetitive jerks	Multifocal spikes seen on EEG

OBJECTIVE FINDINGS

The clinical features of a seizure disorder depend largely on the regions of the brain initially involved and the rate and pattern of spread of the abnormal discharge. The neurologic examination may uncover evidence of a localized brain lesion or an organic disorder. In children, the examination must include looking for developmental delays, adenoma sebaceum (a sign of tuberous sclerosis), and organomegaly (which could indicate a storage disease).

DIAGNOSTIC CONSIDERATIONS

A diagnosis of seizure disorder can have profound medical and psychological implications for a patient. Consequently, careful attention should be given to exploring nonepileptic disturbances that produce abnormal-

TABLE 11-1-2. Causes of Seizure Activity

CAUSE	RESULT
Birth trauma	Anoxia, contusion
Congenital	Abnormal development
Metabolic	Disorders of amino acid or vitamin metabolism, lipidoses, hypoglycemia, hypocalcemia, hyponatremia, uremia
Infection	Encephalitis, meningitis, brain abscess
Perinatal injury	Temporal lobe sclerosis, cerebral palsy
Neoplastic	Primary and metastatic tumors
Vascular	Arteriovenous malformation, arteritis, hematoma, sickle cell disease, postinfarction, hypertension
Postnatal trauma	Anoxia, contusion, penetrating head wound
Toxins or withdrawal	Alcohol, barbiturates, cocaine, lead, organic phosphates, steroids, abrupt medication changes, Reye's syndrome

ities of neurologic function similar to those of seizure disorders. The differential diagnosis should include conversion hysteria (psychogenic origin) as well as cerebrovascular insufficiency (drop attacks) and syncope.

SPECIAL CONSIDERATIONS

The chief issues in managing seizure disorders in children are accurate diagnosis, appropriate selection of an antiepileptic drug, and supportive management to minimize the adverse effects of seizures on maturation. Many children have self-limiting seizures. An accurate diagnosis can prevent the overprescribing of antiepileptics that may have a negative impact on a child's cognitive functioning and academic achievement. Children with seizure disorders have a higher incidence of learning disabilities and other neurologic handicaps than do their peers. Antiepileptic drugs also can contribute to learning problems. Because these problems are so common among children treated for seizure disorders, testing and remedial help for the child should be recommended to the parents.

DIAGNOSTIC TESTS

The use of the encephalogram (EEG) is indispensable in considering a diagnosis of seizure disorder. An EEG can provide a precise definition of the nature of an abnormal neural discharge and often can be used to establish the seizure type. It is best performed on the patient in both the awake and sleeping states, utilizing hyperventilation and phobic stimulation. EEG can detect focal and diffuse brain dysfunction. The two typical patterns to look for are a slowing and the classic epileptiform activity, which is brief and starts and stops abruptly. The number of epileptiform discharges between seizures, referred to as interictal discharges, does not correlate with the frequency of seizures. In fact, the interictal EEG of an awake patient with a seizure disorder may be totally normal. EEG patterns of partial and generalized seizures are typically quite distinct. Partial seizures can produce a focal slowing of the background rhythm, focal spikes, or even sharp waves.

With generalized seizures, EEG tracings may demonstrate a bilateral or widespread spiking and slow wave pattern or a polyspiking and slow wave pattern over the entire frontal and central regions of the brain. Because many epileptiform patterns are confusing and may lead to a misdiagnosis, interpretation of EEG results requires caution and expertise (see Table 11-1-3).

TREATMENT

The management of seizures is based primarily on empirical observations of how certain types of seizures present in relation to the age of the patient and the response of seizure activity to therapeutic intervention. The question of whether to treat with medication is complicated by the fact that the recurrence rate after a single seizure varies from 15 to 60 percent. However, after two seizures, the risk of eventually experiencing a third seizure rises to 85 percent. Therefore, treatment decisions must be individualized to the needs of each patient because the consequences and recurrence rates of seizures are so varied. The aim of treatment is to

TABLE 11-1-3. Diagnostic Tools for Screening Seizure Disorders

Electroencephalogram
Computed tomography and/or magnetic resonance imaging
Fasting blood glucose
Serum urea nitrogen, calcium, and phosphorus
Sedimentation rate
Urinalysis
Positron emission tomography with fluorodeoxyglucose (in surgical candidates)

control seizure activity without drug toxicity. Single-drug therapy is effective in about 50% of those patients.

Pharmacologic Management

The determination of which drug to choose for the initial management of a seizure disorder should be based on two concerns: safety and efficacy. Considerable evidence has demonstrated that the following medications are the most appropriate first-line choices for the specific seizure disorders listed below:

- *Partial seizures:* oxcarbazepine (Trileptal), carbamazepine (Tegretol), valproate (Depakote), or phenytoin (Dilantin)
- *Generalized seizures with convulsions (tonic-clonic or myoclonic):* valproate (Depakote), carbamazepine (Tegretol), or phenytoin (Dilantin)
- *Generalized seizures without convulsions (absence seizures):* valproate (Depakote) or ethosuximide (Zarontin)

Dosing of these medications should follow the manufacturer's guidelines, as outlined in the *Physician's Desk Reference* (PDR). It is important to avoid abrupt cessation of anticonvulsive medication. Many anticonvulsant drugs are available, but those listed above are the mainstay of drug therapy. The safest first-line drug is valproate. When this therapy alone is not effective, phenytoin, carbamazepine, or ethosuximide therapy should be attempted.

Before the initiation of monotherapy with valproic acid or divalproex sodium, a blood count that includes platelets, bleeding time, and liver function should be ordered. This should be repeated after 10 days of therapy and then monthly for the first 6 months of treatment. The dose should be increased gradually from 250 mg/day to 750 mg or even 1500 mg, often in divided doses. Nausea and vomiting usually are a problem only if the dose is increased too rapidly. Gastrointestinal (GI) side effects can be minimized if the medication is taken with meals. Occasional complaints include hair loss, tremors, and weight gain. It is important to avoid abrupt cessation of the medication.

Supportive Measures

Even with adequate seizure control from anticonvulsive therapy, many patients will require concomitant psychological support services such as individual or group counseling. Support materials are available to health care providers and their patients who have a seizure disorder. Help is available from the Epilepsy Foundation of America, 4351 Garden City Drive, Landover, MD 20785, (800) 332-1000.

Patient Education

Patient education should emphasize helping the patient recognize seizure triggers. Although there may be no special triggers in some patients, other patients find that flickering lights (even sunlight), stress, lack of sleep, and lack of food may be associated with a greater likelihood of seizure activity.

The most common cause of an unexpected seizure is failure to take the medication as prescribed. Therefore, an individualized educational plan of care should provide the patient and the patient's family members with informational tools that will enhance their understanding of the patient's seizure disorder. The significance of reminding the patient about the importance of taking all medications appropriately cannot be overemphasized. The risks of driving an automobile and work-related issues also must be reviewed in counseling the patient about his or her seizure risk. The parents of children with seizure disorders must be cautioned against overprotectiveness.

DISPOSITION

Most genetically predisposed seizure disorders are well controlled with the proper medication management, as are most acquired partial seizure disorders. In both children and adults, early initiation of treatment produces the most favorable prognosis as long as there is no underlying progressive structural disease.

COMPLICATIONS AND RED FLAGS

Status epilepticus refers to

- Seizure activity that is so frequent or prolonged that it persists for at least 30 minutes
- Seizure activity occurring with impaired consciousness and without a return of consciousness between seizures

The most frequently occurring type of status epilepticus is generalized convulsive status epilepticus (GCSE). It constitutes a medical emergency that necessitates prompt treatment to avoid neurologic damage. Intravenous diazepam or lorazepam and phenytoin are the first-line therapies for GCSE. Most patients respond to the initial treatment. However, refractory status epilepticus may require pentobarbital, phenobarbital, or inhalational anesthetic agents.

Surgical intervention is appropriate for selected patients who remain intractable after intensive medical therapy. About 10 percent benefit from anterior temporal lobectomy, amygdalohippocampectomy, or corticotomy.

OTHER NOTES AND PEARLS

Refractory complex partial seizures may be due to inadequate doses of anticonvulsant medication, an inappropriate medication choice, or the presence of aggravating factors such as stress, sleep deprivation, menses, and alcohol. Patient noncompliance with taking medication must always be considered if refractory seizures persist. Research is being conducted using biofeedback as a treatment for seizures. In theory, the patient learns how to reproduce the brain waves that seem to prevent seizures. However, some studies indicate that the ability to control seizure activity fades once the biofeedback training is discontinued. For a patient who is a nonresponder to medication, researchers at Johns Hopkins Medical School have conducted an extensive study of a diet called the ketogenic diet. This diet substantially improves seizure control in some children with severe seizures. At least one-third of these children have a marked decrease in or complete cessation of seizure activity. Another one-third of the children on this diet experience a partial or incomplete response, and the remaining one-third receive no benefit from the diet. The high-fat, low-carbohydrate, low-protein diet must be followed with exactness to control seizure activity. It is not recommended without close medical supervision because of the complex protocols and monitoring necessary. Potential health risks associated with the ketogenic diet include weight loss, renal stones, hemolytic anemia, hypoproteinemia, renal tubular acidosis, and elevated hepatic enzymes. For information on the ketogenic diet, contact Johns Hopkins Pediatric Epilepsy Center, 600 North Wolfe Street, Baltimore, MD 21287.

BIBLIOGRAPHY

Browne TR, Holmes GL: *Handbook of Epilepsy,* 2d ed. Philadelphia, Lippincott Williams & Wilkins, 2000.

Devinsky O: Patients with refractory seizures. *N Engl J Med.* 340:1565–1570, 1999.

Engel J, Pedley TA (eds): *Epilepsy: A Comprehensive Textbook.* Philadelphia, Lippincott-Raven, 1997, chaps 1–11, 21–42, 67–69.

Fischer JH: *2000 Guide to Anti-Epileptic Agents.* CNS News, April 2000, pp 10–13.

French JA: Forewarned is forearmed: Knowing mechanisms of antiepileptic drug interactions can improve patient care. *Clin Decision Making Manage Epilepsy* 1(1):1–5, 2000.

Holmes GL: Epilepsy in the developing brain—lessons from the laboratory and clinic. *Epilepsia* 38:12–30, 1997.

Olsen RW, Avoli M: GABA and epileptogenesis. *Epilepsia* 38:399–407, 1997.

Pellock JM: Treatment of seizures and epilepsy in children and adolescents. *Neurology* 51(S4):8–14, 1998.

Ryam SG: Ion channels and the genetic contribution to epilepsy. *J Child Neurol* 14:58–66, 1999.

Sirven JI: Management of epilepsy in older adults. *Clin Geriatr* 8(1):93–100, 2000.

Westmoreland BF: The EEG findings in extratemporal seizures. *Epilepsia* 39(S4):1–8, 1998.

Wyllie E (ed): *The Treatment of Epilepsy: Principles and Practice,* 2d ed. Baltimore, Williams & Wilkins, 1997, chaps 2, 4, 5, 8, 10–12, 21, 22.

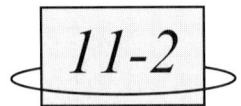

MULTIPLE SCLEROSIS

William A. Mosier

DISCUSSION

Multiple sclerosis (MS) is a slowly progressive demyelinating disease of the central nervous system (CNS). It results in varied neurologic symptoms with periods of alternating remission and exacerbation. The cause is unknown, and current therapy is only marginally effective. The disease generally begins in early adult life. The onset of symptoms rarely occurs before age 15 or after age 40. The name *multiple sclerosis* refers to two features of the disease: *Multiple* indicates that many areas of the brain, spinal cord, and optic nerve are affected, and *sclerosis* suggests that there are hardened plaques in the involved areas.

The course is highly unpredictable. Remissions may last months or years. However, over the course of the disease, the intervals between remissions become shorter.

PATHOGENESIS

The pathologic focus of MS is the fatty myelin coating on nerve fibers in the CNS. MS attacks the myelin, forming plaque in varying locations in the brain, spinal cord, and closely related structures. The prevalence of MS varies from region to region. It appears to be more common in temperate zones. There are an estimated 250,000 cases of diagnosed MS in the United States. The factors that determine susceptibility to MS appear to be acquired before age 15. The incidence of MS is higher in urban settings than in rural areas. It also manifests more frequently among affluent socioeconomic groups. Blood relatives of patients with MS are eight times more likely to develop the disease than is the general population. These epidemiologic factors suggest a viral or altered immune response in a genetically susceptible individual as the probable etiology. MS is the most common demyelinating disease of the CNS.

MICROBIOLOGY

MS attacks the myelin that covers nerve fibers. The damaged myelin cells cause plaques of demyelination with destruction of oligodendroglia, primarily in the white matter of the cervical and dorsal region of the lateral and posterior columns, the optic nerves, and the periventricular areas. Tracts in the midbrain, pons, and cerebellum and gray matter in the cerebrum and spinal cord also may be invaded. Chemical changes in the lipid and protein constituents of myelin have been identified in and around the plaques associated with MS.

SYMPTOMS

The onset of MS is usually insidious. Symptoms often develop over the course of a few days, remain stable for several weeks, and then recede. The most frequently presenting symptoms include

• Paresthesias in one or more extremities, on one side of the face, or in the trunk

• A feeling of clumsiness in or weakness of a hand or leg
• Visual disturbances (e.g., retrobulbar optic neuritis, diplopia, foggy vision, scotomas, partial blindness)

Other symptoms include transient weakness of one or more extremities, minor gait disturbance, limb fatigue, bladder control problems, ocular palsy, dizziness, male impotency, and psychological changes such as mood swings, apathy, and depression. Exposure to excessively warm temperatures tends to exacerbate the symptoms. The symptoms may present for months to years before the disease is diagnosed.

OBJECTIVE FINDINGS

Most neurologic findings are nonspecific, but certain signs are suggestive of MS:

1. *Internuclear ophthalmoplegia.* Paresis of the medial rectus muscle on lateral conjugate gaze but not on convergence can be noted. Nystagmus can be seen in the abducting eye.
2. *Lhermitte's sign.* Neck flexion produces a sensation of an electrical charge that runs down the back and into the legs.
3. *Optic neuritis.* Decreased visual acuity, a defective pupillary reaction to light (Marcus Gunn pupil), edema of the optic disks, and hyperemia all can be early signs of MS. Noted pallor of the temporal half of the disk develops as a later sign of MS (see Tables 11-2-1 and 11-2-2).

DIAGNOSTIC CONSIDERATIONS

Multifocal and recrudescent CNS diseases such as systemic lupus erythematosus (SLE) and Behçet's disease can mimic MS. Additional considerations in the differential must include amyotrophic lateral sclerosis (ALS), arthritis of the cervical spine, a cerebral infarct, CNS abscess or tumor, hereditary ataxia, pernicious anemia, a ruptured intervertebral disk, meningovascular syphilis, cryptococcosis, toxoplasmosis, sarcoidosis, syringomyelia, vascular malformations of the brain or spinal cord, Friedreich's ataxia, leukodystrophy, and neurofibromatosis. When the presenting complaints are vague and there are minimal findings, a diagnosis of conversion disorder (hysteria) may be considered.

SPECIAL CONSIDERATIONS

In the early stages, MS often is mislabeled inaccurately as hysteria. It is important to avoid this mistake. No blood test, x-ray study, or other type of objective examination can determine with total certainty that a patient's presenting complaints are caused by multiple sclerosis. MS is diagnosed by the clinical findings. Laboratory procedures can only lend support for the diagnosis or be used to rule it out.

LABORATORY STUDIES

The only useful laboratory test for MS is an examination of the cerebrospinal fluid (CSF). However, all the abnormalities induced by

TABLE 11-2-1. Neurologic Signs Associated with MS

Abnormal pupillary responses
Abnormal speech patterns
Altered eye movements
Circumscribed sensory disturbances
Limb spasticity
Localized weakness
Overactive tendon reflexes
Paleness of the optic disks
Visual field disturbances

TABLE 11-2-2. Typical Findings on Eye Examination in MS

Centrocecal scotomas

Impaired color vision

Impaired visual acuity

Marcus Gunn pupils

Nystagmus

Optic nerve atrophy

MS are not unique to this disease alone. The characteristic changes in the CSF occurring in MS also may be seen with some infections, other demyelinating diseases, and other CNS diseases of unknown etiology. In MS, proteins associated with the myelin of the CNS, called myelin basic proteins, often are found in higher than normal concentrations. They represent a crude measure of the extent of myelin damage in the CNS. The most characteristic CSF finding in MS is elevated immunoglobulin G (IgG) in 85 to 90% of patients with a definite diagnosis of MS. In over 90% of patients with MS, significant amounts of IgG (as well as IgM and IgA) are present in the form of oligoclonal bands. An elevated kappa-chain content of the CSF may be a better indicator of MS than is IgG (see Table 11-3-3).

RADIOLOGIC STUDIES

Computed tomography (CT) with contrast and magnetic resonance imaging (MRI), especially nuclear magnetic resonance (NMR), can provide assistance in the investigation of MS. Determining that an area of damage is afflicted by demyelination rather than a tumor or damaged blood vessels is better achieved with MRI than with CT. The plaques of demyelination seen in MS patients show up as white patches on both CT with contrast and MRI.

OTHER DIAGNOSTICS

Evoked potential studies are a noninvasive tool to assess nerve fiber conduction in the visual, auditory, and somatosensory pathways. Visual evoked response (VER) testing appears abnormal in 75 to 95% of confirmed cases of MS. Somatosensory evoked potentials will register as abnormal in 70 to 95% of cases. Brainstem auditory evoked response testing will yield abnormal results in 55 to 65% of cases. Test results may uncover unsuspected problems in parts of the nervous system that are still asymptomatic.

TREATMENT

There is no cure for MS. Although spontaneous remissions make treatment efficacy difficult to evaluate, treatments to manage acute exacerbations and complications are utilized. Treatment is aimed at relief of symptoms and prevention of relapse.

TABLE 11-2-3. Findings on Laboratory Tests and Radiologic Studies in MS

TEST	FINDINGS
Cerebrospinal fluid	Abnormal protein composition >55% of time
Computed tomography	White patches notable with high contrast
Magnetic resonance imaging	Areas of abnormal nerve tissue
Evoked potential studies	Pattern shift of brainstem auditory, somatosensory, or visual evoked potentials may appear abnormal in early stages of MS

Pharmacologic Management

Interferon B$_{1b}$ (Betaseron) is an agent that has been approved for use in ambulatory patients with relapsing-remitting multiple sclerosis (RRMS). It tends to reduce the frequency and severity of exacerbations. The recommended dose is 0.25 mg (8 million IU) administered subcutaneously every other day. It is supplied as a lyophilized powder in a single-use vial with a separate vial of sodium chloride to be used as a diluent; it should be stored under refrigeration. The side-effect profile includes "flu-like" symptoms such as fever, chills, and myalgia. Other side effects, such as palpitations, dyspnea, menstrual disorders, possible abnormal liver function, decreased white blood cell count, and depression, also are seen.

Adrenocorticotropic hormone (ACTH) and corticosteroids have been widely used to treat MS since 1970. However, optic neuritis may be the first sign of MS or may occur during an exacerbation. Since optic neuritis can be worsened by corticosteroids such as prednisone, treatment with prednisone during a flare-up of MS is potentially dangerous. Other risks include steroid-induced hypertension and diabetes mellitus.

Muscle relaxants may be helpful in the treatment of the spasticity and muscle stiffness that often develop with MS. The benzodiazepines are used frequently for this purpose. Clonazepam (Klonopin) is usually adequate to improve mobility. It should be noted, however, that after taking a benzodiazepine for several months, a patient will notice withdrawal effects if the drug is discontinued. Insomnia and restlessness are noticed frequently. Therefore, when a patient is in a period of remission, benzodiazepine discontinuation should be done in a tapered manner.

Supportive Measures

Massage and passive range-of-motion exercise of weak limbs can make patients more comfortable. Physical therapy can help preserve as much muscle function as possible and should be emphasized. Most treatment is aimed at relieving symptoms. Wearing braces or using a cane, walker, wheelchair, or battery-powered vehicle may become necessary. Adequate rest and a healthy, well-balanced diet are important. Providing the patient with encouragement and reassurance is essential.

Patient Education

Because living with MS can be difficult, the patient should be encouraged to join an MS support group. The patient also should be counseled about avoiding emotionally and physically stressful situations in an attempt to control symptoms. The patient must be reminded to consult with the health care provider as soon as symptoms become apparent in an attempt to shorten any exacerbation of the disease. The National Multiple Sclerosis Society is an excellent source of current material on MS for patients and providers. Patients should be referred to the society at 205 E 42 Street, New York, NY 10017, (800) 624-8236.

DISPOSITION

In some patients, especially those who develop MS in middle age, there can be a rapid downhill course with recurrent urinary tract infections that can pose a risk of kidney failure. Therefore, a neurology consult should be immediate after the onset of symptoms. The average duration of the disease exceeds 25 years from the time of diagnosis. Thirty percent of patients with MS will relapse in the first year after a remission. Twenty percent will have a relapse within 5 to 9 years. Ten percent may remain in remission for 30 years before the next relapse. Although the course of MS is highly variable and unpredictable, it is important to remember that 70% of patients with MS will lead an active, productive life with prolonged remissions.

COMPLICATIONS AND RED FLAGS

A common complication of MS and of the medications used to treat the associated symptoms is depression. It may result from the stress of the condition, the demyelination process, steroid withdrawal, or a drug reaction. Regardless of the cause, the treatment of choice is antidepressant therapy. Although psychotherapy may be beneficial, an antidepressant drug alone is often sufficient. Fluoxetine (Prozac) is particularly useful because of its benign side-effect profile. A single 20-mg capsule taken each morning with breakfast is often adequate. Widely prescribed alternatives include imipramine (Tofranil) 100 mg at bedtime and amitriptyline (Elavil) 10 to 25 mg tid. However, both imipramine and amitriptyline can interfere with bladder emptying and may contribute to urinary retention if the patient already has bladder problems. As a result of already disturbed functioning of the CNS, an MS patient on an antidepressant must be monitored for abnormal body temperatures or blood pressure problems. A neurologic consultation is always advisable at the onset of an exacerbation of symptoms.

OTHER NOTES AND PEARLS

Many types of treatment have been applied to the management of MS, but few have demonstrated efficacy in clinical studies. Tried and failed therapies include acupuncture, chiropractic, cyclosporine, evening primrose oil, fatty acid supplements, hyperbaric oxygen, megavitamins, and vitamin E. No totally adequate treatment for acute or chronic MS is available. However, research continues in an attempt to find the cause and effective treatments to control, prevent, and reverse this disease. Treatments currently under study include antiviral agents, bee-sting venom, ciliary neurotrophic factor, copolymer-1, cytokines, immunosuppressant drugs, lymphocytapheresis, monoclonal antibodies, oral bovine myeline, prostaglandins, thymectomy, total lymphoid irradiation, 3,4-diaminopyridine, and 4-aminopyridine. The future management of MS may result from research into the molecular genetics of demyelinating diseases. The only certainty at present is that the eventual eradication of MS is expected sooner rather than later.

BIBLIOGRAPHY

Halbreich U: *Multiple Sclerosis: A Neuropsychiatric Disorder.* Washington, DC, American Psychiatric Press, 1997.
Lechtenberg R: *Multiple Sclerosis Fact Book,* 2d ed. Philadelphia, Davis, 1995.
Lublin FD, Whitaker JN, Eidelman BH, et al: Management of patients receiving interferon b-lb for multiple sclerosis: Report of a consensus conference. *Neurology* 46:12–18, 1996.
Richert JR: Demyelinating diseases: Multiple sclerosis, in Kelley WN (ed): *Textbook of Internal Medicine,* 3d ed. Philadelphia, Lippincott-Raven, 1997, pp 2385–2388.

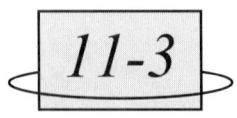

HEADACHES

Andrea G. Weiss

ORGANIC HEADACHES (SECONDARY)

DISCUSSION

Secondary headaches result from symptoms of organic disease as classified by the Headache Classification Committee of the International Headache Society (IHS) in 1988. There are multiple causes of organic headaches (Table 11-3-1).

TABLE 11-3-1. Causes of Headache

Acute-onset headache
  Meningitis
  Intracranial hemorrhage (stroke or ruptured aneurysm)
  Stroke
  Increased intracranial pressure (cerebral edema, hypertensive encephalopathy, hemorrhage)
  Viral illness
  Sinusitis
  Glaucoma
  Metabolic imbalances (hypoglycemia, carbon monoxide poisoning)
  Acute presentation of recurrent headache

Persistent or recurrent headache
  Migraine with or without aura
  Tension-type headache
  Cluster headache
  Postconcussion syndrome
  Intracranial mass or lesion (abscess, neoplasm, arteriovenous malformation, subdural hematoma)
  Cervical muscle strain or spasm
  Temporal arteritis
  Post-lumbar puncture–type headache

PATHOPHYSIOLOGY

The pain from headache can originate extracranially from skin, fat, muscles, blood vessels, periosteal tissues, and fascial regions of the neck. Head pain also can originate intracranially from the great venous sinuses, the dura at the base of the skull, the dural arteries, and the large arteries at the base of the brain. All these regions have pain fibers. The fifth cranial nerve serves most of the facial area and is responsible for pain arising above the tentorium. Actual brain parenchyma, most of the dura, the arachnoid, and the pia mater are incapable of producing pain arising above the tentorium. The ninth, tenth, and eleventh cranial nerves and the upper cervical spinal nerves serve the region below the tentorium; pain often is referred to the neck and the occipital region of the head. The pain-sensitive structures of the head and neck are affected by the following pain-producing mechanisms: distention, dilation, inflammation, tension, and traction.

HISTORY TAKING

An accurate, detailed history is the most important part of the evaluation in distinguishing acute from chronic from recurrent headache. The six principal areas covered in the headache history are

1. Location
2. Character
3. Duration
4. Precipitating and/or aggravating factors
5. Ameliorating factors
6. Medication history

Location

Asking about the location of the head pain is occasionally but not always useful in making a diagnosis. Unilateral headache suggests a migraine, whereas a headache that begins unilaterally and then progresses to a bilateral distribution can be a sign of elevated intracranial pressure (ICP).

Character

Most patients describe their headaches as intense. Asking a patient to provide a description of the pain may be more useful in determining whether it is sharp, piercing, or exploding pain. One should ask if it is made worse by bending forward, having a bowel movement, or coughing. This may be suggestive of an intracranial source. Is the headache occurring in a location typical of prior headaches, and is it usual in character? This information helps differentiate between chronic headaches and those of new onset suggestive of a possible intracranial bleed.

Precipitating, Aggravating, and Ameliorating Factors

Any history suggesting head trauma (recent or in the past) is a "red flag" and warrants methodical investigation. Therefore, one should inquire about associated head trauma or injuries. A history of lethargy, confusion, vomiting, and/or dizziness concomitant with head trauma raises the possibility of a subacute or chronic subdural hematoma. If the headache improves when the patient lies down, this also suggests an intracranial process.

A physician assistant must use a systematic approach to headache assessment to prevent the pitfalls of over-diagnosis and under-diagnosis, which can have life-threatening consequences. As determined from a careful history, the basic critical distinctions between acute versus chronic, episodic versus continuous, and spontaneous versus traumatic headache can aid the clinician in demonstrating rational approaches to the use of further diagnostic tests, appropriate consultation, and ultimately the proper medical management.

PHYSICAL EXAMINATION

The physical examination is an essential part of the evaluation of headache to search for a serious underlying pathology. Despite the advent of sophisticated imaging techniques, the history and physical examination remain indispensable. The blood pressure and temperature should be checked for elevations. The scalp needs to be thoroughly inspected and palpated for any signs of swelling, discoloration, and tenderness. Also, one should palpate for tenderness over the temporal arteries; it is necessary to palpate directly over the temporomandibular joint ligaments to elicit tenderness or an audible pop or click. A sterile gloved finger should be used to probe any scalp lacerations to assess their depth and possible penetration of the skull. Pupils should be assessed for loss of reactivity; a fixed, dilated pupil warrants further investigation into a possible brain abscess or malignancy. Ocular disc margins are examined for clarity; papilledema indicates elevated ICP. One should determine nuchal rigidity on anterior flexion; when present, it is consistent with meningeal irritation. Finally, one should conduct a thorough neurologic examination, looking for ataxia, alterations in mental status (lethargy, confusion, changes in speech and behavior), focal deficits (positive Babinski's sign), and meningeal signs (Brudzinski's and Kernig's signs).

DIAGNOSTIC CONSIDERATIONS

In evaluating a patient with headaches, the issue of the need for an imaging study of the head commonly arises. Mitchell et al.[1] studied the utility of head computed tomography (CT) in patients with headaches, particularly those with abnormal physical examinations or unusual headache characteristics. Only 1% of patients with normal physical examinations had an abnormal CT scan, whereas 10% of patients with abnormal examinations and 12% with unusual histories had abnormal scans. None of the patients with normal examinations and unusual histories had abnormal scans.

Therefore, with the acute onset of headache or a history of a worsening chronic or recurrent headache, emergency CT is the test of choice for prompt detection of potentially life-threatening lesions (an intracranial mass or hemorrhage). If the headache is accompanied by meningeal signs of irritation or evidence of increased ICP, a lumbar puncture and culture should be performed, as well as a complete blood cell count and chemistry profile. Examination of the cerebrospinal fluid (CSF) should follow a CT to rule out an infectious etiology as long as there is no evidence of markedly increased ICP.

A new onset of headache in an elderly patient may represent the onset of temporal arteritis, especially if it is accompanied by palpable tenderness over a temporal artery. An elevated sedimentation rate helps confirm giant cell arteritis. Finally, a neurologic or neurosurgical consultation is recommended in patients with severe headache in whom a definitive diagnosis cannot be established. A consultation also is useful with infection and/or trauma when CT is abnormal and in the presence of altered mental status.

ORGANIC HEADACHES RESULTING FROM MASS LESIONS

DISCUSSION

Mass lesions can cause headache by displacing pain-sensitive structures. Approximately one-third of patients with a mass lesion have headache as an early symptom of the disease. The pain often is reported as being localized to the side of the lesion; however, there are a variety of other presentations, none of which is precisely diagnostic. The headache may be described as mild or severe, persistent or intermittent, sharp or achy, throbbing or pressure-like. Characteristically, the headache remains in one location and becomes progressively worse, lasting for several months. In particular, patients may report that the headache is worse upon awakening. Generally, there are progressive changes in mental status and/or the development of neurologic deficits such as diplopia. Initially these headaches are aggravated by coughing, straining during bowel movements, lying down, and bending over. However, as ICP increases, the headache becomes more generalized and is associated with nocturnal awakening, dizziness, and vomiting (with or without preceding nausea) and can include generalized convulsions. In patients with a brain tumor, headache may be the sole initial complaint, unaccompanied by focal neurologic deficits. However, as the condition progresses, neurologic deficits usually arise.

The following tumors tend to produce general cerebral symptoms or seizures: metastatic carcinoma, glioblastoma multiforme, astrocytoma, oligodendroglioma, meningioma, and primary reticulum cell sarcoma of the cerebrum. The tumors that tend to elevate ICP without conspicuous localizing signs include medulloblastomas, ependymomas of the fourth ventricle, hemangioblastomas, pinealomas, colloid cysts of the third ventricle, gliomas of the tegmentum of the midbrain with blocking of the aqueduct, and craniopharyngiomas.

TREATMENT

Pharmacologic Management

Steroid therapy is initiated before tissue diagnosis in symptomatic patients with a CT or magnetic resonance imaging (MRI) scan that reveals edema surrounding an intracranial mass lesion. Although the information regarding the optimal steroid dose is mostly anecdotal, several guidelines have been established. There is a clear dose-related clinical response to corticosteroids. The majority of these patients respond favorably to dexamethasone 4 to 6 mg given by mouth or parenterally four times daily. In critically ill patients and patients who do not exhibit a favorable response to the initial therapy, one should consider massive doses such as 25 mg four times a day. The benefit for patients receiving this dose is that it allows time for more definitive therapies such as lifesaving surgical decompression. Other interventions, such as radiation, chemotherapy, and surgical intervention, should be sought whenever appropriate.

ORGANIC HEADACHES RESULTING FROM BRAIN ABSCESSES

DISCUSSION

A headache caused by a brain abscess may present as a mass lesion-causing headache, particularly during the latent stages of abscess growth. The formation of a brain abscess involves two stages. Initially a diffuse, poorly marginated area of infection is associated with edema and destruction of brain tissue. Over 4 to 9 days the center of the infection turns into semiliquid pus and necrotic brain tissue. Once this stage is reached, the infection may not be curable by medical therapy (e.g., antibiotics) alone. Encapsulation by gliotic tissue occurs gradually, and a free abscess forms. Lung abscesses, parenteral drug abuse, and parameningeal infections may serve as the source or reservoir for this type of brain infection. The symptoms of a brain abscess manifest as a subacute progression of focal neurologic signs of headache and altered mental status. Seizures occur in 20 to 25% of these patients.

DIAGNOSTIC STUDIES

The definitive diagnosis of brain abscess is made during surgery, although characteristic findings may be seen on MRI or CT. Arteriography is relatively ineffective in localizing a brain abscess.

In patients with suspected brain abscess it is advised to search for parameningeal infection. Adequate views of the mastoids and sinuses are critical, since a brain abscess caused by sinusitis usually occurs adjacent to an infected sinus cavity.

TREATMENT

Treatment consists of surgery with drainage of the abscess cavity by needle aspiration or total excision of the affected region. The best surgical treatment remains controversial; there are advocates of aspiration and defenders of total surgical excision. CT-guided stereotactic biopsy and intraoperative ultrasound make most areas of the brain relatively safe for aspiration. There is good evidence that complete excision of superficial lesions eliminates the risk of recurrence. Antibiotics are used both preoperatively and postoperatively. Antibiotic therapy alone is recommended in patients with multiple or surgically inaccessible lesions and patients who are poor candidates for surgery.

ORGANIC HEADACHES RESULTING FROM SUBDURAL HEMATOMA

DISCUSSION

Headache caused by a subdural hematoma is another type of mass lesion: a collection of blood between the dura and the underlying brain tissue. It is present in 10 to 15% of patients with severe head injuries. Acute subdural hematomas frequently result from high-speed impact accidents and are associated with severe primary brain damage. A subacute subdural hematoma is suspected when, after several days of headache or diminished alertness, deterioration of consciousness develops. Chronic subdural hematomas, in contrast to other forms of hematomas, may follow a trivial trauma that may go unnoticed by the patient and the patient's family members. Commonly, a gradual drift into stupor or coma is preceded by a headache.

DIAGNOSTIC STUDIES

Subdural Hematomas

CT is the test of choice for a subdural hematoma to demonstrate a mass effect and a midline shift beyond the thickness of a hematoma associated with brain injury.

Subacute and Chronic Subdural Hematomas

The CT density of a hematoma changes from hyperdense to isodense to hypodense (relative to brain tissue) as time progresses after a head trauma. In the isodense stages, a sizable hematoma may not be detectable by CT unless intravenous contrast is administered to enhance the vascular membranes. MRI has replaced CT as the study of choice for distinguishing subacute from chronic subdural hematomas. If MRI is not available, contrast CT, nuclear brain scanning, or arteriography can aid in this diagnosis. In the presence of cerebral edema, ICP monitoring is usually necessary during both the intraoperative and the postoperative phases.

Subarachnoid Hemorrhage from Aneurysmal Rupture

Acute rupture of a brain aneurysm produces the sudden onset of a headache that reaches its maximum intensity immediately. It often is accompanied by meningeal irritation and occasionally by an abrupt loss of consciousness. Subarachnoid hemorrhage (SAH) is one of the most common causes of death in apparently healthy young adults. However, SAH also occurs later in life, with the average age being 50 years. While a majority of these cases are caused by the rupture of an intracranial source, SAH also may result from head trauma, venous thrombosis, blood dyscrasias, and a variety of metabolic causes.

In the absence of any rupture, 10 to 15% of patients with an arteriovenous malformation (AVM) may experience chronic headaches characterized by unilateral throbbing-type pain. An acute onset of intense head pain indicates an AVM rupture. Unlike migraine, there are no prodromal or associated symptoms.

TREATMENT

Because even the latest-generation CT scanners are not sensitive enough to detect all SAHs, lumbar puncture remains an essential second step in ruling out SAH. CT is not infallible in detecting blood in the CSF. Lumbar puncture seems to be more sensitive and specific with regard to positive findings. Finally, it should be noted that MRI is no more accurate than CT in ruling out SAH. Angiography may be used, since early surgery (24 to 48 hours) has been demonstrated to be the treatment of choice for accessible ruptured aneurysms with minor neurologic impairment. Surgery is also the treatment of choice for any aneurysm that is surgically accessible. AVMs, however, may or may not be amenable to surgery, since there is a risk of recurrent hemorrhaging from AVMs.

ORGANIC HEADACHES RESULTING FROM STROKE

DISCUSSION

Head pain is frequently a presenting feature of an ischemic (embolic or thrombotic) and hemorrhagic stroke such as primary intracerebral hemorrhage and SAH. Many patients report other neurologic deficits before complaining of a headache because these symptoms (inability to talk or feel an arm or leg) seem more compelling and frightening. Headache may precede, exist concomitantly with, or follow a cerebrovascular accident (CVA; see Chap. 1-3).

On occasion headache may present sooner than the actual signaling of a stroke in evolution. Patients suffering from a stroke involving a large arterial occlusion may surprisingly present with head pain as the sole (initial) symptom. Patients with cortical lesions on CT have been found to have a headache more often than do individuals with deeper infarcts (e.g., SAH versus an ischemic stroke). Headache is more common with posterior circulatory infarcts than it is with anterior circulatory infarcts.

Ischemic strokes present as a primary thrombotic occlusion of a vessel or occlusion of a vessel by fragments from a distant source (embolism). The neurologic deficit associated with an embolism characteristically begins suddenly, with a maximum deficit occurring at the onset. Preceding transient ischemic attacks (TIAs) may occur but are less common than is primary thrombosis. Preceding TIAs are common with thrombotic strokes. This type of stroke also progresses over hours or days, with the neurologic deficit fluctuating or changing in a stepwise fashion, the so-called stroke in evolution. The treatment for stroke is covered in Chap. 1-3.

ORGANIC HEADACHES RESULTING FROM BACTERIAL MENINGITIS

DISCUSSION

Bacterial meningitis from infection or hemorrhage produces pain that is severe, acute in onset, generalized in location, and constant. The headache produced by this condition may be defined as inflammatory. The symptoms may include a severe headache, vomiting, drowsiness, and stupor and have been known to cause coma in extreme cases (see Chap. 9-28).

The causes of bacterial meningitis that vary with age are as follows:

1. *Streptococcus pneumoniae* causes 30 to 50% of cases in adults, 10 to 20% of cases in children, and up to 5% of cases in infants.
2. *Neisseria meningitidis* causes 10 to 30% of cases in adults and 30 to 40% in children up to age 15. It is rare in infants.
3. *Haemophilus influenzae* type B is responsible for 35 to 45% of cases in children but only 1 to 3% in adults. It is rare in infants.

Other pathogens may include *Staphylococcus aureus, S. epidermidis,* group B streptococci, *Escherichia coli,* and other Enterobacteriaceae, such as *Klebsiella, Enterobacter, Proteus,* and *Citrobacter* spp. Other sources of meningitis include *Treponema pallidum, Borrelia burgdorferi,* and *Leptospira interrogans.* Patients with lowered cell-mediated immunity, including transplant recipients, are especially susceptible to intracellular parasites such as *Listeria* spp.

DIAGNOSTIC STUDIES

The following are considered routine tests in all patients with presumptive bacterial meningitis: a complete blood count with differential including a peripheral blood smear, blood cultures, blood urea nitrogen and serum creatinine, serum glucose, electrolytes, and urinalysis. If nephrotoxic drugs are to be used, a baseline serum creatinine clearance is advised. One should obtain a chest x-ray and CT of the head to seek a possible parameningeal focus of infection. After a CT scan, a lumbar puncture needs to be performed to obtain a culture and sensitivities of the organisms in CSF.

TREATMENT

Once the presumptive diagnosis of bacterial meningitis has been made, antibiotic treatment must be initiated immediately. The initial therapy for bacterial meningitis usually includes intravenous ampicillin 12 g/d divided into four doses. If ampicillin-resistant strains of *H. influenzae* are common in a particular geographic area, it is reasonable to add ceftriaxone 4 to 6 g/d divided into two doses. The alternative treatment is chloramphenicol 4 g/d intravenously divided into four doses and erythromycin 4 g/d intravenously divided into four doses. Pediatric treatments and medication doses are beyond the scope of this chapter. Once antibiotic sensitivities are known through lumbar puncture or blood cultures, a more specific antibiotic selection can be made to provide optimum antibiotic availability for the identified pathogen.

OTHER HEADACHE SYNDROMES

CERVICAL ARTHRITIS

Occipital headache associated with pain on movement of the neck may be due to problems in the cervical spine. Arthritic changes can be confirmed by plain x-ray examination of the cervical spine to aid in the diagnosis of cervical arthritis. A trial of aspirin in combination with diazepam can give some relief to these patients. Many patients may also benefit from anti-inflammatory drugs. A cervical collar can be worn during the acute phase, combined with topical therapy such as cold and/or heat applications, in conjunction with physical therapy and cervical traction.

LUMBAR PUNCTURE HEADACHES

The headache that occurs after a lumbar puncture is exacerbated by standing and relieved by lying down. These headaches appear to be caused by persistent leakage of CSF from the subarachnoid space. Management consists of bed rest, analgesics, and hydration. When conservative treatment fails, an epidural blood patch is 90 to 100% effective. In this procedure, autologous blood is injected epidurally at or around the site of the previous lumbar puncture site, effectively tamponading the dural leak. Since the blood spreads both circumferentially and longitudinally along as many as nine spinal segments, the precision of the second puncture is not critical so long as the epidural space is injected.

SINUSITIS

Acute sinusitis is accompanied by a recent history of nasal stuffiness or discharge associated with pain on percussion over the sinuses. These patients often describe frontal headache and increased facial pressure when leaning forward and sometimes note upper tooth pain (see Chap. 3-1).

ACUTE CLOSED-ANGLE GLAUCOMA

The headache associated with a red, painful eye can be produced by acute closed-angle glaucoma. Open-angle glaucoma, which is more common, does not produce headache (see Chap. 14-1).

TEMPOROMANDIBULAR JOINT SYNDROME

Head pain caused by the temporomandibular joint syndrome is characterized by pain on chewing or jaw use with radiation into the ear. These patients may describe joint clicking when yawning as well as jaw restriction.

COLD STIMULUS HEADACHES

A cold stimulus headache results from external exposure to cold or the ingestion of a cold substance ("ice cream headache"). The pain is nonpulsatile and reaches a peak intensity about 25 to 60 seconds after exposure. The great majority of patients with migraine also experience ice cream headache. No treatment is necessary; the headache usually can be avoided by stirring ice cream to a semisolid consistency.

TOXIC HEADACHES

Headaches that are secondary to drugs or environmental exposure are extremely common and often go undiagnosed. Such exposure may aggravate a migraine or tension headache or an unspecified variety of headache. Generally speaking, these headaches tend to be generalized, persistent, and throbbing in nature. Their intensity increases with further exposure to ingestion of the offending agent. Drugs commonly associated with headache include atenolol, nifedipine, cimetidine, ranitidine, and various estrogens. Other implicated substances are nitrates and nitrites, monosodium glutamate, and carbon monoxide.

NONORGANIC BENIGN HEADACHES

DISCUSSION

In 1988, the Headache Classification Committee of the IHS classified headaches into organic and nonorganic disorders. The three primary benign types are tension-type headaches (TTHs), cluster headaches, and migraine headaches with and without an aura.

Headaches do not represent a single disease but instead reflect a diverse set of clinical syndromes that may be interrelated. Therefore, primary (benign nonorganic) headaches cannot be "cured." Many patients seem perplexed at medical providers' inability to stop their head pain. The exact etiology of primary benign headache is unknown.

SYMPTOMS

Depending on the type of nonorganic benign headache, the severity and nature of the pain as well as the degree of incapacity vary from person to person. The onset, frequency, location, character, and duration of the pain are very important to determine and may offer useful diagnostic clues. The pain may have patterns that disturb sleep, worsen with straining or lifting, or are accompanied by other symptoms, such as dizziness, nausea, vomiting, photophobia, phonophobia, strange smells, and scintillating scotomas. Patients may mention certain triggers or patterns of timing that aggravate or ameliorate the head pain.

OBJECTIVE FINDINGS

Most patients with an active headache appear to be uncomfortable and show various signs of being in pain. The presence of high blood pressure and/or fever should alert the clinician to the possibility of an intracranial bleed or infection, such as meningitis. One should note the patient's vital signs and examine for nuchal rigidity. It is necessary to check the patient's pupils and optic discs for irregularities, such as papilledema. One should look for visual field defects, assess facial asymmetry, test the proximal and distal muscles in the upper and lower extremities, and check all deep tendon reflexes, gait, finger-to-nose movements, and rapid rhythmic movements to differentiate between organic and nonorganic disease.

DIAGNOSTIC CONSIDERATIONS

In evaluating a patient with headaches, the issue of the need for an imaging study of the head commonly arises. Mitchell et al.[1] studied the utility of head CT in patients with headaches, particularly those with abnormal physical examinations or unusual headache characteristics. Only 1% of patients with normal examinations had an abnormal CT, whereas 10% of patients with abnormal examinations and 12% with unusual histories had abnormal CT. None of the patients with normal examinations and unusual histories had abnormal head CT scans.

TENSION-TYPE HEADACHES (MUSCLE CONTRACTION)

PATHOPHYSIOLOGY

Stressful events produce a biochemical change in the brain by which serotonin levels are generally reduced. Theoretically, this biochemical change manifests in a depressive state, although the precise biochemical counterpart of depression is not known. In endogenous depression, endorphin levels decrease, facilitating the transmission of pain impulses that can leave the patient more susceptible to pain. Muscles become tonic and contracted. Vasoconstriction occurs, causing an ischemic-type muscle pain with focal tenderness.

SYMPTOMS

Two varieties of TTHs have been identified: episodic and recurrent. The constant bilateral pain form of episodic or acute TTHs typically occurs in the late afternoon, lasting from 30 minutes to several days. It is accompanied by pain that is typically described as constricting in character and bilateral in location and often is associated with anorexia. Physical activity does not exacerbate this type of head pain. Chronic TTHs by definition occur more than 15 days a month for more than 6 months. Unlike the acute form of TTH, chronic TTHs may cause occasional nausea but no vomiting. This type of pain seldom awakens the patient from sleep. TTHs can be precipitated by stress and lack of sleep. Muscle tenderness in the neck and shoulder regions is common. The pain is described as pressure-like, squeezing, or tightening and accumulates throughout the day. Generally, TTHs begin in early adulthood while migraines usually begin in childhood.

OBJECTIVE FINDINGS

Physical examination generally reveals no abnormal findings, with the exception of tenderness and/or palpable muscle spasms at the base of the head, and neck, and/or shoulder region. Also, the patient may complain of pain when asked to perform active range-of-motion exercises of the neck.

TREATMENT

For patients who experience TTHs, pharmacologic treatment considerations include nonsteroidal anti-inflammatory drugs (NSAIDs) alone or in combination with a muscle relaxant. When headaches are not relieved with these agents, consideration of a narcotic is appropriate, to be used on an as-needed basis alone or with an NSAID. Antidepressants also should be considered appropriate treatment; tricyclics tend to work better than the selective serotonin reuptake inhibitors (SSRIs). The side effects of tricyclics, however, may make these agents less appealing for patients to use (see Table 11-3-2).

TABLE 11-3-2. Antidepressants Used for Headache Management

DRUG	ROUTE	DOSE, mg/d
Tricyclic antidepressants*		
Nonsedating types		
Desipramine	PO	5–30
Protriptyline	PO	25–150
Sedating types		
Amitriptyline	PO	10–150
Doxepin	PO	10–150
Imipramine	PO	10–150
Nortriptyline	PO	10–150
Serotonin reuptake inhibitors†		
Fluoxetine	PO	10–80
Sertraline	PO	50–200
Paroxetine	PO	20–60

*Side effects may include drowsiness, dryness of mouth, weight gain, constipation, and urinary retention.
†Side effects may include drowsiness, nausea, sweating, and irritability, but these drugs seem better tolerated than tricyclics.
NOTE: Used in prophylactic doses for migraine and chronic tension-type headaches, particularly but not exclusively those with a depression component.
ABBREVIATION: PO, oral.

CLUSTER HEADACHES

PATHOPHYSIOLOGY

The etiology of cluster headaches is not well understood. Popular theories include a vascular headache disorder and a disturbance of the serotonergic mechanism. This type of headache occurs more commonly in middle-aged men than in women and has no familial predisposition.

SYMPTOMS

The pain is a severe unilateral pain that intensifies around one eye or the temple region. The character of the pain usually is described as sharp and piercing through the affected eye. Episodes last 15 minutes to 3 hours and may recur as many as eight times a day. Headaches often occur 1 or 2 hours after the patient falls asleep, thus awakening the patient from sleep. Associated symptoms may include increased eye lacrimation, rhinorrhea, ipsilateral nasal congestion, redness of the affected eye, and Horner's syndrome (seen in approximately 25% of cluster headache patients). Spontaneous remission may occur, with the patient remaining symptom-free for several weeks before the next recurrence.

TREATMENT

For abortive treatment one should give 2 L oxygen via a mask. Injectable medications such as sumatriptan (Imitrex) and dihydroergotamine (DHE 45) can be administered intramuscularly, intravenously, or subcutaneously; oral and self-injectable forms are available. The contraindications to these medications are discussed below in the section on migraine treatment. Oral ergotamines also may be used. Prophylactic regimens include calcium channel blockers and lithium. Verapamil and lithium carbonate are the preferred treatments for chronic cluster headaches.

MIGRAINE HEADACHES

DISCUSSION

Migraine headache is a familial disorder with autosomal dominant inheritance. These patients tend to be young to middle-aged; 80% have a history of the first attack before age 30 years. About 75% of migraine headaches occur without auras, while 20% occur with auras. Less than 5% are so-called migraine variants, which include hemiplegia with ophthalmologic varieties of ocular dysfunction such as scotomas.

PATHOPHYSIOLOGY

There is a process within both the intracranial and the extracranial vascular structures with phases of vasoconstriction, vasodilation, and inflammation. Vasoconstriction produces anoxia and acidosis and a systemic drop in serum serotonin levels. During this phase a patient may experience neurologic changes called an *aura* that may include several physiologic dysfunctions, such as facial paresthesias and/or partial defects in the visual fields. Anoxia and acidosis cause a local metabolic change and a reaction potentiated by a drop in serotonin that increases cerebral blood flow and causes marked dilation of intracranial and extracranial arteries. Treatment is designed to alter the serotonin receptor reaction in the brain.

SYMPTOMS

Migraine with Aura

Auras are characterized by sensory changes, most often visual symptoms, which range from haziness to shimmering light waves (scintillating scotomas) to bright or dark holes in the visual field and frank hemianopia. Sensory symptoms also may include tingling paresthesias of the face or upper body, with the legs and trunk seldom involved. No aura symptom lasts longer than 60 minutes, and several may occur at once. These symptoms precede a headache by 30 to 60 minutes. Most cases of ophthalmoplegia resolve without residual deficits. Repeated episodes of vasospasm-induced ischemia, however, may produce infarction, thus causing permanent neurologic deficits in the brain. The head pain itself is paroxysmal, unilateral in location, and associated with nausea, vomiting, photophobia, and phonophobia. The medical history and physical examination, including a complete neurologic examination, often do not suggest other disorders.

Migraine Without Aura

Attacks of migraine with an aura last 4 to 70 hours and include at least two of the following characteristics: unilateral location, pulsating quality, moderate to severe intensity, inhibition of daily activities, aggravation by physical activities, and association with at least one of the following signs: nausea, vomiting, phonophobia, and photophobia. The history and neurologic examination do not suggest another secondary, organic headache disorder.

TREATMENT

Nonpharmacologic Therapy

Nonpharmacologic therapy is essential in a motivated patient. Nearly all primary benign headaches are associated with a component of stress or anxiety. Without exploration of these underlying issues, clinicians provide a disservice to patients by often prescribing unnecessary medications. Helpful nonpharmacologic techniques may include psychotherapy, relaxation techniques, massage, relaxation exercises, and biofeedback.

Abortive Therapy

Abortive therapy (Table 11-3-3) involves both oral and injectable deliveries of pharmacologic medications. The oral forms include ergotamines (tablets and suppositories), isometheptene mucate, NSAIDs, phenothiazines, ketorolac, and transnasal butorphanol.

DHE 45 given intramuscularly or intravenously in combination with an antiemetic [prochlorperazine (Compazine) or droperidol (Inapsine)] is another choice for abortive therapy. Side effects may include nausea, vomiting, chest pain, and transient myalgias and arthralgias. This regimen is contraindicated in patients with cardiovascular disease, peripheral vascular disease, and significant liver or renal disease.

When used subcutaneously, sumatriptan works quickly. Side effects may include flushing, chest tightness, chest pain, and transient paresthesias. This medication is contraindicated in patients on monoamine oxidase (MAO) inhibitors, patients with poorly controlled hypertension, and pregnant or nursing women. One should avoid using this drug if ergotamines have been used within the past 24 h. Sometimes, a second injection of sumatriptan has been shown to be effective if the patient's symptoms are partially reduced after the initial injection.

PREVENTION

Preventive therapy is indicated for patients who suffer from debilitating headaches at least 2 to 3 days per month. Pharmacologic interventions may include calcium channel blockers (verapamil and diltiazem), which take 4 to 6 weeks to work. In contrast, beta blockers

TABLE 11-3-3. Abortive Medications for Acute Migraine

DRUG	ROUTE	DOSE, mg	COMMENT
Sumatriptan	SC	6	May repeat once after 1 hour; up to 24 hours; do not use concommitantly with ergot alkaloids; contraindicated in presence of uncontrolled HTN, history of AMI, peripheral vascular disease, pregnancy
	PO	25, 50, 100	As above; response rates somewhat lower than parenteral routes; start with 25–50 mg; if ineffective, increase to 100 mg
Dihydroergotamine	IV, IM, SC		Often coadministered with metoclopramide or any other antiemeted individualized dose to patient, usually in range of 0.5–1.5 mg IV; IM administered in office; SC useful in home
Ergotamine tartrate (with or without caffeine)	SL	2	May repeat twice
	PO	1	With caffeine, 100 mg; oral dose two tablets at onset of headache may repeat one every 30 minutes to 6 max
Isometheptene mucate Dichloralphenazone Acetaminophen	PO	65, 100, 325	Maximum of 5 capsules in 24 hours or 2 stat, repeat 2 capsules in 1hour, then stop
High-dose nonsteroidal anti-inflammatory drugs			See Table 11-3-4; rebound can occur
Adjunctive therapy Phenothiazines	IV	10–12.5 25	Chlorpromazine
	PR		Chlorpromazine

ABBREVIATIONS: AMI, acute myocardial infarction; HTN, hypertension; IM, intramuscular; IV, intravenous; PO, oral; PR, per rectum; SC, subcutaneous; SL, sublingual.

TABLE 11-3-4. Nonsteroidal Anti-Inflammatory Medications Used for Headaches

DRUG	ROUTE	DOSE, mg/d
Naproxen	PO	250–500 bid
Fenoprofen	PO	600 tid
Flurbiprofen	PO	100 bid
Ketoprofen	PO	75 tid

NOTE: Prophylactic doses for daily use in migraine and chronic tension-type headaches.
ABBREVIATION: PO, oral.

TABLE 11-3-5. Beta Blockers Used for Headache Management

DRUG	ROUTE	DOSE, mg/d
Propranolol	PO	60–160
Nadolol	PO	20–120
Timolol	PO	10–20
Metoprolol	PO	100–200
Atenolol	PO	25–100

NOTE: Prophylactic doses for migraine and tension-type headaches. Side effects may include fatigue, depression, diarrhea, and slow heart rate, which may exacerbate underlying asthma and congestive heart failure. One approach recommends beginning at the lowest dose and progressing to the highest dose tolerated before including or switching to additional therapy.
ABBREVIATION: PO, oral.

TABLE 11-3-6. Calcium Channel Blockers Used for Headache Management

DRUG	ROUTE	DOSE, mg/d
Verapamil	PO	120–480
Flunarizine	PO	10
Diltiazem	PO	90–360
Nifedipine	PO	10–30

NOTE: Verapamil and flunarizine seem to be the most effective for migraine. Constipation is the most common side effect.
ABBREVIATION: PO, oral.

(propranolol) have an onset of only 2 to 3 days, but not all patients receive relief from this category of drugs. Tricyclic antidepressants are more effective than SSRIs and work well in patients in whom there is a component of depression and/or anxiety (Tables 11-3-4 through 11-3-6).

NOTES AND PEARLS

The following points should be noted:

- Changing headaches can be a predictor of more serious consequences.
- Any headaches that occur after age 50 are more of a concern than are headaches that begin at an earlier age.
- A headache after age 40 that is abrupt in onset should raise the possibility of an organic cause such as an intracranial hemorrhage.
- A headache that radiates all over the head is usually more innocuous than a headache that remains unilateral and stays in the same location.
- Narcotic medications should be used with caution in patients with chronic headaches. One must be aware of drug-seeking behaviors and other signs of drug dependency.

REFERENCE

1. MITCHELL CS et al: Computed tomography in the headache patient: Is routine evaluation really necessary? *Headache* 33:82–86, 1993.

BIBLIOGRAPHY

Caesar R et al: Acute headache management: The challenge of deciphering etiologies to guide assessment and treatment. *Emerg Med Rep* 16:117–128, 1995.

Dalesso DJ: Diagnosing the severe headache. *Neurology* 44:S6–S12, 1994.

Kumar KL: Recent advances in management of migraine and cluster headaches. *J Gen Intern Med* 9:339–348, 1994.

Morgenlander JC: Lumbar puncture and CSF examination. *Postgrad Med* 95:125–131, 1994.

Pearce JMS: Headache. *J Neurol Neurosurg Psychiatry* 57:134–143, 1994.

Rapoport AM: Update on severe headache. *Neurology* S5, 1994.

Sames TA et al: Sensitivity of new-generation computed tomography in subarachnoid hemorrhage. *Acad Emerg Med* 3:16, 1996.

Weir BK: Headaches form aneurysms. *Cephalalgia* 14:79–87, 1994.

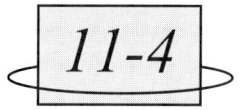

ALZHEIMER'S DISEASE
Freddi Segal-Gidan

DISCUSSION

Alzheimer's disease (AD) affects an estimated 4 million Americans. It is considered to be the fourth leading cause of death among adults, accounting for approximately 120,000 deaths per year. It is a degenerative disorder of the brain involving changes in the number, structure, and function of neurons in the cerebral cortex, producing loss of memory and intellectual function (see Chap. 11-5) along with changes in personality and behavior. The illness lasts on average 8 years, but this varies widely and can reach 15 or more years. There is no known cause or cure, but new therapies to delay the course of the disease are rapidly entering the market. Treatment is aimed at early diagnosis and supportive services for the patient and family.

Advancing age remains the primary risk factor. The incidence of AD is 1 in 100,000 at age 50 and 1 in 1000 at age 70 (Table 11-4-1). AD occurring before age 65 is classified as presenile or early-onset AD. When the disease develops after age 65, it is called senile or late-onset AD. AD affects women almost twice as often as men, though this may be partially due to the longer life span of women. Other risk factors include lower level of education, a family history of AD, a history of head trauma, and trisomy 21 (Down's syndrome). Protective factors that may delay the onset of AD include higher education, estrogen, nonsteroidal anti-inflammatory drugs (NSAIDs), vitamin E, and apolipoprotein E2. AD in persons with a first-degree relative (parent or sibling) with the disease is often referred to as familial AD, while in those without a family history it is termed sporadic AD, although these are somewhat arbitrary classifications.

PATHOGENESIS

The primary feature of AD is loss of neurons in the cerebral cortex. In 1911 Dr. Alois Alzheimer first described the presence of tangled bundles of fibers within the nerve cell (neurofibrillary tangles) and deposits (plaques) over the cortex in the brain of a 59-year-old woman who had died after a 5-year course of progressive dementia and behavioral disturbances. The presence of neurofibrillary tangles and senile plaques in certain regions of the brain remains the basis for a definitive diagnosis of AD, which presently can be made only at autopsy. The deposition of amyloid in the cerebral and meningeal blood vessels (cerebral angiopathy) also is commonly seen pathologically in AD.

SYMPTOMS

The hallmark of AD is the presence of a progressive dementia with insidious onset of no known etiology. Current research suggests that prior to manifestation of clinical symptoms a gradual phase of neuronal degeneration and dysfunction has occurred for a number of years. In early AD there are recent memory problems (forgetfulness),

TABLE 11-4-1. Prevalence of Alzheimer's Disease with Increasing Age

AGE, YEARS	PREVALENCE (%)
60–64	1
65–69	2
70–74	4
75–79	8
80–84	16
>85	30

impaired problem solving, and often difficulty making decisions. Social demeanor is usually preserved, but there may be subtle personality changes. In this stage patients may be aware of their deficits and try to compensate or may withdraw from interactions. They tend to become fearful and anxious and can become depressed.

As the disease progresses, language problems are common, with word-finding difficulty (e.g., "that thing" or "thing you write with" for a pen or pencil) and paraphasic errors ("clock" for "watch," "spoon" for "fork"). Visual-spatial difficulties increase the risk of the patient getting lost, and functional problems require increasing outside supervision. Behavioral problems and personality changes become more common in the middle stages of AD. Wandering, pacing, agitation, and paranoia are more characteristic of AD than of other dementias.

In the latter stages cognitive and functional impairment is profound, requiring supervision and assistance in even the most basic of activities. Severe language problems (aphasia), motor planning (apraxia), and incontinence, particularly of urine, are common. Individuals with AD die *with* the disease, not *from* it. Death associated with end-stage dementia and immobility usually results from accompanying infection (pneumonia, urinary, sepsis).

OBJECTIVE FINDINGS

In the history, the key element is the course of the disease, which is insidious and slowly deteriorating. AD patients typically (though not always) are physically quite healthy, have a sparse past medical history, and take no or very few medications. Mental status testing is essential for documenting the presence of dementia and decline over time. The physical examination is typically normal in AD patients. Increased tone and certain frontal release signs (suck, grasp) are common in the latter stages of the disease.

DIAGNOSTIC CONSIDERATIONS

The clinical accuracy of diagnosis is about 85%. The diagnostic criteria for AD were established in 1984 and are accepted worldwide (Table 11-4-2). A definitive diagnosis of AD can be made only on brain autopsy and requires a preexisting clinical diagnosis of probable or possible AD.

SPECIAL CONSIDERATIONS

The primary population affected by AD is over age 65, although about 10 to 15% of cases occur before that age. Although the diagnostic

TABLE 11-4-2. Criteria for the Diagnosis of Alzheimer's Disease

Clinical diagnosis of probable Alzheimer's disease

> Presence of a dementia by clinical examination and documented by mental status testing
> Deficits in two or more areas of cognition
> Progressive worsening of memory and other cognitive functions
> No disturbance of consciousness
> Onset between ages 40 and 90, most often after age 65
> Absence of systemic disorder or other brain diseases that could account for the progressive deficits in memory and cognition

Clinical diagnosis of possible Alzheimer's disease

> Dementia syndrome in the absence of another neurologic, psychiatric, or systemic disorder sufficient to cause dementia and in the presence of variations in onset, presentation, or clinical course
> Presence of a second systemic or brain disorder sufficient to produce dementia that is not considered to be the cause of the dementia
> A single, gradually progressive severe cognitive deficit in the absence of another identifiable cause

Definitive Alzheimer's disease

> Clinical criteria for probable Alzheimer's disease
> Histopathologic evidence obtained from a biopsy or autopsy of the brain

SOURCE: McKahnn et al, 1984.

criteria set 40 to 90 years as the age limits, rare cases have been diagnosed before age 40, and with the aging of the population, AD is increasingly being diagnosed in persons in the tenth decade and beyond.

LABORATORY TESTS

There is to date no definitive laboratory test for AD. A laboratory evaluation for dementia is essential (see Chap. 11-5) and should be negative. If laboratory abnormalities are identified, they must be addressed and corrected before a clinical diagnosis of AD can be made with any certainty. For instance, previously undiagnosed hypothyroidism must be treated appropriately, thyroid levels must be normalized for several months, and then repeat cognitive testing must be done to establish a persistent and progressive dementia before a clinical diagnosis of AD should be made.

RADIOLOGIC STUDIES

There are no definitive radiologic studies. Serial computed tomography (CT) or magnetic resonance imaging (MRI) of the brain over several years may show evidence of increasing generalized cortical atrophy (ventriculomegaly and enlargement of the sulci). Single-photon emission computed tomography (SPECT) and positron emission tomography (PET) typically show reduced blood flow and metabolism in the temporal and parietal lobes of the brain. It remains uncertain whether these findings are sensitive and specific for AD.

OTHER DIAGNOSTICS

Comprehensive neuropsychological testing may be helpful, especially in the early stages. It can identify specific areas of cognitive decline and their severity. Most AD patients show reduced short-term memory, which is not helped with cues, and deficits in other areas of higher cortical dysfunction, although there may be considerable variation in test results between patients.

TREATMENT

There is no curative or preventive treatment for AD. Guidelines for the appropriate treatment have recently been developed by several different groups (American Psychiatric Association, American Medical Association, California Workgroup on Guidelines for AD). Intervention is aimed at improving function and maintaining maximum independence for as long as possible. Treatment should include not only the patient but also caregivers, whether family, friends, or paid assistance.

Pharmacotherapy

There are currently three medications approved specifically for the treatment of AD: tacrine (Cognex), donepezil (Aricept), and rivastigmine (Exelon). All are cholinesterase inhibitors and have been shown to slow the rate of decline in 15% to 40% of individuals in the early to moderate stages of AD. Donepezil is preferred since it has few side effects and is dosed once daily, making it easier for patients and their caregivers to manage. Tacrine requires dosing multiple times a day with gradual increase in dose and is hepatotoxic. A number of other drugs that may slow the rate of cognitive decline or stop further progression of the disease are undergoing large-scale trials to assess their efficacy and safety but will not be available for 3 to 5 years.

Estrogen, vitamin E, and NSAIDs have recently been shown to have a protective effect on AD. To be effective they need to be used early, prior to the onset of symptoms. Who should take which of these agents, at what dose, and for how long is not well established. (See Chap. 11-5 for a discussion of pharmacologic therapy for behavioral problems associated with dementia.)

TABLE 11-4-3. Resources for Information and Assistance

National Alzheimer's Association
70 E. Lake Street
Suite 600
Chicago, IL 60601
1-800-621-0379

ADEAR (Alzheimer's Disease Education and Referral) Center
PO Box 8250
Silver Spring, MD 20907-8250
1-301-495-3311

Supportive Measures

Individuals with AD should be encouraged to remain as independent as is safely possible. A regular schedule should be maintained to minimize confusion and new learning for a person with AD.

Wandering behavior is seen frequently in patients with AD, although it also may occur with other dementia syndromes. Wandering itself is not a problem, but it presents challenges to the caregiver in regard to the safety of the patient. The goal should be not to stop the wandering (or pacing) but to ensure the safety of the wanderer. Regular physical activity, such as walking and riding a stationary bicycle, may help dissipate excess energy and thus diminish the frequency of wandering. Identification bracelets are an important preventive measure in case the individual becomes lost. Physical and chemical restraints, while frequently used in the past, are not considered appropriate except in extreme cases.

Patient Education

Patients in the early stages should be told about the diagnosis so that they can make appropriate future plans. It is important that the family know what future care the patient wants. The execution of a durable power of attorney for health care if not previously done should be encouraged among those who are cognitively able.

One of the most difficult problems with AD, as with other dementias, is driving (see Chap. 11-5). Clinicians should be aware of state laws regarding reporting requirements. It is debatable whether individuals with early AD still retain the capacity to operate a motor vehicle safely, but those in the middle to later stages are a danger to themselves and others on the road.

The bulk of care for individuals with AD falls on families. Caregivers need accurate information, emotional support, anticipatory guidance, and respite. Placement out of the home in a supportive housing environment or nursing home may have to be considered, even for short periods of time, depending on the patient and family's abilities, resources, and desires. Some AD patients remain at home until death, while others require out-of-home placement early in the course of the disease. The Alzheimer's Association and the Alzheimer's Disease Education and Referral (ADEAR) Center, a service of the National Institute on Aging, are important national resources for families and professionals (Table 11-4-3). Local chapters can provide literature, support groups, and referral to day-care programs, paid in-home aides, and nursing homes. The Internet has become an increasing resource with sites that provide information as well as others devoted exclusively to caregiver issues and support (Table 11-4-4).

TABLE 11-4-4. Internet Sites for Alzheimer's Caregivers Information and Support

Alzheimer's Association	www.alz.org
Caregiver Zone	www.caregiverzone.com
National Family Caregivers Association	www.nfcacares.org

TABLE 11-4-5. Common Causes of Delirium

Medications (prescribed, over-the-counter, illicit)

Infectious (pneumonia, urinary, decubitus)

Cardiovascular (congestive heart failure, myocardial infarction)

Cerebrovascular (cerebrovascular accident, trauma, tumor)

Metabolic (hypo- or hyperthyroid, hypo- or hyperglycemia)

Thermoregulatory (hypo- or hyperthermia)

Psychiatric (bipolar, grief and/or loss, depression)

Environmental (relocation, institutionalization)

DISPOSITION

A diagnosis of AD represents the beginning of an ongoing need for reevaluation and monitoring. Cognitive status should be reassessed at least annually to document a progressive decline consistent with AD. Changes in function should be assessed, and caregivers should be assisted in appropriate ongoing management. The physician assistant may need to suggest out-of-home placement or provide referrals for increased in-home assistance. Intercurrent medical problems should be treated in accordance with the patient's stated wishes.

COMPLICATIONS AND RED FLAGS

AD is a slowly progressive disease of neurodegeneration. Individuals without objective decline over a 1- to 2-year period may be incorrectly diagnosed. Any marked change over a short period (hours or days) in cognition or function may signal a delirium and warrants a complete evaluation for the underlying cause (Table 11-4-5). Seizures or falls in the early stages are extremely rare in AD, although they are common in the late stages of the disease.

AD is a terminal disease, but with good supportive care individuals may maintain quality of life and live for many years. In the latter stages of the disease the patient requires total care, including feeding and turning in bed regularly to avoid pressure sores (see Chap. 2-11). When a patient loses the ability to swallow, the family and the provider face the difficult decision of whether to initiate tube feeding in this terminal stage of AD. The use of nasogastric feeding tubes is only temporary (2 to 4 weeks), and then placement of a permanent gastric feeding tube must be considered.

NOTES AND PEARLS

A genetic link to an increasing incidence of AD has been detected in recent years. Currently markers on four chromosomes (1, 14, 19, and 21) have been shown to be associated with the development of AD. A strong association has been demonstrated between the apolipoprotein E (APO E) E4 allele and the development of late-onset AD. The APO E genetic test is widely available, and its results indicate which allele combination a person has inherited. Higher susceptibility to AD is indicated if the person has one or two E4 alleles. The APO E genotype is only one risk factor and should not be used as a clinical predictor of AD. In the presence of a late-onset dementia, genetic testing for APO E may help confirm a diagnosis of AD, but in the absence of dementia is not predictive.

BIBLIOGRAPHY

Alzheimer's Association: The use of APO E testing in Alzheimer's disease. *Res Pract* 5, 1996.
American Medical Association: *Diagnosis, Management, and Treatment of Dementia: A Practical Guide for Primary Care Physicians.* Chicago, 1999.
American Psychiatric Association: Practice guidelines for the treatment of patients with Alzheimer's disease and other dementias of late life. *Am J Psychiatr* 159(5, suppl):1–39, 1997.
California Workgroup on Guidelines for Alzheimer's Disease Management: *Guidelines for Alzheimer's Disease Management, Final Report published by the group itself* 1998.
Davis KL et al: A double-blind placebo-controlled multicenter study of tacrine for Alzheimer's disease. *N Engl J Med* 327:1253–1259, 1992.
Growdon J: Treatment of Alzheimer's disease. *N Engl J Med* 328:1306–1308, 1992.
Larson EB: Management of Alzheimer's disease in a primary care setting. *Am J Geriatr Psychiatr* 6(2):S34, 1998.
McKahnn G et al: Clinical diagnosis of Alzheimer's disease: Report of the NINCDS-ADRDA Work Group. Department of Health and Human Services Task Force on Alzheimer's Disease. *Neurology* 34:939–944, 1984.
Morris JC: Differential diagnosis of Alzheimer's disease. *Clin Geriatr Med* 10(2):257–275, 1994.
Small GW et al: Diagnosis and treatment of Alzheimer's disease (AD) and related disorders: Consensus statement of the American Association for Geriatric Psychiatry, the Alzheimer's Association and the American Geriatrics Society. *JAMA* 278:1363–1371, 1997.
Whitehouse PJ, Geldmacher DS: Pharmacotherapy for Alzheimer's disease. *Clin Geriatr Med* 10(2):339–350, 1994.

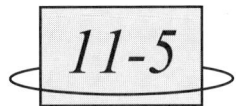

DEMENTIA
Freddi Segal-Gidan

DISCUSSION

Dementia, from the Latin *de mens,* literally means "out of one's mind." It refers to a clinical condition in which there is impairment of memory and other cognitive abilities, resulting in a loss of function. Diagnostic criteria according to the *Diagnostic and Statistical Manual of Mental Disorders,* 4th ed. (DSM-IV) include memory impairment, at least one other area of cognitive decline, and associated functional problems (see Table 11-5-1).[1] Dementia is a syndrome that represents the final common clinical expression of a variety of diseases that damage the brain (Table 11-5-2). Most dementias are irreversible, but there are many conditions with symptoms that may mimic a dementia, especially in the elderly.

Dementias occur at all ages but increase in incidence with increasing age. It is estimated that more than 40 to 50% of individuals over age 85 have cognitive impairment sufficient to meet the clinical diagnosis of dementia. The aging of the population means that there will be a growing prevalence of dementing illnesses with associated increasing costs, direct and indirect, for the care of individuals with these conditions. Early recognition of a dementia is important to prevent excessive morbidity and premature mortality and to give the patient time to make plans for future needs and care.

SYMPTOMS

It may be difficult at times to differentiate the cognitive changes associated with normal aging from those of early dementia. The

TABLE 11-5-1. DSM-IV Criteria for Dementia

A. The development of multiple cognitive deficits manifested by both
  (1) memory impairment (impaired ability to learn new information or to recall previously learned information)
  (2) one (or more) of the following cognitive disturbances:
    (a) aphasia (language disturbance); (b) apraxia (impaired ability to carry out motor activities despite intact motor function); (c) agnosia (failure to recognize or identify objects despite intact sensory function); (d) disturbance in executive functioning (i.e., planning, organizing, sequencing, abstracting)
B. The cognitive deficits in Criteria A1 and A2 each cause significant impairment in social or occupational functioning and represent a significant decline from a previous level of functioning

SOURCE: *American Psychiatric Association.*

TABLE 11-5-2. Causes of Dementia in Adults

Primary degenerative diseases
  Alzheimer's disease
  Pick's disease
  Dementia with Lewy bodies

Cardiovascular disorders
  Vascular disease (multi-infarct)
  Vasculitis

Neurologic diseases with dementia
  Huntington's disease
  Parkinson's disease
  Progressive supranuclear palsy (PSP)
  Amyotrophic lateral sclerosis (ALS)
  Multiple sclerosis (MS)
  Intracranial structural lesions
  Normal pressure hydrocephalus (NPH)
  Tumors
  Subdural hematomas

Metabolic or systemic conditions
  Hypo- or hyperthyroidism
  Hypo- or hyperglycemia
  Sarcoidosis
  Nutritional deficiencies

Infections
  Syphilis
  HIV-AIDS
  Meningitis
  Encephalitis
  Creutzfeldt-Jakob disease
  Brain abscess

Sensory deprivation

Depression

Intoxication
  Drugs and medications
  Alcohol
  Heavy metals
  Carbon monoxide
  Industrial agents (organophosphates)

TABLE 11-5-3. Differentiating Delirium From Dementia

CHARACTERISTIC	DELIRIUM	DEMENTIA
Onset	Abrupt	Gradual
Course	Fluctuating, days to hours	Stable over days to weeks
Duration	Hours to weeks	Years
Alertness	Abnormal: increased or decreased	Usually normal
Attention	Impaired	Usually normal
Orientation	Impaired for time Mistakes unfamiliar for familiar	Impaired
Memory	Immediate and recent memory impaired	Recent impaired; remote intact until late
Thinking	Disorganized	Impoverished
Perception	Illusions, hallucinations	Usually normal
Speech	Abnormal: slow or rapid	Word finding
Sleep-awake cycle	Disrupted	Fragmented sleep
Physical illness	Present	Often absent

stages of dementia individuals require increasing assistance for most basic tasks, such as dressing and bathing; they become incontinent (usually of urine first) and need 24-hour supervision for safety because of their severely impaired memory and judgment. In the terminal stages a dementia patient is bed-bound, requires total care, and may have to be fed.

OBJECTIVE FINDINGS

A comprehensive physical examination, including mental status testing to document cognitive ability, is essential in the diagnosis of dementia. A number of validated, brief screening instruments can easily be mastered and any one of them can be used routinely in the context of a standard history and physical examination (Table 11-5-5). Each instrument tests a variety of cognitive domains and can be used to screen for dementia, but none is diagnostic in and of itself. Referral for definitive neuropsychological testing should be considered for those in the very early stages of a suspected dementia (clinical dementia rating of 0.5), those who score within normal limits but remain suspicious for a dementia, and those with an unusual pattern of decline.

A thorough neurologic examination is required to detect findings of neurodegenerative diseases in which dementia is a component and other conditions that can exacerbate or contribute to an existing dementia.

DIAGNOSTIC CONSIDERATIONS

There are over 60 conditions that can manifest themselves as a dementia or in which a dementia is a primary symptom. The acronym DEMENTIA provides a helpful tool for remembering the causes of dementia that can be reversed or arrested (Table 11-5-6).

Numerous medications, as well as over-the-counter and illicit drugs, can alter cognition and produce an apparent dementia (Table 11-5-7).

Depression is not an uncommon occurrence concurrently with a dementia but also may produce symptoms of cognitive and functional decline that present as a dementia (pseudodementia). Metabolic conditions such as hypo- and hyperthyroidism and hypo- and hyperglycemia can produce alterations in cognition. Common eye and ear disorders, such as cataract and ceruminosis, often come on gradually, are asymptomatic, and may disturb cognition and function.

Nutritional problems, especially malnourishment and vitamin B_{12} deficiency, are known to impair cognition. Trauma, especially subdural

earliest symptoms of dementia often go unrecognized by patients, their families, and health care providers. There is growing evidence that mild, persistent memory loss without involvement of other cognitive areas, called mild cognitive impairment (MCI), may be a risk factor for the development of a dementia. Routine mental status testing among the elderly may help uncover an early dementia months or years sooner than it would otherwise be detected. When symptoms appear suddenly, it is important to differentiate delirium from dementia (Table 11-5-3) in order to initiate appropriate treatment promptly.

The history in a suspected dementia patient should always be confirmed by a collateral source, such as a family member or close friend. An individual may have little or no insight into his or her cognitive impairment. Often it is the family, the employer, or a close relative who notices a change in intellect, behavior, or function and brings the patient to the attention of the health care system. It is important to document the onset of cognitive problems and functional decline: Was there a gradual onset, or did things change over a short period? What activities can the person no longer perform? Most dementias, regardless of etiology, manifest progressive decline in a number of areas that can be monitored over time (Table 11-5-4).

In the early stages there are often difficulties with judgment and more complex problem solving, resulting in problems with tasks such as balancing a checkbook, paying taxes, and cooking. The patient may be apathetic and withdraw from the usual activities and social gatherings. As a dementia progresses, memory problems become more apparent, the ability to function outside the patient's own home declines, and personal care and hygiene may be neglected and require supervision. In the late

TABLE 11-5-4. Clinical Dementia Rating Scale

PROCESS	HEALTHY CDR 0*	QUESTIONABLE DEMENTIA CDR 0.5	MILD DEMENTIA CDR 1	MODERATE DEMENTIA CDR 2	SEVERE DEMENTIA CDR 3
Memory	No memory loss or slight inconsistent forgetfulness	Mild consistent forgetfulness; partial recollection of events; "benign" forgetfulness	Moderate memory loss, more marked for recent events; defect interferes with everyday activities	Severe memory loss; only highly learned material retained; new material rapidly lost	Severe memory loss; only fragments remain
Orientation	Fully oriented to time, place, and person	Fully oriented to time, place, and person	Some difficulty with time relationships; oriented for place and person at examination but may have geographic disorientation	Usually disoriented for time, often for place	Orientation to person only
Judgment, problem solving	Solves everyday problems well; judgment good in relation to past performance	Only doubtful impairment in solving problems, similarities, differences	Moderate difficulty in handling complex problems; social judgment usually maintained	Severely impaired in handling problems, similarities, differences; social judgment usually impaired	Unable to make judgments or solve problems
Community affairs	Independent function at usual level in job, shopping, business and financial affairs, volunteer and social groups	Only doubtful or mild impairment, if any, in these activities	Unable to function independently in these activities though may still be engaged in some; may still appear normal on casual inspection	No pretense of independent function outside home	No pretense of independent function outside home
Home and hobbies	Life at home, hobbies, intellectual interests well maintained	Life at home, hobbies, intellectual interests well maintained or only slightly impaired	Mild but definite impairment of function at home; more difficult chores abandoned; more complicated hobbies and interests abandoned	Only simple chores preserved; very restricted interests, poorly sustained	No significant function in home outside of own room
Personal care	Fully capable of self-care		Needs occasional prompting	Requires assistance in dressing, hygiene, keeping of personal effects	Requires much help with personal care; often incontinent

Clinical Dementia Rating Scale for More Severe Stages of Dementia (Usually Institutionalized)

PROCESS	PROFOUND CDR 4	TERMINAL CDR 5
Speech and language	Speech usually unintelligible or irrelevant; unable to follow simple instructions or comprehend commands	No response; no comprehension
Recognition	Occasionally recognizes spouse or caregiver	No recognition
Feeding	Uses fingers more than utensils; requires much assistance	Needs to be fed; may have nasogastric tube; may have swallowing difficulties
Continence	Frequently incontinent despite assistance or training	Total incontinence
Mobility	Able to walk a few steps with help; usually chair-bound; rarely out of home or residence; purposeless movements often present	Bedridden; unable to sit or stand; contractures

*CDR = clinical dementia rating. Score as 0.5, 1, 2, 3 only if impairment is due to cognitive loss.
SOURCE: Adapted with permission from Hughes CP et al: A new clinical scale for the staging of dementia. Br J Psychiatry 140:566, 1982.

hematomas and intracranial masses, can affect cognition and appear insidiously or abruptly as confusion. Infectious diseases such as pneumonia, urinary tract infections, and syphilis present in the elderly subtly and can produce a delirium that often is mistaken for dementia. In younger individuals HIV-AIDS is increasing as a primary cause of dementia, and with the aging of the population and increasing survival of middle-aged HIV-positive individuals, HIV-AIDS needs to be included as a diagnostic consideration for the elderly, as well. Alcohol use and arteriosclerotic disease (cardiac and cerebral) may be the underlying reason for a decline in cognitive and other functional abilities.

Cerebrovascular disease (vascular or multi-infarct dementia) accounts for about 15% of all dementias in the United States and a considerably higher percentage in other countries (e.g., Japan). These patients usually have a stepwise pattern of decline with periods of stability. They frequently have hypertension, diabetes, peripheral vascular disease, and cardiac problems (arrhythmia, angina, congestive heart failure). In patients with large-vessel disease, cognitive deficits are associated with hemiplegia or aphasia. Small-vessel disease is more difficult to detect, as there may be no or only very subtle neurologic abnormalities on physical examination.

Normal pressure hydrocephalus (NPH) is the most common structural abnormality associated with dementia. It is one of the few surgically correctable causes of dementia. Classically, the patient presents with the triad of early dementia, urinary incontinence, and gait ataxia. Surgical shunting of cerebrospinal fluid can produce a significant improvement in cognition and function and a slowing of further decline, especially when it is done early in the course.

TABLE 11-5-5.   Mental Status Screening Instruments

Folstein Mini-Mental State Exam (MMSE)
Modified Mini-Mental Status Exam (3MS)
Blessed Memory-Information-Concentration Test
Short Portable Mental Status Questionnaire (SPMSQ)
Cognitive Capacity Screening Exam
Kokman Short Test of Mental Status
Cognitive Assessment Screening Inventory (CASI)

Prion diseases are a group of unusual and fatal neurodegenerative diseases caused by transmissible, protein-related infectious agents. Dementia is often the primary presentation of these diseases, which are also referred to as *slow virus diseases.* The most frequent human prion disease is Creutzfeld-Jakob disease (CJD).

Dementia with Lewy bodies (DLB) is an insidious neurodegenerative disease of progressive cognitive impairment leading to dementia as the hallmark feature, much like Alzheimer's disease. Fluctuations in cognition, visual hallucinations, and Parkinsonian motor features (slow, shuffling gait; stiffness; muscle rigidity) early in the course of the disease differentiate it from other dementias.

There are a number of neurodegenerative diseases in which dementia can be a prominent symptom. The most common are Parkinson's disease (see Chap. 11-7), Huntington's disease, and multiple sclerosis (see Chap. 11-02).

SPECIAL CONSIDERATIONS

Undiagnosed or misdiagnosed dementia is a costly illness in terms of both dollars and lives. Not all dementia is Alzheimer's, even in those over age 65. Of dementias in persons over age 65, 40% are due to other causes. Among younger individuals, HIV-AIDS is the fastest-growing cause of dementia.

LABORATORY TESTS

No single test or laboratory formula for detecting and diagnosing a dementia exists. A comprehensive hematologic workup is required to look for possible underlying causes or contributing factors (Table 11-5-8). HIV testing should be done in individuals with dementia and a history of high-risk behavior recently or in the past 5 to 10 years.

An electrocardiogram is important to rule out an underlying myocardial infarction and serve as a baseline for current or future pharmacologic treatment of associated behavioral problems.

RADIOLOGIC STUDIES

The use of brain imaging remains controversial. The American Academy of Neurology has suggested that a neuroimage be obtained at least once in all cases of dementia.[2] Neither computed tomography (CT)

TABLE 11-5-6.   Reversible Causes of Dementia

D	Drugs
E	Emotional and endocrine disorders
M	Metabolic disorders
E	Eye and ear dysfunctions
N	Nutritional deficiencies
T	Tumor or trauma
I	Infections
A	Alcohol, anemia, atherosclerosis

TABLE 11-5-7.   Drugs That Affect Cognition

Antianxiety agents (benzodiazepines)
Antidepressants (lithium, amitriptyline)
Antihistamines (diphenhydramine, hydroxyzine)
Antihypertensives (clonidine, hydralazine, methyldopa, propranolol, reserpine)
Antimicrobials (isoniazid)
Antiparkinsonian drugs (amantadine, bromocriptine, carbidopa)
Antipsychotics (haloperidol, thiothixene, thioridazine, chlorpromazine)
Cardiovascular (atropine, digitalis, diuretics, lidocaine)
H_2 blockers (cimetidine)
Hypnotics (barbiturates, benzodiazepines, chloral hydrate)
Narcotics (codeine, meperidine, morphine, propoxyphene)
Steroids

nor magnetic resonance imaging (MRI) of the brain is diagnostic unless an underlying intracranial structural process is involved. Such imaging is definitely warranted if one suspects a stroke, tumor, or subdural hematoma.

OTHER DIAGNOSTICS

An electroencephalogram (EEG) should be considered if there is the possibility of an underlying seizure disorder but is not routinely recommended. Lumbar puncture is indicated when there is suspicion of a central nervous system infection, a reactive (positive) serum syphilis serology, or hydrocephalus, and when there is a rapidly progressive or unusual dementia. Positron emission tomography and single-photon emission computed tomography scans remain experimental in the diagnostic workup of dementia.

Referral to a psychologist for comprehensive neuropsychological testing may be necessary in the very early stages and for individuals with cognitive deficits that are difficult to assess with screening tests. Psychological referral for assessment and therapy for individuals with depression should be considered. A psychiatric consultation may be required for the associated behavioral problems.

TABLE 11-5-8.   Laboratory Workup for Dementia

Essential
Complete blood count with differential
Electrolytes
Blood urea nitrogen and creatinine
Glucose
Liver function tests
Calcium, magnesium
Protein, albumin
Thyroid-stimulating hormone
Vitamin B_{12}, folate
Syphilis serology
Urinalysis
Chest x-ray
Electrocardiogram
Selective/Optional
Neuroimage of brain (computed tomography or magnetic resonance imaging)
Electroencephalogram
Lumbar puncture
Experimental
Single-photon emission computed tomography
Positron emission tomography
Genetic testing (apolipoprotein E)

TREATMENT

The appropriate treatment depends on an accurate diagnosis of the underlying cause of the dementia. If delirium is suspected as the cause or as a contributing factor, treatment of the delirium should be undertaken aggressively.

Pharmacologic Management

All medications, prescription and nonprescription, that are not absolutely essential should be discontinued. Some medications cannot be stopped abruptly but must be reduced in dose gradually. Alcohol and any illicit drug use must cease for several months before an accurate assessment of cognitive status can be obtained.

Depression, either as the primary underlying diagnosis or as a contributing factor, warrants pharmacologic therapy along with counseling, psychotherapy, and other appropriate activities. Antidepressants with minimal anticholinergic activity should be started at a low dose, with gradual increases every 1 or 2 weeks. If the depressive symptoms include insomnia, nortriptyline and trazodone, which have sedating qualities, can be tried. When there is agitated depression, the selective serotonin reuptake inhibitor (SSRI) agents such as fluoxetine (Prozac), paroxetine (Paxil), and sertraline (Zoloft) may be more appropriate. A practitioner unfamiliar with these medications should consult with or refer to a geriatric psychiatrist for assistance.

Many dementia patients experience disruptive behaviors of agitation, anxiety, aggression, and delusions or hallucinations during the course of illness. These behaviors are very frightening to caregivers and often precipitate institutionalization. It is important to assess whether these behaviors are part of a delirium caused by an underlying acute illness and, if so, to treat the intercurrent illness appropriately and aggressively. Behavioral problems are best managed by environmental manipulation such as taking the individual for a drive or a walk, playing soothing music, and engaging the patient in a distracting activity (puzzles, painting, etc.). When psychotic behaviors persist and present a potential danger, antipsychotics should be considered (Table 11-5-9). The difficulty is that most of these agents can cause increased confusion and agitation or severe lethargy.

Supportive Measures

Many community resources can provide ongoing assistance for an individual with dementia. Senior centers with structured activities may be appropriate for an individual with an early or mild dementia. Adult daycare programs are appropriate for community-dwelling individuals in the mild to moderate stages of a dementia. They provide structured daily activities, socialization, and supervision as well as a respite for caregivers. In-home assistance or out-of-home placement in a supervised living situation may be necessary for a person with a dementia who lives alone. Referral to a hospice for dementia in the terminal stages is appropriate.

Patient Education

Patients and families need accurate diagnostic information to understand the etiology of the dementia. Referral to national associations and their local chapters such as the Alzheimer's Association, Parkinson's Foundation, and Multiple Sclerosis Society is appropriate for individuals with specific dementia diagnoses. Libraries and local bookstores have many books on dementia written for the consumer that can help the family understand the illness better. There are even books that help children deal with a family member with dementia. The American Association of Retired Persons (AARP) and the National Institute on Aging publish free pamphlets about memory loss, aging, and dementia.

Those in the early stages of a dementia who maintain the ability to communicate their needs should be encouraged to discuss their wishes for future care and to complete an advanced directive (preferably a durable power of attorney for health care). The issue of driving

TABLE 11-5-9. Pharmacologic Agents for Behavioral Management in Dementia

Agent	Usual Daily Dose	Indicative Behavior
Haloperiodol	0.5 mg (0.5–3 mg)	Agitation, delusions
Thioridazine	75 mg (10–75 mg) 25 mg (10–75 mg)	Agitation, delusions, insomnia
Risperidone (Risperdal)	1–4 mg (0.5–3 mg bid)	Agitation, delusions
Quetiapine (Seroquel)	25–100 mg (25–150 mg bid)	Agitation, delusions
Buspirone	15 mg (5–40 mg)	Agitation, anxiety
Olanzapine (Zyprexa)	5 mg (2.5–20 mg)	Agitation, anxiety
Trazadone	100 mg (50–400 mg)	Agitation, insomnia
Oxazepam	10 mg (20–60 mg)	Anxiety
Lorazepam	1 mg (0.5–6 mg)	Anxiety
Temazepam	15 mg (15–30 mg)	Insomnia
Nortriptyline	50 mg (50–100 mg)	Depression
Fluoxetine	20 mg (5–40 mg)	Depression
Paroxitine	20 mg (20–50 mg)	Depression
Venlafaxine	75 mg (75–200 mg)	Depression
Citalopram (Celexa)	20 mg (20–40 mg qid)	Depression
Venlafaxine (Effexor)	75–100 mg (37.5–300 mg qid)	Depression
Carbamazepine	600 mg (800–1200 mg)	Agitation
Propranolol	20 mg (60–240 mg)	Agitation

is among the most difficult for these patients, their families, and providers. Individuals with many conditions, including most dementias, that impair the ability to operate a motor vehicle should not drive, as they may be a danger to themselves and others. In many states, such as California, dementia is included in the list of diseases reportable to the department of public health. Often families are relieved and patients are angered when they are informed that a patient should no longer drive. Referral to a driver's assessment program (such as 55 Alive, sponsored by the AARP) or for testing by the state's department of motor vehicles may be necessary to demonstrate the inability of a patient with dementia to operate a car safely.

DISPOSITION

Follow-up depends on the underlying etiology of the dementia. If a structural lesion is found, appropriate referral to a neurosurgeon is required. When a delirium or an intercurrent acute problem is found, it should be treated and followed appropriately. Cognitive status should be reassessed several months after the correction of any underlying problem.

COMPLICATIONS AND RED FLAGS

Regardless of the age of the patient, changes in cognition and function should not be ignored or considered "normal." When cognitive and functional status deteriorates abruptly, hospitalization may be required. When the behavioral problems associated with a dementia are severe, the patient may require psychiatric intervention and hospitalization.

NOTES AND PEARLS

The initial diagnosis of dementia cannot be made in an individual who is comatose, in the postoperative state, or in an emergency room.

Serial examinations over a period of time are the best way to make an accurate clinical diagnosis of dementia. Dementia assessment centers in many metropolitan areas, often affiliated with medical schools, can provide comprehensive assessment and family education and assist in the management of patients with behavioral problems or unusual findings.

REFERENCES

1. American Psychiatric Association: *Diagnostic and Statistical Manual of Mental Disorders,* 4th ed, Washington, DC, American Psychiatric Association, 1994.
2. Corey-Bloom J et al: Diagnosis and evaluation of dementia. *Neurology* 45:211–218, 1995.

BIBLIOGRAPHY

Emergy VA, Oxman TE (eds): *Dementia Presentations, Differential Diagnosis and Nosology.* Baltimore, Johns Hopkins University Press, 1994.
Maletta GJ: Treatment considerations for Alzheimer's disease and related dementing illnesses. *Clin Geriatr Med* 4(4):699–702, 1988.
National Center for Cost Containment: *Dementia Identification and Assessment: Guidelines for Primary Care Practitioners.* Washington, DC, Veterans Health Administration, 1997.
Schmitt FA et al: Cognitive mental status examinations. *Clin Geriatr Med* 5(3):545–581, 1989.
Small GW: Differential diagnosis and early detection of dementia. *Am J Geriatr Psychiatr* 6(2):S26–S33, 1998.

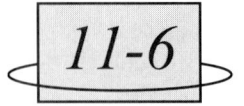

MYASTHENIA GRAVIS

Christopher C. Stephanoff

DISCUSSION

Myasthenia gravis (MG) is the most common of the three disorders that affect the myoneural junction. Each of these disorders presents with varying symptoms of weakness, fatigue, and delayed recovery time, with the characteristic symptoms resulting from transmission abnormalities. As an autoimmune disease, MG manifests when circulating antibodies attack and destroy acetylcholine receptors on the postganglionic membrane of the neuromuscular junction, which is the interface between the nerve and muscle fibers. It functions as a chemical pathway through which an action potential is conducted from the presynaptic to the postsynaptic nerve element. Loss of these receptor sites greatly reduces a neurotransmitter's effectiveness.

Individual nerves originating in the spinal cord and brainstem branch extensively, with each interfacing with and innervating as many as 2000 skeletal muscle fibers at a point termed the synapse (see Fig. 11-6-1). The three basic components of the synapse are the presynaptic membrane, the synaptic cleft, and the postsynaptic membrane. Acetylcholine, a neurotransmitter, is synthesized and stored in vesicles on the presynaptic membrane. If an arriving stimulus possesses sufficient intensity, acetylcholine molecules are released and traverse the synaptic cleft to bind with receptor sites on the postsynaptic membrane. Depolarization takes place at the postsynaptic membrane, causing an influx of sodium and an efflux of potassium ions. The resulting action potential is reproduced along the sarcolemma, producing contraction of the innervated muscle fiber or fibers. Relaxation—cessation of myofibril contraction—takes place when the enzyme acetylcholinesterase destroys acetylcholine molecules. Research has shown that in the synapse, myasthenic patients produce yields and concentrations of acetylcholine that are comparable to those of nonmyasthenic patients. However, in a myasthenic patient, circulating acetylcholine receptor antibodies (AChR-ab) reduce the number of receptor sites on the postsynaptic membrane and bind themselves to those which remain.

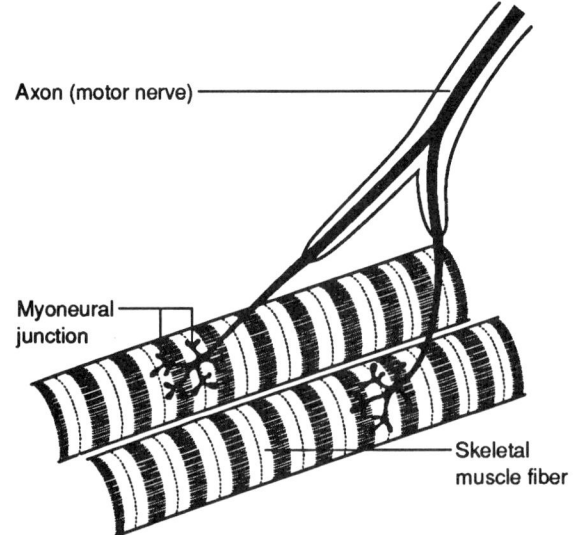

FIGURE 11-6-1. Motor unit. Motor neuron and the muscle fibers innervated by that neuron.

Depolarization thresholds are achieved less frequently, reducing propagated action potentials (see Fig. 11-6-2).

Early muscular weakness and fatigue ensue because fewer muscle fibers are recruited for contraction. Thus, MG patients often describe their symptoms as being more pronounced at the day's end. Although acetylcholine antibodies are known to cause their motor deficiency, the mechanism of action is poorly understood. Also, no direct correlation exists between the number of circulating antibodies and the severity of the disease.

Two pieces of credible evidence support the theory involving acetylcholine receptor antibodies. First, children born to myasthenic mothers have only temporary symptoms of the disease that resolve shortly after birth. Second, plasmapheresis, which is included among the treatment regimens, provides temporary symptomatic relief.[1] Histologically, no changes in muscle parenchyma are seen.

Although MG may manifest at any age and in both sexes, two incidence peaks are seen: young adult females and elderly males. Although these two incidence peaks are recognized, MG is difficult to diagnose in the geriatric population because of comorbid illnesses and vague symptoms. Rates for elderly patients in the seventh decade or beyond range between 13 and 20 percent.[1] The incidence of the disease ranges anywhere from 1 in 10,000 to 1 in 20,000 people. Also, no apparent

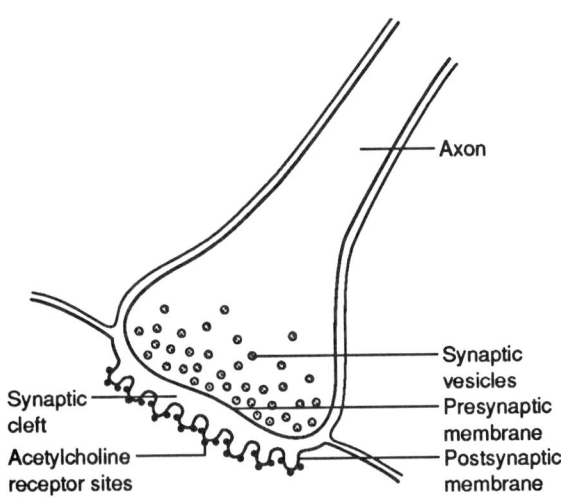

FIGURE 11-6-2. Synapse demonstrating the relationship between neural and muscular structures.

racial or geographic predilections exist. In older patients, it is more common to find an increase in thymus gland masses, whether they are malignant or benign. The significance of this finding lies in the potential for remission or a decrease in symptoms after excision of the tumor.[2–4]

SIGNS AND SYMPTOMS

Muscle weakness, fatigue, and delayed recovery, which increase with exercise and decrease with rest, are the symptoms that most frequently prompt affected individuals to seek medical attention. In most patients, the disease has an insidious course and is manifested initially as impaired ocular movement and eyelid droop (ptosis). In the remainder of MG patients, the onset is abrupt. In less than 20% of MG patients, ocular involvement is the sole manifestation, but most patients have additional striated muscular involvement.

Motor weakness in striated muscles may be exacerbated by certain stressors (illness, menstruation). Other regions of the body with a high incidence of involvement include the muscles of mastication and swallowing, the muscles of respiration, and the proximal skeletal muscles. Paresthesia, or sensory loss, is not evident in a myasthenic patient. The course of the disease is variable in that it may be remitting, static, or progressive.

DIAGNOSTIC STUDIES

Diagnosing MG, as with other disease entities, begins with a detailed medical history and careful physical examination. Too often, MG is a diagnosis of exclusion. Patients presenting with "weakness" as the chief complaint often are thought to be malingering, are not taken seriously, and are believed to have an underlying psychiatric problem.[4] Eliciting a history of extreme end-of-day muscle weakness, diplopia, ptosis, weakness, and fatigue improved by rest provides the clinician with the "keys" to an accurate diagnosis.

Physical diagnostic confirmation should include repetitive exercises directed at reproducing the symptoms stated in the chief complaint. For example, the patient is instructed to maintain an upward gaze for several minutes, and as the levator oculi becomes fatigued, the practitioner looks for the eyelids to begin closing over the eyes. Examining the "cardinal fields of gaze and confrontation" may reproduce diplopia or ocular divergence.[5–8] In patients with difficulty eating and/or drinking, swallowing small sips of water may reproduce the symptoms of drooling and/or choking.[5] Clinicians may employ a variety of tests to achieve an accurate diagnosis.

The infusion of 2 mg of edrophonium chloride (Tensilon) is used often. Tensilon, an anticholinesterase agent with rapid onset and short duration, quickly resolves clinical symptoms and temporarily restores normal muscle function. If the first infusion fails to alleviate or at least improve the symptoms, a second infusion with 8 mg is recommended. Two infusions rather than one of 10 mg are used to prevent potential side effects, such as nausea, diarrhea, salivation, and syncope. Repetitive nerve stimulation (RNS), evaluation of action potentials, and serum analysis of anti-AChR antibodies may be necessary when the results of Tensilon injections are inconclusive.[4]

Electric shocks delivered to a myasthenic patient at a rate of two to three per second will evoke decreased amplitude in action potentials of approximately 10 to 15%.[9] Repeating the RNS while dosing the patient with edrophonium will inhibit this reaction. Serum antibodies are present in approximately 80% of those affected and are considered pathognomonic.[4] In a patient in whom a thymoma is under consideration as the cause, thoracic computed tomography (CT) or magnetic resonance imaging (MRI) is suggested.[10]

TREATMENT

A neurologist should undertake definitive evaluation and care of patients who are thought to be affected with MG. Follow-up depends on the extent of involvement, the course of the disease, and the treatment regimen necessary. In the past, the diagnosis of MG meant almost certain death, usually as a result of respiratory failure.[6]

Today medical and surgical treatment modalities enable most patients to resume fully productive lives. Treatments include anticholinergic medications, thymectomy, immunosuppression, and plasmapheresis. Anticholinergic medications such as oral pyridostigmine improve all the symptoms in some but not all MG patients.

Pyridostigmine is prescribed at a starting dose of 60 mg three to five times daily. The onset of action is 15 to 30 minutes, and it has a duration of 3 to 4 hours. The dosing schedule of the medication should coincide with the times of greatest need.

Surgery may be necessary in patients who are found to have a thymoma, especially those with malignant tumors. Up to 85% of myasthenic patients who undergo thymectomy improve, and approximately 35% can discontinue oral therapy entirely. An improved prognosis is reported when thymectomy is performed within 8 months of symptom onset.[2] Recommendations for thymectomy are questionable in pediatric and geriatric patients, yet this remains the mainstay of treatment in teenagers and middle-aged patients.

Therapy with immunosuppressive agents such as corticosteroids demonstrates a spectrum of symptom remission in nearly all MG patients. Dosing of glucocorticoids should begin between 15 and 25 mg per day, increasing slowly (usually 5 mg every 3 days). Dose increases should continue until an improvement of symptoms or a maximum dose of 50 mg per day is reached. Some authors recommend maintaining the effective level for 1 to 3 months and then modifying the regimen so that patients ultimately receive 100 mg on alternate days. Any patient receiving prolonged glucocorticoid therapy should receive serial follow-up to monitor and treat possible side effects.

Since the circulating antibodies are found in a myasthenic patient's plasma, short-term plasmapheresis may be used in the event of medical procedures or for the prevention of a respiratory crisis. This process involves removing several liters of the patient's blood, centrifuging it to remove plasma that contains the receptor antibodies, and then reinfusing red blood cells with artificial plasma.[4] Another treatment regimen demonstrates that MG patients undergoing inspiratory and expiratory muscle training improve their breathing function and respiratory muscle endurance.[4]

Patient Education

In a myasthenic patient, prevention of symptoms is critical. Avoidance of offending stimuli, ample physical rest, and a healthy diet should be emphasized in counseling sessions. Despite the prevalence of fatigue, treatment protocols are lacking; thus, patients are left to self-manage.[3] Patients are empowered by education. Their active participation provides them with a sense of control in managing the disease. Tailoring a "self-help" protocol to fit their individual needs can be a powerful adjunct to "prescribed" therapies. For example, rest periods during the day give affected skeletal muscle groups the time needed to recoup. Stress management classes may alleviate stress-related fatigue. Dietitians may be consulted to discuss proper diets, including diets high in potassium. Support groups can lend an ear to patients and their caregivers and families.

COMPLICATIONS

Myasthenic or cholinergic crises are conditions that require emergency treatment. A myasthenic crisis results from too little medication and/or too many stressors: infection, injury, or medication changes. A cholinergic crisis, by contrast, is directly related to increased anticholinergic activity, often as a result of overmedication. In both cases, patients frequently present to emergency rooms in varying levels of respiratory failure. Immediate treatment must include airway, breathing, and circulation (ABC) protocols because respiratory failure is the myasthenic complication that is most often responsible for death. Urgent management includes instituting the therapy necessary to correct the underlying cause. Possibilities include reducing or stopping anticholinergic medication, treatment of infections with appropriate antibiotics, pulmonary therapy, and, as was mentioned earlier, plasmapheresis.

REFERENCES

1. Kleiner-Gisman G, Kott HS: Myasthenia gravis mimicking stroke in elderly patients. *Mayo Clin Proc* 73(11):1077–1078, 1998.
2. Nieto IP, Robled JP, Pajuelo MC, et al: Prognostic factors for myasthenia gravis treated by thymectomy. *Ann Thoracic Surg* 67(6):1568–1571, 1999.
3. Grohar-Murray ME, Becker A, Reilly S, Ricci M: Self-care actions to manage fatigue among myasthenia gravis patients. *J Neurosci Nurs* 30(3):191–199, 1998.
4. Weiner P, Gross D, Meiner Z, et al: Respiratory muscle training in patients with moderate to severe myasthenia gravis. *Can J Neurol Sci* 25(3): 236–241, 1998.
5. Andreoli TE, Bennett JC, Carpenter CC: Disorders of myoneural junction and skeletal muscle, in Plum F (ed), *Cecil Essentials of Medicine,* 4th ed, Philadelphia, Saunders, 1997, pp 921–922.
6. Seybold ME: Diseases of the neuromuscular junction, in Stein JH (ed): *Internal Medicine,* 4th ed, St. Louis, Mosby, 1994, pp 1104–1106.
7. Hartung MS: Neurologic disorders with generalized symptomatology: Myasthenia gravis, in Price SA, Wilson LM (eds): *Pathophysiology: Clinical Concepts of Disease Processes,* 4th ed, St. Louis, Mosby, 1992.
8. Bates B: The nervous system, in *A Guide to Physical Examination and History Taking,* 6th ed, Philadelphia, Lippincott, 1995, pp 491–554.
9. Devinsky O, Feldman E, Weinreb H, Wilterdink J (eds): Neuromuscular junction disease: Postsynaptic disease, in *The Resident's Neurology Book.* Philadelphia, Davis, 1997, pp 177–178.
10. Myers AR (ed): Disorders of the neuromuscular junction: Myasthenia gravis, in *National Medical Series for Independent Study,* 3d ed, Baltimore, Williams & Wilkins, 1997, pp 641–642.

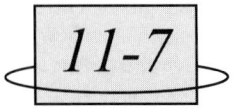

PARKINSON'S DISEASE
Kimberly Brown

DISCUSSION

In 1817, Dr. James Parkinson, a London physician, published his famous "Essay on the Shaking Palsy," in which he described the important and singular condition now known as Parkinson's disease (PD).[1]

Isolated symptoms and features of PD—the characteristic shaking or tremor and the hurrying festination of gait and speech—have been described by physicians back to the time of Galen. However, it was Parkinson who first saw every feature and aspect of the illness as a whole.[2]

PD is a degenerative disorder of the basal ganglia of unknown etiology. It is a relatively common disorder that occurs in all ethnic groups, with an approximately equal sex distribution. The prevalence of PD is reported to be 300 to 350 cases per 100,000 individuals. Approximately 50,000 new cases of PD are diagnosed every year, adding up to greater than one million PD cases. Of affected individuals, 80% are between the ages of 60 and 79. The most common variety, idiopathic PD (Latin paralysis agitans, "shaking palsy"), begins most often between 45 and 65 years of age. Approximately 20% of people older than 65 and more than 50% of those older than 85 have signs of Parkinsonism. A positive family history is present in about 5% of these patients, but genetic factors are not thought to be important determinants of the disease.[3]

The only risk factor associated with PD is advancing age. Aging changes in the basal ganglia may be responsible for noted slower movements, difficulty in coordination, and a decrease in the control of fine motor movements.

PATHOGENESIS

The principal pathologic feature of PD is degeneration of the substantia nigra, particularly the zona compacta. Degenerative changes also are found in other brainstem nuclei, especially the locus caeruleus and the dorsal metanucleus of the vagus. The Lewy body (the pathologic hallmark of PD) is found in degenerating neurons in most cases of idiopathic PD. Pathologic changes occur less predictably in the globus pallidus, striatum, and cortex.

Neurons of the substantia nigra project to the corpus striatum (caudate nucleus and putamen), where they release the neurotransmitter dopamine. Loss of striatal dopamine is the principal biochemical defect in PD. An imbalance of dopamine and cholinergic activity has been proposed to explain clinical phenomena in diseases of the basal ganglia. A relative excess of dopaminergic activity produces involuntary movements; a relative excess of cholinergic activity produces akinesia and rigidity.[3]

Causation is unknown, although it is almost certain that genetic and environmental factors play a role. Stress appears to exacerbate PD but it has not been identified as a causative factor. PD is noted more often in patients with chronic depression. The decreased dopamine in the central nervous system may be a common factor in both PD and chronic depression.[4]

SYMPTOMS AND SIGNS

Diagnosis early in the disease, when the symptoms are mild and may be confined to one side of the body, can pose a problem. However, fully developed PD is unmistakable. Parkinsonism is a clinical syndrome defined by the triad of bradykinesia, rigidity, and resting tremor. The presence of two of three of these cardinal manifestations is required to make the diagnosis. The resting tremor is common and present in about 75% of patients. It characteristically is often the first sign of PD. This tremor involves the face, tongue, and limbs and is often asymmetric. It may begin in one hand and progress to the ipsilateral foot, eventually becoming bilateral. Characteristically, it is usually slower in frequency than essential tremor and has a "pill rolling" motion in the hands at about four to six cycles per second. The tremor is more evident at rest, decreases with voluntary activity, and is absent during sleep.[4] Rigidity, defined as an increase in resistance to passive movement, is responsible for the characteristically flexed posture seen in Parkinson's patients. Cogwheel rigidity refers to the combined rigidity and tremor elicited by extending the flexed forearm or by pronation–supination movements. Bradykinesia (slow movement) and postural instability are also disabling symptoms associated with the disease. The outcome is a slow shuffling gait with a tendency toward propulsion or retropropulsion. Postural instability results from the loss of voluntary movements as well as corrective "righting" reflexes. Absent autonomic righting reflexes may cause the patient to slump over a chair and fall. Patients also describe nightmares; depression; excessive salivation; difficulty turning in bed, buttoning clothes, or cutting food; and problems walking. Orthostatic hypotension, constipation, cognitive impairment, mild intellectual deterioration, micrographia, hypophonia, urinary incontinence, and impotence are symptoms of the more advanced stages of PD.

CLINICAL DIAGNOSIS

The diagnosis of PD is based on a thorough history and physical examination. Neuropsychological testing may help define intellectual impairment. Computed tomography, magnetic resonance imaging, electroencephalogram, and cerebrospinal fluid results are typically normal. Critical evaluation of a patient who is suspected of having PD should include the following checklist:

- Relatively immobile face with widened palpebral fissures
- Variable resting tremor
- Meyerson's sign (repetitive tapping over the bridge of the nose produces a sustained blink response)
- Infrequent blinking
- Rigidity in some or all limbs
- Fixed facial position
- Slowness of voluntary movements
- Seborrhea of face and scalp

• Mild blepharoclonus
• Circumoral tremor

Other findings may include drooling resulting from impairment of swallowing; soft and/or poorly modulated voice; impairment of fine or rapid movements; difficulty walking, with a gait characterized by small, shuffling steps; and difficulty turning and stopping. No alternation in the tendon reflexes or plantar responses is typically noted. Dementia may be present in 15 to 30% of patients (notably, it is more prominent in patients who are not severely affected by tremor).[1]

The differential diagnosis of PD can include those disorders from depression to vascular or frontal disease. If a diagnosis of depression with psychomotor retardation is expected a trial of an antidepressive medication may be conclusive.[5] Drug-induced PD is commonly reversible over the course of several days after withdrawal of the offensive medication. Major tranquilizers including chlorpromazine and haloperidol, antihypertensives including reserpine, and gastrointestinal medications including metoclopramide can commonly cause drug-induced PD.

Huntington's disease, multiple system atrophy (Shy-Drager syndrome), progressive supranuclear palsy (Steele-Richardson-Olszewski syndrome), and Creutzfeldt-Jakob disease all present with features of PD and should be included in the differential diagnosis when bradykinesia and rigidity are apparent.[4]

TREATMENT

Not all patients require treatment. Levodopa is the most effective agent in PD and nonresponse to adequate doses should cast doubt on the diagnosis. Some symptoms, such as pronounced tremor, may require very high dosages before a therapeutic effect is seen.

Once a diagnosis of idiopathic PD is made, therapeutic measures can be aimed at three goals: to restore premorbid levels of neuronal integrity and function, to prevent progression, and to obtain symptomatic improvement.[5]

Pharmacologic Management

In order to treat Parkinson's disease it is necessary to restore the dopaminergic function lost with degeneration of the substantia nigra in the extrapyramidal pathway. The principal pharmacologic agent for treating PD is levodopa, which usually is administered in combination with carbidopa to prevent enzymatic conversion of levodopa to dopamine in peripheral tissues. Combined levodopa/carbidopa has a short half-life of 90 minutes, with the plasma concentration of the drug wearing off in 3 to 4 hours subsequently requiring a minimum of three daily doses. The levodopa/carbidopa combination should be taken without food since the amino acids from ingested proteins interfere with the intestinal absorption of this medication combination. An acceptable response to this formulation can be seen by severely limiting protein intake until dinner. The daily allowance of protein (0.8 g/kg of body weight) can then be provided by dinner and an evening snack.

Five additional categories of pharmacologic treatment exist: dopamine agonists, monoamine oxidase type B (MAO-B) inhibitors, catechol O-methyltransferase (COMT) inhibitors, anticholinergics, and amantadine.

DOPAMINE AGONISTS   Dopamine agonists work on postsynaptic dopamine receptors and are somewhat less effective than levodopa. They produce fewer drug-induced dyskinesias and have a longer half-life than levodopa, thus providing more consistent dopamine-receptor stimulation.

Four dopamine agonists are currently available in the United States:

1. Bromocriptine
2. Pergolide (used in adjunct therapy to treat PD)
3. Pramipexole
4. Ropinirole (used as monotherapy)

All dopamine agonists should be started at a low dose and titrated up, with the average titration taking 6 to 8 weeks.

MONOAMINE OXIDASE TYPE B INHIBITORS   MAO-B is an enzyme responsible for the metabolism of dopamine. Inhibiting MAO-B inhibitors block the path of degradation, causing higher dopamine availability. Selegiline is the only available drug in this group. Effects are milder than levodopa or dopamine agonists.

CATECHOL O-METHYLTRANSFERASE INHIBITORS   COMT inhibitors are the newest group of antiparkinsonian medications. They contribute to the metabolism of levodopa and dopamine peripherally and centrally. Tolcapone, the only drug in this class, allows higher levels of levodopa to cross the blood-brain barrier. It is useful as a supplementary medication for patients who experience waning benefits during intervals in the levodopa/carbidopa cycle. Tolcapone has the potential to cause liver toxicity, so it is important to perform liver function tests on patients every 2 weeks. One should exhaust all other drugs before using tolcapone due to the stringent monitoring requirements.

ANTICHOLINERGICS   This is the oldest group of antiparkinsonian medications. Anticholinergics are most useful in patients with tremor-predominant disease. Elderly individuals are often affected by cognitive side effects, as well as dry mouth, blurred vision, or urinary retention.

AMANTADINE   Amantadine is an antiviral medication. The mechanism of action is not known. Amantadine is used in early tremor-predominant disease and has shown benefits in advanced PD.[7]

Surgical Therapies

Pharmacologic therapy is not the only option in the decision about treatment for a patient with newly diagnosed PD. Neurosurgical procedures were largely abandoned in the late 1960s when levodopa was found to be effective in treating the symptoms of PD. However, with years of exposure, side effects of levodopa as well as the diminished benefit made other treatment modalities more appealing. Surgical therapies are now available including stereotactic thalamotomy as well as a recent renewed interest in the use of stereotactic ventral pallidotomy. The use of pallidotomy appears to be beneficial. Recent studies show that patients were able to resume daily living activities such as dressing, eating, and personal hygiene after surgery. However, caution is to be advised in that some benefits can diminish after 2 years and the long-term effects of the surgery are unknown.

Pharmacologic and/or surgical intervention is just one side of the treatment of the PD patient. Physiotherapy and psychosocial and group support also play a role. Physical therapy or speech therapy helps many patients.[7] Home additions of aids to daily living, such as rails or banisters placed around the home, special table cutlery with large handles, and nonslip rubber mats often can improve the quality of life.[3] Patient information and resources concerning PD are readily available (Table 11-7-1).

TABLE 11-7-1.   Information Sources for Parkinson's Disease

American Parkinson's Disease Association, Inc.
1250 Hylan Boulevard, Suite 4B
Staten Island, NY 10305
1-800-223-2732

National Parkinson's Foundation
1501 Northwest Ninth Avenue
Bob Hope Road
Miami, Fl 33136-1494
1-800-327-4545

Parkinson's Disease Foundation
710 West 168th Street
New York, NY 10032
1-800-457-6676

TABLE 11-7-2. Differential Diagnoses of Parkinson's Disease

DIFFERENTIAL DIAGNOSIS	SYMPTOMS
Advanced age	Mild hypokinesia Slight tremor
Depression	Expressionless face Poorly modulated voice Reduction in voluntary activity
Wilson's disease	Early age at onset Presence of abnormal movements Kayser-Fleischer rings Chronic hepatitis
Huntington's disease	Rigidity Bradykinesia Family history Accompanying dementia
Shy-Drager syndrome	Postural hypotension Anhidrosis Decreased sphincter control Cerebellar neurologic deficits
Steele-Richardson-Olszewski syndrome (supranuclear palsy)	Bradykinesia and rigidity Pseudobulbar palsy Axial dystonia
Creutzfeldt-Jakob disease	Dementia Myoclonic jerking Ataxia Electrocardiogram markings that may mimic atrial flutter

DIAGNOSTIC CONSIDERATIONS

Early-onset PD is difficult to diagnose, particularly if the tremor is minimal or absent. Table 11-7-2 lists the more common differential diagnoses for PD.

NOTES AND PEARLS

Various other therapeutic approaches are being studied. Transplanting substantia nigra tissues from human fetuses into the brains of PD patients has scientific appeal. However, the technique raises many medical ethical questions and continues to be experimental.

Medical treatment of PD patients can be most rewarding because of the noticeable improvement in their ability to perform daily living activities. If initial treatment modalities begin to become less effective neurologic intervention would be warranted.

REFERENCES

1. Olanow CW: A 61-year-old man with Parkinson's disease. *JAMA* 275:716–722, 1996.
2. Sacks OW: *Awakenings.* Garden City, NY, Doubleday, 1973.
3. Aurinoff MJ: Parkinson's disease and other extrapyramidal disorders, in *Harrison's Principals of Internal Medicine,* 14th ed, Fauci AS et al (eds). New York, McGraw-Hill, 1998, pp 2356–2363.
4. Unger J: Diagnosis and management of Parkinson's disease. *Clinical Advisor* 1(3):26–38, 1998.
5. Poewe W: Should treatment of Parkinson's disease be started with a dopamine agonist? *Neurology* 51(suppl 2):S21–S24, 1998.
6. Henderson JM, Dunnett SB: Targeting the subthalamic nucleus in the treatment of Parkinson's disease. *Brain Res Bull* 46(6):467–474, 1998.
7. Simuni T, Stern M: Parkinson's disease: Seven questions physicians often ask. *Consultant* 39(2):367–381, 1999.

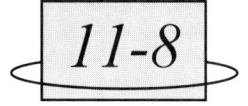

BELL'S PALSY
R. Scott Chavez

DISCUSSION

Bell's palsy is named for Sir Charles Bell, a nineteenth-century Scottish surgeon and physiologist, because of his work on facial palsy. It affects approximately 25 of every 100,000 people annually in the United States. Bell's palsy, a paralysis of the muscles innervated by the seventh cranial nerve, also is known as idiopathic facial paralysis. It is generally unilateral and occurs equally in males and females, with the highest incidence in 20- to 35-year olds. Less than 10% of patients have recurrent episodes. Bilateral Bell's palsy occurs in less than 1% of cases. A positive family history is found in 2 to 14% of these patients.

PATHOGENESIS

Bell's palsy is idiopathic with some degree of genetic predisposition. The facial nerve becomes inflamed within the facial canal, causing total or partial paralysis of the facial muscles. Exposure to cold has been known to precipitate an attack. Some theorists hypothesize that a vasoconstrictor such as endothelin may play a role in the mechanism of the onset of facial nerve paralysis. It is highly unusual to have bilateral paralysis, and other causes should be investigated.

MICROBIOLOGY

Viral factors have been assumed to cause Bell's palsy. Recent research has shown strong clinical evidence that the primary cause of idiopathic Bell's palsy is the herpes simplex virus (HSV-1). Researchers found that nearly 85% of all Bell's palsy patients have this virus. Owing to the growing evidence that Bell's palsy is due to reactivation of HSV, it has been suggested that Bell's palsy be renamed *herpetic facial paralysis.*[1]

SYMPTOMS

A Bell's palsy patient commonly presents with a sudden onset of paralysis of the facial muscles that worsens over 2 to 5 days. Patients who present with many symptoms may have one or many of the following: an abnormal blink, affected taste or speech, an asymmetric smile, buccinator paralysis (food caught in cheek of paralyzed side), drooling of liquids from the corner of a paralyzed mouth, dry eye, excessive perspiration, facial or acoustic pain, a frozen nasalis muscle in the area of the nostrils, hyperacusis (perceiving sounds as unduly loud), inability to whistle or pucker the lips, inability to close the eye, lack of wrinkling on the forehead on the paralyzed side, synkinesis (involuntary movement associated with a voluntary movement), tearing, tightness or swelling of the facial muscle, and/or weakened facial musculature.

OBJECTIVE FINDINGS

The diagnosis of Bell's palsy is made on the basis of a thorough history and clinical examination. The clinician must exclude conditions that can mimic Bell's palsy, such as tumor, trauma, infection, and stroke.

One should assess onset (was it sudden or slow?), involvement (incomplete or complete?), trauma (recent accident or blow to the head?), associated symptoms (any hearing loss, dizziness, tinnitus, abnormalities of taste?), associated pain, medical problems (diabetes, Lyme disease, mumps, tuberculosis, or HIV), medications (thalidomide, isoniazid), immunization history, and any previous history of palsy.

The physical examination should include observation of the patient's general appearance. Anxiety is often present in the early stage. There should be no blebs or skin blisters. The clinician should perform an examination of the upper and lower parts of the face to assess all branches of the facial nerve. The facial nerve is tested by instructing the patient to close his or her eyelids tightly; this is a positive finding when the affected eyelid does not close completely. The patient should be instructed to smile or show the teeth; there will be a unilateral facial paralysis. The patient should lift his or her eyebrows and then lower them. Bell's palsy patients cannot symmetrically lift their eyebrows. The other cranial nerves also should be tested. There may be hypesthesia or dysesthesia of cranial nerves II, V, and IX. There may be some mild periorbital puffiness. Visual acuity should be unchanged. Hearing should be tested with Rinne and Weber. Hearing abnormalities are not seen with Bell's palsy and should be investigated further. Some ear, nose, and throat (ENT) specialists recommend that audiometry should be done to rule out associated cranial nerve VIII involvement. An otoscopic examination should be performed to rule out middle-ear pathology. Taste may not be present over two-thirds of the tongue. There should be no parotid masses. Cerebellar function should be assessed with strength, sensation, and gait intact.

DIAGNOSTIC CONSIDERATIONS

When a patient presents with vesicles along the outer ear canal or behind the ear, the condition is due to herpes simplex and is called the Ramsay Hunt syndrome. Bilateral facial paralysis can be due to Guillain-Barré syndrome or meningitis. Other causes of facial paralysis include multiple sclerosis, sarcoidosis, temporal bone fracture, meningitis, otitis media, a parotid gland tumor, osteoma of the skull, and leukemic or carcinomatous meningitis.

SPECIAL CONSIDERATIONS

The clinician should be especially sensitive to underlying subclinical infections such as tuberculosis and systemic mycoses.

LABORATORY STUDIES

There are no routine laboratory tests for Bell's palsy. Patients should undergo electromyography (EMG) within the first 3 weeks of onset. Serial EMG will determine the extent of recovery of facial motor function.

The literature indicates that laboratory studies to rule out pernicious anemia, diabetes, Lyme disease, and syphilis are appropriate. If it is clinically warranted, a spinal tap may be performed to rule out Lyme disease (see Chap. 9-3). The cerebrospinal fluid will be mildly elevated 33% of the time.

RADIOLOGIC STUDIES

Magnetic resonance imaging (MRI) may be ordered to rule out posterior fossa lesions or tumors; however, a high level of clinical suspicion should dictate its use. A chest radiograph is necessary to rule out sarcoidosis. There are no routine radiologic studies.

OTHER STUDIES

EMG and nerve conduction velocity (NCV) generally are recommended to assess the patient's severity and prognosis. An EMG involves the insertion of a probe into the facial muscles to record muscle activity. An NCV test involves stimulating the facial nerve in front of the ear and measuring the response of the facial muscles. The EMG and NCV should be ordered 7 to 10 days after the onset of facial paralysis.

TREATMENT

Pharmacologic Management

Time is of the essence for a Bell's palsy patient. The symptoms usually appear severe immediately after an attack, and many patients, fearing stroke as a result of unilateral paralysis, rush to the emergency department. Often a dose of steroids is given to reduce swelling and pain; however, the use of steroids remains controversial.

The literature is inconclusive on the utility of steroids in the treatment of Bell's palsy. However, there is widespread agreement in the medical community to use steroids at the onset of symptoms. There is some evidence that steroids may prevent denervation, stop the progression of palsy to paralysis, and shorten the course of the weakness. If steroids are the clinical choice, corticosteroid therapy should begin soon after the onset of the initial symptoms of Bell's palsy. Treatment beyond 4 days after the onset is usually ineffective. For patients seen within 21 days of the onset of weakness, a standard prednisone dose is 1 mg/kg/day for 10 to 14 days followed by a tapering dose.

Antiviral medications such as such as acyclovir (Zovirax) and famciclovir (Famvir) have been shown to be somewhat effective against Bell's palsy. However, for antiviral medications, to be sufficiently effective, they must be administered within 1 to 6 days after an attack.

Surgery

The need for surgical intervention remains controversial, and surgery rarely is advised for Bell's palsy patients. Surgery to relieve pressure on the swollen seventh cranial nerve is thought to confer benefit; however, it is done infrequently and only after a detailed evaluation that strongly suggests a poor outlook for recovery.

The indications in the literature for surgical evaluation include when no recovery is seen after 6 months or 12 months, when other cranial nerves have become affected, when NCV and EMG results are dramatically reduced, when a parotid mass is present, when paralysis is sudden and complete or slowly progressive, or when malignancy or trauma is present.

Supportive Measures

Eye care is essential in Bell's palsy patients. These patients should be given lubricating eyedrops during the day, an ointment at bedtime, and a vaporizer at night. It is important to guard against corneal drying; some clinicians use a transparent eye shield attached to the face with tape to avoid aeration to the eye. The use of a patch is avoided because of the risk of corneal abrasion.

An ophthalmology consultation may be warranted, particularly if the patient reports eye pain. Patients may relieve pain and inflammation with hot and cold hydrotherapy treatments.

Alternative and Complementary Medicine

The use of alternative and complementary medicine remains controversial. Massage therapy has been used to relax muscles and relieve facial pain. Acupuncture has been used to reduce swelling and inflammation. Acupressure has been recommended to relieve symptoms of pain and muscle weakness. Hyperbaric oxygen (HBO_2) has been studied for use in Bell's palsy, and the early results have been promising.

Patient Education

The patient should be given a lot of reassurance and a detailed explanation of the viral disease. The patient's concern about disfigurement and loss of function should be addressed directly with the patient. Often patients think they have had a "stroke."

DISPOSITION

Patients are monitored on an outpatient basis and should be checked monthly for 6 to 12 months. Generally, complete spontaneous recovery can be expected and full function of the facial muscles will be restored.

Approximately 50% of all patients recover within the first 30 days without treatment or intervention. Another 20% recover within 1 to 3 months from the onset of symptoms, while 5% to 10% take 4 to 6 months to recover.

Poor risk factors for complete recovery include age (55 and older), disease (diabetes, hypertension), extent (complete facial weakness), and change in symptoms (excessive tearing or pain). If there is not full recovery by 6 months, the patient's residual paralysis usually will remain without any further spontaneous correction. Treatment for residual paralysis varies. Video photography, motor nerve conduction velocity studies, and blink reflex tests have been employed to scientifically monitor the patient's progress. Facial muscle rehabilitation is helpful on occasion.

COMPLICATIONS AND RED FLAGS

The single most important complication of Bell's palsy is corneal abrasion or ulceration. Appropriate monitoring and eye protection are critical. The use of methylcellulose eyedrops may be helpful. As with the use of any corticosteroids, caution should be taken in administering such medications to patients with diabetes or peptic ulcer disease, pregnant patients, and patients who have received live vaccines (e.g., measles, mumps, rubella, and live oral polio vaccine).

PATIENT RESOURCES

A good Internet support group exists at http://dem0nmac.mgh.harvard.edu/neurowebforum/neurowebforum.html.

American Academy of Otolaryngology
Head and Neck Surgery, Inc.
1 Prince Street
Alexandria, VA 22314
(703) 836-4444

National Organization for Rare Disorders (NORD)
P.O. Box 8923
New Fairfield, CT 06812-1783
(203) 746-6518
http://www.pcnet.com/~orphan

PROVIDER RESOURCES

NIH/National Institute of Neurological Disorders and Stroke
9000 Rockville Pike
Bethesda, MD 20892
(301) 496-5751
(800) 352-9424
http://www.ninds.nih.gov

REFERENCE

1. Furuta Y, Fukuda S, Chida E, Takasu T, Ohtani F, Inuyama Y, Nagashima K: Reactivation of herpes simplex virus type 1 in patients with Bell's palsy. *J Med Virol* 54(3):162–166, 1998.

BIBLIOGRAPHY

Adour KK: Medical management of idiopathic Bell's palsy. *Otolaryngol Clin North Am* 24:663–673, 1991.
Billue JS: Bell's palsy: An update on idiopathic facial paralysis. *Nurse Pract* 22(8):88, 97–105, 1997.
Hughes GB: Practical management of Bell's palsy. *Otolaryngol Head Neck Surg* 102:658–663, 1990.
May M, Klein SR: Differential diagnosis of facial nerve palsy. *Otolaryngol Clin North Am* 24: 613–673, 1991.
Morgan M, Nathwani D: Facial palsy and infection: The unfolding story. *Clin Infect Dis* 14:263–271, 1992.
Morganlander JC, Massy EW: Bell's palsy: Ensuring the best possible outcome. *Postgrad Med* 88:157–164, 1990.
Noone J, Longe S: Bell's palsy in the primary care setting: A case study. *Clin Excell Nurse Pract* 2(4):206–211, 1998.

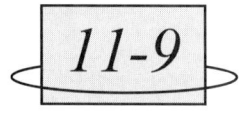

INTRACRANIAL ANEURYSM/INTRACRANIAL ANEURYSMAL HEMORRHAGE

Laura M. Capozzi

DISCUSSION

Intracranial aneurysm is seen in 1 to 6% of adults as a fairly incidental finding at autopsy. However, a feared complication of aneurysm is a rupture resulting in an intracranial subarachnoid hemorrhage. Aneurysms commonly are located at the branching points of the major arteries, traveling through the subarachnoid space at or near the circle of Willis. Cerebral angiography reveals an 0.5 to 1% occurrence of small asymptomatic aneurysms among adults. It has been estimated from autopsy and angiography results that 1 million to 12 million Americans have intracranial aneurysms. The most common type of aneurysm is the saccular, or berry, aneurysm, followed by the fusiform aneurysm. A saccular aneurysm is characterized by a distinct neck and dome within the aneurysm. A fusiform aneurysm presents as a diffuse enlargement of an artery without an identifiable neck; these aneurysms are caused by atherosclerosis, trauma, infection, or tumor. Aneurysms typically rupture at the dome.

Aneurysms are classified by cause, size, site, and shape. These factors in combination are important in determining the treatment.

The majority of intracranial aneurysms are unruptured at autopsy. With the widespread use of diagnostic imaging techniques such as magnetic resonance imaging (MRI) and computed tomography (CT), many unruptured and asymptomatic aneurysms can be diagnosed. The rate of rupture increases with the size of the aneurysm (usually 10 mm or larger) and with advancing age up to the eighth decade; these ruptures occur more often in women than in men.

Epidemiology

The majority of intracranial aneurysms occur in the anterior circulation at the junction of the internal carotid and posterior communicating arteries in the anterior communicating artery complex or at the trifurcation of the middle cerebral artery. Aneurysms of the posterior circulation are found most commonly at the bifurcation of the basilar artery or at the junction of a vertebral artery and an ipsilateral posterior inferior cerebellar artery. Interestingly, multiple aneurysms, usually two or three, are found in 20 to 30% of people with an aneurysm.

Subarachnoid hemorrhage is a common problem associated with intracranial aneurysm. The yearly incidence is about 1 per 10,000 people, and it is associated with high rates of morbidity and mortality. Approximately 12% of these patients die before receiving medical care, and 40% die within 1 month of hospitalization. Among those who survive, 30% have major neurologic deficits. Despite advances in diagnosis and medical or surgical intervention strategies, the fatality rate for aneurysmal subarachnoid hemorrhage has not changed over the past few decades.

Among patients with an aneurysmal subarachnoid hemorrhage, 2% develop a new aneurysm each year. In this patient group, the incidence of aneurysmal rupture is about 6 per 10,000 persons per year. This is substantially higher than the incidence of aneurysmal subarachnoid hemorrhage in the general population.

PATHOGENESIS

Evidence supports the role of genetic factors in the pathogenesis of intracranial aneurysms. These patients are thought to have developmental defects in the arterial wall. Many inherited connective tissue disorders have been associated with intracranial aneurysms, most notably autosomal dominant polycystic kidney disease, Ehlers-Danlos syndrome type IV, neurofibromatosis type I, and Marfan syndrome. Seven to 20% of patients with an intracranial aneurysm have a first- or second-degree relative with a confirmed intracranial aneurysm.

Environmental Risk Factors

Acquired factors also may play an important role in the pathogenesis of intracranial aneurysms. Among the environmental risk factors that may predispose a person to an aneurysmal subarachnoid hemorrhage, cigarette smoking is the only one that has been identified consistently in all the populations studied and is easily the most preventable. The risk of an intracranial aneurysmal hemorrhage is 3 to 10 times higher among smokers than it is among nonsmokers. The risk rises with increases in cigarette pack–years. Cigarette smoking decreases the effectiveness of proteolytic enzymes (proteases) such as elastase. The imbalance in these proteases may result in the degradation of connective tissues, including the arterial wall.

Other Factors

Hypertension frequently is studied in relation to the development and rupture of intracranial aneurysms. Although many studies support the relationship between hypertension and intracranial aneurysm, some do not support an increased risk of intracranial aneurysm in hypertensive patients. Although the incidence of aneurysmal subarachnoid hemorrhage is generally higher in women, before age 50 men are more likely to have an aneurysmal subarachnoid hemorrhage than are women. The use of low-dose oral contraceptives in premenopausal women is thought to decrease the risk of an aneurysmal subarachnoid hemorrhage. Additionally, the risk is lower among women who receive hormone replacement therapy postmenopausally.

Alcohol can lower the risk of an aneurysmal subarachnoid hemorrhage when it is consumed at low levels. However, heavy drinking, especially binge drinking, appears to increase that risk.

Data on hypercholesterolemia as a risk factor for aneurysmal subarachnoid hemorrhage are inconsistent. Pregnancy carries some risk for the rupture of aneurysms that is related to the hemodynamic and endocrine changes that occur. The highest incidence of rupture occurs during the second trimester.

SIGNS AND SYMPTOMS

Although most intracranial aneurysms are asymptomatic until they rupture, the typical presentation is that of a severe headache of acute onset. The headache is often unusual and acute and may precede the rupture by several days or weeks in one-third to one-half of these patients. This prodromal headache often is accompanied by nausea and vomiting, with loss of consciousness at times. This headache may be referred to as a "warning leak" of blood into the wall of the aneurysm or into the subarachnoid space.

Rupture is most common during times of exertion or stress but may occur at any time. Global or focal neurologic abnormalities may be found on physical examination. Meningismus and intraocular subhyaloid hemorrhages are two signs that are helpful in diagnosing a subarachnoid hemorrhage.

The signs of meningeal irritation are secondary to blood byproducts in the subarachnoid space. Neck stiffness therefore may not be noted until several hours after the hemorrhage. Circulation of bloody cerebrospinal fluid down the spinal axis may cause severe low back pain and even bilateral radicular leg pain.

When an intracranial aneurysm becomes large, it may cause a mass effect. The most common symptom associated with a mass effect is headache, and the most common sign is palsy of the third nerve, usually involving the pupillary fibers. This palsy is caused by an aneurysm at the junction of the carotid artery and the posterior communicating artery or an aneurysm in the upper end of the basilar artery. Other signs and symptoms that depend on the location of the aneurysm include brainstem dysfunction, visual field defects, trigeminal neuralgia, cavernous sinus syndrome, seizures, and hypothalamic-pituitary dysfunction.

DIAGNOSTIC CONSIDERATIONS

Intracranial aneurysms are typically asymptomatic unless they cause a mass effect because of their size or location. However, headaches caused by "leaking" intracranial aneurysms must be differentiated from migraines and other types of headaches. The onset of the prodromal headache associated with an intracranial subarachnoid hemorrhage usually does not last longer than 2 weeks. Acute, severe headache in a patient warrants CT scanning in persons who have a family history of intracranial aneurysm or autosomal dominant polycystic kidney disease. In this patient group, the incidence of ruptured intracranial aneurysms is four times higher than it is in the general population.

SPECIAL CONSIDERATIONS

The most important predictor of outcome is the clinical condition the patient exhibits on arrival at the hospital. The scale developed by the World Federation of Neurological Surgeons is the most widely used (see Table 11-9-1). It is based in part on the Glasgow Coma Scale (see Table 11-9-2).

LABORATORY STUDIES

If the symptomatology and signs indicate the likelihood of an intracranial aneurysm with bleeding and if CT is negative, a lumbar puncture should be performed to confirm the presence or absence of xanthochromia or blood. Electrolytes should be monitored to prevent hyponatremia, which can lead to neurologic deterioration.

RADIOLOGIC STUDIES

CT scanning should be the first diagnostic study performed to evaluate the possibility of a subarachnoid hemorrhage. Within the first 24 hours, scanning detects up to 95% of hemorrhages; its sensitivity

TABLE 11-9-1. World Federation of Neurological Surgeons Grading Scale for Subarachnoid Hemorrhage

GRADE	SCORE	MOTOR DEFICIT
I	15	Absent
II	13 or 14	Absent
III	13 or 14	Present
IV	7–12	Absent or present
V	3–6	Absent or present

TABLE 11-9-2.   Glasgow Coma Scale

Eye opening (E)
    4: opens eyes spontaneously
    3: opens eyes to voice
    2: opens eyes to pain
    1: no eye opening

Best motor response (M)
    6: obeys commands
    5: localizes to pain
    4: withdraws to pain
    3: abnormal flexor response
    2: abnormal extensor response
    1: no movement

Best verbal response (V)
    5: appropriate and oriented
    4: confused conversation
    3: inappropriate words
    2: incomprehensible sounds
    1: no sounds

Scores from the three categories are summed to determine the severity of injury:

$$E + M + V = 9 \text{ (comatose)}$$
$$E + M + V = 9\text{--}12 \text{ (moderate head injury)}$$
$$E + M + V = 13\text{--}15 \text{ (minor head injury)}$$

Generally, patients with a World Federation of Neurological Surgeons (WFNS) grade of IV of V have a poor outcome and prognosis despite medical and surgical intervention. Patients with WFNS grades of I and II have a better prognosis, although 30% do not survive until surgery.

decreases to 50% within 1 week. MRI is not sensitive enough in detecting early hemorrhage but may be helpful in detecting subacute or chronic hemorrhage of more than a 2-week duration.

In patients at high risk for aneurysm with subsequent rupture, conventional angiography should be the first diagnostic study performed. The most commonly used imaging techniques are angiography, magnetic resonance angiography (MRA), and helical CT angiography. Helical CT angiography is similar in sensitivity to MRA. They vary in terms of the ability to be a useful diagnostic tool. MRA is the most convenient diagnostic study since it is noninvasive, but it may not be able to detect smaller aneurysms. MRA is the best method for detecting a thrombus (uncommon) within an aneurysm, while CT scanning is preferred to detect calcification within the aneurysmal wall. Helical CT scanning is useful in the presurgical evaluation of patients, since it can show relationships between the aneurysm and structures in the skull.

OTHER DIAGNOSTICS

Lumbar puncture should be performed if an intracranial hemorrhage is suspected but is not revealed by CT. Xanthochromia (yellow discoloration) of the supernatant after centrifuging of the cerebrospinal fluid is diagnostic of a subarachnoid hemorrhage. Xanthochromia is caused by the breakdown of blood products in the cerebrospinal fluid several hours after the initial hemorrhage. Xanthochromia is present in all patients between 12 hours and 2 weeks after a hemorrhage and is detectable for several weeks afterward.

TREATMENT

The goal of treatment is to remove the aneurysm from the intracranial circulation while preserving the parent artery. Removal usually is achieved by surgical resection or endovascular occlusion techniques. Medical treatment includes control of blood pressure and keeping the patient quiet. Pharmacologic treatment includes the use of mannitol to control cerebral edema and calcium channel blockers (e.g., nimodipine) to control arterial vasospasm.

Surgical resection involves the placement of a clip across the neck of an aneurysm. Its proven efficacy makes it the most desirable and definitive treatment. The timing of surgery after an intracranial hemorrhage is controversial. Early surgery within 48 to 72 hours seems preferable, since the incidence of another intracranial subarachnoid hemorrhage is highest during this period. The rate of recurrent hemorrhage varies from 4 to 20% within 24 hours. Additionally, arterial vasospasm occurs after an intracranial subarachnoid hemorrhage, resulting in arterial narrowing, which is a primary cause of cerebral ischemia. Early surgery can prevent this complication. Although the exact cause of the vasospasm is not known, it is related to the amount of blood present in the brain after a hemorrhage. Late surgery performed between days 10 and 14 after an intracranial subarachnoid hemorrhage can be more difficult than early surgery because of secondary brain edema and a tenacious clot around the aneurysm.

Hydrocephalus also may occur during both the early course and the late course in 10 to 30% of these patients. Its presence usually indicates a poor prognosis. Ventricular drainage should be performed to prevent further neurologic deterioration.

Endovascular therapy is becoming a useful treatment modality; it involves the insertion of soft metallic coils within the lumen of the aneurysm. Obliteration occurs through thrombus formation within the entire aneurysm. This technique is most useful for saccular aneurysms.

Of interest is a recent retrospective and prospective study conducted by the International Study of Unruptured Intracranial Aneurysms Investigators, who cautioned about surgical management of patients with unruptured aneurysms less than 10 mm in diameter. Patients without a previous history of ruptured intracranial aneurysms had a very low rate of rupture of 0.05%, consistent with other studies. However, the study found a significantly higher rate of morbidity and mortality associated with surgical repair than was previously reported. The investigators recommended careful evaluation of patients for surgical repair of aneurysms smaller than 10 mm in diameter.

Patient Education

Screening is suggested in patients who have two or more family members who have had an intracranial aneurysm and those with autosomal dominant polycystic kidney disease. Smoking cessation is an absolute necessity for patients who have been diagnosed with an intracranial aneurysm, particularly patients who have had an intracranial subarachnoid hemorrhage. As was mentioned previously, the rate of hemorrhage is directly related to the number of cigarettes smoked, with heavy smokers having a greater incidence of hemorrhage than light smokers.

COMPLICATIONS AND RED FLAGS

The following complications may be seen:

- Acute onset of a severe, often unusual headache, usually with activity
- A family history of intracranial aneurysms or autosomal dominant polycystic kidney disease
- Third cranial nerve palsy involving pupillary fibers and visual field defects

OTHER NOTES AND PEARLS

Physical examination reveals a subhyaloid hemorrhage. These vitreous ocular hemorrhages occur between the retina and the vitreous membrane and are gravity-dependent. As a result, they appear convex at the bottom and flat at the top.

BIBLIOGRAPHY

Fauci AS, Braunwald E, Isselbacher KJ, et al (eds): *Harrison's Principles of Internal Medicine,* 14th ed, New York, McGraw-Hill, 1998.

Meyer FB, Morita A, Puumala M, Nichols D: Subject review: Medical and surgical management of intracranial aneurysms. *Mayo Clin Proc* 70(2): 153–172, 1995.

Schievink W: Medical progress: Intracranial aneurysms. *N Engl J Med* 336(1):28–40, 1997.

Wieber DO: Unruptured intracranial aneurysms: Risk of rupture and risks of surgical intervention: International Study of Unruptured Intracranial Aneurysms Investigators. *N Engl J Med* 339(24):1725–1732, 1998.

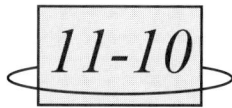

PAIN MANAGEMENT
Meredith Davison

DISCUSSION

Pain provides a mechanism that protects humans from impending harm from the environment. However, beyond the warning purpose, pain becomes meaningless and causes much suffering. The experience of pain is essentially subjective, and individuals display a variety of responses that must be understood to provide effective pain management. The total pain experience involves the pain perception and the associated emotional reactions and physiologic responses. Pain is probably the most common patient problem, the most difficult to assess, and often the most difficult to treat. Pain is commonly the reason people seek health care, but there is much to suggest that health care professionals do not deal adequately with their patients' pain.[1] It is important for the provider to always regard a patient with pain seriously while considering all aspects of the pain, both physiologic and emotional.

Pain is clinically divided into several categories. For example, pain can be either acute or chronic. Acute pain serves to warn the body of possible or real danger. Ordinarily, the pain is sudden and localized and has a short duration, subsiding as healing occurs. It is characterized by sharp painful sensations that can vary in intensity from mild to severe. In contrast to acute pain, chronic pain generally serves no useful purpose and has a long duration of action. It is frequently difficult to localize, with diffuse painful sensations. Chronic pain leads to fatigue and lowers the pain threshold. Pain also can be categorized as somatic or visceral. Somatic pain is a quick response with a sudden onset, while visceral pain tends to linger and ache.

SIGNS AND SYMPTOMS

Patients with acute pain often experience increased heart rate, respiration, blood pressure, peripheral blood flow, muscle tension, palmar sweating, and dilated pupils. These patients also experience anxiety and restlessness. These changes are secondary to activation of the sympathetic nervous system with its release of epinephrine-norepinephrine. The pain is usually obvious in the patient's facial expression, especially with severe pain. Crying, grimacing, and vocalizations may be present in children and some adults.

The signs and symptoms of chronic pain are based on the long-term activation of the autonomic nervous system. The patient may present with sleep disturbances, anorexia, listlessness, apathy, personality changes, irritability, and/or depression. A sense of hopelessness and social withdrawal are also common. A comparison of acute and chronic pain is given in Table 11-10-1.

DIAGNOSTIC CONSIDERATIONS

In patients with acute pain, the primary diagnostic consideration is to ascertain the cause of the pain. After diagnosis of the etiology of the injury or disease process, managing the acute pain can be considered. The specific evaluation of pain should begin with a focused history that includes the following:

• Where does it hurt?
• How badly does it hurt?

TABLE 11-10-1. Characteristics of Acute Versus Chronic Pain

	ACUTE PAIN	CHRONIC PAIN
Purpose	Warning: impending or actual tissue damage	Unclear; often serves no function
Location	Localized	Diffuse
Time course	Transient (<6 months)	Prolonged, sometimes intractable
Signs	Sympathetic stimulation: increased blood pressure, heart rate, muscle tone, respiration, etc.	Sleep disturbances, anorexia, disruption of lifestyle
Characteristics	Sharp, varying intensity, may radiate	Aching, dull, burning, cramping, persistent
Psychological response	Anxiety	Depression, personality changes, anger, helplessness, apathy

• What does the pain feel like?
• What starts the pain and what ends it?
• Does anything cause the pain to change (position, movement, etc.)?
• Is there any time sequence to the pain?
• Was there any trauma or injury that started the pain?

A physical examination should highlight the location of the pain. Check the patient for tenderness, deep palpation, and sensitivity to light touch. Observe for warmth, edema, and possible redness. Ascertain whether any other areas of the body also are experiencing pain or unusual sensations. More focused diagnostic testing may be necessary, depending on the differential diagnosis and the site of the pain.

The diagnostic process involved with chronic pain is more complicated. The first step in the evaluation is to collect information about pain from different modalities, such as the patient interview, questionnaires, behavioral observation, and medical history. At a minimum, information about the precipitating circumstances, alleviating factors, duration of the pain, description of the pain, and previous medical treatments is required. The diagnosis of chronic pain may necessitate the referral of the patient to a facility specializing in the treatment of chronic pain.

TREATMENT

Removing the cause of the pain is always the best treatment. However, since it may take time to eliminate the cause of the pain, other treatment modalities often are used. In some cases, it may be impossible to eliminate the pain; thus medications and nonpharmacologic treatment are relied on frequently. Each type of treatment is discussed briefly below. However, because of the complexity of the pharmacologic actions of analgesics, it is suggested that the reader refer to other sources for a comprehensive discussion of analgesics.

Nonnarcotic Analgesics

Aspirin, acetaminophen, and the nonsteroidal anti-inflammatory drugs (NSAIDs) are collectively referred to as nonnarcotic analgesics. Nonnarcotic analgesics are most useful for the mild to moderate pain associated with headaches, colds, influenza, and muscular aches. Besides analgesic effects, nonnarcotic analgesics have antipyretic and anti-inflammatory actions (with the exception of acetaminophen). These actions enhance their usefulness in treating many conditions with multiple symptoms.

In contrast to narcotic analgesics, which act via the central nervous system, nonnarcotic analgesics have been demonstrated to act peripherally by preventing the formation of prostaglandins. Thus, the pain receptors in the inflamed tissues are not stimulated.

The simplest and most common analgesic is acetaminophen, which is safe, effective, and practically without side effects when used in low doses. The next line of analgesic therapy consists of the other NSAIDs, including aspirin, ibuprofen, and naproxen, as well as a host of others. Common side effects of this group of drugs include gastrointestinal upset and renal dysfunction. Careful assessment of concurrent conditions and other medications may necessitate the use of specific drugs in this class.

Narcotic Analgesics

Drugs similar to morphine that offer pain relief and sedation are referred to as narcotic analgesics. These substances provide effective pain relief without producing a loss of consciousness. The person is aware of pain but is no longer bothered by its intensity.

Narcotic analgesics act by mimicking the action of endorphins, which are endogenous peptides that alter the response to pain stimulation. This class of analgesics inhibits neuronal firing in specific areas of the brain, thus decreasing the release of certain neurotransmitters. Narcotic analgesics can be classified as opiate agonists or opiate partial agonists, depending on their action on opiate receptors in the brain. Opiate agonists have purely stimulant (agonistic) actions, while opiate partial agonists also display an antagonistic property that reduces their abuse potential. Opiate agonists are Schedule II controlled substances because of their abuse potential. Opiate partial agonists are either Schedule IV or Schedule V.

Codeine is the simplest example of a narcotic analgesic; it is easily administered in various combinations with acetaminophen. Codeine is used commonly in intramuscular, subcutaneous, and oral preparations. The effects of codeine are similar to those of other narcotic analgesics. However, the potency of codeine is low, thus limiting its use to less severe pain.

Intermediate-strength narcotics include propoxyphene (Darvon) and oxycodone (Percocet, Percodan). Both of these drugs are more potent than codeine and thus have greater potential for dependence, addiction, and/or abuse. Morphine is the most widely used and one of the most potent narcotic analgesics. The routes of administration are intramuscular, subcutaneous, intravenous, oral, rectal, and epidural. Hydromorphone (Dilaudid) and levorphanol (Levo-Dromoran) are semisynthetic derivatives of morphine that are several times more potent. These potent narcotic analgesics are reserved for severe pain. The common side effects of analgesics are sedation, nausea, and constipation. Habituation to the effectiveness of narcotic analgesics does occur, but usually only after prolonged use. Short-term treatment of acute pain with narcotic analgesics rarely causes any problems or leads to addiction.

Related to narcotic analgesics are the opiate partial agonists, which simultaneously stimulate and block the opiate receptors in the brain. These drugs are valuable in a variety of situations because of their reduced potential for abuse. Examples of drugs in this class include pentazocine (Talwin), nalbuphine hydrochloride (Nubain), butorphanol (Stadol), dezocine (Dalgan), and buprenorphine (Buprenex). All are useful for moderate to severe pain, especially postoperative pain.

Local Analgesics

Injections of local anesthetics such as lidocaine (Xylocaine) and mepivacaine (Carbocaine) can be used to provide pain relief for chronic musculoskeletal pain. Nerve blocks using local anesthetics are also useful for chronic pain such as that from cancer.

Nonpharmacologic Methods

Nonpharmacologic treatment is often useful for the treatment of pain. For example, musculoskeletal injuries respond to cold during the first 24 hours and to heat thereafter. Massage alleviates some pain, and bed rest usually offers relief from mild to moderate pain.

Subjectively experienced pain is never dependent solely on organic dysfunction or tissue damage. The traditional biomedical model of treatment often has failed in the treatment of pain because its focus has been entirely on finding and alleviating the physical cause of pain. However, since the intensity of the pain and its behavioral expression are influenced by many factors, including anxiety level, environmental contingencies, psychological processes, and cultural background, traditional therapies often fail to help a patient with chronic pain.

The role these nonphysical processes play in chronic pain has led to the proliferation of over 1500 multidisciplinary pain clinics in the United States that manage all aspects of pain diagnosis and treatment. Well-designed outcome studies indicate that multidisciplinary pain facilities return chronic pain patients to work permanently as a result of their treatment. Health care providers should refer patients to multidisciplinary pain centers for chronic pain, generally defined as pain that losts for 6 months.

Health providers have not always been effective in dealing with their patients' pain. In general, the reasons for treatment failure relate to overestimating the risk of addiction, poor communication, lack of knowledge of pain management principles, and/or the pharmacologic characteristics of analgesics. Patients have a right to expect that their pain will be controlled, and clinicians should be sensitive to patients' concerns. Table 11-10-2 lists the most common causes of analgesic failure.

SPECIAL CONSIDERATIONS

Pediatrics

Other than modifying the doses of analgesics, there are several guidelines for the management of pain in children:

- Expressions of pain differ according to the age and developmental level of the child. Infants may scream and display muscular rigidity and thrashing of their limbs. Preschoolers often behave aggressively or complain of general malaise. Older children express pain either verbally or behaviorally and may regress to the behavior patterns of a younger child. Adolescents are frequently uncomfortable expressing pain to adults.
- The effects of narcotic analgesics in children may differ from the effects in adults. Be alert for unexpected side effects.
- Narcotic rectal suppositories are useful in children. However, drug absorption is erratic, and the appropriate dose is difficult to choose.

Geriatrics

Guidelines for geriatric patients are as follows:

- Older adults are especially susceptible to respiratory depression, excessive sedation, and the other adverse effects of narcotic analgesics.
- Some older adults may be reticent about complaining of pain and will suffer stoically rather than ask for pain medication. Since pain

TABLE 11-10-2. Common Causes of Analgesic Failure

Overestimating the analgesic efficacy of a drug
Underestimating the analgesic requirement of the patient
Prejudice against the use of analgesics that may prevent objective therapy
Lack of knowledge about analgesic pharmacology
Patient noncompliance because of fear of addiction
Patient not communicating with caregivers for fear of being labeled a drug addict
Patient who wants to please by not complaining
Patient who does not know how or is afraid to communicate with caregiver

SOURCE: Young LY, Koda-Kimble MA (eds): *Applied Therapeutics: The Clinical Use of Drugs,* 6th ed, Vancouver, WA, Applied Therapeutics, 1995, p. 7.4. Used with permission of Applied Therapeutics, Inc.

can have physiologic implications for heart rate and respiration, older patients may need to be given "permission" by the health care provider to use analgesics.

Postoperative Pain

For postoperative pain, the guidelines are as follows:

- The goal is to relieve postoperative pain without excessive sedation. Minimizing pain sensations can facilitate deep-breathing exercises, coughing, and ambulation.
- Patient-controlled analgesia (PCA) is a safe method for postoperative pain management that many patients prefer to intermittent injections. Another method of delivering opiate analgesics is by continuous intravenous infusion. An advantage of this delivery method is better "control" of the pain.

Malignant Disease

For pain from malignant disease, the guidelines are as follows:

- The main consideration in treating the pain associated with chronic malignant disease is client comfort, not preventing drug addiction.
- Cancer pain usually can be controlled with oral pharmacologic management. Antianxiety and antidepressant drugs may allow a reduction in doses of narcotic analgesics.
- Studies have shown that the number of patients who become addicted to drugs is extremely low.
- The progressive pain of cancer is best managed with a step approach, beginning with nonnarcotics and moving toward increasingly potent narcotics.

OTHER NOTES AND PEARLS

Always inquire about self-treatments for pain, including alternative therapies. Many patients will present with a long history of self-medication with analgesics. In addition to NSAIDs that are available without a prescription, patients may have used analgesics from previous prescriptions filled for themselves or others.

When narcotic analgesics are used to relieve the acute, severe pain associated with biliary, renal, or ureteral colic, an antispasmodic drug such as atropine may be needed as well.

Acute toxicity or narcotic overdose can occur from either therapeutic use or abuse. The main goal of treatment is to restore and maintain adequate respiratory function.

Evaluate the need for increased narcotic analgesics to determine whether it is caused by progression of pathologic processes or the development of drug tolerance.

If opiate partial agonists are used by a person who is addicted to narcotic analgesics, remember that the antagonistic property may cause a withdrawal effect.

REFERENCE

1. Martin JJ, Moore GP; Pearls, pitfalls, and updates for pain management. *Emerg Med Clin North Am* 15(2):399–415, 1997.

BIBLIOGRAPHY

American Pain Society. *Principles of Analgesic Use in the Treatment of Acute Pain and Chronic Cancer Pain: A Concise Guide to Medical Practice.* Skokie, IL, American Pain Society, 1992.
Acute Pain Management Guideline Panel: *Acute Pain Management: Operative or Medical Procedures and Trauma: Clinical Practice Guideline.* AHCPR Pub. No. 92-0032. Rockville, MD, Agency for Health Policy and Research, Public Health Service, U.S. Department of Health and Human Services, 1992.
Chang HM: Cancer pain management. *Med Clin North Am* 83(3):711–736, 1999.
Clark BK: Drugs that provide pain relief, in Mathewson-Kuhn M (ed): *Pharmacotherapeutics: A Nursing Process Approach,* 3d ed, Philadelphia, Davis, 1994.
Stacey BR: Effective management of chronic pain: The analgesic dilemma. *Postgrad Med* 100(3):281–296, 1996.
Turk DC: Efficacy of multidisciplinary pain treatment centers in the treatment of chronic pain, in *Pain Treatment Centers at a Crossroads: A Practical and Conceptual Reappraisal Progress in Pain Research and Management.* Seattle, IASP Press, 1996, pp 257–273.

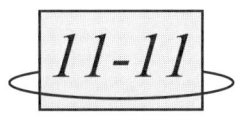

TRIGEMINAL NEURALGIA
Gary J. Bouchard

DISCUSSION

Trigeminal neuralgia (tic douloureux) is the most common syndrome of severe facial pain. The syndrome affects the sensory function of the fifth cranial nerve. The neuralgia is marked by episodes of lancinating pain in one or more of the mandibular, maxillary, or ophthalmic branches of the trigeminal nerve. The cause is unknown, but has been shown in some studies to be associated with anomalous blood vessels compressing the nerve. Trigeminal neuralgia is generally a disease of older persons, but may occur at any age and may rarely affect children. There is a higher incidence in women, with an incidence of 5.9 per 100,000 population per year compared with 3.4 men per 100,000 population per year.

SYMPTOMS AND OBJECTIVE FINDINGS

The patient's description of the pain is the key to an accurate diagnosis of trigeminal neuralgia. The pain is episodic, with paroxysms of pain separated by pain-free intervals. An episode may last from as little as a few seconds to upward of 15 minutes. The frequency of painful episodes commonly ranges from several per day to several per month. The pain-free intervals can be as long as 12 months, but gradually become shorter with time. In general, the intensity of the exacerbations increases with time.

The quality of the pain is sharp and shooting, and patients typically use electrical analogies such as "shock" or "lightning" to describe the pain. The patient's face may be held motionless to avoid exacerbation of the pain, and a contorted facial appearance may be seen (the "tic" in the term "tic douloureux"). The patient can often locate a trigger zone in the lip, cheek, or nose. Stimulation of this area by palpation or by the movements of mastication or facial expression may provoke a typical paroxysm of pain. Bouts of pain have also been provoked by gentle stimuli such as wind or a draft of air.

When asked to indicate the origin of the pain, patients typically will not touch the face but will point to the source with their finger held well above the skin surface. Neuralgia is most common in the second (maxillary) division, the third (mandibular) division is next most common, and involvement of the first (ophthalmic) division is relatively uncommon. The pain may spread to other divisions during an attack; however, the pain does not spread beyond the midline or beyond the distribution of the trigeminal nerve. Bilateral involvement is seen in approximately 5% of cases. The bilateral episodes are rarely simultaneous, more often having a first contralateral episode after several years of ipsilateral recurrences. Bilateral involvement is especially common in patients with multiple sclerosis.

Physical exam is most often normal. A slight sensory deficit to pain and light touch may be present in 15% to 25% of cases. This sensory loss, if present, usually involves a small area and is not noticed by the patient. There is also a risk that a screening neurological exam may miss such a small area of sensory deficit. Sensory loss is not limited to branches directly involved in the present exacerbation of the disease, and may be located in the distribution of an adjacent "silent" branch.

Ipsilateral lacrimation may be present. Motor function is most often normal. A careful oropharyngeal exam is required to rule out dental causes of facial pain. Careful attention should also be paid to the ipsilateral temporomandibular joint for tenderness and decreased range of motion.

DIAGNOSTIC CONSIDERATIONS

Odontalgia is often confused with the facial pain of trigeminal neuralgia, and a thorough oral exam should be performed to rule out dental causes of pain.

Other considerations in the differential diagnosis of trigeminal neuralgia include

Postherpetic neuralgia
Cluster headache
Migraine
Temporomandibular disorders
Temporal arteritis
Glossopharyngeal neuralgia
Acute sinusitis

SPECIAL CONSIDERATIONS

When trigeminal neuralgia occurs in a patient younger than 40 years of age, a specific cause is often found. These include tumors, vascular abnormalities, and demyelinating disease. Trigeminal neuralgia may be the first manifestation of multiple sclerosis. Multiple sclerosis should be considered in younger patients presenting with trigeminal neuralgia.

LABORATORY TESTS

The diagnosis of trigeminal neuralgia is based almost entirely on a patient's history. Laboratory tests are usually noncontributory.

A successful trial of carbamazepine therapy may aid in diagnosis, due to the specific nature of the therapeutic benefit of carbamazepine on neuralgia.

IMAGING STUDIES

Dental radiographs are used to rule out other identifiable causes of facial pain. Magnetic resonance imaging (MRI) can trace the entire length of the trigeminal nerve in a search for tumors, vascular compression, or other abnormalities that may be the cause of the neuralgia. MRI is preferred to computed tomography (CT) due to its superior soft-tissue resolution.

TREATMENT

Carbamazepine is the medical treatment of first choice, and it should be given 200 mg four times daily. Carbamazepine tolerance may develop; the medication may prove less efficacious in the long term and subsequent attacks may be refractory to this treatment. Baclofen in doses of 50 to 60 mg daily is an alternative. Phenytoin in doses of 300 to 400 mg per day may be used as an adjunct to either carbamazepine or baclofen therapy.

Surgical options should be considered in cases of medical treatment failure. These include radiofrequency thermocoagulation or chemical destruction of the trigeminal ganglion with glycerol injection. Surgical procedures are highly efficacious, but there are frequent complications such as sensory loss and recurrence of pain.

COMPLICATIONS AND RED FLAGS

Nutritional status and dental hygiene may be impaired if the painful episodes of neuralgia interfere with eating and routine oral care.

The condition is not fatal; however, there is a small mortality associated with suicide provoked by the presence of gradually worsening chronic pain. The risk of suicide has been greatly reduced with prompt diagnosis and adequate management.

PATIENT EDUCATION

The patient should be informed of the chronic, episodic nature of the condition. It is unrealistic to expect a "cure" in all patients and unwarranted, inappropriate reassurance may damage the patient–provider relationship. Therapeutic optimism tempered with realistic expectations will serve patients best. Self-help and support groups can be of great benefit to a suffering patient.

BIBLIOGRAPHY

Cutrer FM, Moskowitz MA: Headaches and other head pain, in Goldman L, Bennett JC (eds.): *Cecil Textbook of Medicine,* 21st ed, Philadelphia, Saunders, pp. 2071–2072.

Lange DJ, Trojaborg W, Rowland LP: Peripheral and cranial nerve lesions, in Rowland LP (ed.): *Merritt's Textbook of Neurology,* 9th ed, Baltimore, Williams and Wilkins, 1995, pp. 466–467.

Sheremata WA, Honig LS, Bowen B: Multiple sclerosis, in Weiner WJ, Goetz CG (eds.): *Neurology for the Non-Neurologist,* 4th ed, Philadelphia: Lippincott Williams and Wilkins, 1999, pp. 111–1128.

Zakrzewska JM: Trigeminal neuralgia, in Warlow CP, Van Gijn J (eds.): *Major Problems in Neurology,* Volume 28, London, Saunders, 1995.

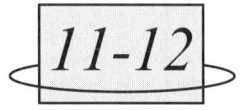

DIZZINESS AND VERTIGO
Gary J. Bouchard

DISCUSSION

Patients may use the term *dizziness* in nonspecific ways to describe symptoms that range from a mild and transient lightheadedness to a severe, intractable spinning feeling. Wherever the patient's sensations fall within this constellation of complaints, there is often great discomfort and anxiety related to these symptoms. The empathetic caregiver who allows a patient to describe his or her subjective sensations accurately and completely will make the most precise and timely diagnosis.

Complaints of dizziness direct the primary care practitioner to several areas of inquiry. These symptoms can be caused by vestibular, visual, or proprioceptive dysfunction. Data obtained in a directed history and physical exam will help to differentiate among these systems.

SYMPTOMS AND OBJECTIVE FINDINGS

It is imperative that the history begin with open-ended questions. A complaint of dizziness requires a request for clarification or more detail. Ask the patient, "What are some other words besides 'dizzy' that can help me understand exactly what you are feeling?" The patient will volunteer the most reliable definition of dizziness for his or her own condition, without cues from the interviewer. The suggestion of a response by the interviewer runs the risk of introducing bias into the subjective data. This is especially damaging to the diagnostic process if responses are suggested to the patient early in the interview.

Other aspects of the patient history contribute to the diagnosis. The timing of the symptoms, especially a history of episodic recurrence, aids in accurate diagnosis. Precipitation factors such as movements of the head or body should be noted. Associated symptoms of hearing loss, tinnitus, nausea, vomiting, and focal neurologic deficits should be discussed with the patient. Underlying medical conditions may mimic dizziness or provoke an exacerbation of vertigo. A careful medication history may reveal the use of pharmaceutical agents that cause vestibular ototoxicity.

The physical exam must include a thorough eye, ear, and neurologic evaluation. Careful testing of the cranial nerves should be undertaken, with attention to visual and auditory function. The eye exam may reveal nystagmus. Proprioception may be impaired. The Romberg test may be abnormal. Impacted cerumen can cause a sensation called "dizziness" by some patients; removing the cerumen will allow for a thorough otoscopic examination and may relieve the symptoms of this small subset of patients.

After the history and physical examination, the interviewer should be able to sort the patient's complaints into the following categories.

Vertigo

Patients with vertigo will tend to use words such as *spinning, tilting, swaying,* or *rotating. Vertigo* is a hallucination of movement. The most common type of vertigo is the patient's sensation that the surroundings are spinning around him or her. A subjective sensation (the feeling that the patient is spinning) is also reported. The sensation most often arises from the semicircular canals. Under normal conditions, the position and linear movement of the head causes distortion of the membranes of the semicircular canals. This will cause hair cells to transmit excitatory or inhibitory impulses to the vestibular nuclei of the pons and medulla. Calcium carbonate crystals or otoliths that are usually embedded in the membrane may occasionally float freely within the endolymph. When free-floating crystals migrate into the posterior semicircular canal, distortion of the membrane by the crystals causes a patient to sense movement when there is none. Central causes of vertigo are also encountered, arising from disease affecting the pons, medulla, or cerebellum.

Vertigo may be further classified into peripheral and central origins. This distinction will help to localize disease to the cochlea, the middle ear, and the eighth cranial nerve (peripheral vestibular system) or to the vestibular nuclei of the pontomedullary junction in the brainstem (central vestibular apparatus). The presence of associated symptoms such as hearing loss and tinnitus are helpful in identifying peripheral origins of vertigo. A central origin of vertigo is suggested by a different set of associated symptoms: diplopia, cortical blindness, homonymous hemianopsia, dysarthria, and motor or sensory deficits of the face and extremities. The character of the patient's nystagmus can also differentiate central from peripheral vertigo. Peripheral nystagmus is unidirectional; the direction of the fast component does not vary with the direction of gaze. Central nystagmus can also be unidirectional but is more commonly multidirectional, with the fast component varying with the direction of gaze. Peripheral nystagmus is inhibited by visual fixation, which can also differentiate it from nystagmus of central origin.

Near-Syncope

Patients with presyncopal episodes will use terms such as *lightheadedness* or *faintness.* This can be associated with generalized weakness, palpitations, diaphoresis, pallor, blurred vision, and a roaring sound in both ears. The symptoms commonly occur with postural changes such as standing. It is associated with a transient hypoperfusion of the brain due to decreased systemic arterial pressure, decreased cardiac output, or cerebral vasoconstriction. A careful cardiovascular exam is indicated, with orthostatic blood pressure measurements and auscultation for carotid bruits and murmurs.

Disequilibrium

Patients within this category complain of impaired balance, lack of coordination, clumsiness, or some degree of disturbance in gait. It is seen only with standing or walking. Symptoms are often described by the patient as being in the lower body or extremities, rather than localized to the head. A variety of neurologic disorders can cause dizziness of this type, including Parkinson's disease, cerebellar ataxia, and frontal lobe neoplasms.

Other Causes

There are other causes of dizziness that do not fit the classifications above. These include hyperventilation syndrome, phobic disorders and other psychiatric illnesses, and a recent change in eyeglasses or contact lenses.

DIAGNOSTIC CONSIDERATIONS

Benign Paroxysmal Positional Vertigo

Benign paroxysmal positional vertigo (BPPV) is the most common cause of vertigo. The patient usually describes episodic, recurring vertigo lasting several minutes or less. Episodes may be as brief as 15 seconds. Specific movements of the head often provoke the attack, usually following a brief delay of several seconds. Patients can often indicate the specific head motion or motions that tend to trigger an attack. Subsequent attacks demonstrate fatigability—assuming an identical head position immediately after an episode causes less intense symptoms than the initial episode. Nystagmus is often associated with BPPV. Hearing loss and tinnitus are not associated with BPPV.

The Dix-Hallpike maneuver is a valuable adjunct to the physical exam. It may reproduce the complaints of vertigo in an asymptomatic patient. The patient is seated, and the examiner rotates the head 45° to the right. The examiner then quickly places the patient into a supine position with the head hanging over the edge of the exam table, with the rightward rotation maintained and the head extended approximately 30°. If no vertigo is seen, the test is repeated with the head rotated 45° to the left.

Labyrinthitis

The second most common cause of vertigo is labyrinthitis, also termed *vestibular neuronitis* or *vestibular neuritis.* Use of the term *labyrinthitis* implies that there is an associated hearing loss. The syndrome is thought to be a sequel of a viral infection. Several household members may be affected concurrently. There is usually no history of episodic reoccurrence. It is gradual in onset, reaches maximal intensity within 1 hour, and resolves within 24 hours. The episode is associated with nausea and vomiting. Hearing loss may or may not be seen. Gait ataxia may be present and may be directed toward the affected side. Nystagmus of peripheral vestibular origin may be seen. There is often a significant phase of disequilibrium that persists after the resolution of the vertigo. The disequilibrium may persist from days to months.

Meniere's Disease

Meniere's disease is associated with excess cochlear production of endolymph, causing endolymphatic hydrops, a characteristic seen in Meniere's disease. The syndrome consists of recurrent episodes of vertigo associated with hearing loss, tinnitus, and a feeling of fullness in the ear. Either ear may be affected initially; the condition may become bilateral as the disease progresses. Low-frequency hearing is lost initially; a more global loss is seen over time. Episodes begin suddenly and characteristically last from 30 minutes to 24 hours. Episodes can be frequent and disabling.

Acoustic Neuroma

Acoustic neuroma is the most common tumor of the cranial nerves. They tend to develop in the area of a nerve near its exit from the acoustic canal. The dizziness of an acoustic neuroma is cerebellar ataxia and described by patients as *imbalance* or *disequilibrium.* The spinning sensation of a classic episode of vertigo is absent. Tinnitus and a progressive loss of auditory acuity usually precede the disequilibrium. There may be deficits in the testing of adjacent cranial nerves, such as facial weakness, decreased facial sensation, and diminished corneal reflex.

Ototoxicity

Many agents cause vestibular toxicity, including aminoglycosides, salicylates, cisplatin, and furosemide. The effects are largely dose related and reversible. Alcohol intoxication will also produce nystagmus and positional vertigo.

Other Diagnostic Considerations

Other conditions that may be associated with dizziness and vertigo include otitis media, migraine, trauma, brainstem dysfunction, multiple sclerosis, diabetes, reactive hypoglycemia, anemia, hypovolemia, hypoxia, hyperventilation syndrome, epilepsy, cardiac dysrhythmias, aortic stenosis, and central nervous system tumors. If all organic causes of dizziness have been ruled out, a psychogenic cause should be investigated.

SPECIAL CONSIDERATIONS

The geriatric patient population is a diagnostic challenge with regard to dizziness. Postural hypotension is common in this demographic group. Polypharmacy with ototoxic drugs may also be seen. All complaints of dizziness in the elderly should be taken seriously and every effort should be made to find a treatable and reversible cause for their discomfort.

LABORATORY STUDIES

Laboratory tests are not helpful in the diagnosis of vertigo. Tests may be ordered to rule out other causes of dizziness such as hypoglycemia, hypoxia, and anemia.

RADIOLOGIC STUDIES

In the presence of focal neurologic findings, computed tomography (CT) or magnetic resonance imaging (MRI) will aid in the further evaluation for space-occupying lesions.

OTHER STUDIES

Electronystagmography (ENG) is occasionally performed in the evaluation of vertigo. ENG can identify vestibular dysfunction but does not always provide a precise diagnosis. Audiologic testing is especially helpful in the diagnosis and follow-up of patients with Meniere's disease. Brainstem auditory evoked potential (BAEP) tests for brainstem dysfunction and electroencephalography (EEG) can rule out epilepsy as a source of dizziness.

COMPLICATIONS

Although 80% of patients with Meniere's disease are in remission at 5 years, there is significant irreversible hearing loss in the majority. Serial audiograms are helpful in identifying these patients. Early definitive treatment can prevent permanent damage to the patient's hearing. Patients with long-standing vertigo may have permanent vestibular damage. This disequilibrium can cause significant gait disturbance. The patient can make up for this deficit with vestibular rehabilitation. In this process, patients learn to rely on visual and proprioceptive cues to maintain balance.

TREATMENT

Symptomatic Therapy

Symptomatic treatment can greatly improve the quality of life of the dizzy patient. Several different classes of medications have antivertiginous effects, including phenothiazines, antihistamines, and benzodiazepines. In the acute phase, promethazine (Phenergan) 25 mg four times daily or diazepam 5 mg four times daily may be helpful, with prochlorperazine suppositories for the control of nausea. For long-term therapy, less-sedating medications are preferred. Meclizine 25 mg four times daily or transdermal scopolamine 0.5 mg every 3 days may prove helpful in such chronic cases. Thiazide diuretics (in tandem with a sodium-restricted diet) have been helpful in the management of Meniere's disease.

Specific Therapy

The Epley positional maneuver has been designed to remove debris from the posterior semicircular canal in cases of BPPV. The patient is seated, and the examiner rotates the head 45° to the right. The examiner then quickly places the patient into a supine position with the head hanging over the edge of the exam table, with the rightward rotation maintained and the head extended approximately 30°. The head is rotated from right to left while still hanging off the edge of the table. The patient then rolls onto the side facing the floor. Finally, the patient sits up. This maneuver may be performed several times, until no vertigo or nystagmus occurs. This brings about a remission in most patients, although recurrences do occur.

Dizziness caused by neoplasm such as acoustic neuroma is an indication for surgical excision. There are also surgical options for Meniere's disease such as labyrinthectomy and vestibular neurectomy. Intratympanic gentamicin has been shown to prevent attacks and preserve hearing.

PATIENT EDUCATION

In addition to any symptomatic treatment, patients should be instructed to lie still with their eyes closed to help end an acute vertiginous episode. Salt restriction to 1 to 2 g of sodium per day has been shown to reduce the frequency of vertigo in Meniere's disease. Vestibular exercises (such as gait exercises that increase reliance on visual and proprioceptive cues) performed twice daily may improve balance and coordination in patients with chronic disequilibrium.

BIBLIOGRAPHY

Adams RD et al (eds): Deafness, dizziness and disorders of equilibrium, in *Adams and Victor's Principles of Neurology,* 6th ed, New York, McGraw-Hill, 1997, pp 294–309.

Baloh RW: Hearing and equilibrium, in *Cecil Textbook of Medicine,* 21st ed, Goldman L, Bennett JC (eds). Philadelphia, Saunders, 2000, pp 2250–2257.

Jensen JM: Vertigo and dizziness, in *Neurology for the Non-Neurologist,* 4th ed, Weiner WI, Goetz CG (eds). Philadelphia, Lippincott Williams & Wilkins, 1999, pp 397–406.

Ruckenstein MJ: A practical approach to dizziness. *Postgrad Med* 97(3):70–81, 1995.

Sloane PD et al: Management of dizziness in primary care. *J Am Board Fam Pract* 7(1):1–8, 1994.

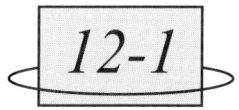

DYSMENORRHEA

Gail Allison

DISCUSSION

The normal menstrual cycle is almost always accompanied by peri-menstrual symptoms, which usually resolve spontaneously and are minimally disruptive. Menstrual cramps begin within approximately 1 to 2 h of bleeding and subside within 24 to 48 h. The intensity of the symptoms varies widely among women. When the symptoms become incapacitating or the patient seeks treatment, the clinical diagnosis is established.

Dysmenorrhea is defined as painful menstruation or difficult menstrual flow. Dysmenorrhea occurs with ovulatory cycles and usually is classified as primary or secondary.[1] *Primary dysmenorrhea* is painful menstruation with an absence of pelvic pathology and is the basic topic of this chapter. *Secondary dysmenorrhea* equates with painful menstrual cramps in the presence of a pathologic condition such as endometriosis, pelvic inflammatory disease (PID), fibroids, salpingitis, or congenital anomalies of the müllerian system.

EPIDEMIOLOGY

Dysmenorrhea is the most common gynecologic complaint and usually begins within 1 to 2 years of menarche. In cross-sectional surveys, 30 to 60 percent of women of reproductive age report experiencing menstrual pain. However, only 7 to 15 percent of those women report severe pain that interferes with daily activity. There is a higher prevalence of dysmenorrhea (ranging from 67 to 72 percent) in young adults age 16 to 24.[2] The rate tends to decrease with age, especially after age 35.[3]

Factors consistently shown to be associated with an increased incidence of dysmenorrhea are earlier age at menarche, longer and heavier menstrual flow, nulliparity, smoking, and a family history of dysmenorrhea in the mother or a sister. Cycle length increases the prevalence of menstrual pain. Oral contraceptive users report less severe pain. Only 31 percent of all women with dysmenorrhea report it to their physicians.[4]

PATHOGENESIS

The synthesis of a number of biochemical agents in the endometrium is accelerated by the rapid decline of progesterone that occurs in the luteal phase just before menstruation. Prostaglandins F_{2a} and E_2, leukotrienes, and possibly prostacyclin have been identified as important contributing biochemical agents. In menstruating women, prostaglandin production increases during the first 2 to 3 days of the menstrual cycle, while women with primary dysmenorrhea produce 8 to 13 times more prostaglandin and at a rate seven times faster than do nondysmenorrheic women. Prostaglandins act directly on the myometrium (uterine musculature), increasing the intensity and frequency of uterine contractions. They cause constriction of the uterine arteries, leading to uterine ischemia, tissue trauma, necrosis, and finally the endometrial shedding of menstruation. The most recent hypothesis states that prostaglandin E_2 may increase the sensitivity of peripheral pain fibers. Psychological factors were long thought to be a primary cause of dysmenorrhea until the discovery of the current biological causes. These factors, including attitudes passed from mothers to daughters, may play a role in women with unresponsive dysmenorrhea and should be considered.

SIGNS AND SYMPTOMS

The diagnosis of primary dysmenorrhea should be one of exclusion. The history includes an onset of problems usually 1 to 2 years after menarche; midline cramping (with or without systemic symptoms), symptoms within the first 24 to 48 h of menses, a duration of 1 to 3 days, and moderate menstrual flow; and no pain at any other time. Constitutional symptoms may include nausea, vomiting, headache, diarrhea, bloating, malaise, fatigue, and/or low back pain. Symptoms are individualized and vary in intensity.

Pelvic and abdominal examination does not reveal any anatomic abnormality or significant pelvic disease.

DIAGNOSTIC CONSIDERATIONS

The most common misdiagnosis for primary dysmenorrhea is secondary dysmenorrhea caused by endometriosis. These symptoms occur 1 to 2 weeks before menses and resolve with the onset of menstruation or shortly thereafter. Women with endometriosis often report dyspareunia; by contrast, women with primary dysmenorrhea rarely report this symptom.

DIAGNOSTIC TESTS

In patients with a suggestive history and a normal pelvic examination, no diagnostic testing is required. A reasonable approach is to proceed with either single or combined therapy through several cycles.

If the patient is unresponsive, further diagnostic testing may be required, including ultrasound and/or laparoscopy. If laparoscopy is negative and treatment is ineffectual, psychological evaluation should be considered as a final assessment.

TREATMENT

Medical management is the mainstay of treatment. For most women, prostaglandin synthetase inhibitors [nonsteroidal anti-inflammatory drugs (NSAIDs)] and/or oral contraceptives provide effective therapy. Surgical therapy is reserved for a small number of women with severe, unresponsive pain. General measures include reassurance that the condition is not caused by pelvic pathology and educational counseling regarding the proper use of NSAIDs or oral contraceptives. One should reevaluate in 1 to 2 months to assess treatment efficacy.

Prostaglandin Synthetase Inhibitor (Antiprostaglandins)

The antiprostaglandins' mechanism of action is to block the synthesis and release of prostaglandins. Antiprostaglandins (NSAIDs) are most effective (up to 80 percent success rate) when taken before the initiation of pain. NSAIDs should be started 1 to 3 days before the onset of menses and continued through day 2 of flow. Generally, these medications are interchangeable with respect to overall effectiveness. The initial choice is best made on the basis of cost, with subsequent modifications based on experience with side effects and effectiveness. Ibuprofen is a good initial choice because it is available in generic form without a prescription, is the least expensive, and is safe. Experience has shown that some women do poorly with one medication in this class but respond positively to another. For this reason, it is acceptable and reasonable to experiment. The major side effects are gastrointestinal (nausea, vomiting, diarrhea), renal (fluid retention, decreased renal function in persons with renal vascular disease), and central nervous system (syncope, sedation). Women with a known allergy to aspirin should not use antiprostaglandins. Table 12-1-1 lists antiprostaglandins and the recommended doses.

Oral Contraceptives

The mechanism of action is probably related to the absence of ovulation and an altered endometrium that inhibits prostaglandin release. Oral contraceptives are the treatment of choice for women who fail treatment on antiprostaglandins. Cyclic administration of any low-dose formulation is acceptable. It is preferable to begin with a monophasic one, since these agents are anecdotally more efficacious than the newer triphasic preparations. If there are other reasons to prefer a triphasic one, a reasonable approach is to try it for a few cycles and then switch to a monophasic one if there is no response. If neither oral contraceptives nor antiprostaglandins are 100 percent effective, combined therapy is an appropriate alternative.

Alternative Therapies

The mainstays of treatment are antiprostaglandins and oral contraceptives; however, alternative therapies are available that are effective to varying degrees. A discussion of dysmenorrhea would not be complete without mentioning the following options:

1. *Exercise.* Helps suppress prostaglandin release and shunts blood away from the uterus. Beta endorphins are released and decrease pain perception.
2. *Local heat (heating pad, hot water bottle, warm bath).* Symptomatic treatment with heat increases blood flow and decreases muscle spasm.
3. *Dietary changes or supplements.* Decrease salt intake and consume foods that contain natural diuretics to decrease water retention. Vitamin E is a mild prostaglandin inhibitor that improves circulation to the uterus by reducing arteriole spasm.
4. TENS *(transcutaneous electrical nerve stimulation).* This technique works by blocking efferent pain stimuli and reducing central awareness of pain. It has been used for many types of musculoskeletal pain. It has limited practical application. It can be expensive, units may not be readily available, and it is inconvenient to carry around a unit for 1 to 3 days. There are no significant side effects.

TABLE 12-1-1. Prostaglandin Synthetase Inhibitors*

DRUG	DOSAGE
Ibuprofen (Motrin)	400–600 mg every 4–6 h
Naproxen (Naprosyn)	500 mg stat, 250 mg every 6–8 h
Ketoprofen (Orudis)	25–50 mg every 6–8 h
Fenoprofen (Nalfon)	200 mg every 4–6 h
Meclofenamate (Meclomen)	100 mg twice daily
Mefenamic acid (Ponstel)	500 mg stat, 250 mg every 6 h
Naproxen sodium (Anaprox)	550 mg stat, 275 mg every 6–8 h

*Individual patients may respond differently to each medication. It is appropriate to use a loading dose on the first day and experiment for effect.

5. *Ovulation suppression.* Suppressing ovulation by using means other than oral contraceptives may be an option for women who are not surgical candidates or in whom other therapies have failed. The practical choice would be depomedroxyprogesterone acetate given intramuscularly. It is relatively inexpensive, provides contraception, and has few side effects; the effect is completely reversible. Ovulation, however, may not resume for several months.
6. *Surgical therapy.* In a few women, medication does not control dysmenorrhea and surgical therapies should be considered. Laparoscopic presacral neurectomy and resection of the uterosacral ligament may become more popular for unresponsive patients. In rare instances, hysterectomy may be considered for women in whom childbearing is no longer desired.

ACKNOWLEDGMENTS

The editor would like to acknowledge the significant contributions of Cheryl Gregorio, the author of this chapter in the first edition of *Primary Care for Physician Assistants.*

REFERENCES

1. Gerbie MV: Complications of menstruation: Abnormal uterine bleeding, in Decherney AH, Pernoll ML (eds): *Current Obstetrics and Gynecology,* 8th ed. New York, McGraw-Hill, 1996.
2. Harlow SD: Menstruation and menstrual disorders: The epidemiology of menstruation and menstrual dysfunction, in Goldman MB, Hatch MC (eds): *Women and Health.* San Diego, Academic Press, 2000.
3. Murphy JR: Dysmenorrhea, in Star WL, Lommel LL, Shannon MT (eds): *Women's Primary Health Care: Protocols for Practice.* Washington, DC, American Nurse's Publishing, 1995.
4. Schroeder B, Sanfilippo JS: Dysmenorrhea and pelvic pain in adolescents. *Pediatr Clin North Am* 46(3):555–571, 1999.

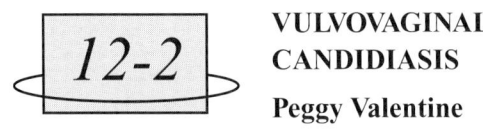

VULVOVAGINAL CANDIDIASIS

Peggy Valentine

DISCUSSION

Approximately 75 percent of women experience at least one episode of vulvovaginal candidiasis in their lifetimes. The majority of cases (80 to 90 percent) are caused by *Candida albicans.* The remaining 10 percent are caused by *C. glabrata* or *C. tropicalis.* The typical complaint includes vulvar pruritus of varied intensity and vaginal discharge. The consistency of the discharge may vary from thin and watery to thick and lumpy ("cottage cheese").

Predisposing factors include pregnancy, oral contraceptives, diabetes mellitus, and recent antibiotic use. During pregnancy and while women are taking oral contraceptives, the high levels of hormones are thought to promote *Candida* growth in the vagina. Vaginal colonization frequently is observed in diabetic women, and antibiotics are thought to eliminate the protective vaginal flora. Wearing poorly ventilated underwear or tight-fitting clothing that increases perineal moisture and temperature is another predisposing factor. It is estimated that 10 to 20 percent of women normally harbor *Candida* species and yeasts without being symptomatic.

SIGNS AND SYMPTOMS

The most common symptom, vulvar pruritus, is present in nearly all symptomatic individuals. Vaginal discharge may vary in quantity and appearance. Other complaints include vaginal soreness, irritation, vulvar burning, dyspareunia, and external dysuria caused by contact of urine with inflamed labia. The symptoms may be exacerbated just before the menstrual period, with some relief at the onset of menstrual flow. Vulvovaginal candidiasis is usually not sexually transmitted, but male partners of affected women may develop balanoposthitis. More frequently, a transient rash, erythema, and pruritus may develop shortly after unprotected sexual intercourse. Same-sex partners can transmit candidiasis by sharing unwashed clothing or sex toys. The symptoms are self-limiting and respond well to topical antifungal agents.

OBJECTIVE FINDINGS

Findings include vulvar erythema and vaginal discharge, which may be watery or thick with clumps like cottage cheese. The discharge often adheres to vaginal mucosa.

DIAGNOSTIC CONSIDERATIONS

A diagnosis can be made when the patient has signs and symptoms of vaginitis, the wet mount demonstrates yeast, and the vaginal yeast culture is positive.

SPECIAL CONSIDERATIONS

Acute vulvovaginal candidiasis occurs frequently among women infected with HIV, but insufficient information exists to determine the optimal management. The current recommended treatment is the same for these patients. Vulvovaginal candidiasis is common during pregnancy. Only topical "azole" therapies should be used (for 7 days) in pregnant women.

LABORATORY TESTS

A wet mount or saline preparation should be done to identify yeast cells or mycelia microscopically. The clinician also should observe for the presence of clue cells and motile trichomonads on the same slide. The use of 10% potassium hydroxide (KOH) is important for revealing the presence of germinating yeast. Vaginal pH is usually normal (4.0 to 4.5); if pH is higher than 5.0, consider bacterial vaginosis, trichomoniasis, or a mixed infection. A vaginal culture should be performed if microscopic findings are negative or inconclusive and vulvovaginal candidiasis is suspected from signs or symptoms. A positive culture, however, does not necessarily mean that *Candida* is responsible for vaginal symptoms.

TREATMENT

Oral or topical azole preparations provide more effective treatment than do simple nystatin preparations. Approximately 80 to 90 percent of patients who complete azole therapy experience relief of symptoms and have negative cultures.

Recommended regimens are either butoconazole 2% cream 5 g intravaginally for 3 days or clotrimazole 1% cream 5 g intravaginally for 7 to 14 days. *Caution:* These vaginal preparations are oil-based and may weaken latex condoms and diaphragms.

Other therapy includes clotrimazole 500-mg vaginal tablet, one tablet in a single application. Single-dose therapy should be reserved for patients with uncomplicated mild to moderate vulvovaginal candidiasis. Multiday regimens (3 and 7 days) are the preferred treatment for severe or complicated cases. An example is miconazole 200-mg vaginal suppository, one suppository for 3 days.

Alternative regimens include oral azole agents such as fluconazole (Diflucan), which may be as effective as topical agents and have high patient acceptance. Use fluconazole 150 mg as a single oral dose. Ketoconazole (Nizoral) 100 mg daily and fluconazole once weekly

for up to 6 months are thought to reduce the frequency of recurrent infections.

PATIENT EDUCATION

Self-medication with over-the-counter (OTC) preparations should be advised only for women who previously have been diagnosed with vulvovaginal candidiasis and have recurrent symptoms.

COMPLICATIONS AND RED FLAGS

Women who experience three or more recurrent episodes of vulvovaginal candidiasis per year should be evaluated carefully. Diabetes mellitus, immunosuppression, the use of broad-spectrum antibiotics, corticosteroid use, and HIV infection may present as recurrent vulvovaginal candidiasis.

BIBLIOGRAPHY

Centers for Disease Control and Prevention: 1998 Guidelines for Treatment of Sexually Transmitted Diseases. *MMWR* 47(RR-1):75–79, 1998.

Mou SM: Gynecologic infections, in Seltzer VL, Pearse WH (eds): *Women's Primary Health Care: Office Procedures and Practice.* New York, McGraw-Hill, 1995, pp 190–191.

Solbel JD: Vulvovaginal candidiasis, in Holmes KK, Mardh P-A, Sparling PF, et al (eds): *Sexually Transmitted Diseases,* 2d ed. New York, McGraw-Hill, 1990, pp 515–522.

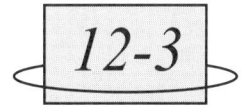

BACTERIAL VAGINOSIS
Peggy Valentine

DISCUSSION

Bacterial vaginosis is the most common cause of malodorous (fishy-smelling) discharge in sexually active women. Vaginal irritation and pain are uncommon, and if they are present, one should rule out coexisting conditions such as trichomoniasis and vulvovaginal candidiasis. No single pathogen is responsible for bacterial vaginosis. An overgrowth of anaerobic bacteria (e.g., *Bacteroides* spp., *Mobiluncus* spp.), *Gardnerella vaginalis,* and *Mycoplasma hominis* replaces the normal lactobacillus vaginal flora. The cause of this vaginal overgrowth is unknown. It remains unclear whether bacterial vaginosis is sexually transmitted, although some studies have demonstrated an increased prevalence among women with multiple sex partners. Treating the male partner has not proved beneficial in preventing recurrence of the disease, and further research is needed to understand the disease course. Bacterial vaginosis has been associated with endometritis, pelvic inflammatory disease (PID), and vaginal cuff cellulitis after invasive genitourinary procedures. There may be a risk of prematurity and chorioamnionitis among pregnant women with this infection.

SIGNS AND SYMPTOMS

The most common symptom is a genital malodor described as "fishy-smelling," and the second most common symptom is increased vaginal discharge. Over half of all women have no symptoms at all. Abdominal pain and pruritus are rarely reported.

OBJECTIVE FINDINGS

Inspection reveals a nonviscous homogeneous white noninflammatory discharge that adheres to the vaginal walls and often is visible on the labia and fourchette. Usually no signs of inflammation are noted. The vaginal pH is usually higher than 4.5.

DIAGNOSTIC CONSIDERATIONS

Clinical and/or Gram stain criteria are used to make the diagnosis. Clinical criteria should include three of the following signs and symptoms:

- Homogeneous, white noninflammatory discharge that adheres to the vaginal walls
- Presence of clue cells on wet mount by microscopic examination
- pH of vaginal fluid higher than 4.5
- Fishy odor of vaginal discharge before or after the addition of 10% potassium hydroxide (KOH) (whiff test)

SPECIAL CONSIDERATIONS

Women of childbearing age who are sexually active.

LABORATORY TESTS

The pH of vaginal secretions is normally less than 4.4. Vaginal pH is best determined by swabbing the lateral and posterior fornices of the vagina and placing the sample directly on pH paper; look for a pH higher than 4.5. One should avoid cervical mucus, since the pH is approximately 7.0. Place a drop of vaginal fluid on a glass slide and add a drop of 10% KOH; a fishy-smelling odor will be released (whiff test). Saline wet mount is done to detect clue cells, usually without polymorphonuclear neutrophils. Take a sample of vaginal fluid with a swab and mix it on a glass slide with a drop of normal saline. Microscopic examination should reveal squamous vaginal epithelial cells covered with many bacteria, giving them a stippled or granular appearance. Since *Gardnerella vaginalis* can be isolated in half of normal women, a specific culture for this organism is not a particularly helpful diagnostic test.

TREATMENT

The primary goal is to relieve vaginal signs and symptoms. Treatment of sexual partners is not recommended, since this does not prevent recurrent infection in women. However, some clinicians empirically treat the partners of patients with frequently recurring bacterial vaginosis. Commercially available lactobacillus preparations have not been shown to be effective.

The treatment of choice is metronidazole (Flagyl) 500 mg PO twice daily for 7 days. Patients should be advised to avoid alcohol during treatment with metronidazole and for 24 h afterward. Metronidazole is contraindicated in pregnancy. HIV-infected patients who have bacterial vaginosis should receive the same treatment regimen as those who are HIV-negative.

Alternative regimens (somewhat less efficacious) include metronidazole 2 g orally in a single dose or metronidazole gel 0.75%, one full applicator (5 g) intravaginally twice daily for 5 days, or clindamycin cream 2%, one full applicator (5 g) intravaginally HS for 7 days (still under investigation). Clindamycin cream is oil-based and therefore may weaken latex condoms or diaphragms; therefore clindamycin 300 mg PO twice daily for 7 days may be given.

PATIENT EDUCATION

The patient should be informed about the diagnosis and the importance of complying with treatment to prevent recurrence. Since bacterial vaginosis is associated with sexual activity, abstinence or condom use is recommended.

DISPOSITION

If the symptoms resolve, follow-up visits are not necessary. Since recurrence of bacterial vaginosis is common, alternative treatment regimens should be used in such cases.

BIBLIOGRAPHY

Centers for Disease Control and Prevention: 1998 Guidelines for Treatment of Sexually Transmitted Diseases. *MMWR* 47(RR-1):70–74, 1998.
Hillier S, Holmes KK: Bacterial vaginosis, in Holmes KK, Mardh P-A, Sparling PF, et al (eds): *Sexually Transmitted Diseases,* 2d ed. New York, McGraw-Hill, 1990, pp 547–555.
Mou SM: Gynecologic infections, in Seltzer VL, Pearse WH (eds): *Women's Primary Health Care: Office Practice and Procedures.* New York, McGraw-Hill, 1995, pp 189–190.

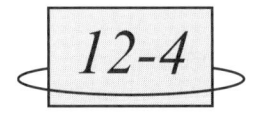

12-4 PREMENSTRUAL SYNDROME
Dana M. Gallagher

DISCUSSION

Premenstrual symptoms are common, affecting up to 75% of menstruating women.[1] Premenstrual syndrome (PMS) is a constellation of physical and/or affective symptoms that recurs cyclically between ovulation and onset of the menses. Premenstrual symptoms abate after menses begins.

In some women, physical symptoms predominate, for example, bloating, tender breasts, and fatigue, whereas others are more bothered by emotional lability and depression. Symptoms may be mild or moderate and may vary in both type and intensity from cycle to cycle. Less than 10% of women suffer severe premenstrual symptoms.[2] Women whose chief complaints are affective are much more likely to have severe PMS than women whose complaints are primarily physical.[3]

PATHOGENESIS

The cause of PMS is unknown, although the patient may recall childbirth or tubal ligation as the event that precipitated her premenstrual symptoms. A variety of possible etiologies have been proposed, including estrogen–progesterone imbalance, vitamin and/or mineral deficiency, neurotransmitter dysfunction, prolactin excess, and psychiatric disorders. To date, none of these theories (either individually or in combination) have been proved.

Since the etiology is unknown and symptom presentation is variable, the treatment is, understandably, individualized.

SYMPTOMS

Physical symptoms can include (but are not limited to) bloating and weight gain, tender breasts, bowel changes, food cravings, headache, and acne. Affective changes can include (but are not limited to) agitation, irritability, rage, crying "for no reason," depression, and homicidal and/or suicidal ideation. Although patients may experience a combination of these, medical intervention is typically sought for relief of one or two particularly disagreeable symptoms.

OBJECTIVE FINDINGS

If the examination takes place during the premenstruum, it may be possible to document physical findings (e.g., to observe a fine tremor of the hand or chart a weight gain or tender breast examination). The patient may be unusually tearful, agitated, or testy during the office visit. Most often, however, there are no objective findings.

DIAGNOSTIC CONSIDERATIONS

Diagnosing PMS requires a minimum of 2 to 3 consecutive months of daily symptom charting by the patient. She must note not only her symptoms but also their cyclicity and severity. It is not uncommon for women to learn during symptom charting that their symptoms are not cyclic. When cyclicity is not verified, another cause should be sought. Since symptom charts make the diagnosis, this documentation is critical, even for the woman who is certain she has PMS. (One of the author's patients documented weekday symptoms that disappeared after she quit her job.)

LABORATORY TESTS

There are no laboratory tests to diagnose PMS. However, laboratory tests may be ordered depending on the patient's presenting complaint. For example:

- A 49-year-old with PMS symptoms should have follicle-stimulating hormone (FSH) levels drawn to screen for menopause.
- A patient complaining of intense premenstrual fatigue should be screened for anemia.
- A patient complaining of depression and sluggishness should be screened for hypothyroidism.

RADIOLOGIC AND OTHER DIAGNOSTIC STUDIES

There are no diagnostic studies for PMS.

TREATMENT

Pharmacologic Management

The selective serotonin reuptake inhibitor fluoxetine (Prozac) has proved helpful in 50% of women with premenstrual affective symptomatology.[3] Dosage is 20 mg orally taken in the morning. In 1999, an advisory panel to the Food and Drug Administration approved fluoxetine for the treatment of severe premenstrual affective symptomatology, "premenstrual dysphoric disorder."[4]

In women with severe affective symptomatology, alprazolam 0.25 mg qid is helpful[3] when used from day 18 of the cycle until menses, with a gradual taper to days 1 and 2 of menses. Taking the drug only during the luteal phase decreases the risk of dependence. Still, alprazolam use should be reserved for those with severe symptoms who do not respond to other regimens.

For women with fluid retention, anecdotal reports support the use of spironolactone 25 mg qid at onset of symptoms.[4]

Although both micronized progesterone 300 mg qid and oral contraceptives have been widely touted for PMS treatment, there is no scientific evidence to support their use.

Supportive Measures

Avoidance of sugar and alcohol may ameliorate premenstrual symptoms of hypoglycemia. Caffeine should be avoided to decrease breast tenderness and irritability. Salt intake can be restricted to decrease the sensation of bloating and fluid retention. Regular aerobic exercise helps fight depression and fluid retention. Recent research has shown that vitamin and mineral regimens may have a positive impact. If the patient requests vitamin supplementation, B complex with B_6 not exceeding 100 mg/d may be used.[5] Calcium 1200 mg/d taken for a minimum of 2 months has been shown to reduce moodiness, bloating, and food cravings.[6]

PATIENT EDUCATION

Self-help books, support groups, and individual, couples, or family therapy may be useful. Offer the patient the option of bringing her spouse or partner to office visits so you can answer questions. Partners frequently have helpful insights about the patient's symptoms and the success of the treatment program. Inform the patient that improvements brought on by diet, exercise, and vitamin supplementation may be subtle over time, not immediate and dramatic. Life-style changes may also be more helpful if observed throughout the cycle rather than in the premenstruum alone.

NOTES AND PEARLS

Once PMS is treated and diagnosed, be sure to evaluate the progress of the patient at intervals. Because of the chronic and somewhat unpredictable nature of the syndrome, the patient continues to be at risk for depression. Should there be a flare-up of symptoms after the patient has responded to treatment, reevaluate the current treatment regimen and look for potential new problems.

REFERENCES

1. Rapkin A, Laughlin D: Guidelines for the diagnosis and treatment of premenstrual syndrome. *Fam Prac Recert* 21(1):42–74, 1999.
2. Tierney LM Jr et al (eds): *Current Medical Diagnosis and Treatment*, 39th ed. New York, Lange Medical/McGraw-Hill, 2000, pp 725–726.
3. Barnhart KT et al: A clinician's guide to the premenstrual syndrome. *Med Clin North Am* 79(6):1458, 1995.
4. Richwine L: Prozac wins panel support for treating severe PMS. *Reuters* July 6, 2000. Food and Drug Administration, US Dept of Health and Human Services; "FDA approve fluoxetine to treat premenstrual dysphonic disorder" attp://www.verify.fda.gov.
5. Wyatt KM et al: Efficacy of vitamin B-6 in the treatment of premenstrual syndrome—Systematic review. *BMJ* 318(7195): 1375–1381, 1999.
6. Thys-Jacobs S et al: Calcium carbonate and the premenstrual syndrome: Effects on premenstrual and menstrual symptoms. *Am J Obstet Gynecol* 179(2):444–452, 1998.

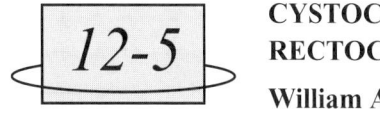

CYSTOCELE AND RECTOCELE
William A. Mosier

DISCUSSION

A *cystocele* is a downward displacement of the bladder that forms a herniation of the anterior vaginal wall below the floor of the bladder. It bulges into the anterior aspect of the vagina. The urinary bladder becomes displaced from weakening of the anterior vaginal wall. Cystoceles can range from mild to severe in their presentation. However, as a rule, they progress slowly.

A *rectocele* is a bulging of the posterior vaginal wall resulting from a herniation of the anterior rectal wall through a relaxed or ruptured vaginal fascia and the rectovaginal septum. In essence it is a rectovaginal sacculation that results from a trauma to the levator muscles and stretching or tearing of the supporting fascia.

PATHOGENESIS

A cystocele results from a loss of support by the structures that are normally responsible for maintaining it. This commonly occurs after childbearing, which can cause permanent stretching of some structures. These structures are typically the pubocervical or paravaginal fascia and the oblique tunnel of the levator sling through which the vagina passes.

A rectocele results from weakened or torn support structures after childbirth and further weakening produced by repeated straining during defecation. A rectocele cannot occur without a definite fascial defect. When not due to the trauma of childbirth, it is due to a congenital or inherent weakness in fascial and muscle supports. No matter what the cause, once the herniation starts, the weakened fascial supports gradually give way.

SYMPTOMS

The severity of complaints varies widely with cystocele. Patients may complain of a sensation of fullness or bulging in their vagina, a bearing-down sensation, urinary stress incontinence, or a vaginal protrusion. The severity of complaints also depends on the degree of prolapse present. A bearing-down discomfort is often aggravated by physical exercise or prolonged standing. If descent of the bladder is extreme, even walking or prolonged sitting may aggravate discomfort. Urinary symptoms are common in patients with a cystocele because of the difficulty in voiding completely. The descent of the bladder can drop its anterior portion below the level of the bladder neck. This creates a mechanical problem that results in difficulty evacuating. This often leads to irritability of the bladder and urinary frequency. Due to sepsis, the patient may experience frequent urinary tract infections.

The symptoms related to having a rectocele are usually few and considerably less severe than those of a cystocele. A slight, or even moderate, rectocele is generally asymptomatic. A patient may have a minimal discomfort during the Valsalva maneuver or may be aware of a bulge in the vaginal vault. Some patients may complain that defecation can be accomplished only with digital pressure applied vaginally against the sacculation. However, symptoms are rarely ever severe enough to require surgical intervention or even a pessary. It is usually an associated cystocele and uterine descent that produce discomfort.

OBJECTIVE FINDINGS

When the vaginal vault is inspected, it is important to distinguish between a cystocele and a rectocele. The distinction between the two is quite obvious.

In the case of a cystocele, a weakness of the anterior vaginal wall causes a visible bulging and is readily palpable. The bulging is usually spherical and often fills the vaginal orifice. On palpation, the mass has a soft consistency and an elastic feel to the touch. A cystocele may be so small that it is not obvious when the patient is in a supine position. Asking the patient to perform a Valsalva maneuver can often make the cystocele more readily palpable.

The diagnosis of a rectocele can also be made via visualization and palpation. A finger placed on the anal canal and pressure exerted toward the upper part of the vagina will make a defect in the posterior vaginal wall obvious. If the patient is asked to perform a Valsalva maneuver, the protrusion of the posterior vaginal wall expands. The defect is usually noted above the anal sphincter.

DIAGNOSTIC CONSIDERATIONS

There are very few pathologic entities that can be confused with a cystocele or rectocele. However, the differential should include enterocele, urethrocele, and vaginal cysts. Gartner's duct cysts, on rare occasion, have been found to dissect beneath the anterior vaginal wall epithelium and assume a cystocele-like position.

TREATMENT

Nonsurgical Management

Nonsurgical intervention should include an attempt to use muscle-strengthening exercises to improve the muscle tone of the levator ani muscles. In the postpartum patient, a pessary may be useful immediately after delivery, especially if the uterus is retroverted and produces strain on the supporting ligaments. A pessary used to elevate the uterus may facilitate the muscles to regain adequate tone. A pessary, however, will not cure a prolapse. It can only prevent it from becoming worse.

For the older patient who is not planning to have any more children and who is an unsuitable candidate for surgical repair, a supporting pessary can be effective if a cystocele is accompanied by a prolapsed uterus. If there is so much relaxation of the support tissue that a prolapse is precipitated by coughing or defecation, a pessary will have no practical usefulness. Pelvic muscle exercises (Kegel exercises) are used to strengthen the muscles surrounding the opening of the urethra, vagina, and rectum. Hormone replacement therapy (HRT) may be useful, especially for postmenopausal women.

Surgical Management

Cystocele and rectocele repairs are considered a regular step in performing vaginal hysterectomies and pelvic floor repairs.

There is usually no urgency for repair of a cystocele. Surgery is indicated if the patient is having the following symptoms:

1. Repeated bouts of cystitis or other chronic urinary tract infections
2. Painful symptoms or a feeling of pressure
3. A cystocele that is growing

When surgery is indicated, the repair is usually done along with other procedures such as a vaginal hysterectomy or pelvic floor repair in conjunction with a urethrocele repair.

The basic surgical technique for cystocele repair is as follows:

1. A midline incision is made through the anterior vaginal mucosa. The incision should extend from the external urinary meatus to the cervix.
2. At the cervix, a transverse incision, through the mucosa over the anterior cervix, is performed that joins with the midline incision to form an inverted T.
3. Dissection is then performed laterally to the margin of the defect.
4. The bladder should be detached from the anterior cervix and elevated with interrupted sutures.
5. Any excess vaginal mucosa should also be excised.
6. Interrupted stitches, using absorbable suture, are then used to approximate the cut edges of the vaginal mucosa to carry out a full-thickness repair.
7. If a layered repair is being performed, then the fascia and mucosa should be approximated separately.

Since a small rectocele usually causes minimal problems for the patient, surgical repair is typically done only when there is prolapse of other pelvic viscera. It is usually recommended that a rectocele be repaired only if there is a significant problem with perineal relaxation. However, a large rectocele should be repaired surgically if the patient has difficulty with fecal elimination specifically caused by the rectocele.

When an abdominal hysterectomy is performed, even an asymptomatic rectocele should be corrected because it is quite common for patients to complain of rectocele symptoms after the removal of the uterus even if they were previously unaware of the presence of a rectocele. When surgical repair of a rectocele is indicated, it is usually done in conjunction with repair of the perineum.

The basic surgical technique for rectocele repair is as follows:

1. A midline incision is usually initiated unless there are lacerations. If lacerations are present, a diamond-shaped area of mucosa is first excised. The incision continues through the vaginal mucosa, stopping posterior to the cervix.
2. A transverse incision is then made, just posterior to the cervix, to meet with the midline incision.
3. Dissection of the vaginal mucosa is then performed laterally until reaching the margin of the defect.
4. Beginning posteriorly, the repair is performed by bringing the diverging fibers of paravaginal fascia to the midline, using absorbable suture.

5. When reaching the perineum, the suturing must accommodate the inclusion of the medial margins of the puborectalis fibers of the levator ani muscles.

6. It is important to remember to restore the triangular shape of the perineum.

SUPPORTIVE MEASURES

No specialized postoperative care is necessary for the patient who undergoes a cystocele or rectocele repair. However, adequate fluids and analgesics should be given, and a low-residue diet and stool softener should be utilized during the initial postoperative period to ensure that no solid material comes through the anus while the tissue is healing. The perineum should be washed (sitz baths) to avoid secondary infection.

PATIENT EDUCATION

Patient education must include a discussion with the patient about family planning. Usually patients should postpone any cystocele or rectocele repair until after they have completed all plans for having any more children. This is due to the probability that subsequent deliveries will destroy surgical repair of a cystocele or rectocele.

Patients should be taught how to perform Kegel exercises. They should be told to contract the pelvic muscles for about 10 to 20 times in a row, at least six times per day.

If a pessary is inserted, patients must be advised that they should not be experiencing any pain or bleeding. They should be instructed to contact the provider if they encounter pain from the use of a pessary.

DISPOSITION

If a patient using a pessary is unable to remove it herself nightly at bedtime and reinsert it each morning, she must be examined at least every 3 months for vaginal irritation. Postmenopausal patients prescribed a pessary should be managed with estrogen therapy in an attempt to improve the resistance and tone of the vaginal epithelium.

COMPLICATIONS AND RED FLAGS

If urinary stress incontinence is present with cystocele, this may be a sign of a coexisting urethrocele or other serious problem. Because of the exposed position and thin overlying vaginal epithelium, a cystocele may ulcerate and cause bleeding or discharge. Urinary retention caused by bladder descent can easily bring on infection. Therefore, checking for cystitis is most important.

When the upper part of the posterior wall rolls out over the perineal body, this is usually not a rectocele but rather an enterocele.

OTHER NOTES AND PEARLS

Always check for a urethrocele. Stress incontinence is the chief symptom of a urethrocele. A rectocele is the least common type of prolapse. When there is a prolapse of the rectum, it is usually associated with a cystocele in uterine descent and a lacerated perineum.

BIBLIOGRAPHY

Baker VV, Deppe G: *Management of Perioperative Complications in Gynecology.* Philadelphia, Saunders, 1997.

Droegemueller W, Sciarra JJ (eds): *Gynecology and Obstetrics,* vol 1. Philadelphia, Lippincott, 1991, pp 61–63.

Lee RA: *Atlas of Gynecologic Surgery.* Philadelphia, Saunders, 1992.

Nichols DH: *Gynecology and Obstetric Surgery.* St Louis, MO, Mosby-Year Book, 1993, chaps 21, 22.

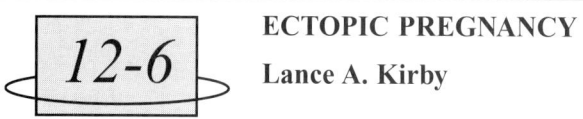

12-6

ECTOPIC PREGNANCY

Lance A. Kirby

DISCUSSION

Ectopic (extrauterine) pregnancy accounts for approximately 2 percent of all pregnancies and remains the most common cause of maternal death in the first 20 weeks of pregnancy. It is responsible for more than 15 percent of all obstetric maternal deaths in the United States. The risk for ectopic pregnancy increases with age: Women 35 to 44 years of age are three to four times more likely than are those 15 to 25 years of age to be at risk. Overall, the risk of maternal death from ectopic pregnancy is 10 times greater than the risk from term childbirth and 50 times greater than that from abortion.

The Centers for Disease Control and Prevention (CDC) began keeping statistics on ectopic pregnancies in 1970, and since that time the incidence has increased fourfold to fivefold. However, the incidence for the maternal mortality rate has decreased sevenfold.[1] Unfortunately, references and investigators rarely agree on many aspects of the descriptions of the women most likely to experience ectopic pregnancies. Pernoll and Garmel[2] report in the lower socioeconomic groups without regard to race, whereas Hickok and Patton[3] report race as a factor, not income.

The primary causes of ectopic pregnancy include conditions that impede or prevent passage of the fertilized ovum through the fallopian tube. Chronic salpingitis and pelvic inflammatory disease (PID) have been implicated. However, the rates for PID and salpingitis have remained stable over the past several years, and tubal histology has been reported as normal in as many as 70 percent of pathologic specimens. Increasing rates of tubal surgeries and assisted reproductive technologies have been suggested as possibilities.

Management has been influenced by the availability of a quick and sensitive test for human chorionic gonadotropin (hCG), technical advancements in ultrasonography, and early diagnostic laparoscopy. It is estimated that early detection is responsible for a 20 percent reduction of rupture before intervention, and the diagnosis is made before rupture in 80 percent of cases.[3] Early detection now allows greater flexibility in management, including extensive use of linear salpingotomy or segmental resection, and nonoperative management.

PATHOGENESIS

Ectopic pregnancy appears to be a process that occurs almost exclusively in humans. The symptoms occur later in the pregnancy, including rupture of the tube and intraperitoneal hemorrhage. The mechanism of pain involves the distention of the fallopian tube as a result of the growing fetus. Although implantation and pregnancy can occur at any point along the reproductive path, approximately 95 percent of these pregnancies implant within the fallopian tube. One important aspect of *all* ectopic pregnancies is the lack of resistance of the endosalpinx to invasion by the trophoblast. The trophoblast implants beneath the endosalpinx in the muscle and connective tissue. Then the trophoblast invades the blood vessels to cause local hemorrhage. A hematoma in the subserosal space enlarges as the pregnancy progresses, with possible bleeding in the distal end of the tube but not out the lumen.

Distention, thinness of the tube, and the trophoblast predispose to rupture.[4] Rupture occurs when the ovum erodes through the tubal wall, and the serosa ruptures when stretched to the breaking point. Other implantation sites, in descending order, are the ovary, abdomen, compound (heterotrophic), and cervix. The tube itself has statistical differences. The closer it is to the ovary, the more likely the implantation will occur, resulting in the highest statistical rate at the ampulla (78 percent). The highest morbidity rate results from cervical pregnancies, which statistically have the lowest implantation rate. Each of the implantation sites may present with its own pathology.

CLASSIFICATION

Ectopic pregnancy may be classified as follows:

Tubal (see sites 1, 2, and 3 in Fig. 12-6-1). A tubal pregnancy may terminate by abortion or missed abortion, extratubal rupture into the broad ligament, or intratubal rupture leading to tubal abortion or the formation of hematosalpinx or pelvic hematocele. Pregnancy may proceed to an advanced stage with or without rupture, but rarely to viability.

Interstitial (see site 4 in Fig. 12-6-1). The pregnancy begins in the portion of the tube that crosses the myometrium; the gestation is similar to intrauterine pregnancies that implant in the cornu or nearby. The ovum may rupture into the uterine cavity. The uterine wall may divide, causing severe destruction of the myometrium, which can result in entrance into the peritoneal cavity.

Abdominal (see site 5 in Fig. 12-6-1). A pregnancy that occurs in the abdomen may rupture into the peritoneal cavity, the retroperitoneal space, or a vital organ. An unrecognizable mass called an adipocere may form, an intraperitoneal abscess may be formed from infected fetal parts, or a lithopedion may be the end result. The pregnancy may continue to an advanced stage.

Ovarian (see site 6 in Fig. 12-6-1). An ovarian pregnancy usually ruptures into the peritoneal cavity. There is a possibility that the rupture contents can dissect into the folds of the ovarian ligament or form a lithopedion. An ovarian pregnancy almost never reaches viability.

Cervical (see site 7 in Fig. 12-6-1). A cervical pregnancy may rupture into the cervical canal and go directly into the vaginal canal. It is rare for a cervical pregnancy to rupture into the base of the broad ligament with an intraabdominal complication of hematoma formation.

ETIOLOGY

Conditions that impede the passage of the fertilized ovum through the tube are tubal factors, zygote abnormalities, ovarian factors, and exogenous hormones.

Tubal Factors

Fifty percent of tubal specimens reveal chronic salpingitis histologically. Other tubal factors include adherent folds of tissue caused by developmental abnormalities (atresia, congenital diverticula, lengthy or tortuous tubes), abnormal tubal anatomy caused by maternal use of diethylstilbestrol (DES) in utero, previous tubal or pelvic organ microsurgery, tubal ligation, and conservative treatment of an unruptured ectopic pregnancy. These conditions are consistent with intrinsic adhesions. Extrinsic adhesions such as peritonitis, transplants, pelvic tumors, and endometriosis have been implicated.

Zygote Abnormalities

Chromosomal defects, gross malformations, and neural tube defect have been reported. An increased incidence of zygote abnormalities has been reported with abnormal sperm counts and spermatozoa.

Ovarian Factors

There is evidence of ectopic development with the fertilization of an unextruded ovum, a transmigrated ovum, post-mid-cycle fertilization, and ovarian enlargement caused by fertility medications.

Exogenous Hormones

The administration of exogenous hormones may play a role in ectopic pregnancies. An increasing incidence of ectopic gestation, varying from 4 to 16 percent, has been reported with progestin-only contraceptives, progesterone secreting intrauterine devices (IUDs), and "morning-after pills"[4] (see Fig 12-6-1).

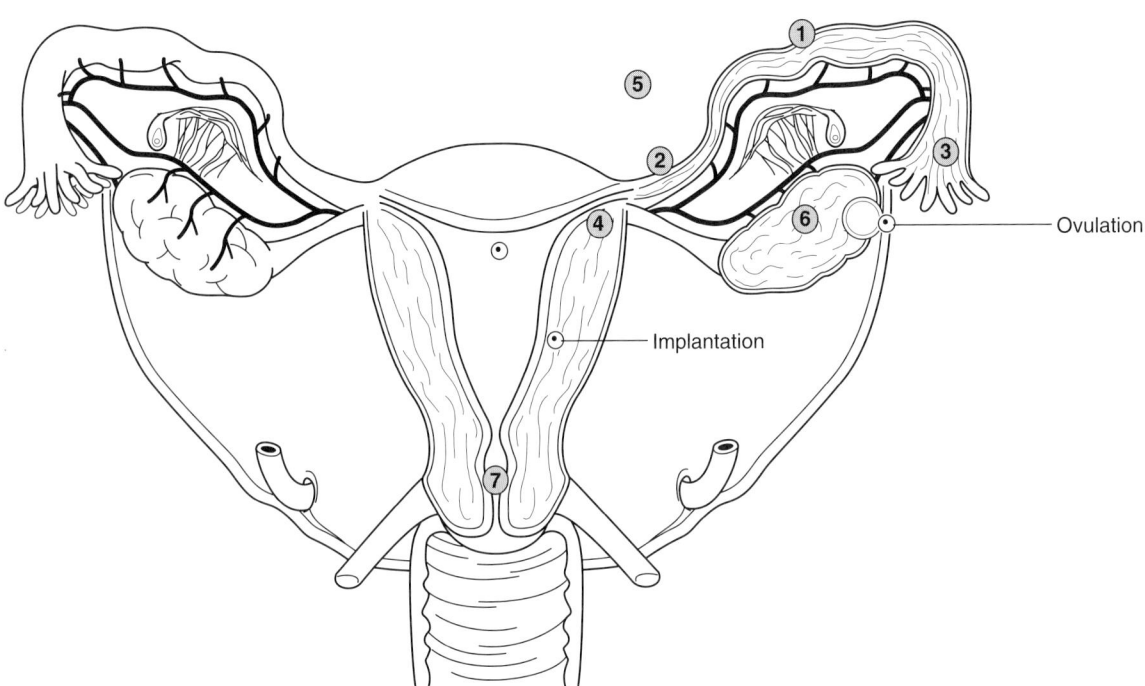

FIGURE 12-6-1. From ovulation to normal implantation, the journey for an ovum can be arduous. At any of these sites the ovum may implant. The most common ectopic sites to the least common in descending order are (1) ampullary, 78%; (2) isthmus, 12%; (3) fimbrial, 5%, (4) interstitial, 2 to 3%; (5) abdominal, 1 to 2%; (6) ovary, ≈ 1%; (7) cervix, 5%. (*From Bates et al.*[5])

SIGNS AND SYMPTOMS

The common symptoms of ectopic pregnancy are summarized in Table 12-6-1. Abdominal or pelvic pain ranging from low-grade soreness to a colicky cramping is generally present even before tubal rupture. With acute rupture, the pain is often sharp and becomes diffuse. Shoulder pain may result from diaphragmatic irritation by a hemoperitoneum. However, there is no specific pain pattern for ectopic pregnancy.

Frequently, patients report normal menstrual cycles, but when questioned further, they often report abnormal timing or flow of "menses." Characteristically, the bleeding is light and results from uterine decidual slough.

The presenting signs of ectopic pregnancy are summarized in Table 12-6-2. The so-called classic triad of ectopic pregnancy—pelvic or abdominal pain, abnormal vaginal bleeding, and an adnexal mass—occurs in only one-third of patients. Note that in the 50 percent of patients with an adnexal mass, one-fifth of those masses are on the side opposite the ectopic pregnancy and usually represent a corpus luteum cyst. Although the uterus may be enlarged as a result of hormonal stimulation, it is not as large as expected for the duration of amenorrhea.[5]

DIAGNOSTIC TESTS

Routine and special examinations are necessary for the timely and ultimately lifesaving diagnosis of extrauterine pregnancy. A pregnancy test must be of primary importance. With the sensitive assays available today, a negative test excludes the possibility of ectopic pregnancy. A positive test focuses on the complications of pregnancy. Quantitative serum β-hCG levels should be followed at 2-day intervals. The levels should increase more than 60 percent within 48 h. The pregnancy is not progressing appropriately if this criterion is not met.

Other hematology tests are usually not helpful in diagnosis but may indicate other complications. Occasionally, the hematocrit may be low, and the complete blood count may identify a blood loss anemia and leukocytosis. The white blood cell count, if elevated, could be an indication of infection, not necessarily ectopic pregnancy. Serum progesterone has been reported to assist in the diagnosis of an abdominal pregnancy.[5] A progesterone level less than 5 ng/mL indicates a nonviable pregnancy. The test identifies only the pregnancy, not the location of the pregnancy.

Pelvic ultrasonography is an excellent adjunct to quantitative hCG. It can image a pregnancy within the uterine cavity reliably but not from outside. Transabdominal ultrasound should identify an intrauterine pregnancy with a serum level of 6000 IU/mL hCG; however, transvaginal ultrasound is more sensitive and reveals an intrauterine pregnancy with 2000 IU/mL hCG.

Culdocentesis is a procedure to determine *ruptured* ectopic pregnancy. It can identify a hemoperitoneum. An 18-gauge needle is inserted into the posterior fornix between the uterosacral ligaments, through the cul-de-sac, into the peritoneal cavity. A negative aspirate (clear peritoneal fluid) indicates no hemorrhage but does not rule out an *unruptured* ectopic pregnancy. A positive aspirate (nonclotting blood) indicates hemorrhage into the abdominal cavity that has undergone fibrinolysis. Clotting blood indicates penetration of a main vessel or rapid blood loss into the abdomen. An empty aspiration is nondiagnostic or equivocal. It simply means that no information was obtained. Unfortunately, "no findings" does not rule in or out an ectopic pregnancy. It must be remembered that culdocentesis is an invasive procedure and as such carries its own inherent risks. It may be argued that equivocal or negative findings do not negate the need to do laparoscopy.

The most accurate method of diagnosis is direct visualization through either laparoscopy or laparotomy. These procedures carry a combined misdiagnosis rate of 2 to 5 percent.

TREATMENT

Traditional therapy consists of surgical removal of the tube. The advent of conservative surgeries has helped maximize preservation of the reproductive organs. Laparoscopic surgery allows for diagnosis and definitive treatment at the same time, with minimal inconvenience with respect to morbidity, cost, hospitalization, and lost work time.

Linear salpingotomy involves opening the tube at the implantation site, removing the pregnancy, and allowing the incisions to heal by secondary intention. "Segmental resection" removes the portion of the tube containing the pregnancy.

In selected cases, nonsurgical (expectant) management is advocated. This allows the pregnancy to regress spontaneously. Regression is documented with serial hCG levels. If trophoblastic function continues, surgery or methotrexate therapy is considered.

Rarely, abdominal pregnancy continues to viable fetal age. The rate of fetus survival is approximately 10 to 20 percent, and more than half of the survivors have significant deformities.[5] The patient is given the option of continuing an abdominal pregnancy or terminating it. Regardless of the choice the patient makes, the placenta is retained in the abdomen to prevent possible hemorrhage. Later the placental remains are resolved (dissolved) with methotrexate. Ovarian pregnancy is dealt with at the time of diagnosis. Cervical pregnancy may be confused with incomplete abortion and may present with uncontrollable bleeding. Hysterectomy may be required for maternal survival.

ACKNOWLEDGMENT

The editor would like to acknowledge the significant contributions to this chapter made by Cheryl Gregorio, the author of "Ectopic Pregnancy" in the first edition of *Primary Care for Physician Assistants*.

REFERENCES

1. Ectopic pregnancy. *MMWR* 44(3):46–48, 1995.
2. Pernoll ML, Garmel SH: Early pregnancy risk, in Decherney AH, Pernoll ML (eds): *Current Obstetrics and Gynecology: Diagnosis and Treatment*, 8th ed. New York, McGraw-Hill, 1994, pp 314–320.
3. Hickok LR, Patton PE: Ectopic pregnancy, in Moor TB, Reiter RC, Rebar RW, et al (eds): *Obstetrics and Gynecology: A Longitudinal Approach*. New York, Churchill Livingstone, 1993, pp 263–272.

TABLE 12-6-2. Signs of Ectopic Pregnancy

SIGN	%
Abdominal tenderness	90
Adnexal tenderness	85
Adnexal mass	50
Uterine enlargement	25
Orthostatic changes	10
Fever	5–10

SOURCE: Audrey and Koh.[6]

TABLE 12-6-1. Symptoms of Ectopic Pregnancy

SYMPTOM	%
Abdominal pain	90
Vaginal bleeding	80
Amenorrhea	75
Dizziness, fainting	25
Normal pregnancy symptoms	15

SOURCE: Audrey and Koh.[6]

4. Pernoll ML, Garmel SH: Early pregnancy risks, in Decherney AH, Pernoll ML (eds): *Current Obstetrics and Gynecology: Diagnosis and Treatment,* 8th ed. New York, McGraw-Hill, 1994, p 315.
5. Bates GW, Barzansky BM, Beckman CRB, et al (eds): Ectopic pregnancy, in *Obstetrics and Gynecology for Medical Students.* Baltimore, Williams and & Wilkins, 1992, p 290–291, 293.
6. Audrey S, Koh MD: Ectopic pregnancy, in Benson RC, Pernoll MM (eds): *Handbook of Gynecology and Obstetrics,* 1st ed. Stamford, CT, Appleton & Lange 1993, pp 99–111.

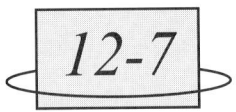

MASTITIS

Dana M. Gallagher

DISCUSSION

Mastitis (breast infection) is characterized by unilateral breast tenderness with localized warmth, swelling, and redness. Mastitis typically occurs after, but is not confined to, the onset of breast-feeding in a first pregnancy. If it is not promptly treated with antibiotics, mastitis can progress to abscess, which necessitates surgical drainage.

PATHOGENESIS

Factors that induce mastitis include poor drainage of a breast duct, the presence of a microorganism, and susceptibility to infection brought on by exhaustion and stress. Rare causes of mastitis include tuberculosis[1] and lupus erythematosus.[2]

Plugged ducts and mastitis must be understood on a continuum and must be differentiated. Plugged ducts occur when the milk flow is obstructed (for example, by tight bras or baby carriers) or after a missed or short feeding. Dried secretions on the nipple can cause backup of milk flow as well. It is incumbent on the mother to watch for the tender lumps that signal plugged ducts and to remove the cause immediately. Mastitis is the end result of plugged ducts.

The most common microbial cause of mastitis is *Staphylococcus aureus; Escherichia coli* is a common culprit as well.[1] Common culprits in mastitis-associated abscesses include *S. aureus* and the anaerobes *Bacteroides* and *Peptostreptococcus.*[3]

SYMPTOMS

A localized area of erythema, heat, swelling, and tenderness is present. Fever [38°C (101°F)], along with intense breast pain and an overall feeling of malaise, is typical.

In contrast to the symptoms of mastitis, plugged ducts are characterized by minor unilateral breast pain without heat or redness. There is no fever, and the woman feels well.

LABORATORY TESTS

The diagnosis of mastitis is made clinically. However, when mastitis does not improve after treatment, cultures of breast milk may be helpful. Before a culture is obtained, the breast and hands should be washed thoroughly; then a midstream clean catch should be manually expressed.

The placement of a purified protein derivative (PPD) may be useful in ruling out tuberculosis as an etiology. Although it is currently rare, as the incidence of tuberculosis rises, this cause of mastitis may become more prominent.

RADIOLOGIC STUDIES

Radiologic studies are not done unless there is no clinical improvement after appropriate antibiotic treatment. If the etiology of an inflamed breast is uncertain, ultrasound and/or a mammogram may be ordered to rule out inflammatory breast cancer.

TREATMENT

Pharmacologic management with dicloxacillin 500 mg orally qid for 10 days should be started immediately. If the patient is allergic, erythromycin (PCE) 333 mg orally tid for 10 days is recommended. The response should be dramatic. The patient should be seen in follow-up within 72 h.

PATIENT EDUCATION

Antibiotics pass through the breast milk but do not harm the baby. Even though the symptoms are likely to improve almost immediately, an entire 10-day course of treatment should be completed. Stopping antibiotic treatment too soon predisposes the woman to recurrent mastitis.[4,5]

Since exhaustion compromises the immune system, rest (especially early in the infection) is important. If the nursing bra is uncomfortable or tight, it should be removed. The mother should nurse frequently, at least every 2 h. Weaning at this time can slow healing and promote breast abscess. Hot moist heat should be applied locally before nursing. Nursing should start on the unaffected side, while the affected side "lets down." If the baby refuses to nurse from the affected side, a breast pump should be used, since drainage is a critical part of treatment. If the baby nurses only casually from the affected breast, drainage should be completed with a breast pump. Acetaminophen can be used to ease pain. The woman should drink plenty of water.

COMPLICATIONS AND RED FLAGS

In the case of an inflamed breast that does not respond to antibiotics within 72 h, the diagnosis should be reviewed. The differential diagnosis includes resistant or atypical microorganisms, breast abscess, and inflammatory breast cancer.

REFERENCES

1. Lawrence RA: *Breastfeeding: A Guide for the Medical Profession,* 4th ed. Chicago, Mosby Year Book, 1994, p 261.
2. Cernea SS, Kihara SM, Sotto MN, Vilela MAC: Lupus mastitis. *J Am Acad Dermatol* 29(2–2):343–346, 1993.
3. Dahlbeck SW, Donnelly JF, Theriault RL: Differentiating inflammatory breast cancer from acute mastitis. *Am Fam Physician* 52(3):930, 1995.
4. Huggins K: *The Nursing Mother's Companion.* Cambridge, MA, Harvard Common, 1986, p 95.
5. Jolley S: *Breastfeeding Triage Tool.* Seattle–King County Department of Public Health, 1996, p 43.

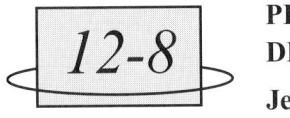

PELVIC INFLAMMATORY DISEASE

Jean M. Covino

DISCUSSION

Pelvic inflammatory disease (PID) is defined as the acute clinical syndrome associated with the ascending spread of microorganisms (unrelated to pregnancy or surgery) from the vagina or cervix to the endometrium, fallopian tubes, and/or contiguous structures.[1] Infections are usually primary and are sexually transmitted. A smaller percentage of cases can be secondary to invasive uterine procedures or to parturition.

Incidence

More than 1.4 million women are diagnosed with PID every year in the United States.[2] Since PID is not a reportable disease in the United States, these numbers may be an underestimate. Recent data concluded that a strategy of identifying, testing, and treating women at risk for cervical *Chlamydia* infection was associated with a reduced incidence of PID[3] (see Chap. 9-6).

Pathogenesis

The pathogenesis of PID is poorly understood. Mechanisms cited as possibly contributing to the canalicular upward spread of microorganisms include changes in cervical mucus, adherence and ascent of spermatozoa, presence of cervical ectopy, intrauterine device (IUD) insertion, menstruation, and vaginal douching.

Microbiology

PID is a polymicrobial infection. Sexually transmitted organisms such as *Neisseria gonorrhoeae* (see Chap. 9-13) and *C. trachomatis* (see Chap. 9-6) account for roughly 80% and 51% of cases, respectively.[2] Other microorganisms implicated in PID include *Mycoplasma hominis, Peptococcus* species, *Mobiluncus* species, *Bacteroides* species, *Haemophilus influenzae, Streptococcus* species, *Gardnerella vaginalis* (see Chap 12-3), *Ureaplasma urealyticum,* and possibly viruses.

Risk Factors

Certain risk factors have been associated with PID and should be sought while taking a history from any woman with lower abdominal pain. These risk factors include age <25 years, multiple sexual partners, presence of an IUD, and recent invasive gynecologic procedure. Also recent data from epidemiologic studies suggests that smoking and use of vaginal douches are associated risk factors.[4,5]

SYMPTOMS

There is no single historic, physical, or laboratory test that is pathognomonic in diagnosing PID. PID is a clinical diagnosis. Symptoms associated with PID include bilateral lower abdominal pain, irregular uterine bleeding, dysuria, and increased or changed vaginal discharge.

OBJECTIVE FINDINGS

Clinical findings associated with PID include temperature >38.0°C (100.4°F), palpable adnexal swelling and/or tenderness, cervical motion tenderness, and an abnormal cervical and vaginal discharge.

LABORATORY FINDINGS

Laboratory studies do not generally add to the accuracy of diagnosing PID. White blood cell (WBC) count and the erythrocyte sedimentation rate (ESR) may or may not be elevated in an acute case of PID. C-reactive protein may be elevated. Vaginal and cervical discharges should be checked by a wet mount examination for the presence of WBCs, since their absence makes the diagnosis of PID less likely. Cervical Gram's stain should be done and checked for >5 WBCs/high-power field and for intracellular gram-negative diplococci. A sensitive urine pregnancy test should be done to rule out ectopic pregnancy. Syphilis serology should be ordered, and HIV testing and counseling should be encouraged since a diagnosis of PID suggests high-risk behavior. Pelvic ultrasound is not useful in diagnosing PID but can help evaluate any pelvic masses.

INVASIVE TECHNIQUES

Invasive procedures are usually not indicated. Culdocentesis, if performed on a woman with PID, shows elevated concentrations of WBCs. Culture of the material is rarely helpful because of contamination by vaginal organisms. If an endometrial biopsy is done, it may suggest histopathologic evidence of endometritis, which correlates well with the presence of salpingitis. Results, however, can take several days. Laparoscopy is the specific means for diagnosing acute salpingitis and is considered the gold standard for confirming the diagnosis. However, the expense and the risk of the procedure must be considered. In most cases PID can be reasonably diagnosed without using the invasive procedures that tend to be reserved for cases where the diagnosis is imperative but remains uncertain (e.g., differentiation of acute appendicitis from PID).

DIAGNOSTIC CONSIDERATIONS

The two most important differential diagnoses that must be considered are ectopic pregnancy and acute appendicitis. Failure to recognize and treat either of these two can have devastating consequences. Other possible differentials include ovarian torsion, ruptured or hemorrhagic ovarian cyst, endometriosis, irritable bowel syndrome, and somatization disorder.

SPECIAL CONSIDERATIONS

Women ages 15 to 24 years who smoke, have multiple sexual partners, and admit to using vaginal douches are at the greatest risk for developing PID. PID in adolescents is more likely to result in infertility and ectopic pregnancy. PID is rare during pregnancy. Patients who are pregnant or HIV-positive with the diagnosis of PID should be hospitalized and treated with parenteral antibiotics.

TREATMENT

All patients with peritoneal signs or abscess formation should be admitted to the hospital and placed on parenteral antibiotics. Criteria for inpatient treatment of PID include:

- Adolescence
- Pregnancy
- Unreliable patient
- Patient who cannot tolerate oral medications
- HIV-positive patient
- No response to outpatient treatment after 72 h
- Uncertain diagnosis

No single therapeutic regimen has been established for persons with PID. When selecting a treatment regimen, health care providers should consider availability, cost, patient acceptance, and geographic differences in antimicrobial susceptibility. Recent studies have demonstrated the presence of bacterial vaginosis–associated bacteria in addition to sexually transmitted organisms and suggest that treatment of acute PID must be broad spectrum in nature and effective against anaerobic bacteria as well as *N. gonorrhoeae* and *C. trachomatis*.[6]

Outpatient Therapy

The 1998 recommendations of the Centers for Disease Control and Prevention for treatment of PID are two types[7]:

- Regimen A calls for ceftriaxone (Rocephin) 250 mg intramuscularly (or any other third-generation cephalosporin) *or* cefoxitin (Mefoxin) 2 g intramuscularly *plus* 1 g of probenecid concurrently *plus* doxycycline 100 mg bid for 14 days.
- Regimen B consists of ofloxacin (Floxin) 400 mg orally bid for 14 days *plus* metronidazole (Flagyl, Protostat) 500 mg orally bid for 14 days.

   Note: Patients who do not respond within 72 h to therapy should be hospitalized. Alternative oral regimens suggested include amoxicillin/clavulanic acid *plus* doxycycline. There is insufficient data to recommend azithromycin as part of treatment regimens.

Inpatient Regimen

There are two treatment options for hospitalized patients:

- Regimen A consists of cefoxitin 2 g intravenously every 6 h *or* cefotetan 2 g intravenously every 12 h *plus* doxycycline 100 mg intravenously or orally every 12 h.
- Regimen B calls for clindamycin 900 mg intravenously every 8 h *plus* gentamicin, loading dose intravenously or intramuscularly (2 mg/kg of body weight), followed by a maintenance dose (1.5 mg/kg) every 8 h.

Inpatient regimens should be continued for at least 48 h after clinical improvement, then followed with doxycycline 100 mg orally bid or clindamycin 450 mg orally qid, to complete a total of 14 days of therapy. Parenteral therapy may be discontinued 24 h after clinical improvement. Azithromycin 500 mg intravenously for 2 days followed by 500 mg orally for a total of 10 days has recently been approved by the FDA. Evaluation and treatment of sex partners of women who have PID are vital to reduce the chance of reinfection.

COMPLICATIONS AND RED FLAGS

The majority of women with acute PID recover completely. However, there are some long-term consequences of this disease. These sequelae include:

- Risk of repeated episodes
- Chronic pelvic pain, usually due to adhesion formation
- Increased risk of ectopic pregnancy due to scarring of the fallopian tubes
- Infertility due to scarring of the fallopian tubes

About 11% of women are infertile after a single episode of PID, 23% after two episodes, and 50% after three or more episodes. The increased risk of infertility and ectopic pregnancy is directly related to the duration of symptoms before treatment.

OTHER NOTES AND PEARLS

Symptoms associated with PID usually occur within 7 days of the beginning of menses. This is probably due to the opening of the cervix at that time. Always do a pregnancy test on any menstruating female patient who presents with lower abdominal pain in spite of when she says her last menses took place. The clinical presentation of PID may help reveal which pathogen is responsible. For example, patients with gonococcal PID often present with an acute onset with temperatures 38.0°C or higher, a palpable adnexal mass, and peritoneal signs. Therapeutic response is rapid. Patients with chlamydial PID often have an insidious onset, complain of irregular bleeding, and have ESR > 30 mm/h. *C. trachomatis* and *N. gonorrhoeae* are often found together in cases of PID, so treatment to cover both organisms is standard procedure. It has recently been suggested that before performing a surgical abortion, treatment of bacterial vaginosis (symptomatic or asymptomatic) should be considered to prevent PID.[8]

REFERENCES

1. Centers for Disease Control: Antibiotics-resistant strains of *Neisseria gonorrhoeae*. Policy guidelines for detection, management, and control. *MMWR* 36:55, 1987.
2. Quan M: Pelvic inflammatory disease: Diagnosis and management. *J Am Board Fam Pract* 7:110–123, 1994.
3. Scholes D et al: Prevention of pelvic inflammatory disease by screening for cervical chlamydial infection. *N Engl J Med* 334:1362–1366, 1996.
4. Marchbanks PA et al: Cigarette smoking as a risk factor for pelvic inflammatory disease. *Am J Obstet Gynecol* 162:639–644, 1990.
5. Scholes D et al: Current cigarette smoking and risks of acute pelvic inflammatory disease. *Am J Public Health* 82:1352–1355, 1992.
6. Sweet RL: Role of bacterial vaginosis in pelvic inflammatory disease. *Clin Infect Dis* 20(suppl 2):S271–S275, 1995.
7. Centers for Disease Control and Prevention: 1998 sexually transmitted disease treatment guidelines. *MMWR* 47(RR-1):75–81, 1998.
8. Joesoef MR, Schmid GP: Bacterial vaginosis: Review of treatment options and potential clinical indications for therapy. *Clin Infect Dis* 20(suppl 1):S72–S79, 1995.

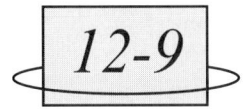

POLYCYSTIC OVARY SYNDROME

Dana M. Gallagher

DISCUSSION

Polycystic ovary syndrome (PCOS) is a common endocrine disorder characterized by hyperandrogenism and chronic anovulation. Hyperandrogenism manifests clinically as hirsutism, acne, and male-pattern alopecia, whereas anovulation encompasses a variety of possible menstrual disruptions, including amenorrhea, oligomenorrhea, dysfunctional uterine bleeding, and infertility. Although some consider obesity to be essential to its diagnosis, approximately one-half of women with PCOS are of normal weight.

Importantly, PCOS is associated with insulin resistance[1] and dyslipidemia.[2,3] In an obese patient, weight loss will improve the entire clinical picture by normalizing insulin and lipid levels and stabilizing menstrual cycling.

PATHOGENESIS

The cause of PCOS is becoming better understood. Historically, PCOS was attributed to a disorder of the hypothalamic-pituitary axis resulting in ovarian hyperandrogenism. More recently, it has been shown that hyperinsulinism is an important precursor to hyperandrogenism, as hyperinsulinism causes the ovaries to increase the production of testosterone. Women with PCOS are at high risk for hypertension, hyperlipidemia, myocardial infarction, and insulin resistance and progression to type 2 diabetes.[4]

SYMPTOMS

The patient presents with a history of menstrual irregularity, often since menarche. She also may be quite concerned about and perhaps ashamed of hirsutism, alopecia, and acne.

OBJECTIVE FINDINGS

Weight should be recorded. Examination of the skin may reveal excessive hair on the face, chin, chest, abdomen, and thighs. Identification of hirsutism should be achieved by both visual examination and palpation, since women typically remove excess hair to appear in public comfortably. Acne and seborrhea may be present; alopecia should be documented. Since these symptoms may be wrongly perceived as a lack of cleanliness or womanliness by the patient, care should be taken during the interview and examination not to shame her with tactless questioning or comments.

The presence of acanthosis nigricans (thick, brown skin in body folds) indicates hyperinsulinemia and also should be charted.

DIAGNOSTIC CONSIDERATIONS

The differential diagnosis includes hyperprolactinemia, acromegaly, and congenital adrenal hyperplasia. These entities can be ruled out through clinical examination, laboratory testing, and imaging studies [prolactin levels, serum growth hormone, and computed tomography (CT) and/or magnetic resonance imaging (MRI)].

LABORATORY TESTS

The following laboratory tests may support a diagnosis of PCOS:

- *Luteinizing hormone (LH) levels.* Hypersecretion is typical, but normal levels do not rule out PCOS.
- *Serum testosterone and androstenedione levels.* Again, hypersecretion is typical, but there may be individual variation.
- *Fasting lipid panel and glucose tolerance testing.* These tests should be performed whenever PCOS is suspected or confirmed. Documenting baseline levels and establishing a surveillance and treatment regimen are critical.

RADIOLOGIC STUDIES

Pelvic sonography is the gold standard for diagnosing PCOS. However, clinical and biochemical markers taken together are highly correlated with ultrasound findings.[5]

TREATMENT

Pharmacologic Management

At this writing, the management of PCOS is starting to resemble the management of diabetes. Emphasis is placed on weight loss through diet and exercise. The successful use of metformin in prompting normal menstrual cycling in research subjects probably will have a profound impact on the treatment of PCOS.[6] Further, in a recent study, the use of the compound *d*-chiro-inositol (which occurs naturally in fruits and vegetables) appeared to normalize insulin and androgen levels in women with PCOS.[7] This may have more specific implications for dietary recommendations in the future.

Depending on the severity of the hirsutism, patients may opt to be treated with spironolactone 25 mg tid-qid[8] or with low-dose oral contraceptives (containing 30 to 35 mg of ethinyl estradiol).[9] Some physicians who have used metformin to treat PCOS note that it ameliorates hirsutism as well.

Patients with acne may respond well to oral contraceptives or can be treated with topical preparations or antibiotics (see Chaps. 2-3 and 12-14). Alopecia may improve after treatment with oral contraceptives. Anovulation (menstrual irregularities) can be cycled with low-dose monophasic oral contraceptives, as was noted above.

Supportive Measures

For hirsutism, patients may pluck excess hair or use depilatories. For more permanent results, referral for hair removal by electrolysis or laser should be made. Vaniqa™ (eflornithine hydrochloride) cream 13.9% applied twice daily to affected areas may prove to be beneficial. With regard to alopecia, changes in hairstyling may camouflage hair loss.

PATIENT EDUCATION

Patients should be informed that acne, hirsutism, and alopecia are slowly changing conditions and that at least 6 months of treatment should be allowed to achieve noticeable improvement. Inform the patient that treatment for PCOS and its associated conditions may be indefinite, as many women relapse after treatment is discontinued. Patients who desire pregnancy should be referred to an infertility specialist for evaluation and treatment. In the event of pregnancy, a woman with PCOS is more likely to develop gestational diabetes and should be monitored accordingly. The use of spironolactone for hirsutism and dermatologic agents such as isotretinoin (Accutane) must be discontinued because of potential teratogenicity. Overweight patients should be encouraged to start a regular program of exercise and weight reduction.

DISPOSITION

Patients should be evaluated at least yearly with a routine gynecologic examination, including laboratory testing for glucose and lipids.

NOTES AND PEARLS

It is likely that increased emphasis will be placed on treating hyperinsulinemia because it underlies the hyperandrogenism, chronic anovulation, and long-term cardiovascular risks associated with PCOS. Since this is a hot area of medical research, watch for late-breaking treatment regimens.

REFERENCES

1. Davidson MB: Clinical implications of insulin resistance syndromes. *Am J Med* 99:420–426, 1995.
2. Wild RA: Obesity, lipids, cardiovascular risk, and androgen excess. *Am J Med* 98(Suppl 1A):1A–27S, 1A–32S, 1995.
3. Bates B: Many young women with PCOS have lipid abnormalities. *Ob Gyn News* August 15, 1996, p 14.
4. Kidson W: Polycystic ovary syndrome: A new direction in treatment. *Med J Aust* 169:537–540, 1998, http://www.mja.com.au.
5. Franks S: Polycystic ovary syndrome. *N Engl J Med* 333(13):853, 1995.
6. Therapy for polycystic ovary syndrome. *PA Today,* January 1999, p. 7.
7. Nestler JE, Jakubowicz DJ, Reamer P, et al: Ovulatory and metabolic effects of *d*-Chiro-Inositol in the polycystic ovary syndrome. *N Engl J Med* 340(17):1314–1320, 1999.
8. MacKay HT: Gynecology, in Tierney LM Jr, McPhee SJ, Papadakis MA (eds): *Current Medical Diagnosis and Treatment,* 38th ed. McGraw-Hill, 2000, p 723.
9. Redmond GP: Androgenic disorders of women: Diagnostic and therapeutic decision making. *Am J Med* 98(Suppl 1A):1A–127S, 1995.

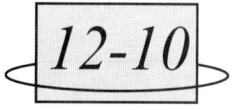

SEXUAL ASSAULT
Jean M. Covino

DISCUSSION

Sexual assault (rape) is a violent crime directed mostly against women. It is defined as act(s) of sexual intimacy performed without the consent of the victim through the use or threat of force or when the victim is unable to give consent because of physical or mental disability.

Incidence

Rape is the most underreported violent crime in the United States. It is estimated that at least 20% of adult women have experienced sexual assault during their lifetimes. Approximately 100,000 cases of rape are reported annually in the United States, and this most likely represents only a small fraction of the actual cases. According to the U.S. Department of Justice, this accounts for approximately 6% of all violent crimes.[1] Note that statistics collected by law enforcement agencies are low estimates since many victims are especially reluctant to report this crime.

Incidence of Sexually Transmitted Infections

The types of sexually transmitted diseases associated with sexual assault are gonorrhea (up to 12%; see Chap. 9-13); trichomoniasis (see Chap. 12-11), monilial vaginitis (see Chap. 12-2), and bacterial vaginosis (see Chap. 12-3) (more than 6% each); *Chlamydia* (more than 4%; see Chap. 9-6); herpes (less than 2%; see Chap. 12-21); and syphilis (less than 4%; see Chap. 9-22). Studies have shown that HIV infections are much less likely to be contracted during an assault.[2]

Epidemiology

Although sexual assault does occur in any age group, victims are more likely to be young, single, female members of minority groups with a low socioeconomic status. Rape is more prevalent in urban areas. More sexual assaults occur during the summer months, whereas the fewest occur during the winter months.

HISTORY AND PHYSICAL EXAMINATION

The history should include a detailed account of the assault and a complete gynecologic history, including the use of any contraceptives. The victim must be asked whether consciousness was lost at any time or whether she or he has defecated, voided, douched, bathed, or showered since the incident. The victim must be questioned regarding the orifice(s) of penetration and whether ejaculation took place.

The physical examination should include general appearance and assessment of psychological and emotional status. The entire body must be checked for signs of trauma, the condition of the external genitalia documented, and a speculum examination performed for women. Pubic hair is combed and cut and fingernail scrapings are collected with standard rape kits. Photographs should be taken if appropriate. Counseling services should be provided and follow-up appointments arranged.

In many areas, usually through emergency departments, specially trained sexual assault medical examiners are available to collect acute forensic evidence. Whenever possible, victims should be referred to these individuals.

SPECIAL CONSIDERATIONS

The very young, very old, and handicapped are particularly vulnerable to sexual assaults. Every state has laws that require the reporting of child abuse. Health care providers should contact their state or local child protective service agency about child abuse reporting requirements in their areas.

LABORATORY TESTS

Initial diagnostic tests for sexually transmitted diseases (STDs) after sexual assault recommended by the Centers for Disease Control and Prevention (CDC) include cultures for *Neisseria gonorrhoeae* and *Chlamydia trachomatis* from any potentially infected sites and wet mount and culture of vaginal swab specimens for *Trichomonas vaginalis* infection. The wet mount can also check for evidence of bacterial vaginosis or yeast. Collect a serum sample to be preserved for subsequent analysis if 12-week follow-up serologic tests are positive (see below).

Follow-up examination 2 weeks after assault should include cultures and wet mount. STD tests should be repeated unless prophylactic treatment has already been provided.

Follow-up examination 12 weeks after assault should include serologic tests for syphilis and HIV infection. If positive, testing of the serum collected at the initial examination will assist in determining whether the infection antedated the assault.

RADIOGRAPHIC AND OTHER DIAGNOSTIC STUDIES

There are no routine imaging studies recommended after a sexual assault unless there are other physical injuries.

TREATMENT

Although not all experts agree, most patients probably benefit from STD prophylaxis because follow-up of patients may be difficult.

Patients may be reassured if offered treatment or prophylaxis for possible infection.[3] The regimen recommended by the CDC includes ceftriaxone (Rocephin) 125 mg intramuscularly stat, plus metronidazole (Flagyl) 2 g orally in a single dose, plus doxycycline 100 mg bid for 7 days or azithromycin 1 g orally in a single dose.[3] The hepatitis B vaccine should be administered with follow-up doses at 1 to 2 and 4 to 6 months after the first dose. Testing for HIV and possible antiretroviral prophylaxis should be offered even though there are no detailed protocols on how to provide this treatment. When the choice is made to take medications to prevent HIV infection, treatment should be initiated as soon as possible, but no later than 72 h following the assault, and should be continued for 28 days.[4] Emergency hormonal contraceptive therapy (e.g., Preven Pack or Plan B) should be offered to postpubertal adolescents and adult women of childbearing age who were raped less than 72 h before examination.

COMPLICATIONS

Aside from obvious physical complications that may occur during a violent attack, health care providers must be aware of the psychological and emotional stress a rape victim undergoes. Eventual psychological manifestations are related to posttraumatic stress disorder. More than half of rape victims experience difficulty in reestablishing sexual or emotional relationships with spouses or other sexual partners. It is very important to offer psychiatric follow-up and counseling to all sexual assault victims.

NOTES AND PEARLS

The majority of rape victims who come to the emergency room do not openly admit to having been sexually assaulted. They may complain of being mugged or may voice concern about HIV or other STDs. Recent data have supported an association of sexual assault history with eating disorder symptoms.[5] Unless the health care provider is thorough in obtaining a sexual history, assault victims will remain unidentified.

REFERENCES

1. Federal Bureau of Investigation: *Uniform Crime Reports for the United States.* Washington, DC, US Department of Justice, 1991.
2. Holmes KK et al (eds): Sexual assault and sexually transmitted diseases, in *Sexually Transmitted Diseases,* 2d ed. New York, McGraw-Hill, 1990.
3. Centers for Disease Control and Prevention: 1998 sexually transmitted diseases treatment guidelines. *MMWR* 47(RR-1):97–102, 1998.
4. Bamberger JD et al: Postexposure prophylaxis for immunodeficiency virus (HIV) infection following sexual assault. *Am J Med* 106(3):323–326, 1999.
5. Laws A, Golding JM: Sexual assault history and eating disorder symptoms among white, Hispanic, and African-American women and men. *Am J Public Health* 86(4):579–582, 1996.

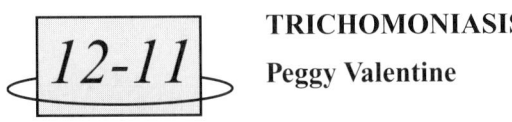

TRICHOMONIASIS
Peggy Valentine

DISCUSSION

Trichomoniasis is a common sexually transmitted infection that is caused by a flagellated protozoan, *Trichomonas vaginalis.* Some infected individuals have no symptoms, but women usually present with a diffuse, malodorous yellow-green vaginal discharge that may be frothy. Vulvar irritation is a common complaint. A "strawberry cervix" is observed in 1 to 2 percent of women on speculum examination and in 50 percent on colposcopy. Women who use barrier methods such as diaphragms and condoms are the least likely to acquire this infection. The majority of men are asymptomatic. Coexistent gonorrhea and other sexually transmitted diseases (STDs) are not uncommon in persons infected with trichomonas. It is therefore important for the clinician to evaluate patients with STDs carefully for other pathogens.

SIGNS AND SYMPTOMS

The infection elicits an acute inflammatory response of the vagina, resulting in a vaginal discharge with polymorphonuclear neutrophils (PMNs). Vaginal discharge, the most common symptom, may be malodorous. Nearly half of affected women complain of pruritus and dyspareunia. Many note a worsening of symptoms after the menstrual period. Lower abdominal pain and tenderness of the adnexa and uterine fundus are uncommon symptoms. The majority of affected men have no symptoms. Those presenting with symptoms may complain of purulent, mucopurulent, or mucoid discharge, occasionally with mild urethral irritation.

OBJECTIVE FINDINGS

Homogeneous discharge varies in amount, is usually green-yellow in color, and is sometimes foamy or frothy. The vaginal mucosa is often erythematous, and occasionally petechiae are noted on the cervix, giving it a strawberry appearance.

DIAGNOSTIC CONSIDERATIONS

The diagnosis is made by observing the motile parasites on wet mount examination. Trichomonads are ovoid and slightly larger than PMNs. It is unfortunate that wet mount does not always reveal trichomonads, and a vaginal culture may be necessary for confirmation of the diagnosis.

LABORATORY TESTS

Using the wet mount, sweep the anterior and posterior fornices with a cotton swab, place a drop of the secretions on a microscopic slide, and mix with one drop of slightly warm saline. Cover with a coverslip and examine under low and then medium magnification. Motile trichomonads confirm the diagnosis; increased numbers of PMNs are usually present. Culture for *T. vaginalis* only if the wet mount is negative and clinical suspicion of trichomoniasis is high.

TREATMENT

Treatment for the patient and partner is recommended. Metronidazole (Flagyl) 2 g orally in a single dose is the recommended regimen. Many patients complain of a metallic taste while taking metronidazole. Metronidazole produces a disulfiram-like (Antabuse) effect, causing nausea and flushing in some individuals, and so alcohol should be avoided. The prothrombin time may be prolonged in patients who take warfarin and metronidazole. Patients who are allergic to metronidazole can be managed by desensitization.

HIV-infected patients who have trichomoniasis should receive the same treatment regimen as those who are HIV-negative.

As an alternative treatment, use metronidazole 500 mg twice daily for 7 days. Metronidazole gel has not been studied for trichomoniasis treatment. There are no effective alternatives to metronidazole therapy. The use of metronidazole is contraindicated in the first trimester of pregnancy but may be considered after the first trimester with a 2-g single dose.

DISPOSITION

Follow-up is unnecessary for men and women who become asymptomatic after treatment.

PATIENT EDUCATION

Sexual partners should be treated. Coitus should be avoided until therapy has been completed by both the patient and the sexual partner and both are without symptoms. To limit the possibility of a recurrence, the patient should be given information about the benefits of a mutually monogamous sexual relationship and the recommendation to use barrier methods.

BIBLIOGRAPHY

Centers for Disease Control and Prevention: 1998 Guidelines for Treatment of Sexually Transmitted Diseases. *MMWR* 47(RR-1):74–75, 1998.

Mou SM: Gynecologic infections, in Seltzer VL, Pearse WH (eds): *Women's Primary Health Care: Office Practices and Procedures.* New York, McGraw-Hill, 1995, p 191.

Pearlman MD, Yashar C, Ernst S, Solomon W: An incremental dosing protocol for women with severe vaginal trichomoniasis and adverse reactions to metronidazole. *Am J Obstet Gynecol* 174:934–936, 1996.

Rein MF, Muller M: *Trichomonas vaginalis* and trichomoniasis, in Holmes KK, Mardh P-A, Sparling PF, et al (eds): *Sexually Transmitted Diseases,* 2d ed. New York, McGraw-Hill, 1990, pp 481–488.

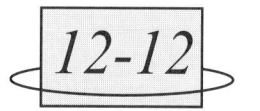

BREAST MASS
Noel J. Genova

DISCUSSION

The evaluation of a breast mass implies separating very common normal "lumps" in women's breasts from cancerous lesions (see Chap. 13-4). Unfortunately, there is no simple method. In many cases, biopsy is the only way to determine whether a breast mass is malignant. The information in this chapter is intended to help clinicians decide if, when, and where to refer a woman who presents with a breast mass. Specialty referral is often needed. Consider the following:

• Mammography has an overall false-negative rate of 10 to 15 percent. Because of the technical limitations of mammography, the false-negative rate in women younger than 50 years old who present with breast mass is higher than the rate for women older than 50.[1]

• Mammography cannot be used at all in pregnant women or women younger than 20 years of age and is difficult to interpret in women younger than 30 to 35 years. Sonography, which can be used in these women, is of little value in diagnosing breast cancer but can be useful in distinguishing cysts from solid masses.[2,3]

• Failure to diagnose breast cancer is a common and costly cause of malpractice claims,[2] especially for women under age 50. Reassurance regarding a lump, thereby avoiding further evaluation, is not helpful to a woman who ultimately learns that the lump was malignant, especially if her prognosis is poor by the time her cancer is diagnosed and treated.

Although evaluation of risk factors is important from a public health and epidemiologic point of view, it is of little diagnostic value in determining whether an individual has breast cancer. With the important exception of increasing age as a risk factor, 75 percent of women with breast cancer do not appear to be at high risk.[1] Although women age 30 to 50 account for many tragic cases of early death from breast cancer, women over age 50 account for 75 percent of breast cancer cases.

DIAGNOSTIC CONSIDERATIONS

Worrisome breast masses generally are described as dominant, firm, and discrete and may or may not be mobile. Bilateral tender masses that resolve spontaneously within a few weeks or months generally are not considered suspicious. The benign masses that are the most difficult to distinguish from cancerous lesions are cysts and fibroadenomas. Both occur very commonly in premenopausal women.

Evaluation of breast masses in women under age 40 is especially challenging. Women in this age group represent only 6.5 to 7 percent of reported breast cancers,[4–6] and so malignancy must be considered when one is evaluating masses that will prove to be fibroadenomas or cysts. Typically, fibroadenomas are firm, have discrete borders, and are freely moveable. Cysts are soft, are often fluid-filled, and may come and go, particularly in relation to the menstrual cycle. Cysts may be diagnosed as benign and treated if needle aspiration yields clear fluid and renders the cyst nonpalpable. Bloody aspirates must be submitted for cytology. Fibroadenomas are solid masses and do not yield fluid with needle aspiration.

Other causes of breast mass are more readily distinguished from breast cancer on history but still must be referred to a surgeon. Breast abscesses, like other abscesses, tend to be red, hot, and tender and may be draining purulent fluid. Lactating women with persistent, painful masses should be referred to a surgeon to rule out a galactocele. Breast trauma may result in fat necrosis.[1]

OBJECTIVE FINDINGS

Although the physical examination has limitations in establishing a diagnosis of breast cancer, having a slightly lower sensitivity than mammography alone,[7] it should be performed by a clinician for all women who present with a breast mass. Breast self-examination should be taught to all women, allowing them to separate normal supportive tissue, ribs, and general premenstrual swelling from discrete masses. Suspicious clinical findings (including nonspontaneous nipple discharge, especially if bloody), whether discovered by the woman or by the clinician, should *never* be disregarded because of a normal mammogram.[6] Cancer cannot be ruled out unless the mass resolves with needle aspiration or is negative on biopsy.

IMAGING

Mammography is helpful as a diagnostic tool (as opposed to a screening tool) only in conjunction with history, physical examination, and fine needle aspiration or biopsy. It also is used to rule out occult cancers, especially those occurring bilaterally, which occur in 3 percent of patients who present with newly diagnosed breast cancer[2] [see Figs. 12-12-1 (Plate 34), 12-12-2 (Plate 35), and 12-12-3 (Plate 36)].

SPECIAL CONSIDERATIONS

Because biopsy is the only truly accurate method for the diagnosis of a breast mass, a primary care clinician must be prepared to refer women with persistent breast masses regardless of negative imaging studies or young age. Communication among providers is critically important to ensure follow-up until there is resolution of the mass or a definitive diagnosis is made.

Patients should be offered all alternatives, with explanations of the risks and benefits of observation, needle biopsy, and excisional biopsy. Considering that there is often no clear-cut "best" time for biopsy, it is helpful if the woman has some input into all decisions made regarding her diagnosis and treatment, if applicable.

Centers specializing in the diagnosis and treatment of breast conditions may have resources that are helpful to both patients and primary care clinicians. Identification of patient education materials, self-help groups, and educators specializing in breast cancer may ultimately be important to women who are referred for the evaluation of a breast mass.

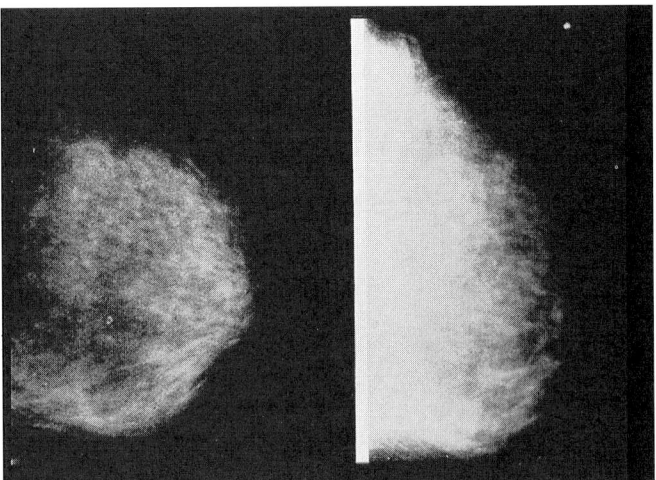

FIGURE 12-12-1 (PLATE 34). Quality assurance for mammography is critical. These images are of the same breast. The image on the left shows a breast that is not properly compressed. It could have mistakenly been read as a dense, glandular breast with no abnormality visualized. The image on the right shows the same breast with proper compression. It is much easier to find a white density indicative of cancer on the right image than on the left image. (*From the American Medical Women's Association for the Breast and Cervical Cancer Education Project for Primary Care Providers, under a cooperative agreement with the Centers for Disease Control and Prevention.*)

FUTURE TRENDS AND CONTROVERSIES

Breast cancer remains a significant cause of death among American women (nearly 45,000 deaths estimated for 1996).[8] It appears that mortality rates from breast cancer are declining among white women, although the cause of this decline is unclear. Genetic testing, which might help identify very young women who are at risk

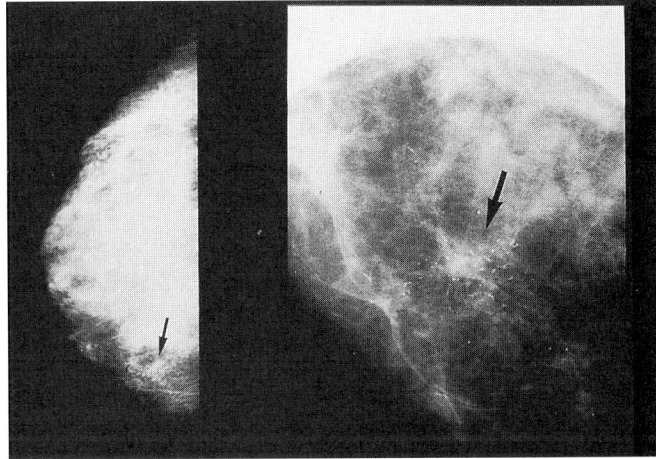

FIGURE 12-12-2 (PLATE 35). The left side contains a density indicated by the black arrow. The cone compression view on the right reveals a finding even more ominous than the original film, illustrating how useful cone compressin mammography can be. This finding represented carcinoma. (*From the American Medical Women's Association for the Breast and Cervical Cancer Education Project for Primary Care Providers, under a cooperative agreement with the Centers for Disease Control and Prevention.*)

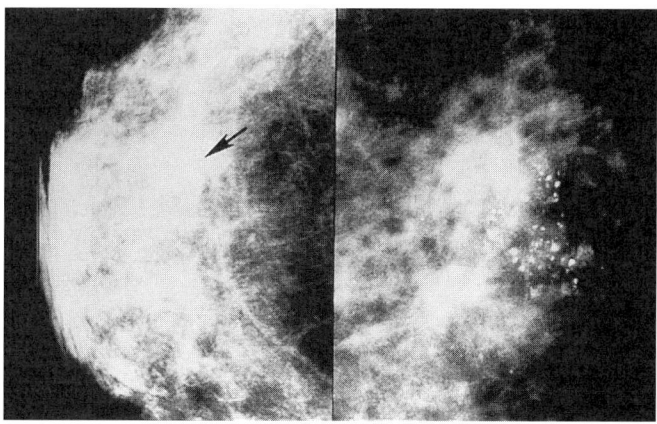

FIGURE 12-12-3 (PLATE 36). On the left side, the radiologist has noted some white specks. These represent microcalcifications in the breast. Imaging them with a magnification view as shown on the right helps identify the sizes and shapes of the calcifications. These are highly suggestive of carcinoma because they are pleomorphic, that is, of different sizes and shapes. In general, cone compression mammography is used to evaluate densities further, and magnification views are done to identify and discern calcifications. (*From the American Medical Women's Association for the Breast and Cervical Cancer Education Project for Primary Care Providers, under a cooperative agreement with the Centers for Disease Control and Prevention.*)

of developing breast cancer, is not ready for use in the general population.[9]

Evaluation of any clinically suspicious breast mass must be done by the primary care clinician in consultation with a surgeon and a radiologist. Many cases, even in the presence of a normal mammogram, require biopsy by fine needle aspiration, core needle biopsy, or open surgical biopsy. The choice of the biopsy method depends on the patient's age, the type of mass, mammographic findings, and the preference of the consulting surgeon.[10]

REFERENCES

1. Carlson KJ, Eisenstat SA, Frigoletto FD, et al: *Primary Care of Women.* Chicago, Mosby, 1995, pp 221, 222, 400, 401.
2. Donegan WL: Evaluation of a palpable breast mass. *N Engl J Med* 327(13):937–939, 1992.
3. *Evaluation of Common Breast Problems: A Primer for Primary Care Providers,* prepared by the Society of Surgical Oncology and the Commission on Cancer of the American College of Surgeons for the Centers for Disease Control and Prevention, Atlanta, 1995.
4. Mitnick JS, Vazquez MF, Kronovet SZ, Roses DF: Malpractice litigation involving patients with carcinoma of the breast. *J Am Coll Surg* 181:315–321, 1995.
5. Morrow M, Wong S, Luz V: The evaluation of breast masses in women younger than forty years of age. *Surgery* 124:634–641, 1998.
6. Osuch JR, Vence LB: The timely diagnosis of breast cancer. *Cancer* 74(1):271–278, 1994.
7. Morris A, Pommier RF, Schmidt WA, et al: Accurate evaluation of palpable breast masses by the triple test score. *Arch Surg* 133:930–934, 1998.
8. American Cancer Society: *Cancer Facts and Figures,* Atlanta, 1996.
9. Langston AA, Malone KE, Thompson JD, et al: BRCA 1 mutations in a population-based sample of young women with breast cancer. *N Engl J Med* 334(3):137–142, 1996.
10. Ballo MS, Sneige N: Can core needle biopsy replace fine-needle aspiration cytology in the diagnosis of palpable breast carcinoma? *Cancer* 78:773–777, 1996.

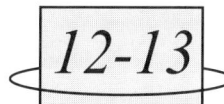

CANCER OF THE CERVIX/ THE ABNORMAL PAP SMEAR

Amelia Naccarto-Coleman

DISCUSSION

Epidemiology

With the introduction of the Papanicolaou (Pap) smear in 1943, the incidence and mortality rate of invasive cervical cancer in the United States has declined more than 50% as the result of regular periodic screening. Carcinoma of the cervix accounts for approximately 16,000 new cases (6% of all cancers) and 5000 cancer deaths in the United States each year. However, in other countries, the prevalence of this disease is highly variable. Worldwide, it continues to be the second most common malignancy in women. These differences are attributed to low socioeconomic status, nonparticipation in screening programs, and several epidemiologic cofactors that have influenced the development of the human papillomavirus (HPV) infection.

Concurrent with the declining mortality rates for invasive carcinoma is the appearance of increasing incidence rates for carcinoma in situ (CIS). This shift has been linked to the efficacy of screening and a trend toward cigarette smoking and earlier sexual activity. Rates for CIS reach a peak during the reproductive years in both black and white women. After the age of 25 years, however, the rates for invasive disease are different. Incidence rates for black women dramatically increase with age; rates stabilize over time for white women.

Overall, more than 25% of invasive cervical cancer occur in women older than 65 years and about 50% of all women who die from cervical cancer are over 65 years of age. These patterns demonstrate the need to reach out to older women, ethnic minorities, poor women, and uninsured women who have not had the benefit of regular screening.

Cervical cancer and its precursors have been associated with several epidemiologic risk factors. These risk factors, as summarized in Table 12-13-1, include early age of first intercourse, early first pregnancy, multiple or high-risk sexual partners, and genital condyloma. Smoking increases cervical cancer risk in a dose-dependent fashion. Immunosuppressed patients are more likely to develop cervical cancer because of impairment of the immune response to HPV. Low-risk groups include nuns and members of some religious groups who are less likely to have multiple sexual partners.

Pathogenesis and Natural History

Unique to cervical cancer is the etiologic relationship between the infectious HPV agent and development of preinvasive and invasive cervical lesions. According to the 1996 National Institutes of Health (NIH) Consensus Statement on Cervical Cancer, HPV DNA is present in more than 93% of all cervical cancer and precursor lesions. More than 70 types of HPV have been identified. However, only 23 of these types actually infect the cervix and out of these, approximately 10 are associated with invasive disease. These 10 are further divided into low-and high-risk categories. Both low-risk (types 6, 11) and high-risk (types 16, 18, 31, and 45) HPV strains account for more than 80% of all cervical intraepithelial neoplasia (CIN). In highly invasive carcinomas, the high-risk types predominate, with HPV-16 in 50% of the cases and HPV-18 in 20%. Approximately 70 to 80% of all cervical cancers are squamous cell (epidermoid). The remaining 20 to 30% are either adenocarcinoma, mixed epithelial, or undifferentiated carcinomas.

Understanding the pathophysiology of the disease is the key to reducing the morbidity and mortality of invasive carcinoma. Cytologic screening assists the practitioner in identifying the precursor lesions that eventually progress to frank carcinoma. This preinvasive stage, detected

TABLE 12-13-1. Risk Factors for Development of Cervical Cancer

High Risk

Early age at first intercourse, especially if younger than 16 years or within 1 year of menarche
Early first pregnancy
Multiple sexual partners
High-risk male partner
History of genital condyloma
Smoking history, dose dependent
Immunosuppression

Increased Risk

History of genital herpes infection
Low socioeconomic status
African American, Hispanic, or Native American race

Possible (or Controversial) Increased Risk

Oral contraceptive use
Vitamin A deficiency

Decreased Risk

Nuns
Barrier contraceptive use
Jewish, Amish, Mormon, or Muslim faith

TABLE 12-13-2. Common Signs and Symptoms of Carcinoma in Situ

Irregular or postcoital vaginal bleeding

Unusually foul-smelling discharge

Suspicious cervical appearance

Dyspareunia

Pelvic pain

Hematuria

by Pap smear screening, provides a unique opportunity to control any further progression of the disease. The entire spectrum of this cellular disorder is manifested by progressive atypical changes in growth and maturation. These morphologic changes are responsible for initiating the process of CIN, defined as the preinvasive phase of cervical cancer.

Cervical epithelium is composed of two different cell types: columnar and squamous. Columnar epithelial cells that are exposed to the vaginal environment are continually replaced or repaired by stratified squamous epithelial cells. This benign regenerative process, called *metaplasia,* is a normal occurrence during a female's neonatal period, adolescence, and first pregnancy. However, certain environmental and hormonal conditions can alter this benign process and result in cellular abnormalities known as dysplasia.

Anatomically, the area most vulnerable to these carcinogenic stimuli is located between the old and the new squamocolumnar epithelial junction called the *transformation zone.* Approximately 95% of all squamous intraepithelial neoplasia develops within this zone. In most cases, the preinvasive stage will either regress entirely or remain static for several years before any further progression occurs. However, when progression does occur, the malignant cells push their way through the basement membrane and gradually invade the cervical stroma. Initially, this process results in microinvasive carcinoma but can evolve into frankly invasive carcinoma over time. Despite negative cytology or cervical biopsy results, a cone biopsy is needed to determine the presence or absence of invasion. Although cervical cancer is primarily a disease of local infiltration, the tendency for lymphatic dissemination is the hallmark. In more extensive disease, infiltration of the underlying tissue extends beyond the pelvic floor to the bladder and the rectum. The more advanced the local disease, the greater the likelihood of lymphatic spread and distant metastases. The International Classification System adopted by the International Federation of Gynecology and Obstetrics (FIGO) is the system most widely used by health care providers to estimate the extent of disease and aid in planning treatment. This clinical staging method is based on physical examination and noninvasive testing.

SIGNS AND SYMPTOMS

Preinvasive stages, such as CIN or CIS, are generally asymptomatic and detected by cytologic findings on routine Pap smears. The most common symptom of invasive carcinoma is abnormal or irregular vaginal bleeding. This can include intermenstrual bleeding, postcoital bleeding, or heavy menstrual bleeding (menorrhagia) (see Table 12-13-2).

Vaginal discharge is the second most common symptom. Preinvasive CIN rarely produces any physical findings, especially if the lesion is endocervical. Cervical lesions and epithelium that appear suspicious, white (leukoplakia), or bloody should be considered for immediate biopsy. Pelvic pain, hematuria, or urinary frequency is usually seen only in advanced stages of the disease.

As the disease progresses, infiltrative cancer can produce cervical enlargement, firmness, and irregularity. Three growth patterns that are clinically seen include exophytic, endophytic, and ulcerative. Exophytic lesions can appear cauliflower-like and bleed easily with palpation. Earlier stages of invasive disease often present with superficial changes that can mistakenly be interpreted as cervicitis or ectropion. Often, there is an associated vaginal discharge that can be bloody, serous, or purulent. Rectovaginal examination is crucial in determining the extent of the involvement. Advanced disease with extensive parametrial involvement may reveal a nodular thickening of the uterosacral ligaments with loss of mobility and fixation of the cervix.

Signs of metastasis can include:

• Enlarged supraclavicular and inguinal nodes
• Unilateral, pitting edema of a lower extremity
• Evidence of disease in the vagina
• Anemia
• Weight loss

SCREENING RECOMMENDATIONS

The Pap smear is the clinician's primary tool in the detection of cervical dysplasia and preinvasive neoplasia. The cervical/vaginal Pap smear examines exfoliated cells from the cervix and the uterus to detect pathologic abnormalities and cellular alterations of the uterine cervix in asymptomatic women. It is never used diagnostically. It has been estimated that with regular screening, the incidence of invasive cervical cancer has decreased as much as 50%. Despite this decline, there is still a large proportion of women who have not had regular Pap smears, especially in elderly black and middle-aged poor women. Some areas report that 75% of women age 65 years or older have not had Pap smears within the previous 5 years. Since 20% of the total number of invasive cervical carcinoma cases occur in women age 65 or older, and 40 to 50% of all women who die from cervical cancer are over 65 years of age, an extra effort targeted at this population is important. Currently, the screening recommendations of the American College of Obstetricians and Gynecologists, American Cancer Society, and the National Cancer Institute are as follows:

• Initiate annual Pap testing at the onset of sexual activity or age 18, whichever comes first.
• After three or more consecutive, satisfactory, and normal examinations, the Pap smear can be performed less frequently at the discretion of the patient and the clinician.
• There is no established upper age limit for testing.

THE PAP TEST

Reliability of the Pap smear to detect abnormalities largely depends on the clinician's technique and/or the laboratory's interpretation. In spite of the best collection techniques, specimen handling, and screening procedures, a 10 to 20% false-negative (missed lesion) rate is still reported. Efficacy is also limited by poor patient compliance, failure to identify high-risk patients, inaccurate or incomplete laboratory reports, and inadequate follow-up. Regardless of the explanation, Pap smear results are reliable only for screening purposes. New technologies developed to improve cervical disease detection include automated computerized analyzers (AutoPap), liquid-based thin-layer cytology (ThinPrep), and tests for the presence of HPV. All abnormal Pap smears require follow-up evaluations and histologic confirmation to make a diagnosis. It is important to note that cytology does not equal histology.

Collection Techniques

The following techniques should be observed to ensure accurate sampling.

BEFORE THE VISIT

- Ideally, patients should be scheduled for routine Pap smears during the proliferative phase of their menstrual cycle, which is the week immediately following their period.
- Ask the patient whether she has noticed an abnormal vaginal discharge or evidence of infection or whether she expects to have her menses during the time of her visit. Avoid sampling if she is menstruating or complaining of a heavy discharge attributable to infection.
- Instruct the patient to avoid intercourse or the use of any intravaginal products for at least 24 to 48 h prior to the examination.

IDENTIFYING INFORMATION

- Label the patient's slide prior to collection.
- Provide the laboratory with a clinical history and any abnormal findings.
- Alert the cytopathologist to patients who present with a history of intermenstrual, postcoital, or postmenopausal bleeding; high risk for cervical pathology; or any visible lesions on examination. Include the last menstrual period (LMP), obstetric history, sexual history, hormonal use, and history of previous Pap smears.

CELLULAR COMPOSITION

- Try to avoid using lubricants of any kind. Moisten the speculum with water or saline if necessary.
- Visually inspect the cervix before collecting a sample and locate the transformation zone.
- Reliable smears must include adequate numbers of squamous epithelial cells sampled from the endocervical canal and the transformation zone.
- Avoid preparing slides with epithelial cells that are obscured by blood, inflammatory cells, or foreign material.
- Sample both the endocervix and ectocervix with a spatula and a cytobrush. Gently cleanse the cervix with a cotton swab to remove any blood, mucus, or discharge. Insert the cytobrush into the cervical canal and rotate it no more than 360°. Spread the material evenly onto a glass slide. Rotate a wooden Ayres spatula around the external os (portio) and then roll onto either the same slide or a second slide.
- Immediately spray the slide with fixative.

QUALITY CONTROL

- Use an experienced, certified, and reputable laboratory that has been endorsed by either the American Society of Cytologists or the College of American Pathologists (or both).
- Inquire about the quality control process including communication and reporting methods, technical equipment, and adequate staffing.

DIFFERENTIAL DIAGNOSIS

The uterine cervix can present with a number of pathologic conditions, including those listed below.

Infections

Commonly associated with acute and/or chronic cervicitis, symptoms usually include a vaginal discharge. Clinicians may choose to perform a KOH prep or wet mount to diagnose *Trichomonas, Candida,* or bacterial vaginosis. Microbiology cultures are useful for diagnosing bacterial infections, and serologic methods aid in the diagnosis of syphilis, herpes, and chlamydial infection. Microscopic features of *Trichomonas, Candida,* and herpes can also be found on Pap smears.

Preinvasive Lesions or Cervical Intraepithelial Lesions

Cervical lesions that are visualized on speculum examination need to be differentiated between early invasive cancer or secondary carcinoma of the cervix and benign conditions such as eversion, polyps, and papillary endocervicitis. Multiple biopsies may be necessary before a final diagnosis can be made. Occasionally, metastatic carcinomas (ovarian, bladder, and breast) have spread to the cervix by direct extension from the uterine corpus or vagina. Lymphomas will also rarely present as a cervical tumor.

Dysplasia and Atypia

Dysplasia and/or atypia detected on Pap smears need to be thoroughly evaluated to rule out invasive carcinoma, infectious processes (other than HPV), cellular reparation, and hormonally induced changes in the postmenopausal patient. The infectious processes that can produce atypical changes include bacterial vaginosis, *Candida, Trichomonas, Chlamydia trachomatis,* and *Neisseria gonorrhoeae.*

Invasive Carcinoma

Microinvasive squamous carcinoma is the earliest invasive form of lesion, defined as less than 3 mm beyond the basement membrane but without invading the lymphatic system. Further extension is staged on the FIGO system and based on the degree and location of invasion.

Miscellaneous

Microglandular endocervical hyperplasia can present with a polypoid mass appearing within the endocervical canal. These lesions are often observed in pregnancy or in women who take oral contraceptives. Endocervical polyps are occasionally seen in women and may present with a history of abnormal bleeding or vaginal discharge. Flat condylomas are seen as a result of an infection with HPV.

DIAGNOSTIC STUDIES AND PROCEDURES

Whenever a clinician receives an abnormal Pap smear report that is suggestive of dysplasia, preinvasive disease (CIS), or invasive carcinoma, the patient is required to undergo a thorough investigation, using the simplest procedure, to confirm an accurate diagnosis. Patients who require further evaluation can be sorted into three distinct groups:

- Patients with unsuspected invasive cancer
- Patients with observable lesions that are amenable to office or outpatient treatment
- Patients who require diagnostic (and often therapeutic) conization.

This process of selecting patients for further studies begins with an analysis of the Pap smear. Colposcopy is the diagnostic test that is used to evaluate any abnormalities that are discovered on the Pap smear or observed on the cervix. Additionally, the diagnostic evaluation of cervical cancer also includes obtaining biopsies of representative areas of the cervix. Several modalities can be used for this procedure including endocervical curettage (ECC), directed biopsies, conization or cone biopsies, and Schiller's test.

Colposcopy

Colposcopic examination uses a vaginal speculum, binocular magnification, and an intense light source to view the uterine cervix. After staining the cervix with a 3% to 5% solution of acetic acid (Schiller's test), a satisfactory examination will identify any lesions or abnormalities and allow the entire transformation zone of the cervical epithelium to be visualized. Abnormal findings that indicate dysplasia and CIS are (1) white epithelium and (2) a mosaic pattern of the surface capillaries. Early stromal invasion is suspected when bizarre capillary configurations are seen. With the exception of pregnancy, whenever these abnormalities are seen, a directed biopsy with evaluation of the endocervical canal by ECC should always be performed. Both specimens need to be submitted separately for pathologic assessment.

Indications for colposcopy include:

1. Pap smears consistent with dysplasia or carcinoma
2. Pap smears consistent with evidence of HPV infection
3. Pap smears reported as atypical squamous cells of undetermined significance (ASCUS) or repeated ASCUS
4. Pap smears with repeated inflammation
5. Abnormal appearance of the cervix
6. Patients with a history of diethylstilbestrol (DES) exposure

Endocervical Curettage and Biopsy

ECC is a general scraping of the interior wall of the cervix and is best performed before taking any biopsies. Do not perform ECCs on pregnant patients. Specimens are submitted separately and labeled as such. In women who present with a dysplastic smear, an estimated 5 to 10% of the results will be positive for dysplasia. Cervical biopsies of defined or well-demarcated lesions are then obtained. Concern is warranted if a significant discrepancy is found between the colposcopic impression, the Pap cytology, and the biopsy histology. Generally, 10% of colposcopies with directed biopsies and ECC would have a discrepancy between the screening Pap and the histologic data from the biopsy and ECC. A difference of one grade is common and acceptable. However, when a two-grade discrepancy occurs, a cone biopsy or conization is needed for further tissue diagnosis (see Table 12-13-3).

Conization

Cervical conization is the most commonly employed modality for diagnostic evaluation if the ECC reveals dysplasia or the colposcopic examination is unsatisfactory. It can be performed by using the cold-knife technique, laser, or a heated wire loop known as the LEEP procedure. Risks include infection, blood loss, anesthesia, and in women who are considering pregnancy, cervical incompetence. The LEEP method claims less marginal tissue destruction, which provides for a more reliable pathologic assessment, less postoperative bleeding, better visualization of the squamocolumnar junction, and greater ease to perform.

TABLE 12-13-3. Indications to Perform a Cone Biopsy or Conization

Two-step discrepancy between cytology and histology
Suspicion of microinvasive carcinoma
Poor cervical visualization
Unsatisfactory colposcopy

Schiller's Test

Schiller's test is nonspecific for cancer but can reveal the presence of immature metaplastic epithelium if nonstaining of the cervix is seen after its application.

CYTOLOGIC CLASSIFICATION: THE BETHESDA SYSTEM

The National Cancer Institute changed the nomenclature for dysplasia in 1988 and developed the current reporting method known as the Bethesda System. Updated in 1992, this system has replaced the earlier interpretations and reflects the current understanding of the development and progression of cervical neoplasia. Comparison of the nomenclature for the CIN and Bethesda classification systems appears in Table 12-13-4. The Bethesda System depends on the pathologist for a diagnosis and appropriate follow-up recommendations. The format of this reporting system includes a statement of specimen adequacy, general categorization, and descriptive diagnosis.

Statement of Specimen Adequacy

- Satisfactory versus unsatisfactory specimens are determined by the presence or absence of both endocervical and metaplastic ectocervical cells.
- Satisfactory smears can be limited by the following four factors:

  1. Lack of metaplastic or endocervical cells
  2. Partially obscuring inflammation, blood, or debris
  3. Drying artifacts
  4. Lack of patient information

- Unsatisfactory implies that either more than 75% of the cells were obscured by blood, inflammation, or debris, or that the slide was broken in transit.

General Categorization

- Within normal limits
- Benign cellular changes
- Epithelial cell abnormality

Descriptive Diagnosis

- Benign cellular changes: infection
- Reactive cellular changes
- Epithelial cell abnormalities

Epithelial cell abnormalities are either of squamous cell origin or glandular origin. This classification introduces the term *squamous intraepithelial lesion* (SIL) to encompass all grades of *cervical intraepithelial neoplasia* (CIN). SIL is further divided into subdivisions of low grade, high grade, atypical, and invasive as listed below in Table 12-13-4.

TABLE 12-13-4. Comparison of Classification Systems

CLASS	CIN	BETHESDA	DESCRIPTION
I	Normal	Normal	Normal
II	HPV	ASCUS	HPV
II	Atypia	ASCUS	Atypia
III	CIN 1	LGSIL	Mild dysplasia
III	CIN 2	HGSIL	Moderate dysplasia
III	CIN 3	HGSIL	Severe dysplasia
IV	CIS	HGSIL	CIS
V	Invasive carcinoma	Invasive carcinoma	Invasive carcinoma

ABBREVIATIONS: CIS, carcinoma in situ; HPV, human papillomavirus.

1. Atypical squamous cells of undetermined significance (ASCUS)
2. Low-grade squamous intraepithelial lesions (LGSIL)
3. High-grade squamous intraepithelial lesions (HGSIL)
4. Squamous cell carcinoma (SCC)

LGSIL includes cellular changes that are associated with HPV infection and CIN 1. HGSIL is associated with CIN 2 and 3. The presence of CIN is strongly suggestive of a history of HPV infection. Some studies demonstrate that lesions reported with mild dysplasia or CIN 1/LGSIL will spontaneously regress without any further intervention. However, because there is no way to predict which lesions will progress, it has become common practice in the United States for all dysplastic Pap smears (CIN) to be followed up with colposcopy and directed biopsy to histologically define and diagnose the level of dysplasia or carcinoma present.

Most of the controversy revolves around the classification of ASCUS. The presence of ASCUS in young women generally indicates the presence of HPV infection. Older women may have a variety of abnormalities. The challenge for the cytopathologist and the clinician lies in the interpretation of the results, which can either be a florid benign reactive process or a preneoplastic one. The major dilemma revolves around the issue of whether a wait and see approach is appropriate for women with ASCUS or LGSIL diagnoses. An upcoming new clinical trial will be testing three different ways to manage these mild cervical lesions as listed below:

1. Observation and follow-up Pap smears every 4 to 6 months
2. Immediate colposcopy and biopsy
3. HPV DNA testing to distinguish between high- and low-risk lesions

MANAGEMENT OF ABNORMAL PAP SMEARS

All abnormal Pap smears require further evaluation. Management is individualized and dependent on the interpretation of the cytologic characteristics of the reporting classification system. Unfortunately, this process is a continuing source of confusion. The Bethesda System has gained widespread acceptance in laboratory and clinical practice today, replacing the outdated CIN grading system and Class system. The responsibility of the treating practitioner, therefore, is to thoroughly understand the cytopathologist's report and interchangeably translate the results to ensure optimal patient care.

Evaluating abnormal Pap smears is a challenging task. It requires a broad knowledge base of the disease process, different nomenclature for multiple classification systems, controversial treatment guidelines for low-grade lesions, competing modalities for diagnostic evaluation, financial restrictions in managed care environments, continuing education on current technologies, sampling techniques and screening methods, educating patients on disease prevention, and communicating test results effectively and reassuringly. Whenever an abnormal Pap smear is suggestive of cervical neoplasia, all patients should be referred for diagnostic evaluation and histologic correlation.

Appropriate guidelines to follow in the management of abnormal Pap smears are listed in Table 12-13-5.

SUMMARY

The role of the physician assistant is extremely important in the screening and evaluation of all Pap smears, regardless of results. Communication is a key element in both preventive education and diagnostic evaluation. Patients should be easily referred for any malignancy and treatment decisions dependent on protocols. As a physician assistant, the provision of compassionate care and understanding; availability for counseling, reassurance, and explanations; and meticulous follow-up or tracking is absolutely imperative for meeting the criteria of optimal patient care.

TABLE 12-13-5. Management of Abnormal Cervical Cytology (Bethesda System)

Atypical Squamous Cells of Undetermined Significance (ASCUS)

• Repeat Pap smear every 4–6 months for 2 years until there are three consecutive negative smears; if a second ASCUS is obtained, consider colposcopy
• If ASCUS is accompanied by severe inflammation, treat the specific infection and repeat in 2–3 months
• ASCUS in a postmenopausal patient should be treated with a course of vaginal estrogen and a repeat Pap smear; consider colposcopy if still abnormal
• If the patient is considered to be at high risk for dysplasia, consider colposcopy

Low-Grade Squamous Intraepithelial Lesion (LGSIL)

• Repeat Pap smear every 4–6 months for 2 years until there are three consecutive negative smears; if a second LGSIL is obtained, consider colposcopy
• Colposcopy with endocervical curettage and directed biopsies as indicated

High-Grade Squamous Intraepithelial Lesion (HGSIL)

• Colposcopy with endocervical curettage and directed biopsies as indicated

Atypical Glandular Cells of Undetermined Significance

Each case must be individualized by the clinical situation and risk factors; options include the following:

1. Repeat Pap smear, using endocervical brush
2. Endometrial biopsy
3. Cone biopsy

PATIENT EDUCATION MATERIALS

"Should I have a Pap Smear?" and "Understanding Your Pap Smear" (free brochures). Send a self-addressed stamped envelope to Pap Smear, American Society of Clinical Pathologists, Box WWW, 2100 West Harrison Street, Chicago, IL 60612-3798.
"Questions and Answers about the Pap Smear." Office of Cancer Communications, National Cancer Institute, Bldg. 31, Rm 10A24, Bethesda, MD 20892; 1-800-4-CANCER.

CLINICAL RESOURCES FOR THE PRACTITIONER

"The Pap Test: Cervical Changes and Health Care," a multimedia teaching module that presents the CIN grading system, metaplasia and dysplasia, causes of cell changes, colposcopy, and treatment options. University of Pennsylvania Cancer Center, Oncolink: http://oncolink.upenn.edu/specialty/gyn_onc/cervical/screening/pap_test.html/.
American College of Obstetrics and Gynecology: http://www.acog.com/.
"Cervical Cancer: A Continuing Medical Education Activity," presented by the National Institutes of Health Foundation of Advanced Education in the Sciences. Participants review detailed statements that represent consensus views from government-sponsored panels of experts. Users send in a posttest and receive a certificate for 1 hour of continuing medical education credit. No fees apply. Free registration at http://text.nlm.nih.gov/nih/cdc/cme/intro102.html.
Gynecology Oncology Tutorials: http://gynoncology.obgyn.washington.edu/Tutorials/Tutorials.html/.

BIBLIOGRAPHY

Beckman CR et al: *Obstetrics and Gynecology,* 3d ed. Baltimore, Lippincott, Williams & Wilkins, 1998.
Brotzman GL, Apgar BS: Cervical intraepithelial neoplasia: Current management options. *J Fam Pract* 39:271–278, 1994.
Consensus Development Conference Statement, Cervical Cancer, NIH 1996, April 1–3; [cited Mar 10, 2001]; 43(1):1–24.
DeCherney AH, Pernoll ML (eds): *Current Obstetric & Gynecologic Diagnosis & Treatment,* 9th ed. New York, Lange Medical/McGraw-Hill, 2001.
Fauci AS et al (eds): *Harrison's Principles of Internal Medicine,* 14th ed. New York, McGraw-Hill, 1998.

Jacobs AJ, Gast MJ: *Practical Gynecology,* 1st ed. New York, McGraw-Hill, 1994.

Kurman RJ, Solomon D: *The Bethesda System for Reporting Cervical/Vaginal Cytologic Diagnoses: Definition, Criteria and Explanatory Notes for Terminology and Specimen Adequacy.* New York, Springer-Verlag, 1992.

Moore JG et al (eds): *Essentials of Obstetrics and Gynecology,* 3d ed. Philadelphia, Saunders, 1998.

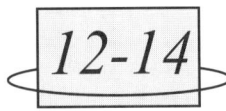

CONTRACEPTION

Lindsey Moser

DISCUSSION

The Centers for Disease Control and Prevention (CDC) has recognized advancements in family planning as one of the 10 most notable public health achievements in the 20th century.[1] In 1960 the FDA approved both the birth control pill and the intrauterine device (IUD). Five years after its introduction the pill became the most popular method of birth control. Today sterilization is the most widely used method.

About one-half of the 6.3 million U.S. pregnancies each year are unplanned,[2] and it is estimated that half of the unplanned pregnancies are due to contraceptive failure. The personal and social costs as well as the medical costs of these unplanned pregnancies make the responsibilities of contraceptive counseling a unique and significant challenge. Giving women and their partners the most up-to-date contraceptive counseling requires expertise and understanding of all current methods, as well as an understanding of the patient's life-style, religious beliefs, comfort requirements, and medical risk. Patients do best with methods they want to use. Table 12-14-1 lists the various contraceptive methods with efficacy and rate of use.[3]

REVERSIBLE METHODS OF CONTRACEPTION

Behavioral Methods

In choosing an appropriate method of contraception, discussions of behavioral control should be offered as a choice. These methods include complete abstinence, "outercourse," withdrawal (coitus interruptus), and periodic abstinence or fertility awareness methods (FAMs). The range of human sexual expression can be introduced to expand patients' understanding beyond intercourse to include other pleasurable intimate activities. This counseling is not only educational but also can be empowering.

These methods offer varying effectiveness and protection against sexually transmitted diseases (STDs) depending on the couple's control and understanding of the methods. Behavioral methods are free from medical or hormonal side effects. They are also accepted by those patients with certain religious values and convictions and are relatively cost free.

Complete and continuous abstinence is defined as refraining from sex play including any genital contact. It is 100% effective against pregnancy and STDs.[4]

Outercourse allows genital sex play without vaginal intercourse. Its effectiveness is nearly 100% against pregnancy with failure possible if preejaculate or semen is spilled on the vulva. Risk of STD transmission is increased with bodily fluid exchange or oral or anal intercourse.

Coitus interruptus or the withdrawal method includes vaginal intercourse but requires the male partner to remove his penis from the vagina before ejaculation. This method requires great self-control, experience, and trust. Its effectiveness is 81 to 96% and transmission of STDs is possible.[4]

Periodic abstinence or FAMs require an understanding of a woman's menstrual cycle and physical signs of ovulation to determine the potential periods of fertility. It requires some instruction and record keeping, checking daily temperatures and cervical mucous, and refraining from genital contact during certain time periods or willingness to use barrier methods. The effectiveness is between 75 and 99% and transmission of STDs is possible.[4]

Barrier Methods

Barrier methods include male and female condoms, vaginal spermicides, diaphragms, and cervical caps. For optimal effectiveness spermicides are best used with a condom, diaphragm, or cervical cap. When used together the effectiveness of barrier methods approaches that of combined oral contraceptives and has the advantage of protection against STDs. The diaphragm and cervical cap require prescriptions, instructions, and fitting by a clinician. Condoms and spermicides have the advantage of availability over the counter, but they eliminate valuable opportunities for clinical intervention to offer education and screening for reproductive health and STDs.

The male condom is available in many sizes, shapes, textures, colors, and even flavors. They are made of latex, nitrile, polyurethane, and animal tissue. They come lubricated and nonlubricated and with or without spermicide. Only water-based lubricants should be used, as oil-based lubricants can deteriorate the condom.

TABLE 12-14-1.   Contraceptive Methods, 1995

METHOD	WOMEN EXPERIENCING UNINTENDED PREGNANCIES IN FIRST YEAR OF USE		COUPLES USING THIS METHOD (%)
	PERFECT USE (%)	TYPICAL USE (%)	
Implant (Norplant, Norplant-2)	0.05	0.05	1.3
Sterilization (male)	0.1	0.15	10.1
Oral contraceptive pill	0.1	5.0	24.9
Injectable (Depo-Provera)	0.3	0.3	2.7
Sterilization (female)	0.5	0.5	25.6
IUD	0.6	0.8	0.7
Condom (male)	3.0	14.0	18.9
Withdrawal	4.0	19.0	2.9
Diaphragm	6.0	20.0	1.7
Spermicides	6.0	26.0	1.3
Periodic abstinence (rhythm method)	9.0	25.0	2.2

SOURCE: Adapted from *Consultant* "Quick Takes" (2000).[3]

The female condom is made of polyurethane (40% stronger than latex) and is designed to cover the cervix, vaginal walls, and perineum. It can be inserted up to 8 h prior to sex and is not recommended to be used concurrently with a male condom. Estimates are about 95% effectiveness when used correctly.[5]

Vaginal spermicides in the form of creams, jellies, foams, suppositories, and the newer gels and vaginal film are sperm-killing substances inserted deep in the vagina before intercourse. The active ingredients are nonoxynol 9 and octoxynol 9, which in the laboratory are lethal to viruses (including HIV) and bacteria and may lower the chance of being infected by an STD by an estimated 25%.[6] Contraceptive effectiveness when used alone ranges from 3 to 21 pregnancies per 100 users.[5] Foams are the most effective spermicide available on the market.[5] The new Bioadhesive Contraceptive Gel provides 24-h effectiveness against pregnancy.[5] The new Vaginal Contraceptive Film (VCF) is a 2-in. square, thin, translucent film undetectable to either partner and can be used alone or with a diaphragm.[5]

The diaphragm and cervical cap are latex products. They must be used with spermicides and inserted prior to intercourse and left in place afterward. The cervical cap has the disadvantage of being more difficult for the patient to insert and is not as commonly available as the diaphragm since fewer practitioners are trained to fit it. It is less effective in women who have given birth. Effectiveness rates in parous women are 60 to 80% versus nulliparous women, 80 to 90%.[4] The diaphragm when properly fitted is 80 to 94% effective in all women.[4]

Future Trends The Today Sponge was reintroduced over-the-counter in 2000. It is made of soft polyurethane foam containing nonoxynol 9. It has active spermicidal action for 24 h after insertion without the need to use additional spermicide. The use-effectiveness rate is 89 to 90%.[7]

Because of their usefulness in preventing the spread of STDs, barrier methods will remain popular. The major problems of latex allergy, breakage, and slippage are being addressed with newer products developed to improve effectiveness. Among others are plans for a disposable diaphragm and polyurethane condoms that transmit heat better and enhance sensation. New formulations of chemical barriers are in development, such as alternatives to nonoxynol 9 that are less irritating to vaginal membranes and provide better protection against HIV and other pathogens (as well as sperm).

Hormonal Methods

Hormonal methods include combined oral contraceptives and the progesterone-only oral contraceptives, including the mini-pill, injectable depo-medroxyprogesterone acetate (DMPA, Depo-Provera), and levonorgestrel subdermal implants (Norplant). Also included are emergency contraception (marketed by brand names Preven and Plan B), the Yuzpe regimen, IUD insertion, Lunelle (monthly estrogen/progesterone injection), and the continued debate over mifepristone (RU-486)

For overall balance of effectiveness, ease of use, cost, and side-effect profile, hormonal methods appear to be the most popular reversible contraceptive methods currently used in the United States.[8] All these methods require prescriptions and monitoring and have significant potential side effects, including death. However, rates of serious complications must be compared with those associated with pregnancy and childbirth, since users of these methods are at risk for pregnancy. Although these methods require clinician visits for use, increasing their cost and decreasing their convenience to the patient, there is a built-in opportunity for reproductive health and cardiovascular screenings, which may be of great benefit to women using these methods.

COMBINED ORAL CONTRACEPTIVES Combined oral contraceptives (birth control pills) have been available for contraceptive use in the United States since 1960. At this point, risks, benefits, and failure rates have been well studied, and statements concerning their use may be made to women with a high degree of certainty. Detailed patient information is provided by the manufacturer with every package of pills that is dispensed. Clinicians prescribing oral contraceptives should be familiar with their product labeling, which includes absolute contraindications, warnings, death rates per 100,000 users per year broken down by age group, benefits, and instructions for use.

All combined oral contraceptives include an estrogen, usually ethinyl estradiol, and progesterone, which vary by product. Dosage of the estrogen component and strength as well as dosage of the progesterone differ from one pill to another. All types of pills utilize 21 "active" pills. Some may contain seven "inactive" pills for improved daily compliance. Exposure to hormones for 3 weeks followed by a 1-week hiatus suppresses ovulation while stimulating the endometrium sufficiently to cause a withdrawal flow or "period" every 4 weeks. Triphasic pills vary the dosage of progesterone within each cycle (increasing the dose incrementally throughout the cycle, mimicking the natural hormonal cycle), whereas monophasic pills contain a consistent dose of progesterone throughout the cycle.

Most women can safely use oral contraceptives. It is the clinician's responsibility to select those women who cannot safely use this method. Education on use and how to manage side effects is vitally important. This includes adjusting the dosages of estrogen and progesterone in a way that minimizes "nuisance" side effects such as weight gain, headaches, irregular vaginal bleeding, and moodiness.

Absolute contraindications[9] to use of oral contraceptives are the following:

- History of cardiovascular disease, including non-pregnancy-related hypertension
- Any type of thrombophlebitis, including pulmonary embolism
- History or suspicion of reproductive organ cancer, including breast cancer
- Liver disease, including current abnormal liver function tests
- Pregnancy
- Smoking beyond age 35 years

Relative contraindications[9] include the following:

- History of migraine headache
- Gallbladder disease
- Family history of cardiovascular disease
- Diabetes
- Smoking before age 35 years
- Hypercholesterolemia
- Depression

Many common major illnesses are not contraindications to pill use, including asthma, congenital cardiac abnormalities, diabetes, and seizure disorders (see "Some Special Considerations," below). In these cases, specialist consultation may be helpful if the clinician who is caring for the woman's reproductive health needs is not the primary provider for the significant illness, as is frequently the case. Bear in mind that these women are frequently advised to avoid pregnancy, at least until their illness is under good control and/or teratogenic medications can be discontinued or changed. Risks of birth control pills must be weighed against the physical and psychological harm that could result from an ill-timed pregnancy.

There are numerous oral contraceptive choices. A clinician should initially base the hormonal dose on the woman's clinical picture and adjust according to the side effects experienced. Adjusting the dosage of estrogen and progesterone to mitigate side effects can be either rational, as in controlling breakthrough bleeding, or trial and error, as in alleviating decreased libido, moodiness, or mild depression. In general, beginning with 20, 30, or 35 μg estrogen is advisable, with an increase in the event of early-cycle (first-week) breakthrough bleeding or a decrease in the event of mild headaches, breast enlargement or tenderness, or weight gain.

Progesterone deficiency, especially in triphasic pills, leads to late-cycle breakthrough bleeding, uterine cramping, and heavy, prolonged periods. Changing to a monophasic pill often improves both symptoms and compliance. Mood changes are best handled by changing the type of progesterone used and adding vitamin B_6 (pyridoxine) 50 to 100 mg orally per day.[10]

Some patients may require several pill changes during their first year using this method, which may be frustrating to both the patient and the clinician. If side effects are not serious and the patient desires to continue oral contraceptives, the clinician can work with the patient to arrive at a dosage that minimizes any undesired effects.

Some Special Considerations Women who have difficulty taking the pill consistently should use an alternative method. This group of women is often thought of as unreliable, but it also includes women who travel frequently for business or work rotating shift schedules.

Antibiotics and anticonvulsant medications may decrease the effectiveness of oral contraceptives. A backup method, usually condoms and spermicide, should be recommended during antibiotic use and for 7 days after antibiotics are discontinued. Concomitant use with anticonvulsants is controversial, with some references advising discontinuation of the pills and others advising use of a pill containing 50 μg of ethinyl estradiol. The latter approach has the advantage of offering a highly effective method for women who must chronically use teratogenic medications. Consultation with a neurologist is wise in these cases.

Potentially serious conditions are possible. These include borderline hypertension, mild dyslipidemia, and migraine headaches. Women must be informed of the risks of continuing oral contraceptive use and closely monitored. Choose an alternative contraceptive method if a preexisting condition is exacerbated. The clinician must offer detailed information and follow-up regarding reasonable alternatives such as an IUD, subdermal implant (Norplant), or elective surgical sterilization.

Patient Education All patients presenting for contraceptive services should have access to appropriate patient education materials. This includes instruction on natural family planning for those couples who desire nonmechanical fertility control methods. Use of oral contraceptive pills must be an informed choice, and the role of patient education in making that choice cannot be overstated.

Finally, as a result of information published in the *Lancet* and the *British Medical Journal* in 1995 and 1996 it appears that oral contraceptives with the third-generation progestin desogestrel and gestodene have an increased risk for venous thromboembolic events as compared with other low-dose oral contraceptive pills.[11,12] Although there is no current plan to remove these pills from the market, patients using desogestrel-containing pills should be informed of the potential increased risk.

Future Trends Because the estrogen in combination pills is required not for the contraceptive effect but to stabilize the endometrium, new trends continue to minimize estrogen doses to lower the risk of thrombotic event. Combination pills containing less estrogen (10, 15, and 20 μg) are being developed and considered for release.[13] A novel estrogen dosing scheme called an "estrophasic" pill was released in 1997. The dose of estradiol increases stepwise throughout the cycle from 20 to 30 to 35 μg. The rationale is to minimize estrogen-related side effects while reducing breakthrough bleeding.[13] The standard 7-day pill-free interval may play a greater role in oral contraceptive failure than previously thought. New shortened pill-free interval pills have been recently released. Pills containing 20 μg ethinyl estradiol and 150 μg desogestrel are taken on days 1 to 21, placebo pills are taken on days 22 and 23, and estrogen-only pills (10 μg ethinyl estradiol) are taken on days 23 to 28. Maintaining hormonal levels with a small amount of estrogen might help to limit follicular development during the placebo interval.[13]

In October 2000 the FDA approved Lunelle, a monthly contraceptive injection. Containing 25 mg medroxyprogesterone acetate (MPA) and 5 mg estradiol cypionate (E_2C), it is the first injectable combination product. The side-effect profile is similar to low-dose oral contraceptives with efficacy comparable to surgical sterilization. Most women who use MPA/E_2C for 6 months or longer report regular menstrual-like bleeding patterns. Restoration of fertility following discontinuation of the product is similar to that observed in oral contraceptives. Initially it would require a monthly visit to a medical office but researchers expect it will eventually be available in a form women can inject themselves.[14]

Oral contraceptives may become even more popular if they are sold over the counter in the United States, as they are in many other countries.[8] Inroads have been made with new TV advertising of birth control pills, more discreet packaging, and easier-to-use methods that limit mistakes. Combination hormonal patches (worn like Band-Aids and changed twice a month),[4] subdermal implants, continuous oral contraceptives, and a once-a-month pill are being developed. A slow-release silicone intravaginal ring may be available soon.[13] A new birth control pill (B-Oval) using a synthetic version of melatonin instead of estrogen is expected to be available soon.[4]

New birth control methods for men that are both reversible and effective have been elusive, but progress is being made. MENT, the androgen 7-alpha methyl-19-nortestosterone, and GnRH, synthetic gonadotropin-releasing hormone, in subdermal implants are being studied. The implants would stay active for approximately 1 year and not affect sex drive. The World Health Organization is also studying injectable testosterone products with duration of action from 1 week to 3 months.[4] A new group of drugs, Gn RH agonists, can be used to prevent the release of follicle-stimulating hormone (FSH) and luteinizing hormone (LH) from the pituitary gland. Blocking the release of these hormones will temporarily suppress ovulation in women and spermatogenesis in men. This may constitute the first potential reversible unisex contraception.[4]

PROGESTERONE-ONLY METHODS With the exception of the minipill, which is slightly less effective than combined oral contraceptives, these methods have two advantages over estrogen-containing pills. First, they have fewer absolute contraindications, and second, their delivery systems do not depend on daily use. These methods, in contrast with combined oral contraceptives, may be used by lactating women, women with a history of cardiovascular disease including hypertension, and smokers older than 35 years.

Absolute contraindications include liver disease (progesterone is metabolized through the liver, and liver function tests should be performed if there is any doubt regarding the woman's hepatic status), current or past thromboembolic disorders, pregnancy, and breast cancer.

Their major disadvantage is irregular bleeding, which ranges from very annoying daily spotting to complete amenorrhea, which may or may not be a perceived advantage for the woman.

Although each of these methods utilizes the same mechanism of action, the delivery systems are completely different, leading to distinct advantages and disadvantages. Contraception via the oral route can be started and stopped easily, providing the option of "trial" use. Its major disadvantage is patient noncompliance.

Injectable DMPA (Depo-Provera) must be given intramuscularly 150 mg every 12 to 13 weeks. There is great variability in duration of absorption, leading to unpredictability regarding abatement of side effects, return of fertility (which can take up to 18 months), and resumption of menses. It should be used with caution in women with depression, since adverse effects may last up to 6 months and be refractory to treatment.

The Norplant system consists of levonorgestrel in six silicone capsules that are placed under the skin of the upper inner arm. It offers highly effective contraception for 5 years. In contrast to Depo-Provera, blood levels of hormone drop rapidly after removal of the implants, allowing for rapid resolution of any adverse effects and almost immediate return to baseline fertility levels. The initial cost to the patient is quite high, and a surgical procedure is required for placement. Surgical removal of the capsules may be difficult and cause scarring.

Special Considerations A frequently encountered concern with Depo-Provera is the management of contraception when either a dose is to be given late or the method is to be discontinued. This is because the woman may remain amenorrheic for many months following even a single shot. If pregnancy can be excluded (by a negative highly sensitive pregnancy test following 2 weeks of abstinence), a repeat shot may be given, or another method, such as combined oral contraceptives, initiated.

Patient Education As with all contraceptive methods, education is essential for success and acceptance of the method. This is particularly true of Norplant, which requires a well-considered 5-year commitment to this method if it is to be cost effective for the patient or third-party payer.

Future Trends Injectable DMPA was introduced into the United States as a contraceptive method in late 1992. It has become quite popular, and the trend is likely to continue. Norplant use has become less popular due to adverse publicity regarding its complications. Manufacturers are working on an improved model, Norplant-2, which has only two rods and is easier to remove. Worldwide large-scale clinical trials are currently ongoing for Implanon, a single implant containing 3-ketodesogestrel, more potent than levonorgestrel and effective for 2 to 3 years.[4] Biodegradable progestin implants that release the hormone gradually into the body for 12 to 18 months are under development.

Intrauterine Devices

Despite being highly effective and requiring no compliance on the part of the contracepting couple after its insertion, the IUD is currently used by only 2% of U.S. women who are at risk for pregnancy. Primary care clinicians who do not insert IUDs should be familiar with their advantages and contraindications and know where to refer those women who desire this method of contraception.

Absolute contraindications to IUD placement include pregnancy, extreme bleeding and cramping with menses that would be worsened with the IUD, risk factors for pelvic inflammatory disease (PID), and sensitivity to its components, particularly copper. The most important relative contraindication to IUD use is nulliparity, since IUD-related infection may lead to future infertility.

The ideal candidate for an IUD is a monogamous woman who has probably completed her childbearing but does not want surgical sterilization for reasons of cost, convenience, or irreversibility. Many of these women choose hormonal or barrier methods of contraception, but some have contraindications to hormonal methods and want the greater effectiveness and spontaneity afforded by the IUD compared with less-convenient barrier methods.

Nulliparous women may find that their contraceptive options are limited. Many clinicians offer IUDs to highly motivated nulliparous women after careful informed consent regarding the possibility of future infertility. IUD candidates must be at low risk for developing PID, namely, having only one partner and no history of sexually transmitted infections. Nulliparous women must also understand that they are at increased risk for other IUD-associated problems, such as increased menstrual pain and cramping, difficulty with insertion, and the possibility of a spontaneous expulsion.

TYPES OF IUDS   Although new devices are being investigated, only two types of IUDs are available in the United States at the time of this writing. The Cu T 380A (ParaGard) is a copper-containing T-shaped IUD. The most popular of the IUDs, it is approved for the duration of up to 10 years after insertion, although data from long-term clinical trials suggest the device provides effective contraception for up to 12 years.[13] It cannot be used in the presence of copper allergy and carries the same warnings and contraindications of any IUD. Progestasert is also T-shaped and slowly releases impregnated progesterone over a 1-year period. It then must be replaced. Theoretically, the release of progesterone increases the efficacy of the IUD and decreases bleeding and cramping.

Future Trends Despite a sudden plunge in popularity after reports of high rates of infection associated with some types of IUDs in the 1970s, this method will continue to be useful in a variety of clinical settings. IUDs with the highest complication rates have been removed

from the market, and many manufacturers have discontinued distribution in U.S. markets. The LNG-20 IUD, available in other countries, releases levonorgestrel directly into the uterus at a constant rate of 20 μg/d for 5 years (maybe longer), and thus decreases the incidence of heavy bleeding and cramping. It is anticipated to be approved by the FDA.[13] The CuFix 330, a "frameless" IUD, supposedly produces less pain and bleeding. It is constructed of a nonbiodegradable polypropylene thread that holds six tiny copper tubes. Results of preliminary testing have been mixed.[13]

Emergency Contraception

Emergency or postcoital contraception is used after sex with a known or suspected birth control failure or sex without the use of birth control. Although not intended for regular use, its place as a backup method for preventing unwanted pregnancy is important. If used correctly only about 2 of 100 women become pregnant after an act of sex.[9] The American College of Obstetricians and Gynecologists estimates that emergency contraceptive pills could prevent 800,000 abortions and 1.7 million unintended pregnancies in the U.S. annually.[15]

The first FDA-approved product, Preven Emergency Contraceptive Kit, contains a pregnancy test and four combination oral contraceptive pills, each containing 0.25 μg levonorgestrel and 0.05 μg ethinyl estradiol. The pregnancy test is done first as Preven is not effective if a woman is already pregnant. Two pills are taken as soon as possible, but within 72 h of unprotected intercourse. The second two pills are taken 12 h later. Initiation of the regime within 24 h of intercourse increases the chance that pregnancy will be prevented. A progesterone-only kit, Plan B, is also available, containing two pills, each with 0.75 μg of levonorgestrel. Both kits are believed to prevent pregnancy in the same way oral contraceptives do, principally by preventing ovulation or fertilization by altering tubal transport of sperm and/or ova. Implantation may also be inhibited by altering the endometrium.[9]

The Yuzpe method introduced in the early 1970s uses varying numbers of birth control pills in brands of oral contraceptive packs. The doses are similar to that of Preven or Plan B and taken in the same way. Typical regimes are as follows: Ovral, 1 dose = 2 white tablets; Lo Ovral, 1 dose = 4 white tablets; Nordette or Levlen, 1 dose = 4 light orange tablets; Triphasil or Tri-Levlen, 1 dose = 4 yellow tablets; Alesse or Levlite, 1 dose = 5 pink tablets; and Ovrette, 1 dose = 20 yellow tablets.[16] Because no studies have been done for pills containing other progestins such as norethindrone, gestodene, or desogestrel, such pills should not be used in routine practice for emergency contraception. Side effects with increased doses of estrogen include marked nausea, vomiting, breast tenderness, and menstrual irregularities. Using an antiemetic with each dose can make the nausea more tolerable. Additional tablets should be provided to replace any lost by vomiting. The commonly experienced nausea with emergency contraception discourages its frequent use as regular birth control.

Copper IUD insertion within 5 days of unprotected intercourse is 99% effective in pregnancy prevention.[4] In cases of rape or a sexual partner at a high risk for STDs, using an IUD may be contraindicated due to the association with PID.

The debate and final approval from the FDA over the antiprogestogen mifepristone (RU-486) rages on. Currently it is licensed only in France, the United Kingdom, Sweden, and China, but it is increasingly available in the United States.[5] In randomized trials comparing emergency contraceptives and RU-486, much lower side effects of nausea, headache, and breast tenderness were encountered and no pregnancies were found with RU-486. There was an increase in menstrual disruption. Compliance is increased, as only one 600-mg dose is required within 72 h of unprotected intercourse. Its efficacy derives from its ability to prevent ovulation and to alter the endometrium, thereby rendering it unsuitable for the establishment of pregnancy.

PERMANENT METHODS OF CONTRACEPTION

Surgical Sterilization

Mechanical interruption of the fallopian tubes in women and of the vasa deferentia in men causes permanent sterilization of the individual with very low failure rates. Primary care clinicians should counsel patients who have clearly come to the decision to have no more children of the availability of tubal ligation and vasectomy options and be familiar with referral sources for these procedures.

Vasectomy is a popular, widely available contraceptive method, often done in the practitioner's office under local anesthesia. The procedure varies, with some clinicians using a "no-scalpel method," while others utilize the traditional approach of small incisions through the scrotum to ligate the vasa deferentia. Success of the procedure in permanently ending the man's fertility approaches 100%, whereas mortality and major morbidity are extremely rare. Common complications, which occur in approximately 1% of procedures, are infection and hematoma. Rigorous attention must be paid to postsurgery sperm analysis, as fertility remains for at least 1 month following the procedure. This is due to sperm remaining in the vasa deferentia after ligation. Some clinicians recommend two analyses for presence and motility of sperm, one done 4 weeks after the vasectomy and the second one done at 6 to 8 weeks. Until infertility is established, couples should continue to use alternative forms of contraception.[17]

Of the two surgical procedures, tubal ligation is a more invasive procedure. It requires more extensive anesthesia and has a greater surgical risk and cost compared with vasectomy. For these reasons, many couples who are making a joint decision regarding family size select a vasectomy. Tubal ligation may be done at the same time as a cesarean birth, but it must be done as a separate surgical procedure following vaginal birth. Vasectomy is also the more reversible of the two procedures, although this varies, and no man should have the procedure done unless he is truly committed to permanent sterilization.

Future Trends A silicone implant into the vas deferens called the Intra Vas Device (IVD) is being studied. Unlike vasectomy, reversal would be simple, cost effective, and with an increased percent of returned fertility. There are also studies of chemical methods for permanent and reversible vasectomy.[4]

Special Considerations

Primary care clinicians may be in better positions than the surgeons performing these procedures to select out patients who are not ready for an irreversible contraceptive method. As with all methods, every option must be discussed with each individual or couple to assure the best contraceptive decision.

ACKNOWLEDGMENT

The editor would like to acknowledge the significant contribution of Noel Genova, author of this chapter in the first edition of *Primary Care for Physician Assistants.*

REFERENCES

1. Medical triumphs: This century's top 10 public health achievements. *Consultant* 39:2449, 1999.
2. Hatcher RA et al: *Contraceptive Technology,* 17th ed. New York, Ardent Media, 1998, p 5.
3. Quick Takes [column]. *Consultant* 40(1):100, 2000.
4. Planned Parenthood: Web page, http://www.plannedparenthood.org/bc/CONTRACHOICES.html.
5. Product Profile: *Advance for Physician Assistants,* April 1999, 55.
6. Hatcher RA et al: *Contraceptive Technology.* 17th ed. New York, Ardent Media, 1998, p 361.
7. Today's Sponge: Informational Web page of Allendale Pharmaceuticals, http://www.todaysponge.com/twentyfour.html.
8. Hatcher RA et al: *Contraceptive Technology,* 17th ed. New York, Ardent Media, 1998, p 405.
9. *Physician's Desk Reference,* 54th ed. Adapted from product labeling information. Montvale, NJ, Medical Economics, 2000.
10. Hatcher RA et al: *Contraceptive Technology,* 17th ed. New York: Ardent Media, 1998, p 443.
11. Jick A, Jick SS, Gurevich V et al: Risk of idiopathic cardiovascular death and nonfatal venous thromboembolism in women using oral contraceptives with differing progesterone components. *Lancet* 346:1589–1593, 1995.
12. Spitzer WO, Lewis MA, Heinemann LAJ, et al: Third-generation oral contraceptives and risk of venous thromboembolic disorders: an international case control study. *Br Med* 312:88–90, 1996.
13. Taylor M: Hormonal contraception and IUDs: What's new, what's next? *Consultant* 40(1), 2000.
14. Shulman LP: Monthly contraceptive injection. *The Female Patient* 25:21–30, 2000.
15. Preven Web page, http://www.PREVEN.com
16. Hatcher RA et al: *Contraceptive Technology,* 17th ed. New York: Ardent Media, 1998, pp 278–279.
17. Smith DR: *General Urology.* Los Altos, CA, Lange Medical, 1984.

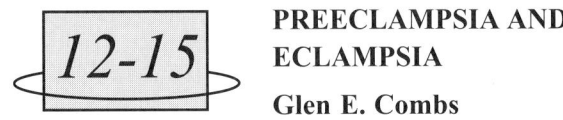

PREECLAMPSIA AND ECLAMPSIA

Glen E. Combs

DISCUSSION

The diagnosis of preeclampsia is made with the occurrence in pregnancy of three major signs: hypertension, proteinuria, and edema. The incidence of hypertension in pregnancy is 14 to 20% in primigravidas and 6 to 7% in multiparas.[1] Twin pregnancies have a higher incidence of preeclampsia than primigravidas. Of all cases of hypertension in pregnancy, 90% are related to preeclampsia. In addition to marked hypertension, patients usually present with proteinuria, excessive sudden weight gain, and edema after the 20th week of gestation. Though elevated blood pressure is an important presenting sign of preeclampsia, it should be emphasized that symptoms including persistent headache, visual disturbances, and continuous epigastric pain are also important diagnostic symptoms of preeclampsia. By the time the patient begins experiencing headache, visual disturbances, or epigastric pain, the condition is usually severe. Therefore monitoring blood pressure and checking for proteinuria and sudden weight gain should become routine for all prenatal office visits to detect early warning signs of preeclampsia. It is recommended that an office visit flowchart illustrating weight gain, presence of proteinuria, and vital signs including blood pressure and pulse rate be kept on all prenatal patients.

The major distinguishing sign that differentiates preeclampsia from eclampsia is the onset of tonic-clonic convulsions. A patient who experiences a seizure is considered eclamptic and should be immediately hospitalized for continuous monitoring and care. Eclampsia is primarily a disease of young primigravida patients, though its incidence is also increased in women older than 35 years. Low socioeconomic status appears to play a significant role in this condition, with low-income nonwhite primigravidas having the highest incidence of eclampsia.

PATHOGENESIS

The actual cause of preeclampsia is unknown. There are multiple theories that have been used to explain the pathogenesis of preeclampsia. One theory suggests that preeclampsia is the result of blood vessel spasm.[2] Vessel spasm ultimately results in systemic problems including hypertension, edema, and proteinuria. Multiorgan vasospastic disease results in decreased sensitivity to angiotensin II and increased thromboxane/prostacyclin ratio and usually begins early in the pregnancy, producing physical signs after the 20th week of gestation. A consequence of vasospasm is cerebral vasoconstriction, which ultimately leads to cerebral edema, hypoxia, and irritation of the cerebral cortex. Severe headache and blurred vision are symptoms of this progressive disease and considered precursors to convulsions and coma.

SIGNS AND SYMPTOMS

The triad of signs for preeclampsia consist of (1) hypertension, (2) sudden weight gain, and (3) proteinuria. Most patients are not aware of two of the major presenting signs, namely, hypertension and proteinuria.

Hypertension

Diastolic pressure is considered a more reliable prognostic indicator than systolic pressure for preeclampsia. Diastolic pressures over 90 mmHg or more should be considered abnormal and warrant further investigation.

Sudden Weight Gain

Weight assessment at each prenatal visit is essential. In most cases, a sudden increase in weight will precede a condition of preeclampsia. Patients who have more than a 2-lb weight gain in any given week or have a 6-lb increase in a month need to be further evaluated for preeclampsia.

Proteinuria

The presence of proteinuria is not unusual in pregnancy. Proteinuria that is 1+ by dipstick by itself is not significant. Two consecutive 1+ or greater protein results in a 6-h interval should be considered abnormal. Urine specimens should be obtained either by clean midstream catch or by catheterization due to the possibility of contamination from vaginal discharge or blood, both of which could give a false-positive result. Proteinuria usually follows the advent of hypertension and sudden weight gain.

Other symptoms that are associated with preeclampsia include headache, abdominal pain, and visual disturbances. Headache pain is usually frontal and is not relieved by ordinary analgesics. A severe headache is an ominous symptom that may precede a seizure. Abdominal pain is usually felt in the epigastric region and in some circumstances localizes in the right upper quadrant as the result of expansion of the liver capsule from edema and hemorrhage. Visual disturbances may include blurring, scotomas, and progressive partial to complete blindness. It is thought that visual disturbances are caused by retinal ischemia, arteriolar spasm, and intraorbital edema. In some rare cases retinal detachments have been observed.

OBJECTIVE FINDINGS

The significant findings of the patient with preeclampsia consist of edema, proteinuria, and hypertension. These signs usually occur following the 20th week of gestation, and any one or a combination of signs may be present. Edema that results in pitting of the face, hands, sacral area, abdominal wall, or legs should be of concern. Specifically, edema that does not disappear after 12 h of bed rest should give reason for further evaluation and diagnostic studies to confirm preeclampsia. Bed rest increases the patient's urinary output and lessens the intravascular dehydration and hemoconcentration.

LABORATORY FINDINGS

In the early stages of preeclampsia, proteinuria may be minimal or not present. In most cases proteinuria develops following hypertension and sudden weight gain. Careful blood pressure measurement, 24-h urine tests for protein and creatine clearance, complete blood cell count (CBC) with platelets, and uric acid are part of the routine laboratory studies needed to monitor the hospitalized patient. Elevated levels of aspartate aminotransferase (AST), bilirubin, and lactate dehydrogenase (LDH) should be anticipated.

OTHER DIAGNOSTIC CONSIDERATIONS

In addition to continuous observation of the mother, ultrasonography should be used to assess fetal growth and size, cardiac activity, amniotic fluid volume, and general well-being. In severe preeclampsia, deterioration of both the maternal and fetal condition should be anticipated. Frequent monitoring of the mother and fetus is of the utmost importance. Maternal evaluation should include a daily platelet count and measurement of liver enzymes. Signs of fetal distress should be further evaluated with a daily biophysical profile.[3]

TREATMENT

Patients with sustained preeclampsia should be hospitalized with strict bed rest throughout most of the day. Treatment should be focused on the prevention of convulsions, control of severe hypertension, the limitation of intravenous fluids, and steps to effect delivery. Delivery of the infant and placenta is considered the only known absolute treatment of preeclampsia and eclampsia. Magnesium sulfate administered intravenously with a loading dose of 4 to 6 g should be initiated followed by 2 g/h for seizure prophylaxis. Patients receiving magnesium sulfate should never be unattended. Blood pressure, urine output, and assessment of reflexes should be measured frequently. Hydralazine (Apresoline) has become one of the frequently used drugs to control severe hypertension (diastolic pressure >100 mmHg).

SUPPORTIVE MEASURES

Managing a patient with preeclampsia involves monitoring vital signs, urine output, and magnesium sulfate serum levels. Ocular fundi should be examined for signs of increased intracranial pressure, and patellar tendon reflexes should be evaluated frequently for hyperreflexia. Hyperreflexia is a sign of cerebral cortex irritability and cerebral edema. In addition, electronic fetal monitoring should be undertaken to evaluate fetal status on a continuous basis.

Magnesium sulfate when administered intramuscularly can be painful, and 1% procaine added to the mixture may help to relieve some of the discomfort associated with the injection. Patients who have had a convulsion should be cared for in a bed with padded side rails, and a padded tongue blade should be immediately available to place in the mouth to prevent tongue biting during a convulsion.

PATIENT EDUCATION

The incidence of sustained hypertension following preeclampsia or eclampsia or in subsequent pregnancies is not high enough to advise against future pregnancies, though women who have had an episode of preeclampsia should be advised to seek early prenatal care on a frequent basis for all future pregnancies. There is some evidence that the prevention or reduction in incidence may be affected with the use of nutritional supplementation of calcium, magnesium, zinc, and fish oils.[4]

Patients should be instructed that excessive weight gain needs to be avoided and that the diet should be well balanced and include approximately 80 to 100 g of protein per day.

COMPLICATIONS

Magnesium toxicity should be monitored in all patients receiving magnesium sulfate. Signs of maternal respiratory distress, semiconsciousness, and loss of deep tendon reflexes are important indicators of magnesium toxicity. At therapeutic levels magnesium sulfate slows neuromuscular conduction and depresses central nervous system irritability. At toxic levels (<9.6 mg/dL) patients may present with slurred speech, somnolence, loss of patellar reflex, paralysis, and respiratory difficulty followed by respiratory arrest. At the first sign of magnesium toxicity, the infusion should be discontinued. If respiratory distress occurs, the patient should be given calcium gluconate intravenously slowly over a 3-min period. Mechanical ventilation may be necessary if the patient further develops respiratory arrest. As a precaution, there should always be ready access to an ampul of calcium gluconate [1 g (10 mL of 10% solution)] and a syringe at the bedside of patients receiving magnesium sulfate. Magnesium sulfate therapy must be monitored with hourly urine output. Urine output should be optimally maintained at 30 mL/h during the periodic infusion of magnesium sulfate. In the event that urine output decreases below 100 mL in 4 h, the dose of magnesium sulfate should be reduced accordingly.

NOTES AND PEARLS

The most important management steps in treating severe preeclampsia include strict bed rest, prevention of convulsions, reduction of maternal high blood pressure, and the quick facilitation of a safe delivery. Once the patient is stabilized, cesarean section or induction should be initiated. Delaying the delivery only puts the mother and fetus at serious risk. In the event that a preterm infant (<36 weeks) is anticipated, the mother should be transferred to a medical facility that has a neonatal intensive care unit to provide adequate support to the newborn.

Eclampsia should be considered a preventable complication of pregnancy.[5] Appropriate prenatal care should identify the patient at risk, and proper treatment should be initiated to prevent eclampsia. It should be acknowledged that eclampsia is the result of failing to diagnosis preeclampsia in a timely way or the result of inadequate treatment. Eclamptic patients should be closely monitored following delivery for blurred vision, severe headache, and scotomas. These symptoms may precede a convulsion, and it is advisable to continue magnesium sulfate therapy for at least 48 h postpartum.

REFERENCES

1. Gabbe SG et al: *Obstetrics: Normal and Problem Pregnancies,* 2d ed. New York, Churchill Livingstone, 1995, p 995.
2. Gant NF, Cunningham FG: *Basic Gynecology and Obstetrics.* East Norwalk, CT, Appleton & Lange, 1993, p 427.
3. Gabbe SG, et al: *Obstetrics: Normal and Problem Pregnancies,* 2d ed. New York, Churchill Livingstone, 1995, pp 1015–1016.
4. Sibai BM et al: *Obstetric and Gynecologic Diagnosis and Treatment,* 8th ed. East Norwalk, CT, Appleton & Lange, 1992, p 386.
5. Gabbe SG et al: *Obstetrics: Normal and Problem Pregnancies,* 2d ed. New York, Churchill Livingstone, 1995, pp 1033–1034.

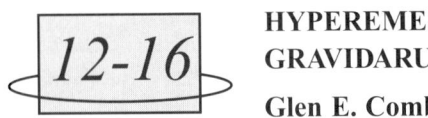

HYPEREMESIS GRAVIDARUM

Glen E. Combs

DISCUSSION

Hyperemesis gravidarum is a condition that consists of protracted vomiting following the first trimester of pregnancy. It is associated with electrolyte imbalance, weight loss, dehydration, and, in some severe cases, hepatic and renal damage. This condition can persist throughout the pregnancy and is considered a challenging management dilemma that may require hospitalization for parenteral fluid and nutrient replacement. Early detection and routine prenatal care can prevent serious complications of this condition.

Some nausea and vomiting during the first trimester of pregnancy is common and is experienced in approximately 70% of all pregnancies.[1] Frequent bouts of nausea and vomiting causing dehydration, ketonuria, significant weight loss, and hypokalemia are generally referred to as hyperemesis gravidarum, which is considered quite rare. Patients with true hyperemesis gravidarum usually require hospitalization to correct fluid and electrolyte imbalance. Negative protein

balance and protracted ketonemia will adversely affect fetal growth and development.

PATHOGENESIS

The cause of pregnancy-related nausea and vomiting is thought to be the result of rapidly rising human chorionic gonadotropin levels associated with the pregnancy. In addition, the emotional feelings coupled with the stress related to the repetitive bouts of nausea and vomiting can exacerbate the condition. The specific cause is somewhat unclear, although relaxation of the smooth muscle of the stomach probably plays a significant role. Steroid hormones associated with pregnancy are also thought to contribute to this condition.

SIGNS AND SYMPTOMS

The major signs and symptoms of hyperemesis gravidarum consist of persistent vomiting, dizziness, presyncope, and signs of dehydration. Depending on the severity of the case, ketonuria and elevated creatinine and blood urea nitrogen (BUN) are also possible.

OBJECTIVE FINDINGS

In addition to the usual signs of pregnancy, patients with hyperemesis gravidarum exhibit signs of postural hypotension and weight loss. In severe cases of persistent vomiting, signs of dehydration are evident, namely, hypotension, dry mucous membranes, and collapsed neck veins.

Ominous findings may consist of hemorrhagic retinitis, liver damage, and central nervous system (CNS) deterioration, which ultimately may lead to coma. Of extreme importance, a finding of hemorrhagic retinitis caused by repetitive vomiting and retching, is a serious sign that carries a 50% mortality rate.[2]

DIAGNOSTIC CONSIDERATIONS

The initial assessment of a pregnant patient with persistent nausea and vomiting should focus on the extent and severity of dehydration. With signs of dehydration, immediate steps should be taken to replenish fluids and nutrients and at the same time correct electrolyte imbalances. Diagnostic concern should be given to the possibility of multiple gestation or molar pregnancy. Certainly other underlying causes need to be excluded, including gastrointestinal problems, diabetes mellitus, peptic ulcer disease, hepatitis, and systemic infection.

Supportive measures that include hospitalization and fetal monitoring should be instituted with the goal of reversing fluid loss and correcting electrolyte imbalances.

LABORATORY TESTS

Pregnancy testing should always be considered in patients of reproductive age who present with nausea and vomiting and have a history of a missed menstrual period or menstrual irregularity. In severe dehydration, hemoconcentration and an elevated BUN or creatine is possible. Electrolyte imbalance including hypokalemia and metabolic alkalosis can accompany severe vomiting. The urine is usually concentrated with an elevated specific gravity and positive for ketonuria. In moderate to extreme cases, the initial baseline laboratory studies should include a pregnancy test, complete blood count, BUN, electrolyte panel, and urinalysis.

OTHER DIAGNOSTIC CONSIDERATIONS

Pregnancy alone is the usual cause of nausea and vomiting, though other conditions need to be considered while making the primary diagnosis of hyperemesis gravidarum. The differential diagnosis should include those conditions that are associated with nausea and vomiting, namely, cholecystitis, gastroenteritis, hepatitis, pancreatitis, peptic ulcer disease, and pyelonephritis. The customary diagnostic workup for these conditions may need to be altered in light of a confirmed pregnancy and potential harm to the fetus. It is important to consider multiple gestation or molar pregnancy as a cause of protracted vomiting, and diagnostic testing as well as ultrasonography may be helpful.

TREATMENT

Unfortunately, it is seldom that symptoms of nausea and vomiting can be completely abated with treatment, though symptoms can be diminished using various treatment modalities singularly or in combination. Conservative treatment for pregnancy-related nausea and vomiting consists of reassurance, psychological support, and avoidance of all foods that trigger nausea. Frequent small meals and light, dry snack foods have proved to be beneficial for some patients. It is important to instruct patients to eat small amounts of foods at frequent intervals. Patients should eat a little less than necessary to feel satisfied, avoiding the feeling of fullness.

Most patients with hyperemesis gravidarum will require hospitalization for treatment and care. Aggressive fluid replacement and the correction of electrolyte imbalances usually relieves or significantly diminishes the symptoms. Low-dose intravenous infusion of promethazine (Phenergan) has proved helpful, using 10 to 25 mg of promethazine per liter of fluid. The patient should be kept off oral foods and liquids and receive 5 to 6 L of intravenous fluid per 24-h period for 48 h following cessation of vomiting.[1] Potassium replacement should be given as needed and monitored closely. Renal function should be assessed for elevated BUN or creatine. All antinauseant drugs should be used sparingly because of the potential adverse effects to the fetus. As a precaution, parental consent should be obtained and documented prior to administration of all medications that may have an adverse effect on the fetus. Parents should have a clear understanding of all potential adverse reactions and possible fetal complications associated with all drug therapy in order to clarify proper informed consent.

SUPPORTIVE MEASURES

High-dose pyridoxine (vitamin B$_6$) therapy has proved helpful in reducing bouts of pregnancy-related nausea and vomiting. A dosage of 10 to 30 mg/d of pyridoxine is the usual amount prescribed. Maternal weight assessment is of importance in managing patients with hyperemesis gravidarum. In most cases the illness is self-limited with good prognosis if weight is maintained at more than 95% of the prepregnancy weight. Frequent feedings of low-fat meals and emotional support are important factors that should become part of the treatment regimen. Reducing pungent odors in the household may very well minimize the unpleasant symptoms of nausea. Some cooking odors can precipitate symptoms and should be avoided.

PATIENT EDUCATION

Nutritional guidance should be part of all preconception counseling appointments in anticipation of pregnancy-related nausea and vomiting. In the event that morning sickness occurs, the patient should be encouraged to eat dry toast or soda crackers prior to getting out of bed and standing. Reassurance should be given that the unpleasant symptoms of nausea usually pass after the first trimester of pregnancy. Patients with persistent vomiting should be encouraged to seek medical attention and should use antinauseant medications only as a final measure.

DISPOSITION

Patients with persistent vomiting and ketonuria should be hospitalized for fluid replacement and correction of electrolyte imbalances. Once the vomiting has been controlled and laboratory values have returned to normal, outpatient therapy may be initiated. Antiemetic suppositories may be of benefit and should be prescribed as needed.

COMPLICATIONS

Complications of hyperemesis gravidarum consist of severe electrolyte imbalances, dehydration, and CNS deterioration. Patients who experience a more than 5% weight loss are at risk for fetal intrauterine growth retardation and possible fetal anomalies.

NOTES AND PEARLS

Making the diagnosis of hyperemesis gravidarum is fairly straightforward, though other causes for vomiting during pregnancy should be explored. Consideration of infection, diabetes mellitus, and gastrointestinal problems should be part of any initial working differential. In addition, molar pregnancy and multiple gestation must be excluded as an underlying cause when completing the initial diagnostic workup.

Hyperemesis gravidarum is a serious condition that requires immediate attention to correct fluid loss and dehydration. Parenteral fluids need to be continued for at least 48 h once the patient has stopped vomiting to lessen the recurrence of symptoms. Maintenance support consists of frequent small low-fat meals plus light, dry snacks. The daily use of pyridoxine (vitamin B$_6$), 10 to 30 mg, may be of some benefit in minimizing the symptoms of nausea and vomiting. Maternal weight loss should be monitored and corrected to avoid potential fetal anomalies. Finally, do not underestimate the importance and benefits of extending emotional support and reassurance to the expectant mother during the remaining time of her pregnancy.

REFERENCES

1. Gabbe SG et al: *Obstetrics: Normal and Problem Pregnancies,* 2d ed. New York, Churchill Livingstone, 1994, pp 127–128.
2. Dambro MR, Fields SA: *Griffith's 5-Minute Clinical Consult.* Baltimore, Williams & Wilkins, 1996, p 507.

MENOPAUSE
Laura Hess

DISCUSSION

During the next two decades, more than 40 million American women will pass through menopause, and by the year 2020, one of every three women will be coping with this significant event in their lives. Menopause is defined as the complete cessation of menstruation caused by loss of ovarian function. The average age of women experiencing menopause is 51 years, with smokers going through menopause 2 to 3 years earlier than nonsmokers. The ovaries actually begin to lose their function over a period of 10 years before a woman stops having regular menses, and this perimenopausal period is often referred to as the climacteric. During this time many women notice changes in their menstrual cycle, such as change in length of cycle or flow pattern. Menopause is not a clearly defined event, but a process that affects a woman physically, mentally, and emotionally.

PHYSIOLOGY

Menopause is associated with a decrease in the density of primordial follicles. During the perimenopausal period, there is great fluctuation in ovarian steroids with production of estradiol in irregular bursts. The glandular secretion of estrogen diminishes steadily, even with regular menstrual cycles, for 5 years preceding menopause. As menopause progresses, the ovary requires higher amounts of follicle-stimulating hormone (FSH) to stimulate estrogen production and ovulation.[1] Oligoovulatory and anovulatory bleeding is common during this time.

Luteinizing hormone (LH) and FSH produced by the pituitary rise during menopause.

SIGNS AND SYMPTOMS

Irregular menstrual bleeding is usually the first manifestation of menopause. After the cessation of menses, vasomotor instability becomes more prominent. Vasomotor symptoms are often a major disruption of a woman's life. The classic "hot flash" is a sudden transient sensation of heat and warmth that occurs most often on the chest, face, and head. It is accompanied by perspiration and can be followed by flushing. Hot flashes may last from 30 s to several minutes, and may occur repeatedly throughout the day and night.[1] Some women are more affected at night and complain of severe sweats and sleep disturbance. Nearly 75% of women experience hot flashes followed by the hot flush and/or night sweats. Women experiencing surgical menopause tend to have more hot flashes than those experiencing natural menopause. The prevalence of hot flashes or flushes is highest the first 2 years after menopause. However, hot flashes can begin well before menopause and last for 10 years following cessation of menses.[1] Although it is unclear exactly what causes the hot flash, researchers have proved repeatedly that estrogen replacement therapy (ERT) can eliminate these troublesome symptoms.

Estrogen is also critical in maintaining vaginal and urethral tone. Women who do not take estrogen often develop symptoms of atrophic vaginitis, such as dyspareunia (painful intercourse) and vaginal irritation. Urethral atrophy can lead to dysuria, nocturia, urinary frequency, and incontinence. Atrophy of the pelvic support from loss of estrogen predisposes to uterine prolapse, cystocele, rectocele, and stress incontinence. These genitourinary changes occur slowly over years following menopause.[2] Treating with estrogen early in menopause prevents or minimizes many of these conditions.

The loss of ovarian hormones is also the major risk factor of osteoporosis (see Chap. 5-2). Estrogen deficiency causes an increased rate of skeletal resorption that is greater than the rise in bone formation, leading to a weakening of cortical and trabecular bone. Bone loss is a subtle, long-term process, with the most rapid loss occurring within the first 3 to 7 years following menopause. The weakened bone cannot tolerate normal stress and may fracture after even minor trauma. Osteoporotic fractures are most common in the spine (vertebral crush fractures), hip (femoral neck or intertrochanteric fractures—see Chap. 10-13), and wrist (Colles' fractures).[3] Currently, osteoporosis contributes to more than 1.5 million fractures in the United States each year. With the population aging, this number is expected to double by the year 2050. Other risk factors for osteoporosis include white or Asian race, body habitus, family history, smoking, alcohol use, physical inactivity or immobilization, medications (steroids, heparin, methotrexate), and certain disease states (hyperthyroidism and hyperparathyroidism). Preventing osteoporosis with ERT may be especially important in women with these concomitant risk factors.

Because osteoporosis can be asymptomatic for decades, it is easy to overlook. Trabecular (spine) fractures begin at approximately age 60, followed by hip (cortical bone) fractures at about age 70. Osteoporosis and the resultant fractures are late physical manifestations of long-term estrogen deficiency following menopause. Early treatment with estrogen not only stops bone resorption but also produces a slight increase in bone density. The closer to menopause that estrogen is initiated, the greater the benefit.

Women frequently attribute their mood swings, irritability, and feelings of agitation to menopause. This area of menopause is challenging for the clinician and patient because the relationship between estrogen loss and certain mood states has not been proved. There is some evidence that estrogen in doses used to control menopausal symptoms can be therapeutic for women experiencing mild symptoms of depression and mood lability. However, hormone replacement therapy (HRT) has not been shown to be beneficial in women with mood disturbances indicating a major depression.[4]

PHYSICAL EXAMINATION

Most menopausal women have unremarkable physical findings. There may be some mild changes in the amount of vaginal secretions, indicating vaginal dryness and causing the woman to complain of dyspareunia. However, within 4 to 5 years after cessation of menses, a significant number of women show signs of atrophy in the vagina and urethra. In those women not using hormones who go on to develop osteoporosis, the physical examination may demonstrate loss of height with kyphotic changes in the spine.

DIAGNOSTIC CONSIDERATIONS

Generally, the clinical manifestations of menopause and the associated age of the patient make it easy to determine that a woman is menopausal. However, other causes of amenorrhea include situational stress, excessive exercise, hypothyroidism, drugs (e.g., oral contraceptives), pituitary disorders such as hyperprolactinemia, and occasionally pregnancy. Polycystic ovary syndrome is an important cause of amenorrhea in younger women characterized by amenorrhea, irregular menstrual cycles, hirsutism, enlarged ovaries, and infertility (see Chap. 12-9). Uterine causes of amenorrhea include endometrial scarring (Asherman's syndrome) as a consequence of septic abortion, overly vigorous curettage, radiation therapy, and cervical stenosis from scarring.[5]

LABORATORY AND RADIOLOGIC STUDIES

An increase of FSH production and decrease in estradiol are the only reliable biochemical markers of menopause. An FSH greater than 30 IU/L defines menopause biochemically. Additionally, the estradiol level is less than 50 ng/dL. In clinical practice, an elevated FSH level is the most important laboratory determinant of menopause. The FSH can be drawn at any point if the clinician needs documentation of menopause. However, complete cessation of menses for more than 6 months with the accompaniment of hot flashes, night sweats, and hot flushes is enough clinical evidence to determine that a woman is experiencing menopause. Checking a serum FSH may be most useful in women who have nonspecific symptoms that may be due to menopause, especially if they have undergone a hysterectomy without oophorectomy.

Bone densitometry of the spine and femoral neck may also be useful in some women to provide a quantitative measurement of bone mineralization. Bone density can be used to predict the risk of osteoporotic fractures of the spine and femoral neck. This test may be particularly helpful in women who are at high risk for osteoporosis.

CARDIOVASCULAR DISEASE AND MENOPAUSE

The potential for dramatically reducing deaths from coronary artery disease was seen as a potential benefit of ERT (see Chap. 1-7). Statistically, coronary artery disease (CAD) is the leading cause of death in women (36% of all deaths in women), far exceeding mortality rates for breast cancer (4%), osteoporosis (2.5%), or diseases of the ovaries and uterus (2%). The incidence of cardiovascular disease sharply rises in women following menopause, eventually matching that in men. The proposed benefits of ERT on the cardiovascular system have been discussed by a number of large-scale epidemiologic trials, including the Framingham Heart Study and the Nurses' Health Study. These studies demonstrated that women taking estrogens had a 50% reduction in cardiovascular disease, with a 35 to 45% reduced total mortality rate.[2]

The Postmenopausal Estrogen/Progestin Intervention (PEPI) trial found that estrogen, with or without a progestin, increased serum levels of high-density lipoprotein (HDL) and lowered levels of low-density lipoprotein. Currently, it is thought that estrogen's positive effect on lipids accounts for 25 to 50% of its cardioprotection, with the remainder due to its direct effect on the blood vessel wall[2] (see Chap. 1-4).

Estrogen reduces the adherence of white blood cells to the vascular epithelium, has an antiproliferative effect on the smooth-muscle cells of the blood vessels, and enhances the normal contraction and relaxation of the blood vessel walls. However, recently the Heart and Estrogen/Progestin Replacement Study (HERS) showed no cardiovascular benefit from HRT in postmenopausal women with documented cardiovascular disease taking estrogen.[6] These results suggest that estrogen-progestin does not reduce overall CAD risk in women with established coronary disease. As a result of this study some suggest the initiation of HRT is not indicated in women with established coronary heart disease (CHD) to prevent heart attacks.

The Women's Health Initiative, a 9-year interventional study of 27,000 women taking either Premarin alone, an estrogen–progestin therapy, or a placebo may answer some of the questions regarding ERT and the heart and will help define the role of HRT in preventing CHD. Results of this 9-year prospective study will be available after 2005.[7]

RISKS AND CONTROVERSIES OF ESTROGEN THERAPY

Endometrial Hyperplasia and Cancer

Estrogen has a potent effect on the lining of the uterus. It has been shown that using unopposed estrogen, meaning estrogen without progesterone replacement, on a woman with an intact uterus increases the risk of endometrial cancer. This risk is proportional to the length of time that a woman is taking estrogen. After 10 to 15 years of unopposed estrogen use, a woman's risk of endometrial cancer is 10 times higher than that of a woman who is not on estrogen.[2] Adding progestin in a cyclic or continuous fashion to the hormone regimen eliminates the risk. Progestins oppose some of the action of estrogens and prevent endometrial hyperplasia. Progestins do, however, mitigate some of the benefits of estrogen by interfering with the elevation of HDL seen with estrogen alone. Because of this the American College of Obstetricians and Gynecologists (ACOG) recommend using the lowest effective dose of progestin. Medroxyprogesterone acetate (MPA) is the most commonly used progesterone in the United States, and the ACOG recommends using 5 mg/d MPA for 12 to 14 days per month or 2.5 mg daily. Findings of the PEPI trial revealed that the use of micronized progesterone (MP) showed less adverse effects on the lipid profiles of women than other progestins.[7]

Breast Cancer

The risk of breast cancer in women taking estrogen is one of the most controversial aspects of HRT (see Chap. 13-4). Some authors believe that estrogen is mitogenic and may accelerate the onset of breast cancer. Taking postmenopausal HRT for 5 years has been linked with an increase in breast cancer risk by 1.3 times; 10 years of HRT use raises the risk to 1.7 times. Others suggest that breast cancer is detected earlier in women taking hormones because regularly scheduled mammograms are done in this population. Several meta-analyses have been done that show a slight overall increase in breast cancer. Yet two recent studies have added even more confusion about the role of estrogen and progestin therapy in the risk of breast cancer. Researchers found that the breast cancer risk for postmenopausal women rose by 24% for every 5 years of use among women on combined estrogen–progestin therapy, compared to only 6% yearly among women on estrogen alone. Another study using data from the National Cancer Institute stated that women on combined HRT had an 8% relative risk increase per year compared to 1% per year on estrogen alone.[8] At this point caution is warranted in interpreting these studies because of flaws in their designs. However, both studies add to a body of data suggesting that postmenopausal estrogen use for more than 5 to 10 years does increase a woman's risk of breast cancer, and adding a progestin increases that risk further.[7] This leaves clinicians with unanswered questions and emphasizes the importance of individualizing treatment by evaluating each woman's symptoms and risk factor profile before initiating ERT. In counseling women, it is important to discuss risk factors

TABLE 12-17-1. Contraindications to Use of Estrogens

Absolute Contraindications
Undiagnosed vaginal bleeding
Suspected or known pregnancy
Active thrombophlebitis or thrombosis
Breast cancer
Estrogen-dependent tumors
Endometrial cancer
Acute liver disease

Relative Contraindications
Chronic liver disease
Gallbladder disease
Hypertriglyceridemia
History of migraines
Endometriosis
Uterine fibroids
History of thrombosis or thrombophlebitis

in relationship to their likelihood of developing a disease. For example, a 50-year-old woman has a 10% lifetime probability of developing breast cancer with a 3% risk of dying of breast cancer. In contrast, this same 50-year-old woman has a 46% chance of developing heart disease with a 31% probability of death related to heart disease.[9]

Other Risks

ERT appears to increase the risk of gallbladder disease in some women, requiring the need for cholecystectomy (see Chap. 6-10). The package insert warns of the risk of thromboembolic disorders; however, this association is based on studies of more potent synthetic estrogens used in oral contraceptives. The relative risk with estrogens used in HRT is quite low. Some absolute and relative contraindications regarding the use of estrogens are found in Table 12-17-1.

TREATMENT

There is no standard treatment regimen for HRT in menopausal women. Each regimen is tailored to fit the individual and focuses on providing the lowest dose of estrogen and progestin to fit the patient's age, risk of bone loss and cardiovascular disease, and symptom profile. Education is necessary to inform the woman of any expected bleeding pattern.

The most common estrogen compounds used for HRT are the natural and equine estrogens such as micronized estradiol, estradiol valerate, estropipate, and the conjugated equine estrogens (CEE). All estrogen preparations are converted to estrone sulfate and rapidly metabolized by the liver. Within 1 week of the start of therapy, there should be a steady state of estrone sulfate in the body and symptom relief should occur. The usual starting dose of CEE (Premarin), estropipate (Ogen), and esterified estrogens (Estratab) is 0.625 mg. Micronized estradiol (Estrace) has a starting dose of 1 mg.[10] See estrogen products listed in Table 12-17-2.

Larger starting doses are often required for women who have had a sudden menopause such as a surgical menopause. Other women who may need higher doses of estrogen are those who smoke more than 15 cigarettes per day, those who abuse alcohol, and those taking psychotropic drugs.

The Selective Estrogen Receptor Modulators

Many women are searching for alternatives to the current therapy for menopausal treatment. The ideal therapy would protect skeletal bone, offer better lipid profiles, antagonize or reduce cell division in the breast and endometrial tissue, reduce genitourinary atrophy, and have minimal side effects. Even though estrogen has many benefits to women, the long-term effects on breast health are still uncertain and compliance is a major problem. About 25% of women never fill their

TABLE 12-17-2. Estrogen Products Used for Hormone Replacement Therapy

BRAND NAME	GENERIC NAME	AVAILABLE DOSAGES
Tablets, Creams, Capsules		
Cenestin	Conjugated estrogens	0.625-, 0.9-, a 1.25-mg table
Estinyl	Ethinyl estradiol	0.20- and 0.05-mg tablets
Estrace	Estradiol	0.5-, 1-, 2-mg tablets 0.01% vaginal cream
Estratab	Esterified estrogens	0.3-, 0.625-, 1.25-, and 2.5-mg tablets
Ogen	Estropipate	0.625-, 1.25-, and 2.5-mg tablets; 1.5-mg/g cream
Ortho-est	Estropipate	0.625- and 1.25-mg tablets
Premarin	Conjugated equine estrogen (CEE)	0.3-, 0.625-, 0.9-, 1.25- and 2.5-mg tablets; 0.625-mg/g cream
Combination Products		
Activella	Estradiol + progestin	Estradiol 1 mg/ norethindone acetate 0.5-mg tablets
Estratest	Esterified estrogen + methyltestosterone	1.25- and 2.5-mg tablets
Estratest HS	Esterified estrogen + methyltestosterone	0.625- and 1.25-mg tablets
Premarin with methyltestosterone	CEE + methyltestosterone	0.625 mg CEE/5 mg testosterone
Premphase	CEE + medroxyprogesterone	0.625 mg CEE(14 tabs) + 0.625 mg CEE/ 2.5 mg progesterone (14 tabs)
Prempro	CEE + medroxyprogesterone	0.625 CEE/2.5 mg progesterone; 0.625 CEE/5 mg progesterone tablets
Patches (Estrogen and Combination Patches)		
Alora	Estradiol	0.05 mg/d, 0.075 mg/d, 0.1 mg/d applied twice weekly
Climara	Estradiol	0.05 mg/d, 0.1 mg/d applied every week
Combipatch	Estradiol + norethindone acetate	Estradiol 0.05 mg + norethindone acetate 0.14 mg/d applied twice weekly
Esclim	Estradiol	0.025 mg/d, 0.0375 mg/d, 0.05 mg/d, 0.075 mg/d applied twice weekly
Estraderm	Estradiol	0.05 mg/d, 0.1 mg/d applied twice weekly
Fempatch	Estradiol	0.025 mg/d applied once or twice weekly
Vivelle	Estradiol	0.0375 mg/d, 0.05 mg/d, 0.075 mg/d, and 0.1 mg/d, applied twice weekly

prescriptions for estrogen and another 25% quit taking their estrogen within the first year of treatment.[11] The most common reasons are fear of breast cancer, abnormal bleeding, and concerns about side effects.

Two selective estrogen receptor modulators are now available for women who cannot take estrogen and are at high risk of osteoporosis. Both tamoxifen and raloxifene (Evista) have been found to increase bone mineral density in women while not stimulating the breast or the uterus. Raloxifene at 60 mg/d has been released for the prevention and treatment of osteoporosis and osteoporotic fractures in women, although it may increase vasomotor symptoms.

Nonhormonal Treatments

Some nonhormonal drug treatments, which may alleviate hot flashes, include the use of clonidine (Catapres) or ergotamine and phenobarbital (Bellergal-S). Synthetic progestins may also offer an alternative for relief of vasomotor symptoms in women for whom estrogen is not appropriate.

For women with an intact uterus, it is necessary to add a progestin to the hormone replacement regimen. MPA is the most widely used progestin for HRT in the United States, although there are a number of progestins available on the market. Progestins do interfere with the positive lipid benefits provided by estrogen, so it is important to use the lowest effective dose. Frequently the use of the progestin can cause some bothersome side effects for women such as bloating, weight gain, irritability, depression, and PMS-like symptoms. The cyclic use of progestins often causes a monthly withdrawal bleed, which is bothersome for some women and a major reason for lack of compliance. By giving a smaller dose of progestin daily, the monthly withdrawal-bleeding pattern is avoided; however, there may be up to 6 months of erratic spotting with the regimen.[11]

Most women are on one of three estrogen–progestin regimens (see Table 12-17-3)[12]:

1. *The cyclic regimen.* This regimen consists of administering estrogen for the first 25 days of the month. A progestin is added on day 14 for a total of 10 to 12 days. Both drugs are stopped from day 26 until the end of the month. Then the estrogen is started again. On this regimen, a woman may expect to have a withdrawal bleed during the hormone-free interval. Withdrawal bleeding occurs in close to 80% of women taking HRT in this fashion. However, over time the bleeding will taper off and often cease.

2. *The continuous regimen.* In this regimen, estrogen is taken every day of the month with no break. Progestin is added from day 1 of the month through day 12, then stopped. A withdrawal bleed is expected shortly after the progestin is stopped. With both the cyclic and continuous regimens, a woman can usually predict when during the month she will have bleeding. The predictability of monthly bleeding is an attractive feature of these methods.

3. *The continuous combined regimen.* Many women would like to eliminate bleeding postmenopausally, so the continuous combined regimen is often chosen and can eliminate bleeding in 60 to 70% of women. With the continuous combined regimen, both estrogen and a low-dose progestin are taken daily. Initially, spotting and irregular bleeding can occur, but after 6 to 9 months more than 50% of women have no bleeding at all. The continuous exposure of the uterus to progestin causes thinning and atrophic changes in the lining of the uterus. Despite the bothersome nature of the early spotting with this regimen, the benefit of not having regular menses makes it an attractive option to many postmenopausal women.

TABLE 12-17-3. Summary of Hormone Replacement Therapy Treatment Regimens

REGIMEN	ADVANTAGES	DISADVANTAGES
Estrogen Alone		
Estrogen daily	Simplest regimen	Only for women who have had hysterectomy or who receive periodic surveillance endometrial biopsy to check for hyperplasia.
Cyclic		
Estrogen on days 1–25; progestin, 5–10 mg, for 10–12 days starting on day 14	The traditional method, which many women are still using	80% of women have withdrawal bleeding, but over time bleeding tapers off.
Continuous		
Estrogen every day; progestin, 5–10 mg, from day 1 to day 12	Simpler than traditional method. Predictable withdrawal bleeding which may be helpful for women early in menopause	As with the cyclic regimen, withdrawal bleeding may continue indefinitely.
Continuous Combined		
Estrogen daily; progestin 2.5 mg daily	Simple regimen After 6–9 months, no more bleeding for 70% of women	Initial bleeding is unpredictable. Women who have ongoing bleeding after 6–9 months may need alternative regimen.

With all these regimens it is critical to educate women on what sort of bleeding pattern to expect. Any abnormality in bleeding patterns usually necessitates an endometrial biopsy to rule out endometrial hyperplasia or cancer. Therefore, education and timely follow-up is necessary to ensure compliance and monitor bleeding patterns.

NOTES AND PEARLS

It is important to document menopause before initiating HRT. Amenorrhea for 12 months and FSH levels >30 MIV/mL indicate a menopausal state. During perimenopause many women complain of symptomatic hot flashes despite having a normal FSH and estradiol level, as well as regular menses. These women are not candidates for HRT but may do well on low-dose oral contraceptives, which both suppress and replace estrogen and, it is hoped, alleviate some of the bothersome symptoms.

A complete history and physical examination should precede the initiation of HRT. Appropriate laboratory tests to order include thyroid stimulating hormone, complete blood cell count, lipid panel, and glucose. Also, a mammogram should be performed. Clinicians should be aware that there is more evidence now demonstrating that ERT is associated with a lower risk of Alzheimer's disease (see Chap. 11-4). There is also some evidence that estrogen helps to preserve the function of the hippocampus, the part of the brain that controls memory. It has also been speculated that ERT decreases colon cancer. More studies are needed to further verify these findings.

REFERENCES

1. Hammond CB: Menopause and hormone replacement therapy—an overview. *Obstet Gynecol* 87:213, 1996.
2. Gallagher J et al: Why HRT makes sense. *Patient Care.* 30:166–192, 1996.
3. Lindsay R: The menopause and osteoporosis. *Obstet Gynecol* 87:16S–19S, 1996.
4. Shenvin BB: Hormones, mood and cognitive functioning in postmenopausal women. *Obstet Gynecol* 87:20S–25S, 1996.
5. Goroll AH et al: Evaluation of secondary amenorrhea, in *Primary Care Medicine,* 3d ed. Philadelphia, Lippincott, 1995, pp 601–607.
6. Hulley S et al: Randomized trial of estrogen plus progestin for secondary prevention of coronary heart disease in postmenopausal women. Heart and Estrogen/Progestin Replacement (HERS) research group. *JAMA* 280:605–613, 1998.
7. HRT 2000: Pause for thought. *Harvard Women's Health Watch.* 7(8), 2000.
8. Schairer C et al: Menopausal estrogen and estrogen-progestin replacement therapy and breast cancer risk. *JAMA* 238:485–491, 2000.
9. Colditz G et al: The use of estrogens and progestins and their risk of breast cancer in postmenopausal women. *N Engl J Med* 332(24):1589–1593, 1995.
10. Brenner PF: The latest on hormone replacement therapy. *Audio Digest* June 15, 1999.
11. Hammond CB: Management of menopause. *Am Fam Physician* 55(5):1667–1673, 1997.
12. Scharbo-Dehaan M: Hormone replacement therapy. *Nurse Pract* (suppl): 115, 1996.

BIBLIOGRAPHY

Grady D et al: Hormone replacement therapy to prevent disease and prolong life in postmenopausal women. *Ann Intern Med* 117:1016–1037, 1992.
Stanford J et al: Combined estrogen and progestin hormone replacement therapy in relation to risk of breast cancer in middle-aged women. *JAMA* 274(2):137–142, 1995.

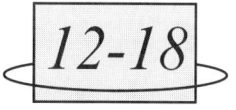

12-18 GESTATIONAL DIABETES
Lori Parlin Palfreyman

DISCUSSION

Gestational diabetes is hyperglycemia that is present only during pregnancy. This definition applies regardless of whether or not insulin is used for treatment. Approximately 90% of all pregnancies complicated by diabetes are due to gestational diabetes. Gestational diabetes most commonly presents early in the third trimester due to exaggerated physiologic changes in glucose metabolism.

It is important to evaluate and treat the condition as soon as possible after diagnosis since adverse fetal consequences occur rapidly after onset. The most common fetal complication is macrosomia that leads to birth trauma due to shoulder dystocia. Unlike other large-for-age infants, newborns of gestational diabetic women have excessive fat deposition on the shoulders and trunk, predisposing them to shoulder dystocia. In addition these infants are more likely to have delayed lung maturity (which normally occurs by 34 weeks' gestation), which can have adverse consequences if early delivery is indicated due to macrosomia.

There are maternal complications as well. Women with gestational diabetes are more likely to develop preeclampsia, which can be life-threatening to both mother and fetus if it progresses into eclampsia. In addition there is increased risk of polyhydramnios that may lead to umbilical cord prolapse when the membranes rupture.

It is important to note that up to 80% of women with gestational diabetes will eventually develop type 2 diabetes. Therefore, it is imperative for all health care providers to follow those women with a history of gestational diabetes and to test them for type 2 diabetes every year after delivery.

CLASSIFICATION

White's classification of diabetes is the classification system most commonly used during pregnancy because it subdivides women according to their degree of hyperglycemia (see Table 12-18-1).

TABLE 12-18-1. White's Classification of Diabetes in Pregnancy

CLASS	ONSET	FASTING PLASMA GLUCOSE	2-HOUR POSTPRANDIAL GLUCOSE	THERAPY
A1	Gestational	<105 mg/dL	<120 mg/dL	Diet alone
A2	Gestational	>105 mg/dL	>120 mg/dL	Diet and insulin

CLASS	AGE OF ONSET	DURATION (YEARS)	VASCULAR DISEASE	THERAPY
B	Over 20	<10	None	Diet and insulin
C	10 to 19	10 to 19	None	Diet and insulin
D	Before 10	>20	Benign retinopathy	Diet and insulin
F	Any	Any	Nephropathy	Diet and insulin
R	Any	Any	Proliferative retinopathy	Diet and insulin
H	Any	Any	Heart	Diet and insulin

SOURCE: From American College of Obstetricians and Gynecologists: Management of diabetes mellitus in pregnancy. *Technical Bulletin* no. 92, May 1986, with permission.

SCREENING AND DIAGNOSIS

In 1998 the American Diabetes Association (ADA) released a recommendation to screen only those women who are at high risk for developing gestational diabetes in order to contain screening costs. The recommendation is to screen women at 24 to 28 weeks' gestation only if they meet at least one of the following criteria[1]:

• 25 years of age or older *or* under 25 years old and obese
• History of diabetes in first-degree relatives
• Member of an ethnic or racial group with high prevalence of diabetes: Hispanic, Native American, Asian, African American, or Pacific Islander

However, the American College of Obstetricians and Gynecologists (ACOG) has criticized these new recommendations, warning that relying on historical and clinical risk factors is uncertain since almost half of all patients with gestational diabetes lack specific risk factors. Therefore, ACOG continues to recommend that *all* pregnant women should be screened between 24 and 28 weeks' gestation.[2]

The best time to screen for gestational diabetes is between 24 and 28 weeks' gestation because insulin response to a glucose load and peripheral insulin resistance start to increase at this time. The patient is given a 50-g oral glucose challenge test (GCT) at any time of day, regardless of previous meal ingestion. A plasma glucose level is checked after 1 h, and the test is positive if the level is greater than 140 mg/dL. If the test is positive, then a 100-g, 3-h oral glucose tolerance test (GTT) is performed. It should be given after 3 days of unrestricted diet and activity. The patient fasts overnight, then comes to the office in the morning and has a fasting plasma glucose level taken. She then drinks the 100-g glucose load and plasma glucose levels are checked at 1 h, 2 h, and 3 h (see Table 12-18-2). The patient is diagnosed with gestational diabetes if two of the values are met or exceeded.

TABLE 12-18-2. American College of Obstetricians and Gynecologists 1994 Criteria for Diagnosis of Gestational Diabetes Using 100-g Oral Glucose Tolerance Test

TIMING OF MEASUREMENT	PLASMA GLUCOSE (mg/dL)*
Fasting	105
1 h	190
2 h	165
3 h	145

*Gestational diabetes is diagnosed when any two values are met or exceeded.
SOURCE: Adapted from American College of Obstetricians and Gynecologists,[2] with permission.

MANAGEMENT

The key to a positive outcome is good glucose control. Upon diagnosis, the patient must receive nutritional counseling and be educated on the use of a glucometer. The goals of diet therapy include providing necessary nutrients to the mother and fetus, controlling glucose levels, and preventing starvation ketosis. An ADA diet is usually begun consisting of approximately 1800 to 2400 kcal. The patient should also check her serum glucose levels four times daily (fasting and 1 h after breakfast, lunch, and dinner). Optimal values are less than 90 mg/dL fasting and less than 130 mg/dL at 1h after meals. Food and serum glucose levels are recorded for 1 week and then are reviewed by the patient's health care provider. If glucose levels are universally high or erratic throughout the week, adjustments in the diet are made. Insulin is added as needed for glucose control only after clear dietary changes are attempted and fail to reduce serum glucose levels.

Exercise, specifically cardiovascular conditioning and non-weight-bearing type, is also encouraged for the gestational diabetic patient because it improves glycemic control when compared with diet alone. Exercises that should be performed are those that encourage the use of upper body muscles and avoid excessive weight-bearing on the trunk or lower body. These guidelines reduce the risk of fetal distress. The exercise needs to be performed three to four times a week for a minimum of 4 weeks before glucose levels are affected.

Further antepartum monitoring depends on the severity of gestational diabetes. Women who are well controlled by diet alone rarely require early delivery or other interventions. There is no consensus on whether or when antepartum fetal testing is necessary for this patient population. Elective induction of labor is controversial unless there is a clear indication of macrosomia via sonogram.

Patients with poor glucose control despite insulin therapy are at the greatest risk for morbidity and mortality. For all insulin-dependent diabetics weekly nonstress tests are begun at 32 weeks' gestation and then increased to biweekly at 36 weeks' gestation. In addition the amniotic fluid index should be monitored via sonogram beginning at 36 weeks' gestation. All insulin-requiring diabetics should be induced at 40 weeks' gestation if spontaneous labor has not occurred. Induction of labor is recommended at 38 weeks in patients with poor glucose control and macrosomia.

POSTPARTUM MANAGEMENT AND PROGNOSIS

Women diagnosed with gestational diabetes are at an increased risk of developing type 2 diabetes in the future, especially if they required insulin during pregnancy. All women diagnosed with gestational diabetes should have a 75-g GTT performed at approximately 6 to 8 weeks postpartum. It is also recommended that dietary management, specifically weight reduction in obese women, can reduce the risk of subsequent overt diabetes. Recurrence of gestational diabetes in subsequent pregnancies is common, with the highest recurrence rates in obese women. Breast feeding is not affected by diabetes and is generally encouraged.

REFERENCES

1. American Diabetes Association: Position statement on gestational diabetes mellitus. *Diabetes Care* 22(suppl 1):S74–S78, 1999.
2. American College of Obstetricians and Gynecologists: Diabetes and pregnancy. *Technical Bulletin* no. 200, Dec 1994, pp 1–8.

BIBLIOGRAPHY

Cunningham FG (ed): *Williams Obstetrics,* 20th ed New York, McGraw-Hill, 1997, pp 1203–1209.
Kaufmann RC, et al: *Obstet Gynecol* 5:734–737, May 1999
Palmer S: Gestational diabetes, in *Current Obstetric and Gynecologic Diagnosis and Treatment,* 8th ed, AH Decherney, ML Pernol (eds). Lange Medical/McGraw-Hill, 1966, pp. 374–378.

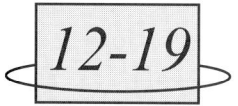

SPONTANEOUS ABORTION
Dana M. Gallagher

DISCUSSION

A spontaneous abortion ("miscarriage") is any pregnancy that ends before the twentieth week of gestation. Miscarriage occurs in approximately 15 to 20 percent of pregnancies, typically before 13 weeks' gestation.[1] Seventy percent of spontaneous abortions probably are due to abnormalities of fetal chromosomes; however, more than half of recurrent miscarriages are of unknown etiology.[2]

Recurrent spontaneous abortion (RSA) is defined as three or more consecutive miscarriages. The risk of RSA is approximately 2 percent.[3]

PATHOGENESIS

Most often, the chromosomal abnormalities that cause spontaneous abortion are not inherited from the parents; they usually occur after the fertilized egg has begun to undergo mitosis. Since an embryo with such defects could not have survived, miscarriage is "nature's way" of ending a nonviable pregnancy.

Other causes of spontaneous abortion include the woman's life-style habits and her medical condition. Bacterial vaginosis[4] and tobacco and cocaine use[5] have been implicated as risk factors for miscarriage. Although the U.S. Food and Drug Administration (FDA) has warned women against the use of caffeine during pregnancy, recent research shows that moderate caffeine intake is unlikely to increase the risk of a miscarriage.[6]

Structural conditions that predispose women to miscarriage include an incompetent cervical os and a septate or bicornuate uterus; adhesions from previous infection or fibroids may interfere with implantation. Hormonal imbalances (commonly, a luteal phase defect) decrease the hospitality of the uterine environment for a developing fetus. Medical conditions, particularly uncontrolled diabetes,[7] hypertension, and lupus erythematosus and other autoimmune disorders, increase the risk of spontaneous abortion as well.

SYMPTOMS

Virtually all women note vaginal bleeding before a spontaneous abortion. Up to 25 percent of all pregnant women bleed sometime during pregnancy, with about half of them suffering miscarriage.[8] There is no pathognomonic bleeding pattern; bleeding may be light or heavy, constant or intermittent, and crampy over the uterus or the low back.

OBJECTIVE FINDINGS

Pelvic examination will reveal an enlarged uterus of a size consistent with the last menstrual period (LMP). Blood may be present in the vaginal vault or at the cervical os. The cervical os should be checked for dilation and for the presence of products of conception. If the cervical os is dilated with pregnancy tissue extruding visibly, miscarriage cannot be stopped ("inevitable abortion").

LABORATORY

A pregnancy test should be run to confirm the pregnancy, especially in cases where the menstrual period has just been missed. Depending on the circumstances of the case, a clinician may wish to check for anemia if bleeding has been heavy or prepare a wet mount if bacterial vaginosis is suspected as a culprit.

DIAGNOSTIC CONSIDERATIONS

Although it is not always used in the case of a very early spontaneous abortion, the more advanced the pregnancy is, the more useful diagnostic ultrasound becomes, as it detects whether there is still a living fetus in the uterus.

TREATMENT

Treatment is dependent on the stage of pregnancy at the time of miscarriage, whether the pregnancy tissue has completely passed, and the medical status of the patient.

In the case of "threatened abortion," where the os is dilated but no pregnancy tissue has been passed, the traditional treatment is bed rest, although there is little evidence that this halts miscarriage once it is in progress. Typically, the woman stays in daily phone contact with the clinician and is advised to call immediately if pain or bleeding increases. If tissue is passed, the woman should be instructed to save it. Visual examination should be made promptly by rinsing the tissue and floating it in water; chorionic villi and sac are detectable even in early spontaneous abortions. Products of conception then should be forwarded to the pathology laboratory for microscopic examination.

In women who are in the process of miscarrying, the chief concern is that the spontaneous abortion be complete; incomplete miscarriage can cause pelvic infection and hemorrhage. Traditionally, women underwent dilation and curettage (D&C) after a miscarriage to ensure that the uterus was completely emptied. Of late, the general thinking is that most cases of spontaneous abortion will end in complete miscarriage without medical intervention[9] or surgical intervention. For cases in which intervention is necessary, research is under way to compare the efficacy of medical versus surgical intervention.[10]

Depending on the patient's circumstances, treatment after a miscarriage may encompass anything from watchful waiting to D&C, a workup for the underlying cause of miscarriage if recurrent, and aggressive management of underlying chronic disease. Because spontaneous abortion can occur over the course of almost two trimesters, in the presence of complex conditions and etiologies, it is recommended that the primary care physician assistant provide treatment in close concert with an obstetrician and/or fertility specialist.

PATIENT EDUCATION

Pregnant women, whether they have ever miscarried or not, will expect anticipatory guidance to avoid spontaneous abortion. It is important to give the usual warnings against smoking, drug use, and excessive caffeine intake.

Contrary to popular lore, miscarriage is not caused by having intercourse or orgasm, working, exercising, or lifting heavy objects. Falling or being badly frightened does not cause miscarriage. A fetus is unlikely to suffer serious morbidity unless the woman is experiencing a life-threatening event herself. Many women are concerned that severe nausea in early pregnancy is a harbinger of miscarriage. It appears that the opposite is true.

It is important to inform the patient that most women who have spontaneous abortions, even if recurrent, go on to have successful pregnancies later. Frequently, women want to know when they can attempt conception again. In the case of an uncomplicated early spontaneous abortion, the woman need wait only one cycle before trying again. In the case of a late-term miscarriage, there is some evidence that waiting 1 year may give the woman time to complete the bereavement process. Research suggests that pregnancy immediately subsequent to late-term miscarriage may interfere with grieving, which may postpone or prolong depression into the next pregnancy.[11] Referrals for support and counseling should be given regardless of the stage at which miscarriage occurred.

NOTES AND PEARLS

Taking a complete menstrual and pregnancy history, including a reproductive review of systems, is key. This should include the woman's wishes about the pregnancy. If, for example, the patient is spontaneously aborting an unwanted 5-week pregnancy, management and follow-up will be focused differently than it would be for a woman who may be undergoing her third miscarriage of a planned pregnancy at 11 weeks. Both of these cases would be handled differently from that of a woman who is miscarrying a pregnancy at 19 weeks. Obviously, there is no cookbook approach to the management of spontaneous abortion; clinical examination, diagnostics, treatment, and follow-up are individualized on a case-by-case basis. Further, although managing early spontaneous abortion before the woman has met her obstetrician is common in many primary care practices, managing a late first-trimester or second-trimester miscarriage is not as typical. Management will be dictated by the supervising physician's comfort with obstetrics and the community standard of care.

REFERENCES

1. Johns Hopkins InteliHealth Web site, http://www.intelihealth.com.
2. Bienstock JL: Hopkins Q&A: Miscarriage causes and prevention still mysterious. Johns Hopkins InteliHealth Web site, http://www.intelihealth. com.
3. Currey R: A woman's grief: The burden of recurrent miscarriage. *PA Today,* December 1999, pp. 21–23.
4. Ralph SG, Rutherford AJ, Wilson JD: Influence of bacterial vaginosis on conception and miscarriage in the first trimester: Cohort study. *BMJ* 319:220–223, 1999.
5. Ness RB, Grisso JA, Hirschinger N, et al: Cocaine and tobacco use and the risk of spontaneous abortion. *N Engl J Med* 340:333–339, 1999.
6. Klebanoff MA, Levine RJ, DerSimonian R, et al: Maternal serum paraxanthine, a caffeine metabolite, and the risk of spontaneous abortion. *N Engl J Med* 341:1639–1644, 1999.
7. The Diabetes Control Complications Trial Research Group: Pregnancy outcomes in the diabetes control and complications trial. *Am J Obstet Gynecol* 174:1343–1353, 1996.
8. The Mayo Clinic Health Oasis Web site, http://www.mayohealth.org/mayo/baby/htm/baby5.htm.
9. Nielsen S, Hahlin M, Platz-Christensen J: Randomised trial comparing expectant with medical management for first trimester miscarriages. *Br J Obstet Gynaecol* 106(8):804–807, 1999.
10. Ballagh SA, Harris HA, Demasio K: Is curettage needed for uncomplicated incomplete spontaneous abortion? *Am J Obstet Gynecol* 179:1279–1282, 1998.
11. Hughes PM, Turton P, Evans CDH: Stillbirth as risk factor for depression and anxiety in the subsequent pregnancy: Cohort study. *BMJ* 318:1721–1724, 1999.

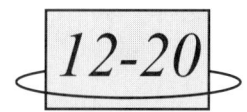

ROUTINE PRENATAL SCREENING
Nina Multak

DISCUSSION

The goal of prenatal care is to prevent and manage those conditions that cause poor pregnancy outcomes. Antepartum surveillance begins immediately following the recognition of missed menses and confirmation of pregnancy. At the first prenatal visit, the health care provider compiles an obstetric and medical database. This database identifies the course of care. Prenatal care is dependent on the individual needs of each pregnant woman. Routine prenatal care is appropriate for healthy women, without preexisting medical conditions, who are 18 to 35 years old.

DIAGNOSIS OF PREGNANCY

Signs, symptoms, and lab tests can suggest and confirm the diagnosis of pregnancy. Symptoms of pregnancy include amenorrhea, urinary frequency, breast engorgement, nausea, vomiting, and fatigue. Signs of pregnancy include presumptive, probable, and positive signs. Presumptive signs of pregnancy include a change in the color of the vulva and vaginal walls to a bluish tinge (Chadwick's sign). Pigmentation of the midline of the abdomen between the symphysis pubis and the umbilicus is known as the *linea nigra.* Increased pigmentation over the bridge of the nose and under the eyes is called *chloasma.* Chloasma is known as the "mask of pregnancy" and is an occasional side effect of oral contraceptives.

Probable signs of pregnancy are related to uterine physical changes. In early pregnancy, the uterus and cervix soften (Hegar's sign). Palpation of fetal parts and ballottement of the fetus are probable signs of pregnancy. Additionally, palpation of uterine contractions is a probable sign of pregnancy.

Detection of fetal heart sounds and fetal movement are positive signs of pregnancy. Doppler devices can detect fetal heart tones between 9 and 12 weeks' gestational age. Stethoscopes can identify fetal heart sounds between 16 and 20 weeks. Primigravidas generally detect fetal movements between 18 and 20 weeks' gestational age, while multiparous women identify fetal movements between 15 and 17 weeks' gestational age.

Lab tests utilized to detect pregnancy include pregnancy tests and diagnostic ultrasound. Urine and serum pregnancy tests measure human chorionic gonadotropin (hCG) produced in the placenta. Urine pregnancy tests become positive approximately 4 weeks' following the first day of the previous menstrual period. Serum pregnancy tests can detect pregnancy before a menstrual period has been missed.

Diagnostic ultrasound enables early and thorough fetal evaluation. Ultrasound is used to assess fetal growth and development. A pregnancy can be detected as early as 3 to 4 weeks' gestational age using transvaginal ultrasound. Cardiac activity in the fetus can be identified at 5 to 6 weeks' gestational age with transvaginal ultrasound.

FIRST PRENATAL OFFICE VISIT

At the first prenatal office visit, a health care provider should take a complete medical history. The medical history should focus on menstrual history, contraceptive use, past medical history, past surgical history, family history, medications, review of systems, and use of tobacco, alcohol, or drugs. The health care provider should obtain the following information during the obstetric history: previous delivery or pregnancy termination, location of delivery, type of delivery (or method of pregnancy termination), duration of labor (recorded in hours), type of anesthesia (note any complications), newborn weight, newborn gender, and fetal and neonatal complications.

The initial evaluation of the newly diagnosed obstetric patient should also include a complete physical exam. The physical exam generally concludes with the pelvic exam. The initial obstetric pelvic exam should focus on the following: signs of sexually transmitted infections, size of uterus, presence of fetal heart tones, presentation of fetus, and examination of bony pelvis.

DIAGNOSTIC CONSIDERATIONS

Ectopic pregnancy and molar pregnancy should be considered in the initial evaluation of the obstetric patient. Ultrasound and beta hCG testing should be used in early pregnancy to rule out these conditions.

SPECIAL CONSIDERATIONS

Patients with medical or obstetric problems may require additional surveillance. Medical problems should be managed by a health care provider throughout the pregnancy. Multiple gestation and other obstetric complications may require additional office visits.

PRENATAL HEALTH CARE OFFICE VISITS

Thorough antepartum surveillance enables health care providers to monitor the progression of pregnancy, provide education, reassure the patient, detect complications, and institute appropriate interventions. The frequency of follow-up visits for the pregnant woman is every 4 weeks through 28 weeks' gestation, every 2 weeks during 29 to 36 weeks' gestation, and weekly for patients over 37 weeks' gestation. If the patient is not 18 to 35 years of age or has medical or obstetric problems, then the intervals for follow-up visits are determined by evaluation of the situation and risk assessment.

The health care provider should evaluate the following at each office visit: blood pressure, weight, urine (identifying the presence of glucose or albumin), edema, fundal height (in centimeters), and fetal heart rate. Following detection of fetal movement by the mother and at each subsequent visit, the mother should be asked about continued fetal movement and signs or symptoms of labor (contractions, fluid leakage, vaginal bleeding). As the estimated date of delivery approaches, the health care provider will perform a cervical exam to evaluate dilation, effacement, and fetal position.

PRENATAL SCREENING TESTS

Table 12-20-1 lists the various prenatal screening tests.

COMPLICATIONS

Complications of pregnancy need evaluation on an individual basis.

OTHER NOTES

The number of women of increased maternal age (>35 years old) having healthy babies is on the rise.

BIBLIOGRAPHY

Beckman CRB et al: *Obstetrics and Gynecology,* 3d ed. Baltimore, Williams & Wilkins, 1998.

TABLE 12-20-1. Prenatal Screening Tests

Amniocentesis	A pocket of amniotic fluid away from fetus and placenta is localized via ultrasound and 10 mL is drawn utilizing sterile technique with a 22-gauge spinal needle. Performed at 16–20 weeks' gestational age. Evaluation for chromosomal disorders and neural tube defects.
Chorionic villus sampling (CVS)	Amniotic fluid sample is taken by ultrasound guidance using a transabdominal or transcervical approach. Performed at 10–12 weeks' gestational age. This method can identify chromosomal abnormalities or biochemical genetic disorders. Neural tube defects cannot be measured with CVS.
24–28 Weeks (When Indicated)	
Gestational diabetes	Screen at 26–28 weeks using a 50-g glucose challenge (nonfasting). Abnormal test is >140 mg/dL. Screen earlier and repeat if risk factors are present. Patient with abnormal screening needs 3-h glucose tolerance test.
32–36 Weeks (When Indicated)	
Group B *Streptococcus* culture	Obtain antepartum lower vaginal culture at 35–37 weeks and treat if positive. Obstetric risk factors associated with neonatal group B *Streptococcus* sepsis: positive vaginal culture, premature delivery, prolonged rupture of membranes, previous baby with group B *Streptococcus* sepsis, or maternal fever.
Nonstress test (NST)	Assess fetal well-being by quantification of fetal activity, done late in pregnancy or earlier if high-risk conditions exist. Electronic measurement of fetal heart rate in response to fetal movement. Patient placed in left lateral decubitus position with transducer on abdomen to record fetal heart rate and movement. A normal or reactive NST occurs when the fetal heart rate increases to a maximum of 156 beats per minute in 15 s after a fetal movement.
Contraction stress test	Assess fetal heart rate in response to uterine contractions. A tocodynamometer and fetal heart rate transducer are placed on the mother's abdomen. Normal test is no change of fetal heart rate in response to contractions. The test is called an *oxytocin challenge test* if oxytocin is required to elicit contractions.
Biophysical profile	Assess fetal well-being via ultrasound. A scored evaluation of fetus including reactive nonstress test, fetal breathing movements, fetal body movement, fetal tone, and adequate amniotic fluid volume.
Fetal lung maturity	Assess fetal maturity through direct measurement and evaluation of pulmonary surfactant. Surfactant production in the fetus increases after 33 weeks' gestational age.

Hacker NF, Moore JG (eds): *Essentials of Obstetrics and Gynecology,* 3d ed. Philadelphia, Saunders, 1998.

Hauth JF, Merenstein GB (eds): *Guidelines for Perinatal Care,* 4th ed. Washington, DC, American Academy of Pediatrics and American College of Obstetrics and Gynecology, 1997.

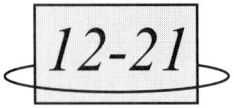

GENITAL HERPES
Nina Multak

DISCUSSION

At least 45 million individuals have been diagnosed with herpes simplex virus (HSV). Control of this disease is difficult as viral shedding occurs when lesions are present as well as during asymptomatic periods. Herpes simplex virus type I (HSV-l) and herpes simplex virus type II (HSV-2), are large, double-stranded DNA viruses. Both viruses cause skin lesions to erupt in various sites on the body, however HSV-2 is the most common cause of genital disease. The virus enters the patient through abraded skin areas and mucosal surfaces. Viral replication occurs in the nerve cell bodies in the ganglia and surrounding neural tissue. The virus then spreads to other areas via peripheral sensory nerves. After the initial infection resolves, the virus can be reactivated via immunosuppression, trauma to the skin or ganglia, and ultraviolet light.

HSV infections can be identified when vesicular lesions on an erythematous base are noted on physical exam. Since HSV lesions may resemble skin ulcerations of other etiologies, it is prudent to utilize laboratory studies to confirm the diagnosis and direct therapy. Laboratory confirmation can provide information that may guide or predict the course of genital HSV infection.

SIGNS AND SYMPTOMS

Table 12-21-1 lists the common signs and symptoms of genital herpes.

OBJECTIVE FINDINGS

Lesions can present in varying stages: pustules, vesicles, or painful erythematous ulcers. Widely spaced, bilateral lesions of the external genitalia are common. Women with genital herpes have frequent involvement of the cervix and urethra. Inguinal lymphadenopathy is frequently noted in patients with a first-episode primary infection.

DIAGNOSTIC CONSIDERATIONS

Table 12-21-2 lists the most common diagnostic considerations for genital lesions.

TABLE 12-21-2. Differential Diagnoses of Genital Lesions

Vesicular and Ulcerative Genital Lesions
Primary syphilis
Secondary syphilis
Chancroid
Granuloma inguinale
Herpes zoster
Lymphogranuloma venereum
Candidiasis
Anal fissure
Rectal fissure
Trauma
Insect bite
Decubitus ulcer
Drug reaction
Skin infection (*Staphylococcus*)

SPECIAL CONSIDERATIONS

Neonatal Herpes

Prevention of neonatal HSV requires prevention of HSV during pregnancy, particularly during the third trimester. When a primary infection occurs during pregnancy, the fetus is at increased risk of acquiring HSV infection and the mother for preterm delivery. Cesarean section is indicated when genital lesions are present in labor. Failure to feed, lethargy, skin lesions, and fever are symptoms characteristic of infection in the neonate. Rash, cerebrospinal fluid abnormalities, and seizures may also be present.

HIV Infection

Patients who are immunocompromised can have severe or prolonged episodes of genital or perianal HSV infection. Lesions identified in HIV-infected patients may be severe, painful, and atypical compared to other patient populations. Suppressive antiviral therapy is frequently effective for HIV-infected patients (see Chap. 9-1).

Allergy, Intolerance, and Adverse Reactions

It is uncommon to have allergic or other adverse reactions to acyclovir, valacyclovir, and famciclovir, the drugs commonly used to treat HSV infection.

LABORATORY STUDIES

Table 12-21-3 lists the laboratory tests for genital herpes.

TABLE 12-21-1. Signs and Symptoms of Genital Herpes

PRIMARY INFECTION	NONPRIMARY FIRST EPISODE	RECURRENT INFECTION
Many grouped vesicles on an erythematous base	Some grouped vesicles on an erythematous base	Singular or grouped vesicles on an erythematous base or no lesions
Systemic symptoms may be present (malaise, fever, myalgia)	Few systemic symptoms present	No systemic symptoms
Localized genital symptoms may be present (pain, dysuria, itching)	Localized symptoms may be present, less severe than primary infection	Localized lesions and symptoms may or may not be present

TABLE 12-21-3. Laboratory Tests for Genital Herpes

NAME	DESCRIPTION
Viral antigen smear	Material from lesion is smeared onto a glass slide, air dried, and transported to a lab facility for evaluation.
Viral culture	Dacron swab is utilized to sample lesion and place in special culture media to send to lab facility. Higher sensitivity in vesicular lesions.
Tzanck smear, Pap smear, Wright's stain	Staining of scraping from lesion base for identification of multinucleated giant cells or intranuclear inclusions of HSV can be done in office. Disadvantages: no differentiation between HSV and varicella zoster; requires experience.
Serology	Can identify asymptomatic carriers. Commercially available tests do not distinguish between the antibodies to the two types of HSV.

TREATMENT

The following treatment guidelines reflect the most recent treatment recommended by the Centers for Disease Control and Prevention.[1]

First Clinical Episode of Infection

During the initial infections episode, one of the following treatment options should be used.

- Acyclovir 400 mg orally three times per day for 7 to 10 days
- Acyclovir 200 mg orally five times per day for 7 to 10 days
- Famciclovir 250 mg orally three times per day for 7 to 10 days
- Valacyclovir 1g orally two times per day for 7 to 10 days

Recurrent Infection (Episodic)

Using one of the following regimens can provide effective treatment for episodic recurrences.

- Acyclovir 400 mg orally three times per day for 5 days
- Acyclovir 200 mg orally five times per day for 5 days
- Acyclovir 800 mg orally two times per day for 5 days
- Famciclovir 125 mg orally two times per day for 5 days
- Valacyclovir 500 mg orally two times per day for 5 days

Frequent Infection Recurrence

Daily suppressive therapy is recommended for patients with six or more recurrences per year. Options are listed below.

- Acyclovir 400 mg orally two times per day
- Famciclovir 250 mg orally two times per day
- Valacyclovir 250 mg orally two times per day
- Valacyclovir 500 mg orally one time per day
- Valacyclovir 1 g orally one time per day

Severe Disease

Patients who have severe disease or who require hospitalization should have intravenous therapy.

[1] These treatment guidelines are reproduced and modified from 1998 guidelines for treatment of sexually transmitted diseases, Centers for Disease Control and Prevention. *MMWR* 47(RR-1), 1998. The material contained within is in the public domain.

- Acyclovir 5 to 10 mg/kg body weight intravenously every 8 h for 5 to 7 days or until clinical resolution is attained

PATIENT EDUCATION

Prevention and control of genital HSV infection can occur through effective education of those at risk for transmitting or acquiring sexually transmitted diseases. The health care provider should include a sexual history as part of the interview, using open-ended questions and a nonjudgmental attitude. When an effective rapport with the patient is facilitated, the health care provider can identify risk factors and effective education can be provided.

Education should include specific information about genital herpes and specific actions that the patient can take to prevent transmitting HSV. Patients should be advised to abstain from sexual contact when lesions are present. Discussion of asymptomatic viral shedding is important. Recommendations to utilize condoms will offer individuals some protection against virus transmission. Patients with active HSV lesions should be encouraged to keep the affected area clean and dry. Patients with HSV and their sex partners should be encouraged to examine themselves for lesions and seek medical attention when lesions appear.

COMPLICATIONS

Herpetic whitlow, HSV infection of a finger, can occur via inoculation of virus from a genital herpes lesion to the hand. Localized tenderness of the affected finger, edema, and erythema are typical signs and symptoms. Lesions of the fingertip (vesicular or pustular), fever, and epitrochlear and axillary lymphadenopathy may be present. Rapid diagnosis speeds the initiation of antiviral therapy and may prevent the need for surgical intervention.

HSV infection of the visceral organs may occur in immunocompromised, burned, or malnourished patients. HSV encephalitis can occur as a result of primary infection; however, it is generally caused by HSV-1. HSV meningitis has been associated with primary genital HSV infection. Additional complications of HSV infection include glomerulonephritis, esophagitis, hepatitis (rare), idiopathic thrombocytopenia, adrenal necrosis, and monarticular arthritis.

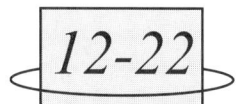

UTERINE FIBROIDS
Dana M. Gallagher

DISCUSSION

Uterine fibroids (leiomyoma, myoma) are benign tumors that grow out of the uterine wall. They can grow from the uterine walls into the uterine cavity (submucous), within the uterine wall itself (intramural), or outward from the uterus toward the abdominal cavity (subserous).

Fibroids can grow in clusters or occur singly. Fibroid size can be quite variable, ranging from a clinically undetectable pea size to visible abdominal distortion by a fibroid larger than a melon.

Myomas are very common. No one knows the exact incidence or prevalence of fibroids; low estimates state that at least 30 percent of reproductive-age women have them.[1] African-American women have a threefold higher risk of fibroids relative to white women, and the age of occurrence is typically earlier. Regarding anecdotal risk estimates, one popular formula is 30 percent of 30-year-olds, 40 percent of 40-year-olds, and 50 percent of 50-year-olds may have fibroids.[2]

PATHOGENESIS

The exact cause of uterine fibroids is unknown. It is clear, however, that the risk for and status of fibroids are positively influenced by the presence of estrogen. At this writing, there is speculation that progesterone also may be a protagonist. Therefore, women who are of reproductive age are at risk for having more and/or larger fibroids compared with postmenopausal women. Fibroids tend to enlarge under the influence of estrogen (both endogenous and exogenous) and regress after menopause. There are conflicting data about whether the use of oral contraceptives accelerates fibroid growth; recent research shows that it probably does not.[3]

There is also speculation that fibroid growth is promoted by basic fibroblast growth factor (bFGF).[4] In women who have fibroids, overactivity of bFGF may prompt excess blood vessel growth, which in turn feeds the fibroid. Because the precise etiology of fibroids is unknown, research is continuing to identify both causation and possible treatments.

SYMPTOMS

For many women, the presence of fibroids is unknown until they are discovered during a pelvic examination or incidentally during surgery or abdominal imaging for other reasons. For others, symptoms of fibroids may include heavier or prolonged periods and postcoital bleeding with subsequent anemia.

Women with large fibroids may complain of abdominal swelling that inflates their clothing size; this may be accompanied by a sensation of lower abdominal pressure or discomfort. Large fibroids also may cause constipation if they press on the rectum or frequent urination if they press on the bladder. Fibroids may be a rare cause of infertility if they impinge on a fallopian tube or of miscarriage if they interfere with implantation.

OBJECTIVE FINDINGS

A uterus with palpable fibroids will feel very firm and enlarged. In describing the uterus, the size should be noted compared to pregnancy in weeks. If the abdominal architecture is distended, this should be noted. If possible, a drawing of the fibroid's location, morphology, and approximate size in centimeters should be made for the chart and updated at annual intervals.

LABORATORY STUDIES

A hematocrit should be obtained and monitored as necessary.

RADIOLOGIC STUDIES

Pelvic sonography will quantify and size fibroids and confirm that there are no other worrisome tumors that are confused with or obscured by fibroids.

TREATMENT

Treatment is for the most part dependent on symptomatology. Most clinicians agree that a woman with small asymptomatic fibroids can reasonably adopt a watch-and-wait stance. The patient may wish to consider treatment if she notes pain, heavy bleeding, or difficulty with the bladder or bowels.

Medical management has focused on decreasing estrogen levels, since high levels seem to contribute to fibroid growth. Gonadotropin-releasing hormone (GnRH) agonists (e.g., Lupron) block the release of follicle-stimulating hormone (FSH) and luteinizing hormone (LH), thus shutting off ovulation and estrogen production. Medroxyprogesterone 150 mg intramuscularly q 28 days, or Danazol 400 to 800 mg daily[5] also may prove useful. Although each of these drugs may show some efficacy in individual cases, all have side effects. Research is under way on the relatively new antiprogestins (notably RU-486).[6]

Hysterectomy traditionally has been the surgical treatment of choice. As women become less willing to part with their uteri, other surgical treatments have become better explored and more accessible. Myomectomy, in which only the fibroid is removed, may be appropriate for women who want to preserve their reproductive capabilities. Myomectomy may, however, weaken uterine integrity and prompt cesarean section in a subsequent pregnancy. Although less generally available, laparoscopy and hysteroscopy have been used for fibroid resection.

Uterine artery embolization is a new nonsurgical approach that is touted for its ability to shrink fibroids by cutting off their blood supply.[7] Early data show that complications are few and fertility may be preserved.

While the "watch-and-wait" treatment option is entirely within the purview of primary care, consider a gynecologic consultation when initiating medical management.

PATIENT EDUCATION

First and foremost, patients need to be reassured that fibroids are common and benign. Women with fibroids should be encouraged to monitor their menstrual bleeding and other symptoms and report any escalation in symptoms promptly.

Many women ask what they can do to shrink fibroids. There is some preliminary evidence that diets high in red meat and ham predispose women to fibroids, while consumption of fish, green vegetables, and fruit may be protective.[8] Since these recommendations are consistent with a heart-healthy diet, there is certainly no harm in the patient's making dietary adjustments.

REFERENCES

1. National Institute of Child Health and Human Development. Uterine fibroids. NICHD Web site, http://www.nichd.nih.gov/publications/pubs/uterine.htm.
2. Mayo Foundation for Medical Education and Research: Uterine fibroids more common than dangerous, 1990. Mayo Web site, http://www.mayohealth.org/mayo/9701/htm/fibroids htm.
3. Chiaffarino F, Parazzini F, LaVecchia C, et al: Use of oral contraceptives and uterine fibroids: Results from a case control study. *Br J Obstet Gynaecol* 106(8):857–860, 1999.
4. WebMD: Uterine fibroids and hysterectomy, March 1999. WebMD Web site, http://webmd.lycos.com/content/dmk/dmk_article_40035.
5. Fibroid tumors. Johns Hopkins InteliHealth Web site, http://www.intelihealth.com.
6. Cramer DW: Epidemiology of myomas. *Semin Repro Endocrinol* 10:320–324, 1992.
7. Johns Hopkins Special Reports: Attacking fibroid tumors, October 19, 1999. Johns Hopkins InteliHealth Web site, http://www.intelihealth.com.
8. Chiaffarino F, Parazzini F, LaVecchia C, et al: Diet and uterine myomas. *Obstet Gynecol* 94(3):395–398, 1999.

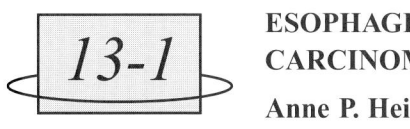

ESOPHAGEAL CARCINOMAS

Anne P. Heinly

DISCUSSION

Compared with other carcinomas, esophageal carcinomas are relatively uncommon in the United States, but they are quite common in other parts of the world, especially China and Japan. An estimated 10,000 cases are reported yearly in the United States, primarily among men over 40 years old. Blacks and Asians seem to have a higher predisposition for this disease, although a specific genetic marker has not been found. Table 13-1-1 reviews the risk factors associated with squamous cell carcinoma, the most prevalent type of esophageal carcinoma. While the incidence of squamous cell carcinoma remains essentially unchanged, adenocarcinoma continues to rise in the United States. It occurs almost exclusively secondary to Barrett's esophagitis, a severe complication of gastroesophageal reflux disease (GERD; see Chap. 6-11). Ten years ago adenocarcinoma accounted for about 10% of esophageal carcinomas; today the incidence is closer to one-third, and the disease is being found earlier in white males.

PATHOGENESIS

Chronic irritation and inflammation provide the setting for both squamous cell carcinoma and adenocarcinoma of the esophagus. The resultant hyperplasia and the subsequent development of atypia are directly related to the tissue's attempt to protect itself from irritation. The most common site of squamous cell carcinoma is the midesophagus, followed by the distal esophagus. The thin layer of squamous epithelium and the absence of a serosa layer allow malignancies to invade the muscular layers readily and, from there, the rich lymphatics of the chest. Unfortunately, the degree of irritation from external sources such as alcohol and tobacco does not provide clues to the timing or extent of injury to the esophagus.

Adenocarcinoma is found primarily in the distal esophagus in association with an incompetent lower esophageal sphincter. The resultant chronic gastric reflux triggers the conversion of the squamous epithelium to a columnar cell-lined esophagus (similar to stomach lining) in an effort to protect itself from the increased acidity. Recently a DNA marker, p53 mutation, has been implicated in the pathogenesis of adenocarcinoma. The presence of the p53 mutation is an early marker that may be predictive of outcome. Studies have revealed patients with negative p53 mutation markers do better postsurgery.[1] There is no doubt that alcohol and tobacco abuse contributes to these changes in association with chronic GERD. Table 13-1-2 reviews esophageal tumors including less common ones.

SYMPTOMS

Esophageal carcinomas present as mechanical obstructions, and thus progressive dysphagia is the first and most classic symptom. Initially the patient has difficulties with solid food, but over time (weeks to months) semisolids and then liquids become difficult. Early clues such as chest fullness or pressure, hiccups, cough, and hoarseness may be interpreted as benign by both the patient and the provider. Odynophagia

(pain on swallowing) eventually occurs as a result of a narrowed, irritated lumen and metastasis to the surrounding nerve plexus. The pain generally is described as constant, deep, and penetrating.

Pulmonary symptoms may bring the patient to a practitioner before dysphagia occurs. Recurrent pneumonia and upper respiratory infections (URIs) are quite common because the tumor mechanically allows aspiration and fistula formations in the pulmonary tree. As the patient's immunologic status diminishes from weight loss, malnutrition, and electrolyte imbalance, the chances of severe pulmonary sequelae increase. Occult bleeding is common and can be readily demonstrated. Gross, profuse bleeding is uncommon but can occur if a major vessel is breached by the tumor.

As may be suspected from the symptoms, esophageal carcinomas generally are found well after they have metastasized. Dysphagia and weight loss are signs of large tumors producing symptoms through a mass effect. This severely affects the prognosis; thus it is imperative that providers listen carefully and associate the possible risk factors so that the patient will have a fighting chance of recovery.

OBJECTIVE FINDINGS

Overt physical signs of esophageal carcinoma are rare. Only general evidence of disease will be present: anemia and weight loss. Careful examination may pick up a supraclavicular nodal enlargement (Virchow's nodes) or unilateral vocal cord paralysis. A thorough physical is mandated to help with the differential diagnosis.

DIAGNOSTIC CONSIDERATIONS

Any disease process that can cause dysphagia should be considered (see Table 13-1-3). Extrinsic compression can occur as well and represents nongastrointestinal sources of dysphagia. The extrinsic type generally is not associated with significant weight loss or anemia.

LABORATORY TESTS

Hypercalcemia and its clinical manifestations are an all too common initial presentation. A patient with elevated serum calcium levels will complain of a rapid onset of spreading weakness, nausea, sedation, and eventual stupor. A hypokalemic alkalosis may occur, and a hypochromic, microcytic anemia associated with chronic blood loss is commonly found. Specific laboratory tests do not exist to diagnose or define esophageal carcinomas. The measurement of CA-19-9 in serum has not been a successful marker.

RADIOLOGIC (IMAGING) STUDIES

The barium swallow remains the gold standard for the initial workup. The double-contrast study is preferred, and the potential findings include nodularity, sudden angularities in contour, stricture formation with lumen stenosis, ulcerations, and rigidity of movement.

Computed tomography (CT) is valuable in looking for metastasis and establishing staging along with a well-performed endoscopic ultrasound. A careful esophagogastroduodenoscopy (EGD) should be performed to confirm the carcinoma by cytology. The tumor also can be visualized for size, location, spread, fistulas, bleeding, and ulcerations. Brush cytology is the recommended method because of its

505

TABLE 13-1-1. Risk Factors for Squamous Cell Carcinoma of the Esophagus

RISK FACTOR	EFFECT
Smoking	Increases GERD, decreases mucosal blood flow, decreases prostaglandin synthesis, interferes with action of H_2 antagonists
Alcohol abuse	Alone, there is a questionable relationship; with tobacco, effects are increased
Chronic candidiasis	Persistent tissue irritation
Chemical ingestion (lye)	Corrosive injury, stricture formation
Achalasia	Relationship unsure; some studies quote 6% increase in cancer rates
Plummer-Vinson syndrome	Webs in upper esophagus associated with iron deficiency; over 90% of cases occur in women
Exposure to radiation	Direct tissue damage, stricture formation

ABBREVIATION: GERD, gastroesophageal reflux disease.

accuracy. Staining the mucosa with Lugol's iodine can define early lesions, and when it is used in conjunction with endoscopic ultrasound, local spread can be clearly defined.

The positron emission tomography (PET) scan is now being used as an adjunct to CT scanning for the staging of metastatic disease. It is not in wide use at this time because of expense and availability.

Once cancer is diagnosed, staging is done to evaluate the extent of invasion and the development of a treatment regimen. Stage 0 is carcinoma in situ, affecting only a single layer of the esophagus. In stage I, the cancer is present in more than one layer but not in lymph nodes. In stage II, esophageal spread is extensive without metastases. Stage III includes the intrusion of the tumor into the chest lymphatics. In stage IV, there are metastases to other organs, such as liver and lung. Unfortunately, most esophageal carcinomas are found in stages III and IV.

TREATMENT

In China and Japan, where early screening is done, therapy is accomplished through the endoscope, using a variety of methods: laser ablation, tumor probe, and sclerotherapy. If the tumor is in stage I or II, a cure is possible. However, in the United States, where practitioners do not screen for esophageal carcinoma, the treatment is only palliative in the vast majority of cases.

TABLE 13-1-2. Esophageal Tumors

TUMOR	DESCRIPTION
Squamous cell carcinoma	Middle to distal esophagus; etiology unknown; risk factors include tobacco, alcohol, lye ingestion, candidiasis; poor prognosis
Adenocarcinoma	Distal esophagus; vast majority result from Barrett's esophagitis (GERD); poor prognosis
Small cell carcinoma	Rare, highly aggressive; survival usually less than a year
Malignant melanoma	Extremely rare; 6-month survival despite surgery
Leiomyosarcoma	Rare, noncancerous malignant tumor; survival after surgery 25%
Leiomyoma	Usually asymptomatic; those with symptoms can be ablated with laser therapy
Lipoma	Fatty, nonmalignant tumor; removed as a polyp if symptomatic

TABLE 13-1-3. Differential Diagnoses of Dysphagia

DIAGNOSIS		SYMPTOMS
Oropharyngeal		
Motor disorders		
	Achalasia	Aperistalsis, esophageal dilation, chest pressure, inability to burp or vomit, weight loss
	Scleroderma	Dysphagia with decreased peristalsis, other systemic manifestations
	Myasthenia gravis	Dysphagia and cough; affects upper esophageal sphincter
	CNS disease	Amyotrophic lateral sclerosis, parkinsonism, Huntington's chorea, polio, cerebrovascular accident: esophageal weakness, aperistalsis, drooling
Structural disorders		
	Zenker's diverticulum	Outpouching through weakened muscular coat usually near the upper esophageal sphincter, regurgitation, halitosis, gurgling, and swelling at the neck
	Chagas' disease	Megaesophagus secondary to trypanosomiasis; seen in children, myxedema, congestive heart failure; restricted to the tropics
Esophageal Body		
Motor disorders		Same as above
Infections (common in immunocompromised patients)		Candidiasis: severe odynophagia, drooling, oral thrush
		Herpes simplex: chest pain, odynophagia, bleeding, nausea/vomiting, leukocytosis
		Cytomegalovirus: serpiginous ulcers, odynophagia, chest pain, hematemesis
Obstructions		Carcinomas
		Reflux esophagitis: inflammation, strictures
		Prolonged nasogastric tube intubation: inflammation, strictures
		Ingestion of corrosives: inflammation, strictures
		"Pill" esophagitis: lodged medication causes inflammation and strictures
Lower esophageal sphincter		All the above and GERD
Extrinsic compression		Substernal thyroid goiter
		Aortic aneurysm (arch or descending)
		Double aortic arch
		Abnormal subclavian arteries
		Mediastinal masses or lymphadenopathy
		Arthritic bone spurs from cervical or thoracic spine

ABBREVIATION: GERD, gastroesophageal reflux disease.

Currently, the only curative procedure for advanced carcinoma is esophagectomy. The most successful procedures involve the middle and distal esophagus. The surgery removes the cancerous section, and the remaining portion or a loop of intestine is anastomosed. This surgery has a grave prognosis, and despite the best efforts, 5-year survival is less than 10%.

Palliative therapies include laser ablation to relieve obstruction, stent placement, and chemotherapy to shrink tumor size (Table 13-1-4). Intratumoral therapy via endoscope with cisplatin/epinephrine injectable gel is becoming a viable adjunct for palliation with fewer side effects than the laser ablation and stenting procedures. Nutritional status must be maintained, and control of nausea, pain, and constipation is essential.

COMPLICATIONS

The most obvious complication of esophageal carcinoma is death. Long-term survival is poor. Complications after esophagectomy are many and include dumping syndrome, GERD, regurgitation, weight loss, muscle atrophy, malnutrition, and psychiatric illnesses.

TABLE 13-1-4. Treatment Options for Esophageal Tumors

TREATMENT	DESCRIPTION
Photofrin	Chemotherapy, twofold therapy, ingestion of porfimer sodium that binds to plasma lipoproteins; in second step nonthermal red laser light is applied to the tumor; the light activates the lipoproteins and kills tumor cells; palliative only, with no extension of life expectancy
Neodymium: YAG laser	Thermal ablation provides palliation and some improvement in survival time
Cisplatin	The most commonly used chemotherapy alone and in combination; remission extremely rare with chemotherapy alone

PATIENT EDUCATION

The best hope in the United States to affect the prevalence of this devastating disease is prevention. Alcohol and tobacco abuse should be stopped. Treatment of Plummer-Vinson syndrome, candidiasis, and GERD is essential. When a diagnosis of esophageal carcinoma is made, it is imperative to inform the patient about all available options and the prognosis. Several studies have shown that skilled clinicians often fall short in explaining a realistic prognosis to their patients.

PEARLS

When a patient comes in with a recurrent dry cough, hoarseness, or persistent URIs, think esophageal cancer after the pulmonary workup. The two systems often produce symptoms that mimic each other, and it takes an index of suspicion to catch esophageal carcinomas early. Keep in mind the risk factors for this consuming disease; the vast majority of cases may be prevented through healthy life-style changes.

REFERENCE

1. Schneider PM et al: p53 mutational status improves estimation of prognosis in patients with curatively resected adenocarcinoma in Barrett's esophagus. *Clin Cancer Res* 6(8):3153–3158, 2000.

BIBLIOGRAPHY

Burdick JS: Esophageal cancer prevention, cure and palliation. *Semin Gastrointest Dis* 11(3):124–133, 2000.
Gamliel Z: Incidence, epidemiology and etiology of esophageal cancer. *Chest Surg Clin N Am* 10(3):441–450, 2000.
Monga SP et al: Intratumoral therapy of cisplatin/epinephrine injectable gel for palliation in patients with obstructive esophageal cancer. *Am J Clin Oncol* 24(4):386–392, 2000.
Rice TW: Clinical staging of esophageal carcinoma. *Chest Surg Clin N Am* 10(3):471–485, 2000.

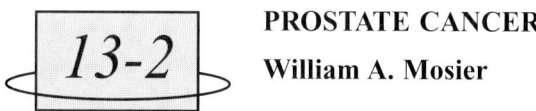

PROSTATE CANCER
William A. Mosier

DISCUSSION

Adenocarcinoma of the prostate is the most common malignant neoplasm in men, accounting for 33% of all cancers diagnosed in men. The risk of acquiring cancer of the prostate (CaP) increases with age. CaP is the second most commonly occurring cancer in American men over age 65 years. Adjusted for age, 80% of all cases of CaP are diagnosed in men over age 65. It is the most frequently diagnosed carcinoma and accounts for about 15% of all deaths from cancer in the United States. One in every six men will eventually be diagnosed with CaP. Metastatic CaP is a leading cause of cancer-related deaths among men. The American Cancer Society (ACS) estimates that from 1980 to 1990 there was a 50% increase in the number of men diagnosed with this condition. This increase in the rate of diagnosis is due to the improved screening tools available and increased awareness of the importance of screening.

Only about 30% of prostatic cancers are potentially curable at the time of diagnosis. In fact, about 50% of all new cases include lymph node involvement or metastases by the time of diagnosis. Two-thirds of all cases of CaP are widespread and incurable by the time they are diagnosed. The resulting malignancy is usually responsive to hormonal manipulation, however. Therefore, the spread of disease can be controlled somewhat. Of tissues removed for the treatment of urinary obstruction resulting from prostatic hypertrophy, 10% are found to have malignant pathology. For an unknown reason, the incidence of CaP is highest among African Americans in spite of the fact that it is rare in Africa. The incidence is lowest among Asians.

Although the etiology is unknown, CaP tends to run in families. Statistics show that 98% of all cases of CaP are adenocarcinomas that arise from the glandular acini and proximal ducts. Less common malignancies of the prostate include neuroendocrine tumors and sarcomas. Even less frequently occurring are transitional cell, squamous cell, and endometrioid carcinomas that originate from the distal ductal elements of the prostate.

PATHOGENESIS

The pathogenesis of CaP is not known. Initiating or promoting factors have not been determined. However, several factors have been suggested as predisposing a man to develop CaP:

• *Genetic factors:* Because of the higher incidence of CaP among relatives of patients with CaP, there may be a yet unidentified genetic factor involved in its pathogenesis.
• *Hormonal factors:* Studies suggest that hormonal factors may be instrumental in the development of CaP as evidenced by the fact that most CaP appears to be dependent on male hormones for growth. What lends strength to this theory is that CaP does not occur in men who have been castrated.
• *Environmental factors:* Environmental factors that have been postulated as influencing the growth of CaP are air pollution, fertilizers and other chemicals, and certain viral infections.

SYMPTOMS

There are no symptoms per se of CaP. However, in the later stages a patient may experience urinary obstruction or bone pain from the spread of the cancer to the low back, pelvis, or thighs. Other symptoms of CaP may include impotence, hematuria, nocturia, a weak or interrupted stream, frequency, urgency, dysuria, and hesitancy. Of course the typical symptoms of cancer may also be present with more advanced CaP, such as nausea and vomiting, weight loss, fatigue, and persistent pain.

OBJECTIVE FINDINGS

Diagnosis is difficult for the detection of early CaP. Screening involves digital rectal examination (DRE) as part of a routine physical examination. Unfortunately, only about 10% of cases of CaP identified as nodules on rectal examination are sufficiently localized for cure. A cancerous prostate may present as a discrete hard nodule or diffuse induration of the prostate on DRE. The diagnostic evaluation of CaP is tied to a staging system that is outlined in Table 13-2-1.

TABLE 13-2-1.   The American Urological Association System for Staging Prostate Cancer

STAGE	DESCRIPTION
A1	A well-differentiated cancer present in no more than three resected chips
A2	A well-differentiated cancer present on more than three resected chips or a not-well-differentiated cancer
B	A well-differentiated nodule detectable on digital rectal examination
C	A local yet extensive tumor that penetrates past the prostate capsule into the seminal vesicles or bladder neck or through the lateral wall of the pelvis (these patients often present with symptoms of urinary obstruction)
D0	Indicates an elevated acid phosphatase level but no physical or radiographic evidence of metastases
D1	Cancer present on histology specimen, and lymph node samples positive below aortic bifurcation
D2	Lymph node involvement superior to aortic bifurcation, or bone, soft tissue, or visceral metastases present

SOURCE: Adapted from the American Urological Association system for staging prostate cancer.

DIAGNOSTIC CONSIDERATIONS

In screening for CaP it is important to consider the possibility of metastases to other tissue, since over 60% of all cases of CaP have metastasized by the time they are diagnosed. When a patient's prostate-specific antigen (PSA) is not elevated, diagnostic considerations should include benign prostatic nodules, prostate stones, nodular whorls of adenoma, and seminal vesicle enlargement.

SPECIAL CONSIDERATIONS

More than 90% of cases of CaP remain latent and never metastasize. The prevalence of the pathology far exceeds its clinical incidence. It is detected in 30% of autopsies done on males who died of unrelated causes. Currently there is no way to definitively determine which cancer will spread and which will not. Therefore, great care must be taken in weighing the potential merits of treatment against the risk of decreased quality of life potentially caused by the side effects of treatment.

LABORATORY TESTS

A laboratory assessment should include a complete blood count, serum acid phosphatase, alkaline phosphatase, lactic dehydrogenase, and renal and liver function tests. The PSA serum level also may be useful as an immunohistochemical marker when the primary site of a prostatic tumor is occult. A PSA level of 4 ng/mL or higher should be considered suspicious of cancer until proved otherwise. An increase in the PSA level generally is correlated with an advanced tumor stage. An elevated PSA after radiotherapy for CaP can predict residual CaP or metastases. After hormonal therapy for metastatic disease has been initiated, PSA may return to normal limits. A persistent decrease in PSA may predict a favorable response to treatment.

Prostatic acid phosphatase is not useful as a screening test in early-stage CaP. However, it may be useful as a marker for treatment response, since it is found to be elevated in many patients with CaP when there is disease outside the prostate capsule.

RADIOLOGIC STUDIES

Computed tomography (CT) and magnetic resonance imaging (MRI) of the pelvis can be useful to detect metastases to pelvic organs and lymph nodes. Skeletal x-ray studies and a radionuclide bone scan are useful for assessing the degree and location of bone metastases. Either renal ultrasonography or intravenous pyelography should be included to assess for hydronephrosis. Despite the value of imaging techniques, they tend to underestimate the severity of tumors about 50% of the time.

OTHER DIAGNOSTICS

Transrectal ultrasonography (TRUS) is a useful screening device for early detection. However, it is not currently recommended for patients with a normal PSA level and a normal DRE.

A transurethral, transrectal, or transperineal ultrasound-guided needle biopsy of the prostate is indicated when there is a suspicion of cancer. It can detect CaP earlier than DRE can.

The level of severity of CaP generally is determined by DRE and the histology of prostate biopsy specimens in conjunction with whether lymph node samples are positive and metastases are identified. Staging is crucial in the investigation and appropriate treatment of CaP. The American Urological Association system for staging CaP is presented in Table 13-2-1.

TREATMENT

The treatment of CaP is dependent on the stage of cancer to which it has progressed:

- If the CaP is confined to stage A1, transurethral resection followed by watchful waiting is a typical therapy. (A serious limitation of watchful waiting is that there is a large margin of error with the currently available prognostic indicators.)
- If CaP is found at stage A2 or stage B, radical prostatectomy or radical radiation therapy is considered. (When the cancer is confined to the prostate, radical prostatectomy can eradicate the tumor in 90% of patients.)
- If the cancer has progressed to stage C, radiation therapy alone is considered the first-line treatment. Once metastases have been confirmed, first-line therapy often is aimed at blocking the synthesis and action of androgens. Androgen deprivation can be achieved by orchiectomy or luteinizing hormone–releasing hormone (LH-RH) analogues, often combined with androgen receptor antagonists (see "Medications," below).
- At stage D1, transurethral prostatectomy (TURP) or radiation is used if the patient is experiencing urinary obstruction. If the patient is asymptomatic at stage D1, watchful waiting or endocrine manipulation is tried. At stage D2, symptomatic patients are first treated with hormonal therapy. If the disease appears refractory to hormonal manipulation, chemotherapy is considered. Palliative radiation therapy may be used for symptomatic areas.
- If a patient at stage D2 is asymptomatic, watchful waiting is considered. A stage D patient with bilateral hydronephrosis or impending spinal cord compression should be considered for orchiectomy. However, in many patients with pain from bone metastases, androgen deprivation produced by medication therapy is equivalent to the androgen deprivation produced by bilateral orchiectomy. The option of adding antiandrogen drugs together with castration, which is called combination androgen blockade (CAB), may lengthen survival and improve the patient's quality of life.

MEDICATIONS

Hormonal therapy (HT) is often considered a first-line treatment for CaP. Some questions that have been raised about HT are as follows:

1. Can HT for CaP prolong patient survival?
2. Can HT improve a patient's quality of life?
3. Is complete androgen blockade superior to androgen reduction therapy?
4. Is preoperative HT more beneficial than postoperative HT?

Although these are unresolved questions, HT is considered a major therapeutic modality.

Typically, therapy for stage D1 or D2 disease consists of androgen deprivation. Because androgen hormones influence CaP, androgen deprivation may improve the symptoms and even cause disease regression. The role of therapy is to reach castration levels of testosterone and dihydrotestosterone. Among the drugs currently used are the following:

- Diethylstilbestrol (DES), an exogenous estrogen
- LH-RH analogues, such as Zoladex (a goserelin acetate implant), that inhibit the release of pituitary gonadotropins
- Antiandrogen blocking agents such as bicalutamide and flutamide (of the two, bicalutamide offers the convenience of once-a-day dosing and is better tolerated)
- Goserelin, a gonadotropin-releasing hormone (GnRH) analogue, which is better tolerated than DES
- Cyproterone acetate (CPA), which has been demonstrated to be an alternative to orchiectomy in advanced cases of metastatic CaP

Second-line agents used in cases of advanced CaP include liarozole, ketoconazole, and aminoglutethimide. A once-a-month injection of the agent Lupron Depot (leuprolide acetate), another GnRH analogue, is also used as a safe and effective alternative to surgical castration.

SUPPORTIVE MEASURES

An increased intake of red meat and dietary fat may be correlated with a higher risk for CaP. Some studies suggest that a diet rich in soy products and vegetables may contain phytoestrogens that can exert a chemopreventive effect on the prostate gland. Decreased levels of vitamin D secondary to insufficient sun exposure and very high levels of vitamin D–binding proteins may also precipitate CaP. Evidence suggests it is appropriate to recommend that patients at risk for developing prostate cancer should ensure they are receiving an adequate daily intake of vitamin E. The antioxidant properties of vitamin E may help fight against the growth of prostate cancer.

PATIENT EDUCATION

All male patients should be instructed about the importance of a yearly DRE after age 40. Men 50 years and older should be reminded to have a PSA test along with the annual DRE. Patients also should be reminded that a high-fat diet and a sedentary life-style are linked to an increased risk of CaP. Choosing the optimal therapy for each patient requires appropriate counseling of patients about the relative risks and benefits of each treatment option. Patients should definitely be counseled about the risks of impotence as a side effect of treatment.

DISPOSITION

Once CaP has been diagnosed, it is imperative to maintain close follow-up. The optimal treatment would provide a complete cure. However, since most cases of CaP have already metastasized by the time of diagnosis, much of the treatment may be palliative. Treatment decisions must be based on the probability of enhancing each patient's quality of life over a potential 10- to 15-year survival period.

COMPLICATIONS AND RED FLAGS

It should be noted that both radical radiotherapy and surgery tend to cause permanent impotence and often cause sphincter problems as well. If flutamide is used for total androgen suppression, liver function tests are required at regular intervals to guard against liver toxicity.

OTHER NOTES AND PEARLS

There are many opinions about how best to treat CaP. However, it is imperative to remember that one is treating people, not just a disease. Therefore, the patient must be drawn into all decision-making about his treatment and consideration must be given as to whether the treatment will truly benefit the individual patient.

Urinary excretion of pyridinoline and deoxypyridinoline appears to be a useful marker for evaluating the activity of bone metastases and their response to hormonal treatment in CaP. Current research is exploring the use of herpes simplex virus thymidine kinase gene transduction followed by ganciclovir (HSV-tk plus GCV) as cytotoxic gene therapy to treat locally advanced or metastatic CaP. Studies are under way in Japan to assess the efficacy of intraarterial chemotherapy for the treatment of advanced CaP, utilizing an implantable injection pump. Prostatic inhibin peptide (PIP) is being researched as a possible additional treatment option. Some studies suggest that vasectomy may be associated with an increased risk of CaP. Studies at the National Cancer Institute are investigating the oral intake of modified citrus pectin as a potential inhibitor of CaP metastases. Other studies suggest a possible relationship between the high consumption of green tea and the low incidence of prostate cancer among Asian men. Advances in gene therapy may represent the best chance for an eventual cure for CaP.

BIBLIOGRAPHY

American Urological Association: Prostate cancer clinical guidelines: Summary report on the management of clinically localized prostate cancer. *J Urol* 154:2144, 1995.

Austin O, Ricer RE: Prostate cancer screening: An appraisal of the PSA test. *Fam Pract Recert* 18:81–91, 1996.

Baffa R et al: A comparative analysis of prostate-specific antigen gene sequence in benign and malignant prostate tissue. *Urology* 47(6):795–800, 1996.

Bauer JJ et al: Prostate cancer: Diagnosis, treatment, and experience at one tertiary-care military medical center, 1989 and 1994. *Mil Med* 161:646–653, 1996.

Campbell MF et al (eds.): *Campbell's Urology.* Philadelphia, Mosby, 1998, pp 111–112, 2491–2493, 2542–2543.

Catalona WJ et al: Use of the percentage of free prostate-specific antigen to enhance differentiation of prostate cancer from benign prostatic disease. *JAMA* 279:1542–1547, 1998.

D'Amico AV et al: Biochemical outcome after radical prostatectomy, external beam radiation therapy, or interstitial radiation therapy for clinically localized prostate cancer. *JAMA* 280:969, 1980.

Fair WR et al: Cancer of the prostate: A nutritional disease? *Urology* 50:840, 1997.

Garnick MB, Fair WR: Prostate cancer: Emerging concepts: Part II. *Ann Intern Med* 125(3):205–212, 1996.

Haas GP, Sakr WA: Epidemiology of prostate cancer. *CA Cancer J Clin* 47:273, 1997.

Ikeda I et al: Pyridimium cross-links as urinary markers of bone metastases in patients with prostate cancer. *Br J Urol* 77(1):102–106, 1996.

Kaplan SA et al: Transurethral resection of the prostate versus transurethral electrovaporization of the prostate: A blinded, prospective comparative study with 1-year follow-up. *J Urol* 159:454, 1998.

Kolvenbag GJ, Blackledge GR: Worldwide activity and safety of bicalutamide: A summary review. *Urology* 47(suppl 1A):70–84, 1996.

Krongrad A et al: Mortality in prostate cancer. *J Urol* 156(3):1084–1091, 1996.

Malkowicz BS, Wein AJ: Prostate cancer, in *Textbook of Internal Medicine,* 3d ed, WN Kelley (ed). Philadelphia, Lippincott-Raven, 1997, pp 1354–1357.

McClain R, Gray ML: Prostate cancer—A primer. *Clinical Advisor* Feb 37–50, 2000.

Millikan R, Logothetis C: Update of the NCCN guidelines for treatment of prostate cancer. *Oncology* 11:180, 1997.

Ragde H et al: Interstitial iodine-125 radiation without adjuvant therapy in the treatment of clinically localized prostate carcinoma. *Cancer* 80:442, 1997.

Rubenstein M: Induction of apoptosis by diethylstilbestrol in hormone-insensitive prostate cancer cells. *J Natl Cancer Inst* 388(13):908–917, 1996.

Williams TR, Love N: Treatment of localized prostate cancer: Choosing the best alternative. *Postgrad Med* 100(3):105–107, 111–112, 118–120, 1996.

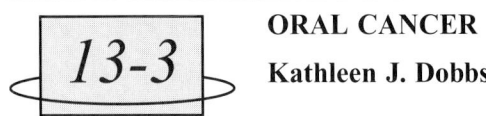

ORAL CANCER

Kathleen J. Dobbs

DISCUSSION

Oral cancers account for less than 5% of all cancers. Though this appears to be a small number, oral cancers have a significant impact on an individual's interaction with the environment. Disfigurement of the face and alterations to speech and eating impact social interaction, distort visual identity, and diminish one's sense of well-being. Early recognition and treatment are essential for optimal outcomes. All health care providers must be cognizant of the presentation of oral cancers.

The oral cavity consists of many structures (see Table 13-3-1).

Each area requires careful examination and consideration. Primary care providers and dentists are best positioned to screen for oral cancers. Discussions on the prognosis and treatment of each specific area within the oral cavity have been the topics of research for years. For the purposes of this chapter, the oral cavity is discussed collectively unless a specific oral cancer needs to be highlighted.

The salivary glands, though not considered as structures of the oral cavity, open into the oral cavity and can be sites for oral cancer, albeit quite rare. The ductal openings of the three largest salivary glands (the parotid, submaxillary, and sublingual) should be examined closely. With a rich blood and lymphatic supply, metastatic spread of all oral cancers to adjacent structures including lymph nodes can occur.

The vast majority of oral cancers are squamous cell. The remaining 5 to 10% includes a variety of cell types such as melanoma, lymphoma, adenocystic carcinoma, adenocarcinoma, and sarcoma.

PATHOGENESIS

The cause of oral cancers remains obscure. However, there are risk factors that show a definite causal relationship. Other risk factors only suggest an increase in the incidence of developing oral cancers.

The combination of large quantities of alcohol and smoking account for approximately three-fourths of all oral cancers in the United States.[1] This additive effect has a greater impact on the disease than either of the risk factors alone. Cancer of the lip may occur in pipe smokers. The popularity of oral tobacco has been followed by an increase in oral cancers, especially the buccal mucosa and floor of the mouth. There is a clear relationship between the common practice of betel nut chewing and development of oral cancers in areas that remain in contact with the quid or chewed mixture. Betel nuts, which are grown in India and Southeast Asia, have appeal for their stimulant effect.

Additional risk factors may include poor dental hygiene, loose or ill-fitting dentures, tertiary syphilis, use of mouthwashes with high alcohol content, genetic predisposition, and previous radiation. The high correlation between lip cancer and sunlight exposure is noted. It is speculated that women may have a lower incidence of lip cancer than men in the same environment secondary to lip protection from lipstick and other protective coverings. In past decades radiation was used as therapy to treat many benign problems such as tonsillitis, enlarged thymus in newborns, chronic sialoadenitis, and acne. There is a correlation between treatment with radiation for benign conditions and cancer in adjacent areas in these individuals.

PRESENTATION

The typical oral cancer patient is a male between 50 and 60 years of age. Despite this propensity, one should be prepared to look for the disease in both younger and older age groups and in both sexes—it is not a rare occurrence. Of all cancers, the incidence in the oral cavity is approximately 5% in men and 2% in women.

Primary care clinicians and dentists are essential to recognizing oral cancers in the early stages. Early detection and treatment significantly improve prognosis and decrease morbidity. Clinical acumen and vigilance may be necessary to appreciate many of the signs and symptoms. Occult oral cancers are possible. Signs and symptoms may be vague or nonspecific within the oral cavity and often present with cervical lymphadenopathy.

Typically oral cancers are symptomatic with patients seeking medical attention for any of the following symptoms: an intraoral mass or distortion in the usual architecture; ulceration, with or without bleeding; pain; halitosis; odynophagia (painful swallowing); dysphagia (difficulty swallowing); trismus; decreased tongue mobility; and loosening of teeth or poorly fitting dentures.

Because of the extensive lymphatic system servicing the oral cavity, any neck mass present for 1 to 2 months should alert the practitioner to look for cancer. An occult oral cancer may be at fault and deserves complete evaluation. This is particularly true if the social history indicates tobacco and alcohol use in the patient.

The presence of lesions in the oral cavity are red flags as well. Leukoplakia and erythroplakia are strong indicators of premalignancy or carcinoma in situ. Leukoplakia appears as white patches in the oral cavity that cannot be removed with scraping. This lesion is thought to be precancerous and should be recognized and evaluated histologically.

TABLE 13-3-1. Structures of the Oral Cavity

ANATOMIC STRUCTURE	LOCATION	PEARLS
Lips	External structures at the entrance of the cavity	Most common site of oral cancer, particularly the lower lip.
Buccal mucosa	Lining of the cheeks, laterally, from maxillary to mandibular gingival borders	Carcinoma is rare. Common site for leukoplakia and *Candida* infection.
Upper and lower alveolar ridges	The mounds in the maxilla and mandible in which the teeth are implanted	Carcinomas are more common in the mandibular vs. maxillary, particularly in the molar and premolar regions. Most arise in edentulous areas. (Lee, 1996)
Retromolar trigone	Area behind the molars adjacent to tonsillar pillars and oropharynx	Bony involvement extension to adjacent structures is common. Difficult to visualize unless mouth is opened wide.
Oral tongue	The anterior two-thirds of the tongue, commonly called the mobile tongue	Second most common site of oral cancer.
Hard palate	Roof of the mouth	Cancers are rare in this area. Most cancers are punched-out ulcerations.
Floor of the mouth	All the tissue located below the oral tongue to the lower alveolar ridges	Considered a "silent area" as it is rarely examined. At this site, cancers typically will develop at the junction of the tongue in the sublingual space.

Erythroplakia is a velvet-like red patch that also cannot be removed by simple scraping. It has greater implications for the development of oral cancer than leukoplakia. It is histologically considered a carcinoma in situ.

Physical examinations of the entire oral cavity and cervical, supra-, and infraclavicular nodes are essential. Inspection and palpation are used to assess oral cancers. A good white light source for inspection allows the examiner to visualize all aspects of the lips and oral cavity, including under the tongue and along the gingival/buccal mucosal border clear back to the retromolar trigone. Patients with dentures or removable orthodontic equipment should have them removed to uncover any lesions or evidence of irritation, especially over the alveolar ridges. With a gloved hand the practitioner must palpate all surfaces of the oral cavity, focusing on changes in consistency or texture. Attention should be given to signs of patient discomfort during palpation. Attention to the opening of the major salivary glands into the oral cavity is mandatory. This can be a site for development of cancer or may be an indicator of diseased salivary glands.

Examination of the tongue requires several maneuvers. The anterior surface is examined with bright light. Over 85% of lingual cancers arise in the lateral margins of the tongue.[2] Induration and ulceration are suggestive of cancer. Grasping the tongue with dry gauze while palpating the tissue with the other gloved hand is very effective for complete examination. Viewing all surfaces of the tongue is crucial.

Neck examination completes the physical examination for oral cancer. The oral cavity has two lymphatic systems draining the area. Neck masses on the ipsilateral side occur most often. Lesions in the midline of the oral cavity drain into both sides, resulting in potentially bilateral lymphadenopathy.

DIAGNOSTIC CONSIDERATIONS

The differential diagnostic considerations in oral cancer vary with the signs and symptoms presented, location of mass or lesion, and concurrent medical problems. Ulcerations of the common aphthous ulcer or canker sore can mimic cancers of the tongue, gingiva, and buccal mucosa. Oral cancers can be confused for the painful and erosive lesions of herpes simplex infection, erosive lichen planus, and benign pemphigus. Oral candidiasis must be differentiated from leukoplakia. Plummer-Vinson syndrome, an iron-deficiency anemia, causes the oral mucosa to have an ash grey color and atrophic changes of the tongue. These atrophic alterations have been implicated in the etiology of cancer of the tongue. Kaposi's sarcoma may also be identified with violaceous macules on the mucosa. Mass lesions such as fibroma and papilloma must be differentiated from malignant oral lesions (see Table 13-3-2).

LABORATORY TESTS

History, physical examinations, and, in many cases, an index of suspicion are the primary diagnostic requirements. Complete blood count

TABLE 13-3-2. Differential Diagnostic Considerations

Aphthous ulcers (canker sore)
Herpes simplex infection (cold sore, fever blister)
Herpes simplex gingivitis (seen in children)
Benign pemphigus
Erosive lichen planus
Plummer-Vinson syndrome (atrophic oral changes)
Oral *Candida* infection
Fibroma
Papilloma (benign neoplasm, cause unknown)

(CBC) with differential count, platelet count, prothrombin time, partial prothrombin time, chemistry profile, and electrocardiogram provide both baseline information and potential clues for further diagnostic workup.

Significant research is being directed toward early detection. Identifying highly sensitive and specific tumor markers for oral cancers is being pursued with vigor. These markers may be used for screening purposes as well as to monitor patients for recurrence. Another area of research is DNA changes; the p53 tumor suppressor gene has received significant attention. Changes in this gene, located on chromosome 17, contribute to the aggressiveness of many head and neck cancers. Tests to detect these p53 gene alterations may allow very early detection of oral and oropharyngeal tumors. These tests may also be used to better define surgical margins and possibly to determine which tumors are most likely to respond to surgery or radiation therapy.[3]

Biopsy is the next essential step. Histologic examination and identification is imperative to confirm the cell type. Tissue may be obtained via fine-needle aspiration biopsy, excisional biopsy, and rarely incisional biopsy of the oral lesion. Cervical or supraclavicular node biopsy is not routinely done for establishing a diagnosis.

RADIOLOGIC STUDIES

Magnetic resonance imaging (MRI) is useful in assessing soft tissue and bone detail. Computed tomography (CT) is often used to define anatomic relationships. Though both imaging studies are useful, CT may be used more often because of cost and availability. Both of these diagnostic studies are very valuable in staging oral cancers. Ultrasonography has limited use; its primary benefits are distinguishing solid from cystic tumors and evaluating neck and thyroid tumors. Chest x-ray, when CT is unavailable, may be used to look for metastasis or a second primary. If oro- or nasopharyngeal lesions are suspected, referral to an otolaryngologist for direct examination of the nasopharynx, oropharynx, and larynx is necessary.

STAGING

The extent of the cancer is categorized into four stages, I through IV, based on a combination of the TNM classifications. *T* indicates the size of the primary tumor, *N* reveals information about nodal involvement, and *M* discloses data on metastases. Stage I has the best outcome for the patient. Stage IV has the highest morbidity and mortality.

Recurrent Oral Cavity Cancers

Return of tumors following treatment has a poor overall prognosis. Treatment will depend on the location and size of the recurrent cancer, as well as prior treatment. Response to treatment for this group is often temporary but may provide symptom relief.

TREATMENT

Once diagnosis and staging have been established, a treatment plan is developed. Quality of life issues must impact on treatment decisions. If cure is the goal, then total eradication of the tumor with the best functional and cosmetic outcome is the strategy. If palliation is the best option, then the priority shifts to limiting the expansion of the mass and providing optimal comfort.

Surgical removal of the tumor and affected lymph nodes, radiation therapy, chemotherapy, or a combination of these modalities are the current methods of treating oral cancer. Referral to a medical oncologist for treatment of oral cancer is important. Often a multidisciplinary team including a medical oncologist; ear, nose, and throat surgeon; dentist; and psychosocial support professionals work together to secure the best possible outcome.

Early cancers of the lip, floor of the mouth, and retromolar trigone are highly curable. The buccal mucosa, tongue, alveolar ridge, and hard palate can be cured if cancer is detected and treated early.[4] Of oral cavity cancer patients, 81% survive 1 year after diagnosis. For all stages (I–IV) combined, the 5-year relative survival is 52%. The 10-year rate is 41%.[5] Recurrence of a second primary after successful treatment of the first cancer can occur. The patient must be monitored periodically for any further cancers.

REFERENCES

1. Day GL: Cancer rates and risks: Oral cavity and pharynx, risks for major cancers, in *Cancer Statistics.* Branch Division of Cancer Prevention and Control, National Cancer Institute, Bethesda, Maryland, 1996.
2. US Public Health Service: Cancer detection in adults by physical examination, *American Family Physician: Put Prevention into Practice.* Washington DC, Volume 51, number 4. March 1995.
3. American Cancer Society: Oral cavity and oropharyngeal cancer facts and statistics, http://www.cancer.org/oral.html, accessed August 2000.
4. National Cancer Institute: CancerNet, Lip and oral cancer, http://www. nci.gov/oral, accessed January 1997.
5. American Cancer Society: Oral cavity and oropharyngeal cancer, http:// www.cancer.org/oral.html, May 2000.

BIBLIOGRAPHY

Alford DR: Department of Otolaryngology and Communicative Sciences, Head and Neck Tumors Core Curriculum Syllabus, http://www.bcm.tmc.edu/ oto/studs/hnt.html, January 1997.
Lee KJ: *Essential Otolaryngology Head and Neck Surgery,* 6th ed. Stamford, CT, Appleton & Lange, 1996.
Schuller DE, et al: *DeWeese and Saunders' Otolaryngology—Head and Neck Surgery,* 8th ed., St. Louis, Mosby, 1994.

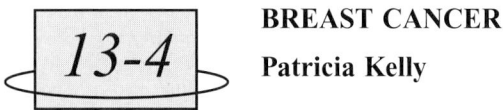

BREAST CANCER

Patricia Kelly

DISCUSSION

The term *breast cancer* refers to a group of neoplasms that usually but not always first present in the female breast. These neoplasms may be ductal (78 percent), lobular (9 percent), associated with other special histologies (12 percent), or inflammatory (1 percent). Breast cancer is often a systemic disease at the time of presentation. Tumor doubling time can vary from 25 to 500 days. Breast cancer is a subtle disease with great variability in its presentation and prognosis.

Prevalence

Breast cancer is the most common lethal malignancy in females. Statistics regarding its incidence can be manipulated to portray breast cancer as an epidemic disease in women of all ages. Slogans such as "One out of eight women will get breast cancer in her lifetime" reinforce this theme. This refers to the statistical chance that a woman living to age 85 has of receiving a diagnosis of this disease. Approximately 12 percent of women will develop breast cancer at some point in their lifetimes; this percentage has increased in recent years and is expected to increase further. The increased incidence, however, is largely a result of a longer life span and greater diagnostic diligence. Since the incidence of breast cancer increases with age, increased longevity inevitably leads to an increased rate of disease.

For this reason, some epidemiologists prefer to identify the probability of developing breast cancer in specified age intervals. When viewed from this perspective, breast cancer risk is more easily understood and less ominous. For example, a 40-year-old woman has a 1 in 77 chance of having breast cancer before age 50. Further, the mortality rate from breast cancer has declined recently; approximately 60 percent of breast cancer victims survive and die of another cause.

Etiology and Risk Factors

New evidence is constantly presented regarding the etiology of and risk factors for breast cancer. Without doubt, there is a genetic component. First-degree relatives of breast cancer patients have a twofold to threefold risk of developing the disease compared with women without affected first-degree relatives. Additionally, the identification of specific genes (*BRCA1, BRCA2*) linked with a marked risk of breast cancer explains the very high incidence of the disease in some family clusters. Relatively few breast cancer patients have these genetic mutations, however.

Women with a history of benign breast disease generally do not have a greater risk of breast cancer, although one type of benign abnormality, hyperplasia with atypia, is associated with a higher risk of subsequent malignancy. High-fat diets have been implicated, but to date there is no evidence that changing to a low-fat diet later in life lowers the absolute risk. Endogenous hormones are implicated in certain groups. Nulliparous women and women who bear the first child after age 31 have a threefold to fourfold increased risk of breast cancer compared with women who have the first child before age 18. However, since most women fall into an intermediate category, the usefulness of this finding is uncertain. Early menarche and late menopause (inferring longer hormone exposure) increase the risk somewhat; however, the parameters have not been defined, and the average age at both of these events changed rapidly during the twentieth century, making epidemiologic correlation difficult.

Low-dose oral contraceptives generally are not thought to increase the risk of breast cancer. Estrogen replacement therapy confers a small risk, since exogenous estrogen can enhance tumor growth. Also, since tumors are not diagnosed when the first cancerous cells form, estrogen replacement may increase the doubling times of certain neoplasms.

It is known that surgical castration (removal of the ovaries) before age 37 without subsequent hormone replacement decreases the risk of breast cancer. This, however, cannot be used as a preventive measure because of the marked increase in cardiovascular disease and osteoporosis that would result.

It appears that increased alcohol intake is associated with increased risk. Even a history of low alcohol intake in large cohorts of women has been only weakly associated with an increased risk of breast cancer. The overall health benefits of low alcohol intake (one drink per day or less) in women are therefore controversial.

Diabetes mellitus also increases the risk, as does age greater than 40 and a previous history of cancer of the ovary, uterus, or colon. Smoking is a weak risk factor. Demographically, Asian women seem to have the lowest risk in the U.S. population.

Because evaluating the risk conferred by one or more of these factors is quite problematic, several "risk-prediction" models have emerged. The most widely used method, developed by Gail and associates, uses the number of affected first-degree relatives, age at menarche, age at first live birth, and number of breast biopsies to calculate risk. Revisions of this model also utilize race and the presence of atypical hyperplasia on breast biopsy. The "Gail model" is most easily calculated by using software available from the National Cancer Institute; a toll-free telephone service for providers is also available. Calculation of risk is important, since it affects screening and preventive measures. For example, the risks of postmenopausal hormone replacement therapy are greater for women who have a substantial risk of breast cancer. Early screening mammography (between ages 40 and 49) would certainly be indicated in higher-risk women. Chemical preventives (tamoxifen) can be utilized in women judged to be at a high risk (>1.7) by the Gail model. Prophylactic mastectomy also can be offered to women at exceptional risk (carriers of *BRCA1* and *BRCA2*). As screening and prevention methodologies improve, accurate calculation and description of risk will become the standard of care.

The following signs and symptoms are significant:

1. Breast lumps are found in the majority of these patients. They tend to be dominant, firm to hard, immobile, irregular, and adherent to skin and/or underlying tissue.
2. Serosanguinous, unilateral nipple discharge should greatly increase the clinical suspicion of a neoplasm.
3. Eczematous skin changes, especially unilateral, can be a sign of breast cancer and warrant further investigation.
4. Any irregularity or "dimpling," induration, or unilateral size change should be explored.
5. Axillary adenopathy that is not otherwise explained is strongly suspicious of breast cancer until another etiology is histologically identified.

Breast pain is seldom a presenting symptom. However, bone pain from previously unsuspected metastatic breast cancer can be the first symptom of disease.

DIFFERENTIAL DIAGNOSIS

"Fibrocystic disease," fibroadenomas, cysts, mastitis, and fibrous tumors often must be evaluated surgically before malignancy can be excluded.

DIAGNOSTIC EVALUATION OF SUSPICIOUS FINDINGS

Mammography is approximately 85 percent sensitive in diagnosing breast cancer. It is less sensitive, however, in women under age 40 and those with dense breast tissue. The specificity of mammography is markedly lower, leading to a great number of invasive procedures, especially for younger patients. The specificity increases in direct proportion to age. A palpable mass that is negative on mammography should always be investigated further.

Surgical Evaluation

The accuracy of fine needle aspiration of solid masses is directly related to the degree of operator and cytopathology experience with this technique. If tissue unequivocally characteristic of a benign entity (such as a fibroadenoma) is found, the sensitivity is higher than 95 percent. The use of large core needle biopsy techniques facilitates adequate tissue sampling and is becoming the standard of care in many localities. However, if insufficient or nondiagnostic tissue is obtained, an excisional biopsy is mandatory. Many surgeons strongly urge excisional biopsy of all solid masses, although the growing popularity of core needle biopsy techniques may challenge this tradition. Cystic structures may be aspirated. Ultrasound may be helpful in differentiating solid masses from cystic masses. If a cyst remains palpable or bloody fluid is obtained, more invasive diagnostic techniques are indicated.

The Positive Biopsy

Staging is necessary to determine the appropriate treatment. The most important element of staging—lymph node status—can be obtained concurrently with mastectomy or local excision (lumpectomy). Further staging studies for all these patients include a complete blood count (CBC), liver function tests, serum calcium, alkaline phosphatase, a chest x-ray, and a mammogram, all obtained preoperatively. Further staging is deferred until the lymph node status is available. If lymph nodes are positive or if the tumor is over 2 cm in size, computed tomography (CT) of the liver, a bone scan, and possibly a bone marrow biopsy are indicated. This further evaluation should be conducted after consultation with a medical oncologist.

Staging of Breast Cancer

The American Joint Committee for Cancer Staging and End-Results Reporting has developed a staging system based on the standard TNM [**T** (tumor size), **N** (node status), and **M** (metastatic disease)] criteria.

True breast cancer is grouped into clinical stages I through IV. Less advanced cancer (smaller tumor size and lack of spread to lymph nodes) generally is staged into the first two groups. More advanced cancer, as indicated by increasing tumor size, invasion of lymph nodes, and/or distant metastatic lesions, is grouped into clinical stages III and IV. There is some overlap; women who have small tumors but one or two positive, small, nonfixed lymph nodes may be classified as stage II. Women with tumors larger than 2 cm, even without positive lymph nodes, are considered stage III, and women with primary tumors larger than 5 cm without evidence of nodal involvement may have stage IV disease and a poorer prognosis.

As a very general rule, women with stage I or stage II cancers have a relative survival rate above 66 percent after 6 years; women with stage III or stage IV cancers have a relative survival rate below 49 percent over the same time period.

Since many oncologists use slightly different staging systems, it is usually most helpful to describe the tumor by size, the number and location of involved nodes, and any metastatic lesions. It is more difficult to predict survival rates with the "intermediate" stages (II and III), and the percentages given above, especially those for stage IIb and IIIa cancers, should be viewed with extreme caution.

There are any number of other variables (hormone receptor status, DNA ploidy, S-stage activity, histologic grade, etc.) that may affect the disease course but that have not been included in a universal staging system. A medical oncologist experienced in breast cancer treatment should evaluate every case individually. Newer prognostic factors, such as estimating the percentage of cells in the S phase of replication, will play a larger role in defining the prognosis in the future.

Breast cancer does not play by the same "rules" as other cancers, and 5 or 10 years of survival is not considered a definitive cure.

TREATMENT
Local Treatment

Breast cancer is frequently a systemic disease at the time of presentation. The standard for surgical treatment at this time is modified radical mastectomy or removal of the tumor with clear margins, node dissection, and postsurgical adjuvant radiation. These treatments are designed to provide local disease control and offer identical outcomes in terms of survival benefit. Current treatment concerns in the United States involve regional variations in the availability of breast preservation surgery and appropriate referrals for radiotherapy, especially in older women. Sentinel lymph node mapping (replacing axillary dissection) is promising but cannot yet be considered the standard of care.

Systemic Treatment

Women generally are traditionally divided into premenopausal and postmenopausal and node-negative and node-positive cohorts for treatment options. There is a consensus that optimal breast cancer treatment involves local and systemic therapies. Systemic adjuvant therapies include hormonal therapy, generally tamoxifen, and combination chemotherapy regimens. Premenopausal women with negative nodes generally are treated with adjuvant chemotherapy if their tumors are larger than 1 cm. Premenopausal women with positive nodes require adjuvant chemotherapy. There has been a recent trend toward treating premenopausal women with 5 years of tamoxifen as well after adjunctive chemotherapy, especially if their tumors are hormone-receptor-positive.

Postmenopausal women who have positive lymph nodes and are hormone-receptor-positive generally are treated with oral tamoxifen

20 mg daily for 2 to 5 years. Depending on age, degree of node positivity, and the size of the tumor, many clinicians also recommend adjuvant chemotherapy for these patients. Adjuvant chemotherapy, which once was reserved for premenopausal women, has been shown to be useful in women up to age 70. Postmenopausal women with hormone-receptor-negative tumors definitely should receive adjuvant chemotherapy. In general, combination hormonal therapy and chemotherapy is more useful than either therapy alone in women with hormone-receptor-positive disease; women with a high risk of recurrence should be provided with this option.

Preoperative chemotherapy or hormonal therapy, with the goal of shrinking the tumor, is useful in increasing the number of women eligible for breast-conserving surgical procedures.

Metastatic disease, if it is life-threatening or symptomatic, should be treated with chemotherapy and hormonal agents if appropriate. For asymptomatic metastatic disease that is hormone-receptor-positive, tamoxifen (or newer hormonal agents) alone may be considered. Radiation can provide palliative control for bone, brain, and chest wall metastases. Hormonal agents (antiestrogens, aromatase inhibitors, gonadotropin-releasing hormone analogues, and progestins) can be used in sequential fashion even after the failure of an initial agent; some patients have a significant response to three or four hormonal compounds used in stepwise fashion.

The standard adjuvant chemotherapy includes cyclophosphamide, methotrexate, and 5-fluorouracil (CMF). There is some evidence that regimens containing doxorubicin (FAC) may offer a slight advantage; however, doxorubicin can cause cardiomyopathy, which is a dose-limiting factor. Cardioprotective drugs that can be administered concomitantly with doxorubicin are proving useful in allowing longer and more intense regimens containing this agent.

Salvage Chemotherapy for Recurrent Disease

Chemotherapy, if it did not previously contain doxorubicin, should now include this agent in combination with other standard agents. The taxanes have been studied extensively and are very valuable in salvage chemotherapy. Newer regimens combine taxanes with doxorubicin. Vinorelbine is a third-line choice. Relatively lengthy remissions can occur with salvage chemotherapy, but a cure is not the goal of this treatment.

There is no current evidence to suggest that very high dose regimens (used with bone marrow augmentation) produce superior results compared with standard chemotherapy.

Newer therapies include specific treatments (monoclonal antibodies) for the overexpressed oncogenes (*HER-2/neu*) apparent in some breast cancers. These therapies can be used alone or in combination with traditional or novel chemotherapeutic agents.

SPECIAL CONSIDERATIONS

With an increase in the incidence of mammography, improvements in technique, and increased radiologist expertise, noninvasive tumors (carcinoma in situ) can now be detected.

Ductal carcinoma in situ is clearly malignant and can be multicentric in more than 50 percent of patients. Because approximately 33 percent of these patients develop invasive carcinoma within 5 years, mastectomy or lumpectomy with radiation therapy usually is indicated. However, some clinicians advocate lumpectomy alone for small, well-differentiated lesions that can be removed with generous margins.

Lobular carcinoma in situ is premalignant, affects primarily premenopausal females, and is commonly bilateral. The risk of developing invasive cancer is high (30 percent over 15 to 20 years), and these patients may benefit from prophylactic bilateral mastectomy. Other options include extremely close follow-up; however, given the 15 percent false-negative rate for mammography, there are risks with this approach that should be understood clearly by the patient and the clinician. Digital mammography and other enhanced imaging techniques may be useful. The efficacy of tamoxifen in prevention is uncertain.

SUPPORTIVE MEASURES

It is very important to convey to breast cancer patients a sense of optimism for the immediate future. Even stage IV disease can be controlled for up to 3 years. The earlier the cancer, the better the prognosis. Breast cancer can have a slow and indolent natural history even without treatment. Cures are possible and even likely in stage I and stage II disease; very long remissions with many cures can be expected in early stage III disease. During disease-free and treatment-free periods, the quality of life is excellent. Many symptoms suffered during chemotherapy can be substantially lessened or prevented by talented clinicians. The newer antiemetic drugs and more sophistication with antiemetic combinations have virtually eliminated acute nausea and vomiting. Pain from metastatic disease can be controlled with sophisticated analgesic regimens and palliative radiation. Quality time is achievable even with advanced metastatic disease.

PATIENT EDUCATION AND PREVENTION

Optimism concerning the treatability of breast cancer is necessary to achieve an acceptable rate of screening. Rates of screening will increase when various health agencies and authorities agree on appropriate screening mammography schedules and adequate reimbursement for these services. There are few or no data to support a baseline mammogram before age 40 in women at average risk. Screening women between ages 40 and 50 can save lives but is costly; the expense of mammography per life saved has been estimated at $100,000.

The current consensus is that annual screening mammography for women 40 through 49 years of age is warranted despite this cost. Women at higher risk (increased disease prevalence decreases false-positive examinations) most clearly benefit. Women who, on the basis of family history, are at very high risk may obtain their first screening mammogram 5 years before the earliest age of diagnosis in their afflicted relative(s).

Women age 50 and over clearly deserve annual screening mammography. Their disease is easier to visualize, and if it is diagnosed at an early stage, their prognosis is generally better than that of premenopausal patients. Future improvements in mammographic technique and interpretation, including digitalized imaging, are very promising.

Breast self-examinations and provider breast examinations are inexpensive; self-examination has been shown to be efficacious in identifying disease at a stage when breast-conserving surgery is an option. No survival benefit from self-breast examination, however, has ever been demonstrated. Surprisingly, routine provider breast examination as currently practiced has a comparatively low positive yield. Increased clinician time spent in breast examination has been shown to improve the diagnostic yield.

Risk prediction modeling using the Gail mode or another standardized method is clearly warranted and virtually free. Risk prediction is most useful in guiding enhanced screening, chemoprevention, or surgical intervention.

Specific recommendations on prevention must be individualized. Tamoxifen has been shown to reduce the incidence of breast cancer. It is now approved for use in women at high risk, as calculated by the Gail model. Concerns regarding tamoxifen include a definite increase in the rate of endometrial cancer. Raloxifene, another selective estrogen receptor modulator, is also under study; this agent does not seem to increase endometrial cancer incidence. Both agents increase the incidence of thromboembolic events, as do other hormone replacement therapies.

DISPOSITION

Follow-up for women with treated breast cancer should be individualized. In general, these patients should be seen at least every 6 months for a physical examination and a thorough review of systems.

Mammograms should be done annually. From a survival standpoint, no routine laboratory test or imaging scan has been shown to be valuable in a patient without symptoms or abnormalities on physical examination, and frequent repeated studies tend to induce anxiety in patients, who fearfully await the results of routine x-rays, CBCs, and chemistry panels.

Other routine health care maintenance should be stressed. Patients should be screened for colon and ovarian cancer regularly; however, optimal schedules have not been demonstrated. Annual pelvic examinations, fecal occult blood testing, and colonoscopy or flexible sigmoidoscopy at regular intervals would be a reasonable approach, since breast cancer patients have an increased incidence of these neoplasms.

BIBLIOGRAPHY

Armstrong K, Eisen A, Weber B: Primary care: Assessing the risk of breast cancer. *N Engl J Med* 342(8):564–571, 2000.

Barton MB, Harris R, Fletcher SW: Does this patient have breast cancer? The screening clinical breast examination: Should it be done? How? *JAMA* 282:1270–1280, 1999.

Hortobagyi GN: Drug therapy: Treatment of breast cancer. *N Engl J Med* 339 (14):974–984, 1998.

Kennedy MJ: Systemic adjuvant therapy for breast cancer. *Curr Opin Oncol* 6(6):570–577, 1994.

Muss HB: The role of chemotherapy and adjuvant therapy in the management of breast cancer in older women. *Cancer* 94(Suppl 7):2165–2171, 1994.

Olivotto IA, Bajdik CD, Plenferleith IH, et al: Adjuvant systemic therapy and survival after breast cancer. *N Engl J Med* 330(12):805–810, 1994.

Osborne CK: Drug therapy: Tamoxifen in the treatment of breast cancer. *N Engl J Med* 339(22):1609–1618, 1998.

Roy JA, Swaka CA, Prichard KI: Hormone replacement therapy in women with breast cancer: Do the risks outweigh the benefits? *J Clin Oncol* 14:997–1006, 1996.

Smith TJ, Hillner BE: The efficacy and cost-effectiveness of adjuvant therapy of early breast cancer in premenopausal women. *J Clin Oncol* 11:771, 1993.

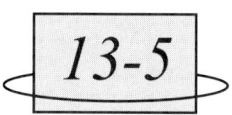

COLORECTAL CANCER
Patricia Kelly

DISCUSSION

Colorectal cancer is the second most lethal cancer in the U.S. population. The number of deaths from colorectal cancer has declined somewhat over the last three decades; this is thought to be secondary to improved screening technique, an increased incidence of screening, and subsequent earlier detection. The absolute incidence also has decreased slightly over the past decade, probably as a result of the removal of premalignant polyps in screened individuals. There were 129,400 reported cases of colorectal cancer in the United States in 1999.

Demographically, this malignancy is slightly more common in the northeastern United States. The risk increases with age; however, younger individuals (age 50 to 70) frequently present with more aggressive disease. There is a roughly 5 percent lifetime prevalence rate in this country.

Heredity is an important risk factor; about 25 percent of cases may be related to genetic causes. As a rule, lifetime prevalence is up to three times higher for persons with a family history of this disease. There are several distinct variants of familial polyposis syndromes, all of which are linked with an increased incidence of colorectal cancer. Some of these syndromes have a familial rate of colorectal cancer higher than 50 percent.

Colorectal cancer has a significantly higher prevalence in Ashkenazi Jews, probably secondary to their increased incidence of *BRCA1* and *BRCA2* mutations. African-Americans, Hispanics, and younger individuals of any ethnicity tend to present with more advanced or aggressive disease. Asian-Americans have disease patterns that resemble those of the white population in the United States. Geographic incidence differentials have led to the study of diet in relation to colorectal cancer risk. It is clear that high-fat, low-fiber diets contribute to the incidence of colorectal cancer. Smoking also increases the risk to two to three times baseline.

Ulcerative colitis markedly increases the risk of colorectal cancer and requires regular screening colonoscopy (see "Screening and Prevention," below). Crohn's disease also may be associated with an increased incidence of this malignancy. Other risk factors include a personal or family history of other cancers, especially reproductive cancers in women. Exposure to asbestos may increase the risk slightly.

Most colorectal cancers start as adenomatous polyps; sessile adenomas also can become malignant. Larger polyps are the most likely to show cancerous changes. Up to 30 percent of persons develop polyps during their lifetimes. The average time from a small polyp to the onset of cancer ranges from 10 to 15 years.

About 98 percent of true colorectal cancers are adenocarcinomas by histology. The distribution of malignant lesions throughout the colon is as follows: 66 percent left colon and 33 percent right colon; about 20 percent of colorectal cancers occur in the rectum. Some patients have disease at more than one site.

SIGNS AND SYMPTOMS

The signs and symptoms are related to the size and location of the neoplasm. Tumors of the left side of the colon may present with changes in bowel habits, flank pain, bleeding, constipation, decreased stool diameter, and obstruction. Right-sided colon cancer results in varying degrees of abdominal discomfort, weight loss, and stools positive for occult blood. Accordingly, hematochezia is more frequently associated with tumors of the descending colon; melena is associated with malignancies of the transverse or ascending colon.

Findings on physical examination may be absent, depending on tumor location and size. Tumor that already has metastasized to the liver may be palpable; infrequently, asymptomatic large colon masses may be palpated through the abdominal wall. Rectal cancer frequently can be detected on digital rectal examination. Stool for occult blood, depending on the technique, may be positive (see "Screening and Prevention," below). Visible bleeding is rarely noted. Weight loss is common in patients with advanced disease.

DIAGNOSTIC CONSIDERATIONS

In symptomatic patients, the causes of abdominal pain must be evaluated systematically. Right-sided pain may prompt consideration of gallbladder disease (see Chap. 6-10). Acute left lower quadrant pain is also seen in diverticulitis, which also can produce bleeding (see Chap. 6-8). Generally, diagnostic studies reveal intracolonic abnormalities that will prompt studies for a definitive diagnosis.

DIAGNOSTIC STUDIES

Laboratory studies should include a complete blood count (CBC) primarily to detect the severity of anemia and a chemistry panel that includes liver function tests to assist in ruling out metastatic disease.

A complete physical examination, including a digital rectal examination with testing of stool for occult blood, should be performed. A carcinoembryonic antigen (CEA) test should be ordered preoperatively if the suspicion of colorectal cancer is strong. It may be included in the initial evaluation or deferred until disease is confirmed by colonoscopy and biopsy.

IMAGING AND ENDOSCOPIC STUDIES

The workup should then progress to a colonoscopy and biopsy for histologic confirmation. If a polyp is discovered and removed, the area should be marked and measured precisely so that further surgery for definitive resection with wide margins may be performed. A CEA is mandatory before the removal of the suspect lesion.

CEA is the best-known marker to follow disease recurrence or progression, and so a baseline level must be established. However, some colorectal cancers do not produce CEA; therefore, a normal CEA should not preclude further evaluation if other findings are suspicious.

If a neoplasm is discovered, it is staged preoperatively and postoperatively. Postoperative staging is of course more definitive. Preliminary (preoperative) treatment planning and final (postoperative) treatment planning are dependent on the stage of the disease.

STAGING OF COLORECTAL CANCER

The most widely used staging system is the modified Duke's-Astler-Coller method (see Table 13-5-1).

Prognosis

A stage A cancer, perhaps represented by a completely excised polyp with tumor limited to the polyp itself, has a 90 to 100 percent 5-year survival rate. Node-negative cancers have 5-year survival rates that range from 55 to 85 percent. Node-positive disease is ominous even without distant metastatic lesions; without local invasion, the 5-year survival rate is between 25 and 50 percent. Locally invasive disease has a 5-year survival rate of 0 to 20 percent, and distant metastatic disease has a median survival rate of 6 to 12 months.

TREATMENT

Unless distant metastatic disease exists, surgery is the initial management of choice. Partial colectomy with wide margins and adjacent lymph node removal is the standard procedure.

Permanent colostomy may or may not be needed but is performed frequently on a temporary basis to permit stool passage postoperatively. Upper and high middle rectal tumors are excised with an anterior resection of the rectum. Abdominal perineal resection generally is used for lower rectal lesions. Obstruction of the left side of the colon requires at least a temporary colostomy with deferred closure. Obstructive tumors of the right side of the colon frequently can be managed by wide resection with immediate anastomosis without the need for even a temporary colostomy. High rectal lesions can be treated

TABLE 13-5-1. Staging of Colorectal Cancer

STAGE	DESCRIPTION
A1	Limited to mucosa; negative nodes
B1	Extension into muscularis propria; negative nodes
B2	Extension through entire bowel wall; negative nodes
B3	Extension into adjacent organs; negative nodes
C1	Positive nodes; lesion limited to muscularis propria
C2	Positive nodes; lesion extends through entire bowel wall
C3	Positive nodes with tumor invasion of adjacent organs (locally invasive)
D	Distant metastatic disease

with the same approach. Perforation secondary to mass obviously requires excision and at least a temporary colostomy.

Adjuvant Chemotherapy and Radiation

Colon cancer with nodal spread is treated with adjuvant chemotherapy with various dosing schemes for up to 1 year. Three large, prospective randomized trials have demonstrated that adjuvant therapy improves the 5-year survival rate approximately 10 to 15 percent. Clinical trials to find the optimal drugs, doses, and length of treatment are ongoing.

Rectal cancer almost always is treated postsurgically with adjuvant radiation therapy and concomitant chemotherapy. For widespread disease, adjuvant chemotherapy may be continued for up to 1 year. This aggressive treatment is necessary because of the technical difficulty of achieving adequate clear surgical margins after resection of a rectal cancer.

Recurrent and metastatic colorectal cancers generally are treated with various chemotherapeutic agents. Long-term remission and survival rates are low, generally with a median survival less than 1 year. A newer chemotherapeutic agent, irinotecan hydrochloride, a topoisomerase 1 inhibitor, has been approved for patients with metastatic colorectal cancer who recur or progress after standard chemotherapy therapy. A 15 percent response rate (complete or partial remission) was noted during premarketing trials, and survival data are being accumulated. This agent has a relatively severe side-effect profile; quality of life must be considered in patients at this stage of illness.

New surgical, intraarterial chemotherapeutic, and cryotherapeutic approaches have been utilized for persons with cancer metastatic to the liver; some palliation may be achieved. With these novel therapies, some patients have 2 or more years of survival.

DISPOSITION

In patients with resected colon cancer, CEA levels should be measured every 3 months for 24 months and every 6 months thereafter. Chest x-rays are recommended annually. Repeat colonoscopy should be performed 6 weeks postoperatively if the patient's condition permits and then annually. Most recurrences occur within 3 years.

Screening and Prevention

Most colon cancers can be prevented by the detection and removal of premalignant lesions. A low dose of aspirin daily may aid in the prevention of colorectal cancer. Low-fat, high-fiber diets may be useful. The cyclooxegenase (COX)-2 inhibitors show promise, as do other NSAIDs (nonsteroidal anti-inflammatory drugs).

Digital rectal examinations should be performed annually in adults over age 40. This test has the advantage of screening for rectosigmoid cancers and prostate abnormalities in men. Annual fecal occult blood testing (age >50) has the potential to decrease colon cancer mortality by one-third to one-half. Efforts to increase the effectiveness of this test are ongoing.

Flexible sigmoidoscopy every 5 years is recommended for individuals older than 50 without other known risk factors; this could reduce the mortality from colorectal cancer by approximately 40 percent. Screening with both fecal occult blood testing and flexible sigmoidoscopy at these recommended intervals could decrease mortality by 65 percent. Alternatively, screening colonoscopy every 10 years starting at age 50 could reduce mortality by 70 percent.

The American Cancer Society currently recommends annual digital rectal examination at age 40 and intensified screening at age 50. Currently, one of the following screening regimens is recommended for individuals over age 49:

1. Annual fecal occult blood test and sigmoidoscopy every 5 years
2. Colonoscopy every 10 years
3. Double-contrast barium enema every 5 years.

The US Preventive Services Task force confines its recommendations to fecal occult blood tests and sigmoidoscopy at the intervals listed above, reserving colonoscopy for persons at higher risk.

Individuals with verified family histories or familial polyposa syndromes require more frequent and more comprehensive evaluations starting at a younger age. Most authorities recommend starting one of the recommended screening regimens in persons with a positive family history at age 40. For aggressive familial syndromes (familial adenomatous polyposis and hereditary nonpolyposis colon cancer), screening starts as early as age 10 and is repeated every 1 to 3 years. These persons generally are followed in specialty settings, as are persons with inflammatory bowel disease. Persons with ulcerative colitis generally are screened with colonoscopy and directed biopsy every 1 to 3 years, depending on the severity and scope of disease and the age of onset.

BIBLIOGRAPHY

Guillem JG, Paty PB, Cohen AM: Surgical treatment of colorectal cancer. *CA Cancer J Clin* 47:113–128, 1997.

Jessup JM, Menck HR, Fremgen A, Winchester DP: Diagnosing colorectal carcinoma: Clinical and molecular approaches. *CA Cancer J Clin* 47:70–92, 1997.

Landis SH, Murry T. Bolden S, Wingo PA: Cancer statistics 1999. *CA Cancer J Clin* 49:8–31, 1999.

Rudy DR, Zdon, MJ: Update on colorectal cancer, *Am Fam Physician* 61:1759–1774, 2000.

U.S. Preventive Services Task Force: Screening for colorectal cancer, in *Guide to Clinical Preventive Services: Report of the U.S. Preventive Services Task Force,* 2d ed. Baltimore, Williams & Wilkins, 1996.

Winawer SJ, Fletcher RH, Miller L, Godlee F, Stolar MH, Mulrow CD, et al: Colorectal cancer screening: Clinical guidelines and rationale. *Gastroenterology* 112:594–642, 1997.

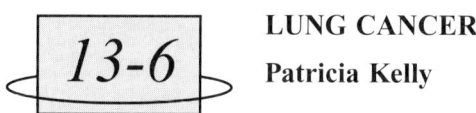

LUNG CANCER
Patricia Kelly

DISCUSSION

Lung cancer is the leading cause of cancer deaths in the United States. Most of these patients die within 1 year of the diagnosis. The peak incidence occurs between ages 55 and 65, although cases occur in smokers as young as 30. This is a disease that is almost completely preventable: Tobacco is the direct cause of approximately 90 percent of lung cancers.

There probably is an enhanced carcinogenic effect of tobacco combined with the pollutants present in modern society. However, tobacco is carcinogenic in and of itself.

Four major histologic types of cancer constitute 95 percent of primary lung tumors:

1. Squamous cell carcinomas
2. Small cell carcinomas
3. Adenocarcinomas
4. Large cell carcinomas

For the purposes of treatment and prognosis, lung cancer is thought of as small cell or non-small cell. Small cell lung cancer generally goes into remission with appropriate chemotherapy, although recurrence within 2 years is the almost absolute rule. If non-small cell lung cancer is diagnosed very early, it potentially can be cured with complete resection. However, at the time of diagnosis, only one in five patients has local, resectable disease. Only 30 to 40 percent of patients with resected local disease, however, survive for 5 years.

SIGNS AND SYMPTOMS

About 10 percent of these patients are asymptomatic and are detected on screening radiography. Others present because of cough, hemoptysis, shortness of breath, weight loss, wheezing, or obstructive pneumonia. Later-stage patients may have lung abscess, tracheal obstruction, esophageal compression, hoarseness, or Horner's syndrome (enophthalmos, ptosis, miosis, and ipsilateral loss of sweat). Patients can develop superior vena cava syndrome with associated swelling of the head and jugular venous distention. Pancoast's syndrome (superior sulcus tumor) involves the eighth cervical and the first and second thoracic nerves, causing shoulder pain and rib destruction. Rapidly progressive bronchoalveolar carcinoma can obstruct the bronchi, causing hypoxemia and death. Metastatic cancer, of course, can produce multiple symptom complexes.

There may be abnormal wheezing, dullness, rales, and rhonchi on lung examination. Of course, these symptoms coincide with the findings of frequently concomitant chronic obstructive pulmonary disease and obstructive pneumonia secondary to a neoplasm. Generally, the patient experiences some weight loss and may have clubbing of the extremities.

DIAGNOSTIC CONSIDERATIONS

Patients with lung cancer may present with paraneoplastic syndromes characterized by anorexia, cachexia, weight loss, decreased immunity, hypercalcemia, hypophosphatemia, hyponatremia, and hypokalemia. Fatigue also may be present and can represent myasthenic Eaton-Lambert syndrome, which is found primarily in patients with small cell lung cancer. Hypercoagulable states also may ensue with all cancers. The syndrome of inappropriate excretion of antidiuretic hormone (SIADH) is found commonly in patients with small cell lung cancer.

LABORATORY STUDIES

No noncytologic laboratory test is diagnostic of lung cancer. Laboratory studies should be reserved for staging.

RADIOLOGIC STUDIES

Chest radiography and, if it is nondiagnostic, computed tomography (CT) are necessary. Chest CT is especially valuable in localizing a tumor for the most important diagnostic test: the confirming biopsy for definitive cytology. CT of the thorax down to the level of the liver and adrenals also assists in staging and in excluding metastatic disease.

BIOPSY

Tissue must be obtained. Histology and the extent of spread determine treatment. Tissue can be obtained from fine needle aspiration, CT-guided biopsy of peripheral lesions, samples from bronchoscopy, nodal biopsy during mediastinoscopy, and video-assisted thoracoscopy. A positive sputum cytology, although diagnostic, is rarely obtainable, and false negatives are the rule.

STAGING OF LUNG CANCER

Non-small cell lung cancers are staged according to the extent and position of nodal spread, the size and degree of invasion of the tumor itself, and any metastatic lesions that are present. Obviously, smaller tumors with absent or limited nodal spread or local invasion may be resectable. Tumors with nodal spread on both sides of the chest and tumors locally invasive to adjacent organs are usually, although not always, not resectable. Tumors with distant metastatic lesions are not resected. If a patient is believed to have a resectable cancer, after consultation with the thoracic surgeon, he or she will require pulmonary function tests and ventilation-perfusion scans to determine whether he or she will have sufficient residual functional lung tissue postoperatively.

Frequently, the question of resectability is resolved only by open surgery. Recently, attempts have been made to "downstage" tumors by giving preoperative chemotherapy and radiation therapy. This is called *neoadjuvant treatment* and can be useful in certain well-motivated patients.

TREATMENT OF NONRESECTABLE LESIONS

Medical oncologists believe that chemotherapy for unresectable non-small cell lung cancer is essentially palliative in nature and may provide only slightly longer survival than do other modalities of palliative care. This difference is small, and the increased survival is measured in months. Some progress has been made by adding cycles of newer agents (docetaxel and paclitaxel) after therapy with standard cisplatin- or carboplatin-based regimens. Gemcitabine and vinorelbine also are undergoing investigation.

Radiation therapy can be used for palliation of hemoptysis, superior vena cava syndrome, and other syndromes that would be amenable to local control. Radiation therapy with curative intent can be offered to patients with earlier stages of lung cancer who decline surgery or are not surgical candidates. The percentage of actual cure with this modality, however, is quite low. Longer courses of radiation therapy than are used for palliation can cause side effects, including radiation pneumonitis and decreased pulmonary function.

TREATMENT OF SMALL CELL LUNG CANCER

Small cell lung cancer is considered limited if the neoplasm is clinically confined to the hemithorax and the associated draining regional nodes at the original presentation. Other patients are considered to have "extensive" disease. Small cell lung cancer is very sensitive to both chemotherapy and radiation and is treated with those modalities sequentially or in combination. The drugs most frequently used for initial treatment are cisplatin-based derivatives and etoposide in combination. Newer agents include epirubicin and irinotecan. Paclitaxel administered in combination with the standard etoposide-cisplatin regimen also has been studied.

Prophylactic whole-brain irradiation is controversial but sometimes is used to prevent the common occurrence of brain metastases. A recent study demonstrated that prophylactic cranial irradiation, which once was out of favor, improves both overall survival and disease-free survival among patients with small cell lung cancer who are in complete remission.

If a patient fails to achieve a complete remission after six cycles of chemotherapy with or without radiation, the chemotherapy is changed to a salvage regimen and radiation therapy is added if it was not utilized previously. Most patients can achieve a complete response, and almost all have a partial response with a survival advantage. However, the disease usually recurs or relapses after 12 to 18 months. At that time, the patient can be treated with chemotherapeutic agents that were not previously used on that particular tumor. It is sometimes possible to induce another complete or partial remission. Entries into clinical trials should be encouraged at this stage, since the optimal salvage regimen has not been established.

Metastatic disease from small cell lung cancer is very amenable to radiation therapy, which should be used on bone and brain lesions.

Pain Management

Pain management is always a concern with any type of lung cancer. Adequate analgesia should be provided to patients who are receiving palliative care and patients who are receiving chemotherapy or radiation therapy but are experiencing pain. Respiratory depression can occur with adequate doses of opioid analgesia; however, this should not prompt the clinician to give a suboptimal dose. The "air hunger" of terminal, end-stage lung cancer also is effectively treated with larger doses of morphine, which reduce anxiety and the subjective feeling of shortness of breath. Patients and their families should receive appropriate education and support from their primary clinicians even after hospice referral. Optimal palliative treatment of end-stage cancer is in and of itself an extremely worthy goal that should be learned and practiced by all clinicians who deal with oncologic patients.

Prevention

Patients (or humans in general) should not be exposed to tobacco products. Children and adolescents must be educated at every opportunity about the dangers of tobacco. Most addicted smokers start smoking before age 18. Therefore, the illegal consumption of nicotine products should be dealt with as firmly as is the illegal consumption of alcohol and illicit drugs. Smoking in all public places should be forbidden. No one should smoke near children or companion animals. Every visit or communication with a smoking patient should include motivation and the offer of a plan for tobacco cessation. Self-help groups, nicotine replacement, adjunctive psychopharmacologic therapy, and strong clinician support are associated with successful cessation attempts. The average former smoker attempts to stop twice before making the successful attempt. One should never give up on smoking patients.

Screening

There is no evidence that screening chest radiography of high-risk patients improves survival. There is no current preventive medicine recommendation for routine chest radiography in the absence of symptoms. However, screening can and does encompass the assessment of all patients for firsthand or secondhand exposure to tobacco and appropriate subsequent education and medical support for smokers and persons exposed to secondhand smoke. Persons who have high-risk environmental exposures (e.g., asbestos) should be cautioned and informed that tobacco is especially risky for them.

There has been recent interest in low-dose, rapid CT scanning in high-risk groups. These tests have been shown to be efficacious in the detection of small, noncalcified nodules and have the potential to markedly increase the number of tumors discovered in the resectable stage. However, false-positive scans are common; diagnostic intervention is expensive, anxiety-provoking, and sometimes risky. Further study is indicated.

BIBLIOGRAPHY

Adelstein DJ: Palliative chemotherapy for non-small cell lung cancer. *Semin Oncol* 22(Suppl 3):35–39, 1995.

Auperin A, Irriagada R, Pignon JP, et al: Prophylactic cranial irradiation for patients with small-cell lung cancer in complete remission. *N England J Med* 341:524–526, 1999.

Belani CP: Paclitaxel and docetaxel combinations in non-small cell lung cancer. *Chest* 117 (4, Suppl 1):114S–151S, 2000.

Elias AD: Future directions in lung cancer research and therapeutics. *Hematol Oncol Clin North Am* 11(3):519–527, 1997.

Green MR, Barkley JE: Intensity of neoadjuvant therapy in resectable non-small cell lung cancer. *Lung Cancer* 17(Suppl 1):S111–S119, 1997.

Henschke CI, McCauley DI, Yankelevitz DF, et al: Early Lung Cancer Action Project: Overall design and findings from baseline screening. *Lancet* 354:86–87, 1999.

Sheperd FA, Dancy J, Ramlau R, Mattson K, et al: Prospective randomized trial of docetaxel versus best supportive care in patients with non-small cell lung cancer previously treated with platinum-based chemotherapy. *J Clin Oncol* 18(10):2095–2103, 2000.

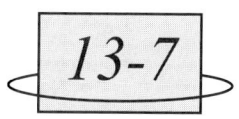

OVARIAN CANCER
Amelia Naccarto-Coleman

DISCUSSION

Ovarian cancer ranks as the number one cause of gynecologic cancer deaths and the fifth leading cause of any cancer-related deaths among women in the United States. An estimated 26,000 new cases were diagnosed in the United States in 1995 and more than 14,000 women died as a result of this deadly disease. Even though the incidence rate is low, overall survival rates, unchanged for over 30 years, remain at 30 to 35% and drop to 4% in women with advanced disease. Widespread screening has been ineffective in detecting this malignancy at its early stages when it is confined to the ovary. Unfortunately, more than two-thirds of these women with documented ovarian cancer have advanced disease (stage III or IV) at the time of diagnosis. Mortality rates are stage-dependent and dramatically increase with age. Worldwide, ovarian cancer accounts for approximately 4% of all cancers in women. With the exception of Japan, this disease is more commonly found in highly industrialized and affluent countries, particularly North America and Western Europe. The incidence of ovarian cancer peaks at two distinct ages: premenarchal and postmenopausal, with the lifetime incidence being 1 in 70 women.

Etiology and Risk Factors

The natural history and etiology of this disease remain unclear. The main theory proposes that incessant ovulation causes repetitive trauma to the ovarian surface, which may lead to the genesis of ovarian neoplasia by disrupting the germinal epithelium, thereby inhibiting repair. Risk factors associated with this hypothesis include advancing age, nulliparity, a history of infertility or delayed childbearing, early menarche, and late menopause. This theory is supported by evidence that shows long-term suppression of ovulation actually decreases the lifetime risk by as much as 50%. Oral contraceptive use, breast feeding, and multiparity have all demonstrated significant protection against the occurrence of ovarian cancer. Women with a family history of ovarian cancer have a significant lifetime risk of developing this disease. Proportionate to the number of first-degree relatives diagnosed with ovarian cancer, the highest risk appears to be in women who have two or more first-degree relatives diagnosed with the disease in two successive generations. This subgroup of familial ovarian cancer is postulated to be an autosomal-dominant inherited trait.

The three hereditary syndromes are:

1. *Site-specific:* families with an increased risk of ovarian cancer only
2. *Breast and ovarian:* families with an increased risk of both breast and ovarian cancers
3. *Lynch type II syndrome:* clustering of endometrial, breast, ovarian, and early-onset colorectal cancers seen within families (also known as family cancer syndrome)

Although age and family history are the two most important risk factors, other considerations currently being investigated are high dietary fat consumption, chemical exposure to talc or asbestos introduced into the peritoneal cavity via perineal dusting, Caucasian race, and most recently, genetic linkages.

PATHOGENESIS

Several different types of ovarian malignancies fall under the disease category of ovarian carcinoma. Each has different characteristics, treatments, and survival rates and can be classified according to their histologic type.

The four major categories are:

1. Epithelial
2. Germ cell tumor
3. Stromal/sex cord tumors
4. Metastatic disease from a distant primary site

Epithelial neoplasms are derived from the peritoneal covering of the ovary and account for more than 60% of all ovarian neoplasms. They are identified by the following subtypes:

1. Serous
2. Mucinous
3. Endometrioid
4. Clear cell
5. Transitional cell
6. Undifferentiated

More than 90% of these tumors are malignant. A subset of ovarian epithelial neoplasia is called *borderline cystadenocarcinoma,* or tumors of low malignant potential. These benign tumors are histologically similar to their malignant counterparts and are clinically important because of the possibility of future transformation.

Germ cell tumors are predominantly seen in younger age groups and rarely after the age of 30 years. They comprise less than 5% of all ovarian neoplasms. Their rapid growth and hemorrhagic nature are associated with acute abdominal symptoms and can easily be confused with appendicitis or pregnancy-associated complications. Prognosis is excellent with a 5-year survival rate exceeding 85%.

Stromal cell tumors are characterized by hormonal production of male, female, and adrenal steroid hormones. They account for less than 5% of all ovarian malignancies and can occur in all age groups. The secretion of large amounts of estrogen is associated with precocious puberty in younger girls and endometrial hyperplasia or vaginal bleeding in postmenopausal females. Prognosis is good with 10- and 20-year survival rates of 90% and 75% respectively after resection.

Metastatic carcinoma can present as bilateral adnexal masses and mimic primary ovarian cancer. This categorization can account for approximately 15 to 20% of all ovarian malignancies and should be a major diagnostic consideration in all ovarian tumors. The most common primary sites are the breast, stomach, colon, and endometrium. Prognosis is dismal with a 5-year survival rate between 5 and 10%.

SIGNS AND SYMPTOMS

Early detection of ovarian cancer is extremely difficult. There are usually no signs or symptoms in the early stages, and in many cases the cancer has spread by the time it is found. The cancer may be present for some time before causing any problems, such as pain or pressure. Even when symptoms do appear, they may be so vague that they are ignored. The keys, therefore, to making a diagnosis of ovarian cancer are a high index of suspicion and familiarity with the epidemiologic risk factors. Symptomatology can include vague abdominal discomfort, painless swelling or bloating of the lower abdomen, dyspepsia, increasing flatulence, early satiety, mild gastrointestinal and bowel disturbances, and nonspecific pelvic discomfort. In the advanced stages of disease, symptoms generally become more specific and are related to the pain and pressure associated with an enlarging mass.

OBJECTIVE FINDINGS

Pertinent features of the physical examination include evaluation of general nutritional status, the supraclavicular lymph nodes, the breasts, and the lungs, as well as abdominal and pelvic examinations. The predominant finding in making a diagnosis is detection of an adnexal mass on bimanual and rectovaginal exam. A pelvic mass is usually palpated on bimanual examination in the advanced stages of the disease. Because of the deep, anatomic location of the ovary, early-stage tumors are usually not detected. Pelvic masses should have their size, consistency, position, and extent of fixation to surrounding structures determined.

The diagnostic evaluation is influenced by the patient's age and menopausal status and the characteristics of the mass on pelvic examination and ultrasonography (see Table 13-7-1). Abdominal swelling or distention due to an ovarian enlargement or accumulation of ascitic fluid appear late in the course of the disease. Other findings might include the effects of functional tumors, which produce steroid hormones, causing postmenopausal bleeding or virilization.

LABORATORY EVALUATION

If an ovarian malignancy is suspected, a general preoperative assessment should be performed including a complete blood count (CBC), differential, platelet count, standard multiphasic chemistry panel with hepatic and renal function tests, serum CA 125 levels, electrocardiogram, and chest x-ray. Elevated CA 125 levels are present in 85% of advanced epithelial ovarian cancers and are useful in monitoring treatment. CA 125 is the only tumor marker approved by the Food and Drug Administration in the United States for assessing women with ovarian cancer. It is approved for only one indication, as an alternative to a second-look operation. Currently, the use of CA 125 as a screening tool is not recommended. However, an appropriate use of CA 125 is in the postmenopausal patient with a pelvic mass who is being referred to a gynecologist or gynecologic oncologist. Other tumor markers for ovarian cancers have been introduced to be used as screening tools alone or in combination; however, these markers seem to be more of a research tool at this time.

IMAGING STUDIES

Sonographic imaging is extremely useful in the evaluation of a pelvic mass. It is more precise in detecting ovarian tumors than is pelvic examination. Ultrasonography is used to estimate ovarian size, complexity, morphology, and the likelihood of malignancy. Color flow Doppler imaging (CDI) studies that evaluate the vascular patterns of adnexal masses show promise in improving the sensitivity and specificity of the radiographic prediction of benign and malignant lesions. Characterization of adnexal masses by computerized tomography (CT) scans and magnetic resonance imaging (MRI) may provide additional clinical information in select instances.

Additional preoperative studies are considered when a malignancy is suspected to evaluate metastatic disease and the patient's general medical condition. These include a chest x-ray to exclude pleural effusion, ultrasound assessment of the abdomen and liver, intravenous pyelogram, and a barium enema if colorectal disease is suspected. Because of the genetic association in familial cancer syndromes, a screening mammogram should also be obtained.

TABLE 13-7-1. Characteristics of a Pelvic Mass

	BENIGN	MALIGNANT
Physical examination	Mobile	Fixed
	Unilateral	Bilateral
	Cystic	Solid or firm
	Smooth	Nodular
Ultrasound	Simple cyst, <10 cm	Solid, >10 cm
	Septations <3 mm	Multiple septations
	Unilateral	Bilateral
	Calcification	None seen
	Gravity-dependent contents	Ascites

OTHER DIAGNOSTICS

Ultimately, evaluation of a suspicious pelvic mass will require an exploratory laparotomy and histologic review to definitively diagnose ovarian cancer. It is the only way to determine whether the tumor is benign or malignant, primary or metastatic. Diagnostic paracentesis is not indicated as a routine procedure because of the high percentage of false-negative results in the presence of widespread intraabdominal disease and the possibility of introducing tumor cells into the peritoneal cavity or implantation of neoplastic cells along the insertion site.

SURGICAL STAGING

Ovarian cancer can spread in three ways: direct extension, exfoliation of malignant cells, and lymphatic spread. Once the diagnosis of ovarian cancer is established, determination of the extent of the disease or stage is made according to the International Federation of Gynecology and Obstetrics (FIGO) system. Comprehensive surgical staging is carried out by meticulous examination of all peritoneal and retroperitoneal surfaces at risk of tumor spread.

DIFFERENTIAL DIAGNOSIS

Epithelial ovarian cancer needs to be distinguished from functional ovarian cysts and benign adnexal masses. This differentiation can be defined by evaluating the characteristics of the mass, the age of the patient, and the radiographic presentation. Benign adnexal masses, as seen on ultrasonography, are generally simple, mobile cysts that are unilateral, under 10 cm in size, and contain septations less than 3 mm in thickness. Malignant masses are often solid, fixed, nodular tumors that are bilateral, contain multiple septations greater than 3 mm in size, and may present with ascites. Other gynecologic causes that simulate this disease are tuboovarian disease, endometriosis, and pedunculated uterine leiomyomas. Nongynecologic causes include inflammatory or neoplastic colonic carcinomas, irritable bowel disease, and hepatic failure with ascites.

TREATMENT

Ovarian cancer is primarily managed by a combination of surgery, chemotherapy, and radiation. Treatment is generally considered in terms of early- or late-stage disease.

Surgery

Primary surgical therapy is indicated in most of the ovarian malignancies, regardless of the stage. This surgery is based on the principle of cytoreductive surgery, or tumor debulking. Tumor debulking reduces the amount of cancer to be treated with chemotherapy or radiation therapy. Surgical intervention is usually aggressive because of direct peritoneal seeding to multiple adjacent structures. In the early stages of disease, however, women who are still in their reproductive years and desire more children have the option to preserve some of their reproductive functions after surgical staging is performed. Treatment goals are optimal debulking of the tumor and accurate surgical staging and diagnosis.

For epithelial ovarian cancers:

- Total abdominal hysterectomy/bilateral salpingo-oophorectomy (TAH/BSO)
- Omentectomy/debulking
- Staging biopsies including nodal sampling if indicated

For ovarian germ cell cancers:

- Salpingo-oophorectomy on the affected side only in patients of reproductive age
- Careful staging and lymph node dissection

For sex cord stromal cancers:

- Adnexectomy of the affected side with surgical staging in patients of reproductive age
- TAH/BSO and surgical staging in postreproductive women

For low malignant potential (LMP) tumors:

- TAH/BSO with optimal staging and debulking in postreproductive women

Chemotherapy

In advanced epithelial ovarian malignancies, systemic chemotherapy is the mainstay of treatment following surgery. It is most effective in patients who have had optimal cytoreduction or in patients who present with minimal disease after resection. Standard initial therapy includes both a platinum agent (either cisplatin or carboplatin) and paclitaxel (Taxol) given intravenously every 3 to 4 weeks for 6 to 12 months. Clinical response rates range between 60 and 70 percent with 5-year survival rates of 10 to 20%. Due to the potential toxicity of these drugs, contraindications include patients with a history of impaired renal function, hearing loss, or neuropathy. All regimens cause some degree of bone marrow suppression but do not warrant the routine use of hematopoietic growth factors or bone marrow transplantation. Neoadjuvant chemotherapy followed by surgery for advanced cases of ovarian cancer is currently being evaluated and compared with conventional cytoreductive surgery followed by chemotherapy to determine quality of life experiences and cost-benefit outcomes. Intraperitoneal chemotherapy in the treatment of ovarian cancers remains to be defined.

Radiotherapy

Postoperative radiation therapy for advanced epithelial ovarian cancer has demonstrated long-term, relapse-free intervals for patients with stage II or III disease. However, whole abdominal irradiation is still controversial and needs further study.

Clinical Trials

Clinical trials are designed to find better ways to treat cancer patients and are based on the most up-to-date information. Patients who do not respond to standard therapy or experience too many undesirable side effects, at any stage, are considered to be appropriate candidates. Treatment centers that are conducting trials on ovarian cancer therapy exist in most parts of the country. Information on the location and availability of these centers can be found by calling the Cancer Information Service at 1-800-4-CANCER (1-800-422-6237).

Follow-up Care

Management is still unclear in patients who are clinically disease-free after primary debulking surgery and chemotherapy. Second-look surgery has traditionally been performed after completion of this regimen to confirm the patient's response to treatment. In some instances, a secondary debulking procedure is used for patients who demonstrate evidence of progressive disease after first-line therapy. Second-look surgery remains controversial and offers no survival benefits or advantages to those patients who have undergone the procedure. Asymptomatic patients are currently monitored every 3 to 4 months with a complete history, physical, rectovaginal pelvic exam, and test of CA 125 levels. CT monitoring is generally recommended at regular intervals. Monitoring CA 125 levels is used to detect early recurrence of disease in women who have had elevated levels prior to surgery. A sevenfold fall in the CA 125 level generally indicates a good response to treatment. However, a normal CA 125 level does not necessarily exclude the presence of disease. In patients who have relapsed after primary therapy, salvage therapy is not curative. In fact, even though the response rate to treatment is very high, there is no evidence that it prolongs survival. When primary treatment consists of platinum chemotherapy, the response to a secondary platinum regimen is based on the interval to relapse. Patients who relapse within 6 months generally have a poor response to platinum-containing regimens. Treatment-free intervals, disease bulk, and serous histology are good predictors of response to salvage therapy. The drug of choice in relapse therapy is paclitaxel. Relapses that occur a second time have almost no possibility for a cure. These patients receive no benefit of survival from the various chemotherapeutic agents and have a response rate of only 15%.

Palliative Therapy

Since the majority of women are diagnosed with advanced stage disease, it is important to keep the patient's quality of life in mind at all times. Supportive measures to control pain, establish good nutritional habits, maintain proper hydration, and relieve additional suffering are critical. Emphasis should be placed on comfort, symptom control, and pain management. Small bowel obstruction is commonly seen with progression of the disease. Gastrointestinal problems can be treated with frequent, small feedings and medication to improve gastric motility. Relief from malignant effusions is achieved by performing paracentesis to draw off as much ascitic fluid as possible. Another problem encountered is pleural effusion, which can be temporarily alleviated by thoracocentesis.

Terminally ill patients may also develop psychiatric problems that can severely alter their quality of life. Women who are diagnosed with this deadly disease suffer from clinical depression and anxiety at higher rates than the general population. Psychiatric symptoms are usually associated with uncontrolled pain, progression of the disease, complications from the illness or treatment, fear of death, or changing social relationships. Supportive psychotherapy and pharmacotherapy should be prescribed for patients who exhibit depression or anxiety. The patient's quality of life is an essential component in determining treatment response and rehabilitation needs. The shorter-acting benzodiazepines, such as lorazepam, alprazolam, and oxazepam, are the preferred choices in the treatment of anxiety. For depression, the use of tricyclics or fluoxetine (Prozac) or sertraline (Zoloft) is extremely beneficial. Pain is best controlled with opioid analgesics.

Death and dying is another area that the health care provider needs to understand in the overall management of the patient with advanced disease. Decisions about advance directives, resuscitation, hospice care, and family matters need to be addressed despite being difficult to initiate. Empathetic listening is helpful in minimizing the fear of abandonment and the fear of death that most patients entertain during the course of their illness. If appropriate, enlisting support from clergy can be beneficial to the patient, family, and medical staff. All of these supportive measures ultimately allow the patient to regain a feeling of control over the remaining portions of her life.

PEARLS

- Reinforce the importance of pelvic (bimanual) examinations in women of all ages.
- Obtain a thorough family history to help identify those patients who are at risk.
- Listen carefully to descriptions of vague, nonspecific, or persistent symptoms.
- Always include a rectovaginal exam in your physical assessment.
- Provide patient education on protective measures and risk factors and stay current on any information pertaining to screening tests.
- Maintain a supportive relationship if the patient is referred for treatment.

RESOURCES

Organizations

- National Cancer Institute (NCI) information resources—Cancer Information Service provides accurate, up-to-date information on cancer to patients, their families, health professionals, and the general public. Information specialists translate the latest scientific information into understandable language and respond in English, in Spanish, or on TTY equipment. Toll-free: 1-800-4-CANCER (1-800-422-6237); TTY: 1-800-332-8615.

Internet

- http://www.nci.nih.gov—NCI's primary Website; contains information about the Institute and its programs.
- http://cancertrials.nci.nih.gov—cancerTrials; NCI's comprehensive clinical trials information center for patients, their families, health professionals, and the general public. Includes information on understanding trials, deciding whether to participate in trials, and finding specific trials, plus research news and other resources.
- http://cancernet.nci.nih.gov—CancerNet; contains material for health professionals, patients, and the public, including information from Physician Data Query (PDQ) about cancer treatment, screening, prevention, supportive care, and clinical trials, and CANCERLIT, a bibliographic database.

BIBLIOGRAPHY

Altchek A, Deligdisch L: *Diagnosis and Management of Ovarian Disorders.* New York, Igaku-Shoin, 1996.

Baker TR, Piver MS: Etiology, biology, and epidemiology of ovarian cancer. *Semin Surg Oncol* 10(4):242–248, 1994.

Beckman RB: *Obstetrics and Gynecology,* 2d ed. Baltimore, Williams & Wilkins, 1995, pp 459–463.

Berek JS, Hacker NF: *Practical Gynecology.* Baltimore, Williams & Wilkins, 1989.

Blackledge GRP et al: *Textbook of Gynecologic Oncology.* London, Saunders, 1991.

Cohen CJ, Jennings TS: Screening for ovarian cancer: The role of noninvasive imaging techniques. *Am J Obstet Gynecol* 170(4):1088–1094, 1994.

Collins WP et al: Screening strategies for ovarian cancer. *Curr Opin Obstet Gynecol* 10(1):33–39, 1998.

DeCherney AH, Pernoll ML (eds): *Current Obstetric and Gynecologic Diagnosis and Treatment,* 8th ed. New York, McGraw-Hill, 1994.

Hacker NF, Moore JG: *Essentials of Obstetrics and Gynecology,* 2d ed. Philadelphia, Saunders, 1992, pp 602–612.

Herbst AL: The epidemiology of ovarian carcinoma and the current status of tumor markers to detect disease. *Am J Obstet Gynecol* 170(4):1099–1105, discussion 1105–1107, 1994.

John EM et al: Characteristics relating to ovarian cancer risk: Collaborative analysis of seven U.S. case-control studies. Epithelial ovarian cancer in black women. Collaborative Ovarian Cancer Group. *J Natl Cancer Inst* 85(2):142–147, 1993.

Osmers RGW et al: Preoperative evaluation of ovarian tumors in the premenopause by transvaginosonography. *Am J Obstet Gynecol* 175(2):428–434, 1996.

Ovarian cancer: Screening, treatment, and follow-up, NIH Consensus Conference. *JAMA* 273:491–497, 1995.

Ovarian cancer: Screening, treatment, and follow-up. NIH Consensus Statement (Online) 1994 April 5–7; [cited 96/18/10] 12(3):1–30.

Ransom SB, McNeeley SG: *Gynecology for the Primary Care Provider.* Philadelphia, Saunders, 1997.

Schwartz PE et al: Neoadjuvant chemotherapy for advanced ovarian cancer: Long term survival. *Gynecol Oncol* 72(1):93–99, 1999.

Shingleton HM et al: *Gynecologic Oncology: Current Diagnosis and Treatment.* London, Saunders, 1996.

Whittemore AS: Characteristics relating to ovarian cancer risk: Implications for prevention and detection. *Gynecol Oncol* 55(3 Pt 2):S15–S19, 1994.

Zuspan FP, Quilligan EJ: *Handbook of Obstetrics, Gynecology, and Primary Care.* St. Louis, Mosby, 1998.

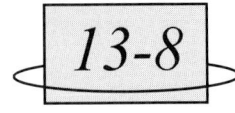

PANCREATIC CANCER
Patricia Kelly

DISCUSSION

Ductal adenocarcinomas account for almost 90% of pancreatic neoplasms. Approximately 60% occur in the head of the pancreas, 9 to 10% in the body, and 7 to 8% in the tail; approximately 20% are overlapping or occur in an unknown subsite. Uncommonly, anaplastic cancers may occur, and rare cases of adenosquamous pancreatic cancers have been reported.

It is well established that there is a 9 in 100,000 incidence of disease in the overall U.S. population. African Americans have an increased risk at 15 per 100,000. Males and females are equally affected. The cause is not known. However, several risk factors have been found:

- Cigarette smoking increases the relative risk to 1.5.
- Diets high in fat and/or meat raise the incidence to an unspecified level.
- Partial gastrectomy increases the risk twofold to fivefold (relative risk 2 to 5).
- It seems likely that diabetes enhances the growth of pancreatic cancer.
- Toxic substances, especially occupational exposure to 2-naphthylamine, benzidine, gasoline derivatives, and DDT and its derivative compounds, can increase the relative risk to between 4 and 7.

Coffee has been investigated extensively, but it has not been demonstrated that any possible human level of coffee intake increases the risk of this cancer.

SIGNS AND SYMPTOMS

Clinical signs of pancreatic cancer include:

- Cachexia
- Low serum albumin
- Palpable abdominal mass
- Jaundice
- Recurrent idiopathic deep-venous thrombosis
- Normal examination (50%)

Common symptoms include:

- Abdominal pain
- Anorexia
- Weight loss
- Early satiety
- Easy fatigability
- Weakness
- Nausea
- Vomiting
- Constipation
- Depression (up to 40%)

Physical Examination

Palpable abdominal masses and/or jaundice should lead the clinician to evaluate the pancreas for a neoplasm.

DIAGNOSTIC STUDIES

Abdominal ultrasound can detect pancreatic cancers in 60 to 90% of cases. Computed tomography (CT) is less operator-dependent and can demonstrate the degree of invasion and lymph node involvement. Spiral CT is quite useful. Up to 20% of pancreatic cancers cannot be found on CT, depending on the sophistication of the equipment and technique utilized. These tumors, unfortunately, represent potentially resectable disease, with lesions less than 2 cm in size. Magnetic resonance imaging (MRI) may offer an advantage when other studies are nondiagnostic.

After noninvasive studies are completed, endoscopic retrograde cholangiopancreatography (ERCP) is utilized to visualize tumors of the pancreaticobiliary junction and obtain biopsies of accessible tumors. For other tumors, percutaneous fine-needle aspiration (CT-guided) is safe. Positive results are diagnostic; negative results with suspicious masses or other studies may require re-biopsy. Tumor markers are not generally useful.

STAGING OF PANCREATIC CANCERS

Staging is most important because only resectable tumors have the possibility of being cured. The TNM system is utilized, with T denoting tumor size:

- T1: tumor that is localized to the pancreas
- T1a: tumor that is less than 2 cm in diameter
- T2: tumor that indicates extension into the duodenum, bile duct, or stomach
- T3: tumor that is unresectable

T2 tumors may be resectable with major surgery [pancreaticoduodenal resection with or without preservation of the pylorus (Whipple procedure with modification)]. Preoperative evaluation with CT, angiography, and laparoscopy is necessary to spare patients with unresectable disease (T3) unnecessary major surgery with significant morbidity and mortality rates. Staging laparoscopy can identify metastatic disease and is quite helpful in treatment planning and prognosis.

TREATMENT AND PROGNOSIS

Less than 20% of pancreatic cancer patients have true resectable disease. Surgery also is utilized for palliation in the relief of jaundice or duodenal obstruction. Even patients with resectable disease who undergo surgery have a 5-year survival rate less than 25%. This rate is improved for a very small subset of patients without any evidence of lymph node involvement; their 5-year survival rate may approach 50%.

The average survival of patients with nonresectable disease is no more than 6 months. The majority of studies have classically demonstrated that the median survival of patients who receive chemotherapy is no better than that of patients who receive the best supportive care. A newer chemotherapeutic agent, gemcitabine, has received approval from the U.S. Food and Drug Administration for use in patients with unresectable pancreatic cancer either as a first-line treatment or for persons who have failed therapy with 5-fluorouracil. Gemcitabine is a nucleoside analogue with antitumor activity. This agent may slightly increase median survival time. Other chemotherapeutic agents are also under study, including paclitaxel.

Radiation therapy combined with chemotherapy for locally advanced but unresectable disease increases the median survival time to approximately 10 months; the side effects are significant, and quality of life must be considered.

Most recently, trials of neoadjuvant (preoperative) chemoradiation treatment of locally advanced disease have been accomplished. This regimen consisted of preoperative fluorouracil and cisplatin combined with radiotherapy and nutritional support via jejunostomy tube, followed by attempted resection. Long-term impact on survival is uncertain, with only 11% of five patients surviving at 5 years. Future studies are planned that combine other chemotherapy agents (paclitaxel and gemcitabine) with radiation in a neoadjuvant fashion prior to attempted surgical resection.

Supportive Measures

Supportive measures include aggressive pain management with narcotics and consideration of percutaneous chemical neurolysis of the celiac ganglion. The patient must be instructed to insist on appropriate doses of analgesics to control pain, since some clinicians may be reluctant to prescribe the large amounts required for patients with advanced disease.

Prevention

Smoking cessation for all patients is a general rule of preventive medicine and may help decrease the incidence of pancreatic cancer. Special attention should be paid to occupational exposures that increase risk to certain solvents (see "Discussion," above).

DISPOSITION

Patients who have had successfully resected disease generally are imaged with abdominal CT every 6 months for at least 5 years. The cost-effectiveness of this approach, however, is questionable since there is no truly effective salvage therapy.

BIBLIOGRAPHY

Jimenez RE et al: Impact of laparoscopic staging in the treatment of pancreatic cancer. *Archives of Surgery* 135:4, 2000.
Prandoni P et al: Deep vein thrombosis and the incidence of subsequent symptomatic cancer. *N Engl J Med* 327:1128, 1992.
Sarcina R: Cisplatin (CDDP), 5-fluorouracil (5-FU) in the treatment of advanced pancreatic adenocarcinoma (meeting abstract). *Ann Oncol* 3(suppl 5):25, 1992.
Tabbarah HJ: Gastrointestinal tract cancers, in *Manual of Clinical Oncology*, DA Casciato, BB Lowitz (eds). Boston, Little, Brown, 1995, pp 145–182.
Tempero M: Dose escalation of gemcitabine in previously untreated patients with pancreatic adenocarcinoma (meeting abstract). *Proc Ann Meet Am Soc Clin Oncol* 13:A660, 1994.
Wanebo HJ et al: Preoperative chemotherapy, radiotherapy, and surgical resection of locally advanced pancreatic cancer. *Archives of Surgery* 135:81, 2000.

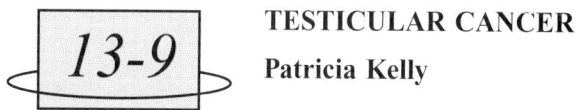

TESTICULAR CANCER
Patricia Kelly

DISCUSSION

Testicular cancer is the most common malignancy in males between 15 and 34 years of age. White people are five to six times more likely to develop testicular cancer than are African Americans. The worldwide incidence of this tumor has doubled in the past four decades. Risk factors include cryptorchidism (ten-fold to forty-fold increase) and testicular feminization syndromes. Ninety-five percent of testicular cancers originate from germ cells. Approximately 40 to 50% of germ cell tumors are seminomas and usually occur in a slightly older age range (30 to 50 years), reaching peak incidence in the fourth decade of life. Another 50% are embryonal carcinomas and teratomas (nonseminomas), which are more frequently found in men between ages 20 and 30, reaching their peak incidence in the third decade of life. In elderly males, lymphomas predominate. More than 90% of patients with the new diagnosis of germ cell cancer of the testicle can be cured. Early diagnosis is the key to effective treatment.

SIGNS AND SYMPTOMS

These patients are frequently asymptomatic and are diagnosed when a small testicular mass is noted during a routine sports or preemployment examination. As testicular self-examination becomes more popular, early detection could increase. The testicular mass may be painless. A painless testicular mass, the classic presentation of a primary malignancy, occurs in the minority of patients, however.

Slightly over 50% of patients present with some degree of mild discomfort or "heaviness," diffuse swelling, or a change in consistency. Unfortunately, common entities such as acute epididymitis (see Chap. 18-4) may mask the palpation of a distinct tumor in up to 25% of patients with an underlying mass. Because testicular discomfort is a common symptom, and epididymitis a common disease, ultrasonography should be performed for all patients who do not respond to antibiotic therapy or who are still symptomatic 2 to 4 weeks after presentation. Other presenting signs and symptoms include gynecomastia and infertility in a small percentage of males. Back pain is most commonly encountered when metastasis has already occurred, especially to the retroperitoneal nodes. Rare patients may have rapid tumor growth with associated necrosis and bleeding that results in flank pain. Patients with nodal metastasis may have palpable contiguous or distant lymph nodes. Patterns of metastatic spread include the interaortocaval nodes, the para-aortic nodes, the retrocrural nodes, and posterior mediastinal adenopathy. Diffuse disease may be found in the lungs and the supraclavicular nodes. Liver, bone, or brain spread may occur.

Uncommonly, extragonadal presentations of primary tumor in the retroperitoneal area and the mediastinum may occur. Extragonadal presentations of primary tumor to the mediastinum may be characterized by shortness of breath, chest pain, or superior vena cava syndrome.

Physical Examination

It is important to palpate the testicle with both hands, using moderate pressure and a "rolling" motion. Any palpable abnormalities, including induration and irregularity, should prompt a further workup.

DIAGNOSTIC CONSIDERATIONS

Hydroceles are not frequently malignant, but approximately 10% of men with testicular cancer have an associated hydrocele. If aspiration of hydrocele fluid yields blood, exploratory surgery is indicated. Transillumination of a suspected hydrocele may aid in the diagnosis but cannot definitively rule out a malignancy. Ultrasound is helpful in this situation. Varicoceles are swollen veins in the spermatic cord; they have a characteristic feel on palpation that has been compared to "a bag of worms." When the scrotum is elevated, venous distention is decreased.

Epididymitis should not exclude suspicion of testicular cancer (see Chap. 18-4). Both can cause pain and testicular swelling. Dysuria and pyuria are more common with epididymitis than they are with testicular cancer. Episodes of recurrent epididymitis with a return to normal testicular examination usually exclude neoplastic disease. Translucent spermatoceles and inguinal hernias generally can be differentiated from testicular cancer on physical examination. Entities such as infectious orchitis, hematoma secondary to injury, and acute testicular swelling, however, generally require surgery to definitively rule out neoplastic disease.

LABORATORY STUDIES

Approximately 50% of testicular tumors in patients between 15 and 34 years of age are nonseminomatous germ tumors. Of these men, 90% will have either positive β-human chorionic gonadotropin (β-hCG) or α-fetoprotein (AFP). β-hCG should never be found in a normal male and strongly implicates testicular cancer. Elevated β-hCG levels appear in 40 to 60% of patients with metastatic nonseminomatous disease. Increased concentrations of β-hCG may also be found in men with seminomatous germ tumors (15 to 20% of patients). AFP

occasionally can also be found with malignant or nonmalignant liver disease, especially hepatocellular carcinoma, but most strongly suggests testicular cancer in a younger age group.

Other laboratory studies are not routinely diagnostically useful, although some clinicians measure lactate dehydrogenase (LDH). Serum LDH levels are increased in approximately 60% of men with nonseminomatous tumors and 80% of those with seminomas.

RADIOLOGIC STUDIES

Although frequently performed, testicular ultrasound is rarely more specific than is physical examination. At this time there is no role for magnetic resonance imaging or computed tomography (CT) of the testes for diagnostic purposes.

EXPLORATORY SURGERY AND HISTOLOGIC DIAGNOSIS

Transinguinal unilateral orchiectomy, with ligation of the spermatic cord at the internal ring, is the diagnostic and initial therapeutic procedure of choice for a suspicious lesion. Routine preoperative laboratory and imaging studies, especially chest x-ray, CT studies, and liver function tests, may suggest metastatic disease. It must be emphasized that any type of needle or partial excisional biopsy is unacceptable and contraindicated. If the lesion is malignant, other diagnostic modalities are used to stage the neoplastic process. Treatment is based on tumor type and the extent of disease spread.

Chest CT and abdominal CT are used to image metastatic pulmonary and retroperitoneal disease. Any palpable upper body lymph node should be biopsied. CT or other imaging studies of the brain are performed if neurologic involvement is likely.

TREATMENT

The prognosis and treatment are dependent on the disease stage and histology of the tumor. Staging of testicular cancer is vital. Briefly, stage I disease involves the testis, epididymis, or spermatic cord only. Stage IIA disease has progressed to the retroperitoneal lymph nodes, with nodes less than 2 cm in size. In stage IIB, retroperitoneal nodes are between 2 and 5 cm in size; stage IIC is characterized by nodes greater than 5 cm. Stage III disease demonstrates metastatic disease outside of the retroperitoneal region. The disease is further formally subdivided to acknowledge the presence or absence of persistently elevated AFP or β-hCG concentrations after surgical intervention has removed all demonstrable malignant tissue.

THERAPY

The therapy of testicular cancer is complex. Early oncologic consultation is very useful, as rapid progress is being made in this area. Clinical trials are suggested for persons with very advanced disease.

Seminomatous Tumors

Radical orchiectomy and node dissection are performed; patients with stage I, IIA, or IIB disease receive retroperitoneal and ipsilateral pelvic lymph node radiation. Since seminomas are exquisitely radiosensitive, these patients do not routinely receive chemotherapy unless relapse occurs. Men with stage IIC disease and higher receive radiation and primary chemotherapy with a regimen that generally contains at least cisplatin and etoposide, and most often bleomycin as well. Higher-risk patients (hepatic, bone, or neurologic metastatic disease, high AFP or β-hCG levels) receive more aggressive regimens containing bleomycin as well as an increased dose of cisplatin. High-dose therapies with stem cell rescue are also under investigation, as are other salvage chemotherapeutic agents.

Nonseminomatous Tumors

Patients with stage I cancer who have no lymphatic, vascular, or other invasion of tumor receive orchiectomy with subsequent surveillance, or orchiectomy with nerve-sparing retroperitoneal lymph node dissection. The complications of this surgical intervention include infertility and retrograde ejaculation. Stage I disease with adjacent tissue invasion requires retroperitoneal lymph node dissection. Patients who appear to have stage I disease surgically, but who demonstrate persistent elevations of β-hCG or AFP, are treated with chemotherapy rather than additional surgery.

Patients with stage II nonseminomatous tumors are treated with orchiectomy as previously described and either retroperitoneal lymph node dissection or chemotherapy. This type of lymph node dissection can be curative. Adjuvant chemotherapy is considered when larger or numerous malignant nodes are discovered. Relapse rates are less than 35% with nodes under 2 cm in diameter. Patients with larger or more numerous (more than six) nodes have a high chance of relapse, but most advance to remission with two cycles of chemotherapy.

Stage IIC and more advanced disease is treated initially with chemotherapy as described previously for seminomatous disease. High-dose chemotherapy, stem cell rescue, and other salvage chemotherapy regimens containing ifosfamide may be utilized for patients who do not have a complete remission with initial chemotherapy or who relapse. Paclitaxel regimens are also under study.

DISPOSITION

Seminomas

Chest x-ray and liver function tests are given twice yearly for 2 years and then annually. Most, although not all, recurrences occur before year 3 of follow-up.

Nonseminomatous Tumors

Lymph node physical examination and markers for all patients who do not receive chemotherapy should be performed monthly for 1 year and then bimonthly for 2 years. A bimonthly chest x-ray should be done.

In patients who are receiving chemotherapy, markers and chest imaging studies should be performed at every clinical decision point regarding the cessation or continuation of chemotherapy, or the patient should be changed to a salvage protocol. When the tumor markers become negative, one should follow as if the patient had initially been a stage I patient and repeat the markers monthly for 1 year and bimonthly for 2 years, with bimonthly chest x-rays.

PROGNOSIS

Both seminomas and nonseminomatous tumors have an excellent prognosis, with a true cure rate greater than 90% when the patient has limited (stages I and IIA) disease. Cure rates are lower with more advanced disease, but significant remissions occur. If the disease does not recur within 5 years, the chances for a true cure are high.

Prevention

Death from testicular cancer is almost totally preventable. Integrating testicular self-examination with interval clinician examination at every routine physical would ensure the early diagnosis of local disease, with an attendant 97 to 98% cure rate.

Patient Education

The diagnosis of testicular cancer in a young male can be psychologically devastating. Thorough discussions concerning the usual efficacy of treatment and an expedited staging evaluation are excellent ways to enhance a patient's coping skills. Men should be reassured that reproductive function and testosterone production will continue in the remaining testicle and that an implant can be inserted at the time of surgery. The specific details of chemotherapy, radiation, and node-dissection surgery can, however, interfere with reproductive function in the long term, although generally not with sexual performance once the course of treatment is complete.

BIBLIOGRAPHY

Bendetto B: Chemotherapy of testis cancer. *Cancer Control Journal* 6(6), 1999.

Bosl GJ, Motzer RJ: Testicular germ-cell cancer. *N Engl J Med* 337(4):242, 1997.

Einhorn LH: Treatment of testicular cancer—A new and improved model. *J Clin Oncol* 8:1777, 1990.

Lowitz BB: Testicular cancer, in *Manual of Clinical Oncology*, DA Casciato, BB Lowitz (eds). Boston, Little, Brown, 1995, pp 228–236.

Vogt HB, McHale MS: Testicular cancer: Role of primary care physicians in screening and education. *Postgrad Med* 92(1):93–96, 99–101, 1992.

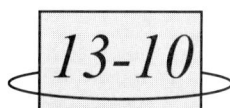

THYROID CANCER
Patricia Kelly

DISCUSSION

Thyroid cancer is a relatively uncommon disease; approximately 18,000 cases were diagnosed in the United States in 1999. Additionally, most thyroid cancers are easily treatable with an excellent prognosis. Thyroid cancers cause only 0.17% to 0.26% (male and female prevalence) of cancer deaths in this country. On the other hand, thyroid nodules can be detected on physical examination in up to 4% of adults. If subjected to ultrasound, up to 50% of middle-aged adults will demonstrate clinically silent nodules.

Between 70 and 80% of the thyroid cancers found in adults are papillary cancers. Among these cases, regional lymph nodes are involved in approximately half the patients. The presence or absence of lymph node metastasis does not alter the prognosis in patients younger than 45 years of age. The mean age at diagnosis with papillary cancer, in a recent large series at the Mayo Clinic, was 44.4 years (Dean, 2000). These patients had a 95.5% 10-year survival rate; thyroid malignancies are indolent cancers with late and infrequent distant metastases, when compared with other head and neck neoplasms. Patients over 45 years of age who have positive lymph nodes or disease outside the thyroid have a poorer prognosis, but comprise only about 20% of patients with disease.

Approximately 20% of thyroid malignancies are follicular; these cancers peak in early middle age. With follicular thyroid cancer, metastasis is usually distant rather than to adjacent lymph nodes. In the Mayo Clinic series, poor prognostic indicators included age greater than 50 years, marked vascular invasion, and metastatic disease at time of diagnosis. Patients in this series with none or one of these indicators demonstrated a 5-year survival rate of 99%; those persons with two or three poor prognostic variables had a 5-year survival rate of 47%.

Medullary thyroid cancer composes a smaller subgroup. Medullary carcinoma is an autosomal dominant disease that may present in a hereditary or sporadic fashion. Between 25 to 50% of patients with medullary cancer present with malignant cervical nodes; between 3 and 10% demonstrate distant metastatic disease. A large series of patients with medullary thyroid cancer in Sweden revealed a 10-year survival rate of almost 70%; other investigators have demonstrated 10-year survival rates of approximately 78% (French Calcitonin Tumor Studies Group).

Approximately 10% of thyroid cancers have very unusual histologies, aggressive courses, and high mortality rates. In general, well-differentiated lesions have an excellent prognosis. On the other hand, anaplastic thyroid carcinoma, though rare, is generally considered incurable.

Risk factors for thyroid malignancy include environmental radiation exposure and, most specifically, neck radiation given for benign conditions. The incidence of papillary thyroid cancer is especially increased in these circumstances. Heredity and congenital risk factors are thought to be rare and do not play a large role in papillary and follicular cancers. However, medullary thyroid cancer is a dominantly inherited syndrome. Iodine deficiency is a risk factor for follicular carcinoma. Females are at increased risk.

SIGNS AND SYMPTOMS

Patients may notice hoarseness or an enlarging neck mass. Rarely, neck pain occurs. Generally, patients are asymptomatic. On physical examination, masses larger than 1 cm usually can be palpated. These patients may have a diffuse enlarged multinodular thyroid, although it is more common to find a single mass. A thorough physical examination of the thyroid gland, asking the patient to swallow during thyroid palpation, is imperative. Adjacent neck structures and lymph nodes also require thorough examination. A palpable thyroid nodule with enlarged lymph nodes and/or fixation to adjacent tissue suggests a malignant process. On the other hand, multinodular goiter suggests a benign process.

DIAGNOSTIC CONSIDERATIONS

Thyroglossal duct cyst remnants may resemble a thyroid nodule, and cervical lymph nodes can be mistaken for an enlarged thyroid or mass.

LABORATORY STUDIES

Chest x-ray, liver function tests, and serum alkaline phosphatase should be obtained to rule out metastatic disease in the lungs, liver, and bones. If alkaline phosphatase is elevated, liver and bone scans and directed plain films of abnormalities on bone scan are indicated. Routine thyroid function tests are usually normal in thyroid cancer patients.

RADIOLOGIC AND IMAGING STUDIES

Thyroid scans reveal nonfunctional "cold" nodules in 9 of 10 of these patients; only 10% of the nodules are malignant. Thyroid ultrasound does not enhance the sensitivity or specificity of the diagnosis.

Thyroid scans should be obtained, however, to exclude functional lesions, although some clinicians omit this step and perform a fine-needle aspiration biopsy, the gold standard of diagnosis. These biopsies have a false-negative rate of 5 to 10%. Since most thyroid cancers are indolent, routine thyroidectomies to reduce this false-negative rate are not recommended.

TREATMENT

Surgical

Total or modified total thyroidectomy is the procedure of choice. Neck dissection is not routinely indicated, since the presence of nodal metastatic disease in patients under 45 years of age does not alter prognosis substantially. Thyroxine is then given to suppress thyroid stimulating hormone (TSH) to subnormal levels and is monitored with routine thyroid function tests, much as it would be in patients with hypothyroidism (see Chap. 5-3).

Patients can receive ablative therapy with iodine 131 postoperatively to destroy any residual thyroid tissue. This treatment has been standard practice for some time, but there are no controlled trials to

validate this belief. Additionally, since most patients with well-differentiated thyroid cancer do quite well, it is not possible to detect the impact of this therapy.

Although most thyroid cancer is indolent, if it does relapse, it is not very amenable to radiation or chemotherapy. These modalities are used primarily for palliation.

SPECIAL CONSIDERATIONS

Hyperparathyroidism can complicate the clinical picture after thyroidectomy unless radioactive ablative therapy is used. Blood calcium levels should be checked 1 week after thyroidectomy, especially if iodine 131 is not utilized or if the signs or symptoms of hypocalcemia appear. These patients may require chronic calcium and sometimes vitamin D supplementation and regular monitoring of blood calcium levels and signs or symptoms of hypocalcemia (see Chap. 5-10).

DISPOSITION

Prognosis

Most fatalities arise from the histologically unusual or rare thyroid cancer variants, including anaplastic giant cell, spindle cell, and Hürthle cell cancer, or advanced medullary cancers.

Patients should be scanned postsurgically; repeat scans should be obtained every 6 months, along with a chest radiogram, for 1 year. Patients then can be followed annually with these imaging studies. Thyroid function studies should be performed every 3 months or as clinically indicated for the first year. After that period, thyroid function studies should be performed as clinically indicated. Thyroid scans must be done in a "hypothyroid" state, and so replacement therapy must be withdrawn 6 weeks before follow-up scans.

Prevention

Known preventive measures include limiting radiation exposure to safe levels and designing garments to shield the thyroid area of persons who could receive repetitive radiologic exposure.

Physical examinations of the thyroid should be performed carefully on all persons, especially those with a history of radiation exposure or iodine deprivation.

BIBLIOGRAPHY

Carlson HE et al: Endocrine neoplasms, in *Manual of Clinical Oncology,* DA Casciato, BB Lowitz (eds). Boston, Little, Brown, 1995, pp 268–287.

Dean DS, Hay ID: Prognostic indicators in differentiated thyroid carcinoma. *Cancer Control* 7(3):229, 2000.

Landis SH et al: Cancer statistics, 1999. *CA Cancer J Clin* 49:8–31, 1999.

McCaffrey, TV: Evaluation of the thyroid nodule. *Cancer Control* 7(3):223, 2000.

Sakiyama R: Thyroid disorders, in *Manual of Family Practice,* RB Taylor. Boston, Little, Brown, 1997, pp 616–621.

Shaha AR. Thyroid cancer: Extent of thyroidectomy. *Cancer Control* 7(3):240, 2000.

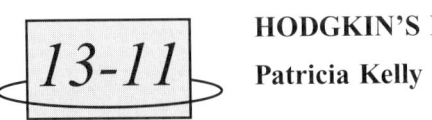

HODGKIN'S DISEASE
Patricia Kelly

DISCUSSION

Hodgkin's disease is a cancer that generally originates in the lymphatic system. It accounts for about 1% of newly diagnosed cancers and is most common in young adults (20 to 30 years of age) and adults above the age of 50. It occurs occasionally in children. Males and females are at essentially equal risk, although some cell types show a male or female preference.

The cause of Hodgkin's disease has not been discovered. Clinically, the disease can present slowly or in a limited area or can progress rapidly and systemically. Current therapy has an approximate 70% cure rate across the board; the stage of disease markedly influences the prognosis. Approximately one-third of patients with advanced Hodgkin's disease succumb to their illness.

Risk factors have not been well delineated. In the United States, the disease found in younger adults seems to be more common with increased affluence and smaller family size. Some researchers have hypothesized that an infectious agent may be responsible; several multiple-sibling episodes have been reported. However, there is no definitive evidence for this hypothesis, and Hodgkin's disease remains a disorder of unknown origin.

SIGNS AND SYMPTOMS

Hodgkin's disease almost always originates in a lymph node. The axial lymphatic system is almost always affected; involvement of peripheral nodes outside the cervical chain is less common. Hodgkin's disease demonstrates contiguous progression throughout the lymphatic tissue. Mediastinal lymph node enlargement is frequently the first sign, encountered on routine chest x-ray. Hilar node involvement often follows. Cervical and supraclavicular adenopathy is common. Retroperitoneal lymphadenopathy is seen late in the course of the disease if it has started above the diaphragm; however, it may be an early sign of disease that originates in the inguinal area. An extranodal site is frequently the spleen. Other extranodal sites are rare at the time of disease presentation but can include the liver and bone marrow.

Constitutional symptoms are present in some cases of Hodgkin's disease (the so-called B symptoms) and are important for diagnosis and staging. These symptoms include persistent fever over 38.5°C (101.3°F), night sweats, and a 10% weight loss over 6 months. The presence of B symptoms confers a worse prognosis.

DIFFERENTIAL DIAGNOSIS

Lymphadenopathy in a young adult should prompt a thorough evaluation. Metastatic cancer to regional lymph nodes should always be ruled out in persons with a single area of nodal involvement. Localized adenopathy of course also can indicate a bacterial infection. HIV, especially in the early stages of seroconversion, can mimic Hodgkin's disease and should be considered in all persons with generalized lymphadenopathy and constitutional symptoms. Serologic tests should be used to rule out viral infection (HIV, Epstein-Barr), which can be confused with the presentation of Hodgkin's disease.

DIAGNOSTIC STUDIES

Physical examination should include palpation of all nodal areas, palpation of the liver and spleen, and a general overview of the patient. Initial diagnostic studies may include a complete blood count (CBC), which can point toward viral or bacterial etiologies; specific serologic studies for virus; a chemistry panel to define hepatic abnormalities that may be present with certain viruses, especially Epstein-Barr and cytomegalovirus; and chest radiography to demonstrate the presence or absence of mediastinal and hilar adenopathy. Skin testing for tuberculosis, which can cause identical constitutional symptoms and sometimes mediastinal adenopathy, is helpful. Mediastinal adenopathy in the absence of peripheral adenopathy strongly argues for a neoplastic origin. If the initial tests are inconclusive for another etiology, the definitive diagnosis is made by means of lymphatic biopsy. Generally, lymph nodes larger than 1 cm that are present for longer than 3 weeks warrant biopsy.

Characteristically, the presence of Reed-Sternberg cells provides conclusive evidence of Hodgkin's disease. These are giant multinucleated cells; however, they may make up less than 1% of the malignant "bulk." There are four common histologic subclassifications of Hodgkin's disease, although a particular histology usually does not alter the prognosis or treatment substantially. Patients with a subtype characterized by lymphocyte depletion have a somewhat worse prognosis; this group is small, however.

After a positive biopsy, initial evaluation should include computed tomography of the thorax, including the pelvis; bilateral bone marrow biopsies; and possibly a lymphangiogram. If there is any suggestion of hepatic or splenic involvement on imaging studies, a laparotomy usually is performed if it will change the proposed treatment. Although it has not been extensively studied, magnetic resonance imaging may be useful in avoiding staging laparotomies.

Staging of Hodgkin's Disease

Following are the stages of Hodgkin's disease:

- *Stage I:* confined to a single lymph node group
- *Stage II:* involves more than one lymph node group but confined to above or below the diaphragm
- *Stage III:* involves nodes on both sides of the diaphragm or involvement of the spleen
- *Stage IV:* indicates hepatic or marrow malignancy

An *A* designation is used for persons with no constitutional symptoms. A *B* designation denotes constitutional symptoms.

TREATMENT AND PROGNOSIS

Surgery is utilized for diagnostic and staging purposes, not for treatment. Radiation therapy is used for most patients with limited (generally stage IA and stage IIA) disease. Radiation fields are dependent on the location of disease.

Chemotherapy generally is utilized for persons with constitutional symptoms and persons with stage III disease or above. Chemotherapy is also effective for stage I and stage IIA disease but is rarely used because of the increased risk and poor tolerance. However, clinical trials are ongoing in an attempt to improve long-term survival. Survival rates for persons with Hodgkin's disease, regardless of extent, who do not have constitutional symptoms are above 80% at 10 years. Patients with stage IIIB and stage IVB disease have a 60 to 80% survival rate. Of persons who receive radiation alone for stage I or stage IIA disease, 75% remain disease-free, and relapses can be managed effectively over 50% of the time with chemotherapy. Persons who have bulky disease, generally stage III and stage IV, especially in the mediastinum, may benefit from combined radiation and chemotherapy. Chemotherapeutic agents have remained relatively stable over the past decade. Most patients are treated with either the MOPP (mechlorethamine, vincristine, procarbazine, and prednisone) regimen or the ABVD (doxorubicin, bleomycin, vinblastine, and dacarbazine) regimen. Some oncologists alternate cycles of the MOPP and ABVD regimens, and there is some trend toward preferring therapies containing doxorubicin (ABVD or ABVD alternating with MOPP).

Persons with extensive or aggressive disease that relapses months after chemotherapy may benefit from high-dose cytotoxic therapy followed by autologous or allogeneic bone marrow or peripheral stem cell transplantation. Fortunately, these patients constitute a minority of all Hodgkin's disease patients.

Recent work has focused on prognostic variables, which might assist clinicians in focusing aggressive therapies on patients most likely to fail conventional treatments. On a recent analysis, seven factors present at time of diagnosis were independent variables predictive of poor outcome: a serum albumin level <4 g/dL, a hemoglobin value <10.5 g/dL, male sex, age >45, stage IV disease, white count ≥15,000/μL, or lymphocyte count <600/μL or 8% of total white cell count.

Prevention and Screening

Since the etiology is not known, there are no specific preventive measures. There is no cost-effective screening test, with perhaps the exception of a thorough lymph node palpation during a routine physical examination. Screening chest radiograms for mediastinal adenopathy are not recommended because of low disease prevalence.

DISPOSITION

Patients are at greatest risk for relapse in the first 3 years. Persons who have received radiation therapy or chemotherapy should be followed carefully. Many oncologists recommend follow-up every 2 months for the first 2 years, then every 3 months for 2 additional years, and then every 6 to 12 months. Examinations should include a standard CBC with sedimentation rate and chemistry panel and a chest radiogram. If mantle radiation was received, routine thyroid function tests are indicated.

COMPLICATIONS AND RED FLAGS

In a primary care setting, it is more common for practitioners to see persons with a history of Hodgkin's disease than to see patients presenting for the initial diagnosis or for oncologic management. Therefore, all providers should be familiar with the sequelae of chemotherapy and radiation treatment.

Elevated thyroid stimulating hormone (TSH) can occur in almost 50% of persons with a history of mantle radiation. Mantle radiation may increase the incidence of lung and breast cancer. Persons who have received gonadal radiation can present with infertility, although the gonads usually are shielded. Men who receive certain types of chemotherapy (the MOPP regimen) will almost always be infertile; sperm banking before therapy should be encouraged. Women, however, can be rendered infertile, especially if they are older than 25 years. Radiation pneumonitis generally is seen in the acute oncologic setting and should not be a concern in primary care. However, cardiac damage, including cardiomyopathy significant enough to require transplantation, can occur after the concomitant use of doxorubicin (Adriamycin) and mantle radiation or high-dose doxorubicin alone. Aseptic necrosis of the femoral heads after the high-dose steroid therapy used in some chemotherapy regimens is not uncommon. Patients treated with certain chemotherapy regimens can develop secondary malignancies a decade after treatment. Acute myelogenous leukemia, epithelial cancers, sarcoma, breast cancer, and other solid tumors have an increased incidence. Some of this can be related to the radiation exposure; the etiology of other cancer incidence increases is unclear.

BIBLIOGRAPHY

Bhatia S et al: Breast cancer and other second neoplasms after childhood Hodgkin's disease. *N Engl J Med* 334(12):745, 1996.
Canellos GP et al: Chemotherapy of advanced Hodgkin's disease with MOPP, ABVD, or MOPP alternating with ABVD. *N Engl J Med* 327(21):1478, 1992.
Devita VT Jr, Hubbard SM: Hodgkin's disease. *N Engl J Med* 328(8):560, 1993.
Hasenclever D et al: A prognostic score for advanced Hodgkin's disease. *N Engl J Med* 339(21):1506, 1998.
Urba WJ, Longo DL: Hodgkin's disease. *N Engl J Med* 326:678, 1992.

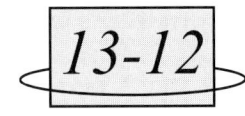

MULTIPLE MYELOMA

Patricia Kelly

DISCUSSION

Multiple myeloma is a type of plasma cell dyscrasia that is characterized by monoclonal production of IgG, IgA, IgD, IgE, or free monoclonal light chain (Bence Jones) protein. Malignant plasma cells gather in the bone marrow and produce these immunoglobulins. It is the most common plasma cell dyscrasia.

Multiple myeloma occurs in 0.00005% of the population and is therefore not a common disease in any age group. It is almost unheard of in persons under age 20 years; the risk increases with age. The highest risk is seen in those age 60 and older; men and women are equally afflicted. African Americans have a higher incidence of this disease and have an earlier age of onset on average. Radiation exposure and chemical exposure (pesticides, petroleum products, and asbestos) seem to increase risk, although the true cause of this disease is unclear. Malignant myeloma causes approximately 1% of all cancer deaths in the western hemisphere.

SIGNS AND SYMPTOMS

The early symptoms are quite nonspecific and include fatigue, weakness, decreased appetite, and sometimes weight loss. Further into the disease course, patients may present with bony pain, frank osteolytic lesions, hypercalcemia, anemia, renal function abnormalities, neurologic symptoms, and repeated bacterial infections.

The physical findings can include skeletal pain on palpation, bruising with petechiae and purpura, epistaxis, numbness, pallor, wasting, and frank neurologic deficits.

Patients with the form of multiple myeloma characterized only by the production of Bence Jones proteins are prone to acute renal failure. Many multiple myeloma patients demonstrate mild to moderate renal insufficiency.

Multiple myeloma patients are functionally immunodeficient and frequently succumb to encapsulated organisms such as *Streptococcus pneumoniae* because they cannot synthesize normal specific antibodies after antigen exposure. On hematologic examination, the complete blood count (CBC) frequently shows a normochromic, normocytic anemia and an elevated sedimentation rate. Leukopenia and thrombocytopenia are seen less commonly. If large numbers of plasma cells are seen in the peripheral blood, very aggressive disease or plasma cell leukemia must be suspected.

In recent years, the presentation of patients with this illness has shifted. Previously, patients were diagnosed primarily with acute disease. Currently, more persons with early, less severe, or localized disease are identified in the clinical setting, indicating improved disease recognition.

LABORATORY AND RADIOLOGIC STUDIES

Routine chemistry and a CBC are indicated. A protein immunoglobulin electrophoresis is also recommended. Approximately 50% of these patients show an IgG spike, 25% demonstrate an IgA spike, and almost 25% demonstrate Bence Jones proteinuria only.

Skeletal lesions are perhaps the most common finding on radiologic examination, which often is prompted by complaints of bony pain. These are osteolytic lesions produced by focal accumulations of plasma cells. The margins of these lesions are sharply defined and sometimes described by radiologists as "punched out." They may be present anywhere but are more common in the skull, ribs, spine, and pelvis.

Diffuse and generalized osteoporosis also may occur even in the absence of characteristic lytic lesions. This frequently leads to pathologic fractures, including compression fractures of the spine that cause neurologic deficits. Hypercalcemia is a common metabolic complication and can be seen on routine chemistry examinations. Increased levels of serum protein are also suspicious for this malignancy.

DIAGNOSTIC CONSIDERATIONS

The characteristic symptoms of multiple myeloma are vague. Laboratory findings on routine chemistry and hematologic tests tend to be equally vague. If the diagnosis is suspected, electrophoresis can guide a clinician to the appropriate diagnosis rapidly. If characteristic lytic lesions or extreme osteoporosis is visualized radiographically, protein electrophoresis should be utilized to exclude multiple myeloma as an etiology before other, more invasive or expensive procedures or imaging techniques are used. Persons with indolent myeloma may demonstrate involvement of the vertebral marrow with magnetic resonance imaging (MRI), facilitating early diagnosis. Multiple myeloma was previously thought to be confined only to the bone marrow, but newer techniques can identify circulating myeloma cells in many patients. The quantity of these cells correlates with disease progression.

TREATMENT

Supportive care of the abnormalities characteristic of multiple myeloma is a cornerstone of treatment. Anemia can be corrected, bony pain can be treated palliatively, and hypercalcemia should be corrected with fluids and/or medication if necessary.

Transfusions of platelets may be appropriate. If renal failure is a prominent component, dialysis should be discussed with the patient as an option.

Immunodeficiencies can be corrected with intravenous gamma globulin; however, this is of limited usefulness. Febrile patients, especially neutropenic febrile patients, should be treated promptly and empirically with a wide-spectrum intravenous antibiotic combination.

New supportive therapies include the use of bisphosphonates to inhibit bone resorption and pamidronate to reduce the incidence of skeletal events. Erythropoietin is useful in anemia therapy and can decrease transfusion requirements.

Oral administration of melphalan, cyclophosphamide, and prednisone is the most common initial chemotherapy. It should be used intermittently and guided by symptomatic improvement. The response to chemotherapeutic agents includes relief of symptoms and improvement in hematologic parameters. For patients unresponsive to initial therapy, various intravenous chemotherapeutic regimens (high-dose melphalan or vincristine, doxorubicin, and dexamethasone combinations) have proved helpful but can induce multiple toxicities. High-dose melphalan treatment has been associated with lethal toxicity in 10 to 20% of patients. Additionally, these more aggressive therapies, though sometimes useful in the induction of a rapid remission, have not demonstrated a clear survival benefit. Results with other novel agents (taxanes, etc.), have not proved beneficial. In extreme cases, younger patients may benefit from bone marrow transplantation.

Autologous stem-cell transplantation has demonstrated utility in patients who have relapsed if they have chemosensitive disease.

Studies concerning the usefulness of interferon α in the treatment of multiple myeloma are ongoing, but its use continues to be controversial. When used, it is generally combined with standard chemotherapy. Investigational therapies include the use of the interleukins and novel monoclonal antibodies. Posttransplantation immunotherapy is also under study.

DISPOSITION

Prognosis

Without treatment, median patient survival is approximately 1 year. Careful, intermittent use of chemotherapy and other symptomatic measures can increase life expectancy significantly to almost 5 years. The natural tempo of each individual's disease greatly influences the prognosis and follow-up. Persons who present with advanced disease (poor performance status, hematocrit less than 30%, severe hypoalbuminemia and leukopenia, or marked renal insufficiency) have a very poor prognosis, with an expected survival of approximately 6 months; treatment may not alter this course substantially. In contrast, some individuals may have a disease course that appears to wax and wane and appear asymptomatic for longer periods. However, progression is the rule, and even if indolent disease is observed, treatment is indicated.

An oncologist will most likely follow these patients. If the primary care practitioner is seen during periods of indolent disease, routine hematologic and serum chemistry testing is appropriate. If disease progression is suspected, repeated immunoglobulin electrophoresis could provide a rough guide to disease progression and help direct oncologic therapy.

Screening and Prevention

Other than an "index of suspicion" on routine clinical encounters, there is no cost-effective screening test for multiple myeloma. Patients over age 50 who present with diffuse multisystem signs and symptoms and have characteristic hematologic and chemistry findings should undergo serum protein electrophoresis to rule out multiple myeloma. Avoiding the environmental hazards, such as pesticides, petroleum products, and radiation, possibly implicated in this malignancy may enhance prevention.

BIBLIOGRAPHY

Alexanian R, Dimopoulos MA: Management of multiple myeloma. *Semin Hematol* 32:20, 1995.
Bataille R, Harousseay J: Multiple myeloma. *N Engl J Med* 336:23, 1997.
Seiden MV, Anderson KC: Multiple myeloma. *Curr Opin Oncol* 6:41, 1994.

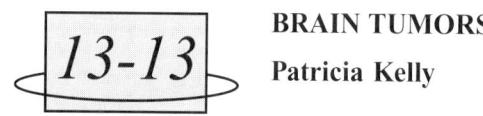

BRAIN TUMORS
Patricia Kelly

DISCUSSION

Primary malignancies of the brain are infrequently encountered in ambulatory practice. However, mass lesions of the head are considered in the differential diagnosis of many nonspecific and common symptoms. The clinician should be cognizant of the incidence of primary neurologic malignancies, associated signs and symptoms, and appropriate referral patterns. Additionally, it is helpful for the provider to be aware of the primary modalities of therapy and the prognosis of these conditions in order to provide appropriate initial patient education and support.

The most common primary malignant brain tumors in adults are gliomas. Gliomas comprise several classes or subsets of brain tumors, including the family of astroglial neoplasms, which is comprised of astrocytomas, anaplastic astrocytomas, and glioblastomas. Oligodendrogliomas are slightly less common. Other common malignant tumors include primary central nervous lymphomas, which are frequently seen in conjunction with HIV infection. In adults, most tumors arise in the cerebral hemispheres. However, in children, many tumors develop infratentorially. Gliomas are not unusual in children and may present in the brainstem. Small cell tumors (medulloblastoma, pineoblastoma, and cerebral neuroblastoma) are also found in the pediatric population. Other childhood brain tumors include ependymomas and craniopharyngiomas, which, although benign, have a great potential for tissue destruction.

Prevalence

Many adult malignancies can eventually spread to the brain; primary cancerous neurologic tumors are less commonly observed. In the United States, the incidence rate for primary malignant brain tumors is 5.8 cases per 100,000 persons per year; 17,400 cases were diagnosed in 1998. Children are also afflicted, although the incidence rate is lower. Primary brain malignancies caused 13,300 deaths in 1998. Lifetime risk is estimated as 0.65% in males and 0.52% in females.

Etiology and Risk Factors

Heredity plays a small role in the etiology of neurologic malignancies; 16% of patients with primary brain tumors have a family history of cancer. Genetic disorders such as neurofibromatosis can predispose patients to astrocytomas, gliomas, and acoustic neuromas; tuberous sclerosis is similarly associated with astrocytomas. Other, more unusual familial syndromes (von Hippel-Lindau disease, Turcot's syndrome, and Li-Fraumeni syndrome) are also linked with various primary brain malignancies. Cranial irradiation, vinyl chloride exposure, and occupational exposure to other aromatic hydrocarbons have been associated with increased incidence of astrocytomas and other malignant tumors of the brain. Tobacco, alcohol, and diet have not been implicated.

SIGNS AND SYMPTOMS

Patient presentation is dependent on tumor location and size. Some patients are asymptomatic. Others have symptoms that are common in many other syndromes: headache, seizure, sensory disturbance or loss, double vision, partial paralysis, paresthesia, numbness, gait disturbance, vertigo, etc. Brain tumors are generally diagnosed after imaging studies are performed during the routine evaluation of neurologic complaints. There are unfortunately no pathognomonic elements of the history and physical examination, since many neurologic disorders cause similar symptoms. Of course, persistent, severe, or worsening headache accompanied by recurring or persisting emesis is particularly worrisome and should prompt appropriate radiologic evaluation and/or specialist consultation. New-onset seizures in adults are very suspicious for intracranial abnormalities and must be thoroughly evaluated. Of course, signs of increased intracranial pressure on physical exam (papilledema), altered mental status, or focal abnormalities on neurologic examination are suggestive of severe intracranial pathology and mandate emergent radiologic evaluation. Brain tumors in children and infants may present with irritability, listlessness, vomiting, and failure to thrive. Older children are more likely to have focal neurologic signs, although many have recurring bouts of headache, nausea, and vomiting without focal deficits.

DIAGNOSTIC CONSIDERATIONS

The differential diagnosis of signs and symptoms of neurologic disturbance includes all space-occupying lesions (primary or metastatic malignancies, benign tumors, and aneurysms), progressive neurologic disorders (e.g., multiple sclerosis) and less ominous entities (e.g., persistent or severe muscle contraction and vascular headaches). Most of these disorders have characteristic signs, symptoms, and patterns of presentation and progression. Since the presentation of intracranial malignancies varies according to tumor location, the diagnosis of a tumor is infrequently based on history or physical examination findings unless the tumor is quite large. Imaging studies, followed by more definitive tissue sampling techniques, are generally required for the diagnosis of smaller lesions.

Diagnostic Evaluation of Suspicious Findings

Computed tomography (CT) and magnetic resonance imaging (MRI) are generally utilized for diagnosis. Plain skull radiographs are not helpful. Lower-grade tumors are best visualized on MRI. Vascular masses are differentiated from tumors through magnetic resonance angiography (MRA). Positron emission tomography (PET) may additionally be useful in the recognition and evaluation of hypermetabolic lesions or lesions that persist after radiation therapy.

The initial challenge in dealing with a suspected brain tumor is to obtain tissue to confirm and further delineate the diagnosis. Biopsy is not a simple technique in neurosurgery and can be made even more difficult when tumors are located in regions where access is technically difficult or dangerous. Advanced imaging technology with guided biopsy techniques, including computerized mapping, robotic operative assistance, and functional intraoperative evoked response monitoring, has markedly advanced best practice in this specialty.

TREATMENT

Surgical resection is generally the initial modality of choice, establishing diagnosis, relieving increased intracranial pressure, and debulking even advanced lesions. Patients greatly benefit from newer computerized imaging, robotic assistance, mapping techniques, and improved intraoperative monitoring modalities.

Laser technology is also utilized to remove tumors from areas previously considered inaccessible to traditional neurosurgical manipulation.

Radiation therapy is generally utilized as well for many, if not most, tumors postresection. In general therapy is, as much as feasible, directed locally at the tumor to avoid the neurologic deficit that occurs with whole brain irradiation. Brachytherapy, or implantation of radioactive materials, is commonly utilized. Stereotactic guidance is used to provide focal irradiation to very discrete areas. Pharmacologic cell sensitizers are sometimes used adjunctively with radiation. Newer modalities permit very precise delivery of high doses of radioactivity, permitting radiotherapy to almost "dissect" away malignant tissue from critical brain areas. Radiation therapy is generally avoided in young children because of the long-term deficits in developmental parameters that can occur and other issues.

Adult tumors are frequently treated with combinations of the nitrosoureas, cisplatin, and procarbazine. Many tumors do not display optimal sensitivity to these agents. In an effort to boost local levels of chemotherapy agents, local stereotactic surgical parenchymal or intraventricular implantation of chemotherapy-impregnated polymer wafers is sometimes utilized. Chemotherapy seems to be slightly more effective against oligodendrogliomas and anaplastic astrocytomas.

As in many malignancies, novel agents are also under study. Tumor-specific monoclonal antibodies hold promise. Early research with gene therapy is also under way. Agents that target growing blood vessels display some early efficacy.

In summary, the treatment of brain tumors is generally multimodal, complex, and rapidly changing. Primary care clinicians may encourage their patients to seek out trials of promising agents. A team of experienced neuro-oncologists, radiation oncologists, and neurosurgeons should direct care.

Special Considerations

In contrast to adults, combination chemotherapy is the standard adjuvant, postsurgical therapy for most pediatric patients, supplanting radiation. Pediatric brain tumors may respond to vincristine, cisplatin, procarbazine, and methotrexate. Radiation, in addition to promoting neurologic deficits in young children, is more likely to lead to secondary malignancies and panhypopituitarism.

Supportive Measures

The diagnosis of a malignant brain tumor is particularly devastating. The therapy is frightening, and the prognosis frequently uncertain or poor. While considerable progress has been made in neurosurgery and neuro-oncology, most adults with brain malignancies will succumb to their disease. Maintaining quality of life throughout treatment should be the shared responsibility of the treatment team, but it often falls on the primary care clinician. Frequent visits and close ties to the primary care team can be useful for the optimal recognition and amelioration of therapeutic side effects. The patient is generally seeing large numbers of specialist physicians and sometimes also engaged in distant consultations or research trials. Coordination of care by the primary clinician is imperative. Family support, with appropriate attention to home environment and significant caregivers, is vital. Treatment for pain, anxiety, or depression also is commonly the domain of the primary care clinician. Aggressive palliative measures are essential for many patients as their disease progresses. Advance directives and other appropriate measures should be addressed as soon as feasible.

DISPOSITION

The 5-year survival rate following diagnosis of a primary malignant brain tumor is approximately 27% for adult patients. Pediatric patients enjoy a slightly higher 5-year survival rate of 59%. In general, the prognosis is poorer with advanced age.

Even when treated optimally, patients must be followed closely for recurrences of residual disease. Second malignancies following radiation therapy can be especially problematic for younger patients. Neurologic function should be closely monitored in the immediate posttherapy phase. Decreased seizure thresholds are quite common and should be considered when other medications are instituted. Primary follow-up will generally be with specialty physicians.

BIBLIOGRAPHY

Black PM: Brain tumors. *N Engl J Med* 324:1471, 1991.

Mack EE: Neurologic tumors, in *Manual of Clinical Oncology,* DA Casciato, BB Lowitz (eds). Boston, Little, Brown, 1995, pp 258–267.

Pollack IF: Current concepts: Brain tumors in children. *N Engl J Med* 331:1500, 1994.

Ries LAG et al (eds): *SEER Cancer Statistics Review,* 1973–1995. Bethesda, MD, National Cancer Institute, 1998.

Shapiro WR: Current therapy for brain tumors. *Arch Neurol* 56:429, 1999.

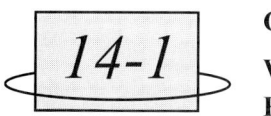

GLAUCOMA
Wesley T. Ota
Francis J. Sousa

DISCUSSION

Glaucoma is a disease of the optic nerve. It is one of the leading causes of blindness in the elderly population. There are two categories of glaucoma: open-angle and angle-closure. The first (90% to 95% of cases) tends to be chronic with slowly progressive visual field loss. This does not become apparent to the patient until late in the course of the disease. Angle-closure glaucoma (5% to 10% of cases) tends to have acute episodes that are symptomatic.

The exact pathophysiology of glaucoma is not well understood. It was previously considered a disease caused by intraocular pressure (IOP) greater than 21 mmHg. Currently, IOP is thought to be only one of multiple risk factors and is not the sole cause of this disease. Other risk factors include a family history of glaucoma, high myopia, African American heritage, and various vascular diseases such as diabetes, hypertension, cardiovascular disease, and migraines. The risk of glaucoma also increases with age, approximately after 40 years. The key point to remember is that individuals can develop glaucoma without having high IOP because of additional known risk factors.

SIGNS AND SYMPTOMS

Open-Angle Glaucoma

This is an asymptomatic disease until very late in the process. It is characterized by progressive, irreversible pericentral and peripheral visual field loss that, when advanced, patients notice as marked peripheral visual field loss. On examination, the eye may appear essentially normal with normal visual acuity, but the optic cup is enlarged, the IOP may be elevated, and visual field testing reveals characteristic visual field loss. Unfortunately, early visual field loss is difficult to detect on routine physical examination. This leaves the primary care provider with screening for elevated pressure and enlarged optic cups as the methods of diagnosis.

Patients older than 40 years, especially if they are African American or have a positive family history, should be screened yearly and referred to an eye doctor if the diagnosis is suspected.

Angle-Closure Glaucoma

This disease presents with ocular pain, decreased vision, halos around lights, and sometimes nausea and abdominal pain. The IOP is usually markedly elevated (greater than 40 mmHg), the conjunctiva is injected, the cornea is cloudy, and the pupil is in the mid-dilated position and minimally reactive. Visual acuity is reduced.

Glaucoma is usually a disease of the elderly, becoming clinically significant after the age of 40. It is most often a bilateral condition that leads to slowly progressive visual loss. In glaucoma, the visual loss is not characterized by visual blurring, but by loss of the peripheral visual field. The disease is usually asymmetric, and the patients become symptomatic only late in the course of the disease.

OBJECTIVE FINDINGS

The objective findings in glaucoma are an enlarged optic cup, progressive visual field defects, and often an increased IOP. Unfortunately, sensitive visual field testing is difficult to perform routinely, making the importance of the optic cup evaluation and measurement of IOP crucial.

DIAGNOSTIC CONSIDERATIONS

The differential diagnosis of glaucoma is that of other diseases causing peripheral visual field loss, including retinitis pigmentosa, tumors, and stroke. The prevalence of this disease is so great that it should be the primary consideration when field loss is being considered.

SPECIAL CONSIDERATIONS

Glaucoma is more common in the elderly, African Americans, persons with vascular diseases or high myopia, and those with a family history of the disease.

TREATMENT

The treatment of glaucoma consists of medications, laser therapy, and surgery.

Open-Angle Glaucoma

The goal of therapy currently involves lowering IOPs to the point that visual field loss is arrested. As discussed, IOP is only one risk factor for glaucoma. Pressure reduction is presently the only treatment modality available. Medications, laser treatment, and surgery are used, generally, in this order. There has recently been emphasis on the treatment of other risk factors previously discussed. Increased vascular perfusion to the optic nerve, neural protection of axons, and genetic mapping have currently been the most recent topics of research.

MEDICATIONS   The agent of first choice depends upon the patient. The following medications are used:

- Beta blockers (timolol, betaxolol, levobunolol) (0.25/0.5%, usually have yellow-top bottles) work to decrease production of the aqueous leading to lower IOPs. Contraindications are asthma, chronic obstructive pulmonary disease (COPD), or any breathing problems; slow heart rate or heart block; and depression.
- Dipivefrin (0.1%, purple-top bottle) decreases production and increases outflow of the aqueous. Contraindications include the fact that dipivefrin may cause chronic follicular conjunctivitis.
- Dorzolamide (2%, orange-top bottle) is a topical carbonic anhydrase inhibitor that decreases production of the aqueous. Contraindications include a sulfa medication allergy.
- Pilocarpine (1%, 2%, or 4%, green-top bottle) increases outflow of the aqueous to lower IOP. Contraindications are that it may cause fluctuations in vision, stinging, or brow ache.
- Apraclonidine (0.5%, white-top bottle) may work on trabecular meshwork to increase aqueous outflow.
- Latanoprost (0.005%, white-top bottle) is thought to work on the uveal-scleral outflow system.

LASER TRABECULOPLASTY   In many patients treatment of the anterior chamber trabecular meshwork with approximately 50 laser burns increases outflow and lowers IOP. This is usually done over 180° of the anterior chamber angle. After 6 weeks, if the pressure is not significantly reduced, the other 180° of the anterior chamber angle may be treated.

Note: (1) The treatment is not a "miracle." It may control pressures in patients that were not controlled on medications alone. (2) Generally, medications must be continued, although laser trabeculoplasty may reduce the number of medications that a patient needs to take. (3) It may have just a transient effect or no effect at all.

SURGERY (TRABECULECTOMY)   If medications or medications in combination with laser do not control the pressure and if visual field loss is progressive, surgery may be required. By far the most common procedure performed is trabeculectomy, in which a new channel or hole for fluid to leave the eye is made, allowing flow of fluid from the anterior chamber to the subconjunctival space.

Also, in some cases tubes with control valves are implanted into the episcleral space. The tube allows flow of fluid from the anterior chamber of the eye to the subconjunctival space, just as the trabeculectomy does.

Angle-Closure Glaucoma

The treatment in this condition is to lower the IOP to a level near normal and then to create an alternative pathway for the aqueous to get to the trabecular meshwork from the posterior chamber without passing through the pupil. After IOP reduction has been achieved the argon laser, or more recently the yttrium-aluminum-garnet (YAG) laser, can be used to make an opening in the iris that allows this flow. The focusing of the laser allows the hole to be made in the iris without harming the cornea or lens.

BIBLIOGRAPHY

Kanski J: *Clinical Ophthalmology,* 4th ed, Boston, Butterworth-Heinemann, 1999.
Newell FW: *Ophthalmology—Principles and Concepts,* 8th ed, St. Louis, Mosby-Year Book, 1996.
Rhee DJ, Pyfer MF (eds): *The Wills Eye Manual—Office and Emergency Room Diagnosis and Treatment of Eye Disease,* 3d ed, Philadelphia, Lippincott Williams & Wilkins, 1999.
Spalton DJ et al (eds): *Atlas of Clinical Ophthalmology,* 2d ed, St. Louis, Mosby-Year Book, 1994.
Stamper RL et al: *Becker-Shaffer's Diagnosis and Therapy of the Glaucomas,* 7th ed, St. Louis, Mosby, 1999.
Vaughan D et al (eds): *General Ophthalmology,* 15th ed, New York, McGraw-Hill, 1998.

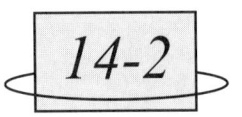

UVEITIS
Wesley T. Ota
Francis J. Sousa

DISCUSSION

Uveitis is inflammation of the uveal tract, the main vascular coat of the eye (the iris, the ciliary body, or the choroid). The disease is usually divided into anterior uveitis (iritis or iridocyclitis) and posterior uveitis (choroiditis). The etiology is often unknown, although trauma, infection, and autoimmune reactions can be related. The inflammation can be acute or chronic, and it often times may recur. The most common form of uveitis is acute, anterior uveitis.

SIGNS AND SYMPTOMS

The classic triad of acute uveitis is redness, pain, and photophobia. The conjunctiva is injected, and often the distribution of the redness is most prominent at the junction of the sclera and cornea known as the limbus. This pattern of redness is often referred to as *ciliary flush.* The pain is an intraocular boring pain that can be throbbing at times. The photophobia is true intraocular pain when the eye is exposed to light (as opposed to glare, when the eye is overwhelmed by glare).

On slit-lamp examination the anterior chamber (AC) has inflammatory cells (clumps of white blood cells) and flare (protein) that has leaked into the AC from the inflamed blood vessels. On the posterior cornea there may be deposits of white blood cells called *keratic precipitates.* The pupil may be small. Vision may be decreased.

SPECIAL CONSIDERATIONS

If acute uveitis is suspected, the patient should be asked about systemic diseases, especially arthritis, bowel disease, and skin disease. Although many different systemic diseases can be associated with uveitis, there are some that are more common: rheumatoid arthritis, ankylosing spondylitis, Reiter's syndrome, ulcerative colitis, and psoriatic arthritis. Sarcoidosis, syphilis, herpetic disease, and other systemic inflammatory problems may also be causes of uveitis.

LABORATORY TESTS

On the first episode of uveitis extensive laboratory testing is usually not indicated. If the history leads the practitioner to suspect a certain disorder, for example, ankylosing spondylitis, then testing may be performed to confirm or disprove this suspicion by obtaining sacroiliac joint x-rays and an HLA-B27 typing.

TREATMENT

The treatment of uveitis should always be under the supervision of an eye doctor. Usually a topical cycloplegic agent (e.g., homatropine 5% drops tid, scopolamine 0.25% drops bid) and topical prednisolone 1% drops every 1 to 4 h are prescribed. Patients are followed regularly by the eye doctor and tapered off the medications as the inflammation resolves.

BIBLIOGRAPHY

Kanski J: *Clinical Ophthalmology,* 4th ed, Boston, Butterworth-Heinemann, 1999.
Newell FW: *Ophthalmology—Principles and Concepts,* 8th ed, St. Louis, Mosby-Year Book, 1996.
Rhee DJ, Pyfer MF (eds): *The Wills Eye Manual—Office and Emergency Room Diagnosis and Treatment of Eye Disease,* 3d ed, Philadelphia, Lippincott Williams & Wilkins, 1999.
Spalton DJ et al (eds): *Atlas of Clinical Ophthalmology,* 2d ed, St. Louis, Mosby-Year Book, 1994.
Stamper RL et al: *Becker-Shaffer's Diagnosis and Therapy of the Glaucomas,* 7th ed, St. Louis, Mosby, 1999.
Vaughan D et al (eds): *General Ophthalmology,* 15th ed, New York, McGraw-Hill, 1998.

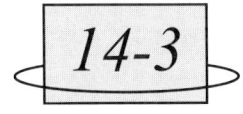

AGE-RELATED MACULAR DEGENERATION
Wesley T. Ota
Francis J. Sousa

DISCUSSION

Age-related macular degeneration (AMD) is one of the leading causes of new blindness in older adults. It is a disorder that involves central vision (visual acuity) and is bilateral, although often asymmetric. The pathophysiology of the condition is not well understood, but it is thought to be a disorder of metabolism of the retina and choroid.

SIGNS AND SYMPTOMS

The symptom associated with AMD is central visual loss. Usually this begins with mild to moderate decrease in visual acuity (20/40 to 20/60), but may progress to marked, severe central visual loss (20/200 to less than 20/400). Fortunately, peripheral vision is spared so that the patient can navigate with mild to moderate difficulty.

There are two forms of the disease: dry and wet.

Dry AMD

This form is characterized by scattered yellow deposits in the macular area (called *drusen*) and associated areas of pigment atrophy (white areas) and pigment clumping (dark areas). Patients with dry form may develop the wet form some time during their disease. The vision loss in these patients is usually very slowly progressive over the course of many years.

Wet AMD

This form is characterized by the above findings as well as by new blood vessels growing under the retina (subretinal neovascularization) which leak and bleed, causing exudate and hemorrhage as well as causing a dark membrane under the retina. Patients with the wet form of the disease often notice an acute change in their vision such as distortion or waviness that was not present days prior.

DIAGNOSTIC CONSIDERATIONS

The differential diagnosis of AMD is that of central visual loss including refractive error, cataract, diabetes, and optic nerve disease. Also, the conditions that can cause macular deposits and/or macular hemorrhage must be considered, such as branch retinal vein occlusion, hypertension, diabetes, bleeding disorders, and arteriosclerosis.

SPECIAL CONSIDERATIONS

AMD should be considered strongly in elderly people with progressive central visual loss.

TREATMENT

The treatment of AMD is based on early diagnosis and patient education. It is crucial that patients play an active role in the daily monitoring of their vision so that they can detect treatable changes.

Most patients do not progress from the dry form to the wet form, but the disability can be devastating to those who do. Daily checking of central visual acuity is important using the Amsler grid. This allows the patient to detect early changes in central vision such as distortion or micropsia (images becoming smaller) that may be the first signs of a subretinal neovascular membrane (SRNVM). If this is detected, a fluorescein angiogram can be performed to diagnose whether the membrane is present and its exact location. If the membrane does not invade the foveal region, it can sometimes be treated with laser photocoagulation. Unfortunately, by the time the diagnosis is made, the disease is often untreatable and will follow its natural course.

Recently, the use of medical therapy including vitamins, zinc, and antioxidants has been proposed as a possible medical therapy to prevent the progression of AMD to the wet stage in which central vision is lost completely due to SRNVM. These regimens are still being studied, and definitive evidence of their effectiveness has not been shown. Protective eyewear against ultraviolet light and smoking cessation are also recommended since these are risk factors that may cause the disease to progress more rapidly.

BIBLIOGRAPHY

Kanski J: *Clinical Ophthalmology,* 4th ed, Boston, Butterworth-Heinemann, 1999.
Newell FW: *Ophthalmology—Principles and Concepts,* 8th ed, St. Louis, Mosby-Year Book, 1996.
Rhee DJ, Pyfer MF (eds): *The Wills Eye Manual—Office and Emergency Room Diagnosis and Treatment of Eye Disease,* 3d ed, Philadelphia, Lippincott Williams & Wilkins, 1999.
Spalton DJ et al (eds): *Atlas of Clinical Ophthalmology,* 2d ed, St. Louis, Mosby-Year Book, 1994.
Stamper RL et al: *Becker-Shaffer's Diagnosis and Therapy of the Glaucomas,* 7th ed, St. Louis, Mosby, 1999.
Vaughan D et al (eds): *General Ophthalmology,* 15th ed, New York, McGraw-Hill, 1998.

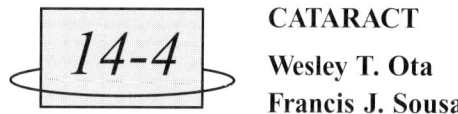

CATARACT
Wesley T. Ota
Francis J. Sousa

DISCUSSION

Cataract is defined as any opacity of the lens of the eye. This means that a cataract is a milkiness of the lens inside the eye, not a growth over the surface of the eye, as many patients may believe. It is one of the leading causes of visual loss in adults. Vision can usually be restored with cataract surgery and intraocular lens implantation.

SIGNS AND SYMPTOMS

Cataract is usually a disease of aging, becoming clinically significant usually after the age of 50 years. It is most often a bilateral condition that leads to slowly progressive visual loss including blurring, distortion, and loss of color perception. Although the disease is bilateral, cataracts are almost always asymmetric so that the patient will complain of one eye being the particularly bad eye.

OBJECTIVE FINDINGS

Cataracts are detected on physical examination with the slit lamp and/or flashlight, but are most commonly and easily found objectively as shadows or black spots in the red reflex with an ophthalmoscope.

DIAGNOSTIC CONSIDERATIONS

The differential diagnosis of cataract includes any cause of progressive visual loss. The most common of these diseases are refractive errors, age-related macular degeneration (AMD) (see Chap. 14-3), diabetic retinopathy with macular edema, and optic nerve disease.

Refractive errors can be detected on physical examination using a Snellen chart and a pinhole. If the vision improves significantly with the use of a pinhole occluder, then the cause of visual loss is probably due to an uncorrected refractive error.

Even though the history of slowly progressive asymmetric visual loss may be very similar in AMD, it can be differentiated from a cataract by the appearance of the macular region of the retina. In AMD the maculae have scattered yellow spots (called *drusen*) and other pigment irregularities, including pigment dropout and pigment clumping. In severe forms of AMD, the maculae may also be found to have exudate and hemorrhage. This form is usually accompanied by severe visual loss.

In diabetic retinopathy, visual loss can also be bilateral and asymmetric. Diabetic visual loss is differentiated by the presence of macular edema. Unfortunately, macular edema is extremely difficult to detect with the direct ophthalmoscope.

The following historical and clinical findings are also important:

- Diabetes history, including diabetic control
- Fluctuations in vision
- The presence of the dot and blot hemorrhages, as well as hard exudates

Optic nerve disease is usually acute, but progressive lesions can present similarly to cataract. To differentiate optic nerve disease, the appearance of the optic nerve head (temporal pallor), the results of pupillary testing (positive afferent pupillary defect), and color vision are used.

SPECIAL CONSIDERATIONS

Although cataract can occur at any age, it occurs most commonly in the geriatric population. Therefore, when evaluating the significance of cataract and the benefits of treatment, it is particularly important to take a detailed history of the patient's visual needs and abilities, as well as disabilities. Systemic diseases must be taken into consideration, and the physical ability of the patient to tolerate surgery must be determined.

TREATMENT

The most common treatment of cataract is surgical removal of the lens with implantation of an intraocular lens. The procedure is performed electively as an outpatient procedure and has one of the highest success rates of any surgery. An increasingly common technique for performing cataract surgery is phacoemulsification. In this procedure, high-frequency sound waves are used to break up and remove the cataract.

Lasers are not used to perform cataract surgery, although many patients will ask about this. Sometimes, after cataract surgery, vision may slowly decrease due to opacification of the posterior capsule. When this occurs, the yttrium-aluminum-garnet (YAG) laser can be used to create an opening in the opacity. This procedure takes just a few minutes to perform as an outpatient procedure and can significantly improve vision.

After cataract surgery, patients are usually placed on a topical antibiotic for 1 to 2 weeks and a topical steroid for 1 to 2 months.

COMPLICATIONS

Although uncommon, infection, bleeding, inflammation, or retinal detachment may occur after the cataract operation, leading to visual loss. In general, anytime a patient complains of pain, redness, or blurred vision after a cataract operation, the surgeon who performed the procedure should be contacted immediately for evaluation and diagnosis.

BIBLIOGRAPHY

Kanski J: *Clinical Ophthalmology,* 4th ed, Boston, Butterworth-Heinemann, 1999.

Newell FW: *Ophthalmology—Principles and Concepts,* 8th ed, St. Louis, Mosby-Year Book, 1996.

Rhee DJ, Pyfer MF (eds): *The Wills Eye Manual—Office and Emergency Room Diagnosis and Treatment of Eye Disease,* 3d ed, Philadelphia, Lippincott Williams & Wilkins, 1999.

Spalton DJ et al (eds): *Atlas of Clinical Ophthalmology,* 2d ed, St. Louis, Mosby-Year Book, 1994.

Stamper RL et al: *Becker-Shaffer's Diagnosis and Therapy of the Glaucomas,* 7th ed, St. Louis, Mosby, 1999.

Vaughan D et al (eds): *General Ophthalmology,* 15th ed, New York, McGraw-Hill, 1998.

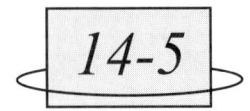

BLEPHARITIS

Wesley T. Ota
Francis J. Sousa

DISCUSSION

Blepharitis is a chronic inflammation of the eyelid margins. There are two categories of blepharitis: seborrheic and staphylococcal. Usually, a combination of both types occurs in most patients.

PATHOGENESIS

Blepharitis is an inflammatory reaction of the eyelids that can be caused by seborrhea, infections, and often a mix of the two. Infections are most commonly caused by the *Staphylococcus* organism, specifically *S. aureus* or *S. epidermidis,* but can be caused by other bacterial, viral, or fungal origins. Seborrheic blepharitis is associated with dermatologic conditions of the scalp and face. This occurs more commonly in elderly persons. More recent studies indicate the inflammatory process is thought to be a delayed or type IV hypersensitivity reaction to the exotoxins of the microorganism. This is a sterile autoimmune response.

The disease starts with telangiectasia and thickening of the eyelids. The chronicity of the disease creates a smoldering low-grade irritation and erythema of the eyelids. Crusting of lipid debris and eczema along the base of the lashes, madarosis (loss of lashes), trichiasis (misdirected lashes), and ulceration develop in the more severe stages of inflammation. Finally, conjunctivitis and keratitis can develop because of the lashes' apposition against the lids. A history of dandruff, atopy, and clogged eyelid glands (chalazia) is common with this disease.

SIGNS AND SYMPTOMS

The most common symptoms of blepharitis are burning and itching sensations of the eyelids and the eyes. Dry eye symptoms are also experienced with lid margin inflammation. There is no effect on vision. Affected patients usually report irritation and crusting worse upon awakening in the morning, but it persists throughout the day. Redness of the eyelid margins and the eye is a common sign of this chronic disease.

OBJECTIVE FINDINGS

Examination of the eyelids reveals accumulation of debris such as scales and crusting on the base of the eyelashes. The eyelashes may be misdirected or missing as the disease becomes chronic. There is often a thickened and hyperemic lid margin because of inflammation. This can sometimes develop into superficial ulcerations. Eczematous skin around the eyes and on the forehead and ears are commonly found with seborrheic blepharitis. The bulbar conjunctiva may be injected as the inflammation spreads to the globe.

DIAGNOSTIC CONSIDERATIONS

Active infection of the eyelid margins can occur from various etiologies, most commonly

- *Staphylococcus*
- Gram-negative microorganisms
- Herpes simplex virus
- *Streptococcus*
- Mites
- Herpes zoster virus

PHARMACOLOGIC TREATMENT

There are no medications that will cure blepharitis. Because it is a chronically occurring disease, only supportive measures are beneficial in keeping the inflammation under control.

SUPPORTIVE MEASURES

The treatment of blepharitis primarily involves eyelid hygiene, as eye drops alone will not resolve the symptoms. The goal is to remove or minimize the offending organism or antigenic cause, thereby reducing the chronic disease process.

Eyelid hygiene should be performed first by placing a warm compress over the eyelid margins for a few minutes to soften and loosen the debris. Next, a cotton-tipped applicator should be dipped into a mixture of half baby shampoo and half water. The upper and lower eyelid margins and eyelash base should be scrubbed with the applicator followed by a rinsing with regular tap water. This should be performed twice a day, and symptoms will diminish in approximately 2 weeks. Because this is usually a chronic problem, lid scrubs should be performed on a regular basis even after the symptoms have resolved. There are commercial lid scrub mixtures that can be purchased that serve the same purpose (Eye-Scrub, Ocusoft). Artificial tears can be used in addition to lid hygiene in order to reduce dry eye symptoms. Cold compresses can be used to decrease inflammation and promote vasoconstriction. Hypertonic saline solution soaks against the eyelid can reduce edema.

Treatment of seborrheic blepharitis should also include dermatologic management of the face and scalp.

PATIENT EDUCATION

Patients should be advised that this is a chronic disease and symptoms will recur unless lid hygiene is done on a regular basis. It is important that the lid scrubs are done properly, emphasizing scrubbing at the base of the lashes, as most failures occur when the skin of the eyelid is scrubbed and not the margins. Symptomatic relief will take approximately 2 to 3 weeks of regular lid hygiene.

DISPOSITION

A follow-up should be done in 1 month to determine whether symptoms and signs have regressed. A review of proper steps in lid hygiene should be emphasized.

COMPLICATIONS AND RED FLAGS

Severe chronic blepharitis can potentially cause corneal ulcerations that can impair vision. Any patient who complains of ocular surface pain should seek consultation by an eye doctor. Primary care providers should not consider using steroids as part of the treatment plan. There can be severely detrimental outcomes if steroids are used inappropriately.

BIBLIOGRAPHY

Arffa RC, Grayson M: *Grayson's Diseases of the Cornea,* 4th ed, St. Louis, Mosby-Year Book, 1997.
Kanski J: *Clinical Ophthalmology,* 4th ed, Boston, Butterworth-Heinemann, 1999.
Kaufman HE et al (eds): *The Cornea,* 2d ed, Boston, Butterworth-Heinemann, 1997.
Newell FW: *Ophthalmology—Principles and Concepts,* 8th ed, St. Louis, Mosby-Year Book, 1996.
Rhee DJ, Pyfer MF (eds): *The Wills Eye Manual—Office and Emergency Room Diagnosis and Treatment of Eye Disease,* 3d ed, Philadelphia, Lippincott Williams & Wilkins, 1999.
Spalton DJ et al (eds): *Atlas of Clinical Ophthalmology,* 2d ed, St. Louis, Mosby-Year Book, 1994.
Stamper RL et al: *Becker-Shaffer's Diagnosis and Therapy of the Glaucomas,* 7th ed. St. Louis, Mosby, 1999.
Vaughan D et al (eds): *General Ophthalmology,* 15th ed. New York, McGraw-Hill, 1998.

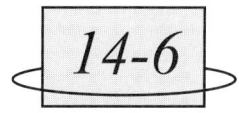

ORBITAL CELLULITIS
Wesley T. Ota
Francis J. Sousa

DISCUSSION

Orbital cellulitis is an acute infection of the orbital tissue of the eye. It is a very ominous infection that requires prompt treatment and hospital admission. It can cause permanent vision loss, intracranial infection, and potentially death if not treated appropriately.

PATHOGENESIS

Orbital cellulitis is an infection that occurs through vascular extensions to the orbit, vascular channels connecting to the adjacent sinuses, or postocular surgery. The most common cause of orbital cellulitis is paranasal sinusitis. The sinuses form the orbicularis oculi muscle except for the lateral aspect. The frontal sinus is found above, the ethmoid and sphenoid sinuses medially, and the maxillary sinus on the floor of the orbit. They are potential entrance ports of mucosal infections. A sheet of fascia called the *orbital septum* is the anterior-most aspect of the orbital cavity. It is a protective tissue that lines the walls of the orbit and extends to the tarsus of the eyelid. The orbital septum inhibits infections entering the orbit from the eyelids. Trauma can cause a break in the skin and create an opening through the orbital septum to cause an orbital cellulitis. Because the venous system of the orbit does not have valves, there are open communications with vessels of the nasal cavity, the face, and the sinuses, potentially leading to infections.

SIGNS AND SYMPTOMS

The common symptoms of orbital cellulitis are acute pain and warmth around the eyes, decreased vision, proptosis, and double vision. There may be signs of a purulent discharge because of the infection, diffuse lid swelling, conjunctival hyperemia, and a febrile illness.

OBJECTIVE FINDINGS

Initially, eyelids are tender, warm, and erythematous. The patient commonly possesses a febrile illness because of the infection and usually presents to the office with a unilateral swollen and closed eyelid. Purulent discharge is often present. The eyelid must be raised in order to determine visual acuity. Vision can be reduced in orbital cellulitis as the disease progresses but is not affected in a similar-appearing inflammation called *preseptal cellulitis.* As orbital cellulitis progresses, the eye becomes more proptotic, ocular motility becomes limited causing double vision, and pain intensifies because of inflammatory reactions.

DIAGNOSTIC CONSIDERATIONS

The organisms most commonly involved with orbital cellulitis are

- *Staphylococcus (aureus, pyogenes)*
- *Streptococcus pneumoniae*
- *Haemophilus influenzae* (most common in children, especially in children under 5 years)

The etiology of orbital cellulitis includes the following:

- Paranasal sinusitis (most common cause)
- Orbital trauma (causing injury to and penetration through the orbital septum)
- Dental infections (through the maxillary sinus)
- Eye surgery complications (retinal reattachment, strabismus)
- Bacteremia

A list of differential diagnoses includes the following:

- Preseptal cellulitis (infection limited anterior to the orbital septum with normal ocular motility and vision, absence of proptosis)
- Orbital pseudotumor (purulent discharge absent)
- Chalazion (localized nodular swelling of the eyelid)

SPECIAL CONSIDERATIONS

The most frequent cause of orbital cellulitis in children is ethmoiditis. The ethmoid air cells are widely open at a young age, predisposing that sinus to nasal infections. A child presenting with fever, a swollen lid, eye pain, and proptosis is highly suspected of orbital cellulitis secondary to an extension of a nasal mucosal infection.

LABORATORY AND RADIOLOGIC STUDIES

Cultures and smears are taken to determine the causative organism and to tailor antibiotic treatment. A consult with an ear, nose, and throat specialist is usually considered. A neurologic consult is obtained if meningitis is suspected.

Computed tomography (CT) scan of the orbit should be performed to detect sinusitis, foreign bodies, and orbital abscesses.

PHARMACOLOGIC MANAGEMENT

The treatment of orbital cellulitis involves the identification of the microorganism and aggressive administration of antibiotics. The patient should be admitted to the hospital for intravenous administration of broad-spectrum antibiotics until improvement. Paranasal sinus decongestion can be reduced with local sprays such as phenylephrine hydrochloride (Neo-Synephrine) or oxymetazoline hydrochloride (Afrin), oral decongestants, and antihistamines.

SUPPORTIVE MEASURES

In cases of corneal exposure due to proptosis, antibiotic ointment (erythromycin, bacitracin) or lubricating ointment (Refresh PM, HypoTears) can be used to prevent exposure keratopathy. A cool compress can be used to decrease the inflammation if the patient is uncomfortable.

PATIENT EDUCATION

The patient should be instructed to complete the antibiotic therapy as prescribed to reduce the risk of recurrence and infection of a more virulent strain.

DISPOSITION

Progress is monitored by body temperature, visual acuity, ocular motility, and degree of proptosis. As definite improvement is seen in the orbital cellulitis, an oral antibiotic regimen can replace the intravenous treatment. The patient is examined every 2 to 4 days until resolution of the infection.

COMPLICATIONS AND RED FLAGS

Orbital cellulitis infection may progress even after aggressive intravenous antibiotic therapy. This can occur with intraorbital abscesses and less commonly with meningitis and cavernous sinus thrombosis. A CT scan of the orbit should be repeated to look for an abscess.

SURGICAL INTERVENTION

Immediate surgical drainage of an abscess should be performed under general anesthesia followed by additional intravenous therapy.

BIBLIOGRAPHY

Kanski J: *Clinical Ophthalmology,* 4th ed, Boston, Butterworth-Heinemann, 1999.
Newell FW: *Ophthalmology—Principles and Concepts,* 8th ed, St. Louis, Mosby-Year Book, 1996.
Rhee DJ, Pyfer MF (eds): *The Wills Eye Manual—Office and Emergency Room Diagnosis and Treatment of Eye Disease,* 3d ed, Philadelphia, Lippincott Williams & Wilkins, 1999.
Spalton DJ et al (eds): *Atlas of Clinical Ophthalmology,* 2d ed, St. Louis, Mosby-Year Book, 1994.
Stamper RL et al: *Becker-Shaffer's Diagnosis and Therapy of the Glaucomas,* 7th ed, St. Louis, Mosby, 1999.
Vaughan D et al (eds): *General Ophthalmology,* 15th ed, New York, McGraw-Hill, 1998.

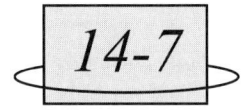

14-7 CORNEAL ABRASIONS AND FOREIGN BODIES

Wesley T. Ota
Francis J. Sousa

DESCRIPTION

Corneal abrasions are superficial irregularities of the cornea caused by a foreign object. The object itself may still be present in the eye, or it may have merely scraped the cornea as in the case of a fingernail or a mascara brush. Pain, photophobia, and redness are the usual symptoms and signs related to the corneal insult.

PATHOGENESIS

The corneal epithelium, the most superficial layer of the cornea, is prone to abrasions by sharp objects or objects with significant force applied to the cornea. The insult causes a disruption of the smooth epithelial surface. Because there are an abundance of pain fibers in the cornea originating from the trigeminal nerve (cranial nerve V), intense pain, redness, and tearing occur with even minor abrasions. The epithelial insult stimulates an inflammatory process of the eye. Because the cornea is essentially avascular, no significant changes are observed. However, the conjunctiva and periorbital area become hyperemic and edematous. Pain thresholds are reduced. All these factors are associated with the release of inflammatory chemical mediators such as prostaglandins, histamine, and bradykinins. The metabolism of the cornea is so high that many superficial corneal abrasions will heal within 1 day as cells multiply and slide over to cover the defect. Deeper or larger abrasions may take 4 to 5 days depending on the severity.

SIGNS AND SYMPTOMS

The hallmark symptom of a foreign body or corneal abrasion is acute pain because of the abundant number of pain receptors in the cornea. As the cornea becomes traumatized, these pain receptors are enhanced which leads to heightened pain. The patient may experience less pain if the eyelid is lifted above the cornea. This can occur because of two reasons: there is minimal contact of the eyelid with the disrupted cornea causing less insult to this area, or the foreign object under the upper lid will not cause additional insult to the cornea as it is raised. Photophobia (pain induced by light), hyperemia, and increased tearing are commonly associated with corneal abrasions and foreign bodies.

OBJECTIVE FINDINGS

Visual acuity can be decreased if the central cornea is affected. The patient commonly presents to the clinic with the eye closed because of pain and sensitivity to light. Profuse tearing is usually associated with corneal abrasions. The bulbar conjunctiva is diffusely hyperemic on external examination. If the patient is unable to open the eye because of pain, a topical ophthalmic anesthetic drop can be used to reduce discomfort so that the eye can be examined. This is recommended as a final resort, as a patient with residual foreign bodies in the eye may be asymptomatic until the anesthetic effect is diminished. This usually occurs after the patient leaves the clinic and has returned home. In cases of disrupted corneal epithelium, the crisp reflection of a penlight will be irregular on external examination. Upon application of a fluorescein strip, the disrupted corneal epithelium will stain green under a cobalt blue or black light. The appearance of the stain may be linear, usually vertically oriented, in foreign body tracks from an object under the upper lid. A pooling of fluorescein will occur around an object embedded in the cornea. Generalized staining will occur in a corneal abrasion with its pattern being dependent on the object that caused the abrasion. For example, a blunt object will cause a wide epithelial stain, whereas a fingernail will cause a narrow and linear stain. The lids should be everted and evaluated if the history and findings support evidence of a foreign body in the eye. The magnification of a biomicroscope (slit lamp) is used for the best evaluation of the cornea. Burton lamps with fluorescein strips, ocular lens loupes, and gross observation are other methods of corneal evaluation.

DIAGNOSTIC CONSIDERATIONS

The differential diagnosis of an acute painful red eye includes the following:

- *Iritis:* injection localized at the limbus, miotic pupil, and decreased vision
- *Angle-closure glaucoma:* diffuse red eye, a mid-dilated pupil, corneal edema, and high intraocular pressures

TREATMENT

Pharmacologic Management

The goal of management of a corneal abrasion is to promote re-epithelialization. The corneal epithelium is the protective layer of the eye. During the interim, the cornea must be protected from bacterial infection entering the disrupted epithelium, and the patient kept comfortable. If there is pain involved with the abrasion, pressure patching the eye for 24 h will increase comfort as well as increase the rate of healing. The patch should be applied with adequate pressure rather than loosely so that the eyeball cannot move and further disrupt the cornea. A topical antibiotic ointment (bacitracin, erythromycin, tobramycin) is used prophylactically under the eye patch to prevent secondary infections. A secondary iritis can develop from spasm of the ciliary body muscle, which is a reflex from eye pain. A topical drop of a cycloplegic agent (scopolamine 0.25%, homatropine 5%, cyclopentolate 1%) is instilled prior to patching to paralyze the muscle and reduce the risk of iritis. This also decreases intraocular pain caused by ciliary muscle spasm. A side effect of this drop is a dilated pupil and should cause

no alarm in follow-up of the patient. If there is a foreign body present in the eye, a sharp object such as a 22-gauge needle or a pin can be used to flick the object off and away from the cornea. A sharp object is used, rather than blunt, in order to reduce further epithelial disruption from iatrogenic causes when attempting to remove the foreign body. There are battery-operated instruments, such as an Alger brush, that have a high spinning tip that can dislodge the foreign body from the eye. If the object is away from the cornea, a blunt object such as a cotton-tipped applicator can be used to remove the foreign body.

SUPPORTIVE MEASURES

Oral analgesics such as aspirin, acetaminophen, and ibuprofen can be considered for the pain. More potent analgesics such as tramadol hydrochloride (Ultram) or acetaminophen with codeine can be used for more severe symptoms.

PATIENT EDUCATION

The patient should be instructed to wear the eye patch continuously overnight without removal until the follow-up appointment. Should pain increase after leaving the office, the patient should contact the office or an eye doctor for evaluation. An eye doctor should see any corneal abrasion that does not appear to be improving on follow-up. Patients with foreign bodies should be instructed to use protective eyewear when engaging in causative activities.

DISPOSITION

Follow-up evaluation of the patient should be performed the next day. The patch should be removed in the office. Visual acuity should be measured. Acuity may be slightly decreased because of residual epithelial disruption or the applied antibiotic ointment. The pain should be significantly less than the previous day. Inspection of the cornea should be performed in the same manner as the initial evaluation. Continue patching with a cycloplegic drop and an antibiotic ointment if significant epithelial disruption still persists, or if the patient is still slightly symptomatic. If significantly resolved, use a broad spectrum antibiotic drop (Polytrim, tobramycin) qid for 3 to 4 days.

COMPLICATIONS AND RED FLAGS

If pain has not decreased, or if there is no improvement of the epithelium, an eye consult is recommended. Additional foreign bodies, secondary infections, or iritis can be the cause of nonresolving symptoms and signs. Corticosteroids should not be used in corneal abrasions as they can allow easier access of bacteria and viruses through the cornea and into the eye.

BIBLIOGRAPHY

Kanski J: *Clinical Ophthalmology,* 4th ed, Boston, Butterworth-Heinemann, 1999.

Newell FW: *Ophthalmology—Principles and Concepts,* 8th ed, St. Louis, Mosby-Year Book, 1996.

Rhee DJ, Pyfer MF (eds): *The Wills Eye Manual—Office and Emergency Room Diagnosis and Treatment of Eye Disease,* 3d ed, Philadelphia, Lippincott Williams & Wilkins, 1999.

Spalton DJ et al (eds): *Atlas of Clinical Ophthalmology,* 2d ed, St. Louis, Mosby-Year Book, 1994.

Stamper RL et al: *Becker-Shaffer's Diagnosis and Therapy of the Glaucomas,* 7th ed, St. Louis, Mosby, 1999.

Vaughan D et al (eds): *General Ophthalmology,* 15th ed, New York, McGraw-Hill, 1998.

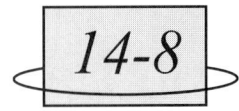

DIABETIC RETINOPATHY

Wesley T. Ota
Francis J. Sousa

DESCRIPTION

Diabetic retinopathy is the retinal manifestation of the systemic disease diabetes mellitus. It is the leading cause of blindness among working-aged adults in the United States. The risk of retinopathy increases with the duration of the disease and the patient's age. Therefore, type 1 diabetics commonly have more complications associated with diabetic retinopathy in their lifetime. The Diabetic Control and Complication Trial (DCCT) found the progression of diabetic retinopathy and other microvascular complications in type 1 diabetics were significantly reduced if the blood glucose levels were in strict control. The United Kingdom Prospective Diabetes Study (UKPDS) found similar results in type 2 diabetics. A hemoglobin A_{1c} level of less than 7% is now considered the recommended target for diabetic patients.

PATHOGENESIS

Diabetic retinopathy is essentially a disease of microvascular occlusion. As vessel walls tend to weaken, some develop microaneurysms while others close off, causing the surrounding tissue to die. The early stage of the disease is called nonproliferative diabetic retinopathy. The initial changes may be invisible but continued deterioration results in visible blood or blood components in the retina such as hemorrhages, hard exudates (lipid accumulation), and edema (serum). Further in the disease process, hypoxia will result in cotton-wool spots (focal infarction).

The disease can progress and lead to a stage called proliferative diabetic retinopathy. Hypoxic tissue will release an angiogenesis factor triggering the growth of new vessels to supply oxygen. This is known as *neovascularization*. These new vessels are fragile and can break, resulting in a vitreous hemorrhage. In conjunction with the neovascularization, there are fibrocytes that proliferate and contain contractile proteins that shrink the fibrovascular stalk growing into the vitreous. They cause traction of the retina that can lead to a retinal detachment or a vitreous hemorrhage.

SIGNS AND SYMPTOMS

There are usually no symptoms in patients with nonproliferative or proliferative diabetic retinopathy. Visual acuity may be decreased if significant leakage of blood vessels occurs in the macula. Many patients will notice daily changes in their vision as their blood sugar fluctuates. This causes changes in the thickness of the crystalline lens of the eye, resulting in non–vision-threatening refractive error shifts. In cases of acute retinal detachments in severe diabetic retinopathy, patients may experience loss of vision, flashing lights, or an increasing number of new floaters in the eye. Vitreous hemorrhages can cause the same symptoms.

OBJECTIVE FINDINGS

Visual acuity may or may not be affected in diabetic retinopathy. Upon fundus examination, hemorrhages (red), exudates (yellow), and cotton-wool spots (white) may be scattered throughout the fundus. Decreased visual acuity and an absence of a red reflex may occur with a retinal detachment or vitreous hemorrhage. A thorough evaluation can be done only through a dilated pupil.

DIAGNOSTIC CONSIDERATIONS

In addition to diabetic retinopathy, hemorrhages in the retina can be caused by a variety of other vascular diseases, most commonly:

- Central retinal vein occlusions
- Branch retinal vein occlusions
- Hypertensive retinopathy
- Blood hyperviscosity syndrome

TREATMENT

Diabetic changes may occur in the peripheral retina, which cannot be seen solely through a direct ophthalmoscope. Diabetic retinopathy is best monitored and managed by eye care practitioners. They have the topical ophthalmic agents available to dilate the eye as well as additional instruments to view the entire fundus. Patients should be asked when their last dilated fundus examination was performed. If they are unsure, ask if they received dark glasses upon leaving the office. Confusion exists if patients are asked if drops were placed in the eye because eye drops that are commonly used to measure intraocular pressures do not dilate the eyes. The following are the recommended guidelines for the frequency of dilated retinal evaluations in diabetics.

1. Type 1 diabetes

- 5 years after diagnosis of diabetes
- At puberty if diagnosis is prior to that
- At least annually thereafter

2. Type 2 diabetes

- Upon diagnosis of diabetes
- At least annually thereafter

Surgical Treatment

Laser instruments are used to cauterize leaking blood vessels or to reduce the oxygen demand of the retina. In cases of retinal detachments or vitreous hemorrhages, surgical vitrectomy and retinal attachment are performed in an attempt to restore as much visual function as possible.

PATIENT EDUCATION

Regulating blood sugar levels to acceptable levels is crucial in reducing the risk of complication of diabetic retinopathy as well as other organ problems. Routine schedules of dilated retinal examinations by eye care practitioners, at least annually, should be emphasized to the patient. Symptoms that require immediate referrals are listed under "Complications and Red Flags" and should be explained to the patient.

DISPOSITION

Proper education should be reviewed emphasizing a dilated fundus examination at least annually and more frequently if recommended by the patient's eye care provider.

COMPLICATIONS AND RED FLAGS

Diabetic retinopathy is the leading cause of blindness among the working-age population in the United States. There are certain symptoms that require immediate referral to an eye doctor. These are symptoms of retinal detachment or vitreous hemorrhage.

The following symptoms warrant immediate eye care practitioner referral:

- New onset of floaters
- Sudden decreased vision (centrally or peripherally)
- Flashes of light

In cases where loss of functional vision has developed, consultation with a low-vision specialist is recommended. They are eye care practitioners who can prescribe magnifiers, telescopes, and other optical and nonoptical aids to assist the patient who has visual impairment related to diabetes or other visually impairing eye diseases.

Diabetes is a disease of multiorgan complications. A team approach and communication among all involved health care providers are crucial in minimizing complications created by this potentially debilitating disease.

BIBLIOGRAPHY

Alexander CL: *Primary Care of the Posterior Segment,* 2d ed, New York, McGraw-Hill, 1998.

Kanski J: *Clinical Ophthalmology,* 4th ed, Boston, Butterworth-Heinemann, 1999.

Newell FW: *Ophthalmology—Principles and Concepts,* 8th ed, St. Louis, Mosby-Year Book, 1996.

Rhee DJ, Pyfer MF (eds): *The Wills Eye Manual—Office and Emergency Room Diagnosis and Treatment of Eye Disease,* 3d ed, Philadelphia, Lippincott Williams & Wilkins, 1999.

Spalton DJ et al (eds): *Atlas of Clinical Ophthalmology,* 2d ed, St. Louis, Mosby-Year Book, 1994.

Stamper RL et al: *Becker-Shaffer's Diagnosis and Therapy of the Glaucomas,* 7th ed, St. Louis, Mosby, 1999.

Vaughan D et al (eds): *General Ophthalmology,* 15th ed, New York, McGraw-Hill, 1998.

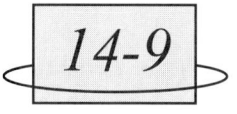

14-9

ENTROPION AND ECTROPION

Wesley T. Ota

Francis J. Sousa

DESCRIPTION

Entropion and ectropion are abnormal appositions of the eyelid margins. *Entropion* occurs when the eyelid margin is turned inward, toward the eyeball. *Ectropion* is the opposite situation, where the eyelid margin is turned outward, away from the eyeball.

PATHOGENESIS

Entropion most commonly occurs due to an involutional change (age). A complex change of the fascia takes place leading to stretching and disinsertion. Cicatricial causes create shrinkage and foreshortening of the conjunctiva resulting in a pulling of the lid margin inward.

In ectropion, the most common cause again is involutional. This results from a lengthening of the lower medial and lateral aspect of the eyelid margin. In cicatricial ectropion, there is a shortening of the laminar portion of the skin on the eyelid. Trauma, such as burns or scars, can cause the shrinkage of this tissue. Palsy of the facial nerve can paralyze the lower lid muscles and give them a laxity, causing ectropion.

SIGNS AND SYMPTOMS

Entropion and ectropion can both cause irritation of the eye. There can be excessive tearing and sensitivity to light, as well as foreign body sensation of the eye. In some occasions, the patient may be asymptomatic. The eye is commonly red because of dryness or irritation.

OBJECTIVE FINDINGS

The diagnosis can be made on the external examination of the eye. In entropion, the entire lid margin, most commonly the lower, is rolled inward toward the eye. A portion or entire row of eyelashes can be hidden since the margin is turned inward. Eyelashes can commonly be seen against the eyeball itself as they are rolled inward. Redness and tearing can occur from irritation of the eyelashes against the cornea producing a foreign body insult. Tear dysfunctions can also occur because of the interruption of the tear layer by the eyelashes and lid margin against the eye.

In ectropion, the lower lid margin droops outward, away from the globe. The pink palpebral conjunctiva is often visible because there is poor apposition of the eyelid to the globe. This does not occur in the upper eyelid as gravitational forces allow the lid to rest upon the eyeball. There is often a false sign of excessive tearing because the tear drainage channel of the lower nasal puncta is not in proper position. Rather than flowing out through the puncta, the tears flow over the lid margin. However, excess tearing and irritation of the eye can occur since the inferior globe and inner eyelids are exposed to air and cause dryness. This can produce a reflex hypersecretion of tears to offset the dry eye. The cornea can show irregularities upon evaluation with fluorescein stain because of exposure to air. As the irregularity progresses, keratinization of the conjunctiva can develop secondary to the chronic severe exposure and dryness.

Visual acuity should not be affected in pure entropion and ectropion conditions. Keratopathy may develop as a secondary complication and should be assessed with a fluorescein strip and a cobalt blue light.

DIAGNOSTIC CONSIDERATIONS

Entropion, or the inward-turned eyelid, can occur from the following etiologies:

- Aging
- Spastic conditions; caused by acute lid swelling; resolves after swelling decreases
- Congenital causes
- Cicatricial causes; caused by trauma, chemical injuries, and inflammatory processes such as trachoma; conjunctiva develops submucosal scarring and vascularization resulting in conjunctival shrinkage and loss of mucus-producing cells

Ectropion, or the outward-turned eyelid, can be caused by the following:

- Aging
- Facial nerve palsy (cranial nerve VII)
- Congenital causes
- Cicatricial causes

The differential diagnosis of entropion includes trichiasis. The same type of symptoms can occur, but the cause is the misdirection of eyelashes toward the globe with a regular lid margin. Trichiasis commonly occurs with chronic inflammation of the eyelids, known as *blepharitis* (see Chap. 14-5).

TREATMENT

Pharmacologic Management

Artificial tears should be used in both situations to keep the eye lubricated. Because of the frequent applications, a preservative-free artificial tear product should be considered. Carboxymethylcellulose 1% (Celluvisc) is often used because of its preservative-free and viscous characteristics. An ocular ointment should be applied at bedtime for lubrication as well. This can be used in place of artificial tear supplements during the day but will impair vision because of its oily properties. In cases of keratopathy, antibiotic ointments (bacitracin, erythromycin) should be applied qid to protect the cornea from secondary infections. Aminoglycoside ointments such as tobramycin (Tobrex) are not recommended because of their toxicity to the cornea during long-term use.

Surgical Intervention

Surgical repair of the lid is required if the condition persists and the patient is symptomatic. A consultation with an oculoplastics surgeon is recommended if this procedure is considered. Spontaneous resolution should be considered prior to surgical intervention in cases such as facial nerve palsy and spastic entropion.

SUPPORTIVE MEASURES

In both situations, taping the eyelid into normal position can minimize secondary ocular symptoms and complications. In entropion, the lid margin should be everted so that the eyelashes are directed away from the globe prior to taping the eyelid. In ectropion, the lid margin should be positioned against the globe before taping. Epilation of the eyelashes in entropion cases significantly decreases the foreign body sensation and corneal complications. Cool soaks can be used in both situations to decrease swelling and inflammation.

PATIENT EDUCATION

Patient education is important in explaining the cause of irritation as well as the management needed to prevent severe ocular complications. The importance of constant lubrication of the eye should be emphasized in order to protect the cornea from scarring that can lead to vision loss.

DISPOSITION

Follow-up should be done as needed in mild cases of entropion or ectropion. If the patient is symptomatic, evaluation should be done in 1 to 2 weeks or sooner if the problem worsens. Patients should be instructed to return if an acute red or painful eye develops. A referral to an oculoplastics surgeon should be considered if the problem could not be managed by supportive measures

BIBLIOGRAPHY

Kanski J: *Clinical Ophthalmology,* 4th ed, Boston, Butterworth-Heinemann, 1999.
Kaufman HE et al (eds): *The Cornea,* 2d ed, Boston, Butterworth-Heinemann, 1997.
Newell FW: *Ophthalmology—Principles and Concepts,* 8th ed, St. Louis, Mosby-Year Book, 1996.
Rhee DJ, Pyfer MF (eds): *The Wills Eye Manual—Office and Emergency Room Diagnosis and Treatment of Eye Disease,* 3d ed, Philadelphia, Lippincott Williams & Wilkins, 1999.
Spalton DJ et al (eds): *Atlas of Clinical Ophthalmology,* 2d ed, St. Louis, Mosby-Year Book, 1994.
Stamper RL et al: *Becker-Shaffer's Diagnosis and Therapy of the Glaucomas,* 7th ed, St. Louis, Mosby, 1999.
Vaughan D et al (eds): *General Ophthalmology,* 15th ed, New York, McGraw-Hill, 1998.

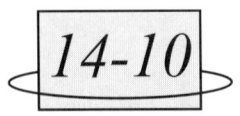

HERPES SIMPLEX KERATITIS

Wesley T. Ota

Francis J. Sousa

DESCRIPTION

The herpesviruses, HSV 1 and HSV 2, are DNA viruses whose natural reservoir is human. The transmission of the virus occurs through direct contact. It is the most ubiquitous communicable infectious virus in humans. Herpes simplex is the leading cause of infectious corneal blindness in the United States.

PATHOGENESIS

Approximately 70% to 90% of the population shows evidence of previous HSV infection by age 15 years and 97% by age 60 years. Primary illness is clinically manifested in only approximately 1% to 6% of the cases. The virus then becomes latent and remains in the trigeminal ganglion. Involvement of the eye is uncommon in primary herpes simplex infections. Almost all herpes simplex keratitis infections present in the recurrent stage and are predominantly of type HSV 1. As the virus replicates on the corneal epithelium, further breakdown of the epithelium occurs. If the infection progresses, deeper corneal tissues become inflamed and can eventually cause an iridocyclitis, an inflammation of the iris and ciliary body.

SIGNS AND SYMPTOMS

The symptoms of herpes simplex keratitis can include tearing, irritation, photophobia, and decreased visual acuity. These symptoms can occur on their own or in conjunction with the others. Hyperemia of the conjunctiva is a common sign of herpes simplex keratitis.

OBJECTIVE FINDINGS

The objective findings of herpes simplex keratitis can vary with each presentation. In primary infections, acute follicular conjunctivitis and preauricular adenopathy are present. There are usually vesicular eruptions of the periocular skin. This should be differentiated from the vesicular eruption of the entire first branch of the trigeminal nerve that occurs with herpes zoster ophthalmicus. There is usually diffuse bulbar conjunctival injection of the affected eye, and corneal sensation is commonly reduced. In recurrent infections, many of these findings may not be present. Often the disease is confined to the cornea. The corneal findings on fluorescein evaluation classically reveal dendritic lesions with minute terminal bulbs at the ends of the branches, but in some cases, the disease may present as minute, diffuse, punctate lesions or as a large geographic lesion.

DIAGNOSTIC CONSIDERATIONS

There are various factors that can induce activation of the herpesvirus, most commonly being:

* Sunlight
* Fever
* Immunodeficiency
* Heat
* Local trauma
* Emotional stress

SPECIAL CONSIDERATIONS

Any person who has a red or irritated eye should be questioned about a previous herpes keratitis, recent trauma, or any predisposition to cold sores. Any dendritic corneal lesion or decreased corneal sensitivity should be considered herpes simplex keratitis until proven otherwise. Pseudodendritic lesions and decreased corneal sensation can occur in herpes zoster ophthalmicus. Pseudodendrites can occur in contact lens wear secondary to contact lens solution preservatives, which create toxicity of the cornea. Although most cases of primary herpes are subclinical, herpes simplex keratitis should be considered in any acute red eye in children or teenagers.

TREATMENT

Pharmacologic Management

Various antiviral agents are presently being used to treat herpes simplex keratitis. The treatment of choice is trifluridine ophthalmic drops 1% (Viroptic) used nine times per day for 10 to 14 days until lesions resolve. The drop usage is then tapered according to corneal findings. Trifluridine, in comparison to the other topically applied antivirals, is

TABLE 14-10-1. Topical Antivirals for Herpes Simplex Keratitis

MEDICATION	DOSAGE	COMMENTS
Trifluridine 1% (Viroptic)	1 gt. q 2 h, max. 9 per day until re-epithe-lialized. Continue additional 1 drop qid for 7 days	Treatment of choice because it has lowest toxicity of topical antivirals.
Vidarabine 3% (Vira-A)	Apply 0.5-in. strip to affected eye q 3 h 5 times per day.	Will impair vision because of ointment form. Can be used h.s. in addition to trifluridine.
Idoxuridine 0.1% sol or 0.5% ung (Herplex, Stoxil)	Sol.: 1 gt. q 1 h during the day and q 2 h h.s. Ung: apply 0.5-in. strip to affected eye q 4 h 5 times per day.	Generally not used unless other antivirals are not ef-fective or create allergic reactions.

ABBREVIATIONS: gt., drop; h.s., at bedtime; sol., solution; ung, ointment.

found to be least toxic to the corneal epithelium. Because the use of drops can be difficult in uncooperative children, a topical ointment, vidarabine 3% (Vira-A), can be applied 5 times per day for 10 to 14 days until lesions resolve. Idoxuridine (Herplex) is not commonly used because of its high corneal toxicity, but it can be applied in case of allergic reactions to the previously discussed medications. The topical ophthalmic form of cidofovir is currently being investigated for the treatment of herpes simplex, varicella zoster, and adenovirus. The use of oral acyclovir (Zovirax) 400 mg orally 5 times per day, valacyclovir (Valtrex) 500 mg orally tid, or famciclovir (Famvir) 500 mg orally bid for 7 days can be taken in cases where topical agents cannot be ap-plied or if bilateral eye infections exist. Acyclovir classification of drugs is contraindicated in pregnant women and persons with renal disease.

SUPPORTIVE MEASURES

Cool compresses can relieve some of the inflammation if the patient is symptomatic.

PATIENT EDUCATION

Patients should be informed about the recurrent nature of the disease and the importance of seeking eye care when significant irritation, redness, or photophobia develops. When seeking eye care for an inflamed eye, the patient should inform the office while making the appointment that there is a history of herpes infection of the eye.

TABLE 14-10-2. Oral Antivirals for Herpes Simplex Keratitis

MEDICATION	DOSAGE	COMMENTS
Acyclovir (Zovirax)	400 mg orally 5 times per day for 7 days	Generically available at reduced price making it cost-effective.
Valacyclovir (Valtrex)	500 mg orally tid for 7 days	Pro-drug of acyclovir but no major benefits except less fre-quent dosage.
Famciclovir (Famvir)	500 mg orally bid for 7 days	Less frequent dosage compared to acyclovir but no other ma-jor advantage. Treatment of choice in herpes zoster be-cause it diminishes the extent of postherpetic neuralgia.

Patients should be educated on the possible causes of recurrence such as stress, trauma, and sun exposure.

COMPLICATIONS AND RED FLAGS

The treatment of ocular herpes infection can be complicated and tricky. An eye doctor who has the proper equipment and time to closely fol-low the patient should manage herpes simplex keratitis and any corneal infections. An iritis can occur in association with herpes simplex ker-atitis, which manifests with symptoms of decreased vision and pho-tophobia. The use of topical steroids is contraindicated in herpes sim-plex keratitis infections as it predisposes the cornea to further breakdown and increased infection. Steroids have been found to inhibit formation of substances needed for the integrity of corneal structure and enhance collagenolytic enzymes, causing thinning and possible perforation of the cornea. Any use of oral, inhaled, or topical corti-costeroids should be discontinued during epithelial infection, if safe to do so. Corneal stroma or uveitic involvement of the eye may require treatment with topical corticosteroids prescribed by an eye doctor.

BIBLIOGRAPHY

Arffa RC, Grayson, M: *Grayson's Diseases of the Cornea,* 4th ed, St. Louis, Mosby-Year Book, 1997.
Kanski J: *Clinical Ophthalmology,* 4th ed, Boston, Butterworth-Heinemann, 1999.
Kaufman HE et al (eds): *The Cornea,* 2d ed, Boston, Butterworth-Heinemann, 1997.
Newell FW: *Ophthalmology—Principles and Concepts,* 8th ed, St. Louis, Mosby-Year Book, 1996.
Rhee DJ, Pyfer MF (eds): *The Wills Eye Manual—Office and Emergency Room Diagnosis and Treatment of Eye Disease,* 3d ed, Philadelphia, Lippincott Williams & Wilkins, 1999.
Spalton DJ et al (eds): *Atlas of Clinical Ophthalmology,* 2d ed, St. Louis, Mosby-Year Book, 1994.
Stamper RL et al: *Becker-Shaffer's Diagnosis and Therapy of the Glaucomas,* 7th ed, St. Louis, Mosby, 1999.
Vaughan D et al (eds): *General Ophthalmology,* 15th ed, New York, McGraw-Hill, 1998.

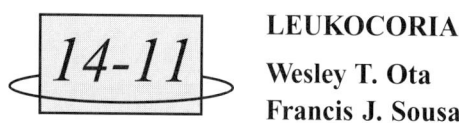

LEUKOCORIA

Wesley T. Ota
Francis J. Sousa

DISCUSSION

Leukocoria means "white pupil." When the normally black pupil is seen as white, or the red reflex as darkened on the ophthalmoscopic examination, the diagnoses of retinoblastoma, congenital cataract, per-sistent hyperplastic primary vitreous, and retinopathy of prematurity should be considered.

RETINOBLASTOMA

Retinoblastoma is the most common intraocular malignant tumor in children. It occurs in about 1 in 20,000 live births, causing about 1% of childhood deaths from cancer. It may present at birth, but usually presents between 8 months and 3 years of age. The genetic etiology of retinoblastoma is very complex. It may occur either as a dominantly inherited disorder or sporadically. About 30% of all cases have a ge-netic basis. Bilateral cases are thought to be genetic, even if the fam-ily history is negative. The disease is hereditary with an autosomal dominant pattern. The disease can be unilateral or bilateral and asym-metric.

OBJECTIVE FINDINGS

Retinoblastoma occurs in small children, making the evaluation of visual acuity difficult. The most common presenting findings are leukocoria and/or strabismus. Ophthalmoscopy reveals often calcified, multifocal retinal tumors in one or both eyes. The eyes are of normal size.

DIAGNOSTIC TESTS

Ocular ultrasound revealing intratumoral calcification is helpful in confirming the diagnosis of retinoblastoma.

SPECIAL CONSIDERATIONS

The early pediatric age group is almost exclusively afflicted. When the disease is bilateral, it is devastating and genetic counseling should be considered.

TREATMENT

Referral to a specialist in eye tumors is strongly recommended. Once the diagnosis of retinoblastoma is confirmed, treatment depends on whether it is unilateral or bilateral. In unilateral cases, the involved eye is enucleated, and careful examination of the other eye is performed regularly to ensure that subclinical involvement does not manifest itself. In bilateral cases, the more seriously involved eye is enucleated and the less involved eye is treated with radiation therapy. Because of the incidence of secondary tumors, especially osteosarcoma, careful follow-up must be part of the long-term management of these patients.

CONGENITAL CATARACT

Congenital cataract is opacity of the lens that is present at birth. It can be unilateral or bilateral, and the etiology is variable, from birth trauma to intrauterine infection. Because vision develops in the first years of life, the visual prognosis in patients with congenital cataracts is very poor.

OBJECTIVE FINDINGS

Visual acuity is generally difficult to evaluate because of the age of these patients. The pupil examination is usually normal, and there is no afferent pupillary defect. On ophthalmoscopy there is a defect in the red reflex, which may present as various degrees of darkness or shadow in the normally orange pupil.

DIAGNOSTIC TESTS

Generally, no special testing is required, but the ophthalmologist may wish to perform an ultrasound examination to evaluate the eye behind the cataract.

SPECIAL CONSIDERATIONS

Because of the age of these patients and their developing vision, it is particularly important to refer them to an eye doctor immediately, since permanent visual loss may develop from amblyopia.

TREATMENT

The treatment of congenital cataracts depends on the severity or density of the opacities in the lenses and the threat to the development of amblyopia. Bilateral congenital cataracts are treated, when indicated, with cataract surgery. Unilateral cataracts have a particularly poor

prognosis, but some studies do show clinical improvement with early surgery.

PERSISTENT HYPERPLASTIC PRIMARY VITREOUS

The vitreous of the normal eye is formed in the prenatal period and is actually the secondary vitreous. The primary vitreous consists of the blood vessels and lymphatics that supply the anterior segment of the eye, including the lens during fetal development. This primary vitreous usually atrophies as the secondary vitreous forms, but in patients with persistent hyperplastic primary vitreous (PHPV) this does not occur properly and the primary vitreous remains. Subsequently the lens is often opaque and the secondary vitreous is not clear.

OBJECTIVE FINDINGS

Vision is usually irreversibly lost in these eyes. The condition is usually unilateral, and the involved eye is smaller (the horizontal corneal diameter can be measured relatively easily). The red reflex is compromised with varying degrees of darkness, depending on the prominence of the PHPV.

TREATMENT

Unfortunately, surgical removal of the opaque vitreous material does not bring the vision back to any significant degree. These eyes are abnormal in other ways, often showing foveal hypoplasia or lack of development of central visions. Therefore, surgical intervention is usually not indicated or beneficial.

RETINOPATHY OF PREMATURITY

Retinopathy of prematurity (ROP) is the condition that was historically known as retrolental fibroplasia (RLF). It is a condition of premature babies who have almost always been on high percentages of inspired oxygen (FIO_2) due to abnormal pulmonary development. In premature babies the retinal blood vessels have not completely formed (especially on the temporal side of the retina). For some reason, when these developing blood vessels are exposed to high FIO_2, they cease growth and new blood vessels form (neovascularization) from the retina out into the vitreous. When this occurs and becomes more severe, the new blood vessels pull the retina off and a total retinal detachment with blindness may result. The condition may be unilateral or bilateral and asymmetric.

OBJECTIVE FINDINGS

These are premature infants. On routine examination of the eyes, the only observation that may be present is a persistent pupillary membrane (persistent tunica vasculosa lentis). This is the group of blood vessels that surround the lens embryologically and atrophy with development.

SPECIAL CONSIDERATIONS

All premature infants, especially those on high FIO_2 for pulmonary dysfunction, should have regular ophthalmologic examinations.

TREATMENT

Fortunately, now that the etiology of ROP is better understood, pediatricians monitor arterial blood gases regularly and attempt to keep FIO_2 as low as possible while still enabling the infant's respiratory system to oxygenate the blood sufficiently. This has greatly decreased the incidence of ROP. Even after the early condition is diagnosed, many cases spontaneously regress and vascularize normally.

For those cases that continue to progress, many different therapies have been attempted. Cryotherapy, scleral buckling, and laser treatment are all modalities that have shown some success, but preventing or reversing the condition is the best alternative in the management of these patients.

BIBLIOGRAPHY

Alexander LJ: *Primary Care of the Posterior Segment,* 2d ed, New York, McGraw-Hill, 1998.

Kanski J: *Clinical Ophthalmology,* 4th ed, Boston, Butterworth-Heinemann, 1999.

Nelson LB, Harley RD: *Harley's Pediatric Ophthalmology,* 4th ed, Philadelphia, Saunders, 1998.

Newell FW: *Ophthalmology—Principles and Concepts,* 8th ed, St. Louis, Mosby-Year Book, 1996.

Rhee DJ, Pyfer MF (eds): *The Wills Eye Manual—Office and Emergency Room Diagnosis and Treatment of Eye Disease,* 3d ed, Philadelphia, Lippincott Williams & Wilkins, 1999.

Spalton DJ et al (eds): *Atlas of Clinical Ophthalmology,* 2d ed, St. Louis, Mosby-Year Book, 1994.

Stamper RL et al: *Becker-Shaffer's Diagnosis and Therapy of the Glaucomas,* 7th ed, St. Louis, Mosby, 1999.

Taylor D, Simmons Hoyt C: *Practical Paediatric Ophthalmology,* 1st ed, London, Blackwell Science, 1997.

Vaughan D, et al (eds): *General Ophthalmology,* 15th ed, McGraw-Hill, New York, 1998.

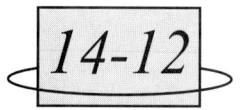

STRABISMUS

Wesley T. Ota
Francis J. Sousa

DISCUSSION

Strabismus is the condition of the eyes when the lines of vision (visual axes) of the two eyes are not aligned simultaneously on the object of regard. By far the most common etiology of strabismus is hereditary or unknown, but it can also occur as a result of trauma, stroke, thyroid disease, tumor, and many other systemic problems. It is most common in young children and requires evaluation by an eye doctor because it can lead to permanent vision loss called *amblyopia.* Visual acuity continues to develop until the age of 8 to 10 years. Until this time strabismus can cause amblyopia, or "lazy eye," to occur.

SIGNS AND SYMPTOMS

The most common presentations of strabismus are *esotropia* (cross-eyed) and *exotropia* (wall-eyed).

Esotropia can be present at birth or shortly thereafter. This is called *congenital esotropia.* It may present later, between ages 6 months and 7 years (usually about 2 to 3 years old) and often has an accommodative component. In either case, one eye may not develop good visual acuity and develop amblyopia.

Exotropia may be present at birth or it may be a progressive problem with age. Often, one of the eyes has a tendency to wander out, and this becomes apparent only when a patient is tired, ill, or compromised in some way. This occasional wandering out is called *intermittent exotropia.* As time goes by, in many of these patients, the eye wanders more frequently and longer in duration. Eventually, it may

lead to the eye being turned outward all the time. This is called *constant exotropia.*

SCREENING ON PHYSICAL EXAMINATION

When performing a physical examination on a child, it is critical to screen for strabismus. This can be done using a variety of methods, but perhaps the two most practical are the Hirschberg light reflex test and the cover-uncover test.

* The light reflex test is performed by shining the penlight simultaneously at both corneas. The light should reflect off each of the two corneas in the same relative location (usually a little to the nasal side of the center of the pupil). If this is the case the eyes are probably aligned properly.
* The better and preferred method for examining for strabismus is the cover-uncover test. This is performed in a well-lit room with the patient fixing his or her gaze at a target, using both eyes. (*Hint:* With young children, it is often handy to carry various finger puppets or other interesting objects so as to assure fixation.) With both eyes attempting to fixate on the object, one eye is covered using an occluder of any kind; often a hand is the least threatening. The eye that is not being covered is observed. If the eye moves, it was not pointed at the object to begin with. If it moves temporally to see the object of regard, the patient is esotropic. If it moves nasally to see the object of regard, the patient is exotropic. Make sure to test each eye.

Regardless of the method used, if there is any doubt as to whether strabismus is present, the patient should be referred to an eye doctor for further evaluation.

TREATMENT

Strabismus should always be treated by an eye doctor. The treatment of strabismus is twofold. The first goal is to preserve or restore the vision in each eye. This is done by evaluating visual acuity and then, if amblyopia is present, patching the good eye. Patching forces the patient to use the amblyopic eye, promoting visual development. Patching must be watched carefully so that there is no regression of vision in the better eye. Also once the vision is restored, it is important not to lose it again from the strabismus.

After any amblyopia has been corrected, the treatment aim becomes cosmetic. When and if the patient or the parents think that it is socially and psychologically important, surgery can be performed to straighten the eyes. This surgery rarely allows the eyes to work together perfectly, but it can do much to make the patient's eye alignment appear normal and it may result in the patient regaining some degree of fusion.

Strabismus can be caused later in life by trauma, stroke, or tumor, among other causes. A late onset of strabismus often causes diplopia. In these patients, the treatment goal is to reduce the double vision. This may be facilitated with surgical procedures, but often prisms in spectacles or an eye patch is preferable.

BIBLIOGRAPHY

Kanski J: *Clinical Ophthalmology,* 4th ed, Boston, Butterworth-Heinemann, 1999.

Rhee DJ, Pyfer MF (eds): *The Wills Eye Manual—Office and Emergency Room Diagnosis and Treatment of Eye Disease,* 3d ed, Philadelphia, Lippincott Williams & Wilkins, 1999.

Stamper RL et al: *Becker-Shaffer's Diagnosis and Therapy of the Glaucomas,* 7th ed, St. Louis, Mosby, 1999.

Vaughan D et al (eds): *General Ophthalmology,* 15th ed, New York, McGraw-Hill, 1998.

Newell FW: *Ophthalmology—Principles and Concepts,* 8th ed, St. Louis, Mosby-Year Book, 1996.

Spalton DJ et al (eds): *Atlas of Clinical Ophthalmology,* 2d ed, St. Louis, Mosby-Year Book, 1994.

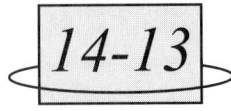

SUBCONJUNCTIVAL HEMORRHAGE

Wesley T. Ota
Francis J. Sousa

DISCUSSION

Subconjunctival hemorrhages are areas of blood located under the conjunctiva. Although it is an alarming visual observation, this is a benign, non–vision-threatening presentation that will gradually resolve in 10 to 14 days. Subconjunctival hemorrhages can occur at any age but more commonly in the elderly population as vascular wall integrity diminishes.

PATHOGENESIS

Subconjunctival hemorrhages develop from an insult to the conjunctival blood vessels of the eye. As a break develops in a conjunctival vessel, blood flows freely through the loose space between the clear conjunctival tissue and the white sclera beneath. Because the conjunctival tissue is strongly attached only to the limbus, where the sclera meets the cornea, an initially focal area of hemorrhage most often spreads and expands prior to its resolution, giving the false suspicion of progression. A traumatic subconjunctival hemorrhage can often obstruct the view of the entire sclera. As the hemorrhage resolves, the color of the blood becomes reddish-brown, the borders become more feathery, and the hemorrhage becomes less dense. Depending on the extent of the hemorrhage, the entire process resolves in approximately 1 to 2 weeks.

SIGNS AND SYMPTOMS

There are generally no symptoms associated with a subconjunctival hemorrhage itself. In some cases, there may be some symptoms of mild irritation. There can obviously be pain secondary to trauma of the eye from which a subconjunctival hemorrhage develops. A red hemorrhage of the bulbar conjunctiva is the only sign alerting the patient to this presentation.

OBJECTIVE FINDINGS

There is no decrease in visual acuity associated with a subconjunctival hemorrhage. On external evaluation of the eye, an area of blood would be observed under the conjunctiva obstructing the view of the sclera. There can be some elevation of the conjunctiva, especially visible at the limbus, as blood fills the loose space below and displaces the conjunctiva forward. There should not be any blood in the anterior chamber, the area behind the cornea of the eye. This would occur in a hyphema, which has an entirely different presentation and is visually compromising.

DIAGNOSTIC CONSIDERATIONS

The etiology of the insult for a subconjunctival hemorrhage can include the following:

- Idiopathic
- Trauma
- Valsalva maneuvers (lifting, sneezing, defecating)
- Bleeding disorders (systemic or secondary to medications)
- Hypertension

A list of differential diagnoses includes the following:

- Hyphema (blood behind the cornea)
- Scleritis (injection and redness of the conjunctiva with no free blood)
- Conjunctival Kaposi's sarcoma (red area usually elevated with a history of AIDS)

LABORATORY TESTS AND WORKUP

Blood pressure should be taken on suspicion of hypertension. A thorough history should be taken regarding trauma, Valsalva maneuvers, and medications. Patients who are on anticoagulants should be questioned on proper medication levels and schedule a follow-up with their internist. Laboratory tests for bleeding disorders should be considered for patients with recurrent presentations.

PHARMACOLOGIC MANAGEMENT

There are no pharmacologic treatments for a subconjunctival hemorrhage.

SUPPORTIVE MEASURES

Artificial tears can be prescribed for patients who have mild ocular irritation. A patient who is on daily aspirin should consider its discontinuation for a few days if safe in order to improve resolution time. Vasoconstrictors have no beneficial effect on subconjunctival hemorrhages.

PATIENT EDUCATION

Because subconjunctival hemorrhages can be quite alarming to patients, reassurance of the benign nature of this condition is very important. If the patient is on anticoagulation or aspirin therapy, questioning about proper monitoring of medication levels is recommended.

DISPOSITION

No follow-up is necessary for a benign subconjunctival hemorrhage. The patient should be reassured of gradual resolution over the next 10 to 14 days. If the presentation does not improve by that time, the patient should contact the office for consultation.

BIBLIOGRAPHY

Newell FW: *Ophthalmology—Principles and Concepts,* 8th ed, St. Louis, Mosby-Year Book, 1996.

Rhee DJ, Pyfer MF (eds): *The Wills Eye Manual—Office and Emergency Room Diagnosis and Treatment of Eye Disease,* 3d ed, Philadelphia, Lippincott Williams & Wilkins, 1999.

Vaughan D et al (eds): *General Ophthalmology,* 15th ed, New York, McGraw-Hill, 1998.

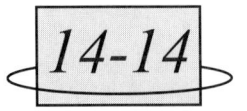

SUDDEN VISUAL LOSS IN ONE EYE

Wesley T. Ota
Francis J. Sousa

DISCUSSION

When any visual loss occurs suddenly and for no apparent reason, the etiology is almost always a vascular compromise. The four major vascular diseases that cause sudden visual loss are:

1. Central retinal artery occlusion (CRAO)
2. Central retinal vein occlusion (CRVO)

3. Anterior ischemic optic neuropathy (AION)
4. Vitreous hemorrhage (associated with diabetes mellitus)

Although the history is very similar in these four conditions, the physical or objective findings make them relatively easy to diagnose and differentiate.

CENTRAL RETINAL ARTERY OCCLUSION

CRAO is an obstruction of the blood flow into the retina of the eye. This causes infarction of the retina and marked visual loss.

OBJECTIVE FINDINGS

Visual acuity is usually lowered to 20/200 or worse. Although the external eye may appear relatively normal, the pupil of the involved eye exhibits an afferent pupillary defect, or a positive swinging flashlight test. The visual fields are markedly constricted. The most dramatic findings will be on ophthalmoscopy, which reveals a pale retina around the optic nerve and macular area except in the immediate fovea, which remains bright red (called a *cherry red spot*); narrowed or irregularly constricted retinal arterioles; an optic nerve that may have somewhat indistinct margins; and perhaps intravascular refractile plaques(s) at the bifurcation of the retinal arterioles (Hollenhorst plaques). This appearance of a pale, poorly vascularized retina with a central red spot is quite distinctive.

The carotid arteries should be palpated to evaluate their pulse and auscultated to evaluate for bruits, which may be associated with carotid obstruction from arteriosclerotic plaques. The status of the heart, such as previous myocardial infarction or valvular heart disease, should also be evaluated as a source of emboli.

SPECIAL CONSIDERATIONS

Often this disease occurs as the result of an embolus from the carotid artery or the heart. It is particularly common in patients with arteriosclerotic vascular disease that is associated with hypertension, diabetes, hypercholesterolemia, and smoking.

TREATMENT

Unfortunately, if these patients do not reach medical care within the first few minutes to hours after the onset of their visual loss, the final visual outcomes are usually very poor.

When the diagnosis is made, probably the most beneficial treatments that carry the lowest risks are having the patient rebreathe into a brown paper bag, which increases the percentage of inspired CO_2 in an attempt to dilate the retinal arterioles, and placing intermittent firm pressure on the eyelids for 10 to 20 seconds with quick release, which increases intraocular pressure and suddenly decreases it in an attempt to loosen the obstruction.

An immediate consultation with an eye doctor for further evaluation and possible treatment is mandatory. Various treatment modalities that are used by specialists include having the patient breathe a 5% CO_2/95% O_2 mixture; performing anterior chamber paracentesis, which involves inserting a needle through the cornea to decompress the globe; and/or giving retrobulbar injections of a vasodilating substance.

Perhaps the most important treatment is to ensure that the underlying diseases are properly addressed and managed by the primary care provider.

CENTRAL RETINAL VEIN OCCLUSION

CRVO is obstruction of the blood flow out of the retina. This causes increased pressure in the venules of the eye, hemorrhage, and varying degrees of hypoxia and ischemia (usually severe).

OBJECTIVE FINDINGS

Visual acuity is usually lowered to 20/200 or worse. Although the external eye may appear relatively normal, the pupil of the involved eye will often exhibit an afferent pupillary defect or positive swinging flashlight test. The visual fields are markedly constricted.

As with CRAO, the most dramatic clinical objective findings are seen on ophthalmoscopy, revealing diffuse hemorrhages throughout the retina involving many different layers of the retina. This is called a *blood and thunder fundus* because of the extent and dramatic appearance of the hemorrhages. The appearance is unique and the diagnosis follows.

SPECIAL CONSIDERATIONS

As with CRAO, these patients often have an extensive history of peripheral vascular disease and diseases that accelerate vascular disease.

TREATMENT

Unfortunately very little can be done to intervene when a CRVO has occurred. Many different therapies have been attempted over the years, including anticoagulation to break up any clot that might be present, but these have proved to be of little or no benefit.

It is important to refer these patients to an eye doctor for thorough evaluation and follow-up. Unfortunately, because of the profound longstanding ischemia, new blood vessel formation (neovascularization) may occur within the first few months. This usually occurs on the iris (rubeosis iridis) and may lead to a very severe form of glaucoma (neovascular glaucoma) that can destroy the little remaining vision and be very painful. Therefore, careful follow-up by the eye doctor is indicated. Usually it is treated medically and with laser therapy to the retina to destroy the ischemic retinal tissue, called *panretinal photocoagulation* (PRP).

ANTERIOR ISCHEMIC OPTIC NEUROPATHY

AION is the obstruction of blood flow through the small arterioles feeding the anterior portion of the optic nerve.

OBJECTIVE FINDINGS

Visual acuity usually is lowered to 20/50 or worse, but this may vary and be less severe. Although the external eye appears relatively normal, the pupil of the involved eye will exhibit an afferent pupillary defect or positive swinging flashlight test. The visual fields show a dense central scotoma.

The most dramatic findings are seen on ophthalmoscopy. The optic nerve is swollen, showing elevation, blurred disk margins, very small or no cup, and obscured vessels on and near the nerve owing to the fluid, and eventually, pallor. This appearance of a pale, swollen nerve with visual loss makes the diagnosis of AION.

SPECIAL CONSIDERATIONS

AION is most often associated with arteriosclerotic disease. An extensive vascular history should be taken and any underlying conditions treated. A special situation that occurs most often in the geriatric age group is AION associated with temporal arteritis. This is important because the diagnosis is easy to miss and must be considered. These patients are usually older than 65 years of age (prevalence accelerates into the seventies, eighties, and nineties) with the clinical syndrome of temporal arteritis or polymyalgia rheumatica. Remember to ask about weight loss, tender temporal headache, jaw claudication, general malaise, fever, night sweats, and proximal muscle myalgias. If the diagnosis is at all suspected clinically, obtaining an erythrocyte sedimentation rate (ESR), which will be elevated in cases of arteritis, and referring the patient for evaluation by a rheumatologist immediately, is indicated. This disease can lead to blindness in the other eye fairly quickly and cause severe systemic problems.

TREATMENT

The treatment of the arteriosclerotic disease is one of controlling the underlying diseases. Extensive research has been done to evaluate the role of steroid use in this disease, and the studies are equivocal.

The arteritic form must be treated aggressively with systemic steroids to control the temporal arteritis, which is a systemic disease. The vision will probably not improve in the affected eye, but the other eye must be spared, as well as the remainder of the body.

Treatment is usually under the management of the rheumatologist and consists of high-dose steroids (prednisone 80 mg/d), which can be tapered as the patient's symptoms improve and the ESR normalizes. The rheumatologist may request a temporal artery biopsy to confirm the diagnosis.

VITREOUS HEMORRHAGE

Vitreous hemorrhage is a usually sudden leakage of blood into the vitreous cavity causing obscuration of the clear vitreous and decreased vision. Although there are many conditions that can cause blood vessels to break and bleed into the vitreous, the most common is diabetes mellitus (see Chap. 14-8, "Diabetic Retinopathy," and Chap. 5-1, "Diabetes Mellitus").

OBJECTIVE FINDINGS

The visual acuity is decreased to varying degrees but may be profound. The external eye is relatively normal in appearance. The pupils are normal. The visual fields are constricted.

The most dramatic physical findings once again are in ophthalmoscopy, which reveals an abnormal red reflex and inability to see the retina clearly or at all. "The patient sees nothing and the clinician sees nothing" would often be an appropriate phrase for this condition.

SPECIAL CONSIDERATIONS

Although diabetes is the most common etiology, consider other causes of neovascularization such as sickle cell disease and previous vascular occlusions of the eye. Also, a retinal tear or detachment may break a blood vessel, causing hemorrhage.

TREATMENT

The initial treatment is to have the patient sit up and stay as relaxed as possible so that the blood can layer in the eye with gravity and allow the source of the bleeding to be identified.

Referral to an eye doctor is mandatory in this condition so that treatment is not delayed. Often a retinal specialist is the best person to manage the problem and treat the underlying condition. In the case of systemic diseases, they must be optimally managed as well.

BIBLIOGRAPHY

Alexander LJ: *Primary Care of the Posterior Segment*, 2d ed, New York, McGraw-Hill, 1998.

Kanski J: *Clinical Ophthalmology*, 4th ed, Boston, Butterworth-Heinemann, 1999.

Newell FW: *Ophthalmology—Principles and Concepts*, 8th ed, St. Louis, Mosby-Year Book, 1996.

Rhee DJ, Pyfer MF (eds): *The Wills Eye Manual—Office and Emergency Room Diagnosis and Treatment of Eye Disease*, 3d ed, Philadelphia, Lippincott Williams & Wilkins, 1999.

Spalton DJ et al (eds): *Atlas of Clinical Ophthalmology*, 2d ed, St. Louis, Mosby-Year Book, 1994.

Stamper RL et al: *Becker-Shaffer's Diagnosis and Therapy of the Glaucomas*, 7th ed, St. Louis, Mosby, 1999.

Vaughan D et al (eds): *General Ophthalmology*, 15th ed, New York, McGraw-Hill, 1998.

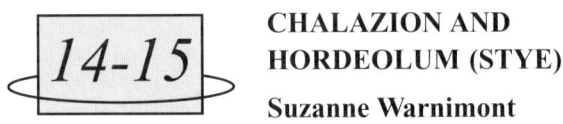

14-15 CHALAZION AND HORDEOLUM (STYE)

Suzanne Warnimont

DISCUSSION

A *chalazion* is a granulomatous inflammation of a meibomian gland of the eye. It is a common non–vision-threatening condition of the eye that can distort vision if the lesion is large enough to press on the cornea.

A *hordeolum* (stye) is a staphylococcal abscess of the meibomian gland (internal hordeolum) or of the glands of Zeis or Moll around the lashes (external hordeolum).

SIGNS AND SYMPTOMS

A chalazion presents as a visible, hard, sometimes tender swelling near the lid margin. The surrounding conjunctiva may be red and elevated.

A hordeolum presents as a red, swollen, tender area on the upper or lower lid margin. An internal hordeolum may point to the internal or external lid; an external hordeolum points externally.

DIAGNOSTIC CONSIDERATIONS

Preseptal cellulitis is associated with an abrasion or site infection and fever. Sebaceous cell carcinoma should be suspected with recurrent chalazion. It causes thickening of both upper and lower lid margins and loss of eyelashes. Biopsy establishes the diagnosis. Pyogenic granuloma may develop after trauma or surgery. Basal cell carcinoma appears dimpled or ulcerated and pearly. A firm appearance increases the likelihood of malignancy (see Chap. 2-7).

SPECIAL CONSIDERATIONS

History should include inquiries regarding a past chalazion excision. Everting the lid may allow better visualization of the nodule caused by a chalazion.

LABORATORY AND RADIOLOGIC STUDIES

There are no appropriate laboratory or radiologic studies for chalazion and hordeolum.

TREATMENT

Chalazion

Use warm compresses for 20 minutes qid with light massage. If the chalazion does not disappear within 3 to 4 weeks of conservative treatment, it may be removed by incision and curettage by an ophthalmologist.

Topical antibiotics (erythromycin ophthalmic ointment bid) may be administered directly behind the lid because penetration through the skin is poor. Steroids may be injected into the lesion, especially if the lesion is near the lacrimal apparatus. Use triamcinolone, 40 mg/mL, 0.2 to 1.0 mL (depending on the size of the lesion), injected into and around the lesion.

PATIENT EDUCATION   If the lesion does not resolve in 3 to 4 weeks with conservative treatment, the patient may choose to have the lesion incised or injected (see above).

COMPLICATIONS OR RED FLAGS   Steroid injection can cause skin depigmentation or localized atrophy at the injection site and should be done only by those skilled with this intralesional procedure.

Hordeolum

Use warm compresses for 20 minutes qid. In the acute stage, antibiotic ointment is instilled into the conjunctival sac with excess rubbed onto the eyelids every 3 hours.

A variety of ophthalmic antibiotic ointments are acceptable, including sodium sulfacetamide (Sulamyd), neomycin sulfate (Neosporin), gentamicin sulfate (Garamycin), and erythromycin.

PATIENT EDUCATION   A nonresponsive lesion may require incision and curettage by an ophthalmologist.

COMPLICATIONS OR RED FLAGS   Hordeolum may lead to diffuse superficial lid infection or preseptal cellulitis.

BIBLIOGRAPHY

Ferri F (ed): *Clinical Advisor.* St. Louis, Mosby-Year Book, 1999, p 236.
Palay DA, Krachmer JH (eds): *Ophthalmology for the Primary Care Physician.* St Louis, Mosby-Year Book, 1997, pp 50–51.
Schachat AP: The red eye, in *Principles of Ambulatory Medicine,* 4th ed, LR Barker et al. Baltimore, Williams & Wilkins, 1995, p 1435.

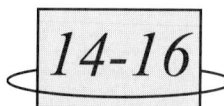

CONJUNCTIVITIS
Wesley T. Ota
Francis J. Sousa

DESCRIPTION

Acute conjunctivitis is a self-limiting inflammation of the conjunctiva, which is the mucous membrane lining of the eye. It is the most common eye disease in the western hemisphere and is determined by the causative agent. The duration of acute conjunctivitis is less than a month.

PATHOGENESIS

One function of the conjunctiva is to protect the eye from foreign objects and infectious organisms. Because it contains a rich vascular supply and many inflammatory cells such as lymphocytes and plasma cells, the conjunctiva often becomes a common site of irritation. Acute conjunctivitis can develop from three main causes: bacterial infections, viral infections, and allergies. This chapter focuses on the discussion of viral infections from the adenoviral strains, although the herpesvirus is another form of infection (see Chap. 14-10).

Conjunctivitis begins with a causative agent that invades the eye. This stimulates the inflammatory cells to migrate to the conjunctival epithelial surface from the stroma. The cells combine with mucus and fibrin and create the exudate that is secreted from the eye. The inflammatory cells involved differ depending on the type of conjunctivitis. Bacterial conjunctivitis has a preponderance of polymorphonuclear cells. Adenoviral infections contain monocytes and lymphocytes, and the majority of cells found in allergic reactions are eosinophils. All of these conjunctivitides are self-limiting because of the high number of lymphocytes to fight the infection, the flushing and diluting action of the tears, and the antigen entrapping capability through the production of exudate.

SIGNS AND SYMPTOMS

The symptoms of conjunctivitis can vary depending on the etiology. A variable amount of diffuse conjunctival redness (hyperemia) is the most obvious sign of conjunctivitis. All types can have symptoms of foreign body sensation, periocular edema, and tearing. The discharge secreted can vary depending on the type of conjunctivitis (see "Objective Findings"). In allergic conjunctivitis, the hallmark symptom is itchiness. Many times, the symptoms of allergic conjunctivitis significantly outweigh the objective findings.

OBJECTIVE FINDINGS

Objective findings are the most important factors in diagnosing the type of conjunctivitis. A purely conjunctival inflammation with no corneal involvement should have no effect on visual acuity. Photophobia can occur when there is corneal involvement.

A bacterial conjunctivitis will present with a purulent or mucopurulent discharge. The discharge is very often greenish-white in color with a sticky consistency. The lashes are matted with this substance as well. There is usually some chemosis of the conjunctiva. Preauricular adenopathy is uncommon in bacterial conjunctivitis. The injection of the conjunctiva is a beefy red color and increases in intensity from the limbus toward the palpebral conjunctiva. The presentation of a bacterial conjunctivitis is initially monocular. The other eye typically becomes involved in approximately 48 h. The infection is self-limiting and commonly resolves in 4 to 7 days with topical antibiotic drops but can resolve without treatment within 10 to 15 days. Acute bacterial conjunctivitis is caused by various microorganisms, most commonly *Staphylococcus aureus, Streptococcus pneumoniae,* and *Haemophilus* spp.

Viral conjunctivitis is generally more common than bacterial conjunctivitis. A viral conjunctivitis has a serous, clear discharge but often will elicit increased tearing. Many viral cases develop occasional mucous strands caused by irritation to the eye. The bulbar conjunctiva is diffusely pink in color versus dark red in bacterial infections. There are follicles, which are lymphocyte germinal centers, present in the inferior palpebral conjunctiva. Preauricular adenopathy is usually present. The history commonly includes a runny nose, upper respiratory infection, or contact with a person who had these symptoms. The onset is commonly unilateral with a duration of 10 to 21 days depending on the adenovirus strain. The conjunctivitis typically worsens for the first 5 to 7 days prior to improving. There is often inoculation of the other eye in approximately 5 to 7 days because of the highly contagious nature of viral infections.

Allergic conjunctivitis presents with a stringy white discharge that has an elastic characteristic. Patients commonly report excessive tearing and itchiness in allergic conjunctivitis as well. There is usually chemosis of the bulbar conjunctiva and often chemosis of the periocular area. Papillae, which are focal areas of serous fluid caused by the inflammatory process, are found in the superior palpebral conjunctiva. The onset of allergic conjunctivitis usually occurs bilaterally as opposed to unilaterally in viral and bacterial infections.

Table 14-16-1 presents the symptoms and signs of acute conjunctivitis.

DIAGNOSTIC CONSIDERATIONS

Acute conjunctivitis can stem from various etiologies, most commonly:

- Bacteria
- Viruses
- Seasonal allergies

TABLE 14-16-1. Categories of Acute Conjunctivitis

CATEGORY	DISCHARGE	ITCHING	PREAURICULAR ADENOPATHY	CYTOLOGY
Viral	Serous, occasional mucous strands	Minimal	Common	Monocytes, lymphocytes
Bacterial	Purulent, mucopurulent	Minimal	Uncommon	Bacteria, PMNs
Allergic	Mucoid, stringy	Severe	Absent	Eosinophils

ABBREVIATION: PMNs, polymorphonuclear neutrophil leukocytes.

- Chemicals
- Hay fever
- Atopy
- Medicamentosa

SPECIAL CONSIDERATIONS

Any inflammation that involves the cornea warrants consultation with an eye doctor. This can be determined by the presence of discharge on the cornea or any irregularity in corneal clarity. The involvement of the cornea would produce a decrease in visual acuity as well. A hyperacute purulent discharge occurs with gonococcal or pseudomonal conjunctivitis. These are serious infections with a severely purulent discharge and the patient should be sent for an eye consult as well. Gonococcal and pseudomonal conjunctivitis can cause corneal perforations and require oral medications and close monitoring. They may require hospitalization. Any person who has a prior history of herpes simplex infection of the eye requires evaluation by an eye doctor (see Chap. 14-10). Any person who has a herpes zoster presentation that affects the first branch of the trigeminal nerve should have an ophthalmology consultation to rule out ocular involvement.

LABORATORY TESTS

Cultures of the conjunctiva are typically not performed in clinical settings unless there is no improvement in the viral infection or acute bacterial infection with antibiotic treatment. Chronic, hyperacute, and neonatal conjunctivitides deserve cultures.

TREATMENT

Pharmacologic Management

The main indication for the treatment of conjunctivitis is to protect the cornea from infection, which can lead to visual compromise. Bacterial conjunctivitis should be treated with a broad-spectrum antibiotic qid for 7 to 10 days. A combination topical drop consisting of trimethoprim and polymyxin B (Polytrim) is an excellent antibiotic. Aminoglycosides, such as tobramycin (Tobrex), can also be used but are known to be more toxic to the cornea on extended use. Sulfacetamide drops are not regularly used in eye care since there is a high resistance to this antibiotic as well as a large population allergic to sulfa medications. Ointments can be applied to the eye for bacterial infections but will impair vision when applied. Because of its prolonged contact time compared to drops, ointments can be considered in difficult cases such as an uncooperative child or an elderly individual who requires assistance in treatment. Ointments can be fairly effective on a bid dose. Tobramycin, erythromycin, and bacitracin are three ophthalmic ointments available for use in the eye.

There are no medical treatments for adenoviral conjunctivitis at the present time. There is current research being performed for a topical form of cidofovir to treat adenovirus infections. Artificial tears can be used to relieve some of the discomfort as well as dilute the antigen. Over-the-counter (OTC) antihistamine-decongestant combinations used qid can minimize redness and decrease irritation as well.

Acute allergic conjunctivitis can best be treated with levocabastine (Livostin), which is a powerful H_1 receptor blocker, used qid for 7 days to minimize itchiness. OTC antihistamine-decongestants (Naphcon-A, Opcon-A, Vasocon-A) can be used qid for mild allergic symptoms. These should not be used on a chronic basis as rebound hyperemic effects will

TABLE 14-16-2. Antibiotics for Bacterial Infections

ANTIBIOTIC	DOSAGE	COMMENTS
Polymyxin B sulfate and trimethoprim (Polytrim)	1 gt. q 3 h × 7 d	Broad spectrum with minimal allergic reactions. Treatment of choice.
Tobramycin sulfate (Tobramycin or Tobrex) sol; Tobrex ung	Sol: 1 gt. q 4 h × 7 d Ung: apply 0.5-in. strip to affected eye qid × 7 d	Broad spectrum with corneal toxicity on chronic use.
Ciprofloxacin (Ciloxan)	1 gt. q 2 h × 2 d, 1 gt. q 4 h × 5 d thereafter	Recommended for severe conjunctivitis if other antibiotics are not effective and for the treatment of corneal ulcers. Temporary white crystalline precipitates can develop with use of this medication.
Ofloxacin 0.3% (Ocuflox)	1–2 gt. q 2–4 h for 2d, then qid for 5 d	Recommended for susceptible infection of the conjunctiva and for corneal ulcers.
Erythromycin (AK-Mycin, Ilotycin)	Apply 0.5-in. strip to affected eye qid × 7 d	Rare allergic or toxic reactions. Excellent as a prophylactic coverage. Used if allergic reactions to other antibiotics occur.
Bacitracin (Bacitracin, AK-Tracin)	Apply 0.5-in. strip to affected eye qid × 7 d	As with erythromycin, used if allergic reactions occur with other antibiotics. Excellent as a prophylactic coverage.

ABBREVIATIONS: gt., drop; sol, solution; ung, ointment.

TABLE 14-16-3. Treatment of Allergic Conjunctivitis

MEDICATION	DOSAGE	COMMENTS
Levocabastine hydrochloride 1% (Livostin), topical antihistamine	1 gt. qid as needed up to 2 wk	Very effective fast-acting treatment of allergic symptoms. Do not use while wearing soft contact lenses.
Naphazoline hydrochloride/pheniramine maleate (Opcon-A, AK-Con A, Naphcon-A), decongestant-antihistamine combination	1 gt. qid as needed	Not intended for chronic regular use as rebound hyperemia may develop. Side effect of pupillary dilation. Contraindicated in patients at risk or with narrow-angle glaucoma.
Naphazoline hydrochloride/antazoline phosphate (Vasocon-A), decongestant-antihistamine combination	1 gt. qid as needed	Not intended for chronic regular use as rebound hyperemia may develop. Side effect of pupillary dilation. Contraindicated in patients at risk or with narrow-angle glaucoma.
Cetirizine hydrochloride (Zyrtec), oral antihistamine	10 mg (1 tab) PO qd	Very fast-acting antihistamine. Has recently been released in the U.S. Minimizes drowsiness. No known adverse reactions. Used in conjunction with macrolide and imidazole derivatives.
Fexofenadine (Allegra), oral antihistamine	60 mg (1 tab) PO q 8–12 h for adults (see insert for children dosage)	Minimizes drowsiness.
Chlorpheniramine maleate (Chlor-Trimeton), OTC oral antihistamine	4 mg (1 tab) PO q 8–12 h	Causes drowsiness.
Diphenhydramine hydrochloride (Benadryl), OTC oral antihistamine	25–50 mg PO tid-qid for adults; 12.5–25 mg PO tid-qid for children over 20 lbs	Causes drowsiness.

ABBREVIATIONS: gt., drop; PO, orally.

often occur. OTC oral antihistamines such as chlorpheniramine maleate (Chlor-Trimeton) or diphenhydramine hydrochloride (Benadryl) can be used as directed. Prescription oral antihistamines (Zyrtec, Allegra) can be considered and have fewer side effects of drowsiness than do OTC antihistamines (see Tables 14-16-2 and 14-16-3).

Supportive Measures

The use of cool compresses can relieve discomfort created by irritation from any of the conjunctivitides. This will decrease the inflammatory process of swelling and pain sensitivity that commonly occurs. If inflammatory symptoms are absent, the use of warm compresses can increase vascular circulation to the affected area in viral and bacterial infections. This will stimulate the body's own immune response to accelerate the recovery time of the infection.

PATIENT EDUCATION

The contagious aspect of bacterial and viral conjunctivitis should be a vital part of patient education. Prior to the antibiotic treatment of a bacterial infection, or during any viral infection, the infection can be transmitted to the other eye as well as other people. Generally, viral infections are more highly contagious than bacterial infections. Patients with bacterial conjunctivitis should be cautioned against social interactions until 24 h after antibiotic treatment. Patients with viral conjunctivitis should be very careful throughout the term of conjunctivitis because

no treatment is available to eradicate the virus. These patients should be informed not to share towels, pillows, or cosmetic eye products with other people. The use of any contact lenses should be discontinued until the conjunctivitis resolves. Allergic conjunctivitis is not a contagious type of inflammation. Most allergic conjunctivitides are caused by seasonal or hay fever stimuli. If this is not the case, the antigen should be identified and avoided in the future.

BIBLIOGRAPHY

Arffa RC, Grayson M: *Grayson's Diseases of the Cornea,* 4th ed, St. Louis, Mosby-Year Book, 1997.

Kanski J: *Clinical Ophthalmology,* 4th ed, Boston, Butterworth-Heinemann, 1999.

Kaufman HE et al (eds): *The Cornea,* 2d ed, Boston, Butterworth-Heinemann, 1997.

Newell FW: *Ophthalmology—Principles and Concepts,* 8th ed, Mosby-Year Book, 1996.

Rhee DJ, Pyfer MF (eds): *The Wills Eye Manual—Office and Emergency Room Diagnosis and Treatment of Eye Disease,* 3d ed, Philadelphia, Lippincott Williams & Wilkins, 1999.

Spalton DJ et al (eds): *Atlas of Clinical Ophthalmology,* 2d ed, Mosby-Year Book, 1994.

Stamper RL et al: *Becker-Shaffer's Diagnosis and Therapy of the Glaucomas,* 7th ed, St. Louis, Mosby, 1999.

Vaughan D et al (eds): *General Ophthalmology,* 15th ed, New York, McGraw-Hill, 1998.

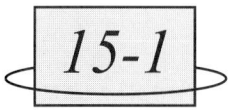

PEDIATRIC NUTRITION
Kimberly Brown

DISCUSSION

Growth may be defined as an increase in size. Physiologic growth depends on a variety of nutrients in the food a child eats. The goal of nutrition is appropriate growth and development along with the avoidance of deficiency states. Requirements vary with stages of development as well as the genetic and metabolic differences that exist among individuals. Nutrient needs also depend on body composition. For example, in full-term neonates, the brain accounts for 10% of body weight and 44% of total energy needs under basal conditions. This indicates that the brain accounts for a high percentage of basal energy requirements.[1]

Nutritional requirements change with the composition of new weight gain. Fat accounts for 40% of weight gain between birth and age 4 months, but only 3% between 24 and 36 months, making constant reassessment of infant and pediatric nutritional intakes important. The stages reviewed in this chapter include infant feeding (e.g., breast feeding versus bottle feeding) and toddler or childhood nutrition to age 12 years. Considerations in early infant nutrition include:

- *Infant feeding:* birth to 1 year
- *Premature infant:* gestation less than 270 days or weight less than 2500 g (5.5 lb)
- *Small for gestational age* (SGA): full-term neonate but experienced intrauterine growth failure and has low birth weight along with general growth retardation

The merits of breast feeding versus bottle (formula) feeding have been largely debated. Epidemiologic research shows that human milk and breast feeding of infants provides advantages with regard to general health, as well as growth and development. There is also strong indication that breast feeding significantly reduces the incidence and/or severity of diarrhea, lower respiratory infection, otitis media, bacteremia, bacterial meningitis, urinary tract infection, and necrotizing enterocolitis.

For bottle-fed babies, the average number of feedings and quantity ingested varies with age (see Table 15-1-1).

There are a number of studies that show a possible protective factor of human milk feeding against sudden infant death syndrome (SIDS), insulin-dependent diabetes mellitus, Crohn's disease, ulcerative colitis, lymphoma, allergic diseases, and other chronic digestive diseases.

There are some contraindications to breast feeding. These include infant galactosemia and maternal illegal drug use, untreated active tuberculosis, and HIV infection.[2] It has been suggested that HIV-positive mothers in developing countries use alternative methods of feeding even though recent evidence suggests that breast feeding may not be a route of transmission.

Additional contraindications to breast feeding include maternal septicemia, nephritis, eclampsia, profuse hemorrhage, chronic poor nutrition, and severe psychological disturbances.[1]

More information regarding the composition of formulas and special formulas for all infants can be found in standard reference texts.

PREMATURE INFANTS

Premature infants require special care in regard to feeding. Extra attention must be paid to the type of milk and the method of feeding. The body composition of premature infants differs from that of full-term infants in that "preemies" have:

1. More water and less protein and minerals per kilogram of body weight
2. Little subcutaneous fat
3. Poorly calcified bones
4. An underdeveloped neuromuscular system, making sucking difficult
5. Inadequate iron stores
6. Limited digestive and absorption abilities[1]

PEDIATRIC NUTRITION AGE 1 TO 2 YEARS

The 1-year-old birthday is a milestone in itself. Major development has occurred since the infant came home from the hospital. One-year-olds use Sippy cups and have become accustomed to a schedule of three meals per day with snacks in between. Independence is being suggested, with toddlers beginning to select foods and feed themselves. Some doubts may arise about whether a balanced diet is being taken. However, children have the ability to select a balanced diet over the course of several days.

A point to emphasize to parents regarding feeding at this time is that the need for kilocalories during this stage decreases. At 1 year of age children need about 1000 kcal, which increases to 1300 to 1500 kcal by age 3 years. It is important to offer a variety of foods in smaller amounts to provide key nutrients. Two to three cups of milk provide protein and iron in this stage. Single foods and finger foods such as raw fruits and vegetables cut into finger-sized pieces can be a great source of nutrition for children who have a decreasing appetite[2] (see Table 15-1-2).

CHILDHOOD NUTRITION TO AGE 12 YEARS

Nutritional habits are formed early in life; therefore, dietary intervention can be effective when started early in childhood.

Dietary Guidelines for Children Age 2 Years and Older

The following recommendations are appropriate for these children:

1. The diet should be nutritionally complete and include a variety of foods.
2. Carbohydrates should provide 60% or more of the daily caloric intake, with at least 30% of the daily caloric intake from complex carbohydrates.
3. A high-fiber diet is encouraged.
4. A low-fat diet is advised.
5. Total fat should constitute less than 30% of caloric intake, with saturated fats and polyunsaturated fats providing less than 10% each. Monounsaturated fats should provide 10% or more of the caloric intake from fats.
6. Cholesterol intake should be less than 100 mg/1000 kcal per day to a maximum of 300 mg per day.

TABLE 15-1-1. Number and Quantity of Feedings per 24 Hours

AGE	AVERAGE QUANTITY IN INDIVIDUAL FEEDINGS (OUNCES)	AVERAGE NUMBER OF FEEDINGS IN 24 h
Birth–2 weeks	2–3	6–10
3 weeks–1 month	4–5	6–10
2–3 months	5–6	5–6
3–4 months	6–7	4–5
4–7 months	7–8	4–5
8–12 months	7–8	3

USEFUL PEDIATRIC NUTRITION CALCULATIONS

Energy Requirements

After age 4 years energy requirements expressed on a body weight basis fall to 40 kcal/kg per day by the end of adolescence. Energy requirements are calculated with a base of 1000 kcal. At age 1 year, it is necessary to add 100 kcal/year. For example, for a child up to age 6 years, a base of 1000 kcal plus 600 kcal (100 kcal/year) equals a 1600-kcal energy requirement for a child age 6 years.

The basal energy requirement for premature infants is 120 kcal/kg per day.[1]

PARENT INFORMATION GUIDELINES

The following outline is helpful in discussions with parents about feeding and nutrition:

- Discuss feeding behaviors in infancy and early childhood bottle feeding.
- Do not place the infant in the crib with his or her bottle.
- Discourage the use of a bottle of milk or juice as a pacifier.
- Explain that the nursing bottle carries a possible risk of otitis media.
- Think about offering a cup of water or juice when appropriate.

The following age milestones should be discussed:

2 to 4 weeks	Use breast or bottle feeding, vitamin D supplementation in breast-fed infants, and fluoride supplementation.
2 to 4 months	Introduce solid foods at 4 to 6 months. Consider an iron supplement in premature infants.
6 months	Solid foods: iron-fortified cereal as well as fruits and vegetables should be added to the diet at this time. Meals may be given two to three times per day. It is acceptable for commercially prepared infant cereals to be the chief source of dietary iron.
12 months	Encourage table foods.

TABLE 15-1-2. Food Choices for Toddlers

VEGETABLES AND FRUITS	BREAKFAST	LUNCH	DESSERT
Apples	Cereal	Pizza	Ice cream
Corn	French toast	Spaghetti	Gelatin
Carrots	Pancakes	Macaroni and cheese	Pudding
Oranges	Eggs	Hamburger	Cookies
Bananas	Bagels	Chicken tenders	
Watermelon		Peanut butter and jelly sandwiches	

18 months	Wean from the use of bottles.
3 years and older	Stress a balanced diet. Avoid low-nutrition foods. However, encourage the child to participate in the selection and preparation of meals and snacks.
5 years and older	Establish a pleasant atmosphere at meal times. Encourage good eating habits. Limit empty carbohydrate foods.
6 years and older	Maintain appropriate weight.

REFERENCES

1. Wilson JD et al (eds): *Harrison's Principles of Internal Medicine,* 13th ed. New York, McGraw-Hill, 1997, pp 780–787.
2. Hathaway WE et al (eds): *Current Pediatric Diagnosis and Treatment,* 12th ed. Norwalk, CT, Appleton and Lange, 1997, pp 238–270.
3. American Academy of Pediatrics: Breast feeding and the use of human milk (position paper). 100(6):1035–1039,1997.

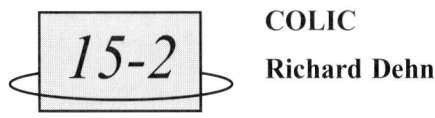

COLIC

Richard Dehn

DISCUSSION

Colic is an infant syndrome of excessive crying in the absence of a physical disorder. It is characterized by lengthy incidents of severely increased crying accompanied by a characteristic "pained" look on the infant's face, abduction of the knees to the abdomen accompanied by abdominal distention, and increased flatus. The crying typically begins in the late afternoon, and efforts to comfort the child are usually ineffective. Infant colic is rarely present before the third week of life and in most cases begins to improve by the fourth month, although occasionally it can last through the first year.

The diagnosis can be challenging, since the crying of normal infants increases from birth until about 6 weeks of age and then gradually decreases until it reaches a steady state at about age 4 months. A normal infant averages about 3 h per day of crying at 6 weeks of age. Parents unaware that this is typical infant behavior may feel that the child is abnormal or that something is wrong.

The general rule for making the diagnosis of infant colic is the rule of threes: a healthy child who cries for a minimum of 3 h per day, at least 3 days per week, for at least 3 weeks.

A prospective study of 1221 families showed a colic incidence of 13% using this criterion. The mean amount of total crying was 241 min per day for the colicky group compared with 112 min per day for the noncolicky group, with a mean age of 5 weeks. The survey also had parents quantify the quality of crying by indicating how many minutes of "colicky" crying (inconsolable crying) the infant exhibited each day. The colicky group was reported to exhibit a mean of 122 min per day of colicky crying compared with a mean of 19 min per day in the noncolicky group.

The crying of a colicky infant is often so distressing to parents that it is hard for them to believe that the child does not have a serious medical malady. In this regard it is imperative that the clinician rule out any pathology that might explain the behavior, thus making colic a diagnosis of exclusion. A careful physical examination and close monitoring of growth parameters are useful tools to help exclude other causes of crying.

The effects of a colicky child on his or her family can be significant. The inconsolable nature of the crying can cause the parents to question their ability to nurture the child, especially when a colicky child is the firstborn. Siblings can find the chaos generated by a colicky child destabilizing at a time when the addition of a new child has already generated family stress. Friends, neighbors, and relatives who normally interact with the parents and siblings find the environment too chaotic for visiting, thus isolating the family. Sleep disturbances created by the inconsolable crying contribute to psychological depression, reducing the family's functional ability to cope with the colicky infant's care demands. Colicky children are at an increased risk for being victims of child abuse. In cases of shaken baby syndrome colic is often present.

PATHOGENESIS

The cause of infant colic is unknown, though many theories exist. Because these children appear to be suffering from gastrointestinal (GI) symptoms (thus the name *colic*), the most popular theory proposes that the crying is due to immaturity of the GI system. As the GI system matures, the painful symptoms resolve, explaining the eventual normalizing of the crying. A few studies have shown that colicky infants have measurable differences in specific organ functions (a recent study showed differences in gallbladder function); however, it is not known whether these differences are the cause of the colic or are secondary to it.

Sensitivity to substances in the diet is also a popular theory. Commonly implicated foods include cow's milk–based formulas, eggs, wheat, and nuts. In bottle-fed infants, eliminating cow's milk–based formulas from the diet can test this hypothesis. In breast-fed infants, the mother must eliminate those foods from her diet. While some infants improve after the dietary changes, the vast majority are unchanged, leading to the conclusion that food sensitivities may be an etiologic factor in only a small percentage of colicky infants.

Another theory is that psychological traits of the parents and their manifestation during pregnancy have a bearing on an infant's coping mechanisms. Several retrospective studies have shown poorer psychological rating scores in the parents of colicky infants than in those of normal infants. However, those studies are not able to show whether the poor scores are a determinant of colicky behavior or a result of it.

Yet another theory is that a colicky infant's neurologic system is immature compared to that of a normal infant and that this affects a colicky infant's ability to make the transition from an awake state to a crying state to a sleep state. A related theory is that colic is caused by lack of establishment of a melatonin nocturnal secretion rhythm that would be maintained by the infant's pineal gland. The hypothesis is that some infants need 12 months to establish a circadian rhythm, having had only 9 months in utero to do so, and thus have 3 months of colic symptoms.

Sensory integration theory hypothesizes that abnormalities in vestibular function decrease an infant's ability to integrate sensory stimulation into appropriate motor responses. Several sensory integration theory researchers have found a positive correlation between a history of infant colic and later sensory integration disturbances such as sensory defensiveness. Treatment of sensory integration disorders involves vestibular stimulation, and this may explain why some colicky infants improve when in motion.

LABORATORY TESTING

Since infant colic is a diagnosis of exclusion, no available laboratory test is useful in making the diagnosis.

TREATMENT

The first step in the treatment of colic is confirmation of the diagnosis and education of the parents about the expected characteristics and time-limited nature of the syndrome. Parents often are relieved to learn that a child does not have a "serious" illness. It is important that the provider evaluate the psychological and social support structure of the family, as family resources are the most important factor in managing colic. The practitioner should carefully monitor the status of the support systems over the course of the syndrome and suggest interventions when necessary. Occasionally the family stresses generated by a colicky infant result in child abuse.

Suggestions for increasing the social and psychological support of affected families include getting friends and relatives to give the parents occasional relief from the overwhelming responsibilities of caring for a colicky infant. Finding good-quality childcare to allow the parents a few hours away from the inconsolable crying is quite valuable. Extra support is also needed for the other siblings, who have temporary feelings of neglect.

Dietary changes can be suggested, keeping in mind that improvement is not a common result. Bottle-fed infants can be switched to soy formula, and the mothers of breast-fed infants can avoid dairy products, wheat, and nuts. Frequent small feedings occasionally improve the abdominal distention; however, it is also important to advise the parents to make sure all the air is expelled from the stomach after feedings. Medications are not useful for controlling colic symptoms. Simethicone has not proved to be any more effective than placebo and aluminum-containing antacids have been implicated in two cases of rickets.

Occasionally exposure to motion improves colicky symptoms. Some infants improve when placed in an infant swing or taken for a car ride. Carrying a child in a front-style infant carrier while walking is sometimes helpful.

However, although a wide range of therapies has been investigated, no one specific treatment regimen has been shown to be more effective than others. Additionally, many of the studies supporting one treatment regimen over another have design and methodology problems, and the results of many studies on colic are conflicting and controversial.

Generally, the overall approach to treatment involves supportive measures directed toward the whole family while monitoring for evidence of child abuse. The guiding philosophy should be one of helping the family survive this difficult self-limited syndrome and preventing long-term residual effects on the individuals in the family.

BIBLIOGRAPHY

Balon AJ: Management of infantile colic. *Am Fam Physician* 55(1):235–242, 245–246, 1997.

Beers MH, Berkow R (ed): *Merck Manual of Diagnosis and Therapy,* 17th ed. Whitehouse Station, NJ, Merck Research Laboratories, 1999, pp 2109.

Botash AS et al: Child abuse, sudden infant death syndrome, and psychosocial development. *Curr Opin Pediatr* 8(2):195–200, 1996.

Crowcroft NS, Strachan DP: The social origins of infantile colic: Questionnaire study covering 76,747 infants. *BMJ* 314(7090):1325–1328, 1997.

Dihigo SK: New strategies for the treatment of colic: Modifying the parent/infant interaction. *Journal of Pediatric Health Care* 12(5):256–262, 1998.

Goldson E: Developmental disorders and behavorial problems, in *Current Pediatric Diagnosis and Treatment,* 14th ed, WW Hay Jr et al (eds). Stamford, CT, Appleton & Lange, 1999, pp 78–79.

Hill DJ: A low allergen diet is a significant intervention in infantile colic: Results of a community-based study. *J Allergy Clin Immunol* 96(61):886–892, 1995.

Lehtonen L: Infantile colic. *Arch Pediatr Adolesc Med* 149(5):533–536, 1995.

Lucassen PL et al: Effectiveness of treatments for infantile colic: Systematic review. *BMJ* 316(7144):1563–1569, 1998.

Lust KD et al: Maternal intake of cruciferous vegetables and other foods and colic symptoms in exclusively breast-fed infants. *J Am Diet Assoc* 96(1):46–48, 1996.

Metcalf TJ: Simethicone in the treatment of infant colic: A randomized, placebo-controlled, multicenter trial. *Pediatrics* (1):29–34, 1994.

Pivnick EK: Rickets secondary to phosphate depletion: A sequela of antacid use in infancy. *Clin Pediatr* 34(2):73–78, 1995.

Raiha H et al: Family life 1 year after infantile colic. *Arch Pediatr Adolesc Med* 150(10):1032–1036, 1996.

Rautava P: Psychosocial predisposing factors for infantile colic. *BMJ* 307(6904):600–604, 1993.

Weissbluth L: Infant colic: The effect of serotonin and melatonin circadian rhythms on the intestinal smooth muscle. *Med Hypotheses* 39(2):164–167, 1992.

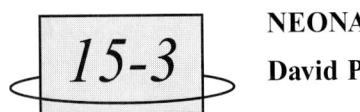

NEONATAL CYANOSIS
David P. Asprey

DISCUSSION

Cyanosis is the visually observable bluish discoloration of the skin or mucous membranes. Cyanosis is either peripheral (acrocyanosis) or central. This distinction is most accurately diagnosed by determining the oxygen level of the arterial blood. If the oxygen level in the arterial blood is below the normal range, it is defined as central cyanosis; if it is within the normal range, the cyanosis is a peripheral cyanosis. While peripheral cyanosis may be a normal physical examination finding, central cyanosis is always considered abnormal and the cause must be identified and treated.

It is important that the clinician be able to distinguish peripheral cyanosis from central cyanosis. Inspection of the mucous membranes is the most reliable method to determine the presence of central cyanosis utilizing the physical examination. Cyanosis that is observable on inspection of the mucous membranes is indicative of central cyanosis. Mild degrees of cyanosis may be very difficult to detect. In order to maximize the examiner's ability to detect the presence of mild cyanosis, the patient should be examined in natural lighting rather than artificial lighting. Utilization of a cutaneous pulse oximeter to measure the patient's oxygen saturation is beneficial when it is available. In patients with normal hemoglobin who have observable central cyanosis, the arterial saturation is typically less than 85%.

SIGNS AND SYMPTOMS

Cyanosis is a common presenting sign in the neonate and when present requires a very thorough investigation for its etiology. Peripheral cyanosis (acrocyanosis) is a common finding in the first 48 to 72 h of life. It is usually a result of slower blood flow through a distal aspect of an extremity resulting in a large arteriovenous oxygen difference. In most instances, peripheral cyanosis alone (without central cyanosis) is not indicative of pathology in the neonate.

Central cyanosis occurs when the absolute concentration of unoxygenated or reduced hemoglobin in the arterial blood exceeds 3g/dL. It is important to recall that the adult and fetal hemoglobin differ in their binding capacity for oxygen. The hemoglobin–oxygen dissociation curve is diagrammed and well described in most standard human physiology texts. In fetal hemoglobin, the curve is shifted to the left, so that at the same oxygen partial pressure the oxygen saturation will be higher in fetal blood than in a child or adult's blood. Consequently, the neonate will develop cyanosis at a lower oxygen partial pressure than older children will.

When the total hemoglobin concentration is low (i.e., anemia) a higher percentage of unsaturated hemoglobin is necessary to develop visible cyanosis. In the normal neonate, the typical hemoglobin concentration is approximately 17 g/dL. In this instance when the oxygen saturation is approximately 82%, more than 3g/dL of unoxygenated hemoglobin is present and cyanosis will result (the oxygen partial pressure necessary to produce cyanosis in this case is approximately 38 to 39 mmHg). Premature infants may have hemoglobin concentrations as low as 12 g/dL or less. In this instance, the level of unoxygenated hemoglobin would need to be 25% (or saturation levels as low as 75%, with an oxygen partial pressure as low as 30 mmHg) to result in a level of reduced or unoxygenated hemoglobin greater than the 3 g/dL necessary to produce visible cyanosis.[1]

Once the presence of central cyanosis is established the potential causes must be considered and the specific etiology identified. Generally, the pathophysiologic mechanisms of cyanosis can be considered to consist of the following five categories: alveolar hypoventilation, right-to-left shunting of blood, ventilation-perfusion inequality, impaired oxygen diffusion, and decreased affinity of hemoglobin for oxygen. In some patients there may be multiple factors present simultaneously, resulting in multiple pathophysiologic mechanisms contributing to the presence of the cyanosis.

Alveolar hypoventilation occurs with conditions that decrease the alveolar ventilation, resulting in an accumulation of carbon dioxide in the alveoli. Consequently, the alveolar oxygen tension is decreased and there will be incomplete oxygenation of arterial blood.

Right-to-left shunting results when a portion of the venous blood is mixed into the arterial system without circulating through the lungs to undergo oxygenation. The admixture of venous blood into the arterial system results in arterial blood supply desaturation. This can occur as a result of intracardiac lesions, extracardiac (vascular) lesions, or by intrapulmonary mechanisms.

Ventilation-perfusion inequality can occur when there is a mismatch between the ventilation and perfusion to each area of the lung. Decreased ventilation with normal or increased perfusion results in incomplete oxygenation of the blood. Admixture of this incompletely oxygenated blood with oxygenated blood will result in a partially desaturated arterial blood supply.

Impairment of diffusion of the gases from the alveoli to the pulmonary capillary blood can result in clinical cyanosis. Any condition that results in accentuated cardiac output may contribute to this problem. The excess volume of blood may result in accelerated blood flow through the pulmonary capillary beds and thus prohibit the full exchange of gases at this level.

Abnormalities of the hemoglobin structure may interfere with its ability to bind with oxygen, resulting in incomplete oxygen saturation. An example of this is methemoglobinemia, which can occur with exposure to oxidants such as nitrates (in untreated water supplies) which are converted to nitrites. The nitrites bind with the hemoglobin, displacing the oxygen molecules.

The most likely causes of central cyanosis in the neonate are either respiratory or cardiac in origin. However, there are numerous potential etiologies for cyanosis and in many instances the degree of cyanosis may be the result of a combination of causes. Table 15-3-1 provides a list of common clinical conditions that may result in central cyanosis in the neonate.

MEDICAL HISTORY

A careful medical history should be obtained for the infant and the mother. The infant's gestational and birth history may provide important diagnostic clues to potential causes of cyanosis. A description of the presentation of the symptoms may also provide important information. Any recent fever or respiratory tract infections should be investigated. The timing and occurrence of the cyanosis, precipitating events, and duration of the cyanosis may provide the clinician with critical clues to the etiology. If the infant is formula fed, an assessment of the water source (untreated water may contain high nitrate levels) is important.

PHYSICAL EXAMINATION FINDINGS

A complete physical examination should be performed with the patient in a quiet, warm environment utilizing natural lighting when possible. The exam should first be conducted with the patient on room air when possible. The clinician should first attempt to distinguish peripheral from central cyanosis. Careful inspection of the skin for plethora may also provide evidence of polycythemia. Observe the capillary refill of the extremities for indications of decreased peripheral blood flow.

Decreased muscle tone, activity, and response to noxious stimuli may suggest central nervous system disease, sepsis, or severe shock. The presence of a murmur, a single second heart sound, and diminished

TABLE 15-3-1.   Common Clinical Conditions Associated with Neonatal Cyanosis

Alveolar Hypoventilation

    Parenchymal disease
        Atelectasis, respiratory distress syndrome—diffuse
        Aspiration syndrome—blood, meconium
        Infection—pneumonia
        Pulmonary hypoplasia
    Space-occupying lesions
        Pneumothorax
        Lobar emphysema
        Diaphragmatic hernia
        Pleural effusion
        Diaphragmatic elevation—ascites, etc.
    Obstructive lesions
        Choanal atresia
        Vocal cord paralysis
        Vascular rings
        Tracheal or bronchial stenosis
    Excessive lung fluid
    Pulmonary hemorrhage
    Diaphragmatic paralysis—phrenic nerve palsy
    Cardiovascular disorders
        Congestive heart failure
        Persistent pulmonary hypertension—persistent fetal circulation
    Central nervous system disorders
        Infection—meningitis
        Hemorrhage—periventricular/intraventricular
        Arteriovenous malformations
        Seizure disorders
        Apnea
    Maternal sedative drugs (magnesium sulfate, opiates)
    Polycythemia
    Methemoglobinemia
    Metabolic
        Hypoglycemia
        Hypocalcemia

Right-to-Left Shunting

    Congenital heart disease (with admixture type defects)
    Parenchymal disease
        Respiratory distress syndrome
        Aspiration syndrome—blood, meconium
        Infection—pneumonia
    Pulmonary hypertension

Ventilation-Perfusion Inequality

    Parenchymal disease
        Atelectasis, diffuse respiratory distress syndrome or localized
            (bronchial mucous plugs)
        Aspiration syndrome—blood, meconium
        Infection—pneumonia
    Polycythemia

Impaired Oxygen Diffusion

    Aspiration syndrome—blood, meconium
    Pulmonary hemorrhage

Decreased Affinity of Hemoglobin for Oxygen

    Methemoglobinemia

SOURCE: Modified from Kitterman.[2]

pulses may be indicative of congenital heart disease. However, it should be noted that significant heart disease may be present in the absence of these findings as well. A careful evaluation of the respiratory system is often the most productive aspect of the physical examination. Note the tracheal position for evidence of pneumothorax or space-occupying lesions. Determine the respiratory rate and pattern and the degree of respiratory effort and observe for evidence of retractions and other signs of respiratory distress (e.g., nasal flaring, grunting).

DIAGNOSTIC CONSIDERATIONS

In many instances the etiology of the cyanosis may be readily apparent. An arterial blood gas should be obtained to assess the severity of the patient's clinical condition, to establish the etiology, and to guide the treatment of the cyanosis. However, differentiating a cardiac cause from a respiratory cause of cyanosis may be rather challenging at times. A particularly useful tool in differentiating respiratory from cardiac causes is an oxygen challenge test. This test is conducted by measuring the arterial partial oxygen pressure on room air. The patient is then administered 90 to 100% oxygen for approximately 15 min and the partial oxygen pressure is repeated. In patients with congenital heart disease and right-to-left shunting, only minimal increases (10 to 15 mmHg) in the partial oxygen pressure will be achieved. However, if the partial oxygen pressure improves considerably (50% or more) while being administered 100% oxygen, a pulmonary etiology is likely. A low partial oxygen pressure with a low or normal partial carbon dioxide pressure is indicative of right-to-left shunting of blood that can occur with congenital heart disease, pulmonary hypertension, and other forms of pulmonary disease.

LABORATORY STUDIES

The following laboratory studies may be useful in assessing patients with cyanosis: a complete blood count to assess the hemoglobin and hematocrit level, cutaneous oxygen saturation monitoring, arterial blood gas to assess the partial oxygen pressure and carbon dioxide levels, electrolyte levels including calcium, and glucose level.

RADIOLOGIC STUDIES

A chest x-ray may be useful in providing diagnostic clues to the etiology of central cyanosis in the neonate. Many findings associated with respiratory disease and in some instances congenital heart disease will have abnormal findings present on the chest x-rays. Observe the x-ray for evidence of pneumonia, infiltrates, space-occupying lesions, air leaks, increased pulmonary blood flow, and cardiomegaly.

OTHER DIAGNOSTIC STUDIES

An electrocardiogram may be useful in establishing the diagnosis of dysrhythmias and some types of congenital heart disease. Echocardiography is an extremely useful and sensitive tool for assessing patients with suspected congenital heart disease. A careful study completed by a skilled pediatric echocardiographer can identify congenital heart disease, persistent fetal circulation, pulmonary hypertension, and the presence of right-to-left shunting through intracardiac and some extracardiac lesions.

TREATMENT

Central cyanosis in the neonate should be treated as a medical emergency. If the specific etiology of the cyanosis is not readily apparent, supportive treatment should be initiated until the etiology can be established and treated appropriately. This treatment includes ensuring the patency of airways, administration of oxygen, ensuring appropriate core body temperature, and correction of abnormal electrolyte, calcium, and hemoglobin levels. In cases of severe cyanosis, intubation and mechanical ventilation may be necessary. In addition, if the oxygen challenge test results in a neonate suggest a cardiac etiology for the cyanosis, consideration should be given to treating the patient with prostaglandin E$_1$ to maintain the patency of the ductus arteriosus. Consultation with a pediatric cardiology clinician or intensivist is recommended before initiating this therapy.

Once a specific etiology has been identified, the treatment should be directed at correcting the underlying clinical condition causing the cyanosis. A full discussion of the treatment options for each of the clinical conditions that may cause cyanosis is outside the scope of this topic. A more detailed discussion of treatment may be found by looking up the specific clinical condition.

PEARLS

When the initial assessment of the patient fails to provide a likely etiology of the cyanosis consider methemoglobinemia. This condition results when infants ingest well water containing high levels of nitrates. The nitrate ion is converted to nitrite in the intestine. After this ion is formed it is absorbed and reacts with hemoglobin to form methemoglobin. Methemoglobin competes with normal hemoglobin for nonreduced oxygen, thus creating cyanosis. A careful history will often reveal that a child has been ingesting water from an untreated well with an excessive nitrate level.

REFERENCES

1. Rudolph AM, Kamei RK: *Rudolph's Fundamentals of Pediatrics.* Norwalk, CT, Appleton and Lange, 1994.
2. Kitterman JA: Cyanosis in the newborn infant. *Pediatr Rev* 4(1):19, 1982.

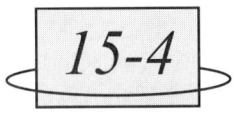

REYE'S SYNDROME

Thomas J. Schymanski

DISCUSSION

Reye's syndrome is an acute and potentially fatal encephalopathy of unknown etiology that is emerging as one of the more common causes of death in childhood. Little is known about the pathogenesis of this syndrome, but it is believed that the major site of injury is the mitochondria. The reasons for this mitochondrial dysfunction are unknown. It is thought to be precipitated by salicylates during episodes of chickenpox or influenza–upper respiratory infection (URI). The circumstances in which salicylates serve as a cofactor (or comitochondrial toxin) in a susceptible host during a viral infection remain to be determined. This most often occurs in children 4 to 12 years old, with a peak incidence at about 6 years of age.

Reye's syndrome is a multisystem disease that affects the liver, brain, heart, kidneys, pancreas, and muscle tissue. Pathologic findings in the brain include cerebral edema with or without herniation; anoxic neuronal changes are most severe in the cerebral cortex. The liver appears swollen and yellow or reddish yellow. Light microscopy reveals a fine vacuolization of the parenchymal cells resulting from intracellular lipid. Glycogen is absent, and there is no evidence of inflammation. Electron microscopy reveals mitochondrial abnormalities consisting of ameboid and spherical structural deformation, loss of dense bodies and cristae, and swelling of the mitochondrial matrix.

The kidneys are pale, with a slight yellowish tinge and a widening of the cortices. Light microscopy reveals fatty degeneration of Henle's loops and proximal convoluted tubules. The glomeruli, vessels, and interstitium appear to be normal. Examination of the heart reveals epicardial petechiae in many cases. Light microscopy reveals oil red O–positive material in the ventricles and especially in the atria. Electron microscopy reveals mitochondrial swelling and fragmentation of the cristae.

Most cases occur in the late fall and winter. Widespread outbreaks have occurred in association with regional influenza epidemics. Varicella virus, the enteroviruses, Epstein-Barr virus, and the myxoviruses have been associated with sporadic cases.

The question remains whether Reye's syndrome is a new disease or whether affected children previously were classified as having "postviral encephalopathy." It is very likely that mild cases are missed

TABLE 15-4-1. Clinical Staging of Reye's Syndrome

GRADE	SYMPTOMS AT TIME OF ADMISSION
I	Usually quiet, lethargic, and sleepy; vomiting, lab evidence of liver dysfunction
II	Deep lethargy, confusion, delirium, combative, hyperventilation, hyperreflexic
III	Obtunded, light coma, with or without seizures, decorticate rigidity, intact pupillary light reaction
IV	Seizures, deepening coma, decerebrate rigidity, loss of oculocephalic reflexes, fixed pupils
V	Coma, loss of deep tendon reflexes, respiratory arrest, fixed dilated pupils, flaccidity and decerebrate (intermittent) posturing, isoelectric EEG

and that these patients recover without any significant medical event. In any case, Reye's syndrome may be the most common potentially lethal virus-associated encephalopathy in the United States.

SIGNS AND SYMPTOMS

The severity of the disease varies greatly but is characterized by a biphasic illness. Initially a viral infection, usually a URI (occasionally exanthematous), is followed on about day 6 by the onset of nausea and vomiting and a sudden change in mental status.

When associated with varicella, the encephalopathy usually develops on the fourth to fifth day of the rash. The changes in mental status may vary from mild amnesia and noticeable lethargy to intermittent episodes of disorientation and agitation that often progress rapidly to deepening stages of coma manifested by progressive unresponsiveness, decorticate and decerebrate posturing, seizures, flaccidity, fixed dilated pupils, and respiratory arrest. Focal neurologic findings are usually not present.

The clinical features are best reflected in the system of clinical staging (see Table 15-4-1); grades I through III represent mild to moderate illness, while grades IV and V indicate severe illness. The majority of affected children have mild illness without progression.

OBJECTIVE FINDINGS

Characteristically, an antecedent viral illness is followed by vomiting and progressive lethargy (noted from the history). Physical examination reveals tachypnea, fever, and lethargy, and stupor and coma are typical findings. Signs of elevated intracranial pressure (ICP) and seizures also may be noted.

DIAGNOSTIC CONSIDERATIONS

The differential diagnosis includes other causes of coma and hepatic dysfunction, such as sepsis or hyperthermia (especially in infants), salicylism, drug ingestion, head trauma, bacterial and viral infections of the central nervous system, and hepatitis.

LABORATORY TESTS AND RADIOLOGIC STUDIES

Elevated serum hepatocellular enzyme assays (serum glutamic-oxaloacetic transaminase, serum glutamate pyruvate transaminase, lactic dehydrogenase) and elevated serum ammonia (arterial) are the laboratory hallmarks; one also may see metabolic acidosis and respiratory alkalosis as well as hypoglycemia and prolongation of the prothrombin time (PT) and partial thromboplastin time (PTT). A liver biopsy generally is performed when the diagnosis is in question but is not essential for the clinical diagnosis. The data gained are crucial in the precise definition of the syndrome. Biopsy should be carried out in atypical or severe cases to rule out other disorders, such as metabolic or toxic liver disease, especially in patients under 1 year of age. Computed tomography may be necessary to rule out an intracranial mass.

TREATMENT

Since the cause of the syndrome is uncertain and widespread metabolic derangements are present, there is no universally accepted therapy. Early diagnosis and prompt institution of intensive supportive care are the mainstays of treatment. Meticulous and constant attention to neurologic, electrolyte, metabolic, cardiovascular, respiratory, and fluid status is essential to cope with rapid changes. Treatment includes intravenous fluid and electrolyte solutions containing glucose, usually 5 to 10% but occasionally up to 50%; the judicious use of nonabsorbable antibiotics (such as neomycin 100 mg/kg per day orally every 6 h); and vitamin K 5 mg/d intravenously or intramuscularly. Increased ICP must be controlled with agents such as mannitol 0.5 to 1 g/kg given intravenously over 45 min and dexamethasone 0.5 mg/kg per day intravenously; close monitoring of ICP may help guide this therapy. Common procedures include monitoring blood gases, blood pH, and blood pressure by means of arterial catheters, inserting an endotracheal tube, and controlling ventilation.

Supportive Measures

The medical professionals who are usually involved in the care of a patient with Reye's syndrome include pediatricians, neurologists, gastroenterologists, and physical and respiratory therapists. The ability to serially monitor arterial blood gases, central venous pressure, and electroencephalography (EEG) plus 24-h intensive care nursing and physician coverage are imperative. Throughout the course of the illness, the primary care provider is an indispensable member of the team, interpreting procedures and progress for the family. After recovery, long-term follow-up by the primary care team is of great importance and involves coordinating care as required for the management of neurologic and psychological sequelae and recognizing and treating patient and family stresses that have resulted from the illness.

Patient Education

Avoid the administration of salicylates in children with a viral illness. Printed patient information can be obtained from the National Reye's Syndrome Foundation, (800) 233-7393 or at http://www.bright.net/~reyessyn/.

Disposition

The overall majority of these patients have mild illness without progression of the condition. The prognosis is related to the degree of cerebral edema and the ammonia level on admission.

Possible neurologic complications include problems with attention, concentration, speech, language, and fine and gross motor skills. These complications necessitate the involvement of medical providers, psychologists, and physical, occupational, and speech therapists.

COMPLICATIONS

Potential complications in addition to the neurologic complications noted above are as follows:

- Aspiration pneumonia
- Respiratory failure
- Cardiac dysrhythmia or arrest
- Diabetes insipidus
- Cerebral edema
- Inappropriate vasopressin excretion

OTHER NOTES AND PEARLS

Reye's syndrome does not always follow a typical clinical pattern. Vomiting may not occur.

BIBLIOGRAPHY

Nelson R et al: *Nelson's Textbook of Pediatrics,* 15th ed. Philadelphia, Saunders, 1996, pp 1144–1155.
Rakel R: *Conn's Current Therapy 1995.* Philadelphia, Saunders, 1995, pp 845–848.
Rakel R: *Textbook of Family Practice,* 5th ed. Philadelphia, Saunders, 1995, pp 388, 462, 644, 1031, 1057.

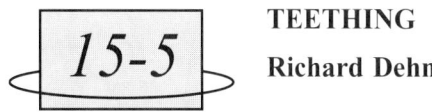

15-5

TEETHING
Richard Dehn

DISCUSSION

Teething is the common term for problems associated with the development and eruption of teeth in children. Teething problems are common in the first 18 months of life, with folklore attributing to teething numerous symptoms, including fever, diarrhea, mouth lesions, rashes, and drooling. In the nineteenth century, teething was thought to be the leading cause of infant death.

In a paper presented at an 1896 meeting of the American Medical Association, Dr. S. W. Foster stated:

"The [teething] child becomes wakeful, restless, and fretful, refuses nourishment; the alimentary canal becomes more active, diarrhea follows, and if relief is not given, relaxation of the vital forces follows, and we have nausea, vomiting, convulsions, paralysis, and not infrequently, death."

The formation of teeth begins in the second gestational month. Primary mandibular and maxillary incisors can appear as early as age 3 months but usually erupt at around 6 months. The lower central incisors often appear first at 5 to 7 months of age, followed by the upper central incisors at 6 to 8 months. The upper lateral incisors usually follow these at 9 to 11 months and the lower central incisors at 10 to 12 months. Generally the first molars appear next at 12 to 16 months, then the cuspids at 16 to 20 months, and finally the second molars at 20 to 30 months. The eruption of all the primary teeth usually is completed by age 3 years. The eruption of permanent teeth commonly begins at about 6 years of age. Medical practice in underdeveloped areas that do not record birth dates sometimes utilizes a method of estimating a child's age by counting the teeth: The age in months equals the number of teeth plus 6 months for children under age 3.

Occasionally children are born with teeth or have the eruption of teeth in the first month of life, and these children often have a family history of early tooth eruption. Some controversy has emerged about whether these teeth should be extracted, since they may lead to tongue lacerations, feeding difficulties, and abrasions to the mother's nipples during breast feeding. Delayed eruption is sometimes present in patients with Down's syndrome, hypothyroidism, hypopituitarism, achondroplastic dwarfism, and other syndromes that involve the delayed development of organ systems.

Typically the pending eruption of a tooth in an infant produces discomfort and tenderness, which lead to irritability and a compulsion by the infant to chew on relatively hard objects. The chewing activity can stimulate increased salivation, which may account for the drooling characteristically described by parents.

Diarrhea often has been associated with teething, but no studies have confirmed a relationship. The development of oral lesions also has been associated with teething, but it is thought that these may be herpetic gingivostomatitis lesions. Fever commonly has been associated with teething; however, studies are unclear about whether there is a relationship. It has been observed that an infant's temperatures are slightly elevated (37 to 38°C or 98.6 to 100.4°F) the day before the eruption of the first tooth, but no studies have shown that teething is associated with greater temperature elevations. The association of fever might be a manifestation of the development of a coincidental viral gingivitis, which might then produce lesions, fever, irritability, drooling, and diarrhea, all of which are folkloric symptoms of teething.

PATHOGENESIS

It is thought that the physical pressure of erupting teeth may create physical pressure on nearby structures. This could produce temporary discomfort and a local sensation of irritability that induces a need to manipulate or stimulate the affected area. Increased chewing resulting from this need can increase salivation, which over time can produce an atopic rash below the lower lip and at the corners of the mouth.

DIAGNOSTIC CONSIDERATIONS

Symptoms attributed to teething by folklore should be considered to be possibly secondary to other causes. Infectious diseases that are common in this age group should be ruled out, along with pathology secondary to trauma. Teething is essentially a diagnosis of exclusion.

LABORATORY TESTS

Since teething is a diagnosis of exclusion, no laboratory testing is useful in making the diagnosis. The diagnosis usually is made in light of the history and physical examination findings, sometimes with additional support from the negative results of laboratory tests used to rule out other disorders.

TREATMENT

The most common treatment for teething is the application of a topical anesthetic (teething gel) to the affected areas. Several compounds are available without prescription that contains ethylaminobenzoate (benzocaine) in a gel formulation that can be applied with cotton, a cotton swab, or a fingertip. For infants and children 4 months to 2 years of age, compounds containing 7.5 to 10% benzocaine can be applied up to four times a day. Products containing 7.5% benzocaine include Anbesol Baby, Num-Zit Gel, Orabase Baby, and Orajel Baby. Products containing 10% benzocaine include Numzident, Orajel, Orajel Nighttime Formula Baby, and Rid-A-Pain. Benzocaine teething gel should be used with caution in infants and young children, since absorption may result in methemoglobinemia. Benzocaine products can produce allergic sensitivity to other local anesthetics, and overuse can suppress the gag reflex and inhibit the swallowing mechanism, with potentially serious results.

Analgesics such as acetaminophen and ibuprofen are considered safer and are thought to be more effective than teething gels for the treatment of teething discomfort. Teething toys are useful mainly for distraction and should be evaluated primarily with safety in mind.

The general approach to the treatment of teething problems first consists of the exclusion of other causes of the symptoms. The expected course of normal tooth eruption should be explained to the parent, and the use of systemic analgesics should be encouraged. The parent should be cautioned about the use of teething gels and encouraged to monitor teething toys and devices for safety. Like many minor childhood problems, teething difficulties eventually go away regardless of what treatment, if any, is provided.

BIBLIOGRAPHY

Castiglia P: Teething. *J Pediatr Health Care* 6(3):153–154, 1992.
Coreil J: Recognition and management of teething diarrhea among Florida pediatricians. *Clin Pediatr* 34(11):591–598, 1995.
Jaber L: Fever associated with teething. *Arch Dis Child* 67(2):233–234, 1992.
King DL: Herpetic gingivostomatitis and teething difficulty in infants. *Pediatr Dent* 14(2):82–85, 1992.
King DL: Teething revisited. *Pediatr Dent* 16(3):179–182, 1994.
Kowitz AA: Paediatric dentistry: Fauchard and before. *Int Dent J* 43(3):239–244, 1993.
Mueller WA, Abrams RB: Oral medicine and dentistry, in *Current Pediatric Diagnosis and Treatment,* 14th ed. WW Hay Jr et al (eds): Stamford, CT, Appleton & Lange, 1999, pp 387–388.

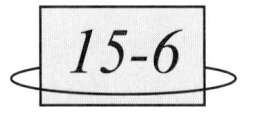

GROWTH AND DEVELOPMENT IN INFANCY AND EARLY CHILDHOOD

Jill Reichman

DISCUSSION

To provide comprehensive health care for infants and children, a clinician needs to monitor their growth and development. Although significant variation in the rate of growth and development may occur among children, an accepted normal range has been established by statistically comparing children of the same age and sex. Growth charts are developed by using available data sources to create percentiles. Plotting growth data for an infant or child allows a clinician to compare that infant or child with the statistical norm and assign a percentile. Conscientious surveillance can identify infants and children who are outside this normal range as well as those who have sudden changes in their growth patterns. Once identified, these children can be closely monitored and referred as needed for further evaluation.

The most basic evaluation of growth and development involves the measurement of height and weight along with head circumference in children age less than 3 years. Using and maintaining data on growth charts help a clinician visually map growth and quickly identify abnormalities and changes in growth curves. Newly revised growth charts were released by the Centers for Disease Control and Prevention (CDC) in June 2000. These revised growth charts better reflect heights and weights for children in the United States. Growth charts are available for recording the length and weight of infants and toddlers age 0 to 36 months and for recording the height and weight of toddlers and older children age 2 to 20 years. A separate chart can be completed to record head circumference in infants and children under age 3 years. All these charts are available with appropriate percentiles for both boys and girls. The newly revised CDC growth charts also include body mass index-for-age (BMI) percentiles for boys and girls ages 2 to 20 years. These BMI charts can be used to identify children and teens who are either overweight or at risk for overweight. Growth charts can be obtained by accessing the CDC Website at www.cdc.gov/growthcharts.

Several other parameters should be evaluated during the routine examination, including neonatal reflexes, gross motor skills, fine motor-adaptive skills, social skills, and language skills. Monitoring developmental milestones in infants and children allows a clinician to screen for children who need further evaluation.

DEVELOPMENTAL MILESTONES

Neonatal Reflexes

Early milestones of development include the appearance and disappearance of neonatal or primitive reflexes. Infants are born with most of the primitive reflexes, which slowly disappear between 5 weeks and 6 months of age. These reflexes are involuntary motor responses

TABLE 15-6-1.   Selected Neonatal Reflexes

REFLEX	DESCRIPTION
Moro (startle)	Occurs when the neck and limbs contract in response to allowing infant's head to fall backward suddenly or when the infant is startled by a sudden noise or jerk. Generally disappears by age 4 months.
Rooting	Elicited in response to touching cheek or corner of mouth and results in turning of head and opening of mouth. Facilitates breast feeding and usually disappears by age 3 to 4 months.
Sucking	Elicited by placing an object in infant's mouth; results in sucking movements of lips. Along with rooting reflex, helps facilitate feeding.
Palmar grasp	Occurs when object or finger is placed in infant's hand, causing infant to grasp object or finger tightly. Usually disappears by age 2 to 3 months.
Tonic neck	Seen in supine infant when head is turned to one side, causing infant to extend extremities on same side and flex extremities on opposite side. Although often present at birth, may not appear until 2 months and usually disappears by 4 months.
Placing	Elicited when dorsal aspect of foot is allowed to touch edge of a table, causing infant to flex at hip and knee and place foot onto tabletop. Disappearance is variable but may occur by 1.5 to 2 months.
Stepping	Elicited when infant is held upright and leaning forward; this causes movements of the legs that look like walking. Usually disappears by 1.5 to 2 months.

SOURCE: Adapted from Berkowitz.[2]

elicited by environmental stimuli. Table 15-6-1 describes some of the reflexes that can be evaluated during a routine examination. The absence or persistence of these reflexes suggests a dysfunction of the central nervous system and requires referral.

Gross Motor Development

Milestones in gross motor development can be observed in a newborn and continue to occur throughout childhood. In the first 2 years of life, gross motor development is dramatic, transforming an infant with little head control into a toddler who runs and jumps. From ages 2 through 6, gross motor development seems less dramatic to the observer, but this is a time when the coordination of gross motor skills is achieved. It is also a time when injuries tend to occur as children venture forth and experiment with new motor skills and abilities. The clinician should be aware of the range of normal abilities and should inform parents about injury prevention. Table 15-6-2 describes the major gross motor milestones as they occur chronologically.

Fine Motor-Adaptive Skills Development

Fine motor skills involve the use of smaller muscles in the hands and fingers and correspond to the development of adaptive skills that require hand-eye coordination. These skills are present in infants but are most notable after age 4 years, when children begin to manipulate small objects easily and perform complicated tasks such as putting together a puzzle. By age 6 years most children can tie their shoes and write their names. Toddlers spend much of their time practicing fine motor skills by using paper and pencils or crayons. Parents should be reminded about the need for supervision of these activities to prevent injuries in young children. Table 15-6-3 describes the major fine motor-adaptive skills in infants and children.

TABLE 15-6-2.   Gross Motor Milestones

AGE	ABILITY
Newborn	Moves head from side to side
1 month	Raises chin, lifts head when prone, makes lateral head movements
2 months	Raises chest with arms when prone
3 months	Holds head steady when upright, sits on lap with support
4 months	No head lag when pulled to sitting, rolls from front to back
5 months	Sits alone momentarily, rolls from back to front
6–7 months	Sits alone steadily
7–9 months	Creeps or crawls, pulls to standing
9–11 months	Cruises, walks when led with support
12–15 months	Stands alone, walks a few steps independently
18 months	Walks backward, walks up stairs with support, starts running
2 years	Runs, jumps down from a low object
3 years	Begins throwing and catching with assistance, walks up stairs using alternating steps, rides a tricycle, begins hopping
4 years	Begins skipping, walks down stairs using alternating steps, refines running and hopping
5 years	Running speed increases; further refines jumping, hopping, and skipping
6 years and older	Skillful hopping and skipping, mature throwing pattern, catches with hands only

TABLE 15-6-3.   Fine Motor-Adaptive Skills

AGE	SKILL
1 month	Hands closed most of the time; can follow object to midline
2 months	Can follow object past midline and vertically
3 months	Hands more often open than closed; can follow object 180°
4 months	Regards hands; reaches for bright object; hands come together; brings objects to mouth
5 months	Grasp now voluntary; combs for objects with hands
6 months	Transfers objects from one hand to other
7 months	Can grasp with three-finger pincer motion
9–12 months	Grasp now two-finger pincer; bangs objects together in midline; releases objects voluntarily; plays pat-a-cake
15 months	Makes tower of three cubes; can draw line with crayon
18 months	Makes tower of four cubes; can scribble
2 years	Makes tower of seven cubes; copies vertical and horizontal lines
3 years	Makes tower of 10 cubes; copies a circle
4 years	Can build bridge from model; copies cross and square; draws person with two to four parts besides head
5 years	Copies triangle; draws person with three parts
6 years	Draws person with six parts; writes name

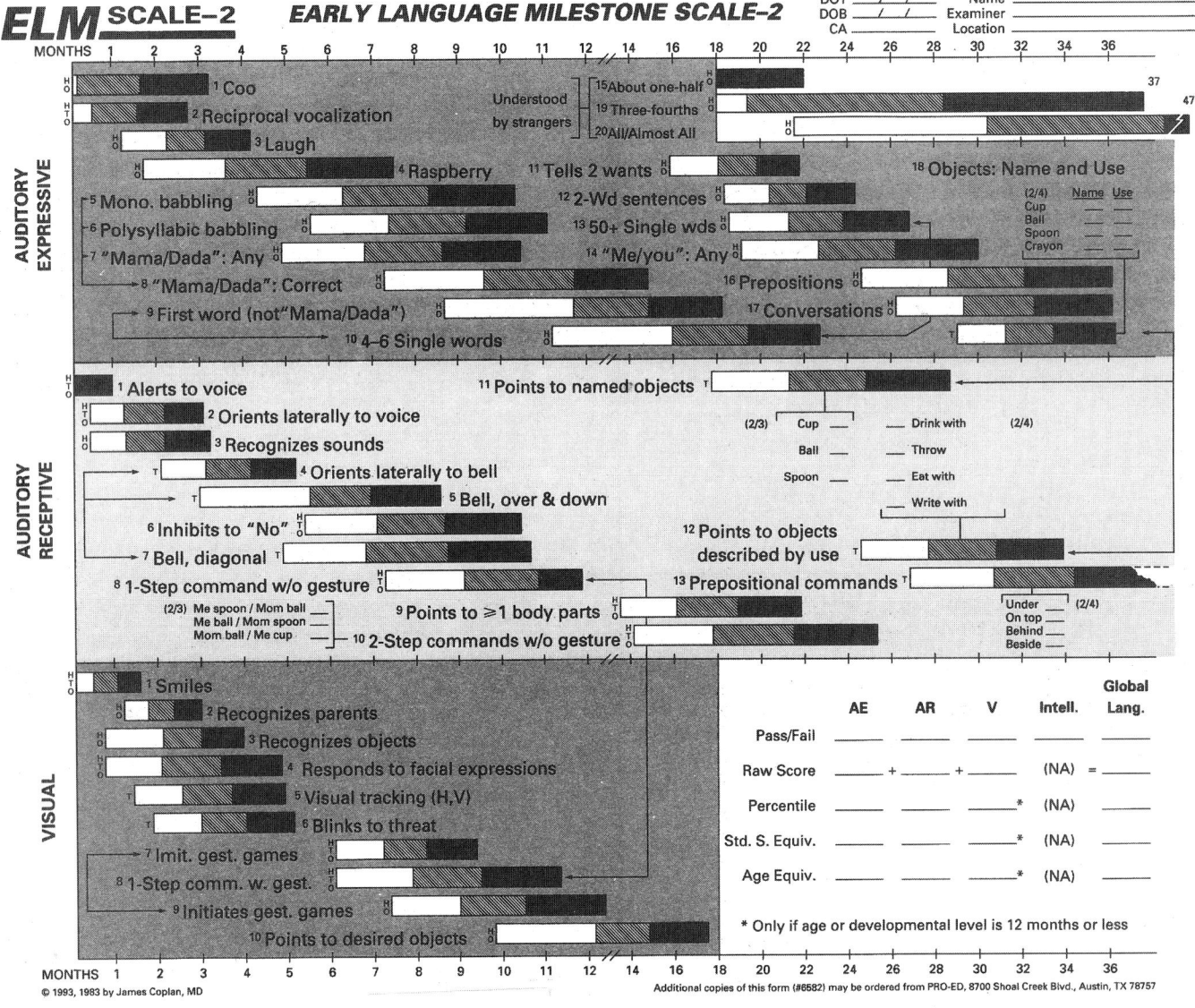

FIGURE 15-6-1. Early Language Milestone Scale–2. (*Continued on next page.*)

Language Development

Like motor skills, speech and language develop with recognizable milestones that can be evaluated by a clinician. In most cases, problems are identified by the parents and brought to a clinician for evaluation. Understanding the range of normal helps a clinician appropriately reassure the parents that the child's development is within the range of normal or, alternatively, initiate a workup and referral for a child with suspected delayed language development. Because delayed language development may be due to hearing impairment, the evaluation of hearing is a critical part of the workup. Careful assessment of language ability may be aided by the use of a screening test such as the Early Language Milestone (ELM) Scale. This allows the screening of language development in children under 36 months of age. The ELM allows a clinician to evaluate expressive, receptive, and visual language through parental reporting and direct observation of the child (Fig. 15-6-1).

The development of language requires three basic abilities: expression, reception, and articulation. Expressive skills can be appreciated very early in life as the vocalizations of infants. Receptive skills involve the ability to hear and react to sound. Later, more sophisticated language skills allow a child to convey meaning and understand language. This can be seen as early as 9 to 12 months of age, when most infants begin to use language meaningfully by saying

"mama" or "dada." These single-word expressions eventually become multiword expressions, whole sentences, and ultimately groups of sentences strung together to express complex ideas. Table 15-6-4 reviews the developmental milestones in language skills as they occur chronologically.

The referral of young children with a suspected delay in language development is aided by the use of tools such as the ELM. There are, however, specific guidelines for referral that should be followed, including the following:

1. Lack of response to sound at any age
2. Lack of babbling by 9 months
3. Inability to understand and/or respond to simple requests by age 2 years
4. Speech predominantly unintelligible by age 3 years
5. Stuttering, poor voice quality, and/or poor ability to articulate after age 5 years

Social Skills Development

Social skills are abilities that allow children to care for themselves and interact with others. As children grow older, some of these skills are molded by cultural or societal norms. These skills, which begin to develop at just a few weeks of age, start as a simple preference for

I. General Instructions

25% 50% 75% 90%   Percentage of Children
Passing Item

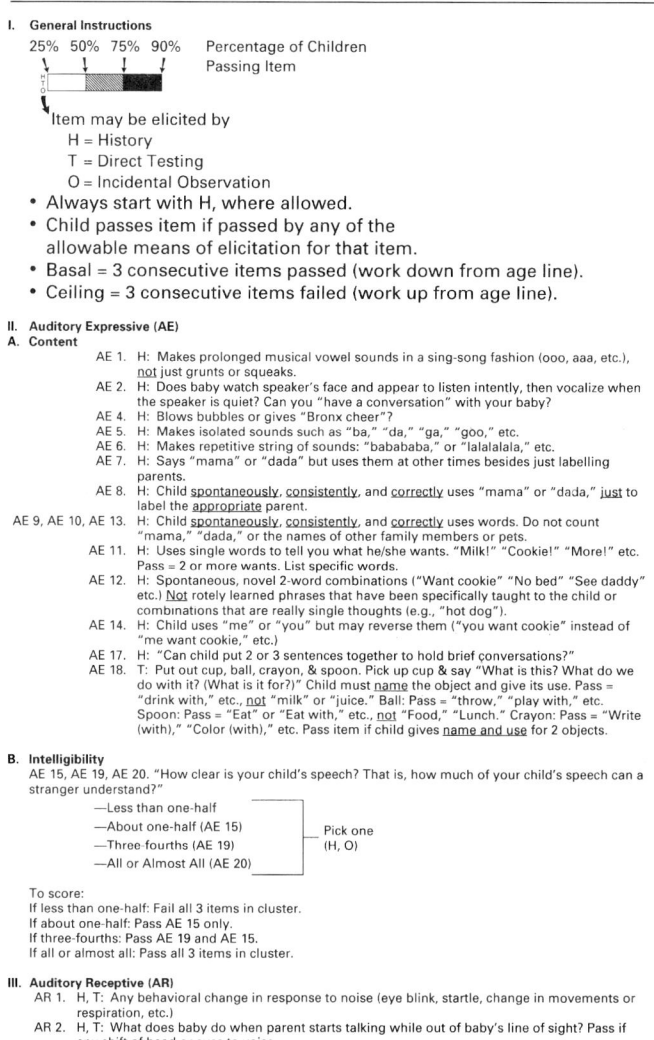

Item may be elicited by
H = History
T = Direct Testing
O = Incidental Observation
- Always start with H, where allowed.
- Child passes item if passed by any of the allowable means of elicitation for that item.
- Basal = 3 consecutive items passed (work down from age line).
- Ceiling = 3 consecutive items failed (work up from age line).

II. Auditory Expressive (AE)
A. Content

AE 1. H: Makes prolonged musical vowel sounds in a sing-song fashion (ooo, aaa, etc.), not just grunts or squeaks.
AE 2. H: Does baby watch speaker's face and appear to listen intently, then vocalize when the speaker is quiet? Can you "have a conversation" with your baby?
AE 4. H: Blows bubbles or gives "Bronx cheer"?
AE 5. H: Makes isolated sounds such as "ba," "da," "ga," "goo," etc.
AE 6. H: Makes repetitive string of sounds: "bababababa," or "lalalalala," etc.
AE 7. H: Says "mama" or "dada" but uses them at other times besides just labelling parents.
AE 8. H: Child spontaneously, consistently, and correctly uses "mama" or "dada," just to label the appropriate parent.
AE 9, AE 10, AE 13. H: Child spontaneously, consistently, and correctly uses words. Do not count "mama," "dada," or the names of other family members or pets.
AE 11. H: Uses single words to tell you what he/she wants. "Milk!" "Cookie!" "More!" etc. Pass = 2 or more wants. List specific words.
AE 12. H: Spontaneous, novel 2-word combinations ("Want cookie" "No bed" "See daddy" etc.) Not rotely learned phrases that have been specifically taught to the child or combinations that are really single thoughts (e.g., "hot dog").
AE 14. H: Child uses "me" or "you" but may reverse them ("you want cookie" instead of "me want cookie," etc.)
AE 17. H: "Can child put 2 or 3 sentences together to hold brief conversations?"
AE 18. T: Put out cup, ball, crayon, & spoon. Pick up cup & say "What is this? What do we do with it? (What is it for?)" Child must name the object and give its use. Pass = "drink with," etc., not "milk" or "juice." Ball: Pass = "throw," "play with," etc. Spoon: Pass = "Eat" or "Eat with," etc., not "Food," "Lunch." Crayon: Pass = "Write (with)," "Color (with)," etc. Pass item if child gives name and use for 2 objects.

B. Intelligibility
AE 15, AE 19, AE 20. "How clear is your child's speech? That is, how much of your child's speech can a stranger understand?"

—Less than one-half
—About one-half (AE 15)
—Three-fourths (AE 19)   Pick one
—All or Almost All (AE 20)   (H, O)

To score:
If less than one-half: Fail all 3 items in cluster.
If about one-half: Pass AE 15 only.
If three-fourths: Pass AE 19 and AE 15.
If all or almost all: Pass all 3 items in cluster.

III. Auditory Receptive (AR)
AR 1. H, T: Any behavioral change in response to noise (eye blink, startle, change in movements or respiration, etc.)
AR 2. H, T: What does baby do when parent starts talking while out of baby's line of sight? Pass if any shift of head or eyes to voice.

AR 3. H: Does baby seem to respond in a specific way to certain sounds (becomes excited at hearing parents' voices, etc.)?
AR 4. T: Sit facing baby, with baby in parent's lap. Extend both arms so that your hands are behind baby's field of vision and at the level of baby's waist. Ring a 2"-diameter bell, first with 1 hand, then the other. Repeat 2 or 3 times if necessary. Pass if baby turns head to the side at least once.
AR 5. T: See note for AR 4. Pass if baby turns head first to the side, then down, to localize bell, at least once. (Automatically passes AR 4.)
AR 6. H: Does baby understand the command "no" (even though he may not always obey)? T: Test by commanding "(Baby's name), no!" while baby is playing with any test object. Pass if baby temporarily inhibits his actions.
AR 7. T: See note for AR 4. Pass if baby turns directly down on diagonal to localize bell, at least once. (Automatically passes AR 5 and AR 4.)
AR 8. H: Will your baby follow any verbal commands without you indicating by gestures what it is you want him to do ("Stop" "Come here" "Give me" etc.)? T: Wait until baby is playing with any test object, then say "(Baby's name), give it to me." Pass if baby extends object to you, even if baby seems to change his mind and take the object back. May repeat command 1 or 2 times. If failed, repeat the command but this time hold out your hand for the object. If baby responds, then pass item V 8 (1-step command with gesture).
AR 9. H: Does your child point to at least 1 body part on command? T: Have mother command baby "Show me your…" or "Where's your…" without pointing to the desired part herself.
AR 10. H: "Can child do 2 things in a row if asked? For example 'First go get your shoes, then sit down'?" T: Set out ball, cup, and spoon, and say "(Child's name), give me the spoon, then give the ball to mommy." Use slow, steady voice but do not break command into 2 separate sentences. If no response, then give each half of command separately to see if child understands separate components. If child succeeds on at least half of command, then give each of the following: "(Child's name), give me the ball and give mommy the spoon." May repeat once but do not break into 2 commands. Then "Give mommy the ball, then give the cup to me." Pass if at least two 2-step commands executed correctly. (Note: Child is credited even if the order of execution of a command is reversed.)
AR 11. T: Place a cup, ball, and spoon on the table. Command child "Show me/where is/give me… the cup/ball/spoon." (If command is "Give me," be sure to replace each object before asking about the next object.) Pass = 2 items correctly identified.
AR 12. T: Cup, ball, spoon, and crayon on table and give command "Show me/where is/give me… the one we drink with/eat with/draw (color, write) with/throw (play with)." If the command "Give me" is used, be sure to replace each object before asking about the next object. Pass = 2 or more objects correctly identified.
AR 13. T: Put out cup (upside down) and a 1" cube. Command the child "Put the block under the cup." Repeat 1 or 2 times if necessary. If no attempt, or if incorrect response, then demonstrate correct response, saying, "See, now the block is under the cup." Remove the block and hand it to the child. Then give command "Put the block on top of the cup." If child makes no response, then repeat command 1 time but do not demonstrate. Then command "Put the block behind the cup," then "Put the block beside the cup." Pass = 2 or more commands correctly executed (prior to demonstration by examiner, if "under" is scored).

IV. Visual
V 1. H: "Does your baby smile—not just a gas bubble or a burp but a real smile?" T: Have parent attempt to elicit smile by any means.
V 2. H: "Does your baby seem to recognize you, reacting differently to you than to the sight of other people? For example, does your baby smile more quickly for you than for other people?"
V 3. H: "Does your baby seem to recognize any common objects by sight? For example, if bottle or spoon fed, what happens when bottle or spoon is brought into view before it touches baby's lips?" Pass if baby gets visibly excited, or opens mouth in anticipation of feeding.
V 4. H: "Does your baby respond to your facial expressions?" T: Engage baby's gaze and attempt to elicit a smile by smiling and talking to baby. Then scowl at baby. Pass if any change in baby's facial expression.
V 5. T: Horizontal (H): Engage child's gaze with yours at a distance of 18". Move slowly back and forth. Pass if child turns head 60° to left and right from midline. Vertical (V): Move slowly up and down. Pass if child elevates eyes 30° from horizontal. Must pass both H & V to pass item.
V 6. T: Flick your fingers rapidly towards child's face, ending with fingertips 1–2" from face. Do not touch face or eyelashes. Pass if child blinks.
V 7. H: Does child play pat-a-cake, peek-a-boo, etc., in response to parents?
V 8. T: See note for AR 8 (always try AR 8 first; if AR 8 is passed, then automatically give credit for V 8).
V 9. H: Does child spontaneously initiate gesture games?
V 10. H: "Does your child ever point with index finger to something he/she wants? For example, if child is sitting at the dinner table and wants something that is out of reach, how does child let you know what he/she wants?" Pass only index finger pointing not reaching with whole hand.

FIGURE 15-6-1. (*continued*). Early Language Milestone Scale–2.

TABLE 15-6-4. Milestones in the Development of Language Skills

AGE	EXPRESSIVE SKILLS	RECEPTIVE SKILLS
0–2 months	Cries, begins gurgling sounds (cooing, vowel-like sounds)	Is aware of sound; turns toward sound; prefers human voice
3–4 months	May start to laugh or chuckle; cooing sustained	Seems to be listening; looks at speaker; reacts differently to different types of speech, e.g., angry versus happy
5–6 months	Cooing includes sounds of consonants, and babbling begins	Responds to own name; begins to understand other familiar words
9–12 months	Sounds start to be repeated, and "words" appear, e.g., *mama, dada*	Responds to *no* or other simple verbal commands by stopping activity or using other gestures to communicate
14–16 months	Vocabulary 10–50 words; speaks using jargon (actual words mixed with nonsense words)	Can point to familiar named objects or body parts
18–24 months	Vocabulary 50–75 words; speaks in two-word phrases, e.g., *my doll, thank you*	Responds to two-step command, e.g., "Come to Mommy and bring the book"; understands complex sentences and simple questions
2–3 years	Fast-growing vocabulary up to 1000 words; speaks in short (three-word) sentences; speech most often intelligible	Can follow a story in a picture book; understands prepositional commands
3–4 years	Vocabulary up to 1500 words; speech intelligible; speaks in four-word sentences	Responds to three-step commands
4–5 years	Language well established; conversation mature; large vocabulary; defines simple words; uses five-word sentences	Responds to four-step commands
5–6 years	Has adult speech pattern; articulation continues to improve	Responds to five-step commands; can follow story told without picture book; begins to understand more subtle nuances of language, e.g., that same word may have two meanings

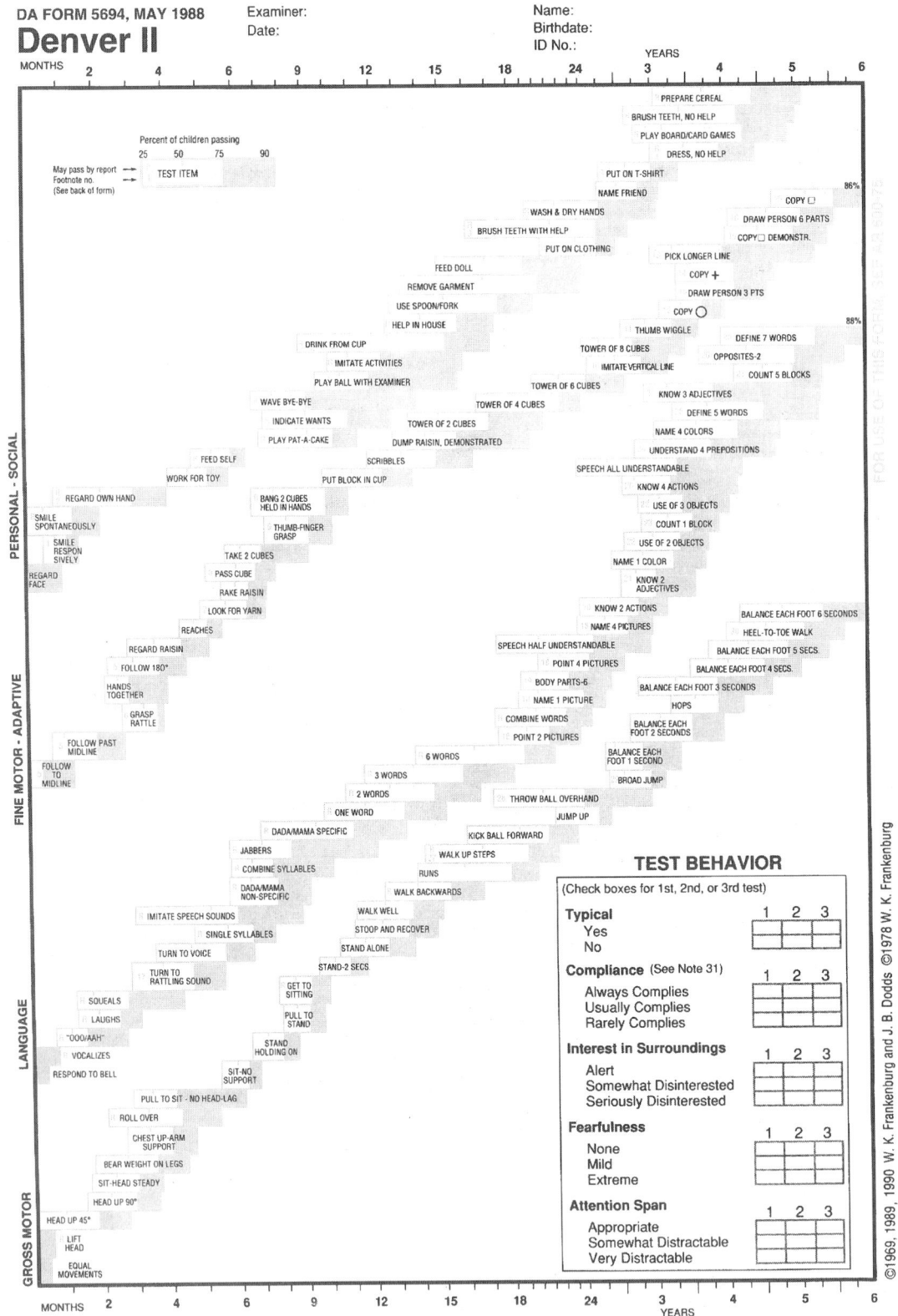

FIGURE 15-6-2. Denver II Developmental Screening Test.

DIRECTIONS FOR ADMINISTRATION

1. Try to get child to smile by smiling, talking or waving. Do not touch him/her.
2. Child must stare at hand several seconds.
3. Parent may help guide toothbrush and put toothpaste on brush.
4. Child does not have to be able to tie shoes or button/zip in the back.
5. Move yarn slowly in an arc from one side to the other, about 8" above child's face.
6. Pass if child grasps rattle when it is touched to the backs or tips of fingers.
7. Pass if child tries to see where yarn went. Yarn should be dropped quickly from sight from tester's hand without arm movement.
8. Child must transfer cube from hand to hand without help of body, mouth, or table.
9. Pass if child picks up raisin with any part of thumb and finger.
10. Line can vary only 30 degrees or less from tester's line. /
11. Make a fist with thumb pointing upward and wiggle only the thumb. Pass if child imitates and does not move any fingers other than the thumb.

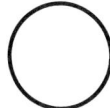

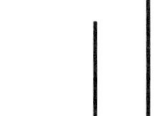

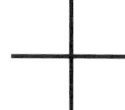

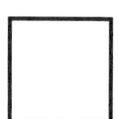

12. Pass any enclosed form. Fail continuous round motions.

13. Which line is longer? (Not bigger.) Turn paper upside down and repeat. (pass 3 of 3 or 5 of 6)

14. Pass any lines crossing near midpoint.

15. Have child copy first. If failed, demonstrate.

When giving items 12, 14, and 15, do not name the forms. Do not demonstrate 12 and 14.

16. When scoring, each pair (2 arms, 2 legs, etc.) counts as one part.
17. Place one cube in cup and shake gently near child's ear, but out of sight. Repeat for other ear.
18. Point to picture and have child name it. (No credit is given for sounds only.)
    If less than 4 pictures are named correctly, have child point to picture as each is named by tester.

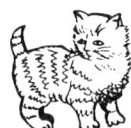

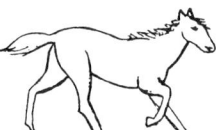

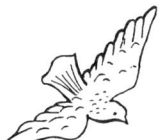

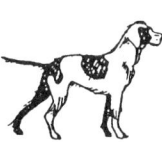

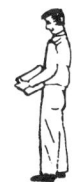

19. Using doll, tell child: Show me the nose, eyes, ears, mouth, hands, feet, tummy, hair. Pass 6 of 8.
20. Using pictures, ask child: Which one flies?... says meow?... talks?... barks?... gallops? Pass 2 of 5, 4 of 5.
21. Ask child: What do you do when you are cold?... tired?... hungry? Pass 2 of 3, 3 of 3.
22. Ask child: What do you do with a cup? What is a chair used for? What is a pencil used for?
    Action words must be included in answers.
23. Pass if child correctly places <u>and</u> says how many blocks are on paper. (1, 5).
24. Tell child: Put block **on** table; **under** table; **in front of** me, **behind** me. Pass 4 of 4.
    (Do not help child by pointing, moving head or eyes.)
25. Ask child: What is a ball?... lake?... desk?... house?... banana?... curtain?... fence?... ceiling? Pass if defined in terms of use, shape, what it is made of, or general category (such as banana is fruit, not just yellow). Pass 5 of 8, 7 of 8.
26. Ask child: If a horse is big, a mouse is __? If fire is hot, ice is __? If the sun shines during the day, the moon shines during the __? Pass 2 of 3.
27. Child may use wall or rail only, not person. May not crawl.
28. Child must throw ball overhand 3 feet to within arm's reach of tester.
29. Child must perform standing broad jump over width of test sheet (8 1/2 inches).
30. Tell child to walk forward, ⊂∞⊃⊂∞⊃⊂∞⊃➔ heel within 1 inch of toe. Tester may demonstrate.
    Child must walk 4 consecutive steps.
31. In the second year, half of normal children are non-compliant.

OBSERVATIONS:

FIGURE 15-6-2. (*continued*). Denver II Developmental Screening Test.

TABLE 15-6-5. An Overview of Social Development in Childhood

AGE	SOCIAL SKILLS	ERIKSON'S DEVELOPMENTAL STAGE
1 month 2 months 6 months 9 months 12 months 18 months	Preference for human face; begins to smile Responds to voice; coos Laughs; interacts with caregiver Prefers mother to others; may show stranger anxiety Plays games; peek-a-boo, pat-a-cake; waves bye-bye on command; may cooperate with dressing; drinks from cup Starts to feed self, with spoon; communicates some needs with gestures and words; hugs and kisses	**Stage 1: Trust versus mistrust (0–1.5 years)** Focus of this stage is trust and social support. Infant learns to trust or mistrust that his or her needs will be met by caregiver. This is determined by consistency of care infant receives from caregiver. Erikson's theory supports idea that this early developmental period sets groundwork for future socialization. Trust is necessary to achieve healthy social interactions. Successful resolution of this stage sets stage for healthy interactions later in life.
2 years 3 years	Cooperates with dressing; communicates verbally with caregivers; helps in bathing self Parallel plays; begins to help with dressing—may button and unbutton; washes and dries hands; may be toilet trained	**Stage 2: Autonomy versus shame and doubt (1.5–3 years)** Focus of this stage is establishment of independence and sense of self. During this phase, much of a child's time is spent practicing self-control. Sense of autonomy and well-being is achieved as child successfully completes this stage. If child feels unsuccessful, he or she is likely to experience feelings of shame. Healthy limits provided by caregiver help the child through this stage.
4 years 5 years	Plays interactively with others; models behavior of others Dresses self; often plays by role modeling; asks questions and when comfortable interacts with others, often enthusiastically	**Stage 3: Initiative versus guilt (3–6 years)** Focus of this stage is learning to care for oneself. During this stage children are eager to learn and begin to understand social rules and appropriate behavior. Successful resolution of this stage helps child be enthusiastic and industrious. Difficulty in this stage can lead to feelings of guilt. As in previous developmental periods, healthy limits set by caregiver help child be successful.

the human face. Later, children shift from playing side by side (parallel play) to engaging in interactive play that requires communication with and consideration of others. Children learn to toilet train, bathe, and dress themselves with the encouragement and modeling of their caretakers.

The psychologist Erik Erikson developed a theory of child development that emphasizes the psychosocial focus of each developmental stage throughout childhood. His theory suggests that at each stage of development a child must successfully navigate a critical period. This accomplishment leads to a healthy sense of self and the development of positive social skills. Table 15-6-5 gives a brief overview of social development in childhood and includes Erikson's stages of psychosocial development.

SCREENING TESTS

There are numerous screening instruments that allow a clinician to look at most or all of the developmental parameters through the use of a single tool. The Denver Developmental Screening Test (DDST), originally published in 1967, has been used worldwide, and it was revised and restandardized in 1989 to make it more accurate. The new Denver II allows a clinician to monitor development in the following areas: gross motor, language, fine motor-adaptive, and personal-social (Fig. 15-6-2). It also includes a test behavior rating scale that offers an opportunity to evaluate variables such as attention span, fearfulness, and compliance.

The authors "emphasize that the Denver II is a screening test, the results of which should be integrated with everything else that one knows about the child, the family, the community, the educational experiences, and the culture in which the child has grown up."[1] The Denver II is not a diagnostic or predictive tool. It is designed to identify children who are not performing as expected for age so that they can be referred for further evaluation.

The Denver II is most effectively administered by a trained clinician. Denver Developmental Materials, Inc., of Denver, Colorado,

offers training materials that include a technical manual and training videotapes. Appropriate training in the administration of the Denver II helps assure the reliability of the test outcome.

Screening is the process by which a clinician can identify children who need further evaluation. Using standardized screening tools, such as growth charts and developmental testing instruments, a properly trained clinician can perform this task with the greatest reliability. In this way, physician assistants can fill a critical role in the early identification and referral of children with suspected developmental delays.

REFERENCES

1. Frankenburg WK et al: The Denver II: A major revision and restandardization of the Denver Developmental Screening Test. *Pediatrics* 89:91–97, 1992.
2. Berkowitz CD: *Pediatrics: A Primary Care Approach.* Philadelphia, Saunders, 1996, pp 49–58.

BIBLIOGRAPHY

Behrman R et al: *Nelson Textbook of Pediatrics,* 16th ed. Philadelphia, Saunders, 2000, pp 23–65.
Bickley L: *Bates' Guide to Physical Examination and History Taking,* 7th ed. Philadelphia, Lippincott, 1999, pp 621–703.
Centers for Disease Control and Prevention: *Advance Data from Vital Statistics and Health Statistics of the CDC/National Center for Health Statistics,* Number 314, June 8, 2000 (revised).
Gormly A: *Lifespan Human Development,* 6th ed. Fort Worth, TX, Harcourt Brace College Publishers, 1997, pp 15–250.
Hay W et al: *Current Pediatric Diagnosis and Treatment,* 14th ed. Norwalk, CT, Appleton & Lange, 1999, pp 1–25.
Rudolph A, Kamei R: *Rudolph's Fundamentals of Pediatrics.* Norwalk, CT, Appleton & Lange, 1994, pp 1–25.
Tanner JM: *Fetus into Man.* Cambridge, MA, Harvard University Press, 1978.
Vaughan V, Litt I: *Child and Adolescent Development: Clinical Implications.* Philadelphia, Saunders, 1990, pp 145–227.
Walker D et al: Early Language Milestone Scale and language screening of young children. *Pediatrics* 83:284–288, 1989.

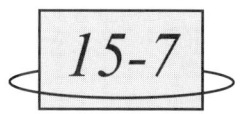

BEHAVIOR PROBLEMS IN CHILDREN AND ADOLESCENTS

Randy Danielsen

DISCUSSION

Despite the occasional horror story regarding children and adolescents, the majority of children and teenagers in America navigate development quite well. It is not uncommon, however, for parents to present to their primary care provider with concerns over the behavior of their child or teenager. Behavioral disorders, including conduct disorder, oppositional defiant disorder, and disorders of attention, are becoming increasingly recognized for their possible association with acts of delinquency.[1]

Conduct disorders carry significant social and monetary costs. These disorders are the most common reason for juvenile referrals in clinical settings, with prevalence estimates ranging from 30 to 50% of clinical populations. Since minor conduct problems disappear with age, it generally is accepted that limited youthful delinquent or resistant behavior is normative and developmentally appropriate. Nevertheless, it is crucial for clinicians to recognize the warning signs of these behavioral disorders and take every opportunity to evaluate their illness and the underlying contributing factors, including home, family, and peers. This is particularly important since many of these youths will not be adequately treated before becoming personally involved with the juvenile justice system, an event that suggests decreased success of treatment. Furthermore, early intervention seems prudent in light of calls for increasingly punitive treatment of juvenile offenders.

In the presence of antisocial acts committed by minors that are severe enough to be the focus of clinical attention, three major diagnoses should be considered. The selection of a diagnosis will of course shape the treatment plan selected. These diagnoses are:

1. Child or adolescent antisocial behavior
2. Oppositional defiant disorder
3. Conduct disorder

The second and third conditions result from a mental disorder. Extreme caution should be used in the diagnosis of disorders associated with children's oppositional and delinquent behaviors. Some authors suggest that these diagnoses are significantly overused and too easily assigned.[2] This observation has serious implications for youth. A label such as *conduct disorder* probably will follow a young person throughout his or her academic career and may influence that person's school performance and attendance. Youths with serious conduct disorders have the potential to be a danger to themselves and/or others and must be identified in order to receive whatever remediation, however limited, may be available. In addition, the early identification of such youths is likely to increase their ability to benefit from treatment.

Antisocial Behavior

The descriptor *antisocial behavior* may be used when a child or teenager needs to receive treatment because of antisocial acts that do not reach the severity levels of more advanced disordered behavior. These behaviors are isolated and singular incidents and do not reflect a pattern of antisocial behaviors. In addition, they are not precipitated by an underlying mental disorder, although they cause significant familial and/or personal disruption. It is important to note that these types of "acting-out" behaviors may indicate a seemingly unrelated problem or stressor in the family or school setting, and a thorough social history is requisite. Thus, the presence of an adjustment disorder with disturbance of conduct should be ruled out on the basis of the recent occurrence of a stressor to which the child has not adjusted.

Impulse control disorders, mood disorders, and attention disorders may produce conduct problems and often co-occur with disorders of conduct (see "Attention Deficit Disorder" Chap. 16-4). Thus, treatment may include alleviating environmental stressors or addressing comorbid psychological problems. The clinician should assess whether the act or acts were committed alone or in a group, and what type or types of delinquent acts were attempted or completed. As a general rule, acts committed alone and acts that include confrontation with or harm to other people should be considered more serious and should alert the clinician to the need for continued monitoring of the patient's behavior.

Oppositional Defiant Disorder

Oppositional defiant disorder is often a precursor of conduct disorder, but there is not a perfect predictive relationship. This disorder is usually present by age 8 years and rarely has an onset after early adolescence. Prevalence estimates range from 2 to 16%. These children are resistant, hostile, and defiant in the home but can display such behavior in other settings. They argue with adults, refuse to comply with rules, and behave in angry, spiteful, vindictive, annoying, and/ or overly sensitive ways. These children often lose their temper and blame others for their problems. To be considered clinically significant, these behaviors must persist for at least 6 months, cause a clear functional impairment, and occur more often than would be expected for the child's age (e.g., children under 3 years of age are frequently, and developmentally appropriately, defiant). Conduct disorder should be ruled out, which includes repeated violations of rules or the rights of others. Mood disorders, psychotic disorders, developmental disabilities, and impulse control problems and attention disorders can mimic or co-occur with oppositional defiant disorder. Furthermore, as with other conduct symptoms, this behavior can result from environmental stressors that may best be detected through a full social history and assessment of a child's current life circumstances and coping resources. Family functioning also must be assessed. Often clinical intervention with the family is necessary, and if the youth is still attending school, behavioral school intervention is warranted.

Conduct Disorder

ETIOLOGY   The development of conduct disorder has been linked to a number of factors, including familial dysfunction,[3] poverty,[4] impulsivity,[5] antisocial attitudes,[6] intellectual limitations,[7] victimization and early childhood trauma,[8] and inadequate prenatal and perinatal care.[9]

Genetic factors have been implicated in the development of conduct disorder. Although these results are suggestive, they are often difficult to interpret since genetic causality overlaps with environmental factors. Neurologic issues appear to contribute to impulse control problems, such as associated attention deficit hyperactivity disorder (ADHD) symptoms. Neurotransmitters have not been conclusively shown to contribute to this disorder; however, youths with conduct disorder tend to have lower overall levels of physiologic arousal,[10] and serotonin levels have been linked to aggression and violent behaviors.[11,12]

PREVALENCE AND ONSET   Conduct disorder may occur as early as age 6 years, but is more likely to be recognized in later childhood and early adolescence. Onset is rare after age 16 years. Prevalence estimates suggest that males under 18 years old are more likely to receive the diagnosis than are females (6 to 16% versus 2 to 9%). In addition, the prevalence of conduct disorder has increased over time, and it occurs more frequently in urban populations.[13] An early onset of delinquent behaviors may predict more severe acts over longer periods of time.[14] Childhood onset (before 10 years of age) or adolescent onset should be diagnostically specified.

COMORBIDITY   Physician assistants should note that children and adolescents with conduct problems are at increased risk for a broad spectrum of health problems and are far more likely to engage in health-deleterious behaviors than are typical youths.

Research indicates that conduct-disordered youngsters are:

- More likely to engage in unprotected sexual activities that could result in early pregnancy and/or sexually transmitted diseases, including HIV infection
- More likely to use and abuse illicit and legal substances
- More susceptible to injury and to being seen in an emergency room
- More likely to fail in school
- More likely to be socially alienated and/or incarcerated
- At higher risk for a variety of mental health problems

SIGNS AND SYMPTOMS

These children view the world as a hostile place. As a result, they may misperceive others' actions as aggressive despite good intentions and react in "justifiably" aggressive ways. The diagnostic criteria stated in the *Diagnostic and Statistical Manual* (DSM-IV) for conduct disorder include a repeated and lasting pattern of behaviors that are violations of the norms and rules of conduct expected for the child's age or that violate the rights of others.[13] To be considered conduct-disordered, a youth must demonstrate three problematic behaviors in the prior 12 months, with at least one behavior occurring in the past 6 months. According to the DSM-IV, the presence of the following behaviors is included in those that should be used to build a case for the treatment of conduct disorder:

1. Aggressive behaviors such as threatening or intimidating people, initiating physical fights, using a weapon with a high level of lethality or injury-causing potential (e.g., gun, knife, broken bottle), physically harming animals and/or people, stealing in the presence of the victim (e.g., face-to-face extortion, mugging, armed robbery), and forcing someone into unwanted sexual activity
2. Destruction of property, including setting intentional fires and perpetrating other types of deliberate damage to property
3. Deceitfulness or theft such as breaking into someone else's car, house, business, or building; stealing an item of value without confronting the victim (e.g., shoplifting); and lying to obtain things or avoid responsibilities (e.g., "conning" others)
4. Serious rule violations, including frequently staying out at night despite parental prohibitions beginning before age 13, running away from home overnight more than once or for long periods, and being truant from school beginning before age 13.

In addition to the exhibition of these types of behaviors, the symptom severity must be of sufficient magnitude to cause serious impairment in the individual's functioning. Often among these youths there is a major discord in the family related to a child's attitudes and behaviors, and school failure, suspension, or expulsion occurs. A substantial proportion of individuals who are diagnosed with conduct disorder are later diagnosed with antisocial personality disorder in adulthood, a disorder that shares with conduct disorder a number of factors, such as lack of empathy or concern for the rights of others, lying, substance abuse, and legal transgressions. In addition, these youths are at risk for adult substance abuse problems.

Male and female patients with conduct problems may or may not present differently. In general, females tend to show internalizing delinquent behaviors, such as substance abuse, early sexual promiscuity, and/or pregnancy. However, more recently females have been showing an increased frequency of committing externalizing acts similar to those of males (e.g., physical fights and interpersonal violence, stealing, weapons use). It is rare to find a youth displaying conduct problems who does not use or abuse mood-altering substances.

What is notable about the types of behaviors considered diagnostic of conduct disorder is the vast range of severity. Clearly, a child who in the last year has verbally intimidated other children, shoplifted a pack of chewing gum, and lied several times to avoid chores has a level of disorder severity different from that of a child who has stolen a neighbor's automobile, set the school gymnasium on fire, and forced a female acquaintance to perform oral sex on him. A clinician must be aware of the broad range of behavior that may support a diagnosis of this disorder and judiciously choose when another diagnosis or no diagnosis is warranted. The general view is that one should use a diagnostic label only when it is fully justified. In the case of conduct disorder, quasi-normative delinquent behaviors that are likely to abate with age must be separated from a repetitive pattern of predatory and/or antisocial behavior in the assignment of a diagnosis. This is a difficult task, and a competent mental health professional can be a useful ally in the diagnostic process. Furthermore, it is helpful to differentiate the disorder as mild, moderate, or severe.

Solitary and Group Activities

A further differentiating factor in understanding conduct disorder may be whether the individual acts delinquently in the presence of others or alone; however, research to date is inconclusive. Clinical views of the solitary versus the group type of violator tend to paint the group type of perpetrator as more likely to be a victim of social facilitation or mob rule who may be swept along with whatever delinquent acts his or her peers are engaged in at the time. Thus, this individual is not a premeditator, and the rewards for the behavior are largely social, consisting of peer recognition and status. Solitary or unsocialized perpetrators, by contrast, are considered more pathologic and as drawing the reward from the commission of the illegal act or the domination or humiliation of another person. However, certain group acts are of such a heinous nature that they suggest the highly pathologic composition of packs of antisocial youth (e.g., "gang" rapes). Both solitary and group-type perpetrators may act impulsively, show little remorse, and lack empathy.

Gangs

Some clinicians believe that all gang members are delinquent or conduct-disordered, but this is not the case. Some youths are nominal members of gangs only, for instance, as a result of their recruitment by a relative who is a member or to be able to use recreational facilities in their neighborhoods that they would otherwise be banned from accessing as nonmembers. Some youths identify with gangs for personal protection. Others find that gangs serve as a surrogate family and/or workplace that provides relatively clear role expectations and support for gang-normative behavior. Problems arise for youths who are engaged in gang-related criminal activity, since the norms of the gang collide with the norms of society. Thus, while gang membership, style of dress, and tattoos may be red flags for potential antisocial behavior and conduct disorder, a thorough psychosocial history using a number of information sources should be used to affirm or disaffirm the practitioner's suppositions.

OBJECTIVE FINDINGS

A full psychosocial history is needed to adequately establish whether a youth is at risk for or can be diagnosed with conduct-related disorders. Psychological testing by a psychologist may be warranted to determine the intelligence level and functional level. It is essential to obtain a history from a parent or caregiver, who may be less likely to "sugar coat" the facts; however, youngsters often hide criminal activity from their parents, and therefore the youth may be the best informant in certain areas of inquiry. These youths are less likely to display attitudinal correlates of opposition or argumentativeness with strangers (such as during a first meeting with a clinician) than with family members, and observation of the patient in other settings and with authority figures is essential to diagnosis and treatment planning. Furthermore, some of these youths have had considerable practice at distorting the truth and are quite successful at hiding their antisocial attitudes and behaviors when it is in their best interest to do so.

Often red flags occur in the individual's story, such as school problems, early and/or frequent sexual activity, early and/or frequent substance abuse, and a clear failure to empathize with others whom they have victimized and/or acknowledge the needs of anyone other than themselves. It is helpful to question the origins of any visible scars or other physical evidence of injuries, which may reveal a history of fighting or abuse. In the examining room, these youths may be disrespectful to the practitioner or may refuse to speak. In addition, the practitioner may feel hostile toward or fearful of them.

Formal measurement of delinquent behavior or prediction of conduct disorders is difficult. The Youth Self-Report Scale and the Child Behavior Checklist teacher- and parent-reported versions may help identify youths who more frequently engage in aggressive and delinquent behaviors, but these scores are not considered clinical cutoff scores.[15]

Documented criminal acts and self-reported and other-reported delinquent acts are often the best clinical indicators of potential conduct problems and are the most accessible to physician assistants. It should be noted that poor early school achievement and prior neglect and/or abuse are seen as being related to later conduct problems.

TREATMENT

Research findings are mixed on the effectiveness of various treatments for disruptive disorders. All treatments must be tailored to the individual child and family. The best treatments probably are multimodal and comprehensive, including the family, children, school, community, and peers.[16] Behavioral, family-based interventions hold promise and need additional evaluation.[16,17] These programs teach parents how to reward positive, prosocial behaviors and remove rewards for problem behavior in a manner that does not provide the child with any power (e.g., the ability to upset parents). Residential treatment often is used for more severe disorders, with varying results. The most effective programs include token economy systems that teach youths how to obtain rewards through their behavior and how to delay gratification and also teach social skills with peers and adults to reduce social rejection.

The Role of the Physician Assistant

It is essential to recall that these patients are children who probably have experienced significant trauma, lack a stable home life, or have been exposed to parental criminal behavior. However, these youths also have the potential to perpetrate serious offenses. Physician assistants (PAs) should encourage parents to constantly evaluate their children or teenagers for indications of healthy or unhealthy functioning. PAs should also use the annual sports physical, routine screenings, or episodic care appointments to provide a professional assessment of the child. The PA can provide these youngsters with much-needed aid. It is important to provide good mental health referrals when indicated (e.g., enough offenses have occurred to warrant concern and impair the youth's ability to function). If the child is already in a group home or another out-of-home court-ordered placement, he or she probably is receiving mental health services in the residential setting. The PA's intervention should vary with the severity of the disorder. Clearly, youngsters who are incarcerated are a different population than youths who infrequently commit less serious offenses. Incarcerated youths are most likely serious violent offenders, repeat offenders of less serious crimes, or both violent and repeat offenders. It is important to be mindful that arrest and/or incarceration typically occur in a youth's life after numerous undetected crimes have occurred, although this is not always the case.

A PA's therapeutic role with such children and adolescents should include:

- Serving as a stable adult figure who shows genuine concern for their welfare
- Serving as an adult figure who keeps his or her agreements and can be trusted

- Serving as an adult who is not easily duped but is willing to believe and trust the youngster within limits
- Modeling and requiring respectful interpersonal behavior
- Indicating to youths that one can and will help them as long as they comply with clinic rules (no smoking on the premises, no stealing supplies, etc.)
- Indicating that they have worth and bolstering their self-esteem
- Empathizing with their difficult experiences
- Empowering them to take control of their futures and change them

It may be useful to discuss with adolescents the career paths they have chosen. If they are engaged in serious offenses, they often spontaneously acknowledge that the path they are now on is likely to lead them to be an exceptional criminal and resident of a penitentiary in adulthood. Most of the time this image does not fit with some of their more positive aspirations. At this point, the practitioner can begin to discuss how to train for a new career if they would like to (e.g., get the GED, look into community college, explore job training programs). The practitioner also must debunk the myth of having a record "wiped clean" at 18 years of age. This is a hope that many of these youths hold dear. Although the opportunity to "stay clean" as an adult and have no record to follow them should be acknowledged, the practitioner must emphasize that the changes that can allow staying clean to happen must occur now. In other words, some youths believe that once their records are expunged, so is their risk of committing crimes. This belief should be challenged, and success should be linked to slow, painstaking behavioral changes. One should support and reward prosocial behaviors and, if possible, allow the child to experience success in his or her contact with the practitioner. These simple steps can be accomplished through verbal praise of appropriate behavior in the waiting and examination rooms and the setting of easily attainable goals that the youth can reach and receive attention for completing. However, each should be an act that the practitioner can easily document when it occurs (e.g., being on time for an appointment). These goals can be set to be progressively more difficult as a relationship develops. A fine line must be observed in developing such goals. The youths must be included in the development of the goals or they are sure to resist and fail. Also, the PA should avoid being too authoritarian with these youths, as this can reduce their responsiveness. However, one should keep in mind that most children who are out of control are desperately seeking structure and guidance. Their acting-out behaviors often require the structure and guidance of the state juvenile justice and/or social services systems. Thus, once a relationship is established, the use of some authority is appropriate.

Simultaneously, the PA should assure the youth that he or she is giving the youth no less than his or her best job despite the discomfort. This is often a rare experience for them with adults.

Children who have had scholastic difficulty must be reintegrated into a targeted, often limited, school setting as quickly as possible,[18] a setting in which they can experience success.

Alternative, safe circumstances must be designed for children in abusive homes and homes in which the parents are partially functional (e.g., poorly managed mental illness in a parent or active addictions). Social services agencies should be notified if there is abuse or neglect.

Pharmacologic Management

The use of medication may be indicated if a youth exhibits certain features, such as hyperactivity, mood fluctuations, and psychotic symptoms. Drug therapy should never be used as an independent treatment without additional interventions.

As was previously noted, youths with conduct problems also often display ADHD symptoms or syndromes. Under these circumstances, the use of stimulant medication can reduce not only inattention but also aggression, oppositional behaviors, and impulsivity. Some research suggests the usefulness of lithium (1 to 6 mg/d) and haloperidol (500 to 2000 mg/d).[19] For youngsters with depressive episodes, antidepressant medications may be indicated.[20] Beta blockers may be indicated for patients with rage reactions or neurologic problems.[21] Carbamazepine may be useful in adolescents with impulsive aggression with emotional irritability or lability, abnormal electroencephalogram, or suggested epileptic symptoms.[22]

There is some risk of misuse or abuse involved in prescribing drugs to youngsters with conduct problems, not only among the youths themselves but often among a patient's peers and family members. Thus, although it has been suggested that certain psychoactive medications may improve conduct problems, caution should be exercised in prescribing pharmacologic agents, and close monitoring by a psychiatrist is recommended, particularly when noncompliance is a problem.

NOTES AND PEARLS

The identification and treatment of conduct problems in youth must be directed by normative developmental expectations of behavior. PAs must guard against the random assignment of such diagnostic labels yet be responsive to troubled youths who need help in reducing delinquent behaviors. The role of the primary care provider should focus on extensive history taking that allows early suspicion, confirmation, and treatment of these disorders. The PA can play an important role in the child's or teenager's development by conducting annual evaluations and engaging the parents in frequent discussions about the child's progress. Positive reinforcement, of both the parent and the child, is essential. When a problem is identified, involving a mental health professional early in the care of both the parents and the child is critical. All treatments for conduct problems should involve the individual youth, the educational system, the family, the medical system, and, if indicated, the legal and social services systems. Pharmacotherapy may be indicated in certain cases.

ACKNOWLEDGMENT

The editor would like to acknowledge Kelly E. Naylor, author of this chapter in the first edition of _Primary Care for Physician Assistants,_ for her significant contributions.

REFERENCES

1. Danielsen RD: Teenage behavioral problems: Identifying troubled adolescents. _Clinician Reviews_ (5):5584, 1995.
2. Lewis DO: Conduct disorder, in _Child and Adolescent Psychiatry: A Comprehensive Textbook,_ M Lewis (ed). Baltimore, Williams & Wilkins, 1991.
3. Farrington DP: The family backgrounds of aggressive youths, in _Aggression and Antisocial Behavior in Childhood and Adolescence,_ LA Hersov et al (eds). Oxford, UK, Pergamon Press, 1978.
4. Fergusson DM et al: The childhoods of multiple problem adolescents: A 15 year longitudinal study. _J Child Psychol Psychiatry_ 35(6):1123–1140, 1994.
5. Pfefferbaum B, Wood PB: Self-report study of impulsive and delinquent behavior in college students. _J Adolesc Health_ 15(4):295–302, 1994.
6. Hoge RD et al: Tests of three hypotheses regarding the predictors of delinquency. _J Abnorm Child Psychol_ 22(5):547–549, 1994.
7. Rantakallio P et al: Juvenile offenders, with special reference to sex differences. _Soc Psychiatry Psychiatr Epidemiol_ 30(3):113–120, 1995.
8. Schwartz IM et al: Is child maltreatment a leading cause of delinquency? _Child Welfare_ 73(5):639–655, 1994.
9. Penzerro RM, Lein L: Burning their bridges: Disordered attachment and foster care discharge. _Child Welfare_ 74(2):351–366, 1995.
10. Raine F et al: Relationships between central and autonomic measures of arousal at age 15 and criminality at age 24 years. _Arch Gen Psychiatry_ 47:1003–1007, 1990.
11. Mann JJ: Psychobiological predictors of suicide. _J Clin Psychiatry_ 48(12): 39–43, 1987.
12. Virkkunnen M et al: Relationship of psychobiological variables to recidivism in violent offenders and impulsive fire setters: A follow-up study. _Arch Gen Psychiatry_ 46:600–603, 1989.
13. _Diagnostic and Statistical Manual of Mental Disorders,_ 4th ed. Washington, DC, American Psychiatric Association, 1994.
14. Tolan PH, Thomas P: The implications of age of onset for delinquency risk: II. Longitudinal data. _J Abnorm Child Psychol_ 21(2):157–181, 1995.
15. Achenbach TM: _The Manual for the Youth Self-Report and 1991 Profile._ Burlington, VT, University of Vermont, Department of Psychiatry, 1991.
16. Henggeler SW, Borduin CM: _Family Therapy and Beyond: A Multisystemic Approach to Treatment of the Behavior Problems of Children and Adolescents._ Pacific Grove, CA, Brooks/Cole, 1990.
17. Patterson GR: _Families: Applications of Social Learning to Family Life._ Champaign, IL, Research Press, 1975.
18. Forehand RL, McMahon RJ: _Helping the Non-Compliant Child: A Clinician's Guide to Parent Training._ New York, Guilford Press, 1981.
19. Campbell SB et al: Behavioral efficacy of haloperidol and lithium carbonate: A comparison in hospitalized aggressive children with conduct disorder. _Arch Gen Psychiatry_ 41:650–656, 1984.
20. Puig-Antich J: Major depression and conduct disorder in prepuberty. _J Am Acad Child Adolesc Psychiatry_ 42:511–517, 1982.
21. Williams DT et al: The effects of propranolol on uncontrolled rage outbursts in children and adolescents with organic brain dysfunction. _J Am Acad Child Adolesc Psychiatry_ 21:129–135, 1982.
22. Evans RW et al: Carbamazepine in pediatric psychiatry. _J Am Acad Child Adolesc Psychiatry_ 26:2–8, 1987.

BIBLIOGRAPHY

Dixon SD, Stein MT: _Encounters with Children. Pediatric Behavior and Development,_ 2d ed. St. Louis, Mosby Yearbook, 1992.
Prothrow-Stith D: _Deadly Consequences: How Violence Is Destroying Our Teenage Population and a Plan to Begin Solving the Problem._ New York, Harper Collins, 1991.

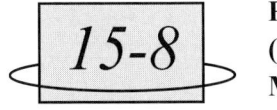

PEDIATRIC INNOCENT (FUNCTIONAL) HEART MURMURS

David P. Asprey

DISCUSSION

The terms _innocent murmur_ and _functional murmur_ refer to the audible sound that results from the flow of blood through a structurally normal heart and vascular system. Primary care clinicians are repeatedly confronted with the diagnostic dilemma of distinguishing innocent heart murmurs from pathologic ones. Pathologic murmurs result from turbulent blood flow created by an underlying cardiac defect. As many as 90% of all children will have an audible heart murmur at some point in time.[1] However, the incidence of congenital heart disease is estimated to be less than 1% (0.8%) of all live births. Consequently, the vast majority of children with murmurs have murmurs that are innocent or functional.

The clinician's responsibility is to screen a child and determine whether his or her murmur is a normal finding or requires further assessment. This further assessment may be accomplished by utilizing additional testing (echocardiography) or by referring the child for evaluation by a pediatric cardiology clinician. As echocardiography has become directly available to primary care clinicians, a debate regarding the cost-effectiveness of ordering an echocardiogram before referral to a pediatric cardiologist compared to direct referral to a pediatric cardiologist has developed. There are data that suggest that referral of children with questionable murmurs to pediatric cardiologists for evaluation is more cost-effective than direct evaluation with echocardiography followed by referral of those with congenital heart disease.[2]

This section focuses on distinguishing innocent heart murmurs from pathologic murmurs. An understanding of the various types of common innocent (normal) murmurs is essential in order to avoid the mistaken diagnosis of organic heart disease. A discussion of the murmurs associated with common congenital heart defects appears in Chap. 1-2.

Distinguishing the innocent murmur from the pathologic murmur indicative of a cardiovascular defect is the main responsibility of the clinician. The five most common innocent heart murmurs in children discussed in this section include:

1. Vibratory or Still's murmur
2. Pulmonary flow murmur
3. Peripheral pulmonary artery stenosis murmur
4. Supraclavicular arterial bruit murmur
5. Venous hum

The unintentional mislabeling of an innocent heart murmur as pathologic may have adverse effects on the psychosocial well-being of the child and his or her family by inducing unnecessary concern about the child. In addition, unnecessarily prescribed subacute bacterial endocarditis (SBE) prophylaxis may result in adverse side effects from the prescribed antibiotics. Finally, misdiagnosis may make following restrictions on physical activities unnecessary, obtaining certain types of employment difficult or impossible, and securing reasonably priced life and health insurance very difficult.

Failing to diagnose a child with congenital heart disease when he or she has a heart defect can be even more problematic. Often children with congenital heart disease are recommended to observe SBE prophylaxis to reduce their risk of acquiring a serious infection of the endocardium. In addition, some children will require medical or surgical treatment of their cardiac defect to prevent irreversible damage (e.g., pulmonary hypertension) from occurring.

Primary care clinicians can effectively distinguish murmurs with a pathologic origin from the innocent variety. The ability to successfully make this distinction with a high degree of accuracy is dependent on the clinician's ability to appropriately utilize the history, physical examination, and laboratory data in a systematic fashion.

SIGNS AND SYMPTOMS

The first and often most important step in distinguishing between innocent and pathologic murmurs occurs by taking a thorough and careful history. Care should be taken to collect a complete and thorough gestational and birth history. This history should include assessing the presence of gestational infections such as rubella, which is associated with patent ductus arteriosus and pulmonic stenosis. Maternal illness such as diabetes can result in increased occurrence of ventricular septal defects and patent ductus arteriosus. Maternal ingestion of medications such as anticonvulsants, amphetamines, progesterone, and estrogen are believed to be teratogenic. Drug and alcohol intake may result in fetal alcohol syndrome, which is associated with ventricular septal defects, patent ductus arteriosus, and atrial septal defects. Birth history should include gestational age (premature infants have a higher incidence of patent ductus arteriosus) and Apgar scores to assess the cardiorespiratory response.

A neonatal history and history of the present illness is also very useful in identifying significant heart disease. Care should be taken to assess the presence of weight gain patterns and development. Failure to adequately gain weight or develop appropriately can be associated with congestive heart failure. A history of difficulty with feeding or fatigue and diaphoresis associated with bottle or breast feeding may also indicate congestive heart failure. The presence of central cyanosis suggests that the patient may have a cardiac defect that allows for desaturated venous blood to mix with oxygenated blood. Tachycardias, shortness of breath, and dependent edema (which may appear on the face or sacrum of infants) are all possible signs of congestive heart failure. Decreased levels of exercise tolerance may be indicative of children with volume overload lesions such as an atrial septal defect or ventricular septal defect. Presence or reports of palpitations, lightheadedness, or syncope may indicate the presence of an arrhythmia. Children with chest discomfort should be assessed for the presence of arrhythmias, mitral valve prolapse, or ischemic heart disease, which is extremely rare in this age group. If any of these findings are identified as abnormal the clinician should investigate each symptom thoroughly and systematically in order to assess its possible association with heart disease.

In addition to the history components mentioned above, collecting a careful family history may provide additional clues to the likely presence of congenital heart disease. Specifically inquire regarding the presence of hereditary diseases often associated with heart disease such as Marfan's syndrome, mitral valve prolapse, Noonan's syndrome, and Williams syndrome. Other common syndromes associated with cardiac defects or abnormalities include trisomy 21 (Down's), trisomy 18, trisomy 13, DiGeorge's, Turner's, and VATER syndromes.

OBJECTIVE FINDINGS

The physical examination is a very powerful tool in distinguishing innocent heart murmurs from pathologic murmurs. Many syndromes are associated with a high incidence of congenital heart disease. Consequently, the general assessment begins with inspection of the patient, which may reveal dysmorphic features and/or the presence of a syndrome associated with congenital heart disease as identified in the previous section. The assessment of the general appearance may also reveal tachypnea or respiratory distress, cyanosis, pallor, or diaphoresis, each of which may be a sign of underlying congenital heart disease.

Palpation should include the precordium and the peripheral pulses. A palpable lift or heave may be indicative of pressure or volume overload cardiac defects such as aortic stenosis, aortic insufficiency, and defects resulting in a large left-to-right shunting of blood (atrial septal defects, ventricular septal defects, or patent ductus arteriosus). Palpation should also be carried out to assess the presence of a thrill. A *thrill* refers to the palpable vibratory sensation that results from turbulent blood flow within the cardiovascular system. Typically the presence of a thrill suggests either obstructive defects (such as pulmonic stenosis, aortic stenosis) or a shunt defect between two chambers with a large pressure difference (such as ventricular septal defect). Peripheral pulses should be carefully assessed for amplitude, intensity, and symmetry. Diminished left arm or leg pulses when compared to the right arm suggest coarctation of the aorta. Bounding pulses suggest the presence of a large patent ductus arteriosus or severe aortic insufficiency.

Finally, because many patients will not have any signs or symptoms of their disease except the presence of a murmur, auscultation of the patient's heart becomes critical to accurately distinguishing between many innocent and pathologic murmurs. Each of the five commonly occurring pediatric innocent murmurs is discussed in the "Diagnostic Considerations" section.

Even in the absence of pertinent findings from the medical history, identifiable syndromes, or dysmorphic features, there are certain auscultatory findings that should be considered abnormal until proven otherwise. These findings include diastolic murmurs, any systolic murmur associated with a thrill, pansystolic murmurs, continuous murmurs that cannot be suppressed (see the discussion on venous hum under "Diagnostic Considerations"), systolic clicks, opening snaps, fixed splitting of the second heart sound, an accentuated P_2 component of the second heart sound, or S_4 gallops. If any of these findings are present the child should be referred to a pediatric cardiology clinician for further evaluation.

DIAGNOSTIC CONSIDERATIONS

It is important to adopt and utilize a systematic approach to performing the auscultatory examination to help ensure that no important information is inadvertently left out. Auscultation of the heart should be performed with the patient sitting, sitting while leaning forward, supine, and in the left lateral decubitus position. In each position the examiner should listen to several heartbeats through a few respiratory cycles at the aortic, pulmonic, tricuspid, and mitral areas at a minimum. In each position the examiner should utilize the diaphragm and bell capabilities of the stethoscope to increase the likelihood of hearing all-important sounds of high and low pitch. At each site the clinician should specifically listen to and assess the first heart sound, the second heart sound, extra sounds in systole (e.g., clicks), extra sounds in diastole (e.g., S_3, S_4, opening snaps), murmurs in systole, and murmurs in diastole.

If a murmur is detected the clinician should note the following characteristics: timing, location of maximal intensity, radiation, intensity (grade), pitch, and quality. If a murmur or extra heart sound is present, special maneuvers such as listening to the change in the timing or quality of the murmur while the patient squats, stands, or performs a Valsalva maneuver may help to distinguish various murmurs.

Innocent heart murmurs have a distinct set of features that with experience the clinician can become very skilled at identifying. Previous studies have shown that pediatric cardiologists can differentiate innocent from pathologic murmurs by clinical exam alone with high degrees of sensitivity and specificity.[2] Each of the five innocent heart murmurs identified in this section have characteristic findings that most clinicians will be able to develop confidence in diagnosing when given adequate experience examining children with murmurs. Table 15-8-1 summarizes the five innocent murmurs, describing their timing, pitch, intensity, location, radiation, quality, and differential diagnosis.[3]

The vibratory or Still's murmur is a low-pitched, vibratory (i.e., with a musical quality) mid-systolic murmur that is heard maximally at the lower left sternal border. This murmur is most prevalent in children between 3 and 6 years of age. Typically it is grade II–III/VI in intensity. This murmur decreases in intensity with the Valsalva maneuver or when the patient is in a sitting or standing position. The intensity will increase with any high-output state such as fever, anxiety, anemia, or exercise. The primary differential diagnosis of this murmur is a small ventricular septal defect or subvalvular left ventricular outflow tract stenosis such as a subaortic membrane or idiopathic hypertrophic subaortic stenosis.

The pulmonary flow murmur is an early- to mid-systolic ejection murmur that is middle- to high-pitched and is heard maximally at the upper left sternal border. It is usually grade I–II/VI in intensity and is louder during inspiration and when the patient is in a supine position. Typically this murmur is present in older children between the ages of 8 and 14 years. It will increase in intensity during times of increased cardiac output. This murmur usually has very little radiation. The primary differential diagnosis of this murmur is pulmonic stenosis (generally associated with a pulmonic click in valvular pulmonic stenosis) or atrial septal defect that is associated with a fixed, split second heart sound.

The peripheral pulmonary artery stenosis murmur is most common in the newborn period and especially the premature infants or infants with low birth weight. This is a short, mid-systolic murmur that is generally of middle pitch and intensity, seldom louder than grade II/VI. This murmur is usually transient and will resolve spontaneously by approximately 6 months of age. The murmur will often be heard loudest over the lung fields rather than the heart and will radiate throughout the lung fields. There should be no ejection click present with this murmur. The primary differential for this murmur is supravalvular stenosis, which is very rare in isolation. If the murmur does not diminish in intensity or resolve by 6 months of age, another cause for the murmur should be sought.

The supraclavicular arterial bruit murmur is a harsh, relatively low-pitched (best heard with the bell) systolic murmur that is usually heard maximally just above the clavicles and typically is louder on the right side. This murmur is usually grade II–III/VI in intensity and can be made softer by hyperextending the shoulders during auscultation. This murmur is generally present in older children but is reported in children of all ages. The primary differential diagnosis for this murmur is that of supravalvular aortic stenosis. The examiner should be certain to check for the presence of a suprasternal notch thrill. The presence of this type of thrill suggests a pathologic cause of the murmur.

The venous hum murmur is a common, continuous murmur that is present at either the upper right or upper left sternal border and is usually grade II–III/VI in intensity when the child is in a sitting position. It results from the turbulence created by venous return from the head and neck through the jugular vein. This murmur can be decreased in intensity or even obliterated by having the child rotate his or her head to a position of maximal rotation in either direction, by digital compression of the jugular venous system just above the clavicles, or by placing the patient in a supine position. This murmur is common among children between 3 and 8 years of age. The primary differential diagnosis of this murmur is patent ductus arteriosus. The murmur associated with patent ductus arteriosus is continuous and heard maximally at the upper left sternal border; however, this murmur is neither reduced in intensity nor eliminated by the maneuvers described above.

LABORATORY STUDIES

In most children with murmurs laboratory data is of little benefit. Electrocardiograms (ECGs) may provide additional information about the heart and the likelihood of a heart defect. However, some studies have indicated that ECGs do not help clinicians distinguish between innocent and pathologic murmurs.[4]

RADIOLOGIC STUDIES

Likewise there is considerable debate regarding the usefulness of the chest x-ray in distinguishing innocent heart murmurs from pathologic murmurs.[5] Many pediatric cardiology clinicians will perform chest x-rays only on children less than 2 years of age who are referred for an initial evaluation of a murmur.

OTHER DIAGNOSTIC STUDIES

Echocardiograms are utilized only in those situations in which pathology is suspected or in cases when the diagnostic evaluation does not provide a clear differentiation of the patient's condition.

TREATMENT

Patients diagnosed with innocent heart murmurs have a normal heart, therefore no treatment is necessary.

Patient Education

Educating the patient and his or her parents about the meaning of an innocent heart murmur is extremely important. It is a natural reaction for parents to assume that if their child has a murmur that there is something wrong with his or her heart. It is important that the clinician assure the patient and the family that this is a normal finding. Parents can be advised that many times the murmur resolves on its own as the child gets older, but that if it doesn't it is of no consequence because the child's heart is normal. If the patient was started on SBE prophylaxis, care should be taken to inform the family that it is not indicated in patients with innocent heart murmurs. It may be useful to explain to the child and the family that anything

TABLE 15-8-1. Clinical Characteristics of Innocent Heart Murmurs

TYPE OF INNOCENT MURMUR	TIMING	PITCH	INTENSITY	LOCATION	RADIATION	QUALITY	DIFFERENTIAL DIAGNOSIS	MISCELLANEOUS COMMENTS
Vibratory or Still's murmur	Mid-systolic ejection	Low frequency	Typically grade II–III/VI	2d or 3d left ICS	No significant radiation	Musical or vibratory	IHSS, small VSD, PS	Usually louder with patient supine or with inspiration
Pulmonary flow murmur	Early to mid-systolic	Mid to high frequency	Typically grade I–II/VI	2d or 3d left ICS	Slight radiation to lung fields through PA branch arteries	Blowing	ASD, PS	Accentuated by states of increased cardiac output
Peripheral pulmonary artery stenosis murmur	Short mid-systolic	Mid to high frequency	Typically grade II/VI	2d left ICS	To lung fields and axilla bilaterally	Typically soft	ASD, PS	Typically present in the newborn period only
Supraclavicular arterial bruit murmur	Early systolic	Low frequency	Typically grade II–III/VI	Supraclavicular fossa bilaterally	To carotid artery area	Harsh	AS	May be reduced by having the patient hyperextend his or her shoulders
Venous hum	Continuous	High frequency	Typically grade II–III/VI	May be bilateral, supraclavicular to 1st or 2d ICS	None	Soft	PDA	Suppressed by laying patient supine or digital compression of the neck veins

ABBREVIATIONS: AS, aortic stenosis; ASD, atrial septal defect; ICS, intercostal space; IHSS, idiopathic hypertrophic subaortic stenosis; PA, Pulmonary artery; PDA, patent ductus arteriosus; PS, pulmonic stenosis; VSD, ventricular septal defect.

573

that results in increased cardiac output (anxiety, fever, etc.) will make the murmur louder and that clinicians unfamiliar with the child's examination may interpret the intensity of the murmur as a sign of heart disease.

Disposition

No follow-up is necessary for patients diagnosed with an innocent heart murmur.

PEARLS

Often it will be very challenging to obtain an adequate period of quiet time to perform a complete cardiac exam including the auscultation of potentially subtle sounds in small children. If unable to perform an adequate cardiac examination due to the activity level of the child, clinicians should schedule another appointment for the child or ask the parents to drop into the clinic at a time when the child is sleeping. Absence of evidence does not always equate with evidence of absence (in other words, unless you have been able to listen carefully and convince yourself that the sounds in question are not present, it is not wise to assume that they do not exist).

REFERENCES

1. Harris, J. Peter: Evaluation of heart murmurs. *Pediatr Rev* 15(12):490–493, 1994.
2. Danford DA et al: Cost assessment of the evaluation of heart murmurs in children. *Pediatrics* 91(2):365–368, 1993.
3. Asprey D: Evaluation of children with heart murmurs, in *Lippincott's Primary Care Practice,* Vol 2, No. 5, 1998, pp 508–513.
4. McCrindle BW et al: Cardinal clinical signs in the differentiation of heart murmurs in children. *Arch Pediatr Adolesc Med* 150(2):169–174, 1996.
5. Birkebaek NH et al: Diagnostic value of chest radiography and electrocardiography in the evaluation of asymptomatic children with a cardiac murmur. *Acta Paediatr* 84(12):1379–1381, 1995.

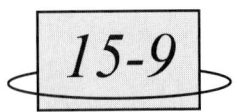

PEDIATRIC ARRHYTHMIAS

David P. Asprey

DISCUSSION

Cardiac arrhythmias are a relatively common problem among children. Potential etiologies of the arrhythmia are congenital, toxin induced, medication or drug induced, and the sequela of surgical repair of congenital heart disease. When evaluating children with a suspected arrhythmia, the distinguishing features are the presence of significant symptoms and the presence of a structural heart disease. The majority of children who have an arrhythmia but no underlying heart disease or significant symptoms do not require treatment. Conversely, children with an arrhythmia who have a structurally abnormal heart or have significant symptoms should seek immediate evaluation and treatment. Typically, serious symptoms (lightheadedness, near-syncope, syncope, and chest pain) occur as a result of diminished cardiac output that may be secondary to tachycardia, profound bradycardia, or cardiac standstill.

In this chapter the discussion of the various pediatric arrhythmias is divided into the following categories: sinus rhythm variations, atrial originating arrhythmias, ventricular originating arrhythmias, and atrioventricular conduction disturbances.

SINUS RHYTHM VARIATIONS

Several physiologic variations of sinus rhythm exist and occur commonly in the pediatric population.

Sinus Arrhythmia

Sinus arrhythmia is a physiologic, phasic variation in the timing of the impulse that is discharged from the sinoatrial (SA) node. The result is a rhythm that appears to change rate from beat to beat. Because the discharged electrical impulse is traveling through the normal conduction mechanism, it results in normal sinus rhythm. The observable variations in the heart rate correlate with the respiratory cycle. While this finding may occur with respiratory distress or increased intracranial pressure, it is most often associated with a normal heart. This variation of sinus rhythm does not require treatment.

Sinus Bradycardia

Sinus bradycardia occurs when the underlying rhythm of the heart is sinus but the heart rate is lower than the normal range for the patient's age. The normal resting heart rates are age dependent; as a rule the normal newborn range is 110 to 150 beats per minute, 2 to 3 years is 85 to 125 beats per minute, 4 to 6 years is 75 to 115 beats per minute, and over 6 years of age is 60 to 100 beats per minute. Sinus bradycardia may result from athletic conditioning, vagal stimulation, increased intracranial pressure, hypothyroidism, hypoxia, and hyperkalemia and as a side effect to drugs such as digitalis and β-adrenergic blockers. If marked bradycardia is present, adequate cardiac output may not be maintained, resulting in the development of symptoms. Typically, in otherwise healthy children, sinus bradycardia is without significance and does not require treatment.

Sinus Tachycardia

Sinus tachycardia occurs when the underlying rhythm of the heart is sinus but the rate exceeds the upper limits of the established normal range for the child's age. Causes of sinus tachycardia include anemia, hypovolemia, anxiety, fever, congestive heart failure, and catecholamines. The treatment of sinus tachycardia involves treating the underlying cause.

ATRIAL ORIGINATING ARRHYTHMIAS

Several abnormal heartbeats or rhythms originate from the atrium: *Wandering atrial pacemaker* refers to the phenomenon that occurs when the origination point of the electrical impulse within the atrium varies from one beat to the next beat. This is manifested in the electrocardiogram (ECG) by a changing P-wave axis and morphology. This is a normal finding and is not usually associated with cardiac disease; consequently, no treatment is indicated.

Premature Atrial Contractions

Premature atrial contractions (PACs) occur when the SA node or another region of the atrium generates an organized atrial contraction that occurs earlier than anticipated in the cardiac cycle. Often the electrical impulse is generated from an area of the atrium other than the SA node, thus the morphology and axis of the P wave are abnormal. In most instances, the QRS complex will be normal in duration and morphology as the conduction of the electrical impulse through the ventricles occurs via the normal mechanism. A distinguishing feature of PACs when compared to other premature beats is that there is an incomplete compensatory pause. PACs may be a normal finding in newborns or children. In addition, they may occur as a result of trauma to the atrium (e.g., cardiac surgery, catheter stimulation) or in response to drug toxicity or inflammation. Isolated PACs are not hemodynamically significant and often go unnoticed by the patient. No treatment is required unless they are determined to be the result of a correctable, underlying etiology.

Supraventricular Tachycardia

Supraventricular tachycardia (SVT) is the most common tachyrhythmia to occur in children. It is characterized by a regular and very rapid heart rate that may range from 180 beats per minute to nearly 300 beats per minute. Both the onset and cessation of SVT tend to be abrupt. Consequently, a careful history to elicit the onset and cessation is useful in establishing this diagnosis. Episodes of SVT may last as little as a few seconds to as long as several hours. Some children will be unaware of the rapid heart rate and others will describe their heart as racing or fluttering. Very small children may even describe their chest as "hurting" because of a lack of understanding or ability to describe what they are experiencing. Rarely will this arrhythmia result in significant symptoms associated with decreased cardiac output. The ECG reveals a normal (narrow) QRS complex with regular R-to-R intervals.

While the specific etiology of SVT is often undetermined, the most common mechanism is reentry within the atrioventricular (AV) node. SVT occurs when a premature atrial beat is conducted through the AV node via a bypass tract. As the impulse proceeds through the ventricle and back to the AV node, the impulse is transmitted back up to the atrium in a retrograde manner through the AV node bypass tract. This impulse is then transmitted through the atrium and back to the AV node, and an accelerated rhythm occurs.

The specific cause of SVT is not identifiable in greater than 50% of the cases that occur in children. Wolff-Parkinson-White syndrome may be present in as many as 20% of all children with SVT; however this diagnosis can only be established from an ECG taken when the child is not experiencing tachycardia. SVT is associated with Ebstein's anomaly of the tricuspid valve and corrected transposition of the great arteries. SVT may be precipitated by caffeine ingestion and sympathomimetic amines commonly utilized in decongestants. If SVT is sustained for long periods of time, it may result in congestive heart failure secondary to diminished cardiac output.

The treatment regimen of SVT that is not associated with significant symptoms is conservative initially. This regimen will first include vagal stimulation. In infants and small children, brief and sudden submersion of the face in ice water (diver's reflex) will abort the episode of SVT in up to as many as 80% of the cases. Older children may be taught how to perform self-administered vagal stimulation maneuvers such as carotid massage, Valsalva maneuver, and drinking ice water among others. If these conservative treatments are unsuccessful, pharmacologic treatment should be initiated. Adenosine is most effective in the acute setting when the mechanism of SVT is presumed to be a result of an AV reentry bypass tract. It is administered rapidly as an intravenous bolus followed with a saline flush. The starting dose is 50 μg/kg and is increased in 50-μg/kg increments every 1 to 2 min up to a maximum of 250 μg/kg. Once the SVT is interrupted, digitalization may be necessary to prevent reoccurrence. Other treatments include primary digitalization, propranolol, or verapamil. In addition, transesophageal-pacing wires may be utilized to achieve overdriving of the rhythm and subsequent conversion to sinus rhythm. Finally, in acute symptomatic cases cardioversion may be indicated.

Atrial Flutter

Atrial flutter is characterized by a very fast atrial rate that is described as a "sawtooth" pattern on the ECG. The atrial rate may approach 300 beats per minute with varying ventricular response rates from 2:1 to 5:1. The resulting ventricular response may be quite irregular. Most patients who are old enough to verbalize their symptoms will describe palpitations and occasionally lightheadedness.

The causes of atrial flutter include myocarditis, digitalis toxicity, congenital heart disease that results in atrial dilation, and atrial trauma due to surgery or other intracardiac interventions. Digitalization acts to decrease the ventricular response rate. Cardioversion may be necessary to convert some cases of atrial flutter. Anticoagulation therapy is indicated before cardioversion in order to prevent systemic embolization.

Atrial Fibrillation

Atrial fibrillation is also characterized by a very rapid atrial rate between 300 and 500 beats per minute. Unlike atrial flutter there is no distinct "sawtooth" pattern representing the atrial activity on the ECG. However, like atrial flutter an irregular ventricular rate is typically present. The causes of atrial fibrillation are the same as those associated with atrial flutter. Likewise, the treatment of atrial fibrillation is the same as that for atrial flutter. It should be noted that even when cardioversion is initially successful, it will often convert back to atrial fibrillation.

VENTRICULAR ORIGINATING ARRHYTHMIAS

Premature Ventricular Contractions

Premature ventricular contractions (PVCs) occur when an ectopic focus within the ventricles generates an electrical impulse that results in the contraction of the ventricles at a point earlier than expected in the cardiac cycle. With a PVC the electrical impulse is generated in and transmitted through the myocardium of the ventricle and is not transmitted through the normal His-Purkinje conduction system. Consequently, the transmission of the impulse is slower and thus the morphology of the QRS complex is widened. It is important to realize that some patients will have a wide QRS from a bundle branch block or other conduction abnormality, making it difficult to identify conduction abnormalities. A distinguishing feature of PVCs compared to PACs with aberrancy (which appear as a widened QRS) is that a patient with a bundle branch block experiencing PVCs will usually have a full compensatory pause, while PACs will have an incomplete compensatory pause.

PVCs may be classified into different categories based on the uniformity of the QRS complexes and their relationship to other PVCs. If each of the PVC complexes appears the same throughout the tracing they are described as uniform or unifocal, implying that the electrical impulse generating the PVC is consistently arising from the same area within the ventricular myocardium. Conversely, if each of the PVC complexes is different in appearance they are described as multiform or multifocal PVCs. This pattern implies that the electrical impulses generating the PVCs are arising from different areas within the ventricular myocardium each time.

PVCs may vary in their timing and relationship to other PVCs. A single PVC on a tracing without other PVCs on the strip being reviewed is described as an *isolated PVC*. If the PVC alternates with a normal QRS complex, so that every other beat is a PVC, this is described as *bigeminy*. If every third complex is a PVC, this pattern is known as *trigeminy*. When two PVCs occur in succession this is referred to as a *couplet*.

PVCs may be a normal finding in the newborn or child. In addition, they may occur as a result of trauma to the ventricle (e.g., cardiac surgery, catheter stimulation), myocarditis, cardiomyopathy, myocardial ischemia, drug toxicity, or inflammation. Isolated PVCs are not hemodynamically significant and are usually undetectable to the patient. Occasional PVCs are believed to be benign in children, particularly if they are suppressed by exercise and are uniform or unifocal.

In children without underlying congenital heart disease, occasional uniform PVCs do not warrant extensive investigation. Children and infants with frequent PVCs, bigeminy, or trigeminy should be evaluated with ECG, echocardiogram, and exercise stress testing. If each of these tests is normal no further evaluation is indicated. If these tests are abnormal or unavailable, referral to a pediatric cardiology clinician should be considered. Children and infants with ventricular couplets, triplets, or multiform PVCs should undergo evaluation including ECG, echocardiogram, exercise stress testing, and 24-hour Holter monitoring. No treatment will be required for PVCs unless they are associated with significant symptoms or are the result of a treatable underlying etiology. When indicated, pharmacologic treatment options include lidocaine as an intravenous bolus and beta blockers among others. Agents that are known to prolong the QT interval should be avoided.

Ventricular Tachycardia

Ventricular tachycardia (VT) is quite rare in the pediatric age group. It is described as three or more PVCs in succession with a rate greater than 120 beats per minute (normally 120 to 200 beats per minute). The QRS complexes in VT are wide and have a characteristic morphology analogous to that of the QRS complex associated with PVCs. The presence of sustained VT is a medical emergency. Sustained VT is usually an unstable condition that has the potential to progress to ventricular fibrillation. Torsade de pointes is a characteristic type of VT that on ECG will appears as VT with a rapidly changing QRS morphology and amplitude.

The presence of VT is always abnormal. It is usually associated with abnormalities of the ventricular myocardium such as myocarditis, cardiomyopathy, and myocardial tumors or in conjunction with severe forms of congenital heart disease. Torsade de pointes may be associated with long QT syndrome and drugs that prolong the QT interval. Symptoms associated with VT usually occur as a result of decreased cardiac output.

Treatment of VT in the acute symptomatic setting (patient unconscious or profoundly symptomatic) should include synchronized cardioversion using approximately 1 joule/kg. In the conscious patient, a lidocaine bolus given intravenously at a rate of 1 mg/kg over the course of 1 to 2 min followed by an intravenous drip will often be effective. Bretylium tosylate given at 5 mg/kg intravenously over the course of 10 min may also be effective. In all cases of confirmed VT the clinician should strive to identify the underlying cause and treat any correctable causes.

Ventricular Fibrillation

Ventricular fibrillation (VF) is very rare in children and infants and occurs when the electrical activity of the heart fails to generate a synchronized contraction of the ventricles. Consequently, the cardiac output is dramatically decreased and is typically incompatible with life. The ECG will show only fine variations in the amplitude of the baseline waveform and often appears as artifact electrical activity. When specific waveform activity correlating with the ventricular contractions is identifiable, it is typically very rapid and of varying morphology.

VF is an emergency and if untreated is fatal due to inadequate cardiac output. It may occur as a result of myocardial ischemia, electrolyte imbalance, myocarditis, digitalis, quinidine, catecholamines or other drug toxicities, and as a result of some postoperative states. Because this rhythm is fatal, immediate treatment with cardiopulmonary resuscitation (CPR) and electrical defibrillation (2 joules/kg) are required. When the onset of VF is witnessed, a precordial thump may be administered immediately as the first-line attempt to reestablish sinus rhythm. However, if an initial attempt is unsuccessful, CPR should be started immediately until cardioversion can be performed.

ATRIOVENTRICULAR CONDUCTION DISTURBANCES

AV block can occur at different regions within the normal conduction system, resulting in varying degrees of heart block. Heart block is divided into three broad categories known as first degree, second degree, and third degree.

First-Degree Heart Block

First-degree heart block occurs when there is a delay in the conduction of the impulse generated in the SA node (or other region of the atrium) and its transmission to the ventricles, resulting in ventricular contraction. This manifests itself on the ECG as a prolongation of the PR interval beyond the upper limits normal for age. Normal PR intervals are age- and heart rate–dependent; normal ranges should be determined by consulting published standardized tables.

Causes of first-degree heart block include idiopathic in healthy children and infants, certain forms of congenital heart disease, acute rheumatic fever, cardiomyopathies, cardiac surgery or trauma, and digitalis toxicity. There is no hemodynamic compromise associated with first-degree heart block and no treatment is necessary.

Second-Degree Heart Block

Second-degree heart block occurs when some of the atrial electrical impulses do not result in a ventricular contraction. Thus, the ECG will demonstrate some P waves that are followed not by a QRS complex but by another P wave. There are three different forms of second-degree heart block that are well described. Mobitz type I is also known as Wenckebach phenomenon and manifests itself on the ECG tracing by a PR interval that becomes increasing prolonged until the P wave fails to produce a QRS (dropped beat) and is eventually followed by the succeeding P wave. This form of second-degree heart block suggests AV node disease. Patients identified with this condition should undergo 24-h Holter monitoring. Treatment includes correction of the underlying condition.

MOBITZ TYPE II SECOND-DEGREE HEART BLOCK
Mobitz type II second-degree heart block is characterized on the ECG by consistent PR intervals but has occasional P waves which do not result in QRS complexes, thus a beat is dropped and the P wave is followed by the subsequent P wave. The conduction through the AV node is either normal or the impulse is blocked completely. This block is believed to occur at the level of the His bundle. In addition, this form of second-degree heart block may progress to third-degree or complete heart block. Patients with this condition should undergo periodic 24-h Holter monitoring to determine whether periods of bradycardia or third-degree heart block are occurring.

SECOND-DEGREE HEART BLOCK WITH A 2:1 OR 3:1 AV BLOCK
The final type of second-degree heart block is described by its ratio of P waves to QRS complexes. This form manifests itself by a series of P waves followed by a QRS complex. Thus, it may be described as second-degree heart block with a 2:1 or 3:1 AV block. This form of second-degree heart block usually occurs at the level of the His bundle. These patients should be followed with periodic 24-h Holter monitoring. Treatment involves correction of underlying problems.

Causes of all three types of second-degree heart block are similar and include idiopathic in healthy children, cardiac ischemia, myocarditis, cardiomyopathy, cardiac surgery, and digitalis and other drug toxicities.

Third-Degree or Complete Heart Block

Third-degree or complete heart block occurs when the atrial activity and ventricular activity are functioning completely independent of each other. Because the atrial activity is not influencing the ventricular response, the ventricular response rate may become quite slow due to its lower rate of automaticity. Third-degree heart block may be congenital or acquired. Congenital causes are seen in infants with some forms of congenital heart disease and infants who are born to mothers with systemic lupus erythematosus. The most common etiology of acquired third-degree heart block includes cardiac surgery and myocardial ischemia. Children with third-degree heart block should undergo periodic 24-h Holter monitoring to assess the low heart rates and presence of prolonged pauses that typically occur during sleep. Treatment may require permanent pacemakers in symptomatic patients or patients with congestive heart failure.

BIBLIOGRAPHY

Behrman RE et al: *Nelson's Textbook of Pediatrics,* 15th ed. Philadelphia, Saunders, 1996.

Park MK: *The Pediatric Cardiology Handbook,* 2d. ed. St. Louis, Mosby-Year Book, 1997.

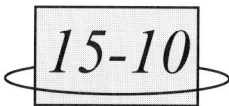

THE NEWBORN PERIOD

Virginia Schneider

DISCUSSION

The newborn period consists of only the first 28 days of life, while infancy lasts until the end of the first year. Some special considerations are in order when dealing with newborn infants which set them apart from older infants and young children. The objective of this chapter is to familiarize clinicians with basic newborn care and common problems associated with this age group.

History

The baby at birth has no history of his or her own apart from the history of the mother, the family, and the events of the prenatal period. It is important to ask about the pregnancy and any illnesses or complications; the mother's general health, especially the presence of chronic illnesses; and the route of delivery, intrapartum anesthesia, and delivery complications. In addition to the pregnancy and delivery, the family history should be reviewed, especially for inherited diseases and the health status of other siblings. Table 15-10-1 lists significant historical factors that require further investigation.

Size and Gestational Age

All babies have weight, length, and fronto-occipital circumference (FOC) measured at birth, and these measures are plotted on a growth chart. In order to determine whether the newborn has grown normally in utero, the baby's gestational age must also be determined. There are many methods for determining gestational age, each with varying accuracy. Maternal dates based on the last menstrual period (LMP) are still the most accurate method even among women who are vague historians. Generally, the mother's dates are confirmed for accuracy by performing an examination for gestational age (Ballard exam). If

TABLE 15-10-1. Maternal and Family History Information that Requires Investigation

Chronic maternal diseases	Fetal distress or meconium passage
Viral illness or high fever during pregnancy	General anesthesia delivery
Bleeding or threatened abortion	Shoulder dystocia or breech presentation
Sexually transmitted diseases	Preterm or postterm delivery
Severe maternal anemia	Siblings with major health problems
Poor maternal weight gain	Patterns of health problems in families
Pregnancy-induced hypertension	More than 2 spontaneous abortions
Gestational diabetes	Unexplained mental retardation or early death in family
Emergency cesarian section	

TABLE 15-10-2. Methods for Determining Gestational Age

Mother's dates based on last normal menstrual period
Early fetal ultrasound measurements (before 12 weeks)
Date of quickening
Fundal height
Fetal heart tones
Ballard examination of the infant

there is some discordance between the two measures, the prenatal history may provide other clues to establish the correct gestational age. Table 15-10-2 lists various methods for determining gestational age.

Why is establishing gestational age and evaluating growth so critical? Most newborns are born at term and are normally grown—they are average for gestational age (AGA). A few are born prematurely (<37 completed weeks gestation), postterm (>42 weeks gestation), small for gestational age (SGA; less than the tenth percentile of growth for age), or large for gestational age (LGA; greater than the ninetieth percentile of growth for age). An FOC measurement less than the tenth percentile for age is termed *microcephaly* and is particularly significant even if other measures are normal. Each of these deviations from normal has its own particular problems associated with it (see Table 15-10-3). All these newborns require more stringent evaluation and observation. Abnormally grown children may have medical and developmental problems related to the cause. Knowing the baby is abnormally grown is an important step toward identifying potential problems.

Physical Examination

The physical examination of a newborn is not significantly different from the examination of a child or adult. Most physical examination texts cover the topic thoroughly and accurately. A few tips: Do try to make a general assessment before you disturb the baby very much. Most babies are healthy, and a sick infant will often immediately appear so if you observe the color, movement, cry, and breathing for a few moments. The baby's state may profoundly influence the results of your examination. A crying baby may appear tachypneic. A sleeping baby may appear to have poor muscle tone. A baby who has just eaten may not exhibit some neurologic reflexes. The examination of a newborn who is getting sick changes rapidly, sometimes from a few questionable symptoms to profound shock over the course of an hour. Frequent reassessment of any abnormal findings is an important component of caring for newborn infants.

Weight and Feeding

It is normal for a term infant to lose up to 10% of birth weight within 1 week of life. At the 2-week visit, the baby should be back to birth weight. Reassure the parents this pattern is normal. Preterm infants may lose 15 to 20% of birth weight because water comprises a greater percentage of their body composition.

Breast feeding is one of the most important contributions a mother can make to her baby's general health. Most women have already made the decision about how they will feed their baby by the time they deliver (many by the time they conceive). Still, always encourage a mother to breast feed and give her whatever expert assistance is available. Breast feeding is not an instinct; it is a learned skill. Most women fumble and stumble getting breast feeding established, even mothers who have previously breast fed.

The only way to make milk is to put the baby to the breast. Breast feeding should be initiated as soon after delivery as the baby is interested. Water test feeds are not essential—breast milk aspirated into the lungs is not significantly more irritating than water. Generally, feedings should occur on demand, but in the first few days breast feeding should

TABLE 15-10-3. Complications and Causes Associated with Abnormal Growth Parameters

GROWTH	COMMON CAUSES	POTENTIAL COMPLICATIONS
Premature	Infection Multiple gestation Fetal anomalies	None to major organ failure due to immature development
Postmature	No specific causes	Placental insufficiency leading to asphyxia
Large for gestational age	Maternal diabetes Genetic syndromes Constitutional or familial	Delivery trauma including fractures Erb's palsy Birth asphyxia
Small for gestational age	Placental insufficiency most commonly due to maternal age or illness Chromosomal abnormalities and other genetic syndromes Congenital infections Multiple gestation Constitutional or familial	Varies widely depending on cause from none (familial) to severe mental retardation and death (chromosomal syndromes, congenital infections)
Microcephaly	Chromosomal abnormalities and other genetic syndromes Congenital infections Congenital central nervous system malformations	Varies depending on the cause from mild retardation to vegetative state and death

be attempted every 2 to 3 hours if the baby does not wake to feed. Breast-fed babies should be seen in the office within a few days of discharge to make sure the baby is adequately hydrated, voiding and stooling well, and to ensure any jaundice is within reasonable limits.

Some cheerless statistics: 50 to 90% of mothers attempt breast feeding in the hospital, but less than 40% are breast feeding by the 2-week visit. Less than 20% are breast feeding by the 2-month visit (in spite of the recommendation by all major medical groups that breast feeding should be the only source of nutrition for infants through 4 to 6 months of age and should be continued for the first 12 months of life). If the mother must bottle feed, she should start with a test feeding of water (formula is more irritating when ingested into the lungs). Feedings should be on demand, not scheduled. The average baby takes 7 to 8 ounces the first day (60 mL/kg per day), working up to an average of 20 ounces by day 5 (180 mL/kg per day). The goal is to deliver approximately 120 kcal/kg per day for routine body functions and adequate growth.

Voiding and Stooling

By 24 h, the baby should urinate and stool at least once (if none is recorded, check the delivery records for passage at birth). While occasionally it is normal for stooling and voiding to be delayed, the baby may need to be evaluated for renal and gastrointestinal (GI) anomalies.

There should be at least six wet diapers per day after the first 24 h, and at least one should be soaked. This may be reduced to four to five if highly absorbent disposable diapers are used. Stooling occurs with nearly every feed. The consistency in the beginning is black-green and sticky like tar (*meconium*), changing to yellow, seedy, cottage cheese consistency by day 3. This is not diarrhea as many new mothers may report. Stool of breast-fed babies may have this appearance or may appear green-tinged and runny. Breast-fed babies after the first 2 weeks may fall into a pattern of very infrequent stooling (up to once a week) because the milk components are so well absorbed. A baby with constipation has hard, pellet-like, infrequent stools. Straining, making funny noises, and turning red in the face is common and, if accompanied by stools of normal consistency, is generally not constipation.

Preventive Care in the Newborn Period

Several measures are taken to prevent potential complications for nearly all newborns (see Table 15-10-4). At birth, most infants receive a vitamin K injection to prevent hemorrhagic disease of the newborn, antibiotic or silver nitrate eye drops to prevent ophthalmia neonatorum, and antibacterial treatment to the umbilical cord. Either at birth or in the first weeks of life, most infants also receive the first hepatitis B vaccination. Infants of mothers who are positive for hepatitis B surface antigen (HBsAg) also need to receive hepatitis B immunoglobulin (HBIG) in the first 12 to 24 h of life. This prevents maternal-fetal transmission of the virus in 95 to 98% of cases. Breast feeding is still recommended for infants of HBsAg-positive mothers.

TABLE 15-10-4. Routine Interventions During the Newborn Period

INTERVENTION	TIMING	RATIONALE
Vitamin K prophylaxis	Birth	Maternally transferred clotting factors disappear by 48 h. Gut colonization of the baby is required to produce vitamin K and takes 48–72 h. The potential production delay may result in poor clotting and hemorrhage. Injection of vitamin K is given prophylactically.
Eye prophylaxis	Birth	GC and *Chlamydia* may be asymptomatic in the mother. GC ophthalmia can cause blindness if untreated in the newborn. Erythromycin ointment, tetracycline ointment, or silver nitrate drops are instilled prophylactically to reduce incidence.
Hepatitis B vaccine	First 2 weeks	Administered in three vaccines over the first year of life to reduce the risk of hepatitis B infection and possible chronic hepatitis.
Newborn screening	First 2 weeks	A panel of tests performed to screen newborns for serious diseases that are often asymptomatic and may cause damage to the infant that is irreversible (see text).

Laws in all states mandate newborn screening. A small amount of blood is collected on filter paper sheets from which multiple tests can be performed. Which tests are performed and their required timing varies state to state. Screening is commonly done for diseases that are asymptomatic in the first weeks of life and for which early identification and intervention will prevent serious, irreversible long-term complications. The most commonly screened-for diseases and their approximate incidence are galactosemia (1:35,000), phenylketonuria (1:15,000), hypothyroidism (1:4000), and hemoglobinopathies including sickle cell disease (1:15).

Umbilical Cords

Normal umbilical cords contain two arteries and one vein. A two-vessel cord may be associated with genetic syndromes. Because of cord bacteria colonization and subsequent white blood cell phagocytosis, a normal cord separates in 7 to 14 days. Worry about a cord still attached at 30 days—it may indicate an immunologic problem. Teach parents to thoroughly clean around the cord insertion site with alcohol several times a day until it separates to prevent infection. Be concerned about a red, smelly, or weepy cord or cellulitis of the surrounding skin. This may indicate omphalitis, infection of the cord. The vessels in the cord track directly into the systemic circulation, so suspicion of this disease requires hospitalization and parenteral antibiotics. Umbilical hernias generally close spontaneously by school age. They rarely incarcerate, but clinicians should discuss signs and symptoms with parents. It is important to pay attention to the parent who complains of a persistently malodorous or moist umbilicus. The omphalomesenteric duct is supposed to close in fetal life, but occasionally it doesn't, leaving a tract between the bowel and the skin. Closure is a simple procedure.

Circumcision

Although there is a potential for certain medical benefits, such as a mild decrease in urinary tract infections and penile cancer and a decrease in sexual partners' risk of cervical cancer, routine neonatal circumcision is not essential to the child's well-being. Other than religious beliefs and parental preferences, circumcision is considered a cosmetic procedure. There is a 0.2 to 0.6% complication rate for the procedure, ranging in severity from simple local irritation and bleeding to necrosis and penile sloughing.

Contraindications to the procedure are any congenital genital abnormality (because the tissue may be needed for the surgical repair of the anomaly) or a family history of bleeding disorders. If an informed decision for circumcision is made, procedural anesthesia should be provided.

Early Discharge

Early discharge (24 to 36 h after delivery) is becoming a routine part of the normal delivery hospitalization. To assure the health and safety of the mother and infant, do a careful assessment of the infant by physical exam; assess feeding, voiding, and stooling patterns; recheck family history for previous infant problems; and assess home and family support systems. The American Academy of Pediatrics recommends an office or home visit 48 h after discharge to reassess the newborn.

MAJOR NEWBORN PROBLEMS

Bacterial Sepsis

During the newborn period, the infant is an immunocompromised host and is at risk for infection. Most bacterial exposure occurs during passage through an infected birth canal. Infants are also exposed to pathogens in utero (ascending genital infections) and occasionally through bloodborne transmission (malaria).

TABLE 15-10-5. Sepsis Risk Factors

Premature or prolonged rupture of membranes
Prolonged labor
Maternal fever ≥100.4°F during labor or up to 24 h postpartum
Maternal chorioamnionitis
Maternal group B streptococci colonization
Unsterile delivery (toilets)
Serious maternal infections (meningitis)
Prematurity
An "open" birth defect (meningomyelocele)

Infants are frequently evaluated for sepsis based on the presence of risk factors as well as actual symptoms. The presence of any of the sepsis risk factors listed in Table 15-10-5 means the baby should be considered for a sepsis workup even if the baby looks perfectly healthy. Infants can transition from looking well to being critically ill in a few hours. Signs and symptoms in the infant are often vague and nonspecific (see Table 15-10-6). A sepsis workup generally includes complete blood count with differential and platelets; electrolytes; blood culture; cerebrospinal fluid for cell count, glucose, protein, and culture; and urinalysis and urine culture if the baby is greater than 3 days old. Antibiotic treatment is initiated while awaiting test results. Infants less than 72 h old are typically given ampicillin and gentamicin to cover maternally acquired infections (group B streptococci, *Enterococcus, Escherichia coli*). After 72 h of life, antibiotic choice depends on whether the baby is at home or is still hospitalized. Treatment continues until cultures are negative, 48 to 72 h minimum.

Congenital Infections

A number of agents can infect the fetus through the mother and cause severe damage to the developing fetus. Presenting signs vary, but common features are growth retardation, decreased FOC or microcephaly, and jaundice with hepatitis. The most common and severe make up the common abbreviation *TORCHS*—toxoplasmosis, rubella, cytomegalovirus, herpes, and syphilis. Congenital rubella, a common infecting agent in the past, causes congenital cataracts, growth retardation, mental deficiencies, and hepatitis. Toxoplasmosis is relatively uncommon in the United States. It is transmitted through contact with cat feces, undercooked pork, and contact with infected soil.

TABLE 15-10-6. Common Signs and Symptoms of Sepsis in Newborns

Temperature instability
Poor perfusion
Lethargy/poor tone
Irritability
Diarrhea
Cyanosis
Apnea
Tachypnea
Poor feeding
Full anterior fontanelle
Seizures

TABLE 15-10-7. Comparison of Types of Jaundice

	PHYSIOLOGIC JAUNDICE	EXAGGERATED PHYSIOLOGIC JAUNDICE	PATHOLOGIC JAUNDICE
Onset	After 24 h of life	After 24 h of life	Often before 24 h of life
Causes	Increased fetal red blood cell life span Increased fetal red blood cell breakdown Enterohepatic shunting Immature liver function	Decreased elimination from delayed feeding and stooling Increased production from bruising, cephalhematomas, or polycythemia Hypoglycemia or hypothermia early in the hospital course	Rh incompatibility ABO incompatibility Other hemolytic anemias Congenital viral infections Bacterial sepsis Galactosemia

Cytomegalovirus is currently the most common of the congenital viral infections and is believed to be the leading cause of congenital deafness. Herpes and syphilis are usually diagnosed through maternal history or positive serology.

Jaundice

Physiologic jaundice (jaundice that begins after the first 24 h of life with a bilirubin level that does not exceed 12.9 mg/dL) is the most common cause of neonatal jaundice and occurs in 50% of babies. More recent information indicates that bilirubin levels up to 15 mg/dL in a healthy term infant may be compatible with physiologic jaundice. Normal physiologic jaundice can also be "exaggerated" to higher bilirubin levels by many nonpathologic factors. Physiologic jaundice resolves by 2 weeks, and any jaundice persisting beyond that time must be investigated. Jaundice in the first 24 h of life should always be considered abnormal until proven otherwise (see Table 15-10-7).

Evaluation of *any* jaundiced infant should include:

- Family history of jaundice or hemolytic disease
- Review of the hospital record for predisposing factors
- Careful review of the feeding history
- Review of the chart for any other symptoms reported by family or staff
- Careful physical examination
- Lab evaluation for maternal blood type, infant blood type, and direct Coombs' test

Hypoglycemia and Glucose Screening

Glucose screening is recommended routinely within the first 30 min of life for LGA infants, SGA infants, infants of diabetic mothers (IDMs), preterm infants, and infants with any symptoms of illness. Hypoglycemia is typically defined as a serum blood glucose less than 40 mg/dL. Signs and symptoms of hypoglycemia in an infant include jitteriness, poor feeding, tachypnea, apnea, cyanosis, seizures, poor perfusion, irritability, and lethargy. *Hypoglycemia is a medical emergency.* When in doubt, treat and get help. Always notify the supervising physician. General treatment guidelines are listed in Table 15-10-8.

TABLE 15-10-8. Treatment Guidelines for Hypoglycemia in Infants

CONDITION	TREATMENT
Asymptomatic, glucose 40–80 mg/dL	Feed formula or breast milk
Asymptomatic, glucose 20–40 mg/dL	Oral feeding or IV glucose
Asymptomatic, glucose <20 mg/dL	IV push 5 mg/kg glucose and start glucose drip
Symptomatic, glucose 40–80 mg/dL	Oral feeding or IV glucose
Symptomatic, glucose <40 mg/dL	IV push 5 mg/kg glucose and start glucose drip

BIBLIOGRAPHY

Bordley WC et al: Newborn screening fact sheet. *Pediatrics* 98(3):467–472, 1996.

Committee on Genetics, American Academy of Pediatrics: Issues in newborn screening. *Pediatrics* 89(2):345–349, 1992.

Guidelines for Perinatal Care. Elk Grove Village, IL, American Academy of Pediatrics, 1997.

Maisels J: Clinical rounds in the well baby nursery: Treating jaundiced newborns. *Pediatr Ann* 24(10):547–552, 1995.

Oski FA et al: *Principles and Practice of Pediatrics,* 2d ed. Philadelphia, Lippincott, 1994.

Provisional Committee for Quality Improvement and Subcommittee on Hyperbilirubinemia, American Academy of Pediatrics: Management of hyperbilirubinemia in the health term newborn. *Pediatrics* 94(4):685–702, 1994.

Schneider VF, Cabrera-Meza L: *Rudolph's Brief Atlas of the Newborn.* Toronto, Decker, 1995.

Taeusch HW et al: *Schaefer and Avery's Diseases of the Newborn,* 7th ed. Philadelphia, Saunders, 1995.

Task Force on Circumcision, American Academy of Pediatrics: Circumcision policy statement. *Pediatrics* 103(3):686–693, 1999.

Internet Resource

American Academy of Pediatrics: www.aap.org.

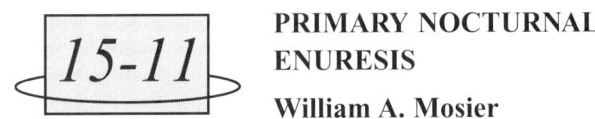

15-11 PRIMARY NOCTURNAL ENURESIS

William A. Mosier

DISCUSSION

Nocturnal enuresis, better known as bed-wetting, is more common than most people realize. It is a disorder that affects an estimated 7 million children and adolescents annually in the United States. It is often assumed to be the result of emotional problems. However, that is rarely the case. In fact, it is the enuresis itself that can lead to low self-esteem, resulting in psychological problems. Bed-wetting is caused by neither emotional nor behavioral problems. Nocturnal enuresis is a condition that usually stems from biologic causes. After the age of 6 years, bed-wetting becomes a medical condition. Approximately 90% of all enuretic children go undiagnosed and untreated by a health care provider. Because of the social stigma attached to bed-wetting, children and their families are frequently too ashamed and embarrassed to discuss it with non-family members. Thinking that there is no solution, bed-wetting often remains "in the closet"—becoming a family's well-guarded secret. Although 66% of parents actively worry about their child's bed-wetting and 61% view it as a significant problem, only 33% consult a health care provider.

The term *enuresis* can be applied to a number of different symptomatologies. The following terms are used to differentiate the various forms of enuresis:

- *Diurnal enuresis:* daytime urinary incontinence
- *Nocturnal enuresis:* nighttime urinary incontinence

• *Primary enuresis:* child has never achieved continence for an extended period of at least 6 months
• *Secondary enuresis:* child has maintained continence for at least a 6-month period, then reverted to incontinence (causes of secondary enuresis may include urinary tract infections, neurogenic bladder and associated spinal cord abnormalities, and posterior urethral valve in boys or ectopic ureter in girls)
• *Primary nocturnal enuresis* (PNE): involuntary nighttime urinary incontinence in an individual who has never been routinely dry at night more than twice monthly for more than 6 months past the age of 5 years

Children who experience both daytime and nighttime incontinence present a problem very different than simple nocturnal enuresis. Though enuresis can present in various forms, several studies suggest that the vast majority of enuretics (over 80%) are actually afflicted with only PNE. The strongest evidence suggests that the most common cause of PNE is a lack of nocturnal secretions of antidiuretic hormone (ADH).

Epidemiology

By 36 months of age, 60% of all children have voluntary sphincter control and are able to maintain nighttime continence. The prevalence of bed-wetting among 5-year-olds is about 20%. The proportion of children who continue to experience involuntary bed-wetting declines with age at a rate of about 15% per year of age. By age 6, at least 10% of all children have still not achieved nocturnal continence. By age 10, the prevalence of bed-wetting is about 5%. Even at age 18, there is still no less than 1% of the population that continues to have nighttime incontinence. A child with one parent having a positive family history for PNE stands a 44% chance of also having the condition. A child with both parents having a positive family history for PNE will have a 77% chance of being a bed-wetter. This statistic alone represents a three out of four chance that a child will be a bed-wetter. Although some studies dispute the finding that bed-wetting is more common in boys than in girls, the stronger evidence suggests that it is, though the ratio is difficult to assign with certainty.

PATHOGENESIS

Though considerable disbelief remains about the basic cause of PNE, ample evidence is available to resolve confusion concerning the origin of PNE. One only need rely on evidence from research rather than misguided misconceptions. Although the pathophysiology of enuresis is multifactorial, the principal cause of PNE is relatively straightforward. The origin of PNE appears to be an inadequate increase in ADH occurring during the typical hours of nighttime sleep (8:00 P.M. to 8:00 A.M.). There are other possible causes of nocturnal enuresis; however, most are extremely rare. In rare cases enuresis may be due to small bladder capacity, nonresponsiveness to the sensation of a full bladder, poor bladder muscle control, or a sleep disorder.

The incidence of enuresis caused by an abnormality of bladder function and size is very low. Children with a small bladder capacity typically experience daytime as well as nighttime symptoms. Less rare, but still uncommon, is enuresis caused by a urinary tract infection (UTI). Evidence-based medicine reveals that the most convincing research suggests persistent bed-wetting, beyond the age of 3 years, rarely signals a kidney or bladder problem. Other studies have confirmed that there is no correlation between enuresis and specific sleep stages. In fact, individuals with PNE have been found to have a normal sleep pattern. The preponderance of research demonstrates that there is no correlation between abnormal sleep patterns are PNE.

Research also demonstrates that the vast majority of enuretics have a nighttime bladder capacity that equals or exceeds daytime bladder capacity. These individuals also tend to urinate on a full bladder. There-

fore, the odds of a small bladder size being the cause of PNE are quite unlikely.

Research supports that:

1. It is a serious misconception to believe that PNE is caused by drinking too much water or other fluid before bedtime (this may be an intervening variable, but it is not a causal factor).
2. PNE does not result from too deep a sleep pattern that makes the child unable to arouse when the urge to urinate occurs (children with PNE have normal sleep patterns).
3. A child with PNE is not "too lazy" to get up in the middle of the night to use the toilet (motivation levels of children with PNE manifest as age appropriate).
4. Bed-wetting does not manifest as a result of emotional scars, like divorce or the death of a loved one.

All commonly held beliefs linking PNE with bedtime fluid intake, excessively deep sleep, laziness, and emotional problems as etiology are false. What research does indicate is that more than 90% of bed-wetters carry a gene that is responsible for this condition. In fact, a gene marker associated with PNE has been located on chromosome 13. Studies suggest that the gene is a dominant gene. This theory is reinforced by the evidence that family history is a significant factor in the predisposition for manifesting the symptoms of PNE. The supposed mystery behind "spontaneous resolution" of PNE can be accounted for by delayed maturation of the central nervous system, which corrects the lack of adequate ADH secretion by the hypothalamus that occurs in PNE during the evening hours (from 8:00 P.M. to 8:00 A.M.).

The Role of ADH in PNE

The most convincing evidence points to a deficiency in the nighttime secretion of ADH as the principal factor responsible for PNE. Medical evidence has shown that a child who is still bed-wetting at age 6 years almost always is a child whose body produces extra urine during the typical bedtime hours. Research has demonstrated that a bed-wetting child most probably does not produce enough ADH to control the nighttime flow of urine. The human body produces ADH to help concentrate urine at night so that the bladder won't overflow during sleep. Non-bed-wetting children and adults have an increase in ADH that controls the nighttime production of urine. Bed-wetting children lack this increase in ADH and therefore experience a build-up of urine in the bladder at night. This build-up can lead to uncontrollable "accidents" (PNE).

Examination of plasma ADH levels remains constant in enuretics, while, as previously stated, nonenuretic children have an increase of ADH levels during the night. Since, in most bed-wetters, there is an inadequate rise in the nocturnal secretion of this endogenous regulator of urine output, the result is an overproduction of nighttime urine. By contrast, in non–bed-wetters, the nocturnal increase in ADH decreases the nighttime production of urine. Additional research suggests that heredity plays a significant role in this hormone malfunctioning. Current evidence suggests that the activation of ADH is delayed in bed-wetters beyond the age of 36 months, which results in an overproduction of urine during the night.

SYMPTOMS

The only real presenting complaint symptomatic of PNE is a nighttime urinary incontinence in a child or adolescent who has never been routinely dry at night for more than 6 months beyond the anticipated age of successful toilet training (36 months).

OBJECTIVE FINDINGS

The first step in the evaluation of enuresis is to take a careful history. The history should include questions about any previous urinary tract infection (UTI) and urinary habits, a history of bed-wetting in other family members, history of the child's voiding pattern, and whether there has been any previous work-up or treatments. The inquiry about a family history of bed-wetting is the single most important component of the history taking. In fact, the strongest evidence for PNE is a positive family history of PNE.

The initial evaluation should also include a complete physical examination of the abdomen, genitalia, inspection of the lower back for spinal abnormalities, as well as an observation of voiding. A complete neurologic evaluation should be performed and should include examination of the peripheral reflexes, perineal sensation, analysis of sphincter tone and an observation of gait. A urinalysis of a midstream urine specimen should be done to rule out a UTI or other possible pathology. A culture should be ordered if the urinalysis is positive for a UTI. The diagnosis of PNE is essentially one of exclusion. If the physical examination is normal and the urinalysis and culture are negative, no further evaluation is necessary. Taking a complete history, performing a thorough physical examination, and ordering a urinalysis will usually be all that is necessary to rule out other conditions.

DIAGNOSTIC CONSIDERATIONS

The majority of children with PNE are healthy. Therefore, other signs of pathology will rarely be seen. Diagnostic considerations will be no more complicated than to rule out other potential causes of the child's incontinence. The differential should include epispadia, spinal lesions, or distended bladder. Anatomical abnormalities of the urinary tract, such as an epispadiac urethra, a posterior urethral valve, or a bladder abnormality must always be considered, even though such abnormalities are extremely rare. The urinalysis should include urine specific gravity and dipstick tests to rule out diabetes insipidus. A urine culture should only be included if the urinalysis results are positive for a urinary tract infection.

SPECIAL CONSIDERATIONS

The most important consideration in the evaluation of patients with PNE is the perceived severity of the problem within the patient's family. The stigma of bed-wetting can be the catalyst for considerable pain and suffering for the child with PNE. The most important reason for considering intervention for PNE is to minimize damage to a child's self-esteem. Other prominent concerns include: guilt and an inability to participate in activities involving nights away from home, such as overnight scouting events and sleepovers with friends. The impact of involuntary bed-wetting on a child's self-esteem may lead to behavior problems and may also interfere with age-appropriate peer activities.

Medical intervention that provides a safe and rapid control of PNE can have a positive effect on self-esteem and free a child to participate more fully in peer activities.

LABORATORY TESTS AND RADIOLOGIC STUDIES

Urodynamic and radiologic studies are not useful in diagnosing PNE. In fact, in the absence of symptoms of a UTI, radiologic evaluation is not recommended for children with PNE. However, if a child has a history of UTIs or symptoms consistent with a UTI, ultrasonography and voiding cystourethrography are indicated.

TREATMENT

The attitude of the patient and his or her parents is the most important factor to consider in selecting the appropriate treatment for a child with PNE. Although growing up means eventually growing out of bed-wetting, it is possible to shorten the duration of this embarrassing problem with safe treatment that will promote a healthier and happier childhood. Children should be assured that there is effective treatment

available that can help them cope successfully with their bed-wetting. When bed-wetting becomes a problem for a child and his or her family, the first step is to agree to approach the problem as a treatable condition and then to decide on a specific course of treatment. To ensure a successful response to treatment, the home environment must provide consistent support for the child's goal—to maintain a dry bed.

The rationale for providing treatment for PNE is multifaceted. Effective treatment removes the burden of having to clean up after a bed-wetting episode. It also eliminates the potential for family conflict stemming from the occurrence. Successful treatment can have a profoundly powerfully protective effect on a child's self-esteem and self-confidence. Since the rate of spontaneous resolution of PNE is only about 15%, being patient until this occurs may not always be in the best interest of the child, especially in view of the self-esteem factors overshadowing the physical signs of bed-wetting.

The key elements of a successful intervention to treat PNE are:

1. A supportive attitude, on the part of the parents and the health care provider, toward the child.
2. An understanding of the nature of the condition by both the health care provider and the parents.
3. Cooperation of the child.

Treatment options for PNE consist of both nonpharmacological and pharmacological approaches or a combination of both. The five most common approaches to the treatment of PNE are:

1. Conditioning therapy (utilizing moisture-sensitive alarms—generally referred to as sleep alarms).
2. Motivational therapy (utilizing emotional support, reassurance, guilt removal, and a reward system).
3. Bladder-stretching training (utilizing exercises to assist with the ability to retain urine for longer periods).
4. Water and stimulant abstinence.
5. Pharmacologic therapy.

The efficacy of the various treatments is quite variable, and some are considerably labor intensive, rendering them impractical for the average family.

Conditioning Therapy

Conditioning therapy primarily consists of the use of signal alarm devices. This approach utilizes a moisture-sensitive device, placed near the child's genital area, which triggers an alarm when it senses moisture. In theory, the alarm will awaken the child so that he or she will use the toilet. However, many children will sleep through the alarm or not get up to urinate when they do hear it. Some alarms are so loud that even though they do not arouse the child, other family members are awakened, thus potentially causing additional family stress, compounding the already strained family situation. Various types of alarm devices are available. Although some models can be quite costly, the average cost for an alarm device is about $55.00.

The alarms utilize either a sound or vibratory device. Alarm devices are effective about 70% of the time.

The drawbacks are that sleep alarms may:

- take six months to gain adequate control
- cause an interruption in normal sleep pattern
- cause sleep loss (for the child *and* the parents)
- not be suitable for use with children under age seven years of age.

Alarms may have a substantial negative impact on self-esteem, especially for those children who have to wait until age 7 to begin treatment. Even though 7 out of 10 children will eventually respond to the treatment, there is a 30% relapse rate. Another important consideration is that, to be successful, the use of an alarm system requires the cooperation and motivation of both the child and his or her family. An alarm system requires that the parents consistently monitor the child's progress. It also requires long-term commitment. If and when a relapse does occur, the alarm system can always be restarted. However, this will require a repeat of the same cooperation and time-intensive commitment that was previously utilized to control the nighttime enuresis. If this method is applied consistently, though, a favorable response will generally result.

However, there is an effect from the use of alarm-system–conditioning therapy that is often disregarded. When a child is abruptly awakened from a deep sleep during the night simply to use the toilet, over time, an unnatural preoccupation with sphincter control can result. This effect may involve a neurotic obsession that makes the child extra-vigilant of his or her bodily functions. The end result could be that the individual grows up having a difficult time achieving relaxation to cope with the inevitable stressors that life presents.

Motivational Therapy

Motivational therapy consists of providing the child with emotional support in order to protect the child's self-esteem and to alleviate the child's feelings of guilt. The use of motivational therapy requires that parents never demonstrate impatience with reference to a child's incontinence. This may be a very unrealistic expectation. However, without this component being in place, motivational therapy will not work.

This method utilizes a chart or diaries to identify dry nights from wet nights and a reward system (often stickers) that will, in theory, reinforce a child for remaining dry. The problem with this method is that the nights when a child has a relapse, he or she may experience feelings of inadequacy and a sense of failure. This will, in turn, have a negative impact on self-esteem. The resolution rate for this technique is 25%. Even though the resolution rate with this method is low, there can be as much as a 70% decrease in wet nights; though the relapse rate is at least 5%. Because of a relatively substantial decrease in symptoms, on the surface this method can appear to be an appropriate first-line intervention. However, because of the necessity of long-term follow-up and the need for consistent encouragement from parents, this method is not a practical intervention for first-line therapy. An important consideration in relation to the use of this method is that it can backfire, resulting in a negative impact on self-esteem, due to feelings of guilt that the child may experience on those nights when he or she "fails" to stay dry.

A substantial decrease in wet nights can help to decrease the frequency of morning cleanups that result from wet nights. However, it does not alter the fact that a large percentage of children will experience self-doubt after each wet night, once they learn that a reward is only given for dry nights. Because the typical child with PNE is at considerable risk of suffering from low self-esteem, each time the child has a setback while utilizing this method, an even greater risk of damage to self-esteem may result. This technique is also very difficult for parents to apply consistently. However, without consistent implementation, this method will not render positive results. Another risk of utilizing this method is that it can precipitate a tendency, on the child's part, to lie and to claim that he or she was dry when, in reality, this was not the case. A child may be tempted to do so just to receive the anticipated reward.

The probability that this will happen requires that the parents check the bed themselves each morning. Unfortunately, because of this necessity, a vicious cycle of sneaking leading to mistrust, leading to more sneaking and more mistrust may be reinforced. This can tend to nurture an unhealthy relationship between parent and child.

Bladder-Stretching Exercises

Bladder-stretching exercises have been demonstrated to have as much as 40% effectiveness. Although urodynamic studies do not demonstrate that children with PNE have a reduced bladder capacity, the use of bladder-stretching exercises is still advocated by some. The technique requires the child to "practice" holding his or her urine for progressively longer periods of time, during the day. However, its usefulness is limited as a treatment because it may take more than a year before adequate "stretching" of the bladder occurs. Because the process can be very uncomfortable for the child, the strong patient commitment required for this method to work is difficult to sustain.

Water and Stimulant Abstinence

Water and stimulant abstinence has demonstrated only limited success in controlling the symptoms of PNE. This approach consists of avoiding the drinking of water, or of any other liquids, at least four hours prior to going to bed. Caffeinated beverages and chocolate should especially be avoided with this intervention strategy. Although abstention from the use of caffeinated substances is relatively easy to ensure in this approach, if a child is thirsty prior to going to bed, it is not always easy for parents to not permit a child to have "a little" water prior to going to bed. This factor alone limits the effectiveness of this approach.

Other Therapeutic Approaches

Therapies that have been tried and do not demonstrate any consistent efficacy are: hypnotherapy, diet therapy, psychotherapy, chiropractic treatments, homeopathy, and acupuncture. Hypnotherapy, though providing potentially a successful short-term response, does not demonstrate sustained effectiveness.

Diet therapies demonstrate very inconsistent response rates. It is also important to note that if the origin of PNE was related to diet, rather than a genetic predisposition, other children in the family of a child with PNE would also be afflicted with the condition. However, this is frequently not the case. In the case of psychotherapy, since young children are not good candidates for psychotherapeutic interventions, it has limited usefulness in the treatment of PNE beyond helping a child to cope with the emotional stress and self-esteem issues induced by feeling inadequate due to chronic bed-wetting. In reference to chiropractic treatments and acupuncture, some anecdotal information has claimed efficacy; however, neither intervention has demonstrated any consistent evidence-based efficacy.

Pharmacologic Therapy

Due to the fact that PNE can cause significant stress for a child and his or her family, pharmacologic treatment is the initial treatment chosen by over 51% of primary care providers. Though none of the pharmacologic treatments result in a cure for PNE, they can provide a rapid intervention, until such time as the child is able to achieve dry nights without medication.

The pharmacotherapy most frequently used as first-line treatment for PNE is desmopressin acetate. Fifteen years of treating PNE with desmopressin acetate, has demonstrated its safety for the long-term control of the symptoms of PNE. Desmopressin acetate can effectively correct the ADH deficit that, in most children with enuresis, is the major cause of PNE. Desmopressin acetate is effective for consistent control of PNE until the child's nighttime ADH levels remain adequate on their own. In double-blind, randomized trials, this therapy has demonstrated as much as a 70% long-term response rate. Desmopressin acetate can help control PNE rapidly, usually within one to three days of therapy. Without any apparent health risks, desmopressin acetate can even be combined safely with other techniques to enhance efficacy. Controlled clinical trials have demonstrated that the incidence of adverse events, as well as the side-effect profile, is comparable to that of a placebo.

Treatment with desmopressin acetate must be administered on a nightly basis in order to maintain effective control over nighttime incontinence. At six-month intervals the medication can be decreased gradually to assess whether or not nighttime ADH levels have increased to the point that the medication is no longer needed. Although the cost of the medication is comparatively high ($50–$100 dollars per month), the cost of low self-esteem and feelings of guilt and shame can carry an emotional expense that may far outweigh the financial cost of the medication. Desmopressin acetate is available in tablet form or as a nasal spray. Due to its convenience, most families prefer the tablet form. The starting dose of desmopressin acetate is 0.2 mg (1 tablet) administered at bedtime. The dose may be titrated up to 0.6 mg (3 tablets) until a desired response is achieved. The tablet and the spray are interchangeable; however, due to the possibility of inadequate absorption in children with nasal congestion, tablets may be more appropriate for children with allergies or frequent colds.

Imipramine is also used with relative success, to treat many cases of enuresis. Although it can be toxic in excessive doses, many enuretics can be well controlled with safe doses of 25 to 75 mg/HS. Since no deaths from the use of imipramine have been recorded, at doses of less than 150 mg, it is prudent to limit doses to no higher than 75 mg/hs to avoid any risk of complication. It is hypothesized that imipramine effectiveness can be attributed to a mild effect on the nighttime secretion of ADH. Double-blind controlled trials have demonstrated a long-term effectiveness rate of 25%. No optimal duration of treatment has been determined.

Anticholinergic medications will only be mentioned because of their history of use in attempting to treat PNE. The mechanism of action of anticholinergic medications such as oxybutynin and hyoscyamine is as a relaxant of smooth muscle tissue that can decrease the ability of the bladder to contract; thus allowing it to hold more urine. Although the use of anticholinergic medications for treating other conditions has well-documented efficacy, there is only limited anecdotal evidence that medications such as oxybutynin and hyoscyamine are useful in the treatment of PNE as stand-alone therapy.

Sometimes combinations of therapies are necessary for the effective treatment of resistant cases of PNE. Desmopressin acetate has at various times been used in combination with hyoscyamine, oxybutynin, imipramine, conditioning therapy, motivation therapy, and even water and stimulant avoidance intervention when any one of these therapies alone has not adequately resolved the symptoms of PNE. Although some children seem to have difficulty achieving and maintaining dry nights, with proper educational training of both the child and the parents, the success rate can be greatly enhanced.

The key to achieving a successful response rate to PNE interventions is frequent follow-up visits. These visits are essential to reinforce family follow-through.

Supportive Measures

Most children eventually outgrow bed-wetting. However, it is not uncommon for bed-wetting to go on until a child is 9 or 10 years old. Occasionally, it will last through the teenage years. It is important to reassure the patient and his or her family that he or she is not "bad" or "a big baby" just because of the bed-wetting. Children should be helped to understand that PNE is a medical condition that is probably inherited from one of their grandparents; just like the color of their eyes and hair or the shape of their nose. Providing positive emotional support to a child and reminding parents of the importance of being patient about "accidents" are absolutely necessary in helping a child to build self-acceptance and self-confidence in spite of his or her bed-wetting.

Besides following a health care provider's treatment recommendations, parents can provide additional support measures useful in helping a child to feel that he or she can have an active role in solving a bed-wetting problem. Parents can be encouraged to implement the following:

1. Parents should help children not to feel guilty when they have an accident, by encouraging the children to talk about their feelings openly. Parents should comfort their bed-wetting child by reminding the child that their love is not contingent on whether or not the child wets the bed and to make the child realize that they know that any "accident" was not the child's fault.
2. Parents should help their children to avoid caffeinated beverages and chocolate within four hours of bedtime. This may help prevent some "accidents."
3. Parents should help their child to avoid drinking any liquids after supper.
4. Parents should ensure that their child uses the toilet before going to bed.
5. Parents should teach their child to clean up when such "accidents" do occur. They should also ensure that all cleanup is handled in a "matter-of-fact" manner. The child should be responsible for changing wet pajamas and sheets and even for putting the wet clothing in the washer and dryer.
6. Using a diary to monitor progress toward achieving consistently dry nights can be useful if the child and parents are consistent in its use.
7. Parents should be encouraged to ask the child's health care provider about how to get a copy of the Disney video, *Bed-Wetting: Jasper to the Rescue.* (These videos are available, at no charge, from Phone-Poulenc Rorer Pharmaceuticals.)
8. Parents should be encouraged to use the Internet to find additional support material about primary nocturnal enuresis. One useful E-mail site is: http://www.drynights.com

Patient Education (and Tips to the Patient's Parents)

The psychological and emotional impact of bed-wetting on the child and his or her family can be devastating. Some parents blame themselves and think that they have somehow failed in their parental role. How parents handle their response to bed-wetting will have a dramatic impact on their child's sense of self-worth for the rest of his or her life. Most parents see bed-wetting as a behavioral problem. It is important to help parents understand that children do not wet the bed on purpose. Parents must be helped to understand that bed-wetting is not something their child is doing out of spite or something that he or she can voluntarily control. Tragically, one out of every three parents will punish their child for involuntary incontinence. It is absolutely vital for parents to understand that they should not reprimand their child for bed-wetting. Some parental behavior can actually make enuresis more difficult to manage. Inappropriate parental interventions occur because parents misunderstand the cause of bed-wetting. Parents must be helped to understand that belittling the child about the odor of urine in the bedroom, scolding the child about wet sheets and mattress, or withdrawing privileges because of bed-wetting are all inappropriate interventions. It is absolutely essential that parents understand that a child should not be punished for bed-wetting. Family members should focus on providing support and positive reinforcement for dry nights rather than punishment for wet nights. Bed-wetting is no joking matter for the child that must endure it. The impact of bed-wetting on a child and his or her family goes far beyond the physical discomforts resulting from wet sheets and smelly pajamas. Bed-wetting can negatively affect a child's emotional development. Bed-wetting can be one of the most embarrassing and emotionally uncomfortable episodes of an individual's growing-up years. Too often, the bed-wetter must endure the condescending label of "baby." He or she is teased without mercy, made fun of, and even yelled at in front of friends and family.

Bed-wetting can produce a sense of guilt and failure that leads to a toxic shame that affects the child's psychosocial development and academic performance, and that also strains family relations. The stigma of being a bed-wetter can be worse than almost any other trauma of childhood. Even though the frustration and extra burdens on the family that are caused by the bed-wetting can seem overwhelming, parents must be helped to understand that bed-wetting is not their child's fault. Parents must be helped to understand that bed-wetting is not the result of anything that anyone has done wrong.

DISPOSITION

Overcoming a child's bed-wetting problem will require a cooperative effort between the child, his or her parents, and the health care provider. A lack of understanding about the causes of enuresis frequently leads to a mishandling of the problem by the bed-wetting child's parents. Therefore, helping parents to understand that neither they nor the child are responsible for the bed-wetting phenomenon will help parents to better cope with PNE. With adequate emotional support and the proper medical treatment, most children will be able to control their bed-wetting, feel less anxious about it, and gain a happier and healthier self-image. The physician assistant's role is to share in the education of the family about PNE, its cause, and safe interventions available to treat it.

COMPLICATIONS AND RED FLAGS

When bed-wetting continues beyond age 6 years, it may have a profoundly negative impact on both the bed-wetting child and his or her family. The bed-wetting child may feel very isolated. The child's self-esteem may become challenged and a growing lack of patience on the part of the child's parents may complicate the situation. The vast majority of parents respond to bed-wetting with anger, blaming their child and attempting to solve the problem with punishment and ridicule.

The problem with using this approach is that it may result in emotional scars that become quite pronounced as the bed-wetting child matures. Despite its widespread occurrence, parents are typically reluctant to talk about bed-wetting in the family. It is often a topic of considerable embarrassment for many parents. The whole family may consider bed-wetting with such frustration and confusion that the issue becomes shrouded in secrecy. Unsure what others will think, the family may even be afraid to share "the secret" with their health care provider.

OTHER NOTES AND PEARLS

Bed-wetting is, of course, normal during infancy and the toilet-training period. However, if the bed-wetting continues after age 6 years and produces a stress on the family that is causing a negative impact on the child's self-esteem and considerable disruption to the family, intervention is appropriate. Therefore, it is prudent to perform routine screening of all children during well-child checkups, as well as when a child is brought to a health care provider for urgent care. PNE can be a source of considerable distress for children and adolescents afflicted with it. A child may view it as a personal defect. It can negatively impact psychological well-being, causing significant damage to self-esteem. The reaction from parents and other family members may even compound the problem. Embarrassed and discouraged, parents may be unwilling to ask for medical advice. For this reason, medical intervention is indicated when parents and/or the child are disturbed by the physical manifestations of PNE to the point that they seek professional help. The type of intervention offered will depend upon the provider's understanding of the negative consequences of this condition. For this reason, a thorough knowledge of the underlying disorder and the appropriate evidence-based intervention strategies for controlling the symptoms will be a PA's best way of maintaining preparedness for providing the support families need when they request help for this frustrating condition.

BIBLIOGRAPHY

Cendron M: Primary nocturnal enuresis: Current. *Am Fam Physician* 59(5):1205–1214, 1999.

Eiberg H et al: Assignment of dominant inherited nocturnal enuresis (ENURI) to chromosome 13q. *Nat Genet* 10:354–364, 1995.

Garber KM: Enuresis: An update on diagnosis and management. *J Pediatr Health Care* 10:202–208, 1996.

Mosier WA: Desmopressin acetate: Treatment of choice in the management of primary nocturnal enuresis. *2nd International Children's Continence Symposium: Proceedings.* Rome, International Children's Continence Symposium, 31:57, 1993.

Mosier WA: Update on childhood enuresis. *The Clinical Advisor for Physician Assistants* 1(4):32–38, 1998.

Norgaard JP, Djurhuus JC: The pathophysiology of enuresis in children and young adults. *Clin Pediatr* July(suppl):5–9, 1993.

Norgaard JP: Urodynamics in enuresis 1: Reservoir function pressure-flow study. *Neurourol Urodyn* 8:119–124, 1998.

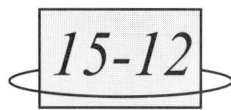

PEDIATRIC ORTHOPEDIC DEFORMITIES OF THE LOWER EXTREMITIES AND FEET

Ricky Kortyna

DISCUSSION

Abnormal positioning of the lower extremities or the feet is a common reason for parents to bring a child to the office for evaluation. While a significant number of these cases require no treatment, a few are harbingers of potentially serious conditions (see Table 15-12-1). It is up to the health care provider to determine whether the variation is physiologic or pathologic.

ABNORMALITIES OF THE LOWER EXTREMITIES

Genu Varum (Bowlegs)

Physiologic genu varum refers to the normal bowing of the lower extremities. This is a common finding in newborns and may persist up to 18 months of age.[1] The etiology of this is secondary to in utero positioning in which the hips are flexed, abducted, and externally rotated.[2] Obese black children who walk early are at high risk.[3] However, when the parents notice bowlegs in a child, it is up to the health care provider to determine whether the etiology is physiologic or pathologic from such entities as rickets, achondroplasia, or asymmetric growth of the growth plate. If the bowing is rapid and progressive it most likely represents a pathologic condition. On examination, a standing height must be obtained as well as a recorded measurement of the distance between the knees. The angle between the knees will decrease from an average of 15° at birth to 10° at 1 year of age to neutral alignment by 2 years of age if it is physiologic in etiology.[2] Radiographs are not needed if pathologic considerations are not being considered. There is no treatment as this condition generally corrects itself: "orthopedic" shoes and wedges do not help. If, however, the bowing either

TABLE 15-12-1. Red Flags for Pediatric Orthopedic Problems

Progressive bowing of the legs
Bowing that does not resolve by 2 years of age
Persistent internal tibial torsion after 7 years of age
Anterolateral bowing of the tibia
Cavus deformity at any age
Toe-walking after 3 years of age

progresses or does not resolve by the age of 2 years, then radiographs of the lower legs and a metabolic workup should be considered.

Genu Valgum (Knock Knees)

Minimal genu valgum is normal after 2 years of age, with a mean of about 12° by age 3 years, with a decrease to 7 to 9° by age 8 years.[3] This mild variation is secondary to overcorrection of genu varum.[2] The child may place one leg in front of the other when standing in an attempt to place the feet together.[4] Those children with deformities over 20° may require bracing and, if this is not effective, either growth plate stapling or osteotomy in an attempt to prevent long-term patellofemoral problems such as degeneration.

Tibia Vara (Blount Disease)

The bowing of the lower legs in this condition is due to abnormal growth of the medial tibial growth plate.[5] It is most frequently seen in blacks, those of Mediterranean descent, and obese children. The infantile form occurs in the first 3 years of life and may be difficult to differentiate from physiologic genu varum. The juvenile form generally occurs after 6 years of age. Either one or both legs may be affected but up to 50 to 80% are bilateral, depending on the age of the child. The frequency of bilateral involvement drops as the child ages.[2] The child should be examined both supine and standing with the patellae pointing forward in order to best assess the severity of bowing. Standing anteroposterior radiographs with the patellae pointing forward allow for a more accurate measurement of the deformity. On radiographs, peaking of the proximal medial tibia epiphysis, abnormalities of the proximal medial growth plate, and an angle of greater than 11° between the tibial metaphysis and diaphysis may be seen.[5] Long-leg bracing when the patient is weight-bearing is possibly effective; nighttime bracing is not. This disease may resolve spontaneously, with bracing, or in the more severe cases, with surgical realignment. The indications for surgical intervention include age of 4 years or greater, failure of orthoses, and a more severe deformity. Proximal tibial and fibular osteotomies are the procedures of choice.[2]

Internal Tibial Torsion

This condition gives the appearance of bowing of the lower extremity as the tibia is rotated along its longitudinal axis. It is the most common cause of inward-pointing toes in children between the ages of 1 and 3 years.[3] (Another consideration for this appearance in a child over 3 years of age is internal femoral torsion.[6]) Internal tibial torsion is due to in utero positioning and may be seen with metatarsus adductus (discussed below).[2] The parents become aware of this condition when the child begins to walk and they notice either a wide-based gait, bowing of the legs, or toeing-in. Examination with the child in the seated position with the legs together and the knees bent over the table highlights the feet pointing inward. Examination of the child in a standing position reveals the patellae pointing straight ahead or slightly outward while the feet point inward. This condition often corrects itself, and no treatment is needed if the child is under 3 years of age. After the age of 3 years, pediatric orthopedists are divided as to the effectiveness of bracing.[2,3,7] If there is not spontaneous improvement by 7 years of age, surgical intervention with tibial realignment is indicated.

External Tibial Torsion

This common condition is always associated with a calcaneovalgus foot and is due to in utero positioning. The combination of the calcaneovalgus foot with external tibial torsion in the normally externally rotated hip produces toeing-out. Serial visits for measurements are needed, but this condition generally resolves spontaneously.[2]

Anterolateral Bowing of the Tibia

This condition is serious as it may represent the presence of congenital pseudoarthrosis of the tibia, a finding often associated with neurofibromatosis. The parents will bring the child into the office because of "bowlegs." Anterolateral bowing is unilateral and associated with a leg length discrepancy. Examination includes measurement of leg length, palpation of the lower extremities, and a careful search for café au lait spots. Radiographs are obtained, which may show a radiolucent area in the apex of the bowed tibia or narrowing of the medullary canal. Fractures are common and must be corrected surgically. Unfortunately often these fractures don't heal properly (pseudoarthrosis), and varied nonconventional treatments have been tried with mixed success. Some children have required amputation.[8] These children should be followed every 6 months to look for recurrent fractures or to determine leg length discrepancies.

Posteromedial Bow of the Tibia

This condition is usually present at birth, is unilateral, and is benign. The general appearance at birth is with the dorsum of the foot resting on the front of the tibia. The foot, which is free of pathology, can be flexed to the neutral position. The tibia is angled posteriorly. This may resolve spontaneously, but some orthopedic surgeons recommend either stretching exercises or serial casting.[8] The tibial deformity resolves by 4 years of age. These children need to be followed on a serial basis as they may develop a leg length discrepancy of up to 5 cm.[9]

Rickets

Rickets, inadequate mineralization of the bone matrix secondary to abnormal calcium and phosphorus metabolism, may cause bowing of the legs. The etiology of rickets is most often due to a deficiency of vitamin D but an additional consideration is hypophosphatemic rickets, an X-linked dominant inherited condition in which the children are short and have decreased serum phosphorus levels secondary to chronic renal tubular wasting of phosphate.[8] Examination of the legs reveals bowing. Treatment involves correction of the underlying metabolic etiology. Bracing may be effective for mild to moderate deformities, but, again, there is controversy.[9] If there is severe deformity of the legs and the underlying etiology has been treated, osteotomies are done in order to achieve adequate correction. Preferably this is done after skeletal maturity is reached.

ABNORMALITIES OF THE FEET

Metatarsus Adductus

This term refers to excessive in-turning of the forefoot in relation to the rest of the foot, resulting in a C-shaped foot. It occurs in 5/1000 live births and is the most common foot deformity of the newborn.[10] This deformity is thought to be the result of "uterine packing," uterine positioning, an excessively large fetus, or twinning. It occurs equally in males and females and is bilateral in half of the cases.[2] On examination the foot will have a C shape and the ankle will dorsiflex beyond neutral. There may be a deep crease of the medial border of the foot. If the ankle does not dorsiflex, clubfoot should be suspected. The examiner may be able to gently correct the deformity by pushing the affected portion laterally. Metatarsus adductus may be either flexible, meaning that the examiner can correct the deformity, or rigid, meaning that it cannot be corrected. While examining the feet, the examiner must also examine the hips as developmental dysplasia of the hips is associated with this deformity. In a child who is walking, toeing-in will be seen as will abnormal wear of the shoes.[2] Radiographs are not needed. A simple way to follow the progression of this condition is to obtain serial photocopies of the feet by standing the child on a photocopy machine.[11] If the metatarsus adductus is flexible, it will spontaneously improve. Stretching exercises may be of benefit. For the rigid metatarsus adductus, stretching and serial castings are used; in rare cases, surgery is needed. Shoe wedges are not effective,[12] although this is controversial.[2]

Clubfoot (Equinovarus Foot or Talipes Equinovarus)

Clubfoot is an inward turning of the foot that is easily recognized in the newborn. In fact, it is often discovered on prenatal ultrasound. It is more common in males, may be an inherited trait, and has an overall incidence of 1/1000.[10] When it does occur in females the deformity tends to be more severe.[8] If one foot is involved, it appears smaller and shorter than the noninvolved foot. The heel also appears smaller or absent and has a downward and inward rotation. This is a rigid deformity that cannot be corrected by the examiner. The components of clubfoot include plantar flexion of the ankle, inversion of the heel, midfoot cavus, and adduction of the forefoot.[4,11] Both feet may be affected with either symmetric or asymmetric involvement. On examination, one must search for neurocutaneous markers such as midline capillary hemangiomas, dermal-dural sinus tracts, or hair tufts since these may signal myelomeningocele (spina bifida). Both legs must be examined in their entirety as there may be a leg length discrepancy. Atrophy of the involved gastrocnemius is seen, especially when the child begins to walk; this is secondary to fibrosis. Radiographic evaluation is useful to determine the degree of clubbing, but care must be taken in interpretation since there is minimal calcification of the bones shortly after birth.[8] Treatment begins shortly after birth and consists of stretching exercises, serial casting, taping, and/or bracing. These treatments may be enough to correct the deformity but often they are not entirely successful, and the malposition returns. Failure of nonoperative treatment occurs most often in female patients. If that is the case, then surgical correction via soft tissue releases is required.[2] Even with surgery, the rate of recurrence is nearly 10% within 3 years.[10] These children require at least biannual evaluations by a pediatric orthopedic surgeon and may require shoes of different sizes if the affected foot does not grow at the same rate as the noninvolved foot.[13] Parents need to be educated that the presence of clubfoot does not prohibit the child from crawling or walking.

Calcaneovalgus Feet

This is common in the newborn and is due to in utero positioning. The foot is hyperdorsiflexed and the forefoot abducted. As mentioned previously, this is seen with external tibial torsion. The newborn will have an extremely externally rotated foot and the dorsum of the foot can easily be brought up to touch the tibia. The differential includes vertical talus, which is a rigid deformity. Roentgenographs may be needed to differentiate calcaneovalgus deformity from vertical talus. In calcaneovalgus the x-rays are either normal or demonstrate a mild hindfoot valgus appearance versus an equinus rocker-bottom deformity in vertical talus. No treatment is needed for calcaneovalgus feet since this spontaneously resolves by 6 months or, at the latest, 2 years of age.[2]

Congenital Vertical Talus

This deformity is visible at birth. When viewed from the side the sole of the foot appears convex, hence giving rise to the name *rocker-bottom foot*.[10] The heel is fixed downward as in clubfoot but the forefoot is displaced upward and laterally. The deformity is bilateral in half of the cases. It may occur alone or be associated with other deformities such as arthrogryposis and myelomeningocele. Therefore examination should include the search for neurocutaneous markers as discussed above. Treatment is begun shortly after birth with simple stretching exercises and serial casting. Even with treatment there will

still be limited range of motion.[14] This is not a problem provided the foot can be placed in a position that allows the child to wear shoes. If shoe wearing is not likely to occur because of the rigidity of the deformity, surgical intervention is required.

Flat Feet

Flat feet should not be diagnosed prior to 6 years of age because of the presence of the fat pad. After the age of 6 years the diagnosis can be made, but if the foot is flexible—the arch returns when the child is not weight-bearing—then it is of no consequence. If there is a history of a recent onset of flat feet, trauma, or severe pain, then the etiology needs to be further explored. Rigid flat feet may also be caused by tarsal coalition, vertical talus, a tight Achilles tendon, arthritis, or neuromuscular imbalance from varied etiologies.[3] Examination begins with observing shoe wear—with flat feet the wear is abnormal and occurs on the inner or medial side of the shoe.[15] Examination is done with the child walking around the room. With weight-bearing the foot is flat and the heel is in a valgus position. Both of these findings reverse when the child is no longer weight-bearing. Radiographs are needed in those children with foot pain or limited range of motion.[16] Asymptomatic patients do not need radiographs or treatment. Symptomatic patients with rigid flat feet may respond to orthotics. Surgery, either soft tissue reconstruction or osteotomies, is rarely indicated.[3]

Cavus Feet

In contradistinction to a flat foot, a cavus foot has an abnormally high arch. If there is not a history of cavus deformity then an underlying neuromuscular problem such as spinal cord pathology should be strongly considered. This condition rarely shows up in children under 8 years of age.[10] Because of the unusual shape of the foot these children have a difficult time being fitted properly for shoes, tend to prefer shoes with a high heel, toe-walk, and often complain of anterior ankle pain.[10,11] In addition to the high arch, other findings include a varus angulation of the hindfoot, adduction of the forefoot, and clawing of the toes. Calluses beneath the metatarsal heads are not uncommon. There may be weakness of the extensor hallicus longus and the anterior tibialis.[4] Not only must the spine be examined for neurocutaneous markers, but a complete neurologic examination of the lower extremities, looking for weakness, atrophy, and absent reflexes, is indicated. Radiographs of both the spine and feet are needed, and, if there are suspicions of underlying spinal cord pathology, an MRI of the spinal cord is required. Neuro-electrical studies such as nerve conduction velocity (NCV) and electromyography (EMG) are frequently obtained. These children need to be seen by both orthopedics and neurology/neurosurgery. Underlying spinal cord pathology must be treated. If there is no spinal cord pathology then a custom-made orthosis will help. Should the deformity progress, the child will have an increasingly difficult time finding shoes and will be subject to repeated ankle injuries.[17] If this is the case, a hindfoot fusion (triple arthrodesis) with potential tendon transfers is the surgical treatment of choice.[10]

Tarsal Coalition

Tarsal coalition refers to a congenital connection between two or more tarsal bones. The connection or coalition may be fibrous, cartilaginous, or bony and most frequently involves the calcaneus and navicular laterally and the talus and calcaneus medially. Symptoms occur in early adolescence with foot pain and stiffness. Examination shows a valgus heel and decreased subtalar motion. Radiographs or CT are needed to confirm the anatomic location of the coalition. Conservative treatment consists of casting, and if this is not effective, then surgical correction of the coalition is done.

Toe Deformities

Extra toes (polydactyly) are noticed at birth and, if merely attached by a tag of skin, are immediately amputated. However, if the attachment is via cartilage or bone, then delayed surgical treatment is indicated. Fusion of the toes (syndactyly) is generally a benign cosmetic problem, but health care practitioners must be aware of the association with varied syndromes, including Down's, fetal hydantoin, and Apert's syndrome.[2] Acrosyndactyly is the joining of the tip of the toes with an unjoined open web. This is seen with oligohydramnios and soft-tissue constriction bands. Since this is almost always asymptomatic, there is no treatment.[8]

OTHER PEDIATRIC ORTHOPEDIC CONDITIONS

Toe Walking

Under the age of 3 years, toe walking is generally considered to be normal: beyond then it requires evaluation. It may affect either or both feet and the etiologies include cerebral palsy, spinal cord pathology, leg length discrepancy of any etiology, muscular dystrophy, cavus foot deformities, contractures, and habitual behavior. Since toe walking is seen only when children are able to walk, it is important to ask the child to demonstrate if he or she can walk normally. Examination focuses on the gait, with the child undressed down to diapers or underwear. Range of motion of the hip, knee, and ankle are performed to determine if contractures are present. Care must be taken to thoroughly evaluate the Achilles tendon to eliminate contractures there. Bilateral toe walking is most likely due to cerebral palsy, contractures, and habit. Unless spinal cord pathology is suspected, there is little need for radiographs. Neuroelectrical studies and creatine phosphokinase are obtained to rule out muscular dystrophy. Children who toe walk often need a neurology consult to help determine the underlying cause. After the workup has been completed, stretching, serial casting, and orthosis are offered. If toe walking is secondary to leg length discrepancy, then the underlying cause of the discrepancy must be evaluated. Those with discrepancies under 2 cm are not treated, 2 to 5 cm are treated with shoe inserts, and those over 5 cm by surgical lengthening of the femur or tibia.[18]

RED FLAGS

Table 15-12-1 on page 585 lists the common "red flags" when dealing with a child with orthopedic problems of the lower extremities and feet.

REFERENCES

1. Raggio CL: Physiologic genu varum, in Pizzutillo PD (ed): *Pediatric Orthopedics in Primary Care,* New York, McGraw-Hill, 1997, p. 239.
2. Thompson GH: Common orthopedic problems of children, in Behrman RE, Kliegman RM (eds): *Nelson Essentials of Pediatrics,* Philadelphia, Saunders, 1998, pp 746–781.
3. Sponseller PD: Bone, joint, and muscle problems, in Johnson KB, Oski FA (eds): *Oski's Essential Pediatrics,* Philadelphia, Lippincott-Raven, 1994, pp 155–169.
4. Ward WT, et al: Orthopedics, in Zitelli BJ, Davis HW (eds): *Atlas of Pediatric Physical Diagnosis,* St. Louis, Mosby-Wolfe, 1997, pp 625–682.
5. Staniski D: Tibia vara (Blount's disease), in Pizzutillo PD (ed): *Pediatric Orthopedics in Primary Care,* New York, McGraw-Hill, 1997, pp 241–242.
6. Ellert RE, Georgopoulos G: Orthopedics, in Hay WW et al. (eds): *Current Pediatric Diagnosis and Treatment,* Stamford CT, Appleton and Lange, 1997, pp 704–723.
7. Raggio CL: Internal tibial torsion, in Pizzutillo PD (ed): *Pediatric Orthopedics in Primary Care,* New York, McGraw-Hill, 1997, pp 243–244.
8. Rab GT: Pediatric orthopedic surgery, in Skinner HB (ed): *Current Diagnosis and Treatment in Orthopedics,* Norwalk, CT: Appleton and Lange, 1995, pp 512–554.
9. Stanitski D: Posteromedial bow of the tibia, in Pizzutillo PD (ed): *Pediatric Orthopaedics in Primary Practice,* New York, McGraw Hill, 1997, pp 249–250.
10. Rab GT: Pediatric orthopedic surgery, in *Current Diagnosis and Treatment in Orthopedics,* HB Skinner (ed). Norwalk, CT, Appleton and Lange, 1995, pp 512–554.
11. Aronsson DD et al: Pediatric orthopedics, in *Essentials of Musculoskeletal Care,* W Greene (ed). Rosemont, American Academy of Orthopedic Surgeons, 1997, pp 547–668.
12. Raggio CL: Metatarsus adductus, in *Pediatric Orthopaedics in Primary Practice,* PD Pizzutillo (ed). New York, McGraw-Hill, 1997, pp 269–270.
13. Nogi J: Clubfeet, in *Pediatric Orthopaedics,* PD Pizzutillo (ed). New York, McGraw-Hill, 1997, pp 271–272.
14. Nogi J: Congenital vertical talus, in *Pediatric Orthopaedics in Primary Practice,* PD Pizzutillo (ed). New York, McGraw-Hill, 1997, pp 273–274.
15. Dise TL: Flatfeet and tibial torsion, in *Saunders Manual of Pediatric Practice,* L Finberg (ed). Philadelphia, Saunders, 1998, pp 988–989.
16. Horn BD: Flat feet, in *Pediatric Orthopaedics in Primary Practice,* PD Pizzutillo (ed). New York, McGraw-Hill, 1997, pp 275–276.
17. D'Astous J: Cavus foot, in *Pediatric Orthopaedics in Primary Practice,* PD Pizzutillo (ed). New York, McGraw-Hill, 1997, pp 277–280.
18. Thompson GH: Toe-walking (equinus gait), in *Pediatric Orthopaedics in Primary Practice,* PD Pizzutillo (ed). New York, McGraw-Hill, 1997, pp 297–300.

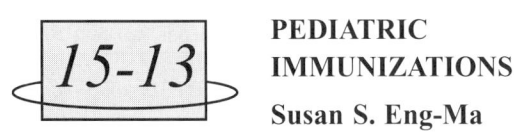

15-13 PEDIATRIC IMMUNIZATIONS
Susan S. Eng-Ma

DISCUSSION

Immunity from infectious diseases can be acquired passively or actively. Passive immunity is protection transferred from another person as antibodies and is temporary, while active immunity is protection produced by one's own immune system. The objective is for vaccines to produce protection without generating disease. Vaccinations allow for group immunity to be achieved in order to potentially eradicate childhood diseases.

The vaccine era started in 1796 in England when Dr. Edward Jenner injected someone with material from a cowpox lesion and called the procedure a *vaccination* (Latin *vacca,* "cow"). Since then many vaccines have been developed and used to decrease morbidity and mortality from infectious diseases. Today, vaccinations protect children against many of the deadly diseases of childhood—polio, measles, chicken pox, diphtheria, tetanus, mumps, rubella, and pertussis. Recently, vaccines for hepatitis B, *Haemophilus influenzae* type b, varicella, pneumococci, and rotavirus have been added to this list. Children should begin their first series of immunizations during the first months of life, and for complete protection, immunizations should be finished within a certain time. One of the most significant public health accomplishments of the twentieth century has been the extensive utilization of immunizations to prevent life-threatening infectious disease. Childhood immunization rates have increased dramatically in just the last few years through concerted national, state, and local governmental efforts.

IMMUNIZATION SCHEDULES AND RECENT UPDATES

Immunization recommendations are constantly changing. Each year the Advisory Committee on Immunization Practices (ACIP), the American Academy of Pediatrics (AAP), and the American Academy of Family Physicians (AAFP) jointly develop their annual Recommended Childhood Immunization Schedule (Fig. 15-13-1). Major changes in the last few years include:

- All routine childhood polio vaccinations in the United States are now the injectable IPV (inactivated polio vaccine).
- Rotavirus vaccine, approved for use in 1998, has been withdrawn from the market due to an increased incidence of intussuception in recently immunized infants.

Vaccines[1] are listed under routinely recommended ages. Bars *indicate range of recommended ages for immunization. Any dose not given at the recommended age should be given as a "catch-up" immunization at any subsequent visit when indicated and feasible* Ovals *indicate vaccines to be given if previously recommended doses were missed or given earlier than the recommended minimum age.*

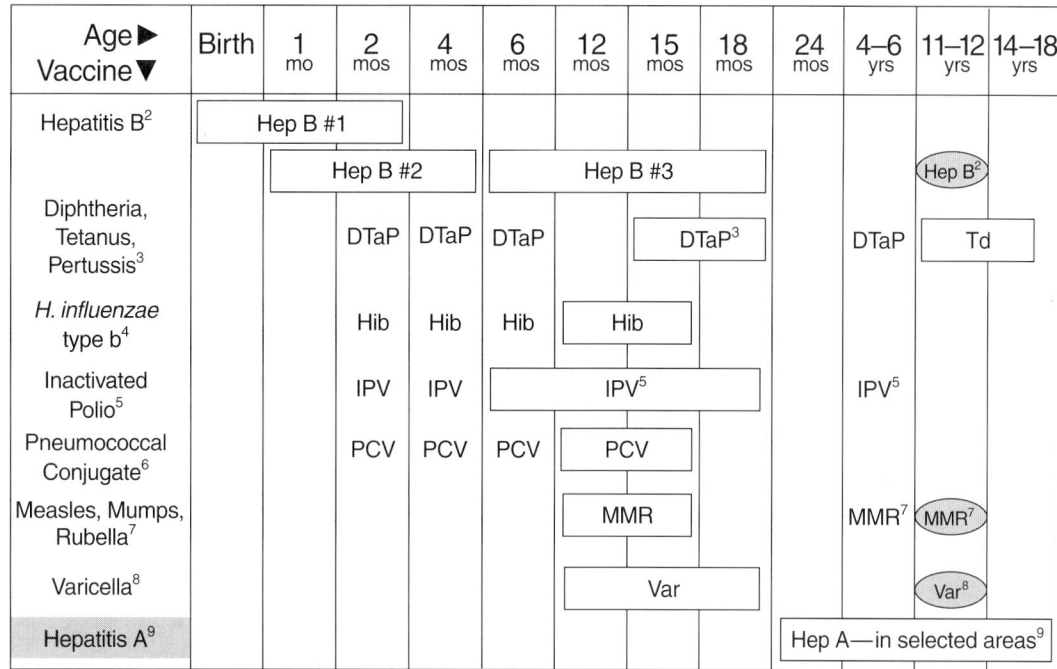

Approved by the Advisory Committee on Immunization Practices (ACIP), the American Academy of Pediatrics (AAP), and the American Academy of Family Physicians (AAFP).

[1] This schedule indicates the recommended ages for routine administration of currently licensed childhood vaccines, as of 11/1/00, for children through 18 years of age. Additional vaccines may be licensed and recommended during the year. Licensed combination vaccines may be used whenever any components of the combination are indicated and its other components are not contraindicated. Providers should consult the manufacturers' package inserts for detailed recommendations.

[2] **Infants born to HBsAg-negative mothers** should receive the 1st dose of hepatitis B (Hep B) vaccine by age 2 months. The 2nd dose should be at least 1 month after the 1st dose. The 3rd dose should be administered at least 4 months after the 1st dose and at least 2 months after the 2nd dose, but not before 6 months of age for infants.
Infants born to HBsAg-positive mothers should receive hepatitis B vaccine and 0.5 mL hepatitis B immune globulin (HBIG) within 12 h of birth at separate sites. The 2nd dose is recommended at 1 to 2 months of age and the 3rd dose at 6 months of age.
Infants born to mothers whose HBsAg status is unknown should receive hepatitis B vaccine within 12 h of birth. Maternal blood should be drawn at the time of delivery to determine the mother's HBsAg status; if the HBsAg test is positive, the infant should receive HBIG as soon as possible (no later than 1 week of age).
All children and adolescents who have not been immunized against hepatitis B should begin the series during any visit. Special efforts should be made to immunize children who were born in or whose parents were born in areas of the world with moderate or high endemicity of hepatitis B virus infection.

[3] The 4th dose of DTaP (diphtheria and tetanus toxoids and acellular pertussis vaccine) may be administered as early as 12 months of age, provided 6 months have elapsed since the 3rd dose and the child is unlikely to return at age 15 to 18 months. Td (tetanus and diphtheria toxoids) is recommended at 11 to 12 years of age if at least 5 years have elapsed since the last dose of DTP, DTaP, or DT. Subsequent routine Td boosters are recommended every 10 years.

[4] Three *Haemophilus influenzae* type b (Hib) conjugate vaccines are licensed for infant use. If PRP-OMP [PedvaxHIB® or ComVax® (Merck)] is administered at 2 and 4 months of age, a dose at 6 months is not required. Because clinical studies in infants have demonstrated that using some combination products may induce a lower immune response to the Hib vaccine component, DTaP/Hib combination products should not be used for primary immunization in infants at 2, 4, or 6 months of age, unless FDA-approved for these ages.

[5] An all-IPV schedule is recommended for routine childhood polio vaccination in the United States. All children should receive four doses of IPV at 2 months, 4 months, 6 to 18 months, and 4 to 6 years of age. Oral polio vaccine (OPV) should be used only in selected circumstances. [See *MMWR* May 19, 2000/49(RR-5);1–22.]

[6] The heptavalent conjugate pneumococcal vaccine (PCV) is recommended for all children 2 to 23 months of age. It also is recommended for certain children 24 to 59 months of age. [See *MMWR* Oct. 6, 2000/49(RR-9);1–35.]

[7] The 2nd dose of measles, mumps, and rubella (MMR) vaccine is recommended routinely at 4 to 6 years of age but may be administered during any visit, provided at least 4 weeks have elapsed since receipt of the 1st dose and that both doses are administered beginning at or after 12 months of age. Those who have not previously received the second dose should complete the schedule by the 11 to 12-year-old visit.

[8] Varicella (Var) vaccine is recommended at any visit on or after the first birthday for susceptible children, i.e., those who lack a reliable history of chickenpox (as judged by a health care provider) and who have not been immunized. Susceptible persons 13 years of age or older should receive 2 doses, given at least 4 weeks apart.

[9] Hepatitis A (Hep A) is shaded to indicate its recommended use in selected states and/or regions and for certain high risk groups; consult your local public health authority. [See *MMWR* Oct. 1, 1999/48(RR-12);1–37.]

For additional information about the vaccines listed above, please visit the National Immunization Program Home Page at http://www.cdc.gov/nip/ or call the National Immunization Hotline at 800-232-2522 (English) or 800-232-0233 (Spanish).

FIGURE 15-13-1. Recommended Childhood Immunization Schedule, United States, January–December 2001.

• The heptavalent conjugate pneumococcal vaccine (Prevnar) is recommended for all children 2 to 23 months of age as well as certain children 24 to 59 months of age.

Hepatitis B virus (HBV) infects more than 350 million people worldwide, especially in Southeast Asia, China, and Africa. It is estimated that some 1.25 million Americans are infected with chronic HBV, with many reproductive-age women among those infected. With the recent influx of immigrants from the parts of the world listed above it is paramount to address the vertical transmission that may occur between a mother and her newborn. Although hepatitis B surface antigen (HBsAg) is part of routine prenatal evaluations, an infected pregnant woman's infant will need to receive 0.5 mL of hepatitis B immuno-globulin within 12 h of birth. Chronic HBV may develop in up to 90% of infants and 30 to 60% of young children infected with the virus, compared with 5 to 10% of adults. Asian American children are 20 times more likely than other American children to be infected with HBV, with vaccination rates ranging from 10 to 71% for various Asian ethnic groups in different geographic locations. At present, the use of the hepatitis vaccine remains controversial because of recent claims that it may trigger demyelinating diseases.

Please refer to the respective chapters for further discussion on the following topics: diphtheria (Chap. 9-10), tetanus (Chap. 9-23), pertussis (Chap. 9-18), measles (Chap. 9-16), mumps (Chap. 9-17), rubella (Chap. 9-21), varicella (Chap. 9-26), and influenza (Chap. 9-15).

CHILDHOOD IMMUNIZATION INITIATIVE

The goal of immunization programs is to provide immunity from vaccine-preventable diseases to as many children as possible, while minimizing cost and the occurrence of unfavorable reactions. The Centers for Disease Control and Prevention started the Childhood Immunization Initiative (CII) in 1993 in an effort to increase vaccination levels and to decrease vaccine-preventable diseases of preschool-aged children. It also ensures that state and local health agencies perform regional evaluation of coverage. One of the objectives for Healthy People 2000 is to have 90% of the nation's children completely vaccinated by their second birthday. The CII's goal to increase vaccination coverage levels among children aged 2 years to ≥90% by 1996 was met and exceeded. Standards for Pediatric Immunization Practices from the National Vaccine Advisory Committee are listed in Table 15-13-1. By adopting these standards, clinicians can enhance the delivery of immunizations by improving the quality and quantity of services. Significant monetary commitment by the government will reduce the cost to families for vaccines, and increased community participation, education, and partnership will provide greater access. Continued surveillance of the diseases and vaccinations will prove to be invaluable in the widespread delivery of immunizations.

RECENT EPIDEMICS

Often childhood diseases are mistakenly perceived as mild. Undervaccination happens because of ignorance of the threat of target diseases. The horrors and ravages of diseases like polio, measles, and tetanus have not been part of our recent memory; therefore, the lack of experience with these diseases has promoted a sense of complacency and a lack of urgency to vaccinate.

An epidemic starts when a large group of inadequately immunized preschool-aged children is exposed to an infectious disease. Despite long records of the safety and success of established vaccines, there are still many children who remain unvaccinated and are susceptible to vaccine-preventable diseases. In 1993, only 65% of 2-year-olds in the United States were fully immunized.

The resurgence of measles during 1989 through 1991 happened because of inadequate vaccinations of preschool-aged children by the recommended ages. This resurgence was characterized by a shift in the

Table 15-13-1. Standards for Pediatric Immunization Practices

1. Immunization services are readily available.
2. There are no barriers or unnecessary prerequisites to the receipt of vaccines.
3. Immunization services are available free or for a minimal fee.
4. Providers utilize all clinical encounters to screen and, when indicated, vaccinate children.
5. Providers educate parents and guardians about immunization in general terms.
6. Providers question parents or guardians about contraindications and, before vaccinating a child, inform them in specific terms about the risks and benefits of the vaccinations the child is to receive.
7. Providers follow only true contraindications.
8. Providers administer simultaneously all vaccine doses for which a child is eligible at the time of each visit.
9. Providers use accurate and complete recording procedures.
10. Providers should coschedule immunization appointments in conjunction with appointments for other child health services.
11. Providers report adverse events following vaccination promptly, accurately, and completely.
12. Providers operate a tracking system.
13. Providers adhere to appropriate procedures for vaccine management.
14. Providers conduct semiannual audits to assess immunization coverage levels and to review immunization records in patient populations they serve.
15. Providers maintain up-to-date, easily retrievable medical protocols at all locations where vaccines are administered.
16. Providers should practice patient-oriented and community-based approaches.
17. Properly trained persons must administer vaccines.
18. Providers need to receive ongoing education and training regarding current immunization recommendations.

age distribution of measles from predominantly school-aged children to predominantly preschool-aged children. In 1991, more than 2000 cases and 9 deaths from measles were reported to the New York City Department of Health.

VACCINE SAFETY

From 1980 to 1996, there were 134 cases of oral polio vaccine (OPV)-associated paralytic polio in the United States; hence, the new recommendation to abandon this commonly used oral vaccine. Naturally, the concern for the safety of the vaccine is an important consideration. Children should be immunized with vaccines that are safe and effective, and the benefits of the vaccine should outweigh the risks of natural disease. The concern over whole-cell pertussis vaccine is not completely unfounded; therefore acellular pertussis vaccine became available in 1996.

The U.S. Department of Health and Human Services' Vaccine Adverse Events Reporting System (VAERS) performs ongoing surveillance of adverse events that require medical attention occurring 30 days following immunizations. These reports are entered into the VAERS database and are not necessarily proof of causality until further investigation.

CONTRAINDICATIONS

Clinicians should note the following contraindications to vaccination.

• When reviewing a child's history, it is important to note whether there was a prior allergic or severe anaphylactic reaction to any vaccine since this contraindicates that particular vaccine.

- Anaphylactic allergy to the following substances contraindicates use of the vaccine indicated in parentheses: baker's yeast (HBV); gelatin (varicella, measles-mumps-rubella [MMR]); neomycin (MMR, IPV, varicella); or streptomycin (IPV).
- If there is any history of encephalopathy within 7 days of the previous dose of DTP, do not give DTP or DTaP. Moreover, if after the previous dose of DTP or DTaP there was a fever ≥105°F, collapse or shocklike state, or persistent, inconsolable crying lasting ≥3 h within 48 h of administration, take precautions to weigh the risks and benefits of giving this vaccine. The same precautions for DTP and DTaP would apply if a previous administration resulted in convulsions or seizures within 3 days or Guillain-Barré syndrome within 6 weeks or if there is any underlying neurologic disorder.
- For a child who is HIV-positive, poliovirus vaccine live oral (OPV) and varicella are contraindicated. For a child with a household contact who is HIV-positive or immunodeficient secondary to medications or illness, only OPV is contraindicated. For a child who may be immunodeficient because of steroids or other congenital factors, MMR, OPV, and varicella are all contraindicated.
- If a child recently received immunoglobulin, the administration of MMR and varicella should be considered by weighing the risks and benefits.
- Precaution should be taken when giving MMR if there is a history of thrombocytopenic purpura.
- Finally, when evaluating a child with multiple symptoms, one must think about all of the symptoms and if any one of them is a contraindication, do not vaccinate.

PATIENT EDUCATION

While knowing true contraindications for administering a vaccine is crucial, it is important to educate patients and dispel common misconceptions about vaccinations. Providing copies of the Vaccine Information Sheets to guardians of vaccine recipients can be helpful in answering questions they may have. Providing the National Immunization Information Hotline numbers [800-232-2522 (English) and 800-232-0233 (Spanish)] can be an invaluable resource to parents and caregivers to alleviate any concerns. Proper referrals to resources permit parents and guardians to explore and share their fears and experiences.

The following Internet resources may also be helpful:

- Immunization Action Coalition and Hepatitis B Coalition: http://www.immunize.org
- National Immunization Program: http://www.cdc.gov/nip
- CDC Website on state and local health department: http://www.cdc.gov/nip/publications/VIS/default.htm
- CDC Vaccine Safety Website: http://www.cdc.gov/nip/vacsafe/hottopics/hepb

FUTURE DEVELOPMENTS

Combination vaccines that contain multiple antigens to prevent different diseases or to protect against multiple strains of infectious agents causing the same disease are needed to minimize the number of injections children need to receive. Although the combination vaccine of DTaP–*H. influenza* type b has not been currently approved for infants less than 12 months of age, combination vaccines can ultimately relieve the burden of additional visits to meet the increased demands of completing immunization requirements. Additional visits may become a barrier to comprehensive vaccine records. Although new combination vaccines have been licensed, caution must be taken with possible decreased immunogenicity and increased costs of products because of research and development.

Lastly, there is exciting research and investigation into inserting recombinant proteins into transgenic plants such as bananas so that they are edible vaccines. Current investigational vaccines also include meningococcal conjugates, combination products, and live-attenuated influenza. Many of these will be available in the next few years.

BIBLIOGRAPHY

American Academy of Pediatrics Committee on Infectious Diseases: Prevention of rotavirus disease: Guidelines for use of rotavirus vaccine. *Pediatrics* 102:1483–1491, 1998.

Centers for Disease Control and Prevention, Advisory Committee on Immunization Practices: Pertussis vaccination: Use of acellular pertussis vaccines among infants and young children. *MMWR* 46(RR-7), 1997.

Centers for Disease Control and Prevention: Combination vaccines for childhood immunization. *MMWR* 48(RR-5):1–15, 1999.

Centers for Disease Control and Prevention: Status report on the Childhood Immunization Initiative: National, state, and urban area vaccination coverage levels among children aged 19–35 months—United States, 1996. *MMWR* 46(29):657–671, 1997.

Centers for Disease Control and Prevention: Notice to readers. Recommended childhood immunization schedule—United States, 1999. *MMWR* 48:8–16, 1999.

Centers for Disease Control and Prevention, US Department of Health and Human Services: National Immunization Program. Public Health Service. Guide to Contraindications to Childhood Vaccinations, 1998.

Johnson KB, Oski FA: *Oski's Essential Pediatrics,* 2d ed. Philadelphia, Lippincott-Raven, 1997.

Zimmerman RK et al: Hepatitis B virus infection, hepatitis B vaccine, and hepatitis B immune globulin. *J Fam Pract* 45:295–315, 1997.

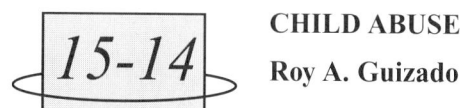

CHILD ABUSE
Roy A. Guizado

DISCUSSION

Child abuse has traditionally been thought to be physically or mentally violent in nature. Unfortunately, it has encompassed many more areas such as neglect, abandonment, and withholding of medically indicated treatment. Current literature renames child abuse as *child maltreatment,* and it is defined as any act or failure to act by a parent or caretaker that results in death, serious physical or emotional harm, sexual abuse (exploitation), or imminent risk of serious harm to a child. According to the 1996 Child Abuse Prevention and Treatment Act (CAPTA), a child is a person who has not reached the age of 18 years.[1]

The four major types of maltreatment are *physical abuse, child neglect, sexual abuse,* and *emotional abuse.*[2]

1. Physical abuse is marked by physical injury secondary to beating, kicking, hitting, biting, burning, or shaking of a harmless child. A parent or caretaker who overdisciplines through physical punishment may be guilty of physical abuse.
2. Child neglect is the failure to provide for a child's basic needs and can be physical, educational, or emotional. Physical neglect includes refusal or delay in seeking adequate health care, abandonment, inadequate supervision, and not allowing a runaway to return home. Educational neglect includes chronic truancy, failure to enroll a child in school, and failure to attend to special educational needs. Emotional neglect is characterized by inattention to a child's need for affection, poor psychological care, spousal abuse in the child's presence, and/or granting permission for a child to take drugs or alcohol.
3. Sexual abuse includes fondling a child's genitals, intercourse, rape, sodomy, exhibitionism, child prostitution, and production of child pornography.
4. Emotional abuse is defined as acts or omissions by caretakers and parents that result or could result in behavioral, cognitive, emotional, or mental disorders of a serious nature.

In 1999, the U.S. Department of Health and Human Services (DHHS) released *Child Maltreatment 1997: Reports from the States to the National Child Abuse and Neglect Data System.*[3] The report reflected that 984,000 children were abused or neglected in 1997. This is slightly less than the number of cases reported in 1996 (1,030,751). Historically, the rate of maltreatment had been on the rise, especially from 1990 to 1996. The 1997 results revealed neglect as the main form of maltreatment, while 24% was physical abuse, 13% sexual abuse, 6% emotional abuse, and 2% medical negligence.

In 1997, more than half of the abuse and negligence cases involved children 7 years old and younger; 25% were younger than 4 years. The 8- to 11-year-old age range accounted for 22% of abuse and neglect cases, while the 12- to 18-year-old group accounted for 25%. Children over 8 years old had a higher proportion of physical, sexual, and emotional abuse than children 7 years old and younger. In regards to gender, the percent of maltreated females was 52% compared to 47% males. Of sexual abuse victims, 77% were females and 23% were male. Analyzing victim statistics based on ethnicity, 64% were white, 23% were African/black Americans, 10% were Latin Americans, 2% were Native American Indian or Alaskan Native, and 1% were Asian or Pacific Islanders. Another study, the National Incidence Study of Child Abuse (NIS-3), released in 1996 showed a 25% increase of maltreatment of children from families with an annual income below $15,000 as compared to families with an annual income above $30,000.[4] A 1999 study done by the National Center of Addiction and Substance Abuse reported children of substance-abusing parents were three times more likely to be abused and more than four times likely to be neglected.

The 1997 DHHS report revealed a staggering 75% of the abusers were parents while other relatives accounted for 10%.[3] Caretakers such as foster parents, child-care providers, and staff accounted for 2% of abusers, with the remaining 13% categorized as non-caretakers or unknown.

Professionals such as educators, law enforcement officers, medical and mental health workers, and social service workers generated 81% of alleged maltreatment reports. Parents, other relatives, or the children themselves accounted for 9% of the cases reported. Friends or neighbors reported 8% of the cases. The final 2% of the reported cases were from anonymous or other sources.

PHYSICAL ABUSE

Location of Injuries

By nature, children tend to move in a forward direction whether to explore or for locomotion. Most accidental injuries occur on the anterior aspect of the body, the palmar aspects of the hands, or over bony prominences. Areas that should raise suspicion for maltreatment include buttocks, genitalia, back, abdomen, flank regions of the body, and the lateral aspect of the face. The palms and backs of the hands are common sites for abuse, but as previously mentioned, they can also be areas of normal accidental injury.[5,6]

History

If a child admits he or she is being battered or abused, the decision for the health care provider has already been made. This patient needs to be reported as a victim to the child protective services (CPS) agency or the appropriate authorities for that particular region. If there are any injuries unusual for a specific age group, maltreatment should be suspected. An example of this is the parent who states his or her 3-month-old was trying to pull up into a seated position on the couch and accidentally rolled off and hit her head on the floor. The explanation sounds reasonable, but not feasible for two reasons. According to the revised Denver Developmental Screening Test, most infants do not roll over until 4 months of age. Also, most infants will not pull themselves up to a seated position until 5 months of age. For this child to be rolling over and trying to pull herself up into a seated position is developmentally impossible. Abuse should be suspected. The health care practitioner should review previous records if possible to establish a history of previous, recurrent, or unexplained injuries, all of which could suggest some sort of abuse.

Folk medicine practices can border on physical abuse and should be identified to educate parents. Some of the more common practices are coining and spooning, seen in a variety of Asian cultures. Cupping is common in Russian and Latin American cultures, and the fallen fontanelle (*caida de mollera*) is seen in Mexican and Latino cultures.[5]

The history should also focus on the caretaker. Some indicators that suggest child abuse include:

• An unreasonable explanation
• The story changes from one person to the next
• A history of previous abuse
• A delay in seeking health care for the child
• A history of substance abuse
• Blaming of another party (e.g., sibling) for an injury

Weaker indicators for child abuse include:

• Parent/caretaker is hostile without a reason
• Parent/caretaker is inflexibile or passive and dependent
• Parent/caretaker has too high expectations of a child
• Parent/caretaker is a hospital or health care practitioner "shopper"

Types of Injures

DAMAGE TO SKIN AND SURFACE TISSUES   Bruises are common on the frontal plane of a child. If abuse is suspected, the entire skin surface should be inspected. In a maltreated child, bruises in varying stages of healing are commonly seen over the back, buttocks, neck, upper lip oral mucosa, genitals, and lateral face. Look for discerning characteristic patterns such as an outline of a hand or fingertips, rings, paddles, hangers, looped objects, linear markings like that of a strap or belt, or circumferential markings. These may be a clue to the instruments used in physical abuse and are solid evidence of abuse.

There are many accidental burns that are not considered abuse. The difficulty is determining which burns are accidental and which ones are abusive. One differential consideration is the cause of the burn. Common sources of burns that may not be abusive include burns from vaporizers, swimming pool deck tiles overheated secondary to sun exposure, hot water heaters, and hot floor grates. Irons, hair curlers, hair curling irons, and hot water accounts for over half of all the accidental burn injuries.

Some burn patterns are considered abusive. Scald and immersion burns are characterized by "stocking" or "glovelike" burn patterns. They are usually full thickness. Less frequently seen is the "donut-shaped" burn, which is caused by immersion of a child's buttocks into scalding water. The portion of the buttocks that come into contact with the vessel that holds the water is spared full-thickness burns, while the rest of the buttocks are severely burned. Burns in which flexion areas are spared should be suspicious for immersion abuse.

Flow patterns of hot liquid can be studied to help detect abusive splash burns. The typical shape of a splash burn is a "V" or arrow sign. These arrow signs can be used to determine the position of the child and the direction of travel of the hot liquid. This, in conjunction with the history, will help determine whether abuse can be considered.

As with bruises, discernment of patterns may be useful in identifying abuse. Circular burns are consistent with cigarette butts, linear marks can be seen with space heaters and heating grates, steam iron marks can be triangular or linear. Branding-type burns are abusive. Special attention should be focused on circumferential burns of the neck, torso, and extremities since these markings can be consistent with rope burns.[7]

Human bites are always intentionally inflicted and are strong evidence of abuse. Human bites have three components to be identified. The first is the bite mark itself, characterized by teeth imprints, which can be irregular in size, shape, and position. The second component is the suck mark, caused by the suction used to draw the skin into the mouth, which is characterized by a central area of bruising or contusion. The last component is the thrust mark, caused by the tongue that is pushed against the skin trapped by the teeth. It is also characterized by a central area of contusion. The practitioner should try to document bite marks via photography, and salivary swabs should be done in acute cases.[8]

DAMAGE TO THE CENTRAL NERVOUS SYSTEM

Head injuries account for the most common cause of death resulting from child abuse. Subdural hemorrhages account for 90% of all fatal head injuries. Lack of external lesions, e.g., hematomas, bruising, and lacerations, does not rule out internal injury. In addition to the usual physical examination (including level of consciousness, ophthalmic examination, and a thorough neurologic examination), other diagnostic modalities, such as x-rays, computed tomography (CT), and magnetic resonance imaging (MRI), should be used to evaluate possible trauma. Most head injuries are due to blunt trauma, secondary to object impact, such as boards, hammers, or stab wounds.

Shaken infant syndrome is responsible for approximately half of the nonaccidental deaths of children and is a hallmark for abuse. The pathophysiology is due to a sudden acceleration/deceleration syndrome causing the brain to impact on the skull. This results in damage to vessels, contusion, or laceration of the brain. Some indicators of this syndrome include decreased levels of consciousness, finger imprint bruising on the arms or trunk, retinal hemorrhages, and subdural hemorrhages. Other symptoms include vomiting, neurologic signs, blindness, paralysis, and learning problems.

DAMAGE TO OTHER INTERNAL ORGANS

Chest and abdominal injuries associated with blunt force can be associated with abuse. Frequently, this type of injury is due to a punch or kick to the epigastric area. Generally in the abused child, the time of presentation after the injury is delayed. Many children have scars or resolving bruises over the abdomen and chest, and old rib fractures are commonly seen. Males are two to three times more often seen for this type of injury than females. Previous history usually shows multiple visceral and intestinal injuries. In child abuse, the most common organ injured is the liver. Spleen injury is more commonly associated with accidental injuries. Laboratory studies including SGOT, SGPT, amylase, stool guaiac, hemoglobin, hematocrit, and urine analysis should be ordered for children with chest and abdominal injuries. These studies are the basis for the use of further diagnostic modalities such as plain x-rays, CT scans, and MRIs.

DAMAGE TO THE SKELETAL SYSTEM

Fractured bones are common in growing children. Some areas of fracture deserve the attention of health care providers as possible sites for abuse. Epiphyseal fractures occurring at the ends of long bones, the scapular acromial process, and the end of the clavicles are skeletal areas associated with child abuse. Multiple posterior rib fractures, fractures in various stages of healing, oblique and spiral fractures of long bones, vertebral fractures, and depressed skull fractures are also suspect for child abuse. The health care provider can use multiple diagnostic modalities to aid in the diagnosis of maltreatment such as plain films, CT scans, nuclear medicine, MRI, and ultrasound.[5]

NEGLECT

Neglect, as previously defined, has three categories—physical, educational, and emotional. The physical environment encompasses the fundamental needs of a child: adequate sanitary shelter free of structural and environmental hazards, inaccessibility to chemicals and drugs, and adequate nutrition, clothing, hygiene, and most importantly, supervision. Education is needed to provide the child with socialization skills and responsible behavior needed for future life. Emotional security must be provided through support and encouragement to alleviate feelings of abandonment on both the physical

and mental levels. It is difficult, if not impossible, to place certain signs and symptoms for this abuse. If through history any of these conditions come to light, it should be reported to the appropriate local authority. In some children and infants, a nonorganic failure to thrive may be the only symptom for neglect. When these children are hospitalized, it is common to see a rapid positive response to nutrition and a nurturing environment.

SEXUAL ABUSE

Sexual abuse has three individual categories—assault, incest, and exploitation. Exploitation includes child prostitution and child pornography. The children experiencing exploitation are in the greatest need for psychiatric intervention. The areas of assault and incest are self-explanatory. Risk factors for sexual abuse include living apart from both parents, poverty, family alcohol and/or drug abuse, and exposure to prostitution.[5]

Sexual abuse must be reported if a patient discloses abuse. Sexual abuse should be considered in children who present with stained or bloody underwear, any unexplained genitourinary injury or disease unusual for their age, young pregnant girls, and children with a sexually transmitted disease (STD). If a history reveals that a child has detailed age-inappropriate understanding of sexual behavior, inappropriate aggressiveness or unusual sexual behavior with others or toys, or compulsive masturbation, then sexual abuse should be considered. Some symptoms of abuse in younger children include enuresis, fecal soiling, eating disorders, compulsive behavior, school and learning problems, and sleeping disturbances. Older children may exhibit withdrawal, depression, poor hygiene or excessive bathing, poor social skills, delinquent behavior, alcohol or drug abuse, school problems, fire setting, sudden acquisition of money or gifts, or fear of home life.

As with all types of abuse, the history and physical exam is important. Good rapport, which allows opportunities to provide reassurance, should be developed with the child. A thorough review of the medical records should also be completed. In cases of sexual abuse, another professional should be in the room during the examination. Documentation should be provided for the demeanor of the patient as well as a complete physical with emphasis placed on the genital examination. Physical symptoms that should be documented are signs of other forms of abuse, scars from other injuries, difficulty in walking or sitting due to ano/genital pain, genital secretions and discharge on the patient and patient's clothing, STDs, and physical trauma or irritations to the ano/genital area. Physical trauma includes foreign bodies, lacerated and torn vaginal opening, swollen inflamed penis or scrotum, and bite marks.

A rape examination kit with detailed instructions, to ensure the chain of evidence, should be obtained from the local authorities. The exam is best handled by those who have been trained to deal with sexual assault and proper collection of evidence. Some laboratory studies that should be considered include HIV; hepatitis B and C; gonorrhea and chlamydia cultures of the rectum, throat, and vaginal/urethral areas; herpes simplex cultures; and tests for syphilis and trichomonas. Human papillomavirus examination should be considered. An appropriate follow-up such as a referral to a regional sexual abuse center for further physical and psychological intervention is indicated.

EMOTIONAL MALTREATMENT

Emotional maltreatment is difficult to diagnose. It is even more difficult for the health care provider to intervene since emotional maltreatment takes place over a long period of time. In this type of abuse the parent/caretaker ignores the child and fails to provide stimulation and responsiveness. The child's sense of needs and worth are rejected. Sometimes the child will be purposely isolated from the family, depriving the child of human contact. This type of abuse can also be seen by the parent/caregiver who terrorizes a child through verbal abuse or creation of a fearful climate or an environment without security. Parents can reinforce destructive antisocial behavior that can lead to abnormal interactions within the social environment. Overpressuring a child causes him or her to grow up too fast emotionally. Overachievement in academics and motor skills may cause feelings of never being good enough.

Some signs and symptoms of emotional maltreatment are an impaired ability to enjoy life, refusal to self-defend, sexual precociousness, cheating, stealing, blaming others, low self-esteem, extreme behaviors, and apathy. Cognitive signs of emotional abuse include a decreased attention span, hyperactivity, language delay, motor delay, lack of curiosity, and learning disorders. Some physical symptoms seen in emotional maltreatment are characterized by a nonorganic failure to thrive, awkwardness, eating disorders, chronic loose stools, poor energy levels, increased accidents, and sleep disorders.

The history may reveal parents and/or caretakers who seldom share positive emotions with the child. Sometimes the child will be humiliated in public or constantly yelled at. The child may be overly punished and never realize what appropriate behavior is. The parent/caretaker will use the child as a scapegoat or threaten the child with violence. It is common for such individuals to have antisocial behaviors themselves.

Overall, the final consequences of emotional maltreatment are costly. Children will suffer psychiatric disorders such as depression and borderline personality disorder. Self-destructive and antisocial behaviors will surface. Language and other cognitive delays may occur. Low self-esteem will develop, and the child may never adapt to the current society's expectations.

The physical exam is limited for evaluation of emotional abuse. If such abuse were suspected, appropriate referral to a regional abuse center or psychiatrist would be indicated.

REPORTING

Each state mandates what needs to be reported and by whom. It would be fair to say that every state requires child abuse to be reported. There is a criminal penalty in each state for failure to report. Some states have civil penalties as well. Each practitioner needs to become familiar with the local statutes and laws governing child abuse and maltreatment. Reports are generally made to one of four agencies—social services agencies, police departments, health departments, and juvenile courts. Some states provide immunity to people who report child abuse. Health care practitioners should check with their state government to see whether immunity is granted.

PREVENTION

Prevention can occur if parents and caretakers have the needed resources, education, and community services to properly parent a child. There is no one special program that is more effective than others, but health care providers should be aware of what can be made available to their patients, the family, and the parents/caretakers should abuse be observed. Historically, parents who have utilized educational and child abuse preventive services have improved their parenting skills and have higher school completion rates and higher employment rates.

REFERENCES

1. Child Abuse Prevention and Treatment Act (CAPTA). *Public Law* 104-235, Section 111; 42 U.S.C. 5106g. Amended October 1996.
2. National Clearinghouse on Child Abuse and Neglect Information: *Child Maltreatment Fact Sheet.* 1997.
3. US Department of Health and Human Services, National Center on Child Abuse and Neglect: *Child Maltreatment 1997: Reports from the States to the National Child Abuse and Neglect Data System.* Washington, DC, Government Printing Office, 1999.
4. National Clearinghouse on Child Abuse and Neglect Information: *Third National Incidence Study of Child Abuse and Neglect: Final Report* (NIS-3). Washington, DC, Government Printing Office, 1996.
5. Monteleone JA, Brodeur AE: *Child Maltreatment—A Clinical Guide and Reference,* 2nd ed. St. Louis, G.W. Medical Publishing, 1998.
6. Bickley L. The physical examination of infants and children, in *Bates' Guide to Physical Examination and History Taking,* 7th ed. Philadelphia, Lippincott, 1999, p 621.
7. Hobbs CJ, Wynne JM: *Physical Signs of Child Abuse—A Colour Atlas.* Philadelphia, Saunders, 1996.
8. Monteleone JA: *Recognition of Child Abuse for the Mandated Reporter,* 2d ed. St. Louis, G.W. Medical Publishing, 1996.

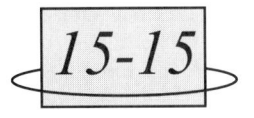

ADOLESCENT VIOLENCE
Theresa Horvath

DISCUSSION

Interpersonal violence is an especially grave concern for adolescents living in the United States. Firearm injuries are the second leading cause of death for those aged 15 to 24 years.[1] Sixty percent of all students in a nationwide survey reported engaging in a physical fight, and over half have carried a weapon.[2] Young males between the ages of 15 and 19 represent a particularly high-risk subgroup.

Identifying teenagers at risk to either perpetrate or become victims of violent injury is an important task for clinicians working among adolescents. Although morbidity and mortality from firearm injury are the most serious consequences of violent behavior, teenagers also suffer emotional and physical consequences from more covert and pervasive forms of violence. The combined effects of how families control anger, a low threshold for taking risks, and peer and community pressure can make acting violently more common for adolescents than for constituents of other populations. As violent behavior spans all geographic regions of the country, it is necessary to become familiar with all forms of violence and the particular ways that they affect teenagers

One distinct area in which adolescents confront violence is in school. School violence is a particularly serious problem not only because of the longstanding problem of fighting and weapon carrying that occurs within some inner-city schools but also because of recent, well-publicized, multiple-victim shootings in suburban and rural schools. The multiple-victim assaults, such as those in Columbine High School in Littleton, Colorado, and Westside Middle School in Jonesboro, Arkansas, have been particularly ghastly, and they have captured media attention in a way that other types of adolescent violence have not. Yet inner-city violence affects not only high schools but whole communities. Sixty-five percent of urban teenagers in one small study report that they personally have known someone who had been shot.[3] Along with the victims, witnesses, family members, and most members of the community are in some way affected, as weapon carrying and violence contribute to a general awareness that the community in which one lives and goes to school is not safe.

In contrast, nonurban multiple-victim violence occurs in middle-class or affluent communities where violence has not typically been thought to be part of the environment. The victims, including the witnesses and community members, are utterly unprepared for such incidents. Rather than contributing to an overall perception of deterioration within a neighborhood, multi-victim shootings destroy the sense of safety that community members have taken for granted. Since these events are highly publicized, the incidents of violence in suburban schools also shatter the security throughout the country to the extent that adolescents and adults fear an attack may occur in their hometown. However, in sheer numbers, it is inner-city violence that affects the greatest number of adolescents and remains the largest problem to address.

Much of adolescent violence is hidden. The potential for violence exists in many aspects of everyday life and can be inflicted by those most trusted by a teenager. Fighting among peers in dating situations can not only result in date rape but in other forms of violence as well; many teenagers throughout the country report that their last fight was with a romantic partner. In addition, adult coaches may endorse violence within team athletics and this behavior may manifest in verbally and physically menacing behavior directed toward the community at large. Coaches can be the most important role models for an adolescent male, and the sanction of violence by these mentors can greatly impact decision-making for these students. Violent family lives can predispose young people to perpetuate violence toward each other. And most important, self-inflicted violence is a hidden problem of enormous magnitude. The underlying factors such as depression or victimization, which place teenagers at risk for suicide, are often overlooked or ignored. All of these forms of violence have one thing in common: they are preventable if physician assistants and other health care providers are sensitive to warning signals, can screen for hidden signs, and have referral mechanisms available once an adolescent is determined to be at risk.

There are a number of distinct behaviors that can be screened for to reduce the injury rates among teens. Some of them include weapon carrying, multiple-victim shootings, suicidal ideation, dating violence, violent behavior in team sports, family violence, and high-risk behaviors including substance abuse.

Weapon Carrying

Carrying a weapon is the most dangerous predictor of violence. One-third of all students in a nationwide survey reported carrying some type of weapon to school, with 14% of all students nationwide specifically carrying a gun. These students were most likely to be male and nonwhite.[2] Although these statistics were gathered nationally, homicides among young African American men overwhelmingly occur within the inner cities of New York, Florida, Michigan, Missouri, California, and the District of Columbia.

Some students report that they carry a gun only for protection, with the hope that they will never have to use it. Some feel that carrying weapons will protect them from being victimized, or they may choose to carry weapons as a result of having been attacked in the past. Prior victimization leads to a greater possibility of further victimization. It also increases the likelihood that the victim will act violently against others.[4] The distinction between the victim and perpetrator often is not great, and an escalating cycle of self-assertion, fear, preemptive aggression, and revenge leads to increasingly greater levels of violence, sometimes culminating in homicide.[3]

Most adolescents who are victims of violent injury have histories that contribute to violence, such as participation in theft, destruction of property, and suspension or expulsion from school. The most significant predictor of violent behavior is the use of, and most especially selling, illicit drugs.[4] Although many teenagers use guns to carry out criminal activity, gun-carrying adolescents are more likely to use their firearms to resolve relatively minor interpersonal disputes. Disagreements over money, esteem, and lovers are likely catalysts for gun- or knife-related violence. These three areas of conflict can define the most important parameters of some teenagers' lives, and the threat of loss of any one of them can be more devastating than almost any other aspect of their identity.

Witnessing violent acts, especially knife or gun violence, will predispose adolescent males to carry weapons. As these acts are fairly common in some communities, there is a dose-related effect with increasing exposure to violence leading to more young people carrying weapons, resulting in the community perception that the neighborhood is unsafe, leading to more weapon carrying. What results is a vicious cycle, referred to as the *contagion model of violence*. A community standard for carrying weapons evolves, leading to some young members choosing to own a gun because so many peers do.

While gun carrying also exists among adolescent females, it is not nearly as prevalent as among males. Nationally, 4.7% of girls carry weapons as opposed to 21.3% of boys. Young African American women have the highest rates of gun carrying among females (6.7%). Rates of gun carrying decrease with each successive grade in high school, a trend similar to adolescent boys.[2] Interestingly, adolescent girls do not fit the contagion model of violence in the same way as boys. Teenage young women who witness violence are more likely to experience posttraumatic stress disorder rather than to arm themselves.

Multiple-Victim Shootings

Since February 1996, there have been a number of highly publicized and sensational student school attacks. These shootings occur most often in suburban or rural areas of the United States and highlight the scores of similar attacks nationwide. Since these incidents and the adolescents who perpetrated them are discrete, common features and risk factors have been sought to identify others who may consider such violent acts.

The profiles of the young men who engage in multi-victim shootings differ greatly from their urban peers. While urban violence will encompass a large number of adolescents, some with relatively few risk factors, nonurban violence most often occurs among teenagers who have multiple behavioral, familial, and psychological problems. Most have troubled family relationships and lack supervision. Poor coping or social skills, as well as various degrees of social isolation and rejection by peers, are common among these teens. Many have had bouts of uncontrolled anger or depression, and a recent stressful event or loss of status can trigger high-risk adolescents to become violent.

In one study of ten of the most famous multi-victim attacks, it was found that, unlike urban adolescents, few of these adolescent boys had brought weapons to school, nor was substance abuse common among them. Impulsivity, hyperactivity, and previous mental health treatment were similarly infrequent.[5] Yet all of them had blamed others for their problems, had threatened violence, and had a detailed plan for the attacks. They were all strongly interested in weapons and, with one exception, all had communicated violent intentions to others. All of the adolescents had access to firearms, were fascinated with weapons and explosives, and all but one had a preoccupation with violent media or music. While there is not any one factor that could have predicted these acts of violence, most adolescents with inclinations toward attacking their classmates have a large number of unresolved school, peer, familial, social, and personal behavior problems. While many young people have some of the same characteristics as this small subgroup of teenagers, it is the confluence of factors that these young men share that placed them at high risk for acting on their violent impulses.

Of all the missed opportunities to identify these young men as community risks, the chief one was the lack of attention to their threats. Each threat of violence among adolescents must be taken seriously and evaluated, in much the same way as with those who threaten suicide. A primary health care provider such as a physician assistant can diagnose violent ideation, and he or she can initiate a team approach among psychiatrists, social workers, and developmental specialists that may result in the most effective intervention.

Adolescent Suicide

Adolescent suicide is a grave problem. Teenage suicide is the third leading cause of death among people aged 15 to 24. It is estimated as many as 5000 teenagers a year may successfully end their lives. A recent nationwide study reported that 15.7% of high school students attempted suicide within a 12-month period. These attempts were most likely to be among females, the majority of whom were white, although rates among African Americans are increasing. Furthermore, 7.4% of all students surveyed nationally reported they had injured themselves significantly enough to warrant medical treatment during a suicide attempt.[2] Two-thirds of suicidal teenagers in another study did not disclose a history of self-harm to anyone and therefore did not receive treatment for their wounds nor for their underlying distress (see Chap. 16-7).

Access to firearms has a strong relationship to successful suicide. Whereas guns are used in 60% of all suicides, among adolescents firearms account for nearly 70%.[6] The mere presence of a gun in the home increases the likelihood of attempted suicide fivefold overall and makes it twice as likely that a teenager will kill him- or herself. Both adolescent and adult women are more likely to attempt suicide, while men are more successful at committing suicide. Men favor handguns as a means of suicide, while women tend to overdose medication or die from self-inflicted lacerations. Other methods of suicide are less common among both men and women.

As with adults, adolescents suffering from depression, alcohol or drug use, or emotional and psychiatric problems are at higher risk for suicide than others. A history of sexual abuse is strongly correlated with successful suicide among both adolescent and adult women and may be the most significant single risk factor for females.

Teenagers have two risk factors that are unique.

1. Parents and other adults may be less likely to heed warning signs and more likely to attribute depressive symptoms to the normal moodiness of adolescents. Serious depression is likely to go unnoticed and untreated in these cases.
2. The impulsive nature of teenagers may make it more likely that a passing suicidal ideation will be carried out, especially if that teen has access to firearms.

Teens may not have the life experience to understand that difficult times will pass, making them more disinclined to withstand periods of hopelessness and despair. Teens are also more likely to confide their feelings of desperation and pessimism, which affords more opportunities for counseling, mental health intervention, and support once they are identified as being at risk. Identification of suicidal ideation is the crucial first step in this process.

Violence among Romantic Partners

Dating violence has been an underreported form of adolescent aggression. It is estimated that 20 to 60% of all adolescents have experienced some sort of violence from a romantic partner.[7] While sexual assault and violence have most often been associated with inner cities, large studies in nonurban areas show significant amounts of dating violence as well. In fact, teenagers living in rural areas are at risk for violence in a romantic relationship at rates comparable to those of college freshmen.

Studies of teenagers have found as many as 17% of college men admitted to coercing a partner to perform sexual favors, and 33% report that they do not take no for an answer while on a date.[7] Dating violence can often be as severe as sexual assault but is more likely to manifest in unwanted kissing or fondling, or in physical fighting to resolve interpersonal differences. The most frequent manifestation of abuse in dating relationships is verbal abuse. Although verbal abuse is not as serious as physical abuse, it has been shown among adults that verbal abuse can begin a cycle that escalates into battery.

Studies of violence among adult romantic partners report that women are most likely the victims of these encounters. Among teenagers, however, girls and boys have equal rates of instigating fighting, and teenage males are also susceptible to coercion and fear in dating relationships. A main difference is that females are more likely to perpetrate fighting behavior, while males perpetuate more sexual violence. Young women report date violence more frequently than young men, which may skew the true incidence of abuse concerning men. Violence in dating relationships among adolescents is highly predictive of a continuation of that behavior into adulthood.[8]

Alcohol and drug use have been cited as the chief risk factors for romantic violence. Fighting among partners is also more likely among adolescents with poor school performance, multiple dating partners, and exposure to others forms of violence within the family or community. Young women victims of date rape tend to have

histories that include pregnancy, past experiences of forced sex, attempted suicide, or high-risk sexual behavior. Teenage females who lack self-confidence and self-esteem are at high risk for becoming victimized, for not reporting a violent incident once victimized, and for being unable to end a violent relationship, thus perpetuating their victimization.

Young men who experience dating violence tend to have male sexual partners and have a history of forced sex or physical violence in the past. The risk for dating violence among adolescent women who have women sexual partners has been inadequately studied.

African Americans are reported to have higher rates of dating violence among teenagers than do other racial groups. This is true for all types of violent injury. Yet when variables such as income, gender, and exposure to violence are controlled, racial differences do not emerge as significantly.[4]

The Culture of Violence—Team Athletics

Team sports, especially contact sports such as ice hockey, football, and rugby, are played with a modicum of gratuitous physical violence or intimidation. Even the team members of sports with incidental contact such as soccer, basketball, water polo, and lacrosse have counted on these tactics to gain a competitive advantage. Attempts by high school athletes to intimidate or even hurt members of the opposing team may be modeled on professional sportsmen who use these methods.[9] Some coaches, too, see intimidation of umpires and referees as part of their role in supporting their teams. This intimidation may extend to confrontations with other coaches as well. Forcefully advocating for advantage may make the other coach and team members feel disrespected and may divert their concentration from the competition. But more importantly, coaches who use verbal and physical intimidation sanction this behavior among young athletes.

That high school coaches are uncritical of intimidation and violence as tactics is further complicated by the esteem in which young men participating in team sports are held. Some high schools rely on winning team sports to foster school spirit among the rest of the student body and a good reputation within the community. Athletes, especially good athletes on good teams, are held in very high regard not only by their peers but by adults as well.

This status gives some young men a sense of invincibility that may extend into social relationships. A style of verbal and physical intimidation can characterize their peer interactions, including dating relationships. In some communities, this behavior is tolerated as part of an athletic persona, which may encompass a group identity as well. Assaulting peers who are deemed to be threats or outsiders, destroying property, and abusing women may constitute aspects of this identity. Yet high school athletes may escape scrutiny because of the protection their adult supporters afford. This complicated web may have a profound impact on the culture of violence within a school or community and may present a challenge for those who attempt to advocate for the victims of this type of violence.

Violence in Families

The effects of physical abuse on children are well known. These youngsters suffer a myriad of emotional and physical problems and are at great risk for becoming perpetrators of child abuse and other battering as adults. Less is known about children who witness domestic violence between their parents or against other child members of their family. This is important because far more children witness domestic violence than are direct victims of it.

Many of the sequelae of child abuse appear in child witnesses as well. Conduct disorder, antisocial behavior, self-injury, anxiety, low self-esteem, and poor problem-solving skills are all seen in these youngsters. Moreover, the psychologic effect of witnessing a close family member, such as a mother, being physically abused is greater when the witness knows the perpetrator. In situations where a child watches one parent abuse the other, or either parent or a caretaker abuse another child, posttraumatic stress disorder is likely to result. These children are at increased likelihood to further suffer the effects of, for example, a parent who is unsupportive, less nurturing, and emotionally unavailable as a result of spousal abuse.

Children who witness domestic violence are at greater risk of becoming abusive adults. Furthermore, there are strong indications that both male and female adolescents growing up in such families will become either victims or perpetrators of violence, and in some cases, both.[7] Male children raised by adults with poor parenting skills may develop an inability to relate in romantic relationships. Moreover, unskilled parenting has been further shown to predispose a young man to engage in verbal and physical abuse of female peers. The lack of male role models at home can precipitate this problem as well. Other family issues such as moving from a primary residence more than twice within 4 years, low educational level of the parents, and low family income can also put a teen at risk for violence.

High-Risk Behaviors and Violence

A number of high-risk behaviors such as drinking alcohol, using illicit drugs, and early age at first sexual intercourse have all been associated with adolescent violence. The use of psychoactive substances such as alcohol and drugs plays a role in diminishing inhibitions, which enables some teenagers to act violently. Such substances also distort cognitive perception. Illegal drugs play an additional role in fostering interpersonal violence as the supply and distribution of illegal drugs increase the opportunities for violent encounters. The money needed to support a drug habit may result in stealing, which again increases the potential for violence. Lastly, a history of arrest is the single best predictor of gun carrying among adolescent men. Most all of those with drug-related arrests have been subsequently found to carry guns. Although these risk behaviors are harmful on their own, when they are linked to other behaviors they are highly predictive of violence. Tobacco use, for instance, has been shown to correlate with interpersonal violence among adolescents, especially when it is part of a syndrome that includes illegal drug use, delinquency, early sexual intercourse, and dropping out of school.[10] The risk of becoming a victim in a sexual relationship is related to early experience of sexual intercourse, especially for females. This risk is compounded when associated with attemped suicide, use of injectable drugs, riding in a car with a drunk driver, a history of pregnancy, or a history of forced sex.[8]

Easy access to guns is also cited as a risk factor, especially for teenage suicide and nonurban school assaults. "Easy access" refers to unlocked guns in the teenager's home or guns that the teens themselves own. The type of gun is also a risk. Handguns are most often used in suicide, while assault weapons, especially rapid-firing weapons and rifles, are used in multi-victim shootings. Although teenagers in urban areas are less likely to have access to a gun at home, those who carry weapons agree that a gun can be obtained in inner cities with relative ease. Adults have less control over the gun use of city teens as a result. But among teenagers who have access to their parents' firearms, a single-firing weapon or rifle should be the only weapon kept in the home.

SCREENING

Developing good screening tools is essential for all physician assistants and other health care providers who treat adolescents.

History

There are a number of important areas to address in the medical history for all adolescents:

- PREVIOUS HOSPITALIZATION FOR TRAUMA: Nearly 44% of assault-related trauma victims have subsequent reinjury and readmission. Prior assault-related injury victims have a 20% chance of becoming a homicide victim.[6]
- PREVIOUS SUICIDE ATTEMPT OR SUICIDAL IDEATION: A history of depression, including the coping mechanisms used by the adolescent when depressed, should be screened. Remember that a history of poorly explained trauma may be a hidden suicide attempt.
- USE OF TOBACCO, ALCOHOL, AND OTHER DRUGS: A careful history of the conditions under which these substances are used is important, as the linking of these behaviors is predictive of violence. For example, does the patient ride in a car with a drunk driver? Does he or she drink and drive?
- SEXUAL ACTIVITY: Early experience with first intercourse, a history of forced sex, multiple same-sex partners for males and opposite-sex partners for females, and a history of pregnancy are all associated with violence.
- FIGHTING: How often and under what conditions does the patient fight? Are weapons involved? It is important to specifically ask about fighting in dating relationships, as many teens don't consider romantic fighting as violence.
- WEAPON OWNERSHIP: If anyone in the family owns a weapon, where is it kept? Under what conditions is it used? Are there small children who may have access to it? Gun safety counseling may be necessary for the whole family.
- ARREST: A history of prior arrest is strongly predictive of subsequent weapon carrying.
- ANGER REACTION: How does the patient express his or her anger? A teenager may not consider hitting someone, especially a family member or partner, as fighting, especially if it is common practice within the home.
- FAMILY HISTORY: Does anyone in the family hit anyone else? Has the patient ever been beaten by a family member? How many times has the family moved? What is the composition of the family? Whom does the patient consider his or her chief support?
- SCHOOL HISTORY: How well does the patient do in school? Has he or she ever been suspended? Does he or she have friends at school? Is there a student or teacher with whom he or she is particularly angry? Does the patient have a plan for revenge?

Physical Examination

Clinicians examining adolescents should evaluate the following:

- GENERAL APPEARANCE: Is the patient well groomed? Are there physical deformities or stigmata that might make the patient more vulnerable to abuse? For example, does the patient stutter?
- AFFECT: Does the patient seem immature for age? Depressed? Is he or she confrontational with providers or parents? Does the patient act inappropriately or is he or she ill-tempered? Are there signs of drug use such as agitation or constricted or dilated pupils? Is there an odor of alcohol, tobacco, or marijuana on the patient?
- SKIN: Are there fresh signs of bruising? Ask about all old scars. Look for signs of intravenous drug use.
- GYNECOLOGIC AND GENITOURINARY ISSUES: Is there evidence of high-risk sexual behavior such as signs of a sexually transmitted disease? Does he or she choose to engage in sexual intercourse?

INTERVENTION

The goals of intervention should be twofold:

1. Identify adolescent patients at risk for serious injury.
2. Help adolescents make choices that decrease their risk of future harm from violence. Information from counseling and referral agencies should be gathered before a violence-screening program is

initiated and checked periodically for accuracy of the information. Identify the nearest adolescent medicine practice and learn what services it offers. Find the nearest adolescent psychiatry service for treatment of depression and attempted suicide. Is there an accessible substance abuse rehabilitation center that provides specialized care to adolescents? Determine what alternatives are available for patients who are in imminent danger from their family, peers, or romantic partners.

Helping adolescents to alter their self-destructive behaviors and to make life-sustaining choices is a difficult and often frustrating task, but there are advantages a physician assistant and other clinicians have that may lead to success. First, the initial encounter with an adolescent patient may be in an emergency setting. A frightening experience that resulted, or nearly resulted, in harm may spur the patient to recognize his or her danger. For adult as well as adolescent patients a near-disaster may be the impetus needed to motivate a positive change in behavior.

For physician assistants who care for adolescents as part of an ongoing primary care practice, developing a good relationship with young patients will foster the roles of mentor and role model. Building trust and having patience are the keys to building such a relationship. For that reason, it is very important to be nonjudgmental and act as a patient advocate. Negotiating the needs of the patient when they conflict with those of parents or school officials, accepting patients as they continue to engage in self-destructive behavior, and finding the areas of common ground rather than engaging in conflict with them will help this process.

Becoming involved in community organizations that address the problems of adolescent violence is another way to intervene. Physician assistants have joined teams of emergency medicine doctors or trauma surgeons who provide education to adolescents concerning the dangers of violence. Some have joined organizations advocating gun control. Still others have joined community groups that provide services such as tutoring, sports, or counseling to teenagers. Lastly, school-based health centers, facilities that provide medical care to students in the school, can afford the opportunity to address the problem of adolescent violence on multiple levels for physician assistants who work in high school centers. The ability to treat adolescents by themselves and in their environment fosters relationships with them built on trust. With no parental figure to rely on, the development of adult decision-making skills is implicit. Moreover, physically being in the school every day allows access to the adolescent community, which is often hidden from health care providers and other adults. Social involvement both within the school and in the neighborhood is attainable when the provider is an integral part of the community of adolescents.

REFERENCES

1. Hoyert DL et al: Deaths: Final data for 1997. *National Vital Statistics Reports* 47(19):1999.
2. US Department of Health and Human Services: Youth risk behavior surveillance—National Alternative High School Youth Risk Behavior Survey, United States, 1998. *MMWR* 48(SS-7): 1999.
3. Freudenberg N et al: Coming up in the boogie down: The role of violence in the lives of adolescents in the South Bronx. *Health Education & Behavior* 26(6):788–805, 1999.
4. Fein JA, Mollen CJ: Interpersonal violence. *Curr Opin Pediatr* 11:588–593, 1999.
5. Verlinden S et al: Risk factors in school shootings. *Clin Psych Rev* 20(1):3–56, 2000.
6. Christoffel KK et al: Youth violence prevention: The physician's role. *JAMA* 283(9):1202–1203, 2000.
7. Grausz HM, Pelucio MT: Adolescent violence. *Emerg Med Clin North Am* 17(3):595–602, 1999.
8. Kreiter SR et al: Gender differences in risk behaviors among adolescents who experience date fighting. *Pediatrics* 104(6):1286–1292, 1999.
9. Sheilds EW: Intimidation and violence by males in high school athletics. *Adolescence* 34(135):503–521, 1999.
10. Lowry R et al: School violence, substance use, and availability of illegal drugs on school property among US high school students. *J Sch Health* 69(9):1999.

BIBLIOGRAPHY

Howard KA et al: Beliefs about the risks of guns in the home: Analysis of a national survey. *Injury Prevention* 5(4):284–289, 1999.
Ordinas P et al: Parental influences on students' aggressive behavior and weapon carrying. *Health Education & Behavior* 26(6):774–787, 1999.
Rodriguez MA, Gorovitz E: The politics and prevention of gun violence. *Western Journal of Medicine* 171:296–297, 1999.

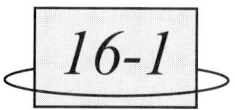

EATING DISORDERS: ANOREXIA AND BULIMIA

Meredith Davison

DISCUSSION

Both anorexia nervosa and bulimia nervosa are eating disorders with potentially serious medical complications; they primarily affect adolescent girls and young women. Although eating disorders are more prevalent in societies that place a high value on slimness as a characteristic of beauty, they occur in all socioeconomic classes and major ethnic groups. Anorexia nervosa is characterized by fear of obesity, distorted body image, obsession with thinness, and eventually, secondary physiologic abnormalities. Bulimia nervosa occurs when individuals consume large quantities of food in a short period of time and then self-induce vomiting or abuse laxatives to compensate. Since these eating disorders are often seen in the same individual, some believe the two are different manifestations of the same underlying entity. About 40% to 50% of anorexics have a history of binge eating. However, each disorder is described separately in the *Diagnostic and Statistical Manual of Mental Disorders, Fourth Edition (DSM-IV)*, and bulimia is further divided into purging and nonpurging types (see Tables 16-1-1 and 16-1-2).

ETIOLOGY

The exact cause of anorexia nervosa and bulimia is unknown. Current understanding suggests that multiple psychological, biologic, and cultural factors are involved in an interactive fashion. Individuals may have a physiologic/genetic predisposition and early childhood experiences that interact with current societal influences. Both of these eating disorders tend to cluster in families with other psychopathologic conditions, particularly emotional disorders and alcohol abuse.

EPIDEMIOLOGY

The worldwide incidence of anorexia nervosa is estimated to be 1 per 100,000 but in western countries the incidence in white adolescent females may be as high as 1 per 200. Evidence suggests that anorexia nervosa has increased during the last 20 years. Anorexia nervosa occurs predominantly in females, with a sex distribution of approximately 10:1. Age of onset is usually between 10 and 25 years.

Risk factors for anorexia nervosa include female, slightly overweight, white, adolescent, feelings of low self-esteem, achievement-oriented middle- to upper-income family, a culture that equates female beauty with thinness, and an intense interest in diet and physical fitness. Females account for 90 to 95% of anorexia nervosa cases, although there is evidence of an increased prevalence in males.

The onset of bulimia is similar to that of anorexia nervosa, usually during late adolescence or early adulthood. The lifetime prevalence of bulimia is estimated to be between 2 and 4% of adolescent women in western industrialized societies but less than 1% for males. Risk factors for bulimia are similar to those of anorexia nervosa. In addition, some studies suggest a possible genetic predisposition for the development of bulimia since a higher concordance rate has been found in monozygotic twins. Bulimia also tends to cluster in families with other psychopathologic conditions, particularly affective disorders and alcohol abuse. Other physiologic changes that develop in the course of the eating disorder may exacerbate the condition. Recent studies suggest some bulimia patients may have impaired satiety responses. Pain thresholds may also be altered. These changes suggest some underlying abnormalities in biologic processes may predispose to the development of this disorder and its maintenance.

SIGNS AND SYMPTOMS

The most common presenting signs and symptoms of anorexia nervosa are weight loss, amenorrhea, hyperactivity, social isolation, depression, and preoccupation with food. Symptoms secondary to weight loss include hair loss, yellow skin, fatigue, and gastrointestinal (GI) complaints (nausea, vomiting, constipation, bloating, epigastric pain). Most patients with bulimia exhibit relatively normal body weight, and the marked physical changes associated with starvation found in anorexia nervosa are not present. The most obvious sign of bulimia is episodic binge eating. The patient also senses a lack of control over eating during the binge episode. Characteristics of binge eating include eating the food very quickly, frequently without chewing; eating large amounts of food that is high in calories; frequently experiencing guilt and remorse after the episode; and hiding the binge episodes.

OBJECTIVE FINDINGS

Most objective findings in anorexia nervosa result from weight loss and are similar to the findings in starvation. They include decreased weight, decreased temperature, hypotension, bradycardia, edema, dry skin, a yellowish skin discoloration, nail changes, lanugo hair, systolic murmurs, and short stature.

Patients with bulimia ordinarily present with weakness and fatigue, swelling of hands and feet, headaches, abdominal fullness, and nausea. Other signs include skin changes, primarily on the hand secondary to self-induced vomiting, enlargement of the salivary glands, and dental erosions. Dental erosions occur on the lingual, palatal, and posterior occlusal surfaces of the teeth. Recurrent vomiting causes decalcification of the dental surfaces exposed to the vomitus. Dental fillings or amalgams often project above the surface of the teeth. Females with both anorexia nervosa and bulimia frequently present with either primary or secondary amenorrhea, depending on their age.

Psychosocial features of patients with eating disorders frequently include low self-esteem, depression, perfectionistic attitude, overachieving, and social withdrawal. These patients also display a disturbed body image in which the body size is overestimated, as well as a misperception of physical sensations. They often deny fatigue following excessive exercising and have a distorted awareness of hunger.

Families of patients with eating disorders generally present with obvious economic, social, and academic success. Beneath the family facade, there may be issues of overprotectiveness, rigidity, emotional coldness, and lack of communication. Although a typical family pattern predisposing to the development of eating disorders has not been discovered, the eating disorder itself often disrupts the family.

TABLE 16-1-1.   *DSM-IV* Characteristics of Anorexia Nervosa

Diagnostic Criteria

1. Refusal to maintain body weight at or above a minimally normal weight for age and height (e.g., weight loss leading to maintenance of body weight less than 85% of that expected; or failure to make expected weight gain during period of growth, leading to body weight 85% of that expected).
2. Intense fear of gaining weight or becoming fat, even though underweight.
3. Disturbance in the way in which one's body weight, size, or shape is experienced, undue influence of body weight or shape on self-evaluation, or denial of the seriousness of the current low body weight.
4. In postmenarcheal females, amenorrhea, i.e., the absence of at least three consecutive menstrual cycles. (A woman is considered to have amenorrhea if her periods occur only following hormone, e.g., estrogen, administration.)

Types

Restricting type: During the current episode of anorexia nervosa, the person has not regularly engaged in binge eating or purging behavior (i.e., selfinduced vomiting or the misuse of laxatives, diuretics, or enemas).
Binge-eating/purging type: During the current episode of anorexia nervosa, the person has regularly engaged in binge eating or purging behavior (i.e., self-induced vomiting or the misuse of laxatives, diuretics, or enemas).

SOURCE: *From American Psychiatric Association, pp 544–545. Used with permission.*

DIAGNOSTIC CONSIDERATIONS

The diagnosis of eating disorders is based on the criteria in the *DSM-IV* (see Tables 16-1-1 and 16-1-2). Differential diagnoses include other behavioral disorders associated with weight loss, such as severe depression, psychological reactions to food, and psychotic disorders. Physical disorders to be ruled out are inflammatory bowel disease, diabetes mellitus, malabsorptive states, hypo- and hyperthyroidism, brain tumors (especially of the fourth ventricle), collagen vascular disease, and Addison's disease.

SPECIAL CONSIDERATIONS

Males

Although less common, anorexia nervosa does occur in males and the signs and symptoms resemble those in females. Some have suggested

TABLE 16-1-2.   *DSM-IV* Characteristics of Bulimia Nervosa

Diagnostic Criteria

1. Recurrent episodes of binge eating. An episode of binge eating is characterized by both of the following:
   A. Eating, in a discrete period of time (e.g., within any 2-hour period), an amount of food that is definitely larger than most people would eat during a similar period of time and under similar circumstances.
   B. A sense of lack of control over eating during the episode (e.g., a feeling that one cannot stop eating or control what or how much one is eating).
2. Recurrent inappropriate compensatory behavior to prevent weight gain, such as self-induced vomiting; misuse of laxatives, diuretics, enemas, or other medications; fasting; or excessive exercise.
3. The binge eating and inappropriate compensatory behaviors both occur, on average, at least twice a week for 3 months.
4. Self-evaluation is unduly influenced by body shape and weight.
5. The disturbance does not occur exclusively during episodes of anorexia nervosa.

Types

Purging type: During the current episode of bulimia nervosa, the person has regularly engaged in self-induced vomiting or the misuse of laxatives, diuretics, or enemas.
Nonpurging type: During the current episode of bulimia nervosa, the person has used other inappropriate compensatory behaviors such as fasting or excessive exercise, but has not regularly engaged in self-induced vomiting or the misuse of laxatives, diuretics, or enemas.

SOURCE: *From American Psychiatric Association, pp 549–550. Used with permission.*

that male adolescents with anorexia nervosa may present with more severe medical abnormalities because of a delay in establishing the diagnosis. An increase in bulimia has been recently reported in males, especially those who try to maintain specific weights for sports events (e.g., wrestling).

Young Children

A recent review of anorexia nervosa in children under 13 years of age found that younger children had a higher severity of illness, a delay in diagnosis, and a higher incidence of family psychiatric history. Since bulimia tends to have a slightly later onset than anorexia nervosa, it is seldom observed in children.

LABORATORY TESTS

The evaluation of anorexic patients should include complete blood count and platelet count, erythrocyte sedimentation rate (ESR), blood urea nitrogen (BUN), and creatinine, urinalysis, serum electrolytes, liver function tests, serum calcium and phosphate, serum albumin, carotene, thyroxine, and a chest x-ray. Other tests that may be of interest are stools for occult blood and fat, upper GI tract series and small bowel series, barium enema, and a computed tomography or magnetic resonance imaging scan of the head. Fluid and electrolyte abnormalities are frequently revealed by laboratory tests. Metabolic alkalosis, hypochloremia, and occasionally hypokalemia are most commonly seen.

NUTRITIONAL ASSESSMENT

The nutritional assessment of anorexia nervosa should involve weight, height, triceps circumference, skin folds, midarm circumference, and a calculation of percentage body fat.

TREATMENT

For all eating disorders the goal of treatment is stabilization of medical and nutritional problems, management of psychosocial problems in the patient and her or his family, and reestablishment of healthy eating habits.

Medical Management of Anorexia Nervosa

Treatment of eating disorders first focuses on normalization of the nutritional status, particularly in patients with severe symptoms of malnutrition. Hospitalization should be considered in patients who have the following:

• Severe medical complications
• Severe depression, particularly with the risk of suicide
• Mental instability, including failure to comply with outpatient treatment
• Severe binging and/or purging behavior

Oral feeding to increase weight should be tried first. Some patients, however, will require nasogastric feeding or intravenous hyperalimentation. Following diagnosis and stabilization in the hospital, long-term therapy should focus on both individual and family psychotherapy.

Pharmacotherapeutics

Antidepressant drugs have been frequently used in the treatment of eating disorders, but controlled trials suggest that they are not effective in treating the primary symptoms of anorexia nervosa. In adult patients with bulimia nervosa, however, psychopharmacologic therapy is moderately effective. These drugs appear to have a potent and significant suppressant effect on binge eating and purging behavior. Studies suggest that individuals who are not depressed at baseline may respond equally well to antidepressant treatments. Fluoxetine hydrochloride

(Prozac), a serotonin reuptake inhibitor, is the drug of choice. Although antidepressants can be quite useful, research indicates that relapse is high with discontinuation of the drugs. The combined use of psychotherapy with antidepressants may be the best treatment for bulimia.

Antidepressants have also been found to be effective in treating the depression often associated with anorexia nervosa. Antidepressant medications can be of help in medically stable anorexics.

PSYCHOTHERAPY

The treatment of eating disorders is difficult at best. Treatment begins with an open acknowledgment to the patient and family that, although the striving for thinness and control is obviously very important, it has serious dangers, including physical illness, psychologic morbidity, and even death.

The most effective psychotherapy approach is cognitive behavioral therapy techniques delivered in either group or individual formats. The core cognitive distortion in eating disorders is the patient's belief that the only way to feel good about her or his own competence is to be in rigid control of body weight. There are a number of common elements in successful treatment programs:

- There is a strong emphasis on nutritional counseling.
- Behavioral techniques are used to control binge eating and challenge irrational beliefs.
- Alternative ways to deal with disruptive emotions, such as anger and depression, are taught.
- Family treatment accompanies individual psychiatric care. The focus is on decreasing parental overprotectiveness, fortifying intergenerational boundaries, and minimizing the child's role as a peacemaker in the family.

PROGNOSIS

The course and outcome for eating disorders are highly variable. It is currently estimated that about half of patients with anorexia nervosa or bulimia nervosa will have a full recovery. About one in five have no improvement with the rest having partial recovery. Various studies have found that the percentage of former eating disorder patients who were eating normally at follow-up ranges from 15 to 82%, depending on the length of follow-up and the patient's initial symptoms. Depressive symptoms were still commonly reported. Factors related to a good prognosis for anorexia nervosa are young age of onset, high educational achievement, supportive family, an improvement in body image after weight gain, and good initial ego strength. A poor prognosis is associated with late age of onset, premorbid obesity, self-induced vomiting or purging, laxative abuse, long duration of disorder, low social class, disturbed parental relationship, marked depression, and obsessive behavior.

Generally, bulimia appears to have a better outcome than anorexia nervosa. There is a correlation with severity of the disorder and outcome, in that individuals with greater eating pathology require more intensive therapeutic interventions. Cognitive-behavioral therapy is reported to the more effective than medications, although adjunct medication appears to enhance the behavioral therapy. Follow-up studies report that self-induced vomiting and laxative abuse are still present in some bulimics even after improvement was shown.

OTHER NOTES AND PEARLS

- The most important ingredient in the diagnosis of eating disorders is a high degree of suspicion.
- These patients usually present with a lack of insight into the severity of their weight loss, sometimes still maintaining that they are overweight.
- The patient may wear loose, baggy clothes to hide the extent of her emaciation.

- As many as 50% of anorexic patients have an associated major depressive syndrome.
- Bulimia nervosa may increase the risk of miscarriage while premature birth and prenatal death have been associated with anorexia nervosa.
- Suicide is a chief contributor to the high mortality rate among patients with anorexia nervosa.

BIBLIOGRAPHY

American Psychiatric Association: Diagnostic and Statistical Manual of Mental Disorders, 4th ed, Washington, DC, American Psychiatric Association, 1994.

Becker AE et al: Eating disorders. *N Engl J Med* 340(14):1092, 1999.

Casper RC: Recognizing eating disorders in women. *Psychopharmacol Bull* 34(3):267, 1998.

Gilbert IC et al: Anorexia nervosa outcome: Six-year controlled longitudinal study of 51 cases including a population cohort. *J Am Acad Child Adoles Psychiatry* 33:729, 1994.

MacKenzie R, Neinstein LS: Anorexia nervosa and bulimia, in *Adolescent Health Care: A Practical Guide,* 3d ed, Neinstein LS (ed). Baltimore, Williams & Wilkins, 1996, pp 564–593.

Olivardia R et al: Eating disorders in college men. *Am J Psychiatry* 152:1279, 1995.

Peterson CB, Mitchell JE: Psychosocial and pharmacological treatment of eating disorders: A review of research findings. *J Clin Psychol* 55:685, 1999.

Steinhausen HC, Seidel R: Outcome in adolescent eating disorders. *Int J Eat Disord* 14:487, 1993.

Yates A: Biological considerations in the etiology of eating disorders. *Pediatr Ann* 21:739, 1992.

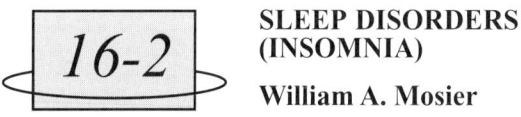

SLEEP DISORDERS (INSOMNIA)

William A. Mosier

DISCUSSION

Sleep is a complex physiologic function. The variations in depth and length are markedly pronounced. The range of sleep period, in healthy adults, is 4 to 10 hours. Insomnia can be defined as an involuntary sleeplessness severe enough to interfere with daytime alertness and energy level. Insomnia should be thought of as a symptom of some other underlying problem and not a disease in itself. There is an increased rate of mortality in individuals who sleep fewer than 4 hours or more than 10 hours per night.

Throughout the life span, total sleep time, in a 24-hour period, declines. It is highest during infancy and declines with age. The average newborn sleeps 18 hours per day. The average total sleep time in an elderly individual is 6.5 hours. Of all the factors that can modify normal sleep architecture, age is the strongest influence; however, contrary to common perception, the need for sleep does not significantly decrease with age. However, because of changes in individual circadian rhythms, a decrease in sleep regulation may occur with advancing age.

Individuals deprived of sleep for as little as 60 hours tend to experience increased fatigue and irritability and decreased concentration. With longer periods of sleep deprivation, illusions and even hallucinations can impair consciousness. One of three Americans reports difficulty sleeping. About 40 million Americans (9%) suffer from chronic sleep disorders. Insomnia is the most commonly reported symptom of premenstrual syndrome (PMS), and 40% of women experiencing menopause suffer from insomnia for 2 to 5 years after the onset of menopause.

Insomnia is generally classified into two categories: primary (no apparent cause) and secondary (a cause can be identified). Sometimes insomnia is classified as transient (lasting only a few nights), short-term (lasting up to 3 weeks), or long-term (lasting more than 3 weeks).

TABLE 16-2-1.   Common Sleep Problems

Chronic insomnia
Narcolepsy
Sleep apnea
Sleepwalking
Changes with advanced age
Body clock disorder (e.g., jet lag)
Disturbances caused by shift work changes
Restless leg syndrome
Periodic leg movement disorder

The three most commonly occurring insomnia patterns are the following:

1. Sleep-onset insomnia (taking more than 30 minutes to fall asleep)
2. Sleep-maintenance insomnia (frequent waking during the night)
3. Early-morning awakening (having a pattern of awakening about 2 hours prior to normal waking time)

Other sleep disturbances are sleep apnea, narcolepsy, body clock disorder, changes due to aging, periodic limb movement disorder, problems caused by shift work, restless leg syndrome, and sleepwalking (see Table 16-2-1).

Approximately 50% of patients presenting with the complaint of insomnia have previously been diagnosed with a psychiatric disorder. Only about 15% of individuals diagnosed with psychiatric disorders have no sleep complaints. The most common psychiatric disorders associated with sleep complaints are depression and anxiety disorders. Alcohol and other drug abuse disorders (including tobacco use) reflect a positive relationship to increased rates of insomnia. Approximately 90% of patients hospitalized for depression demonstrate sleep disturbance verified by electroencephalogram (EEG). In fact, 90% of all patients diagnosed with major depression complain of insomnia. Less than 10% complain of hypersombulance. Approximately 25% of patients complaining of chronic insomnia are diagnosed with an anxiety disorder.

Psychophysiologic or chronic primary insomnia (also referred to as *conditioned* or *learned insomnia*) usually involves difficulties in both sleep onset and maintenance of sleep. Conditioned insomnia usually results from a somatized anxiety-tension state and poor sleep hygiene.

PATHOGENESIS

The sleep-wake cycle is controlled by the circadian system. This internal biologic clock is thought to be located in the suprachiasmatic nucleus (SCN) of the hypothalamus. Two of the neurotransmitters that promote sleep associated with slow-wave sleep activity are serotonin and γ-aminobutyric acid (GABA). The human body moves through five stages during a normal sleep period. The typical sleep period consists of four to six sleep cycles. Each cycle lasts about 90 minutes in the nonelderly adult. A cycle consists of two different types of sleep: non–rapid eye movement (NREM) sleep and rapid eye movement (REM) sleep.

NREM sleep is divided into four different stages:

1. *Stage I* is a brief transition from wakefulness to sleep. It is characterized by slow, rolling eye movements identifiable on electrooculogram (EOG); low-voltage, mixed frequency EEG activity; and moderately high-amplitude discharges recorded on electromyogram (EMG). Stage I sleep tends to increase in the elderly.
2. *Stage II* generally constitutes the onset of true sleep. It is characterized by a moderately low-voltage EEG interspersed with brief, high-voltage discharges (referred to as *K complexes*), as well as vertex waves interspersed with low- to moderate-amplitude discharges (referred to as *sleep spindles*).

3. *Stage III* is considered deep sleep. It is characterized by high-amplitude background activity of delta and theta waves, as well as K complexes and sleep spindles.
4. *Stage IV* is also referred to as a deep sleep phase. It is characterized by high-voltage delta waves.

Eye movements are infrequent or totally absent during stages III and IV. Low-voltage muscle potentials occur during stages II, III, and IV. The secretion of growth hormone (GH) is elevated during NREM sleep. The immune system is also more active during this slow-wave sleep. Stage III and stage IV tend to decrease in the elderly.

Stage V (REM) sleep is the stage at which dreams that can be remembered occur. Heart rate, blood pressure, and respirations are similar to waking state during REM sleep. It is characterized by an abrupt change in EEG pattern; it appears as a low-voltage, fast-frequency activity resembling the pattern observed during wakefulness or stage I sleep. It may resemble a sawtooth wave pattern of moderately high amplitude or a triangular-shaped waveform. REM sleep demonstrates an absence of deep tendon reflexes. During REM sleep there is also a markedly suppressed or totally absent EMG activity. Positron emission tomography (PET) studies indicate that the brain's use of glucose during REM sleep is within the same range as that recorded during wakefulness. REM sleep constitutes about 25% of a person's total sleep time.

Patients manifesting generalized anxiety disorder (GAD) typically demonstrate the following:

- Prolonged sleep onset latency (time from laying down to sleep until actual onset of sleep)
- Increased stage I and II sleep
- Decreased slow-wave sleep
- Lower REM sleep percentage

The sleep architecture associated with major depression includes the following:

- Shortened REM sleep latency (time from sleep onset to the onset of REM sleep)
- Increased REM sleep density (frequency of eye movements)
- Reduced total sleep time
- Reduced sleep efficiency
- Increased awakenings
- Decreased slow-wave sleep
- Increased duration of the first REM sleep period

The only apparent gender difference associated with insomnia is a decreased slow-wave sleep pattern identified in men diagnosed with major depression.

SYMPTOMS

Insomnia associated with mood disorders is common. The presenting complaints may be problems of sleep onset, middle-of-the-night awakenings, and/or early-morning awakenings. [It is useful to remember that all three of these presenting disturbances may commonly occur in patients meeting the *Diagnostic and Statistical Manual of Mental Disorders,* fourth edition (*DSM-IV*) criteria for major depression.] Because of the sleep maintenance difficulties involved with insomnia, many patients also complain of daytime fatigue and lethargy.

OBJECTIVE FINDINGS

Asking the patient detailed questions about the quality and quantity of sleep can greatly assist in getting an accurate picture of the origin of the insomnia. The following questions are useful to ask:

1. How long does it take you to fall asleep once you have gone to bed?
2. Do you remain asleep all night?
3. Do you awaken feeling well rested in the morning?

TABLE 16-2-2. Medications Known to Produce Insomnia

OTC AGENTS	PRESCRIPTION AGENTS	
Alcohol	Antiparkinsonian agents	NSAIDs
Caffeine	Amantadine HCl	Flurbiprofen
Cough, cold, allergy	Diphenhydramine HCl	Indomethacin
preparations	Pergolide mesylate	Ketoprofen
Actifed	Cardiovascular agents	Naproxen
Alka-Seltzer Plus	Acebutolol	Psychotropics
Benadryl	Atenolol	Alprazolam
Benylin Cough	Betaxolol	Clozapine
Belix	Captopril	Isocarboxazid
Comtrex	Diltiazem HCl	Muscle relaxants
Contac	Guanfacine HCl	Cyclobenzaprine
Coricidin	Metoprolol	H_2 blockers
Dimetapp	Nifedipine	Ranitidine
Drixoral	Pindolol	Asthma preparations
Robitussin Night	Propranolol HCl	Aminophylline
Relief	Conjugated estrogens	Theophylline
Sudafed		
Triaminic		

ABBREVIATIONS: HCl, hydrochloride; NSAIDs, nonsteroidal anti-inflammatory drugs; OTC, over-the-counter.

DIAGNOSTIC CONSIDERATIONS

A patient with a presenting complaint of insomnia should be screened for the other core symptoms of major depressive disorder. When differentiating between depression and anxiety, it is helpful to remember that the anxious patient may have more difficulty falling asleep, whereas the depressed patient may fall asleep more readily but experience early morning awakenings. If the depression and anxiety screening prove negative, then thyroid disorders should be ruled out. If untreated, hyperthyroidism may cause irritability, tension, and insomnia. The chemical replacement therapy for hypothyroidism can also produce symptoms of insomnia. Cystitis in women and benign prostatic hypertrophy (BPH) in men can cause nighttime awakening and disrupt restful sleep, resulting in fatigue the following day. Other organic causes of insomnia can be angina, arthritis, asthma, back pain, chronic sinusitis, diabetes, dementia, epilepsy, heart disease, and ulcers. Some medications can produce a side effect of insomnia, including some antidepressants, tranquilizers, diuretics, and even some high-potency vitamin supplements (see Table 16-2-2).

SPECIAL CONSIDERATIONS

Age-related changes in sleep physiology correspond to patient complaints of disrupted sleep. Sleep disorders are particularly prevalent among the elderly. Approximately half of all individuals over the age of 65 suffer from insomnia. Although they constitute only 25% of the U.S. total population, persons over 50 years of age account for 50% of all prescribed sleep medications. Insomnia in the elderly is usually secondary to some other underlying condition or event. Taking a complete medical, psychiatric, and medication history is necessary to evaluate insomnia in any patient, but especially in an elderly patient. Although transient insomnia can be resolved when the stressors are removed or modified, chronic insomnia requires a comprehensive evaluation and treatment plan to address the underlying causes.

DIAGNOSTIC TESTS

Diagnosis is usually based on symptoms that can be identified from taking a thorough history. However, it is sometimes helpful to have the patient undergo sleep studies in a sleep laboratory to aid in the search for an underlying cause of the insomnia. In psychophysiologic insomnia, sleep EEG studies typically demonstrate delayed sleep onset or frequent nocturnal awakenings but otherwise no specific changes

in sleep architecture or REM sleep abnormalities. However, in insomnia associated with depression, early-morning awakenings (at least 2 hours before the usual time for awakening) as well as the typical REM sleep findings associated with depression are useful for identifying depression-based insomnia. (See "Pathogenesis," above, for EEG findings associated with depression.)

TREATMENT

The goal of treatment should be uninterrupted sleep and improved daytime function. Short-term use of the sedative-hypnotic drugs may be useful. However, long-term use can be habit forming, lead to decreased efficacy, and result in rebound insomnia. By matching specific drugs to specific sleep problems, treatment for insomnia can be tailored to each patient's needs. Insomnia is best managed by treating the underlying disorder. It must be emphasized that alteration of sleep is a hallmark symptom of affective disorders such as depression. Therefore, treatment with antidepressants and careful monitoring is warranted as first-line treatment for insomnia if depression is suspected. When no underlying condition can be uncovered, treatment should begin with behavior modification strategies followed by conservative use of medication only when necessary.

Regardless of their effect on depression, antidepressants can differ greatly in their effects on sleep. Research substantiates that both sedating and nonsedating antidepressants can decrease insomnia as a result of decreasing a patient's overall symptoms of depression. Antidepressants that produce an immediate prolongation of REM sleep latency, a reduction of total REM sleep time, and a reduction of total REM density appear to provide a better clinical response to the treatment of insomnia. Antidepressants that tend to stimulate REM sleep at the onset of sleep episodes and stimulate shorter REM sleep episode duration are associated with an increased risk of insomnia relapse. If a mood disorder or anxiety disorder is the underlying cause of the sleep disturbance, medications most often utilized are tricyclic antidepressants, buspirone, selective serotonin reuptake inhibitors (SSRIs), and sedative hypnotics.

Sedative-hypnotic agents should generally be limited to 7 to 10 days of use. Reevaluation of the patient is recommended if treatment continues for more than 3 weeks.

The benzodiazepines can be useful in the treatment of insomnia because they seem to bind to the omega receptors, which are part of the GABA receptor complex. The benzodiazepines along with the first of a new class of nonbenzodiazepine sleep agents commonly prescribed for insomnia are listed in Table 16-2-3 along with their half-lives, common dosages, and typical onset of action. The benzodiazepines are only a temporary solution to the problem of insomnia. They should be prescribed only for the shortest possible time. It should also be remembered that because they cause depression to the central nervous system, eventually they may worsen the insomnia. Contrary to common perception, a benzodiazepine with a longer half-life may

TABLE 16-2-3. Common Sleep Agents Used to Treat Insomnia

DRUG	HALF-LIFE	DOSAGE	ONSET OF ACTION
Benzodiazepines			
Quazepam (Doral)	2–4 days	7.5–15 mg	Intermediate
Flurazepam (Dalmane)	2–3 days	15 mg	Intermediate
Estazolam (ProSom)	14 h	1 mg	Fast
Temazepam (Restoril)	10–20 h	15 mg	Intermediate
Lorazepam (Ativan)	12–18 h	0.5–1 mg	Intermediate
Oxazepam (Serax)	5–10 h	10–15 mg	Intermediate
Triazolam (Halcion)	2–4 h	0.25 mg	Fast
Nonbenzodiazepines			
Zolpidem tartrate (Ambien)	2.5 h	5–10 mg	Fast
Zaleplon (Sonata)	1 h	5–20 mg	Fast

actually be safer, as evidenced by a decrease in observed rebound. Quazepam (Doral) has not been documented as demonstrating rebound phenomena. However, extreme care must be taken to monitor for the effects that long half-life may have, such as impairment of daytime function if dosed too high. Nonbenzodiazepine hypnotic agents are now available for treating patients with sleep disorders. The first of these newer agents to become available was zolpidem tartrate (Ambien). It is the first of a new class of imidazopyridine agents chemically distinct from benzodiazepine. Zolpidem tartrate is indicated for the short-term treatment of insomnia. An improvement over the benzodiazepine hypnotics, zolpidem tartrate tends to preserve the deep sleep of stage III and IV NREM sleep.

A more recent addition to the nonbenzodiazepine agents is zaleplon (Sonata). Clinical trials uncovered no evidence of tolerance over 4 weeks of treatment. It has a shorter half-life than any of the other sleep agents, thus allowing for rapid clearance. Clinical studies assessing for residual effects have failed to demonstrate evidence of drug-related daytime drowsiness with this agent.

SUPPORTIVE MEASURES

Relaxation therapy, such as muscle relaxation techniques, biofeedback, breathing exercises, and meditation, have been found to be useful for enhancing sleep induction ability. Stimulus-control therapy is also a valuable adjunct treatment to improve sleep hygiene. Patients should be taught techniques to refine their bedtime habits. A patient who is unable to fall asleep should get out of bed and go do another activity until tired. The patient should be instructed about the importance of discontinuing the drinking of coffee and other caffeinated beverages. The use of tobacco and alcohol should also be discouraged. Patients should be reminded that these substances actually interfere with normal sleep patterns and can cause a person to awaken during the night. Sugary snacks and heavy, late-evening meals can stimulate metabolism, making it difficult to fall asleep and/or sleep restfully. Moderate daily exercise reduces anxiety and therefore may improve a patient's sleep pattern as well.

PATIENT EDUCATION

Patients should be instructed to avoid the habit of watching television or reading a book in bed if they have difficulty falling asleep. Taking the time to teach healthy bedtime habits can help patients understand the relationship between sleep hygiene and the inability to fall asleep. Patients should also be instructed about how the abuse of sleeping pills can actually cause insomnia to worsen.

DISPOSITION

When prescribing a hypnotic for the treatment of insomnia, use the lowest possible dose, dispense a limited number of doses, monitor for side effects, monitor for cognitive or behavioral changes, monitor for effectiveness, and plan for a follow-up office visit in 2 to 3 weeks.

COMPLICATIONS AND RED FLAGS

Short-term memory problems and rebound insomnia can be side effects of the benzodiazepines. It is important to remember that the helpful effects of the benzodiazepines may diminish over time. The risk of addiction is a major concern if the dose must be increased to control the insomnia. Mixing the benzodiazepines with alcohol can result in death. Although triazolam (Halcion) is currently available in the United States, it is associated with rebound insomnia and amnesia. It has been removed from the market in the United Kingdom based on the recommendations of the Committee on Safety of Medicines in the United Kingdom. Therefore, it should probably not be considered as a first-line choice.

OTHER NOTES AND PEARLS

Sleep complaints should not be automatically treated with hypnotic agents. Careful evaluation of each patient's insomnia must be performed to uncover and treat any underlying condition, such as a mood disorder. In general, hypnotics should be prescribed for the short term only. In cases of chronic insomnia they should be combined with other therapeutic approaches. Because REM latency appears to be reduced in individuals suffering from depression, the following question is postulated: Is insomnia a consequence of depression, an indicator of vulnerability to depression, or a predictor of depression in individuals at risk for manifesting depression? Not every patient with insomnia has major depressive disorder. However, if a patient complains of insomnia, it is most prudent to inquire about other core symptoms of depression before prescribing a sedative hypnotic. The old adage, "The anxious patient can't fall asleep; the depressed patient can't stay asleep" is probably an oversimplification. However, any sleep disturbance is a possible marker for underlying anxiety or depression.

BIBLIOGRAPHY

Almeida OP et al: Sleep complaints among the elderly—Results from a survey in a psychogeriatric outpatient clinic in Brazil. *Int Psychogeriatr* 11:47–56, 1999.

Ancoli-Israel S: Insomnia in the elderly—A review for the primary care practitioner. *Sleep* 23(S1):S23–S30, 2000.

Bonnet MH, Arand DL: Hyperarousal and insomnia. *Sleep Medicine Reviews* 1(2):97–108, 1997.

Kupfer DJ, Reynolds CF: Management of insomnia. *N Engl J Med* 336:341–346, 1997.

Morin CM et al: Behavioral and pharmacological therapies for late-life insomnia—A randomized controlled trial. *JAMA* 281:991–999, 1999.

National Center on Sleep Disorders Research: *Insomnia: Assessment and Management in Primary Care* (National Institute of Health Publication #98-4088). Washington, DC, US Department of Health and Human Services, 1998, pp 7–14.

Ohayon MM: Prevalence of DSM-IV diagnostic criteria of insomnia: Distinguishing insomnia related to mental disorders from sleep disorders. *J Psychiatr Res* 31:333–346, 1997.

Richardson GS: Managing insomnia in the primary care setting: Raising the issues. *Sleep* 23(S1):S9–S12, 2000.

Roth T et al: Sleep disorders, in Quan M (ed.): *Clinical Cornerstone 2000* 2(5):1–54.

Simon GE, VonKorff M: Prevalence, burden, and treatment of insomnia in primary care. *Am J Psychiatry* 1997;154(10):1417–1423.

Thase ME, Neylan TC, Mellman T: The Effects of Depression on Sleep. *Primary Psychiatry* April 2000;(S4):57–63.

Zammit G, Wiener J: Quality of life assessment in people with insomnia. *Sleep* 1999;22:S379–S385.

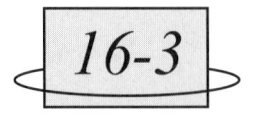

ANXIETY AND PANIC DISORDERS

Don St. John
Sarah Clarke

DISCUSSION

Anxiety disorders are the most prevalent psychiatric disorders, affecting 12% of the population at any given time. Patients with anxiety-related complaints represent 20% to 30% of patients in a primary care setting. The majority of patients with anxiety disorders are seen in a medical setting, especially in primary care. Because patients often present with somatic complaints, this diagnosis is often missed.

Table 16-3-1 lists the anxiety disorders described in the *Diagnostic and Statistical Manual of Mental Disorders,* fourth edition (*DSM-IV*).

TABLE 16-3-1. Anxiety Disorders

Panic disorder with or without agoraphobia

Agoraphobia without panic disorder

Generalized anxiety disorder

Social phobia

Specific phobia

Obsessive-compulsive disorder

Adjustment disorder with anxiety

Acute stress disorder

Posttraumatic stress disorder

Substance-induced anxiety disorder

Anxiety disorder due to a general medical condition

SOURCE: *From American Psychiatric Association.*

There are a number of factors involved in the etiology of anxiety disorders, ranging from psychosocial (e.g., adverse early environment) to behavioral (e.g., learned response) to biologic and genetic (e.g., abnormalities of the locus coeruleus).

SYMPTOMS

The symptoms of anxiety vary according to the specific disorder, but there is much overlap of symptoms as well as comorbidity. General symptoms of anxiety include a sense of apprehension, worry, tension, uneasiness, emotional lability, and hypervigilance. Somatic symptoms include palpitations, chest pain, nausea, dizziness, motor tension (tremor, twitches, muscle aching), insomnia, and autonomic hyperactivity (diaphoresis, tachycardia, diarrhea). The possibility of an anxiety disorder should be considered and communicated to the patient early in the evaluation of such symptoms.

Anxiety may also contribute to the morbidity of medical conditions such as chronic obstructive pulmonary disease, coronary artery disease, gastrointestinal ulcers, ulcerative colitis, asthma, hypertension, urticaria, and seizure disorders. Some anxiety disorders (e.g., panic disorder) mimic physical conditions, and physical disorders (e.g., hyperthyroidism) and certain substances (e.g., caffeine) often give rise to anxiety symptoms. Table 16-3-2 gives a differential to consider when evaluating anxious patients.

TREATMENT CONSIDERATIONS

Although many anxiety disorders are acute reactions to circumstances, others are chronic disturbances with a fluctuating course. Long-term treatment may be required for patients who fail to achieve full resolution of symptoms with brief interventions. Psychopharmacologic management varies according to the specific disorder being addressed. Attention must be paid to development of coping skills and improvement of social support systems and interpersonal relationships. Depression is frequently comorbid with all anxiety disorders, especially in the presence of chronic and severe symptoms and other comorbidity, such as low assertiveness, highly generalized anxiety, and severe agoraphobia.

SPECIAL POPULATIONS
Children

Symptoms of anxiety in children include physiologic hyperarousal, hypervigilance, and temperamental fearfulness, often demonstrated by behavioral restraint. Pediatric patients who develop an anxiety disorder may be irritable as infants, shy and fearful as toddlers, and cautious, quiet, and introverted during school years. Separation anxiety and school refusal (phobia) are associated with the develop-

TABLE 16-3-2. Differential Diagnoses of Anxiety Disorders

Cardiac

Ischemic heart disease
Mitral valve prolapse
Dysrhythmias
Pericarditis

Endocrine and Metabolic

Hyperthyroidism
Hypoglycemia
Pheochromocytoma

Gynecologic

Menopause
Premenstrual syndrome

Neurologic

Transient ischemic attacks
Cerebrovascular accident
Psychomotor epilepsy
Postconcussion syndrome
Delirium

Nutritional

Deficiencies of thiamine, pyridoxine, folate, iron

Respiratory

Asthma
Chronic obstructive pulmonary disease

Pharmacologic

Caffeine
Alcohol use or withdrawal
Sympathomimetics
Yohimbine
Amphetamines
Cocaine
Benzodiazepine withdrawal
Corticosteroids
Illicit drugs, especially marijuana, phencyclidine, and organic solvents

ment of adult anxiety disorders. Children with anxiety are more likely to develop anxiety and other psychiatric disorders in adult life.

Behavioral inhibition is a strong predictor of the later development of anxiety. Parental anxiety may be a marker for at-risk children. Children appear to respond to psychopharmacologic management as adults do, though studies of specific agents are few. Other therapy methods used in children include contingency management, in vivo exposure, and cognitive restructuring. Involvement of parents is important in treating children with anxiety disorders.

Elderly

Anxiety disorders are common in the elderly, often in association with physical illness. Psychopharmacologic treatment must begin with low doses, gradually increasing to therapeutic response, as tolerated by the individual patient. Benzodiazepines (BZDs) should be avoided in patients with dementia because of the risks of confusion, incoordination with falls, paradoxical reactions, and behavioral disinhibition. Many drugs have altered metabolism and are likely to accumulate in elderly patients. Buspirone, trazodone, selective serotonin reuptake inhibitors (SSRIs), and beta blockers have been effective in this special group of patients.

GENERALIZED ANXIETY DISORDER

PREVALENCE AND ETIOLOGIC FACTORS

Personal susceptibility and life stressors appear to play an important role in the etiology of generalized anxiety disorder (GAD). GAD tends

TABLE 16-3-3. Benzodiazepines

DRUG	HALF-LIFE, h	DOSE EQUIVALENT, mg	ONSET	DOSAGE RANGE, mg/d
Low-potency				
Diazepam	20–50	5	Fast	2–40
Chlordiazepoxide	5–30	25	Slow	10–40
Clorazepate	36–200	3.75	Intermediate	7.5–60
Prazepam	48–78	10	Slow	20–60
Oxazepam	5–10	30	Slow	40–120
High-potency				
Alprazolam	12–15	0.25	Fast	0.75–8
Clonazepam	18–50	0.5	Slow	1–8
Lorazepam	10–20	1	Fast	1–10

to occur in persons with high levels of trait anxiety, that is, temperamental tendencies to react to stressful circumstances with anxiety symptoms. Primary care practitioners, not psychiatrists, usually see patients with GAD. Lifetime prevalence is 8.5%; 1-year prevalence is 3%. Women are twice as likely to develop GAD as men.

SIGNS AND SYMPTOMS

GAD symptoms often begin gradually and early in life. Despite an early onset, often in childhood, the average age of presentation for treatment may be years later. GAD tends to run a chronic or recurrent course.

Symptoms include chronic worrying out of proportion to the situation (the principal feature of GAD), difficulty concentrating, dizziness, insomnia (especially difficulty falling asleep), unrestful sleep, emotional tension, easy distractibility, irritability, and restlessness. Physical symptoms include dry mouth, palpitations, flushing, frequent urination, headache, and fatigue.

Signs may include diaphoresis, tachycardia, and diffuse muscular tension. Discrete episodes or attacks of anxiety are absent.

The worry of GAD is diffuse, unfocused, and ongoing. Patients tend to believe they have little control over situations, especially aversive situations. Patients also tend to selectively attend to threatening or potentially threatening information in both their internal and external environments.

DIAGNOSTIC CONSIDERATIONS

Differential diagnosis includes many physical conditions. A representative list can be found in Table 16-3-2. Patients with hyperthyroidism may have a fine tremor and heat intolerance (see Chap. 5-4). Hypoglycemia tends to be episodic, predictably occurs several hours after meals, and is reversed by glucose ingestion. A history of head trauma with amnesia surrounding the event may suggest postconcussion syndrome. Patients with delirium exhibit an altered level of consciousness and cognitive dysfunction.

Many psychiatric disorders have prominent anxiety symptoms. A diagnosis of GAD is usually not made in the presence of another diagnosed primary anxiety disorder. In other anxiety disorders, the focus of anxiety is on the principal feature of the disorder. Panic attacks are discrete episodes of intense anxiety. There is a specific focus of anxiety in specific phobic disorders. Anxiety occurs in social contexts with social phobia. A hypochondriacal patient fears disease and exaggerates the danger of physical signs and symptoms.

One-third of patients with GAD have other axis I disorders, most commonly depressive disorders and substance abuse. There may be considerable symptom overlap between depression and GAD. Schizophrenic patients may display disorganized thinking and constricted affect and may be distrustful if paranoid. Twenty-five percent of patients have comorbid panic disorder and/or major depressive disorder. Ninety percent of elderly patients with GAD may have comorbid depression. GAD symptoms are often prodromal to panic disorder. Substance abuse is common in patients with GAD and may begin as a form of self-treatment. Axis II disorders are also commonly present.

TREATMENT

Pharmacologic Management

Patients with GAD may require long-term pharmacotherapy, since symptoms tend to recur with medication discontinuation. BZDs are the treatment of choice for acute and time-limited therapy, though there are many patients who may require chronic use. BZDs are especially effective in patients who have panic attacks. Tolerance to the adverse effects (especially drowsiness, dizziness, and slowed responses) often develops after 6 to 8 weeks of treatment. However, impairment of short-term memory and learning sometimes persists. Because of this, BZD use may interfere with psychological therapy. BZD use is also associated with a higher dropout rate from concurrent psychological therapy. Abuse tends to occur in those patients who abuse other drugs, especially alcohol. Escalation of dosage initiated by the patient should alert the practitioner to potential for abuse. As the patient responds, the BZD dose may be slowly tapered and discontinued. The half-life of longer-acting agents may be prolonged in elderly patients. Table 16-3-3 lists commonly used BZDs with dosage ranges. Table 16-3-4 lists significant potential drug interactions.

All of the currently available antidepressants appear to be effective for the treatment of GAD, especially for more severe or chronic symptoms or when dependence is a concern. Tricyclics have been studied the most. Of the newer antidepressants, venlafaxine XR is the most extensively studied, with demonstrated efficacy in alleviating both psychic and somatic symptoms of anxiety with relatively fast onset of action. Serotonergic drugs, especially fluoxetine, may initially increase anxiety symptoms. Beginning with low doses and gradually increasing to dosages used to treat depression may be helpful in developing tolerance to side effects. Among the SSRIs, fluvoxamine appears to be the most sedating, followed by paroxetine, sertraline, and fluoxetine, which tends to be more activating. Bupropion is likely to worsen anxiety symptoms, especially at the onset of therapy, but can be an effective treatment.

TABLE 16-3-4. Potential Benzodiazepine Drug Interactions

All may potentiate CNS depression when used with any other CNS depressant.

Diazepam
  Theophylline and rifampin may decrease effects.
  Cimetidine, valproate, and fluoxetine may increase effects.

Chlordiazepoxide
  Effects of levodopa increased.
  May increase serum levels of phenytoin.
  May alter levels of anticoagulants.

Prazepam
  Cimetidine and MAOIs may potentiate.

Alprazolam
  Effects of digoxin may be potentiated.
  May increase levels of imipramine and desipramine.
  Potentiated by other drugs metabolized by CYP450 enzyme system 3A4.

ABBREVIATIONS: CNS, central nervous system; MAOIs, monoamine oxidase inhibitors.

Buspirone has been shown to be as effective as tricyclics in the treatment of GAD and, at higher dosages, may also be effective in treating comorbid depression. Buspirone is well tolerated by most patients and has few significant drug interactions. Patients who have been previously treated with BZDs tend not to respond as well to buspirone. As with antidepressants, it often takes 2 to 6 weeks before effectiveness is realized, and onset of action may be gradual. Buspirone cannot be used on an as-needed basis, does not treat BZD withdrawal symptoms, and cannot be directly substituted for BZDs. Buspirone may be used to augment the action of antidepressants, though concurrent use of serotonergic agents may lead to a serotonin syndrome if instituted too rapidly. Side effects are uncommon and usually remit with continued use. Dizziness may occur 30 to 60 minutes after a dose and usually does not last longer than 20 minutes Headache may occur and responds to over-the-counter analgesics. Other possible side effects include drowsiness, nausea, insomnia, and nervousness (especially when first instituted). As with all serotonergic agents, buspirone should not be given with monoamine oxidase inhibitors (MAOIs) because of the possibility of serotonin syndrome.

Beta blockers have been used to treat the peripheral autonomic symptoms of anxiety, especially tachycardia and tremor. Antihistamines may be used short-term for the elderly, with appropriate caution regarding sedation and potential anticholinergic effects. Recent clinical trials with hydroxyzine have demonstrated its efficacy in GAD. Antipsychotics should be avoided because of potentially serious adverse reactions, such as tardive dyskinesia, and the dysphoria often associated with their use. Caffeine and alcohol, as well as illicit drugs, should be avoided during treatment of GAD.

Psychological Therapies

The patient should be informed of the fluctuating and chronic nature of GAD and the tendency for symptoms to wax and wane in response to stressors. Patients may find anxiety support groups helpful. Some patients respond to specific bibliotherapy recommendations.

Many patients find supportive counseling effective in treating their anxiety symptoms. Patients may be aided in identifying stressors and developing more effective means of coping with the stresses of their lives. Nondirective forms of therapy are often not as effective as more directive forms such as cognitive-behavioral therapy (CBT). Insight-oriented therapy may be helpful for some patients in exploring the meaning and function of anxiety in their lives.

Specific interventions include relaxation training, meditation, imagery, social skills training, problem-solving training, and biofeedback. Relaxation is used to reduce arousal and should be practiced daily. Patients should be encouraged to enter situations where avoidance has taken place, using their relaxation skills to manage situation-specific anxiety.

In cognitive therapy, patients are taught to identify, evaluate, and modify chronically worrisome and danger-related thoughts and behaviors and develop more rational responses. Anxious thoughts are replaced by more positive, realistic, and functional thoughts.

PANIC DISORDER

PREVALENCE AND ETIOLOGIC FACTORS

Panic disorder (PD) is believed to be a genetically influenced disease in which biologic factors play an important role. Biologic factors may include abnormalities involving the nucleus coeruleus, dorsal raphe nucleus, hippocampus, cerebral noradrenalin system, and cerebral serotonergic system. Findings of 20% of patients with a first-degree relative with panic, and monozygotic/dizygotic concordance of 5:1, point to a genetic component. Psychological etiologic factors may include anxious attachment caused by aberrant family patterns, repression of unconscious conflicts, and childhood trauma.

Childhood anxiety may predispose to the development of PD. Half of patients have a history of a childhood anxiety disorder, especially separation anxiety and school phobia. Patients appear to have a pre-existing tendency to fear and misinterpret physical and emotional sensations. Exposure to frightening situations, scary stories, the sudden loss of a loved one, poor parental relationships, and threats of harm during childhood may also predispose to the development of PD.

Women are two to three times as likely to develop PD as men, with a lifetime prevalence rate of 2% to 3% for women and 0.5% to 1.5% for men.

PD usually begins in the late teens and early twenties, with 20% to 40% of patients having their first attack before age 20. PD rarely begins before age 12 or after age 40. Median age of onset is 25 for men, 28 for women. Initial attacks commonly follow an adverse life event. Occasionally attacks occur in thyroid disorders, the immediate postpartum period, or with use of marijuana, cocaine, or amphetamines. Late-onset PD is unusual and presents with fewer panic symptoms, less avoidance, and less somatization.

Caffeine may cause attacks in some patients. Shame may prevent patients from seeking evaluation and treatment in western cultures, which value self-reliance and view fear as weakness.

SIGNS AND SYMPTOMS

Though PD and agoraphobia may be independent syndromes, they are treated as related and similar syndromes in this section.

The key characteristic of PD is recurrent panic attacks with subsequent fear of recurrence. Symptoms include palpitations, tachycardia, diaphoresis, tremor, shortness of breath or choking sensation, hyperventilation, chest pain, nausea and abdominal pain, dry mouth, dizziness, weakness, presyncope, paresthesias, chills or hot flashes, and derealization or depersonalization. Many of these symptoms can be attributed to adrenergic excess. During attacks, patients irrationally fear losing control, going crazy, or dying. Panic attacks have a sudden onset, peak within minutes, and last 5 to 30 minutes. Attacks occur without warning or in agoraphobic situations. Panic attacks often awaken patients from sleep, resulting in anticipatory bedtime anxiety and insomnia.

The initial panic attack is usually well remembered and alarming. Patients may display increased general anxiety and apprehensive preoccupation with everyday difficulties prior to the initial attack. Each attack magnifies fear of future attacks. Patients begin to worry about the implications or consequences of a panic attack, especially public humiliation, and anxiety rises in anticipation of future attacks. Significant behavioral changes (primarily avoidance) may occur in response to repeated attacks. Left untreated, PD progresses from limited-symptom attacks to full panic attacks, hypochondriasis, limited phobic avoidance, extensive phobic avoidance, and then development of secondary depression. The disorder may evolve rapidly, over days to weeks, or slowly, over months to years.

Agoraphobia is fear of being in a place or situation where escape may be difficult, or a fear of separation from one's source of security. This fear leads to phobic avoidance of places and situations where attacks have occurred in the past or where the patient fears an attack may occur. Agoraphobic patients commonly avoid crowded places, travel, and being alone. Some eventually become housebound.

Patients with PD often have self-perceptions of poor physical and/or emotional health and may complain of marital and financial concerns not apparent to others. They often view themselves as overanxious, emotionally overly dependent on others, unassertive, and lacking self-confidence. They may express shame and humiliation regarding their dependence, especially if housebound. Their sense of security may be fragile and closely bound to their family environment. Patients are often fearful of the medical profession and medications, with heightened sensitivity to adverse medication effects. Patients often have good work records and maintain their marriages, though sexual adjustment tends to be poor and there is a higher rate of divorce and separation among patients with panic disorder.

DIAGNOSTIC CONSIDERATIONS

Panic attacks may occur in other disorders, such as depression (where 20% of patients have panic attacks without panic disorder), other anxiety disorders, and certain personality disorders, especially borderline personality disorder.

The most common complications of PD are depression and substance abuse, especially alcohol dependence; 70% of patients may develop a secondary depression. These patients tend to respond better to antidepressants than to BZDs. About 15% to 30% of patients abuse drugs, especially alcohol and BZDs. Patients with PD are also at increased risk for committing suicide and for sudden death due to coronary artery disease. There may be an increased risk of peptic ulcer disease and hypertension among patients diagnosed with PD. Dependent personality traits are common among patients with PD, as is social phobia.

PD is not a diagnosis of exclusion. When symptoms are of recent onset, however, other treatable disorders should be ruled out before making the diagnosis of PD. Evaluation should include a complete history and physical examination and may include a complete blood count, general blood chemistry screen, electrolytes, thyroid function studies, serum cortisol, electrocardiogram, and pulmonary function studies. The differential diagnoses can be found in Table 16-3-5.

TREATMENT

The goal of treatment is the cessation of panic attacks. A 70% reduction in symptoms constitutes a good response to treatment. Patients often respond best to a combination of medications and psychological therapy. Patients should be informed about the diagnosis and prognosis, especially the propensity for fluctuation in the course of the disorder. Many patients respond well to self-help materials. The National Institute of Mental Health has educational materials and may be reached at 1-800-64-PANIC. Drug therapy may facilitate cognitive-behavioral therapies; however, BZDs may reduce motivation for exposure and other psychological therapies. Because PD is chronic, patients often require long-term treatment.

Pharmacologic Management

Patients with PD are often sensitive to medication effects. They may also fear that medication will lead to loss of control. Drugs should be started at low doses and very gradually increased to therapeutic doses as tolerated. Elderly patients may require half the usual starting dose used for younger patients. Patients should be warned against sudden discontinuation of drugs. No medication should be discontinued until the patient has been panic-free at least 6 months. The most common reason for treatment failure is use of inadequate dosages for inadequate lengths of time.

Antidepressants are effective in treating PD. Patients should be warned that symptoms may temporarily increase the first 1 to 2 weeks of therapy and with each dose increase. Patients should remain on medication for at least 6 to 12 months, then may be very slowly tapered (over a 1- to 5-month period) to the least effective dose that prevents relapse. More detailed information on antidepressants can be found in Chap. 16-5.

All the tricyclics are equally effective in treating PD. Nortriptyline tends to have the fewest anticholinergic side effects. Protriptyline may be activating to some patients. Tricyclics may be given in divided doses or once daily, usually at bedtime. Three to four weeks at a therapeutic dose may be needed to attain an antipanic effect. Remission may be maintained at a dosage lower than that initially needed to attain cessation of panic symptoms.

TABLE 16-3-5. Differential Diagnoses of Panic Disorder

Cardiopulmonary

  Pulmonary embolus
  Dysrhythmia
  Supraventricular tachycardia (sudden increase then decrease in heart
    rate, with other symptoms secondary to tachycardia)
  Silent myocardial infarction (especially in diabetics)
  Mitral valve prolapse
  Angina
  Hypoxia
  Asthma

Neurologic

  Temporal lobe epilepsy, partial complex seizure disorder (sudden
    paroxysmal episodes of fear with derealization, depersonalization,
    nausea, and behavioral automatisms) Meniere's disease
  Transient ischemic attack or cerebrovascular accident
  Atypical migraine
  Small tumor of the temporal lobe (rare)

Endocrine

  Pheochromocytoma (rare, with marked episodic elevation of blood
    pressure and vasomotor lability)
  Hypoglycemia (probably overdiagnosed)
  Hyperthyroidism, especially thyrotoxicosis
  Carcinoid syndrome
  Diabetes mellitus
  Addison's or Cushing's disease

Psychiatric

  Posttraumatic stress disorder
  Separation anxiety
  Social phobia
  Generalized anxiety disorder
  Nightmare
  Sleep terror disorder
  Personality disorder, especially borderline, dependent, avoidant
  Adjustment disorder with anxious mood

Drug-induced

  Caffeine
  Aminophylline or theophylline
  Sympathomimetic agents
  Monosodium glutamate
  Psychostimulants and hallucinogens
  Thyroid supplementation
  Antipsychotics
  Hydroxyzine
  Levodopa
  Nicotine

Drug Withdrawal

  Alcohol, antihypertensives, barbiturates, nicotine, benzodiazepines,
    tricyclic antidepressants

Other

  Severe pain
  Severe anemia
  Labyrinthitis
  Chronic fatigue syndrome

Serotonergic agents are useful in treating PD. As of this writing, citalopram, paroxetine, and sertraline have been approved for use in PD, though fluoxetine and fluvoxamine may be used as well. Patients with panic disorder may be more sensitive to activating side effects, especially with fluoxetine, though many patients find this drug effective.

MAOIs affect both the noradrenergic and serotonergic systems and are effective in treating panic disorder, but many patients are reluctant to take them because of the restrictive diet and potential side effects. Bupropion, which may be activating, may worsen panic symptoms.

BZDs are often started to provide rapid (often within a week) relief of symptoms. Table 16-3-3 lists BZDs used in the United States, their potency, and dosage ranges. Table 16-3-4 lists some important drug interactions. Therapeutic efficacy is equal to that of antidepressants when adequate doses are used, and all of the BZDs appear to be equally effective. Shorter half-life agents may be associated with interdose rebound or breakthrough panic attacks during sleep.

Once the patient has been panic-free for at least 3 months, the BZD may be slowly tapered and discontinued. Patients should be warned of a possible temporary increase in anxiety with each dosage reduction. Often the last reductions are the most difficult. Although BZDs are most often used short-term, some patients require more long-term use. Driving ability may be impaired the first 1 to 2 weeks of therapy, but tolerance to sedative effects often develops rapidly. BZD use should be monitored closely or avoided in the elderly because of memory impairment and increased risk of falling. Physical dependence may occur in as little as 1 to 2 weeks, especially with higher doses, and patients should be warned of serious withdrawal symptoms with sudden discontinuation. As a rule, patients with PD do not develop psychological dependence and often take less than an effective dose because of fear of addiction.

Buspirone is not effective for treatment of PD, though it may be helpful in treating other comorbid or underlying anxiety disorders and may augment the effectiveness of antidepressants.

Psychological Therapies

Up to 15% of patients are panic-free following CBT. The risk of relapse is lower following CBT than after medication treatment alone. Techniques used include somatic management (breathing and other relaxation training), distraction, exposure (to both internal and external cues), cognitive restructuring (confronting catastrophic thinking and overestimation of danger), and relapse prevention (preparation for potential panic-evoking situations). Patients respond best once symptoms have been partially controlled by medications. Some patients find supportive and interpersonal therapy helpful. These therapies can be expensive and are not always covered by insurance. Qualified professionals may not be easily accessible. Individual and group therapy appear to be equally effective.

PROGNOSIS

As a rule, the earlier treatment is instituted in the disease process, the better the outcome. A substantial minority of patients achieve remission by the end of the first year of treatment, but relapse is frequent following medication discontinuation, and many patients require long-term maintenance treatment. Poor response is associated with psychiatric comorbidity, especially personality disorders, avoidance behaviors, anxiety sensitivity, and a history of childhood anxiety.

OBSESSIVE-COMPULSIVE DISORDER

DISCUSSION

The exact etiology of obsessive-compulsive disorder (OCD) is unknown but appears to involve abnormal serotonin neurotransmission and basal ganglia dysfunction. OCD appears to be a genetic disorder with 70% concordance of monozygotic twins and 50% concordance of dizygotic twins. There is a 25% chance that a first-degree relative will also have OCD.

About 2% to 3% of the U.S. population develops OCD. Males and females are at equal risk, though males tend to develop the disorder earlier than females. Avoidant and dependent personality disorders are common among OCD patients but tend to improve with treatment of OCD symptoms. Failure to marry and an inability to sustain interpersonal relationships are common.

SIGNS AND SYMPTOMS

Obsessions are persistent, disturbing thoughts or impulses that the patient experiences as intrusive or inappropriate and finds illogical, but irresistible. Obsessions go beyond excessive worries about real-life problems and are recognized by patients as products of their own mind. Patients consider their obsessions absurd and actively attempt to resist them. Patients often attempt to ignore or suppress obsessional thoughts or neutralize them with other thoughts. There is often some form of pathologic doubting behind obsessions.

Compulsions are repetitive, purposeful, intentional behaviors or mental acts that a patient feels driven to perform in response to obsessions and according to rules that must be rigidly applied. They are aimed at preventing or reducing the distress of obsessions or preventing some dreaded event or situation.

Obsessions and compulsions must cause marked distress, markedly interfere with the patient's functioning, and be significantly time-consuming to be pathologic. Most patients recognize that they are excessive and/or unreasonable. Attempts to resist the obsessions and compulsions may produce extreme anxiety. Common types of obsessions and compulsions are listed in Table 16-3-6.

Two-thirds of patients with OCD have the onset of significant symptoms before age 15, with onset typically during adolescence or early adulthood. About 5% of patients with OCD have a comorbid tic disorder, and 50% of patients with Tourette's syndrome have comorbid OCD, especially males. OCD is generally a chronic disorder in which symptoms tend to develop quickly (in fewer than 30 days) and then may fluctuate, worsening with stressors.

Patients should be informed that OCD is a lifelong illness, with symptoms waxing and waning throughout their lifetime. Because of embarrassment or fear of "being crazy," many patients do not volunteer OCD symptoms but present with anxiety or depressive symptoms, which are common in OCD. All patients with anxious or depressive symptoms should be specifically asked about obsessions or compulsions so treatment may be directed toward the primary problem.

DIAGNOSTIC CONSIDERATIONS

The differential diagnosis includes "normal" routines or rituals (e.g., perfectionistic behaviors, habits of dressing or grooming a certain way), which are not distressing or time-consuming; excessive and/or impulsive gambling, eating, or sexual behaviors; major depressive disorder; organic mental disorders (e.g., brain tumor, head injury); Tourette's syndrome; schizophrenia; and obsessive-compulsive personality disorder. All but the last two may be comorbid with OCD. Schizophrenic

TABLE 16-3-6. Types of Obsessions and Compulsions

Cleaning	The patient fears contamination and has cleaning compulsions.
Checking	The patient demonstrates repetitive checking (such as door locks, the stove or oven, or other appliances) secondary to pathologic doubting.
Doubting/sinning	The patient fears something terrible may happen if everything is not perfect. Some patients may become paralyzed into inaction.
Counting/arranging	The patient compulsively arranges things into very specific patterns or obsessively counts (such as crossing a threshold only after taking a specific number of steps or not speaking until the number of words spoken by another party are counted). Patients often display magical thinking and superstition.
Hoarding	The patient believes something terrible may happen if something is discarded and may save unusual items, such as wrappers or used gum.

delusions are not recognized by the patient as excessive or unreasonable and are usually not considered by the patient as illogical.

Of patients with OCD, 80% develop a secondary depression. These patients tend to present with the depressive symptoms. Also, 13% of patients with OCD have a comorbid eating disorder, and 15% have comorbid trichotillomania, which is often resistant to pharmacologic management.

TREATMENT

Pharmacologic Management

Effective psychopharmacologic agents increase serotonin activity. Currently available drugs are the SSRIs (i.e., fluvoxamine, fluoxetine, paroxetine, sertraline, citalopram), venlafaxine, and clomipramine, all of which appear to be equally effective in the treatment of OCD. Patients may respond best to dosages that are higher than generally used to treat depression, titrated rather rapidly. An adequate trial, 4 months in the upper dosage range, should be undertaken before considering changing to a different agent. Since a given patient may respond to one SSRI over another, a different agent should be tried if there is no response to the first.

Clomipramine reaches steady-state plasma levels in 1 to 3 weeks. Blood levels are accurate and may be used to ensure adequate dosage and compliance if the patient has not responded or to rule out toxicity if the patient has excessive side effects. Tobacco, alcohol, and antipsychotics may raise the level of clomipramine's major metabolite. Common side effects include dry mouth, dry skin, and constipation. Orthostatic hypotension, sexual dysfunction (loss of libido, anorgasmia, and/or erectile dysfunction), tremor, ataxia, rigidity, dizziness, sedation, and headache may also occur. Clomipramine may be given once daily or in divided doses.

A good pharmacologic response is 50 to 70% improvement in symptoms. Response is measured by the patient's spending less time with symptoms, finding it easier to ignore symptoms, and experiencing less distress. Those who respond usually do so within 4 months of initiation of treatment. Any improvement occurring after the initial 4 months tends to be slight and very gradual. Although 70% of patients show some response to pharmacologic treatment, most will have residual symptoms.

Patients should be informed that medications might need to be taken lifelong, since symptoms tend to rapidly recur with discontinuation. Most patients require the initial treatment dose for long-term use.

Augmentation may be considered for patients who respond poorly or not at all to single agents. Patients with comorbid tic disorders and schizotypal personality disorder may respond to augmentation with a neuroleptic. Other augmentation strategies include lithium, pindolol, trazodone or nefazodone, risperidone, olanzapine, quetiapine, and fenfluramine. Women tend to respond best if estrogen levels are stabilized. Cingulotomy has been used successfully in some patients with severe, treatment-resistant OCD.

Psychological Therapies

Patients respond best when a combination of CBT and medications are used. Techniques include graded exposure, response prevention, and thought stopping. Only clinicians experienced in the psychotherapy of OCD should administer these interventions. Support groups provide education and destigmatize patients.

PHOBIC DISORDERS

ETIOLOGY AND PREVALENCE

Current ideas regarding the etiology of phobic symptoms include the use of repression and displacement as defense mechanisms, learned behavior, and classic conditioning. Agoraphobia and specific phobias are two to three times more prevalent in women than men. Social phobia appears to affect the sexes equally. Social phobias tend to begin during adolescence.

SIGNS AND SYMPTOMS

A phobia is an irrational dread of and compelling desire to avoid a specific object, situation, or activity. The fear is excessive and disproportionate to any actual danger, always anticipated, and never spontaneous. Apart from contact with the feared stimulus, the patient is usually free of symptoms. Anticipatory anxiety quickly develops, followed by avoidant behaviors, often taken to extremes. Phobic symptoms become a phobic disorder when they cause undue distress and impair a patient's functioning. Patients rarely present for treatment of phobic symptoms.

Common specific phobias include fear of animals, storms, heights, flying, and closed places. Phobias usually have their onset in childhood or early adolescence and cease within 5 years in 50% of patients. Specific phobias tend to remit spontaneously with age. If they persist into adulthood, they may become chronic, but are rarely disabling. Certain phobias may interfere with medical care, such as fear of needles or blood, or claustrophobia, which may interfere with computed tomography (CT) scans, magnetic resonance imaging (MRI), and other specialized medical procedures.

Social phobia is the excessive fear of embarrassment in social situations and of being scrutinized and judged by others. Social phobia is more than merely a fear of public speaking and may generalize to many or all social encounters. The mean age of onset is 15 to 19 years. Social phobia has a lifetime prevalence of 13%, making it the third most common mental disorder. Patients may fear and avoid eating and writing in public, or use of public toilets. In such situations, patients fear being unable to perform and embarrassing themselves. Substance abuse, mood disorders, and suicidal ideation and attempts may occur. Sixteen percent of relatives of social phobics are also diagnosed with social phobia. Unfortunately, without early therapy, social phobia runs a chronic and unremitting course throughout the patient's lifetime.

DIAGNOSTIC CONSIDERATIONS

Patients with schizophrenia often have negative symptoms similar to social phobia prior to the onset of positive symptoms. Patients with paranoid delusions fail to see the irrationality of their fears. Patients with clear OCD and phobic symptoms are given only the OCD diagnosis. Patients who avoid social situations as a result of posttraumatic stress disorder (PTSD) have a specific and identical past stressor. Depression may be comorbid or secondary to phobic disorders. The fears some depressed patients demonstrate may initially appear to be phobias but clear as the depression clears. Phobias are common in patients with borderline, paranoid, and avoidant personality disorders. Patients with avoidant personality disorder display a general discomfort in social situations and require continual reassurance. They do not identify fears of scrutiny and judgment as the cause of their social avoidance.

TREATMENT

Beta blockers have been used to treat "stage fright" when given in single doses an hour before performance. BZDs may also be used as needed for anticipated stressful social situations, though their use may interfere with psychotherapy, especially exposure techniques. MAOIs work well for social phobias, as do the SSRIs; paroxetine was recently approved for the treatment of social phobia. The tricyclic antidepressants may be somewhat less effective than the MAOIs and the SSRIs in treating social phobia. Patients with social phobia are prone to developing dependence on alcohol or sedative drugs, especially if psychotherapy is not concurrently used. Buspirone has not demonstrated efficacy in treating phobic disorders. Medications are not effective in treating specific phobias.

The most effective treatment of specific phobias is psychotherapy. Exposure is essential to successful therapy and includes such techniques as flooding, graduated exposure, and systematic desensitization. Relaxation training is usually the first step in treatment. Patients with social phobia often benefit from assertiveness training, social skills training, and cognitive therapy for their dysfunctional thoughts. Cognitive therapy is most effective when the fear of negative evaluation is targeted. Utilizing a combination of techniques tends to be more effective than using one technique alone.

POSTTRAUMATIC STRESS DISORDER

ETIOLOGY

By definition, PTSD follows a severe and extraordinary stressor. The stressor need not be a single event (e.g., a natural disaster such as a tornado or earthquake), but may be repetitive and/or ongoing severe traumas such as military combat or past childhood sexual abuse.

The most common cause of PTSD for men is military experience. Increased risk of developing PTSD is associated with young age, less military training, prior emotional or physical abuse, and the presence of psychiatric symptoms prior to the stressor. For women the most common causes of PTSD are rape and sexual and physical abuse. Increased risk of developing PTSD symptoms is associated with the use of physical force, display of a weapon, and physical injury.

SIGNS AND SYMPTOMS

PTSD symptoms may begin hours, months, or even years following the stressor. The stressful event is one in which the patient experiences, witnesses, or is confronted with actual or threatened death or serious injury, producing intense fear, helplessness, and/or horror. The event is usually beyond the ordinary traumas of human experience. Dissociative symptoms often appear after the event and include a subjective sense of numbing and detachment, a reduction in the awareness of one's surroundings, derealization, depersonalization, and dissociative amnesia surrounding the event. The event is then persistently reexperienced in recurrent images, thoughts, dreams, affect, or a sense of repeatedly reliving the experience. Stimulation of any of the senses may cause this reexperiencing, such as sound (e.g., a helicopter used in battle), smell (e.g., the cologne of one's attacker), touch (e.g., cold metal reminiscent of a gun used), or sight (e.g., dark clouds present just prior to a tornado).

As a result, the patient may begin to avoid all stimuli that may arouse recollection of the trauma. The patient eventually develops persistent symptoms of anxiety, hypervigilance, and increased arousal. These symptoms must cause the patient significant distress or impairment of function to be pathologic.

PTSD tends to occur in two stages:

1. In the avoidance phase, the patient may experience psychic numbing, minimization of the effect of the experience, affective detachment, poor interests, and a constricted affect.
2. During the reexperiencing phase, the patient may demonstrate hypervigilance, intrusive memories, poor sleep, poor concentration, rumination, and affective instability.

Occupational or interpersonal impairment is common in patients suffering with PTSD. Substance abuse, mood disorders, panic attacks, or phobic disorders may also develop in response to PTSD symptoms.

Acute PTSD lasts less than 3 months. Chronic PTSD lasts longer than 3 months. Delayed-onset PTSD does not emerge until at least 6 months after the trauma, and may even emerge years later, such as with childhood sexual abuse. This last type carries the worst prognosis.

The intensity of the physiologic response to the original trauma appears to be the most significant predictor of poor outcome and chronic course. Ongoing life stressors may slow recovery. A protracted course may also be associated with dissociative symptoms, emotional constriction, and drug abuse.

DIAGNOSTIC CONSIDERATIONS

Acute stress disorder is diagnosed when PTSD symptoms occur within 4 weeks of the event but last only 2 days to 4 weeks. The type of event and symptoms are otherwise the same as with PTSD. Schizophrenic patients may experience hallucinations or delusions, but without a past identified stressor. Dissociative disorders occur more often as a result of childhood abuse and may represent a special type of PTSD. Dissociation may also be a symptom associated with borderline personality disorder. Up to 85% of patients with borderline personality disorder have a history of childhood sexual abuse. An adjustment disorder may occur in response to more ordinary trauma (death of a loved one, loss of a significant relationship, etc.), in which the patient demonstrates a brief but strong affective response. Other considerations include temporal lobe epilepsy, malingering, other anxiety disorders (especially panic disorder), major depressive disorder, and compensation neurosis. Substance abuse commonly develops in response to PTSD symptoms and may worsen symptoms during acute intoxication or a "bad trip."

TREATMENT
Pharmacologic Management

Any of the antidepressants may be used for symptom control, but SSRIs are currently considered first-line therapy due to their safety and tolerability. Some clinicians have found the MAOI phenelzine especially useful. Carbamazepine or valproic acid may be used for behavioral control, especially irritability and aggression. Beta blockers, trazodone (especially in divided doses), and buspirone may also be used for anger management. Trazodone (25 to 100 mg) may be useful for treating insomnia. BZDs should be used with caution since they may cause disinhibition or lead to dependence.

Psychological Therapies

Immediate debriefing following a severely traumatizing event may be helpful in preventing the development of PTSD. Such debriefing should include repetitive disclosure of the event in detail, exploration of troubling reactions, identification of coping strategies, exploration of feelings about leaving the disaster site, and a specific and workable plan of transition and referral.

Support groups may be helpful to reinforce normal reactions; address common fears, concerns, and traumatic memories; increase the capacity to tolerate disturbing emotions; and share coping strategies. Cognitive-behavioral techniques, such as exposure and cognitive restructuring, may be helpful. Psychodynamic therapy has been helpful for some patients.

BIBLIOGRAPHY/RECOMMENDED RESOURCES

American Psychiatric Association: *Diagnostic and Statistical Manual of Mental Disorders,* 4th ed, Washington, DC, American Psychiatric Association, 1994.
Andreasen NC, Black DW: *Introductory Textbook of Psychiatry.* Washington, DC, American Psychiatric Press, 1995.
Baughan DM: Barriers to diagnosing anxiety disorders in family practice. *Am Fam Pract* 52(2):447–450, 1995.
Coryell N, Winokur G: *The Clinical Management of Anxiety Disorders.* New York, Oxford, 1991.
Davis M: *The Relaxation and Stress Reduction Workbook.* Oakland, CA, New Harbinger, 1995.

Feighner J: Overview of antidepressants currently used to treat anxiety disorders. *J Clin Psychiatry* 60(suppl 22):18–22, 1999.

Katon N: *Panic Disorder in the Medical Setting.* National Institute of Mental Health, DHHS Pub No (ADM) 89-1629. Washington, DC, US Government Printing Office, 1989.

McGlynn TJ, Metcalf HL: *Diagnosis and Treatment of Anxiety Disorders: A Physician's Handbook,* 2d ed, Washington, DC, American Psychiatric Press, 1991.

Noyes R, Holt CS: Anxiety disorders, in *The Medical Basis of Psychiatry,* 2d ed, Winokur G (ed). Philadelphia, Saunders, 1994, pp 139–160.

Pollack MH, Otto MW (eds): Anxiety disorders: Longitudinal course and treatment. *Psychiatr Clin North Am* 18:4, 1995.

Weinstein RS: Panic disorder. *Am Fam Pract* 52(7):2055–2063, 1995.

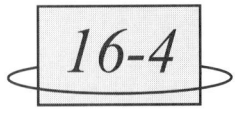

ATTENTION DEFICIT DISORDER

Anita D. Glicken

DISCUSSION

Attention deficit disorder (ADD), which has a subtype that includes hyperactivity (ADHD), is the most commonly diagnosed childhood mental disorder. Recent estimates suggest that between 3% and 9% of children have the disorder, accounting for one-third to one-half of all child mental health referrals. In population-based studies, boys are three times more likely than girls to have the disorder; however, the ratio is 6:1 in clinical studies. The majority of children with ADHD demonstrate hyperactive and impulsive motor behavior. Much less frequently (one in seven children with ADHD), inattention may be the predominant symptom without increased motor behavior. Symptoms are often first identified in the preschool years, exhibited in a variety of settings, and consistent over time.

ETIOLOGY

During the past 10 to 15 years, multiple causes have been suggested for ADHD, which was originally labeled *minimal brain dysfunction* (MBD). There is some evidence that these children do demonstrate a greater incidence of neurologic "soft signs." For example, they may experience increased difficulty with fine and gross motor coordination or balance. This has led researchers to explore prenatal and postnatal risk factors in these children such as maternal age, cigarette smoking, alcohol consumption, and length of labor, all of which may also increase the occurrence of soft neurologic damage. At this time, however, no consistent association with ADHD has been demonstrated.

During the 1970s, the popular media supported the notion that food additives or sugar might play an important role in the etiology of ADHD. Many studies have addressed this possibility and the findings remain controversial. Additional avenues of exploration examine how acquired problems, such as otitis media, may be related to ADHD. Others continue to explore localized areas in the central nervous system or the role of neurotransmitter mechanisms. The latter research is due, in part, to the fact a number of these children have a positive response to stimulant medication. Although no definitive answer has emerged on the etiology of ADHD, recent studies suggest it may be an inherited disorder.

SIGNS AND SYMPTOMS

The core clinical features of ADHD include impulsivity, distractibility, inability to sustain attention and/or concentration, and developmentally inappropriate activity levels. The *Diagnostic and Statistical Manual of Mental Disorders,* fourth edition (*DSM-IV*) criteria for ADHD are summarized in Table 16-4-1.

TABLE 16-4-1. Summary of *DSM-IV* Criteria for Attention-Deficit/Hyperactivity Disorder

- Six (or more) identified symptoms of either inattention, hyperactivity/impulsivity, or both that have been present for 6 months and are maladaptive and inconsistent with developmental level

- Inattention includes symptoms such as poor attention to detail, frequent forgetfulness, distractibility, difficulty organizing tasks and responsibilities, and difficulty in maintaining attention or sustained mental effort in play, school, or work situations

- Hyperactivity/impulsivity includes symptoms such as frequent motor restlessness, excessive talking, difficulty remaining seated when necessary, interrupting others, and difficulty taking turns

- Some symptoms must be present before the age of 7 years

- Impairment from symptoms must be present in two or more settings (e.g., school and home)

- Must be evidence of clinically significant impairment in social, academic, or occupational functioning

SOURCE: From American Psychiatric Association.

OBJECTIVE FINDINGS

There are no consistent, specific neurologic or physical findings that establish a diagnosis of ADHD, although it should be noted that some children do demonstrate neurologic soft signs. Recent authors have suggested that a positive response to methylphenidate is indicative of a diagnosis. However, a positive response to stimulants should not be used to establish a diagnosis, as these effects are nonspecific.

DIAGNOSTIC CONSIDERATIONS

The *DSM-IV* criteria are helpful in the differential; however, diagnosis is often confounded by several factors. This includes the commonality between these psychiatric criteria and descriptions of normal childhood behaviors. ADHD also has a comorbidity with a number of other childhood disorders, including oppositional defiant disorder; conduct disorder, mood disorders, anxiety disorders, and learning problems. These comorbid conditions and associated problems with academic and social functioning add to the complexity of diagnosis and treatment for ADHD.

SPECIAL CONSIDERATIONS

The majority of the literature on ADHD focuses on the school-age child. However, it is often the developmental issues of preschoolers and adolescents that make diagnosis and treatment difficult. Caution should be exercised in diagnosing a child under the age of 5 years with the disorder since overactivity and inattention are normal in 3- and 4-year-olds. Because of these normal developmental trends, 12-months' duration of symptoms should be observed for this age group, rather than the 6 months recommended in the *DSM-IV.*

Adolescents with ADHD are often under-diagnosed. They typically demonstrate impaired concentration and attention as well as difficulty structuring time and activities. These behaviors may be misinterpreted as normal developmental behavior. Additional confusion also exists related to those adolescents previously diagnosed with ADHD as a child. Although there is considerable research that demonstrates that ADHD may decrease in only one-third of children during adolescence, many health care providers and educators still believe that ADHD disappears with puberty. ADHD in adults has only recently become an area of interest and is also often misdiagnosed. Comorbid disorders among adults may include antisocial personality disorder and substance abuse.

LABORATORY TESTS AND OTHER DIAGNOSTICS

No laboratory or radiologic studies can be used at this time to identify ADHD. Several behavioral rating scales, which have proved effective in gathering a thorough clinical history and observational data from families and schools, are widely available. The Connor's Parent Rating Scale requires approximately 10 minutes to complete and consists of 48 items. Another commonly used scale is the Child Behavior Checklist (CBCL). The CBCL is broader than the Connor's scale and assesses nine domains of childhood psychopathology. In addition to identifying ADHD, the CBCL also uncovers childhood depression and somatization. Separate self-report measures are also available for adolescents and teachers. The Child Attention Problems instrument assesses classroom behavioral changes in children on stimulant medication.This scale, as well as the Iowa Connor's Teacher Rating Scale, may aide in the recognition of ADHD in adolescents.

TREATMENT

Treatment for ADHD is multifaceted and includes medication, counseling, cognitive therapy and behavior management, school-based interventions, family therapy, and social skills training in various combinations.

Psychostimulants remain the most common treatment for ADHD. Approximately 70% of ADHD children treated with stimulants show significant decreases in inattention, hyperactivity, and impulsivity. Methylphenidate hydrochloride (Ritalin) and dextroamphetamine (Dexedrine) are the most commonly prescribed drugs. Dextroamphetamine increases dopamine and norepinephrine neurotransmission and inhibits monoamine oxidase activity, while methylphenidate releases stored dopamine, decreases dopamine reuptake, and inhibits monoamine oxidase activity. The two drugs, equally effective in therapeutic doses, demonstrate a behavioral effect within 0 to 60 minutes, usually lasting 3 to 6 hours. Most patients will require a second dose at noon and recent reports suggest that methylphenidate should optimally be administered three times a day. The sustained-release forms have a greater delay in the onset of action and their effect does not last as long as a second dose of standard medication, but they eliminate the problems associated with drug administration during the school day. This may reduce the likelihood of stigmatization and teasing by classmates, which are contributory factors for nonadherence. The recommended starting dose for methylphenidate is 5 mg and for dextroamphetamine it is 2.5 mg. For young children, one-half of this amount is recommended, and the dextroamphetamine elixir may simplify use. The effective daily dose of the stimulant medication varies. The recommended average daily dose of methylphenidate ranges from 10 mg to 40 mg.

The third available stimulant is magnesium pemoline (Cylert). It is occasionally prescribed for patients who do not respond to methylphenidate. Like the slow-release drugs mentioned above, it has a longer half-life and is generally given only in the morning. Pemoline is absorbed and metabolized at varying rates. As a result, behavioral changes may not be seen for up to 2 weeks and the medication often exhibits a small acute effect and a substantial delayed effect. The initial daily dose is 18.75 mg, with weekly increments of 18.75 mg up to 75.0 mg daily. Older children and adolescents may require a slightly higher dose. Patients receiving pemoline should be monitored for possible liver toxicity every 6 months, as 1% to 2% of patients may develop hepatotoxicity. It should be noted that all medications have side effects, and most are dose-related. Possible adverse effects include insomnia, anorexia, irritability, nausea and vomiting, mood alterations, and an increase in heart rate or blood pressure.

Alternative medications should be considered for children and adolescents when the adverse effects of stimulant treatment are not tolerable. Tricyclic antidepressants are the most frequent alternative. Imipramine (Tofranil or Janimine), desipramine (Norpramin), and amitriptyline (Elavil) are believed to potentiate adrenergic synapses by blocking uptake of dopamine at nerve endings and increasing local dopamine levels. Their most common side effect is drowsiness, which can be mitigated by giving the medication at bedtime. While the

clinical onset of the effects of the drug can be slower, possible advantages are a longer duration of action, the feasibility of a single dose, absence of symptom rebound or insomnia, and less risk of abuse or dependence. Onset of the drug action is gradual and it may be several weeks before significant changes are seen. The initial dose for all three drugs is 25 to 50 mg per day up to 5 mg/kg per day. Doses in excess of 3.5 mg/kg have been associated with mild diastolic hypertension, tachycardia, and electrocardiograph conduction anomalies. Plasma levels must be monitored to avoid toxicity.

Several other medications have also been found useful in managing the impulsivity, hyperactivity, or distractibility of ADD. These include carbamazepine, bupropion, nomifensine, fluoxetine, and clonidine. Clonidine (Catapres), an antihypertensive drug in adults, according to teachers' and parents' ratings was found to be as effective as methylphenidate in decreasing motor activity, improving frustration tolerance, and enhancing cooperation and compliance. Clonidine may be a suitable option for children with ADHD who have a poor response to stimulants, tic disorders, extreme overactivity, oppositional or conduct disorder, or hyperarousal. A combination of clonidine and methylphenidate is often considered for those children who do not respond to either drug alone and seems to be particularly effective for those children who are easily distracted and hyperaroused.

There is strong evidence that stimulant medication has short-term benefits in normalizing many of the clinical symptoms of ADHD. Pharmacologic treatments appear less reliable in producing any long-term benefits. Also, stimulants appear to have unreliable therapeutic effects on many of the secondary problems of children with ADHD such as academic or emotional difficulties. These considerations have led several authors to suggest that sound clinical practice in the treatment of ADHD should include multimodal treatment strategies that combine multiple forms of intervention. Interventions include an individualized approach for the ADHD child and family that incorporates judicious use of stimulant medication along with psychosocial interventions. Psychosocial interventions might include social skills and cognitive training, parent training and home-based programming, and classroom-based behavior modification techniques, as well as individual and family counseling. The National Institute of Mental Health (NIMH) has recently launched a 5-year multisite, multimodal treatment study of children with ADHD and its associated comorbid conditions and social-emotional and academic impairments. The findings of this important project should shed some light on the synergistic or additive effects of stimulant and psychosocial treatments.

PATIENT EDUCATION

Parents of children with ADHD need to recognize that their child's inattentiveness and distractibility are not willful behaviors and are generally beyond the child's control. This recognition may help the parent depersonalize the child's behaviors and assist them in supporting treatment endeavors. Families of all individuals with ADHD need education about the disorder and a clear explanation of treatment options. Individuals and families should also be informed of their legal rights with respect to the Americans with Disabilities Act (ADA, PL 101-336) and the Individuals with Disabilities Education Act (IDEA, PL 101-476). Although IDEA does not at this time possess a separate classification for ADD, many states have chosen to include children with that diagnosis for special education and related services. These laws promote the rights of persons with disabilities. For example, ADA's definition of disability, which includes ADD, may assist an individual in obtaining reasonable accommodations in an employment setting.

DISPOSITION

Proactive and thoughtful management allows most patients with ADHD to be treated successfully by their primary care provider. Children being treated with medication for ADHD should be closely followed with periodic data gathered from teachers and parents. Observational data should be utilized for adjusting dosages. All patients should be carefully monitored for previously noted side effects. Patients should have their height and weight checked regularly, and heart rate and blood pressure should be monitored during treatment, particularly after an increase in dosage.

COMPLICATIONS, RED FLAGS, AND INDICATIONS FOR REFERRAL

With many patients the clinical indications for ADHD are ambiguous. Parents and teachers supply much of the data through verbal reports, which may be distorted by those individuals' own needs. Further confusion may result when a diagnosed child does not respond to medication. A physician assistant may also suspect a comorbid disorder or learning disability. Referral to a mental health professional for differential diagnosis, including psychoeducational assessment, may help detect learning disabilities or a comorbid condition.

Medical providers should be aware that methylphenidate and dextroamphetamine are controlled substances and potential drugs of abuse. They also have illicit street value if sold. Requests for dosage adjustments, early refills, and replacement of lost or stolen medication should alert the prescriber to the possibility of medication abuse. Other family members may be using these drugs for their stimulant effects.

OTHER NOTES AND PEARLS

A multidimensional, systematic approach to the differential diagnosis of ADHD is critical prior to the implementation of any treatment regimen. Since normal children demonstrate improved attention with methylphenidate, a drug response should not be the sole criteria for diagnosis. The use of drugs alone, without other kinds of therapy, often is inadequate to resolve educational difficulties or social skills deficits. Important questions remain unanswered with respect to which subgroups of individuals with ADHD will receive differential benefit from particular treatments. Optimal results will be achieved by those medical providers who thoughtfully integrate current knowledge, skills, and experience with available treatment methodologies and resources in a consistent and compassionate manner. Future research should prove critical in improving the efficacy and efficiency with which this disorder is treated.

BIBLIOGRAPHY

American Psychiatric Association: *Diagnostic and Statistical Manual of Mental Disorders,* 4th ed, Washington, DC, American Psychiatric Association, 1994.

Block SL: Attention-deficit disorder: A paradigm for psychotropic medication intervention in pediatrics. *Pediatr Clin North Am.* 45(5):1053–1083, 1998.

Cyr M, Brown CS: Current drug therapy recommendations for the treatment of attention deficit hyperactivity disorder. *Drugs* 56(2):215–223, 1998.

Elia JE et al: Treatment of attention-deficit hyperactivity disorder. *N Engl J Med* 340(10):780–788, 1999.

Goldman LS et al: Diagnosis and treatment of attention deficit/hyperactivity disorder in children and adolescents. *JAMA* 279(14):1100–1107, 1998.

Richters JE et al: NIMH collaborative multi-site multimodal treatment study of children with ADHD: I. Background and rationale. *J Am Acad Child Adolesc Psychiatry* 34(8):897–1000, 1995.

Searight HR et al: Attention-deficit/hyperactivity disorder: Assessment, diagnosis, and mangement. *J Fam Pract* 40(3):270–279, 1995.

Spencer T et al: Pharmacotherapy of attention-deficit hyperactivity disorder across the life cycle. *J Am Acad Child Adolesc Psychiatry* 35(4):409–442, 1996.

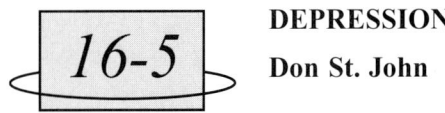

DEPRESSION
Don St. John

DISCUSSION

Depression is a serious medical condition with significant morbidity and mortality, resulting in more disability than nonpsychiatric illnesses such as coronary artery disease, chronic lung disease, and diabetes mellitus. The cost of health care doubles for a patient who is depressed—especially if elderly. About 25% of high users of primary care services meet criteria for a major depressive disorder, two-thirds of which have a previous history of a major depressive episode. Eventually 15% of depressed patients complete a suicide.

Most depressed patients are seen exclusively in a primary care setting. However, both patients and providers rarely volunteer a psychiatric explanation for their medical symptoms. Unfortunately, most patients seen in a primary care setting who are depressed are incorrectly diagnosed, untreated, or inadequately treated.

ETIOLOGY

Depression appears to be a final common pathway syndrome with several potential and interacting etiologic factors. The stress diathesis model probably best explains the etiology of depression.

Twin and adoption studies demonstrate a genetic component to affective disorders. Possible biologic factors include a deficit of norepinephrine at central nerve terminals (the catecholamine hypothesis), abnormal serotonin function, dysregulation of the acetylcholine system, increased cholinergic sensitivity, and abnormalities of the hypothalamic-pituitary-adrenal axis.

Cognitive factors include significant tangible loss or expectation of loss (especially early in life), events that lower self-esteem, depressed close family members, severe punishment or overprotection by parents, strict parental rules, extremely critical parenting, and isolation from others. Behavioral factors include learned helplessness and modeling by depressed family members.

Psychodynamic factors include anger turned inward and early severe loss. Adverse life events may precipitate a depressive episode, especially separation from important persons.

RISK FACTORS

Comorbid psychiatric and nonpsychiatric medical problems and various medications may increase the risk of a patient developing depression (see Table 16-5-1). There is a strong relationship between economic stress and depressive disorders. Depression is twice as common in urban areas as in rural areas. An increased risk is associated with loss of either parent in the first 5 years of life, poor or absent support network, and a history of sexual, physical, or emotional abuse, especially early in life. Also at risk for developing depression are young women with children and minimal support, and women widowed when young or middle-aged. Factors that tend to protect one from depression include the presence of a strong support system and close, confiding relationships.

EPIDEMIOLOGY

Depression is one of the most common mental disorders in the general population and the most common disorder seen by psychiatrists. At any given time, 5% of the US population meet criteria for a major depressive disorder. In the United States, 5 to 12% of men and 10 to 25% of women will develop a major depressive episode at some time in life. The incidence of depression appears to be increasing for each decade since World War II, with a progressively earlier age of onset. The lifetime prevalence of dysthymia may be

TABLE 16-5-1. Physical Illnesses Associated with Depression

Metabolic
  Dehydration
  Azotemia, uremia
  Acid-base disturbance
  Hypoxia
  Hypo- and hypernatremia
  Hypo- and hyperglycemia
  Hypo- and hypercalcemia

Endocrine
  Hypo- and hyperthyroidism
  Addison's disease
  Cushing's disease
  Hypo- and hyperparathyroidism
  Diabetes mellitus

Neurologic
  Sleep apnea
  Parkinson's disease
  Seizure disorders
  Amyotrophic lateral sclerosis
  Multiple sclerosis
  Brain tumors
  Dementia
  Meningitis
  Neurosyphilis
  Normal pressure hydrocephalus
  Cardiovascular accident
  Transient ischemic attack
  Traumatic brain injury

Oncologic
  Pancreatic cancer
  Central nervous system tumors
  Leukemia
  Lung tumors
  Occult carcinomas

Infections
  AIDS
  Postviral syndrome
  Lyme disease
  Syphilis
  Influenza
  Hepatitis
  Pneumonia
  Urinary tract infection
  Endocarditis
  Tuberculosis
  Brucellosis

Cardiovascular
  Congestive heart failure
  Myocardial infarction

Pulmonary
  Chronic obstructive lung disease
  Malignancy

Gastrointestinal
  Malignancy
  Liver failure
  Irritable bowel syndrome
  Chronic abdominal pain

Genitourinary
  Renal failure
  Urinary incontinence

Musculoskeletal
  Arthritis
  Osteoporosis
  Polymyalgia rheumatica
  Paget's disease

Collagen
  Vascular
  Systemic lupus erythematosus

Hematologic
  Anemias

Other
  Thallium toxicity
  Mercury toxicity
  Deficiencies of vitamin B_{12}, thiamin, folic acid

from 3% to 13%, making it the fourth most common psychiatric disorder in the United States.

SIGNS AND SYMPTOMS

The basic abnormality in depression is an abnormal alteration in mood. Depressed mood must be present most of the day, every day for at least 2 weeks, and significantly interfere with functioning (social, occupational, etc.) to make a diagnosis of major depressive disorder. The primary depressive symptoms may be remembered by the mnemonic *SIG: E-CAPS* ("prescribe energy capsules"), as shown in Table 16-5-2.

Affective symptoms of depression include a pervasive mood disturbance (crying, brooding, sadness, irritability, etc.), dysphoria, and anhedonia. Cognitive symptoms include disturbances in perception of one's self, world, and future (Beck's cognitive triad), inappropriate ("false") guilt, sense of inferiority and worthlessness, thoughts of death and suicide, ruminative or obsessive thoughts, excessive fears, and self-reproach. Somatic symptoms include insomnia (initial, middle, and/or terminal) or hypersomnia, fatigue and anergia, changes in appetite and weight, pain, diminished libido, and difficulty concentrating. Behavioral symptoms include psychomotor agitation (such as purposeless pacing, wringing hands) or retardation (characterized by speech latency or catatonia), poor eye contact, tearfulness, speech latency, social withdrawal, low frustration tolerance, and suicide attempts.

For many patients symptoms are worse in the morning, with improvement throughout the day. Anxiety (see Chap. 16-3) is commonly present in depressive disorders. Suicidal ideation is more likely to be passive (wishing one were dead) than active (planning and/or carrying out a suicide attempt).

Somatic symptoms also include heightened sensitivity to pain, headache, back and neck pain, vague abdominal pain, fatigue, and sexual problems. Numerous and persistent physical complaints, inappropriate requests for urgent attention, high frequency of patient contacts (e.g., appointments and phone calls), unexpected emotions displayed during an appointment, and excessive anxiety regarding a significant other are clues that depression may be a significant factor behind presented somatic symptoms. Table 16-5-3 lists general guidelines to enhance the detection of depression, and Table 16-5-4 gives some sample diagnostic questions.

An abnormal suppression of cortisol secretion following dexamethasone administration may be present. About half of patients show a blunted response of thyroid-stimulating hormone (TSH) to thyrotropin- releasing hormone administration. Electroencephalogram (EEG) abnormalities include decreased delta sleep, decreased rapid eye movement (REM) latency, and increased REM density.

SPECIFIC FEATURES

Vegetative symptoms are more prominent for patients with *melancholia*. Common symptoms include anhedonia for all activities, diurnal variation of symptoms (worse in the morning, improving throughout the day), terminal insomnia (early morning awakening), psychomotor retardation or agitation, anorexia and weight loss, and excessive guilt.

TABLE 16-5-2. Primary Depressive Symptoms That Make Up the Mnemonic *SIG: E-CAPS*

Sleep
Interests
Guilt
Energy
Concentration
Appetite
Psychomotor agitation or retardation
Suicidal ideation

TABLE 16-5-3. Enhancing the Detection of Depression

1. Make early eye contact.

2. Clarify the presenting complaint.

3. Use active listening skills.
   a. Paraphrase the feelings and thoughts the patient is communicating.
   b. Validate the patient's feelings and perspective.
   c. Be vigilant to both verbal and nonverbal cues of depression.
   d. Confirm nonverbal cues of depression with the patient.
   e. Ask open questions.

4. Attend to what the patient believes to be important.

5. Directly inquire about the patient's feelings.

6. Normalize feelings and reactions when appropriate.

7. Avoid negative questions.

8. Avoid leading questions.

9. Express concern or sympathy when appropriate.

10. Maintain a nonjudgmental attitude.

11. Use supportive statements that are factual and believable.

12. Clarify expectations, both yours and the patient's.

13. Inquire about family, home, and work in the context of the presenting symptoms.

Melancholia tends to respond better to somatic therapies and may be more prominent in older patients.

Up to half of depressed patients develop *psychotic symptoms,* such as delusions and hallucinations. Patients usually do not volunteer psychotic symptoms, fearing they are "going crazy" and will be "locked up" or "put away." Delusions or hallucinations are usually mood-congruent (content consistent with depressive themes). Relapse and recurrence tend to be more common and symptom severity tends to be greater when psychotic symptoms are present. A patient who has had psychotic symptoms during a depressive episode is more likely to develop them during future episodes. Neuroleptics are usually required with an antidepressant for treatment.

TABLE 16-5-4. Examples of Diagnostic Questions

"Are you depressed?" "Have you been bothered by feeling down, depressed, or hopeless?" and "Have you been bothered by little interest or pleasure in doing things?" are as sensitive as the Beck Depression Inventory for screening for depression.

"Many people who are depressed no longer enjoy things they used to enjoy, such as hobbies, interacting with friends, and sex. This is a common symptom of depression. What do you normally enjoy doing? What do you still enjoy? What have you lost interest in?"

"How are you getting along with your spouse . . . coworkers . . . friends?"

"Have you noticed a change in your appetite?"

"How have you been sleeping?"

"Have you noticed any change in your energy level?"

"Have you felt more fidgety or is it difficult to sit still? Have you felt slowed down?"

"Sometimes persons who are depressed have unusual thoughts, very confused thoughts, and even hear voices or see things that aren't really there. Have you had any of these experiences?"

"Many people who are depressed have thoughts that life is no longer worth living and may think about committing suicide. These thoughts can be very distressing. Have you been struggling with thoughts like these?"

This list is not all-inclusive. Mark Zimmerman's *Interview Guide for Evaluating* DSM-IV *Psychiatric Disorders and the Mental Status Exam,* Psych Products Press, is a more thorough yet quick and easy-to-use interview guide, with specific questions arranged according to *DSM-IV* criteria.

Motor immobility or excessive motor activity (purposeless), extreme negativism or mutism, peculiarities of voluntary movement (such as posturing), stereotypical movements, echolalia, and echopraxia are *catatonic features* sometimes present. Depression with catatonic features tends to respond better to electroconvulsive therapy (ECT).

Atypical features include increased appetite and weight gain, hypersomnia, leaden paralysis, and sensitivity to interpersonal rejection. Most patients with dysthymia have atypical depressive symptoms. Women comprise 90% of patients with atypical features. Atypical symptoms may be more difficult to treat and tend to respond poorly to tricyclic antidepressants (TCAs) and ECT, responding better to serotonergic agents and best to monoamine oxidase inhibitors (MAOIs).

Postpartum blues is common (50 to 80%), occurs within the first 2 weeks postpartum, lasts less than 2 weeks, does not meet full criteria for major depressive disorder, and responds to reassurance. Pharmacotherapy is usually not necessary. However, the presence of postpartum blues increases the risk of developing postpartum depression.

The clinical features and treatment of *postpartum depression* (a depressive episode occurring within 4 weeks of parturition) do not differ from the treatment of depressive disorders that occur at any other time of life. Risk factors for the development of postpartum depression include stressful life events (other than the childbirth), unemployment, marital conflict, and absence of a good social support system. Postpartum onset of depression may increase the risk of developing a bipolar disorder. Untreated postpartum depression is associated with disturbances in cognitive and emotional development for the child that remain for at least age 4 to 5 years.

Symptoms of *postpartum psychosis* resemble mania and delirium. More than half of these patients meet full criteria for a major depressive disorder. Postpartum psychosis is rare (1 to 2 per 2000 births), develops rapidly within 1 to 2 weeks of parturition, and requires immediate psychiatric intervention because of potential danger to the child and mother. Patients often have a history of a bipolar disorder.

The *Diagnostic and Statistical Manual of Mental Disorders,* fourth edition (*DSM-IV*), does not list *seasonal affective disorder* (SAD) as a separate diagnosis, but "with seasonal features" may be added as a modifier to an affective diagnosis when a pattern of a temporal relationship between symptoms and season exists. Approximately 5% of the population experiences depressive symptoms during the winter months, another 10 to 20% presenting subsyndromal symptoms. Seasonal symptoms are more common in young adults and women. Symptoms tend to be atypical. Over 90% of patients experience depression during the winter, but some patients suffer their depressive symptoms consistently during the summer months. Seasonal depression may respond to phototherapy.

Depression is *masked* when the patient does not complain of a depressed mood, but otherwise meets full criteria for a depressive disorder. Masked depression is especially common in the elderly, who are more likely to present somatic symptoms and expect to feel depressed as a "normal" part of aging.

By definition, patients with a *bipolar disorder* suffer at least one manic or hypomanic episode and at least one depressive episode (see Chap. 16-6). Patients with bipolar depression tend to be depressed longer, relapse more frequently, display more depressive symptoms (especially atypical), have more severe symptoms, develop psychotic symptoms, are more likely to commit suicide, and are more incapacitated by the depression. Other more common characteristics include seasonal variations, postpartum symptoms, and sensitivity to changes in time zone, sleep/wake cycle, diet, exercise, and work schedules. The presence of both manic and depressive symptoms is termed *mixed bipolar affective disorder.* As a rule, patients with a bipolar diagnosis will require treatment with a thymoleptic (mood stabilizer).

Dysthymic disorder is common, affecting 3% of the population, and is frequently not recognized by primary care practitioners and patients. Persistence of depressed mood is the most discriminating feature of dysthymia. Depressed mood is present most of the day, for more days than not, for at least 2 years. Onset is insidious, usually during adolescence. Fewer vegetative symptoms are present, and so-cial-motivational and cognitive symptoms are more prominent. Many patients will say they have always felt depressed, describing them-selves as chronically unhappy, miserable, irritable, and angry. Patients with dysthymia are high utilizers of medical services. Comorbid psy-chiatric and medical problems are the rule. The course tends to vary, dependent on environmental stressors. Only 50% of patients fully re-cover, and 70% will eventually develop major depressive disorder, which decreases recovery to only 33%.

A patient who experiences a major depressive episode while also meeting criteria for dysthymia has *double depression.* Treatment re-sistance and high relapse rates are characteristic. Most patients will require lifelong therapy.

Many patients may not meet full *DSM-IV* criteria for a depressive disorder yet suffer significant social, occupational, and family im-pairment from depressive symptoms. Patients with *subsyndromal de-pression* commonly present in primary care settings with somatic symptoms. Subsyndromal depression is associated with higher rates of lost workdays, health services utilization, and suicide. Patients of-ten meet full criteria for another psychiatric disorder, especially ob-sessive-compulsive disorder, generalized anxiety disorder, panic dis-order, personality disorders, and substance abuse. Subsyndromal symptoms should be treated as aggressively as a depressive disorder meeting full diagnostic criteria.

Depressed mood is an expected and common symptom of uncom-plicated *bereavement;* however, 10% of grieving patients will eventu-ally meet full criteria for a major depressive disorder. Grief-related de-pressive symptoms that result in significant impairment of function should be treated as a major depressive disorder, even if full criteria are not met. Treatment of depressed mood does not interfere with the grieving process.

Depression that develops in response to or during the course of an-other illness may be a *secondary depression* due to that illness and not a separate, comorbid illness. Characteristics of a secondary de-pression include absence of family history of affective disorders, greater cognitive impairment, and poorer response to treatment. Tables 16-5-5 and 16-5-1 list drugs and nonpsychiatric illnesses that have been associated with depression. A direct causal relationship is often difficult to determine.

COURSE OF DEPRESSION

The onset of depression usually occurs after puberty, with a median age of onset of 37 years. Age of onset tends to be earlier when a positive family history of affective disorders or alcoholism is present. Untreated episodes last 3 to 9 months, with 85% remitting within 1 year. Up to 80% of patients eventually fully recover from a depressive episode. Pre-dictors of a favorable prognosis include absence of stressful life events and presence of a positive social support, especially intimate friendships.

Episode length tends to remain constant for an individual patient. Longer episodes are associated with delay in treatment, older age, lower socioeconomic status, and prior history of a long episode. Women tend to have more episodes than men. Of patients with unipolar depression, 10 to 15% will eventually have a manic or hypomanic episode, con-verting their diagnosis from a unipolar to a bipolar disorder.

Half of patients never have another episode. For the other half, de-pression recurs or becomes chronic, with the chance of recurrence in-creasing dramatically with each subsequent episode: 12% of patients with major depressive disorder fail to recover within 5 years, 7% within 10 years. *Recurrence* is defined as a new depressive episode following a period of at least 2 months without depressive symptoms. Each recurrence results in decreasing length between episodes and increasing treatment resistance. The risk of recurrence is greatest the first 4 to 6 months following recovery and decreases with time.

TABLE 16-5-5. Medications Associated With Symptoms of Depression

Antihypertensives
    Reserpine (15%)
    Propranolol (8%)
    Methyldopa
    Clonidine
    Hydralazine
    Guanethidine

Psychotropics
    Sedatives
        Barbiturates
        Benzodiazepines
        Meprobamate
    Antipsychotics
    Hypnotics

Antiparkinsonian
    Levodopa

Analgesics
    Narcotics/opiates
    Indomethacin

Cardiovascular
    Digitalis
    Diuretics
    Lidocaine
    Antiarrhythmic agents

Oral hypoglycemic agents

Antimicrobials
    Sulfonamides
    Interferon α
    Isoniazid

Steroids
    Corticosteroids (20%)
    Estrogens (90% of women with depression
        secondary to estrogen have pyridoxine deficiency
        and respond to supplementation)

Others
    Cimetidine
    Cancer chemotherapeutic agents
    Stimulant withdrawal
    Smoking cessation

Increased risk of recurrence is associated with dysthymia, substance abuse, comorbid anxiety and personality disorders, older age of on-set, and greater number of previous episodes.

Predictors of *relapse* (redevelopment of a major depressive episode following a partial response to treatment) include greater number of prior episodes, secondary depression, and increased length of prior episodes. A patient is *refractory* to treatment when symptoms persist despite an accurate diagnosis, patient compliance, and treatment at an adequate dosage for an adequate time period (at least 6 to 8 weeks for most drugs). Depression is *chronic* when full criteria for major de-pressive disorder are present continuously for at least 2 years. Each new depressive episode increases the risk of chronicity by 15%.

COMPLICATIONS AND RED FLAGS

The most serious complication of depression is suicide, which occurs in 15% of depressed patients. Risk of suicide is especially high shortly after discharge from inpatient treatment (see Chap. 16-7).

Of the top 10 major medical disorders, depression and cardiac dis-ease have the most negative impact on social, occupational, family, and physical functions. Patients with depression are four times more likely to die from physical illness. Depressed patients are at greater risk for developing substance abuse problems.

Patients show impaired judgment and may make poor decisions when depressed. Occupational and academic failures are common. Complications extend beyond the depressed patient, with 40% of children of depressed patients developing long-lasting major impairments.

DIAGNOSTIC CONSIDERATIONS

Other Psychiatric Disorders

Depression is commonly comorbid with and may develop as a secondary illness during other psychiatric disorders, especially substance abuse, panic and other anxiety disorders, and cluster B personality disorders. The presence of comorbid psychiatric disorders tends to result in more severe symptoms and treatment resistance.

Anxious and depressive symptoms commonly co-occur. Anxious patients tend to fear and believe they have no hope for the future, whereas depressed patients are more generally hopeless. Anxiety tends to worsen throughout the day, whereas depression tends to be worse in the morning, improve during the day, then become worse again in the evening. Patients with comorbid anxiety disorders tend to respond better to antidepressants than anxiolytics, such as benzodiazepines.

Patients with avoidant, dependent, and borderline personality disorders commonly develop depressive disorders. Depressed patients often respond to the medical interview through a general negative bias, which can give the impression of long-standing symptoms and inaccurately suggest the diagnosis of a personality disorder. The diagnosis of a personality disorder should be suspended until depressive symptoms have abated and characterologic traits can be better assessed. Pervasiveness of symptoms throughout late adolescence and adulthood is the key feature of a personality disorder. Patients with personality disorders often lack effective coping skills, are more vulnerable to environmental stressors, and are at higher risk for experiencing stressful life events.

Depressive symptoms are commonly present in patients with somatoform disorders, such as somatization disorder, chronic pain, etc. Because somatizing patients tend to complain of somatic symptoms over mood symptoms, the presence of depression may be masked by the somatic complaints. Patients with somatization disorders somatize whether they have a depressed mood or not, whereas depressed patients somatize only when depressed. Reframing somatic symptoms as "signals" of depression may help the patient accept a diagnosis of depression.

A diagnosis of depression should be deferred until a substance-abusing patient has been drug-free for at least 4 to 6 weeks. Depression is more likely primary when there is a positive family history for affective disorders; depressive symptoms were present prior to substance use, persist during abstinence, and are chronic; and

profound suicidal ideation is present. Though ongoing substance abuse significantly increases treatment resistance, it is not necessarily a contraindication to antidepressant therapy. A dual diagnosis is made when substance abuse coexists with another psychiatric disorder (see Chap. 16-10).

Depression may be misdiagnosed as dementia in elderly patients (pseudodementia). Depressive symptoms tend to be more acute, are worse in the morning, and involve both recent and remote memory problems. Depressed patients often have a past history of depressive episodes and demonstrate more self-reproach. Depressed patients have normal psychometric testing, selectively remember negative events, and show concern for their memory loss (demonstrate insight into their disorder). Dementia has a more insidious onset with no self-reproach; it is worse at night and presents with recent memory loss greater than remote memory problems (see Chap. 11-5). Table 16-5-6 contrasts symptoms of depression with those of dementia and delirium.

The negative symptoms of schizophrenia (apathy, flat affect, anhedonia, avolition, low social drive, etc.) may be misdiagnosed as depression. Patients who are depressed complain of dysphoria, whereas the emotional experiences and expressions of schizophrenic patients are more restricted. Delusions and hallucinations occurring in the context of an affective disorder tend to be briefer and less bizarre than those of schizophrenia. The appearance of depressive-like symptoms in a patient with schizophrenia usually signals worsening of the schizophrenia; however, depression can co-occur with schizophrenia, especially following an active psychotic episode (postpsychotic depressive disorder of schizophrenia).

Five percent of women develop premenstrual dysphoric disorder. Symptoms occur 7 to 10 days premenstrually and resolve within a few days of menses. Use of daily mood charts can help identify this pattern.

The presence of family violence must be directly queried since it is usually not volunteered and must be addressed for safety reasons. Depression has been triggered by attempts to stop smoking. Caffeine withdrawal can look like depression with symptoms including somnolence, lethargy, and headache.

Nonpsychiatric Medical Disorders

Tables 16-5-1 and 16-5-5 list nonpsychiatric medical problems and medications, respectively, that may cause, mimic, precipitate, mask, aggravate, or interfere with the treatment of depression. Comorbidity is the rule for depressed patients and results in poorer function and lower recovery rates. Risk factors for comorbid depression include recent stress, presence of six or more physical symptoms, higher symptom severity, lower overall rating of health, practitioner perception of encounter as difficult, and age less than 50 years. Hospital utilization

TABLE 16-5-6. Differentiating Among Depression, Dementia, and Delirium

DEPRESSION	DEMENTIA	DELIRIUM
Depressed mood is prominent symptom	Mood typically not depressed	Rapid mood variation
Acute onset	Insidious onset	Acute onset
Symptoms of short duration	Symptoms of longer duration	Symptoms of brief duration
History of depression	No history of depression	No history of depression
Patient complains of cognitive deficits	Patient lacks insight into cognitive deficits	Disorientation
Little effort at tasks	Patient struggles with tasks	Diminished alertness
Symptoms worse in the morning	Sundowning present	Waxing and waning level of consciousness
"I don't know" as typical answer	May confabulate answers	Nonauditory perceptual disturbances
Variable performance on neuropsychological tests	Poor performance on neuropsychological tests	Variable performance on neuropsychological tests
Guilt	Absence of guilt	Absence of guilt
Loss of both recent and remote memory	Memory loss greater for recent events	Quite variable memory disturbance

is increased even 4 years after discharge from inpatient treatment of a medical problem when a comorbid psychiatric condition exists. The mortality rate for depressed patients hospitalized for a variety of medical problems is twofold even 2 years following the hospitalization.

Patients with comorbid depression and breast cancer show an increase in mortality. Patients with chronic depression are at increased risk of developing cancer. Depressed women are at increased risk for falls and fall-related fractures. Cell-mediated immunity is decreased in depressed patients and returns to normal with effective treatment.

Depression is especially common in patients with diabetes mellitus, chronic obstructive pulmonary disease (COPD), myocardial infarction, chronic fatigue syndrome, and HIV infection. About 25 to 50% of patients develop depression after a stroke, and in some patients, depression appears to be causally related to the brain injury. One-third of patients with Parkinson's disease develop depression (see Chap. 11-7). Elevated TSH is more common in depressed patients, and some treatment-resistant depressed patients have subclinical hypothyroidism (see Chap. 5-3). Patients with two or more pain complaints are six times more likely to be depressed; those with three or more are eight times more likely to be depressed.

Patients who develop depression following a myocardial infarction are at increased risk for subsequent morbidity and mortality. Depression is also an independent risk factor for coronary artery disease up to 10 years after a depressive episode.

SPECIAL POPULATIONS

Adolescents have fewer introspective abilities and tend to have more acting-out behaviors when depressed. Obtaining clinical information and support from significant others (parents, teachers, adult leaders, friends) is important when working with adolescents.

Studies estimate that 45% of hospitalized elderly patients are depressed, though only half receive treatment. Similarly, 40% of depressed nursing home patients are diagnosed with depression, and of these, less than 25% receive adequate treatment. There is a strong correlation between the presence of depressive symptoms and mortality in elderly women.

Elderly patients may present with memory problems, worry and nervousness, anhedonia (when asked), stooped posture, psychomotor retardation, failure to follow treatment guidelines, lack of interest in personal care, and functional impairment disproportionate to the extent of medical illnesses.

Elderly patients have the highest rates of suicide (most of whom were not diagnosed), especially single, elderly white males. They also have higher rates of masked depression and become functionally more impaired and impaired faster than younger patients. Depression risk increases with concomitant medical illnesses, and the elderly have higher rates of primary medical problems. Elderly patients have more losses and fewer individual and social resources.

Depression in older patients is as treatable as for younger patients, though they have increased sensitivity to medication side effects and may require more time to respond to antidepressants. The cognitive impairment of pseudodementia does respond to appropriate antidepressant therapy.

EVALUATION

A thorough medical history and physical exam are essential to rule out primary and comorbid conditions. Further diagnostic studies are guided by history and physical findings. Acknowledge and validate the patient's feelings of hopelessness, guilt, and negative self-evaluation, then develop hope that depression can be effectively treated. Maintain a warm, approachable, nonthreatening, and nonrushed attitude. Depressed patients have a negative cognitive bias and will easily recognize frustration and hopelessness in the provider.

There are many structured interview and self-rating scales that may be used to diagnosis and monitor depression (see Fig. 16-5-1). Common ones include the Beck Depression Inventory, Hamilton Depression

TABLE 16-5-7. Potential Indications for Inpatient Treatment of Depression

High immediate risk of suicide or homicide
Poor capacity to comply with treatment
Lack of adequate psychosocial support system
Need for concurrent treatment of substance abuse
Serious complicating medical or psychiatric condition requiring close medical supervision
Failure to respond to outpatient treatment
Inability to care for basic needs
Initiation of electroconvulsive therapy

Rating Scale, Zung Depression Scale, Geriatric Depression Scale, and Structured Clinical Interview for the Diagnostic and Statistical Manual (SCID). Such scales may be useful screening tools, but they cannot substitute for the clinical interview in making the diagnosis of a depressive disorder. Table 16-5-4 gives some examples of helpful diagnostic questions to use.

Identify specific symptoms to target for treatment. In psychiatry, treatment options are often more driven by symptoms than diagnosis. Documentation of symptom improvement by using a validated rating scale (Table 16-5-1 is a rating scale developed and used by Mark Zimmerman and the author) may be helpful in demonstrating patient response to managed care companies. Inform the patient of common depressive symptoms to alleviate the common fear of "going crazy." Specifically ask about psychotic symptoms, which are usually not volunteered, and normalize them as a common symptom of depression. Previous manic symptoms must be specifically requested because bipolar disorders usually require a thymoleptic (see Chap. 16-6).

Inquire about suicidal ideation at each visit (see Chap. 16-7). Obtain information about previous depressive episodes, course, treatment response, and family history, which may guide in determining a specific treatment regimen. Evaluate potential sources of strength and support in the patient's environment, which may need to be addressed during the treatment phase. Table 16-5-7 lists some indications of the possible need for inpatient treatment. Table 16-5-8 lists some indications for referral to a psychiatric specialist.

Plan frequent and regular follow-up to ensure adequate response and return to baseline functioning. Response of somatic symptoms, reflective of the depression, parallels the response of the depression. Daily mood charts can be helpful in determining treatment response, especially since recall is colored by current mood.

TREATMENT

Depression is a treatable disorder, and treatment can be lifesaving. Effective treatment can be found for most patients. Patients should be advised that many treatment options exist and that recovery is the rule. The goal of treatment is symptom remission. Use of standardized treatment guidelines and protocols by primary care providers improves both the

TABLE 16-5-8. Indications for Psychiatric Referral

Lack of skill or confidence in diagnosis or treatment of depression
High risk of suicide
Failure to respond to adequate antidepressant treatment trials (especially if patient's condition continues to worsen)
Consideration of need for inpatient treatment
Concern regarding drug interactions
Consideration of unusual doses or combinations of psychiatric drugs
Consideration of using a monoamine oxidase inhibitor

Name: _____   Date: _____

INSTRUCTIONS: This scale includes questions about symptoms of depression. For each item please indicate how well it describes you during the **PAST WEEK,** INCLUDING TODAY. Circle the number in the column next to each question that best describes you.
Please give this to the practitioner you are seeing today. Thank you.

---

0 = not at all true   1 = rarely true   2 = sometimes true   3 = often true   4 = almost always true

---

During the PAST WEEK, INCLUDING TODAY...

1.	I felt sad or depressed	0 1 2 3 4
2.	I had crying spells	0 1 2 3 4
3.	I felt blue or down in the dumps	0 1 2 3 4
4.	I did not laugh as much as usual	0 1 2 3 4
5.	I was not interested in my usual activities	0 1 2 3 4
6.	I did not get pleasure from the things I usually enjoy	0 1 2 3 4
7.	My appetite was poor and I didn't feel like eating	0 1 2 3 4
8.	My appetite was much greater than usual	0 1 2 3 4
9.	I had difficulty sleeping	0 1 2 3 4
10.	I was sleeping too much	0 1 2 3 4
11.	I felt physically slowed down, like my body was stuck in mud	0 1 2 3 4
12.	My energy level was low	0 1 2 3 4
13.	I felt tired and worn out	0 1 2 3 4
14.	I had a low opinion of myself	0 1 2 3 4
15.	I felt guilty	0 1 2 3 4
16.	My self esteem was low	0 1 2 3 4
17.	I thought I was a failure	0 1 2 3 4
18.	I thought I was worthless and no good	0 1 2 3 4
19.	I thought I was inferior to other people	0 1 2 3 4
20.	I thought I was useless	0 1 2 3 4
21.	I had problems concentrating	0 1 2 3 4
22.	I had more difficulties making decisions than usual	0 1 2 3 4
23.	I wished I was dead	0 1 2 3 4
24.	I thought that others would be better off if I was dead	0 1 2 3 4
25.	I thought that life was not worth living	0 1 2 3 4
26.	I thought about killing myself	0 1 2 3 4
27.	I thought the future looked hopeless	0 1 2 3 4
28.	I am having sexual problems	0 1 2 3 4
29.	I used alcohol or street drugs	0 1 2 3 4
30.	I am having difficulty affording treatment or medication	0 1 2 3 4

FIGURE 16-5-1. Depression scale.

TABLE 16-5-9. Comparison of Antidepressants

DRUG	USUAL DOSE mg/d ETC.	DOSE RANGE mg/d ETC.	HALF-LIFE h ETC.	P-450 SYSTEM
Amitriptyline	150–300	75–300	9–46	3A4 2D6
Nortriptyline	75–150	40–150	18–56	3A4 2D6
Protriptyline	15–40	15–60	54–198	3A4 2D6
Imipramine	150–300	75–300	6–28	3A4 2D6
Desipramine	150–300	75–300	12–28	3A4 2D6
Clomipramine	150–300	100–300	15–62	3A4 2D6
Trimipramine	150–200	75–300	16–40	3A4 2D6
Doxepin	150–300	75–400	8–25	3A4 2D6
Trazodone	200–400	50–600	6–13	3A4
Nefazodone	300–500	200–600	3–18	3A4
Amoxapine	200–300	75–600	9–14	
Maprotiline	150–225	75–225	27–50	
Fluoxetine	5–20	10–80	48–96	2D6 2C9 3A4
Sertraline	50–100	25–200	26	2D6
Paroxetine	20–30	10–60	20	2D6
Fluvoxamine	50–150	50–300	20	1A2 2C9 3A4
Citalopram	20–40	20–60	33	2C19 2D6
Venlafaxine	75–225	150–375	4–10	
Mirtazapine	15–45	15–45	20–40	2D6 1A2 3A4 2C9
Bupropion	150–300	150–450	10–21	
Phenelzine	60–90	30–90	2	
Tranylcypromine	30–60	30–60	2	
St. John's wort	900	300–1000	25	
Hypericin	1.0	0.4–2.7	25	

detection and treatment of depressive disorders, to a degree comparable to that of psychiatric specialists. Pharmacotherapy and psychotherapy are both effective treatments for depression. A combination of medication and psychotherapy is more effective than either treatment alone.

Practitioners should take a collaborative approach with patients to empower the patient and challenge dependency and hopelessness. The depression should be validated at the same time that the patient is encouraged that efforts are being made toward achieving remission of symptoms. Depression should be framed as a medical illness and not a characterologic weakness. Understanding cultural differences in the expression and experience of mood and depression assists in assessing treatment response. Patients should be informed that response to treatment tends to be "sawtoothed," not linear.

Significant others should be involved in monitoring and providing support. Increasing contact with others may help to stimulate a socially withdrawing patient. Structure and security should be provided in the environment, and the patient should be discouraged from making major life decisions while actively depressed.

Compliance is improved when the patient is advised to take medications daily and continued even if the patient is feeling better, instructed that an antidepressant must be taken for 2 to 4 weeks to notice an effect, and given specific instructions about potential medication problems and how to deal with them. Written handouts can be valuable tools, but they must be reviewed with the patient in the clinical setting.

Pharmacologic Management

About 60 to 75% of patients achieve complete remission with pharmaco- logic therapy alone. Less than 30% fail to respond to antidepressants. Good response is associated with vegetative symptoms, hypersomnia, melancholia, acute onset, absence of family dysfunction, history of prior response to antidepressants, and family history of mood disorders. Antidepressants previously effective for the patient and family members are more likely to be effective for the current episode. Medications are often chosen by side effect profile, safety in overdose, cost, ease of administration, and potential drug interactions. Table 16-5-12 gives suggestions for choice of antidepressant.

Response may not be seen for weeks after achieving therapeutic doses. Patients with psychotic depression may require higher doses of antidepressants, usually in combination with an antipsychotic. Antidepressants (especially the TCAs) used to treat bipolar depression may lead to induction of mania or increased cycling. Antidepressants with potential for toxicity should be given in limited quantities to patients at risk for suicide or with a history of impulsivity. Most pharmaceutical companies have patient assistance programs that provide medications at little or no cost to patients who are unable to afford their medications. A listing of such programs can be found at www.needy-drugs.com.

Approximately 70% of patients respond to the first antidepressant given; however, 60 to 75% of patients fail to achieve complete remission of symptoms. An adequate treatment trial is 6 weeks at full therapeutic dose. If a patient fails to respond to the first drug, an antidepressant with a different mechanism action may be considered.

There is a 50% chance of relapse if antidepressants are discontinued before 6 months, so therapy should be continued for at least 9 to 12 months. When discontinuation is considered, it should occur

TABLE 16-5-10. Comparison of Antidepressants: Side Effects

DRUG	ANTICHOLINERGIC	DROWSINESS	INSOMNIA	HYPOTENSION	WEIGHT GAIN	CARDIAC	GI DISTRESS
Amitriptyline	++++	++++	0	++++	++++	+++	0
Nortriptyline	+	+	0	++	+	++	0
Protriptyline	++	+	+	++	0	++	0
Imipramine	+++	+++	+	++++	+++	+++	+
Desipramine	+	+	+	++	+	++	0
Clomipramine	+	++	+	++	++	++	0
Trimipramine	+	++++	0	++	+++	++	0
Doxepin	+++	++++	0	++	+++	++	0
Trazodone	0	++++	+	+	0	+	+
Nefazodone	0	++	+	+	−	+	+
Amoxapine	++	++	++	++	+	+++	0
Maprotiline	++	++++	0	0	++	+	0
Fluoxetine	0	0	++	0	−	0	+++
Sertraline	0	+	++	0	+/−	0	++
Paroxetine	0	+	++	0	+	0	++
Fluvoxamine	0	++	++	0	−	0	++++
Citalopram	0	+	++	0	0	0	++
Venlafaxine	+	++	+	+	0	+	+
Mirtazapine	+	++++/++	+	++++	++	++	++
Bupropion	0	−	++	0	−	+	+
Phenelzine	+	+	++	++	++	0	+
Tranylcypromine	+	+	++	++	++	0	+
St. John's wort	0	−+	0	0	−	0	+
Hypericin	0	−+	0	0	−	0	+

gradually. A longer period of treatment should be considered when history of recurrence, greater severity, later age of onset, and longer depressive episodes are present. Maintenance regimens are often the same as those needed to achieve remission. Lifelong maintenance should be considered after three episodes because of the 90% risk of relapse. About 10% of patients prove resistant to all antidepressants.

Patients with psychotic symptoms may require higher than usual doses of antidepressants and usually require an antipsychotic as well. Once psychotic symptoms are absent and the depression is responding well to treatment, the antipsychotic should be tapered off. However, some patients will require a maintenance antipsychotic. The newer "atypical" antipsychotics appear to have a lower rate of tardive dyskinesia as a side effect, have fewer side effects, and may have additional antidepressant effects.

All antidepressants have been associated with the onset of a manic episode and increased cycling in patients with a bipolar disorder. It is unclear whether the episode is triggered by the antidepressant or sequentially follows a depressive episode. The TCAs are more likely to induce mania. Bupropion has the lowest incidence of associated mania and may decrease rapid cycling. Because of this potential risk, consideration should be given to tapering off an antidepressant once the symptoms have been well controlled (6 to 12 weeks if depression typically follows mania or 6 to 12 days if mania typically follows depression for a given patient). Many patients will require maintenance antidepressants, but some can be maintained on a thymoleptic alone. Most patients with a bipolar disorder will require treatment with a thymoleptic (see Chap. 16-6).

Tables 16-5-9 through 16-5-11 provide comparisons of dosing, side effects, drug interactions, etc. for the antidepressants available in the United States at the time of this writing. Table 16-5-13 lists potential drug interactions through the CYP-450 system. Table 16-5-14 lists therapeutic plasma levels of the antidepressants whose levels have been found to be clinically relevant.

SELECTIVE SEROTONIN REUPTAKE INHIBITORS Selective serotonin reuptake inhibitors (SSRIs) are the drugs of first choice for treating depression because of their efficacy, tolerable side-effect profile, once-daily dosing, and relative safety in overdose. Despite their high cost, they may be more cost-efficient than TCAs because they are so well tolerated and do not require serum levels for dosing. Unlike TCAs, increasing the dose of an SSRI does not necessarily lead to an enhanced therapeutic effect.

There appear to be more similarities than differences among the five current choices. SSRIs appear to be more effective in treating women, premenstrual dysphoric disorder, dysthymic disorders, and atypical symptoms (especially irritability, anger, and fatigue) than are TCAs. SSRIs are also the first drugs of choice for treating anxiety disorders, especially obsessive-compulsive disorder, and impulsivity.

All but sertraline demonstrate nonlinear pharmacokinetics. All but fluoxetine take 2 to 4 weeks to attain a steady state. Each SSRI is chemically distinct, and response or nonresponse to one SSRI does not necessarily predict response or nonresponse to another. A partial treatment response can often be enhanced by increasing the dose. When a patient fails to respond to an adequate trial of one SSRI, another may be substituted without a wash-out period, except for fluoxetine, which requires a 2- to 4-week wash-out to avoid developing a serotonin syndrome.

Potential side effects include headache, nervousness, insomnia, drowsiness, fatigue, anorexia, weight loss, tremor, nausea, dry mouth,

TABLE 16-5-11. Comparison of Antidepressants: Neurotransmitter Systems Affected

DRUG	NORADRENALINE	SEROTONIN	DOPAMINE	HISTAMINE	α-ADRENOCEPTOR BLOCKADE
Amitriptyline	*	**		**	*
Nortriptyline	**			*	*
Protriptyline	****				
Imipramine	**	**		*	*
Desipramine	****				
Clomipramine	*	**			*
Trimipramine	****	**		*	*
Doxepin	*	**		****	*
Trazodone		*		**	*
Nefazodone	*	**	*		*
Amoxapine	**	*	**		*
Maprotiline	**			**	*
Fluoxetine		**			
Sertraline		**	***		
Paroxetine	*	****			
Fluvoxamine		**			
Citalopram		****			
Venlafaxine[a]	**	**	*		
Mirtazapine[b]	**	**		H$_1$***	***
Bupropion	*		**		
Phenelzine	**	**	*		
Tranylcypromine	**	**	*		
St. John's wort	*	*	*		

[a]Tends to be serotonergic at low doses, noradrenergic and mildly dopaminergic at high doses.
[b]Histamine blockade tends to predominate at low doses.

diarrhea, constipation, sweating, inhibited libido, anorgasmia, and impotence. All but the last three side effects tend to be transient, often improving as the antidepressant effects become noticeable. A slight increase in bleeding and bruising (increased bleeding time) may occur, especially when taken concomitantly with a nonsteroidal anti-inflammatory agent. An increase in prothrombin time may occur with concurrent warfarin therapy. Cardiovascular side effects (other than mild bradycardia) are rare and usually the result of drug interactions.

Sexual side effects may be dose-related and are transient in only a minority of patients. Most patients will not volunteer sexual problems and must be directly queried during follow-up encounters. Adverse sexual effects of the SSRIs is an important cause of noncompliance with pharmacotherapy. Treatment approaches for SSRI-induced sexual dysfunction include using a shorter-acting agent and taking drug holidays (not effective for fluoxetine because of its very long half-life), as-needed sildenafil or yohimbine, or addition of bupropion, buspirone, cyproheptadine, trazodone, or amantadine. Spontaneous orgasm has been rarely reported as an SSRI-induced side effect.

SSRI-induced insomnia may be treated by administering the antidepressant in the morning, lowering the dose, adding a hypnotic agent (especially low doses of trazodone), or switching to a less-stimulating antidepressant. Patients with AIDS appear to be sensitive to developing akathisia, especially with fluoxetine. SSRIs may stimulate respiratory drive in patients with chronic pulmonary disease. Syndrome of inappropriate antidiuretic hormone (SIADH) has been reported with SSRI use. Withdrawal symptoms are unusual (rare with fluoxetine) and include gastrointestinal distress, visual problems, fatigue, palpitations, dizziness, paresthesias, anxiety and panic, irritability, and vivid dreams.

Serotonin syndrome may occur with concomitant use of other serotonergic agents. Signs and symptoms include confusion, agitation, anxiety, headache, dizziness, hyperthermia, diaphoresis, tachycardia, hypertension, dilated pupils, tachypnea, nausea, myoclonus, hyperreflexia, muscle rigidity, restlessness, tremor, and seizure. This is often misdiagnosed as escalation of psychiatric symptoms.

SSRIs need to be completely washed out before switching to an MAOI because of the potential for a hypertensive reaction, especially with fluoxetine, which can take as long as 6 to 7 weeks to clear. They may also inhibit the metabolism of TCAs and carbamazepine, resulting in toxicity.

TRICYCLIC ANTIDEPRESSANTS The tertiary amine TCAs (amitriptyline, imipramine, doxepin, and trimipramine) are less well tolerated than the secondary amine TCAs (nortriptyline, desipramine, and protriptyline). TCAs are highly lipophilic and 63 to 98% protein bound. The dose-response curve is usually linear.

Except for nortriptyline (which is twice as potent) and protriptyline (which is five times as potent), dosing may begin at 25 to 75 mg, given once daily at bedtime, then increased by 25 mg every 1 to 2 days until intolerable side effects develop, 150 mg is reached, or the patient demonstrates a positive response. Protriptyline should be given in the morning because of potential activation. Plasma levels may be obtained 7 days after the patient has been on a fixed dose (see Table 16-5-14). Plasma levels can be helpful in patients who are having more side effects than expected, fail to respond to a usual therapeutic dose, or are on another medication that may alter TCA levels. Plasma levels are obtained 12 hours after the last dose.

TABLE 16-5-12. Choosing an Antidepressant

DISORDER	SSRI	TCA	MAOI	TRAZO	NEFAZ	MIRTAZ	BUPRO	VENLA	AMOX	MAPR
Anxiety	+	+	+		+	+	−			
OCD	+	2				+			+	
Bingeing	1						+			
Atypical	+	−	+				+			
Dysthymia	+	−	+				+			
Agitation	+			+	+	+				
ADHD	3						+			
Melancholia		+								
Bereavement		+								
Substance abuse	+									
Premenstrual	+						+			
Delusions		−							+	
Schizophrenia		−							+	
Children		−								
Seizure							−			−
Chronic pain		+								
Migraine	+	+	+		+	+				
Fibromyalgia		4				+				
Gastric hyperacidity		5								
Obesity	6						+			
Narcolepsy		+		+						
Diabetes		+	−							
CAD	+	−	−	−			+			−
Liver disease					−		−			
Hypertension								−		
Glaucoma, closed angle		−								

+ = Consider using
− = Avoid or use with caution
1 = Fluoxetine
2 = Clomipramine
3 = Fluoxetine
4 = Usually smaller than antidepressant doses
5 = Doxepin
6 = Fluoxetine, fluvoxamine

ABBREVIATIONS: Disorders: OCD, obsessive-compulsive disorder; ADHD, attention-deficit/hyperactivity disorder; CAD, coronary artery disease. Medications: SSRI, selective serotonin reuptake inhibitor; TCA, tricyclic antidepressant; MAOI, monoamine oxidase inhibitor; Trazo, trazodone; Nefaz, nefazodone; Mirtaz, mirtazapine; Bupro, bupropion; Venla, venlafaxine; Amox, amoxapine; Mapr, maprotiline.

Lower starting doses should be considered for women, who tend to be more sensitive to side effects. Ingestion of food has no effect on bioavailability. Obese patients may require higher doses. TCAs are excreted in breast milk. TCAs are also used to treat anxiety, chronic pain, headache, fibromyalgia, gastric hyperacidity (especially doxepin), and narcolepsy.

Predictors of good response to TCAs include insidious symptom onset, upper socioeconomic class, presence of biologic symptoms (anorexia, weight loss, middle and late insomnia, psychomotor disturbance), and orthostatic hypotension in response to treatment. Predictors of poor response include the presence of neurotic, hypochondriac, and hysterical traits; history of multiple prior episodes; presence of delusions; and atypical symptoms (hypersomnia, hyperphagia, profound anergy, mood reactivity, rejection sensitivity, and nocturnal worsening of mood). Switching to another TCA in response to an adequate but ineffective TCA trial is usually not helpful.

The tertiary amines have more histaminic (e.g., weight gain, drowsiness) and anticholinergic (e.g., dry mouth, constipation, blurred vision, urinary retention) effects than the secondary amines. Anticholinergic side effects may be treated with bethanecol 10 to 30 mg once to twice daily. Galactorrhea and a fine resting tremor may also occur. Dry mouth may be treated by increasing fluid intake, chewing sugarless gum, sucking on sugarless candy, using saliva substitutes, rinsing with 1% pilocarpine three to four times daily, or taking pilocarpine 5 mg orally thrice daily. Weight gain is common and may be prevented or treated with regular exercise.

Sexual dysfunction (anorgasmia, impotence, and painful ejaculation) is common with TCA use. TCAs may impair pulmonary toilet in patients with chronic respiratory disorders. Potential cardiovascular side effects include orthostatic hypotension, tachycardia, prolonged ventricular conduction, prolonged PR interval, and an antiarrhythmic effect. Nortriptyline appears to have significantly fewer cardiovascular

TABLE 16-5-13.   Drug Interactions Related to the Cytochrome P-450 System

ENZYME	SUBSTRATE	INHIBITOR	INDUCER
CYP1A2	Acetaminophen *Amitriptyline* Caffeine *Clomipramine* Clozapine *Fluvoxamine +++* Haloperidol *Imipramine* Olanzapine Ondansetron Propranolol Tacrine Theophylline Verapamil Warfarin	*Bupropion +* Cimetidine Ciprofloxacin Diltiazem Erythromycin Fluoroquinolones *Fluoxetine ++* *Fluvoxamine +++* Grapefruit juice *Mirtazapine +* *Nefazodone +* *Paroxetine ++* *Sertraline +* Tacrine *Venlafaxine +*	Charbroiled meat Cruciferous vegetables Omeprazole Phenobarbital Phenytoin Rifampin Tobacco
CYP2B6	*Bupropion +* Cyclophosphamide Orphenadrine		
CYP2C9/10	Diclofenac Ibuprofen Mefenamic acid Naproxen Phenytoin Piroxicam Tolbutamide *Tricyclic antidepressants* Warfarin	Amiodarone Cimetidine Disulfiram Fluconazole *Fluoxetine +++* Fluvastatin *Fluvoxamine +++* Itraconazole Ketoconazole Metronidazole Ritonavir *Sertraline +* Trimethoprim-sulfamethoxazole	Barbiturates Rifampin
CYP2C19[a]	Alprazolam *Citalopram +* *Clomipramine* Diazepam *Imipramine* Lansoprazole Omeprazole Phenytoin Propranolol	Felbamate Fluconazole *Fluoxetine ++* *Fluvoxamine +++* Omeprazole Ritonavir *Sertraline ++* *Venlafaxine +*	
CYP2E1	Acetaminophen Ethanol Isoniazid	Disulfiram	Ethanol Isoniazid
CYP2D6	*Citalopram +* Clozapine Codeine Dextromethorphan Haloperidol Encainide Flecainide *Fluoxetine* Haloperidol *Maprotiline* Metoprolol Mexiletine *Mirtazapine +* *Nefazodone +* Ondansetron Oxycodone *Paroxetine +++* Perphenazine Propranolol Risperidone Tacrine Terfenadine Thioridazine Timolol	Amiodarone *Bupropion +* Cimetidine Fentanyl *Fluoxetine +++* Fluphenazine *Fluvoxamine +* Haloperidol *Mirtazapine +* *Nefazodone +* *Paroxetine +++* Perphenazine Propoxyphene Quinidine *Sertraline +* Thioridazine *Venlafaxine +* Yohimbine	Rifampin

(Continued)

TABLE 16-5-13. (Continued)

ENZYME	SUBSTRATE	INHIBITOR	INDUCER
	Tramadol *Tricyclic antidepressants* ++ *Venlafaxine* + Verapamil		
CYP3A4	Acetaminophen Alprazolam Amiodarone Astemizole *Bupropion* + Carbamazepine Cisapride Clarithromycin Clonazepam Codeine Corticosteroids Cyclosporine Dextromethorphan Diazepam Diltiazem Disopyramide Erythromycin Estradiol Ethinyl estradiol Felodipine Fentanyl Glyburide Ketoconazole Lansoprazole Lidocaine Loratadine Lovastatin Midazolam *Mirtazapine* + *Nefazodone* +++ Nifedipine Omeprazole Ondansetron Progesterone Protease inhibitors Quinidine *Sertraline* ++ Sibutramine Sildenafil Simvastatin Tamoxifen Terfenadine Theophylline Triazolam *Tricyclic antidepressants* ++ *Venlafaxine* + Verapamil Warfarin	Cimetidine Ciprofloxacin Clarithromycin Diltiazem Erythromycin Fluconazole *Fluoxetine* ++ *Fluvoxamine* +++ Grapefruit juice Itraconazole Ketoconazole *Nefazodone* +++ Omeprazole *Paroxetine* + Protease inhibitors Quinidine *Sertraline* ++	Barbiturates Carbamazepine Glucocorticoids Phenytoin Rifabutin Rifampin

*a*18% of patients of Japanese descent and 19% of African American descent are poor metabolizers.

side effects. Heart failure can slow TCA clearance, leading to toxicity. Diabetic patients may be more sensitive to hypotensive side effects because of autonomic insufficiency. Doses of 35 to 50 mg/kg are usually fatal.

TCAs are demethylated by the CYP-450 3A4 system and hydroxylated by CYP-450 2D6. Table 16-5-13 lists some important drugs metabolized by the P-450 system. Increased plasma levels are increased with aging, smoking, liver disease (especially alcoholic), and use of oral contraceptives, methylphenidate, chloramphenicol, haloperidol, phenothiazines, cimetidine, disulfiram, and SSRIs (especially fluoxetine). Decreased plasma concentrations occur with smoking, acute alcohol ingestion, and use of barbiturates, carbamazepine,

chloral hydrate, phenytoin, and trihexyphenidyl. TCAs should be avoided in patients with closed-angle glaucoma. They may lower the seizure threshold at the upper therapeutic dosage range.

Discontinuation of TCAs should be gradual because significant withdrawal symptoms occur in 70% of patients with abrupt discontinuation. Withdrawal symptoms ("afebrile flu") begin 24 hours after the last dose, last up to 14 days, and include nausea, headache, giddiness, coryza, chills, weakness, musculoskeletal pain, and increased dreaming and nightmares.

TRAZODONE Trazodone is compatible with most other antidepressants, although serotonin syndrome is a potential complication when

TABLE 16-5-14. Therapeutic Plasma Levels

Well-Established Therapeutic Levels

Nortriptyline: 50–150 ng/mL
Amitriptyline: 80–250 ng/mL (amitriptyline + nortriptyline)
Desipramine: 125–300 ng/mL
Imipramine: 150–250 ng/mL (desipramine + imipramine)

Less-Well-Established Therapeutic Levels

Clomipramine: Up to 700 ng/mL (clomipramine + desmethylclomipramine)
Doxepin: 150–250 ng/mL (doxepin + desmethyldoxepin)
Trimipramine: 150–250 ng/mL
Fluoxetine: 200–700 ng/mL (fluoxetine + norfluoxetine)

used with other serotonergic agents. Trazodone is frequently used to treat insomnia because of its short half-life and sedating side effect, and it may block other SSRI-induced side effects as well. It may also augment the effectiveness of other antidepressants, especially the SSRIs. Trazodone may also be used to treat agitation, anger, and narcolepsy.

Other side effects include orthostatic hypotension (usually lasts 4 to 6 hours and abates with continued use), exacerbation of preexisting myocardial irritability, headache, nausea, dry mouth, constipation, reversible hepatotoxicity (first few weeks), and increased libido. A unique and potentially serious side effect is priapism, usually the first few weeks of treatment, occurring in 1 in 6000 men when dosed greater than 150 mg/d. An overdose of 16 to 17 grams may be fatal. Trazodone is highly protein bound.

NEFAZODONE Nefazodone is chemically similar to trazodone but has additional neurotransmitter activity (antagonism of 5-HT$_2$ receptors), which may make it more effective as an antianxiety agent. It has also been used to treat agitation, headache, and fibromyalgia. Nefazodone demonstrates nonlinear pharmacokinetics at doses greater than 200 mg/d. It is highly protein bound. Food may delay absorption. Usually 300 mg/d are required for efficacy.

Side effects are dose-dependent and diminish over the first 6 weeks of use. Nefazodone is less sedating than trazodone. Nefazodone may seriously interact with MAOIs because of its serotonergic activities. Adverse side effects include headache, drowsiness, dizziness, hypotension (especially orthostatic), dry mouth, nausea, constipation, diarrhea, increased appetite, pharyngitis, blurred vision, and visual trails (in 5% of patients). It does not appear to have adverse sexual effects and has not been associated with priapism.

VENLAFAXINE Venlafaxine is unique in that it increases both synaptic norepinephrine and serotonin by inhibiting reuptake, and it has some dopaminergic effect. It may be a better antidepressant for patients showing only partial response to SSRIs, though its effectiveness may diminish within 3 months of use. One-third of previously treatment-resistant patients respond to venlafaxine, but half of these eventually relapse. Venlafaxine may also be used to treat anxiety and attention-deficit/hyperactivity disorder.

Venlafaxine is only 30% protein bound, extensively metabolized in the liver, and cleared by the kidneys. Therefore, the dosage may need to be lower for patients with liver or renal dysfunction. Food has no effect on absorption. Antidepressant effect tends to be strongest at doses over 200 mg/d.

Potential side effects include dizziness, insomnia, nervousness, headache, somnolence, dry mouth, nausea, constipation, anorexia or increased appetite, yawning, sweating, and anorgasmia. Most side effects are dose-dependent. Nausea is quite common, occurring in 44% of patients when the drug is first instituted and with dosage increases. Dividing doses and giving the medication after a low-fat meal may alleviate side effects. Hypertension occurs in 10% of patients and is both dose- and age-dependent. The incidence of nausea and hypertension may be less with the long-acting form. As with TCAs, abrupt discontinuation may lead to withdrawal symptoms, such as headache,

nausea, dizziness, insomnia, and anxiety. Use with MAOIs may be associated with a hypertensive crisis.

BUPROPION Bupropion is a unique antidepressant agent that structurally resembles the amphetamines and tends to be more activating than other antidepressants. It is primarily dopaminergic, with some noradrenergic effect. Maximum daily dose is 450 mg because of the potential for seizure induction, and it must be given in divided doses, with the doses 6 hours apart. No more than 200 mg should be given in one dose. Bupropion does not appear to induce rapid cycling in bipolar disorders. It is also effective in treating attention-deficit disorder in adults, smoking cessation, premenstrual dysphoric disorder, and binging and purging, though use in bulimia has been associated with increased seizure risk, probably related to nutritional deficiencies (see Chap. 16-1).

Bupropion induces its own metabolism as well as the metabolism of other hepatically metabolized agents, such as carbamazepine. Dosage should be decreased in the presence of liver disease, as it is extensively metabolized during the first pass through the liver. It increases REM sleep.

Adverse effects include dry mouth (14%), nausea and vomiting, rash, orthostatic hypotension, hypertension, excitement and agitation, seizures (in 0.4%, especially in patients with a history of seizure disorder), weight loss (30%, dose-dependent), and increased sexual interest. No cardiovascular side effects have been identified. Anxiety may escalate early in therapy because of its stimulating properties. Bupropion should be administered early in the day because of frequent insomnia as a side effect. Bupropion could worsen psychotic symptoms and has been associated with psychotic side effects. Patients tolerate the sustained-release preparation much better than the immediate-release form.

The risk of bupropion-induced seizure in the absence of additional risk factors is 0.05% at 400 mg/d of the sustained-release preparation. The risk for the original immediate-release formulation is 0.4% at 450 mg/d, 2.3% at 600 mg/d, and 2.8% at 900 mg/d.

Adding bupropion to an SSRI is a common augmentation strategy, but may increase the risk of seizure and delirium. Patients with AIDS may also be at greater risk for seizure. Other potential drug interactions may occur with warfarin, phenytoin, carbamazepine, phenobarbital, and cimetidine. Bupropion may stimulate respiratory drive in patients with chronic pulmonary disease. It does not appear to have a withdrawal syndrome.

MIRTAZAPINE Mirtazapine is a strong blocker of α-adrenoceptors, resulting in increased noradrenalin and serotonin activity. Mirtazapine stimulates 5-HT$_1$ and blocks 5-HT$_2$ and 5-HT$_3$, resulting in an overall serotonin agonist effect. Its anxiolytic effect at 15 mg/d equals that of diazepam at 10 mg/d. Mirtazapine may also be used to treat agitation, headache, and obsessive-compulsive disorder.

Mirtazapine demonstrates linear pharmacokinetics and is 85% protein bound. A lower dose should be considered for elderly patients, who may develop higher plasma concentrations.

Potential side effects include dry mouth, drowsiness (especially at 15 mg/d), increased appetite and weight gain, orthostatic hypotension, slightly increased heart rate, transient and benign elevation of liver function tests, and increased cholesterol and triglycerides. Most side effects are mild and transient. Agranulocytosis and neutropenia have been reported as a potential rare side effect. Cognitive and motor performance may significantly deteriorate when mirtazapine is taken with alcohol or a benzodiazepine.

MONOAMINE OXIDASE INHIBITORS The MAOIs (phenelzine and tranylcypromine) are generally avoided by nonpsychiatric practitioners because of the dietary and pharmacologic restrictions required to prevent hypertensive crises. However, they are highly effective and well-tolerated antidepressants, regardless. MAOIs have also been used to treat social phobia, panic disorder, headache, narcolepsy, and bulimia.

Inhibiting monoamine oxidase results in a serotonin and noradrenalin agonist effect. MAOIs demonstrate linear pharmacokinetics.

TABLE 16-5-15. Medications and Foods to Avoid While Taking a Monoamine Oxidase Inhibitor

Drugs

    Serotonin reuptake inhibitors
        Fluoxetine (Prozac), paroxetine (Paxil), Sertraline (Zoloft), fluvoxamine (Luvox), venlafaxine (Effexor), buspirone (BuSpar).
    Cyclic antidepressants
        Amitriptyline (Elavil), nortriptyline (Pamelor), protriptyline (Vivactil), clomipramine (Anafranil), imipramine (Tofranil), desipramine (Norpramin), trimipramine (Surmontil), amoxapine (Asendin), doxepin (Adapin, Sinequan), maprotiline (Ludiomil), trazodone.
    Stimulants and decongestants
        Amphetamines, ephedrine, epinephrine, norepinephrine, isoproterenol, methylphenidate (Ritalin), phenylephrine, phenylpropanolamine, pseudoephedrine, etc. Some of these medications are commonly found in over-the-counter cold preparations and appetite suppressants. Includes decongestant nasal sprays.
    Dextromethorphan
        Found in many over-the-counter cold preparations.
    Synthetic narcotics
        Meperidine (Demerol), buprenorphine (Buprenex), propoxyphene (Darvon), fentanyl (Duragesic), nalbuphine (Nubain), butorphanol (Stadol), etc.
        Carbidopa-levodopa (Sinemet), reserpine, risperidone (Risperdal), St. John's wort.
    Barbiturates
        May cause excessive sedation.
    Diabetic medications
    Medications used to treat diabetes may result in excessively low bloodsugar.
    Herbal remedies
        Ginkgo biloba may interfere with effectiveness.

Foods

    Cheeses
        All cheeses (including sour cream) except cream cheese, American cheese, ricotta, cottage cheese, and yogurt.
    Drinks
        Beer, sherry, Chianti and other red wines, all distilled alcohols.
    Yeast/protein extracts
        Yeast is safe when baked, e.g., in bread.
    Meats
        All smoked or pickled meats, including fish and other seafood.
        Beef or chicken livers.
        Fermented sausages.
        Bologna, pepperoni, salami, summer sausage.
    Fruits
        Avocados, figs, raisins, banana peel.
    Fermented bean curd
        Soybeans, soy paste, soy sauce.
    Fava or broad beans.
    Large amounts of caffeine or chocolate.
    Other
        High-protein foods that have undergone degeneration (e.g., old leftovers).

They are usually given twice daily. At least a 2-week wash-out is required when changing between an MAOI and most of the other antidepressants. Onset of action may be longer than that for other antidepressants. MAOIs are lethal when an overdose is taken.

MAOIs are especially effective for atypical depression, especially atypical features (symptoms worse in the evening, initial insomnia, increased appetite and weight gain, hypersomnia), dysthymia, anxiety (especially with agoraphobia), and bipolar depression. Abrupt discontinuation may lead to vivid and frightening dreams, so gradual withdrawal is usually recommended.

Side effects include sedation or stimulation, orthostatic hypotension (primarily the first two months of treatment), hepatic damage, muscle tension, myoclonic jerks, and acute hypertensive crisis associated with certain foods and medications (see Table 16-5-15). Peripheral neuropathy, ataxia, hyperacusis, irritability, and seizures may occur if the patient is also pyridoxine deficient, so many practitioners recommend vitamin supplementation. Orthostatic hypotension can be relieved by dividing the dose, giving it once daily at bedtime, or by increasing sodium intake. Sedation may be avoided by giving the full dose at bedtime, and stimulation may be avoided by giving once daily before 5:00 P.M. The sexual dysfunction associated with MAOIs can be treated with bethanechol 10 mg, 30 min prior to intercourse.

Symptoms of a hypertensive crisis include a soaring blood pressure, severe headache, chest pain, fever, and vomiting. The hypertension has been treated with sublingual nifedipine, but this is controversial. Hypoglycemia may occur when given with insulin and oral hypoglycemic agents. Use with succinylcholine may lead to prolonged muscle relaxation.

Withdrawal symptoms following abrupt discontinuation are common and include vivid and frightening dreams, headache, hypotension, weakness, insomnia, anxiety, delirium, hallucinations, and paranoia. Onset is in days, with duration of up to 5 days.

AMOXAPINE Amoxapine inhibits reuptake of both noradrenalin and serotonin, with significant dopamine-blocking properties (similar to haloperidol), and is metabolized by the liver. Side effects are common and include anticholinergic symptoms, hypotension, sedation, seizures, extrapyramidal symptoms, tardive dyskinesia, and hyperprolactinemia. Since the development of better-tolerated antidepressants, amoxapine is rarely used.

ST. JOHN'S WORT St. John's wort is an herb commonly used in Europe to treat mild to moderate depression. The mechanism of action is unknown. It appears to inhibit noradrenalin and serotonin reuptake, increase dopamine and nocturnal melatonin, and inhibit prolactin. Hypericin (one chemical present in St. John's wort) is an MAOI, but not at clinical doses. Its effectiveness in treating mild to moderate depression may be comparable to phototherapy and standard antidepressants. It is also as effective as diazepam for treating anxiety.

St. John's wort demonstrates almost a linear dose-response curve. It is dosed at 900 mg/d of the extract or 0.9 mg/d of hypericin. Six to eight weeks may be required for effectiveness. Symptoms responsive to St. John's wort include depressed mood, sleep latency, fear, and somatic complaints. St. John's wort is very well tolerated, with no reported significant drug interactions or toxicity. Because it is not regulated by the FDA in the United States, purity and potency may vary from batch to batch and company to company. Long-term side effects and risk of relapse is not known. Valerian root may potentiate the antidepressant effect.

REBOXETINE Reboxetine represents a new class of antidepressants that are not yet available in the United States. It is a selective noradrenalin reuptake inhibitor and seems to be especially helpful for treating low motivation and energy, rejection sensitivity, and social isolation. It is dosed at 8 to 10 mg/d, 4 to 6 mg/d for the elderly. Side effects include constipation, insomnia, dry mouth, sweating, headache, and hypotension.

STRATEGIES FOR TREATMENT RESISTANCE An adequate treatment trial is 6 to 8 weeks at full dose (or serum levels for TCAs). When a patient fails to respond to a treatment trial, medication compliance problems, hypothyroidism (including subclinical), presence of a sleep disorder, substance abuse, estrogen deficiency, and other primary or comorbid conditions should be ruled out. Treatment options include increasing dose to the upper range (see Table 16-5-9), drug substitution, antidepressant combinations, augmentation, and addition of other treatment methods (e.g., phototherapy or psychotherapy). Consider changing to an antidepressant of a different class if there is no response to an adequate trial, though changing among the SSRIs may be effective.

If there has been incomplete response, consider combining antidepressants. An SSRI may be combined with a TCA (with caution, as TCA blood levels can be significantly elevated with concomitant SSRI use). Mirtazapine, trazodone, or nefazodone may be added to an SSRI.

Combining an SSRI (or TCA) with bupropion is becoming increasingly popular; however, this combination may lower the seizure threshold.

AUGMENTATION   Augmentation may also be considered for patients who demonstrate a partial response to an adequate antidepressant trial. Augmentation is often preferred over switching antidepressants for patients who develop a recurrence while on a maintenance antidepressant regimen because of a potentially quicker response and avoidance of symptom escalation during an antidepressant switch. Of the augmenting agents discussed below, no one is more efficacious than another. Some patients can discontinue the augmenting agent after 2 to 4 months, but most will need to continue the augmenting agent indefinitely with the primary antidepressant.

Lithium has the largest body of evidence for augmentation. It has an antidepressant effect when used as monotherapy, but because of its adverse effects profile and difficulty of use, its main use in the treatment of affective disorders is as a mood stabilizer and as an augmenting agent. (See Chap. 16-6 for more information about lithium.) About 70% of bipolar patients and 50% of unipolar patients respond to lithium augmentation. Predictors of good response include presence of bipolar symptoms, family history of bipolar disorder, mood lability, history of postpartum depression, hypersomnia, hyperphagia, and early age of onset. About 75% of patients who partially respond on a TCA demonstrate a 50% or better improvement in symptoms within 48 hours of adding lithium. Half of partially responding patients on an SSRI demonstrate symptomatic improvement. Use with bupropion may lower the seizure threshold.

Buspirone is a serotonergic antianxiety agent which may be used to augment the effect of SSRIs, TCAs, and bupropion, especially in the presence of concurrent anxiety symptoms (see Chap. 16-3). It has antidepressant properties when used as monotherapy at high doses.

Stimulants are generally not effective first-line agents for the treatment of depression, but they can be effective for augmentation. They are especially useful in elderly and medically ill patients and for symptoms of lethargy and lack of motivation. Response may often occur within 1 to 4 days, and abuse is rare when used for augmentation.

Triiodothyronine (T_3) is effective as an augmenting agent for patients with normal thyroid indices (replacement with thyroxine is used for patients with clinical or subclinical hypothyroidism). Effectiveness for augmentation is best documented with the TCAs. T_3 may be used in augmentation for both unipolar and bipolar (in either phase) disorders. Onset of TCA antidepressant action may be accelerated when T_3 is started simultaneously with the TCA. Usual dosage is 0.05 mg/d. There appears to be no dose-response relationship. Response may occur within 2 to 4 weeks.

The beta blocker pindolol also has $5-HT_{1A}$ antagonist activity and has demonstrated effectiveness as an augmenting agent in some studies. Concomitant use at the start of an antidepressant trial may result in a quicker therapeutic response. It is dosed at 5 to 20 mg/d.

Neuroleptics (antipsychotics) are usually required when psychotic symptoms are present. Because patients with affective disorders may be at higher risk for developing tardive dyskinesia, and because of the well-tolerated side-effect profile, the atypicals (olanzapine, risperidone, and quetiapine) are preferred. Olanzapine has demonstrated antidepressant activity as monotherapy for patients without psychotic symptoms.

Thymoleptics (mood stabilizers) such as carbamazepine, valproic acid, lamotrigine, gabapentin, and topiramate have shown some efficacy as augmenting agents, even for unipolar depression. Clonazepam may be helpful for patients with comorbid anxiety. Patients with postpartum and perimenopausal depressive symptoms may respond to estrogen. Other augmentation strategies include moclobemide (a reversible MAOI-A), selegiline (a reversible MAOI-B), inositol, bromocriptine, mifepristone, dexamethasone, dehydroepiandrosterone, corticotropin-releasing factor, substance P, and antiglucocorticoids (e.g., metyrapone, aminoglutethimide, ketoconazole). There are numerous other agents currently under investigation for the treatment of depression. Consultation with a provider familiar with these new agents is indicated prior to their use.

OTHER CONSIDERATIONS

Pregnancy and Nursing   No antidepressant has FDA approval for use during pregnancy. However, the risks of untreated depression during pregnancy are well documented. For many patients the benefits of antidepressant pharmacotherapy outweigh the potential risks. All psychotropic drugs are highly lipophilic, therefore crossing the blood-brain barrier and probably the placenta as well. No evidence has been documented of teratogenicity in all but the MAOIs. The concentration of antidepressants in breast milk varies. Irritability, colic, and poor feeding have been reported in nursing infants of mothers taking antidepressants. ECT (see below) also appears to be safe during pregnancy. (See Cohen and Altshuler for a more thorough discussion.)

Elderly Patients   Treatment response may be slower in elderly patients. The elderly are more sensitive to medication side effects, may develop higher drug levels, and metabolize many drugs slower. Initial dosage should be lower for elderly patients and increases should be more gradual. The number of agents used should be limited and the medication regimen simple. Avoid treating medication-related side effects with another drug. Have the patient bring all medications (including over-the-counter and "natural") to each appointment. Patients with late-onset depression require lifelong pharmacotherapy.

Other Somatic Treatments

ECT is the gold standard for the treatment of depression, with 80% of patients responding, often rapidly and dramatically. Current indications include severe depression, treatment resistance, psychotic depression, high suicide risk, the presence of cardiovascular disease precluding use of antidepressants, and pregnancy. ECT causes short-term memory loss and confusion. There is no evidence of permanent brain damage or permanent memory loss. Patients are at high risk for relapse if maintenance antidepressant pharmacotherapy is not instituted during or immediately following an ECT series.

Phototherapy is effective for both treatment and prevention of seasonal depression and is only effective when used during the winter months. The usual "dose" is 10,000 lux for 30 to 45 minutes. It is usually used in the morning, but some patients use a "booster dose" in the late afternoon. Patients respond within 1 to 2 weeks, and efficacy tends to remain stable over time. An adequate treatment trial is 2 weeks. The only adverse effect is a slight risk for precipitation of mania. Continued use of phototherapy during the high-risk seasons decreases the risk of recurrence.

Sleep deprivation (patient remains awake from 2:00 A.M. through 10:00 P.M.) can have immediate, but short-term antidepressant effects, often effective in 1 to 3 nights. Patients with atypical symptoms and sensitivity to changes in sleep/wake cycle, work schedule, and time zone tend to respond the best.

Transcranial magnetic stimulation has demonstrated effectiveness in some small studies. The mechanism of action may be similar to ECT. No anesthesia is required. Side effects include headache, discomfort at the site of stimulation, and seizures when high intensities and frequencies are used.

Psychotherapy

Cognitive-behavioral and interpersonal psychotherapy have demonstrated effectiveness equal to pharmacotherapy in the treatment of mild to moderate depression, though individual response varies widely. Formal therapy may be time-consuming, expensive, not covered by third-party payers, and not widely available, especially in rural areas.

Intense exploration into personal problems during an acute depressive episode is contraindicated, as it may heighten negativity and hopelessness. Patients with melancholic features and psychotic symptoms and patients with poor insight may not respond as well to psychotherapeutic techniques. Therapeutic factors associated with effectiveness include an active and directive therapist, focus on current problems, emphasis on changing current behavior, self-monitoring of change and progress, use of homework, and a predetermined number of sessions.

COGNITIVE-BEHAVIORAL THERAPY Cognitive-behavioral therapy (CBT) has been the most studied psychotherapy technique in the treatment of depression. Cognitive interventions include identifying dysfunctional automatic thoughts, challenging cognitive distortions, cognitive restructuring, and problem solving. Common cognitive distortions present in depressed patients include all-or-nothing thinking, over-generalization, selective abstraction, emotional reasoning, personalization, disqualifying the positive, jumping to conclusions, magnification or minimization, labeling, and arbitrary inferences (i.e., mind reading, fortune telling). CBT also decreases the likelihood of relapse and residual symptoms.

Behavioral interventions include activity scheduling, development of mastery and pleasurable activities, graded task assignments, and assertiveness training. Clinicians specifically trained in these techniques should perform formal CBT.

INTERPERSONAL THERAPY In interpersonal therapy, patients are assisted in developing functional strategies to deal with specific problem areas such as grief, interpersonal disputes, role transitions, and interpersonal deficits. Attention is placed on relationships, using the therapeutic relationship as an example.

OTHER THERAPY APPROACHES Family therapy enhances support and compliance. Marital therapy may be helpful for support and in mild depression associated with marital strife. Dysthymia tends to respond best to social skills training, problem solving, and a focus on the present. Group therapy appears to be as effective as individual therapy and is more cost-effective.

BIBLIOGRAPHY/RECOMMENDED READINGS

American Psychiatric Association: *Practice Guidelines for Major Depressive Disorder.* 1996.

Beck AT et al: *Cognitive Therapy of Depression.* New York, Guilford, 1979.

Cohen LS, Altshuler LL: Pharmacologic management of psychiatric illness during pregnancy and postpartum period. *Psychiatr Clin North Am* 4:21–60, 1997.

Hornig-Rohan M, Amsterdam JD: Treatment-resistant depression. *Psychiatr Clin North Am* 19:2, 1996.

Keller MB: Mood disorders. *Psychiatr Clin North Am* 19:1, 1996.

Paykel ES: *Handbook of Affective Disorders.* New York, Guilford, 1992.

Sansone RA, Sansone LA: Dysthymic disorder: The chronic depression. *Am Fam Physician* 53(8):2588–2594, 1996.

Stuart MR, Lieberman JA: *The Fifteen Minute Hour: Applied Psychotherapy for the Primary Care Physician,* 2d ed, Westport, CT, Praeger, 1993.

US Department of Health and Human Services: *Clinical Practice Guidelines for Recognition and Treatment of Major Depression.* 1993.

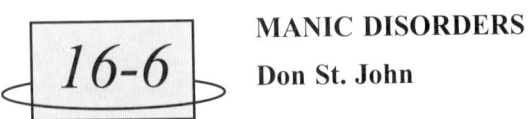

MANIC DISORDERS
Don St. John

DISCUSSION

Mania is the defining symptom of bipolar affective disorders (BPADs), which have a 1% lifetime prevalence and equal distribution in men and women. Age of onset is usually late adolescence to the middle of the fourth decade. An affective disorder is present in first-degree relatives more than 50% of the time.

The *Diagnostic and Statistical Manual of Mental Disorders,* fourth edition (*DSM-IV*) criteria for a manic episode are

1. A distinct period of abnormally and persistently elevated mood, lasting at least 1 week.
2. Three or more of the following symptoms:
   a. Inflated self-esteem
   b. Decreased need for sleep
   c. More talkative than usual or pressured speech
   d. Flight of ideas
   e. Distractibility
   f. Increase in goal-directed activity or agitation
   g. Excessive involvement in pleasurable activities
3. Sufficient severity to cause marked impairment of functioning.

Manic patients without psychotic symptoms have *classic mania.* *Hypomania* (mild euphoria or irritability, expansive speech, reduced sleep) is characterized by the same criteria as mania but is not severe enough to cause marked impairment of functioning. *Cyclothymia* is characterized by numerous episodes of alternating depression and hypomania, to a less severe degree than hypomania. Of patients with cyclothymia, 15 to 50% will eventually develop BPAD type I (alternating periods of depression and mania) or II (alternating periods of depression and hypomania).

SIGNS AND SYMPTOMS

A manic patient's mood is always and persistently elated, angry, and/or irritable. The affect is hyperreactive and labile. This mood elevation is usually not recognized as abnormal by the patient, both during and after the episode.

Grandiose ideas and delusions are common. Predominant themes may be religious, sexual, financial, political, and persecutory. Often one or two themes predominate. Eutonia (a subjective sense of well-being), inflated self-esteem, and grandiosity are frequently present. Thought and perception appear to the patient to be unusually sharp and brilliant.

A significant decrease in need for sleep is often present, and the patient may find very brief periods of sleep refreshing. Speech may be pressured, loud, rapid, and difficult to interrupt. The patient may switch topics abruptly and even talk when alone.

The patient may be easily distractible, rapidly going from one activity to another. Decreased attention occurs to both internal and external cues. Increased goal-directed behavior and thoughts are distinguishing symptoms of mania.. There is often an increase in energy with psychomotor hyperactivity or agitation. Weight loss may occur in response to both increased physical activity and inattention to nutritional needs. Disinhibition may be exhibited by increased sexual talk or behavior, overly familiar and demanding demeanor toward others, over-spending, fast driving, and aggression.

From 20 to 80% of acutely manic patients develop psychotic symptoms. Delusions are usually of grandeur but may be paranoid as well. Delusions tend not to be fixed and persistent as in schizophrenia, though 10% of patients may exhibit continued delusional thinking 2 years after the manic episode. Hallucinations, usually auditory, tend to reflect prevailing delusions.

The manic patient usually demonstrates poor insight, both during and after a manic episode. Mania may last a few days to months, with an average duration (untreated) of 3 to 6 months. Mania often follows a depressive episode. Mania can be precipitated by drug withdrawal (especially rapid discontinuation of lithium), stressful life events (especially if associated with sleep deprivation), antidepressant pharmacotherapy (though this is controversial), seasonal changes (mania is more likely during the spring months), sleep deprivation, hormonal changes (especially the postpartum period), and light exposure.

Atypical symptoms include dysphoria, rapid-cycling, mixed manic and depressed symptoms, and lithium unresponsiveness. Mania of organic etiology is more likely to present in an atypical manner.

COURSE OF ILLNESS

Without treatment, a manic episode lasts 6 to 24 weeks. The average lifetime number of episodes is 9 to 10. There is an 85% risk of relapse after the first manic episode, 50% risk during the first year. Episodes may recur every 2 years, with the interepisode interval progressively diminishing with each subsequent episode. Half of patients may experience subsyndromal interepisode symptoms, which is a predictor of high risk for relapse. One-tenth of patients will be continuously manic for 7 years, one-third for 2 to 4 years. Mixed mania (both manic and depressive symptoms) is associated with a high risk for suicide.

Elderly patients may demonstrate more cognitive impairment, slower flight of ideas, and less grandiosity. They often do not exhibit the full manic syndrome as younger patients do. They are also often less responsive to treatment.

DIAGNOSTIC CONSIDERATIONS

Distinguishing an acute manic episode from an acute psychotic episode as in schizophrenia, and especially schizoaffective disorder, can be difficult. Patients with BPAD tend to have normal personality and general functioning between discrete episodes of mania, as opposed to the persistent presence of negative symptoms (social withdrawal, lack of motivation, poverty of speech, etc.) characteristic of schizophrenic patients. The triad of manic mood, rapid or pressured speech, and hyperactivity is a robust finding in mania. There is more disturbance of mood, more overactivity and physical agitation, and more elation with mania. A manic episode tends to have an abrupt onset. There is less formal thought disorder in mania, and delusions and hallucinations tend to reflect the mood disturbance. Affective and schizophrenic family histories tend to be distinct.

There is a significant overlap of symptoms for patients with BPAD type II and borderline personality disorder, making distinction difficult. Truly manic patients have a more abrupt onset and offset of mood changes and manic behavior, with more stable premorbid and interepisode periods, than patients with personality disorders, who tend to exhibit much more affective instability and hyperreactivity. The interpersonal relating style of a personality-disordered patient remains constant, whereas, with bipolar disorder, interpersonal dysfunction clears between episodes. Symptoms of attention-deficit/hyperactivity disorder tend to be more chronic, with less clear onset and offset of symptoms, absence of expansive mood, clear presence during childhood, and lack of psychotic symptoms.

Mania is more likely to be secondary or organic if the first episode occurs after age 40 or before puberty, and if a family history of affective disorders is absent. The mood tends to be more irritable than expansive, patients are less likely to be psychotic, and patients tend to respond better to antiseizure medications than lithium. Table 16-6-1 lists drugs and illnesses that have been associated with manic symptoms.

Evaluation of a first episode of mania may include thyroid function studies, complete blood count, blood glucose, drug and alcohol screen, head scan (computed tomography or magnetic resonance imaging, as indicated by historical and physical findings), electroencephalogram, and a thorough physical examination, with special attention to the neurologic exam, to rule out secondary causes.

Comorbidity

Higher rates of obsessive-compulsive disorder occur in bipolar patients. Comorbid impulse control disorder may predate the formal diagnosis of BPAD.

Patients with BPAD have the highest rate (more than half) of comorbid drug and alcohol abuse of all psychiatric disorders. They tend to develop alcohol dependence rather than abuse. Alcohol abuse and dependence predict a poor response to lithium.

TREATMENT

Mood Stabilizers (Thymoleptics)

Lithium is most effective for the treatment of classic mania, resulting in improvement in 70% of manic patients, with average doses of 1200

TABLE 16-6-1.   Secondary Causes of Mania

Pharmacologic

  Amphetamines
  Anabolic steroids
  Anticholinergics
  Baclofen
  Bromide
  Bromocriptine
  Caffeine
  Calcium replacement
  Captopril
  Chloroquine
  Cimetidine
  Clarithromycin
  Cocaine
  Corticosteroids
  Disulfiram
  Hallucinogens
  Heterocyclic antidepressants
  Hydralazine
  Isoniazid
  Khat
  Levodopa
  Methylphenidate
  Metrizamide
  Monoamine oxidase inhibitors
  Opiates
  Procarbazine
  Procyclidine
  Sympathomimetics
  Yohimbine

Infectious

  Neurosyphilis
  Encephalitis
  Influenza
  Lyme borreliosis
  AIDS

Endocrine

  Addison's disease
  Cushing's disease
  Hyperthyroidism
  Hypothyroidism
  Postpartum
  Menses-related

Neurologic

  Multiple sclerosis
  Huntington's chorea
  Wilson's disease
  Head trauma
  Complex partial seizures
  Diencephalic and third ventricle tumors
  Cerebrovascular events
  Migraine
  Neoplasms

Nutritional

  Deficiencies of
    Vitamin B_{12}
    Folate
    Niacin
    Thiamin

Other

  Systemic lupus erythematosus
  Rheumatic chorea
  Light therapy
  Polycythemia
  Electroconvulsive therapy
  Treatment-resistant obstructive sleep apnea

to 2400 mg/d. Twelve-hour blood levels should be targeted at 0.9 to 1.4 mg/dL during an acute episode. Steady state is achieved in 4 to 5 days. Lithium clearance is increased during acute mania, so levels may rise as the patient responds to treatment. Relapse is less likely if therapeutic levels of lithium are continued during the maintenance phase of treatment. Once the patient is stable, the dose may be given once daily, usually at bedtime. Elderly patients may respond to a lower dose.

Side effects include tremor, nausea and vomiting, diarrhea, cognitive dulling, polyuria, and polydipsia. Lithium may exacerbate psoriasis. Long-term use of lithium can result in significant weight gain, decreased renal function, and hypothyroidism. Significant drug interactions may occur with thiazide diuretics, nonsteroidal anti-inflammatory agents, angiotensin converting enzyme (ACE) inhibitors, and some antipsychotics. Signs of lithium toxicity include tremor, nausea and vomiting, diarrhea, and confusion. There is a 4 to 12% risk of a congenital malformation when taken during pregnancy. Predictors of poor response to lithium include atypical presentation, history of more than three lifetime manic episodes, and prior poor response to lithium. Three weeks at a therapeutic serum level constitutes an adequate therapeutic trial.

Valproic acid and divalproex appear to be more effective for atypical and rapid-cycling mania, and overall as effective as lithium. Valproic acid may be started at 750 mg/d in divided doses and increased 250 to 500 mg/d until a 12-h therapeutic level of 50 to 120 μg/mL is achieved. Once the patient is stable, valproic acid may be administered once daily, usually at bedtime. Valproate may also be initiated at 20 mg/kg per day. Steady state occurs in 2 days. Benign liver function studies elevation occurs in 5 to 15% of patients and does not predict hepatic failure, which is a rare complication.

Potential side effects include nausea, sedation, tremor, and rarely blood dyscrasia. A few patients will gain weight while taking valproate. Alopecia may occur, which is temporary and reversible, even if the patient remains on the medication. Neural tube defects have been reported in infants of mothers taking valproic acid. Drug interactions may occur with some neuroleptics, tricyclic antidepressants, aspirin, erythromycin, and fluoxetine.

Carbamazepine is also more effective than lithium for atypical symptoms and rapid cycling, and overall as effective as lithium. Carbamazepine is given at 400 to 1000 mg/d to a therapeutic 12-h serum level of 6 to 12 μg/mL. Steady state is achieved in 3 to 4 days. Carbamazepine induces its own metabolism, so blood levels must be checked regularly and the dosage adjusted as indicated during the first several months of use.

Potential side effects include weight gain, nausea, sedation, ataxia, anticholinergic effects in elderly patients, and temporary and reversible alopecia. Benign liver function studies increases occur in 5 to 15% of cases. About 10 to 20% of patients will develop a decrease in white blood cell count, which is not predictive of aplastic anemia or agranulocytosis, rare side effects. Carbamazepine also induces the metabolism of several other drugs, especially antipsychotics. Carbamazepine may also lower the effectiveness of oral contraceptives. Neural tube defects and neonatal hemorrhage have been associated with carbamazepine use during pregnancy.

Recent studies indicate that other antiseizure medications, such as gabapentin, lamotrigine, and topiramate, are effective, with favorable side-effect profiles, low toxicity, and an absence of need for therapeutic drug levels.

Antipsychotics

High- and low-potency antipsychotics and atypical antipsychotics (risperidone, olanzapine, quetiapine, and clozapine) appear to be equally effective as the thymoleptics described above in treating the symptoms of flight of ideas, delusions, psychomotor agitation, and combativeness. Patients may require high doses. Patients with affective disorders may be at increased risk for developing tardive dyskinesia so

discontinuation of an antipsychotic (especially the typicals) should follow symptom resolution and adequate thymoleptic therapy. The attempted taper should be very gradual. However, some patients may require maintenance treatment with an antipsychotic. The atypicals appear to be related to a lower risk of tardive dyskinesia and should be considered first. Depot neuroleptics have been used successfully in patients who have mainly manic episodes (rather than depression) and have been difficult to manage.

Benzodiazepines

Benzodiazepines are useful in decreasing psychomotor agitation, aggression, and logorrhea. They tend to normalize sleep, which in itself is therapeutic during a manic episode. Tapering of these drugs should be considered as behavior normalizes; however, continued use is associated with a lower relapse rate in some patients. Clonazepam 1 mg every 4 to 6 hours or lorazepam 2 to 4 mg orally or intramuscularly every 2 hours are typical doses.

Other Drugs

Other drugs reported as effective in treating manic symptoms in small studies and case reports include verapamil, nimodipine, clonidine, fenfluramine, thyroid supplementation, choline, donepezil, and omega-3 fatty acids.

Electroconvulsive Therapy

Electroconvulsive therapy (ECT) is highly effective in treating mania and may be considered when mood stabilizers are relatively contraindicated, such as during pregnancy, in the elderly, in patients with epilepsy, and in patients with cardiovascular disease. Remission or significant clinical improvement occurs in 80% of patients, including 50 to 60% of patients who have failed to respond to standard thymoleptic pharmacotherapy. Lithium should be discontinued prior to ECT treatments, as concomitant use may be associated with a higher risk of organic brain syndrome. Concurrent use of antiseizure medications and benzodiazepines may interfere with effectiveness. Maintenance ECT has been effective in controlling otherwise intractable bipolar illness but is little studied.

Other Treatment Considerations

Psychosocial management is not possible during an acute manic state because of the absence of insight. Patients should be protected from the consequences of their behaviors. Avoid confining manic patients in a small space. Restrict telephone use to avoid excessive charges. Maintain the environment with as little stimulation as possible. Set limits in a nonambivalent and firm manner.

Antidepressants (especially tricyclic antidepressants) should be discontinued unless past history suggests otherwise. Sleep should be induced quickly to prevent escalation of manic symptoms. Clinicians should be aware of the potential for aggressive and assaultive behaviors, especially when the patient exhibits suspiciousness, agitation, and excitement.

Inpatient treatment should be considered when the patient is unable to cooperate with treatment, at risk for suicidal or homicidal behavior, pregnant, lacks an adequate social support system, or when protection from the consequences of poor judgment is necessary. The patient may be discharged when there has been a significant reduction in symptoms, good social support, and a commitment to continued treatment.

Mood stabilizers should be continued on an outpatient basis for at least 4 to 6 months, usually at the dose (or blood level) required for control of acute symptoms. Indefinite continuation of mood-stabilizer therapy should be considered after three or more episodes of depression and mania, one severe episode, or three hypomanic episodes. Most patients will require two or more medications for maintenance.

The presence of good social support between episodes decreases the risk of relapse. Educating the patient and significant others regarding treatment and course of illness can enhance treatment compliance.

COMPLICATIONS

Complications are primarily social, with increased marital discord and divorce and significant business difficulties. Finances may be severely exhausted through spending sprees. Sexual indiscretions increase the risk of sexually transmitted diseases and may further damage the patient's significant relationships. Death from physical exhaustion or dangerous activities may occur. Acutely manic patients are at high risk for both suicide and homicide.

BIBLIOGRAPHY

American Psychiatric Association: *Diagnostic and Statistical Manual of Mental Disorders,* 4th ed, Washington, DC, American Psychiatric Association, 1994.

Brown ES, Suppes T: Bipolar disorders. *Psychiatr Clin North Am Ann Drug Ther* 5:145–160, 1998.

Wender SF: An update on the diagnosis and treatment of mania in bipolar disorder. *Am Fam Physician* 51(5):1126–1136, 1995.

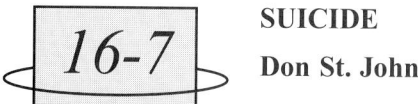

SUICIDE

Don St. John

DISCUSSION

Suicide is a growing problem worldwide. At least 20% of the population has seriously considered or attempted suicide. Approximately 1% of the population will complete a suicide. There are 30,000 suicides per year in the United States, 1000 per day in the world. In the United States, suicide is the eighth leading cause of death overall, the second leading cause of death in the 15- to 24-year-old age group, and the leading cause of death in lock-ups. There has been a gradual increase in the suicide rate during this century, though little variation in the past 15 years. The suicide rate for adolescents tripled between 1952 and 1992. There are significant differences in the suicide rate internationally. Suicide rates tend to diminish during war, rise during times of economic stress, increase with media coverage of suicide, and peak during the spring.

The method of suicide is determined by availability and cultural acceptability. Firearms are the preferred method in the United States. Hanging is the preferred method in locked inpatient psychiatric units, and jumping for other inpatient units. Patients who choose overdosing tend to take whatever medications they can find, prescription and nonprescription, with no particular drug class preferred. The meaning of suicide varies by culture.

Baechler has defined the act of suicide as "when people are using their own deaths instrumentally to try to solve their problems of living." Suicide is an outcome behavior, not a specific disorder, which involves a continuum or spectrum of behaviors, from consideration to ideation, planning, attempting, and completion. Survivors (those with a significant relationship with the victim) may be considered the final phase.

Completed suicide is the final act that results in the death of the victim. Attempted suicide (*parasuicide,* suicide gesture) does not result in death. Some patients perform self-harm behaviors with no intent of causing death. Reasons for *self-harm* may include trying to "feel something" (e.g., during dissociative episodes), releasing tension, punishing self or others, attention-seeking, vengeance, or escape (e.g., taking a larger than therapeutic dose of medications to induce a

TABLE 16-7-1. Contrast Between Typical Suicide Completers and Attempters

	COMPLETER	ATTEMPTER
Sex	Male	Female
Age	Older	Younger
Impulsivity	Low	High
Substance use	High	Very high
Method	Firearms, hanging	Overdose, cutting oneself
Motivation	Self-directed	Interpersonal-directed
Note	Often	Sometimes
Chance of discovery	Low	High
Suicidal preoccupation and intent	High	Low
Plan	Well-planned	Impulsive

prolonged and deep sleep). A *survivor* is one who had a significant relationship with the victim.

The rate of attempted suicide rate is 10 times that of completed suicide. Attempts may be a "cry for help" or used as a cathartic (to provide relief from a stressful situation), and are more likely in women who tend to be impulsive. Attempts are often associated with substance use. The most common attempted method is drug ingestion (overdose). A personality disorder (especially cluster B) is present in 40% of attempters. The motivation behind an attempt is often interpersonal and meant to affect other individuals, make a statement, or create some change in a relationship. Table 16-7-1 contrasts typical characteristics of patients who attempt versus complete suicide.

Patients commit suicide for a variety of reasons. Some feel so hopeless and have such psychic pain that they can see no alternative solution to the situation. These patients tend to be depressed and chronically ill (especially with poorly treated pain). Some younger patients with toxic pride are unable to cope with feelings of perceived failure, such as the straight-A medical student who obtains his first "C" and is then unable to face family and friends. Such students are often disconnected from the institution.

Histrionic or impulsive patients may commit suicide to punish themselves, obtain revenge or attention, provide stimulation and excitement, or symbolically kill or punish themselves or others. They may not intend to actually die, but sometimes their plans to be found, or their understanding of the lethality of the method, are inaccurate.

Some patients turn to suicide as a "rational" solution to a terminal or progressive illness, to provide ultimate relief from suffering. Suicide that occurs in response to poorly managed pain demonstrates the failure of the medical profession to adequately manage pain. Some suicides may be altruistic.

Psychotic patients may commit suicide in response to a command hallucination or delusion, though this is rare. Risk-taking and self-neglect are other causes of suicide.

RISK ASSESSMENT

It is not possible to predict with any clinically useful degree of accuracy the risk of an individual patient committing suicide, despite the availability of several assessment tools and the large body of data concerning suicide risk factors. However, an individual's risk factors need to be identified and addressed to lower both the chronic and acute risk of completing a suicide.

Suicidal behavior fits the stress–diathesis model well. Suicide appears to be the final outcome of a complex interplay of genetics, environment, circumstances, and coping efficacy. Typically multiple stressors accumulate over time, putting a patient at increasing chronic, and eventually acute, risk for suicide.

Risk factors can be distal and predisposing or proximal and precipitating. The treatment outlined in this chapter addresses proximal factors. Suicide prevention addresses more distal factors, and is addressed under the realm of public health.

Sex

Eighty percent of suicide completers are male. Two thirds of patients who complete a suicide are white, male, and unmarried. Males tend to use more lethal methods, though females (especially those over age 65) are using increasingly lethal methods, such as firearms. The suicide rate for females is higher in cultures where women's social status is extremely low.

Age

Patients under 19 and over 45 years of age represent the highest risk groups. Adolescent suicide may be associated with public shame, family conflict, exposure to violence (especially a suicide in the family), and a depressed father. Men over 65 have the highest suicide rate. Ninety percent of older males will complete a suicide during their first attempt. They may be socially isolated and lonely. The majority have seen a primary care practitioner within 30 days of the event, usually presenting vague somatic complaints. When depression is present, one-third are not treated, and most of those who are identified and treated, are treated inadequately. This older, at-risk group may be more sensitive to the normal losses associated with aging, and often have lifelong evidence of poor adaptive skills.

History of Suicide Attempts

Past history of suicide attempt(s) is the most robust predictor of suicide. Thirty to forty percent of suicide victims have a past history of at least one attempt. The risk of completion is 1% within 1 year of an attempt. Ten to fifteen percent of attempters will eventually complete a suicide during their life.

Family History of Suicide

Up to 11% of suicide victims have a first-degree relative who committed suicide. Exposure to suicide in the family is associated with increased risk, perhaps by modeling suicide as an acceptable problem-solving method. Exposure of adolescents to the suicide of a family member, friend, or high-profile celebrity is associated with a stronger attraction to death and acceptance of suicidal behavior. There is some evidence that impulsivity and aggression, which is associated with increased risk, may be genetic.

Presence of a Psychiatric Disorder

More than 90% of completers have a major psychiatric illness, usually depression, at the time of the suicide. Fifteen percent of patients with unipolar depression will eventually complete suicide, which is five to seven times the risk in the general population. The most at-risk period may be just as the patient begins to respond to treatment, especially the first 3 months following discharge from an inpatient unit. Only 50% of patients had been diagnosed with depression, and most of those diagnosed were inadequately treated at the time of the suicide. Adequate treatment of depression is the single most effective intervention in the prevention of suicide. Risk for suicide is not correlated with symptom severity. Nineteen percent of patients with a bipolar disorder will eventually commit suicide, usually during a mixed manic state.

Forty percent of schizophrenic patients attempt suicide, and 30% of these patients succeed with their first try. Ten to fifteen percent of all patients with schizophrenia eventually complete a suicide. The suicidal schizophrenic patient tends to be young, male, white, single, unemployed, and socially isolated, with a chronic and relapsing illness and high expressed emotion in the family. The suicide is usually committed during the first 5 years of the illness, during a relatively nonpsychotic phase. Suicide in response to command hallucinations is rare.

The majority of suicidal patients with personality disorders also have a current axis I depressive or substance abuse disorder at the time of the suicide. Suicide is rare in cluster A disorders. The suicide rate for patients with cluster C disorders does not differ from the general population. Patients with borderline personality disorder are at highest risk, with 15% eventually completing a suicide.

Substance Abuse

Substance abuse tends to act as a proximal or precipitating factor. Forty percent of suicide victims have alcohol in their blood at the time of death. Victims tend to use substances to disinhibit themselves prior to the act. Eighteen percent of all alcoholics eventually commit suicide, usually late in the disease process. Alcoholics who have been excluded from their marriages and families are at particularly high risk.

Hopelessness

A sense of hopelessness is the most robust psychological factor present in suicidal patients. The patient may perceive no other viable solution for the precipitating problem, and recognize no reason to live. Cognitive disorders associated with hopelessness include dysfunctional assumptions, dichotomous thinking, cognitive rigidity, poor problem-solving abilities, a negative self-concept and traumatizing self-denigration, a sense of isolation, poor concept of future, and the use of aggression in problem-solving.

Psychosocial Stressors

A current psychosocial stressor alone is rarely responsible for a completed suicide. Other chronic factors are usually also present. Stressors which may be precipitating factors include a disrupted close interpersonal relationship, recent bereavement (especially of a spouse), and unemployment or retirement. Chronic stressors include residence in a violent area, low socioeconomic status, social isolation (e.g., a recent geographic move, separation, divorce, or widowhood), loss of a parent during childhood, and the presence of chronic, severe, and debilitating medical problems.

Suicidal Ideation

Chronic suicidal ideation is highly associated with suicide risk. Up to 75% of victims give some clue just prior to the act, usually a veiled verbal warning, such as "Its not worth it . . . I'm a burden . . . I've had enough . . . thanks for trying." The majority of suicide victims have visited a health care practitioner within a month of committing suicide. The patient may demonstrate an attitude of finality at the end of the encounter (e.g., saying "Good-bye" instead of "See you next month"). Intent and lethality are strongly correlated; unfortunately, the majority do not explicitly communicate their intent. A rather abrupt appearance of an attitude of peace and calm displayed by a chronically suicidal patient may be a warning sign that the patient has finally accepted suicide as the method to deal with life's problems. One in six leave a note.

The more lethal and detailed the plan, the greater the risk of completion. Access to and familiarity with the chosen method also increases the risk of a completed suicide. Adolescents are at increased risk of copying a suicide that is praised or glorified.

TABLE 16-7-2. Signs of Possible Increased Suicide Risk in Children and Adolescents

- Change in eating and sleep habits
- Frequent physical complaints
- Persistent boredom, difficulty concentrating, decline in schoolwork
- Diminished interest in pleasurable activities
- Unusual neglect of personal appearance
- Marked change in personality
- Violent actions, rebellious behavior, running away
- Preoccupation with death and suicide
- Verbal hints of suicide
- Voices being "rotten inside"
- Intolerance of praise or rewards
- Puts affairs in order
- Sudden cheerfulness in the midst of depression
- Withdrawal from friends, family, and activities
- Drug and alcohol use

Coping Skills

Patients with poor coping skills are at increased chronic risk. Perfectionism and cognitive rigidity, poor problem-solving abilities, aggressive and impulsive personality traits, and a negative self-concept interfere with a person's ability to cope with life stressors and consider healthy choices. Patients at risk may have a poor concept of the future, equate rejection with abandonment, and indirectly express effect.

Other Risk Factors

The presence of a firearm in the home is an independent risk factor. Risk increases around anniversaries of important losses. Other risk factors include unemployment and diagnosed cancer or HIV infection. Patients who grew up under negative parenting style, absent father, or childhood sexual abuse are at increased risk. Table 16-7-2 lists possible signs of increased risk in children and adolescents.

Protective Factors

Patients with strong religious beliefs and practices are at lower risk, sometimes in response to fears of negative eternal consequences. Social group norms against suicide are protective. Males who are married are also at lower risk. Other protective factors include presence of a strong social support system, personal sense of self-efficacy, well-developed coping skills, good social competencies, the presence of loved objects (such as children in the home or cherished pets), empathy toward potential survivors, and a perceived future, especially specific near-future events the patient is interested in.

INTERVENTION

The ultimate goal of intervention is to protect the patient from self-harm. However, suicides will occur, despite our best efforts. Intervention can occur at the primary/preventative level (reducing risk factors and enhancing protective factors for the entire population), secondary level (reducing risk factors in populations determined to be at increased risk), or tertiary level (crisis intervention for a specific patient determined to be at acute risk). This chapter will focus on intervention at the tertiary level.

Crisis intervention involves assessing risk factors, physically interfering with the patient's chosen method, enhancing ethical and moral barriers to committing suicide, addressing underlying distress, developing a good social support system, and giving the patient hope that the current suicidal crisis will pass. Intervention assists the patient to choose to live

by enhancing a sense of self-control and personal effectiveness. Past failures and losses are not addressed during the crisis intervention phase.

Characteristics of the Practitioner

Effective intervention begins with the establishment of a trusting and collaborative therapeutic relationship. Take an active, problem-solving stance. Approach patients with confidence, empathy, support, and a nonjudgmental attitude. Promote an open and honest discussion about the patient's suicidal thoughts, letting him or her know you take the suicidal feelings seriously. Maintain a low threshold to refer. Similar to all potential emergency situations, suicidal crises should be prepared for in advance. Referral sources should be identified and available before a crisis occurs.

Clinicians should understand their limits of training and experience, as well as their comfort level with suicidal patients. Maintain awareness of your countertransference (the feelings invoked in you by working with the patient) by asking such questions as "How am I reacting . . . to what am I reacting . . . what are my feelings telling me about this patient?"

Open and Thorough Discussion

All depressed patients should be screened for suicidal ideation. Most patients are ambivalent about suicide, and are relieved to be able to discuss their suicidal thoughts and feelings. Exposing and discussing this ambivalence are important in establishing alternative solutions. Embrace the patient's sense of hopelessness, acknowledging the patient's psychic pain and choice of suicide as only one option. Some sample questions to use are listed in Table 16-7-3.

Assess the patient's degree of intent. Is it definite or conditional? Most patients with suicidal ideation have no intent of ever following through with a suicide attempt. Some patients may deny intent to maintain access to the opportunity to attempt suicide.

Assess the meaning suicide has to the patient. Determine what unexpressed beliefs, attitudes, or expectations maintain the desire to die. Death may be viewed positively and not feared—for example, perceiving suicide as a chance for rebirth or reunion with someone who has previously died. Seek possible fantasies of revenge, control, or sacrifice.

Evaluate the patient's plan. How specific is it? What accessibility does the patient have to the needed instrument(s)? How plausible and lethal is it? What preparations has the patient made, such as taking out a new insurance policy or gathering the instruments needed for the suicide. Assess the patient's judgment and degree of impulsivity.

Patients tend to choose the same methods used during previous attempts. Determine the patient's understanding of the lethality of past attempts, and past responses to similar stresses. Establish past reasons, degree of isolation, precautions made against discovery, timing, and anticipatory acts (e.g., giving away possessions).

Is there a psychiatric disorder that requires treatment? Is the patient using alcohol or illicit substances? What situational and social factors are contributing to the suicidal ideation?

Finally, what protections can be mustered to immediately lower the acute risk? What reasons does the patient have to live? What deterrents are there to committing suicide? What adaptive capability does the patient have? What resources and supports are available to this particular patient?

Challenging the Option

The goal of crisis intervention is to decrease the suicidal potential by the end of the encounter. The motive for the patient's suicidal ideation should be challenged and hopefully destroyed.

Accept the person and the pain, but not suicide as the preferred method of coping. Any ambivalence the patient demonstrates should be capitalized on. Make the patient aware of factors being ignored in the seemingly hopeless situation. Be aware that a depressed affect biases the memory to selectively recall in a negative and hopeless manner.

TABLE 16-7-3. Interviewing the Potentially Suicidal Patient

Presence of Suicidal Ideation

Does it ever seem like life is not worth living anymore?
Have you ever felt so bad you thought life was not worth living?
Have you been thinking about hurting yourself or taking your life?
Many patients who are depressed think about suicide. Have you had
    thoughts like this?
How bad do you feel?
Do you wish you were dead?

Intent

How strong are these feelings?
What would have to happen for you to commit suicide?
What would have to happen for you to decide not to commit suicide?
Under what conditions would you seriously consider suicide?
What's preventing you from committing suicide?
Why commit suicide now?

Meaning

What is the problem you are trying to resolve by committing suicide?
What will suicide do for you?
What do you hope to accomplish by committing suicide?

Plan

If you were to commit suicide, how would you do it?
What have you done in past suicide attempts?
What preparations have you made?

Past History

How have you coped with this stress before?
Have you ever tried to kill or hurt yourself before?
Have you ever attempted or seriously considered suicide before?
How close have you come to attempting suicide in the past?
What happened?
What were you hoping to accomplish?
How did others react?

Protective

Who else needs to know you are thinking about suicide?
Who else have you told about these thoughts?
What is preventing you from committing suicide?
Who can be with you during this stressful time?
Will you work with me to diminish these thoughts?
Will you be safe?

Other

How much alcohol have you been using the past month?
What street drugs are you using?

Cognitive distortions (such as futility and hopelessness regarding a specific situation, a sense of inadequacy and failure as a human being, and an intense feeling of guilt for real or imagined wrong) should be realistically and gently, but firmly, challenged. Identify negative thinking and reframe in a more positive and realistic manner. Keep alert to such distortions as over-generalizations, exaggerations, and selective abstractions. Help patients to reality-test their appraisal of the situation and reinterpret their experiences more realistically.

Confidentiality

General rules of medical confidentiality may not apply when the patient's life is in danger. Patients should be informed of the limits regarding confidentiality. The patient should be informed when the patient's clinical condition is discussed with other health care providers, family, and friends. The patient should be reassured that this is for his or her safety. Permission for such information sharing should be requested, but is not required during an acute suicide intervention.

Help patients organize their thinking and behavior. The practitioner may need to be quite directive and even paternalistic. If the suicidal threats are obviously being used in a manipulative manner, the suicidal talk may need to be confronted and challenged.

Support Systems

Organize a supportive environment. This may be done on an outpatient basis if safety can be assured. The ultimate safe and supportive environment may be the inpatient psychiatry ward, though safety can never be completely guaranteed. Involve supportive family and friends. Give precise instructions to the patient's social network regarding care and supervision. Have someone stay with the patient until the suicidal crisis has passed. Do not allow the patient to be alone, even in the health care facility.

Identify the patient's personal strengths and emphasize them to the patient. If the patient is to be treated as an outpatient, provide a 24-hour emergency telephone number.

There is no research evidence that suicide contracts are effective at lowering the rate of suicide, and they do not provide legal protection, but they do promote collaboration. The contract should stipulate that the patient will call the 24-hour number (which is written on the contract) if there is any escalation of suicidal thoughts, especially intent and planning. The contract should be in force for a specified and brief time period, renewable at the end of the period. The patient should call in daily to review safety procedures. Family and friends should be involved in both the negotiation and fulfillment of the contract. A patient's refusal to contract indicates a significant acute risk. Contracts are contraindicated for psychotic and impulsive patients.

Inpatient Treatment

Most patients with suicidal thoughts can be treated on an outpatient basis. There is little evidence that an inpatient approach diminishes the risk of suicide in the community. Inpatient treatment interferes with the patient's normal activities and sense of autonomy, institutionalizes the "sick role," and can interfere with the therapeutic relationship (especially if involuntary).

Indications for inpatient treatment can be found in Table 16-7-4. Hospitalization (especially if involuntary) should be promoted as a show of concern, not a threat or punishment. Patients do commit suicide even when hospitalized on locked units.

It is important to know the policies of each institution and the laws of your state regarding involuntary commitment before you find yourself in such a situation. If commitment is necessary, it should be carried out as rapidly as possible. The risk of suicide and need for suicidal precautions must be clearly communicated to each professional treating the patient, and the reasons for suicidal precautions (and involuntary commitment) must be clearly and thoroughly documented in the patient's medical record.

Other Considerations

Consultation is strongly recommended when dealing with a suicidal patient. Underlying conditions, especially depression, should be adequately treated. The patient should be kept busy to diminish anxious ruminating. Benzodiazepines can be used to acutely diminish the anxiety associated with suicidal ideation. Firearms should be removed from the patient's environment, and any other preferred method should be contained. All

TABLE 16-7-4. When to Admit a Suicidal Patient

- Need to shelter patient from self-harm
- Need to develop supports sufficient to justify outpatient treatment
- Need to examine the patient in a nondrugged state
- Need to observe the patient to adequately determine the risk of a suicide attempt
- Need to remove the patient from a stressful situation
- Need to stabilize the patient's emotional state
- Need to reassess outpatient treatment

medications (including over-the-counter) should be kept and dispensed by a responsible adult. Contagion can be reduced by avoiding publicity.

When foreseeability is present, failure to protect the patient from self-harm may lead to the demise of the patient, as well as a lawsuit. An error of fact (failure to obtain necessary data) increases legal liability, but an error of judgment—if based upon an adequate risk assessment and made in good faith—is not usually grounds for legal liability. Most states provide immunity from legal action if involuntary commitment proceedings and breach of ordinary confidences are performed in good faith. Use the same usual and reasonable degree of care given to all patients and document, document, document. Any corrections made in the medical record must be dated and signed. Documented late entries into the record are legally acceptable, but the medical record must never be altered.

Prevention

Because suicide is a rare event in a large at-risk population, the efficacy of prevention methods can be difficult to assess. Primary and secondary prevention aims to lower antecedent conditions, decrease the acquisition of vulnerabilities, change the processes that eventually lead to suicide, and enhance protective factors. Reduction of availability of means can reduce risk in a community, such as removal or locking of firearms in the home.

Survivors

Six other people are intimately affected by each suicide. The grief associated with losing a loved one to suicide is especially difficult to bear. Survivors often feel totally rejected by the victim and shamed by the stigma. There is often much guilt and unreasonable responsibility taken for the event. Intense anger at both self (for failure to prevent) and the victim is common, but difficult to reckon with. Survivors also may develop preoccupation with suicidal thoughts, and fear their own potential self-destructive impulses. Symptoms of post-traumatic stress disorder are common. Management includes trauma mastery, grief resolution, and family and group therapy, and should be carried out by a professional with specific training and experience in this area.

Personal Impact

Working with suicidal patients is one of the greatest stresses identified by providers. The emotional reaction to loss of one's patient to suicide is similar to the grief experienced with loss of a close family member. Reactions are similar to those of survivors, but are often not acknowledged and dealt with because they are "part of the job." Feelings of personal and professional inadequacy, blame, and fear of litigation or loss of professional standing can significantly hamper working through the grief, and result in depressive and anxiety disorders.

SELECT BIBLIOGRAPHY

Bongar B, ed. *Suicide: Guidelines for Assessment, Management, and Treatment.* New York, Oxford, 1992.

Dattilio FM, Freeman A, eds. *Cognitive-Behavioral Strategies in Crisis Intervention.* New York, Guilford Press, 1994.

Freeman A, Reinecke MA. *Cognitive Therapy of Suicidal Behavior.* New York, Springer, 1993.

Mann JJ, ed. Suicide. *Psychiatr Clin North Am* 20:3;1997.

Maris RW, Berman AL, Maltsberger JT, Yufit RI, eds. *Assessment and Prediction of Suicide.* New York, Guilford Press, 1992.

Silverman MM, Maris RW, eds. *Suicide Prevention: Toward the Year 2000.* New York, Guilford Press, 1995.

St. John D. The Suicidal Patient: Identifying, evaluating, and intervening. *J Am Acad Phys Asst* 9:58–76; 1996.

Tanney B, Tierney R, Lang W. *The Suicide Intervention Handbook.* Calgary, Living Works Education, 1994.

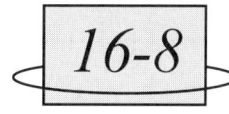

PSYCHOTIC DISORDERS: SCHIZOPHRENIA

William A. Mosier

DISCUSSION

When the psychotic disorders were first described in the 1800s, they were thought to be a single entity and were given the one label—schizophrenia. At that time, it was assumed that all psychotic symptoms had the same etiology and pathophysiology. It is now recognized that schizophrenia is better understood as a disease process involving behavior, emotion, movement, perception, and thought—rather than as one disease entity.

Although traditionally the definition for psychosis relied primarily on a description of presenting symptoms, current efforts include addressing the underlying elements of the brain abnormalities responsible for the varied symptoms. Viewing the psychotic disorders, such as schizophrenia, as variations of a complex clinical syndrome, is a more realistic way to picture this grossly misunderstood phenomenon.

Psychosis Defined

The term *psychosis* is referred to as "a loss of ego boundaries" or "a gross impairment in reality testing" that is manifested as delusions and/or hallucinations that are not accompanied by insight. According to the *Diagnostic and Statistical Manual of Mental Disorders,* fourth edition (DSM-IV), there are three broadly defined uses of the term "psychosis" that address different aspects of its expression. The term *psychotic* refers to delusions, hallucinations, disorganized speech, and/or disorganized or catatonic behavior. These criteria are found in the following disorders: schizophrenia, schizophreniform disorder, schizoaffective disorder, brief psychotic disorder, psychosis due to a general medical condition, and substance-induced psychotic disorder.

The term *psychotic* is often used interchangeably with the term *delusion* in disorders such as delusional disorder and shared psychotic disorder. The *International Classification of Diseases and Related Health Problems,* tenth edition (ICD-10), identifies several conditions under the umbrella of psychotic disorders (Table 16-8-1).

The different psychotic disorders can be distinguished, one from the other, by specific behavioral criteria. DSM-IV provides descriptions and diagnostic criteria for the various expressions of psychosis. (See Tables 16-8-2 to 16-8-10 for the essential features of each disorder.)

Schizophrenia

The use of the term *schizophrenia* should be reserved only for psychiatric disturbances lasting at least 6 months that include a minimum of two of the following: delusions, hallucinations, disorganized speech, grossly disorganized or catatonic behavior, or negative symptoms (see "Symptoms" later in the chapter).

TABLE 16-8-1. Categories of Psychosis

Schizophrenia
Schizophreniform disorder
Schizoaffective disorder
Schizoid personality disorder and schizotypal personality disorder (see Chap. 16-9)
Delusional disorders
Acute and transient psychotic disorders (brief psychotic disorders)
Psychotic disorders resulting from a medical condition
Substance-induced psychotic disorder

TABLE 16-8-2. DSM-IV Criteria for Schizophrenia

A. *Characteristic symptoms.* Two (or more) of the following, each present for a significant portion of time during a 1-month period (or less if successfully treated): (1) delusions, (2) hallucinations, (3) disorganized speech (e.g., frequent derailment or incoherence), (4) grossly disorganized or catatonic behavior, and (5) negative symptoms (i.e., affective flattening, alogia, or avolition).

Only one criterion A symptom is required if delusions are bizarre or hallucinations consist of a voice keeping up a running commentary on the person's behavior or thoughts, or two or more voices conversing with each other.

B. *Social/occupational dysfunction.* Since the onset of symptoms, one or more major areas of functioning such as work, interpersonal relations, or self-care are markedly below the level achieved prior to onset of symptoms. When onset is observed during childhood or adolescence, determination is based on failure to attain expected level of interpersonal, academic, or occupational achievement.

C. *Duration.* Continuous signs of the disturbance persist for at least 6 months. The 6-month period must include at least 1 month of symptoms (or less if successfully treated) that meet criterion A, and may include periods of prodromal or residual symptoms. During these prodromal or residual periods, the signs of the disturbance may be manifested by only negative symptoms or two or more symptoms listed in criterion A present in an attenuated form (e.g., odd belief, unusual perceptual experiences).

D. *Schizoaffective and mood disorder exclusion.* Schizoaffective disorder and mood disorder with psychotic features have been ruled out because either (1) no major depressive, manic, or mixed episodes have occurred concurrently with the active-phase symptoms; or (2) if mood episodes have occurred during active-phase symptoms, their total duration has been brief relative to the duration of the active and residual periods.

E. *Substance/general medical condition exclusion.* The disturbance is not due to the direct physiological effects of a substance (e.g., a drug of abuse, a medication) or a general medical condition.

F. *Relationship to a pervasive developmental disorder.* If there is a history of autistic disorder or another pervasive developmental disorder, the additional diagnosis of schizophrenia is made only if prominent delusions or hallucinations are also present for at least a month.

Additional classification can be applied based on the longitudinal course of the condition. These classifications can be applied only after at least 1 year has elapsed since the initial onset of active-phase symptoms. The classifications are as follows:

1. Episodic with inter-episode residual symptoms (episodes are defined by the reemergence of prominent psychotic symptoms)
2. Episodic with no inter-episode residual symptoms
3. Continuous (prominent psychotic symptoms are ongoing)
4. Single episode but with only partial remission

As a diagnosis, schizophrenia can be differentiated into five subtypes. DSM-IV criteria are used to identify each subtype (Table 16-8-3).

Schizophreniform Disorder

The term *schizophreniform disorder* is generally a provisional one. Because the diagnosis of schizophrenia requires that the criteria for diagnosis must have been present for at least 6 months prior to diagnosis, schizophreniform disorder refers to symptoms that have been observed for at least 1 month but less than 6 months. Once symptoms advance beyond 6 months, the diagnosis should be changed to schizophrenia (Table 16-8-4).

Schizoaffective Disorder

Ongoing psychotic features, occurring with concurrent depressive, manic, or mixed manic-depressive symptoms, characterize schizoaffective disorder. The criteria for both schizophrenia and a mood disorder must be met. If symptoms of a mood disorder are not consistently seen superimposed over the symptoms of psychosis, the diagnosis of schizoaffective disorder cannot be applied (Table 16-8-5).

TABLE 16-8-3. Schizophrenia Subtypes

Paranoid Type

Characterized by delusional thinking and/or hallucinations. Paranoid schizophrenia is the second most common type of schizophrenia observed, with auditory hallucinations being the most common hallucinations presented. Criteria are

• Preoccupation with one or more delusions or frequent auditory hallucinations.
• None of the following are observable: disorganized speech, disorganized or catatonic behavior, flat or inappropriate affect.

Disorganized Type

Characterized by a flat affect, disorganized pattern of speech, and odd behavior. Criteria are

• Disorganized speech and mannerisms with flat or inappropriate affect.
• Criteria for catatonic type are not met

Catatonic Type

Characterized by bizarre motor symptoms. Criteria consist of at least two of the following:

• Stupor or motoric immobility
• Excessive and purposeless motor activity
• Mutism, maintenance of a rigid posture, or motiveless resistance to verbal commands

Undifferentiated Type

Characterized by the display of symptoms from more than one of the other three types. (The majority of patients with schizophrenia are of this type.) Criteria consist of criterion A from Table 16-8-1, but are exclusive of criteria for paranoid, disorganized, or catatonic types.

Residual Type

Characterized by the absence of delusions, hallucinations, disorganized speech, and grossly disorganized or catatonic behavior. Criteria consist of continuing evidence of the negative symptoms of schizophrenia or at least two symptoms from criterion A for schizophrenia present (e.g., odd beliefs or bizarre perceptions).

TABLE 16-8-4. DSM-IV Criteria for Schizophreniform Disorder

• Criteria A, D, and E of schizophrenia are met.

• An episode of the disorder (including prodromal, active, and residual phases) lasts at least 1 month but less than 6 months.

• A good prognosis exists when there is evidence of at least two of the following:

Onset of psychotic symptoms occur within 4 weeks of the first noticeable change in usual behavior or functioning.
Patient experiences confusion or perplexity at the height of the psychotic episode.
Premorbid social and occupational functioning was within normal limits.
There is an absence of blunted or flat affect.

Delusional Disorder

A delusional disorder is characterized by the presence of non-bizarre delusions that persist for more than 1 month. Non-bizarre delusions consist of fears of situations that, although not probable, could conceivably occur in real life. The diagnosis of delusional disorder

TABLE 16-8-5. DSM-IV Criteria for Schizoaffective Disorder

• An uninterrupted period of illness during which there is a major depressive episode, a manic episode, or a mixed episode concurrent with symptoms that meet criterion A for schizophrenia. *(To meet the criteria for major depressive episode a pervasive depressed mood must be present.)*

• Delusions or hallucinations for at least 2 weeks in the absence of prominent mood symptoms.

• Symptoms that meet criteria for a mood disorder are present for a substantial portion of the total duration of the active and residual periods of the illness.

• The disturbance is not due to the direct physiologic effects of a substance (e.g., a drug of abuse, or medication) or a general medical condition.

TABLE 16-8-6.   DSM-IV Criteria for Delusional Disorder

- Nonbizarre delusions (e.g., being followed, poisoned, infected, loved at a distance, deceived by a spouse or lover, or having a disease), of at least 1-month duration.

- Criterion A for schizophrenia has never been met.

- Apart from the impact of the delusion(s) or its ramifications, functioning is not markedly impaired and behavior is not obviously odd or bizarre.

- If symptoms of a mood disorder have occurred concurrently with delusions, their total duration has been brief relative to the duration of the delusional periods.

- The disturbance is not due to the direct physiologic effects of a substance (e.g., a drug of abuse, a medication) or a general medical condition.

TABLE 16-8-7.   Typical Delusional Subtype Themes

Erotomanic type	Delusions that another person, usually of higher status, is in love with the individual
Grandiose type	Delusions of inflated self-worth, power, knowledge, identity, or special relationship to a deity or famous person
Jealous type	Delusions that the individual's sexual partner is unfaithful
Persecutory type	Delusions that the person (or someone to whom the person is close) is being malevolently treated in some way
Somatic type	Delusions that the person has some physical defect or general medical condition
Mixed type	Delusions characteristic of more than one of the above types but no one theme predominates

cannot be used if the individual being assessed has ever met criterion A for schizophrenia (Table 16-8-6).

Except for the direct impact the delusional thoughts may have on daily living, psychosocial functioning tends not to be markedly impaired. However, interpersonal functioning is more likely to be impaired than occupational functioning (Table 16-8-7).

Brief Psychotic Disorder

Brief psychotic disorder is characterized by a sudden onset of psychotic symptoms that last less than 1 month, after which the individual makes a full recovery. A history of a preexisting personality disorder may predispose a person to brief psychotic disorder. Evidence suggests that this disorder is very uncommon (Table 16-8-8).

Psychotic Disorder Due to a General Medical Condition

Psychotic disorder due to a medical condition is characterized by delusional thoughts or hallucinations that directly result from the physiologic effects of a specific medical condition. Examples are a psychotic disorder due to a brain tumor or Alzheimer's type dementia. A clue to identifying this type of psychotic disorder is its atypical presentation (e.g., presence of visual or olfactory hallucinations). See Table 16-8-9.

TABLE 16-8-8.   DSM-IV Criteria for Brief Psychotic Disorder

- Presence of one (or more) of the following symptoms: (1) delusions, (2) hallucinations, (3) disorganized or incoherent speech, or (4) grossly disorganized or catatonic behavior.

- An episode lasts at least 1 day but less than 1 month, with eventual full return to premorbid level of functioning.

- The disturbance is not better accounted for by a mood disorder with psychotic features, schizoaffective disorder, or schizophrenia and is not due to the direct physiologic effects of a substance (e.g., a drug of abuse, a medication) or a general medical condition.

TABLE 16-8-9.   DSM-IV Criteria for Psychotic Disorder Due to a General Medical Condition

- Prominent hallucinations or delusions.

- Evidence from history, physical examination, or laboratory findings indicates that the disturbance is the direct physiologic consequence of a general medical condition.

- The disturbance is not better attributed to another mental disorder.

- The disturbance does not occur exclusively during the course of a delirium.

TABLE 16-8-10.   Diagnostic Criteria for Substance-Induced Psychotic Disorder

- Hallucinations or delusions are present, where the patient has no insight that they are substance induced.

- There is evidence from the history, physical examination, or laboratory findings that the symptoms from criterion A for schizophrenia developed during, or within 1 month from, substance abuse, resulting intoxication, or withdrawal; or medication use is etiologically related to the psychosis.

- The disturbance is not better accounted for by a psychotic disorder that is not substance induced, and there is no history of recurrent non–substance-related episodes of psychotic behavior.

- The disturbance does not occur exclusively during the course of a delirium.

- This diagnosis should be made only when the symptoms are in excess of those usually associated with the intoxication or withdrawal syndrome, and when the symptoms are sufficiently severe to warrant independent clinical attention.

Substance-Induced Psychotic Disorder

Substance-induced psychotic disorder is characterized by delusions or hallucinations that are a direct result of drug abuse, a legally prescribed medication, or exposure to a specific toxin. This psychotic disorder is distinguishable from other psychotic disorders by its timing in relation to the precipitant and only when the patient has no history of any other psychotic disorder. See Table 16-8-10.

EPIDEMIOLOGY

Prevalence

The prevalence of psychotic disorders does not tend to vary from one geographical location to another. The prevalence generally ranges from 3 to 10 per 1000 persons. Although a higher prevalence of schizophrenia has been reported in Sweden (17/1000), a tendency for individuals with psychotic disorders to gravitate toward environments that lend themselves to a more austere lifestyle could account for this statistic. A higher prevalence of individuals with psychotic disorders is seen in urban as opposed to rural settings, which on the surface would seem to contradict the previous sentence. However, this "social drift" is thought to be due to an urban environment being more accommodating for individuals to maintain a socially withdrawn lifestyle and yet still obtain access to modern conveniences.

Although an underlying genetic vulnerability probably exists from birth, it rarely manifests prior to puberty. Lifetime risk of developing a psychotic disorder appears to be equal for men and women. However, the peak age of onset is between 15 and 25 for males and 25 and 35 for females. The course of the disease is extremely variable. An interesting note is that the intensity of psychosis often, but not always, diminishes with age.

Incidence

The incidence of psychotic disorders ranges from 10 to 70 per 100,000 people. The only geographical variance is that which was noted under "Prevalence." The lifetime risk is approximately 2%. The high-risk period for expressing psychotic symptoms seems to be between the ages of 20 and 40. Age of onset tends to be earlier for men than for women. There are no apparent cross-cultural differences in risk of developing psychotic disorders. However, epidemiologic studies consistently demonstrate that lower socioeconomic status is associated with the psychotic disorders. This is assumed to be due to the fact that as the untreated patient's symptoms worsen, they are less able to complete an education and hold down a job, thus resulting in a decline in socioeconomic status. Individuals with psychotic disorders are more likely to be unmarried. It is estimated that 50% of all homeless people suffer from a psychotic disorder. Epidemiologically, both genetic and environmental factors play a significant role in the manifestation of psychosis. Even though environmental factors might explain how psychosis manifests under curtain circumstances, a hereditary susceptibility provides the most probable underlying susceptibility.

PATHOGENESIS

Risk Factors

The development of the symptoms of psychosis cannot be attributed to one isolated cause. Three interrelated factors are involved in the etiology of psychotic disorders. A genetic predisposition and neurodevelopmental factors interacting with environmental influences are all significant in the pathogenesis of psychotic disorders (Table 16-8-11).

GENETIC PREDISPOSITION   The influence of heredity has been widely studied. Twin studies reveal as much as a 50% concordance rate for monozygotic twins. Dizygotic twins share only a 10% increased risk of both manifesting symptoms of one of the psychotic disorders when a positive family history for the disorder exists. There is a 10% increased risk for developing a psychotic disorder if the disorder exists in a first-degree relative. Children of parents who manifest symptoms of psychotic disorders have a 40% chance of developing a psychotic disorder. If neither biological parent carries the predisposition for a psychotic disorder, their offspring has a 1% risk of developing a psychotic disorder.

Although a genetic influence over psychotic disorders is undeniable, which gene or genes are involved and the heterogeneity of the transmission are still in question. The fact that there is not a 100% concordance in monozygotic twins demonstrates that certain nonhereditary factors must also be involved in the pathogenesis of the psychotic disorders in individuals who are genetically vulnerable.

NEURODEVELOPMENTAL VULNERABILITY   Considerable research supports the correlation between congenital influences on the development of neurotransmitter and other CNS structural abnormalities and an increased vulnerability for manifesting psychotic disorders.

ENVIRONMENTAL INFLUENCES   Birth complications and autoimmune compromise secondary to maternal infection during pregnancy (causing a prenatal exposure to the influenza virus) has also been implicated in the etiology of psychotic disorders. A disproportionately larger percentage of individuals suffering from psychotic disorders has been found to have a history of birth trauma, fetal distress, low birthweight, malnutrition, and prenatal hypoxia than the population at large (Buka et al., 1993; Waltrip et al., 1990). Possibly the most significant issue related to environmental influences is that psychosis cannot be caused

TABLE 16-8-11.   Risk Factors for Psychotic Disorders

- Genetic predisposition (heredity)

- Neurodevelopmental vulnerability
  CNS structural abnormalities
  Neurotransmitter abnormalities

- Environmental influences
  Autoimmune mechanisms
  Prenatal infection secondary to maternal infection
  Other pregnancy and birth complications

by interpersonal conflict or emotional trauma. However, environmental factors can trigger a psychotic episode in a predisposed individual.

Neurotransmitters Involved in Psychotic Disorders

The psychotic disorders are a disorder of brain neuronal circuits. The neurotransmitters implicated in psychotic disorders are dopamine, serotonin, acetylcholine, and norepinephrine. The action of dopamine in the neuroanatomy of the psychotic disorders most probably results in an excess of dopamine in the limbic system and basal ganglia pathways, resulting in what is referred to as the "positive symptoms" of psychosis, and a dopamine deficiency in the mesocortical pathways, resulting in what is referred to as the "negative symptoms" found in the psychotic disorders (Davis et al., 1991; Weinberger et al., 1992).

Serotonergic neurons have a modulating effect on dopaminergic neurons. An excess of serotonergic activity in the frontal cortex may result in inhibition of dopaminergic pathways increasing the negative symptoms of psychotic disorders. Fluctuations in norepinephrine may interfere with a balanced flow of dopamine in the brain. The amino acids glutamate and aspartate have also been implicated in the pathogenesis of psychotic disorders. The symptoms resulting from neurotransmitter abnormalities are mediated through four different dopaminergic pathways: The mesocortical, mesolimbic, nigrostriatal, and tuberoinfundibular tracts. The mesocortical tract is associated with cognition, communication, and social responsiveness. Decreased dopamine activity in this area results in the "negative" symptoms of psychosis (see "Symptoms," next). The mesolimbic tract is responsible for memory, emotional arousal, motivation, thought processing, and motor activity. Overactivity of dopamine in this area results in expression of the "positive" symptoms of psychosis (see "Symptoms," next).

An important consideration in understanding the pathogenesis of psychosis is that there have been reports of progressive cerebral tissue loss after repeated psychotic relapses. In essence, each time an individual experiences a psychotic episode, it is a neurochemical catastrophe that causes atrophy to the superior temporal gyres. The possible mechanism may be neurotoxicity due to glutamate, free-radical damage due to impaired antioxidants, hypercortisolemia-induced atrophy, or apoptosis secondary to increased brain catecholamines. But whatever the cause, at a cellular level, psychosis is actually neurotoxic to brain tissue (Knoll et al., 1998; Nasrallah, 1993).

SYMPTOMS

There is no one single defining feature of the psychotic disorders. Each patient presents with a unique combination of multiple symptoms. The range of symptoms that characterize the psychotic disorders stem from three functional areas. The patient's cognitive, emotional, and motor activity will determine how a person manifests his or her psychosis. The so-called positive symptoms include delusions, disorganized speech, disorganized thinking, grandiosity, hallucinations, hostility, inappropriate (bizarre) behavior, suspiciousness, and uncooperativeness. The so-called negative symptoms include alogia, anhedonia, avolition, blunted affect, emotional withdrawal, inappropriate affect, lack of spontaneity, poverty of thoughts, and social withdrawal (Tables 16-8-12 and 16-8-13).

OBJECTIVE FINDINGS

The clinical features of the psychotic disorders identified in DSM-IV can be used as the basis for making the diagnosis of a psychotic

TABLE 16-8-12.   Positive Symptoms of Psychosis

Hallucinations (auditory, visual, somatosensory)

Delusions (paranoid or nonparanoid)

Bizarre behavior

Disorganized speech

TABLE 16-8-13. Negative Symptoms of Psychosis

Social withdrawal

Apathy

Lack of motivation

Impaired attention

Failure to express complex conceptual thoughts

Inappropriate expression of emotions or gestures

Anhedonia

disorder. The presence of hallucinations or certain types of delusions is generally diagnostic of a psychotic disorder. However, if a developmental disorder such as autism is present, the diagnosis of a psychotic disorder is inappropriate.

Assessment of psychosocial functioning is critical to an accurate diagnosis of a psychotic disorder. Interview with family members to obtain as accurate a history as possible is particularly useful.

DIAGNOSTIC CONSIDERATIONS

The differential diagnosis for psychotic disorders includes anxiety disorders (Chap. 16-3), depression with psychotic features (Chap. 16-5), bipolar disorder (Chap. 16-6), nonpsychotic personality disorders (Chap. 16-9), substance-induced psychosis, and psychosis resulting from a medical condition. The medical conditions that are most often associated with psychotic symptoms include advanced Parkinson's disease (Chap. 11-7), dementia (Chap. 11-5), AIDS (Chap. 9-1), autoimmune disease, brain trauma, brain tumors (Chap. 13-13), endocrine or metabolic disturbances, paresis, multiple sclerosis (Chap. 11-2), stroke (Chap. 1-3), and temporal lobe epilepsy (Chap. 11-1). Steroid-induced psychosis, called, "roid rage," is an important diagnostic consideration. Other substance abuse disorders should also be ruled out. Psychotic episodes may be triggered by drugs such as amphetamines, LSD, and marijuana (Chap. 11-10). In the elderly population, delirium and/or dementia-related diseases can manifest as confusion and/or agitation that may be misdiagnosed as a psychotic disorder (Table 16-8-14).

SPECIAL CONSIDERATIONS

The psychotic disorders rarely present in isolation. They most often present with other mental disorders or general medical conditions, most common of which are substance abuse, depression, obsessive-compulsive disorder, and generalized anxiety disorder. The most common substance

TABLE 16-8-14. Substances That Can Induce a Dose-Related Psychosis

Alcohol

Amphetamines

Beta blockers

Bupropion

Carbamazepine

Cocaine

Corticosteroids

Hallucinogens

Indomethacin

Marijuana

Phenytoin

Procainamide

abuse disorders include nicotine addiction and alcohol abuse. Any patient with a comorbid substance abuse problem must have treatment for substance abuse fully integrated into treatment for the psychotic disorder. The symptoms of psychosis can be exacerbated by the use of some prescription and even over-the-counter medications.

The human immunodeficiency virus (HIV) has been associated with the development of psychosis in approximately 10% of HIV/AIDS patients (see Chap. 9-1).

DIAGNOSTIC STUDIES

There is no standard set of laboratory tests for identifying any of the psychotic disorders. Any test that might be selected should be based on the history and presenting symptoms. Tests are more useful for ruling out other medical conditions or for identifying any comorbid medical conditions. Reasonable testing could include CBC, endocrine tests, hepatic function tests, and urinalysis. Electroencephalogram and neuroimaging techniques may be useful to search for underlying conditions such as a brain tumor, multiple sclerosis, a subdural hematoma, or even neurosyphilis. Other useful screening tools include *neuropsychological testing.* Neuropsychological testing, typically administered by a psychologist, can be useful to evaluate the patient's cognitive functioning, level of disability from a psychotic disorder, degree of disorganized thinking, and skewing of thought patterns.

TREATMENT

Since 1955, the focus of care for individuals with psychotic disorders has shifted from long-term institutionalization to short-term community hospital treatment for stabilization of symptoms with ongoing outpatient management of the patient's symptoms. The burden of care for many patients with a psychotic disorder has shifted to the family. Unfortunately, the family is often not equipped to handle the burden adequately. Patients without a family support system often become homeless as a consequence of their deteriorating condition. Due to the frequent lack of adequate support systems available, outpatient treatment of the patient with a psychotic disorder, especially during times of breakthrough psychotic episodes, can be an extremely challenging strain on the health care system. The optimal long-term management of persons with psychotic disorders consists of two distinct strategies: pharmacologic treatment and behavior management training. Pharmacologic treatment refers to the specific drug interventions that may be necessary to assist the patient in controlling the symptoms of psychosis. Behavioral treatment refers to the specific social skills training that will be useful in assisting the patient to acquire or regain social competence and independent living skills.

Pharmacologic Management

The objectives of antipsychotic drug therapy are to block psychotic symptoms, prevent relapse, and enhance efficacy of nonpharmacologic interventions for control of psychotic behavior.

FIRST-LINE TREATMENT: *ATYPICAL NEUROLEPTICS (SECOND-GENERATION ANTIPSYCHOTICS)* Since the mid-1990s, the atypical neuroleptics have become available for the treatment of the psychotic disorders. The relative safety and efficacy of these newer medications has made them the first-line treatment for the psychotic disorders. The relatively lower incidence of side effects has also helped to improve patient compliance. The currently approved atypical neuroleptics include clozapine, Olanzapine, Quetiapine, and Risperidone. The improved profile may be due to selectivity for dopamine receptors (D3 to D6) in the limbic system and frontal cortex, rather than D2 receptors in the striatum, which is the site of selective activity of the conventional neuroleptics. Moreover, the atypical neuroleptics also block serotonin 5HT2 receptors. This effect lowers the risk of

TABLE 16-8-15. Advantages of the Atypical Neuroleptics

- Lower incidence of EPS
- Lower risk of tardive dyskinesia
- Improved ability to treat the negative symptoms of psychotic disorders
- Improved ability to block the positive symptoms in previously refractory patients
- Improved cognitive functioning compared to conventional neuroleptics

extrapyramidal symptoms (EPS) and improves treatment outcome by decreasing the so-called negative symptoms of psychosis.

As previously stated, the symptoms resulting from neurotransmitter abnormalities are mediated through four different dopaminergic pathways, the mesocortical, mesolimbic, nigrostriatal, and tuberoinfundibular tracts. The ideal medication to treat the symptoms of psychosis would only block certain activity in the mesolimbic tract and not interfere with any other pathway. For example, if a medication blocks dopamine in the tuberoinfundibular tract, there can be a resulting endocrine response leading to an increase in prolactin release. When there is a blockade of dopamine in the nigrostriatal tract, there can be a resulting increase in unwanted neurologic reactions such as EPS. However, blockade of 5-HT2a in this area can counteract this effect, actually decreasing EPS (Table 16-8-15).

SECOND-LINE TREATMENT: *CONVENTIONAL NEUROLEPTICS (FIRST-GENERATION ANTIPSYCHOTICS)*   The advent of chlorpromazine and the other conventional neuroleptics in the 1950s had a profound positive effect on the successful management of the psychotic disorders. The therapeutic effect of the conventional neuroleptics is thought to be due to the blockade of dopamine (D2) receptors in the striatum of the mesolimbic tract. However, their dopamine blockade in the nigrostriatal tract has also been implicated in the development of EPS. The older, so-called conventional neuroleptics include the phenothiazines (chlorpromazine, fluphenazine, mesoridazine, perphenazine, prochlorperazine, thioridazine, and trifluoperazine) and the thioxanthene compound thiothixene. The older conventional neuroleptics have a range of side effects that severely limits their usefulness and aggravates the problem of patient compliance. The relatively high side-effect profile as noted in Table 16-8-16 has limited the usefulness of the older neuroleptic medications.

Efficacy of Medication Intervention

TYPICAL VERSUS ATYPICAL NEUROLEPTICS   Generally speaking, the newer atypical neuroleptics have three major advantages over the older typical neuroleptics:

1. The atypical neuroleptics act not only on the positive but also the negative symptoms of psychosis.
2. The lower incidence of motor disturbances provides for a greater safety profile.
3. Low side-effect profile encourages better patient compliance to continuing on medication.

TABLE 16-8-16.   Disadvantages of the Older "Conventional" Neuroleptics

- Many potential drug–drug interactions
- Anticholinergic side effects: delirium, drowsiness, dry mouth, irritability, memory impairment, tachycardia, and urinary retention
- Extrapyramidal side effects: sedation, seizures, tardive dyskinesia, lack of control over the negative symptoms of psychosis (resulting in limiting effectiveness of behavior management training interventions)
- Decrease of dopamine in the mesolimbic pathway (resulting in an actual increase in the negative symptoms of psychosis)

TABLE 16-8-17.   Spectrum of Clinical Responses Seen in Neuroleptics Due to Specific Receptor Activity

Alpha adrenergic	Miosis, orthostatic hypotension, reflex tachycardia
Dopamine-2	EPS, prolactin elevation
Histamine-1	Sedation, weight gain, hypotension
Muscarinic	Blurred vision, cognition and memory clouding, constipation, dry mouth, sinus tachycardia, urinary retention
5-HT-2a (Serotonin)	Decreased negative symptoms of psychosis, decreased EPS

The older conventional or typical neuroleptics block A9 receptors of the nigrostriatal pathway, which is linked to EPS. The atypical (newer and safer) neuroleptics are more active at A10 receptors in the mesocortical and mesolimbic tracts, which produce a lower incidence of EPS.

SIDE-EFFECT PROFILES   The broad range of side effects associated with the neuroleptic agents is generally due to the affinity of the neuroleptics for histamine-1, muscarinic, alpha-adrenergic, and dopamine-2 receptors. The incidence and severity are dose related, although EPS have occurred at relatively low doses. The degree to which any one neuroleptic agent causes the various side effects identified is determined by the pharmacokinetics unique to the medication and the biochemical uniqueness of each patient (Table 16-8-17).

Psychotherapy and Behavior Management Training

The psychotic disorders are now officially recognized as brain diseases and not psychological disorders. However, not all patients with a psychotic disorder will have a robust response to drug therapy. Because of this and the fact that the manifesting symptoms of a psychotic disorder can have a profoundly devastating emotional effect on a patient, medication management should be integrated with psychotherapeutic interventions. These interventions should include cognitive-behavioral approaches that incorporate social skills training, stress management, and medication compliance issues. Referral to a mental health facility that uses these approaches in an outpatient group therapy setting can provide patients with the support structure necessary for encouraging medication compliance and practicing techniques to enhance self-control.

Supportive Measures

Referral for assistance with activities of daily living and help with independent living skills is important. Patients also benefit greatly from support group activities that include discussion and role-playing of socially competent conflict resolution, criticism management, decision-making practice, and assertiveness training. It is important to assess the ability of the patient's family to manage the stress produced by the patient's level of functioning. The family's ability to cope with the patient's condition will significantly effect the patient's ongoing response to treatment.

Patients and their families should be encouraged to seek additional support for coping with the psychotic disorders. Some resources are

- National Institute of Mental Health: *http://www.nimh.nih.gov*
- National Mental Health Consumer Self-Help Clearinghouse, (800) 553-4539
- National Alliance for the Mentally Ill, (800) 950-6264 or on the Internet at *http://www.nami.org*
- National Mental Health Association, (800) 969-6642 or on the Internet at *http://www.nmha.org*

PATIENT EDUCATION

It is important to identify psychotic disorders as brain abnormalities that are not the result of "bad" parenting. Help patients and their families to see the condition as "nobody's fault." Patient education should include helping all parties involved to understand the nature of psychotic disorders, their treatment, and coping strategies for effectively dealing with the symptoms.

DISPOSITION

Prognosis

Given our better understanding of the nature of the psychotic disorders that has occurred over the past 100 years, there has been a significant change in treatment strategies. These changes have greatly improved patient outcome in terms of quality of life. Over 300 outcome studies document that, though far from perfect, one out of three patients with a diagnosed psychotic disorder may remain stable and avoid major relapsing episodes. The prognosis is directly related to receiving the proper medication or medications and compliance with the medication regimen, once stabilization is achieved.

Screening and Prevention

In the case of a psychotic disorder being caused by a specific medical condition such as Alzheimer's disease, screening for dementia can be useful for the purpose of ensuring early intervention to treat psychotic symptoms that can manifest due to dementia. Because a psychotic disorder may be substance induced, screening for substance abuse should be an ongoing concern to the primary care PA. It is also important to be aware of drug–drug interactions and the potential toxic levels of certain drugs that might produce a medication-induced psychosis. With timely monitoring of these medications, preventable complications can be avoided.

The most important issue in regards to prevention is not in terms of preventing the disease but rather in preventing relapse. To do so requires a concerted effort to encourage patients to remain compliant with taking their medication (or medications) at the appropriate dose, for an extended period of time—often for the rest of their lives.

COMPLICATIONS AND RED FLAGS

The major complicating factor influencing the course of a patient's psychic symptoms is noncompliance with treatment. Therefore, it is extremely important to help the patient realize that to achieve his or her personal goals will require compliance with treatment.

OTHER NOTES AND PEARLS

Monitoring the patient, on an ongoing basis, for tardive dyskinesia is absolutely essential. Routinely evaluating the patient for prodromal signs of relapse will minimize exacerbation of symptoms and full-blown psychotic episodes. When noncompliance is suspected, depot-jectable neuroleptics should be considered to control psychotic behavior.

The selection of the most appropriate neuroleptic for any one patient must take into consideration several factors. Efficacy for treating both the negative as well as the positive symptoms of psychosis is of paramount importance when attempting to plan for the long-term management of patients suffering from any one of the psychotic disorders. The reduced incidence of side effects found with the newer agents is a crucial factor to consider when dealing with the issue of patient compliance to the medication plan.

A major step in understanding psychotic disorders is to move away from the myths about the psychotic disorders that are commonly held.

- *Myth 1: Bad parenting causes psychosis.* Fact: This has been proven not to be the case! In fact, families of individuals with a psychotic disorder can be an important link to a more successful treatment outcome.

- *Myth 2: Schizophrenics (individuals with a psychotic disorder) have a "split personality."* Fact: Multiple personality disorder (its existence is hotly debated) is an entirely different phenomenon.

- *Myth 3: All psychotics are violent.* Fact: Individuals receiving the proper treatment for their psychosis are no more likely to become violent than any other person in the general population.

Manifesting symptoms of the psychotic disorders may be episodic, occurring in cycles. Because the psychotic disorders affect the way a person thinks, feels, and acts, without treatment, individuals with a psychotic disorder may have problems keeping a job or developing healthy relationships with others. The proper diagnosis and management of the psychotic disorders is medically challenging. Careful clinical evaluation is required. With the proper intervention, individuals afflicted with a psychotic disorder can lead healthy, fulfilling lives.

REFERENCES

Addonizio G, Susman VL. Neuroleptic malignant syndrome. In: Shriqui CL, Nasarallah HA, eds. *Contemporary Issues in the Treatment of Schizophrenia.* Washington, DC, American Psychiatric Press, 1995, pp. 551–574.

American Psychiatric Association. Practice guidelines for the treatment of patients with schizophrenia. *Am J Psychiatry* 154 (suppl 4):1–63; 1997.

American Psychiatric Association. *Diagnostic and Statistical Manual of Mental Disorders,* 4th ed (DSM-IV). Washington, DC, APA, 1994.

American Psychiatric Association. *Tardive Dyskinesia: A Task Force Report of the American Psychiatric Association.* Washington, DC, APA, 1992.

Anderson C, Chakos M, Mailman R, Lieberman J. Emerging roles for novel anti psychotic medications in the treatment of schizophrenia. *Psychiatr Clin North Am* 21:151–179; 1998.

Bachrach LL. What we know about homelessness among mentally ill persons: An analytic review and commentary. In: Lamb HR, Bachrach LL, Kass FI, eds. *Treating the Homeless Mentally Ill.* Washington, DC, American Psychiatric Press, 1992, pp. 13–40.

Baldessarini RJ. Drugs and the treatment of psychiatric disorders. In: Hardman JG, Limbird LE, eds. *Goodman & Gilman's The Pharmacological Basis of Therapeutics,* 9th ed New York, McGraw-Hill, 1996, pp. 399–430.

Bollini P, Pampallona S, Orza MJ, et al. Antipsychotic drugs: Is more worse? A meta-analysis of the published randomized control trials. *Psychol Med* 24:307–316; 1994.

Breir A, Wokowitzx OM, Pickar D. Stress and Schizophrenia. In: Tammings CA, Schultz SC, eds. *Schizophrenia Research. Vol I. Advances in Neuropsychiatry and Psychopharmacology.* New York, Raven, 1991, pp. 141–152.

Buka SL, Tsuang MT, Lipsitt LP. Pregnancy/delivery complications and psychiatric diagnosis: A prospective study. *Arch Gen Psychiatry* 50:151–156; 1993.

Cancro R, Lehmann HE. Schizophrenia: Clinical features. In: Kaplan HI, Sadock BJ, eds. *Comprehensive Textbook of Psychiatry.* 7th ed. Baltimore: Lippincott/Williams & Wilkins, 2000, pp. 1169–1194.

Carpenter WT, Buchanan RW. Schizophrenia. *N Engl J Med* 330:681–688; 1994.

Corbett R, Camacho F, Woods AT, et al. Antipsychotic agents antagonize noncompetitive N-methyl-D-aspartate antagonist-induced behaviors. *Psychopharmacology* 120:67–74; 1995.

Craig TKJ, Timms PW. Homelessness and schizophrenia. In: Hirsch SR, Weinberger DR, eds. *Schizophrenia.* Oxford, Blackwell Science, 1995, p. 664.

Davis KL, Kahn RS, Ko G, et al. Dopamine in schizophrenia: A review and re-conceptualization. *Am J Psychiatry* 148:1474–1486; 1991.

Gerlach J. Oral versus depot administration of neuroleptics in relapse prevention. *Acta Psychiatr Scand* 89(suppl 382):28–32; 1994.

Goff DC, Shader RI. Non-neurologic side effects of antipsychotic agents. In: Hirsch SR, Weinberger DR, eds. *Schizophrenia.* Oxford, Blackwell Science, 1995, p. 577.

Hegarty JD, Baldessarini RJ, Tohen M, et al. One hundred years of schizophrenia: A meta-analysis of the outcome literature. *Am J Psychiatry* 151:1409–1416; 1994.

Javitt DC, Zukin SR. Recent advances in the phencyclidine model of schizophrenia. *Am J Psychiatry* 148:1301–1308; 1991.

Jibson MD, Tandon R. A summary of research findings on the new anti psychotic drugs. *Essential Psychopharmacol* 1:1; 1996.

Kane JM. Drug therapy—schizophrenia. *N Engl J Med* 334:34–41; 1996.

Knoll JL, Garver DL, Rambug JE, et al. Heterogeneity of the psychosis: Is there a neurodegenerative psychosis? *Schizophrenia Bull* 24:365–379; 1998.

Liberman RP, Van Putten T, Marshall BD, et al. Optimal drug and behavior therapy for treatment-refractory schizophrenic patients. *Am J Psychiatry* 151:756–759; 1994.

Marder SR. Schizophrenia: Somatic treatment. In: Kaplan HI, Sadock BJ, eds. *Comprehensive Textbook of Psychiatry.* 7th ed, Baltimore, Lippincott/ Williams & Wilkins, 2000, pp. 1199–1205.

Marder SR, Meibach RC. Risperidone in the treatment of schizophrenia. *Am J Psychiatry* 151:825–835; 1994.

Marder SR, Van Putten T. Anti psychotic medications. In: Schatzberg AF, Nemeroff CB, eds. *Textbook of Psychopharmacology.* Washington, DC, American Psychiatric Press, p. 257, 1995.

Mass JW, Contreras SA, Miller AL, et al. Studies of catecholamine metabolism in schizophrenia/psychosis, 1. *Neuropsychopharmacology* 8:97–109; 1993.

McEvoy JP, Scheifler PL, Frances A, eds. The expert consensus guideline series: Treatment of schizophrenia—1999. *J Clin Psychiatry* 60(suppl 11):12–33; 1999.

McGlashan TH, Krystal JH. Schizophrenia-related disorders and dual diagnosis. In: Gabbard GO, ed. *Treatments of Psychiatric Disorders,* 2nd ed, Washington, DC, American Psychiatric Press, 1995, pp. 1039–1074.

Meltzer HY. Treatment of the neuroleptic-nonresponsive schizophrenic patient. *Schizophr Bull* 18:515–542; 1991.

Nasrallah HA. Neurodevelopmental pathogenesis of schizophrenia. *Psychiatr Clin North Am* 16:269–280; 1993.

Norquist GS, Karno M. Schizophrenia: Epidemiology. In: Kaplan HI, Sadock BJ, eds. *Comprehensive Textbook of Psychiatry.* 7th ed. Baltimore, Lippincott/ Williams & Wilkins, 2000, pp. 1110–1116.

Outcasts on Main Street: Report of the Federal Task Force on Homelessness and Severe Mental Illness. Washington, DC, US Department of Health and Human Services, Interagency Council on the Homeless, 1992.

Peuskens J. Risperidone in the treatment of patients with chronic schizophrenia: A multinational, multicenter, double-blind, parallel-group study versus haloperidol. *Br J Psychiatry* 166:712–726; 1995.

Pickar D. Prospects for pharmacotherapy of schizophrenia. *Lancet* 345:557; 1995.

Rifkin A. Pharmacologic strategies in the treatment of schizophrenia. *Psychiatr Clin North Am* 16:351–363; 1993.

Sande MA, Volberding PA. *The Medical Management of AIDS,* 3rd ed, Philadelphia, Saunders, 1992.

Schatzberg AF, Nemeroff CB, eds. *Textbook of Psychopharmacology.* Washington, DC, American Psychiatric Press, 1995.

Schooler NR, Keith SJ, Severe JB, et al. Maintenance treatment of schizophrenia: A review of dose reduction and family treatment strategies. *Psychiatr Q* 66:279–292; 1995.

Shriqui CL, Nasrallah HA, eds. *Contemporary Issues in the Treatment of Schizophrenia.* Washington, DC, American Psychiatric Press, 1995.

Small JG, Hirsch SR, Arvanitis LA, et al. Quetiapine in patients with schizophrenia. A high- and low-dose double-blind comparison with placebo. Seroquel study group. *Arch Gen Psychiatry* 54:549–557; 1997.

Straube ER, Oades RG. Genetic studies. *Schizophrenia: Empirical Research and Findings.* San Diego, Academic Press, pp. 361–384, 1992.

Tienari P, Kaleva M, Lahl I, et al. Adoption studies on schizophrenia. In: Eggers C, ed. *Schizophrenia and Youth: Etiology and Therapeutic Consequences.* Berlin, Springer-Verlag, 1991, pp. 42–51.

Tollefson GD, Beasley CM, Tran PU, et al. Olanzapine versus haloperidol in the treatment of schizophrenia and schizoaffective and schizophreniform disorders: Results of an international collaborative trial. *Am J Psychiatry* 154:457–465; 1997.

Waltrip RW, Carrigan DR, Carpenter WT. Immunopathology and viral reactivation: A general theory of schizophrenia. *J Nerv Ment Dis* 178:729–738; 1990.

Waring EM. The psychobiology of first-episode schizophrenia. *Can J Psychiatry* 40(suppl 2):S33–S37; 1995.

Weinberger DR, Berman KF, Suddath R, et al. Evidence of dysfunction of a prefrontal-limbic network in schizophrenia: A magnetic resonance imaging and regional cerebral blood flow study of discordant monozygotic twins. *Am J Psychiatry* 149:890–897; 1992.

Zisook S, Heaton R, Moranville J, et al. Past substance abuse and clinical course of schizophrenia. *Am J Psychiatry* 149:552–553; 1992.

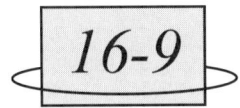

PERSONALITY DISORDERS

16-9

Don St. John

DISCUSSION

The Diagnostic and Statistical Manual of Mental Disorders, fourth edition (DSM-IV) defines *personality traits* as "enduring patterns of perceiving, relating to, and thinking about the environment and oneself that are exhibited in a wide range of social and personal contexts." A diagnosis of a personality disorder is entertained when the patient demonstrates an "enduring pattern of inner experience and behavior that deviates markedly from the expectations of the individual's culture, is pervasive, and inflexible, has an onset in adolescence or early adulthood, is stable over time, and leads to distress or impairment" (DSM-IV). The DSM-IV does not refer to personality dimensions. This chapter will follow the convention of referring to specific personality disorders as categories that are either present or absent.

Personality disorders become evident in early adulthood. Although personality traits may become exaggerated under stress, a diagnosis of a personality disorder is given only when symptoms are persistently maladaptive. Longitudinal evaluation using all available data is the best approach to diagnosing a patient with a personality disorder.

In diagnosing a personality disorder, the clinician must take into account cultural, ethnic, and social background. Personality features also vary in severity. The defining behaviors and thought patterns must not be due to other psychiatric and nonpsychiatric conditions or substance use.

Behaviors and cognitions related to a personality disorder usually disturb others more than the patient. Clues to the presence of a personality disorder include difficulties in the therapeutic relationship, aberrant expectations of others by the patient, and clinician (and other staff) frustration and negative feelings toward a patient. The presence of childhood conduct problems is an independent predictor of personality disorder in all clusters.

The diagnosis *personality disorder due to a general medical condition* is used when an enduring and maladaptive personality change is secondary to medical conditions. Unlike the other personality disorders, this is placed on axis I of the psychiatric five-axis diagnostic scheme. Table 16-9-1 lists some medical conditions that can cause personality change.

AXIS II PERSONALITY DISORDER CLUSTERS

Personality disorders are placed on axis II of the psychiatric five-axis diagnostic system. Placement on axis II does not imply that these disorders are less likely than axis I disorders to be etiologically related to biologic and psychosocial risk factors, or that the axis II disorders are less likely to be genetically related to one or more axis I disorders. There is also no inherent assumption that medications and psychotherapy will fail to have a positive impact. Personality traits that do not reach the threshold of a specific diagnosable disorder may be listed on axis II as "traits" of that disorder.

Personality-disordered patients meet criteria for an average of three personality disorder diagnoses. Most patients with significant personality pathology are diagnosed with a mixed personality disorder, because they are not diagnosable by specific DSM-IV categorical criteria.

DSM-IV organizes personality disorders into three main clusters, based on descriptive similarities (Table 16-9-2). In clinical practice,

TABLE 16-9-1. Medical Causes of Personality Change

Apathy	Concussion, brain tumor, frontal lobe pathology, cerebral vascular accident (CVA), Huntington's disease, hyperparathyroidism, adrenal insufficiency
Disinhibition	Frontal lobe tumor or injury (especially right), CVA, Huntington's disease, Wilson's disease, syphilis, epilepsy
Irritability	Pernicious anemia, Wilson's disease, Huntington's disease, adrenal insufficiency or excess, brain injury, hyperprolactinemia
Mood lability	Brain injury (especially right cerebrum and frontal lobes), CVA, migraine (episodic mood changes), hypercortisolism, acromegaly, Huntington's disease
Aggression	Brain tumor or injury (especially frontal lobe)
Obsessive-compulsive	Chronic fatigue syndrome, epilepsy, frontal lobe pathology
Suspiciousness	Hypothyroidism, brain injury, partial complex seizures
Dependent	Chronic fatigue syndrome

Substance abuse, brain injuries, and brain tumors may result in a variety of personality changes

the clusters have come to be used as a diagnostic shorthand (e.g., a patient who allows others to make most of his or her decisions, is highly anxious in social situations, and is overly sensitive to criticism may be described as having "cluster C features." The diagnosis "personality disorder, NOS (not otherwise specified)" is used when a personality pattern meets general criteria for a personality disorder, with traits of different personality disorders present, but symptoms do not meet the full criteria for any of the personality disorders individually.

PREVALENCE

Ten to fifteen percent of the general population meets the full criteria for a personality disorder. Personality disorders are diagnosable in 50% to 75% of patients in an outpatient psychiatric clinic, and 40% to 77% of patients on an inpatient psychiatric unit. Of those seen in an outpatient psychiatric clinic, 7% meet the criteria for cluster A, 63% for cluster B, and 30% for cluster C diagnosis.

ETIOLOGY

The etiology of personality disorders appears to be multifactorial, and the diathesis–stress model is most applicable. Personality traits—such as impulsivity, aggression, reward dependence, and harm avoidance—

appear to be significantly heritable. Environmental factors may amplify temperamental dispositions.

CATEGORICAL PERSONALITY DIAGNOSIS: CLUSTER A

Paranoid Personality Disorder

PREVALENCE Patients with paranoid personality disorder (paranoid PD) are likely to come into the medical care system not because they recognize and desire assistance with their problems, but because of litigation issues such as a disability or a malpractice claim. The prevalence of paranoid PD is reported to be 0.5% to 2.5% in the general population, 10% to 30% among those in inpatient psychiatric settings, and 2% to 10% in outpatient mental health clinics.

DIAGNOSIS The most distinctive feature is pervasive suspiciousness. Patients with paranoid PD assume others are exploiting, harming, or deceiving them. Patients rarely acquire insight. Arguments and conflicts with medical practitioners are common. The patients tend to socially isolate themselves and are hypervigilant of their environment.

They misread the actions of others and magnify minor slights. As a result, they tend to distrust the practitioner's motives. They usually have no long-term interpersonal relationships of any depth. Because of their suspicious nature and perception of attacks on their character that are not apparent to others, they tend to be highly litigious. These patients often have difficulty dealing with the medical profession, because they detest dependency. Circumstances placing the patient in a dependent position may even result in psychotic symptoms. They have difficulty sharing personal information, fearing it may be used against them, and tend to deny any difficulties they may be having.

They frequently read demeaning or threatening meanings into the remarks and actions of others, and are unable and unwilling to perceive reality as others do. They tend to bear grudges and are unwilling to forgive, difficult to get along with, and argumentative and complaining. They tend to elicit a hostile response in others. They have inflexible and constricted coping skills. Alcohol and substance abuse and dependence are common.

Symptoms wax and wane according to stress. Patients commonly include clinicians in their delusional systems. Delusions tend to be systematic, rational, and convincing. They may experience brief psychotic episodes (minutes to hours), which may eventually meet criteria for delusional disorder or schizophrenia.

TREATMENT Paranoid PD carries a poor prognosis. At best, therapy may control or modulate, but not reverse the basic personality pattern. Avoid challenging paranoid ideas, but do not falsely agree with or confirm paranoid beliefs. Avoid confronting delusions, which only tends to increase anger and distrust.

TABLE 16-9-2. Comparison of Personality Disorders

CLUSTER A (ODD, ECCENTRIC)			CLUSTER B (DRAMATIC, EMOTIONAL, ERRATIC)				CLUSTER C (ANXIOUS, FEARFUL)		
PARANOID	SCHIZOID	SCHIZOTYPAL	ANTISOCIAL	BORDERLINE	HISTRIONIC	NARCISSISTIC	AVOIDANT	DEPENDENT	OBSESSIVE-COMPULSIVE
Pervasive suspiciousness	Detached relationships	Social deficits	Disregard for rights of others	Affective lability	Excessive emotionality	Grandiosity	Social inhibition	Excessive need to be cared for	Perfectionism
	Restricted emotions	Cognitive and perceptual distortions	Violation of rights of others	Chronic dysphoria	Provocative interpersonal style	Excessive need to be admired	Feelings of inadequacy	Submissive and clinging behavior	Mental and interpersonal control
		Eccentric behavior		Unstable relationships	Attention seeking	Lack of empathy	Hypersensitivity to negative evaluation	Fear of separation	Excessive orderliness
				Impulsivity					

Take a professional, but not over-friendly, stance. Attend to and be empathic toward patient fears, even if the patient appears irrational. Maintain a comfortable interpersonal distance. Because of their litigious nature, keep meticulous records. A supportive approach may reduce suspiciousness, quick temper, and volatility. Help the patient identify potential rewards of getting along with others.

Outline detailed treatment plans, and give advance information about potential risks. Explain each step of any procedure to the patient, and document all interactions in detail. Give the patient as much control over treatment as possible. Avoid elective (especially cosmetic) surgical procedures. Specific psychotherapeutic interventions include improving coping skills and assertiveness training. Low-dose neuroleptics may be helpful for psychotic breaks, and to decrease paranoia.

Schizoid Personality Disorder

DIAGNOSIS Individuals meeting criteria for schizoid personality disorder (schizoid PD) are infrequently seen in clinical settings, seeking treatment only during crisis or because of the concerns of others. Generally they delay seeking care.

The essential feature of schizoid PD is detachment from social relationships and restricted emotions in interpersonal settings. Patients with schizoid PD neither desire nor enjoy close relationships, tend to choose solitary activities, and are labeled as loners. They take pleasure in few, if any, activities, and prefer mechanical or abstract activities. They appear indifferent to the praise or criticism of others, and are oblivious to the subtleties of social interaction. They may appear emotionally cold and detached, with flat affect, and rarely reciprocate gestures or facial expressions. A patient with schizoid PD may feel threatened by an illness that forces interaction with others such as health care providers.

These patients show little interest in sexual experiences with others, and usually don't marry. Patients with schizoid PD have poor insight and low motivation to change. Brief psychotic episodes (minutes to hours) may occur in response to stress. These personality traits are often present in childhood, but are not necessarily lifelong. Alcohol and drug use may co-occur.

Differential diagnosis includes autism and avoidant personality disorder. Patients with autism have more severe social impairment and stereotypical behaviors and interests. Patients with avoidant personality disorder fear social situations, while schizoid patients have no desire for social interaction.

TREATMENT Patients with schizoid PD respond best to a supportive stance, and appreciate efforts to ensure privacy. Clinicians should focus on the more technical, not interpersonal, elements of treatment. Specific interventions that may be helpful include crisis intervention and social skills training. Patients may respond to a group therapy setting to enhance social image, motivation, and interpersonal skills. Pharmacotherapy is used only for specific targeted symptoms. Stimulants may enhance energy and affect.

Schizotypal Personality Disorder

PREVALENCE Patients with schizotypal personality disorder (schizotypal PD) may seek treatment in a primary care setting for anxiety and depression, and over half have a history of major depressive disorder. They tend to present because of occupational or social problems, or the concern of others.

Schizotypal PD has been reported to occur in approximately 3% of the general population and may be slightly more common in males. Schizotypal PD is believed to be genetically related to schizophrenia, because a small proportion of patients do eventually meet full criteria for schizophrenia. There is considerable co-occurrence with schizoid, paranoid, avoidant, and borderline personality disorder.

DIAGNOSIS The essential feature of schizotypal PD is the presence of social and interpersonal deficits with cognitive or perceptual distortions and eccentricities of behavior. Diagnostic criteria include ideas of reference; odd beliefs or magical thinking; unusual perceptual experiences; odd thinking and speech; suspiciousness or paranoia (similar to paranoid PD); inappropriate or constricted affect; social isolation similar to schizoid PD; lack of social skills; odd, eccentric, or peculiar behavior or appearance; lack of close friends other than first-degree relatives; and excessive social anxiety.

Schizotypal PD can be distinguished from paranoid PD and schizoid PD by the presence of eccentricity and cognitive/perceptual distortions. It is differentiated from mild autism by a more severe lack of social awareness and the absence of stereotypical behaviors.

TREATMENT Clinicians may need to give advice to these patients more than with others, especially since they seem to have difficulty generalizing information. A supportive approach, to enhance self-worth, can be helpful. Social supports should be strengthened to discourage isolation. Respect the patient's sensitivities. Identify and encourage areas of positive interest. Avoid probing into personal matters, which may be experienced as painful or terrifying.

The psychotherapeutic approach used with patients with schizophrenia (e.g., reality-testing, social skills training, attention to interpersonal boundaries, and psychoeducation) may be helpful. Interactions should be well structured. Institutional treatment may actually increase symptoms and should be avoided when possible.

Individuals with schizotypal PD may respond to the same neuroleptic medications used to treat schizophrenia. When used, neuroleptics should be given in low doses. Patients tend to be very sensitive to medication side effects, especially during quiescent periods. Selective serotonin reuptake inhibitors may be helpful for treating anxiety and depressive symptoms.

CATEGORICAL PERSONALITY DIAGNOSIS: CLUSTER B

Antisocial Personality Disorder

PREVALENCE Patients with antisocial personality disorder usually present for treatment as an ultimatum from others (often in the context of a legal investigation), for depressed mood, or for treatment of substance abuse. Patients may complain of dysphoria, anxiety, and an inability to tolerate boredom.

The overall prevalence of antisocial PD in community samples is about 3% in males and 1% in females. Prevalence estimates in clinical settings varies from 3 to 30%, depending on the predominant characteristics of the populations being sampled. Even higher prevalence rates are associated with prison settings, with up to 80% of men and 65% of women meeting full criteria. Half of patients in alcohol treatment and the majority of heroin and other drug addicts meet full criteria. Seventy-five percent of patients with antisocial PD will spend one or more years behind bars. Forty percent of boys and 25% of girls with childhood conduct disorder are eventually diagnosed with antisocial PD. There seems to be little variation in prevalence across ethnic groups.

DIAGNOSIS The essential diagnostic feature of antisocial PD is a disregard for and violation of the rights of others. This begins in childhood or early adolescence and continues into adulthood. Older terms for antisocial PD include psychopathy and sociopathy.

Antisocial PD cannot be diagnosed until a patient reaches the age of 18 years. Childhood conduct disorder (CD) must be present prior to age 15 for the diagnosis to be made. CD is characterized by a persistent pattern of behaviors in which the basic rights of others, or major age-appropriate societal rules, are violated. A patient meets criteria for antisocial PD only if the essential personality features are inflexible, maladaptive, and persistent.

Antisocial patients fail to conform to social norms of lawful behavior. Their demeanor may be arrogant, with an inflated self-appraisal. They lack empathy, while maintaining an intellectual understanding of right and wrong. Even though a personality disorder may be behind an individual's illegal behavior, patients with antisocial PD are accountable for their actions, as they lack only the will to obey rules.

Malingering may bring the antisocial patient to the attention of health care professionals. Deceitfulness, repeated lying, use of aliases, and conning and manipulating others for personal profit or pleasure are common. They are often compulsive or pathologic liars, knowing what is and is not a lie. Because of their deceitfulness, clinicians need information from others for diagnostic and assessment purposes. The history obtained from family members is usually more accurate than that from the patient.

Relationships are superficial, short-lived, and bereft of trust. They treat others as objects, and believe they have no obligation to society or others. They are impulsive, which can result in irresponsible and dangerous health behaviors, acting with no consideration of consequences.

Irritability and aggressiveness result in repeated fights and assaults. They have a reckless disregard for the safety of self or others, as indicated by fast and dangerous driving, unsafe sexual behavior, and substance use.

Affect dysregulation is associated with antisocial PD in women, especially poor anger modulation. Women may express the disorder primarily through promiscuous sex or emotionally manipulative relationships. These symptoms and behaviors make differentiation from borderline personality disorder difficult.

Patients with antisocial PD are consistently irresponsible. They fail to sustain consistent work or honor financial obligations. Sexual relationships are often irresponsible and exploitative. Many are incompetent as parents, and child neglect and abuse is a very real danger. They fail to learn from past actions.

A lack of remorse is very characteristic of patients with antisocial PD. They may blame the victims of their behavior for consequences, and fail to compensate or make amends. Patients do not regard their behaviors as problematic.

COURSE   The course of the disorder is difficult to predict for any given individual. Behaviors may become less evident and even remit at an average age of 35 years. Remission is more likely in the patient who remains married, has strong family ties, and is involved in the community.

COMORBIDITY   Common comorbid conditions include pathologic gambling, depression, attention-deficit hyperactivity disorder (ADHD), somatization disorder, factitious disorder, malingering, and paraphilias. Patients with antisocial PD are more likely to have learning disorders, and score 10 points lower than the general population on IQ testing. Many will also meet criteria for borderline, histrionic, and narcissistic personality disorder.

ETIOLOGY   Males in families of patients with antisocial PD are more likely to have antisocial PD, substance abuse, ADHD, and learning disabilities. Females in the same families are more likely to have depression or somatization. The presence of antisocial PD in a parent predicts oppositional defiant disorder in boys.

A combination of environmental and genetic factors may be required for antisocial PD to develop, especially for women. Poverty, substandard housing, bad neighborhoods, parental abuse and neglect, inadequate nutrition and medical care, absence of parent(s), and erratic or inappropriate discipline are environmental factors associated with antisocial PD. Physiologic findings in patients with antisocial PD include low central nervous system serotonin, excessive testosterone, and frontal lobe pathology.

TREATMENT   Developing rapport can be very difficult. Clinicians should avoid power struggles. To avoid being perceived as judgmental, define antisocial behavior as a disorder to the patient. Carefully and respectfully investigate the concerns and motives they bring to medical encounters. Communicate directly, and avoid being punitive. Set clear limits on indicated medical procedures.

There is no proven treatment for antisocial PD; however, patients and their significant others can benefit from certain general therapies, such as anger management and problem solving. Patients must be invested for treatment to be effective. Focus on the disadvantages of antisocial behavior to the patient, and the personal advantages to changing behaviors. Treat coexisting disorders. A milieu treatment program may be of benefit. Inpatient settings are usually not helpful.

Patients with antisocial PD tend not to respond as well to antidepressants. There are a variety of drugs that can be used to curb aggression, including lithium, buspirone, SSRIs, and anticonvulsants. Avoid the use of benzodiazepines, which may decrease impulse control and lead to addiction.

Borderline Personality Disorder

PREVALENCE   Of all the personality disorders, patients with borderline personality disorder (borderline PD) are the most commonly seen and most disruptive patients in a primary care setting. Borderline PD is a common psychiatric disorder, affecting 2 to 8% of the general population, 10% of patients treated in an outpatient mental health setting, and 20% of patients in an inpatient psychiatric setting. Although it is diagnosed more commonly in women (75% of patients), many males with borderline PD may be misdiagnosed with an antisocial personality disorder, because male psychiatric patients tend to have more antisocial characteristics. Patients may present to a psychiatrist for suicidal ideation and behavior, self-mutilation, and mood disturbance and to primary care practitioners with somatic complaints, chronic pain, medication sensitivity, and drug-seeking.

DIAGNOSIS   The core dimensions of the disorder include affective lability and chronic dysphoria, unstable relationships, and behavioral impulsivity. Sensitivity to perceptions of abandonment is the most sensitive and specific criteria for borderline personality disorder, and may be the primary basis for relational instability. Labeling an adolescent with borderline PD should be avoided, as many of the characteristics of borderline PD are "normal" during adolescence.

The patient's frantic efforts to avoid real or imagined abandonment result in excessive dependency and intolerance for being alone. They may have extreme reactions to seemingly minor incidents, such as having an appointment changed or waiting beyond the scheduled appointment time. Attempts to foster autonomy may be interpreted by the patient as imminent abandonment. Apparently clinging behaviors such as bringing up a dramatic complaint (e.g., chest pain) at the end of an appointment and requesting to personally speak to one specific clinician are common. Pleas for help are made through frequent crises, purposely simulating or complicating medical conditions, and active interference with treatment and recovery.

Patients consume a disproportionate amount of time and may make excessive demands for prompt, simplistic solutions to problems, medications, excuses (e.g., work and school), disability, and frequent and unnecessary phone calls and appointments. They then respond to limit setting as reflecting a lack of empathy and understanding on the part of the practitioner.

Patients with borderline PD display a pattern of unstable and intense interpersonal relationships characterized by alternating extremes of idealization and devaluation. An inexperienced clinician may experience extreme frustration when a patient rapidly changes from overdependence to angry rejection. Angry outbursts and suicidal behaviors may occur in response to seemingly minor stressors such as the clinician announcing that he or she will be on vacation for a few days.

A therapeutic relationship may develop very rapidly, often after one or two meetings, with the patient degrading past clinicians. Boundary violations such as excessive interest in clinician's personal affairs, seductive behaviors, premature familiarity with provider and other staff, making special requests, and giving expensive gifts are typical behaviors.

They usually have a very poor or absent social support system, and often use only professionals (who are safe) for support. They tend to feel safer with a pet. Splitting is common because of an inability to integrate contradictory experiences, ideas, representations. This is often evident when there is strong disagreement among staff members, with certain staff strongly defending the patient. They are hypervigilant to any indication of untruthfulness or exploitation by a professional.

Another feature of borderline PD is the markedly and persistently unstable self-image or sense of self. This results in frequent and significant changes in values, goals, career, and sexual orientation, and contradictory self-representations. Patients complain of chronic feelings of emptiness, and may complain of boredom, constantly seeking something to do.

Potentially self-damaging impulsivity may be evident by excessive spending, unsafe sexual behaviors, substance abuse, reckless driving, binge eating, or gambling. Such behaviors are often in response to a relationship problem or other stressor. Uncontrolled impulsivity is a poor prognostic indicator.

The consequences of recurrent suicidal behavior, gestures, or threats, and self-mutilating behaviors, are common to those working in an emergency or critical care setting. Patients often have an ever-present wish to not be alive. Patients will not volunteer, and even deny, suicidal and self-harm thoughts because of fears of involuntary hospitalization. The risk of a completed suicide is 8 to 10%. Self-harm behaviors (e.g., cutting, burning, biting, bruising, head banging, hair pulling, recklessness) are not suicide attempts, but performed to counter emotional numbness, punish the self, relieve stress, manipulate others, seek attention, communicate intense emotions, carry out vengeance, escape a situation, or just out of habit.

The basic mood is dysphoria. Patients may appear fine to others, while complaining of extreme depression and anger. Affective instability due to a marked reactivity of mood commonly results in an erroneous diagnosis of a bipolar disorder; conversely, patients with bipolar disorders, especially bipolar II disorder, are often diagnosed with borderline PD, despite the absence of the other diagnostic criteria for this disorder.

Inappropriate, intense anger or difficulty controlling anger (e.g., frequent displays of temper, constant anger, recurrent physical fights) has lead to the term "borderline rage." They often turn their anger and rage upon themselves in self-harm behaviors. Patients may threaten lawsuits in response to apparently minor incidents. Transient paranoid ideation or severe dissociative symptoms often occur in response to stress, as a coping mechanism. Patients may complain of losing time, and may be diagnosed by others with "multiple personality disorder." The intermittent presence of psychotic-like symptoms (hallucinations, ideas of reference, paranoid ideation, derealization or depersonalization, distortions of reality) resulted in the term "borderline," to signify that these patients vacillate between neurotic and psychotic symptoms. Clinicians may have difficulty obtaining a cohesive history because of lapses of memory during dissociative episodes.

COURSE   The course of illness varies considerably among patients. There is some evidence of borderline PD "burning out," or presenting with less dramatic behaviors, after age 35 to 40, but some patients continue with pervasive dysfunction. Impulsivity tends to decrease with age, but dysphoria and the sense of inner chaos often persist. Some patients deteriorate in their 40s and 50s. Often patients demonstrate a pattern of undermining themselves, especially just before a goal is to be realized, and tend towards recurrent job loss, interrupted education, and broken marriages. Poor outcome is associated with self-damaging acts, inappropriate anger, and substance abuse. A good outcome is associated with higher IQ and shorter length of hospitalizations.

COMORBIDITY   Patients diagnosed with borderline personality disorder often meet the criteria for other personality disorders, especially antisocial, histrionic, schizotypal, and avoidant personality disorders. Most patients also meet criteria for at least one axis I disorder, including mood, somatoform, substance abuse, dissociative, generalized anxiety, panic, and schizoaffective disorders. The features of borderline PD overlap extensively with post-traumatic stress disorder.

ETIOLOGY   There is no consensus regarding etiology. Psychoanalytic theories of the etiology of borderline personality run the gamut from overprotective mothering to maternal neglect, and there is some empirical support for these explanations. Other proposed environmental factors include a seriously deficient maternal presence characterized by irregular parental control, parental inconsistency, histrionic and exhibitionist parental models, serious childhood abuse characterized by a childhood environment of trauma, early separation or loss, abnormal parenting, early, prolonged, betrayal, and an invalidating childhood environment.

Patients with borderline PD appear to have a biological vulnerability to stress. Borderline personality disorder is five times more likely to be present in first-degree relatives. There is also evidence that personality dimensions and traits, such as affective dysregulation and impulsive aggression, appear strongly inheritable. Family history and biological data do not support borderline personality disorder as a mood-spectrum disorder. There appears to be little difference in prevalence cross-culturally.

Early sexual abuse is present in 70 to 85% of patients, and tends to occur early, by a primary caregiver, and is ongoing and serious. However, only 20% of such sexually abused children eventually develop borderline personality disorder.

TREATMENT   There is no specific pharmacotherapeutic agent for the treatment of borderline personality disorder. Patient response to treatment tends to be nonspecific, with patients often showing only modest improvement over placebo (20 to 30%). Patients often fail to notice a response to medications, while others may report significant improvement. Assessment of response to any treatment program should be assessed by considering the level of functioning and the report(s) of significant others.

Treatment is determined by first identifying target symptoms. The duration of treatment is clinically defined. The potential for dangerous overdose should be taken into consideration. Unusual side effects and drug reactions are not uncommon. Patients with histrionic features are especially sensitive to side effects. There are both pros and cons to the options of splitting psycho- and pharmacotherapy between different practitioners versus having one practitioner handle both.

Avoid prescribing to placate a patient, hostile prescribing (e.g., using a neuroleptic to mute the patient), withholding medications due to negative countertransference or fear that a drug may reduce the patient's investment in therapy, or dogmatically not prescribing because of a past history of substance abuse.

The presence of a comorbid: axis I disorder has no relationship to response to antidepressants. Response tends to be nonspecific, with improvement noticed for a variety of symptoms. Antidepressants tend to promote more contained responses to stress. Serotonergic agents may be helpful for the treatment of anger, affective reactivity, depressed mood, impulsivity, self-harm behaviors, irritability and aggression, rejection sensitivity, and mood lability. Monoamine oxidase inhibitors may be used for treating impulsivity, anger, and atypical depressive symptoms. However, patients may not comply with the required dietary restrictions. Patients tend to respond poorly to tricyclic antidepressants.

Antipsychotics may be useful for anger/hostility, aggression, impulsivity, racing and psychotic thoughts, paranoia, dissociation, ideas of reference, anxiety, and depression. Use of antipsychotics may decrease suicidal behavior. Antipsychotics may have an antidepressant effect as well with these patients.

Mood stabilizers (thymoleptics) tend to decrease impulsivity and mood lability. Lithium may be effective for impulsivity, aggression, and mood lability. Carbamazepine or valproic acid may be used to treat aggression, anger, irritability, impulsivity, mood lability, and dissociation.

Benzodiazepines may be helpful for hostility, suspiciousness, cognitive disturbance, sleep, and anxiety, but they can cause behavioral disinhibition. Patients may claim improvement in their mood while significant others report a significant increase in symptoms. These patients are also at high risk for abuse and dependence.

Stimulants may be helpful for concomitant ADHD-like symptoms, and may be effective in treating aggression, impulsivity, and occasionally violence. Naltrexone may decrease self-harm thoughts and behaviors.

The therapeutic relationship is central to effective therapy. Psychotherapy can be effective if it maintains a cognitive-behavioral approach, focuses on teaching coping skills, helps the patient develop tolerance to emotional intensity, is structured, and has clearly identified boundaries and limits. Therapy is longer term than with other disorders. Group therapy can be quite effective, if it is very structured and takes a psychoeducational approach. Psychoanalytic therapy is poorly tolerated and probably contraindicated.

Hospitalization is used primarily for asylum and respite from intense emotions or interactions. Inpatient treatment should be brief and goal-oriented, and serves not as a cure but as a life preserver.

Histrionic Personality Disorder

PREVALENCE Patients with histrionic personality disorder usually present to the primary care setting with multiple exaggerated somatic complaints. Their dramatic presentation may appear out of proportion to the actual seriousness of their medical or emotional problem. Prevalence of histrionic PD is estimated at 2 to 3% in general population studies, and 10 to 15% in inpatient and outpatient mental health settings when assessed with a structured interview.

DIAGNOSIS The essential features of the disorder are excessive emotionality, a provocative interpersonal style, and attention-seeking behaviors. These patients are uncomfortable in situations where they are not the center of attention. They are at increased risk of suicidal gestures to obtain attention and caregiving.

Attempts to control and obtain attention from others often takes the form of exaggerated compliments, gifts, flirtatiousness, or requests for special treatment (e.g., extra time during appointments). They may give dramatic descriptions of symptoms, and present new symptoms at each visit to maintain the clinician's attention. Patients may be inappropriately sexually seductive or provocative in behavior and dress. Often same-sex relationships are impaired. Because these patients use physical appearance to draw attention to them, patients may become overly concerned that a medical problem will destroy their attractiveness.

They frequently respond to stressors through somatic complaints. These patients are suggestible, and may give answers they believe the clinician wants to hear. Excessively impressionistic speech that is lacking in detail poses a challenge to obtaining a good medical history.

Individuals with histrionic personality disorder consider their interpersonal relationships as more intimate than they actually are. They often address professionals by their first names, even after only one visit, and behave in an excessively familiar manner.

COMORBIDITY Common associated disorders include somatization; conversion; a major depressive disorder; and borderline, narcissistic, antisocial, and dependent personality disorders.

TABLE 16-9-3. Working with Patients Who Somatize

1. Rule out diagnosable medical illness.
2. Acknowledge symptoms as real. Then reframe somatic complaints as an expression of stress (e.g., "your body's way of telling you you're stressed").
3. Provide limited reassurance.
4. Explicitly state the limits on your own behaviors (e.g., what you are and are not willing to do), and outline these limits at the outset of treatment.
5. Be conservative with medical management:
   - Avoid both over- and under-responding to medical problems.
   - Avoid responding to presented crises as emergencies, if they are not true emergencies.
   - Avoid extensive diagnostic testing.
6. Schedule frequent, regular, brief, structured appointments, during which presented symptoms are addressed, but the focus of the encounter is on life stressors and the patient's level of functioning.
7. Simultaneously attend to both medical symptoms and current stressful psychosocial situations.
8. Lower treatment expectations.
9. The treatment goal is to manage, not cure or control, medical complaints.
10. Focus on the patient's level of functioning (social, occupational, etc.) when assessing treatment response.
11. Limit the number of providers involved in the patient's care.
12. Have the patient see the same practitioner, nurse, receptionist, and examining room for familiarity (for the patient) and control of splitting (for the staff).
13. Encourage collaboration.
14. Monitor drug use closely, and limit prescription amounts and refills.
15. Know what over-the-counter drugs the patient is taking.
16. Avoid polypharmacy.

TREATMENT When working with histrionic patients, the clinician should emphasize objective issues and avoid emotional issues. Interpersonal boundaries should be clearly established. Treatment goals should be specific and behaviorally oriented. Scheduling appointments at regular intervals can reduce disruptive phone calls and "emergency" visits. Table 16-9-3 lists other general ways of working with somaticizing patients. Antidepressants can be effective for depressive symptoms.

Narcissistic Personality Disorder

PREVALENCE Patients with narcissistic personality disorder may present to the primary care setting with depressive symptoms. Such individuals are not likely to seek psychiatric help unless they have received a severe challenge to their sense of superiority. More often the patient presents at the insistence of a significant other, especially if sustained grandiosity has led to hypomanic-like symptoms, such as decreased need for sleep, increased activity level, and grandiosity.

The prevalence of narcissistic personality disorder is less than 1% in the general population and 2 to 16% in clinical populations. Fifty to seventy-five percent of patients diagnosed with narcissistic personality disorder are male.

DIAGNOSIS The essential features of narcissistic personality disorder are grandiosity, excessive need for admiration, and lack of empathy. Patients may overestimate their abilities, and are sensitive to criticism. They are preoccupied with fantasies of unlimited success, power, and beauty, whether true vocational function is high (demonstrating ambition and confidence) or low (demonstrating unwillingness to risk).

In the clinical setting, these patients will often describe the many important people they know and imply that the clinician is not prestigious enough to treat them. They will often demand to have "the expert" clinician and "only the best" treatment. Developing an illness can be frightening and threatening, as it means they are vulnerable, and not special. They often deny an illness and minimize symptoms, leading to noncompliance. This sense of entitlement may lead to lawsuits and frequent changes of providers. Their sense of entitlement results in excessive and often unrealistic demands and an expectation to be catered to. They have a lack of sensitivity to the needs of others. Individuals with this disorder may become frustrated and angry when they do not get the recognition or special treatment they believe they deserve and may react with rage or counterattack. Patients require excessive admiration and attention, because of the presence of a fragile self-esteem.

COMORBIDITY Common comorbid conditions include anorexia, substance abuse (especially cocaine), and histrionic, borderline, antisocial, and paranoid personality disorders.

TREATMENT Acknowledge the patient's strengths and allow the patient to maintain a sense of competence by channeling his or her "skills" to deal with medical problems. Work towards collaboration in treatment. Set limits appropriately and empathetically. Depressive symptoms may respond to pharmacotherapy.

CLUSTER C

Avoidant Personality Disorder

PREVALENCE Patients with avoidant personality disorder may present physical symptoms as a reason for avoiding others and social activities. The prevalence of avoidant personality disorder is between 0.5% and 1% in the general population and about 10% in outpatient mental health clinics; it is diagnosed with equal frequency in males and females.

DIAGNOSIS The essential features of avoidant personality disorder are social inhibition, feelings of inadequacy, and hypersensitivity to negative evaluation. In contrast to patients with many other personality disorders, individuals with avoidant personality disorder frequently have sufficient insight to provide the clinician with the criteria necessary to make the diagnosis.

Because of fears of rejection, patients avoid occupational activities requiring interpersonal contact. They assume others will be critical, and they avoid group activities. Patients show restraint within intimate relationships because of their fear of shame, and are preoccupied with being criticized or rejected in social situations. They are usually isolated with a poor social support network. They may avoid novel situations and many medical treatments because of their unusual reluctance to take personal risks, and fear of embarrassment.

COMORBIDITY Mood and anxiety disorders, cluster A personality disorders, and borderline personality disorders are common. Social phobia may be difficult to differentiate from avoidant personality disorder. Avoidant personality disorder is essentially a problem of relating to persons, and social phobia is primarily a problem of performing in social situations.

TREATMENT The symptoms of avoidant personality disorder may improve with time. The clinician should take a supportive and empathic stance. Anxious and depressive symptoms should be treated, following standard treatment regimens. Beta blockers may be useful to lower autonomic excitation.

Dependent Personality Disorder

PREVALENCE Dependent personality disorder is among the most frequently reported personality disorders in clinical and nonclinical populations. It is diagnosed 2.5 to 4 times more often in women than in men.

DIAGNOSIS The essential feature of dependent personality disorder is an excessive need to be taken care of that leads to submissive and clinging behaviors and fears of separation. Patients with dependent PD have difficulty making decisions without excessive advice and reassurance from others. They take a passive and helpless stance, and shift the responsibility for problem solving to the clinician, with numerous requests for advice and reassurance. Patients with dependent PD move others to assume responsibility for major areas of their lives. Interpersonal relationships are insecure, clinging, jealous, and possessive. They may over-disclose details of their personal life to obtain the support of the clinician.

They have difficulty expressing disagreement, due to their fear of losing support or approval, and will even agree to things they believe are morally wrong or illegal. These patients are highly motivated to please authority figures, and usually comply well with treatment regimens, but may not report side effects, ineffectiveness, or other difficulties. Patients may become emotionally labile when frustrated, and angry outbursts may occur if not attended to.

Individuals with dependent personality disorder feel uncomfortable and helpless when alone. Suggestions for more autonomous functioning may be rejected due to a lack of confidence in their ability, as they are convinced that they are unable to function independently. Patients with dependent PD will urgently seek another relationship when a close one ends, and are indiscriminate when choosing a partner or friend. Patients may go to excessive lengths to obtain nurturance and support, even to the point of staying with an abusive partner.

They may present submissive and dependent behaviors designed to elicit care-giving or dramatic and urgent demands for medical attention. Patients may even contribute to an illness in order to encourage medical procedures as a means to obtain attention. They may come to the treatment setting following the loss of a relationship that previously supported them or when a relationship becomes increasingly emotionally and/or physically abusive.

COMORBIDITY Patients with dependent PD are at increased risk for mood, anxiety, and adjustment disorders, and for substance abuse. Dependent PD tends to co-occur with borderline, avoidant, and histrionic PD. Chronic physical illness or separation anxiety in childhood or adolescence may predispose to the development of dependent PD.

TREATMENT A primary objective for treatment is to foster independence without forcing the patient. Consistent and explicit limits to clinician availability must be set. Frequent periodic appointments may be scheduled for reassurance. Others should be enlisted to provide support for the patient, especially nonprofessionals. Antidepressants may be helpful for depressive and anxious feature.

Obsessive-Compulsive Personality Disorder

PREVALENCE The prevalence of obsessive-compulsive PD is 1% in community samples and 3 to 10% in individuals presenting to mental health clinics. The disorder is diagnosed about twice as often in males. To some extent, the traits of obsessive-compulsive PD are adaptive in certain situations and occupations. It is only when they reach the level of significant functional impairment in work and interpersonal relationships that they constitute a disorder.

DIAGNOSIS The essential feature of obsessive-compulsive personality disorder is a preoccupation with perfectionism, mental and interpersonal control, and orderliness at the expense of flexibility, openness, and efficiency. This personality disorder is associated with less functional impairment than the others. Despite the similarity in names between obsessive-compulsive disorder (axis I) and obsessive-compulsive personality disorder (axis II), the majority of patients with axis I obsessive-compulsive disorder do not meet the criteria for axis II obsessive-compulsive personality disorder, and most individuals with obsessive-compulsive personality disorder never develop obsessive-compulsive disorder.

The meaning of illness to a patient with obsessive-compulsive PD is that there is not enough order in the patient's life, blaming self for symptoms. They are preoccupied with details and rules to the extent that the major point of the activity is lost. Because of a strong drive to maintain a sense of control, patients may fear relinquishing control to health care providers.

Patients with obsessive-compulsive PD are detailed historians. They also may ask repetitive questions and pay excessive attention to details regarding an illness or treatment plan. The perfectionism of obsessive-compulsive PD interferes with task completion. Patients are excessively careful and repetitious, poorly allocating their use of time. Decision-making is very difficult without rules.

Patients may be excessively devoted to work and productivity to the exclusion of leisure and friendships. Activities such as vacations are formally organized. Affection is expressed in a highly controlled or stilted fashion, and relationships are functional, formal, and serious. These patients can be very compliant with a well-organized and detailed treatment plan. They also demonstrate a good placebo response.

Patients with obsessive-compulsive PD are over-conscientious; scrupulous; inflexible in morals, ethics, and values; self-critical; and rigidly deferential to authority. They have difficulty discarding worthless objects, and are labeled as "pack rats" by others. They may be reluctant to delegate tasks or work with others, unless things are done the patient's way, which includes very rigid and detailed instructions. Patients may adopt a miserly spending style, often living below their economic ability.

TREATMENT   Give clear and thorough explanations of diagnostic and treatment options. Avoid vague and impressionistic explanations. Anticipate possible special concerns. Avoid overemphasizing uncertainties about treatment. Treat the patient as an equal partner in medical care, and encourage self-monitoring.

Others

The DSM-IV includes two additional criteria sets in the appendix as disorders needing further study. The essential feature of *depressive personality disorder* is a pervasive pattern of depressive cognitions and behaviors. The usual mood is unhappy, dejected, and gloomy. The patient's self-concept is centered on low self-esteem. The patient may be critical and derogatory of self, brooding, and given to worry. Overall attitude is negativistic and pessimistic.

The essential feature of *passive-aggressive personality disorder* (or negativistic personality disorder) is a pervasive pattern of negativistic attitudes and passive resistance to demands for adequate performance in social and occupational situations. Patients passively resist fulfilling routine tasks, especially work situations. They tend to externalize blame. Overall attitude is sullen and argumentative. Resistance to treatment may take the form of procrastination, forgetfulness, stubbornness, and intentional inefficiency, especially if the patient perceives the clinician as an authority figure.

GENERAL TREATMENT CONSIDERATIONS

The primary goal of treatment of patients with personality disorders is to improve patient function and quality of life. The approach is pragmatic and focused on the present, giving attention to skill acquisition. Help patients understand any unfavorable consequences of their behaviors, and encourage learning different, less dysfunctional responses. A clinician can increase hope by reducing and identifying realistic expectations. Patients with personality disorders do not purport to be difficult, but they can be disruptive and take a considerable amount of clinical time from a medical practice. Personality-disordered patients are best treated by a team whose members communicate well with one another. Limit the number of staff who interact with the patient. Maintain a clear understanding of patient and practitioner roles, and respect and maintain appropriate interpersonal limits.

Deal with potential countertransference problems with regular consultation with a peer or supervisor. Clinicians working with personality-disordered patients should maintain balanced and healthy personal lives to avoid unmet personal needs that can make a clinician vulnerable to unhealthy countertransference behaviors, such as boundary violations.

Unlike many other medical therapies where treatment is determined by diagnosis, personality disorders are treated by identifying and targeting specific symptoms/behaviors for treatment. Medications often have nonspecific effects on patients with personality disorders. Such patients are also more sensitive to medication side effects.

Patients with personality disorders show a poorer response to pharmacotherapy, are at higher risk for suicide, and are more sensitive to the adverse effects of life stressors. Degree of recovery is less and slower than with patients without an axis II diagnosis. Patients with cluster C disorders respond better than those with cluster B disorders. Patients with cluster A disorders respond poorly to therapy. There is often little correlation between self-reported and other-reported treatment outcomes.

The presence of a personality disorder increases a patient's susceptibility to depression. Treatment of axis I disorders does positively impact axis II pathology. A combination of psychotherapy and pharmacotherapy is usually employed. Substance abuse problems must be addressed early.

Selective serotonin reuptake inhibitors may be used for aggression and impulsivity. Mood stabilizers may be effective for affective regulation. Low-dose neuroleptics (especially the newer atypicals) may be used for cognitive–perceptual abnormalities. Naltrexone has demonstrated effectiveness in decreasing self-harm behaviors. Stimulants may be cautiously used for cognitive dysfunction. Because of the long-term nature of symptoms and potential for abuse, benzodiazepines should be avoided.

Effective psychotherapy focuses on the present, a supportive collaborative relationship, and skill acquisition. Therapy with personality-disordered patients will be longer, and change is slower and less perceptible than with axis I disorders. Group and individual approaches appear to be equal in effectiveness. Cognitive-behavioral methods are often used for affect management and to strengthen adaptive behaviors.

RECOMMENDED READINGS

American Psychiatric Association. *Diagnostic and Statistical Manual of Mental Disorders,* 4th ed, Washington, DC, APA, 1994.

Black D: *Bad Boys, Bad Men: Confronting Antisocial Personality Disorders.* New York, Oxford University Press, 1999.

Millon T, Davis RD. *Disorders of Personality: DSM-IV and Beyond,* 2nd ed, New York, Wiley, 1995.

Paris J: *Borderline Personality Disorders: A Multidimensional Approach,* Washington, DC, American Psychiatric Press, 1994.

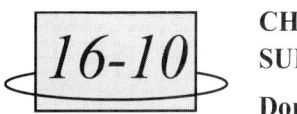

CHEMICAL DEPENDENCY/ SUBSTANCE ABUSE

Donna L. Tully

DISCUSSION

For the past century, Americans have often thought of drugs as a foreign problem for which other countries are largely to blame.[1] However, according to the Robert Wood Johnson report on substance abuse in 1993, chemical dependency is America's leading health problem. More deaths and disabilities result from substance abuse annually than from any other preventable cause. This report also links serious crimes, homicides, motor vehicle accidents and deaths, and high divorce rates among the myriad destructive results of substance abuse in our nation.[2]

The term "addiction" is not used in the current *Diagnostic and Statistical Manual of Mental Disorders,* fourth edition (DSM-IV)[3] in part because of the stigma ascribed to people with chemical dependencies, "addicts." This prejudice can and oftentimes does influence medical providers and health care delivery systems, further inhibiting access to quality, compassionate care for this group of patients who have a multitude of medical problems. Substance dependency is defined in DSM-IV as "a maladaptive pattern of substance use, leading to clinically significant impairment or distress, as manifested by three (or more) of the following, occurring within the same 12-month period of time":

1. Tolerance.
2. Withdrawal.
3. Taking the substance in larger amounts and over a longer period of time than intended.
4. Persistent desire or unsuccessful efforts to cut down or control substance use.
5. A great deal of time spent to obtain the substance or recover from its effects.
6. Important social, occupational, or recreational activities are given up due to substance use.
7. Continued use despite knowledge of the recurrent physical or psychological problems caused by the substance.

The major drugs of abuse can be classified as follows: CNS depressants, CNS stimulants, nicotine, opioids, inhalants, hallucinogens, psychomimetics, and anabolic steroids.[4] In this chapter the drugs that will be discussed in the most detail are also those most commonly seen clinically and associated with problems of abuse: alcohol, nicotine, cocaine, marijuana, heroin, and amphetamines.

EPIDEMIOLOGY

Since 1971, the annual National Household Survey on Drug Abuse[5] has been the primary source of estimates of the prevalence and incidence of illicit drug, alcohol, and tobacco use in the United States. The 1998 survey states that an estimated 13.6 million Americans, age 12 years and older, reported current use of illicit drugs. This figure is a 54% decrease in illicit drug use as compared to 1979. The peak year for drug use since this survey began (27 years ago) was 1979. In 1998, 4.1 million Americans (of a total 13.6 million self-reported illicit drug users) met the diagnostic criteria for drug dependence. Of this group, 27% were 12 to 17 years old. Marijuana continues to be the most frequently used illicit drug in the United States with 60% of all illicit drug users reporting use of only marijuana. It is also the most popular illicit drug among adolescents, with the current prevalence of 8.3% of all American youths.

Cocaine users totalled approximately 1.8 million Americans in 1998 and the youth rate was 10.8% (12 to 18 years old). This recent rate is similar to high initiation rates of cocaine in the early 1980s when cocaine use was at its peak incidence.

Hallucinogen use by new users reached an estimated 1.1 million Americans in this survey. Four drug categories accounted for 90% of hospital admissions for substance abuse diagnoses: alcohol (48%), cocaine (15%), opiates (primarily heroin, 16%), and marijuana (13%). Methamphetamines and its derivatives made up about 5% of hospital admissions for drug-related problems.

Alcohol use, which is legal at and above age 21 in the United States, was reported by 19.1% of the population. Some 33 million Americans (or 31.7%) reported binge drinking and 12 million (13.8%) were classified as heavy drinkers. Among adolescents (12 to 17 years), the rate of alcohol use in 1998 was 19.9%, a relatively stable figure since 1992. Illegal or underaged drinking rates have not changed significantly since 1994. The rate of binge drinking (31.7%) and heavy alcohol abuse

(13.8%) among young adults (18 to 25 years) has remained similar to rates observed in 1996.

ETIOLOGY

The causes for drug addiction are complex and appear to be multifactorial, involving some combination of genetic/biochemical factors as well as social, psychological, and environmental factors. There are currently two major theories for drug-taking (and potential drug dependency): drug reward versus withdrawal reversal. Drug reward appears to be primary in supporting the chronic, relapsing nature of most drug dependency including alcohol and nicotine. There is increasing research evidence to implicate the dopamine system in the meso-limbic region of the brain with the rewarding effects of abusing opioids (such as heroin and morphine), alcohol, nicotine, and psychostimulants (such as cocaine, amphetamines, and their derivatives). Activation of the dopaminergic pathway mediates drug reward, subjectively pleasurable, which is the critical component of the drug reinforcement properties. With repeated drug use, this system becomes increasingly sensitized to the effects of the drug. The researchers who support the dopamine theory postulate that drug-seeking and taking is a primary drive state similar to seeking food and sex. They state this explains the extreme difficulties in psychopharmacologic treatment of drug binge use and relapses. In short, these drugs stimulate their own continued use. Stopping their use can become analogous to giving up food or sex.

The theory of negative reinforcement states that drug seeking and taking occurs not because of the induced positive reward state, but rather to reverse the discomfort and negative withdrawal symptoms that come from not using the drug(s). Although each drug has its set of particular withdrawal symptoms, some symptoms are seen in most drugs that cause dependency, such as anxiety, anhedonia, dysphoria, depression, and craving more use of the discontinued drug.

Genetics seem to play an important, though not universal, role in determining who develops alcoholism. The heritability factor for alcoholism is estimated to be 50 to 60%, meaning that for all of the factors that influence the probability of developing alcohol dependence, at least half can be directly attributed to genetics.[2] The best predictor of future alcohol dependence among adolescents is a family history of alcoholism. About half of all hospitalized male alcoholics have a family history of alcoholism. Alcohol metabolism is a major biological determinant that can influence drinking behavior. The vulnerability for development of alcoholism is affected by the genetic variation of the production of two principal enzymes involved in ethanol metabolism: alcohol dehydrogenase and aldehyde dehydrogenase. Some ethnic populations carry genotypes that confer partial immunity (not full immunity as once thought) against developing alcohol dependence.[6] Neurobiochemically, alcohol and some other addictive drugs may be more rewarding for those who are born with or require greater dopamine release in anticipation of drug availability. However, in a milder type of alcoholism (type I), only 20% of all causes are estimated to be due to hereditary factors, thus highlighting environmental factors (such as low socioeconomic class) also as important etiologic agents. When alcoholism occurs in familial patterns, the disease tends to begin young in life, and have a history of frequent relapses and a bleaker prognosis for treatment success.

A large body of literature, including clinical studies, suggests that abnormalities in serotonin, a central neurotransmitter that regulates moods and sleep, also plays a vital role in the regulation of alcohol intake and the development of alcoholism. Neuroendocrine studies have provided evidence that the serotonin system is altered in the brains of patients with alcohol abuse as well as those with depression and suicidal and impulsive behaviors. Current research with cocaine is also demonstrating that cocaine alters the metabolism of serotonin, dopamine, and other key neurotransmitters. The clinical implications of this research remains to be further elucidated.

POPULATIONS AT HIGH RISK

Populations of people at higher than average risk for developing chemical dependency include youths (teens and preteens, especially gay and lesbian adolescents), chronically mentally ill patients (dually diagnosed), elderly men, people with chronic disabilities, and the homeless (who often fit several of the other categories) (Table 16-10-1).[7]

The highest rate for initiation into alcohol and marijuana use is between 15 and 18 years of age. However, children who begin drug use before they reach adolescence are at a greater risk for developing chemical abuse problems than their older peers who begin substance experimentation in later teen years. These younger children often have one or more of the following traits: short attention span, significant shyness, and antisocial behaviors and/or engaging in acts of severe aggression. Other personality traits associated with preadolescent substance use include rebelliousness, resistance to traditional authority figures, a strong need for independence, low self-esteem, and feeling a lack of control over one's life.[2] Other high-risk factors for drug use by teens include having an alcoholic/drug-addicted parent(s), child abuse/neglect, physical abuse, depression, suicidality, pregnancy, and physical handicaps. It must be noted, however, that teenage alcohol and/or drug use does not predict future chemical dependency. The best-found predictors of substance abuse problems as adults were deviant adolescent behaviors and use of drugs (including alcohol) as teenagers. A highly predictive risk factor for future alcohol, cannabis, and polysubstance use disorders in young adults was a lifetime of daily cigarette smoking among adolescents. Earlier smoking onset was highly correlated with future substance abuse, while smoking cessation for over a year was associated with lower rates of future alcohol problems in particular.[8] As compared with the general population, individuals with mental illnesses show an increased incidence of substance abuse. Individuals with schizophrenia or with bipolar disorder are at more than four times the risk of having a drug abuse disorder. At some point in their lifetimes, 47% of patients with schizophrenia, 56% of those with bipolar disease, 27% of people diagnosed with major depression, and 24% of patients with any type of anxiety disorder have met the criteria for one or more substance abuse disorders.[9]

TABLE 16-10-1.   Risk Factors for Alcohol Abuse

Absence of aldehyde dehydrogenase (enzyme that produces flushing or palpitations with alcohol ingestion)

Aggressive behavior, oppositional defiant disorder, conduct disorder, or school-based problems

Alcohol use by peer group

Chronic anxiety

Easy accessibility to alcohol

Family history

Feelings of desperation

Feelings of resentment

Genetic predisposition to alcohol dependence

History of learning disabilities, attention-deficit/hyperactivity disorder, impulsiveness, reckless behavior

Low self-esteem

Low tolerance for stress

Neurotransmitter deficit (e.g., serotonin)

Pessimistic attitude

Poor interpersonal skills

SOURCE: *The Physicians' Guide to Helping Patients with Alcohol Problems.* Rockville, MD, National Institute on Alcohol Abuse and Alcoholism, 1995. NIH pub. no. 95-3769.

It is estimated that there are one-half million elderly alcoholics in the United States and an additional 5% to 10% are heavy consumers of alcohol.[10] Elderly males are also in the highest risk category in the United States for depression and suicidality.

RISKS ASSOCIATED WITH DRUG ABUSE

Chemical dependency is associated with many physical, psychological, social, occupational, and legal problems. Among a few of the long list of potential medical complications of substance abuse are infections (hepatitis, HIV and related infections), liver failure, cirrhosis, gastrointestinal (GI) bleeding, renal failure, congestive heart failure, anxiety, depression, suicide, sexually transmitted diseases, unwanted pregnancy, septic arthritis, endocarditis, osteoarthritis, trauma and subsequent injuries, seizures, coma, and death from overdoses. For more specific health consequences listed by drug and category, see Table 16-10-2.

SIGNS AND SYMPTOMS

Five classic hallmarks of behavior in a person with chemical dependency include drug craving, drug relapse, increasing desire for the drug with concurrent decreasing pleasure from it, spontaneous remissions, and compulsive use, regardless of the negative withdrawal symptoms and/or consequences of continued use.

Early warning signs of substance abuse/addiction vary from the subtle to the obvious. Due to the common defense mechanisms of denial and minimization in substance abusers, family members and friends may become acutely aware of these warning signs much sooner than the chemically dependent person himself of herself. Obtaining historical information from the patient's support system of friends and family, whenever possible, becomes a key factor in assessing for chemical dependency. Table 16-10-3 lists the early warning signs of possible drug addiction.

Each drug category has its own associated specific signs and symptoms. The five drug classes described next were chosen because these are currently the major drugs of abuse seen in clinical practices in the United States.

Central Nervous System Depressants

Central nervous system (CNS) depressants include the sedatives: alcohol, barbiturates, benzodiazepines, and other chemically similar compounds. Some of the mild effects of alcohol intoxication include slightly decreased alertness and fine lateral nystagmus, while moderate levels of intoxication manifest with slurred speech, ataxia, sedation, and coarse nystagmus. High levels of alcohol consumption can progress to respiratory depression, coma, and even death.

CNS Stimulants

The prototypes of the CNS stimulant category are cocaine and amphetamines (and its derivatives). The physical effects of cocaine, a strong stimulant, include immediate euphoria, hyperactivity, grandiosity, elevated vital signs (blood pressure, pulse, and temperature), dilated pupils, loss of appetite, insomnia, and anxiety. High doses and/or prolonged use of cocaine can trigger aggressive paranoia, nasal septum collapse (if snorted), seizures, cardiorespiratory arrest, and death.

The effects of amphetamines are qualitatively similar to cocaine but more prolonged. Chronic, heavy use of methamphetamines causes a rapidly developed tolerance to the drug, seizures, and a paranoid psychosis that is difficult to treat.

Opioids

Heroin, the only illegal opioid, is a highly addictive narcotic. Reported signs and symptoms of heroin use include euphoria, drowsiness, "nodding off," constricted pupils, nausea and vomiting, and respiratory depression. Many health-related problems to heroin use involve drug

TABLE 16-10-2.   Effects and Health Consequences of Substance Abuse

DRUG	INTOXICATING EFFECTS	HEALTH CONSEQUENCES
Alcohol	CNS depression, sedation, lack of coordination, altered mood Blood alcohol 150-200 mg/dl Legal driving level <100 mg/dl most states (Some have changed limit to <80 mg/dl) 12–24 hours after use stops: weakness, sweating, hyperreflexia, GI symptoms, seizures, hallucinations, delirium fremens	Cirrhosis, peripheral neuropathy, dementia, cardiomyopathy, CHF, arrhythmia, pancreatitis, gastritis, thiamin deficiency **Women:** Adverse health effects develop sooner with less consumption than men **Pregnant women:** FAS with 7–14 drinks/week; more risk early in pregnancy or with binge drinking; FAS: fetal growth retardation, facial deformities, CNS dysfunction (microcephaly, mental retardation, behavior problems); any alcohol may cause risk **Adolescents and young adults:** Contributes to leading cause of death (MVA) and other problems (injuries, homicides, suicides, unsafe sex, legal problems) **Elderly:** Slowed metabolism: Elevated alcohol with less drinking; isolation, falls, malnutrition, dementia, self-neglect, suicide
Marijuana	Euphoria, increased taste perceptions, relaxation, drowsiness	Asthma, bronchitis, memory impairment, pharyngitis
Cocaine, amphetamine	Stimulates CNS: Euphoria, hyperactivity, alertness, grandiosity, anger, impaired judgment, altered pulse, blood pressure Other symptoms: Perspiration, chills, paranoia, seizures, chest pain, myocardial infarction, arrhythmia Acute withdrawal: Depression, suicidal ideation Withdrawal: Fatigue, unpleasant dreams, psychomotor retardation or agitation, increased appetite	Chronic use: Fatigue, social withdrawal, weight loss Snorting: Nasal mucosal irritation, perforated nasal septum Short-acting: Rapid dependence Dependence: Large amounts of money for repetitive use, prostitution; increased incidence of STDs Amphetamine: Diaphoresis, flushing, hyperreflexia, insomnia, irritability, restlessness, tachycardia Chronic use: Confusion, depression, headache, paranoia
Opioids	CNS depression: Drowsiness, decreased vital signs, dry mouth, constipation, euphoria, flushing, itchy skin	Tolerance within 2–3 days after prescribed use Withdrawal within 4–6 hours: CNS hyperactivity, anxiety, increased respiration, yawning, perspiration, lacrimation, rhinorrhea. Dependence associated with high death rate from overdose, injuries, violence **Men:** Erectile dysfunction **Women:** Irregular menses **Pregnant women:** Withdrawal in newborn
Phencyclidine hydrochloride (PCP)	Ataxia, disinhibition, euphoria	Panic attacks, sweating, sensitivity to sensation Hallucinations, flashbacks, panic attacks, psychosis
Hallucinogens	Altered visual perception	IDU: Shared needles, hepatitis B, hepatis C, hepatitis D, HIV, septicemia, bacteria endocarditis, localized cellulitis

*Adapted from Schonberg S: *Substance Abuse: A Guide for Health Professionals.* Elk Grove Village, IL, American Academy of Pediatrics/Pacific Institute for Research Evaluation; and from Ask K, Schik M, Schwartz M: Helping the teenage drug user. *Patient Care* 23(20):614-272, 1989.
ABBREVIATIONS: CHF = congestive heart failure; CNS = central nervous system; FAS = fetal alcohol syndrome; GI = gastrointestinal; HIV = human immunodeficiency virus; IDU = injection drug use; MVA = motor vehicle accident.

contamination and uncertain dosage levels (due to variability in street drug purity) and complications from nonsterile "works" (needles/syringes). These include HIV, hepatitis, skin abscesses, phlebitis, and necrotizing fasciitis.

Hallucinogens

Psychomimetics and hallucinogens are a diverse category for drugs that alter perceptions and/or mimic psychotic states. Drugs included in this broad category are cannabis (marijuana), lysergic acid diethylamide (LSD), and phencyclidine (PCP). Marijuana, the most commonly used drug in this class, will be highlighted here. Observable signs of use include a mildly dissociated, dreamy mental state, dilated pupils, elevated pulse rate, and dry mouth. Toxic dose levels of cannabis can produce disorientation, rotary nystagmus, tachycardia, and ataxia. Daily or chronic use is associated with lung damage.

Nicotine

For a complete discussion of the signs and symptoms of nicotine, see Chap. 16-12.

HISTORY OF SUBSTANCE USE

A comprehensive history of substance use/abuse is the first step to an accurate assessment of patients with potential chemical dependency. Optimally the health history will be taken in a quiet, uninterrupted space with the medical provider demonstrating a genuinely empathetic, respectful demeanor. This approach will not only yield the most accurate information, but may also help to decrease patient defensiveness and build rapport and trust between the patient and provider. The following information is recommended to screen all patients in their health habit/drug use history: substances used (currently and in the past), amount taken (per day, week, month), route(s) of drug administration, age of first use, signs and symptoms of tolerance, withdrawal, and any complications or new symptoms when using the drug. Also specifically ask about prior attempts to quit, professional treatment (both inpatient and ambulatory) programs, and how they felt about those treatment experiences. If not mentioned by the patient, directly ask about prescription medications taken longer than recommended or in larger doses than originally prescribed.

Obtaining a two-generation family history of substance abuse/addiction can be very helpful for future predictive value, especially in high-risk adolescents. Within the history questions, providers should

TABLE 16.10-3. Some Early Warning Signs of Possible Drug Addiction

Uncomfortable without alcohol or drugs

Increased confidence when using a substance

Lying about drinking or drug use and amounts

Drinking or using alone

Increasing number of problems at home, work, or school

Inability to quit or control drug use on one's own

Frequent absences from work or school, or inability to maintain obligations

Financial problems or unexplained wealth

Memory changes or loss (blackouts)

Multiple incidents with the legal system, medical problems, or accidents

Unpredictable moodiness and lability: depression, anxiety, paranoia, agitation, and irritability

query patients about those perceptions concerning the consequences that drug use has on their level of daily functioning as well as the impact on relationships at work, home, and socially. Many substance abusers will not be as aware of the detrimental effects of their drug use as family members, coworkers, and friends may be. Whenever possible, and with the permission of the patient, interviewing the patient's key support system members will clarify the drug history and often provide a more objective view. The frequently present (unconscious) defense mechanisms of denial and minimization prevent the chemically dependent person from providing an accurate history, whether or not they are seeking help for their drug use. Family members may also be needed for medical/substance use histories when patients are acutely intoxicated or in withdrawal states and mentally incapable of providing accurate information.

To assist in the history-taking process of screening for alcoholism, several well-validated and reliable tools are available. The four-question CAGE interview tool may, in fact, also be a better predictor for alcoholism than current laboratory tests. It can be easily adapted to screen for other drugs of abuse as well.[11] CAGE is a mnemonic that stands for these four questions:

C: Have you ever felt the need to Cut down on drinking (or drug use)?
A: Have you ever felt Annoyed by criticisms of drinking (or drug use) by others?
G: Have you ever had Guilty feelings about drinking (or drug use)?
E: Have you ever taken a morning Eye opener (or used drugs to get started in the A.M.)?

The sensitivity of the CAGE instrument for identifying lifetime alcohol problems in health care setting patients ranges from 60 to 95%, with a wide specificity range of 40 to 95%.[12] To identify potential alcohol abuse/dependency or current dangerous drinking patterns, medical providers can augment the 4-question CAGE tool[13] with the 10-question AUDIT (Alcohol Use Disorder Identification Test).[14] This alcohol-screening instrument (Table 16-10-4) has a greater sensitivity and specificity (both at 96%) than the CAGE tool.[15]

Another popular reliable screening tool for alcoholism is the 25-item Michigan Alcohol Screening Test (MAST), which has a reported sensitivity of 90 to 98%. Since historically alcohol questionnaires have been shown to be less sensitive with elderly patients, the MAST now has a 24-item age-appropriate clinical interview tool for patients over 65, the MAST-Geriatric (Table 16-10-5).

OBJECTIVE FINDINGS

Physical examination findings vary not only with the drug(s) used, but also with the route of administration. For examples, cutaneous abscesses (from "skin popping"), intravenous (IV) needle track marks, and inflamed or scarred veins can often be found with intravenous use of heroin, cocaine, PCP, methamphetamine, and barbiturates. Nasal lesions including a perforated septum can occur with chronic cocaine use. Hepatomegaly and ascites are found with chronic alcohol abuse, presenting as a swollen, enlarged liver or a small, scarred liver depending upon the stage of cirrhotic disease. In patients who present with frequent accidents or head trauma, consider underlying substance abuse.

Laboratory tests to date are not sensitive or specific enough to routinely screen asymptomatic patients for signs of substance abuse/dependency. Thus the use of laboratory tests needs to be individualized and matched with the presenting history and clinical findings. The most useful and cost-effective routine lab tests include syphilis serology, cholesterol screening, urinalysis dipstick, and tuberculin skin testing. Syphilis and tuberculosis are appearing with increasing frequency in narcotic addicts.[4]

In 75% of chronic abusers or heavy users of alcohol, elevated liver enzymes, particularly serum AST (aspartate aminotransferase), GGT (gamma glutamyltransferase), and ALT (alanine aminotransferase) can substantiate the clinical suspicions of medical providers about a patient's alcohol abuse. Remember, however, that there are many other causes of elevated GGT besides alcoholism, such as metabolic diseases (diabetes mellitus, hyperlipidemia) and prescription medications (anticonvulsants, tranquilizers). These objective laboratory results provide objective data that patients often need before they are ready to acknowledge and begin to change their patterns of alcohol consumption. Routine hepatitis serologic screening is expensive and has a low yield unless preceded by abnormal liver function tests. Carbohydrate-deficient transferrin has 58 to 70% sensitivity and 82 to 98% specificity in detecting heavy alcohol use.[16] A complete blood count (CBC) can demonstrate macrocytic anemia as well as a potential gastric bleed, both found with chronic alcohol abuse.

With IV drug users, it is a reasonable approach to obtain a one-time baseline renal function test to screen for glomerular nephropathies associated with IV drug use. Routine, every 6 months, HIV testing for IV drug users is part of the harm-reduction guidelines in many clinical sites. Testing for STDs and pregnancy should be considered as clinically warranted.

DIAGNOSTIC SCREENING: SERUM AND URINE TOXICOLOGY TESTING

To detect alcohol abuse, a blood level of 300 mg/100 mL or higher is a useful indicator, while a serum blood alcohol of 100 mg/100 mL or higher during a routine medical visit is the usual cutoff level for acute intoxication.

Urine drug toxicology results vary with factors such as a patient's age, type of drug ingested, and excretion rates by the body of different drugs. Positive urine drug tests occur, on average, within 1 to 4 days after the most recent drug dose, with chronic marijuana use extending for the longest time after use, up to 14 days. Direct witnessing of urine sample collection can help to decrease the number of falsely negative drug screens. False-positive urine drug tests can be minimized by running a second confirmatory test on the same urine sample.

Many emergency rooms, urgent care centers, and other acute medical settings routinely screen for drugs and alcohol in patients presenting with the following presenting problems: motor vehicle accidents, suicide attempts, seizures, unexplained syncopal episodes, acts of violent behavior, and unexplained cardiac arrhythmias.

TREATMENT

Once the medical provider has diagnosed substance abuse or chemical dependency, the next step is to engage the person in the process

TABLE 16-10-4. AUDIT Questionnaire

Directions: For each of the following questions, please check (✓) the box next to the most appropriate response.*

1. How often do you have a drink of alcohol?
- ☐ 0 Never
- ☐ 1 Monthly or less
- ☐ 2 2 to 4 times a week
- ☐ 3 2 to 3 times a week
- ☐ 4 4 or more times

2. How many drinks containing alcohol do you have on a typical day when you are drinking?
- ☐ 0 1 or 2
- ☐ 1 3 or 4
- ☐ 2 5 or 6
- ☐ 3 7 to 9
- ☐ 4 10 or more

3. How often do you have 6 or more drinks on one occasion?
- ☐ 0 Never
- ☐ 1 Less than monthly
- ☐ 2 Monthly
- ☐ 3 Weekly
- ☐ 4 Daily or almost daily

4. How often during the last year have you found that you were not able to stop drinking once you have started?
- ☐ 0 Never
- ☐ 1 Less than monthly
- ☐ 2 Monthly
- ☐ 3 Weekly
- ☐ 4 Daily or almost daily

5. How often during the last year have you failed to do what was normally expected from you because of drinking?
- ☐ 0 Never
- ☐ 1 Less than monthly
- ☐ 2 Monthly
- ☐ 3 Weekly
- ☐ 4 Daily or almost daily

6. How often during the last year have you needed a first drink in the morning to get yourself going after a heavy drinking session?
- ☐ 0 Never
- ☐ 1 Less than monthly
- ☐ 2 Monthly
- ☐ 3 Weekly
- ☐ 4 Daily or almost daily

7. How often during the last year have you had a feeling of guilt or remorse after drinking?
- ☐ 0 Never
- ☐ 1 Less than monthly
- ☐ 2 Monthly
- ☐ 3 Weekly
- ☐ 4 Daily or almost daily

8. How often during the last year have you been unable to remember what happened the night before because of drinking?
- ☐ 0 Never
- ☐ 1 Less than monthly
- ☐ 2 Monthly
- ☐ 3 Weekly
- ☐ 4 Daily or almost daily

9. Have you or someone else been injured as a result of your drinking?
- ☐ 0 No
- ☐ 1 Yes, but not last year.
- ☐ 2 Yes, during the last year.

(Continued)

TABLE 16-10-4. (Continued)

10. Has a relative, friend, doctor, or other health worker been concerned about your drinking or suggested you cut down?
- ☐ 0 No
- ☐ 2 Yes, but not last year.
- ☐ 4 Yes, during the last year.

Record sum of individual item scores here: ☐

*In determining the responses categories it has been assumed that one "drink" contains 10 g alcohol. In countries where the alcohol content of a standard drink differs by more than 25% from 10 g, the response category should be modified.

Very High	(26–40)
High	(17–25)
Medium	(8–16)
Low	(1–7)
No problem	(0)

of acknowledging his or her disease and the resulting medical, psychological, and social problems that have been caused by the unhealthy relationship to alcohol or drugs. Only by fully engaging the patient in this process of acknowledgment can providers hope to be successful in working cooperatively with patients toward the long and often painful process of necessary behavioral changes to achieve sobriety and recovery. When this step of engaging patients is skipped, the result can be frustration, anger, and often failure to assist patients in achieving sobriety. Depending upon the medical provider's personality, beliefs and biases about substance abuse, and experiences with drug abuse (personal as well as professional), he or she may employ a variety of strategies to convince patients to choose abstinence. These strategies range from gentle persuasion using logic or firm limit-setting, to scare tactics with medical facts and statistics. All of these approaches will ultimately fall on deaf ears and have a low success rate until the patient is able to acknowledge the drug problems and is ready to actively take steps to change years of ingrained behavior and attitudes. Proshaska and DiClemente[17] studied this process of making significant behavioral changes. They identified six key stages of change that most people go through as they attempt lifestyle changes (Table 16-10-6). Understanding the stages of change that most people (not just addicts) progress through before achieving lasting success in altering lifestyle behaviors can augment patience and diminish frustration for both providers and patients and family members.

Another major area of predictable frustration in the treatment of people with addictions is dealing with relapses, that is, returning to substance abuse after some period of abstinence. Although many people view a relapse as a treatment failure of the patient and/or medical system, relapses are actually a very common event in the process of making behavioral changes. Experienced providers in the field of chemical dependency recognize that there is no perfect way to achieve the ultimate goal of abstinence and therefore educate patients and their families and support systems about realistically anticipating occasional relapses into compulsive drug use. This educational approach can minimize the normal reactions of shame, guilt, blame, and anger that often accompany a relapse, which can isolate patients who then may not return for needed ongoing medical treatment.

Inpatient Versus Outpatient Triage

Once both the patient and the health provider have reached agreement about the diagnosis of chemical dependency and the agreement of the patient to receive help, a collaborative decision must be reached about whether to initiate inpatient or outpatient treatment. Here are a few

TABLE 16-10-5. Michigan Alcoholism Screening Test—Geriatric Version (MAST-G)

1. After drinking have you ever noticed an increase in your heart rate or beating in your chest? 1. __ __
2. When talking with others do you ever underestimate how much you actually drink? 2. __ __
3. Does alcohol make you sleepy so that you often fall asleep in your chair? 3. __ __
4. After a few drinks have you sometimes not eaten or been able to skip a meal because you didn't feel hungry? 4. __ __
5. Does having a few drinks help decrease your shakiness or tremors? 5. __ __
6. Does alcohol sometimes make it hard for you to remember parts of the day or night? 6. __ __
7. Do you have rules for yourself that you won't drink before a certain time of day? 7. __ __
8. Have you lost interest in hobbies or activities you used to enjoy? 8. __ __
9. When you wake up in the morning do you ever have trouble remembering part of the night before? 9. __ __
10. Does having a drink help you sleep? 10. __ __
11. Do you hide your alcohol bottles from family members? 11. __ __
12. After a social gathering have you ever felt embarrassed because you drank too much? 12. __ __
13. Have you ever been concerned that drinking might be harmful to your health? 13. __ __
14. Do you like to end an evening with a nightcap? 14. __ __
15. Did you find your drinking increased after someone close to you died? 15. __ __
16. In general, would you prefer to have a few drinks at home rather than go out to a social event? 16. __ __
17. Are you drinking more than in the past? 17. __ __
18. Do you usually take a drink to relax or calm your nerves? 18. __ __
19. Do you drink to take your mind off your problems? 19. __ __
20. Have you ever increased your drinking after experiencing a loss in your life? 20. __ __
21. Do you sometimes drive when you have had too much to drink? 21. __ __
22. Has a doctor or nurse ever said he or she was worried or concerned about your drinking? 22. __ __
23. Have you ever made rules to manage your drinking? 23. __ __
24. When you feel lonely does having a drink help? 24. __ __

SCORING: 5 OR MORE "YES" RESPONSES IS INDICATIVE OF A DRINKING PROBLEM.

SOURCE: *Blow et al: Alcohol Clin Exp Res 16(2):372, 1992.*

suggested triage questions:

- Does the patient request and have a strong desire to be admitted to a hospital detox or chemical dependency treatment center?
- Is there a current history of daily substance abuse or frequent switching to multiple, addictive drugs?
- Has the patient experienced many prior treatment failures, especially as an outpatient?
- Is there a sober (or non–chemical-abusing) stable support system of family members or friends to assist this person day-to-day in efforts to stay sober?

TABLE 16-10-6. Prochaska and DiClemente's Stages of Change

Precontemplation: Client is unaware of any problems (denial) and is not considering change.

Contemplation: Client acknowledges problems/concerns but is ambivalent about making a change.

Determination: Client is committed to making a change in the near future, but still considering what to do.

Action: Client is actively seeking steps to change, but has not yet reached a stable state.

Maintenance: Client has achieved initial goals and is working to maintain goals.

Relapse: Client has experienced a recurrence and must decide what to do next.

SOURCE: Prochaska J, DiClemente C. In search of how people change: Applications to addictive behaviors. *Am Psychologist* 47:1102–1114; 1992.

- Does this patient have a chaotic lifestyle at home or in the streets as a homeless person?

The current criteria for inpatient or residential treatment for chemical dependency developed by the American Psychiatric Association and the American Society of Addiction Medicine also include the coexistence of severe medical or psychiatric conditions, risk of harm to self or others (danger of suicide or homicide), and a social or family environment that interferes with successful recovery.[13]

Although the process of medical/physical detoxification may take only a few days or weeks, depending upon the drug(s), the ongoing process of sobriety is an endeavor that requires months or even years. A successful, long-term recovery program surrounds the patient with a stable, nonaddicted community of formal (professionally trained providers) and informal (family, friends) supports. Long-term residential programs are good resources for homeless patients or those whose primary social network consists entirely of drug users. These programs offer a drug-free therapeutic living environment that is staffed by counselors and successfully recovering people who act as positive role models. The average optimal involvement in residential care is approximately 6 months.[4]

It is recommended that primary care medical providers become well acquainted with their local public and private chemical dependency resources and personnel, in both the inpatient and outpatient arenas, in order to offer their patients a variety of individualized treatment options. These experts can also conduct a thorough assessment of their own and assist in your decision about treatment disposition. Most county mental health departments offer chemical dependency programs that provide a comprehensive substance abuse intake free of charge, although there may be a long wait for an intake appointment. They also maintain current directories of available openings in the full range of facilities for detox, short-term, and residential rehabilitation. These directories include useful information such as cost, length of stay, acceptable third-party payments, languages spoken, and programs designed for high-risk, high-recidivism target populations.

For patients who do not require inpatient treatment, or refuse to be admitted as inpatients, many facilities offer similar services at lower cost for partial hospitalization or day/evening treatment programs. These options can allow employed patients the ability to continue to work in their daytime jobs while attending evening treatment programs. This is a particularly relevant option; according to the 1999 Substance Abuse and Mental Health Services Administration (SAMHSA) study, 70% of drug and heavy alcohol users, ages 18 to 49, work full time.[5] After-care meetings, run by chemical dependency program staff members, provide ongoing weekly or monthly support for program graduates toward maintaining their new, chosen lifestyles of abstinence.

Both inpatient and outpatient chemical dependency programs emphasize patient and family education, teaching addicted patients new, more effective coping strategies for managing life stressors, improving interpersonal communication skills, and finding community resources to widen their social activities and circle of non–drug-addicted associates. Treatment techniques may include supportive couples/family therapy, specific short- and long-term goal setting, cognitive and behavioral treatments, and pharmacologic medical therapies.

Once a detox or rehabilitation program is chosen, the facility usually requires medical clearance by the referring medical provider before patient admission is allowed. Acute health problems must be identified and at least stabilized before the patient enters programs, especially where minimal medical staffing support or medications are available on site. Clarify the level of medical care in inpatient chemical treatment facilities before admitting patients with significant coexisting medical and/or psychiatric diagnoses.

Outpatient Treatment

The role of the primary care provider for patients who can be managed as outpatients can be envisioned as the coordinator of ongoing services provided by a team of specialists in managing the chronic, often relapsing condition of chemical dependency. Using an empathetic but firm approach, the PA can provide the treatment for coexisting medical, nutritional, and common psychiatric diagnoses as well as management of pain concerns with limited, judicious use of controlled substances such as narcotics and sedative-hypnotics. Primary care providers also can anticipate and offer patients and their families individual-specific community resources for individual, couples, and family counseling, relapse monitoring and prevention, and free community-based self-help programs such as AA, Alanon, Alateen, and NA.[18]

Pharmacologic Treatment

Pharmacologic treatment of chemically dependent patients includes not only prescribing drug regimens during inpatient detox (beyond the scope of this chapter) but also the outpatient use of medications such as methadone, an opioid agonist, and naltrexone, an opioid antagonist, to block the acute effects of opioids and also to reduce alcohol cravings. Other medications (such as SSRIs) for these patients are used to address the dysthymic states that predated drug abuse or persist after drugs or alcohol are discontinued. Common symptoms in early recovery such as persistent insomnia and acute anxiety/panic episodes also may need medical attention with pharmacologic interventions.

Methadone is the most well known and perhaps most effective pharmacological agent for the treatment of opiate dependency. This outpatient medication still provokes controversy among both medical and lay communities. However, when properly administered and monitored, usually through licensed methadone maintenance centers, methadone has been shown to successfully replace heroin abuse and reduce related criminal activities including high-risk behaviors such as injection drug use. Naltrexone, while a potent opiate antagonist, has a low compliance rate among opiate addicts and therefore is not routinely used for maintenance therapy of abstinence from heroin. One possible explanation for the compliance problem may be the lack of any morphine-like subjective effects, which can help retain opiate-dependent patients in treatment. Naltrexone is contraindicated in patients with liver failure or acute hepatitis because of its dose-related hepatotoxicity. Research suggests promise for treating opiate-dependence with a new medication called buprenorphine.

The opioid antagonist naltrexone has also been proved to be clinically effective in decreasing patients' alcohol consumption. Studies have shown that alcohol-dependent patients who receive a daily dose of 50 mg of naltrexone have reduced episodes of heavy drinking and a lower relapse rate than patients on a placebo medication.[19] Acamprosate, an extensively studied drug in Europe, is currently undergoing

U.S. drug research trials for its role in abstinence maintenance in alcoholic patients. Research is also being conducted for its future effectiveness in combination with naltrexone.[20]

FOR MORE INFORMATION

Alcoholics Anonymous Central Office in local telephone white pages for meetings schedules for AA, NA, ALANON, ALATEEN, and other free 12-step self-help groups: www.alcoholics-anonymous.org

Centers for Disease Control and Prevention. *Morbidity & Mortality Weekly Reports:* www.cdc.gov

Haight-Ashbury Free Clinic, San Francisco, has an excellent medical providers' handbook about street drugs: *Uppers, Downers and All-Arounders* by D. Inaba (July, 2000): www.hafci.org

Hazelton Institute in Minneapolis. Excellent audiovisual materials, videotapes, and written patient-education pamphlets at: www.hazelton.org

National Institute on Drug Abuse (NIDA) under the National Institutes of Health in Rockville, MD (NIH): www.nida.nih.gov/NIDAHome1.html

Substance Abuse and Mental Health Services Administration (SAMHSA): www.samhsa.gov

BIBLIOGRAPHY

1. *Keeping Score: Drug Strategies.* Washington, DC, 1995.
2. Miller N. *The Principles and Practice of Addictions in Psychiatry.* Philadelphia, Saunders, 1997, p. 57.
3. American Psychiatric Association. *Diagnostic and Statistical Manual of Mental Disorders,* 4th ed, Washington, DC, American Psychiatric Association, pp. 175–272.
4. Buttaro T, Bailey P,Sandberg-Cook J, Trybulski J. *Primary Care: A Collaborative Practice.* St. Louis, Mosby, 1999, pp. 1096–1103.
5. *HHS National Household Survey on Drug Abuse.* Substance Abuse and Mental Health Services Administration, August 18, 1999.
6. Chen Y, Lu R, Peng G, et al. Alcohol metabolism and cardiovascular response in an alcohol patient homozygous for the ALDH 2*2 variant gene allele. *Alcohol Clin Exp Res* 23:1853–1860, 1999.
7. Mosier W. Alcohol addiction: Identifying the patient who drinks. *JAAPA* 12:24–56, 1999.
8. Lewinsohn P, Rohde P, Brown R. level of current and past adolescent cigarette smoking as a prediction of future substance abuse disorders in adulthood. *Addiction* 94:913–921, 1999.
9. Fuller P, McCrone S. The identification and treatment of patients with a dual diagnosis of psychiatric disorder and substance use disorder: A primary care problem. *Am J Nurse Practitioners* 1999, pp. 13–26.
10. Ham R, Sloane P. *Primary Care Geriatrics,* 3rd ed, St. Louis, Mosby. 1997, p. 367.
11. Beresford P, Blow F, Hill E, et al. Clinical practice: Comparison of CAGE questionnaire and computer assisted lab profiles in screening for covert alcoholism. *Lancet* 336:482–485, 1990.
12. Liskow B, Campbell J, Nickel E, et al. Validity of the cage questionnaire in screening for alcohol dependence in a walk-in triage clinic. *J Stud Alcohol* 56:277–281, 1995.
13. O'Connor P, Schottenfeld R. Patients with alcohol problems: A review article. *N Engl J Med* 2:592–600, 1998.
14. Saunders J, Aasland O, Babor T, et al. Development of the Alcohol Use Disorders Identification Test (AUDIT): WHO collaborative project on early detection of persons with harmful alcohol consumption. *Addiction* 88:791–804, 1993.
15. Ewing J. Detecting alcoholism: The CAGE questionnaire. *JAMA* 252:1905–1907, 1984.
16. Lesch O, Walter H. Carbohydrate-deficiency transferrin as a marker of alcohol intake. *Alcohol* 31:265–271, 1996.
17. Prochaska J, DiClemente C. In search of how people change: Applications to addictive behaviors. *Am Psychol* 47:1102–1114, 1992.
18. Felix-Ortiz de la Garza M, Sorensen J. Self-help group for drug-addicted clients: Assisted implementation in outpatient treatment. *J subst Abuse Treat* 12:259–268, 1995.
19. Cowen M, Lawrence A. The role of opioid–dopamine interactions in the induction and maintenance of ethanol consumption. *Prog Neuropsychopharmacol Biol Psychiatry* 23:1171–1212, 1999.
20. Dale D, Federman D. Naltrexone, acamprosate help patients avoid relapse. *Clin Advisor* 22:80–81, 1999.

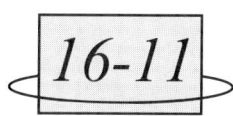

TOBACCO ABUSE
Virginia M. Hass

DISCUSSION

Tobacco abuse is the leading cause of preventable morbidity and mortality in the United States, causing more than one of every six deaths annually. In 1990, over 400,000 individuals died as the result of tobacco-related illnesses, and the four leading causes of death in the United States (heart disease, cancer, cerebrovascular disease, and chronic obstructive pulmonary disease) are all related to both primary and secondary tobacco exposure.

Tobacco abuse occurs in many forms, including cigarette and cigar smoking, snuff, and chewable tobacco. The common thread in all of these forms of tobacco abuse is nicotine addiction. Disturbingly, several recent studies have demonstrated the highly addictive nature of nicotine, indicating that nicotine is as addictive as other drugs of abuse, with the transition from experimentation to dependence occurring as frequently among smokers as it does with cocaine, alcohol, or heroin. However, over 70% of smokers surveyed indicated that they have attempted to quit or have considered quitting. Therefore, primary care providers are in the position to positively influence the lives and health of not only persons addicted to tobacco, but the lives and health of their families as well, through primary, secondary, and tertiary prevention.

EPIDEMIOLOGY

Despite an overall decline in the past three decades, more than one in four Americans still use tobacco. Fifty-four million are cigarette, pipe, and/or cigar smokers; and 12 million use "smokeless tobacco" (snuff or chew). These numbers reflect a decrease of almost 40% in the prevalence of tobacco use among adults since the mid-1960s. Unfortunately, tobacco use, particularly cigarette smoking, has continued to climb among certain populations. These include women, African Americans, Hispanic males, less-educated individuals, and adolescents. Additionally, adolescents make up the fastest-growing group of smokeless tobacco users. This trend among adolescents is particularly disturbing, as recent research indicates that smoking begins primarily during childhood and adolescence, with over 80% of smokers reporting that they began smoking before age 18. The Centers for Disease Control and Prevention reported in 1998 that 36% of high school students were current cigarette smokers. These statistics have significant implications for primary prevention of nicotine addiction.

TRENDS AND PATHOPHYSIOLOGY IN TOBACCO-RELATED DISEASE

Nicotine Dependence

Nicotine dependence underlies tobacco abuse for the vast majority of persons who smoke, chew, or use snuff; and any effort to treat tobacco abuse must address this problem. Nicotine is a central nervous system stimulant, the effects of which can be felt within seconds of ingestion. Nicotine stimulates the release of norepinephrine in the locus ceruleus, activating higher cortical functions such as alertness, concentration, and memory. In the mesolimbic system, nicotine stimulates the pleasure-reinforcing areas of the brain through the release of dopamine.

Symptoms of nicotine dependence are similar to the symptoms of any addiction. They include craving for the substance, inability to refrain from use despite adverse effects or inappropriate settings, and experiencing withdrawal symptoms that are relieved by the substance. Additionally, many persons afflicted with nicotine dependence will use the substance within minutes of awakening each day.

Table 16-11-1. Toxic Effects of Tobacco Use on the Cardiovascular System

STRUCTURE/EFFECT	MECHANISM OF INJURY
Acceleration of atherosclerosis and peripheral vascular disease	Direct toxic effects on vascular endothelium
Coronary and peripheral vasoconstriction	Direct stimulation of arterial smooth muscle, resulting in vasospasm
Coronary artery thrombosis and thromboembolic stroke	Increased platelet aggregation and adherence to vascular endothelium
Lipid profile	Reduction of high-density lipoprotein (HDL) levels
Hypertension	Strongly associated with the development of hypertension, though mechanism not entirely clear
Myocardium	Increased myocardial oxygen demand

The withdrawal syndrome described in smokers and users of other forms of nicotine includes anxiety, nervousness, insomnia, mild tachycardia, hunger and weight gain, craving for nicotine, and decreased alertness and attention span.

Cardiovascular Disease

Cardiovascular disease remains the leading cause of death in the United States, and is strongly influenced by tobacco abuse. Smoking has direct toxic effects on the cardiovascular system, increasing the risk of coronary heart disease, aortic aneurysm, and cerebrovascular and peripheral vascular diseases, including Buerger's disease, a disorder seen almost exclusively among smokers (Table 16-11-1).

Chronic Lung Disease

Although the precise mechanisms by which chronic lung disease occurs as the result of smoking are not precisely understood, cigarette smoking is directly related to many such illnesses, including chronic bronchitis, emphysema, and COPD. Furthermore, numerous studies have demonstrated higher rates of respiratory symptoms (cough, frequent upper respiratory infection, wheezing, shortness of breath) and an acceleration of age-related decline in pulmonary function among smokers than nonsmokers. The progression of chronic lung disease in smokers has been hypothesized, and is outlined in Table 16-11-2. (See Chap. 17-11-1.)

Lung Cancer

Smoking accounts for between 80 and 90% of all lung cancers, the leading cause of cancer death among both men and women in the United States. The relative risk of lung cancer is directly proportional to both the duration and intensity of smoking. Current smokers of one or more packs per day are 14 times more likely to develop lung cancer than nonsmokers; and the relative risk of lung cancer remains higher in former smokers than among those who had never smoked, even after 15 years of abstinence. Additionally, morbidity and mortality due to lung cancer appears to be more closely related to the number of cigarettes smoked per day than to the total number of years smoked. Put in practical terms, the smoker who has accumulated 30 pack-years (calculated by multiplying the number of packs/day times the number of years smoking) by smoking 3 packs/day for 10 years has a higher relative risk of lung cancer than the smoker who has consumed 1 pack/day for 30 years. Other factors influencing the development of lung cancer include depth of inhalation and use of filtered or mentholated cigarettes.

In the last 15 years, overall rates of lung cancer deaths have declined, following the decline in smoking in the general population.

TABLE 16-11-2. Progression of Chronic Lung Disease in Smokers

STAGE OF DISEASE PROCESS	PHYSIOLOGIC CHANGES	SYMPTOMS AND SIGNS
Early	Chronic inflammation of airways and alveoli due to chronic irritant exposure (i.e., chemicals and tars in cigarette smoke) Increased sputum production	Chronic cough ("smoker's cough")
Middle	Chronic hyperresponsiveness of airways results in bronchial narrowing	Wheezing shortness of breath
Late	Chronic inflammation results in destruction of alveoli and lung parenchyma Hyperinflation of the lungs (emphysema)	Barrel chest

However, because there is a long latency period between exposure and the development of smoking-related lung cancer, the death rate from lung cancer is expected to continue to rise among those groups in which smoking rates continue to climb (listed earlier). (See Chap. 13-6.)

Oropharyngeal Effects

Cancers of the oral cavity, oropharynx, and esophagus have been linked to the use of all forms of tobacco (cigarettes, pipes, cigars, and "smokeless" tobaccos); and the risk of all forms of oropharyngeal cancer is increased among smokers who regularly use alcohol. The National Cancer Institute has reported that approximately 75% of oropharyngeal cancers can be linked to this deadly combination. Other tobacco-induced mucosal conditions are listed in Table 16-11-3.

Other Cancers

Tobacco use is associated with an increased risk of numerous nonrespiratory forms of cancer. Carcinomas of the pancreas, bladder, and cervix have been associated with cigarette smoking. (See Chaps. 13-8 and 12-13.)

Poor Pregnancy Outcomes

The correlation between cigarette smoking and adverse pregnancy outcomes has been well established. Women who smoke prior to or during pregnancy have higher rates of infertility, ectopic pregnancy, low birth-weight infants, spontaneous abortion, preterm labor, and placental abnormalities. Suggested pathophysiologic changes responsible are outlined in Table 16-11-4. The association between tobacco use and infertility has implications for counseling women regarding smoking cessation during the preconception period as well as during pregnancy.

Other Effects

Users of tobacco products have a higher incidence of dyspepsia, gastritis, and duodenal and gastric ulcers. Additionally, these conditions are less responsive to therapy in those who smoke. Smoking is also associated with premature aging of the skin, with facial wrinkling around the mouth and eyes a prominent feature. The pathophysiology for these changes in not clear.

SPECIAL CONSIDERATIONS

The impact of tobacco use and smoking is not uniform among all populations. Smokers who are exposed to other inhaled environmental toxins, particularly asbestos or uranium, appear to have an increased risk of lung cancer. Comorbid conditions such as diabetes accelerate the cardiovascular changes associated with smoking.

Gender and Racial Differences

Gender and racial differences in lung cancer prognosis are also evident. Women have a lower relative risk (RR) of lung cancer mortality than do men, among both moderate and heavy smokers, and see greater

TABLE 16-11-3. Oropharyngeal Conditions Associated with Tobacco Use

CONDITION	DESCRIPTION	MALIGNANT POTENTIAL
Leukoplakia	A white patch or plaque on the oral mucosa that cannot be wiped off and cannot be classified as any other disease. Lesions may be small to extensive.	
Homogeneous	Uniformly white appearance with smooth or corrugated surface.	Low risk
Nonhomogeneous	Mixed white and red appearance.	High risk
Erythroleukoplakia	Whitish lesion with bright red velvety plaques and irregular outline.	Highest risk
Homogeneous erythroplakia	Bright red velvety plaques that cannot be characterized as any other condition.	High risk
Snuff dipper's pouch	White or white/red adherent lesion, classified by degree of severity. Degree 1: Slight superficial wrinkling of mucosa, whitish to pale gray. Degree 2: Obvious wrinkling w/o mucosal thickening, distinct white to gray, occasionally red coloring. Degree 3: Deeply wrinkled, obviously thickened mucosa, distinct white or gray color changes. Degree 4: Heavy wrinkling and thickening, white yellowing to brown color.	Most lesions will regress if smokeless tobacco use is stopped.
Smoker's palate	Diffuse palatal keratosis with chronic inflammation. Coloration ranges from gray-white to red.	Low risk
Smoker's melanosis	Melanin pigmentation in the attached gingiva. Occurs in 5% to 10% of smokers.	None known; reversible with smoking cessation
Effects on dental health	Staining, periodontal disease, gingival recession and bleeding, halitosis, and tooth loss are all more frequent among tobacco users than nonusers.	—

TABLE 16-11-4. The Impact of Tobacco Use Upon Female Fertility and Pregnancy

OUTCOME	ASSOCIATED PATHOPHYSIOLOGIC CHANGES
Infertility	Direct hormonal effect (increased estrogen metabolism), impaired fallopian tube motility, impaired embryonic implantation, alteration in immunity leading to increased risk of pelvic inflammatory disease (hypothesized)
Ectopic pregnancy	Impaired fallopian tube motility
Spontaneous abortion	Impaired placental function, fetal nicotine toxicity (hypothesized)
Low birth weight	Impaired maternal weight gain due to decreased appetite, fetal nicotine toxicity, fetal carbon monoxide toxicity, fetal hypoxia due to carbon monoxide toxicity and/or nicotine-induced vasoconstriction of umbilical arteries
Placental abnormalities (abruption, previa)	Abruption is related to nicotine-induced vasoconstriction. Cause of increased incidence of placenta previa unclear, may be related to impaired implantation

improvements in relative risk reduction after smoking cessation. For women who quit smoking, the RR = 1.1 after 6 years for those who smoked less than 1 pack/day, and the RR = 2.4 after 15 years for those smoking more than 1 pack/day. For men who quit smoking, the RR never reaches the same level of reduction, remaining 3.3 in those smoking less than 1 pack/day and 5.3 in those smoking more than 1 pack/day, even after 15 years. African Americans have a poorer prognosis for lung cancer mortality than whites. Patterns of tobacco use, access to medical care, and possibly genetic factors all appear to be related.

Tobacco Abuse Among Children

Primary prevention is the most effective means of stopping tobacco-related morbidity and mortality. Over 3000 children *per day* begin using tobacco, and over 60% of current users report starting by age 14. Furthermore, tobacco use may be an early indicator of other high-risk behavior, and is considered by some to be a "gateway" drug to further drug and alcohol use. The National Institutes of Health (NIH) recommend five "A's" for primary intervention with children, tailored to three age groups: infants and preschool children, school-age children, and adolescents. This primary prevention plan includes the following:

- Anticipate the risk for tobacco use at each developmental stage.
- Ask about exposure to tobacco smoke and tobacco use at each visit.
- Advise all smoking parents to stop and all children not to use tobacco products.
- Assist children in resisting tobacco use; assist tobacco users in quitting.
- Arrange follow-up visits as needed.

Passive Tobacco Exposure

The effects of passive smoking should not be underestimated. Studies have demonstrated a direct relationship between second-hand smoke exposure and development of the disease processes mentioned. Additionally, children exposed to passive smoke have a higher incidence of otitis media, URI, and asthma than their non–smoke-exposed counterparts. (For more information on otitis media, see Chap. 3-2.)

SYMPTOMS AND OBJECTIVE FINDINGS

Early in the disease process, tobacco abuse most commonly presents in the context of a smoker or other tobacco user who presents for a problem unrelated to smoking. Later, the patient may also present with secondary disease processes either directly or indirectly related to the tobacco abuse, such as COPD, cardiovascular disease, respiratory and nonrespiratory cancers, and dyspepsia. See the chapters relating to

these disease processes for specific discussion of their symptoms and signs.

Because 25% of Americans use tobacco, it is imperative to screen every patient for tobacco use. Screening may be quickly and simply accomplished by asking patients if they currently smoke or have ever smoked. Exposure to passive smoke should also be assessed, particularly among children. Nonsmokers can be identified and their decision not to smoke supported, particularly among children and adolescents. Both current and former smokers need to be monitored for health risks related to their smoking history. Identification of current tobacco users also allows the health care provider to assess their readiness to quit and to offer assistance. Former smokers can be congratulated on their success and monitored for relapse.

Current smokers will often continue to smoke despite adverse symptoms such as dyspepsia, cough, or frequent URI. Because many smokers will not volunteer their smoking status, health care providers must specifically ask when patients present with such problems.

DIAGNOSTIC CONSIDERATIONS

There are no specific laboratory or diagnostic tests for tobacco use, although carbon monoxide measurement has been used in research to verify whether a study participant smokes. Additionally, carboxyhemoglobin levels, as measured in arterial blood gases, will be elevated in an individual who smokes. However, neither of these tests is as useful as a careful history in screening for tobacco abuse.

The U.S. Preventive Services Task Force (USPSTF) has published guidelines that may be used to screen for smoking-related illnesses. See the chapters relating to these disease processes for specific discussion of screening recommendations. Additionally, the USPSTF recommends regular patient counseling to prevent tobacco use, with the following listed as "A" recommendations (i.e., there is good evidence to support the recommendation that the condition be specifically considered in periodic health examinations):

- Obtain complete history of tobacco use, and assess nicotine dependence among users, from all adolescent and adult patients.
- Counsel all tobacco users on cessation on a regular basis.
- Counsel all pregnant women and smokers with children living at home on the harmful effect of smoking on fetal and child health.
- Repeated messages over long periods of time are associated with the greatest success in helping patients quit.
- Prescription of nicotine substitutes as an adjunct for selected patients.

TREATMENT

"Nicotine dependence is a serious and complex chemical addiction, and most people who suffer from the affliction cannot become abstinent of nicotine without intensive assistance" (Love, 1998, p. 46). With these words of guidance, it becomes clear that a comprehensive, biopsychosocial approach is essential to the successful treatment of nicotine addiction. Such a comprehensive approach includes medical, psychological, and pharmacologic support.

Medical Management

The management of tobacco abuse in primary care begins with screening as discussed earlier. Once the tobacco user is identified, the key to successful intervention is determining the patient's readiness to quit. Change theory describes a model of stages, upon which interventions may be based:

- *Precontemplative.* The individual is not ready to consider smoking cessation.
- *Contemplative.* The individual is ambivalent about smoking cessation, with no stop date set, but is ready to plan to quit within the next 6 months.

- *Preparation.* The individual has made definite plans for smoking cessation and has set a stop date within the next month.
- *Action.* The individual has quit within the last 6 months.
- *Maintenance.* The individual has been tobacco-free for more than 6 months.

Patients may be counseled about tobacco cessation at any of these stages, with the message tailored to their level of readiness. Suggested approaches for each stage are outlined in Table 16-11-5.

Pharmacotherapeutics

Prescription of adjunct pharmacologic therapy may facilitate tobacco cessation, but should not be used as the sole therapy. Supportive measures (discussed below) are crucial to effective smoking cessation plans. Most nicotine replacement therapies are available over the counter. However, pregnant women; children; and people with heart disease, poorly controlled hypertension, asthma, or allergy to adhesive should consult their health care provider prior to using these drugs. All brands of nicotine replacement and bupropion (Zyban) marketed for smoking cessation come with patient education materials. Pharmacotherapeutic approaches to smoking cessation are listed in Table 16-11-6.

Supportive Therapy

MOTIVATIONAL INTERVIEWING Motivational interviewing—in which the health care provider expresses empathy, clarifies discrepancies, avoids arguments, and supports the patient's self-efficacy—helps patients build commitment and readiness to quit using tobacco.

TABLE 16-11-5. Suggested Stage-Appropriate Interventions for Smoking Cessation

STAGE OF CHANGE READINESS	SUGGESTED INTERVENTIONS
Precontemplative	Avoid lecturing on smoking cessation Provide clear, personalized information on why tobacco cessation is important to the patient's health Let patients know help is available when they are ready Follow up at each visit
Contemplative	Spend time exploring patient motivations for tobacco cessation Listen and respond to "both sides" of their arguments for and against quitting Offer information regarding options to assist in tobacco cessation
Preparation	Concentrate efforts on patient in this stage Capitalize on patient readiness to quit Provide specific information about how to quit, which methods to use, and available support groups
Action	Ask patients about any continued struggle with cravings, medication use and effectiveness, continued support, ways to handle stress and relapse Reinforce and congratulate patients on continued abstinence
Maintenance	Continue to reinforce success and assess for relapse, which may occur after years of abstinence Offer assistance with tobacco cessation again, if needed

TABLE 16-11-6. Pharmacologic Agents Used as Adjunctive Therapy in Smoking Cessation

AGENT	DOSING INFORMATION	RATIONALE/COMMENTS
Nicotine replacement therapy		Nicotine replacement therapy of all types reduces the symptoms of withdrawal, provides nicotine intake independent of environmental triggers, and allows tobacco users to focus on behavioral therapy Concurrent use of tobacco products and nicotine replacement therapy is contraindicated due to risk of nicotine toxicity and coronary ischemia
Nicotine gum (Nicorette)	Gum, 2-mg and 4-mg sticks (OTC)	Must be chewed slowly and intermittently, parked as a lozenge between chewing to enhance absorption Use of 4-mg sticks is recommended in heavy smokers ($\geq$1.5 packs/day) Underdosing is associated with higher failure rates Usual duration 8–12 weeks, with tapering use throughout this period Side effects: GI upset, diarrhea, mouth sores, headache (with incorrect chewing)
Nicotine patch (Habitrol, Nicotrol, Nicoderm CQ)	Transdermal, 16- and 24-h duration, dose varies with brand (OTC)	Patients who awaken with nicotine craving should use a patch with 24-h duration Start with the highest-dose patch, unless patient smokes <10 cigarettes/day, has known CHD, or weighs <100 lbs Underdosing is associated with higher failure rates Usual duration 8–12 weeks, with tapering dose at 4–6-week intervals Side effects: local cutaneous reactions, itching, dizziness, and allergic reaction to adhesive
Nasal spray (Nicotrol NS) and oral inhaler (Nicotrol inhaler)	Nasal spray, 0.5 mg/spray (R_x) Oral inhaler, 80 puffs over 20 min delivers 2 mg of nicotine (R_x)	Can be used alone or in combination with the gum or patch Nasal spray useful for immediate relief of severe cravings Oral inhaler useful for patients who miss handling cigarettes Usual duration: Nasal spray, 6–8 weeks, tapered gradually. Oral inhaler, 3–6 months, tapered gradually Side effects: Nasal spray, hot sensation in nose/throat, sneezing, coughing, rhinorrhea, and watery eyes. Not recommended for patients with chronic sinus disorders or asthma. Oral inhaler, local irritation of mouth and throat, rhinitis, headache, GI upset
Bupropion SR (Zyban)	Oral sustained-release tablet, 150 mg	Reduces craving for tobacco No risk of nicotine toxicity, may be safer in pregnancy and patients with CHD Contraindicated in patients with history of seizure disorder or eating disorder Start 2–4 weeks prior to stop date: 150 mg qd for 3 days, then increase to 150 mg bid Modest effect (reduction) on weight gain associated with smoking cessation, may be important to people who fear weight gain Usual duration 12 weeks, not necessary to taper May be used in conjunction with nicotine replacement therapy Side effects: Increased risk of seizures (1 per 1000), nervousness, rash, dry mouth, insomnia, difficulty concentrating, and constipation

BEHAVIORAL THERAPY   Behavioral therapy includes specific actions aimed at (1) increasing patient awareness of triggers to use tobacco and (2) beginning to reduce tobacco use. Examples include keeping a smoking diary, tapering the number of times per day tobacco is used, limiting tobacco use to specific locations or times of day, and removing ashtrays.

Other behavioral therapies reviewed by the AHCPR included hypnosis and acupuncture. Although there is anecdotal support of these therapies, controlled studies did not demonstrate that any of them were more effective than placebo in achieving abstinence.

CREATING A PLAN   Creating a tobacco cessation plan includes setting a stop date, planning for how to cope with cravings and stress, identifying support, and specific pharmacologic therapy to be used, if any. Just a few of the possible actions to be taken are outlined in Table 16-11-7.

PROGNOSIS

Benefits of Cessation

For all smokers with comorbid diseases, the primary intervention should be smoking cessation. For smokers with cardiovascular disease, smoking cessation reduces the overall risk of morbidity and mortality, rapidly reduces the risk of myocardial infarction, and improves the benefits of concurrent therapy. Similar reduction in risk is seen in individuals with cerebrovascular disease who stop using tobacco.

Smoking cessation remains the single most effective means of preventing chronic lung disease and preserving and improving pulmonary function in those with established lung disease. The Cardiovascular Health Study found that smokers who quit before the age of 40 had no detectable difference in lung function compared with those who never smoked. Furthermore, the earlier the smoker quit after the age of 40, the greater the preservation of pulmonary function when compared with nonsmokers. Those who continued to smoke had lung function similar to nonsmokers who were 10 to 20 years their senior. A longitudinal study of smokers with early COPD demonstrated more rapid than normal age-related decline in pulmonary function among those who continued to smoke than in those who quit, with the use of an inhaled bronchodilator having no significant effect on the loss of lung function. Reductions in relative risk of smoking-related diseases are presented in Table 16-11-8.

Relapse Prevention

As with any other addiction, relapse remains a possibility, even after years of abstinence. Over 85% of tobacco users will relapse at least once after they quit. It is important that health care providers be prepared to identify relapse and offer continued support. Factors contributing to the relapse should be explored, and specific strategies tailored to the individual's triggers. If pharmacotherapy was not used during previous smoking cessation attempts, it should be offered with the next attempt.

Important errors by health care providers in primary and secondary prevention of tobacco abuse include

- Failure to identify all smokers in the practice.
- Failure to arrange adequate follow-up for tobacco users who want, or are attempting, to quit.
- Failure to prescribe or use adequate doses of nicotine replacement therapies.
- Failure to intervene during severe illness related to smoking—a time when patients may be more responsive to tobacco cessation intervention.
- Failure to recognize comorbid conditions influencing tobacco abuse (e.g., other substance abuse, psychiatric illness).

Fortunately, it is never "too late" for a patient to quit using tobacco. Even those with significant morbidity related to their addiction will see improved health benefits with cessation of tobacco use. In summary, permanent abstinence is possible, and the sooner one quits using tobacco, the better. Primary health care providers are in a position to help all tobacco users in their clinical practices reduce or eliminate their dependence upon tobacco.

PEARLS

Patient Education Materials

- You can quit smoking. *Fam Prac Recert* 21:127–128, 1999.
- Clearing the Air: How to Quit Smoking and Quit for Keeps. National Cancer Institute website, 1999. *http://rex.nci.nih.gov/NCI_pub_index/pub_index_doc.html*

Resources for Health Care Professionals

The following organizations have multiple publications for health care professionals on tobacco abuse and related illness, as well as ways to incorporate prevention, screening, and smoking cessation activities into practice:

- American Lung Association: *http://www.lungusa.org* or (212) 315-8700.
- American Cancer Society: *http://www.cancer.org* or (404) 320-3333.
- National Cancer Institute: *http://rex.nci.nih.gov* or (800) 4-CANCER.

TABLE 16-11-7.   Sample Tobacco Cessation Plan

TIME PRIOR TO QUIT DATE	ACTION
Up to 6 months	Set a stop date, and tell someone close to you about the plan If possible, "buddy up" with a friend or family member who is also quitting Start keeping a tobacco use diary Begin to change your smoking routines When you want to use tobacco, wait a few minutes, and try substituting another activity
Up to 3 months	Switch to a brand of tobacco you find unpleasant Make smoking unpleasant—smoke only in areas you find uncomfortable, for example, outside on a cold day Change to a lower-tar, lower-nicotine brand of tobacco
1 month prior	See your health care provider for prescription(s) to be used in smoking cessation. If bupropion will be used, start now Practice going without cigarettes—stop carrying them with you Think of quitting in terms of 1 day at a time, not forever Clean your clothes to get rid of the tobacco smell Join a smoking cessation support group
On the stop date	Throw away all tobacco, matches, and ashtrays Visit the dentist to have your teeth cleaned Make a list of things you would like to purchase, estimate the cost in terms of your tobacco product, and put the money aside each day to buy these items Keep very busy on the big day—plan for activities you enjoy Remind your family and friends that you've quit and ask for support
Immediately after quitting	Cultivate a fresh nonsmoking environment around yourself—clean the carpets, drapes, etc. Spend as much time as possible in places where smoking is not allowed Drink lots of liquids, but try to avoid alcohol, coffee, or other beverages you associate with tobacco use Use substitutes for playing with something in your hand or your mouth—play with a pencil, chew gum, etc.

TABLE 16-11-8. Reduction in Relative Risk of Morbidity and Mortality After Smoking Cessation[a]

TIME SINCE SMOKING CESSATION	LUNG CANCER MORTALITY				MYOCARDIAL INFARCTION		CORONARY HEART DISEASE MORTALITY	
	MEN		WOMEN		MEN	WOMEN	BOTH SEXES	WOMEN
PACKS/DAY	<1	≥1	<1	≥1	n/a	n/a	n/a	n/a
Current smokers	nd	nd	nd	nd	2.9	3.6	2.02	4.0
<12 months	16.8	23.4	3.4	21.1	2.0[b]	2.6[b]	1.57[b]	3.1[b]
12–23 months	16.7	25.3	9.0	18.2				
24–35 months	19.7	20.5	2.5	13.2	1.1	1.3	1.41[c]	2.04[c]
>35 months	8.6	14.2	1.1	12	1	1.0		
>10 years	6.3	13.6	1.1	2.9	nd	nd	0.99	1.04
>15 years	3.3	5.3	1.6	2.4	nd	nd	nd	nd

n/a = not applicable; nd = data not available.

[a] Data from Hays, et al., 1998

[b] Data reflects 1 to 23 months

[c] Data reflects 24 months to 10 years

BIBLIOGRAPHY

Cromwell J, Bartosch WJ, Fiore MC, et al. Cost-effectiveness of the clinical practice recommendations in the AHCPR guideline for smoking cessation. *JAMA* 278:1759, 1997.

Dale LC, Hurt RD, Hays JT. Drug therapy to aid in smoking cessation. *Postgrad Med* 104:75, 1998.

Eberman KM, Patten CA, Dale LC. Counseling patients to quit smoking. *Postgrad Med* 104:89, 1998.

Facts and Comparisons. *Drug Facts and Comparisons.* 1993. Updated monthly.

Glynn TJ, Manley MW. *How to Help Your Patients Stop Smoking.* NIH pub. no. 98-3064, 1998.

Hays JT, Dale LC, Hurt RD, et al. Trends in smoking-related diseases. *Postgrad Med* 104:56, 1998.

Love N. The ultimate "penicillin" for lung cancer. *Postgrad Med* 104:45, 1998.

Mayhew MS, Grandjean CK. Smoking deterrents. In: Edmunds MW, Mayhew MS, eds. *Pharmacology for the Primary Care Provider.* St. Louis, Mosby, 2000.

Mecklenburg RE, Greenspan D, Kleinman DV. *Tobacco Effects in the Mouth.* NIH pub. no. 96-3330, 1996.

United States Preventive Services Task Force. *Guide to Clinical Preventive Services,* 2nd ed, Philadelphia, Lippincott, 1996.

Wadland WC, Stoffelmayr B. Cigarette smoking. In: Weiss BD, ed. *20 Common Problems in Primary Care.* New York, McGraw-Hill, 1999.

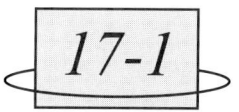

ASTHMA

David A. Luce

DISCUSSION

Asthma is a respiratory disease with the hallmark of intermittent, reversible obstruction of the airways. The resulting airflow obstruction usually results in cough, wheezing, dyspnea, and chest tightness. Although the disease has several precipitating characteristics, increased recognition of the role of airway inflammation is revolutionizing asthma management.

Since 1979 asthma prevalence in the United States and the rest of the world has been increasing. Approximately 10 million people, 3 to 5 percent of the U.S. population, have asthma. In spite of vastly improved pharmacologic treatment, there is a disturbing trend in rising numbers of outpatient visits, hospitalizations, and asthma-related deaths. Although the trend is partially due to better reporting and more accurate diagnoses, the cause remains unknown.

Patients at increased risk of dying from asthma include elderly persons; African Americans; those with previous life-threatening, acute asthma episodes or an asthma-related hospitalization within the past year; those with poor general medical care or lack of access to medical care; and those with psychological or psychosocial problems. The primary-care clinician must look for those patients to prevent unnecessary asthma-related deaths.

Asthma is one of three diseases under the broad, umbrella classification of chronic obstructive pulmonary disease (COPD). However, COPD usually refers to the other two, emphysema and chronic bronchitis. Emphysema and chronic bronchitis symptoms are much more chronic and demonstrate little reversibility. Cigarette smoking is almost always causative for emphysema and chronic bronchitis, and the underlying pathologic changes occur in the lung parenchyma.

Although significant overlap exists among these three diseases, asthma differs substantially from the other two. Mild to moderate asthma symptoms are usually episodic and reversible. Cigarette smoking is not a primary etiologic factor but it is a trigger and the pathogenesis occurs in the airways themselves.

Asthma's basic pathophysiologic changes occur in the airways. Those changes fall into three categories:

- Airway inflammation. This is more evident in severe asthma but plays a role in all cases.
- Airway obstruction. Extensive narrowing and marked restriction of airflow; reverses spontaneously or with treatment.
- Airway hyperresponsiveness. Exaggerated response to a multitude of stimuli such as allergens, environmental irritants, viral infections, cold air, or exercise.

The pathophysiologic process of airway hypersensitivity, inflammation, and obstruction is uniform in all types of asthma. However, there are several different ways to classify the disease. For example asthma is often classified as acute or chronic, and as mild intermittent, mild persistent, moderate persistent, or severe persistent. Asthma is also classified as intrinsic or extrinsic. Extrinsic asthma results from inhaled allergens triggering IgE-mediated airway reactions. Intrinsic asthma results from other nonallergic stimuli. See Table 17-1-1 for the asthma subsets.

SIGNS AND SYMPTOMS

The most common symptoms are episodic wheezing, cough, chest tightness, and dyspnea. Symptoms are often more prevalent at night and most severe in the early morning hours due to circadian changes in bronchomotor tone and airway reactivity. As an attack becomes more severe and prolonged, fatigue and sweating become evident.

OBJECTIVE FINDINGS

Diffuse wheezing on auscultation is the most common physical finding in bronchospasm. Tachypnea and tachycardia may be evident. Prolonged expiration is present on auscultation. More severe episodes result in use of accessory muscles in breathing, intercostal retractions, hyperresonance, and distant breath sounds. Ominous findings during a severe attack include increasing fatigue, diaphoresis, pulsus paradoxus (>25 mm Hg), diminishing wheezing, inaudible breath sounds, and cyanosis.

DIAGNOSTIC CONSIDERATIONS

It is important to differentiate asthma from several other diseases and clinical entities in which wheezing occur. The differential diagnosis of asthma includes COPD, alpha$_1$-antitrypsin deficiency or cystic fibrosis, left ventricular failure, pulmonary embolism, and anatomic upper airway obstruction such as abscess, tumor, or epiglottitis. Large airway obstruction as in bronchogenic carcinoma or foreign-body aspiration, functional upper airway obstruction, drug side effects, parasitic infections such as *Strongyloides,* and bronchopulmonary aspergillosis may also cause similar symptoms.

SPECIAL CONSIDERATIONS

The diagnosis and management of asthma in infants and young children is often much more difficult because pulmonary function tests are not feasible. A nebulizer or a spacer with a facemask is necessary to deliver inhaled medications to young children. Coexisting respiratory or cardiac conditions often complicate the diagnosis and management of asthma in elderly patients. Many medications exacerbate asthma symptoms in older patients. Asthma medications are also likely to produce troublesome side effects in the elderly. Pregnant patients should understand that most asthma medications are relatively safe and that poorly controlled asthma greatly increases the risk of perinatal mortality, prematurity, and low birthweight.

Asthma patients have a greater risk of complications during and after major surgical procedures. They should have thorough, preoperative clinical assessment including pulmonary function testing. If FEV$_1$ values are below 80 percent of a patient's prior personal best results, they should receive a short course of oral corticosteroids prior to the procedure. If they have taken systemic corticosteroids within the last 6 months, they should receive intravenous or oral corticosteroids the night before, the day of, and the day after surgery.

LABORATORY TESTS

During acute episodes of bronchospasm the total white blood cell count is often elevated. Eosinophilia is almost always present in patients with asthma unless they are taking or have recently taken

TABLE 17-1-1. Asthma Subsets

Exercise-induced asthma (EIA)	Bronchospasm beginning 5 to 10 min after beginning aerobic activity
Sampter's triad or triad asthma	Patients with a combination of asthma, aspirin sensitivity, and nasal polyps
Drug-induced asthma	Asthma precipitated by many common inhaled and oral agents such as aspirin, other nonsteroidal anti-inflammatory drugs (NSAIDs), beta blockers, histamine, methacholine, acetylcysteine, aerosolized pentamidine, and any other nebulized medication
Occupational asthma	Asthma caused by exposure to specific offending agents in the workplace. Causes such as laboratory animals and over 200 other sensitizing agents are commonly present in workplace environments
Baker's asthma	A form of occupational asthma caused by flour in small bakeries
Cardiac asthma	Wheezing of congestive heart failure (CHF) probably due to vasodilation in the small airways
Status asthmaticus	Severe, acute asthma exacerbation unresponsive to aggressive, emergency treatment

systemic corticosteroids. Microscopic examination of the sputum may show eosinophils, mucus casts of the small airways (Curschmann spirals), or Charcot-Leyden crystals from eosinophilic cellular matter. Early in an asthmatic episode the arterial blood gases reveal respiratory alkalosis and hypoxemia. Normalizing p_{CO_2} or developing respiratory acidosis are ominous signs and may indicate impending respiratory failure and the necessity for mechanical ventilation.

RADIOLOGIC STUDIES

In order to rule out other possible causes of bronchospasm, it is essential to order a routine, baseline chest film on every patient with asthma. It is also critical to identify treatable, complicating conditions such as pneumonia or pneumothorax. However, it is not necessary to get a chest x-ray every time a patient has an uncomplicated, acute episode of wheezing, as it usually shows only hyperinflation.

OTHER DIAGNOSTICS

Routine pulmonary function testing in asthma is rapidly becoming as important as routine capillary blood glucose monitoring in diabetes. Because the severity of bronchospasm often does not correlate with the intensity of symptoms or the degree of wheezing on auscultation, pulmonary function tests yield objective, "hard" data for much more effective diagnosis and management. The forced vital capacity (FVC) and the forced expiratory volume after 1 second (FEV_1) are excellent indicators of airflow obstruction and reversibility. A decreased mid-expiratory flow rate (MMEF or FEF_{25-75}) is very specific for narrowed small airways and points toward an asthmatic process rather than an obstructive, large-airway, or parenchymal process. The peak expiratory flow rate (PEFR) is also a reliable indicator of airway function and is easy to measure at home.

A patient with suspected asthma and consistently normal pulmonary function tests should undergo methacholine or histamine bronchial provocation testing to confirm the diagnosis. Skin testing or RAST testing in a patient with extrinsic allergic asthma will often identify the offending allergens.

TREATMENT

Medications: Patients and clinicians need to be aware that the majority of metered-dose inhalers (MDIs) still contain chlorofluorocarbons (CFCs) as the propellant. However, because of the potential hazards that CFCs have due to depletion of the atmospheric ozone layer, new MDIs are being manufactured with non-CFC propellant systems. Clinicians should educate patients on the new delivery systems and their proper use. Each patient's therapy should be unique and specific. Aggressive therapy to achieve initial control of asthma symptoms is the immediate goal of therapy. Then, the long-term goal is stepping down to the least amount of medication that prevents symptoms that interfere with a normal, active lifestyle and that maintains optimum measures of pulmonary function.

There are two general classes of asthma medications, long-term control and quick-relief medications. The best classification system in managing chronic asthma involves a stepwise approach, adding first-through fourth-line agents as severity increases:

Step 1. Mild intermittent asthma (symptoms ≤2 times/week, nocturnal symptoms ≤2 times/month, a peak expiratory flow rate [PEFR] or FEV_1 ≥80 percent of predicted with <20 percent PEFR variability). An as-needed beta$_2$-agonist MDI works very well as the first-line, reliever agent.

Step 2. Mild persistent asthma (symptoms ≤2 times/week, nocturnal symptoms >2 times/month, a PEFR or FEV_1 ≥80 percent of predicted with 20 to 30 percent PEFR variability). A daily anti-inflammatory medication is a good second-line agent after the beta$_2$-agonist. Either of the mast-cell stabilizers (milder, few side effects) sodium cromolyn or nedocromil, an inhaled corticosteroid (more potent, more side effects, starting dosage of 200 to 800 μg/day), or an oral leukotriene inhibitor is an appropriate maintenance, controller medication.

Step 3. Moderate persistent asthma (symptoms daily, nocturnal symptoms >1 time/week, a PEFR or FEV_1 60 to 80 percent of predicted with 20 to 30 percent PEFR variability). Corticosteroid MDI dosage should increase to 800 to 2000 μg/day. A sustained-release oral theophylline; an oral, long-acting beta$_2$-agonist; an inhaled, long-acting beta$_2$-agonist; an anticholinergic MDI; or an oral leukotriene inhibitor is the appropriate third-line agent. Patients on theophylline should have serum concentrations between 5 and 15 μg/mL.

Step 4. Severe persistent asthma (symptoms continuous, nocturnal symptoms frequent, a PEFR or FEV_1 ≥60 percent of predicted with >30 percent PEFR variability). Corticosteroid MDI dosage should increase to >800 to 2000 μg/day. A sustained-release theophylline; an oral, long-acting beta$_2$-agonist; an inhaled, long-acting beta$_2$-agonist; an anticholinergic MDI; or an oral leukotriene inhibitor; supplements as-needed, short-acting beta$_2$-agonists. Long-term oral corticosteroids daily or every other day in the lowest possible daily dosages are a fourth-line agent.

Exercise-Induced Asthma (EIA)

A beta$_2$-agonist, cromolyn sodium, or nedocromil metered-dose inhaler (MDI) 15 to 20 min prior to exercise is effective in EIA, a relatively mild form of asthma. When a single agent alone fails to prevent wheezing on exertion, a beta$_2$-agonist and cromolyn sodium or nedocromil is a potent combination.

Acute Asthma Exacerbations

An inhaled, short-acting beta$_2$-agonist via MDI or nebulizer is the first agent in the office or emergency department for acute episodes. More severe episodes require higher doses. A patient should start oral or parenteral corticosteroids as quickly as possible, because these

TABLE 17-1-2. Asthma Medications

DRUG	DOSAGE BRONCHODILATORS	COMMENTS
Beta₂-Adrenergic Agonists		
Albuterol (Proventil, Ventolin, Volmax)	MDI: 1–4 puffs every 4–6 h	The most widely used of the beta₂-agonists; available in a chlorofluorocarbons (CFC)-free MDI (Proventil HFA)
	Nebulized solution (0.5%): 0.5 mL with 2.5 mL normal saline every 4–6 h	Patients can use home nebulizers, young children can use masks
	Unit dose solution (0.083%): one dose (3 mL) every 4–6 h	For use in home nebulizers
	Powder (Ventolin Rotacaps): Inhale one capsule every 4–6 h	For use with a plastic Rotahaler; device is breath-actuated
	Tablets and syrup: 2–4 mg orally every 6–8 h	Proventil Repetabs 4 mg every 12 h; Volmax 4 or 8 mg every 12 h
Bitolterol (Tornalate)	MDI: 2–3 puffs every 6–8 h	Slightly longer duration of action than albuterol
	Nebulized solution: 1.25 mL every 6–8 h	
Levalbuterol (Xopenex)	Nebulized solution: 0.63 to 1.25 mg/3 mL every 6–8 h	
Metaproterenol (Alupent)	MDI: 1–4 puffs every 3–4 h	Shorter duration of action but more rapid onset of action
	Nebulized solution: 0.3 mL with 2.5 mL normal saline every 3–4 h	For use in home nebulizers
	Unit dose solution: One 2.5 mL dose every 4–6 h	For use in home nebulizers
	Tablets and syrup: 10–20 mg orally every 6–8 h	CNS symptoms such as nervousness and tremor are common with the oral preparations
Pirbuterol (Maxair, Maxair Autohaler)	MDI: 2 puffs every 4–6 h	Most cardioselective of the beta₂-agonists; autohaler is breath-actuated
Salmeterol (Serevent, Serevent Diskus)	MDI: 2 puffs every 12 h	Longest-acting beta₂-agonist for maintenance; has a longer onset of action and should not be used for acute therapy; also available as a dry powder MDI
Terbutaline (Brethaire) (Brethine, Bricanyl)	MDI: 2–3 puffs every 4–6 h	
	Tablets: 2.5–5 mg orally 3 times a day	Nervousness and tremor are common in the oral preparations
	Subcutaneous injection: 0.25 mg SC; may repeat once in 30 min	Less cardioselective than other beta₂-agonists; slower onset of action and fewer side effects than SC epinephrine
Other Sympathomimetics		
Epinephrine	Subcutaneous injection: 0.3–0.5 mL 1:1000 solution SC; may repeat once in 30 min	No more effective than inhaled beta₂-agonists; alpha and beta stimulation cause tremor, nervousness, palpitations, and vomiting
Anticholinergics		
Ipratropium bromide (Atrovent, Combivent)	MDI: 2–4 puffs every 6 h	Particularly useful in COPD; helps dry secretions; very few side effects; available in combination with albuterol as MDI (Combivent)
	Combivent: 2 puffs q 6 h	
	Unit dose solution: One 2.5 mL dose every 6–8 h (may be mixed with albuterol nebulized solution)	
Theophyllines		
Theophylline, oral (several brands, short- and long-acting)	Sustained-release tablets and capsules; short-acting tablets and capsules: 200–600 mg orally every 8–12 h	Used for maintenance therapy; serum theophylline levels must be maintained between 5 and 15 μg/mL; available in 24-h preparations
Aminophylline	Intravenous injection: Loading dose of 6 mg/kg over 10 min in patients who haven't received theophylline in past 24 h	Not recommended in initial, acute emergency care; may be useful in acute care of hospitalized patients when inhaled beta₂-agonists haven't been effective

Anti-Inflammatory Agents

	Corticosteroids	
Beclomethasone dipropionate (Beclovent, Vanceril, Vanceril Double Strength)	MDI: 2–4 puffs every 6–12 h	Rinsing mouth after use and spacer devices help prevent oral candidiasis

(Continued)

TABLE 17-1-2.   (Continued)

DRUG	DOSAGE BRONCHODILATORS	COMMENTS
Corticosteroids		
Budesonide (Pulmicort, Turbuhaler)	Inhalation powder MDI: 1–2 puffs once or twice daily	Rinsing mouth after use and spacer devices help prevent oral candidiasis
Flunisolide (AeroBid, AeroBid-M)	MDI: 2–4 puffs every 12 h	Rinsing mouth after use and spacer devices help prevent oral candidiasis
Fluticasone propionate (Flovent 44 μg, 110 μg, 220 μg)	MDI: 88–880 μg twice daily	Available in 3 dosage strengths; rinsing mouth after use and spacer devices help prevent oral candidiasis
Hydrocortisone sodium succinate	Intravenous injection: 4 mg/kg every 6 h	Treats the late-phase asthmatic response and usually does not act immediately
Methylprednisolone sodium succinate	Intravenous injection: 0.5–1 mg/kg every 6 h	Treats the late-phase asthmatic response and usually doesn't act immediately
Prednisolone liquid (Prelone, 15 mg/5 mL, Pediapred, 5 mg/5 mL)	Oral liquid: 40–60 mg every 24 h for acute exacerbations	
Prednisone	Tablets: 40–60 mg every 24 h for acute exacerbations	Should be used for very short courses of 7–10 days. Long-term use only when absolutely necessary and at the lowest dose possible daily or every other day.
Triamcinolone acetonide (Azmacort)	MDI: 2–6 puffs every 6–12 h	Rinsing mouth after use and spacer devices help prevent oral candidiasis
Leukotriene Inhibitors		
Montelukast (Singulair)	Tablets: 10 mg once in the P.M.	Indicated for the prophylaxis and chronic treatment of asthma in adults and children 6 or older
Zafirlukast (Accolate)	Tablets: 20 mg twice daily	Indicated for the prophylaxis and chronic treatment of asthma in adults and children 7 or older; use with caution in patients on oral warfarin anticoagulant therapy as prothrombin times (PT) will increase
Zileuton (Zyflo Filmtabs)	Tablets: 600 mg 4 times daily	Indicated for the prophylaxis and chronic treatment of asthma in adults and children 12 or older; contraindicated in patients with active liver disease or elevated liver enzymes
Mast Cell Stabilizers		
Cromolyn sodium (Intal)	MDI: 2–4 puffs 4 times daily	Not effective in acute episodes, but may be used 15–20 minutes prior to exertion to prevent EIA
	Nebulized solution: 20 mg 4 times daily	For use in home nebulizers
Nedocromil sodium (Tilade)	MDI: 2 puffs 4 times daily Nebulized solution: 11 mg 4 times daily	For use in home nebulizers

medications take several hours to take effect (they treat the late-phase response). Subcutaneous epinephrine and intravenous aminophylline offer no advantage over inhaled beta$_2$-agonists and add little to initial outpatient management unless anaphylaxis is present. More severe episodes require oxygen. Monitoring should be close and regular (hourly PEFR or FEV$_1$, pulse oximetry, arterial blood gases, and a chest x-ray if underlying pulmonary pathology is suspected). Admission to the intensive care unit may be necessary if an episode is not resolving or if there are signs of increasing respiratory effort or fatigue.

See Table 17-1-2 for adult medication regimens. Pediatric dosages are lower and must be adjusted.

SUPPORTIVE MEASURES

Preventive measures such as decreasing exposure to allergens and irritants in the outdoors, indoors, and workplace environments are crucial. Eliminating exposure of infants and young children to passive smoking may decrease asthma morbidity. Helping patients to avoid starting or to quit active smoking is vital. Improved maternal care, smoking cessation, and improved nutrition will help avoid prematurity and small size at birth (a risk factor for developing asthma during childhood or adolescence). Preventive measures to decrease the frequency of viral respiratory infections leading to recurrent bronchitis or bronchiolitis may make the development of asthma less likely in young children. Patients with persistent asthma should be given an annual influenza vaccine.

PATIENT EDUCATION

Education in asthma self-management empowers a patient to achieve the optimum level of wellness. The primary responsibility for patient education rests with the principal primary care clinician and other members of the health care team. Because improving compliance and guiding self-management are so essential to improved outcomes, many local and national organizations and support groups promote asthma education as well. Patients with mild to moderate asthma should participate in active lives at school, home, and work, including sports and recreation. High-quality training in proper inhaler technique, slow inhalation of MDIs over 4 to12 seconds (depending on lung volume), is critical to the medication's adequate deposition in the small airways.

Learning to keep a daily record of PEFRs with a home peak flow meter can greatly increase asthma control. Any drop in the PEFR is an early warning of decreasing pulmonary function. A patient should be given a written treatment plan for daily self-management and a written action plan for management of exacerbations. A patient can add or increase prescribed medications according to a prearranged plan using an asthma management zone system. Knowing whether a patient is in the "green, yellow, or red zone" enables the clinician to monitor and adjust the care plan. This prevents prolonged exacerbations that cause missed days from school and work or hospitalization.

DISPOSITION

Regular, follow-up visits facilitate monitoring progress and assessing home PEFR results and symptom records to adjust the care plan. In the allergic patient who has documented positive results on skin testing or RAST testing, immunotherapy may make a marked improvement.

COMPLICATIONS AND RED FLAGS

Asthma that does not respond to aggressive medical management should stimulate the search for underlying causes and possible specialty evaluation. Patients who require continuous oral steroids, or those who may benefit from immunotherapy, should also be referred to a specialist in asthma care. During acute exacerbations, increasing symptoms and signs of respiratory fatigue indicate the need for hospitalization for continuous monitoring.

OTHER NOTES OR PEARLS

Asthma severity cannot be assessed by signs and symptoms alone; objective measurements of lung function are essential. Thorough, ongoing education and training in proper MDI technique, spacer devise use, and home peak-flow monitoring empower patients to self-manage their asthma and literally change their lives. Aggressive use of short courses of oral corticosteroids avoids prolonged exacerbations, missed school and work, hospitalizations, and asthma deaths. Because of the uncertainty of high-dose, inhaled corticosteroid long-term effects on growth, children with mild to moderate persistent asthma deserve an initial trial of inhaled cromolyn sodium or nedocromil as an anti-inflammatory agent.

BIBLIOGRAPHY

Fishman MC, Hoffman AR, Klausner RD, Thaler MS. *Medicine,* 4th ed. Philadelphia, Lippincott-Raven, 1996.

McPhee SJ, Ganong WF, Lange JD. *Pathophysiology of Disease: An Introduction to Clinical Medicine,* 3rd ed. Stamford, CT, Appleton & Lange, 2000.

National Asthma Education and Prevention Program. Expert panel report 2. *Guidelines for the Diagnosis and Management of Asthma.* Bethesda, National Institutes of Health, 1997, pub. no. 91-4051.

Stobo JD, Hellmann DB, Ladenson PW, et al. *Principles and Practice of Medicine,* 23rd ed. Stamford, CT, Appleton & Lange, 1996.

Tierney LM Jr, McPhee SJ, Papadakis MA. *Current Medical Diagnosis and Treatment,* 39th ed. New York, Lange Medical/McGraw-Hill, 2000.

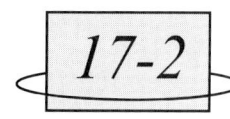

ACUTE BRONCHITIS
Maureen MacLeod O'Hara

DISCUSSION

Acute bronchitis in a previously healthy individual is defined as an inflammation of the large airways of the tracheobronchial tree caused by an infectious agent. The large airways of the lower respiratory tract are defined as the part of the trachea below the vocal cords to the intermediate bronchi. Infection of the smaller airways is termed *bronchiolitis* and is considered a disease of infants. The anatomic dividing line between the upper and lower respiratory tract is the vocal cords, which are above the cricoid cartilage (Fig.17-2-1).

ETIOLOGY AND EPIDEMIOLOGY

Acute bronchitis is the ninth most common ambulatory illness in the United States and is most prevalent during the winter and early spring. This coincides with the peak incidence of viral respiratory illness, the most common cause of acute bronchitis. The most common viruses responsible for this infection include adenovirus, influenza virus A and B, coronavirus, rhinovirus, respiratory syncytial virus, and parainfluenza virus. Bacterial pathogens that are less prevalent include *Haemophilus influenzae, Mycoplasma pneumoniae, Moraxella catarrhalis, Chlamydia pneumoniae, Chlamydia psittaci, Streptococcus pneumoniae, Staphylococcus aureus,* and pneumococci. *Bordetella pertussis* and *Corynebacterium diphtheriae* are considerations in nonimmunized children. The lower respiratory tract is usually sterile in healthy individuals, and the mechanism of infection is considered to be aspiration of organisms from the nasopharynx. Inhalation is not a usual route of entry for organisms into the lower respiratory tract, except for *Legionella pneumophila* and *Mycobacterium tuberculosis.* Reflux from the stomach and subsequent aspiration may be a source of enteric pathogens. Acute bronchitis usually follows an upper respiratory illness (URI), which can strike anyone over age 1 year.

SYMPTOMS

The chief complaint is a cough preceded by the signs and symptoms of a URI, such as nasal congestion with discharge, sore throat, malaise, muscle aches, headache, slight fevers, chills, and sneezing for a few days to 2 weeks. Patients complain of a productive or nonproductive cough, and possible hemoptysis secondary to the productive cough. Purulent sputum is suggestive of bacterial infection. Persistent fevers lasting more than 3 to 5 days may indicate pneumonia. Dyspnea is a rare complaint. Generally speaking, bacterial illness is characterized by fevers of 38.9°C (102°F) or more and chills, whereas viral illness tends to be milder.

OBJECTIVE FINDINGS

In addition to the finding of URI, the lung examination may demonstrate scattered rhonchi or possibly crackles and wheezes. Children may have hyperemic pharynx and tonsils, and injected tympanic membranes.

LABORATORY FINDINGS

Chest x-ray is usually normal and is obtained to rule out pneumonia. A complete blood count (CBC) is not obtained routinely, but may show increased white cells, especially if the patient has a URI or pneumonia. Sputum Gram stain may demonstrate many polymorphonuclear cells and can be misleading because of the presence of normal flora. Culture and sensitivity are reserved for hospitalized patients and usually are not obtained for outpatients.

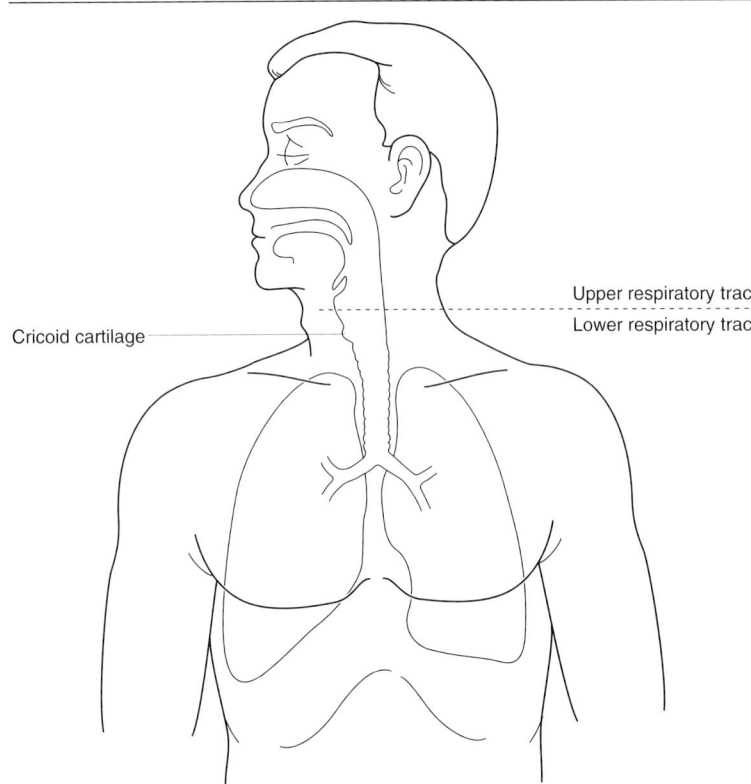

FIGURE 17-2-1. The anatomic dividing line between the upper and lower respiratory tracts is the vocal cords, which are above the cricoid cartilage.

Cricoid cartilage

Upper respiratory tract

Lower respiratory tract

DIFFERENTIAL DIAGNOSIS

The differential diagnosis includes bronchiectasis, pneumonia, asthma, chronic bronchitis, tuberculosis, cystic fibrosis, aspiration, retained foreign body, inhalation of noxious agents, and lung cancer. Recurrent episodes of bronchitis in children may indicate asthma and should be evaluated.

TREATMENT

Treatment generally includes rest, cough suppressants for sleep (medications containing benzonatate, dextromethorphan, or codeine), oral hydration (3 to 4 L/day to thin mucous secretions), and antipyretic measures. Expectorants (guaifenesin) may or may not be helpful. Because of the inflammation of the airways, inhaled bronchodilators may be helpful for dyspnea or persistent dry cough. If patients are suffering from a URI, decongestants may be helpful, but should be avoided at bedtime. Decongestants have a stimulating effect and the postnasal drainage my exacerbate cough response. Patients can expect to be symptomatic for 1 to 2 weeks, although a dry cough may persist for 3 to 6 weeks.

There is a new class of antiviral agents on the market called neuraminidase inhibitors. These agents are available in inhaled, oral, and intranasal forms and claim to be active against influenza types A and B (see Chap. 9-15). Previous influenza agents, amantadine and rimantadine, were effective only for type A. Studies show that neuroaminidase inhibitors shortened influenza cases by a few days and must be given almost at the onset of symptoms (within 30 to 48 h) to have optimum effectiveness.

Meta-analysis of antibiotic treatment for acute bronchitis found that antibiotics did not shorten the course of the illness in patients who did not have an underlying chronic pulmonary disease. However, if a bacterial etiology is suspected, antibiotics are indicated for 5 to 10 days. For both adults and children, amoxicillin, cephalosporins, and erythromycin are effective choices. Antibiotics helped patients when the therapy was directed against specific bacteria. Bacterial pathogens were found in up to 25 percent of patients. Patients who are more at risk—such as those with asthma, smokers, and those with chronic bronchitis, diabetes, congestive heart failure, and immunosuppression—should be considered for antimicrobial therapy.

PATIENT EDUCATION

Patients who smoke are at risk for recurrence of acute bronchitis and possible chronic bronchitis. This may provide another opportunity to encourage smoking cessation. Because influenza A and influenza B are implicated as a cause of bronchitis, consideration should be given to annual influenza vaccination in the fall. Studies have shown effectiveness of vaccinating populations from ages 15 to 64, as well as the elderly over age 65.

BIBLIOGRAPHY

Berkow R, ed. *Merck Manual of Diagnosis and Therapy,* 16th ed. Rahway, NJ, Merck, 1992.

Cho-Chou K, Jackson LA, Campbell LA, et al. *Chlamydia pneumoniae* (TWAR). *Clin Microbiol Rev* 8:451–461;1995.

George RB, Light RW, Matthay MA, Matthay RA, eds. *Chest Medicine: Essentials of Pulmonary and Critical Care Medicine,* 3rd ed. Baltimore, Williams & Wilkins, 1995.

Griffith HW, Dambro MR, Griffith J. *The 5-Minute Clinical Consult.* Philadelphia, Lea & Febiger, 1994.

Henry D, Ruoff GE, Jackson R, et al. Effectiveness of short-course therapy (5 days) with cefuroxime axetil in treatment of secondary bacterial infections of acute bronchitis. *Antimicrob Agents Chemother* 39:2528–2534; 1995.

Hueston WJ. Albuterol delivered by metered-dose inhaler to treat acute bronchitis. *J Fam Pract* 39:437–440;1994.

Labus JB. *The Physician Assistant Medical Handbook.* Philadelphia, Saunders, 1995.

Loughlin GM, Eigen H, eds. *Respiratory Disease in Children: Diagnosis and Management.* Baltimore, Williams & Wilkins, 1994.

Mainous AG, Zoorob RJ, Hueston WJ. Current management of acute bronchitis in ambulatory care: The use of antibiotics and bronchodilators. *Arch Fam Med* 5:79–83;1996.

MIST (management of influenza in the Southern Hemisphere trialists) study group. Randomized trial of efficacy and safety of inhaled Zanamivir in treatment of influenza A and B virus infections. *Lancet* 352:1977–1981; 1998.

Murray JF, Nadel JA. *Textbook of Respiratory Medicine,* 2nd ed, vol 1. Philadelphia, Saunders, 1994.

Myint S, Taylor-Robinson D, eds. *Viral and Other Infections of the Human Respiratory Tract.* London, Chapman & Hall, 1996.

Neuzil KM, Reed GW, Mitche, EF, Griffin MR. Influenza-associated morbidity and mortality in young and middle-aged women. *JAMA* 281:901–907; 1999.

Nolan TE. Upper respiratory and pulmonary problems. *Clin Obstet Gynecol* 38:147–155;1995.

Read RC. Treating influenza with Zanamivir. *Lancet* 352:1872–1873;1998.

Roche Pharmaceuticals. Introducing the first neuraminidase inhibitor in pill form: Tamiflu (oseltamivir phosphate). Promotional letter sent to providers. New Jersey, Roche Laboratories, 1999.

Smucny JJ, Becker LA, Glazier RH, et al. Are antibiotics effective treatment for acute bronchitis? A meta-analysis. *J Fam Pract* 47:453–460; 1998.

Thom DH, Grayston JT, Campbell LA, et al. Respiratory infection with *Chlamydia pneumoniae* in middle-aged and older adult outpatients. *Eur J Clin Microbiol Infect Dis* 13:785–792;1994.

Vogel F. A guide to the treatment of lower respiratory tract infections. *Drugs* 50:62–72;1995.

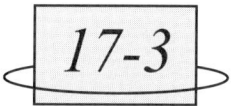

BRONCHIECTASIS

Catherine J. Heymann

DISCUSSION

The word *bronchiectasis* is derived from the Greek *bronchos* ("windpipe") and *ektaus* ("extension" or "stretching"). It is an abnormal, irreversible structural deformity of the medium-size and large bronchi that results in decreased mucus clearance, ciliary dysfunction, and dilated bronchi. Increased, pooled, and often purulent secretions produce the primary symptom: a chronic productive cough. Pooled secretions become a breeding ground for the growth of pathogens, culminating in recurrent pulmonary infections that are difficult to resolve and often involve unusual or resistant organisms.

Bronchiectasis may be acquired, congenital, or primary. Acquired bronchiectasis is either focal or diffuse in distribution and usually is acquired in childhood through recurrent pulmonary infections before the bronchial tree is fully developed. The current use of antibiotics for respiratory infections and immunizations for pertussis, measles, and influenza has significantly reduced the incidence of acquired bronchiectasis in the United States. Bronchiectasis acquired in adulthood is unusual and results from a severe necrotizing pulmonary infection such as tuberculosis. Primary congenital bronchiectasis is rare and results from genetically induced developmental abnormalities of the bronchial tree. However, several genetic disorders are associated with the development of primary bronchiectasis, including cystic fibrosis (50 percent of all cases),[1] primary ciliary dyskinesia (PCD), alterations in the immune system, yellow nail syndrome, congenital tracheobronchial anomalies, alpha₁-antitrypsin deficiency (AAD), and reactive airway disease (RAD).

PATHOGENESIS

Bronchiectasis begins with bronchial tube and/or interstitial tissue inflammation that is initiated by an infection at the epithelial surface. Once it has been initiated, the process is perpetuated by interaction between inflammatory, immune, and resident cells of the airway, resulting in airway damage, hyperactivity, tissue reorganization, and/or obstruction of the bronchi and the adjacent tissue. The walls of the bronchi become dilated and show inflammatory damage, chronic inflammation, increased mucus production, loss of cilia function, and decreased mucus clearance. Adjacent or distal to the bronchi, there may be alveolar, interstitial tissue, cartilage, muscle, or elastic tissue damage. Normal components of lung tissue are replaced by fibrous material, causing traction on the bronchial walls, further dilation of the bronchi, and loss of lung volume. As the disease progresses, increased vascularity of the bronchial walls may result in an anastomosis between pulmonary veins and arteries. Ultimately, right-to-left shunts may occur, causing hypoxia, cor pulmonale, and pulmonary hypertension.

Acquired Bronchiectasis

Bronchiectasis usually results from repeated infective episodes that cause direct bronchial destruction or mechanical obstruction before the bronchial tree has fully matured. Modern antibiotics, immunizations, and diagnostic techniques have reduced the incidence of acquired bronchiectasis in childhood. Rare causative agents of bronchiectasis in adults include RAD, severe infection, obstruction (foreign body, tumor, lymph node enlargement), inhaled irritants (cigarette smoke, immunologically active substances such as silica, talc, Bakelite, and asbestos), and aspiration of gastric contents.

Primary Bronchiectasis

Primary bronchiectasis is often comorbid with congenitally acquired diseases. Damage to the immature bronchi usually results from altered host defense mechanisms that are unique to the specific genetic abnormality.

Cystic fibrosis (CF) is an autosomal recessive genetic disorder that manifests itself in childhood or infrequently in adolescence or early adulthood. The lungs of a newborn with CF are normal, but soon deteriorate as a result of diffuse destruction of the small bronchi from abundant, very viscous secretions (see Chap. 7-1).

Primary ciliary dyskinesia (PCD) is an autosomal recessive disorder with incomplete penetrance that produces an abnormal ultrastructure of the cilia and poor mucociliary transport in all bodily systems. PCD produces a diffuse bronchiectasis from recurrent upper and lower respiratory infections. PCD may be present in up to 11 percent of children who present with chronic respiratory diseases. Young's syndrome and Kartagener's syndrome are subgroups of PCD, with the primary site of cilia dysfunction in the sinuses or genital tract and less frequently affecting the bronchial tree.

Immunodeficiency states may result in an abnormal response to a pathogen or allergen, causing bronchial damage through an accelerated infectious inflammatory response and decreased clearance of bronchial secretions. Immunodeficiencies include panhypergammaglobulinemia, common variable immune deficiency, and selective IgA, IgM, and/or IgG deficiencies.

AAD is a genetic disorder that classically presents as emphysema, cirrhosis, and/or pancreatitis in adolescence or early adulthood. Damage to tissues is caused by an imbalance between protease and protease inhibitors, causing a reduction in tissue elasticity.

Yellow nail syndrome is thought to be a congenital hypoplasia of the lymphatic system characterized by primary lymphedema, exudative pleural effusion, and thick, curved yellow-green nails. Up to 40 percent of patients develop bronchiectasis.[1,2]

Congenital tracheobronchial anomalies include tracheobronchomegaly and a complete or partial absence of bronchial cartilage beyond the segmental bronchi (Williams–Campbell syndrome).

The pathology of any underlying abnormality that results in the chronic pulmonary changes associated with bronchiectasis must be considered in selecting treatment options.

Microbiology

The pathogens associated with the development or exacerbation of bronchiectasis are numerous and may be related to comorbid diseases. Necrotizing pneumonia from *Klebsiella,* staphylococci, influenza virus, fungi, anaerobes, atypical mycobacteria, or mycoplasma may be responsible for bronchiectasis. Severe pneumonia may complicate measles, pertussis, or adenovirus infections, causing significant pulmonary damage and bronchiectasis, especially in children. In third-world countries, tuberculosis is the most common infection that initiates the pulmonary damage that causes bronchiectasis (see Chap. 9-31).

Allergic bronchopulmonary aspergillosis (ABPA) is an allergic reaction to a fungus in the bronchial lumen and a rare cause of acquired bronchiectasis.

Aspergillus fumigatus is the most common pathogen isolated. Histoplasmosis (see Chap. 9-32), coccidioidomycosis (valley fever) (see Chap. 9-7), cryptococcosis (see Chap. 9-8), blastomycosis, paracoccidioidomycosis (South America), and mucormycosis are less common and are found in specific geographic regions or immunologically compromised patients. In early CF, *Staphylococcus aureus* is a common pathogen. Later in the disease, *Pseudomonas aeruginosa* and *Pseudomonas cepacia* are more frequently isolated.

SYMPTOMS

A persistent cough, often with purulent mucus production, is the most frequently reported symptom. Occasionally a dry chronic cough that is intermittently productive is the presenting complaint. Hemoptysis occurs infrequently but may be substantial (>200 to 600 mL/24 h). A few patients remain asymptomatic. With progression of the disease, disabling dyspnea, fatigue, weight loss, anemia (or polycythemia), cyanosis, clubbing of the nails, and hemoptysis may occur.

A fever with increased or a new onset of hemoptysis and/or purulent sputum indicates an infectious exacerbation of the underlying process or an adjacent pneumonia.

OBJECTIVE FINDINGS

Chest auscultation is quite variable. Abnormal inspiratory and/or expiratory rales and low-pitched expiratory rhonchi are common over the affected area. Fine inspiratory crackles may denote infection, interstitial disease, early pneumonia, or chronic heart failure. Coarse inspiratory crackles are indicative of late pulmonary disease and/or pneumonia. Diminished breath sounds and dullness to percussion may be noted over areas of severe inflammation, pooled secretions, or mucus plugging. Egophony (A to E sounds) and decreased tactile fremitus can be appreciated in areas of consolidation. Diaphragmatic movement and chest contour may be unchanged. Later signs of bronchiectasis include clubbing and cyanosis, but these signs usually do not appear until large areas of the bronchi and lung parenchyma are involved. Signs and symptoms of cor pulmonale or right ventricular failure are seen with massive lung involvement, pulmonary fibrosis, and arteriovenous shunting.

DIAGNOSTIC CONSIDERATIONS

A chronic cough defined by persistent or recurrent coughing can last for weeks or months. Establishing the cause of a chronic cough is essential in guiding therapy. Is the cough the result of an acute illness, a complication of another disease, bronchiectasis, or all three? The differential diagnosis for a persistent cough is large (Table 17-3-1).[1–5]

SPECIAL CONSIDERATIONS

Damage to the bronchi and the adjacent interstitial tissue may be initiated in childhood by viral or bacterial pneumonia, adenoviruses,

TABLE 17-3-1. Differential Diagnosis of Chronic Cough

Angiotensin-converting enzyme inhibitor: adverse reaction
Chronic sinusitis and/or rhinitis
Congestive heart failure
Cystic fibrosis
Esophageal disease
  Esophageal reflux
  Achalasia
  Zenker's diverticulum
Inhaled irritants (e.g., smoker's cough)
Mechanical irritants (e.g., postnasal drip)
Pericardial inflammation
Postbronchitis syndrome
Psychogenic throat clearing
Chest cough
Psychogenic cough
Pulmonary abscess
Pulmonary emboli
Pulmonary sequestration
Reactive airway disease
Respiratory infections
Tracheobronchial neoplasms
Tracheobronchial obstruction

foreign body obstruction, asthma, and influenza. With more children in day-care settings, exposure to potential pathogens has increased. Immunizations and appropriate antibiotic therapy for community-acquired infections constitute good preventive medicine.

LABORATORY STUDIES

Multiple causes of bronchiectasis and the necessity of treatment for any contributing disease provide a plethora of laboratory tests to utilize. Testing for an infective process includes a complete blood count (CBC) with differential to detect a "left shift" and a Gram stain of sputum with culture and sensitivity to identify an offending pathogen. Normochromic, normocytic anemia of chronic disease and polycythemia of chronic hypoxia also may be noted on a CBC.

Tests for genetic disorders that may induce bronchiectasis are more expensive and complicated. CF is diagnosed through a sweat chloride test (quantitative pilocarpine iontophoresis), with a result of above 60 mEq in a child or 80 mEq in an adult considered abnormal. Primary ciliary dyskinesia can be diagnosed by abnormal cilia ultrastructure with electron-microscopic studies. Congenital immunologic deficiencies can be diagnosed by testing IgA, IgM, IgE, and IgG subclasses.

ABPA is recognized by "golden plugs" with hyphae in sputum, peripheral eosinophilia, rapid to intermediate skin reactivity to *Aspergillus* antigen, precipitating antibodies to *Aspergillus* antigen, and/or a markedly elevated IgE level. One should consider ABPA if a patient presents with pulmonary infiltrates and/or central bronchiectasis and a clinical history of asthma. AAD is diagnosed by alpha$_1$-trypsin phenotype and quantitation. Because this is a genetic disorder, all family members should be tested.

RADIOLOGIC STUDIES

High-resolution thin-section (1.5-mm) computed tomography (CT) has been reported to have high sensitivity (96 percent) and specificity (93 percent) in the diagnosis of bronchiectasis.[2] CT has replaced bronchography in most circumstances as the "gold standard" for diagnosis. The appearance of thick-walled circular cavities with or without fluid ("honeycombing") or thin parallel lines ("tram tracks") is diagnostic. Chest radiography can be normal in the early stages of disease, but the later stages may show changes similar to those seen on CT. The distribution of affected lung tissue may be an indicator of the contributing diagnosis in bronchiectasis (Table 17-3-2).[1,2]

TABLE 17-3-2. Diagnostic Clues by Distribution of Bronchiectasis

Upper Lobes
Allergic bronchopulmonary aspergillosis
Tuberculosis
Histoplasmosis
Histocytosis X
Cystic fibrosis

Middle Lobes
Tuberculosis
Cancer
Middle lobe syndrome

Lower Lobes
Primary ciliary dyskinesia
Swyer–James syndrome
Cancer
Sequestration
Cystic fibrosis
Diffuse bronchiolitis
Infections
Immune deficiencies

In Kartagener's syndrome, a subclass of PCD, radiography also reveals dextrocardia and situs inversus.

Classically, three variations of bronchiectasis may be seen on x-ray or CT. Varicose bronchiectasis demonstrates an irregular, beaded pattern of dilated bronchi resembling varicose veins. Cystic or saccular bronchiectasis displays large sacs without recognizable structures distally. Cylindrical bronchiectasis shows dilated bronchi with blunt end-points where mucus obstructs the airway. Determination of the specific type of bronchiectasis has limited clinical significance and no impact on treatment modalities.

OTHER DIAGNOSTICS

Pulmonary function testing (PFT) may demonstrate obstructive or combined restrictive-obstructive disease that may improve with bronchodilators. If obstruction is suspected, fiber-optic bronchoscopy may visualize a foreign body, a tumor, or another localized tracheal or endobronchial abnormality. In severe disease or an acute exacerbation, oximetry helps define the degree of O_2 saturation and hypoxia. Arterial blood gases and assessment of P_{CO_2} define lung ventilatory function and CO_2 retention.

TREATMENT

The major goals of treatment for bronchiectasis include

1. Detecting and treating any underlying cause
2. Improving clearance of tracheobronchial secretions
3. Controlling or preventing recurrent infections
4. Reversing airflow obstruction
5. Controlling or preventing complications

Treatment modalities encompass medications, chest physical therapy, patient education, and infrequently surgical resection or transplantation.

Pharmacologic management includes the use of antibiotics for acute infections, prophylactic antibiotics to prevent recurrent infections, and medications to manage restrictive-obstructive airway disease. Pathogens are usually mixed gram-negative and gram-positive, necessitating the use of a broad-spectrum antibiotic. Appropriate empiric antibiotic therapies are listed in Table 17-3-3.[1,2,6]

Further treatment should be guided by the isolation and identification of an organism or organisms by sputum smear, culture, and sensitivity. If no specific pathogen can be identified, alternating cycles of two or three antibiotics may be employed for 2 to 4 weeks. Because

TABLE 17-3-3. Selection of Antibiotics for Initial Treatment of Bronchiectasis

Amoxicillin 500 mg tid

Ampicillin 250–500 mg qid

Tetracycline 250–500 mg qid

Trimethoprim (160 mg)–sulfamethoxazole (800 mg) 1 tablet q 12h

Amoxicillin–clavulanate 500 mg tid

the most common pathogen for CF patients with recurrent infections is *P. aeruginosa* or *P. cepacia,* the initial therapy may consist of a quinolone (dose must be individualized) combined with an aminoglycoside (dose must be individualized) until another pathogen is isolated.

If restrictive and/or obstructive airway disease is present, additional pharmacologic treatments may include a combination of a beta agonist, theophylline, ipratropium bromide, and oral or inhaled corticosteroids. The use of these therapies is covered in Chapter 17-1.

Bronchopulmonary aspergillosis requires glucocorticoids to reduce bronchial inflammation. Prednisone (0.5 mg/kg per day) is preferably given in a single morning dose to reduce the incidence of adrenal suppression. Several weeks of therapy may be needed before one can taper to alternate-day dosing and discontinue the steroids. The addition of bronchodilators is useful, especially in acute episodes. No antibiotics are needed unless a secondary infection is suspected.

AAD can be treated effectively with gene therapy and should be referred to a qualified specialist. Gene therapy is now in clinical trials for CF patients.

Supportive measures include chest physical therapy and expectorants to facilitate the clearance of tracheobronchial secretions. Traditional chest physical therapy (PT) includes postural drainage, clapping, and vibration. CF patients may require chest PT one or more times per day chronically. Bronchiectasis patients without CF may need chest PT only on an intermittent basis.

Patient education should include cautions against smoking, secondhand smoke, exposure to known inhalant irritants and asthmatic triggers, and the use of antitussives or sedatives (which depress pulmonary function). Advice regarding a healthy diet, exercise, and stress reduction is an important component of patient education.

Disposition includes follow-up on a routine basis for basic medical care, monitoring for any deterioration in pulmonary status, and reevaluation of the treatment plan. At the first signs and/or symptoms of an upper respiratory infection, intensive antibiotic therapy should be instituted. A follow-up visit should be scheduled within 7 to 10 days to assure resolution of the infection. Routine influenza immunizations and one-time Pneumovax are appropriate for patients with compromised pulmonary status.

COMPLICATIONS AND RED FLAGS

Intensive management of upper respiratory infections and bronchiectasis may prevent or slow the progression of the disease and reduce the severity of complications such as protracted dyspnea, cyanosis, respiratory acidosis, obstruction, recurrent pneumonia, chronic infections, cor pulmonale, pulmonary hypertension, and pulmonary fibrosis. Infection in bronchiectasis patients rarely results in septicemia or a localization of an abscess at a remote site (e.g., brain).

Hemoptysis may be massive and life-threatening. Surgical resection of areas of bleeding pulmonary tissue may be required. Surgery or heart–lung transplantation may be considered if a patient has disabling hypoxia and/or significant localized disease.

NOTES AND PEARLS

Low-grade bronchiectasis probably is underdiagnosed. A chronic cough or bronchial infection that does not clear with standard therapy is a red flag for further evaluation. The threshold for suspicion of bronchiectasis should be lowered in patients with risk factors for pulmonary disease or congenital or acquired diseases associated with bronchiectasis. As with any chronic disease capable of disabling a patient without optimal control, an evaluation and a consultation with a specialist (pulmonologist) are desirable.

REFERENCES

1. Fauci AS, Braunwald E, Isselbacher KJ, et al, eds. *Harrison's Principles of Internal Medicine,* 14th ed. New York, McGraw-Hill, 1998.
2. Marwah OS, Sharma OF. Bronchiectasis. *Postgrad Med* 97:149–159; 1995.
3. Adler SN, Lam M, Gasbarra DB, Conners AF. *A Pocket Manual of Differential Diagnosis,* 3rd ed. Boston, Little, Brown, 1994.
4. Greenberger NJ, Agee KR, King TM, Newson M. *The Medical Book of Lists,* 3rd ed. St Louis, Mosby Year Book, 1990.
5. *Drug Facts and Comparison,* 50th ed. New York, Wolter Kluwer, 1996.
6. Chesnutt MS, Prendergrast TJ. Lung, in: Tierney LM, McPhee SJ, Papadakis MA, eds. *Current Medical Diagnosis and Treatment,* 39th ed. New York, McGraw-Hill, 2000, pp. 289–290.

BIBLIOGRAPHY

Barker AF. Bronchiectasis. *Semin Thorac Cardiovasc Surg* 7:112–118; 1995.
Berge E, Os I, Skjorten F, Svalander C. Alpha₁-antitrypsin deficiency—not only pulmonary and hepatic involvement. *Tidsskr Nor Laegeforen* 115:8232–8236; 1995.
Curiel DT, Pilewski JM. Gene therapy approaches for inherited and acquired lung disease. *Am J Respir Cell Mol Biol* 14:1–18; 1996.
Knoell DI, Wewers MD. Clinical implications of gene therapy for alpha I-antitrypsin deficiency. *Chest* 107:535–545; 1995.
Lee PH, Carr DH, Rubens MB, et al. Accuracy of CT in predicting the cause of bronchiectasis. *Clin Radiol* 50:839–841; 1995.
Patrick H, Patrick F. *Common Med Probl Ambulatory Care* 79:361–372; 1995.
Rabassa AA, Schwartz MR, Ertan A. Alpha I-antitrypsin deficiency and chronic pancreatitis. *Dig Dis Sci* 40:1997–2001; 1995.
Ray D, Saha K, Date A, Jairaj PS. Raised serum IgE levels in chronic inflammatory lung diseases. *Ceylon Med J* 40:14–18; 1995.
Reiff DB, Wells AU, Carr DH, et al. CT findings in bronchiectasis: Limited value in distinguishing between idiopathic and specific types. *Am J Roentgenol* 165:261–267; 1995.
Shelhamer JH. Airway inflammation. *Ann Intern Med* 123:288–304; 1995.
Tasaka S, Kanazawa M, Mori M, et al. Long-term course of bronchiectasis and bronchiolitis obliterans as late complication of smoke inhalation. *Respiration* 62:40–42; 1995.

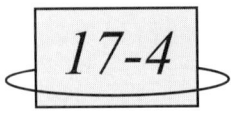

LARYNGOTRACHEOBRONCHITIS (CROUP)

Greg J. Mete, Sr.

DISCUSSION

Croup or infectious laryngotracheobronchitis is a common disease seen in primary care. It is usually a benign, self-limiting viral disease that responds to conservative treatment in a majority of cases, but the health care provider must be aware of the potential for episodes serious enough to cause respiratory distress. Croup is an acute viral illness that is one of the most common forms of airway obstruction in children. Infectious croup is seen in the pediatric age ranges of 6 months to 6 years, though it is most often seen below 3 years of age. Spasmodic croup appears to be similar to infectious croup but may have a different etiologic process. Croup usually starts as an upper respiratory infection that spreads to the larynx and trachea, with subsequent subglottic mucosal swelling and secretions. This illness is predominately seen in the fall and winter.

PATHOGENESIS

The dominant etiology of this illness is the parainfluenza virus type 1 (though types 2 and 3 have been implicated). Other organisms include respiratory syncytial virus, influenza, rubeola virus, adenovirus, and *Mycoplasma pneumoniae.* It is spread by direct contact and males are affected more than females by 3:2 ratio. Children with recurrent croup may have the potential for structural anomalies or other processes such as gastroesophageal reflux disease (GERD) or asthma. In one study, up to 50 percent of hospitalized patients with croup were found to have GERD. Patients hospitalized three or more times with croup were shown to have a high association with GERD. There may be a correlation with recurrent croup and the development of asthma.

SIGNS AND SYMPTOMS

Croup is normally preceded by an upper respiratory infection (URI) and then spreads to the larynx and trachea, which causes subglottic mucosal swelling and secretions that cause the characteristic "seal" bark and inspiratory stridor. The cricoid cartilage prevents distention of the subglottic region so dyspnea can occur. Fever is usually low grade or absent. A high fever should alert the astute clinician of the potential for epiglottitis, a serious life-threatening condition. The clinical triad for croup is a barking cough, inspiratory stridor, and a hoarse voice. There are varying degrees of cough, stridor, and dyspnea, but stridor on inspiration is the hallmark of croup, and this indicates that there is an obstruction above the larynx. Patients who have mild disease may just have stridor on exertion, and if the disease worsens, symptoms may progress to stridor at rest, respiratory retractions, tachypnea, and in severe cases cyanosis and apnea.

OBJECTIVE FINDINGS

During the initial presentation the patient may appear quiet in the caregiver's lap but may become more symptomatic if the child gets irritated during the exam. Exposure to humidified air will often decrease the symptoms so the child may improve by the time he or she reaches the clinician's office. Resting respiratory rate may vary from normal (16/min) to over 50/min. Breath sounds may be essentially clear with only upper airway stridor. Use of respiratory accessory muscles indicates significant obstruction and air hunger. Although rare, cyanosis is a definite sign of a child in respiratory distress. The child may have a tachycardia and appear pale. The posterior pharynx may appear red with slight edema and clear drainage. The neck examination may reveal mild lymphatic enlargement in the anterior chain.

DIFFERENTIAL DIAGNOSIS

The biggest concern when seeing a child with stridor is to differentiate between croup and epiglottitis. Epiglottitis is cellulitis of the upper airway and is caused most often by *Haemophilus influenzae* type B. Even though epiglottitis is relatively rare since the inception of the *Haemophilus influenzae* B (HIB) vaccine, it can still occasionally be seen. Other causes include *Staphylococcus aureus, Streptococcus pneumoniae, Streptococcus pyogenes* (group A beta-hemolytic streptococcus), and rarely group C beta-hemolytic streptococcus.

Other important considerations in the differential diagnosis of stridor include bacterial tracheitis, spasmodic croup, pharyngeal abscess, and foreign body aspiration. Bacterial tracheitis is an acute bacterial infection of the upper airway, and although it does not affect the epiglottis, it can cause just as severe respiratory distress. Initially bacterial tracheitis may present like viral croup, but it is postulated that bacterial colonization occurs, resulting in moderate leukocytosis, high fever, and purulent secretions that may cause airway obstruction and the absence of epiglottitis. *Staphylococcus aureus* is the most common cause of this disease, although *Haemophilus influenza,* group A *Streptococcus pyogenes,* and *Neisseria* have been reported. Treatment includes hospitalization and management similar to epiglottitis to include airway management and the use of antibiotics.

Spasmodic croup appears to be similar to infectious croup but may have a different etiologic process. It has shorter episodes, usually resolves spontaneously, occurs mainly at night, and usually there is no fever or antecedent URI. The etiology of the disease may be allergy related, although some suspect either a viral or psychogenic origin.

LABORATORY TESTS

Diagnostic procedures are not normally indicated in classic croup, because it is almost always a clinical diagnosis and laboratory tests do little to add to its diagnosis in the office. Pulse oximetry may be recorded in the office to document oxygen saturation in room air if warranted. A pulse oximetry reading below 90 percent may indicate a need for hospitalization. Hospitalized patients may require monitoring of their arterial blood gases. Leukocytosis may be seen in the latter stages of progressive croup.

RADIOLOGIC STUDIES

X-rays are only needed for atypical presentations such as rapid onset, drooling, or respiratory compromise such as one would see in epiglottitis. If radiographic images are ordered, they should include either an AP of the neck or a PA chest x-ray to look for a "steeple" sign. The steeple sign is narrowing of the subglottic region of the proximal trachea that can be seen with infectious croup (Fig. 17-4-1). If the provider is concerned about epiglottitis, a lateral neck x-ray will be

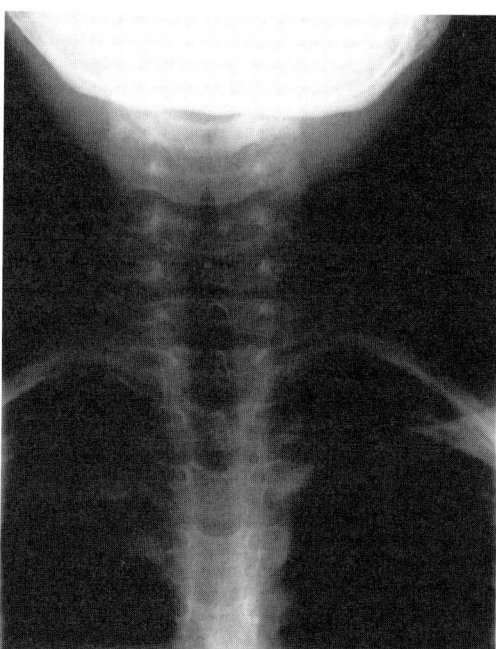

FIGURE 17-4-1. AP of the neck of a 9-year-old boy with recurrent LTB. Notice the steeple sign at the subglottic juncture. The patient, at the time of this x-ray, presented with severe respiratory stridor and the characteristic brassy, seal-like cough. (*Photo courtesy of Greg Mete. Used with permission.*)

needed to rule out the ominous "thumb" sign, which is hypertrophy of the epiglottis and dilation of the hypopharynx. The steeple sign is not always present and is only seen in only about 50 to 60 percent of cases.

TREATMENT

The mainstay in the treatment of croup consists of supportive measures such as reducing fever, ensuring adequate hydration, steam inhalation, and humidified air. These are tried and proven measures and are usually all that is necessary in the treatment of croup. Other methods such as keeping the child calm, placing the child on the caregiver's lap in the bathroom while running the shower at full blast, and/or exposing the child to cool night air, are part of the conservation measures that suffice in most cases. Cool mist vaporizers can be helpful, but remind the caregiver to change the water and clean the machine daily. Acetaminophen can be helpful for fever reduction and pain relief.

Other treatment options include the use of mist aerosols, racemic or L-epinephrine, and the possible use of parenteral, inhaled, or oral steroids. Antihistamines, decongestants, and antibiotics have no proven place in uncomplicated croup and should be avoided, as should cough suppressants such as codeine. Initial treatment after the immediate evaluation can begin with mist aerosols (normal saline in a nebulizer). Children that respond to mist aerosols will probably do so later at home with conservative therapy.

Racemic epinephrine (RE) has been credited over the years with reducing subglottic inflammation and is a sympathomimetic amine (with both D and L isomers) with a dual affinity for both alpha and beta receptors. Within the respiratory tract it has vasoconstrictor (alpha) properties that reduce edema. It also has bronchodilator (beta) properties that decrease airway smooth muscle spasm. These combined pharmacologic effects result in enlargement of the airways and assist with removal of secretions. Traditionally it was felt that if a child received racemic epinephrine, he or she should be admitted to the hospital for observation due to potential rebound effect that can be seen 2 to 3 hours after administration. There is also some controversy regarding if the rebound phenomenon actually exists. Some authorities feel that the return of symptoms may just be the natural progression of the disease after the RE wears off and not caused by the treatment. Some authors are now recommending that if a child is observed for 3 to 4 hours after being treated with both racemic epinephrine and dexamethasone, the patient may be discharged, provided he or she shows substantial improvement in croup scores. Patients must also have reliable caregivers at home and be well hydrated, and strict oral and written return precautions must be given and adhered to.

Of course, releasing to home a child treated with racemic epinephrine must be done on a case-by-case basis, but it appears that appropriately observed children *who substantially improve* after their observation period may be discharged to home. A child requiring two or more racemic inhalation treatments during the 3-to 4-hour observation period needs to be hospitalized. The dosage for racemic epinephrine is 0.05 mL/kg per dose (max 0.5 mL) of 2.25% solution in 3 mL of normal saline every 1 to 2 hours. Many clinicians are considering using L-epinephrine in lieu of racemic epinephrine. The dosage for nebulized epinephrine is 0.5 mL/kg of 1:1000 (1 mg/mL) in 3 mL normal saline. The maximum dose for children age 4 or less is 2.5 mL, and 5.0 mL for children over 4.

Although still controversial, steroids either alone or combined with racemic epinephrine are being used by more providers in more serious cases of croup. These patients being treated with steroids still require close observation and return precautions. Many authors now recommend the use of steroids in the outpatient setting for the nonimmunocompromised patient with mild to moderate croup as long as an observation period is included and the patient improves before being discharged to home. Many experts have recommended the use of steroids such as inhaled budesonide and systemic steroids such as parenteral or oral dexamethasone.

If steroids are elected, dexamethasone is given orally or parentally as a single dose, or repeated in 12 hours of 0.5 to 1 mg/kg up to 10 mg. Dosing of a single IM dose ranges from 0.6 mg/kg to as low as 0.15 mg/kg. It has been reported that both inhaled and systemic steroids might start to work in little as 1 hour. Inhaled steroids such as budesonide are being studied, but may not be available in all areas in the United States. In the outpatient setting, oral dexamethasone may be preferable because the parent and child will more likely tolerate this versus a painful shot. Dexamethasone elixir, however, is only available in 0.05 mg per teaspoon, and the potential volume of the medication must be taken into consideration when considering oral versus an intramuscular injection. Children suspected of having or being exposed to varicella or who are immunocompromised should avoid steroids. Children whose symptoms worsen need to be hospitalized, and those with impending respiratory compromise will potentially require an artificial airway. All hospitalized children with croup should receive steroids. Consider an evaluation by pediatrics, otolaryngology, or anesthesia for all hospitalized patients. Most children luckily have a relatively uneventful course with croup and will be able to be monitored on an outpatient basis and recover within a few days. Consultation with an otolaryngologist should be made in children who present atypically or have recurrent symptoms.

PARENT EDUCATION

Croup although usually self-limiting and responsive to supportive care, can worsen and in some cases progress to respiratory distress. Due to this, careful return precautions must be given to the parents of a child being released to home. Increased respiratory difficulty requires more observation and possible admission to a hospital. Warn parents to be aware of lethargy, refusing to take adequate fluids, and stridor at rest that is worsening. Children who develop a high temperature, start drooling, or look toxic and are laboring, need immediate attention and must go to the nearest emergency department.

PEARLS

The history will be very important in diagnosing this condition. The most important historical determinations regarding stridor are patient age and the duration of symptoms. Croup is usually seen in patients over 6 months and usually lasts for 3 to 7 days. Bronchiolitis is usually seen in children less than 2 years of age. Children who have been symptomatic over a prolonged period may have a congenital cause of stridor such as tracheomalacia. Rapid onset in children over 6 months should make one suspicious of epiglottitis.

REFERENCES

Folland DS. Treatment of croup, sending home an improved child and relieved parents. *Postgrad Med* 101:271;1997.

Geelhoed GC. Croup. *Pediatr Pulmonol* 23:370–374; 1997.

Kunkel NC, Baker MD. Use of racemic epinephrine, dexamethasone, and mist in the outpatient management of croup. *Pediatr Emerg Care* 12:156–159;1996.

Ledwith CA, Shea LM, Mauro RD. Safety and efficacy of nebulized racemic epinephrine in conjunction with oral dexamethasone and mist in the outpatient treatment of croup. *Ann Emerg Med* 25:3:331–337;1995.

Nicolai T, Mutinus EV. Risk of asthma in children with a history of croup. *Acta Paediatrica* 85:1295–1299;1996.

Waki EY, Madgy DN, Belenky WM, Gower VC. The incidences of gastroesophageal reflux in recurrent croup. *Int J Pediatr Otorhinolaryngol* 32:223–232;1995.

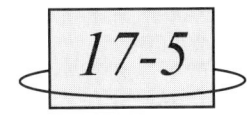

PNEUMOTHORAX

Barry A. Cassidy

DISCUSSION

The pathophysiology and consequences of pneumothorax are better understood after review of the mechanisms of respiration. For the lung to exchange gases properly, it must be capable of expanding. Lung inflation is maintained by a negative pressure differential between the pleural space and the alveoli. Downward contraction of the diaphragm creates a bellows-like effect that increases the area of the lung, passively moves air into the lung, and generates a negative pressure differential between the lung and the outside atmosphere.[1]

The visceral pleura and parietal pleura separate alveolar tissues from the chest wall. During embryologic development, the pleura envelops the lungs, separating them from the heart and mediastinum, and then folds back on itself, covering the chest wall cavity and creating the pleural space. Pleural fluid in the intact pleural space allows the visceral pleura and parietal pleura to move on each other without friction.[2]

Any mechanism (external or internal) that interrupts the integrity of the pleural space, allowing air to enter, disrupts the negative pressure differential between the lungs and the outside atmosphere and results in a pneumothorax (air in the thorax). Pneumothorax is a common entity and is characterized as primary (spontaneous and not related to an underlying lung disorder) or secondary (related to an underlying lung disorder).

A high degree of suspicion for pneumothorax can be based on the patient's situation:

1. Penetrating trauma to the chest can cause a pneumothorax.
2. Patients, particularly smokers, with chronic obstructive pulmonary disease (COPD) develop spontaneous ruptures of blebs, resulting in secondary pneumothorax.
3. Iatrogenic pneumothorax occurs secondary to the attempted insertion of central venous lines, after lung biopsies, and after chest surgery.
4. Patients receiving positive-pressure ventilation from a ventilatory treatment such as intermittent positive-pressure breathing (IPPB) or intubated and on a positive-pressure ventilator are prone to develop pneumothorax.

Less likely etiologies of pneumothorax include menstruation (catamenial), blunt trauma from diving injuries or being near large explosions, pressurization changes during descent in an airplane, and deceleration injuries from automobile accidents. Spontaneous secondary pneumothorax is reported to occur in anywhere from 2.5 to 18 per 100,000 persons and is more commonly found in males than in females. The burden falls on the clinician to determine how the air got into the pleural space and what, if anything, should be done about it.

Understanding the mechanism of injury helps prevent a clinician from making the life-threatening mistake of missing a tension pneumothorax or performing a needless and dangerous invasive procedure. In most cases, the clinician relies on the chest x-ray to diagnose pneumothorax and determine a therapeutic plan. However, a chest x-ray can be a major cause of misdiagnosis. The following scenarios have all happened to this author.

• In an emergency department, a chest x-ray clearly showed a large tension pneumothorax. A chest tube was placed by a first-year resident. The physical findings, however, did not fit the noncommunicative patient's presentation (the x-ray technician put the wrong name on the x-ray; the patient in the room across the hall had the tension pneumothorax).

• A patient with chronic bullous emphysema had an overpenetrated x-ray that appeared to show a significant pneumothorax. The house staff was poised to place a chest tube, but the attending physician asked that CT be performed because the patient was stable (the CT revealed that the area in question was a large bulla, not a pneumothorax).

- An intubated unconscious patient on a ventilator developed respiratory distress. The supine portable chest x-ray revealed what appeared to be a collapsed lung with the edges of the pleura visible and no visible lung markings peripheral to the pleura. The placement of a chest tube did not improve the patient's condition, and air was not seen in the air leak chamber when the tube was inserted (in reality, what appeared to be pleura was actually a fold in the bed sheet; the patient improved with vigorous suctioning of the endotracheal tube).

It is imperative to make sure the patient's presentation fits the x-ray. The patient's history often reveals the disease process. For instance:

- Trauma to the chest can lead to the suspicion that the integrity of the parietal pleura has been compromised.
- A history of emphysema with acute respiratory distress may lead to the assumption that the integrity of the visceral pleura has been compromised as a result of a ruptured bleb.
- A history of bullous emphysema with chronic dyspnea alerts the practitioner to watch for large bullae that may masquerade as a pneumothorax.
- A large area of radiolucency of the left lung field with no evidence of atelectatic lung near the inferior mediastinum may represent severe gastric distention into the thorax with displacement of the lung into the apex of the thoracic cavity.

OBJECTIVE FINDINGS

Although the physical examination of a patient with a pneumothorax follows a logical pathway, it is not pathognomonic. In the presence of pneumothorax, one might predict such things as asymmetric chest expansion, tympany on percussion, absent breath sounds, and significant dyspnea if the pneumothorax is substantial in size. However, many of these findings can be present with other conditions, such as large bullae, atelectasis, a pulmonary embolus, lobar consolidation, effusion, and a hiatal hernia.

The chest x-ray serves as the most valuable tool in making the diagnosis of pneumothorax. If the patient is stable, an end-expiration view will show the smaller pneumothorax better than will an end-inspiration view. Lateral decubitus views help find an anterior air collection often missed on the anteroposterior (AP) and posteroanterior (PA) chest x-ray views and differentiate pneumothorax from skin folds in obese patients. Experienced clinicians, however, do not underestimate the importance of historic and physical findings.

DIAGNOSTIC CONSIDERATIONS

On inspection, the patient's general status reveals much about the seriousness of the disease process. Severe dyspnea, tachypnea, tachycardia, jugular venous distention, extreme agitation, asymmetric chest expansion, tracheal deviation, poor oxygen saturation, signs of cyanosis, and hemodynamic instability in patients who are at high risk for pneumothorax (sustained recent chest trauma, postcentral line insertion, on a ventilator or with chronic pulmonary disease) are symptoms highly indicative of tension pneumothorax.

A tension pneumothorax occurs when air is allowed to enter the pleural space but cannot leave (creating a one-way-valve situation). In this setting, pressure continues to increase, causing collapse of the ipsilateral lung, depression of the diaphragm, shifting of the mediastinum, obstruction of the inflow of blood (vena cava) into the right atrium, decreased cardiac output, cardiac arrhythmias, and ultimately electromechanical disassociation. Thus, a tension pneumothorax is a medical emergency and requires immediate treatment. The placement of a chest tube to water-seal suction is the treatment of choice;

however, if the materials are not immediately available, placement of a large-bore (12- to 14-gauge) Intracath needle into the chest wall (generally the second intercostal space in the midclavicular line) will temporarily release the pressure of a tension pneumothorax until the pleural space can be controlled with a chest tube. A plastic Intracath needle should be used so that the sharp needle bore can be removed before it punctures the expanding lung after insertion.[3]

SPECIAL CONSIDERATIONS

The insertion of a needle is not an innocuous procedure, and the clinical index of suspicion of tension pneumothorax should be high before the procedure is done. If a pneumothorax is not present (particularly in a patient with emphysematous disease), the insertion of a needle into the chest wall can puncture the lung, probably create an air leak resulting in a pneumothorax, and potentially infect the pleural space, possibly leading to the development of an empyema.

Patients on ventilators who have a sudden desaturation of blood and develop dysrhythmias recalcitrant to DC cardioversion should be suspect for possible pneumothorax (the dead air space will not conduct the electric current).

RADIOLOGIC STUDIES

Pneumothorax on chest x-ray is often reported in terms of a percentage of thoracic space filled by lung. A 10 percent pneumothorax implies that 90 percent of the lung remains inflated while the remaining 10 percent of the thoracic cavity is filled with air. This method of measurement is somewhat arbitrary and has led some researchers to suggest that a pneumothorax should be reported in terms of actual measurement of the area of air seen on the AP or PA and lateral (LAT) chest films (e.g., 2 cm by 10 cm). This method seems preferable, particularly if a physician assistant is describing x-ray findings on the phone.

Unfortunately, the standard chest x-ray can be inaccurate in determining the true size of particularly smaller pneumothoraces. Patients in this group who are clinically stable should have CT examinations to determine the true size of the existing pneumothorax.

TREATMENT

Roentgenographic findings of pneumothorax can be coincidental. Patients admitted to the hospital may be found to have small pneumothoraces; others are found on routine chest x-rays for workups of coughs or illnesses. The difficulty for the clinician is to decide what, if any, therapy to offer the patient. The cause, size, and changes of the pneumothorax determine in large part what treatment will be given.

Treatment for spontaneous pneumothorax can be thought of in a linear therapeutic progression from noninvasive to significantly invasive procedures directly related to the severity of the pneumothorax.

The first modality to employ is supplementation of oxygen. Oxygen supplementation creates a gas pressure gradient between the pleural space and the tissue capillaries surrounding the plural space that enhances the absorption of pleural nitrogen. Supplemental oxygen administration has been reported to increase the basal resolution rate three to four-fold.[4,5] Administration of oxygen via nasal cannula at 3 to 4 L/min is a valuable therapeutic modality.

A second level of therapeutic consideration involves simple observation. While a simple "watch and wait" approach is inexpensive and attractive in small pneumothoraces of less than 15%, caution is warranted. O'Rourke and Yee looked at a series of 40 patients with small spontaneous pneumothoraces and 9(23%) of the patients required chest tube insertions for progression of the pneumothorax. Seven of these nine patients had underlying chronic obstructive pulmonary disease.[6]

Simple aspiration of the pneumothorax can be accomplished with a small catheter (often IV catheter) between the fourth and fifth intercostal space over the superior rib margin in the anterior axillary line. A three-way stopcock and a large syringe are used to remove the air in the pleural space. A number of commercial kits exist that include one-way valves such as the Heimlich valve. There is debate as to whether simple aspiration is as effective as chest tube insertion.[7] However, if the pleural space cannot be controlled, then one is forced to insert a chest tube.

The mode of injury always warrants one's attention. For instance, a patient who develops a pneumothorax after an attempted invasive procedure (e.g., placement of a central venous line) probably will get a chest tube. Certainly this type of patient must be watched closely. The cause of such a pneumothorax is the needle puncturing the lung. The hole in the lung allows air to leak into the pleural space, and if this is allowed to continue, the increased pressure will collapse the lung. The pleural space cannot seal a break in the integrity of the pleura if the visceral and the parietal pleura are not in contact. Therefore, air leaks that occur from the lung parenchyma itself usually require the placement of a chest tube. Once the negative pressure is reestablished in the pleural space by means of water-sealed suction, the pleura can heal itself.

One should note the type of air leak present in the air leak chamber after the insertion of a chest tube. An air leak (bubbles in some systems and fluttering valves in others) should be present upon expiration. (The air leak chamber consists of several small columns of water in most pleural drainage systems, and should not be confused with the single water seal chamber that indicates centimeters of water pressure and slowly bubbles.) If a continuous air leak is present (on both inspiration and expiration), one should first look for a major system leak in the tubing. If no system leak is found, a thoracic surgeon should be called immediately, as there is a massive hole in the lung or a bronchial leak. This can be extremely critical, particularly if the patient has undergone recent thoracic surgery.

Sometimes small leaks can occur that manage to seal themselves. In this situation, the size of the pneumothorax remains the same and the patient can be observed without the placement of a chest tube as long as no significant increase in the pneumothorax occurs. When the source of the air leak is stopped, the remaining air in the pleural space is reabsorbed in a matter of a day to weeks.

A spontaneous pneumothorax should be watched closely. If the area of air seen on the chest x-ray is small and the leak continues, a chest tube should be placed. Ironically, a larger pneumothorax (provided that there is no tension pneumothorax) adds to the safety of the chest tube placement, as the air collapses the lung and protects the examiner from hitting the lung with the instruments. A trocar (a heavy metal skewer with an angled point) is inserted into some chest tubes and used to push through the pleura. Many physicians feel that trocar chest tubes are dangerous, particularly in the hands of an inexperienced user. A much safer means of insertion involves cutting down with a scalpel to the chest wall in a controlled manner, taking a Kelly clamp or scalpel, puncturing or cutting the pleura, introducing a finger to widen the incision, and then inserting the chest tube; this method protects any nearby organs and those stuck to the chest wall. A great deal of damage can be done if one is not familiar with chest tube insertion.

Patients on ventilators who develop pneumothorax probably will need the placement of a chest tube. The positive pressure probably will cause a continuous air leak, and placement of the chest tube will be essential. Generally, chest tubes placed while a patient is on a ventilator are left in until the ventilator is removed or the amount of positive pressure can be decreased significantly. Chest tubes that have been in place for an extended period may become clogged with fibrous material and become nonfunctional. There is no advantage to leaving a nonfunctioning chest tube in place.

A stable outpatient who complains of shortness of breath or an episode of sharp pleuritic chest pain and is found to have a pneumothorax can pose a treatment dilemma. Not all patients require chest tubes. Patients with recurrent pneumothorax should be referred to a thoracic surgeon. Treatment of recurrent pneumothorax can be accomplished by the instillation of a chemical irritant. These agents work by causing a chemical irritation of both the visceral and the parietal pleura. This inflammatory reaction induces the formation of adhesions that hold the pleural spaces together and cause eventual obliteration of the pleural space. Unfortunately, chemical pleurodesis, although very easy to perform, particularly with a chest tube in place, causes severe pain to the patient. There are a variety of "cocktails" to do chemical pleurodesis, such as doxycycline, talc, and cisplatin. Parental tetracycline hydrochloride is often referred to in the literature, but it is no longer commercially available in the United States. Most chemical pleurodesis compounds contain a local anesthetic such as lidocaine. Regardless of the type of local anesthetic used, this remains a very painful procedure. Ironically, the more the procedure hurts, the more likely it is that the lung will remain adherent. Ample premedication should be given, and the patient should be warned that the procedure will be painful.

In most cases, chest tubes are left in until 12 to 24 h after the air leak stops. Some patients may have persistent air leaks, and their chest tubes are left in place for 3 weeks. At the end of the 3-week time frame, most lungs become adherent to the chest wall.

Some clinicians remove the chest tube after chemical or mechanical pleurodesis and insert a new chest tube if the lung collapses. Compliant patients may be sent home with continuous air leaks after the placement of a Heimlich tube (a "flutter" valve attached to the chest tube that lets air exit the pleural space and not reenter it) and followed on an outpatient basis until the air leak stops.

Mechanical pleurodesis is another alternative and can be accomplished via thoracoscopic surgery or through the traditional thoracotomy incision. The pleura is rubbed briskly with Brillo-type pads or with instruments that irritate it. This requires a general anesthetic but is much more comfortable for the patient. Once pleurodesis has been performed (either chemical or mechanical), the lung should become adherent to the chest wall. This adds risk and difficulty to any future lung surgery. The patient should be told to inform future physicians that pleurodesis has been performed.

REFERENCES

1. Witten ML. General overview of the pulmonary system, 1996. *http://www.physiol.arizona.edu*
2. Lewis CE, Colt HG. Pleural effusion from diagnostic thoracentesis to thoracoscopy. *Phys Assist* 20:68–83; 1996.
3. Pluth JR. Personal communication, July 12, 1996.
4. Northfield TC. Oxygen therapy for spontaneous pneumothorax. *BMJ* 4:86–88; 1971.
5. Chadha TS, Cohn MA. Noninvasive treatment of pneumothorax with oxygen inhalation. *Respiration* 44:147–152; 1983.
6. O'Rourke JP, Yee ES. Civilian spontaneous pneumothorax: Treatment options and long-term results. *Chest* 96:1302–1306; 1989.
7. Baumann MN, Strange C. Treatment of spontaneous pneumothorax. *Chest* 112:789–804; 1997.

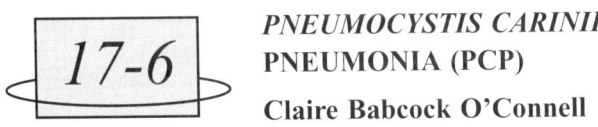

PNEUMOCYSTIS CARINII PNEUMONIA (PCP)

Claire Babcock O'Connell

DISCUSSION

Controversy over the classification of *Pneumocystis* still exists; most microbiologists will classify the organism as a fungus, but many clinicians believe it to be a protozoan. Regardless, *Pneumocystis carinii* pneumonia (PCP) remains an important respiratory condition and the most common AIDS-defining illness in HIV disease. The first cluster of opportunistic respiratory disease in gay men in San Francisco and

New York in the early 1980s proved to be PCP. The incidence and mortality of PCP has declined since the development of advanced diagnostic and therapeutic methods. Despite this, it remains the most common threat to patients with HIV and has a mortality rate of 10 to 20 percent; when untreated, PCP is uniformly fatal in HIV-positive patients.

Pneumocystis carinii is a ubiquitous microbe and infection in humans is common. Serologic studies show that virtually all children have been exposed to the organism within the first few years of life. Inhalation of the cyst form is the most common route of transmission. Disease in immunocompetent persons is rare. It is not known whether the infection lies dormant or if new infection triggers disease in the immunosuppressed host. Outbreaks in late winter or following epidemics of other respiratory illnesses, and clusters of infection in groupings of immunosuppressed hosts, suggests that the organism is spread human to human.

The organism exists in the lungs in three forms: the trophozoite, the cyst, and an intermediate form known as precyst. All three forms can be viewed with special staining. Propagation is slow causing the accumulation of foamy alveolar exudates. Cell membrane permeability becomes altered leading to impaired gas exchange and a reduction in diffusing capacity and lung compliance. Pneumocystis therapy is also associated with a release of tumor necrosis factor-a and interleukins from the alveoli, which causes a further inflammatory reaction. Alveolar hypertrophy, interstitial edema, and fibrosis occur, which further degrades respiratory function.

More than 90 percent of infections with PCP occur with CD4+ T-cell counts below $100/mm^3$. PCP is also encountered in patients with higher T-cell counts if the count has been rapidly declining or in the presence of other opportunistic infections such as thrush.

SYMPTOMS

PCP typically presents with a chronic, nonproductive cough and dyspnea. The onset is insidious, and fever is common. Fatigue and weight loss are not unusual. The symptoms are usually very subtle, but the presentation can be quite variable. Symptom duration does not correlate with severity or prognosis.

OBJECTIVE FINDINGS

The lung exam in patients with PCP is generally normal. Some patients (<40 percent) may have rales, usually late in the course of the illness. Cyanosis, tachypnea, retractions, and wheezing are less common and often indicate severe disease.

Arterial blood gases reveal hypoxemia and respiratory alkalosis. Pulmonary function testing confirms hypoxemia in almost all patients. Level of hypoxemia is often used as an indicator of disease severity. Pao_2 is below 80 mm Hg in over 80 percent of cases. Other abnormalities include an increased alveolar–arterial oxygen gradient and reduced carbon monoxide diffusing capacity.

Bronchoalveolar lavage is very sensitive and has become the cornerstone of diagnosis. Sampling from involved sites carries a very high yield of organisms. Transbronchial biopsy and sputum induction may also aid in the diagnosis of PCP.

DIAGNOSTIC CONSIDERATIONS

The differential diagnosis of PC includes many other respiratory pathogens and conditions. Many other diseases may be evident concurrently. Table 17-6-1 is a list of conditions commonly seen in HIV-positive patients that should be included in the differential.

LABORATORY TESTS

CD_4+ T-cell counts below $100/mm^3$ are typical with PCP pneumonia. Elevated lactic dehydrogenase (LDH), although nonspecific, can

TABLE 17-6-1. *Pneumocystis carinii* Pneumonia Differential Diagnoses in HIV-Positive Patients

Mycobacterium tuberculosis
Haemophilus pneumoniae
Cryptococcus neoformans
Invasive CMV pneumonitis
Kaposi's sarcoma
Streptococcus pneumoniae
Staphylococcus aureus
Mycobacterium avium
Legionella pneumophila
Coccidiomycosis
Nocardiosis
Mycoplasma pneumoniae
Blastomycosis
Histoplasmosis
Aspergillosis
Lymphoid interstitial pneumonitis
Other mycobacterial species
Carcinoma
Chlamydia spp.
Toxoplasmosis
Strongyloides spp.

be used to aid in the differentiation of PCP from other respiratory illnesses in HIV-positive patients. Very high levels of LDH are correlated with increased risk of death. Therapy against PCP can be monitored through decreasing LDH values. Arterial blood gases reveal hypoxemia and hypocapnia; these findings exacerbate with exertion.

RADIOLOGIC STUDIES

The typical chest x-ray in PCP demonstrates a bilateral interstitial infiltrate, although the radiographic appearance of PCP can be highly variable. The changes are usually initially seen in the perihilar area and spread to the lower and then the upper lobes. The apices are typically spared unless the patient has received aerosolized pentamidine treatment. The infiltrate is typically diffuse, although specific areas of infection may be seen. Nodules, cavitary lesions, and pleural effusion may occur but, if found, should prompt definitive diagnosis to prevent a misdiagnosis.

Gallium scans may show increased uptake in areas of infection, especially in patients suspected to be infected but present with normal chest x-rays. However, scans are not specific for PCP and the rate of false positives is high. Computed tomography will also reveal diffuse alveolar infiltrates and bronchial wall thickening.

DIAGNOSIS

Identification of the organism is necessary for definitive diagnosis. The cyst and precyst forms are easily identified from induced sputum or bronchoalveolar lavage specimens using special stains (Giemsa, cresyl echt violet, methenamine silver). Diff-Quik and Papanicolaou stains help to identify trophozoites. Immunofluorescence and polymerase chain reactions are also helpful for identifying both the cyst form and trophozoite. Induced sputum specimens that are negative do not rule out the diagnosis in patients suspected to have PCP.

Repeat sputum or bronchoscopy is recommended. There is presently no useful technique to culture the organism.

TREATMENT

Pharmacologic Management

PCP is treated with trimethoprim/sulfamethoxazole (TMP/SMX; Bactrim, Septra). Mild to moderate disease is commonly treated with 15 mg/kg per day TMP and 75 mg/kg per day SMX in 3 or 4 divided doses orally for 21 days. If the patient is unable to tolerate oral drugs, the same dose is given IV, or IV pentamidine and can be given as a single dose of 4 mg/kg per day for 21 days.

Clinical improvement of PCP in HIV-positive patients is usually slow and radiographic evidence of improvement is delayed. Often, patients show a worsening of clinical status in the early part of treatment due to the increasing inflammatory reaction in the lungs. If no improvement is seen at the end of one week of treatment, alternative therapies should be considered. CDC recommended alternatives include dapsone, trimethoprim plus dapsone, or dapsone plus pyrimethamine plus leucovorin. Atovaquone is better tolerated but less effective. Aerosolized pentamidine was used commonly as an alternative to TMP/SMX but is not often recommended due to its propensity to cause refractory apical illness.

The most frequent side effect of TMP/SMX is a delayed rash that is usually mild and can be treated with antihistamine. The most serious side effect of TMP/SMX is neutropenia. Development of neutropenia is dose dependent; therefore it is recommended that the lowest dose possible be given. Other side effects include fever, abnormal liver enzymes, and GI symptoms. Desensitization therapy for individuals sensitive to TMP/SMX is highly successful. Pentamidine can cause rales, neutropenia, renal toxicity (especially if given with aminoglycosides or amphotericin B), hypotension, hypoglycemia, nausea/vomiting, arrhythmias, and pancreatitis. Dapsone may cause nausea/vomiting, rash, fever, hemolysis, and methemoglobinemia.

Adjunctive corticosteroid (prednisone 40 mg PO bid followed by systemic weaning) is recommended for moderate to severe disease. Mortality is significantly reduced if steroid therapy is instituted with 72 hours of initiating the anti-PCP regimen. Studies have shown that steroid therapy results in improved survival, a reduction in respiratory failure (ARDS), and less pulmonary damage due to the anti-inflammatory action of steroids. If steroid therapy is administered to a patient who has been misdiagnosed with PCP and in fact has a fungal infection, the patient may initially show improvement, but the condition will ultimately worsen. Steroids have the potential to exacerbate tuberculosis, Kaposi's sarcoma, and other bacterial pneumonias, but if used for the recommended short term this has not been a problem clinically.

Supportive Measures

Adequate oxygenation and hydration are very important to ensure a good response to treatment, especially in patients with severe PCP or evidence of chronic obstructive pulmonary disease. Hydration is especially important if the patient is treated with pentamidine. Many patients will benefit from continuous positive airway pressure in an ICU setting. Maintenance of electrolyte balance and good nutritional intake is also beneficial.

PATIENT EDUCATION AND DISPOSITION

Patients should be instructed to seek medical care and treatment for any change in respiratory status. Prophylaxis is recommended for any HIV-positive patient with a history of prior PCP, unexplained fever, esophageal thrush, or a CD_4+ T-cell count below $200/mm^3$. Prophylaxis is most commonly with TMP/SMX in a single dose (160 mg TMP/800 mg SMX). Recent studies have shown a dose given 3 times per week may be equally effective. The alternative prophylactic regimen is dapsone 100 mg PO qid. Dapsone 50 mg PO qid with pyrimethamine 50 mg PO once weekly may be more effective than dapsone alone. Further alternatives include aerosolized pentamidine 300 mg/month via nebulizer or atovaquone 1500 mg/day PO.

Several studies have shown success with stopping PCP prophylaxis if the CD4+ count rises above $200/mm^3$ while the patient is maintained on highly aggressive antiretroviral therapy (HAART). The study period has been relatively short term but results are promising. Presently, USPHS experts are considering a recommendation to discontinue primary PCP prophylaxis in patients whose CD4+ count remains above $200/mm^3$ for 3 to 6 months while being maintained on HAART. Any patient with a history of PCP would not discontinue secondary prophylaxis.

COMPLICATIONS

Pneumothorax and cavitation were commonly encountered in patients treated with aerosolized pentamidine but also may be seen in HIV-positive patients with their first bout of PCP. Extrapulmonary *Pneumocystis* may be seen in up to 3 percent of patients. Frequent sites of infection include the external ear, mastoid, choroid, skin, small bowel, peritoneum, liver, spleen, thyroid, lymph nodes, and the blood. Disseminated infection has been documented with organisms also found in the pancreas, stomach, adrenal glands, heart, kidneys, and central nervous system. Lesions outside of the lung are frequently calcified, symptoms are nonspecific, diagnosis is difficult, and prognosis is poor. Death is a result of multiple organ failure.

BIBLIOGRAPHY

Chaisson R, Bishai W. The management of *Pneumocystis carinii,* toxoplasmosis, and HSV infections in patients with HIV disease. *Medscape, HIV Clinical Management Series,* vol.7, 1999.

Dobkin JF. Opportunistic infections and AIDS. *Infect Med* 12:58–70;1995.

Goldman L, Bennett JC, eds. *Cecil Textbook of Medicine,* 21st ed. Philadelphia, Saunders, 2000.

Muma R. *HIV Manual for Health Care Professionals.* Norwalk, CT, Appleton & Lange, 1994.

Powderly WG. Opportunistic infections. Medscape, *HIV/AIDS,* 1999, p. 5.

Ungvarski PJ, Flaskerud JH. *HIV/AIDS: A Guide to Primary Care Management.* Philadelphia, Saunders, 1999.

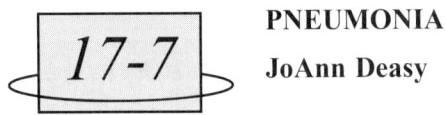

PNEUMONIA

JoAnn Deasy

DISCUSSION

Pneumonia is an infection of the lower respiratory tract characterized by inflammation and consolidation of lung tissue. The alveoli fill up with exudate, resulting in the exclusion of air and solidification of part of the lung. Pneumonia may be caused by a wide spectrum of infectious disease agents. Those agents gain entry to the lower respiratory tract most often through the inhalation of aerosolized material or the aspiration of upper airway normal flow. Less frequently, infectious disease agents may be seeded in the lungs through the blood (hematogenous spread). Only a hundred-thousandth of an inch separates the air environment in the lungs from the bloodstream.

PATHOPHYSIOLOGY

The surface area of the lungs is approximately 150 m², almost the size of a tennis court. Each day over 10,000 L of air passes in and out of the respiratory tract. This air contains particles from the environment. Normally, the lungs are quite resistant to infection. Pneumonia occurs when the offending microbe overwhelms the host's defenses. When a person is challenged with an infectious disease agent, the outcome depends on microbial virulence, the quantity of infectious inoculum, and host susceptibility.

The alterations in host defense that may predispose a person to pneumonia occur at different levels. Protective defense mechanisms include nasal clearance, which removes organisms through sneezing and blowing anteriorly and posteriorly; also, the nasopharynx traps particles, which are then swallowed. The larynx expels many particles via the cough reflex. The beating mucociliary action of the tracheo-bronchial tree moves particles toward the oropharynx, where they are then swallowed or expectorated. Bacteria or other particles making their way to the alveoli are phagocytized by alveolar macrophages. Respiratory secretions contain antimicrobial substances. General immune defenses such as antibodies, leukocytes, and the local blood supply are also protective against pneumonia.

If the protective barriers are passed and microbes make their way to the lungs, some organisms produce a typical inflammatory response to the alveoli while others may produce tissue destruction and cavitation. Viruses generally produce inflammation between the alveoli as opposed to directly in the air spaces. Influenza viruses and viruses that cause the "common cold" impair host defenses by damaging respiratory epithelium and cilia, resulting in an increased frequency of pneumonia after these viral infections. Acute pneumonia that develops in nonhospitalized patients is referred to as community-acquired pneumonia (CAP). Pneumonia acquired in the hospital (nosocomial pneumonia), may be caused by more virulent bacterial strains, and the patient may have coexisting illnesses and impaired immune defenses.

COMMUNITY-ACQUIRED PNEUMONIA

Lower respiratory tract infection is the number one cause of death from infectious diseases in the United States. The clinical picture of community-acquired pneumonia (CAP) varies from mild disease to severe involvement requiring hospitalization. In 1993 the American Thoracic Society (ATS) published CAP guidelines that categorized patients with CAP by age, presence of coexisting medical illnesses, and severity of the pneumonia. This approach stratifies patients in terms of mortality risk and is used to determine whether the patient should be treated on an outpatient basis, as an inpatient, or in the intensive care unit. In 1997 the Infectious Diseases Society of America (IDSA) published guidelines for management of CAP. The IDSA guidelines put greater emphasis on diagnostic studies as compared to the ATS guidelines and address the role of new quinolones in the treatment of CAP.

Symptoms

The symptoms that are suggestive of pneumonia are fever, chills, pleuritic chest pain, dyspnea, cough, and sputum production. Ten to thirty percent of patients with pneumonia complain of headache, nausea, vomiting, abdominal pain, diarrhea, myalgia, and arthralgia.[1] In the elderly (over 65 years of age), the classic symptoms of pneumonia are less commonly noted; instead, nonrespiratory symptoms such as confusion and other mental status changes may predominate. If a fever is present in the elderly, it is usually a low-grade fever. In children, upper respiratory symptoms usually precede fever and cough.

Objective Findings

Vital signs that are predictive of pneumonia include fever higher than 37.8°C (100°F), pulse rate over 100 beats per minute, and respirations more than 25 per minute. The presence of crackles on auscultation of the chest and locally decreased breath sounds are strongly associated with pneumonia. In the elderly, an increased respiratory rate may be the only objective finding.

Hospitalization

The majority of patients with CAP are treated as outpatients (about 75 percent). The decision to hospitalize is based on clinical judgment. Certain risk factors, physical findings, and laboratory findings are associated with a complicated course and may be indications for hospitalization. These factors include age over 65; coexisting illnesses such as chronic obstructive pulmonary disease (COPD), diabetes mellitus, congestive heart failure (CHF), or alcoholism; respiration rate greater than 30/min; diastolic BP below 60 mm Hg; altered mental status; evidence of respiratory distress ($P_{O_2} < 60$ mmHg); and lack of a support system.

Laboratory and Radiologic Studies

The chest x-ray is considered the gold standard for the diagnosis of pneumonia. The presence of a new or progressive infiltrate supports the diagnosis. Because opacity on chest radiography may represent infection, blood, edema fluid, malignancy, or inflammation caused by noninfectious processes, the radiograph must be interpreted in conjunction with the medical history and the physical examination findings.

In addition to the chest x-ray, diagnostic tests that may be performed in the outpatient setting include a complete blood count (CBC), looking for leukocytosis and a shift to the left, and a sputum Gram stain. The Gram stain should be examined for the presence of neutrophils and the identification of the predominant bacteria. The presence of large numbers of squamous epithelial cells suggests that the specimen represents saliva rather than sputum. Pulse oximetry can be done as a measure of oxygenation. Oximetric Sa_{O_2} levels below 91 percent indicate poor oxygen delivery in patients without long-standing pulmonary disease. In a patient who is hospitalized with pneumonia, two sets of blood cultures should be done. Although the yield is low, a positive culture usually indicates the etiology of the pneumonia and is a marker of more serious disease. In addition to the studies already mentioned, a sputum culture, blood chemistries (BUN, glucose, and sodium), and arterial blood gas determinants should be obtained in the hospitalized patient. HIV serology and a test for legionnaire's disease are suggested in at risk populations. If a specific etiology of the pneumonia is suspected, other organism-directed tests can be done.

Microbiology

Streptococcus pneumoniae is the most common cause of CAP in all age groups. From a historical perspective, *S. pneumoniae* was the first recognized pathogen for CAP and the associated symptoms of high fever, chills, chest pain, and purulent sputum were termed "typical pneumonia." This term was subsequently extended to other bacterial pneumonias. Individuals presenting with subacute illness, nonproductive cough, diarrhea, or other symptoms were said to have "atypical pneumonia," which implies infection with *Mycoplasma pneumoniae*, *Chlamydia pneumoniae*, *Legionella* species, or viruses. Recent analysis of published data shows that there is considerable overlap of clinical symptoms and radiographic findings among etiologic pathogens. A classification of typical versus atypical may be overly simplistic. This does not diminish the importance of a thorough history and physical examination in an attempt to ascertain the most likely etiology, because in some cases the clinical features may strongly suggest a specific etiology. Table 17-7-1 presents what have been described as the characteristic clinical findings associated with various etiologic agents of CAP.

A study looking at 316 consecutive patients hospitalized with suspected CAP was able to make a microbiologic diagnosis in

TABLE 17-7-1.   Selected Etiologic Agents of Pneumonia

Streptococcus pneumoniae (Pneumococcus)

Onset of pneumonia often abrupt with sudden chill, fever, cough, and pleuritic chest pain. Rust-colored or yellow sputum. May follow upper respiratory infection.
Gram stain: Gram-positive diplococci.
CXR: Lobar consolidation.
Treatment: Penicillin, macrolide or doxycycline. *Other:* Quinolone.[a]

Mycoplasma pneumoniae

Characteristics: Onset gradual with nonproductive cough. May be associated with sore throat and earache. More prevalent in younger age groups.
Gram stain: Polymorphonuclear neutrophils (PMNs), no predominant bacteria.
Lab: Complement fixation test: rise in specific antibody.
CXR: Patchy infiltrates.
Treatment: Macrolide or doxycycline. *Other:* Quinolone.[a]

Haemophilus influenzae

Characteristics: May follow URI. More common in older age group (less than 60 years) and those with chronic cardiopulmonary disease.
Gram stain: Gram-negative coccobacilli.
CXR: Lobar consolidation.
Treatment: Second-generation (or third) cephalosporin or amoxicillin–clavulanic acid. *Other:* Quinolone[a] or azithromycin.

Moraxella catarrhalis

Characteristics: More common in elderly with preexisting lung disease and immunocompromised persons. Presents with cough, weakness, and dyspnea.
Gram stain: Gram-negative diplococci or coccobacilli. Most strains produce beta-lactamase.
CXR: Patchy infiltrate or lobar consolidation.
Treatment: Second-generation cephalosporin or amoxicillin–clavulanic acid. *Other:* Quinolone.[a]

Klebsiella pneumoniae

Characteristics: More common in the elderly, alcoholics, diabetics, and nosocomial setting. Presents with fever, chills, purulent sputum, and pleuritic chest pain.
Gram stain: Plump gram-negative rods.
CXR: Lobar consolidation.
Treatment: Cephalosporin plus aminoglycoside.

Staphylococcus aureus

Characteristics: Uncommon. Occurs in debilitated persons, nosocomial setting, and after influenza infection. High fever, chills, cough, pleuritic chest pain. High mortality rate.
Gram stain: Gram-positive cocci in clumps.
CXR: Patchy infiltrates.
Treatment: Vancomycin or cephalosporin.

Chlamydia pneumoniae (TWAR Agent)

Characteristics: Affects young adults. Clinical presentation similar to *Mycoplasma* spp.
Gram stain: Not helpful.
Lab: Serologic studies available.
CXR: Patchy or interstitial infiltrate.
Treatment: Tetracycline.

Legionella pneumophila

Characteristics: Associated with environmental water sources. No person-to-person transmission. More common in elderly, smokers, and alcoholics. Dry cough; gastrointestinal and CNS symptoms may be present. Progresses to respiratory failure in 30 percent of patients.
Gram stain: Few polymorphonuclear neutrophils, no predominant bacteria.
Lab: Various studies available, including direct immunofluorescent stain of sputum, rise in antibody titer, urine antigen test.
CXR: Patchy or lobar consolidation.
Treatment: Macrolide or quinolone.[a]

Pneumocystis carinii

Characteristics: Found in persons with AIDS and other immunosuppressive states. Sudden onset of fever, cough, dyspnea, and tachypnea is typical (see Chap. 17–6).
Gram stain: Not helpful. Special stains of sputum or bronchoalveolar lavage fluid may identify cysts.
CXR: Diffuse interstitial and alveolar infiltrates.
Treatment: Trimethoprim–sulfamethoxazole or pentamidine.

Aspiration Pneumonia

Characteristics: Predisposing factors include neurologic damage, esophageal diseases, alcohol or drug abuse. Etiology includes anaerobes and aerobes. Slow onset, less fever. Weight loss, malaise, and fatigue common.
Gram stain: Mixed flora.
CXR: Dependent segments of lung most often involved. Lung abscess may form.
Treatment: Must include anaerobic coverage.

NOTE: CXR = chest x-ray.
[a]Quinolone: Levofloxacin (Levaquin), sparfloxin (Zagam), grepafloxacin (Raxar), trovafloxacin (Trovan).

71 percent of included cases. In approximately 25 percent of cases, more than one organism was identified. *S. pneumoniae* was the most common diagnosis (39 percent), followed by *Mycoplasma pneumoniae* (16 percent), *Haemophilus influenzae* (11 percent), *Legionella* sp. (11 percent), influenza A virus (5 percent), *Chlamydia pneumoniae* (3 percent), *Moraxella catarrhalis* (3 percent), *Staphylococcus aureus* (3 percent), *Enterobacteriaceae* (2 percent), *Pseudomonas* sp. (1 percent), and other organisms (5 percent).[2] The epidemiology of *Legionella* seems to vary with the geographic location.

Treatment

Antibiotics are the mainstay of treatment for CAP. The ideal way to treat pneumonia would be to know the causative infectious disease agent and direct treatment against that agent. However, even among hospitalized patients in whom extensive studies are done, in as many as 50 percent of pneumonia patients, no etiologic agent is identified. Therefore, treatment is usually empirical. Empirical treatment should be based on (1) the severity of illness, (2) the most common pathogens in published studies, and (3) the age of the patient and coexisting morbidities. For outpatient management, a macrolide, fluoroquinolone, or doxycycline is recommended. Alternative options include a second-generation cephalosporin or amoxicillin/clavulanate; however, these will not be active against atypical agents. When prescribing a macrolide, clarithromycin or azithromycin are preferred if *H. influenzae* is suspected. Erythromycin has a limited spectrum of activity and significant gastrointestinal side effects. The newer macrolides, clarithromycin and azithromycin, are better tolerated but more expensive. In addition to antibiotics, outpatients should be encouraged to maintain a good fluid intake, monitor their temperature, and rest. The overuse of cough suppressants should be avoided.

For hospitalized patients not requiring intensive care, a beta-lactam with or without a macrolide is recommended or a fluoroquinolone alone. Severe pneumonia requiring hospitalization in an intensive care unit is usually treated with a macrolide or a fluoroquinolone plus ceftriaxone or cefotaxime. In patients with structural lung disease, antipseudomonal coverage must be considered; and in aspiration pneumonia, anaerobic coverage is necessary. If diagnostic testing reveals the etiology of the pneumonia, a change can be made to a narrower-spectrum antibiotic. The presence of bacterial resistance to commonly used antibiotics can complicate treatment. The problem of increasing drug resistance of *S. pneumoniae* is of particular importance and must be followed carefully by clinicians. If *S. pneumoniae* is resistant to both penicillin and cephalosporins, then vancomycin, imipenem, or one of the new quinolones is an appropriate antibiotic choice.

The new quinolones—grepafloxacin, sparfloxacin, levofloxacin, and trovafloxacin—were introduced in 1997. The latter two are available both orally and intravenously. These agents show enhanced in vitro activity against *S. pneumoniae* (including penicillin-resistant strains), and are effective against *H. influenzae, M. catarrhalis,* and atypical bacterial pathogens.

Generally, pneumonia is treated for 10 days. Patients with *M. pneumoniae* and *Legionella* spp. may require 14 to 21 days of therapy. Azithromycin can be used for shorter courses because of its long half-life. Most hospitalized patients are started on intravenous therapy. When a patient shows clinical improvement, he or she may be switched from parenteral to oral therapy. In most cases, this occurs on day 3 of hospitalization. The decision is based on patient factors, pathogen characteristics, and antibiotic properties.

Disposition

Patients with pneumonia who receive outpatient treatment should return to the clinic for a recheck or receive a phone call 2 to 3 days after starting antibiotic therapy. Patients who are not improving at 72 h or are actually deteriorating should be reevaluated. The antibiotic regimen may need to be changed, or the patient may be a candidate for hospitalization. In previously healthy persons, fever is generally gone in 2 to 4 days and leukocytosis resolves by day 4 or 5 of therapy. It is not unusual for abnormal physical findings to persist for 7 days. Cough and fatigue may persist for several weeks. Radiographic resolution of pneumonia lags behind clinical resolution. In younger (less than 50 years of age) and previously healthy patients, x-ray resolution of pneumonia occurs within 4 weeks.

Patients should be seen at the end of treatment to confirm the clinical cure. This is an appropriate time to administer pneumococcal vaccine. The chest x-ray should be repeated 4 weeks after the initiation of therapy to confirm resolution.

Diagnostic Considerations

Bronchitis, especially in persons with chronic lung disease, may present similarly to pneumonia. Other infectious processes, such as *Mycobacterium tuberculosis* and fungal infections, may mimic CAP. A number of noninfectious processes may present a picture that is clinically similar to pneumonia, including congestive heart failure, pulmonary fibrosis, pulmonary emboli, pulmonary edema, and myocardial infarction.

Complications and Red Flags

Infectious complications include meningitis, arthritis, endocarditis, pericarditis, peritonitis, and empyema. Noninfectious complications include renal failure, heart failure, multisystem organ failure, and adult respiratory distress syndrome (ARDS; see Chap. 17-13).

Prevention

Streptococcus pneumoniae vaccine is a capsular polysaccharide vaccine that contains the 23 most prevalent types. It is recommended for all persons over 65 years of age and all patients over 2 years of age who have chronic disorders of the pulmonary or cardiovascular system as well as some other chronic diseases, such as diabetes. Persons with compromised splenic function or splenectomy and those who are HIV-positive also should be vaccinated. Yearly influenza vaccine should also be administered to those at risk for pneumonia. Attention to smoking cessation, avoidance of alcohol abuse, and promotion of good nutrition addresses host defense impairment.

HOSPITAL-ACQUIRED (NOSOCOMIAL) PNEUMONIA

Discussion

Hospital-acquired (nosocomial) pneumonia is defined as a pneumonia occurring more than 48 hours after admission to the hospital. Colonization of the pharynx is promoted by instrumentation of the upper airway in a hospitalized patient as well as by the use of broad-spectrum antibiotics that change the flora and promote the emergence of resistant organisms. Inhalation of contaminated aerosols and hematogenous dissemination of microbes also may play a role in the development of nosocomial pneumonia. It is especially common in patients who require intensive care and mechanical ventilation. Host factors such as advanced age, comorbidities, and immunosuppression also promote nosocomial pneumonia.

The bacteria most often responsible for hospital-acquired pneumonia include gram-negative rods, *Streptococcus* spp. and *Staphylococcus* spp. *Pseudomonas aeruginosa* and *Acinetobacter* sp. are responsible for nosocomial pneumonia in the most debilitated patients. Nosocomial pneumonia may represent a polymicrobial infection.

Signs and Symptoms

Fever and purulent sputum are the clinical findings most often associated with nosocomial pneumonia.

Laboratory and Radiologic Studies

The minimum workup usually includes a complete blood count for leukocytosis, a chest radiograph for a new pulmonary infiltrate, two blood cultures for bacteremia, and a sputum Gram stain and culture. Thoracentesis for pleural fluid examination should be performed in patients with pleural effusion when nosocomial pneumonia is suspected.

Treatment

Treatment is empiric and should be started as soon as nosocomial pneumonia is suspected (after blood cultures) because of the high mortality rate associated with hospital-acquired pneumonia. There is no consensus about the best antibiotic regimen. A third-generation cephalosporin with antipseudomonal coverage combined with an aminoglycoside is often used.

REFERENCES

1. Marrie TJ. State of the art clinical article: Community-acquired pneumonia. *Clin Infect Dis* 18:501–515;1994.
2. Neill AM, Martin IR, Weir R, et al. Community acquired pneumonia—aetiology and usefulness of severity criteria on admission. *Thorax* 51:1010–1016;1996.

BIBLIOGRAPHY

Bartlett JG, Breiman RF, Mandell LA, File TM. Guidelines from the Infectious Diseases Society of America. Community acquired pneumonia in adults: Guidelines for management. *Clin Infect Dis* 26:811–838;1998.

Niederman MS, Bass JB Jr, Campbell GD, et al. Guidelines for the initial management of adults with community acquired pneumonia: Diagnosis, assessment of severity, and initial antimicrobial therapy. American Thoracic Society, Medical Section of the American Lung Association. *Am Rev Respir Dis* 148:1418–1426;1993.

Rakel RE. *Conn's Current Therapy 2000.* Philadelphia, Saunders, 2000.

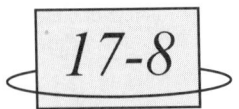

PULMONARY EMBOLUS

Barry A. Cassidy

DISCUSSION

In 1969 at the old Duke University Hospital, one could find pasted to the ceiling of an internal medicine ward a simple note that stated, "Think PE." The note was a tribute to the evasive quality of the often deadly disorder known as pulmonary embolism (PE). Almost 30 years later, the diagnosis of PE remains a practitioner's nightmare. By definition, an embolus constitutes a moving thrombus, and in the case of PE, the embolus occurs on the right side of the closed cardiovascular circulation circuit.

The circuit can be viewed as having two sides: the low-pressure right side and the high-pressure left side. Anatomically, the low-pressure right-sided venous system begins at the level of the postcapillary venule and terminates at the distal branches of the pulmonary arterial system. The left-sided system (in this description, it actually starts at the postalveolar pulmonary venous system) can be conceptualized as starting in the high-pressure left ventricle and terminating at the precapillary arterioles.

Conceptualizing a closed right-sided and left-sided vascular system helps one view embolic events on the basis of their expected anatomic end-point symptomatology (right-sided events terminate in the central venous circulation, the right side of the heart, or the lung parenchyma, whereas left-sided events manifest in any organ system, including the heart, brain, abdominal viscera, mesentery, and extremities).

ETIOLOGY AND RISK FACTORS

Both sides of the closed cardiovascular system can develop thrombi that are susceptible to embolism. Many factors increase the risk of thrombus formation in the right-sided circulation:

- Hypercoagulable states, particularly carcinogenic states[1]
- Pregnancy and oral contraceptives[2,3]
- Recent surgical procedures with general anesthesia, particularly orthopedic, neurosurgical, and gynecologic surgery[2]
- Recent major trauma (head injuries, spinal cord injuries, complex pelvic fractures, and hip fractures; long bone fractures are also a common source of fat emboli)[4]
- Atrial fibrillation causing the formation of a clot in the right atrium[5]
- Right ventricular myocardial infarction[5]
- Immobilization, particularly casting of the lower extremities and also including long airplane flights[6]
- Nonthrombotic embolization occurring in the right-sided circulation from amniotic fluid emboli–posttherapeutic abortion, fat emboli, after a long bone fracture, and iatrogenic air emboli secondary to invasive venous procedures[7]

Thrombosis formation is inversely proportional to flow; thus, the slower the flow state (pressure of flow), the higher the risk of thrombosis. Consequently, the low-pressure right-sided circulation is more susceptible to thrombosis formation than is the high-pressure left side. Any condition that causes venous stasis increases the likelihood of thrombus formation. Clinicians can heighten their awareness of the possibility of PE by thinking physiologically. For instance, inflammatory processes in the venous system that result from trauma or infection affect flow through the veins and set the stage for thrombus development.

The most likely origin of PE is the deep venous system of the extremities and the veins in the pelvic area. One can be misled and feel secure that deep venous thrombosis is not present in the setting of a superficial phlebothrombosis or thrombophlebitis. However, it has been pointed out that the presence of superficial venous disease must be considered a risk factor for deep venous thrombosis and should be treated as such.[8] Although emboli arising from the superficial venous system are filtered out before they get into the deep system, one is obligated to make sure that the underlying process causing the superficial venous abnormality is not present in the deep venous system. The risk of developing PE from lower-leg deep venous thrombosis is less than it is from thrombosis above the knee, but there is a significant relationship between the two entities. If left untreated, 20 percent of lower leg thromboses eventually will extend into the proximal system.[9]

PREVALENCE

Galvin and Choi[10] estimated that 500,000 patients suffer annually from PE and that 10 percent (50,000) of those patients die. A multicenter study done at the Henry Ford Heart and Vascular Institute looked at the prevalence of acute PE among 51,645 patients hospitalized over a 21-month period. Four hundred four autopsies were performed in this group of patients, and PE was observed in 14.6 percent (59) of the autopsies. Among patients at autopsy who died from PE, the diagnosis was unsuspected in 70 percent.[11] Morpurgo and Schmid[12] similarly found in 92 postmortem examinations revealing PE that 72 percent of the cases were not diagnosed before death.

Morgenthaler and Ryu[13] from the Mayo Clinic did a retrospective study of 2427 autopsies performed over a 5-year period in an attempt to determine the clinical characteristics of hospitalized patients who died of confirmed PE at autopsy. Ninety-two patients (3.8 percent) were judged to have died of PE, among whom 11 patients (12 percent) had no risk factors for PE. Prophylaxis against thromboembolism was instituted in slightly less than half the 92 patients (46 percent); presumably, the others were undiagnosed or were not suspected of having PE before death. Classic symptoms were often absent: Dyspnea was reported in 59 percent, chest pain in 17 percent, and hemoptysis in 3 percent. PE was entertained as a diagnosis in 49 percent.[13] Giuntini and associates[1] suggested that venous thromboembolism is the third most common acute cardiovascular disease after cardiac ischemic syndromes and stroke.

SIGNS AND SYMPTOMS

The classic triad of hemoptysis, pleuritic chest pain, and dyspnea occurs in less than 20 percent of patients with PE.[10] One might incorrectly assume that those who develop hemoptysis, pleuritic chest pain, and dyspnea are more likely to die. In fact, the classic symptoms occur when the PE is located in the very periphery of the pulmonary arteries, where the mortality rate is the lowest. However, the classic symptoms should be considered a "heralding sign" for the major embolus that frequently follows.

The diagnosis of PE is based more on suspicion than on purely quantitative facts.[14] Swan and associates at the University of Arizona Health Sciences Center did an interesting study that supports the infrequency of symptoms in PE. They studied the use of thrombectomy with deliberate pulmonary embolization of thrombus after initial thrombolysis for occluded hemodialysis catheters. Thirty-one patients with 43 acutely thrombosed prosthetic hemodialysis fistulas were treated with thrombolysis and/or thrombectomy. Perfusion lung scans were obtained in 22 patients. Forty-one of the 43 patients (95 percent) had no clinical signs or symptoms, yet 59 percent of the lung scans were consistent with PE.

Over the years, authorities have speculated reasonably that symptoms with PE are more likely if the embolus is more peripherally located. One confusing factor in PE is that it occurs as a comorbid partner of many serious illnesses. The diagnosis of PE does not lend itself to a laundry list of signs and symptoms. When a patient experiences hemodynamic difficulties, begins acting strangely, becomes dyspneic with or without chest pain, or in general experiences a major change in clinical status, one should think of PE. Once the question has been raised, one should establish a strategy for ruling out the possibility that PE exists.

DIAGNOSTIC CONSIDERATIONS

The best way to diagnose PE is to be able to see its presence. Consequently, the best test is autopsy or surgery, followed by pulmonary angiography. Since deep venous thrombosis (DVT) is the most common source of PE, venography is an invasive yet helpful diagnostic test. The risk of invasive procedures is real, but those procedures are warranted when the suspicion of PE is high; they become less attractive when the suspicion is moderate to low. The goal has been to find a noninvasive or minimally invasive test to stratify the likelihood of PE as a diagnosis.

Holbert and coworkers[15] proposed that spiral computed tomography, particularly for patients with cardiopulmonary disease, helps confirm the diagnosis of PE in the emergency setting. Looking at risk factors, diffusion of gases, and functional abnormalities is helpful when PE becomes a diagnostic consideration.

Risk Factors

Listing risk factors helps an examiner quantitate the suspicion of possible PE. For instance, a previous history of PE, recent trauma to an extremity, birth control pills, smoking history, a history of cancer, a recent operation, superficial thrombophlebitis, and invasive central venous lines in place, separately or combined, allow a graphic representation of one's suspicions.

Diffusion of Gases

Blood gas diffusion as measured by arterial blood gases (ABGs) provides helpful but not absolute data. Large (or multiple) PEs block O_2 diffusion, and one would expect a lowering of the Pa_{O_2}. Calculation of the expected Pa_{O_2} requires knowing the concentration of oxygen and the barometric pressure in the site where the test is being performed. Once the expected Pa_{O_2} is calculated, it can be compared to the measured Pa_{O_2} of the patient. (The patient's normal baseline ABG must be known to determine whether any change has occurred.) This yields the A–a (alveolar-arteriolar) gradient that is reported on most ABG reports.* An A–a gradient below 15 to 20 suggests that gas diffusion is impaired. The ABG findings commonly found in PE patients are a low measured $Pa_{O_2} < 60$ mmHg and a low $P_{CO_2} < 40$ mmHg with resultant respiratory alkalosis. The lowering of the P_{CO_2} probably is related in part to the tachypnea that results from dyspnea or pain.

ABGs unfortunately are of indiscriminate predictive value in permitting the exclusion of PE. Stein and associates[16] used data from the National Heart, Lung and Blood Institute's Prospective Investigation of Pulmonary Embolism Diagnosis (PIOPED) to study 768 patients (438 with and 330 without prior cardiopulmonary disease) and looked at the predictive value of diagnosing PE on the basis of the results of those patients' ABGs. Their conclusions showed that PE could not be excluded in more than 30 percent of patients with no prior cardiopulmonary disease and in no more than 14 percent of patients with prior cardiopulmonary disease.[16] There is a place, however, for the measurement of blood gases to determine the possibility of PE. Abnormal ABGs in concert with other tests can increase suspicion, leading to more definitive invasive tests.

The chest x-ray affords an indirect anatomic view of the status of the lung parenchyma. Once thought to be of little value in the diagnosis of PE except to exclude other cardiopulmonary disorders, the chest x-ray gives a great deal of information to a skilled radiographer. Chest x-ray findings (present in more than 80 percent of patients with known PE[7]) generally are not specific to PE but are found in other disorders as well. Chest x-ray findings that are fairly specific to PE (Westermark's sign, dilation of the pulmonary artery, and Hampton's hump, a triangular or rounded pleural-based infiltrate with its apex toward the hilum) are not likely to be appreciated by a nonradiologist. This points out the idea that the evaluation of suspected PE should be multidisciplinary in nature. One pitfall that is germane to primary practitioners is that radiographic changes may take 12 to 24 h to manifest and therefore may not show on the initial chest x-ray.

The lung scan and ventilation-perfusion ($\dot{V}/\dot{Q}$) scan probably offer the most suggestive information among all noninvasive studies. Worsley and Alavi[17] reviewed data from the PIOPED study regarding $\dot{V}/\dot{Q}$ scan interpretation. A helpful fact concluded from this study was that a normal $\dot{V}/\dot{Q}$ scan excludes the diagnosis of PE. Second, scans that are highly suggestive have definite clinical value and should be responded to accordingly. However, the intermediate group of $\dot{V}/\dot{Q}$ scans requires additional supporting data to warrant more invasive diagnostic procedures.[17]

Functional Abnormalities

Large proportions of patients who develop PE do so from DVT of the lower extremities. The relationship of DVT to PE is so significant that several authorities believe that although separate, both entities should be treated as if PE were an extension of DVT.[9,18–21] Patients at high risk for PE and those with complaints of DVT should have noninvasive ultrasound evaluation of the lower extremities. Positive ultrasonography results in the lower extremities indicate immediate treatment to prevent or limit PE. When clinical suspicion for PE is high, pulmonary angiography should be considered.

The D-dimer test has received interest as a possible predictor of PE. When fibrin monomers bond to form a thrombus, factor XIII acts to bond their D domains. This bond is resistant to plasmin, and thus this degradation fragment is the D-dimer. Elevated levels of D-dimer indicate that fibrinogen has been acted on to form a fibrin monomer and that this monomer was lysed by plasmin. D-dimer fragments can be measured easily in plasma. Unfortunately, there is not universal acceptance of the reliability of D-dimer as a prognostic test for PE.[22,23]

*The formula for calculating the A–a gradient is $(F_{I_{O_2}})$ (barometric pressure -47) $-$ [(1.2) measured Pa_{CO_2})].

Venography is the gold standard for diagnosing DVT. Unfortunately, it is a very uncomfortable procedure and is reserved as a last option. Similarly, the true gold standard for diagnosing PE is pulmonary arteriography. The pulmonary angiogram is invasive, although it is not as painful to the patient as a venogram, and carries a number of risks: Anaphylaxes may delay the onset of treatment and increase pulmonary pressures, and the manipulation of the heart may cause ventricular fibrillation. The angiogram helps determine whether an operation is an option (particularly in large "saddle emboli") and answer the question of whether the PE is significant. The angiogram is particularly helpful in the setting of moderate- to high-probability $\dot{V}/\dot{Q}$ scans when comorbid conditions can account for filling defects on the scan.

Other Diagnostic Considerations

The electrocardiogram (ECG) has been reported to have a number of findings attributable to PE. The usefulness of the ECG as a predictor of PE is dubious, since PE is so often associated with other cardiopulmonary disorders. The classic ECG findings in PE are S_1-Q_3-T_3 (an S wave in lead 1, a Q wave in lead 3, and a T-wave abnormality in lead 3), sinus tachycardia, nonspecific ST-T wave changes, right or left bundle branch block, atrial fibrillation, and premature atrial contractions or premature ventricular contractions.

TREATMENT

The treatment of PE falls into two categories: (1) attempting to prevent PE and (2) responding to PE. Patients who are at high risk and develop DVT should be treated immediately with anticoagulation, hospitalization, and bed rest. Patients who develop PE also should be anticoagulated but may require much more supportive treatment and are best managed in an intensive care unit.

Types of Anticoagulation

The gold standard for therapy for PE is heparinization. Historically, unfractionated heparin has been used intravenously to achieve immediate anticoagulation. Generally, patients are given a bolus of 5000 to 10,000 units of heparin and are maintained at 800 to 1000 units/h titrated on the basis of activated partial thromboplastin time (aPTT) values obtained every 4 to 6 h (aPTT values are kept to 1.5 to 2.5 times the normal baseline).

The aPTT reagents have been found to have a fair amount of variability. Gibaldi and Wittkowsky[24] suggested that practitioners base their titration of heparin on serum concentrations of heparin of 0.2 to 0.4 U/mL. Heparin's advantage over other anticoagulants lies in its relatively immediate onset of action. However, it has additional advantages in the setting of PE. Heparin has both anti-inflammatory and vasodilatory effects on arteries. The exact nature of these effects is not clearly understood, but some studies suggest that heparin may exert its anti-inflammatory effects by inhibiting the passage of leukocytes through the subendothelial basement membrane.[25] The effectiveness of heparin therapy is well known. Agnelli[26] reported a 60 to 70 percent reduction in the incidence of fatal PE in heparin-treated patients. Generally, heparin is administered for 4 to 7 days, and an oral anticoagulant [warfarin (Coumadin)] is started concurrently once the heparin dose has been stabilized. Warfarin takes 36 h to begin exerting its anticoagulant effects; consequently, it is not an adequate choice for immediate treatment. Once the warfarin is stabilized, the heparin can be discontinued. Anticoagulation should continue for 3 to 6 months, depending on the individual case.

Unfortunately, there are times when heparin is contraindicated or patients prove to be resistant to its effects. Agnelli reviewed a cause of heparin resistance as follows:

Unfractionated heparin presents an aspecific "nonfunctional" binding to plasma proteins such as fibrinogen, factor VIII, vitronectin, and fibronectin. This aspecific binding limits the anticoagulant effect of unfractionated heparin and is responsible for the heparin resistance observed in some patients with pulmonary embolism as well as of the high intersubject variability of the heparin-induced anticoagulant effect.[26]

A problem related to heparin that is particularly germane in today's cost-conscious atmosphere is that patients must be hospitalized to be anticoagulated safely with heparin. Some promising studies indicate that subcutaneous (SQ) heparin may be as effective as intravenous heparin. Berkowitz[27] at Duke University reviewed the surgical literature in 1995 and reported that SQ heparin is as efficacious as intravenous heparin. Hass did a comprehensive review of multiple trials comparing the efficacy of low-molecular-weight heparin (LMWH) versus unfractionated heparin (UH) for the treatment of DVT. She found that LMWH was as efficacious as UH and had a superior benefit-to-risk ratio. LMWH similarly has been shown to be as effective as UF in the treatment of PE in two good-sized randomized studies.[28,29] LMWH can be given in fixed subcutaneous doses without the need for frequent checks of aPTT. Two additional large clinical trials suggest that LMWH in the treatment of DVT in the home is just as efficacious and safe as UH treatment in the hospital.[30,31] Koopman and colleagues[30] cautioned that patients be followed closely when treated at home with 24-h medical consultation available. When a significant embolus has occurred or a significant DVT exists, one should be cautious about deviating from the known and acceptable community standard. Clinicians may be pushed to try alternative treatment plans for patients with suspected PE, but the condition requires constant professional surveillance, and to do otherwise would be unwise.

Other forms of long-term anticoagulation were offered in the past. The combination of warfarin and aspirin has been promoted because of its dual action on the clotting mechanism. This combination is used particularly in neurologic disorders that feature both platelet emboli and thromboemboli. The combination has the advantage of preventing thrombus formation and platelet aggregation but has distinct disadvantages, including potential hemorrhage and compliance difficulties. Lotke and associates[32] at the University of Pennsylvania did a prospective randomized study of 388 patients having total hip or knee replacement surgery. They found no difference between the aspirin and warfarin groups in regard to the incidence of changes in $\dot{V}/\dot{Q}$ scans or bleeding complications.[32]

Postoperative complications of PE have been addressed by preventing the stasis of blood in the lower extremities through the use of elastic support stockings or pneumatic compression stockings (PCS); others have used SQ heparin administration every 12 h as prophylaxis. Data from St. Luke's Hospital in Chesterfield, Maryland, support the concept that SQ heparin and PCS used together are superior to those agents used individually.[33]

Patients at high risk for or with documented large DVT can be treated with the insertion of a filter in the inferior vena cava. Trauma patients at high risk for PE may be considered for the prophylactic insertion of vena caval filters.[34] Patients admitted to the hospital for PE should be administered oxygen even if the Pa_{O_2} is <160 mmHg. Oxygen has a salutary effect on pulmonary hypertension, which is a consequence of PE. This is important to remember, as justification probably will be needed for insurance purposes. It is recommended that one make a statement to that effect in the chart to avoid unnecessary hassles.

Thrombolytic therapies such as urokinase and streptokinase have been utilized for years at major centers for PE documented by angiography.[5] They have caused problems of significant bleeding and have not gained favor as a routine therapy for PE.

Future Therapies

Patients allergic to heparin, those who fail heparin prophylaxis, and those who have contraindications to anticoagulation present serious management problems. New investigations show promise for the drug Ancrod, which is a fibrinogen-depleting agent produced from snake venom.[35] New experimental drugs such as CGP-39393, which is a recombinant hirudin, show great promise as prophylactic agents for the prevention of postoperative thromboembolism.[36] Recent studies suggest that r-hirudin is as effective and safe as UH for treatment of thrombosis.[37] Future studies are anticipated that will compare r-hirudin to LMWH.

Improved protocols for the use of thrombolytics such as tissue plasminogen activator, alteplase, anistreplase, urokinase, and streptokinase may yield improved strategies for the management of PE. The use of these agents in other countries has been encouraging. Simpler forms of administration, control of posttherapeutic bleeding problems, and decreasing costs will make these agents beneficial and practical for use in the United States.[38]

Finally, there probably will be a small place for surgery as an option for treating patients with acute PE, particularly those who are hemodynamically unstable and cannot wait for other therapies and agents to act. Thoracic and cardiovascular surgery consultations[39] should be obtained as quickly as possible in this select group of patients. Finally, Anderson and colleagues[40] noted in a small study of five critically ill patients that the late pulmonary dead space fraction (Fd_{late}), a noninvasive CO_2 expirography bedside calculation, was 89 percent specific for detecting PE. Further research is under way and should lead to a reliable inexpensive noninvasive bedside technique to help diagnose PE in critically ill patients.

REFERENCES

1. Giuntini C, Di Ricco G, Marini C, et al: Pulmonary embolism: Epidemiology. *Chest* 107(Suppl 1):3S–9S, 1995.
2. Rosenow EC: Venous and pulmonary thromboembolism: An algorithmic approach to diagnosis and management. *Mayo Clin Proc* 70(1):45–49, 1995.
3. World Health Organization: Venous thromboembolic disease and combined oral contraceptives: Results of an international multicentre case-control study. *Lancet* 346(8990):1575–1582, 1995.
4. Hofmann S, Huemer G, Kratochwill C, et al: Pathophysiology of fat embolisms in orthopedics and traumatology. *Orthopade* 24(2):84–93, 1995.
5. Spittell JA, Pluth JR: Pulmonary embolism, in Juergens JL, Spittell JA, Fairbairn JF (eds): *Peripheral Vascular Diseases,* 5th ed. Philadelphia, Saunders, 1980, p 757.
6. Levy Y, George J, Shoenfeld Y: The occurrence of thromboembolic events following airplane flights—"the economy class syndrome." *Isr J Med Sci* 31(10):621–623, 1995.
7. Baer GR: The approach to diagnosis of pulmonary embolism. *Physician Assist* 6:21–50, 1996.
8. Guex JJ: Thrombotic complications of varicose veins: A literature review of the role of superficial venous thrombosis. *Dermatol Surg* 22(4):378–382, 1996.
9. Hull RD, Pineo GF: Prophylaxis of deep venous thrombosis and pulmonary embolism, *Med Clin North Am* 82(3):477–493, 1998.
10. Galvin JR, Choi BS: *Electronic Differential Multimedia Laboratory.* Iowa City, University of Iowa College of Medicine, Department of Radiology, 1995.
11. Stein PD, Henry JW: Prevalence of acute pulmonary embolism among patients in a general hospital and at autopsy. *Chest* 108(4):978–981, 1995.
12. Morpurgo M, Schmid C: The spectrum of pulmonary embolism: Clinicopathologic correlations. *Chest* 107(Suppl 1):18S–20S, 1995.
13. Morgenthaler TI, Ryu JH: Clinical characteristics of fatal pulmonary embolism in a referral hospital. *Mayo Clin Proc* 70(5):417–424, 1995.
14. Swan TL, Smyth SH, Ruffenach SJ, et al: Pulmonary embolism following hemodialysis access thrombolysis/thrombectomy. *J Vasc Intervent Radiol* 6(5):683–686, 1995.
15. Holbert JM, Costello P, Federle MP: Role of spiral computed tomography in the diagnosis of pulmonary embolism in the emergency department. *Ann Emerg Med* 33(5):520–528, 1999.
16. Stein PD, Goldhaber SZ, Henry JW, Miller AC: Arterial blood gas analysis in the assessment of suspected acute pulmonary embolism. *Chest* 109(1):78–81, 1996.
17. Worsley DF, Alavi A: Comprehensive analysis of the results of the PIOPED Study: Prospective investigations of pulmonary embolism diagnosis study. *J Nucl Med* 36(12):2380–2387, 1995.
18. Hirsh J, Hoak J: Management of deep vein thrombosis and pulmonary embolism, *Circulation,* 93:2212–2245, 1996.
19. Turkstra F, Koopman MMW, Buller HR: The treatment of deep vein thrombosis and pulmonary embolism. *Thromb Haemost* 78(1):489–496, 1997.
20. Hass SK: Treatment of deep venous thrombosis and pulmonary embolism. *Med Clin North Am* 82(3):495–510, 1998.
21. Egermayer P, Town GI: The clinical significance of pulmonary embolism: Uncertainties and implications for treatment—a debate. *J Intern Med* 241:5–10, 1997.
22. Becker DM, Philbrick JT, Bachhuber TL, Humphries JE: D-dimer testing and acute venous thromboembolism: A shortcut to accurate diagnosis? *Arch Intern Med* 156(9):939–946, 1996.
23. Van Beek EJ, Schenk BE, Michel BC, et al: The role of plasma D-dimers concentration in the exclusion of pulmonary embolism. *Br J Haematol* 92(3):725–732, 1996.
24. Gibaldi M, Wittkowsky AK: Contemporary use of and future roles for heparin in antithrombotic therapy. *J Clin Pharmacol* 35(11):1031–1045, 1995.
25. Bartlett MR, Cowden WB, Paris CR: Differential effects of the anti-inflammatory compounds heparin, mannose-6-phosphate, and catanospermine on degradation of the vascular basement membrane by leukocytes, endothelial cells, and platelets. *J Leukoc Biol* 57(2):207–213, 1995.
26. Agnelli G: Anticoagulation in the prevention and treatment of pulmonary embolism. *Chest* 107(Suppl 1):39S–44S, 1995.
27. Berkowitz SD: Treatment of established deep vein thrombosis: A review of the therapeutic armamentarium. *Orthopedics* 18(Suppl):18–20, 1995.
28. The Columbus Investigators: Low-molecular weight heparin in the treatment of patients with thromboembolism. *N Engl J Med* 337:657, 1997.
29. Simonneau G, Sors H, Charbonnier B, et al: A comparison of low-molecular weight heparin with unfractionated heparin for acute pulmonary embolism. *N Engl J Med* 337:663, 1997.
30. Koopman MMW, Prandoni P, Piovella F, et al: Treatment of venous thrombosis with intravenous unfractionated heparin administered in the hospital as compared with subcutaneous low-molecular-weight heparin administered at home. *N Engl J Med* 334:682, 1996.
31. Levine M, Gent M, Hirsh J, et al: A comparison of low-molecular weight heparin administered primarily at home with unfractionated heparin administered in the hospital for proximal deep-vein thrombosis. *N Engl J Med* 34:677, 1996.
32. Lotke PA, Palevsky H, Kennan AM, et al: Aspirin and warfarin for thromboembolic disease after total joint arthroplasty. *Clin Orthop* (324):251–258, 1996.
33. Ramos R, Salem BI, De Pawlikowski MP, et al: The efficacy of pneumatic compression stockings in the prevention of pulmonary embolism after cardiac surgery. *Chest* 109(1):82–85, 1996.
34. Rogers FB, Shackford SR, Ricci MA, et al: Routine prophylactic vena cava filter insertions in severely injured trauma patients decrease the incidence of pulmonary embolism. *J Am Coll Surg* 180(6):641–647, 1995.
35. Cole CW, Shea B, Bormanis J: Ancrod as prophylaxis or treatment for thromboembolism in patients with multiple trauma. *Can J Surg* 38(3):249–254, 1995.
36. Eriksson BI, Ekman S, Kalego P, et al: Prevention of deep-vein thrombosis after total hip replacement: Direct thrombin inhibition with recombinant hirudin, CGP39393. *Lancet* 347(9002):635–639, 1996.
37. Crowther MA, Ginsberg JS: Direct thrombin inhibitors in venous thromboembolism, in Sasahara A (ed): *New Therapeutic Agents in Thrombosis and Thrombolysis.* New York, Marcel Dekker, 1997, p 159.
38. Goldhaber SZ: Contemporary pulmonary embolism thrombolysis. *Chest* 107(Suppl 1):45S–51S, 1995.
39. Marder VJ: Thrombolytic therapy: Overview of results in major vascular occlusions. *Thromb Haemost* 34(1):101–105, 1995.
40. Anderson JT, Owings JT, Goodnight JE: Bedside noninvasive detection of acute pulmonary embolism in critically ill surgical patients. *Arch Surg* 134:869–875, 1999.

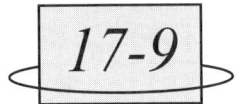

PLEURISY
Randy Trudeau

DISCUSSION

Pleurisy is a term used to describe inflammation or irritation of the pleura—a thin two-layer membrane that lines the lungs and the chest cavity. The parietal pleura lines the inner surface of the chest wall, diaphragm, and mediastinum, while the visceral pleura covers the outer surface of the lungs and lines the fissures.

ETIOLOGY

Pleurisy is not a disease but a manifestation of a disease or diseases. Pleural inflammation may be caused by many different etiologic factors including trauma, infection, irritation, and neoplastic processes. Pleural trauma is most notably caused by rib fractures. Infection is most commonly related to pneumonia, either viral or bacterial. Irritant substances include noxious agents that affect the pleura via the bloodstream or lymphatics or by crossing the conductive respiratory tissue. Examples include asbestos-related diseases, pleural effusions secondary to tuberculosis, drug ingestion, and collagen vascular disease. Neoplastic cells can invade the pleura in a similar fashion.

PATHOPHYSIOLOGY

Typically, the pleura first becomes congested and edematous. This is followed by cellular infiltration and fibrous exudates that develop on the pleural surface. Exudates may be absorbed or organized into fibrous tissue, resulting in pleural adhesions. Pleural exudate follows as a result of an outpouring of fluid rich in plasma proteins from damaged vessels. Occasionally some diseases (e.g., coxsackievirus B causing pleurodynia) may run their course without significant exudation of the fluid from the inflamed pleura, thus leaving a dry and fibrous pleurisy.

SIGNS AND SYMPTOMS

The onset is usually sudden, but this may be variable, depending on the etiology. Pain, which is the dominant symptom, may vary from vague discomfort to an intense stabbing sensation. Aggravating factors include deep inspiration, coughing, laughter, and any activity that results in sudden movements of the thoracic cavity. The discomfort usually occurs over the area of pleural inflammation and can be accentuated by moving the affected side.

The pain associated with pleurisy results from inflammation of the parietal pleura, which is innervated by the intercostal nerves. The pain, however, can be referred to distant regions. Irritation of the posterior and peripheral portions of the diaphragmatic pleura, which is supplied by the lower sixth thoracic nerve, may cause pain referred to the lower chest or abdomen and may mimic an intra-abdominal process. The phrenic nerve innervates the central portion of the diaphragmatic pleura; thus, pain may be referred to the neck or the ipsilateral shoulder. The visceral pleura is supplied by the visceral afferent nerves and is mostly anesthetic; therefore, it does not produce sharp and localized pain.

PHYSICAL EXAMINATION

The physical examination of the pleura seeks evidence of pleural adhesions, increased pleural thickness, pleural inflammation, or the presence of air or excessive fluid in the pleural cavity. Respirations may be noted to be shallow and rapid. The patient may splint the affected side.

A pleural friction rub is pathognomonic in pleurisy, although it is often absent or heard only 24 to 48 h after the onset of pain. This friction rub varies from intermittent sounds that may simulate crackles to fully developed harsh grating, leathery, or creaking sounds synonymous with respiration. Pleuritis, which is adjacent to the heart (pleural pericardial rub), varies with cardiac pattern as well as respiration, and the clinical picture varies with the underlying disease.

If fluid develops at the site of inflammation between the two membranes, the liquid is called a *pleural effusion.* As a pleural effusion develops, pleuritic pain usually subsides; however, increasing dyspnea may be noted. Accompanying the dyspnea, percussion dullness, decreased or absent breath sounds, absent tactile fremitus, and egophony at the upper border of the fluid are noticeable. If superficial tenderness to light palpation is present, it may be of musculoskeletal origin. Fever generally is not present unless the primary etiology is an infectious source.

LABORATORY STUDIES

The diagnosis of pleurisy is generally one of exclusion. Diagnostic studies focus more on the cause of the pleurisy. A complete blood count (CBC) will help the evaluation for acute infectious problems. The erythrocyte sedimentation rate (ESR), although nonspecific, may help in determining inflammatory or metastatic causes. Blood urea nitrogen and creatinine are elevated in uremic pleurisy.

RADIOLOGIC STUDIES

Chest x-rays are of limited value in diagnosing pleurisy. Pleural lesions generally cause no shadow; however, pleural effusions, though typically small, may confirm that acute inflammation of the pleura is present. The x-ray is useful to rule out a potential pneumonia, evaluate trauma to the chest wall, and rule out neoplasms or associated pulmonary or chest wall lesions. A ventilation-perfusion (VQ) scan may be ordered if a pulmonary embolus is considered in the differential diagnosis.

DIAGNOSTIC CONSIDERATIONS

The following diagnoses and conditions can result in pleurisy:

Chest wall trauma: rib fracture
Neoplasm: primary lung cancer or metastases
Vascular: pulmonary embolus
Metabolic: uremia
Infection: pneumonia or influenza
Abdominal disease
Intercostal neuritis
Herpetic neuritis
Myocardial infarction
Spontaneous pneumothorax
Pericarditis
Chest wall lesions
Inflammatory: SLE or rheumatoid arthritis

TREATMENT

Treatment of the underlying disease is essential. If no underlying cause is found, treatment is aimed at relieving the discomfort. Although controversial and not recommended by all practitioners, chest pain may be relieved by wrapping the entire chest with two or three 6-inch-wide nonadhesive elastic bandages. The bandages should be removed several times a day, and the patient should be encouraged to take deep breaths. This maneuver is an attempt to expand the patient's lungs fully and prevent atelectasis. Pain from coughing can be relieved by having the patient hold a pillow firmly against the chest wall when coughing.

Idiopathic pleuritic pain may be controlled with the use of acetaminophen, although nonsteroidal anti-inflammatory drugs (NSAIDs) may be preferable because of their anti-inflammatory effects. Codeine-containing analgesics (30 to 60 mg every 4 to 6 h) are useful in combating more severe pain. It is important to consider the cough suppressant properties of codeine when using this analgesic. A patient taking narcotics should be urged to breathe deeply and cough when pain relief from the drug is maximal. Antibiotics and aqueous aerosol inhalations along with bronchodilators should be considered where there is associated bronchitis and to prevent a complicating pneumonia.

COMPLICATIONS

Complications include scarring from adhesions at the site of inflammation, lung collapse or compression secondary to effusion or fibrosis, impaired breathing secondary to lung collapse or decrease in vital capacity, and pneumonia, which may be a cause of pleurisy or a complication of the pain of pleurisy, producing insufficient coughing that suppresses the expulsion of bronchial secretions.

SPECIAL CONSIDERATIONS

The patient should notify the office if he or she develops increased fever or pain, prolonged or worsening dyspnea, cough that becomes dry and nonproductive, changes in nail beds, or bloody sputum.

BIBLIOGRAPHY

Berkow R, Fletcher AJ. *The Merck Manual,* 17th ed. Merck, 2000.
DeGowin RL. *DeGowin and DeGowin's Diagnostic Examination,* 6th ed. New York, McGraw-Hill, 1994.
Fauci AS, Braunwald E, Isselbacher KJ, et al, eds. *Harrison's Principles of Internal Medicine,* 14th ed. New York, McGraw-Hill, 1998.
Griffith AW. *Instructions for Patients,* 5th ed. Philadelphia, Saunders, 1995.
Labus JB. *The Physician Assistant Medical Handbook.* Philadelphia, Saunders, 1995.

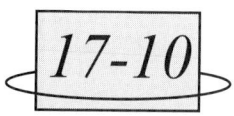

OCCUPATIONAL PNEUMOCONIOSIS
Pamela Moyers Scott

DISCUSSION

Occupational pneumoconiosis (OP) is a chronic lung disease caused by the inhalation of dust particles through exposure at work. The name of the specific occupational pneumoconiosis is derived from the etiologic dust. The three most common forms are silicosis, coal worker's pneumoconiosis (CWP), and asbestosis, which are caused by exposure to silica (or quartz) dust, coal dust, and asbestos fibers, respectively.

Other occupational pneumoconioses and offending dusts include berylliosis (beryllium), byssinosis (cotton), bagassosis (pressed stalks of sugarcane), baritosis (barium sulfate), siderosis (iron sulfate), stannosis (tin oxide), and farmer's lung (moldy hay).

Accurate information on the true incidence of individuals affected with occupational respiratory diseases is difficult to obtain because of inconsistent and voluntary reporting, misdiagnoses as other forms of respiratory illness, and individuals with mild disease who do not access the health care system. In 1986, the U.S. Department of Labor estimated that annually, in the United States, 65,000 individuals develop an occupational respiratory disease and 25,000 die from it.[1]

With more emphasis on prevention, these statistics should decrease. For example, from January 1992 to June 14, 1997, there were only 1914 cases of CWP, the most prevalent worldwide disease caused by mineral dusts, reported in the United States,[2] and the annual death toll from silicosis in this country has decreased to 250 deaths annually.[2,3]

Millions of Americans are exposed to potentially disease-producing dusts regularly through their employment. The individuals who will develop a disease process and the severity of the disease cannot be determined in advance. Several variables determine the toxicity of inhaled dust. These variables include the physical, chemical, and mechanical properties of the dust particles, including their size, shape, penetrability, concentration, solubility, form, acidity, fibrogenicity, and antigenicity.[4] Additionally, the individual worker's immune status and ventilation rate and depth are important factors.[4]

SIGNS AND SYMPTOMS

Initially, all affected individuals with OP are generally asymptomatic. As the disease progresses, a mild productive cough and exertional dyspnea occur. These symptoms may continue to worsen until the patient experiences dyspnea at rest. Signs and symptoms associated with complications from OP may be the presenting complaint (e.g., pneumonia, cor pulmonale, congestive heart failure).

OBJECTIVE FINDINGS

Early in the course of the disease, the physical examination is generally unremarkable. Depending on the severity of the OP and the presence of complicating disease processes, the patient may have any of the following: diminished breath sounds, rhonchi, wheezing, rales, fever, edema, jugular vein distention, clubbing, cyanosis, and varying degrees of dyspnea. No physical findings are specific for occupational pneumoconiosis.

DIAGNOSTIC CONSIDERATIONS

The differential diagnosis includes any chronic respiratory condition, such as emphysema, chronic bronchitis, asthma, and lung cancer.

SPECIAL CONSIDERATIONS

Cigarette smoking appears to have an additive detrimental effect on the development and progression of the disease.

LABORATORY STUDIES

There are no specific laboratory tests to diagnose occupational pneumoconiosis. However, if patients are on a theophylline preparation, periodic serum levels are necessary. A complete blood count (CBC) may be useful in individuals suspected of having a coexisting infection or polycythemia.

RADIOGRAPHIC STUDIES

Early in the course of the disease, the chest x-ray (CXR) is often normal. However, pulmonary function abnormalities may be demonstrated in the absence of radiographic findings. The first visible finding of occupational pneumoconiosis on CXR is the presence of small (<5 mm), round parenchymal opacities (see Fig. 17-10-1). If the disease progresses, these nodules coalesce, forming larger irregular lesions referred to as progressive massive fibrosis (PMF) (see Fig. 17-10-2). An accurate occupational history is the only definite means to distinguish the various occupational pneumoconioses from one another, and the radiographic evidence is virtually identical. However, some features are more suspicious for specific disease processes. Asbestosis is more often associated with the following: pleural plaques (see Fig. 17-10-3), an indistinct cardiac border (ground-glass appearance), and coalescence of parenchyma and obliteration of the acinar units (honeycombed lung). Hilar lymph node calcification may produce the characteristic eggshell pattern of silicosis.

OTHER DIAGNOSTICS

Pulmonary function testing (PFT) can reveal an obstructive, restrictive, or mixed pattern. An obstructive pattern is defined as normal or decreased forced vital capacity (FVC) associated with decreased forced expiratory volume (FEV). A restrictive pattern is characterized by decreased FVC and normal or increased FEV. A mixed pattern

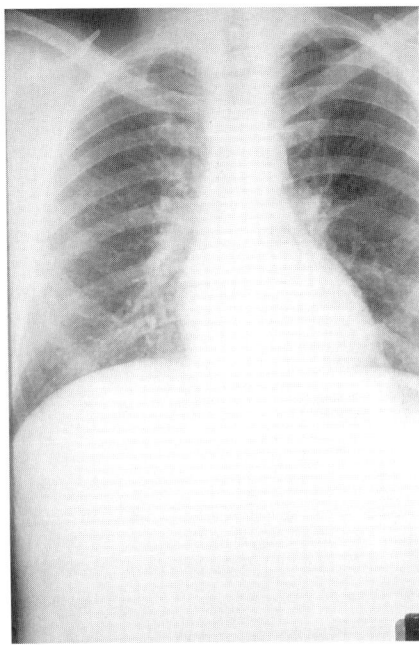

FIGURE 17-10-1. Simple occupational pneumoconiosis evident by the appearance of small, round parenchymal opacities.

reveals a normal or decreased FVC and FEV, depending on the specific occupational disease that is present. Coal worker's pneumoconiosis is seen initially as an obstructive pattern, whereas asbestosis and silicosis are initially restrictive.

Oxygen saturation as determined with a pulse oximeter is decreased in accordance with the severity of the pulmonary impairment.

Arterial blood gases (ABGs) also reveal hypoxemia that is consonant with the severity of the pulmonary impairment.

TREATMENT

Pharmacologic Management

First-line treatment of occupational pneumoconiosis generally consists of inhaled beta agonists such as pirbuterol (Maxair), albuterol (Ventolin, Proventil), and metaproterenol (Alupent). Generally, these drugs are delivered by a metered-dose inhaler (MDI) at a dose of two inhalations qid. Individuals with less severe disease may benefit from using these medications on an as-needed basis only. However, if the patient requires them more than two or three times a week, he or she probably will benefit from using them regularly to prevent bronchospasms instead of treating them when they occur. Regardless, individuals who use beta-

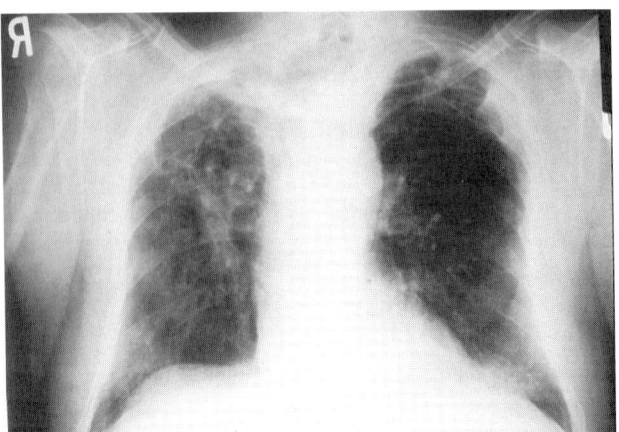

FIGURE 17-10-2. Complicated occupational pneumoconiosis evident by the appearance of progressive massive fibrosis and bullous formation.

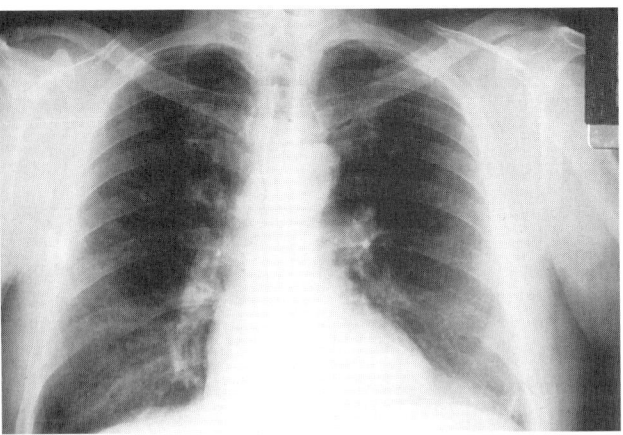

FIGURE 17-10-3. Probable asbestosis based on the presence of bilateral pleural thickening along with the parenchymal opacities.

agonist MDIs must be cautioned never to exceed the recommended dose because of the potential for cardiac arrhythmias.

Salmeterol (Serevent) is the only currently approved long-acting beta agonist MDI available in the United States. The dose is two inhalations bid. Salmeterol has the same potential for fatal cardiac arrhythmias as the shorter-acting preparations and is not indicated for the relief of acute symptoms.

Since many individuals have difficulty using MDIs properly, breath-activated devices are available to enhance patients' ability to receive an accurate dose of medication: pirbuterol (Maxair Autohaler), albuterol (Ventolin Rotacaps), and salmeterol (Serevent Diskus). Many of the beta agonists are also available in a solution with normal saline for delivery by an ultrasonic nebulizer. Spacers also appear to be effective in enhancing the delivery of the desired MDI dose to the lungs.

An ipratropium bromide (Atrovent) MDI or nebulizer solution is also useful in treating OP. The usual dose of the MDI is two inhalations qid. Because ipratropium induces bronchodilation through a mechanism different from that of the beta agonists, it can be used alone or in combination with those agents.

Although it is an effective bronchodilator, theophylline is not used as much today as it was in the past because of its side-effect profile, potential for toxicity, and potential for drug interactions as well as the need for serum monitoring. Oral beta agonists are also available; however, they are used infrequently because the topical inhaled formulations tend to be much better tolerated. Examples include albuterol (Volmax, Ventolin) and terbutaline (Brethine).

Corticosteroids are occasionally beneficial in the treatment of OP by decreasing the amount of inflammation in the airways. Whenever possible, inhaled medications are preferred because they reduce significantly, if not eliminate entirely, the possibility of serious side effects. Inhaled corticosteroids include triamcinolone (Azmacort), beclomethasone (Beclovent, Vanceril), and fluticasone (Flovent). Fluticasone is also available in a breath-activated device (Flovent Rotadisk).

Home oxygen is necessary when the oxygen partial pressure (P_{O_2}) is less than 55 percent and in individuals with severe complications such as pulmonary hypertension, right-sided congestive heart failure, and cor pulmonale. Depending on the severity of the disease, the dosing schedule can be continuous (24 h/day), at night (8 to 10 h/day), or as needed. Care must be taken not to exceed 2 L/min via nasal cannula because the respiratory drive of OP patients could be based on O_2, not CO_2, and higher flow rates could result in respiratory depression and arrest.

SUPPORTIVE MEASURES

All individuals with OP should drink at least 8 to 10 8-oz glasses of water a day. This will keep them adequately hydrated as well as serve as a mucolytic.

Individuals with mild disease who continue to work should be moved to an area of reduced dust exposure and/or use protective equipment regularly. Additionally, they should have annual chest x-rays and PFTs to monitor the progression of the disease process.

Immunizations

All patients with OP should receive the influenza vaccine annually. They should receive immunization against pneumococcus at least once and boosters at 5-year intervals if they are considered to be at high risk for fatal pneumococcal disease. Additionally, they should receive a tuberculin purified protein derivative (PPD) skin test annually.

Patient Education

Once OP is diagnosed, the worker must take measures to reduce exposure to prevent the disease from progressing. Depending on the type of dust involved and the particular work environment, workers may have legal rights to help them accomplish this. Smoking cessation is essential.

Prevention

It is currently believed that practically all dust-induced respiratory disease can be prevented.[3,5] Improved prevention occurs when employers, employees, and health care providers work together to minimize the effects of occupational dusts. These efforts should include emphasizing the hazards of the job, encouraging the use of protective equipment and procedures, and stressing the importance of regular medical screenings.

Screening Asymptomatic Workers

Individuals in high-risk occupations should receive preplacement chest x-rays and PFTs; information and advice on smoking cessation; annual medical, respiratory symptoms, and work history questionnaires/updates; PFTs at 1- to 3-year intervals,[2] and chest x-rays every 3 to 5 years.[2]

Disposition

Follow-up of a patient with OP depends on the severity of the disease and the associated complications. All these individuals should be seen at least annually for a history and physical update, chest x-ray, PFT, PPD, influenza vaccine, and appropriate health maintenance and education.

COMPLICATIONS AND RED FLAGS

Complications from any occupational pneumoconiosis may include PMF, cor pulmonale, right-sided congestive heart failure, pulmonary hypertension, chronic bronchitis, pneumonia, tuberculosis, and death. Specifically related to CWP is Caplan's syndrome, which is characterized by PMF and rheumatoid arthritis. Chronic lymphocytic alveolitis and lung cancer have been reported in individuals with silicosis. Asbestos exposure has been linked with many carcinomas, including lung, laryngeal, renal, and gastrointestinal cancers, as well as mesotheliomas.

REFERENCES

1. Anderson M: Introduction to occupational lung disease, in American Lung Association: *Occupational Lung Diseases: An Introduction,* New York, American Lung Association, 1986, pp 1–7.

2. U.S. Department of Labor: *Mine Safety and Health Administration: Dust—What You Can't See CAN Hurt You.* Washington DC, U.S. Department of Labor, 1999, pp 1–24.

3. U.S. Department of Labor, National Institute for Occupational Safely and Health: *A Guide to Working Safely with Silica,* Washington, DC, U.S. Government Printing Office, 1997, pp 2–3.

4. Speizer F: Environmental lung diseases, in Fauci AS, Braunwald E, Isselbacher KJ, et al (eds): *Harrison's Principles of Internal Medicine,* 14th ed. New York, McGraw-Hill, 1998, pp 1429–1436.

5. American Lung Association: *Facts about Dust Diseases: Lung Hazards on the Job.* New York, American Lung Association, 1988, pp 2–7.

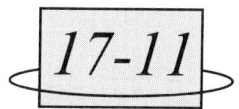

CHRONIC OBSTRUCTIVE PULMONARY DISEASE: EMPHYSEMA AND CHRONIC BRONCHITIS

Maureen MacLeod O'Hara

EPIDEMIOLOGY

The term *chronic obstructive pulmonary disease* (COPD) refers to the obstructive airflow disorders emphysema and chronic bronchitis. Up to 70,000 patients a year die from COPD, making it the fourth leading cause of death in the United States. It accounts for more than 14 million office visits and 2 million hospitalizations annually. The National Heart, Lung, and Blood Institute estimate that the annual cost of treatment for COPD is $18 billion. Approximately 2 million Americans have emphysema, and 14 million have chronic bronchitis. COPD is approximately three times more prevalent in white persons and approximately two times more prevalent in men. The incidence in women seems to be increasing as a result of higher numbers of women smokers in recent years.

Cigarette smoking is the primary risk factor for both emphysema and chronic bronchitis 80 to 90 percent of the time. These patients give a history of symptoms for 10 to 15 years and a history of smoking one or more packs per day for 25 years or more. It is not clear, however, why only 10 to 15 percent of smokers eventually develop COPD. In 1990, 28 percent of men and 22 percent of women over age 20 (i.e., 45 million people) smoked cigarettes in the United States. According to a 1995 study by the Centers for Disease Control and Prevention, 29 percent of boys and 26 percent of girls age 12 to 21 smoke, and so the potential for developing respiratory diseases remains significant. Pipe and cigar smokers along with those who have quit smoking, have a higher rate of COPD than do nonsmokers but a lower rate than those who still smoke cigarettes.

The risk of developing COPD is approximately 10 to 30 times greater in smokers than in nonsmokers, indicating that there are risk factors for nonsmokers to develop COPD, including respiratory problems as children (viral infections and asthma), exposure to environmental or occupational dust, air pollution, and secondhand smoke. Among COPD cases, 0.5 to 2 percent are due to alpha$_1$-antitrypsin deficiency, suggesting a genetic predisposition. Alpha$_1$-antitrypsin deficiency should be suspected in persons who develop emphysema in their late thirties to early forties. If patients develop COPD from any of these factors and smoke cigarettes, the disease process may accelerate.

Survival rates for severe COPD are estimated to be 50 percent after 5 years and 25 percent after 10 years. After the first episode of respiratory failure, 66 percent of these patients die within 2 years.

PATHOPHYSIOLOGY

Emphysema is defined as "abnormal stretching and destructive changes in the alveoli" by the American Thoracic Society (ATS) and is a pathologic diagnosis that is made at autopsy. It is an assumed diagnosis in a living patient. Emphysema affects lung parenchyma distal to the terminal bronchioles and is characterized by destruction of alveolar walls and an abnormal, irregular enlargement of air spaces.

This progressive destruction from the peripheral to the terminal airways accounts for the loss of alveolar capillary surface area and a disturbance in the capacity of the lungs to diffuse gases. Since there is a loss of both air space and blood vessels, emphysema demonstrates less of a ventilation-perfusion mismatch than does chronic bronchitis.

Elements in cigarette smoke are known to stimulate elastase enzymatic activity, causing degenerative changes in elastin and alveolar structures. These elements also interfere with antielastase activity and the repair process of elastin fibers. These substances also cause the release of cytotoxic oxygen radicals from white blood cells in lung tissue. The destruction of alveolar walls causes a loss of elasticity and an increase in lunge compliance, resulting in obstruction of expiratory airflow. Because of this increased compliance, the work of ventilation is less intensive and may result in less CO_2 retention early in the disease process.

There are several patterns of tissue destruction in emphysema. In centrilobar or centriacinar emphysema, the most severe destruction appears in the central portion of the lobule or acinus with sparing of the alveolar ducts and alveoli (see Fig. 17-11-1). Centrilobular emphysema is most often seen in the apex but spreads to the base of the lobe as the disease progresses. Mild destruction in the apices causes little or no lung dysfunction. Centrilobular is the most common type of tissue destruction and is seen most often in smokers.

Panlobular or panacinar emphysema affects the terminal bronchiole with its alveolar ducts and alveolar sacs, causing air trapping, and seems to be more prominent in portions of the lower lobes. Centrilobular and panlobular emphysema may coexist in the same lung. Paraseptal emphysema involves destruction of the alveolar ducts and sacs as well as the interlobar walls. It is more common in the peripheral lobules.

Bullous emphysema involves large cystic areas of destruction where air spaces have a diameter greater than 1 cm, giving an appearance of Swiss cheese. By comparison, normal lung tissue appears to have a fine texture similar to that of bread. The air spaces or bullae gradually increase in size from the forces of the elastic recoil of other areas with greater elasticity, causing a loss of lung parenchyma volume.

Chronic bronchitis is a clinical diagnosis and is defined by the ATS as "excessive sputum production with chronic or recurring cough on most days for a minimum of 3 months of the year for at least 2 consecutive years." It includes smooth muscle hypertrophy, inflammation, mucosal edema, narrowing of airways, goblet and squamous cell metaplasia, mucosal plugging of small airways (less than 2 to 3 mm), and peribronchial fibrosis. As chronic bronchitis worsens over time, the airflow resistance (obstruction), which starts in the small airways, comes to involve larger peripheral airways as well.

The obstruction of small airways from any of the causes mentioned above results in CO_2 retention and hypoxemia from ventilation-perfusion mismatch. Hypoxemia and acidemia (from respiratory acidosis) cause constriction of pulmonary arteries and increased pulmonary arterial pressure, leading to pulmonary hypertension. *Cor pulmonale* is a term used to describe right ventricular enlargement caused by a disease of the lung. COPD is an underlying cause of pulmonary hypertension. Emphysema contributes to pulmonary hypertension by increasing vascular resistance from the loss of capillary beds. Chronic bronchitis contributes to pulmonary hypertension as a result of hypoxemia and acidemia. In advanced disease, cor pulmonale manifests more often in chronic bronchitis-dominant patients as polycythemia and evidence of fluid retention, such as dependent edema and jugular venous distention.

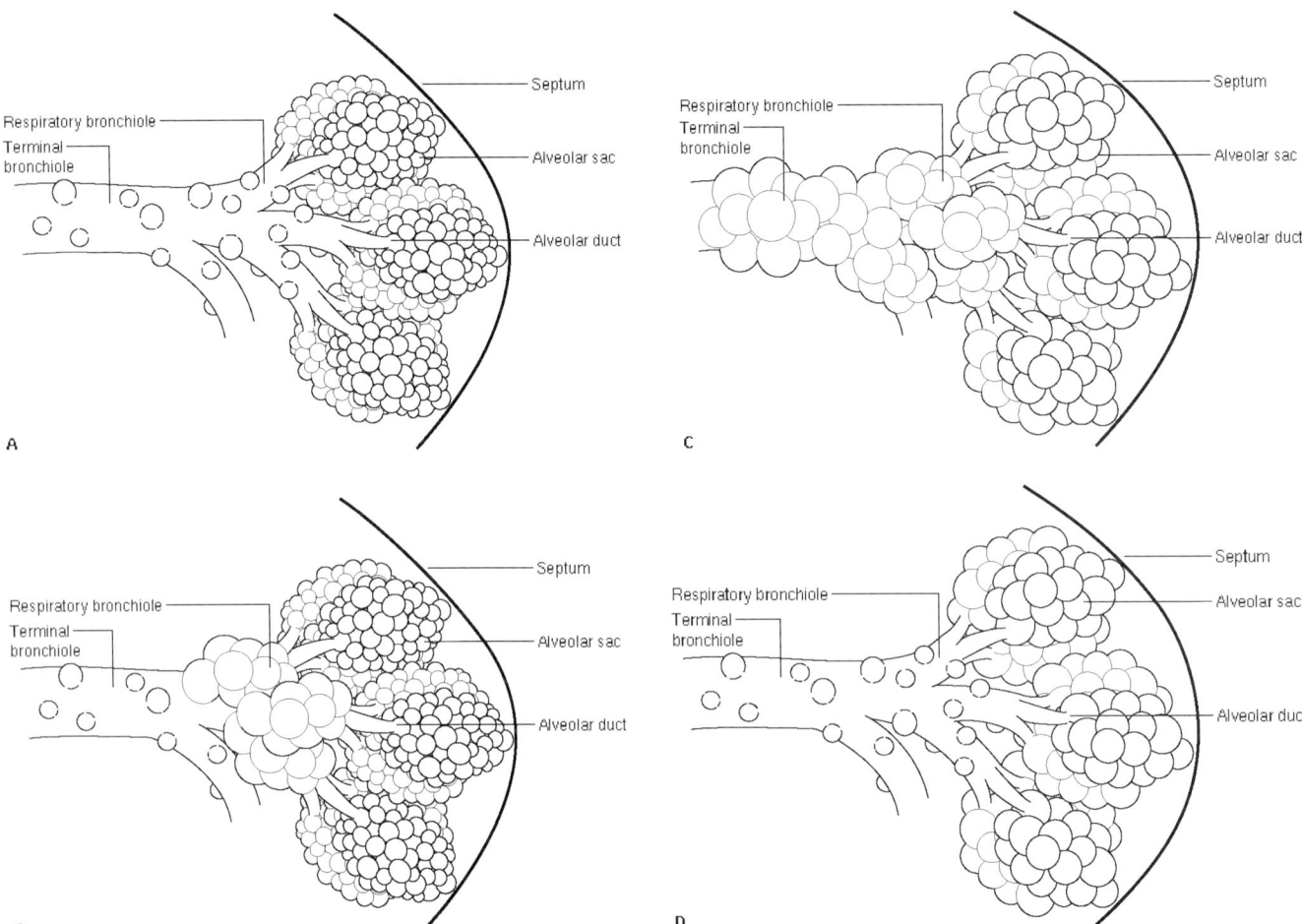

FIGURE 17-11-1. Tissue destruction in emphysema. *A.* Normal acinar (lobar) unit. *B.* Centriacinar (centrilobular) emphysema. *C.* Panacinar (panlobular) emphysema. *D.* Paraseptal emphysema. (*From Calverley and Pride, 1995; George et al, 1995; West, 1987.*)

ASSESSMENT

COPD presents a diagnostic challenge for clinicians since approximately one-third of office visits are for respiratory complaints. Patients may have a predominance of emphysema or chronic bronchitis but usually have a mixture of both diseases. The diagnosis is based on the history, physical examination, and laboratory findings, since there is not a single pathognomonic hallmark for COPD.

CLINICAL FINDINGS

History

Early detection of COPD is difficult because of its slow, progressive, insidious nature. Symptoms may be present for several years before patients seek treatment. Coughing and wheezing are early symptoms and may be overlooked or dismissed as "smoker's cough," since dyspnea may not be present. Practitioners may not note the connection between a series of respiratory infections and the onset of COPD. Also, clinicians may not have the opportunity to see trends developing if patients do not maintain long-term therapeutic relationships as a result of changes in health insurance carriers or loss of coverage. Patients may complain of cough, wheezing, or recurring respiratory infections that may be attributed to disease entities other than COPD, but it is shortness of breath (dyspnea) or, more specifically, dyspnea on exertion, described as "breathlessness," that usually causes patients to seek medical attention. Patients may describe breathlessness while performing activities of daily living such as cleaning, making the bed, and dressing. Dyspnea is a late symptom and usually indicates 20 to 30 percent irreversible lung tissue destruction (see Table 17-11-1).

Physical Examination

Depending on the severity of the progression of the disease process and the relative degrees of predominance of emphysema and chronic bronchitis, the physical findings vary. Physical examinations may be normal for many years, but the most prominent feature of the physical examination is prolonged expiration. A simple measure of obstruction can be obtained by having the patient take a deep breath and forcefully exhale as fast as possible. Using a peak flowmeter as a device for the patients to blow into or listening to the trachea with a stethoscope, the practitioner times the length of the exhalation. Longer than 4 to 6 s is considered abnormal and indicates obstruction. The Snider match test is a screening test that is considered positive if the patient is unable to blow out a match held 15 cm from the mouth.

Type A, or emphysema-predominant, patients usually are able to maintain adequate oxygenation for a longer time during their disease. This slows the onset of the pulmonary hypertension and right-sided heart failure that are common in chronic bronchitis. These patients are labeled "pink puffers" because of their pursed-lip breathing, pink skin color, and thin body habitus. Type B, or chronic bronchitis-dominant, patients are often cyanotic from decreased oxygen saturation and being overweight, giving them the label "blue bloaters."

Pedal edema is common in type B patients because of pulmonary hypertension. COPD patients become dyspneic almost immediately upon lying down, whereas patients with congestive heart failure become orthopneic in a few hours. Pitting edema that does not clear with leg elevation should make one suspicious of right-sided heart failure. Digital clubbing is unusual in COPD patients and may indicate a neoplasm, infection, or interstitial lung disease (see Table 17-11-2).

LABORATORY FINDINGS

Pulmonary Function Tests

Pulmonary function tests (PFTs) are used to characterize the pattern of the airway defect, quantify the airway obstruction, assess the reversibility of the airway obstruction, and monitor the progression of the disease. In normal lungs, vital capacity (VC), or the total amount of air a person can exhale after a maximal inspiration, exceeds the residual volume (RV), or the amount of air that remains in the lung after a full exhalation, by a ratio of 3:1. COPD causes difficult and incomplete emptying of the lungs, resulting in an increase in RV and a decrease in VC so that the ratio approaches 1:1 (see Fig. 17-11-2). Any reduction of VC will impair the ventilatory capacity of the lungs. Spirometry employs a machine to measure lung volumes, flow rates, and diffusion capacity, providing information about lung function. The values given in this chapter are approximations of normal and abnormal, since lung function has been shown to vary with age, gender, race, height, and weight. Normal values are individualized for each patient on the basis of these variables and are reported as predicted normal values (PNV). Variations from PNV are considered abnormal for the patient.

The volume of air forcefully exhaled in 1 s is called the one-second forced expiratory volume (FEV_1). In obstructive disease, the rate of exhalation slows because of narrowing of the airways. FEV_1 may be prolonged as much as 15 to 20 s compared to a normal value of 3 s. The airway obstruction component of chronic bronchitis is considered reversible if the FEV_1 improves at least 15 percent or 200 mL

TABLE 17-11-1.   History Questions and Usual Responses

HISTORY QUESTION	EMPHYSEMA	CHRONIC BRONCHITIS
Quantity and length of smoking Date of cessation	One or more packs per day for 25 years or more	
Cough Productive/nonproductive Sputum color Noninfected Infected	Minimal Scant sputum	Almost daily Thick, copious: 2 oz to 1 cup per day, worse in morning White, tan, gray Yellow, green, brown, red
Frequency of respiratory infections	Occasional	Frequent
Dyspnea	Frequent	Intermittent
Wheezing	Minimal	Frequent
Hemoptyses	Rare	Occasional
Weight change	Loss	Gain
Duration of symptoms before office presentation	10 to 15 years	10 to 15 years
Age at presentation of complaints	50–55	35–40

SOURCE: Griffith et al, 1994; Hahn, 1996; Johannsen, 1994; Kelley, 1994; Labus, 1995; Peterson et al, 1995; Scientific American, 1995.

TABLE 17-11-2. Usual Physical Findings

	TYPE A: EMPHYSEMA-PREDOMINANT, "PINK PUFFER"	TYPE B: CHRONIC BRONCHITIS-PREDOMINANT, "BLUE BLOATER"
General	Thin, cachectic, pursed-lip breathing, accessory muscle use, barrel chest	Obese, cyanotic
Vital signs	Tachypnea (>18 respirations/min), occasional tachycardia (>100 beats per min)	
Cardiovascular	Cor pulmonale rare	Cor pulmonale common Jugular venous distention, right-sided heart failure, right ventricular heave (pulmonary hypertension), S_3 murmur (tricuspid insufficiency)
Gastrointestinal		Hepatomegaly, ascites (right-sided heart failure)
Pulmonary	Dyspnea, prolonged expiration, minimal wheeze, hyperresonant to percussion, decreased breath sounds, reduced diaphragmatic excursion, low position of diaphragm	Minimal dyspnea, prolonged expiration, coarse rhonchi, wheeze, minimally decreased breath sounds
Extremities		Pedal edema

SOURCE: Braunwald et al, 1988; Griffith et al, 1994; Hahn, 1996; Johannsen, 1994; Labus, 1995; Scientific American, 1995.

after the administration of an aerosol bronchodilator. It is not unusual for nonsmokers to lose 20 to 25 mL of FEV_1 per year, while heavy smokers may lose 40 to 50 mL per year. Nonsmokers who have alpha$_1$-antitrypsin deficiency may lose 80 mL of FEV_1 per year, while smokers with alpha$_1$-antitrypsin deficiency may lose 150 mL per year. Forced vital capacity (FVC) is the total air forcefully exhaled. The normal value of the ratio of FEV_1 to FVC is 75 to 80 percent. A reduced FEV_1 with a reduced FEV_1/FVC ratio is considered the most indicative of obstructive disease. Forced expiratory flow ($FEF_{25-75\%}$) measures the flow of air in the middle of an exhalation. This is helpful information, since the obstructive process affects the small airways first, and their collapse can be detected by the low flow volume. Total lung capacity (TLC) is the amount of air in the lungs after a full inspiration (RV + VC). In emphysema, the TLC may actually increase as a result of hyperinflation from the increased lung compliance and loss of elastic recoil. An increased RV/TLC ratio may indicate air trapping. Functional residual capacity (FRC) is the amount of air remaining in the lung after a normal resting expiration. It is a measure of the balance between lung elastic recoil and chest wall recoil. FRC increases in emphysema as the elastic recoil of the lung decreases and gives an indication of the severity of hyperinflation. In chronic bronchitis, the mechanism for increased FRC is increased airway resistance from mucus plugging and inflammation. FRC also increases with an increase in the respiratory rate. Hyperinflation increases the work of breathing as inspiratory capacity is reduced by an increase in RV. This is demonstrated by an increase in breathlessness. There are several methods to measure FRC with spirometry; the most common techniques use helium or nitrogen gas. Inspiratory and expiratory lung

volumes also may be recorded by flow-volume loops in a graphic presentation. These loops have characteristic shapes that depend on the type of respiratory disorder.

The spirometer can measure the inequality of ventilation by analyzing the nitrogen concentration expressed as the percentage of nitrogen per liter of expired air, called a single-breath nitrogen test (SBN_2). In normal subjects, the inspired oxygen will attempt to equilibrate with the nitrogen from the dead spaces of the lung. In persons with obstructive disease, the dead spaces may be larger and unevenly distributed so that the inspired oxygen is not sufficient to dilute the nitrogen from the poorly ventilated areas of the lung, causing the nitrogen concentration to be increased. Helium is another gas that can be used to make these measurements.

In spirometry, reduced diffusing capacity of the lung for carbon monoxide (DL_{CO}) is a measure of ventilation. DL_{CO} is decreased more in emphysema than it is in chronic bronchitis because of the destruction of the pulmonary capillaries in the alveolar walls. In chronic bronchitis, DL_{CO} is reduced by the thickening of tissues in the small airways (see Table 17-11-3 and Fig. 17-11-3). If patients with COPD continue to smoke, their PFTs should be checked every 1 to 2 years to measure the decline. In patients who are nonsmokers, the interval can be longer. When FEV_1 falls to less than 50 percent of the predicted normal value, an arterial blood gas should be obtained.

Arterial Blood Gas

Hypoxemia with or without carbon dioxide (CO_2) retention is common in COPD because of the uneven ventilation-perfusion of the lung. Emphysema-predominant patients typically have mild to moderate hypoxemia with oxygen tension (Pa_{O_2}) levels of 65 to 70 mmHg and normal CO_2 tension levels (Pa_{CO_2}) of 35 to 40 mmHg. Chronic bronchitis-predominant patients typically have severe hypoxemia with Pa_{O_2} levels of 45 to 60 mmHg and hypercapnia with Pa_{CO_2} levels of 50 to 60 mmHg. Some patients can compensate for the increased CO_2 retention. Their kidneys can slowly retain bicarbonate so that the pH remains constant. Compensated respiratory acidosis can be seen in patients when FEV_1 drops below 1.0 L/s. Arterial blood gas (ABG) should be checked yearly once Pa_{O_2} falls to 55 mmHg or FEV_1 drops to 1.0 L/s (see Table 17-11-4).

Pulse Oximetry

Pulse oximetry can be used to periodically check oxygen saturation (Sa_{O_2}). Oximetry is an indirect measure of Sa_{O_2} with an accuracy of 3 to 5 percent for Sa_{O_2} values greater than 70 percent at sea level. An Sa_{O_2} of 90 percent approximates a Pa_{O_2} of 60 mmHg. Sa_{O_2} should be

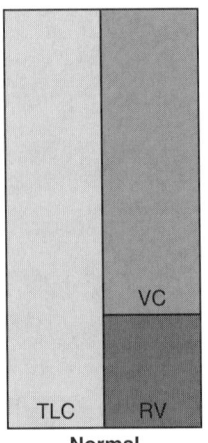
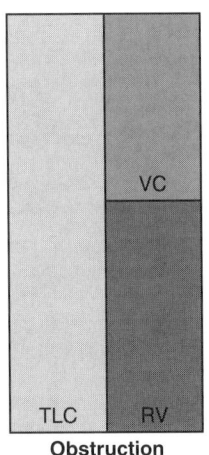

Normal   **Obstruction**

FIGURE 17-11-2. Lung volumes. (*From Fishman et al, 1985; O'Hara, 1995.*)

TABLE 17-11-3. Pulmonary Function Values

MEASUREMENT	NORMAL	MILD	MODERATE	SEVERE
FEV$_1$	4 L/s	1.2 to 1.5 L/s (may be dyspneic)	1.0 L/s (may be sedentary) <1.0 L/s (may show signs of hypoxemia, hypercapnia, cor pulmonale)	≤500 mL/s (may be bed-bound)
		≥50% PNV	39–49% PNV	<35% PNV
FEV$_1$/FVC	75–80%	60%		
FVC	5 L/s		Decreased	
FEF$_{25-75\%}$	3.5 L/s		Decreased	
TLC	6.58 to 9.25 L		Increased in emphysema	
RV/TLC	30–40%			
DL$_{CO}$			Decreased in emphysema > chronic bronchitis	
Single-breath nitrogen washout			Increased nitrogen concentration	

SOURCE: Fishman et al, 1985; Hahn, 1996; Johannsen, 1994; O'Hara, 1995a; West, 1987.

95 percent or more for adequate tissue oxygenation. Pulse oximetry should not be used to replace ABG but to monitor patients, keeping in mind that it gives no information about Pa$_{CO_2}$.

Electrocardiogram

The electrocardiogram (ECG) is normal early in the course of the disease. Later in the course of the chronic bronchitis component, there may be right axis deviation (QRS axis +90 degrees and +180 degrees), tall R waves in lead V$_1$ or V$_2$ (≥6 mm), and deep S waves in V$_5$ or V$_6$ (≥10 mm). During exacerbations, tall P waves (≥2.5 mm) may be seen. There is not a good correlation, however, between these findings and pulmonary hypertension or cor pulmonale. Only one-third of COPD patients are found to have hypertrophy of the right ventricle at autopsy.

Complete Blood Count

The complete blood count is usually normal but may show polycythemia later in the course of chronic bronchitis-predominant disease as a result of hypoxemia. The hemoglobin may drop below 16 percent from oxygen desaturation, and the hematocrit may be elevated to 50 to 60 percent in chronic bronchitis patients. The hematocrit value is usually three times the hemoglobin value.

Age	86 years	Room temp/pressure	23° C/760 mmHg			
Gender/race	F/black	Height	64 in./163 cm			
Weight	125 lb/57 kg	Spirometry and lung volumes at BTPS				

			Pre ℞			Post ℞		
			Predicted	Best	%Predicted	Best	%Predicted	%Change
	SPIROMETRY							
FVC		Liters	2.35	1.22	52*	1.32	56*	8
FEV$_1$		Liters	1.56	0.70	45*	0.70	45*	0
FEV$_1$/FVC		%	80	57		53		
FEF$_{25\text{ to }75\%}$		L/sec	1.08	0.32	30*	0.30	28*	−6
PEF		L/sec	5.08	2.36	46*	2.73	54*	−16

			Pre ℞					
			Predicted	Average	%Predicted			
	LUNG VOLUMES							
VC		Liters	2.35	1.22	52*			
TLC		Liters	4.69	4.76	102			
RV		Liters	2.08	3.54#	170*			
RV/TLC		%	44	74#				
FRC N$_2$		Liters	2.94	3.69	126			
	DIFFUSION							
DL$_{CO}$		mL/min/mmHg	15.3	6.5#	43*			

* = Outside normal range.

\# = Outside 95% confidence interval.

Calibration: Predicted: 3.30 Actual: Expired 3.37 Inspired 3.28

BTPS = Body temperature, ambient pressure and saturation with water vapor; PEF = Peak expiratory flow.

FIGURE 17-11-3. Example of a pulmonary function test.

TABLE 17-11-4. **Values of Arterial Blood Gases and Hemoglobin and Hematocrit**

Arterial measurements	Normal range on room air at sea level	
Pa_{O_2}	80–100 mmHg	
Pa_{CO_2}	35–45 mmHg	
pH	7.35 to 7.45	
Oxygen saturation (Sa_{O_2})	96 to 100%	
Venous measurements		
Hemoglobin	Men 16 g/dL ± 2	Women 14 g/dL ± 2
Hematocrit	47% ± 5	42% ± 5
Definitions		
Adequate hemoglobin saturation	$Pa_{O_2} > 60$ mmHg	
Hypercapnia	$Pa_{CO_2} > 45$ mmHg	
Hypoxemia	$Pa_{O_2} < 60$ mmHg	

SOURCE: O'Hara, 1995a.

IMAGING

Chest X-Ray

X-ray abnormalities may be minimal and can be negative in up to one-third of these patients. Typical findings in emphysema-predominant patients are overinflation, flat diaphragm, low position of the diaphragm at or below the seventh rib, and increased retrosternal air space. Retrosternal air space is defined as an increase in radiolucency of 2.5 cm or more between the sternum and the most anterior margin of the ascending aorta on the lateral view. Chronic bronchitis is difficult to see on x-ray and may be suggested by cardiac enlargement, lung field congestion, increased lung markings, and thickening of bronchial walls (parallel or tram lines). The chest x-ray is useful in ruling out other respiratory diseases (see Fig. 17-11-4).

Computed Tomography

Computed tomography (CT) is exceptional for showing anatomic details and particularly useful in demonstrating lung parenchyma and interstitial disease. CT provides direct visualization of emphysematous areas without interference from overlapping structures so that a pathologic diagnosis of emphysema can be made in a living patient. This is helpful when early diagnosis is useful, such as in the diagnosis of alpha$_1$-antitrypsin deficiency, and to demonstrate extensive upper lobe emphysema when a patient does not have PFT abnormalities.

DIFFERENTIAL DIAGNOSIS

Other bronchopulmonary diseases can coexist or be confused with COPD. The differential diagnosis includes upper airway obstruction (neck mass, upper airway narrowing), tuberculosis, lung cancer, cystic fibrosis, asthma, acute bronchitis, pneumothorax, bronchiectasis, chronic pulmonary embolism, and heart failure.

TREATMENT

Bronchodilators

Inhalation of bronchodilators is the first-line treatment for COPD. This is the recommendation of the ATS. Recent studies have shown that improvement in FEV_1 was significantly higher and exacerbations of COPD were lower when patients used a combination therapy of anticholinergic agents and beta-adrenergic agonists than when they used either drug alone.

Anticholinergic Agents

Inhaled anticholinergic agents cause bronchodilation by inhibiting the release of acetylcholine from the vagus nerve in respiratory smooth muscle. They are considered first-line therapy for emphysema. Anticholinergic agents have a slightly later onset of action than do beta-adrenergic agonists (BAAs), approximately 45 min, and a duration of 6 to 12 h. Ipratropium bromide (Atrovent) is available in metered-dose inhaler (MDI) form. The use of a spacing device allows the patient to inhale the aerosolized particles from a reservoir to improve delivery of the medication. Atropine sulfate and glycopyrrolate (Robinul) are used for nebulization. Nebulization is another delivery method for inhalation therapy. Nebulizer treatment takes 5 to 15 min and is a more expensive delivery method than MDI mainly because of the greater amount of medication required in solution for aerosolization. The advantages of this delivery method are greater deposition of medication in the large and small airways and ease of use, especially by the elderly, for whom inspiratory effort and coordination of the puff from the inhaler may be a problem.

The side effects of anticholinergic agents are minimal but include dry mouth, flushing of the skin, blurred vision, tachycardia, and urinary retention. Atropine seems to dilate large airways more effectively than do BAAs, primarily because of the greater number of cholinergic (muscarinic) receptors in the central airways compared with the peripheral airways. BAAs, seem to have better dilatory effects on small airways because the density of the beta$_2$ receptors increases as the peripheral airways narrow. This may account for the synergistic effects of BAAs and anticholinergic agents. As was stated above, studies show that stable COPD patients do better with routine doses of both drugs administered together two to four times a day. Inhalers are now available that contain the combination of both anticholinergic agents and BAAs. Also, anticholinergic solutions and BAAs may be mixed together in the chamber of a hand-held nebulizer for ease of delivery (see Table 17-11-5).

Beta Agonists

Inhaled beta-adrenergic agonists are used to reverse bronchospasm, addressing the chronic bronchitis component of COPD. Short-acting inhaled BAAs such as albuterol sulfate (Proventil, Ventolin) and metaproterenol sulfate (Alupent) have few side effects of skeletal

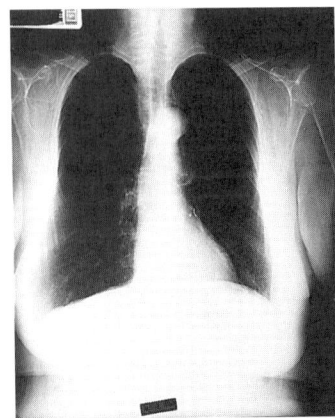

FIGURE 17-11-4. Example of a chest x-ray in a 65-year-old white female with COPD.

TABLE 17-11-5. **Anticholinergic Drug Dosing**

MEDICATION	ROUTE	DOSING
Atropine sulfate	Nebulizer	1–3 mg in 3 mL normal saline q 6 to 8 h (can be mixed with BAA dose)
Glycopyrrolate (Robinul)	Nebulizer	0.2–1.0 mg in 3 mL normal saline q 6 to 10 h (can be mixed with BAA dose)
Ipratropium bromide (Atrovent)	MDI	2 puffs qid (18 μg/puff)

SOURCE: O'Hara, 1995b.

TABLE 17-11-6. Beta Agonist Medications

MEDICATION	ROUTE	DOSE
Short-acting		
Albuterol sulfate (Proventil, Ventolin)	Oral	2–4 mg tid to qid
	0.5% solution	0.5 mL in 3 mL normal saline q 4 to 6 h
	MDI	2 puffs qid (90 μg/puff)
Metaproterenol sulfate (Alupent, Metaprel)	Oral	20 mg tid to qid
	5% solution	0.3 mL in 3 mL normal saline q 4 to 6 h
	MDI	2 puffs qid (650 μg/puff)
Terbutaline sulfate (Brethine, Bricanyl)	Oral	5 mg tid
	MDI	2 puffs qid (200 μg/puff)
Long-acting Salmeterol xinafoate (Serevent)	MDI	1 puff bid (42 μg/puff)

SOURCE: O'Hara, 1995b.

muscle tremor, palpitations, nervousness, tachycardia, and hypertension because less is absorbed into the systemic circulation. They can be self-administered conveniently with an MDI. The onset of action occurs within minutes, and the duration is 3 to 6 h. Oral BAAs have more systemic side effects and are used by patients who cannot handle the use of an MDI.

Salmeterol xinafoate (Serevent) is a long-acting selective inhaled beta$_2$ receptor agonist that was introduced into the United States in 1994 for chronic asthma. Patients with stable moderate to severe COPD have shown benefit from salmeterol. For breakthrough symptoms, rescue medication with a short-acting inhaled BAA up to eight puffs per day can be used in acute exacerbations. Patients must understand that salmeterol is used only for chronic treatment (see Table 17-11-6).

Methylxanthenes

Theophylline is a weaker bronchodilator than BAAs, but there is evidence that it has some anti-inflammatory properties as well as the ability to improve respiratory muscle strength, increase diaphragmatic contractility, increase right and left ventricular contractility, act as a pulmonary vasodilator to decrease pulmonary hypertension, and increase cardiac output. Even at therapeutic levels (10 to 20 mg/L), theophylline has a significant potential for adverse effects and drug interactions and should be monitored for toxicity. One should check levels 2 to 5 days after a change in dose or when symptoms of toxicity are present, in particular nausea, vomiting, tachycardia, hypertension, and tremor. Theophylline is considered an adjunct with routine doses of anticholinergic agents and BAAs in the treatment of stable COPD patients and is particularly useful for nocturnal dyspnea (see Table 17-11-7).

Corticosteroids

Corticosteroids are accepted for use in acute asthma. Recent studies show less efficacy for COPD. However, for patients with a greater predominance of the chronic bronchitis component, corticosteroids may be helpful in reducing inflammation in the airways. Patients who have a demonstrable improvement in FEV$_1$ with corticosteroids may benefit from this adjunctive treatment.

Corticosteroids are available in varying potencies and formulations that are based on a comparison to hydrocortisone. Because of the variety of responses to corticosteroids, there are several approaches to their use. Oral prednisone is four times more potent than hydrocortisone in regard to anti-inflammatory action and can be used for acute exacerbations of chronic treatment in conjunction with bronchodilators and theophylline. Patients can be given a challenge of 40 to 60 mg of oral prednisone per day; if at the end of 2 to 3 weeks FEV$_1$ im-

TABLE 17-11-7. Theophylline Side Effects, Interactions, and Dosing

Side effects
Headache
Anxiety
Tremulousness
Hypokalemia
Hypercalcemia
Nausea
Vomiting
Gastroesophageal sphincter relaxation
Tachycardia
Arrhythmias
Levels > 40 mg/L
Seizures
Death
Drug interactions
Erythromycin
Cimetidine (Tagamet)
Phenytoin (Dilantin)
Quinolones (e.g., Cipro)
Propranolol (Indural)
High-dose allopurinol
Rifampin
Barbiturates
Lithium
Dosing
Sustained-release products
Theo-Dur 200–300 mg qh or bid
Slo-bid 200–300 mg qh or bid (check levels appropriately)

SOURCE: Johannsen, 1994; O'Hara, 1995b.

proves 20 to 30 percent compared to baseline, consideration should be given to long-term therapy. Patients can be tapered from 40 to 60 mg per day to 20 mg over 1 to 2 weeks and then to less than 10 mg daily (5 to 7 mg per day or 15 to 20 mg on alternate days). The side effects of prednisone may develop if the daily dose is higher than 10 mg for longer than 3 weeks (see Table 17-11-8). Studies show that the improvement in FEV$_1$ may last as long as 6 months, after which a decline is seen. The annual decline in FEV$_1$ with corticosteroids, however, is slower than it is with bronchodilator treatment alone.

Inhaled corticosteroids (ICSs) can be used alone or in conjunction with oral prednisone. The advantage of ICSs is that they have the anti-inflammatory potency of oral corticosteroids with minimal systemic side effects. The maximum dose of ICSs is about 1.5 to 2.0 mg per day, which is equivalent to 10 mg of oral prednisone. The therapeutic effects of ICSs begin in 6 to 12 h, and maximum efficacy is achieved in 2 to 4 weeks. If patients respond well to ICSs, it may be

TABLE 17-11-8. Corticosteroid Side Effects

Short course (>10 mg for less than 3 weeks)
Increased appetite
Acne
Fluid retention
Mood alterations
Hyperglycemia in susceptible persons
Long-term effects (>10 mg for longer than 3 weeks)
Hypertension
Diabetes mellitus in predisposed persons
Osteoporosis
Cushingoid obesity
Poor wound healing
Personality changes
Glaucoma
Cataracts
Dyspepsia
Suppression of the hypothalamic-pituitary-adrenal axis

SOURCE: O'Hara, 1995b.

TABLE 17-11-9. Inhaled Corticosteroid Dosing

METERED-DOSE INHALER	DOSE
Beclomethasone dipropionate (Beclovent, Vanceril; inhaler includes spacer)	4 puffs (42 μg/puff) bid to qid
Dexamethasone sodium phosphate (Decadron)	3 puffs (84 μg/puff) bid to qid
Flunisolide (Aerobid)	2 puffs (250 μg/puff) bid to qid
Triamcinolone acetonide (Azmacort; inhaler includes spacer)	4 puffs (100 μg/puff) bid to qid

SOURCE: O'Hara, 1995b.

possible to lower the dose of oral corticosteroids or withdraw them altogether (see Table 17-11-9).

For acute exacerbations, a short course of oral prednisone can be helpful for patients with or without long-term low-dose oral prednisone or ICS treatment. The onset of action takes a few hours, but the effects of one dose may last 16 to 36 h. A short course may prevent a relapse (see Table 17-11-10).

Patients can be started on bronchodilators, theophylline, and corticosteroids individually or in combination, depending on which symptoms of emphysema or chronic bronchitis predominate. Medications can be maximized in a stepwise fashion. Patients may feel better on a regimen containing a combination of medications, although there may not be a significant improvement in FEV_1.

Other Anti-Inflammatory Agents

Cromylin sodium (Intal) and nedocromil sodium (Tilade) have been used in the treatment of asthma. Their use may be helpful in conjunction with respiratory tract allergies in association with COPD, but their use in the treatment of COPD has not been proved effective.

Mucokinetics

Mucokinetic agents may be helpful for patients with chronic bronchitis predominance. They facilitate mucociliary clearance by increasing mucus production while decreasing the viscosity and tenaciousness of mucus. Oral iodides have antiallergic and anti-inflammatory properties. They serve as an expectorant by stimulating the vagal-gastropulmonary reflex and as a mucolytic by splitting mucoproteins. Guiafenesin is a common iodinated glycerol that is available in liquid or tablet form. It also can be found in combination with other ingredients for cough and rhinorrhea. BAAs and the methylxanthenes also have mucociliary clearance properties (see Table 17-11-11).

TABLE 17-11-10. Oral Prednisone Burst

No previous oral prednisone use: 30 mg/d for 1 to 2 weeks
Previous oral prednisone use: 60 mg/d for 1 to 2 weeks
With or without previous oral prednisone use 40–60 mg/d for 5 to 7 days 40–80 mg/d for 5 to 7 days, then taper
Tapering suggestions 40 mg 40 × 2 days, 30 × 2 days, 20 × 2 days, 15 × 2 days, 10 × 2 days, 5 × 2 days 60 mg 60 × 1 day, 50 × 1 day, 40 × 1 day, 30 × 1 day, 20 × 1 day, 15 × 1 day, 10 × 2 days, 5 × 2 days

SOURCE: O'Hara, 1995b.

TABLE 17-11-11. Mucokinetic Drugs

DRUG	ROUTE	DOSE
Guaifenesin	Tablets	200–400 mg q 4 h up to 2400 mg/24 h
Organidin NR	Elixir, 1.2%	1 teaspoon qid
Humibid LA	Tablets	600 mg, 1 or 2 bid up to 2400 mg/24 h

SOURCE: *Physicians' Desk Reference,* 1995.

Oxygen

Supplemental oxygen (O_2) therapy has been shown to improve survival and quality of life. Patients at rest with a Pa_{O_2} less than 55 mmHg with or without signs of cor pulmonale or a Sa_{O_2} less than 88 percent benefit from supplemental O_2. Low-flow O_2 by nasal cannula of 1 to 3 L raises Pa_{O_2} to 60 to 80 mmHg and Sa_{O_2} to approximately 90 percent. Patients are encouraged to use the O_2 15 to 24 h a day because survival is improved so significantly with continuous use. O_2 helps reduce hypoxemia, which in turn reduces pulmonary hypertension. The purpose of supplemental O_2 therapy is to enhance physiologic delivery of O_2 to the tissues. There are concerns that O_2 therapy will cause Pa_{CO_2} to increase, blunting the chemoreceptors for respiratory drive. It is theorized that the increase in Pa_{CO_2} is due to the increased ventilation of the anatomic dead space. If the Pa_{CO_2} stabilizes and does not lead to an increased respiratory acidosis, it is considered more dangerous to withdraw or withhold O_2 than to prevent the increasing Pa_{CO_2}. Only hypoxemia is treated; hypercapnia is not treated but is monitored for respiratory acidosis.

Patients who desaturate during exercise to less than 88 percent also benefit from supplemental O_2. It is documented that COPD patients desaturate when sleeping, especially during rapid eye movement (REM) sleep and may experience periods of apnea. The supine position increases hypoxemia and decreases the respiratory drive. Sleep studies have shown diaphragmatic pauses and irregular breathing in association with REM sleep. Sa_{O_2} may drop 10 to 50 percent for more than 30 min during REM sleep (see Table 17-11-12).

Diuretics, Digitalis, and Phlebotomy

Patients with COPD may exhibit pedal edema even without right-sided congestive heart failure. Diuretics may provide symptomatic relief. Digoxin is a weak inotropic stimulant for the right ventricle and should be used in patients with both right and left ventricular failure. In the past, phlebotomy was used in patients whose hematocrit was above 55 to 60 percent. It was thought that the increase in blood viscosity contributed to right-sided heart strain. Now supplemental O_2 therapy is used.

TABLE 17-11-12. Indications for Oxygen Therapy

Continuous therapy
  At rest on room air
    Pa_{O_2} 55 mgHg*
    Pa_{O_2} 55–59 mmHg with peripheral edema (cor pulmonale), polycythemia (hematocrit > 55%), congestive heart failure
    Sa_{O_2} < 88%*
    Hematocrit > 55%

Intermittent therapy
  Nocturnal hypoxemia
    Pa_{O_2} < 55 mmHg*
    Sa_{O_2} < 88%*
  Exercise-induced hypoxemia
    Pa_{O_2} < 55 mmHg*
    Sa_{O_2} < 88%*

*Will be reimbursed by Medicare.
SOURCE: Fei and Murata, 1994; Scientific American, 1995.

Antibiotics

COPD patients are at risk for lower respiratory infections as a result of reduced mucociliary clearance. These patients probably are afflicted more often with viral illness that goes on to become secondarily superimposed with bacterial infections. COPD patients should be considered for antibiotic treatment for 7 to 10 days when there is an increase in dyspnea, increased sputum production, and purulent sputum. The organisms most often recovered from the sputum of COPD patients are *Haemophilus influenzae* and *Streptococcus pneumoniae*. *Mycoplasma pneumoniae* and *Moraxella (Branhamella) catarrhalis* are also common. The literature shows an improvement in acute exacerbations in ambulatory patients with antibiotic treatment, but antibiotic prophylaxis consisting of 1 week of oral medication per month is considered controversial. If sputum cultures are not taken, consideration for empirical treatment should be given on the basis of the common organisms, and if there is no improvement in 2 days, one should consider a broader-spectrum agent to cover the less common organisms, such as *Enterobacteriaceae* and *Pseudomonas* species (see Table 17-11-13).

Antiviral Treatment

The original antiviral agent, amantadine (Symmetrel syrup 50 mg/5 mL, 100 mg bid), may help decrease the severity of the symptoms of influenza A. There is a new class of antiviral agents on the market called neuraminidase inhibitors. It is reported to be effective against influenza types A and B and is available in oral, intranasal, and inhaled forms. Studies have shown that symptoms of the flu are shortened by a few days. The medication must be given within 30 to 48 h of the onset of symptoms to be effective. Studies in the elderly have been limited, and at this point, more studies will need to be done to confirm its efficacy in patients with COPD.

Vaccinations

It is recommended that patients with COPD have influenza vaccinations annually to prevent lung damage from viral infections. Pneumovax 23 (Merck) is a pneumococcal vaccine that is effective against 23 types of pneumococcal strains that are responsible for 85 to 90 percent of

TABLE 17-11-13. Examples of Antibiotic Coverage and Dosing for Outpatients

DRUG	BRAND NAME	DOSE	COVERED ORGANISMS OR PARTICULAR INDICATION
Penicillins			
Penicillin*	Pen V	250 mg tid or 500 bid	*S. aureus, S. pneumoniae, S. pyogenes, S. viridans* group
	Bicillin C-R	2.4 million units IM, then use oral agent	Same as penicillin
	Wicillin	1.0 million units IM, then use oral agent	Same as penicillin
Ampicillin		250–500 mg qid	Same as pencillin, some gram-negatives, *H. influenzae* (not β-lactam-producing)
Amoxicillin		250–500 mg tid	Same as ampicillin
Amoxicillin/clavulanate potassium	Augmentin	250–500 mg tid	Same as pencillin, *H. influenzae* (β-lactam-producing), *M. catarrhalis*
Cephalosporins			
First generation			
Cefadroxil	Duricef	500 mg bid	*S. aureus, S. epidermidis, S. pneumoniae, S. pyogenes, M. catarrhalis*
Cephalexin	Keflex	250–500 mg qid	Gram-positives, some gram-negatives
Second generation			
Cefaclor	Ceclor	250–500 mg tid	*S. pneumoniae, S. pyogenes, H. influenzae, M. catarrhalis,* some gram-negatives
Cefuroxime	Ceftin	250–500 mg tid	Same as cefaclor
Third generation			
Cefixime	Suprax	400 mg qd	Gram-positives, *H. influenzae, M. catarrhalis,* gram-negatives (including *Pseudomonas aeruginosa*)
Ceftriaxone	Rocephin	1 to 2 g IM, then use oral agent	Gram-positives, *H. influenzae, M. catarrhalis,* gram-negatives (± *P. aeruginosa*)
Macrolides			
Erythromycin		250 mg qid or 500 mg bid	Beta-hemolytic streptococci, *S. aureus, S. pneumoniae, S. pyogenes, S. viridans,* ±*H. influenzae, Legionella pneumophilia, M. catarrhalis, M. pneumoniae*
Clarithromycin	Biaxin	250–500 bid	Erythromycin-resistant organisms, β-lactam-producing *H. influenzae, M. catarrhalis*
Azithromycin	Zithromax	500 mg day 1; 250 mg days 2 through 5	Same as clarithromycin
Tetracyclines			
Tetracycline		500 mg bid to qid	Gram-positives, *H. influenzae, M. pneumoniae, M. catarrhalis*
Doxycycline	Vibramycin	100 mg bid	Same as tetracycline
Quinolones			
Ciprofloxacin	Cipro	500–750 mg bid	Gram-positives, resistant gram-negatives, methicillin-resistant *S. aureus, P. aeruginosa*
Ofloxacin	Floxin	400 mg bid	Same as ciprofloxacin
Sulfa			
Trimethoprim-sulfamethoxazole	Bactrim	Double-strength bid	Gram-positives, *Diplococcus pneumoniae, S. pneumoniae,* gram-negatives (except *P. aeruginosa*), *H. influenzae, L. pneumophilia, M. catarrhalis*

*All medications given orally unless indicated.
SOURCE: Dantzker et al, 1995; Johannsen, 1994; Sanford et al, 1995.

pneumococcal infections. The recommendation is that COPD patients be vaccinated at least once and that consideration be given to revaccination every 5 to 10 years.

Antiprotease Therapy

Alpha$_1$-antitrypsin deficiency is an inherited disorder that causes destruction of interstitial elastin fibers in alveolar walls by elastase. The deficiency can be detected by serum levels of alpha$_1$-antitrypsin below 11 μM. The ATS recommends recombinant antiprotease replacement therapy consisting of injections of purified alpha$_1$-antitrypsin weekly (60 mg/kg) or monthly (250 mg/kg) for selected candidates. This therapy is costly and controversial and is under clinical investigation.

Pulmonary Rehabilitation

Pulmonary rehabilitation is a multidisciplinary approach. The goal is to maximize functional capacity in activities of daily living and quality of life. It includes respiratory therapy, physical therapy, nutrition, psychology, and social work. Secondary goals of pulmonary rehabilitation are to increase exercise tolerance, teach respiratory muscle training techniques, teach energy conservation techniques, provide psychosocial support, and give the patient information about the disease process, the use of medications, and smoking cessation. The best candidates for rehabilitation are those who are motivated to improve their health status. All patients can benefit from pulmonary rehabilitation, but those with mild to moderate disease probably benefit the most.

SURGICAL TREATMENT

Lung Transplantation

The first successful single-lung transplantation was performed in 1983 for pulmonary fibrosis. Since that time, single-lung transplantation has been used for patients with end-stage emphysema. The majority of transplant patients are those with alpha$_1$-antitrypsin deficiency. Since they are younger than patients with smoking-induced COPD, in general, they are better surgical candidates. Bilateral lung transplants have been performed in patients with chronic bronchitis. In spite of problems with the availability of donors, postoperative infections, organ rejection, and immunosuppression, survival rates have been reported to be as high as 93 percent at 1 year, 74 percent at 3 years, and 50 percent at 5 years. Significant improvement in pulmonary function has made lung transplantation a viable therapeutic option for end-stage disease.

Reduction Pneumoplasty

Reduction pneumoplasty or bullectomy is another treatment option for bullous emphysema. The procedure was introduced in the 1950s. It was reintroduced in 1994 with modern surgical techniques and has gained some popularity. The volume of one lung or both lungs is reduced by 20 to 40 percent in the hyperinflated areas. Respiratory mechanics are improved because the chest wall and diaphragm return to a more normal position. The FEV$_1$/FVC ratio is greatly improved, Pa$_{O_2}$ is increased, Pa$_{CO_2}$ is decreased, and up to half of these patients do not need supplemental oxygen. Mortality rates have been reported as 3 to 15 percent at 2 years. Survival rates are higher than they are with lung transplantation because there are fewer postoperative complications. Despite the enthusiasm for this procedure, it is not performed as often as it might be because of the cessation of payment for the procedure by the Health Care Financing Administration (Medicare) in 1996.

ACUTE RESPIRATORY FAILURE

Acute respiratory failure is defined as a decrease in Pa$_{O_2}$ of 10 to 15 mmHg from baseline ABG values or an increase in Pa$_{CO_2}$ with pH $\leq$7.3 (acidemia). Hypoventilation at the level of the alveoli and pulmonary capillaries is the mechanism of failure in obstructive disease, causing an increase in the ventilation-perfusion mismatch. These patients may complain of headache, visual disturbance, memory loss, confusion, and palpitations. Reversal of hypoxemia corrects the acidemia. Respiratory failure calls for admission to an intensive care unit. The criteria for intubation and mechanical ventilation include altered mental status, labored breathing (tachypnea >30 breaths per minute), hypoxemia not responsive to O$_2$ therapy, and rising hypercapnia. The mortality rate in patients who undergo mechanical ventilation for any reason is as high as 38 percent.

PATIENT EDUCATION

Smoking Cessation

Since there is no cure for COPD, quitting smoking is the number one intervention to help slow the deleterious effects and reduce the complications of COPD. Nicotine substitution in gum or patch form is available to help patients with smoking cessation. Health care providers should encourage smoking cessation at every opportunity, realizing that patients may fail at quitting smoking several times before achieving success. Consider antidepressant therapy for patients who are trying to quit.

TABLE 17-11-14. Instructions for Using Metered-Dose Inhalers

WITHOUT SPACER	ALTERNATIVE METHOD WITHOUT SPACER	WITH SPACER
1. Put inhaler together and shake canister		Put inhaler together with spacer and shake canister
2. Take cap off and close lips around mouthpiece. Be sure tongue is away from opening. Hold canister with index finger on top and thumb on bottom	Take cap off and hold mouthpiece approximately 1 in (3 cm) from open mouth. Hold canister with index finger on top and thumb on bottom	Close lips around tubing of spacer mouthpiece. Be sure tongue is away from opening. Hold canister with index finger on top and thumb on bottom
3. Exhale completely through mouth		
4. Begin to inhale slowly and squeeze canister		
5. At end of inhalation, hold breath for 4 to 10 s if possible		
6. Wait 1 min before inhaling any more puffs		
7. Use bronchodilators before using inhaled corticosteroids		
8. Rinse out mouth after steroid use		

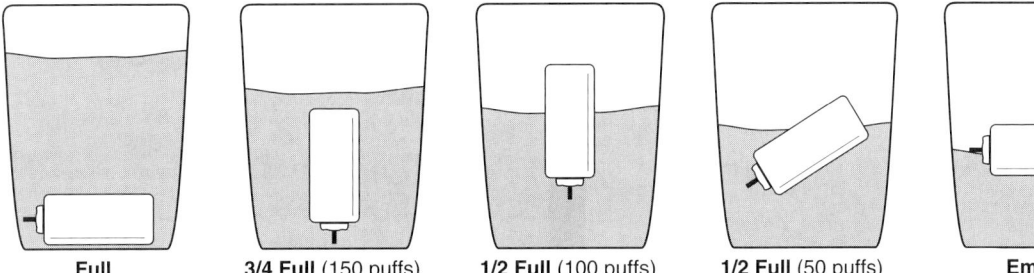

| Full | 3/4 Full (150 puffs) | 1/2 Full (100 puffs) | 1/2 Full (50 puffs) | Empty |

FIGURE 17-11-5. Method of estimating the amount of medication in an inhaler canister. (*From Dantzker et al, 1995; Pagliaro and Pagliaro, 1986.*)

Environmental Concerns

Patients with hypoxemia should avoid high altitudes, which may lower Pa_{O_2} levels. Patients should live at altitudes lower than 3500 to 4000 ft and may need supplemental O_2 when traveling at high altitudes. Extremes of temperature and humidity may exacerbate airway hyper-reactivity and bronchospasm. Patients should be advised to use air-conditioning in the summer and humidifiers in the winter. Particulate matter from air pollution or ozone (more than 0.12 parts per million) may irritate the airways. Patients should be advised to curtail outdoor activities on days of poor air quality. Efforts should be made to eliminate allergens from a patient's environment.

Advance Directives

All Medicare and Medicaid providers are required to inform all patients about their right to make choices regarding health care under provisions of the Self-Determination Act, which became effective on December 1, 1991. Discussion should be initiated regarding do not resuscitate orders and a living will or durable power of attorney for health care when patients are not critically ill. Patients can designate another person to make health care decisions if they are incapacitated and/or can document their wishes regarding resuscitation and life support measures.

Exercise

Exercise should be encouraged to maintain cardiovascular fitness and skeletal muscle tone. Walking is recommended. Exercise also raises self-esteem, increases the capacity to maintain the activities of daily living, reduces breathlessness, and increases exercise capacity.

Nutrition

The work of breathing imposes high metabolic demands and requires high caloric expenditure. There can be an increase in resting energy expenditure of 10 to 20 percent without the matching caloric intake to counteract weight loss. The loss of more than 50 percent of ideal weight puts a patient at risk for nutritional deficiencies and decreased muscle strength of the diaphragm. A high-fat, high-protein (20 percent of total calories), low-carbohydrate diet is recommended because of the increased CO_2 from the by-products of the breakdown of carbohydrates. Adequate hydration of 2 L of water per day helps keep mucus secretions thin even in persons with right-sided heart failure.

Depression

Depression is seen in 42 percent of patients with COPD. It is described as an adjustment disorder with depressed mood because of identifiable stressors. These patients exhibit low self-esteem and lack confidence and spontaneity. The tricyclic antidepressant medications have been shown to produce improvement in patients with depression and COPD. The tricyclics have atropine-like properties that promote bronchodilation and decrease obstruction. Nortriptyline and desipramine have been used commonly.

Follow-up

One must make sure that patients understand the correct technique for the use of inhalers (see Table 17-11-14). Patients can estimate how much medication is in the canister by putting it in a glass of water. When it is empty, it floats (see Fig 17-11-5). Patients should be seen in the office at least every 6 months for follow-up even if they are feeling well. It should be discussed in advance what patients should do in case of an acute exacerbation in terms of additional (rescue) medications or if they should go to the office or emergency department for treatment.

REFERRAL TO A PULMONARY SPECIALIST

There are no hard and fast rules about referring patients to a pulmonary specialist. The history, physical examination, and initial studies of chest x-ray and PFTs should be obtained. It is recommended that patients be referred to a pulmonologist whenever a provider becomes uncomfortable with the treatment regimen. Evaluation of patients for alpha$_1$-antitrypsin deficiency, CT scan, lung transplantation, or reduction pneumoplasty falls into the sphere of care of the specialist.

BIBLIOGRAPHY

Anderson KD: Change in quality of life after lung volume reduction surgery. *Am J Crit Care* (8)6:389–396, 1999.

Braunwald E, Isselbacher KJ, Petersdorf RG, et al (eds): *Harrison's Principles of Internal Medicine,* 11th ed. Companion Handbook. New York, McGraw-Hill, 1988.

Campbell S: For COPD: A Combination of ipratropium bromide and albuterol sulfate is more effective than albuterol base. *Arch Intern Med* 195:156–160, 1999.

Calverley PMA, Pride NB (eds): *Chronic Obstructive Pulmonary Disease.* London, Chapman & Hall, 1995.

Chapman KR: *Undertreatment of Chronic Obstructive Pulmonary Disease.* 1999 annual meeting symposium highlights. Yardly, PA, Medical Association Communications, 1999.

Dantzker DR, MacIntyre NR, Bakow ED: *Comprehensive Respiratory Care.* Philadelphia, Saunders, 1995.

Fei RL, Murata GH: Contemporary management of the patient with chronic obstructive pulmonary disease. *Compr Ther* 20(5):277–281, 1994.

Fishman MC, Hoffman AR, Klausner RD, Thaler MS: *Medicine,* 2d ed. Philadelphia, Lippincott, 1985.

Friedman M, Serby CW, Menjoge SS, Wilson D, Hilleman DE, Witek TJ: Pharmacoeconomic evaluation of a combination of ipratropium plus albuterol compared with ipratropium alone and albuterol alone in COPD. *Chest* 115:635–641, 1999.

Griffith HW, Dambro MR, Griffith J: *The 5 Minute Clinical Consult.* Philadelphia, Lea & Febiger, 1994.

Hahn MS: Chronic obstructive pulmonary disease: Understanding this progressive illness. *AdPA,* April 1996, pp 15–19.

Johannsen JM: Chronic obstructive pulmonary disease: Current comprehensive care for emphysema and bronchitis. *Nurs Pract* 19(1):59–67, 1994.

Kelley WN, (ed): *Essentials of Internal Medicine.* Philadelphia, Lippincott, 1994.

Labus JB: *The Physician Assistant Medical Handbook.* Philadelphia, Saunders, 1995.

Niewoehner DE, Erbland ML, Deupree RH, Collins D, Gross NJ, Light RW, et al: Effect of systemic glucocorticoids on exacerbations of chronic obstructive pulmonary disease. *N Engl J Med* 340(25):1941–1947, 1999.

O'Hara MM: Understanding asthma: Why it happens and how to assess your adult patient. *J Am Acad Physician Assist* 8(3):20–35, 1995a.

O'Hara MM: Understanding asthma: New priorities in treatment. *J Am Acad Physician Assist* 8(7):60–78, 1995b.

Pagliaro AM, Pagliaro LA: *Pharmacologic Aspects of nursing.* St. Louis, Mosby, 1986.

Pauwels RA, Löfdahl C-G, Laitinen LA, et al: Long-term treatment with inhaled budesonide in persons with mild chronic obstructive pulmonary disease who continue smoking. *N Engl J Med* 340(25):1948–1953, 1999.

Peterson M, Rahr R, Blessing D, Ayachi S: Chronic obstructive pulmonary disease: Improving the outcome. *Physician Assist* 19(11):39–53, 1995.

Physicians' Desk Reference, 49th ed. Montvale, NJ, Medical Economics, 1995.

Sanford JP, Gilbert DN, Sande MA: *The Sanford Guide to Antimicrobial Therapy.* Dallas, Antimicrobial Therapy, 1995.

Scientific American Medicine. SAM-CD, Jan. 1996. Online Computer Services. *Chronic Obstructive Diseases of the Lung.* New York, Scientific American, 1995.

West JB: *Pulmonary Pathophysiology: The Essentials,* 3d ed. Baltimore, Williams & Wilkins, 1987.

Young J, Fry-Smith A, Hyde C: Lung volume reduction surgery (LVRS) for chronic obstructive pulmonary disease (COPD) with underlying severe emphysema. *Thorax* 54:779–789, 1999.

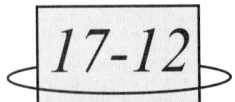

SARCOIDOSIS

Susan S. Eng-Ma

DEFINITION

The term *sarcoidosis* derives from Greek roots meaning "the formation of abnormal flesh." Sarcoidosis is a chronic multisystem inflammatory disorder of unknown cause that is characterized by the accumulation of noncaseating granulomas in multiple organs, especially the lungs, and in the lymph nodes in the mediastinum and hilar regions. Any organ system can be affected, giving sarcoidosis protean clinical presentations.

EPIDEMIOLOGY

There appears to be a higher incidence of sarcoidosis in the winter and early spring months than in the rest of the year. Sarcoidosis affects people of all ages, races, and genders worldwide. Typically, patients are between ages 20 and 40 at diagnosis and were previously healthy, although the disease may occur at any age. Race and gender appear to affect the incidence. The disease prevalence is accepted as being much higher among those of African-American or northern European descent, whereas sarcoidosis of childhood is more common among whites. In the United States, sarcoidosis has an age-adjusted annual incidence of 35.5 per 100,000 for blacks and 10.9 per 100,000 for whites. It is seen more often in women than in men.

ETIOLOGY

It has been about a century since one of the first descriptions of sarcoidosis by Boeck, but its cause remains unknown. Historically, cases of sarcoidosis were noted to cluster geographically as well as temporally. This information, coupled with the antigen-stimulated phenotype sometimes seen in T cells derived from patients with sarcoidosis, has suggested the possibility of an infectious cause of the disease. The role of T cells in propagating the inflammatory response may be just as significant as their ability to discern specific antigens. Mycobacteria

species, particularly those without cell walls, continue to be very suspicious as the infectious cause of sarcoidosis. Some authorities suspect that human herpes virus 8 plays a highly suspected role in the disease; this is still under investigation.

DIFFERENTIAL DIAGNOSIS

Other diseases to be considered generally include infectious diseases such as tuberculosis and fungal infections, infection with mycobacteria other than tuberculosis (MOTT), hypersensitivity pneumonitis, berylliosis, pneumoconioses, foreign body granulomatosis, and lymphomas.

CLINICAL MANIFESTATIONS

Many patients with sarcoidosis may be asymptomatic at presentation, with only hilar adenopathy found on routine chest radiographs. In symptomatic patients, an insidious onset of symptoms from pulmonary, ocular, or cutaneous involvement is usual. Symptomatic patients may present with the gradual progression of cough, dyspnea on exertion, retrosternal chest pain, and occasional wheezing. More advanced disease with mycetomas or endobronchial disease may even present with hemoptysis. Some patients may present with nonspecific constitutional symptoms of fatigue, weakness, malaise, fever, and weight loss. A variety of typical clinical manifestations are listed in Table 17-12-1.

Individuals may present acutely with the triad of polyarthralgias, erythema nodosum, and uveitis along with bilateral hilar and often paratracheal adenopathy. When this is accompanied with a fever, it is suggestive of Lofgren's syndrome, which has a good prognosis. Sarcoidosis can present as an acute arthropathy that involves the PIP and large joints. It frequently presents as a migratory arthritis and a chronic arthritis also can develop.

CLINICAL EVALUATION

Since the causative agent is unknown, sarcoidosis remains a diagnosis of exclusion. Meticulous history taking with an emphasis on

TABLE 17-12-1. Clinical Manifestations of Sarcoidosis

ORGAN SYSTEM	SIGNS AND SYMPTOMS
Intrathoracic: lungs and/or lymph nodes (90%)*	Asymptomatic nonproductive cough, shortness of breath, chest pain, wheezing, radiographic abnormalities
Ocular (20–30%)	Iridocyclitis, chorioretinitis, keratoconjunctivitis, glaucoma, cataract, blindness, Heerfordt's syndrome†
Cutaneous (20–30%)	Erythema nodosum, lupus pernio, nodular or flat plaques, subcutaneous nodules
Reticuloendothelial system	Peripheral lymphadenopathy (40%), hepatosplenomegaly (20%)
Musculoskeletal (10–15%)	Polyarthritis, bone cysts, myositis
Myocardial (5%)	Palpitations, syncope, dizziness, chest pain, arrhythmia, sudden death
Nervous system (5%)	Seizures, basal granulomatoid meningitis, hypothalamic hypopituitarism or hypothyroidism, cranial nerve palsies, hydrocephalus
Exocrine glands (4%)	Painless swelling of the parotid glands, keratoconjunctiva sicca††
Renal	Hypercalcemia (10–20%), hypercalciuria (20–25%), nephrocalcinosis

*Percentage of patients with involvement.
†Anterior uveitis, parotid gland enlargement, facial palsy, fever.
‡Lacrimal gland enlargement, xerostomia, xerophthalmia.

occupational and environmental exposure coupled with a thorough physical examination concentrating on the lung, skin, eye, liver, and heart is of the utmost importance.

The initial evaluation should include pulmonary function tests, ophthalmologic evaluation with slit-lamp examination, electrocardiography, liver function tests, and serum calcium levels to provide baseline information. Elevated levels of serum calcium are related to the increased activity of the macrophages within the granulomas, which produces more 1,25-dihydroxyvitamin D. Such laboratory tests may reveal abnormalities significant of occult multiorgan system involvement. Tuberculin skin testing with controls usually is performed, and cutaneous anergy to recall antigens such as tuberculin, *Candida,* and mumps is typical.

Associated laboratory abnormalities include hypercalcemia, hypercalciuria, and elevated liver enzymes, especially alkaline phosphatase. Polyclonal hypergammaglobulinemia often can occur in 25 to 80 percent of all cases, and leukopenia can exist in 5 to 10 percent. An increase in serum angiotensin converting enzyme (ACE) is noted in laboratory studies; ACE comes from the cell membrane of epithelioid cells of the sarcoid granuloma, and its synthesis is controlled by T lymphocytes. ACE once was felt to be helpful in the diagnosis of sarcoid but now is considered too nonspecific to be useful.

Pulmonary function testing usually reveals a primarily restrictive picture with decreased lung volumes, increased elastic recoil (decreased compliance), and a decrease in diffusion capacity (DL_{CO}). Reduced expiratory flow rates indicative of airflow obstruction occur in about 20 percent of these patients.

RADIOGRAPHIC IMAGING

Several radiographic patterns of pulmonary involvement have been described, and chest radiographs may be normal or show bilateral hilar or mediastinal adenopathy with or without pulmonary parenchymal involvement. The upper lobes of the lungs tend to be more involved than are the lower lobes. The clinical "staging" of chest radiographs is shown in Table 17-12-2. Frequently, a progression from one "stage" to another is not systematically recorded.

Computed tomography of the chest is most useful in the workup of sarcoidosis when the findings on chest x-ray are atypical or when there is a need for better definition of mediastinal lymph node involvement. High-resolution computed tomography (HRCT) is more sensitive than x-rays in appreciating the presence of nodules in the parenchyma and their exact position in relation to the pleura and vessels. CT is most useful in the evaluation of advanced sarcoidosis because of its ability to visualize bullae, infection, bronchiectasis, vascular obstruction, and mycetoma formation but cannot be used as a diagnostic tool.

OTHER DIAGNOSTIC STUDIES

The bronchoalveolar lavage differential cell count of sarcoidosis typically shows increased proportions of total and CD4 T-lymphocyte

TABLE 17-12-2. Chest Radiographic Stages in Sarcoidosis

DESCRIPTION	FREQUENCY OF PRESENTATION, %
0: Normal chest radiograph	10
I: Bilateral hilar adenopathy; paratracheal adenopathy possible	50
II: Adenopathy with pulmonary parenchymal involvement	30
III: Pulmonary parenchymal involvement without adenopathy	10*
IV: Pulmonary fibrosis with honeycombing	

*Frequency combined for stages III and IV.

cells compared with other interstitial lung diseases and can support the diagnosis of sarcoidosis but is not diagnostic in itself. The need for tissue diagnosis should be determined clinically, and if required, transbronchial biopsy of the lung is preferred to open lung biopsy. Biopsy of the tissue for sarcoidosis should be obtained from an obviously involved organ or tissue. For example, liver and conjunctival biopsies should be done only when those organs are clearly involved clinically. The finding of noncaseating granuloma on a lung biopsy specimen is highly suggestive of the diagnosis of sarcoidosis.

The Kveim-Siltzbach skin test, in which homogenates of human sarcoid cells and tissue are injected intradermally to induce granuloma formation, has been used with variable results. It is not widely available and has not been standardized with U.S. Food and Drug Administration (FDA) approval. Gallium 67 scans once used were to evaluate for the disease but have been noted to be nonspecific; radioactivity has resulted in decreased clinical utility.

TREATMENT

Treatment is nonspecific. Patients initially should be observed for a period of no less than 6 months, with possible spontaneous recovery. Corticosteroids are indicated to ameliorate rapidly progressive pulmonary impairment; cardiac, neurologic, ocular, or splenic involvement; and hypercalcemia. Relapse is common when treatment is discontinued, but it remains unclear whether therapy actually alters the course or the eventual outcome of disease. The current protocol for therapy is debatable. For patients with non-life-threatening disease, it is recommended that 30 to 40 mg daily for 8 to 12 weeks be given, with gradual tapering to 10 to 20 mg every other day over a 6- to 12-month period. Observe for potential relapse and reinstitute therapy as needed. It is controversial to keep patients on therapy for 1 year or longer since complications may arise. For patients with potentially life-threatening organ involvement, a maximum dose of 1 mg/kg is suggested.

Alternative agents such as methotrexate and azathioprine appear to be promising in patients with refractory disease and those who cannot tolerate the side effects of corticosteroids. The clinical usefulness of cyclophosphamide, chlorambucil, hydroxychloroquine, and cyclosporine remains to be determined since their use has been limited and anecdotal.

Surgery is reserved for patients with severe organ (lung, heart, or liver) damage, although reoccurrence of sarcoidosis has been noted in some patients even with the use of corticosteroids and immunosuppressive medications.

TREATMENT WARNING

Any sign or symptom suggestive of adrenal insufficiency should be evaluated on an emergency basis. Moreover, a potential complication for patients on long-term steroid therapy is glucocorticoid induced osteoporosis. It is essential to provide proper nutritional counseling, calcium supplements, estrogen replacement therapy, and weight-bearing exercises to prevent bone loss. Early monitoring can minimize unnecessary bone loss with the use of dual energy x-ray absorptiometry on a regular basis.

NOTES AND PEARLS

The following points should be considered:

- Patients may have typical clinical and/or radiographic features but atypical presentations and may have symptoms that mimic those of other disorders, such as tuberculosis and malignancy.
- For reasons that have not been identified, the pancreas is not involved in sarcoidosis, and so diabetes mellitus is not a complication of sarcoidosis.
- Patients who have onset at a later age with multisystem involvement and stage III radiographic findings often have a worse prognosis compared with those with acute Lofgren's syndrome.

• The typical clinical presentation of a young, previously healthy African-American woman should alert providers to be highly suspicious of the disease.

PATIENT EDUCATION AND SELF-CARE

Patients should be well informed about the disease, its possible course and prognosis, and complications and side effects from the medications. Patients should be warned about abrupt discontinuation of steroid therapy. Proper referrals to support groups and other resources will permit patients to explore and share their experiences:

• Sarcoidosis National Network, American Lung Association, 1726 M Street, NW, Suite 902, Washington, DC 20036, (202) 785-3355
• American Lung Association, 1740 Broadway, New York, NY 10019-4374, (212) 315-8700 or (800) LUNG-USA, http://orchin.uc.edu/htdocs/ala/sarcoidosis.html
• Sarcoid Research Institute, 3475 Central Avenue, Memphis, TN 38111, (901) 766-6951
• Sarcoid Research Institute, http://www.netten.net/soskelnt
• Sarcoidosis Worldwide Support Group, http://members.aol.com/swsg2/index,htm
• National Jewish Medical and Research Center, http://njc.org/MSUhtml/MSU/Sarcoidosis.html

BIBLIOGRAPHY

Goldman L, Bennett JC: *Cecil Textbook of Medicine,* 21st ed. Philadelphia, Saunders, 2000.

Hurst JW (ed): *Medicine for the Practicing Physician,* 4th ed. Stamford, CT, Appleton & Lange, 1996.

Johns CJ, Michele TM: The clinical management of sarcoidosis: A 50-year experience at the Johns Hopkins Hospital. *Medicine Baltimore* 78(2):65–111, 1999.

Jones RE, Chatham WW: Update on Sarcoidosis. *Curr Opin Rheumatol* 11:83–87, 1999.

Newman LS, Rose CS, Maier LA: Sarcoidosis. *N Engl J Med* 336(17):1224–1234, 1997.

Singleton JK, Sandowski SA, Green-Hernandez C, et al: *Primary Care,* 1st ed. Philadelphia, Lippincott Williams & Wilkins, 1999.

Stobo JD, Hellmann DB, Ladenson PW, et al: *Principles and Practice of Medicine,* 23rd ed. Stamford, CT, Appleton & Lange, 1996.

Tierney LM Jr, McPhee SJ, Papadakis MA: *Current Medical Diagnosis and Treatment,* 38th ed. Stamford, CT, Appleton & Lange, 1999.

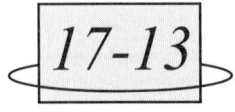

ACUTE RESPIRATORY DISTRESS SYNDROME

Timothy F. Quigley

DISCUSSION

Acute respiratory distress syndrome (ARDS), formerly known as adult respiratory distress syndrome, is characterized by sudden respiratory failure, acute onset of severe hypoxemia, dyspnea, bilateral generalized pulmonary infiltrates, and normal pulmonary capillary wedge pressure.[1] ARDS usually follows a catastrophic clinical event, especially sepsis, major trauma, multiple transfusions, aspiration of gastric contents, drug overdose, smoke inhalation, near drowning, or pancreatitis, among others.[2] Table 17-13-1 outlines many of the causes of ARDS. In 5 to 10 percent of patients with ARDS, the precipitating event is unknown.[3]

The annual incidence of ARDS is 5 to 10 per 100,000 population,[4] with the greatest risk factors including sepsis, pneumonia, trauma, and gastric content aspiration.[3] The mortality rate for ARDS has often been higher than 50 percent,[2] and death usually is due to multiple organ failure. That mortality rate has declined gradually in recent years, prob-

TABLE 17-13-1. Etiology of ARDS

Sepsis and shock
Major trauma
Aspiration of gastric contents
Near drowning
Multiple blood transfusions
Diffuse pneumonia
Acute pancreatitis
Drug overdose
Inhalation of gas and/or smoke
Disseminated intravascular coagulation

ably as a result of more effective supportive measures. There is still no definitive therapy for ARDS.

PATHOGENESIS

The pathophysiology of the lung injury with ARDS differs, depending on the causes, but common elements of the syndrome are damage to the epithelial cells of the pulmonary capillaries and alveoli that causes alveolar flooding, inactivation of surfactant and pulmonary edema, infiltration with inflammatory cells that leads to hyaline membrane formation, and eventual fibrosis and reduced lung compliance. The severe hypoxemia seen in ARDS results from the impaired ventilation of the collapsed alveoli and venoarterial shunting.[2]

In sepsis-precipitated ARDS, the mechanism of lung injury is presumed to be microorganisms or their endotoxic products circulating in the pulmonary circulation. Aspirated gastric contents cause a chemical burn to the pulmonary parenchyma, damaging the alveolar epithelium and leading to ARDS. Major trauma, especially long bone fractures, may release fat emboli that are directly toxic to the pulmonary capillary endothelium. In the case of acute pancreatitis, high circulating levels of lipase and amylase are presumed to cause direct pulmonary parenchymal damage.[2]

SIGNS AND SYMPTOMS

Since ARDS is a clinical syndrome with a wide variety of causative factors, the underlying illness or injury complicates the clinical presentation. The first symptom of ARDS is dyspnea, which usually is seen 24 to 72 h after the precipitating event. The patient may become increasingly dyspneic in the face of worsening hypoxemia as the syndrome progresses.

OBJECTIVE FINDINGS

In addition to respiratory distress and tachypnea, ARDS patients often develop tachycardia. Pulmonary auscultation may reveal bilateral crackles. Clinical findings may become more evident as the syndrome follows its course of increasing alveolar flooding. Refractory hypoxemia that is not responsive to supplemental oxygen is characteristic of ARDS. The diagnostic criteria for ARDS are listed in Table 17-13-2.

DIAGNOSTIC CONSIDERATIONS

Since ARDS is a syndrome, not a specific disease, the usual definition of the differential diagnosis does not strictly apply. ARDS should, however, be differentiated from pulmonary edema of cardiac origin because there is a definitive treatment available for that disorder.[1] Congestive heart failure should be excluded clinically (see Chap. 1-1). Hantavirus pulmonary syndrome (HPS) causes acute respiratory

TABLE 17-13-2. Diagnostic Features of ARDS

Catastrophic precipitating event (see Table 17-13-1)

Acute onset 24 to 72 h after event

Dyspnea, tachypnea

Tachycardia

Auscultation: bilateral crackles

Radiography: bilateral diffuse pulmonary infiltrates

Decreased P_{O_2}

Normal or decreased P_{CO_2}

Normal pulmonary capillary wedge pressure

Absence of cardiogenic pulmonary edema

failure and is characterized by fever, hypotension, thrombocytopenia, increased hematocrit, hemoptysis, and pleuritic chest pain.[3]

LABORATORY TESTS

The clinical features noted above and arterial blood gases showing hypoxemia ($P_{O_2} < 50$) with a normal to decreased P_{CO_2} characterize ARDS. A complete blood count may reveal elevated white blood cell counts associated with bacterial infection, while blood cultures may demonstrate sepsis. Amylase and lipase levels are elevated in patients with acute pancreatitis. A toxicology screen may confirm a suspected drug overdose.[5]

RADIOLOGIC AND IMAGING STUDIES

Chest radiographs may not show changes during the earliest periods of hypoxemia and dyspnea but within a short time will reveal diffuse bilateral infiltrates that become confluent, the so-called white-out characteristic of ARDS. Unless there is comorbid heart disease, the heart size should appear normal.[2]

Computed tomography (CT) of the thorax is not essential but may provide important diagnostic information about the underlying illness or pulmonary complications, such as abscess, pneumothorax, and surgical emphysema.[4]

OTHER DIAGNOSTICS

The insertion of a pulmonary artery (Swan-Ganz) catheter is not essential but may be valuable in distinguishing ARDS from cardiogenic pulmonary edema. There will be a normal pulmonary capillary wedge pressure (PCWP) with ARDS but a high PCWP in the case of pulmonary edema of cardiac origin.[2] The routine use of a Swan-Ganz catheter in ARDS is not recommended.[1]

TREATMENT

There is no specific therapy for ARDS, but the basis of treatment remains aggressive supportive measures, treatment of the underlying condition, and avoidance of complications.

The primary supportive measure is directed at correcting the gas-exchange abnormalities. Some patients stabilize their hypoxemia with supplemental oxygen alone, but most ARDS patients require intubation and mechanical ventilation with positive end-expiratory pressure (PEEP).

Other supportive measures that usually are provided in an intensive care unit under a specialist's direction include enteral nutrition and careful fluid management. Some patients require diuretics for elevated intravascular volume, packed red blood cells to main-

tain adequate hemoglobin levels, and/or antimicrobial treatment for sepsis.[1]

Some pulmonologists use the prone position in ARDS patients for ventilation support, improved postural drainage, increased ventilation, and removal of secretions. In patients who are unresponsive to the usual supportive care, some specialists administer inhaled nitric oxide (NO), which acts as a vasodilator, improving arterial oxygenation and reducing the amount of mechanical ventilation needed. Because of uncertainty about the long-term effects of NO, its use generally is restricted to patients who are refractory to the more routine supportive measures.[4] Corticosteroid therapy has been used in ARDS treatment, but clinical trials have not proved its efficacy.[3]

DISPOSITION

The course of ARDS is variable, lasting from a few days to a few months. The 50 percent mortality rate in ARDS has declined somewhat in recent years, presumably as a result of aggressive supportive care and treatment of complications. Multiple organ failure is the usual cause of death.[1] The highest mortality rate, about 90 percent, is seen in patients with sepsis syndrome. The primary determinants of the outcome are development of infection, advanced age, degree of precipitating illness, and extent of pulmonary fibrosis.[3]

Survivors of ARDS generally show substantial improvement in pulmonary function and quality of life 1 year after presentation. Increased time on mechanical ventilation, however, is associated with more impairment of pulmonary function.[6]

COMPLICATIONS AND RED FLAGS

If no underlying process is discovered to precipitate ARDS, a careful search for occult sources of sepsis should be undertaken. Pulmonary barotrauma with pneumothorax is a significant complication of patients with ARDS, presumably because of overdistention of already weakened lung structures through high PEEP and mechanical ventilation.[3]

NOTES AND PEARLS

Suspect ARDS in a hospitalized patient with significant noncardiac illness or injury who develops a sudden onset of extreme dyspnea and refractory hypoxemia 12 to 72 h after the onset of the illness.

Clinical trials are under way in efforts to reduce the high mortality rate in patients with ARDS. Therapies under investigation include ketoconazole, corticosteroids late in the course of ARDS, N-acetylcysteine, prostaglandin E, nonsteroidal anti-inflammatory drugs (NSAIDs), neutrophil inhibitors, human recombinant interleukin-1 receptor antagonists, small tidal volume mechanical ventilation, and nitric oxide.[1]

REFERENCES

1. Chestnut MS, Prendergrast TJ: Acute respiratory distress syndrome, in Tierney LM, McPhee SJ, Papadakis MA (eds.): *Current Medical Diagnosis and Treatment 2000,* 39th ed. New York, McGraw-Hill, 2000, pp 348–350.
2. Weinberger SE: *Principles of Pulmonary Medicine,* 3d ed. Philadelphia, Saunders, 1998, pp 335–347.
3. Steinberg KP, Hudson LD: Approach to the management of the patient with acute respiratory distress syndrome, in Kelley WN (ed.): *Textbook of Internal Medicine,* 3d ed. Philadelphia, Lippincott-Raven, 1997, pp 1937–1942.
4. Wyncoll DL, Evans W: Acute respiratory distress syndrome. *Lancet* (354): 497–501, 1999.
5. Jenkins TW: Adult respiratory distress syndrome in Labus JB (ed): *The Physician Assistant Medical Handbook.* Philadelphia, Saunders, 1995, pp 744–746.
6. Hudson LD, Steinberg KP: Epidemiology of acute lung injury and ARDS. *Chest* (116):74S–82S,1999.

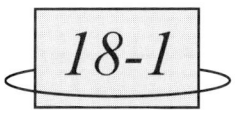

ACUTE RENAL FAILURE
Donald J. Sefcik

DISCUSSION

Normally, the kidneys receive approximately 1700 L of blood flow and produce 180 L of glomerular filtrate and 1200 mL of urine each day as they remove metabolic nitrogenous by-products and regulate the volume and composition of body fluids. When an abrupt decline in renal function occurs, the body's fluid milieu is disrupted and various clinical changes ensue.

Acute renal failure (ARF), a clinical condition characterized by an abrupt increase in plasma nitrogenous compounds [blood urea nitrogen (BUN) and creatinine], may manifest as a nonspecific entity or a complex array of signs and symptoms. The clinical picture tends to manifest as alterations in body fluid volume and solute composition. Early recognition and intervention have a profound impact on the long-term prognosis.

Asymptomatic elevations of BUN and creatinine (azotemia) and symptomatic renal failure (uremia) may evolve during oliguria (less than 400 mL of urine output/24 h) or with a normal urine output.

For diagnostic purposes, renal failure traditionally is discussed from a physiologic perspective. The three major classes of renal failure are categorized as

- *Prerenal:* affecting perfusion to the kidney
- *Postrenal:* affecting urine outflow distal to the kidney
- *Renal:* an intrinsic, pathophysiologic alteration within the kidney

PATHOGENESIS

The insults to the kidney that elicit renal failure are diverse. The common factor is an alteration in the ability of the kidney to remove nitrogenous compounds from plasma. Renal impairment usually is defined as a glomerular filtration rate (GFR) approximately 40 to 50 percent of normal, renal insufficiency occurs when GFR is approximately 20 to 40 percent of normal, and renal failure develops at a GFR less than 10 percent of normal. As GFR declines, BUN and creatinine accumulate and electrolyte alterations (hyperkalemia, hyperphosphatemia, and hypocalcemia), body fluid shifts (third spacing of fluids), hypertension, and an acid-base imbalance (acidosis) tend to develop.

Prerenal renal failure, the most common type (55 percent of all cases of renal failure), occurs secondary to a reduction in renal perfusion. This may be caused by volume depletion, vasodilation, and reduced cardiac output (see Table 18-1-1).

Intrinsic renal failure (40 percent of all cases of ARF) results from processes that cause injury to the kidney or nephron. The term *acute tubular necrosis* (ATN) often is used in reference to intrinsic renal failure. However, many cases of ARF, regardless of etiology, are not associated with necrosis of the tubule, and this description should be reserved for histologic diagnosis. The causes include ischemia, nephrotoxins, interstitial nephritis, and miscellaneous systemic disorders (see Table 18-1-1).

Postrenal renal failure (5 percent of all cases of ARF) generally results from an obstructive process. Common sites of obstruction include the bladder outlet, the ureter, and the urethra (see Table 18-1-1).

SYMPTOMS

Generally, the degree of symptomatology reflects the severity of renal impairment. The inability of the kidney to regulate body fluid volume, electrolytes, and acid-base balance produces the clinical picture of ARF. Early symptoms noted by these patients may include fatigue, nausea, swelling, anorexia, shortness of breath, and a reduction in urine output.

The early presentation of ARF is nonspecific. In addition to the general symptoms noted above, patients may have complaints that can help the clinician determine the cause of renal failure. For example, abdominal discomfort may be a result of bladder distention in patients with bladder outflow obstruction. Flank pain may be noted in patients with hydronephrosis secondary to ureteral obstruction. Fever and rashes may be seen in patients with some immunologic disorders associated with intrinsic renal diseases.

The diagnosis of renal failure is not generally difficult once serum chemistries have been obtained. Eliciting the type of ARF—prerenal, postrenal, or renal—poses a more difficult diagnostic challenge to a clinician (see Table 18-1-1).

OBJECTIVE FINDINGS

ARF may progress through a series of phases. Commonly, an oliguric phase occurs during which GFR is reduced, BUN and creatinine rise, and problems of fluid overload and electrolyte imbalance develop. This may be followed by a diuretic phase that can last from days to weeks. Early in this phase, urine output begins to increase, followed by a reduction in BUN and creatinine. Before the advent of dialysis, urine output could exceed 3 or 4 L per day during the recovery phase. A major emphasis in the treatment of ARF is preventing the complications that may develop.

BUN and creatinine tend to increase more than 10 mg/dL and 0.5 mg/dL daily, respectively. Simultaneously, these patients tend to develop hyperkalemia, hyperphosphatemia, hypocalcemia, fluid overload, and acidosis. As the ARF syndrome progresses, pulmonary edema, cardiac dysrhythmias, vomiting, and hypertension may develop.

If the condition becomes protracted, additional clinical manifestations, including dermatologic (pruritus and uremic frost), cardiac (pericarditis and congestive heart failure), neurologic (headaches and neuropathies), osteodystrophic (osteoporosis and osteomalacia), and hematopoietic abnormalities (anemia and bleeding tendencies), may develop.

Physical findings on examination may include orthostatic hypotension, tachycardia, tachypnea, rales, jugular venous distention, peripheral edema, rashes, hypertension, flank tenderness, bladder distention, and prostatic hypertrophy, depending on the underlying pathology that initiated the ARF.

DIAGNOSTIC CONSIDERATIONS

The first problem facing a clinician is distinguishing a patient with ARF from a patient with chronic renal failure (CRF). Generally, patients with azotemia and anemia (commonly normocytic, normochromic) have a more protracted type of renal failure (CRF). When prior laboratory tests are available for comparison, the knowledge that the azotemia is of recent onset is invaluable in making the determination that a patient has ARF.

TABLE 18-1-1. Major Classes of Acute Renal Failure

Prerenal types (perceived as hypoperfusion)
  Hypovolemia
    Hemorrhage (acute blood loss)
    Inadequate intake
    Excessive output (vomiting, diarrhea, perspiration, etc.)
    Third spacing of bodily fluids
  Reduced cardiac output
    Myocardial disease and/or injury (intrinsic heart problem)
    Obstruction to cardiac filling (pericardial tamponade, etc.)
    Obstruction to cardiac outflow (valvular defects, etc.)
  Loss of vascular tone
    Pharmacologic drug use (vasodilators)
    Sepsis
    Anaphylaxis

Renal types (intrinsic renal disorders)
  Ischemia
    Renal arterial obstruction and/or stenosis
    Hypoperfusional states
  Glomerular disorders and/or injuries
    Glomerulonephritis
    Vasculitis
  Acute tubular disorders and/or injuries
    Toxins (drugs, especially aminoglycosides, contrast agents, etc.)
    Ischemia
  Interstitial nephritis
    Immune-mediated (drugs, especially β-lactam antibiotics)
    Infectious
    Idiopathic

Postrenal types (obstructive processes)
  Ureteral
    Bilateral (uncommon: tumor, stones, etc.)
    Unilateral (if only one functional kidney)
  Bladder
    Prostate enlargement (benign hypertrophy, tumor, etc.)
    Miscellaneous outlet obstruction
      Tumor
      Stone
  Urethral
    Stenosis (stricture, etc.)
    Extraurethral (fibrosis, etc.)

LABORATORY TESTING

When one is confronted with a patient in ARF, the ultimate diagnostic challenge is to determine the underlying process that initiated the azotemia. Initially, a thorough history and physical examination (H&P) are performed to begin the search. With azotemia, the first goal is to separate patients who have a chronic form of renal failure from those with true ARF. A recent baseline laboratory is invaluable in this endeavor. Generally, during ARF, creatinine rises at a rate of 0.5 to 2.5 mg/dL per day. Once an ARF syndrome is established, the following guidelines may offer direction in delineating the cause.

Although often considered paramount in the management of ARF, quantification of the urine volume provides minimal information about the etiology. This is the case because ARF may demonstrate oliguria, polyuria, or normal urine output during various phases of its evolution. Of greater value in determining the etiology of the ARF process are an examination of the urine, especially the sediment, and selected serum chemistries.

Although it is not definitive, certain implications may be drawn from some findings on urinalysis. Sediment devoid of cellular elements is seen characteristically in both prerenal and postrenal ARF. In some lower genitourinary and prostatic disorders, however, hematuria and pyuria may be seen. Typically, cellular casts tend to be associated more commonly with intrinsic renal disorders. Proteinuria, depending on quantity, may be a manifestation of glomerular filtration abnormalities or may be seen in tubular injury as a result of an ischemic or nephrotoxic insult.

During the initial assessment (H&P), one should search for clues to assist in determining the cause of renal failure. If the bladder is distended, a Foley catheter may demonstrate a urinary bladder outflow obstructive process. Renal ultrasound or computed tomography (CT) may show signs of ureteral distention or obstruction. Renal failure indexes, a combination of urine and serum chemistries, may be valuable in differentiating prerenal from renal causes of azotemia and should be reviewed next (see Table 18-1-2). The combination of an elevated ratio of plasma BUN to plasma creatinine (>20), a low fractional excretion of sodium (FENa <1 percent), low urinary sodium (<20 meq/L), and elevated urinary osmolality (>500 mosmol/kg) suggests a prerenal ARF situation. Often, however, the distinction is not well demarcated, and overlap exists between prerenal and renal ARF indexes.

Attention must be directed to the electrolytes, since hyperkalemia, hypocalcemia, hyperphosphatemia, and hypermagnesemia tend to occur. The serum pH also should be monitored, as metabolic acidosis is a common occurrence.

TREATMENT

The goals of therapy are to (1) remove any possible causes, (2) minimize additional renal injury, and (3) prevent and/or treat complications. Hospitalization of patients with ARF must be considered.

One should begin with the removal of any drugs that may be nephrotoxic or may reduce renal perfusion. If necessary, volume expansion with isotonic saline may be employed; however, it is necessary to avoid volume overload. A diuretic such as furosemide may convert oliguric to nonoliguric renal failure. Fluid balance is easier to manage in nonoliguric patients. One must avoid potentially harmful contrast agents such as intravenous pyelography dyes. Drug levels are monitored as warranted, and drug doses are adjusted as necessary.

In all patients, meticulous attention to fluid status is critical. Serial monitoring of daily weights, fluid intake and urine output, blood pressure, electrolytes, BUN, creatinine, and hemoglobin should guide management. Dialysis is indicated in some cases of ARF (see Table 18-1-3).

Hyperkalemia, hypocalcemia, pulmonary edema, cardiac dysrhythmias, and other miscellaneous complications should be anticipated, prevented when possible, and treated as indicated.

COMPLICATIONS AND RED FLAGS

During the treatment of renal failure, one should monitor the patient for signs of volume overload. Daily weights and attention to the patient's fluid intake and output (I&O) are important parameters. As ARF resolves, hypokalemia must be anticipated, especially if the patient demonstrates significant diuresis during recovery. Gastrointestinal bleeding may occur.

TABLE 18-1-2. Commonly Used Renal Failure Indexes That Assist in Differentiating Prerenal from Intrinsic (Renal) Azotemia

INDEX	PRERENAL (INTRINSIC)	RENAL
Urinary sodium (mmol/L)	<10	>20
Urinary specific gravity	>1.020	<1.010
Plasma BUN/plasma creatinine	>20	<10
Urine osmolality (mosmol/kg H_2O)	>500	<300
FENa* (fractional excretion of sodium)	<1	>1

$$FENa = \frac{(\text{urinary sodium} \times \text{plasma creatinine}) \times 100}{(\text{plasma sodium}) \times (\text{urinary creatinine})}$$

*Many consider FENa to be an extremely sensitive indicator in determining whether ARF is prerenal or renal.

TABLE 18-1-3. Indications for Dialysis in Patients with Acute Renal Failure

Significant symptomatic pulmonary edema (secondary to volume overload)

Hyperkalemia (not responsive to more conservative approaches)

Toxic drug levels (amenable to correction by dialysis)

Azotemia

Pericarditis

Altered mental status (confusion, coma)

Significant acid-base disturbances

Bleeding (suggestive of platelet dysfunction)

Fluid overload

A dreaded complication is infection, which may occur in up to 75 percent of these patients. When infection occurs, it is the cause of death in as many as 75 percent of patients who die during the course of renal failure.

PROGNOSIS

Death may occur in up to 65 percent of patients with ARF, with infection being the most common cause. The typical patient with ARF begins to show signs of improvement after about 10 days. Most cases tend to resolve over a 3- to 4-week course. Resolution often manifests as a daily increase in urine output as renal function returns toward baseline.

Of the three broad classifications of ARF, intrinsic renal failure tends to have the most variable outcome. The majority of patients who survive a course of ARF recover enough renal function to live a normal life.

NOTES AND PEARLS

The nutritional support of the patient should be monitored. Limiting dietary proteins reduces the magnitude of the azotemia. Sodium and daily fluid intake should be monitored to avoid fluid overload. Drugs that are cleared renally often require dose adjustments, and their plasma levels should be observed closely.

BIBLIOGRAPHY

Brady HR, Brenner BM: Acute renal failure, in Fauci AS, Braunwald E, Isselbacher KJ, et al (eds): *Harrison's Principles of Internal Medicine,* 14th ed. New York, McGraw-Hill, 1998, pp 1504–1513.

Mitch WE: Acute renal failure, in Bennet JC, Plum F: *Cecil Textbook of Medicine,* 20th ed. Philadelphia, Saunders, 1996, pp 552–556.

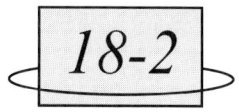

BENIGN PROSTATIC HYPERPLASIA

William A. Mosier

DISCUSSION

The term *benign prostatic hyperplasia* (BPH) refers to a noncancerous abnormal enlargement of the prostate gland. The prostate gland begins to undergo hyperplastic changes during the third decade of life. Most men begin to experience some symptoms of prostate gland enlargement by age 50, but significant problems are not common before age 60. As many as 90 percent of men between ages 70 and 90 have symptoms of BPH. The normal prostate is soft and pliable and is about the size of a walnut. When the prostate becomes hypertrophic, it often becomes rigid. This can constrict or even totally occlude the urethra. The result can be urinary retention, which eventually can lead to

azotemia and irreversible bladder dysfunction. Fortunately, the condition does not progress to the severe form in most patients. It is estimated that only about 5 percent of men who undergo consideration for treatment present with severe manifestations of BPH. An estimated one in four men will require treatment for BPH symptoms by age 80.

PATHOGENESIS

The etiology is not totally understood. However, it is thought to be related to the impact of the aging process on the hormone testosterone. An estrogen-dominant environment also plays a significant role in the development of BPH.

BPH is potentially dependent on estrogen for its development. Studies have confirmed that the ratios of estradiol (E2) to total testosterone (total T) and E2 to free testosterone (free T) are correlated significantly with prostate size. Blocking of the aromatization of testosterone to estrogen in the prostate stroma hypothetically can reverse or at least halt the progression of the disease. Studies have demonstrated that circulating autoantibodies to prostate specific antigen (PSA) exist in the serum of patients with BPH but not in the serum of patients without BPH. A possibly related factor that is considered controversial is that BPH may be associated with a diminished sex life with few or no ejaculations. This observation is based on studies that have indicated that the occurrence of BPH is higher among groups that average fewer ejaculations per month than are reported by control groups.

PATHOPHYSIOLOGY

Possibly originating within the periurethral glands, fibroadenomatosis nodules form around the periurethral region of the prostate. The hyperplastic process may form along the lateral walls of the prostate or may include tissue at the inferior margin of the vesicle neck. The tissue tends to be glandular with varying amounts of fibrous stroma.

SYMPTOMS

The symptoms of BPH begin when the enlarged gland interferes with the draining of the bladder through the urethra by blocking the passage of urine. This is caused by tensing of the enlarged muscle of the prostate gland around the urethra. Common complaints include progressive urinary frequency, urgency, nocturia, hesitancy, a feeling of a full bladder without being able to urinate, impotence, blood in the semen or hematuria, dripping or dribbling, and intermittency with a low-pressure flow that results in decreased force and size of the urinary stream (see Table 18-2-1).

TABLE 18-2-1. Commonly Occurring Symptoms of BPH

Starting and stopping of stream during urination

Sensation of incomplete emptying

Weak and diminished stream

Straining to urinate

Bladder distention

Intermittency

Impotence

Frequency

Hematuria

Hesitancy

Dribbling

Nocturia

Urgency

Dysuria

OBJECTIVE FINDINGS

Enlargement of the prostate, which can be verified on digital rectal examination, is not a prerequisite for the development of BPH symptoms. Clinically significant BPH may present with minimal or no detectable prostatic enlargement. However, when prostatic enlargement is detectable, it often presents with a rubbery consistency and a loss of the median furrow.

DIAGNOSTIC CONSIDERATIONS

When an enlarged prostate is encountered in men under age 40, venereal disease must be considered. Another important differential to screen for is cancer of the prostate. An indurated and tender prostate encountered on digital rectal examination is suggestive of prostatitis. A hard, nodular prostate usually is indicative of carcinoma or, rarely, prostatic calculi. Although much less common, obstructive causes of voiding difficulties that should be considered are urethral stricture, malfunctioning anterior or posterior urethral valves, müllerian duct cysts, and dysfunction of the bladder neck or external sphincter that does not allow for appropriate relaxation during voiding. Nonobstructive causes of voiding difficulty that should be considered are neurogenic bladder caused by detrusor denervation or irritation and parasympatholytic or sympathomimetic medications that may cause incomplete voiding.

SPECIAL CONSIDERATIONS

It is important to avoid all instrumentation until after a patient has made a committment to receive definitive treatment, since any manipulation may provoke increased trauma, obstruction, and infection. The risk of obstruction caused by an enlarged prostate constricting or totally closing off the flow of urine through the urethra at the bladder neck is of major concern. The risk is increased by alcohol consumption, cold moist weather, smoking, emotional stress, and the use of drugs such as antihistamines, atropine, beta-adrenergic blockers, calcium channel blockers, and muscle relaxants.

OTHER DIAGNOSTIC TOOLS

When a patient is committed to treatment for the relief of symptoms, the following diagnostic tools may be useful in disclosing the severity of BPH. Maximum urinary flow rate and residual volume may help provide a urodynamic analysis of the severity of the symptoms. An intravenous urogram (IVU) may be useful in determining whether the terminal portions of the ureters are displaced upward or whether there is a defect at the base of the bladder. IVU is also useful in ruling out hydronephrosis and dilated ureters. A postvoiding cystogram can indicate the amount of residual urine. If the BPH is severe, catheterization after voiding can measure the residual urine and also drain it. This can be necessary for stabilizing renal function and managing a urinary tract infection. Cystoscopy is useful in estimating gland size and differentiating an obstruction that may be present, such as vesicle neck contracture or prostatitis. PSA is not sufficiently accurate to distinguish between BPH and cancer of the prostate.

TREATMENT

An asymptomatic, moderately enlarged prostate does not require treatment. When treatment is initiated, it is usually at the request of a patient who is experiencing problems with urination. When the complaints are minimal, medication may be the first line of therapy to alleviate the symptoms. Safe, effective medications are available to treat BPH.

When a urinary tract infection or bladder outlet obstruction complicates BPH, the initial treatment must be directed toward the eradication of infection and the stabilization of renal function.

Some of the more common intervention strategies for treating BPH are

- Pharmacologic therapy (antiandrogens or alpha$_1$-adrenergic inhibitors)
- Prostatic incision (transurethral incision of the prostate)
- Prostatectomy (open or transurethral)
- Prostatic stents
- Thermotherapy
- Balloon dilation

Medications

Three classes of medications have proved useful in treating uncomplicated cases of BPH: antiandrogens such as 5α-reductase inhibitors, long-acting selective alpha$_1$-adrenergic inhibitors, and muscarinic receptor antagonists.

ANTIANDROGENS Because the nodular changes in the prostatic epithelium and stroma that manifest as BPH are androgen-dependent, one treatment approach is to attempt to regulate the amount of androgen available to the prostate. The 5α-reductase inhibitor agent finasteride (Proscar) is used to interfere with the conversion of testosterone to dihydrotestosterone. The goal is to decrease androgen bioavailability to the prostate tissue. It may require 6 months or more for the benefits of finasteride to become observable, and a significant percentage of patients may not respond. Studies suggest that the most favorable response occurs in men with larger prostates.

ALPHA$_1$-ADRENERGIC INHIBITORS Hyperplasia of the prostate is primarily a phenomenon of the stroma, as opposed to the epithelial tissue, in the majority of males. The smooth muscle of the stroma receives adrenergic innervation. For this reason, the antihypertensives that function as selective alpha$_1$-adrenergic inhibitors may be useful for relaxing the smooth muscle of the prostate and the bladder neck. The mechanism by which this occurs is directly related to the fact that alpha$_1$-adrenoceptors are densely distributed in the prostate and bladder neck but only sparsely distributed in the body of the bladder. Therefore, selective alpha$_1$-adrenoceptor blocking agents such as doxazosin (Cardura), tamsulosin (Flomax), and terazosin (Hytrin) are able to relax the smooth muscle of the prostate and bladder neck without interfering with bladder contractility. The usual onset of action with graduated dosing is at least 2 weeks. Many patients can maintain the benefits of treatment over time. However, some patients develop a tolerance to the treatment after as little as 6 months of therapy.

MUSCARINIC RECEPTOR ANTAGONISTS Symptomatic relief of urinary frequency, urgency, and/or urge incontinence in patients with normal renal function can be achieved with the muscarinic receptor antagonist tolterodine tartrate. It can be effective alone or when given in combination with an alpha$_1$ blocker and/or a 5α-reductase inhibitor.

ALTERNATIVE THERAPIES In addition to the pharmacologic agents that are available, certain alternative herbal remedies have demonstrated efficacy in controlled trials. Saw palmetto (*Serenoa repens*) extract is an over-the-counter supplement commonly found in pharmacies and health food stores. Saw palmetto is a lipid-soluble extract from the nonedible berry of a variety of palm tree that grows close to the ground, similar to a bush. The plant's berries contain the active agent beta-sitosterol, which has demonstrated 5α-reductase-inhibitory activity. Randomized, double-blind trials with patients with BPH have demonstrated a statistically significant decrease in the symptoms of BPH compared with placebo.

Surgery

It can take as long as 20 years after the diagnosis before BPH becomes sufficiently troublesome to warrant surgical intervention. The indications for surgery include urinary retention, chronic urinary tract infections, recurrent prostate infections, persistent bleeding from the prostate, swelling or destruction of the kidney caused by urinary obstruction (revealed on x-ray), and kidney failure. The surgical procedures utilized are relatively simple. The two most widely used prostatectomies are

- *Open surgical procedure.* This approach involves removing the entire prostate through a lower abdominal incision.
- *Transurethral resection of the prostate (TURP).* TURP is considered the mainstay of urologic treatment for BPH. As the name implies, a resectoscope is passed through the urethra via the penis until it reaches the bladder neck. An electric cutting loop then is used to resect the enlarged tissue. The procedure is also done using a modified electrovaporizing loop.

Alternative procedures with flowery or fishy names such as TULIP and TUNA hold promise for simpler, safer, and more efficacious treatment for BPH. Some of these procedures are

- *Transurethral incision of the prostate (TUIP).* This procedure is similar to TURP except that rather than removing any tissue, small incisions are made in the prostate to relieve pressure on the urethra.
- *Transurethral needle ablation of the prostate (TUNA).* This procedure usually is performed using only topical urethral anesthesia, has half the cost of TURP, and promises to be the treatment of choice in the near future.
- *Transurethral ultrasound-guided laser-induced prostatectomy (TULIP).* This is one of the first laser systems designed to treat BPH. Although it has many advantages over TURP, its two biggest disadvantages are that (1) prolonged catheterization during the postoperative phase is required and (2) since no tissue is obtained, no histology sample is available to rule out prostate cancer.
- *Transurethral laser ablation of the prostate (TULAP).* This is a commonly practiced form of transurethral laser surgery.
- *Visual laser ablation of the prostate (VLAP).* Although VLAP may not always result in as complete a removal of prostatic tissue as is achieved with TURP, it is associated with a lower morbidity rate, a shorter procedure time, and shorter hospitalization.
- *Endoscopic laser ablation of the prostate (ELAP).* The side effects of urinary tract infections and dysuria may be more common with this procedure; however, the need for blood transfusions appears to be less common than it is with TURP.
- *Transurethral microwave thermotherapy (TUMT).* This procedure can be implemented by using either a high-energy or a low-energy thermotherapy protocol. It is both outpatient-based and anesthesia-free. The low-energy protocol is most beneficial in patients with a relatively small prostate.
- *Endoscopic roller ball electrovaporization of the prostate (EREV).* This is experimentally considered a safe, effective, and economic alternative to the standard TURP. It is performed using a modified TURP.

These techniques have been developed in an attempt to overcome some of the drawbacks of TURP (see "Complications and Red Flags," below). The approaches that utilize laser energy direct a fiber, via cystoscopy, into the prostate, using heat to shrink the gland. The procedure is quicker to perform than a TURP and causes virtually no bleeding.

SUPPORTIVE MEASURES

Hot sitz baths can help relieve discomfort. It is important for the patient to drink at least eight glasses of fluid a day to promote urine production and bladder flushing. The patient also should be reminded to avoid alcohol, coffee, smoking, and spicy foods that tend to irritate the bladder.

PATIENT EDUCATION

Patient education should include a reminder of the importance of a yearly rectal examination for all male patients over age 40. If BPH has been diagnosed, a rectal examination may be indicated semiannually. The patient also should be cautioned about taking cold and allergy medications that may contain anticholinergic or sympathomimetic agents that can aggravate BPH and cause further urinary retention. Patients should be encouraged to continue an active sex life or masturbate into their advanced years. Patients should be discouraged from engaging in sexual stimulation and arousal without ejaculation. Maintenance of physical fitness should be emphasized.

DISPOSITION

Since BPH develops over a protracted period, any diagnosed case of BPH should be monitored with semiannual examinations. When in doubt, a urology consultation should be requested.

COMPLICATIONS AND RED FLAGS

The complications of severe untreated BPH include hydronephrosis, profuse hematuria, urinary retention, and urinary tract infections. A complaint of a burning sensation on urination with chills and fever should be assumed to be a urinary tract infection until proved otherwise. Prolonged urinary retention may lead to progressive renal failure and azotemia. Although it is well known that the open surgical procedure can result in significant sexual dysfunction, outcome studies have identified a much higher mortality and morbidity rate after TURP than was previously recognized. Studies now indicate that two-thirds of all men who undergo a TURP will experience diminished or absent ejaculation and that 5 percent will become impotent.

OTHER NOTES AND PEARLS

The availability of a self-administered questionnaire concerning BPH symptoms that a patient could complete would be a valuable adjunct to standard diagnostic procedures. The International Continence Society (ICS) has developed such a tool, the ICS male questionnaire. It is considered to have a high level of validity and reliability as well as being easy for patients to complete.

An emerging treatment for BPH is transurethral microwave thermotherapy. This is a technology that not only is less costly and less invasive but also causes no identifiable adverse effects on sexual function. Various other strategies for managing BPH are being studied, such as lasers, electrocautery, and ultrasonics. However, their ability to maximize efficacy and minimize side effects has not been clearly established. A medication called Cernilton is being considered for the treatment of BPH.

BIBLIOGRAPHY

Anderson RJ: Primary care management of benign prostatic hyperplasia. *Hosp Pract,* March 15, 1998, pp 11–21.

Boyle P, Gould AL, Roehrborn CG: Prostate volume predicts outcome of treatment of benign prostatic hyperplasia with finasteride: Meta-analysis of randomized clinical trials. *Urology* 48(3):398–405, 1996.

Catalona WJ, Partin AW, Slawin KM: Use of the percentage of free prostate-specific antigen to enhance differentiation of prostate cancer from benign prostatic disease. *JAMA* 279:1542–1547, 1998.

De Wildt MJ, Debruyne FM, de la Rosette JJ, et al: High-energy transurethral microwave thermotherapy: A thermoablative treatment for benign prostatic obstruction. *Urology* 48(3):416–423, 1996.

Donovan JL, Abrams P, Peters TJ, et al: The ICS-BPH study: The psychometric validity and reliability of the ICS male questionnaire. *Br J Urol* 77(4):554–562, 1996.

Elhilali MM, Ramsey EW, Barkin J, et al: A multicenter, randomized, double-blind, placebo-controlled study to evaluate the safety and efficacy of terazosin in the treatment of benign prostatic hyperplasia. *Urology* 47(3):335–342, 1996.

Girman CJ, Kolman C, Liss CL, et al: Effects of finasteride on health-related quality of life in men with symptomatic benign prostatic hyperplasia: Finasteride Study Group. *Prostate* 29(2):83–90, 1996.

Hill M, Hampl R, Petrik R, Starka L: Concentration of the endogenous antiandrogen epitestosterone and androgenic C19-steroids in hyperplastic prostatic tissue. *Prostate* 28(6):347–351, 1996.

Horton R: Benign prostatic hypertrophy, in Kelley WN (ed.): *Textbook of Internal Medicine,* 3rd ed. Philadelphia, Lippincott-Raven, 1997, pp 2542–2543.

Issa MM: Transurethral needle ablation of the prostate: Report of initial United States clinical trial. *J Urol* 156:426–427, 1996.

Lepor H, Shapiro E, Wang B, Liang YC: Comparison of the cellular composition of benign prostatic hyperplasia in Chinese and Caucasian-American men. *Urology* 47(1):38–42, 1996.

Lepor H, Williford WO, Barry MJ, et al: The efficacy of terazosin, finasteride, or both in benign prostatic hyperplasia: Veterans Affairs Cooperative Studies Benign Prostatic Hyperplasia Study Group. *N Engl J Med* 335(8):533–539, 1996.

Matzkin H, Cytron S, Simon D: Is there an association between cigarette smoking and gland size in benign prostatic hyperplasia? *Prostate* 29(1):42–45, 1996.

Meade WM, McLoughlin MG: Endoscopic roller ball electrovaporization of the prostate—the sandwich technique: Evaluation of the initial efficacy and morbidity in the treatment of benign prostatic obstruction. *Br J Urol* 77(5):696–700, 1996.

Mosier WA, Schymanski TJ, Walgren KD: Benign prostatic hyperplasia: Focusing on primary care. *Clinician Rev* 8(7):55–75, 1998.

Roehrborn CG, Siegel RL: Safety and efficacy of doxazosin in benign prostatic hyperplasia: A pooled analysis of three double-blind, placebo-controlled studies. *Urology* 48(3):406–415, 1996.

Simpson RJ, Fisher W, Lee AJ, et al: Benign prostatic hyperplasia in an unselected community-based population: A survey of urinary symptoms, bothersomeness and prostatic enlargement. *Br J Urol* 77(2):186–191, 1996.

Span PN, Benraad ThJ, Sweep CG, Smals AG: Kinetic analysis of steroid 5-alpha-reductase activity at neutral pH in benign prostatic hyperplastic tissue: Evidence for type I isozyme activity in the human prostate. *J Steroid Biochem Mol Biol* 57(1–2):103–108, 1996.

Zippe CD: Benign prostatic hyperplasia: An approach for the internist. *Cleve Clin J Med* 63(4):226–236, 1996.

Zlotta AR, Peny MO, Matos C, et al: Transurethral needle ablation of the prostate: Clinical experience in patients in urinary acute retention. *Br J Urol* 77(3):391–397, 1996.

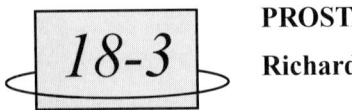

PROSTATITIS

Richard Dehn

DISCUSSION

Prostatitis is a broad diagnostic term that encompasses four different entities: acute bacterial prostatitis, chronic bacterial prostatitis, chronic nonbacterial prostatitis, and prostatodynia. These four diagnostic entities require different therapeutic responses, making a correct initial diagnosis important.

Acute bacterial prostatitis presents with fever and dysuria. Pain often is reported in the suprapubic, perineal, or sacral region. Symptoms of obstruction may develop as prostatic edema increases. On physical examination, the patient is often febrile and the prostate is extremely tender, enlarged, and indurated. Urinalysis shows pyuria, and microscopic examination of expressed prostatic secretions, if obtainable, shows increased leukocytes.

Chronic prostatitis is a chronic inflammation of the prostate. In chronic bacterial prostatitis, the cause of the inflammation is bacterial.

In chronic nonbacterial prostatitis, the cause of the inflammation can be a nonbacterial infectious agent, but it has been hypothesized that in some cases an autoimmune mechanism may be responsible. With chronic prostatitis, the patient experiences some of the symptoms of acute prostatitis without the fever and septic characteristics. The symptoms can vary from minimal to incapacitating and can include irritative voiding discomfort, perineal pain, and obstructive symptoms. Occasionally the patient will report hematuria or hematospermia. Physical examination of the prostate is generally normal. The organisms most commonly found to cause chronic bacterial prostatitis are aerobic gram-negative enteric bacteria, but occasionally enterococci are involved. Chronic nonbacterial prostatitis can be caused by the organisms *Chlamydia trachomatis* and *Ureaplasma urealyticum* but also can be caused by a noninfectious inflammatory process. It is thought that in some cases external urinary sphincter dysfunction can produce a chronic chemical irritation that causes inflammation. The ratio of bacterial to nonbacterial cases of chronic prostatitis is 1:14. Most nonbacterial cases occur in younger men, and most bacterial cases involve older patients.

Prostatodynia is a syndrome of chronic prostatitis symptoms without objective evidence of prostatic inflammation. Approximately one-third of patients who present with symptoms of chronic prostatitis have no objective evidence of prostatic inflammation, and it is thought that these cases are caused by a nonprostatic organ system pathology that produces referred symptoms.

The gold standard for determining prostatic inflammation is a microscopic analysis of expressed prostatic secretions. Inflammation is suspected if more than 10 leukocytes per high-power field (hpf) are observed.

PATHOGENESIS

Bacterial processes are thought to enter through the urinary tract. Recurrent chronic bacterial infections probably are related to problems of sphincter function. Chronic nonbacterial prostatitis and prostatodynia can be caused by a wide variety of pathologies, including processes outside the genitourinary system.

LABORATORY TESTING

With acute bacterial prostatitis, urinalysis shows pyuria and the microscopic examination of expressed prostatic secretions, if obtainable, shows increased leukocytes (>10/hpf). Care should be taken in massaging the prostate, since an overly vigorous examination may cause septicemia. A complete blood count (CBC) usually will show elevated white blood cells with a shift to the left, and the urine culture usually will be positive. A culture of the prostatic secretions also will be positive.

In chronic bacterial prostatitis, the urinalysis is usually negative, although the microscopic examination of expressed prostatic secretions will show increased leukocytes (>10/hpf). A culture of the prostatic secretions usually will be positive. CBC will be normal unless it is confounded by another systemic illness.

In chronic nonbacterial prostatitis, the urinalysis is usually negative, although the microscopic examination of expressed prostatic secretions will show increased leukocytes (>10/hpf). A culture of the prostatic secretions will be negative. CBC will be normal unless it is confounded by another systemic illness.

In prostatodynia, the urinalysis is usually negative and the microscopic examination of expressed prostatic secretions will show fewer than 10 leukocytes per high-power field. A culture of the prostatic secretions will be negative. CBC will be normal unless it is confounded by another systemic illness.

Prostate specific antigen (PSA) is elevated significantly in acute bacterial prostatitis, but after resolution of the infection, levels return to baseline. Levels should be normal in patients with chronic prostatitis or prostatodynia. Elevations in the absence of acute prostatitis should be investigated.

Transrectal prostatic sonography may be of some value in differentiating chronic prostatitis from prostatodynia. It sometimes is possible to visualize evidence of inflammation; however, such evidence should be considered persuasive and not necessarily diagnostic.

A difference in the pH of the expressed prostatic secretions that varies with the diagnosis has been observed in patients with prostatitis. In a study of 40 men with clinical prostatitis, the mean pH was found to be 7.6 in those with chronic bacterial prostatitis, 7.1 in those with chronic nonbacterial prostatitis, and 6.5 in those with prostatodynia.

DIAGNOSTIC CONSIDERATIONS

Acute and chronic infections in the genitourinary system should always be considered, such as cystitis, pyelonephritis, epididymitis, and urethritis. Anal disease and diverticulitis can present with prostatic symptoms. Prostatic cancer and bladder cancer should be ruled out in older patients with negative cultures who complain of chronic voiding symptoms.

TREATMENT

An acute bacterial prostatitis patient is usually septic enough to warrant hospitalization. After collection of culture specimens, antibiotics should be started. Fluoroquinolones are the drugs of choice, either ciprofloxacin (Cipro) 200 mg intravenously every 12 h or ofloxacin (Floxin) 200 mg intravenously every 12 h. A less expensive alternative to this regimen is ampicillin 1 g intravenously every 6 h and gentamicin 1.0 to 1.5 mg/kg of body weight intramuscularly every 12 h. Rapid improvement usually results from these therapies, and after the patient has been afebrile for 24 to 48 h, he should be switched to an oral antibiotic and the treatment should be continued for at least 1 month to prevent chronic prostatitis. At the end of the treatment regimen, the urine should be cultured and the prostatic secretions examined to confirm a successful outcome.

The treatment of chronic bacterial prostatitis involves a long course of antibiotic therapy. Trimethoprim-sulfamethoxazole (Bactrim DS, Septra DS) bid, ciprofloxacin (Cipro) 250 mg tid, and ofloxacin (Floxin) 200 mg bid are all acceptable regimens. Antibiotics should be continued for at least 6 weeks and possibly up to 12 weeks. If symptoms persist, suppressive therapy is helpful for the control of symptoms but is not curative.

Patients with chronic nonbacterial prostatitis should be placed on a course of doxycycline (Vibramycin) 100 mg bid or erythromycin 500 mg qid for 14 days. If the patient fails to respond to this regimen, urodynamic testing should be considered. Sphincter spasticity may be improved by treatment with an alpha-adrenoceptor antagonist. Terazosin (Hytrin) can be started at 1 mg daily and increased up to 10 mg, or Doxazosin (Cardura) can be started at 1 mg daily and increased to 8 mg. This class of drugs can produce postural hypotension; therefore, the patient should be cautioned and advised to take the drug at bedtime. Continued symptomatology requires further consideration of pathology in other nearby structures, especially those of the genitourinary system. Occasionally improvement is attained with nonsteroidal anti-inflammatory drugs. The use of transurethral microwave thermotherapy has been investigated and has shown promise in chronic nonbacterial prostatitis patients who are resistant to other therapies. Prostatodynia treatment is similar to the treatment of chronic nonbacterial prostatitis that is not responsive to antibiotics.

BIBLIOGRAPHY

Chandiok S: Prostatitis—clinical and bacterial studies. *Int J STD AIDS* 3(3):180–190, 1992.

Klimberg IW: Prostatitis, in Rakel RE (ed): *Conn's Current Therapy 2000,* Philadelphia, Saunders, 2000, pp 685–687.

Neal DE Jr: Use of terazosin in prostatodynia and validation of a symptom score questionnaire. *Urology* 43(4):460–465, 1994.

Nickel JC: Transurethral microwave thermotherapy for nonbacterial prostatitis. *J Urol* 155(6):1950–1954, 1996.

Presti JC, Stoller ML, Carroll PR, Urology, in Tierney LM Jr, McPhee SJ, Papadakis MA (eds): *Current Medical Diagnosis and Treatment,* 39th rev. ed. New York, McGraw-Hill, 2000, pp 926–928.

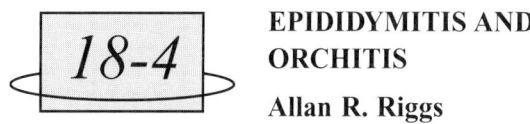

18-4 EPIDIDYMITIS AND ORCHITIS

Allan R. Riggs

EPIDIDYMITIS

DISCUSSION

Although epididymitis and orchitis can occur simultaneously, they are usually separate infections and are discussed separately in this chapter.

Acute epididymitis is an inflammation of the epididymis, a tube-like structure on the posterior surface of the testis. This condition, which usually is seen in adult men, is the most common emergency involving the scrotum. Epididymitis causes more than 20 percent of urologic hospital admissions. Most cases of epididymitis result from retrograde infection from the urethra. The infecting organism transits the reverse pathway of the sperm; that is, the organism travels from the urethra to the prostatic urethra, to the ejaculatory duct, to the vas deferens, to the tail of the epididymis, and finally to the body and head of the epididymis. Occasionally the infection may spread to the testis (epididymoorchitis) or the spermatic cord. Most cases of epididymitis are caused by bacteria, but other etiologies include viruses (e.g., mumps), chemical agents (e.g., urine), nonspecific causes[1] and trauma.

The cause of epididymitis usually varies with the patient's age. In infants and children younger than 5 years old, epididymitis usually results from an anatomic abnormality such as a posterior urethral valve or an ectopic ureter or from a neurologic or functional abnormality. The inflammatory agent is usually a coliform or pseudomonad bacterium or a chemical agent such as urine.[1] *Haemophilus influenzae* type B can be a cause of epididymitis in prepubertal boys, and dysfunctional voiding problems can be the etiology in boys 10 to 15 years of age.[1]

In sexually active males under age 35, epididymitis usually is caused by a sexually transmitted organism and is associated with urethritis. In males over age 35, epididymitis usually is caused by coliform bacteria and is associated with prostatitis, urinary tract infections, and urinary tract instrumentation.

Microbiology

The microbiology of epididymitis in infants and young and prepubertal boys was discussed above. In heterosexual males under age 35, epididymitis usually results from urethritis caused most frequently by *Chlamydia trachomatis* (up to 70 percent of cases) and less commonly by *Neisseria gonorrhoeae*. Both organisms may infect some patients. Since 30 to 50 percent of urethritis cases have no specific etiology, it is possible that an unknown pathogen that causes nonchlamydial, non-*Ureaplasma* urethritis also causes nonspecific epididymitis.

Homosexual males who participate in unprotected anogenital intercourse have developed epididymitis, usually from coliforms, with one case resulting from *H. influenzae* infection.[2] In males over age 35, the causative agents are usually gram-negative urinary tract pathogens such as *Escherichia coli* and *Pseudomonas aeruginosa*.[1] Less common infectious etiologies of epididymitis include *Streptococcus faecalis, Ureaplasma urealyticum,* viruses, and spirochetes.[2] Chronic epididymitis can be caused by *Treponema pallidum* and *Mycobacterium tuberculosis.*

SYMPTOMS

The presenting symptoms include a dull aching pain and swelling in the epididymis. The pain may radiate into the spermatic cord and the lower abdomen and flank. The pain of epididymitis may start slowly and increase over hours to days, in contrast to the pain of testicular torsion, which has an abrupt onset. A patient with epididymitis may report that lying down decreases the pain, whereas the pain of testicular torsion persists regardless of position. The presenting symptoms of nausea and vomiting have a positive predictive value of 96 percent and 98 percent, respectively, for a spermatic cord torsion, and so those symptoms suggest torsion instead of epididymitis.[3] The patient also may complain of urethral discharge, dysuria, and pain at the tip of the penis. Fever may be present. The symptoms may result from a physical strain such as heavy lifting or trauma or from sexual activity with a full bladder.[4] Providers should have a high index of suspicion with a pediatric patient because an embarrassed child may complain of lower abdominal or inguinal pain instead of scrotal pain. The clinician should confirm the history with the patient and do a thorough genitourinary exam.[5]

OBJECTIVE FINDINGS

First observe the patient to assess his level of discomfort. Then perform a general abdominal examination with emphasis on bladder distention and flank tenderness. Check the inguinal regions for redness, swelling, obvious hernias, and tenderness. Tenderness of the spermatic cord in the groin is typical of epididymitis but is not typical of testicular torsion.[5] Physical examination of the testes and scrotum is best performed with the patient standing. Early in the disease, the epididymis may be firm, swollen, tender, and discrete from the testis, but as the infection persists, both the epididymis and the testicle become one swollen, tender mass. Elevation of the testis usually relieves the pain (a positive Prehn's sign), whereas this maneuver usually increases the pain of testicular torsion. Because this sign is known to be unreliable, it should not be the sole basis for the diagnosis.[6] The cremasteric reflexes should be checked, since a positive reflex usually indicates epididymitis or appendiceal torsion, whereas a negative reflex usually indicates testicular torsion. Unfortunately, the absence of a cremasteric reflex can be a normal finding in some infants and teenagers.[7] Bluish discoloration (blue dot sign) of the scrotum over the upper pole is an indication of appendiceal torsion instead of epididymitis.[5] Transillumination with a penlight helps differentiate hydrocele, which presents as a reddish glow. Rectal examination may reveal a tender prostate, and the patient may have a fever.

If the diagnosis is uncertain on physical examination, other studies (e.g., ultrasound) should be performed.

DIAGNOSTIC CONSIDERATIONS

The most common differential diagnosis that needs to be ruled out quickly to save the testicle is testicular torsion. Although usually seen in prepubertal males, torsion occasionally is seen in young adults. It is suggested by a sudden, severe onset along with a negative urinalysis and increased pain with testicle elevation.

Torsion of the epididymal appendages, which also usually is seen in prepubertal males, is another consideration. Other differential diagnoses within the scrotum include orchitis, testicular tumor, hematocele, spermatocele, varicocele, congenital hydrocele, and incarcerated inguinal hernia.

Diagnostic considerations involving the scrotal wall include gangrene of the scrotal skin, Fournier's gangrene, abscess of the scrotal wall, fungal infection, trauma, urinary extravasation, and edema from cardiac, hepatic, or renal failure.[8]

SPECIAL CONSIDERATIONS

Patients undergoing immunosuppressive therapy and patients with AIDS are at risk for developing tuberculosis. Therefore, when these patients present with epididymitis, the clinician should consider *M. tuberculosis* as a possible etiology.[8] *Aspergillus fumigatus* is another atypical organism that has caused epididymitis and orchitis in AIDS patients.[9] Be alert for the possibility of unusual pathogens in an immunosuppressed patient with epididymitis.

A drug-induced epididymitis has been reported in patients on the antiarrhythmic drug amiodarone (Cordarone). Another etiologic risk factor for epididymitis is an intact foreskin. A 1998 study showed high statistical significance in the relationship between epididymitis and being uncircumcised.[10]

LABORATORY STUDIES

In the sexually acquired form of epididymitis, Gram staining of the urethral smear may show gram-negative intracellular diplococci that are consistent with gonorrhea. The patient should not urinate for at least 2 h before the urethral swab is obtained. A urethral smear with white blood cells and no bacteria usually indicates a chlamydial infection. Urinalysis with pyuria only also may indicate chlamydial infection. It is best to get a first void urine specimen (the first 50 mL of voided urine after 2 h of continence) to identify pyuria caused by urethritis. Culture or nonculture tests for *N. gonorrhoeae* and *C. trachomatis* should be obtained.

In epididymitis that is not sexually acquired, the urinalysis usually shows bacteriuria, pyuria, and varying amounts of hematuria. Urine culture will show the causative bacterium.

The complete blood count in epididymitis may show increased white blood cells (WBCs) with a shift to the left, but one study stated that the WBC count is not helpful and should not be ordered routinely.[5] If there are suspicions of epididymitis from syphilis or tuberculosis (e.g., chronic epididymitis), a Venereal Diseases Research Laboratories (VDRL) and/or a microhemagglutination assay for antibodies to *Treponema pallidum* (MHA-TP) test and a tuberculin skin test will be helpful.

RADIOLOGIC STUDIES AND OTHER IMAGING STUDIES

In selected cases in which urinary tract abnormalities may be a factor, for example, in young boys and elderly men, an intravenous pyelogram (IVP) and a voiding cystourethrogram (VCUG) should be obtained. Scrotal ultrasound may help differentiate epididymitis from testicular torsion. Color Doppler ultrasound evaluates testicular blood flow and thus may be helpful in differentiating early testicular torsion from epididymitis. This procedure can be difficult, and the accuracy is dependent on the operator.[11] One must use caution in the interpretation because if the problem is a late torsion, there will be falsely increased blood flow because of inflamed scrotal vessels.

In patients with epididymitis, technetium 99m (^{99m}Tc) pertechnetate testicular scanning shows increased perfusion through the spermatic cord vessels and increased uptake in the region of the epididymis. In contrast, there is decreased uptake of ^{99m}Tc with early torsion. Several hours after the torsion, a halo of increased uptake may surround the torsed testicle, indicating attempted collateral circulation.[4]

One must bear in mind that both technetium testicular scanning and Doppler ultrasound can have false-positive and false-negative results.

OTHER DIAGNOSTICS

Doppler stethoscopes have been suggested as a helpful adjunct to physical examination in a primary care office, but one article stated that Doppler stethoscopes have not been useful and thus are not indicated as a diagnostic tool.[5]

If the diagnosis of epididymitis is in doubt, a prompt urologic consultation should be made for surgical exploration of the scrotum. In young boys and elderly men with bacteriuria, cystoscopy should be performed after treatment to rule out an obstructive etiology of the epididymitis.[2]

TREATMENT

Pharmacologic Management

Since most cases of epididymitis have an infectious etiology, antibiotics should always be used (see Table 18-4-1). One should start the initial antibiotics on the basis of clinical clues (e.g., sexually transmitted disease–acquired) and Gram staining of the patient's urethral smear and/or urine.

A patient with epididymitis secondary to sexually transmitted urethritis should be treated with ceftriaxone 250 mg intramuscularly and doxycycline 100 mg orally bid for 10 to 14 days to cover *N. gonorrhoeae* and *C. trachomatis,* respectively.

Young boys with bacteriuria, elderly men with bacteriuria, and homosexuals with epididymitis resulting from anogenital intercourse should be treated for coliform infection. Outpatient therapy should be started with a broad-spectrum antibiotic such as trimethoprim-sulfamethoxazole or a quinolone, although quinolones are contraindicated in patients 17 years of age and younger. The appropriate length of treatment for coliform epididymitis is unknown and may need to be protracted, since relapse after 7 to 10 days can occur. One recommendation suggests ofloxacin 200 or 300 mg twice a day for 10 to 21 days for enteric epididymitis.[7] If the patient is systemically ill, he should be admitted for intravenous aminoglycoside therapy.[2]

One should consider antibiotics that cover tuberculous and fungal organisms in patients with concurrent epididymitis and HIV infection.

Nonsteroidal anti-inflammatory drugs may be helpful, but steroids have not been found to be useful. Antipyretics such as acetaminophen are helpful. In patients with severe pain, an anesthetic block of the spermatic cord with 1% lidocaine can be performed.[8]

Supportive Measures

Symptomatic treatment includes intermittent ice applications, sitz baths, bed rest, and scrotal elevation with a towel. The latter two treatments help with maximal lymphatic drainage. Athletic supporters may constrict and should be avoided.

Patient Education

With sexually acquired epididymitis, patient education should emphasize safe sex practices such as using condoms and limiting the number of partners. The patient should be tested for and educated about other sexually transmitted diseases and should notify his partners about receiving therapy. With epididymitis that is not sexually acquired, the patient should be advised to avoid activities that may bring on epididymitis (e.g., heavy lifting) and to seek medical care at the first symptoms of prostatitis and/or urinary tract infection. In treating epididymitis, a clinician has a golden opportunity to educate patients about testicular self-examination.

Disposition

The patient should be reevaluated if there is no improvement in 48 h. It is necessary to advise the patient that swelling and discomfort may linger for weeks or months even though the infectious agent has been eliminated. If fever persists after adequate antibiotics, an abscess may be present. The abscess is evaluated with ultrasound and then treated with surgical drainage and/or epididymoorchiectomy.[8]

Uncomplicated epididymitis usually requires 10 to 14 days of treatment, but if there is concurrent bacterial prostatitis, antibiotics should be continued for 4 weeks. The follow-up for epididymitis is done at 1 month.[8]

COMPLICATIONS AND RED FLAGS

The complications of epididymitis include testicular necrosis, testicular atrophy, abscess, and infarction. Some amount of atrophy occurs in approximately two-thirds of cases of acute epididymitis, whereas abscess and infarction are relatively rare, with a 5 percent incidence of each one. Infertility may occur in up to 50 percent of patients with

TABLE 18-4-1. Antibiotics for Acute Epididymitis

ANTIBIOTIC	DOSE	BACTERIUM	COMMENTS
Ceftriaxone (Rocephin)	250 mg IM in a single dose	*N. gonorrhoeae*	*Caution:* Accompanying renal and hepatic impairment. PCN allergy
Doxycycline (Doryx)	100 mg PO bid for 10–14 days	*C. trachomatis*	Photosensitivity
Ofloxacin (Floxin)	300 mg PO bid for 10 days	*N. gonorrhoeae* *C. trachomatis*	Alternative regimen per CDC.[12] Ofloxacin contraindicated for persons ≤17 years of age
Sulfamethoxazole 800 mg, trimethoprim 160 mg (Bactrim DS)	1 DS tablet PO bid × 10 days (pediatric dose as calculated)	Coliform (e.g., *E. coli*)	For young boys and older men with pyuria and bacteriuria. Treat for 4 weeks if bacterial prostatitis is suspected
Cipofloxacin (Cipro)	250 mg PO bid × 10 days	Coliform (e.g., *E. coli*)	For older men with pyuria and bacteriuria. Treat for 4 weeks if prostatitis is suspected. Contraindicated for persons ≤17 years of age
Aminoglycoside [e.g., gentamicin (Garamycin)]	1.5 mg/kg q 8 h IV for at least 5 days, then switch to an oral antibiotic	Coliform (e.g., *E. coli*)	For systematically ill patients who require hospitalization. Reduce dose for renal impairment. Watch for nephrotoxicity and neurotoxicity

NOTE: DS = double strength; PCN = penicillin; CDC = Centers for Disease Control and Prevention.

bilateral epididymitis. Some patients may experience treatment failure or recurrence of epididymitis.

The two red flags are testicular torsion and testicular cancer. One should consider torsion if a patient presents with a sudden onset of acute testicular pain, especially if the patient is age 15 or younger and epididymitis cannot be confirmed by physical examination and laboratory testing. A urologic consultation is indicated, since surgical exploration is needed within 4 to 6 h after the onset of the torsion to save the testicle (see Chap. 18-7).

A testicular tumor is another indication for a urologic consultation. Testicular cancer usually presents with asymptomatic swelling, but pain is a presenting symptom in approximately 20 percent of these patients. Since swelling and pain are classic symptoms of epididymitis and epididymoorchitis, a follow-up evaluation to rule out a hidden malignancy should be performed after the resolution of these infections (see Chap. 13-9).

Other reasons for a urologic consultation include a suspected abscess, lack of response to treatment, and an unsure diagnosis of the problem. When in doubt, it is best to consult.

ORCHITIS

DISCUSSION

Orchitis is an inflammation of the testis that usually results from hematogenous spread during a systemic bacterial or viral illness. Orchitis may be a complication of epididymitis (epididymoorchitis). Additional etiologies include syphilis (gumma of the testis), tuberculosis, and granuloma, which is thought to result from an autoimmune process directed against spermatozoa. Rarely, orchitis can occur secondary to Behçet's disease.[13] Many viruses can cause orchitis, and viruses are the most common etiology of acquired testicular failure in adults.[14] Orchitis results from the virus actually infecting testicular tissue, not from secondary inflammation. In mumps infection, orchitis is the most common complication, occurring in up to 25 percent of adult men[6] (see Chap. 9-17). Among these men, approximately 66 percent develop unilateral orchitis and the other 33 percent have bilateral orchitis. Orchitis usually follows parotitis by 3 to 4 days, but it may precede or start on the same day as parotitis. After mumps, the testes may return to normal size and function or may atrophy secondary to the effect of the virus on the seminiferous tubules, along with ischemia caused by pressure and edema against the inelastic tunica albuginea. Atrophy, which usually is detectable 1 to 6 months after the acute infection resolves, does not always correlate with the severity of orchitis or the development of infertility.[14]

Microbiology

The bacterial causes of orchitis are the same organisms that cause epididymitis. In sexually active males under age 35, one should treat for chlamydia and gonorrhea. In young boys, older men, and homosexuals, coliform bacteria are the likely cause of orchitis. Although rare, syphilis and tuberculosis, especially in immunocompromised patients and chronic cases, must be considered.

The viral etiologies include mumps virus, echovirus, lymphocytic choriomeningitis virus, and group B arboviruses.[14] Rarely, the Epstein-Barr virus can cause orchitis as a complication of infectious mononucleosis[15] (see Chap. 3-3).

SYMPTOMS

Orchitis presents with testicular pain and swelling, high fever, chills, headache, nausea, and vomiting. Fever may be between 103 and 106°F (39.4 and 41.1°C) with shaking chills.[16]

OBJECTIVE FINDINGS

On physical examination, the patient may have fever. The scrotum is usually erythematous, swollen, and edematous. Occasionally, epididymitis is present without orchitis and is palpable as a swollen, tender cord.[16] A hydrocele may be seen with transillumination. If the patient has orchitis caused by mumps, the parotid glands may be swollen.

DIAGNOSTIC CONSIDERATIONS

The differential diagnoses are the same as those for epididymitis and within the scrotum include testicular torsion, testicular cancer, hematocele, spermatocele, varicocele, congenital hydrocele, and incarcerated inguinal hernia. Diagnostic considerations involving the scrotal wall include gangrene of the scrotal skin, Fournier's gangrene, abscess of the scrotal wall, fungal infection, trauma, urinary extravasation, and edema. Testicular inflammation also can occur with pleurodynia, leptospirosis, melioidosis, relapsing fever, chickenpox, brucellosis, and lymphocytic choriomeningitis.[16]

SPECIAL CONSIDERATIONS

As with epididymitis, patients undergoing immunosuppressive therapy and patients with AIDS are at risk of developing orchitis from *M. tuberculosis.*

For unknown reasons, prepubertal males with parotitis do not seem to get orchitis.

LABORATORY STUDIES

For a patient with a suspected bacterial orchitis, the clinician should follow the same laboratory protocols used with epididymitis: Gram stains, cultures, and immunologic tests for *N. gonorrhoeae, C. trachomatis,* coliforms, *M. tuberculosis,* and *T. pallidum* (see the laboratory studies section for epididymitis, above).

In viral orchitis, one should attempt to make a definitive diagnosis by culturing the virus from blood, urine, throat swab, cerebrospinal fluid (CSF) and/or secretions from Stensen's duct. A rapid diagnosis of mumps can be made by immunofluorescent testing to detect viral antigen in the oropharyngeal cells.[16] Serologic tests such as enzyme-linked immunosorbent assay (ELISA) can be used to determine acute infection. Acute and convalescent sera should be obtained 2 to 3 weeks apart. A fourfold increase in titer confirms a recent infection.

With mumps orchitis, the complete blood count (CBC) may show a leukocytosis with a shift to the left. In contrast, mumps without orchitis may show a normal CBC or a mild leukopenia with a lymphocytosis. The erythrocyte sedimentation rate may rise with mumps orchitis. Serum amylase also is elevated. Plasma testosterone is low during acute orchitis but returns to normal after the illness.[16]

RADIOLOGIC STUDIES AND OTHER IMAGING

Radiologic studies usually are not indicated unless urologic abnormalities are thought to be a causative factor in orchitis. If that is the case, one should obtain an IVP and a VCUG. Scrotal ultrasound may help differentiate orchitis from epididymitis and testicular torsion. Doppler ultrasound, which evaluates testicular blood flow, may help differentiate orchitis from testicular torsion, as may ^{99m}Tc pertechnetate testicular scanning.

OTHER DIAGNOSTICS

Doppler stethoscopes have been suggested as a helpful adjunct to physical examination in a primary care office, but one article stated that Doppler stethoscopes have not been useful and thus are not indicated as a diagnostic tool.[5]

TREATMENT

Pharmacologic Management

If the orchitis is thought to be of bacterial etiology, one should start antibiotics on the basis of clinical clues (e.g., sexually transmitted disease–acquired) and Gram staining of the patient's urethral smear and/or urine. Orchitis secondary to a sexually transmitted infection should be treated with ceftriaxone 250 mg intramuscularly and doxycycline 100 mg orally bid for 10 to 14 days. Orchitis secondary to a urologic abnormality should be treated with a broad-spectrum antibiotic such as trimethoprim-sulfamethoxazole or a quinolone. If the patient is sick enough for hospitalization, an intravenous aminoglycoside should be used until cultures and sensitivities come back.

In the rare case of syphilitic orchitis, one should use penicillin or erythromycin. In tuberculous orchitis, four antituberculous drugs may be needed, especially if multiple-drug-resistant *M. tuberculosis* is a possibility (see Chap. 9-31).

The treatment of viral orchitis is mainly palliative. Although this has not been proved in controlled studies, glucocorticoids seem to be of some benefit in decreasing fever and testicular pain and swelling. One should start with 60 mg of prednisone and taper the dose over the next 7 to 10 days.[16] When 1 % lidocaine is injected into the spermatic cord, it provides quick pain relief and may decrease testicular damage by improving the local blood supply. Acetaminophen and nonsteroidal anti-inflammatory drugs (e.g., ibuprofen) help with the pain and fever.

In a patient with bilateral mumps orchitis, interferon α2b may be helpful in preserving fertility.[17]

Supportive Measures

Symptomatic treatment includes bed rest, scrotal elevation, ice compresses, and sitz baths.

Patient Education

If orchitis is secondary to a sexually acquired infection, the patient should be educated about safe sex practices and advised to have his partner(s) get treatment. Testicular self-examination should be taught. If a patient presents with orchitis secondary to mumps, he should be reassured that physical activity did not bring on the orchitis. Although it is too late for a patient with mumps orchitis, other patients should be educated about prevention with the mumps vaccine.

DISPOSITION

A patient should be reevaluated in 24 to 48 h if the symptoms are worsening. A patient with mumps orchitis should be advised that the swelling, pain, and tenderness will persist for 3 to 7 days and then gradually decrease, especially when the fever breaks. A reasonable follow-up is 1 month.

COMPLICATIONS AND RED FLAGS

The complications of orchitis include atrophy and subnormal sperm counts and/or sterility. Unilateral atrophy occurs in a third of cases of mumps orchitis, and bilateral atrophy occurs in a tenth of cases.[14] If no significant atrophy has occurred, sterility is uncommon. However, if there is bilateral atrophy after mumps, below-normal sperm counts and/or sterility are very common.[16] Another complication is pulmonary infarction that is thought to be due to thrombosis of the veins in the prostatic and pelvic plexuses, which occurs with the testicular inflammation. Priapism can be an uncommon complication.[16]

As in epididymitis, the red flags are for testicular torsion and cancer.[12] Providers should always consult a urologist if these diagnoses are suspected or if there are other complications or concerns that are beyond one's skills, knowledge, and experience.

REFERENCES

1. Bukowski TP, Lewis AG, Reeves D, et al: Epididymitis in older boys: Dysfunctional voiding as an etiology. *J Urol* 154(2):762, 1995.
2. Slanetz PA, Whitman GJ, Chew FS: Epididymal abscess. *AJR* 165(2):376, 1995.
3. Jefferson RH, Perez LM, Joseph DB: Critical analysis of the clinical presentation of acute scrotum: A 9-year experience at a single institution. *J Urol* 158:1199, 1997.
4. Presti JC Jr, Stoller ML, Carrol PR: Urology, in Tierney LM, McPhee SJ, Papadakis MA (eds): *Current Medical Diagnosis and Treatment,* 39th ed. Lange/McGraw-Hill, 2000, p 917.
5. Galejs LE, Kass EJ: Diagnosis and treatment of the acute scrotum. *Am Fam Physician* 59(4):818, 1999.
6. Burgher SW: Acute scrotal pain. *Emerg Med Clin North Am* 16(4):789, 1998.
7. Joly-Guillau ML, Lasry S: Practical recommendations for the drug treatment of bacterial infections of the male genital tract including urethritis, epididymitis and prostatitis. *Drugs* 57(5):748, 1999.
8. Cendron M, Sant GR: Testicular disorders and disorders of the scrotal contents, in Nobel J (ed): *Textbook of Primary Care Medicine,* 2d ed. St. Louis, Mosby Yearbook, 1996, p 1805.
9. Hood SV: Prostatitis and epididymo-orchitis due to Aspergillus fumigatus in a patient with AIDS. *Clin Infect Dis* 26(1):229–231, 1998.
10. Bennett, RT, Gill B, Kogan SJ: Epididymitis in children: The circumcision factor? *J Urol* 160:1842–1844, 1998.
11. Mettler FA: *Essentials of Radiology.* Philadelphia, Saunders, 1996, p 246.
12. Centers for Disease Control and Prevention: 1998 Guidelines for treatment of sexually transmitted diseases. *MMWR* 47(RR-1):87, 1998.
13. Callejus-Rubio JL, Ortego N, Piez A et al: Recurrent epididymo-orchitis secondary to Behçet's disease. *J Urol* 160:496, 1998.
14. Griffin JE, Wilson JD: Disorders of the testes, in Fauci AS, Braunwald E, Isselbacher KJ, et al (eds): *Harrison's Principles of Internal Medicine,* 14th ed. New York, McGraw-Hill, 1998, p 2093.
15. Weiner RL: Orchitis: A rare complication of infectious mononucleosis. *Pediatr Infect Dis J* 16(10):1008, 1997.
16. Ray CG: Mumps, in Isselbacher KJ, Braunwald E, Wilson JD, et al (eds): *Harrison's Principles of Internal Medicine,* 13th ed. New York, McGraw-Hill, 1994, p 830.
17. Casella R, Leibundgut B, Lehmann K, et al: Mumps orchitis: Report of a mini-epidemic. *J Urol* 158:2160, 1997.

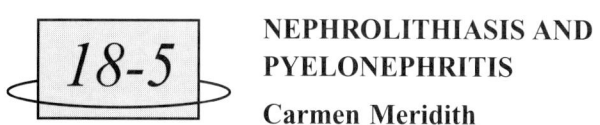

NEPHROLITHIASIS AND PYELONEPHRITIS

Carmen Meridith

NEPHROLITHIASIS

DISCUSSION

Renal colic caused by renal lithiasis (renal calculi, kidney stones) has been called the worst of all acute pains. Stones usually form in the renal pelvis, and the symptomatology is caused by the passage of a stone through the ureter. Bladder stones are less common but may present with hematuria and intermittent urinary obstruction.

Stones form because of the concentration of crystals in the urine, frequently as a result of a metabolic derangement caused by diet, an internal disorder, or even the environment (see Table 18-5-1). A past history of stones, gout, or hypercalcemia should be sought in evaluating the patient.

Geography, weather, and the mineral content of the local drinking water are factors to consider. Certain areas of the United States (the south, southwest, and west) have higher numbers of cases, but even in colder climates, such as that in the northeast, drinking water can cause local incidence patterns that vary from town to town. Kidney stones are rare in children and adolescents. The incidence of renal

TABLE 18-5-1. Dietary Habits and Conditions Associated with Renal Stones

Diet
Calcium intake
Dairy products
Calcium supplements
Purine-containing foods (protein-rich food; metabolite is uric acid)
Meat (especially red meat)
Fish
Poultry
Oxalate
Cola
Chocolate
Cranberries
Tea
Vitamin C (more than 1000 mg daily)
Diseases and conditions
Urinary tract infection
Gout
Inflammatory bowel disease
Pregnancy

stones peaks between ages 30 and 50 and is somewhat higher in men. There is a 3:1 male:female incidence. July, August, and September are the months with the highest incidence. Other risk factors include a sedentary life-style, professional and managerial occupations, calcium, oxalate- and phosphate-rich foods, and low urinary volumes.

The stones generally are formed of calcium oxalate, calcium phosphate, cystine, and uric acid. When associated with infection, struvite (staghorn) stones form and can be quite large, encompassing the whole renal pelvis. Most renal stone are calcium stones (usually composed of calcium phosphate, calcium oxalate, or a mixture of both, which is the most common form).

There are three theories for the formulation of stones:

1. *Nucleation theory.* Presence of crystal or foreign body in urine supersaturated with crystallizing salt
2. *Stone matrix theory.* Protein matrix formation serving as the framework for crystal deposition
3. *Inhibitor of crystallization theory.* Absence or low concentration of certain crystal inhibitors

Stones less than 5 mm usually can be passed without difficulty. Stones between 5 and 10 mm can pass approximately 50 percent of the time. Stones larger than that cause many complications, including partial or complete obstruction of the ureter and ureter lacerations. Larger stones require some type of intervention, which may include percutaneous ultrasonic lithotripsy, extracorporeal shock-wave lithotripsy, an ultrasonic transducer passed into the ureter during cystoscopy, a basket passed through a cystoscope, and nephrolithotomy. Lithotripsy is much less invasive and is replacing surgery.

SIGNS AND SYMPTOMS

The initial symptom is usually an intermittent, excruciating unilateral flank pain (renal colic) that is acute in onset and has no prodrome. This pain may radiate into the ipsilateral lower abdominal quadrant, the scrotum, or the labia; this may be a clinical indication that the stone has passed to the lower third of the ureter. Once the stone passes into the bladder, frequency, urgency, and dysuria often occur, mimicking a urinary tract infection.

Gross hematuria may be seen. Patients can present either with pain and no hematuria or hematuria and no pain but usually have both to a remarkable degree. The urinalysis is usually free of casts and white blood cells (WBCs) unless there is concomitant infection such as a urinary tract infection or pyelonephritis. Symptoms of vagal stimulation, including nausea and vomiting, bradycardia, and even fainting, can occur. (Some patients may have tachycardia from pain instead of bradycardia.)

DIAGNOSTIC CONSIDERATIONS

Many diseases and conditions can mimic renal stones. Table 18-5-2 lists the most common diagnostic considerations.

LABORATORY STUDIES

Laboratory studies should include a hemogram, urinalysis with culture, serum chemistry, and a 24-h urine specimen to assess calcium, phosphorus, uric acid levels, and creatinine clearance. The urinalysis (UA) probably will show hematuria, either microscopic or frank blood. The UA also may show leukocytes when a stone is associated with a urinary tract infection (UTI). A urine culture can identify urea-splitting organisms commonly associated with struvite stones, such as *Proteus* spp. The stone, if passed, should be retained and sent to the laboratory for analysis.

A metabolic evaluation should be considered for patients who present with new stone formation within 1 year of the preceding stone. This may include measurement of urine and serum content of calcium, phosphorus, uric acid, creatinine, citrate, and so on. A parathyroid hormone level and a fasting calcium-loading test are very helpful. It is important to differentiate between resorptive, renal, and absorptive hypercalciuria.

RADIOLOGIC AND IMAGING STUDIES

About 90 percent of renal stones are radiopaque and are visible on a KUB (kidneys, ureters, and bladder) view. An intravenous pyelogram (IVP) usually is obtained to evaluate renal function and ascertain the degree of obstruction. The iodine-based IVP dye is very hyperosmolar and causes diuresis, which is often both therapeutic and diagnostic. One should avoid an IVP if there is an iodine allergy, however. Many clinicians are now choosing to use spiral computed tomography (CT) to confirm the diagnosis. Ultrasound is another diagnostic option that can show the location and size of the stone, as well as the condition of the kidneys. Ultrasound is especially useful in a patient who is pregnant or anuric or has chronic renal failure.

TREATMENT OF URETERAL STONES

Smaller stones are likely to pass. Typically, 31 to 93 percent pass spontaneously, and 90 percent pass if they are in the distal ureter and are less than 4 mm in diameter; about 50 percent will pass if they are in the distal ureter and are 4 to 5.9 mm in diameter. Expectant therapy includes hydration, analgesia, and plain films at 1- to 2-week intervals (for calcified stones).

TABLE 18-5-2. Diagnostic Considerations for Renal Stones

Aneurysm of the abdominal aorta
Acute pyelonephritis
Biliary colic
Appendicitis
Pancreatitis
Bowel obstruction
Pelvic inflammatory disease
Diverticulitis
Gastroenteritis
Perforated ulcer

Manipulative or surgical treatment may be indicated if there is fever and UTI, severe colic, complete obstruction, or impaction of stone. Manipulative therapy includes endoscopic instruments; distal stones are best managed in this manner. Extracorporeal shock-wave lithotripsy (ESWL) is moderately successful. In percutaneous ultrasonic lithotripsy, a nephroscope is inserted through nephrostomy tract and an ultrasound probe is used to fragment the calculus. Laser lithotripsy using a ureteroscope is another method of lithotripsy. Surgical measures are used rarely since the various forms of lithotripsy are usually clinically successful.

Pharmacologic Management

Pain control is an essential component of treatment. Ketorolac (Toradol) 60 mg given intramuscularly acts on the smooth muscle of the ureter and diminishes spasms and is an effective analgesic for renal stones. Narcotic analgesics such as meperidine (Demerol) 50 to 100 mg intramuscularly and morphine 10 to 15 mg intramuscularly also can be used. Nausea and vomiting may need to be controlled before imaging studies are performed. Control usually can be achieved with promethazine rectal suppositories or intramuscular promethazine. These medications also have a desirable relaxant effect.

Most patients can be managed on an outpatient basis. With adequate pain control, rest, sufficient oral (6 to 8 oz of water per hour) or intravenous (normal saline) hydration, and straining of the urine, 90 percent of stones can be passed successfully. Overhydration should be avoided as it can damage the kidneys.

Patient Education

Appropriate dietary modifications, if indicated, should be encouraged, including decreased animal protein, increased fruits and vegetables, decreased dairy products, and decreased sodium.

Disposition

A referral should be made to a urologist for follow-up. The stone, if obtained, should be analyzed for its composition, and a more thorough workup can be done if it is clinically warranted.

COMPLICATIONS AND RED FLAGS

Hospitalization is mandatory when the following conditions are present:

- Adequate analgesia requiring intravenous agents
- Persistent vomiting or ileus
- Coexisting pyelonephritis
- Documented or suspected renal dysfunction [elevated blood urea nitrogen (BUN) or creatinine, bilateral ureteral stones, oliguria or anuria, hydronephrosis]

Drug Seekers

In the outpatient setting, providers should be aware of the "well-dressed patient from out of town who presents with classic renal 'colic' and requests a narcotic only "until the stone passes." Often this patient has an "allergy to nonsteroidal anti-inflammatory drugs and only Demerol will work." The patient also may solicit a written prescription for preferred narcotics. This is the classic presentation of a drug-seeking patient. These clever patients always have gross or microscopic hematuria, which usually is added to the urine by pricking their fingers.

PYELONEPHRITIS

DISCUSSION

Infection of the kidneys is an acute disorder and can vary from mild symptoms to sepsis. In young, previously healthy adults, pyelonephri-

tis frequently follows a UTI, especially when there is a delay in seeking care.

Etiology

Pyelonephritis involves both the parenchyma and the pelvis. The organisms involved include the aerobic gram-negative bacteria: *Enterobacteriaceae*, *E. coli* (most common), *Proteus* spp. (important; produces urease), *Klebsiella* spp, *S. epidermidis*, *S. saprophyticus*, *S. aureus*, *Streptococci* group D (enterococci), and *Staphylococcus* spp. (infection by hematogenous spread and can cause bacteriuria and renal abscesses).

Pathology

The kidneys may be enlarged secondary to inflammation from multiple subcapsular abscesses. This usually is seen in the cortex and can result in pus-filled collecting tubules.

Pathogenesis

Usually ascending infection and hematogenous spread are uncommon, and lymphatic spread rarely occurs. The female predisposition is due to a short urethra and the close proximity of the anus, vaginal introitus, and periurethral areas, which leads to bacterial colonization.

Males are less susceptible. Ascension of infection depends on establishing infection in bladder; microbial virulence factors; vesicoureteral reflux, the most important quality of ureteral peristalsis; and susceptibility of renal medulla to infection.

SIGNS AND SYMPTOMS

The symptoms may include an abrupt onset of shaking chills, moderate to high fever, a constant ache in the loin, irritative voiding symptoms, malaise, nausea, vomiting, and diarrhea. Flank or back pain, dysuria, and tachycardia may be seen. On examination, the patient will have costovertebral (CVA) tenderness, fever, and a corresponding rapid pulse and may appear sick or "toxic-looking."

DIAGNOSTIC CONSIDERATIONS

Pyelonephritis can mimic many abdominal diseases and conditions (see Table 18-5-3).

SPECIAL CONSIDERATIONS

Infants and children should always be screened for pyelonephritis and urosepsis when they present with fever, vomiting, or lethargy. The elderly may present with a vaguely altered mental status or an abdominal complaint. Immunocompromised patients who present with fever should have a urinalysis as part of the workup. Pregnant women with fever or vomiting should always be screened for pyelonephritis.

TABLE 18-5-3. Diagnostic Considerations for Pyelonephritis

Renal calculi
Appendicitis
Diverticulitis
Pancreatitis
Cholecystitis
Obstructive uropathy (stricture, etc.)
Pelvic inflammatory disease (especially *Chlamydia*)

LABORATORY STUDIES

The patient will present with leukocytosis, polymorphonuclear neutrophils (PMNs), bands, and an increased erythrocyte sedimentation rate (ESR). Urinalysis will exhibit heavy pyuria, bacteriuria, proteinuria, and hematuria. Leukocyte casts and glitter cells (large PMNs containing cytoplasmic particles) are also present. The urine culture will be positive. Blood cultures may be indicated, depending on the severity of the infection.

RADIOLOGIC STUDIES

Plain films can show obliteration of renal outline, edema, and calcifications.

TREATMENT

Specific Measures

Hospitalization usually is considered for more seriously ill patients. Empirical antibiotics are recommended until culture results are available.

If the patient is hospitalized, intravenous ampicillin 1 g every 6 h and gentamicin 1 mg/kg every 8 h often are used for up to 3 weeks.

If the patient is not hospitalized, a single oral drug is used. The choices include

- Trimethoprim-sulfamethoxazole (Bactrim DS or Septra DS) 160 and 800 mg bid for 21 days
- Ciprofloxacin (Cipro) 500 mg bid for 21 days
- Ofloxacin (Floxin) 200 to 300 mg bid for 21 days

Supportive Measures

Supportive measures include analgesics, antipyretics, and hydration. Patients who fail to respond may require excretory or retrograde urography to rule out obstructive uropathy, which can lead to irreversible renal damage.

Prevention

It is very important to prevent damage to an immature kidney in the pediatric population. All UTIs must be evaluated thoroughly and treated. It is also important to identify any underlying abnormalities.

Patient Education

When treated in the outpatient setting, patients need to understand the importance of taking medication as directed.

DISPOSITION

At least one follow-up visit is recommended 1 or 2 weeks after antibiotics are finished for a repeat urine culture.

COMPLICATIONS AND RED FLAGS

Hospitalization is required if a patient appears septic, has a chronic underlying disease such as diabetes, has intractable nausea and vomiting, or is very young or very old. Important considerations for other patients include being pregnant, male gender (young adult), and immunocompromised or immunosuppressed patients (HIV, transplants, cancer, etc.). If a patient does not improve in 48 to 72 h, renal calculi, abscess, and necrosis need to be considered.

ACKNOWLEDGMENT

The editor would like to acknowledge the contribution of Michaela O'Brien-Norton, the author of this chapter in the first edition of *Primary Care for Physician Assistants.*

BIBLIOGRAPHY

Coe FL, Favus MJ: Nephrolithiasis, in Fauci AS, Braunwald E, Isselbacher KJ, et al: *Harrison's Principles and Practice of Internal Medicine,* 14th ed. New York, McGraw-Hill, 1998, pp 1569–1574.

Howes DS: Urinary tract infections, in Tintinalli JE, Ruiz E, Krome RL: *Emergency Medicine.* New York, McGraw-Hill, 1996, pp 527–532.

Peacock WF: Urologic stone disease, in Tintinalli JE, Ruiz E, Krone RL: *Emergency Medicine.* New York, McGraw-Hill, 1996, pp 549–553.

Presti JC, Stoller ML, Carroll PR: Acute pyelonephritis urinary stone disease, in Tierney LM, McPhee SJ, Papadakis MA (eds.): *Current Medical Diagnosis and Treatment,* Lange/McGraw-Hill, 2000, pp 924–933.

Stamm WE: Urinary tract infections and pyelonephritis, in Fauci AS, Braunwald E, Isselbacher KJ, et al: *Harrison's Principles and Practice of Internal Medicine,* 14th ed. New York, McGraw-Hill, 1998, pp 817–824.

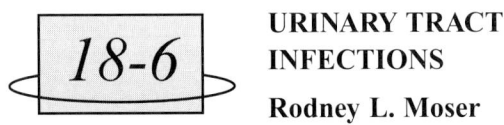

URINARY TRACT INFECTIONS

Rodney L. Moser

DISCUSSION

Urinary tract infections (UTIs) are among the most common bacterial infections seen in a primary care practice, especially in females of all ages. There are between 6 million and 7 million office visits annually in the United States for acute, uncomplicated UTIs, with an annual health cost that exceeds $1 billion.

There is a 50-fold increase in UTIs in adult women after they become sexually active. UTIs frequently occur in children, especially girls over age 1. Before age 1, UTIs are twice as common in boys; this is due to obstructive anomalies such as urethral stenosis. UTIs in healthy adult males are relatively uncommon compared to those in women and are related predominantly to prostate infections, although elderly men often have UTIs that result from urinary tract obstructive syndromes. Because of bacterial colonization under the foreskin, there appears to be a slightly higher incidence of UTIs in uncircumcised males in comparison to circumcised males.

UTIs are subdivided into upper and lower tract infections. Upper tract infections include pyelonephritis (see Chap. 18-5), and lower tract infections include cystitis, urethritis, and prostatitis (see Chap. 18-3). Urethritis is an infection of the urethral opening that is seen primarily in adolescence and is associated with sexually transmitted diseases such as chlamydia (see Chap. 9-6). Cystitis is an infection of the bladder. Pyelonephritis is an infection of the renal parenchyma with systemic involvement (see Chap. 18-5). Infection in any part of the urinary tract may spread to another part (e.g., cystitis can spread in an ascending fashion and lead to pyelonephritis). Most infections are of the ascending type. Anatomic defenses against ascending infections include acidic urine, large and dilute volume, complete bladder emptying, and a tract free of any obstruction.

All UTIs have a pathologic number of microorganisms causing infection and symptomatology. The urine is considered sterile until it is contaminated with pathogens at the distal urethra. Bacteriuria is detected in over 1 percent of all females. Virtually any organism introduced into the urinary tract can cause infection. The majority of these infections are caused by fecal flora (see Table 18-6-1). In acute uncomplicated infections, a single coliform pathogen (*Escherichia coli* is responsible for over 90 percent of first infections) is usually responsible. These infections are typically sensitive to a large number of broad-spectrum antibiotics.

Acute UTIs can cause inflammation of any part of the urinary tract, resulting in intense hyperemia and often bleeding. Renal infections are the most serious complication type of UTI and require more aggressive management. Pyelonephritis is discussed in Chap. 18-5.

TABLE 18-6-1. Common Microorganisms That Cause Urinary Tract Infections

ORGANISM	PERCENT OF CASES
Escherichia coli	75–90
Enterobacter	2–5
Klebsiella	2–5
Proteus	1–2
Miscellaneous*	3–4

Pseudomonas, Staphylococcus epidermidis, Chlamydia, Ureaplasma/Mycoplasma, and others.

SIGNS AND SYMPTOMS

In lower tract infections in women and older children (cystitis), a sudden or gradual onset of dysuria (burning), frequency, and urgency is considered classic. These patients also complain of lower abdominal (suprapubic and/or bladder) discomfort and foul-smelling turbid urine. A particularly annoying symptom is strangury, or the voiding of tiny drops of urine, accompanied by urethral spasm.

Gross hematuria is not an unusual presenting sign. Fever and other constitutional symptoms are variable but relatively uncommon in simple cystitis. There is no true costovertebral angle (CVA) tenderness in lower tract infections, although referred low back discomfort is possible.

The symptoms of upper tract involvement are more systemic and include CVA (flank) pain and tenderness, abdominal pain, voiding symptoms (dysuria, frequency, and urgency), fever and/or chills, tachycardia, headache, malaise, and vomiting.

UTIs may be asymptomatic in the elderly, diabetic patients, and persons with diminished mental abilities. In children, the signs and symptoms appear to be age-related. Infants may present with irritability, fever, poor feeding, and even failure to thrive. All infants with a fever of undetermined origin should have a urinalysis and blood and/or urine cultures. In children over age 3 or 4, the symptoms are more classic.

A large number of dysuric patients do not have a UTI, and this may explain the many negative cultures seen in "classic" patients. Many women with characteristic symptoms do have corresponding bacterial colony counts consistent with a UTI. Urethritis secondary to sexual trauma and vaginitis, particularly monilial, are likely diagnostic considerations. In little girls, dysuria can be caused by a variety of local irritants, such as soaps (bubble baths), detergents, fabric softeners (especially the drier sheet type), poor hygiene, masturbation, and pinworms. Children who are sexually abused often present with UTIs or UTI symptomatology.

DIAGNOSTIC CONSIDERATIONS

In adult women, vaginitis (particularly monilial) is the most common comorbid finding (see Chap. 12-2). Vaginal yeast infections can cause profound urethral irritation and dysuria. Other vaginal infections, such as bacterial vaginosis and trichomoniasis, can present with dysuria (see Chaps. 12-3 and 12-11). Sexually transmitted diseases such as chlamydia, gonorrhea, and herpes simplex infections should be considered, especially in heterosexually active women with negative or borderline bacteriuria or negative urine cultures.

Since UTIs correlate with sexual activity, urethral microtrauma during coitus can be responsible for UTI-type symptoms (honeymoon cystitis). Since many women with classic UTI symptoms avoid a careful examination, these findings often are missed. Colposcopy, if available, may reveal tiny periurethral fissures.

SPECIAL CONSIDERATIONS

In the pediatric population, a standard urologic recommendation is that all boys regardless of age and all girls under age 6 have a thorough workup after just one confirmed UTI. In girls over age 6, a workup usually is done after a second UTI (see "Radiologic and Imaging Studies," below), depending on the clinical judgment of the provider.

UTIs are more common in sexually active women who use diaphragms and/or spermatocides for contraception (see Chap. 12-14). They are also more common in diabetic patients, immunocompromised patients, the elderly (especially those who are bedridden), and spinal cord patients (especially those who use intermittent self-catheterization or indwelling catheters).

Pregnant females may have asymptomatic bacteriuria up to 15 percent of the time. If untreated, a simple UTI has a 20 to 40 percent chance of developing into pyelonephritis, which can lead to a premature birth and other perinatal complications.

LABORATORY STUDIES

A complete urinalysis (chemical dipstick and microscopy) is a quick and cost-effective study that frequently can be done in the office. The specimen must be a fresh, clean midstream catch. One should avoid accepting specimens brought from home in plastic containers and baby food jars. Urine is a good culture medium for bacteria, even at room temperature. The urinalysis should be done within an hour, or the specimen should be refrigerated and done within 18 h. Specimens obtained by straight catheterization or percutaneous suprapubic aspiration are also appropriate. Pediatric specimens obtained in sterile bags with an adhesive back applied over the genitalia (Tin-Kol bag) frequently are contaminated with skin flora and fecal material.

Since many patients with a history of UTIs tend to medicate themselves with old antibiotics or phenazopyridine hydrochloride (Pyridium), a careful medication history is essential. Chemical dipsticks test a variety of items from pH to nitrites. Increased nitrites in the urine are a suggestive marker for a UTI.

Microscopy of fresh centrifuged or uncentrifuged urine will quickly reveal pyuria or bacteriuria. More than 10 white blood cells (WBCs) per high-power field are considered abnormal; however, many active UTIs have "packed fields" of WBCs and red blood cells (RBCs). The degree of pyuria and bacteriuria does not necessarily correlate with the severity of the symptoms. The presence of leukocyte casts indicates parenchymal involvement. If the urinalysis is normal, the patient should be examined carefully for other diagnostic possibilities.

Urine cultures, including sensitivity assessments, are needed for chronic or recurrent infections but need not be done routinely in uncomplicated cases. The urine culture will be positive for the causative organism, but colony counts exceeding 10^5/mL are not essential to confirm the diagnosis.

RADIOLOGIC AND IMAGING STUDIES

Uncomplicated, infrequent UTIs do not require radiologic or imaging studies in most cases. If clinically warranted (pyelonephritis, recurrent infections, etc.), renal imaging studies, including a voiding cystoureterogram (VCUG) and renal ultrasonography, are the standard workup. Computed tomography (CT) also may be useful in selected patients. Intravenous pyelography is used infrequently in the evaluation of UTIs in children unless there is a strong possibility of structural anomalies. A 99m-DMSA renal scan is useful only in acute infections.

Cystoscopy often is done to detect abnormalities of the urethra or bladder.

TREATMENT OF UNCOMPLICATED INFECTIONS

Pharmacologic Management

Although 1-day and 3-day regimens often are touted as being more cost-effective, having fewer side effects, and leading to better patient compliance, they should be limited to very select uncomplicated patients with initial UTIs.

A variety of antibiotic choices are available to treat UTIs. Treatment with short-term antimicrobial therapy (1 to 3 days) is appropriate for uncomplicated cystitis in women. Two tablets of trimethoprim-sulfamethoxazole 160/800 given as a single dose is a very cost-effective alternative to longer-duration therapy.

The following regimens also are used and are considered standard oral regimens for adult, nonpregnant women[1]:

- Nitrofurantoin monohydrate macrocrystals (Macrobid) 100 mg bid for 7 days
- Cephalexin 250 to 500 mg qid for 1 to 3 days
- Ciprofloxacin (Cipro) 250 to 500 mg bid for 1 to 3 days
- Norfloxacin 400 mg bid for 1 to 3 days
- Ofloxacin 200 mg bid for 1 to 3 days

Treatment of Pregnant Females

Pregnant females are given nitrofurantoin monohydrate macrocrystals (Macrobid) 100 mg bid for 7 days. Penicillin and cephalosporins are also safe and effective. Aminoglycosides, tetracycline-type medications, and quinolones should be avoided. Sulfonamides should not be used in the last 6 weeks of pregnancy.

Treatment of Children

For uncomplicated infections in children older than 2 months of age who are not vomiting, oral sulfisoxazole (Gantrisin) or trimethoprim-sulfamethoxazole (Bactrim, Septra) suspension in doses based on weight can be given.

For children under 2 months, parenteral antibiotics starting with ampicillin and gentamicin or cefotaxime should be used, depending on the urine culture. Any child, regardless of age, who appears toxic should be admitted and placed on parenteral antibiotics pending clinical improvement.

Older children can be treated with antibiotic therapy similar to that used for adults, with the dose adjusted for weight.

NOTES AND PEARLS

Tired of waiting all day for an infant or toddler to urinate into a bag? Try a few minutes of rhythmic "tapping" (like percussion) over a full bladder, about once a second. This may stimulate urination in a few minutes or so. Have the parent hold a sterile urine cup to catch the flow. Give it a try.

REFERENCE

1. Tierney LM, McPhee SJ, Papadakis MA: *Current Medical Diagnosis and Treatment,* New York, McGraw-Hill, 2000, pp 922–926.

BIBLIOGRAPHY

Fauci AS, Braunwald E, Isselbacher KJ, et al (eds): *Harrison's Principles of Internal Medicine,* 14th ed. New York, McGraw-Hill, 1998.

Hay WH, Hayward AR, Sondheimer JM (eds): *Current Pediatric Diagnosis and Treatment,* 15th ed. New York, McGraw-Hill, 2000.

Hanno PM, Wein AJ: *Clinical Manual of Urology,* 2d ed. New York, McGraw-Hill, 1994.

Wasson J (ed): *The Common Symptom Guide,* 4th ed. New York, McGraw-Hill, 1996.

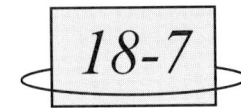

TESTICULAR TORSION
Stephanie D. Bowlin

DISCUSSION

Testicular torsion is defined as a twisting of the spermatic cord of the testicle that usually occurs only on one side. The spermatic cord is a tube attached to the upper pole of the testes. It contains the vas deferens (which transports sperm), blood vessels, nerves, and muscle. Torsion of the testis or cord results from bilateral maldevelopment of fixation between the enveloping tunica vaginalis and the posterior scrotal wall.[1,2] As the cremaster muscle contracts, testicular torsion occurs. The damage to the testicle is sometimes irreversible. Torsion is most common in adolescents age 12 to 20 because of maximum hormone stimulation, but all ages can be affected.[3]

SIGNS AND SYMPTOMS

Often there is a history of participation in a sports event or some type of strenuous activity or of trauma just before the appearance of pain associated with testicular torsion. However, a number of patients are sleeping when the pain presents. The pain is unilateral, acute, and severe and is felt in the lower abdomen, the inguinal canal, or the testis. The pain can be constant or intermittent. Pain is not affected by posture because torsion is an ischemic episode, and the area becomes inflamed only after the testis has infarcted. Patients also may complain of symptoms of gastroenteritis and return to the clinic 1 to 2 days later with full-blown torsion. It is evident whether the patient had torsion when he presented; however, torsion should be considered when an adolescent male presents with lower abdominal pain. On physical examination, the scrotum is red, swollen, elevated, and tender to the touch. Nausea and vomiting may be present, and if the pain is severe, the heart rate will be increased.

DIAGNOSTIC CONSIDERATIONS

On appearance, testicular torsion may be difficult to distinguish from torsion of the appendix testis or appendix epididymis and epididymitis (see Chapter 18-4). To distinguish torsion of the testis from torsion of the appendages or epididymis, a small palpable lump on the superior pole of the testis or epididymis is occasionally discernible. It may appear blue when the skin is pulled tautly over it (blue dot sign).[4] This sign is pathognomonic of torsion of the appendix testis or epididymis. Patients with these processes are not usually in the 12- to 20-year-old age group, and their pain may be relieved by placing the patient in the supine position and elevating the scrotum above the pubic symphysis (Prehn's sign).[5] In testicular torsion, however, Prehn's sign increases the pain of the torsion. If a diagnosis of torsion of the appendages can be confirmed by color flow Doppler ultrasound, immediate surgery may not be necessary. Other diagnostic considerations that present similarly include orchitis, testicular tumor, inguinal hernia, hydrocele, variocele, spermatocele, and groin pain and/or strain. Transillumination of the scrotum with a penlight may aid in ruling out some of these differential diagnoses.

RADIOLOGIC AND IMAGING STUDIES

There are no readily available clinical or laboratory parameters to judge either the degree or the duration of testicular ischemia.[2] However, evaluation by color flow Doppler ultrasound is useful because this study includes a thorough assessment of intratesticular blood flow. The results may show an altered testicular echo texture, which is indicative of testicular infarction.[5] In epididymitis, testicular blood flow is usually normal. While Doppler ultrasound may be useful, the accuracy of the diagnosis is limited by its availability and the operator's experience in interpreting the images.[2] Testicular isotope scanning is also effective in assessing an acute scrotum, although some providers feel that this test produces unnecessary delays in treatment and increases the cost to patients.

TREATMENT

This is a urologic emergency. No matter how long the patient has been symptomatic or what the presenting physical examination suggests, if testicular torsion cannot be excluded by history and physical examination, an emergency urologic referral should be made for scrotal exploration. Surgery is the definitive diagnostic test and the procedure of choice.[5] Surgery is performed to untangle the twisted cord and attach the affected testicle to the inside scrotal wall, thereby preventing recurrence. Surgical repair should be performed within 3 to 4 h after symptoms begin.

While awaiting transportation of the patient to the operating room, the health care provider should attempt manual detorsion of the affected testis. The majority of testes will twist in a lateral to medial fashion; therefore, detorsion should be performed with a medial to a lateral motion (the detorsion procedure has been described as "opening a book"). The patient should be informed that the detorsion procedure is painful and that local anesthesia will not be used; when the procedure is complete, the elimination of pain will indicate a successful treatment. The use of anesthesia would mask the pain. A worsening of the patient's pain indicates that detorsion should be performed in the opposite direction. Any relief of pain is considered a positive result and may convert an emergent procedure to an elective one.

PATIENT EDUCATION

Inform the patient and parents that if one testicle is removed, the remaining healthy testicle should provide sufficient hormones for normal male maturation, sexual functioning, and reproduction. After surgery, wrap ice packs in plastic and apply them to the affected side to relieve swelling and pain. Apply for 5 to 10 min and repeat as needed. Resume activity gradually. Wear an athletic supporter or a cup for protection during sports activities. Use pain medication as prescribed. Patient follow-up is indicated if fever, chills, or excessive bleeding from the surgical site occurs.

REFERENCES

1. Griffith HW: *Complete Guide to Symptoms, Illness and Surgery.* Putnam Berkley Group, electronic rights by Medical Data Exchange, 1995.
2. Tintinalli JE, Ruis E, Krome R (eds): Renal and genitourinary disorders, in *Emergency Medicine,* 4th ed. New York, McGraw-Hill, 1996; pp 535–537.
3. Health Library: http://thriveonline.aol.com/assets/health.lookrule.gif.
4. Tierney L, McPhee S, Papadakis M (eds): *Current Medical Diagnosis and Treatment,* 39th ed. New York, Lange Medical/McGraw-Hill, 1995; pp 919–920, 928–929.
5. Older R, Watson L: Ultrasound diagnosis of testicular torsion: Beware the swollen epididymis. *J Urol* 157:1369–1370, 1997.

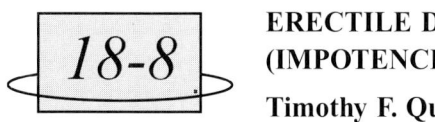

ERECTILE DYSFUNCTION (IMPOTENCE)
Timothy F. Quigley

DISCUSSION

Erectile dysfunction (ED) is defined as "the inability to achieve or maintain an erection satisfactory for sexual intercourse."[1] The term *impotence* has fallen into disfavor because of the associated negative connotations. With the introduction of sildenafil (Viagra) in March 1998, there has been increased public attention to and patient demand for evaluation and treatment of ED. As many as 34 percent of men age 40 to 70 years old have experienced some degree of ED in their lifetimes.[2] The prevalence increases to more than 50 percent in men over age 70.[3] Current treatment is successful more than 95 percent of the time.[4]

PATHOGENESIS

Normal male erection requires an intact neurovascular system, including the autonomic and sympathetic nerve supply to the penis. Erection is caused by an increase in arterial flow, relaxation and engorgement of the cavernosal smooth muscle, compression of the venules that limit outflow, and contraction of the bulbocavernosus and ischiocavernosus muscles.[5] The relaxation of the corpus cavernosum is mediated by several neurotransmitters, including nitric oxide, acetylcholine, vasoactive intestinal polypeptide, and prostaglandins.[1]

While most cases of ED were considered to be of primarily psychogenic origin until recently, experts now estimate that up to 80 percent of cases of ED have an organic cause. Table 18-8-1 lists the most common causes of ED,[7] particularly aging; vascular disease, including hypertension and dyslipidemia; endocrinologic disease such as diabetes mellitus and thyroid dysfunction; medication side effects, especially from antihypertensives and antidepressants; hormonal disorders such as hypogonadism; pelvic trauma, including prostate surgery; substance abuse, including alcohol and tobacco; and affective disorders such as anxiety and depression.[8]

SIGNS AND SYMPTOMS

A complete medical and sexual history is required for the clinical evaluation of ED. The presence of ED may be the first indication of significant health problems such as diabetes, hypercholesterolemia, and neurologic disease. A complete history may reveal reversible causes of ED such as hormonal and thyroid disorders. Since ED frequently results from age-related diseases, medication side effects, and endocrinologic and vascular diseases, the clinician should ask these patients if they are encountering any sexual problems.

A gradual onset of erectile difficulties generally is associated with organic disease, while a sudden onset suggests a psychogenic origin. Patients should be asked about their past medical history, surgical history, substance abuse, current medications, and psychosocial history and past sexual functioning. Table 18-8-2 outlines the important items to cover in the evaluation of ED. If a patient consistently has nocturnal or morning erections, is able to masturbate to ejaculation, or has had recent relationship difficulties, one should suspect psychological causes of ED.[8]

OBJECTIVE FINDINGS

The physical examination should focus on the evaluation of the endocrinologic, vascular, and neurologic systems. Table 18-8-3 outlines the basics of a physical examination of a patient who presents with ED.

The endocrinologic examination should focus on signs of hypogonadism, abnormal genital development, and penile deformities. The vascular examination should focus on signs of hypertension, atherosclerosis, and peripheral vascular disease. The neurologic examination may include genital and perineal sensation. A prostate examination is routine in this clinical evaluation, since the age group most frequently affected by ED is at high risk for prostate cancer.

DIAGNOSTIC CONSIDERATIONS

A complete sexual history should distinguish ED from other male sexual dysfunctions, such as loss of libido, premature ejaculation, and anorgasmia.

TABLE 18-8-1. Common Etiologies of Erectile Dysfunction

Vascular
  Atherosclerosis
  Hypertension
  Hyperlipidemia
  Smoking
  Blunt trauma
  Surgical trauma
  Pelvic irradiation

Neurologic
  Alzheimer's disease
  Parkinson's disease
  Cerebrovascular accidents
  Neurologic tumors
  Multiple sclerosis
  Herniated disk
  Amyotrophic lateral sclerosis
  Spina bifida
  Peripheral neuropathies

Psychological
  Stress
  Anxiety
  Depression
  Performance anxiety
  Relationship conflict
  Sexual abuse
  Fear of sexually transmitted diseases
  Religious conflict

Endocrine
  Hypogonadism
  Cushing's disease
  Primary testicular failure
  Thyroid disease
  Hyperprolactinemia

Medications
  Antihypertensives
    Beta-blockers
    Alpha antagonists
    Diuretics
  Antidepressants
    Selective serotonin reuptake inhibitors
    Tricyclics
    Monoamine oxidase inhibitors
  Anxiolytics
  Cimetidine
  Lipid-lowering agents
  Nonsteroidal anti-inflammatory drugs
  Cytotoxic agents
  Corticosteroids
  Antipsychotics

Substance abuse
  Tobacco
  Alcohol
  Heroin
  Marijuana

Penile disorders
  Priapism
  Peyronie's disease

SOURCE: Onel and Albertsen.[6]

Libido (sexual desire) is usually intact in a patient with ED unless prior failure of sexual performance or medication side effects have caused secondary loss of desire. Premature ejaculation rarely has an organic cause, and the patient's history may reveal sexual inexperience, unreasonable performance expectations, or emotional disorders.[5] Anorgasmia in the presence of normal libido and erection may be caused by medication side effects, especially those of selective serotonin reuptake inhibitors and antihistamines.

TABLE 18-8-2. Medical and Sexual History in Erectile Dysfunction

History of present illness
  Onset and duration of erectile difficulties
  Degree of dysfunction: partial or complete
  Presence of nocturnal or morning erections
  Ability to masturbate

Medical history
  Vascular disease
  Endocrinologic disease
  Hormonal disease
  Surgical history

Medication use
  Antihypertensives
  Antidepressants
  Hormones
  Other medications (See Table 18-8-1)

Substance abuse history
  Tobacco
  Alcohol
  Other drugs of abuse

Mental health history
  Anxiety/depression
  Relationship difficulties
  Past sexual abuse

SOURCE: Guay et al.[3]

LABORATORY STUDIES

The history, the patient, and the clinical setting should guide the extent of diagnostic testing. The goal of laboratory studies should be to identify previously unrecognized systemic diseases. A routine urinalysis, complete blood count (CBC), chemistry panel, and lipid panel may reveal common metabolic disorders such as diabetes, renal insufficiency, and dyslipidemia. Testing of thyroid-stimulating hormone (TSH) may detect unrecognized thyroid disease. The role of more extensive endocrinologic testing (e.g., serum testosterone or prolactin) is controversial since the incidence of endocrinopathy in patients who present with erectile dysfunction is around 2 percent.[7] Prostate specific antigen (PSA) testing may help detect an occult prostate malignancy.

OTHER DIAGNOSTICS

More extensive diagnostic testing may be reserved for patients who require invasive treatments, and many of the more specialized tests are performed under the supervision of a urologist with expertise in ED. Table 18-8-4 outlines specialized tests for ED.

TABLE 18-8-3. Physical Examination of a Patient with Erectile Dysfunction

Endocrinologic examination
  Palpate thyroid gland for hypertrophy
  Evaluate breasts for gynecomastia
  Examine quality of axillary and pubic hair
  Palpate for fibrous penile plaques
  Palpate testicles for atrophy, size, and descent

Vascular examination
  Take blood pressure
  Palpate peripheral pulses

Neurologic examination
  Assess anal sphincter tone
  Test bulbocavernosus reflex
  Test cremasteric reflex
  Observe gait

Other
  Palpate prostate for hypertrophy, inflammation, malignancy

TABLE 18-8-4. Specialized Tests for Erectile Dysfunction

Nocturnal studies
  Portable home monitor records penile rigidity during sleep
  Nocturnal tumescence testing performed in sleep laboratory

Vascular erectile testing
  Duplex Doppler ultrasonography records arterial and venous flow
  Dynamic infusion pharmacocavernosometry
  Dynamic infusion pharmacocavernosography

Pharmacologic testing
  Penile injection of vasoactive substance will induce erections with intact
    vascularity

Radiologic testing
  Pelvic arteriography before vascular reconstructive surgery

Hormonal testing
  Total and free serum testosterone levels
  Gonadotropins
  Gonadotropin-releasing hormone
  Prolactin level

SOURCE: Jordon.[1]

TREATMENT

Until 1998, there were limited options for therapy for ED. Now there are a variety of effective treatments that have proved successful for the vast majority of patients with organic ED. These treatment options include oral medication, urethral suppositories, injectable vasoactive substances, vacuum erection devices, and vascular surgery. Patients who suffer from psychogenic ED may benefit from psychotherapy, including behaviorally oriented sex therapy.[5]

Treatment of a diagnosed medical condition such as diabetes, hypertension, or atherosclerosis is the first therapeutic step, but control of these chronic diseases does not ensure the return of normal erectile function.[8] Treatment of hypogonadism or hypothyroidism may help reverse ED, as may discontinuance of medications with unwanted side effects. Patients who continue to smoke should be counseled about smoking cessation techniques and benefits.

Medication

Sildenafil (Viagra) is the first oral medication approved by the U.S. Food and Drug Administration (FDA) for the treatment of ED. Since its introduction in March 1998, the availability of this treatment has radically changed the treatment of ED, and primary care providers, not specialists, are now treating ED. Clinical practice has shown that the efficacy of sildenafil is about 50 percent.[9]

Sildenafil causes relaxation and engorgement of the cavernosal smooth muscle but does not have a direct effect on arousal, ejaculation, or orgasm. It is efficacious in men with both psychogenic and organic causes of ED.

Table 18-8-5 summarizes the mode of action, dosage, side effects, interactions, and contraindications of sildenafil. Of particular concern is the absolute contraindication to administering sildenafil to a patient who is concurrently taking any nitrate-containing medications. The additive effect of the nitric oxide release with sildenafil combined with nitrate medications can cause severe hypotension and sudden cardiac death.[10]

Yohimbine, an alpha-adrenergic blocker, has been used in the pharmacologic treatment of ED for decades, but its efficacy has been limited to patients whose ED is of psychogenic origin.

Table 18-8-6 lists several alternatives to sildenafil for the treatment of ED. Pharmacologically, some patients benefit from urethral suppositories or penile injection therapy. Patients with hypogonadism should be considered for testosterone supplementation.

TABLE 18-8-5. Sildenafil (Viagra) Summary

Mode of action: Sildenafil inhibits the conversion of cyclic guanosine monophosphate (cGMP) in the corpus cavernosum, increasing the availability of cGMP. The inhibition of this enzyme causes relaxation of the cavernosal smooth muscle and the resultant erection. This inhibitory action of sildenafil is mediated by the neurotransmitter nitric oxide

Metabolism: Sildenafil is metabolized hepatically in the P450 and 2C9 routes

Absorption: Peak plasma concentration in median 60 min

Dosage: 50 mg taken 1 h before anticipated sexual activity. May be increased to 100 mg if needed. Starting dose of 25 mg recommended for patients more than 65 years old and patients with renal or hepatic impairment. Should not be used more than once every 24 h and should not be used with other drugs for erectile dysfunction[8]

Adverse effects: Headache, flushing, dyspepsia, change in perception of color (bluing)[8]

Contraindications: Absolutely contraindicated in patients taking oral nitrate medication and patients who use illicit recreational drugs that contain amyl nitrite ("poppers"). Use cautiously in patients with active coronary ischemia, congestive heart failure, borderline low blood pressure, or retinitis pigmentosa, along with patients on complicated multidrug antihypertensive program and patients taking drugs that are metabolized by or inhibit cytochrome P450 enzyme 3A4[10]

Drug interactions: Cimetidine, erythromycin, and possible other inhibitors of cytochrome P450 isoenzyme 3A4 may decrease sildenafil clearance

Efficacy: Clinical efficacy around 50%. Limited efficacy after radical prostatectomy. Virtually no efficacy if nonnerve-sparing procedure.[9] Best results with ED caused by anxiety and/or mild ED[3]

Nonpharmacologic Treatment

Vacuum erection devices represent a noninvasive treatment approach, while penile prostheses and vascular surgery are more invasive procedures that are utilized primarily by urologic surgeons[9] (see Table 18-8-6).

TABLE 18-8-6. Alternative Treatments for Erectile Dysfunction

PHARMACOLOGIC TREATMENTS

Urethral suppositories: Alprostadil, in pellet form, causes smooth muscle relaxation and subsequent erection. Placement of restrictive band at base of penis reduces venous outflow. Clinical efficacy in organic dysfunction is about 25%. Adverse effects include localized burning, hypotension, and syncope

Penile injection therapy: Before introduction of sildenafil (Viagra), injection therapy was the most popular therapy for ED. Using fine 27- to 30-gauge needle, the patient injects alprostadil (Caverject) at the dorsolateral base of penis, causing erection in 5 to 10 min. Efficacy is about 80 percent. Side effects include fibrosis, pain, and priapism

Testosterone supplementation: Used for hypogonadism and/or low libido. Topical patches or intramuscular injections increase serum concentrations of testosterone. Risks include stimulation of occult prostate cancer, exacerbation of sleep apnea, and polycythemia[9]

NONPHARMACOLOGIC TREATMENTS

Vacuum erection devices (VEDs): Patient inserts penis into a cylinder connected to a vacuum pump, which causes venous engorgement and erection. A restrictive band at the base of the penis traps the venous blood. Side effects include ischemia if ring is in place longer than recommended. The penis is colder because of the venous blood trapping, and this coldness is sometimes objectionable to the man's partner[6]

Penile prostheses: Surgical implantation of semirigid rods, inflatable saline-filled rods, or hinged rods is an alternative for patients who do not succeed with less invasive treatments. Risks include device malfunction and infection

Vascular surgery: Arterial bypass surgery often is reserved for select young men with pelvic or perineal trauma. Long-term efficacy is poor[3]

FOLLOW-UP

Short- and long-term follow-up care of patients receiving treatment for ED is important. Patients may have questions about the medications or devices they are using, and positive reinforcement may be valuable. In addition, progression of the underlying disease may cause treatment failure and necessitate the trial of a different mode of therapy.[3]

COMPLICATIONS AND RED FLAGS

Because of the potential for sudden severe hypotension in patients who take nitrates in addition to sildenafil, emergency care providers should ask all men with chest pain if sildenafil has been taken before administering sublingual nitroglycerin. Under no circumstances should sildenafil be prescribed to a cardiac patient who is taking long- or short-acting nitrates.

Priapism, a prolonged painful erection, is an uncommon but dangerous side effect of sildenafil, urethral suppositories, and penile injection therapy. Emergency treatment includes aspiration of blood from the corpora, injection of phenylephrine, and in severe instances surgical treatment.[8]

NOTES AND PEARLS

Recent advances in the treatment of ED have meant an improved quality of life for many affected men. An unprecedented number of men are now presenting in the primary care setting seeking treatment. While the development and marketing of sildenafil (Viagra) have increased public awareness of this disease, there are several other available options if sildenafil is not successful. Providers should avoid rushing to prescribe sildenafil without investigating for more serious acute, chronic, reversible, or comorbid conditions.

Unfortunately, there is a high dropout rate with all available therapies because of cost, side effects, inconvenience, and poor patient acceptance.[1] Two new medications—oral phentolamine and sublingual apomorphine—are in phase III clinical trials and soon may be available in the United States.[9]

REFERENCES

1. Jordan GH: Erectile function and dysfunction: How it works and what can be done when it doesn't. *Postgrad Med* 105(2):131–147, 1999.
2. Laumann EO, Paik A, Rosen RC: Sexual dysfunction in the United States: Prevalence and predictors. *JAMA* 281(6):537–544, 1999.
3. Guay AT, Levine SB, Drogo K, et al. New treatments for erectile dysfunction. *Patient Care,* March 15, 1998, www.patientcareonline.com.
4. Bachmann GA, Coleman E, Driscoll CE, et al: Patients with sexual dysfunction: Your guidance makes a difference. *Patient Care,* April 15, 1999, pp 99–123.
5. Presti JC, Stoller ML, Carroll PR: Urology, in Tierney LM, McPhee SJ, Papadakis MA (eds): *Current Medical Diagnosis and Treatment 2000,* 39th ed. New York, McGraw-Hill, 2000, pp 936–938.
6. Onel E, Albertsen PC: Management of Impotence. *Clin Advisor,* April 1999, pp 27–37.
7. Burnett AL: Erectile dysfunction: A practical approach for primary care. *Geriatrics* 53(2):34–48, 1999.
8. Viera AJ, Clenney TL, Shenenberger DW, et al: Newer pharmacologic alternatives for erectile dysfunction. *Am Fam Physician* 60(4):1159–1166, 1999.
9. Morgentaler A: Male impotence. *Lancet* 354:1713–1718, 1999.
10. Kloner RA, Zusman RM: Cardiovascular effects of sildenafil citrate and recommendations for its use. *Am J Cardiol* 84:11N–17N, 1999.

INDEX

Page numbers followed by the letters *f* and *t* indicate figures and tables, respectively.

Digitalis
  for chronic obstructive pulmonary disease
    (COPD), 698
  overdose of, 165
Digoxin, 2, 3*t*
Dihydroergotamine (DHE 45), 441, 442*t*
Dimenhydrinate
  for labyrinthitis, 126, 126*t*
  for Ménière's disease, 129, 129*t*
Diphenhydramine (Benadryl)
  for allergic rhinitis, 123*t*, 124
  for arthropod infestations, 66
  for common cold, 134
  for conjunctivitis, 550, 551*t*
  for contact dermatitis, 56
Diphtheria, 315–317, 331
  diagnosis of, 316–317
  general considerations in, 315–316
  pathogenesis of, 316
  signs and symptoms of, 316
  treatment of, 317
  vaccination against, 317
Diphtheria, tetanus, and acellular pertussis
    (DTaP) vaccine, 317
Diphtheria antitoxin, 317
Dipivefrin, 533
Diploid cell vaccine, human (HDCV), 334
Disease-modifying antirheumatic drug
    (DMARD), 382
Disequilibrium, 463
Disruption, 274*t*
Diuretics
  for chronic obstructive pulmonary disease
    (COPD), 698
  for congestive heart failure, 2, 3*t*
  for cor pulmonale, 21
Diverticular disease, 212–214, 213*f*, 213*t*
Diverticulitis
  diagnostic considerations, 259, 260*t*, 264
Dizziness and vertigo, 462–464
  complications of, 464
  diagnostic considerations for, 463–464
  laboratory and radiologic studies for, 464
  patient education in, 464
  special considerations for, 464
  symptoms and objective findings of, 462–463
  treatment of, 464
Donepezil (Aricept), 444
Donovanosis (granuloma inguinale), 321–322
Dopamine agonists, 453
Dornase alfa (Pulmozyme), 272
Dorzolamide, 533
Double crush syndrome, 402
Down syndrome, 276
Doxazosin, 713
Doxepine, 426
Doxycycline
  for chlamydia, 311
  for epididymitis, 715*t*
  for Lyme disease, 307
  for lymphogranuloma venereum, 347
  for pelvic inflammatory disease (PID), 475, 476
  for proctitis, 254
  for prostatitis, 713
  for syphilis, 340
Dressler's syndrome, 32
Drug addiction, 651–658. *See also* Substance abuse
Drug overdose. *See* Poisoning and drug overdose
Drusen, 535
DTP (diphtheria, tetanus, pertussis) vaccine, 331
Ductal adenocarcinoma, 522–523

Duodenal ulcer, 260*t*, 261
Dysmenorrhea, 465–466
Dysplasia, 274*t*, 483
Dysthymic disorder, 616–617

Ear infection, inner, 124–126. *See also* Labyrinthitis
Early language milestone scale, 562, 562*f*–563*f*
Eating disorders, 599–601
  diagnostic considerations in, 600, 600*t*
  etiology and epidemiology of, 599
  general considerations for, 599
  laboratory studies and nutritional assessment for, 600
  prognosis for, 601
  psychotherapy for, 601
  signs, symptoms, and objective findings of, 599
  treatment of, 600–601
Eclampsia, 490–491
Econazole, 106*t*
Ecthyma, 89–92
  complications in, 92
  diagnostic and laboratory tests for, 91
  general considerations for, 89
  signs, symptoms, and objective findings of, 89–91, 91*f*
  treatment of, 91–92
Ectopic pregnancy, 471–473
  classification of, 472, 472*f*
  diagnostic considerations for, 307, 542
  etiology of, 472, 472*f*
  general considerations for, 471
  pathogenesis of, 471–472
  signs and symptoms of, 473, 473*t*
  treatment of, 473
Ectropion, 541–542
Eczema, atopic, 66–67
Eczema herpeticum, 66
Effusion, of knee, 414, 415
Efudex (5-fluorouracil), 88
Elbow dislocations, 376
Elbow pain, 364–365, 364*f*, 365*f*
Elderly patients
  anxiety and panic disorders in, 605
  appendicitis in, 265
  depression in, 619
    treatment of, 629
  hip fractures in, 406, 408
  Michigan Alcoholism Screening Test (MAST) for, 655, 657*t*
  pain management for, 460–461
  sleep disorders of, 603
Electrocautery, 87, 88
Electroconvulsive therapy, 632
Electrolyte balance disorders, 147–151
  of calcium, 149–150
  of magnesium, 150–151
  of phosphorus, 150
  of potassium, 148–149, 148*t*, 149*t*
  of sodium, 147–148, 147*t*
Electromyogram, 402–403
Elimite (permethrin 5%), 65
Emphysema, 691–693, 692*f*, 693*t*
Encephalitis, viral, 306*t*
Endocervical curettage, 484, 484*t*
Endometrial cancer, 494–495
Endometrial hyperplasia, 494–495
Enteritis, 264
Enterobiasis, 317–318
Enterobius vermicularis, 317–318
Enterohemorrhagic *Escherichia coli*, 352–353
Entropion, 541–542

Enuresis, nocturnal, 580–585. *See also* Primary nocturnal enuresis
Epicondylitis, 364–365, 364*f*, 365*f*
Epidermolysis bullosa, 69
Epidermophyton, 50
Epididymitis, 713–716
  complications in, 715–716
  diagnostic considerations in, 714
  general considerations for, 713–714
  laboratory and radiologic studies for, 714
  symptoms and objective findings of, 714
  treatment of, 715, 715*t*
Epiglottitis, 155–157
  complications in, 157
  vs. croup, 674
  diagnostic considerations in, 155–156
  disposition of, 157
  general considerations for, 155
  laboratory and radiographic studies for, 156, 156*f*
  signs, symptoms, and objective findings of, 155
  treatment of, 156
Epilepsy (seizure disorders), 431–433
  complications of, 433
  diagnostic considerations for, 432, 432*t*
  general considerations for, 431, 432*t*
  pathogenesis of, 431, 432*t*
  signs, symptoms, and objective findings of, 431–432
  treatment and disposition of, 432–433
Epinephrine
  for anaphylaxis, 173
  for asthma, 667*t*
  for laryngotracheobronchitis (croup), 675
Epistaxis, 142–143, 143*t*
Equinovarus foot, 587
Erectile dysfunction, 723–726
  complications in, 726
  diagnostic considerations in, 723–724, 724*t*, 725*t*
  follow up for, 725
  general considerations for, 723
  laboratory studies for, 724
  pathogenesis of, 723
  signs, symptoms, and objective findings of, 723
  treatment of, 725, 725*t*
Erysipelas, 70
Erythema chronica migrans, 98
Erythema infectiosum (fifth disease), 111
Erythema multiforme, 77–78
Erythema nodosum, 78–79
Erythromycin
  for acne, 108*t*
  for bacterial meningitis, 439
  for cellulitis, 70
  for chalazion, 548
  for chlamydia, 311
  for conjunctivitis, 550, 550*t*
  for diphtheria, 317
  for lymphogranuloma venereum, 347
  for mastoiditis, 137
  for pertussis, 331
  for prostatitis, 713
Escherichia coli, 352–353
Esophageal carcinomas, 505–507
  complications of, 506
  diagnosis of, 505–506, 506*t*
  general considerations in, 505
  pathogenesis of, 505, 506*t*
  patient education in, 506
  risk factors for, 505, 506*t*

ISBN 0-07-137014-5

90000

9 780071 370141

MOSER/PRIMARY CARE PA